D1558371

# CLINICAL INFECTIOUS DISEASES

## A Practical Approach

# CLINICAL INFECTIOUS DISEASES

## A Practical Approach

*Editor in Chief*
**RICHARD K. ROOT, M.D.**

*Editors*
**FRANCIS WALDVOGEL, M.D.**
**LAWRENCE COREY, M.D.**
**WALTER E. STAMM, M.D.**

New York Oxford
OXFORD UNIVERSITY PRESS
1999

Oxford University Press

Oxford New York
Athens Auckland Bangkok Bogotá Buenos Aires Calcutta
Cape Town Chennai Dar es Salaam Delhi Florence Hong Kong Istanbul
Karachi Kuala Lumpur Madrid Melbourne Mexico City Mumbai
Nairobi Paris São Paulo Singapore Taipei Tokyo Toronto Warsaw

*and associated companies in*
Berlin Ibadan



Published by Oxford University Press, Inc.
198 Madison Avenue, New York, New York 10016



The science of medicine is a rapidly changing field. As new research and clinical experience broaden our knowledge, changes in treatment and drug therapy do occur. The author and the publisher of this work have checked with sources believed to be reliable in their efforts to provide information that is accurate and complete, and in accordance with the standards accepted at the time of publication. However, in light of the possibility of human error or changes in the practice of medicine, neither the author, nor the publisher, nor any other party who has been involved in the preparation or publication of this work warrants that the information contained herein is in every respect accurate or complete. Readers are encouraged to confirm the information contained herein with other reliable sources, and are strongly advised to check the product information sheet provided by the pharmaceutical company for each drug they plan to administer.

Library of Congress Cataloging-in-Publication Data
Clinical infectious diseases : a practical approach /
edited by Richard K. Root . . . [et al.].
p. cm. Includes bibliographical references and index.
ISBN 0-19-508103-X
1. Communicable diseases. 2. Anti-infective agents.
I. Root, Richard K.
[DNLM: 1. Communicable Diseases. 2. Anti-Infective Agents—therapeutic use.
WC 100 C6417 1998] RC111.C563 1998
616.9—dc21 DNLM/DLC for Library of Congress 98-14548

1 3 5 7 9 8 6 4 2
Printed in the United States of America
on acid-free paper

# Preface

*Clinical Infectious Diseases: A Practical Approach* is structured to give the interested reader comprehensive yet practical information about the etiology, pathogenesis, clinical presentation and diagnosis, therapy, and prevention of all significant infectious disease entities. Designed to present material at a level of comprehension somewhere between general medical texts and more encyclopedic infectious disease texts, the book is accessible to a wide range of specialists and generalists at all levels of expertise.

We recognize that approaches to the diagnosis, management, and prevention of infectious diseases are becoming increasingly international in scope. This is most true in the developed world, as technologies for the diagnosis of infections, and the medications to treat them, become more universally available. With this point in mind, and building on our own areas of interest, we recruited authors from many different continents who are known for their strong reputation in a particular field. In writing their chapters, we asked for a consensus of treatment options if possible, noting the variability of approaches when appropriate. Differences in the availability of antibiotics, in diagnostic approaches in Europe and North America, and in geographic-specific epidemiology are also noted.

A brief history of infectious diseases and an overview of the infectious process proceed to four introductory sections (Parts I–IV) that provide basic ideas and principles critical to the reader's understanding and management of all types of infectious disease. The main body of the text is then devoted to the clinical evaluation and management of infectious disease syndromes, organized primarily by the location of disease manifestation (Part V), and by particular patient group (Part VI). A separate section at the end of the book is devoted to the Human Immunodeficiency Virus (Part VII).

Part I introduces the basic pathophysiologic mechanisms used by different classes and species of organisms to cause infection, important concepts in infectious disease epidemiology, and information about the host's response to infection. Part II is devoted to methodology, with chapters on radiologic and laboratory techniques that evaluate responses to infection and detect the presence of infectious organisms. Part III introduces general principles of antimicrobial action and usage, featuring a series of chapters on individual antimicrobial agents. It concludes with specific recommendations for administering antimicrobial agents by specific causative organism and site of infection. A tabular format facilitates ease of access to this information. Part IV is devoted to immunologic approaches for the management and prevention of infection. As well as classic chapters on active and passive immunization, an entire chapter is devoted to the expanding experimentation and use of immunomodulatory agents in clinical practice.

Armed with the information gained from these initial sections, the clinician should be properly equipped to tackle the problems posed by patients who present with the various infectious disease syndromes found in Parts V, VI, and VII. In Part V, the focus is not on lengthy descriptions of the microbiology of infectious diseases, but on the review of infectious disease syndromes by organ system, because this is the way the majority of patients present before an etiologic diagnosis is known. For example, information on tuberculosis is found in the chapter on "Cavitary Pulmonary Disease," varicella is found under "Infections with Rash," brain abscesses are discussed in the chapter on "Focal Central Nervous System Infections," and syphilis is discussed in the chapter on "Genital Ulcer Disease." To facilitate understanding, each chapter has a similar organization: Introduction, Etiology, Epidemiology, Host Defenses, Pathogenesis, Clinical Presentation, Diagnosis, Treatment, and Prevention. Extensive cross-referencing to the introductory chapters, as well as to other clinical chapters, avoids excessive repetition that would add significantly to the size of the text. Part VI emphasizes the unique aspects of epidemiology and altered host defenses that are characteristic of different groups of patients at increased risk for specific infections. Discussions focus on patients who are post-surgery; have extensive body burns, multiple trauma, or prosthetic devices; and those made immunodeficient by disease, malnutrition, or immunosuppressive therapy. Given the increasing prevalence of world travel, chapters also address the care of patients returning from trips to tropical and developing countries with specific symptom complexes, such as diarrhea, fever, or eosinophilia.

Because of the importance of HIV infection worldwide and the rapidly burgeoning flow of information about it, Part VII is devoted to this single disease entity. Separate chapters deal with its epidemiology and prevention, pathogenesis, immunology, clinical manifestations, antiretroviral therapy, therapy for opportunistic infections, and vaccine development.

In all of these chapters, the reader will find practically oriented *annotated* reading lists that cite the key papers in a given specialty, allowing for a more targeted search for additional information. The almost uniform availability of electronic literature search methods has made a more cumbersome approach unnecessary.

In summary, while we recognize that clinicians have an expanding choice of textbooks in the Infectious Disease field, we offer our book for several features that should make it particularly useful:

- An underpinning of relevant basic and clinical science of infectious diseases
- A practical review of antimicrobial agents and immunization or immunomodulation approaches
- A focus on patients and the way they present
- The use of tables to summarize diagnostic and therapeutic information and to facilitate clinical management
- What we believe are consensus approaches to clinical management among all developed countries.

**Richard K. Root, M.D. Seattle, Washington, USA**
Dr. Root has a long-standing interest in host-defense mechanisms against infection, in particular phagocytic cells and the pathogenesis of fever, as well as severe infections such as pneumonia, sepsis, and septic shock.

**Francis Waldvogel, M.D. Geneva, Switzerland**
Besides his broad impact as one of the founding fathers of the International Society of Infectious Diseases, Dr. Waldvogel has made seminal contributions to understanding the pathogenesis of staphylococcal diseases, and more specifically to the interactions between these organisms and phagocytes in bone and foreign-body infections.

**Lawrence Corey, M.D. Seattle, Washington, USA**
Dr. Corey, a clinical virologist, is best known for his outstanding epidemiologic and clinical work focusing on human herpesvirus infections, and in HIV infection.

**Walter Stamm, M.D. Seattle, Washington, USA**
Dr. Stamm has made major fundamental and practical contributions to the understanding of sexually transmitted diseases, in particular those caused by chlamydial species, and in the epidemiology, pathogenesis, and treatment of urinary tract infections and of nosocomial infections.

# Acknowledgments

All reference texts are the product of the efforts of many people and services beyond those represented by the Editors and Authors. The Editor in Chief would like to recognize the major contributions made to the editing process by Christine List-Root. The organizational backbone that she developed and pursued, frequently contacting the international pool of authors, was absolutely essential to the creation of a book of this type. She was ably assisted in this process by Betsy Zickler, whose years of experience in the publication field were indispensable.

At Oxford University Press-USA, several editors deserve mention for their important role in this process: Donald Jackson, former Vice President for Medical Publishing, Beth Barry, former Editor for Clinical Medicine, and most recently and importantly, Lauren Enck, current Editor for Clinical Medicine. She in particular is to be commended for her tenacity and vigor in bringing this project to its final fruition. Her expertise and critical assessments have been essential to the completion of this text. Special thanks also go to Nancy Wolitzer, who assisted in the editing and production of the volume.

Finally in the creation of this book we acknowledge the truth of an old statement: "Behind every successful man there stands a surprised woman!" We lovingly acknowledge the importance of the support given to us by our wives, Marilyn, Ann, Amy, and Peggy. Whatever successes that we have had in our professional endeavors we owe in large part to their balancing influences in our lives.

# Contents

Contributors, xiii

1. Historical Notes on Infectious Disease, 1
   HAROLD P. LAMBERT
2. Infectious Diseases: An Overview, 7
   RICHARD K. ROOT

## Part I Pathophysiology of Infectious Diseases

3. Microbes and Virulence Factors: Bacteria, 19
   DAVID A. RELMAN
4. Pathophysiology of Viruses and Viral Diseases, 27
   DAVID M. KOELLE AND LAWRENCE COREY
5. Parasitic Protozoa and Helminths, 37
   ADEL A. F. MAHMOUD
6. Fungi and Fungal Diseases, 43
   JOHN E. EDWARDS, JR. AND PETER G. PAPPAS
7. Epidemiology in Clinical Infectious Diseases, 53
   RICHARD A. GOODMAN AND JAMES M. HUGHES
8. Epidemiology and Control of Infectious Diseases in Health Care Facilities, 61
   HUAN J. CHANG AND WILLIAM R. JARVIS
9. Host Responses to Infection: Fever, Hyperthermia, and Hypothermia, 71
   RICHARD K. ROOT
10. The Acute Inflammatory Response, 83
    JAN VERHOEF
11. The Specific Immune Response, 91
    JOHN M. DWYER

## Part II Diagnostic Methods in Infectious Disease

12. Modern Imaging Techniques in Infectious Disease, 111
    ERIC J. STERN, HANH V. NGHIEM, JOHN F. HIEHLE, JR., AND DAVID H. LEWIS
13. Hematologic Alterations in Infectious Disease Patients, 121
    PHOTIS BERIS AND FRANCIS A. WALDVOGEL
14. Metabolic and Endocrine Alterations in Infectious Disease Patients, 133
    FRANCIS A. WALDVOGEL
15. Specimen Management and Rapid Detection of Infectious Agents, 137
    FRED C. TENOVER
16. Clinical Bacteriology, 145
    JAMES J. PLORDE
17. Clinical Virology, 159
    RHODA L. ASHLEY
18. Clinical Mycology, 169
    MICHAEL A. PFALLER
19. Clinical Parasitology, 181
    JAMES J. PLORDE
20. Rickettsia and Chlamydia, 195
    W. CONRAD LILES AND WALTER E. STAMM

## Part III Antimicrobial Drugs: Principles and Usage

21. Mechanisms of Antimicrobial Action and Resistance, 209
    GEORGE A. JACOBY
22. Pharmacology of Antimicrobials, 217
    SANDRA L. PRESTON AND GEORGE L. DRUSANO
23. Antimicrobial Toxicities and Drug Interactions, 225
    JAMES E. LEGGETT AND SUSAN R. RABER
24. Selection of Antimicrobials for Treatment, 233
    JAY P. SANFORD AND RICHARD K. ROOT
25. Outpatient Parenteral Therapy of Serious Infections, 241
    ALAN D. TICE

26. Control of Antimicrobial Usage, 245
PETER G. DAVEY

27. Penicillins, 249
CATHERINE M. CRETICOS AND JOHN N. SHEAGREN

28. Cephalosporins, 257
JAMES B. MALOW AND JOHN N. SHEAGREN

29. Other Beta-lactam Antibiotics: Penems, Carbapenems, and Monobactams, 265
PIERRE TATTEVIN, GUILLAUME BRETON, AND CLAUDE CARBON

30. Aminoglycosides, 273
DAVID N. GILBERT

31. Glycopeptides, 285
ADEL S. SULAIMAN, ROBERT M. RAKITA, AND BARBARA E. MURRAY

32. Macrolides and Clindamycin, 291
HOWARD S. GOLD AND ROBERT C. MOELLERING, JR.

33. Tetracyclines and Chloramphenicol, 299
THOMAS M. HOOTON

34. Fluoroquinolones, 305
RALF STAHLMANN AND HARTMUT LODE

35. Sulfonamides and Trimethoprim, 313
STEPHEN E. SANCHE AND ALLAN R. RONALD

36. Miscellaneous Antibacterial Drugs, 319
GORDON DOW AND ALLAN R. RONALD

37. Antimycobacterial Drugs, 327
CHARLES A. PELOQUIN AND MICHAEL D. ISEMAN

38. Antimicrobial Therapy for Bacterial Diseases, 337
DAVID H. SPACH AND W. CONRAD LILES

39. Antiviral Drugs and Therapy, 349
CATHERINE DIAMOND AND LAWRENCE COREY

40. Antiparasitic Drugs and Therapy, 365
KEITH B. ARMITAGE

41. Antifungal Drugs, 389
PETER G. PAPPAS AND JOHN E. EDWARDS, JR.

42. Selection of Antifungal Drugs for Deep Mycoses, 397
PETER G. PAPPAS AND JOHN E. EDWARDS, JR.

## Part IV Vaccines and Immunomodulatory Agents

43. Principles of Vaccine Development and Immunoprophylaxis, 407
GORDON L. ADA

44. Passive Immunoprophylaxis and Treatment, 411
JAMES E. PENNINGTON

45. Specific Vaccines, 415
PAUL T. HEATH AND E. RICHARD MOXON

46. Growth Factors, Immunomodulators, and Cytokines, 427
BRIGITTA U. MUELLER AND PHILLIP A. PIZZO

## Part V Infectious Disease Syndromes

47. Approach to the Patient with Fever: Acute Febrile Illness, 439
ETHAN RUBINSTEIN AND DAVID HASSIN

48. Fever in Hospitalized Patients, 449
DAVID N. SCHWARTZ AND ROBERT A. WEINSTEIN

49. Fever of Unknown Origin, 459
RICHARD K. ROOT AND ROBERT G. PETERSDORF

50. Bacteremia, Sepsis, and Septic Shock, 471
GIORGIO ZANETTI, JEAN-DANIEL BAUMGARTNER, AND MICHEL-PIERRE GLAUSER

51. Infections with Rash, 483
MORTON N. SWARTZ

52. Cellulitis and Abscesses, 501
DENNIS L. STEVENS

53. Infectious Diseases with Lymphadenopathy, 505
IVOR BYREN

54. Upper Respiratory Tract Infections, 513
CHARLES B. SMITH

55. Bronchitis and Bronchiectasis, 523
CHRISTOPH M. TANG AND CHRISTOPHER P. CONLON

56. Acute Pneumonia, 529
FENG YEE CHANG AND VICTOR L. YU

57. Cavitary Pulmonary Disease, 539
JOHN L. JOHNSON AND JERROLD J. ELLNER

58. Diffuse Pulmonary Infiltrates and Acute Respiratory Distress Syndrome, 557
KENNETH P. STEINBERG

59. Pleurisy and Empyema, 565
HARTMUT LODE, TOM SCHABERG, AND J. ELLER

60. Intraoral Infections, 573
JOHN S. GREENSPAN AND DEBORAH GREENSPAN

61. Diarrhea and Gastroenteritis, 581
HERBERT L. DUPONT

62. Hepatitis, 589
MARGARET C. SHUHART AND ROBERT L. CARITHERS, JR.

63. Pyogenic Biliary Tract and Hepatic Infections, 597
JAN V. HIRSCHMANN

64. Infectious Complications of Pancreatitis, 605
E. PATCHEN DELLINGER

65. Peritonitis and Intraabdominal Abscesses, 613
E. PATCHEN DELLINGER

66. Infective Endocarditis, 621
ADOLF W. KARCHMER

67. Intravenous Catheter-Related Infections, Suppurative Thrombophlebitis, and Mycotic Aneurysms, 637
DANIEL P. LEW AND JACQUES SCHRENZEL

68. Myocarditis and Pericarditis, 643
A. MARTIN LERNER

69. Urinary Tract Infections, 649
Walter E. Stamm

70. Genital Herpes, Syphilis, and Genital Ulcer Disease, 657
H. Hunter Handsfield

71. Urethritis, Epidydimitis, Orchitis, Prostatitis, 669
Kimberley K. Fox, Susan F. Isbey, Myron S. Cohen, and Culley C. Carson III

72. Vulvovaginitis, Cervicitis, and Pelvic Inflammatory Disease, 681
Joanne E. Embree and Robert C. Brunham

73. Meningitis, 689
Young S. Kim and Martin G. Taüber

74. Encephalitis, 703
R. Tyler Frizzell and Richard J. Whitley

75. Infections Associated with Myelopathy, Radiculopathy, and Neuropathy, 715
Christina M. Marra

76. Focal Central Nervous System Infections, 723
Allan R. Tunkel and W. Michael Scheld

77. Ocular and Periocular Infections, 733
Annabelle A. Okada and Ann Sullivan Baker

78. Osteomyelitis, 741
Jon T. Mader, Mauro Ortiz, and Jason H. Calhoun

79. Infectious and Postinfectious Arthritis, 757
MeKonnen Abebe, Lee D. Kaufman, and Benjamin J. Luft

80. Myositis and Fasciitis, 767
Dennis L. Stevens

81. Chronic Fatigue Syndrome, 773
Dedra S. Buchwald

## Part VI Infections in Special Patient/Risk Groups

82. Postsurgical Wound Infections, 783
Ronald Lee Nichols

83. Burn Infections, 789
Roberta Mann, Baiba J. Grube, David M. Heimbach

84. Infections Complicating Traumatic Injury, 795
Wayne N. Campbell

85. Prosthetic Device Infections, 801
Werner Zimmerli

86. Infection in the Immunodeficient Patient, 809
Michel Aoun and Jean Klastersky

87. Infection in the Organ Transplant Recipient, 821
Robert H. Rubin and Nina E. Tolkoff-Rubin

88. Hematopoietic Stem Cell Transplantation, 829
Raleigh A. Bowden

89. Infection in the Malnourished Patient, 839
Philippe Lepage, Achim Schwenk, Patrick De Mol, and Jean-Paul Butzler

90. Intravenous Drug Abuse and Infection, 849
Christian Ruef

91. Alcohol Abuse, Host Defenses, and Infection, 853
Rob Roy MacGregor

92. Fever in Travelers to Tropical Countries, 859
W. Conrad Liles and Wesley C. Van Voorhis

93. Endemic and Traveler's Diarrhea in Tropical Countries, 875
Herbert L. DuPont

94. Eosinophilia in Travelers to Tropical Countries, 881
Adel A. F. Mahmoud

95. Infections after Animal Bites and Scratches, 885
Stephen J. Gluckman

96. Ectoparasite-Related Diseases, 891
David H. Spach and Karen M. Van de Velde

## Part VII Human Immunodeficiency Virus and AIDS

97. Epidemiology and Prevention, 905
François Crabbé, Marie Laga, and Peter Piot

98. AIDS Pathogenesis: Molecular Biology and Virology of HIV, 915
J. Michael Kilby and George M. Shaw

99. AIDS Immunology, 927
Sharon A. Stranford and Jay A. Levy

100. Clinical Manifestations of HIV Infection and AIDS, 937
Ann C. Collier, Christina M. Marra, and Lili A. Sacks

101. Antiretroviral Therapy, 959
Lawrence Corey

102. Therapy of Opportunistic Infections, 965
Jason I. N. Tokumoto and Harry Hollander

103. Vaccines, 977
Dani P. Bolognesi

Index, 981

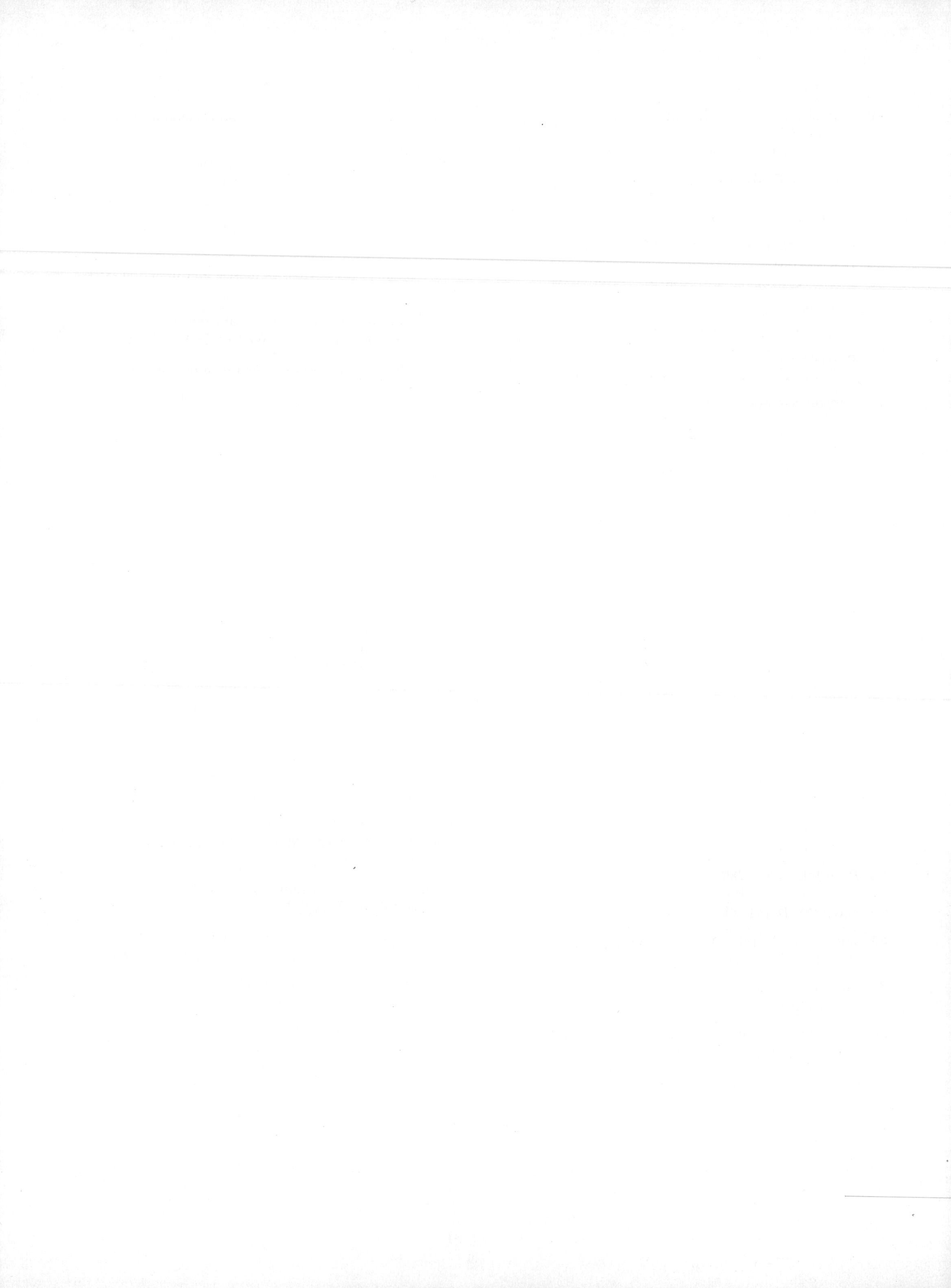

# Contributors

*Italic numbers at end of entries are chapter numbers.*


**MEKONNEN ABEBE, M.D., M.P.H.**
Department of Medicine
State University of New York Stony Brook School of Medicine
Stony Brook, NY
*79*

**GORDON L. ADA, D.SC.**
Division of Immunology and Cell Biology
John Curtin School of Medical Research
Australian National University
Canberra City, Australia
*43*

**MICHEL AOUN**
Laboratory of Microbiology and Infectious Diseases
Department of Medicine
Institut Jules Bordet
Brussels, Belgium
*86*

**KEITH B. ARMITAGE, M.D.**
Assistant Professor of Medicine
Case Western Reserve University School of Medicine
Cleveland, OH
*40*

**RHODA L. ASHLEY, PH.D.**
Professor of Laboratory Medicine
University of Washington School of Medicine
Children's Hospital and Medical Center
Seattle, WA
*17*

**ANN SULLIVAN BAKER (DECEASED)**
Infectious Disease Unit
Massachusetts Eye & Ear Infirmary
Boston, MA
*77*

**JEAN-DANIEL BAUMGARTNER, M.D.**
Chief, Service of Internal Medicine
Hôpital de zone
Morges, Switzerland
*50*

**PHOTIS BERIS, M.D.**
Head, Clinical Hematology Unit
Hôpital Cantonal Universitaire
Geneva, Switzerland
*13*

**DANI P. BOLOGNESI, PH.D.**
Director, Center for AIDS Research
Duke University Medical Center
Durham, NC
*103*

**RALEIGH A. BOWDEN, M.D.**
Fred Hutchinson Cancer Research Center
Seattle, WA
*88*

**GUILLAUME BRETON, M.D.**
Chef de Clinique-Assistant
Hopitaux de Paris
Paris, France
*29*

**ROBERT C. BRUNHAM, M.D.**
Head, Section of Infectious Diseases
Head, Department of Medical Microbiology
University of Manitoba School of Medicine
Winnipeg, Canada
*72*

**DEDRA S. BUCHWALD, M.D.**
Associate Professor
University of Washington School of Medicine
Department of Medicine
Harborview Medical Center
Seattle, WA
*81*

**Jean-Paul Butzler, M.D., Ph.D.**
Professor and Chairman
Department of Clinical Microbiology
St. Pierre University Hospital
Brussels, Belgium
*89*

**Ivor Byren, M.R.C.P.**
Consultant in Genitourinary Medicine
Honorary Consultant in Infectious Diseases
Infectious Diseases Department
Nuffield Department of Medicine
John Radcliffe Hospital
Oxford, United Kingdom
*53*

**Jason H. Calhoun, M.D.**
Professor of Orthopedic Surgery
Chief of Orthopedic Surgery
Adjunctive Member, Marine Biomedical Institute
University of Texas Medical Branch
Galveston, TX
*78*

**Wayne N. Campbell, M.D.**
Infectious Diseases Department
Department of Traumatology
R. Adams Cowley Shock Trauma Center
University of Maryland Medical Center
Baltimore, MD
*84*

**Claude Carbon, M.D.**
Professor, Internal Medicine Unit
Hopital Bichat
Paris, France
*29*

**Robert L. Carithers, Jr., M.D.**
Professor of Medicine
University of Washington School of Medicine
Seattle, WA 98195
*62*

**Culley C. Carson, III, M.D.**
Professor and Chief of Urology
University of North Carolina School of Medicine
Chapel Hill, NC
*71*

**Feng Yee Chang, M.D.**
Associate Professor of Medicine
National Defense Medical Center
Chief, Division of Infectious Disease and Tropical Medicine
Tri-Service General Hospital
Taipei, Taiwan
*56*

**Huan J. Chang, M.D.**
Robert Wood Johnson Clinical Scholars Program
University of Chicago School of Medicine
Division of Rheumatology, Department of Medicine
University of Illinois-Chicago School of Medicine
Chicago, IL
National Centers for Infectious Disease
Hospital Infections Branch
Atlanta, GA
*8*

**Myron S. Cohen, M.D.**
Chief, Division of Infectious Diseases
Department of Medicine
Professor of Medicine, Microbiology and Immunology
The University of North Carolina at Chapel Hill
Chapel Hill, NC
*71*

**Ann C. Collier, M.D.**
Professor of Medicine
University of Washington School of Medicine
Harborview Medical Center
Seattle, WA
*100*

**Christopher P. Conlon, M.D.**
Nuffield Department of Medicine
John Radcliffe Hospital
Oxford, United Kingdom
*55*

**Lawrence Corey, M.D.**
Professor of Medicine and Laboratory Medicine
Department of Medicine and Laboratory Medicine
University of Washington School of Medicine
Head, Program in Infectious Diseases
Fred Hutchinson Cancer Research Center
Seattle, WA
*4, 39, 101*

**François Crabbé, M.D., M.P.H.**
Institute of Tropical Medicine
Antwerp, Belgium
*97*

**Catherine M. Creticos, M.D.**
Section of Infectious Diseases
Illinois Masonic Medical Center
Chicago, IL
*27*

**Peter G. Davey, M.D.**
Department of Pharmacology
Ninewells Hospital and Medical School
Dundee, Scotland
*26*

**E. Patchen Dellinger, M.D.**
Professor of Surgery
Vice-Chair, Department of Surgery
Chief, Division of General Surgery
University of Washington Medical Center
Seattle, WA
*64, 65*

**Patrick De Mol, M.D., Ph.D.**
Head, Department of Microbiology
Centre Hospitalier Universitaire de Liège
Liège, Belgium
*89*

**Catherine Diamond, M.D.**
Department of Medicine
University of Washington Medical Center
Fred Hutchinson Cancer Research Center
Seattle, WA
*39*

**GORDON DOW, M.D.**
Section of Infectious Diseases
The Moncton Hospital
Moncton, Canada
*36*

**GEORGE L. DRUSANO, M.D.**
Professor and Director
Division of Clinical Pharmacology
Department of Medicine
Albany Medical College
Albany, NY
*22*

**HERBERT L. DUPONT, M.D.**
Chief, Internal Medicine
St. Luke's Episcopal Hospital
Houston, TX
*61, 93*

**JOHN M. DWYER, M.B.B.S., PH.D., F.R.A.C.P.**
Professor & Chairman
Department of Medicine
University of New South Wales
Chairman, Section of Clinical Immunology
Prince of Wales Hospital
Randwick, Australia
*11*

**JOHN E. EDWARDS, JR., M.D.**
Professor of Medicine
University of California-Los Angeles School of Medicine
Chief, Division of Infectious Diseases
Harbor-UCLA Medical Center
Torrance, CA
*6, 41, 42*

**DR. J. ELLER**
Freie Universitat Berlin
City Hospital Zehlendorf
Heckeshorn, Germany
*59*

**JERROLD J. ELLNER, M.D.**
Professor of Medicine and Pathology
Vice-Chair, Department of Medicine
Case Western Reserve University School of Medicine
Tuberculosis Research Unit
University Hospitals of Cleveland
Cleveland, OH
*57*

**JOANNE E. EMBREE, M.D.**
Pediatric Infectious Disease Specialist
University of Manitoba School of Medicine
Winnipeg, Canada
*72*

**R. TYLER FRIZZELL, M.D., PH.D.**
Assistant Professor
Idaho Neurological Surgery, P.A.
Boise, ID
*74*

**KIMBERLEY K. FOX, M.D., M.P.H.**
Assistant Professor of Medicine
University of North Carolina School of Medicine
Chapel Hill, NC
*71*

**DAVID N. GILBERT, M.D.**
Regional Director, Postgraduate Medical Education
Providence Health System
Director, Earle A. Chiles Research Institute
Providence Portland Medical Center
Professor of Medicine
Oregon Health Sciences University
Portland, OR
*30*

**MICHEL-PIERRE GLAUSER, M.D.**
Head, Department of Infectious Diseases
University Hospital
Lausanne, Switzerland
*50*

**STEPHEN J. GLUCKMAN, M.D.**
Associate Professor of Medicine
University of Pennsylvania School of Medicine
Director, Infectious Diseases Clinical Services
Hospital of the University of Pennsylvania
Philadelphia, PA
*95*

**HOWARD S. GOLD, M.D.**
Division of Infectious Diseases
Department of Medicine
Beth Israel Deaconess Medical Center
Instructor in Medicine
Harvard Medical School
Boston, MA
*32*

**RICHARD A. GOODMAN, M.D., M.P.H.**
Associate Director, Epidemiology Program Office (EPO)
Editor, *Morbidity and Mortality Weekly Report (MMWR)* Series
Centers for Disease Control and Prevention
Atlanta, GA
*7*

**DEBORAH GREENSPAN, B.D.S., SC.D.**
Professor of Clinical Oral Medicine
Department of Stomatology, and Clinical Director, Oral AIDS Center
School of Dentistry
University of California-San Francisco
San Francisco, CA
*60*

**JOHN S. GREENSPAN, B.SC., B.D.S., PH.D., F.R.C.PATH.**
Professor and Chair, Department of Stomatology
Director, Oral AIDS Center
School of Dentistry
Professor, Department of Pathology
Director, AIDS Clinical Research Center
School of Medicine
University of California-San Francisco
San Francisco, CA
*60*

**Baiba J. Grube, M.D.**
Department of Surgery
City of Hope National Medical Center
Duarte, CA
*83*

**H. Hunter Handsfield, M.D.**
Director, STD Control Program
Seattle-King County Department of Health
Harborview Medical Center
Professor of Medicine
University of Washington School of Medicine
Seattle, WA
*70*

**David Hassin, M.D.**
Department of Internal Medicine
Hillel Yaffe Medical Center
Hadera, Israel
*47*

**Paul T. Heath, F.R.A.C.P., M.R.C.P.C.H.**
Research Fellow
Oxford Vaccine Group
Department of Paediatrics
John Radcliffe Hospital
Oxford, United Kingdom
*45*

**David M. Heimbach, M.D., F.A.C.S.**
Professor of Surgery
University of Washington School of Medicine
Director, University of Washington Burn Center
Harborview Medical Center
Seattle, WA
*83*

**John F. Hiehle, Jr., M.D.**
Department of Radiology
Crozer-Chester Medical Center
Upland, PA
*12*

**Jan V. Hirschmann, M.D.**
Professor of Medicine
University of Washington School of Medicine
Assistant Chief, Medical Services
VA Medical Center
Seattle, WA
*63*

**Harry Hollander, M.D.**
Professor of Clinical Medicine
Director, Categorical Medicine Residency
University of California-San Francisco School of Medicine
San Francisco, CA
*102*

**Thomas M. Hooton, M.D.**
Associate Professor, Department of Medicine
University of Washington School of Medicine
Medical Director, Harborview Medical Center HIV/AIDS Clinic
Seattle, WA
*33*

**James M. Hughes, M.D.**
Director
National Center for Infectious Diseases
Centers for Disease Control and Prevention
Atlanta, GA
*7*

**Susan F. Isbey, M.D.**
Instructor, Department of Medicine
University of North Carolina School of Medicine
Chapel Hill, NC
*71*

**Michael D. Iseman, M.D.**
Chief, Clinical Mycobacterial Service,
Division of Infectious Disease
National Jewish Medical and Research Center
Professor of Medicine, University of Colorado School of Medicine
Denver, CO
*37*

**George A. Jacoby, M.D.**
Head, Infectious Disease Section
Lahey Clinic
Burlington, MA
*21*

**William R. Jarvis, M.D.**
Acting Director, Hospital Infections Program
Centers for Disease Control
Atlanta, GA
*8*

**John L. Johnson, M.D.**
Assistant Professor of Medicine
Division of Infectious Diseases
Case Western Reserve University
Tuberculosis Research Unit
Cleveland, OH
*57*

**Adolf W. Karchmer, M.D.**
Chief, Division of Infectious Diseases
Beth Israel Deaconess Medical Center
Professor of Medicine, Harvard Medical School
Boston, MA
*66*

**Lee D. Kaufman, M.D.**
Associate Professor of Medicine
Chief, Division of Rheumatology
State University of New York at Stony Brook
Stony Brook, NY
*79*

**J. Michael Kilby, M.D.**
Assistant Professor of Medicine
University of Alabama Medical Center
Birmingham, AL
*98*

**Young S. Kim, M.D.**
Merck & Company, Inc.
West Point, PA
*73*

**Jean Klastersky, M.D.**
Professor and Chief of Medicine
Laboratoire de Microbiologie et Department des Maladies Infectieuses
Service de Medicine
Interne et laboratoire D'Investigation
Institut Jules Bordet
Brussels, Belgium
*86*

**David M. Koelle, M.D.**
Assistant Professor, Departments of Medicine and Laboratory Medicine
University of Washington School of Medicine
Associate in Clinical Research
Fred Hutchinson Cancer Research Center
Seattle, WA
*4*

**Marie Laga, M.D., Ph.D.**
Institute of Tropical Medicine
Antwerp, Belgium
*97*

**Harold P. Lambert, M.D., F.R.C.P.**
Visiting Professor, London School of Hygiene and Tropical Medicine
London, United Kingdom
*1*

**James E. Leggett, M.D.**
Assistant Director, Medical Education
Providence Portland Medical Center
Associate Professor, Oregon Health Sciences University
Portland, OR
*23*

**Philippe Lepage, M.D., Ph.D.**
Head, Department of Pediatrics
Centre Inter-Universitaire Ambroise Pare
Mons, Belgium
*89*

**A. Martin Lerner, M.D., F.A.C.P.**
Clinical Professor of Internal Medicine
Wayne State University School of Medicine
Attending Physician
William Beaumont Hospital
Royal Oak, MI
*68*

**Jay A. Levy, M.D.**
Professor of Medicine
Department of Medicine
Division of Hematology/Oncology
University of California-San Francisco School of Medicine
San Francisco, CA
*99*

**Daniel P. Lew, M.D.**
Professor, Department of Medicine
Head, Infectious Diseases Division
Geneva University Hospital
Geneva, Switzerland
*67*

**David H. Lewis, M.D.**
Associate Professor of Radiology
University of Washington School of Medicine
Department of Nuclear Medicine
Harborview Medical Center
Seattle, WA
*12*

**W. Conrad Liles, M.D., Ph.D.**
Assistant Professor of Medicine, University of Washington
Chairman, Infection Control Committee
Co-Director, Infectious Diseases and Tropical Medicine Clinic
University of Washington Medical Center
Seattle, WA
*20, 38, 92*

**Hartmut Lode, M.D.**
Professor of Medicine
Freie Universitat Berlin
Chief, Chest and Infectious Disease Dept.
City Hospital Zehlendorf
Berlin, Germany
*34, 59*

**Benjamin J. Luft, M.D.**
Professor and Chairman
State University of New York Stony Brook
Department of Medicine
Stony Brook, NY
*79*

**Rob Roy MacGregor, M.D.**
Professor of Medicine
Department of Internal Medicine
University of Pennsylvania School of Medicine
Philadelphia, PA
*91*

**Jon T. Mader, M.D.**
Professor, Division of Infectious Diseases, Department of Internal Medicine
Chief, Hyperbaric Facility
Marine Biomedical Institute
The University of Texas Medical Branch
Galveston, TX
*78*

**Adel A.F. Mahmoud, M.D., Ph.D.**
Professor and Chairman, Department of Medicine
Case Western Reserve University School of Medicine
Physician in Chief, University Hospitals of Cleveland
Cleveland, OH
*5, 94*

**James B. Malow, M.D.**
Assistant Professor of Medicine
Rush Medical College
Director, Section of Infectious Diseases
Illinois Masonic Medical Center
Chicago, IL
*28*

**Roberta Mann, M.D., F.A.C.S.**
Medical Director, Torrance Memorial Burn Center
Torrance, CA
*83*

**Christina M. Marra, M.D.**
Associate Professor
Department of Neurology and Medicine
University of Washington School of Medicine
Harborview Medical Center
Seattle, WA
*75, 100*

**Robert C. Moellering, Jr., M.D.**
Physician in Chief
Beth Israel Deaconess Medical Center
Shields Warren-Mallinckrodt Professor of Medical Research
Harvard Medical School
Boston, MA
*32*

**E. Richard Moxon, F.R.C.P., F.R.C.P.C.H.**
Action Research Professor of Pediatrics
Oxford Vaccine Group
Department of Pediatrics
John Radcliffe Hospital
Oxford, United Kingdom
*45*

**Brigitta U. Mueller, M.D.**
Assistant Professor of Pediatrics
Harvard Medical School
Department of Medicine
Children's Hospital
Boston, MA
*46*

**Barbara E. Murray, M.D.**
Professor and Director
Division of Infectious Diseases
University of Texas Medical School at Houston
Houston, TX
*31*

**Hanh V. Nghiem, M.D.**
Associate Professor of Radiology
University of Washington School of Medicine
Department of Radiology
University of Washington Medical Center
Seattle, WA
*12*

**Ronald Lee Nichols, M.D.**
William Henderson Professor of Surgery
Professor of Microbiology and Immunology
Department of Surgery
Tulane University School of Medicine
New Orleans, LA
*82*

**Annabelle A. Okada, M.D.**
Department of Ophthalmology
Tokyo Medical College Hospital
Tokyo, Japan
*77*

**Mauro Ortiz, M.D.**
Department of Internal Medicine
Tulane University Medical Center
New Orleans, LA
*78*

**Peter G. Pappas, M.D.**
Associate Professor of Medicine
University of Alabama School of Medicine
Birmingham, AL
*6, 41, 42*

**Charles A. Peloquin, Pharm.D.**
Director, Infectious Disease Pharmacokinetics Laboratory
National Jewish Medical and Research Center
Adjoint Associate Professor of Pharmacy and Medicine
University of Colorado
Denver, CO
*37*

**James E. Pennington, M.D.**
Senior Vice President, Clinical Research
Shaman Pharmaceuticals
South San Francisco, CA
*44*

**Robert G. Petersdorf, M.D.**
Professor of Medicine Emeritus
University of Washington School of Medicine
Distinguished Professor Veterans Administration
Seattle WA
*49*

**Michael A. Pfaller, M.D.**
Professor of Pathology
Director, Medical Microbiology Division
University of Iowa College of Medicine
Iowa City, IA
*18*

**Peter Piot, M.D., Ph.D.**
Executive Director, UNAIDS Program
Geneva, Switzerland
*97*

**Phillip A. Pizzo, M.D.**
Thomas Morgan Rotch Professor and
Chair, Department of Pediatrics
Harvard Medical School
Physician-in-Chief and Chair
Department of Medicine
Children's Hospital
Boston, MA
*46*

**James J. Plorde, M.D.**
Professor of Medicine and Laboratory Medicine
University of Washington School of Medicine
Director, Microbiology Laboratory, VA Medical Center
Seattle, WA
*16, 19*

**Sandra L. Preston, Pharm.D.**
Assistant Professor of Medicine
Department of Medicine
Albany Medical College
Albany, NY
*22*

**SUSAN R. RABER, PHARM.D.**
Assistant Professor, College of Pharmacy
Oregon State University
Clinical Pharmacist, Providence Portland Medical Center
Portland, OR
*23*

**ROBERT M. RAKITA, M.D.**
Associate Professor of Medicine
Division of Infectious Diseases
University of Texas Medical School at Houston
Houston, TX
*31*

**DAVID A. RELMAN, M.D.**
Assistant Professor of Medicine, Microbiology and Immunology
Stanford University School of Medicine
Staff Physician, Veterans Affairs Palo Alto Health Care System
Palo Alto, CA
*3*

**ALLAN R. RONALD, M.D.**
Head, Section of Infectious Diseases
St. Boniface General Hospital
Winnipeg, Canada
*35, 36*

**RICHARD K. ROOT, M.D.**
Professor and Vice-Chairman
Department of Medicine
University of Washington School of Medicine
Chief, Medical Service
Harborview Medical Center
Seattle, WA
*2, 9, 24, 49*

**ROBERT H. RUBIN, M.D.**
Gordon and Marjorie Osborne Chair of Health Sciences and Technology
Director, Harvard MIT Center for Experimental Pharmacology and Therapeutics
Chief of Transplantation Infectious Disease
Massachusetts General Hospital
Boston, MA
*87*

**ETHAN RUBINSTEIN, M.D.**
Professor & Director
Infectious Diseases Unit
Sheba Medical Center, Tel Aviv University School of Medicine
Tel-Hashomer, Israel
*47*

**CHRISTIAN RUEF, M.D.**
Division of Infectious Diseases and Hospital Epidemiology
University Hospital of Zurich
Zurich, Switzerland
*90*

**LILI A. SACKS, M.D.**
Departments of Internal Medicine
Swedish Hospital & Providence Hospital
Seattle, WA
*100*

**STEPHEN E. SANCHE, M.D., F.R.C.P.C.**
Division of Infectious Diseases
Royal University Hospital
Saskatoon, Canada
*35*

**JAY P. SANFORD, M.D. (DECEASED)**
Clinical Professor of Internal Medicine
University of Texas Southwestern Medical Center
Dallas, TX
*24*

**TOM SCHABERG, M.D.**
Director, Chest Clinic Unterstedt/Rotenburg
Rotenburg, Germany
*59*

**W. MICHAEL SCHELD, M.D.**
Professor of Medicine and Neurosurgery
University of Virginia Health Sciences Center
Charlottesville, VA
*76*

**JACQUES SCHRENZEL, M.D.**
Infectious Diseases Division
Geneva University Hospital
Geneva, Switzerland
*67*

**DAVID N. SCHWARTZ, M.D.**
Assistant Professor of Medicine
Rush Medical College
Senior Physician, Division of Infectious Diseases
Cook County Hospital
Chicago, IL
*48*

**ACHIM SCHWENK, M.D.**
Klinik I für Innere Medizin
Universitat Koln
Koln, Germany
*89*

**GEORGE M. SHAW, M.D., PH.D.**
Professor of Medicine
University of Alabama School of Medicine
Birmingham, AL
*98*

**JOHN N. SHEAGREN, M.D.**
Professor, Rush Medical College
Chairman, Department of Internal Medicine
Illinois Masonic Medical Center
Chicago, IL
*27, 28*

**MARGARET C. SHUHART, M.D.**
Assistant Professor of Medicine
University of Washington School of Medicine
Harborview Medical Center
Seattle, WA
*62*

**Charles B. Smith, M.D.**
Professor of Medicine and Associate Dean
University of Washington School of Medicine
Chief of Staff
VA Puget Sound Heath Care System
Seattle, WA
*54*

**David H. Spach, M.D.**
Associate Professor of Medicine
Division of Infectious Diseases
University of Washington School of Medicine
Harborview Medical Center
Seattle, WA
*38, 96*

**Ralf Stahlmann, M.D.**
Professor of Pharmacology and Toxicology
Freie Universitat Berlin
Fachbereich Humanmedizin
Universitatsklinkum Benjamin Franklin
Institut fur Klinische Pharmakologie und Toxikologie
Berlin, Germany
*34*

**Walter E. Stamm, M.D.**
Professor of Medicine
Head, Division of Allergy & Infectious Diseases
University of Washington School of Medicine
Seattle, WA
*20, 69*

**Kenneth P. Steinberg, M.D.**
Assistant Professor of Medicine
Division of Pulmonary and Critical Care Medicine
University of Washington School of Medicine
Harborview Medical Center
Seattle, WA
*58*

**Eric J. Stern, M.D.**
Associate Professor of Radiology
University of Washington School of Medicine
Department of Radiology
Harborview Medical Center
Seattle, WA
*12*

**Dennis L. Stevens, M.D.**
Professor of Medicine
University of Washington School of Medicine
Seattle, WA
Chief, Infectious Diseases
Veterans Affairs Medical Center
Boise, ID
*52, 80*

**Sharon A. Stranford, Ph.D.**
Division of Hematology/Oncology
Department of Medicine
University of California-San Francisco School of Medicine
San Francisco, CA
*99*

**Adel S. Sulaiman, M.D.**
Millard Fillmore Hospital
Buffalo, NY
*31*

**Morton N. Swartz, M.D.**
Professor of Medicine
Harvard Medical School
Chief, Jackson Firm, Medical Service
Department of Medicine
Massachusetts General Hospital
Boston, MA
*51*

**Christoph M. Tang, M.R.C.P., Ph.D.**
MRC Clinician Scientist
Department of Paediatrics
John Radcliffe Hospital
Oxford, United Kingdom
*55*

**Pierre Tattevin, M.D.**
Interne des Hopitaux
CHU Bichat-Claude Bernard
Paris, France
*29*

**Martin G. Taüber, M.D.**
Professor, Chief of Infectious Diseases
Co-Director, Institute for Medical Microbiology
Berne, Switzerland
*73*

**Fred C. Tenover, Ph.D.**
Chief, Nosocomial Pathogens Laboratory Branch
Centers for Disease Control and Prevention
Atlanta, GA
*15*

**Alan D. Tice, M.D., F.A.C.P.**
Clinical Associate Professor
University of Washington School of Medicine
Seattle, WA
Infections Limited, P.S.
Tacoma, WA
*25*

**Nina E. Tolkoff-Rubin, M.D.**
Chief, Hemodialysis and CAPD Units
Director, End Stage Renal Disease Program
Massachusetts General Hospital
Associate Professor of Medicine
Harvard Medical School
Boston, MA
*87*

**Jason I.N. Tokumoto, M.D.**
University of California-San Francisco School of Medicine
San Francisco, CA
*102*

**Allan R. Tunkel, M.D., Ph.D.**
Professor of Medicine
Associate Chair for Education
Allegheny University of the Health Sciences
Philadelphia, PA
*76*

**Karen M. Van de Velde, M.D.**
Santa Fe, NM
*96*

**Wesley C. Van Voorhis, M.D., Ph.D.**
Associate Professor of Medicine
Adjunct Associate Professor of Pathobiology
University of Washington School of Medicine
Seattle, WA
*92*

**Jan Verhoef, M.D., Ph.D.**
Professor and Head
Eijkman-Winkler Institute for Microbiology, Infectious Diseases & Inflammation
University Hospital Utrecht
Utrecht, The Netherlands
*10*

**Francis A. Waldvogel, M.D.**
Professor of Medicine
Chairman, Department of Internal Medicine
Hôpital Cantonal Universitaire de Genève
Geneva, Switzerland
*13, 14*

**Robert A. Weinstein, M.D.**
Professor of Medicine
Rush Medical College
Chairman, Division of Infectious Diseases
Cook County Hospital
Chicago, IL
*48*

**Richard J. Whitley, M.D.**
Loeb Eminent Scholar Chair, Pediatrics
Professor of Pediatrics, Microbiology and Medicine
University of Alabama at Birmingham
Children's Hospital
Birmingham, AL
*74*

**Victor L. Yu, M.D.**
Professor of Medicine
University of Pittsburgh School of Medicine
Chief, Infectious Disease Section
VA Medical Center
Pittsburgh, PA
*56*

**Giorgio Zanetti, M.D.**
Division of Infectious Diseases
Department of Internal Medicine
University Hospital
Lausanne, Switzerland
*50*

**Werner Zimmerli, M.D.**
Professor of Medicine
Head, Division of Infectious Diseases
University Hospitals Basel
Basel, Switzerland
*85*

# CLINICAL INFECTIOUS DISEASES

## A Practical Approach

# 1

# Historical Notes on Infectious Disease

HAROLD P. LAMBERT

The observation that some illnesses seem to spread through populations and that those who recover may no longer be susceptible must be as old as human communities. The idea that such illnesses might be spread by minute living creatures, the concept of a "contagium vivum," was formulated by a number of thinkers, most notably by a Veronese physician, Frascatoro. Writing in 1546, he explicitly distinguished between contagion by direct contact, by infected material, and at a distance. As so often happens in the history of science, such insights long preceded the technical advances that allowed them to be tested, and it was more than a century later when the secretive and meticulous draper of Delft, Anton van Leeuwenhoek (1632–1723) constructed the minute simple microscopes with which he achieved magnifications of up to ×300. The microscopic world was revealed. Leeuwenhoek certainly saw protozoa, including *Giardia* in his own diarrheal stool, and equally certainly saw bacteria. Compound microscopes did not surpass the precision of his observations until the middle decades of the eighteenth century, when the problem of chromatic aberration had been solved, and staining methods and oil-immersion lenses developed. By then the microbial world was richly populated, and small organisms as causes of disease were established in two infections, both of them fungal: muscardine of silkworms and a human skin disease, favus.

## Infection and the Microbial World

Despite these advances, the question of spontaneous generation was still central and unresolved. Argument raged between the protagonists of the germ theory of disease and the miasmatists, who held that epidemics of infectious fevers were caused by exhalations produced from putrid animal and vegetable matter. Indeed, the great movements for sanitary reform in the burgeoning cities of Europe and North America were made when miasmal theory was generally in the ascendant, and by many who firmly disbelieved in the germ theory of disease. How, a miasmatist would have asked, can a theory of contagion be alleged when, as in typhus and typhoid, the main epidemic fevers of the time, a direct chain of spread is often inapparent? A microbial theory was hard to maintain in the absence of several crucial elements of microbial ecology yet to be discovered: subclinical infection, the carrier state, and the role of vectors. The debate was, of course, much more complicated than a simple opposition would suggest, and underlying it were deeply held beliefs, present in most cultural systems, about the nature of contagion and pollution. Nevertheless, despite these conceptual difficulties, spontaneous generation was refuted by the experiments of Spallanzani (1729–99) and others, and finally buried by Louis Pasteur (1822–95).

Pasteur's involvement in the question of spontaneous generation was intimately connected with current differences of opinion on the nature of fermentation. The prevalent view, that fermentation was a chemical process and that yeast was not a living material, had already, in the 1830s, been called into question by several workers who observed the multiplication of yeast cells by budding. Pasteur showed that fermentation depended on living organisms, that these organisms could be found in the air, and that the chemical reactions found during fermentation were specific to the organism involved. These findings were not lost on those concerned with infectious disease, since the parallels among fermentation, putrefaction, and infection had often been noted. Joseph Lister, then working at the Glasgow Royal Infirmary and already deeply interested in the pathology of wound infection, seized on Pasteur's findings as the clue to reducing the appalling toll of surgical sepsis, which, following the discovery of general anesthesia, remained the chief barrier to advance in surgery. His introduction of antiseptic surgery was eagerly copied throughout the surgical world, until supplanted by aseptic surgery by the 1890s. Even before Pasteur and Lister, the role of attendants in the spread of puerperal fever had been suggested by several authors in the eighteenth century, most famously by Semmelweiss in Vienna and by Oliver Wendell Holmes at Harvard.

The concepts underlying a modern theory of infection, the end of spontaneous generation, the variety and ubiquity of the microbial world and the idea of specific microbial agents as causes of specific infections, were now in place. It needed only further technical advance to pave the way for the explosion of knowledge of the microbial etiology of infectious disease that took place in the last two decades of the nineteenth century. In this a central figure was Robert Koch (1843–1910); his development of solid media, pour plates, improved staining methods, and techniques of sterilization for bacteria enabled huge and rapid advances in microbiology. Those made by Koch himself and his collaborators began with his work on anthrax and his analysis of the conditions in which spores were formed. Among his later discoveries, his work on tuberculosis and cholera is most well known, but equally important were his studies that established the bacteriology of wound infection. Once the causal organisms of many important infectious diseases had been identified, understanding of host–parasite interactions was much advanced when discrete serological groups were recognized among many species. Especially important was the discovery of the carrier state, so crucial for understanding the behavior of typhoid, of diphtheria, and of streptococcal and meningococcal disease. The biggest fundamental advance, following Griffith's description of pneumococcal transformation in 1928, was the pivotal finding by Avery, Macleod and McCarty (1944) that the transforming principle is DNA. From this, and the breaking of the genetic code in 1952 by Watson and Crick, the whole era of molecular genetics takes its origin.

## Immunity and Immunization

The erratic interactions of concept, observation, experiment, and medical practice are vividly illustrated in the history of immunization. Just as the spread through populations of some diseases had been observed, so it was also noted that those who recovered were often no longer susceptible, and could be employed in handling patients without danger. The direct application of this observation had long been made in a number of Far Eastern countries in the form of variolation to protect against smallpox. Material from a patient with a mild attack could protect against more dangerous forms of the disease. Attenuated material was no doubt developed empirically, but the process was not without risk, either of severe or fatal smallpox from the inoculation, or lack of protection from an overattenuated preparation. Contacts, too, were at risk of developing smallpox. Despite this, enthusiastic advocacy by Lady Mary Wortley Montagu, who saw its benefits in Constantinople, led to the introduction of variolation in England. Variolation became acceptable after it was performed on children of the royal family, following a number of preliminary trials on condemned criminals (who were pardoned in exchange for their cooperation) and orphan children. Similarly in New England, Cotton Mather's enthusiasm led to its use by his friend Dr. Boyston in the Boston epidemic of 1721. Inoculation came to be fairly widely practiced in the latter half of the eighteenth century, although never on a mass scale, until it was supplanted by Jennerian vaccination.

A belief that an attack of cowpox protected against smallpox was fairly prevalent in rural areas, and several people had the idea of inoculation with cowpox. Benjamin Jesty, a farmer in Dorset, inoculated his wife and sons in this way. Edward Jenner (1749–1823) did a similar thing, taking material from the vesicles on the hands of Sarah Nelmes, a dairy maid with cowpox, and inoculating an eight-year-old boy, James Phipps. He went on to show, six weeks later, that inoculation with smallpox did not "take," and after a few similar observations, that the cowpox material could be passed from person to person without losing effect. The Royal Society refused his communication, telling him that he ought not risk his reputation by putting forward such an outlandish idea. In spite of this setback, Jenner published his findings in 1798, and vaccination, as the new method was called, rapidly came into widespread use in many countries. Its early protagonist in America was Benjamin Waterhouse, professor of physic at the new medical school at Harvard College.

All this, with its effects in mitigating one of the most prevalent and most feared scourges of human populations, took place more than half a century before the germ theory of infection was developed, and for this we return to the wily chemist from the Jura, Louis Pasteur. In a famous series of experiments, he found that a culture of the organism causing fowl cholera (*Pasteurella septica*) left in a cupboard during the summer holidays was no longer virulent. He used this accident to establish that animals which had been injected with the old culture were now resistant to infection by a fresh strain, itself shown to be virulent on injection into a new batch of fowl. From this came the concept of attenuation, and its use in inducing resistance to infection. There followed its application by Pasteur to immunization against anthrax in animals and, in 1885, to immunization against human rabies. In honor of Jenner, Pasteur called this process vaccination. These early successes all involved the use of living organisms, but almost immediately the American bacteriologists Salmon and Theobald Smith (1859–1934) developed a killed and effective vaccine from the Salmonella causing hog cholera. The problems of standardization and storage are generally much less difficult with killed than with live vaccines, and their work initiated an explosion in vaccine development. Important milestones in the evolution of vaccination against diseases of humans are shown in Table 1.1.

**Table 1.1** Major developments in vaccination

| | Bacterial infections | | Viral infections | |
|---|---|---|---|---|
| Date | Attenuated | Killed or component | Attenuated | Killed or component |
| 1721 | | | Variolation in Europe and America | |
| 1798 | | | Cowpox | |
| 1885 | | | Rabies | |
| 1888 | | Diphtheria | | |
| 1896–97 | | Typhoid; cholera; plague | | |
| 1927 | BCG | Tetanus; pertussis | | |
| 1936 | | | | Influenza Yellow fever |
| 1955 | | | | Poliomyelitis |
| 1958–60 | | | Poliomyelitis | |
| 1963–70 | | | Measles Mumps Rubella | |
| 1970s | | Meningococcus; pneumococcus | | |
| 1980–present | | *H. influenze* B | | Hepatitis A and B |

## Theories of immunity

The principles of immunization, and their first fruits in the prevention of human and animal disease, were established before any coherent theory of mechanism was evolved. This soon followed, and the latter years of the century were marked by a vigorous controversy between the protagonists of humoral and those of cellular theories. Briefly, cellular theory originated with Elie Metchnikoff (1845–1916), working then in Odessa but later at the Institut Pasteur in Paris, whose work on the comparative pathology of inflammation convinced him that phagocytosis was the crucial mechanism of defense against infection. Humoral theory began with the work of Nuttall in England, who showed the bactericidal effect of normal serum on anthrax bacilli. Studies of mechanism and advances in vaccination now converged with the crucial studies of von Behring and Kitasato in Koch's laboratory in Berlin. Taking up the discovery, by Roux and Yersin at the Institut Pasteur, that the pathology of diphtheria could be reproduced by a bacteria-free filtrate of a culture of the organism, they showed, for both diphtheria and tetanus, that injected culture filtrates would immunize animals against the disease, and that the immunity induced could be passively transferred by injecting their serum into other animals.

Various properties of immune serum—agglutination, precipitation, and the intricacies of complement lysis—were soon analyzed, but the crucial advances in understanding were made in the 1890s by Paul Ehrlich (1854–1915). He clearly distinguished between active and passive immunity, devising methods of standardizing toxins and antitoxins that were the direct forerunners of modern biological standardization. His receptor (or side chain) theory of the nature of toxin–antitoxin binding, with its concept of specificity mediated by interlocking surface configurations of antigen and antibody molecules, is a remarkable anticipation of modern immunological understanding. The bitter dispute between the exponents of humoral and cellular mechanisms was partly resolved by Wright and Douglas (1903); their demonstration of opsonization showed that cellular and humoral factors were complementary. Another of those tantalizing hiatuses in the history of infectious disease then appears, perhaps because pursuit of the basis of serological specificity was a more immediately productive line of research than difficult cellular studies. So it was that the first half of the twentieth century saw an enormous expansion of work on serological specificity, on allergy, and on the biochemical basis of antigen–antibody interaction, but only fragmentary progress on cellular and functional aspects. Only in the decades following the Second World War were lymphocyte physiology, the genetic basis of antibody diversity, and the mechanisms of antigen recognition revealed. Metchnikoff's vision of defense against infection in a larger biological and evolutionary setting, dormant for half a century, at last came into its own.

## Specific Therapy

The fits and starts of progress are nowhere better exemplified than in the early history of antimicrobial drugs. During the 1870s several workers in different counties observed inhibition of bacteria by molds in culture; two of them, William Roberts and John Tyndall, both specifically mention the inhibitory effect of a *Penicillium*. Almost at the same time Pasteur himself, working with Joubert, observed bacterial antagonism and expressed the hope that the phenomenon might prove useful in therapy. Of the various leads from this work on fungal–bacterial and bacterial–bacterial interactions, one aroused special interest. This was pyocyanase, a cell-free extract of *Ps. pyocyanea*, which was used to treat infected wounds and was produced commercially for a time. These early leads all foundered on the twin problems of toxicity and instability, and no more was heard of antibiosis as a prospect in therapeutics until the development of penicillin 40 years later.

Progress in chemotherapy also suffered frustrations and delays, following its vigorous activity in the first decade of the new century. There had, indeed, been empirical discoveries before; ipecacuanha for amebiasis, Peruvian bark (quinine) for malaria, and mercury for syphilis. It was Ehrlich who gave chemotherapy a rational basis. His work on differential staining led remarkably early (1891) to the treatment of malaria by methylene blue, but more systematic work a decade later examined the effect of a series of arsenical compounds on experimental trypanosomiasis in mice. The fact that, at the time, the recently discovered cause of syphilis, *Treponema pallidum*, was thought to be a protozoon, led to its inclusion in Ehrlich's experiments, and so eventually to the cure of syphilis by salvarsan, first administered to humans in 1909. A few years before the same line of inquiry had led to the use by Koch of another arsenical, atoxyl, in the treatment of trypanosomiasis, soon abandoned because its administration was sometimes complicated by optic atrophy.

Salvarsan, despite its formidable toxicity, marked a revolutionary advance in chemotherapy, but its introduction was followed by another of those frustrating pauses, almost as long as that preceding the general use of penicillin. Between 1909 and 1935 the common bacterial infections remained unassailable, although two more antiprotozoal agents were developed, suramin for trypanosomiasis and mepacrine (atebrin) for malaria. In Germany the search for chemotherapeutic activity in synthetic dyes, following directly in the tradition of Ehrlich, had continued and in 1935 Domagk reported that one of them, prontosil red, cured streptococcal infection in mice. Again, a major advance followed a false premise, for, as was quickly shown by Tréfouël and colleagues in Paris, the activity resided not in the dye but in the sulphonamide moiety of the compound. Early skepticism about the discovery was overcome as a result of the favorable results achieved in puerperal sepsis by Colebrook at Queen Charlotte's Maternity Hospital in London and by the work of Perrin Long at Johns Hopkins Hospital in Baltimore. Sulphanilamide itself was soon supplanted by other more effective and less toxic compounds, and a flood of publications recorded the first effective treatments for many bacterial infections, most notably pneumococcal pneumonia, meningococcal meningitis, and streptococcal puerperal sepsis. The gradual increase of confidence in the new therapies is exemplified in published work on meningococcal infection during the late 1930s. Sulphonamides were at first used together with antimeningococcal serum, the only specific treatment then available, then tentatively as sole treatment. When it was shown that chemotherapy alone was as good as or better than combined therapy, serum was abandoned.

The story of penicillin is too well known to need repeating in detail. Fleming, at St. Mary's Hospital in London, unaware of the much older observations on inhibition of bacteria by *Penicillium* species, noticed lysis of staphylococcal colonies in the vicinity of a contaminant fungus later identified as *Penicillium notatum.* He established the range of antibacterial activity of crude extracts, and showed that the extracts were nontoxic by injection in mice, and nonirritant on infected surfaces in man and on the human conjunctiva. Efforts at further development foundered on problems of purification and stability until the team in Oxford led by Florey and Chain succeeded in producing enough material, albeit still in relatively crude form, for limited clinical trial. The first papers describing the remarkable effects of penicillin on streptococcal and staphylococcal infections were published in 1940. The focus now shifted to the United States, and the development of large-scale manufacture enabled the wide use of penicillin in the later stages of World War II. The expansion of penicillin derivatives with selective actions and pharmacological properties followed the isolation of 6-aminopenicillanic acid in England in 1957, with the resulting family tree of compounds now available.

Nearly 20 years elapsed between the discovery of the cephalosporins in 1948 and their first clinical applications. Brotzu, a bacteriologist and public health official in Sardinia, pursuing his ingenious idea that the disappearance of typhoid bacilli from sewage might result from antibiotic action, isolated a mold, identified as *Cephalosporium acremonium*, from a sewage outfall. The culture was sent to Oxford, where Abraham and his colleagues isolated three new antibiotics from it. One of these, cephalosporin C, was the source of the nucleus from which the first commercially produced cephalosporins were eventually derived.

During the 1940s several other antibiotics were discovered, some of them from fungal and others from bacterial sources, but were too toxic for systemic use. In 1944, however, Waksman isolated streptomycin from the soil fungus *Streptomyces griseus*. Its dramatic benefits in tuberculosis, the first treatment of this infection to produce unequivocal benefit, were soon vitiated by the rapid emergence of drug resistance, then restored as combination therapy with PAS and isoniazid replaced single drug treatment. The subsequent decades have seen continuous development of antimicrobial chemotherapy, so that appropriate agents are now available and active against most bacterial and fungal—and some viral—infections. The evolutionary adaptability of microorganisms has, however, been emphasized by the apparently inexorable advance of antibiotic resistance, which has rendered many previously valuable drugs useless. Some important findings in the development of chemotherapy are listed in Table 1.2.

Antiviral agents arrived late in the history of chemotherapy. Indeed, it was generally held that the intimate association between virus and host cell made it impossible to develop specific therapy. The first step was the discovery that thiosemicarbazones, already known as antituberculous agents, were active against vaccinia virus. By 1963 one of these compounds, methisazone, had been shown to be modestly effective in the prevention of smallpox in contacts of the disease. Within a few years several different lines of attack were developing: the interferons, interferon inhibitors, amantadine, and especially idoxuridine. The last agent was especially important as the first of the many nucleosides now in general use. The advent of HIV/AIDS gave a vigorous impetus to the development of new antiviral agents, especially to those active against retroviruses. These include nucleoside analogue and nonnucleoside analogue reverse transcriptase inhibitors, and the protease inhibitors. Given in various combinations, these compounds have already led to a dramatic improvement in the outlook for patients with HIV/AIDS; it is still too early to judge their influence in the long term. Many important viral diseases of man and animals still remain beyond the reach of chemotherapy.

## Viral Infections

The meaning of the word *virus* has shifted several times since it was first used, but here it is confined to its modern connotation. The origin of virology lies in the development of efficient filters, in connection both with pure water supplies and in the course of the technical developments in bacteriology during the 1890s. The modern era began with tobacco mosaic disease and the discovery, independently by Ivanovski in Russia and by Beijerinck in Holland, that the agent passed through porcelain filters and mul-

**Table 1.2** Major developments in antimicrobial chemotherapy

| | Antibiotics | Synthetic compounds |
|---|---|---|
| 1929–40 | Penicillin | |
| 1935 | | Prontosil red. Sulphanilamide |
| 1939 | Griseofulvin | |
| 1944 | Streptomycin | |
| 1946 | | Para-aminosalicylic acid |
| 1948 | Cephalosporins<br>Chloramphenicol | |
| 1952 | | Isoniazid |
| 1956 | Vancomycin | |
| 1957 | Rifamycin<br>Kanamycin | |
| 1960 | Fusidic acid | |
| 1962 | | Nalidixic acid (quinolones) |
| 1963 | Gentamicin | Idoxuridine |
| 1972 | Rosaramycin | |
| Recent | Numerous new beta-lactams, macrolides, and peptides | Fluoroquinolones.<br>New antivirals, including acyclovir, ribavirin, zidovudine anti-retroviral agents. |

tiplied in infected tissues. There followed vigorous argument about the nature of the mysterious process. Was the agent a small bacterium or, as Beijerinck contended, some fluid material able to replicate only in living tissue? Matters were advanced by Loeffler and Frosch, who, attempting to produce a vaccine against foot and mouth disease by filtered vesicle fluid, found that the calves became infected by the filtrate. Other filterable infective agents were soon discovered—myxomatosis and, confusingly, the agent of bovine pleuropneumonia of cattle. The latter, as we now know, is a Mycoplasma and not a virus. All this was achieved by 1900; by 1920 viruses of plants, insects, and animals including man, tumor viruses, and bacterial viruses had all been discovered.

The first half of this century saw the discovery of numerous new viral causes of infection, concurrent with a gradual refinement of the techniques for their study, particularly the development of high-speed centrifugation, electron microscopy, and refinements in protein chemistry. Above all, tissue and cell-culture techniques were developed, enabling the production of viral vaccines. Advances in understanding viral pathogenesis did not, however, derive as much from the discovery of new human viruses, important as these were, as from the study of bacteriophages, which became a central focus of research during the 1930s and 1940s. Eugene and Elisabeth Wollman, who both died in Auschwitz, began to elucidate the nature of lysogeny; their work was completed when it was finally shown that the DNA of the bacteriophage, not its protein, is inserted into the host cell and initiates viral multiplication. Later, the phenomenon of viral latency became important in human viral disease, both in DNA viruses like herpes simplex, and with some of the RNA viruses, the genome of which becomes incorporated into that of the host cell.

The years following World War II saw the identification of viruses causing some of the most prevalent of human diseases, including the chief exanthemata of childhood, the common cold, and many forms of hepatitis. From the viewpoint of preventive medicine, pride of place in a rich harvest must surely go to Enders, Robbins and Weller at the Children's Hospital in Boston, who, by growing poliovirus in non–nervous system tissue, enabled vaccination against poliomyelitis to be realized. Live attenuated and killed viral vaccines are now part of the essential armory of any public health system.

## Tropical Diseases

The discovery of the etiology of the great infective scourges of the Tropics are epics of infectious-disease history, with their stories of scientific ingenuity, resolution, and personal courage and sacrifice. Yellow fever makes a bridge between the history of virology and that of tropical protozoal diseases. Although somewhat neglected in the excitements of the discoveries of insect transmission, as early as 1901 the US Government Commission headed by Walter Reed showed that yellow fever could be transmitted to volunteers injected with blood from patients which had passed through a bacteriological filter. So this ancient disease, with its huge historic impacts, was one of the first human diseases for which a viral cause was established, and also one of the first for which proof was provided of a separate invertebrate cycle involved in transmission. The stories of parasitic and protozoal disease, which are beyond the scope of the present discussion, here overlap, since the evidence on insect transmission and separate life cycles was emerging virtually simultaneously in the last decade of the nineteenth century for malaria in Algeria, India, and Italy, and for yellow fever in the Americas.

The long history of yellow fever, its apparently mysterious and capricious behavior and its toll of human life is well known. The modern era begins with Carlos Finlay in Cuba, and his careful deductions from epidemiological evidence that the disease is transmitted by the mosquito, and specifically *Aedes aegypti*. The clinching evidence came from the epic work of the Commission, at the turn of the century, during which one of its members, Lazear, died of accidentally acquired yellow fever. Curiously, in spite of Reed's early and successful transmission of a filterable agent, the causal agent of yellow fever remained in dispute for another quarter of a century. For a long time the chief contender was Noguchi's "*Leptospira icteroides*." Famous for his studies on spirochetes, scrub typhus, and trachoma, Noguchi died from yellow fever in 1928 during an expedition to West Africa in pursuit of his agent. So, too, did Adrian Stokes the previous year, having proved the viral etiology of the disease in the course of his transmission experiments with rhesus monkeys.

Elucidation of bacterial and rickettsial diseases associated with arthropod transmission was achieved in a different sequence. The association of plague with rats had long been recognized and the causal bacillus was found by Kitasato and Yersin in 1894, but the mechanics of transmission by the rat flea was not worked out until 1914. The same era saw the solution of the biology of typhus, its spread by lice, and the discovery of its etiological agent, *Rickettsia prowazeki*.

## The Modern Era

The understanding of the biology of infectious disease that gradually emerged during the nineteenth and early twentieth centuries changed and refined public health practice. Some epidemic diseases, such as chicken pox and diphtheria, are contagious; others, such as yellow fever, are not. Control of cholera requires not just clean-looking water, but bacteriological filtration, while quarantine is not likely to do much as a control measure. But the greatest impact of advances in preventive medicine came from the development of safe and effective vaccines against many important viral and bacterial diseases, and in therapeutics from the development of chemotherapy against many microbial scourges of man and animals.

These basic concepts and their practical applications were all firmly in place by the middle of the twentieth century. New diagnostic techniques continued to be developed, new agents of infection discovered, and new therapies introduced, but in retrospect the midcentury appears as something of a plateau in comparison with both the heady days of the turn of the century and with the revolution in molecular biology of the last two decades.

The spectacular progress in molecular biology has affected all aspects of infectious diseases. In epidemiology especially, molecular methods have led to a quantum leap in understanding of such important topics as the spread of antibiotic resistance and the nature of the mechanisms involved. Infectious diseases research has been transformed by molecular methods, and new organisms—for example, hepatitis C virus—are now being identified by the use of these methods when traditional methods of culture and inoculation in experimental models have failed. The study of microbial pathogenesis, so long in the doldrums, has taken on a new lease of life. Genetically engineered vaccines show vast potential; those for protection against hepatitis B have been in production for some years and many other vaccines based on recombinant technology are under development. Nevertheless, important discoveries are still made by traditional techniques, as witnessed by the model investigations that unraveled the etiology and epidemiology of Lyme disease. The continual discovery of new agents and new mechanisms of infectious disease makes it clear that the future of this field of study is certain to be as exciting as the past.

## ANNOTATED BIBLIOGRAPHY

Garrison FH. An Introduction to the History of Medicine, 4th ed. WB Saunders, London and Philadelphia, 1929.

Lechevalier HA, Solotorovsky M. Three Centuries of Microbiology. Dover Publications, Toronto and London, 1974.

*A short text linking numerous passages from classical papers in microbiology, giving a vivid and realistic picture of the development of the subject.*

Pelling M. Contagion/germ theory/specificity. in: *Companion Encyclopaedia of the History of Medicine*, Bynum WF, Porter R, eds. Routledge, London, 1993.

*Clear account of the intricacies of this fundamental topic in the history of infectious diseases. The two volumes of this encyclopedia contain many other essays relevant to the history of infectious disease.*

Porter R. The Greatest Benefit to Mankind: A Medical History of Humanity from Antiquity to the Present. Harper Collins, London, 1997.

*A large one-volume history, conventionally arranged but far from conventional in its awareness of the social context in which medical advances take place. Full of fascinating material and eminently readable.*

Shryock RH. The development of Modern Medicine: An Interpretation of the Social and Scientific Factors Involved, 2nd ed., University of Wisconsin Press, Madison, WI, 1947, reprinted 1979.

*An excellent short book that puts medical history into a wider setting; especially good on the American experience.*

Singer C, Underwood E. A Short History of Medicine. Oxford University Press, London, 1962.

*Of the two standard texts, Garrison is centered on biography, with accounts of a vast number of important medical figures. Singer is more descriptive of trends and movements in medical history.*

# 2

# Infectious Diseases: An Overview

RICHARD K. ROOT

We live in a sea of microorganisms. Not only can they be found in every part of our environment, but billions colonize our skin and inhabit our gastrointestinal and respiratory tracts. The vast majority of these organisms live a quiet and sometimes symbiotic existence on and in our bodies, kept in check by a complex array of host defense mechanisms. On rare occasions a new microbe, or even sometimes one that had been living quietly as part of our colonizing flora, aggressively attempts to invade or alter the host using various attacking mechanisms. The resulting struggle between host and invader may be experienced as fever, other manifestations of the inflammatory response, or organ malfunction. This constitutes an *infectious disease.* The outcome may range from complete resolution to death of the host, or chronic infection, either overt or latent (Fig. 2.1). Latent infection and asymptomatic carriage represent immunologic stalemates. This chapter will review some of the major steps and factors in the establishment and resolution of infectious disease, as well as its diagnosis, treatment, and prevention.

## Microbial Factors

### Virulence

A wide variety of bacteria, viruses, fungi, protozoa, helminths, and sometimes arthropods can infect man. Their capacity to cause disease during this process is a function of their *virulence.* Virulence is an operational term since it rests on the interaction between microbial factors and the defenses of the host. A change in either can lead to the expression of disease. For example, organisms of normally low virulence—i.e., not usually capable of causing disease in a normal individual—may become dangerous pathogens when immunity is compromised. These organisms are usually labeled as *opportunistic pathogens.* The microbial factors that determine virulence are those that allow the organism to colonize, proliferate, invade, or otherwise modify host tissues and organs.

### Epidemiological factors

Before an organism can infect, the host and organism must meet and the organism must establish a residence. Infectious-disease epidemiology is concerned in part with the study and determination of the outcome of this meeting. All etiologic agents have some habitat or *reservoir* where they normally reside and multiply. In the case of some organisms, man himself may provide this habitat. The place from which an organism is transmitted to the host is termed the *source;* this may in some cases be distinct from the reservoir. An infecting agent may come from an *endogenous* source, i.e., be part of the flora normally colonizing the skin or mucous membranes, or may be *exogenous*, i.e., acquired from the environment. In a sense, all organisms acquired after birth are exogenously acquired, but those that are capable of colonizing the normal host for long periods of time without causing disease are termed endogenous *normal flora* (Table 2.1).

Mechanisms by which an organism may be acquired exogenously from a source include direct or indirect contact, from a vehicle, by airborne spread, or by contact with specific insects or animals. *Indirect contact* involves that with objects or surfaces that may be contaminated with infectious secretions. These objects are termed *fomites* (Latin for "tinder"). A vehicle usually refers to food or water, or in some cases blood or intravenous infusions, that may have the capacity to infect multiple recipients. Airborne transmission occurs when organisms can travel long distances on droplet nuclei or dust particles and be acquired by the host. Insects or animals can serve as the means of transmitting organisms from a reservoir to a host—in some cases, malaria is an example—insects may be both reservoir and source. Knowledge of infectious-disease transmission is often crucial to understanding its development, whether it represents a danger to others, and how it may be prevented. Chapters 7 and 8 deal in detail with epidemiological factors in the transmission and control of infectious diseases.

### Colonization

An infectious disease may or may not develop after contact between a microbe and a host. In many cases a period of *colonization* of the host by the organism on mucosal, skin, or wound surfaces precedes active infection. Whether or not infection subsequently develops is the result of the interplay between the virulence factors of the microbe and the defense mechanisms of the host. Typically colonization first takes place at the original site of contact; this is termed the *portal of entry.* Whether or not colonization occurs is a function of the infecting dose of microbes, their ability to *adhere to* host epithelial cells or other tissues—or to survive in surface secretions—and competition from already established flora.

Many microorganisms have developed unique structures or secrete certain substances to promote attachment. Specific molecules on the organisms that are responsible for attachment are termed *adhesins;* these are usually glycoproteins that can bind to cellular surface receptors or to extracellular matrix materials. In bacteria, adhesins are often localized to surface filamentous structures (pili, fimbriae) and bind with high affinity to host cell-surface glycoproteins or gangliosides. The virulence of *Neisseria gonorrheae* and many enteric or urinary pathogens is highly dependent on pili, which promote adherence in the face of opposing urinary or fecal flow. In the mouth viridans streptococci produce dextrans that glue them to tooth surfaces (or to cardiac

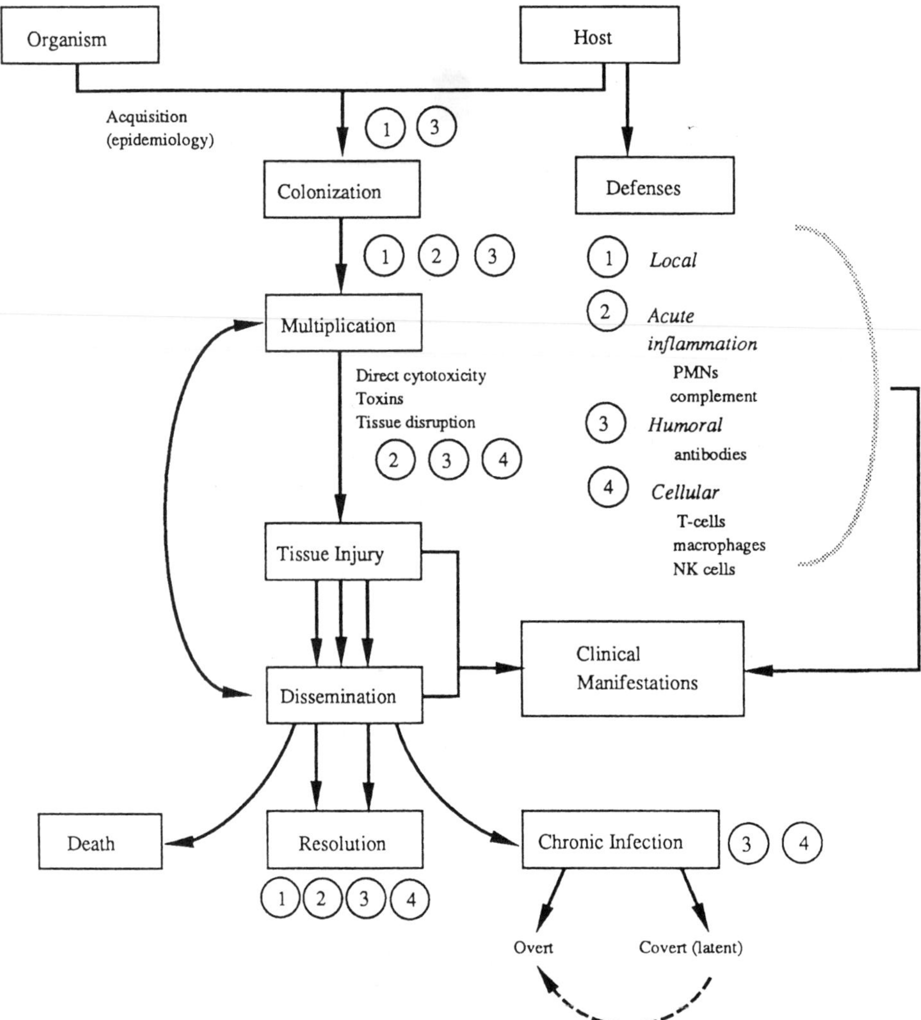


**Fig. 2.1** Schematized interplay between microorganisms and host factors that lead to infection, infectious disease, and resolution. The circled numbers indicate sites at which the designated host responses may interrupt or modify the pathogenesis of disease. [Source: Used with permission from Heinzel FP, Root, RK. Introduction of infectious diseases: Pathogenic mechanisms and host responses. In Harrison's Principles of Internal Medicine, 12th Edition, Wilson, JD, et al., eds. McGraw Hill, New York, 1991.]

valves). Coagulase-negative staphylocci can secrete a complex proteoglycan surface slime that promotes adherence to prosthetic devices. Newer approaches to the development of antimicrobials are using compounds to inhibit bacterial adherence.

## Multiplication

Following colonization, many pathogens undergo multiplication as a necessary preliminary to invasion or production of tissue or organ-altering toxins. Multiplication can take place only if there is an appropriate supply of nutrients, moisture, and, in the case of strictly aerobic organisms, oxygen. In addition, it will be affected by the prevailing pH, the ionic strength, and competing flora in the immediate environment. These conditions may be dramatically changed by the health of the host, which may lead to modifications in the production of cellular attachment receptors or by antibiotic therapy. Colonization of the nasopharynx of severely ill patients by gram-negative bacteria and multiplication of *Clostridium difficile* in the colon following antimicrobial treatment that reduces competing flora are important clinical examples of these phenonoma.

## Invasion and dissemination

Most infectious diseases become clinically evident only when organisms invade locally or disseminate and produce tissue injury or organ dysfunction. These can be the result of direct actions of the microorganisms or their toxins or the host inflammatory or immune responses. Once local defenses are breached, the acute inflammatory response attempts to localize the infection to the entry site. Secondary sites of inflammatory defense are at the level of the lymphatic system or in the bloodstream. Each of these sites may become clinically inflamed and injured during the process (see Chapter 10).

Once disseminated, some organisms may proliferate only in specific sites or organs, whereas others may invade widely and exhibit multiple metastatic sites of infection. An example of specific tissue and organ tropism is the propensity of polioviruses to cause anterior horn cell destruction and paralysis, as well as aseptic meningitis following dissemination from the gastrointestinal tract (see Chapter 76). *S. viridans* in the bloodstream can adhere specifically to cardiac valves damaged by preexistent rheumatic heart disease and cause endocarditis with or without multiple secondary sites of infection (see Chapter 66). Other organisms generate an overwhelming septic response in the host, leading to widespread organ dysfunction and death unless effective treatment can be provided (see Chapter 50).

The factors that govern tissue tropism are being characterized for an increasing number of organisms, as are virulence factors that are responsible for invasion and dissemination. For example, recent evidence indicates that pathogenic pneumococci utilize receptors for platelet-activating factor on respiratory cells to adhere to and invade these cells. Once they have accessed the local lymphatics and bloodstream their antiphagocytic capsule plays a major role in resisting their removal by phagocytosis. This capsule is also important in resisting phagocytosis in the alveoli and in the subarachnoid space where these organisms can multiply freely. Much of the resulting tissue injury is mediated by the frustrated acute inflammatory response. Other organisms possess digestive enzymes, which are important in the invasive process. These may be simple proteases (e.g., from schistosome larvae) or complex mixtures of proteases, lipases, lecithinases, collagenases, and hyaluronidases that are both cytolytic and digest extracellular matrix, facilitating spread through host tissues. *Staphylococcus aureus*, *Streptococcus pyogenes*, *Pseudomonas aeruginosa*, and *Clostridium perfringens* are organisms that secrete tissue-necrotizing enzymes or toxins with these properties.

For obligate intracellular parasites, which include some bacteria, all viruses, and many protozoans and fungi, cellular invasion is a necessary prelude to their survival and proliferation. Many of these organisms possess surface molecules that facilitate binding and entry into their target cells. A good example is the human immunodeficiency virus, whose surface glycoproteins gpl20 and gp40 promote specific binding to the CD4 proteins displayed on T-helper lymphocytes with subsequent fusion and entry. Other organisms gain access by phoagocytosis into macrophages, where they resist the normal killing mechanisms, in some cases by inhibiting lysosomal fusion with phagosomes (tubercle bacilli and *Toxoplasma gondii*). Sheltered from antibodies and other inflammatory cells in this intracellular haven, they can subvert a supply of cellular nutrients to promote their proliferation and survival. Chlamydia and rickettsia contain surface proteins that can induce their phagocytosis by their normally nonphagocytic target cells (see Chapter 20). This intracellular residence also makes it difficult to eradicate these organisms by immune mechanisms (cellular cytotoxicity and macrophage activation) or antimicrobials that cannot penetrate and maintain their activity in this location.

## Microbial toxins

Microbial toxins may be proteins secreted or released from microbes that can alter cellular, tissue, or organ function at some distance from the site of organism multiplication. Invasion of host tissues is not a necessary requirement for their action. The most striking examples include the Clostridial toxins that cause neurological dysfunction in tetanus and botulism, and the toxin released by *Corynebacterium diphtheria* that is both cytolytic and neurolytic, giving rise to the characteristic local asphyxiating membrane and the distal myocarditis and neuritis. The actions of these toxins can be neutralized by antibodies either produced by the host during the protective immunization process or by passive administration of antisera. A second group of extracellular

**Table 2.1** Bacteria commonly found on heathy human body surfaces

| Bacteria | Skin | Conjunctiva | Upper respiratory tract | Mouth | Lower intestine | Genitourinary tract: External genitalia | Genitourinary tract: Anterior urethra | Genitourinary tract: Vagina |
|---|---|---|---|---|---|---|---|---|
| AEROBIC AND FACULTATIVELY ANAEROBIC | | | | | | | | |
| Staphylococci | + | + | + | + | ± | + | ++ | + |
| Streptococci | | | | | | | | |
| Viridans | ± | ± | + | ++ | + | + | ± | + |
| Group A | | | ± | ± | | | | |
| Group D | | | ± | + | + | + | + | + |
| *S. pneumoniae* | | ± | + | + | | | | |
| Neisseriae | | ± | ± | + | | | + | ± |
| Corynebacteria | + | + | + | + | + | + | + | + |
| Haemophili | | ± | + | + | | | | |
| Enterobacteriaceae | | | ± | ± | ++ | + | + | ± |
| ANAEROBIC | | | | | | | | |
| Clostridia | | | | ± | ++ | | ± | ± |
| Propionibacteria | ++ | | + | ± | ± | | ± | |
| Actinomycetes | | | + | + | ± | | | |
| Lactobacilli | | | | + | + | | ± | ++ |
| Bifidobacteria | | | | + | ++ | | | ++ |
| Bacteroides | | | + | ++ | ++ | + | + | + |
| Fusobacteria | | | + | ++ | + | + | + | ± |
| Cocci | | | | | | | | |
| Gram-positive | + | | + | ++ | ++ | + | ± | + |
| Gram-negative | | | + | ++ | + | | ± | + |

Key: ±, irregular; +, common; ++, prominent.

Source: Used with permission from Washington, JA. Diagnosis of infectious diseases. In Infectious Diseases, 1st Edition, Gorbach et al., eds. WB Saunders Co., Philadelphia, 1992, Table 14.1.

protein toxins are those produced by *S. aureus* or *S. pyogenes* that can bind to specific structural peptides on host T-cell receptors (V beta peptides that are genetically determined) and macrophage class II histocompatibility antigens and induce massive release of cytokines. This property has classified these toxins as *superantigens*, a property that is discussed in detail in Chapter 11.

Finally, other microbial toxins are structural in nature and may be released only during organism multiplication or destruction. Termed *endotoxins*, these complex lipopolysaccharide molecules which make up the outer envelope of gram-negative bacteria are capable of eliciting the large array of host inflammatory and cytokine responses that contribute dramatically to the phenonomology of sepsis and septic shock (see Chapter 50).

## The Host Defense Systems

In order to cope with the surrounding microbial horde, we have evolved a complex series of defense mechanisms that range from the immediate and nonspecific to the delayed and highly specific. It is the interaction between these defense mechanisms and the virulence factors of microbes that determines both the clinical manifestations and outcome of infection.

### Local defenses

The first barrier to invading microbes is provided by the integrity of the epidermis and mucosal epithelium. These physical barriers may be able to hold organisms in check without the involvement of the inflammatory or immune defenses. On the skin they can be assisted in this process by antibacterial fatty acids secreted by sebaceous glands. In the mouth saliva contains several antibacterial enzymes (lysozyme and lactoperoxidase), as does mucus in the respiratory tract. Saliva and mucus may also contain IgA antibodies against some organisms to which the host has been previously exposed; these act to inhibit attachment to host epithelial cells.

In the proximal respiratory tract rhythmically beating cilia sweep the mucus blanket out of the airways. When cilia are impaired by exposure to respiratory viruses, alcohol, or cigarette smoke, secondary bacterial infections may ensue. In the stomach the acid pH kills many organisms, in particular the anaerobic species swallowed in saliva; gastric bacterial counts are dramatically reduced.

Urine and vaginal secretions also contain antibacterial factors that together with flow keep organism counts down or eradicate them completely. In the gut intestinal motility is another process that regulates the type and amount of flora. When motility is impaired by ileus, the counts of anaerobic organisms in the small bowel rise sharply.

### Acute inflammatory defenses

Unfortunately the local defense systems may be easily breached either traumatically, including by the well-meaning insertion of intravenous lines or urinary catheters, or by the invasive properties of the organisms themselves. When this occurs the second line of defense is provided by phagocytic cells, principally *polymorphonuclear leukocytes (PMN) and macrophages*, that work in concert with the complement system to attempt to localize and eradicate the invaders. If the host has been previously exposed to the offending microbes, both phagocytes amd the complement system can be aided and focused in their actions by the presence of opsonizing or bactericidal antibodies. In their absence activation of the complement system occurs by the less efficient alternative pathway. Similarly, without opsonizing antibodies phagocytes must use less effective receptors for binding and internalizing organisms (see Chapter 10).

The bone marrow normally produces and releases about 10 billion neutrophils per day in the average adult. When challenged by infection it may rapidly increase its production of PMN by ten- to 15-fold in response to increased elaboration of specific *colony-stimulating factors (GCSF and GMCSF)*. In concert, production of complement components also increases as part of the acute phase response in inflammation. The production of GCSF, GMCSF, and complement components is increased by the inflammatory cytokines tumor necrosis factor (TNF), interleukin-1 (IL-1), and interleukin-6 (IL-6) released from macrophages and T lymphocytes stimulated by exposure to microbial virulence factors or phagocytosis. These events amplify the effectiveness of the acute inflammatory response until specific immune factors can intervene.

Once PMN are released from the bone marrow they spend a relatively short time in the circulation (6–12 hours) before exiting between endothelial cells in postcapillary venules in a process known as *diapedesis*. Microbial factors and the inflammatory cytokines promote the adherence of PMN to the endothelial cells and diapedesis in reponse to chemotactic factors produced at a site of inflammation or infection. The basic mechanisms involved in these events are discussed in Chapter 10.

PMN are the first phagocytes (other than resident tissue macrophages) to reach a site of inflammation or microbial invasion where they ingest and attempt to kill the offending agents. The killing process is achieved usually within the phagolysosomes of PMN by the coordinated production of toxic oxygen products during a stimulated burst in oxygen consumption and the secretion of a host of lysosomal enzymes and peptides with microbicidal activity. Not surprisingly, some organisms, particularly those that can survive within an intracellular location, can resist killing by detoxifying the oxidants (catalase and superoxide dismutase) or inhibiting phagolysosomal fusion. Likewise, the processes of oxidant production and phagolysosomal fusion are not so precise that all the toxic compounds are contained within phagosomes. Their leakage into normal tissues along with lysosomal proteases, lipases, and nucleic acid hydrolases contributes to the tissue injury and cytotoxicity characteristic of inflammation. Once they have phagocytized their target particles and have completed their metabolic burst and lysosomal degranulation, PMN die within hours. Their average survival in tissues is about 3 to 5 days.

Macrophages are derived from circulating monocytes that are also produced and released from the bone marrow. While not as highly mobile as PMN or able to be increased numerically within hours of exposure of the host to an inflammatory or infectious stimulus, they have other unique properties that are indespensable to long-term defense against intracellular pathogens and to the specific immune response. The supply of tissue macrophages is replenished from monocytes that leave the circulation, usually several days after entry from the bone marrow. Macrophages concentrate in some organs responsible for scavenging microbes from the blood (liver and spleen) or from the airways (alveolar macrophages). They are also found in abundance in the skin and draining lymph nodes. While their phagocytic and microbicidal activities reduplicate the actions of PMN, macrophages are not destroyed by these events but can live for months to years in their resident tissues. Furthermore, their microbical activities can be markedly enhanced following exposure to cytokines released by T lymphocytes during the specific immune response, in particular *gamma interferon.* This process is known as *macrophage activation.* Finally, macrophages have critical accessory cell functions for the specific immune response by serving as antigen-presenting cells to T and B lymphocytes.

Eosinophils are also phagocytic cells; however, they are not as adept at the process as either macrophages or PMN, and they contain a different array of intralysosomal compounds. Some of these compounds—e.g., major basic protein—are toxic to metazoan parasites such as schistosome larvae. Eosinophilia is a characteristic feature of infection with metazoan parasites.

Together with circulating antibodies the complement system plays a key role in so-called *humoral immune defenses.* This system of more than 25 proteins and regulators can be rapidly activated either by antibodies bound to antigens (in particular, IgM or IgG antibodies) by the *classical pathway* or by specific microbial factors in the absence of antibodies by the *alternative pathway.* These factors are surface molecules and can include polysaccharides, peptidoglycans, or lypopolysaccharides (endotoxins). In general, activation by the alternative pathway is slower and less efficient than that by the classical pathway.

Biologic activities of the complement system include vasodilation and increasing capillary permeability (C3a and C5a), opsonization (C3b and C3bi), PMN chemotaxis (C5a), and lytic destruction of gram-negative bacteria and selected other organisms by its terminal membrane attack complex (see Chapter 10).

When either the complement system or PMN are impaired by disease or, sometimes, therapy, the result is a significantly increased susceptibility to bacterial infections. In the case of the complement system these are usually organisms that are killed by its bactericidal action (*Neisseria* and *Hemophilus* species). When PMN are impaired quantitatively or qualitatively, pyogenic bacteria and opportunistic fungi become more frequent and dangerous pathogens (see Chapter 86).

## Specific immunity

The host defense systems become much more focused and efficient in their ability to eradicate or contain organisms when specific immune mechanisms become active. This process may take days to weeks to become effective unless the antigens presented by the invaders have been previously encountered and the memory capacity of the immune system is stimulated. Antigenic memory is contained within specifically selected T lymphocytes that can rapidly proliferate and secrete cytokines to rearm cytotoxic or antibody-producing cells within several days. The specificity of the immune response is provided in the variable regions of receptors on CD4-positive T lymphocytes that can recognize up to a billion different epitopes. This recognition is followed by the production of highly specific antibodies or cytotoxic T lymphocytes or arming of macrophages to inactivate or eradicate both extracellular and intracellular pathogens. The mechanisms involved in activation of the immune system and the cooperative role played between macrophages and other antigen-presenting cells, specific cytokines, and T and B lymphocytes are discussed in detail in Chapter 11.

In brief, a central mechanism in the development of specific immunity is the activation of T lymphocytes leading to their proliferation and the secretion of cytokines that both amplify and regulate the process. Microbial antigens must be presented to T cells (and in some cases to B cells directly) by *antigen-presenting cells* that are macrophages or modified macrophages called dendritic cells. T cells recognize both the antigen through the complementary structure of its *T cell antigen receptor* and the "self" nature of the presenting cell by its unique class II *major histocompatibility complex* (*MHC*), which is intimately involved in the presentation. Successful presentation and recognition then leads to clonal proliferation of the recipient lymphocytes and their secretion of amplifying and regulating cytokines, among which interleukin-2 (IL-2) plays a key role. Ultimately these cytokines stimulate clonal proliferation of T cells with either cytotoxic or regulatory (i.e., *helper* or *suppressor*) activities and B cells that form specific antibodies against the offending antigen. Besides the generation of an expanded and specific cytotoxic T-cell repertoire, activation of macrophages is accomplished by exposure to gamma interferon produced in increased amounts during the immune response process. Finally, other proinflammatory cytokines formed and released by macrophages or lymphocytes during this process play a major role in the induction of fever, acute-phase protein production, leukocytosis, and many other clinical manifestations of infection (see Chapters 9, 10, and 50).

## Role of antibodies in infection

*Antibodies* are bifunctional glycoproteins termed *immunoglobulins* and are produced by mature B cells. They can bind with high specificity to microbial antigens or infected cells displaying these antigens at their variable, or *Fab*, region, by means of complementary charge and recognition of molecular topography. The constant portions of the antibody molecule, in particular the *Fc regions*, are responsible for harnessing many of its biological activities, including *activation of the complement system*, *antibody-dependent cellular cytotoxicity* (*ADCC*) and *opsonization* of organisms for phagocytosis. Antibodies can also *neutralize* viruses or toxins by blocking binding to their target cells and inhibit microbial adherence at colonizing sites by binding to adhesins. When confronted with new antigens antibody production is not easily detected until 5 to 7 days later; if there are memory responses, circulating antibodies may appear against invading organisms or their toxins in 2 to 3 days.

The constant portions of immunoglobulin molecules also define their *isotype*, or class, and their distribution within the body. IgM antibodies are large pentamers, highly efficient in complement fixation. They are largely confined to the circulation, where they participate in complement-mediated opsonization and clearance or bactericidal activities. IgG antibodies are distributed throughout the fluid compartments of the body and are found in small concentrations in secretions. They are most active in opsonization, neutralization, and ADCC. IgA antibodies are concentrated on mucosal surfaces and in secretions. Much of their activity appears to be centered on blocking microbial adherence, as well as multiplication and invasion from these surfaces. IgE antibodies are present in small amounts in plasma and can trigger immediate hypersensitivity reactions when bound to their specific antigens and IgE receptors on basophils and mast cells. The role of IgD immunoglobulins in host defense requires further clarification,

Besides their protective role, antibodies may participate in some of the deleterious consequences of infection and inflammation. When antigen–antibody complexes appear in the circulation they can deposit in glomeruli, where they play a pathogenetic role in glomerulitis, or in joints, where they trigger inflammatory responses leading to arthritis. ADCC may be a mechanism by which virus-infected cells are eradicated, thereby contributing to organ injury. When antibody formation is impaired, particularly that of IgG, the result is recurring and life-threatening bacteremias as well as sinopulmonary infections with encapsulated bacteria. These can be prevented or reduced by periodic administration of IgG (see Chapter 44).

### Cellular immunity

This is the host response that is mediated by macrophages, cytotoxic and other T lymphocytes, and their soluble products called *cytokines*. PMN, antibodies, and the complement system are well designed to eradicate pathogens when they are in the extracellular location. Once organisms become intracellular these defenses are not nearly as effective and cellular immune mechanisms are called into play for this purpose. In contrast to antibody production, it may take weeks for cellular immunity to be fully expressed.

Intracelluar organisms may be eliminated by enhanced phagocytic and microbicidal activity by macrophages (an event known as *macrophage activation*), or the action of specific cytotoxic T lymphocytes. In addition, other cytotoxic lymphocytes, known as natural killer (NK) cells, which do not contain T-cell receptors or require MHC recognition for proliferation, may be stimulated by cytokines to show enhanced killing of virus-infected cells. During the course of eradication of intercellular organisms the cytotoxic process may injure or eradicate the infected host cell as well. Thus, it appears that much of the hepatocyte injury that occurs with hepatitis B infection is due to cytotoxic T-lymphocyte action (see Chapter 62).

## The Outcomes of Infection

Each event in the pathogenesis of an infectious disease involves a complex interplay between microbial virulence factors and the host defenses. The scenario that develops as the disease unfolds is often a highly changing one as first the microbe and then the host defenses change positions and strategies. To survive as successful parasites microbes have devised a number of mechanisms to counteract host defenses; these may be more or less prominent during different stages of the infectious process.

For example, at the very time that host defense mechanisms are becoming amplified and focused, microbial virulence factors may counteract their effectiveness and turn the potential benefits of the inflammatory response into harmful host tissue injury. Thus, encapsulated organisms such as the pneumococcus can stimulate a strong inflammatory response yet escape effective phagocytosis until modified by antibiotic treatment or coated with opsonizing antibodies. Staphylococci and pyogenic streptococci make toxins that destroy PMN or inhibit phagocytosis by binding opsonizing immunoglobulins in nonfunctional forms. Intracellular staphylococci and other catalase and superoxide dismutase–positive organisms can detoxify oxidants generated by phagocytes during the respiratory burst. Other organisms that have a propensity to invade the bloodstream can resist the lytic action of the complement system despite triggering its biologic activities. Still others seize upon the act of their phagocytosis to gain entry into macrophages where they not only resist killing but may use the cells as vehicles to ferry them into priveleged sites like the central nervous system. Intracellular pathogens are largely protected from the actions of PMN, antibodies, and complement despite stimulating their activation and production. These events can contribute to the inflammatory manifestations of infection while failing to eradicate the offenders. Later in the infectious process, when specific immunity is established, some organisms such as borellia or HIV can change their surface coats, rendering specific antibodies formed against an earlier version ineffective and contributing both to chronicity and relapses of infection.

The outcome of an infection is determined by the final balance between host immunity and microbial virulence factors (Fig. 2.1). When treatment of infection is given it is to suppress the microbe while hopefully giving the host defenses the upper hand. At one extreme the infection may lead to the *death* of the host, an event that may also prove suicidal to the organism unless it can be transmitted to a new host. At the other extreme, the organism may be eradicated during *resolution* of the infection, and because of the development of an effective immune response and immunological memory the host is protected for life against reinfection by the same organism. The natural history of most of the viral childhood exanthems before the advent of specific immunization followed this course.

When there is an equal balance between host immunity and the microbe, a situation of *chronic disease* may develop. This is the case for much of the course of HIV infection or many chronic parasitic infections. Sometimes host immunity may succeed only in suppressing the overt clinical manifestations of infection while the pathogen lurks in a *latent state*, only to reappear at a later time when immunity wanes or is suppressed by malnutrition or drug treatment. Reactivation of tuberculosis or the development of Herpes zoster infection in the elderly patient are examples of this phenonomen. Finally, in some patients invasive infection may resolve but the organism continues to proliferate on a mucosal site and a chronic *carrier state* is established.

## Clinical Manifestations of Infection

The characteristic clinical manifestations of infection—fever, chills, myalgias, sweats, anorexia, fatigue, weakness, and weight loss—have been known since antiquity, as have signs of inflammation and infectious skin lesions. By the end of the nineteenth century, physicians knew that many infections were accompanied by leukocytosis and changes in serum proteins as expressions of the acute-phase response. The twentieth century has witnessed an explosion of the understanding of the spectrum of infectious diseases to include malignancies, immunosuppression, chronic arthritides, dementias, and, most recently, peptic ulcer disease. Not all of these stimulate the cardinal signs of fever and inflammation. Nevertheless, when these signs are present they signal the likely presence of infection and the need for a diagnostic workup for this possibility. Furthermore, they become useful markers to follow once treatment is initiated.

It is now known that the production of fever and the other signs of inflammation during infection signals an interactive role among specific microbial factors, host cells, and humoral proteins. The act of phagocytosis or the binding of endotoxin to CD14 proteins on monocytes and macrophages can trigger the formation and release of the potent proinflammatory cytokines IL-1 and TNF. These cytokines not only act as pyrogens but can initiate and amplify the specific immune response (IL-1) and stimulate the formation of secondary proinflammatory cytokines, interferon gamma, and IL-6, as well as colony-stimulating factors that enhance myelopoiesis. Working collectively, this group of molecules plays a central role in the development of most of the clinical features of both acute and chronic infections (see

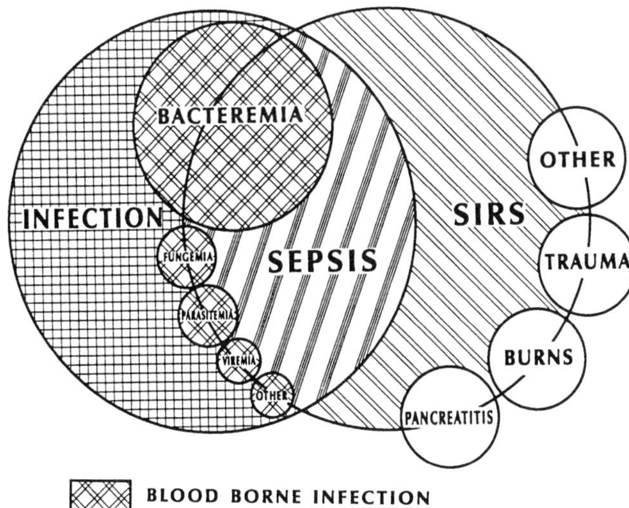


**Fig. 2.2** The interrelationship between systemic inflammatory response syndrome (SIRS), sepsis, and infection. [Used with permission from Bone RC, Balk RA, Cerra FB et al ACCP/SCCM Consensus Conference. Definitions for sepsis and organ failure and guidelines for use of innovative therapies in sepsis. Chest 1992; 101:1644–1655.]

Chapters 9, 10, 11, 46, and 50). A host of secondary molecules, including the kinins, coagulation proteins, prostanoids, and nitric oxide, serve as the immediate effectors of the actions of the inflammatory cytokines. Not surprisingly, the stimuli that trigger such a potent inflammatory system also initiate the simultaneous production of regulators. These include specific inhibitors such as IL-1 receptor antagonist protein and soluble TNF receptors, as well as the counter-regulatory cytokines IL-4, IL-10, transforming growth factor beta (TGF beta), and products of the actions of inflammatory cytokines that inhibit their continuing synthesis, prostaglandin E1 and the glucocorticoids.

The balance of the actions within this cornucopia of mediators has a major effect on determining the clinical expression of many infectious diseases as well as their outcome. In judging the seriousness of illness as a measure of the intensity of the inflammatory response and as a prognostic indicator investigators in critical care medicine have recently come up with the concept of a "*sepsis score.*" Such patients who manifest signs of sepsis, in particular *septic shock*, have more severe and generalized illness and are more likely to die from the infection than those who are not septic (see Chapter 50). They have also been demonstrated to have higher levels of inflammatory cytokines in their circulation, in particular TNF and IL-6, at the time of their presentation. The concentrations of these cytokines have been correlated prognostically with both the development of septic shock and survival from severe infection. The conceptual relationsips between infection and sepsis are portrayed in Figure 2.2, and discussed more thoroughly in Chapter 50.

Clearly, inflammatory responses to infection are not all deleterious. The proliferation of lymphocytes in response to cytokines is augmented at febrile body temperatures, as are chemotaxis and some of the phagocytic activities of PMN. Enhanced myelopoiesis and formation of complement factors supply an army of cells and key proteins for the inflammatory defenses. Inflammation-induced hyperemia augments the delivery of leukocytes and humoral factors to a site of infection. Increased capillary permeability promotes the entry of key serum proteins into an infected site. Reductions in serum iron can remove an essential element for the proliferation of some pathogens. Support for the beneficial role of the inflammatory cytokines in infection comes from experiments that demonstrate the unchecked spread of certain intracellular infections, such as listeriosis, when TNF action is specifically inhibited, or the increase in resistance to challenge with infectious agents when animals are pretreated with this cytokine.

## Diagnosis and Treatment of Infectious Diseases

Faced with a patient with a suspected infectious disease, the clinician has several objectives. First, the organ system that is involved with the illness must be defined. Second, the severity and tempo of the illness must be gauged, initially by the clinical signs and later by obtaining certain laboratory data if illness severity warrants it. Third, an effort must be made to determine the nature of the infecting agent. Fourth, a decision regarding treatment with specific antimicrobials must be reached. Finally, the need for and type of supportive care must be estimated. This approach requires obtaining a careful history and performing an appropriate physical examination as well as judicious use of laboratory data (see Chapter 47). It also requires a knowledge of which pathogens are likely to cause particular infectious syndromes and the availability of specific treatment.

Identifying the possibility of an infectious disease process is not usually difficult if the illness has an acute onset and is accompanied by systemic signs such as fever, chills, anorexia, and malaise. Fever, however, may not be a major manifestation of most minor infectious illnesses, or of infections in the elderly or patients taking medications with an antipyretic action, and it may not be prominent in chronic infectious diseases. Thus, a high level of suspicion regarding infection must be entertained in these situations.

Likewise, identifying the involved organ system or site is fairly easy in patients with rhinorrhea and cough, or sore throat, or nausea and vomiting and diarrhea, or flank pain and dysuria, or severe headache, or cellulitis or a swollen tender joint. It may be more difficult in patients with diffuse systemic involvement or chronic febrile illnesses without focal signs. In these latter patients, imaging and laboratory studies play a more important role in establishing specific organ involvement with disease (see Chapter 49). Because certain agents predictably cause infections in different organ and tissue sites, it is useful to *classify the illness*, if possible, as pneumonia, gastroenteritis, meningitis, diffuse sepsis, etc. Furthermore, this classification will help guide further diagnostic and therapeutic efforts. To assist in this process, the clinical portions of this text are organized syndromically and by organ system.

The *tempo of disease* is important to assess along with its severity, since these will determine the speed at which diagnostic studies should be obtained and whether treatment must be promptly administered or could be delayed until a specific pathogen is identified. Besides the pace of the disease, the adequacy of the patient's host defense mechanisms and his ability to withstand infection are other critical factors to consider in these decisions.

The next major focus of evaluation of the patient with suspected infectious disease is to determine if there are any unusual *exposures or risk factors* for certain types of infections. The previously health patient with a cough, headache, and pulmonary infiltrate who has cared for a sick parrot is likely to have a much different cause for his pneumonia (*Chlamydia psittaci*) than another patient with similar symptoms who is neutropenic from cytotoxic chemotherapy and has no exposure to sick birds (an aerobic gram-negative rod or opportunistic fungus). Thus, it is important to inquire about occupational and travel history, sexual and other personal habits, previous history of infections, other illnesses, and medications, besides possible exposures to other ill persons or sources for transmission of infection

Once these elements of history and physical examination have been obtained, the further diagnostic workup can center on necessary imaging studies to *define organ involvement* (see Chapter 12), hematological and other laboratory studies to *characterize the intensity and nature of the inflammatory response*, and possible metabolic or organ dysfunction (see Chapters 13 and 14). A list of suspected pathogens can be assembled from the nature of the infection—e.g., pneumonia or urinary tract infection—and specific laboratory studies carried out to attempt identification. Chapters 15 to 20 present the microbiologic diagnosis of infectious diseases by pathogen group to be coupled with the approaches outlined in each of the syndromic chapters. As a general point it is usually preferable to carry out these diagnostic studies *before* administering therapy in all but the most benign and self-limited illnesses. In these, a broad and unnecessarily costly diagnostic evaluation is not indicated.

Almost all patients with an infectious disease appreciate or need some treatment directed at their *supportive care*. This may range from giving fluids and antipyretics for fever or decongestants for rhinitis to massive fluid replacement for septic shock or oxygen therapy for pneumonia. These therapeutic approaches are discussed in detail in the appropriate chapters.

The decision whether or not to use specific antimicrobial therapy rests on the severity of the illness, the nature of the patient's host defense mechanisms, and the likelihood that the suspected or proven pathogen is susceptible to available treatment (see Chapter 24). In general, once a decision has been made to administer an antimicrobial the choice should be made based on efficacy, relative toxicity, and cost. Efficacy is a function not only of the results of in vitro testing but the likelihood that the patient will cooperate with therapy, and that the drug will reach the site of infection in vivo and be active at that site. Furthermore, in the case of nosocomial pathogens that may be resistant to first-line antimicrobials a knowledge of their likely antibiotic susceptibilities for the particular hospital is indespensable in making good treatment choices.

## Prevention of Infection

As is true of any disease, prevention is far preferable to treatment and cure. For centuries quarantine and avoidance of spoiled foods, visibly polluted water sources, and dwellings inhabited by sick people were the only means of preventing the acquisition and spread of certain infectious diseases. The notion that severe disease could be prevented by previous exposure to a milder form of a similar disease—i.e., *immunity*—did not achieve credence until the landmark studies by Lister in the late 1700s demonstrating protection from smallpox in individuals previously infected by an inoculation of fluid from a cowpox lesion (*vaccination*). The next two centuries saw immunization become a mainstay in the prevention of an increasing array of life-threatening toxogenic or highly contagious and disabling infectious diseases. It has also become a marker of the efficacy of both primary care and the adequacy of public health measures in communities and countries. Recent outbreaks of measles, diphtheria, and tetanus signal the breakdown of these systems in several highly developed countries.

Not only are effective vaccines a far cheaper, more cost effective way of dealing with infectious diseases than the use of increasingly expensive antimicrobials, but experience has shown that with the exception of influenza virus, which mutates yearly, most immunizing epitopes on bacterial toxins or capsules or whole viruses are quite stable. This is a far different situation than exists with many antimicrobials in which rapidly developing resistance by an increasing number of major pathogens presents a serious problem for worldwide public health and the management of infectious diseases (see Chapter 26). Thus, knowledge of the patient's immunization status and keeping it current are major obligations for the primary-care physician. Furthermore, immunization status must be considered in the evaluation of patients with suspected infectious diseases.

*Active vaccines* (i.e., those capable of inducing a humoral or cellular immune response by the host) may consist of killed or attenuated whole organisms, inactivated toxins ("toxoids"), or subunit antigens that play a key role in pathogenicity (see Chapters 43–45). To be effective in preventing disease, they should be given before exposure has occurred. With most active vaccines, protection lasts for years after completion of an immunizing course. *Passive vaccines* are usually immunoglobulin preparations containing antibodies against active virulence factors of the agent and can be given after exposure has occured (e.g., rabies or tetanus immune globulins). They can also be used prophylactically for a period of anticipated exposure (e.g., pooled human immune serum globulin for hepatitis A prevention). The duration of their protective effect is only as long as adequate levels of the administered antibodies remain in the body—i.e. about 20 to 30 days (see Chapter 44).

Other means to avoid infection include the standard use of aseptic procedures in surgery, the careful debridement of traumatic wounds (see Chapter 82), and the application of isolation procedures in the hospital setting (see Chapter 8). Prophylactic antimicrobials can be successfully employed to prevent wound infections, endocarditis, or secondary infection after exposure to communicable and potentially highly lethal agents such as *Neisseria* meningococcus (see Chapter 73).

Finally, in patients with known defects in host defense immunological restoration is being used to prevent infection. Monthly administration of immune serum globulin to patients with IgG deficiencies reduces sinopulmonary infections and septicemias (chapter 44). Daily use of recombinant cytokines (GCSF or interferon gamma) for patients with PMN disorders has reduced the frequency of pyogenic bacterial and opportunistic fungal infections (see Chapter 46). For patients who have severe combined immunodeficiencies or other genetic disorders of immune function, both bone-marrow transplantation and gene therapy have been dramatically employed as treatments (see Chapter 86).

### ANNOTATED BIBLIOGRAPHY

Bone RC, Balk RA, Cerra FB et al. ACCP/SCCM Consensus Conference: Definitions for sepsis and organ failure and guidelines for the use of innovative therapies in sepsis. Chest 1992; 101:1644–1655.

*An attempt to quantify the manifestations of the systemic inflammatory response and to differentiate infectious from other causes in response to infection. The definitions from this conference have been employed to standardize clinical studies of responses to treatment of infection and sepsis.*

Gorbach SL, Bartlett JG, Blacklow NR, eds. Infectious Diseases. WB Saunders, Philadelphia, 1992.

*This first-edition comprehensive treatise on clinical infectious diseases uses a format that is similar to the Mandell et al. text cited next but augments and supplements information in several different areas. It is well referenced and is due for an update in the near future.*

Mandell GL, Bennett JE, Dolin R, eds. Principles and Practice of Infectious Diseases, 4th ed. Churchill-Livingston, New York, 1995.

*This encyclopedic book is considered by many to be the most authoritative reference on the epidemiology and clinical manifestations of infectious diseases, the organisms that cause them, and the host defenses that protect against them. It is very well referenced and has been updated every four to five years.*

Wilson MB, ed. World Guide to Infections. Oxford University Press, New York, 1992.

*A concise but comprehensive text that details the major infectious diseases and their manifestations as seen in different locales in the world. It is particularly useful for a rapid review of potential infectious disease problems encountered in developing countries.*

# I

# PATHOPHYSIOLOGY OF INFECTIOUS DISEASES

# 3

# Microbes and Virulence Factors: Bacteria

DAVID A. RELMAN

An understanding of the processes by which bacteria cause disease requires an appreciation of both participants, pathogen and host, as well as the manner by which the two relate and respond to each other. Hence, a discussion of either one alone is inadequate. Nonetheless, a brief presentation of basic bacterial structure, taxonomy, and the principles of pathogenicity may be useful at the outset of this discussion. Novel scientific methods, technical approaches, and an integration with cell biology, structural biology, and immunology have revolutionized our view of bacterial pathogenesis, as well as the manner in which we ask questions and then set out to answer them.

## Bacterial Structure, Taxonomy, and Pathogenicity

Bacterial classification of prokaryotes has traditionally relied heavily on a few prominent morphologic features. One of these features, the cell wall, fulfills a critical function in providing structural stability and a barrier through which the external environment can be selectively sampled. Peptidoglycan is a network of polysaccharide chains cross-linked by short peptides. It is the principal structural component of the cell wall lying just external to the cytoplasmic membrane, and is specific to bacteria. Bacteria can be divided into those that have a relatively thick peptidoglycan layer interspersed with teichoic or lipoteichoic acids and coated with surface proteins, and those that have a thinner peptidoglycan layer linked by lipoproteins to a phospholipid–lipopolysaccharide bilayer outer membrane. This outer membrane contains surface proteins as well as integral proteins, some of which act as receptors, porins, and active transporters. The thick cell wall of the first type retains the crystal violet-iodine complex of the Gram's stain; these organisms are classified as gram-positive. The organisms with the second cell wall type retain only the red saffranin counterstain; they are classified as gram-negative. Bacteria with alternative cell wall structures (e.g., *Rickettsia*, spirochetes) or no cell wall (e.g., *Mycoplasma*) may stain poorly or not at all with the Gram procedure. Some of the components of the bacterial cell wall and the mechanisms for its synthesis and assembly offer unique and useful targets for antibacterial agents. Other structural or functional features that are relatively specific to bacteria include some outer-surface organelles such as pili, certain metabolic and secretion pathways, and the bacterial versions of some housekeeping enzymes.

Contrary to traditional teachings, phenotypes such as cell wall structure and Gram-staining characteristics are not reliable criteria on which to base taxonomy or organismal classification. Emphasis instead has turned in recent years to the use of certain genetic sequences as reflections of chromosomal or organismal evolutionary history. The sequences of the bacterial 16S and 23S rRNAs (and their genes) have been particularly reliable in this regard. Based on the comparative analysis of rRNA sequences, the phylogeny of the Bacteria (domain) has been revised (see Fig. 3.1). One of the most interesting findings is that the gram-negative organisms, the organisms with rodlike structures, and the anaerobic organisms are not phylogenetically coherent groups—i.e., these phenotypes are scattered across many evolutionary branchings. On the other hand, the gram-positive organisms belong to a single broad cluster, and the spirochetes are also a discrete evolutionary group. The close phylogenetic relationship between all mitochondrial ribosomal DNA sequences and the rickettsia-like organisms (not shown) suggests that the mitochondrion may have arisen from an ancestor shared by these obligate intracellular bacteria.

Because bacteria are haploid, they need to protect their genome and thus tend not to share their DNA with others. The observation that most pathogenic bacteria have clonal population structures is consistent with this concept. On the other hand, when one examines the genetic basis of pathogenicity a number of somewhat surprising findings emerge. First of all, two highly related organisms may display entirely different capabilities as pathogens. For example, among the two pairs of highly related bacteria—*E. coli* K12 and the enterohemorrhagic *E. coli*, and *Listeria innocua* and *L. monocytogenes*—the latter member of each pair is much more virulent in humans. Second, virulence-associated genes appear to be transmitted widely among members of the same bacterial species and even across genus boundaries. The genetic structure of virulence determinants provides an explanation: they are often found on transposable or transmissible genetic elements—i.e., plasmids, bacteriophages, and transposons. Among the many examples, the *Yersinia* cytolysins and tyrosine phosphatase are encoded by a virulence plasmid, and the diphtheria toxin gene and the cholera toxin gene cassette are carried by bacteriophages. Furthermore, chromosomal genes associated with bacterial virulence are not randomly distributed within the genome; instead, they are often found in discrete segments of the bacterial chromosome—i.e., "pathogenicity islands." For example, many of the *Salmonella* invasion and virulence genes are located within approximately 40 kb segments of the chromosome that are missing from the corresponding portion of the nonpathogenic *E. coli* chromosome. In some cases, the different guanine-cytosine composition of these segments in comparison with the overall chromosomal composition, and the finding of transposable elements at the ends of these segments, suggests that they may have arisen in one species and then become shared among others. These findings suggest that the evolution of bacterial virulence, when viewed from a distance, may have occurred more in leaps and bounds, rather than as a gradual process.

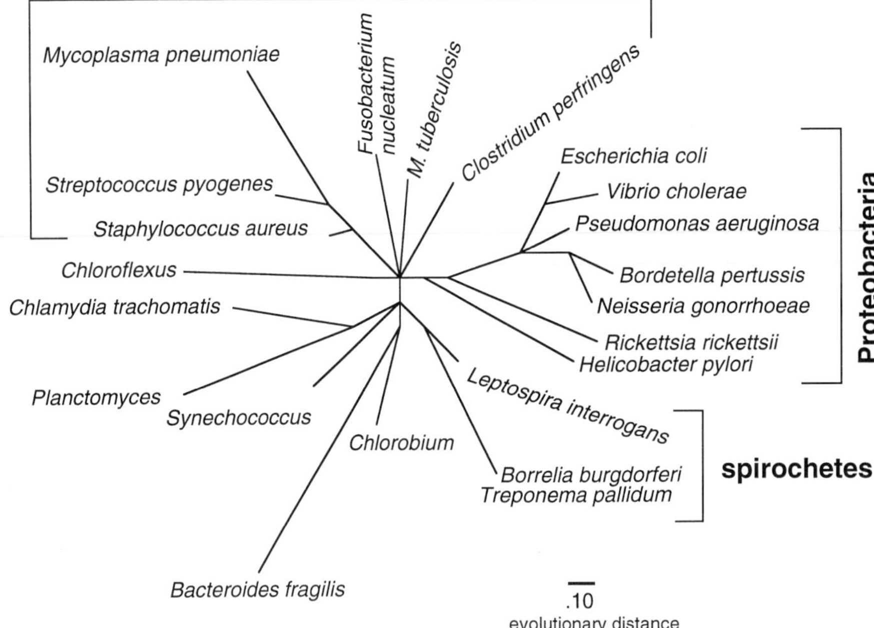


**Fig. 3.1** Phylogenetic tree of the domain Bacteria, based on comparative analysis of small subunit ribosomal DNA sequences. Evolutionary distance is proportional to the sum of the line-segment lengths that connect any two organisms (substitutions per nucleotide position).

## General Mechanisms of Bacterial Pathogenesis

### Pathogenic strategies

The primary goal of a bacterium is to replicate—i.e., make more bacteria. Some organisms accomplish this mission primarily within a human host. When the strategy for multiplication involves replication in a privileged niche or in a normally sterile site, or when the strategy results in substantive cellular or organismal pathophysiology, then disease is the outcome. Damaged or altered host tissues may offer a bacterium novel receptors, nutrients, colonization sites, access to distant sites, and a mechanism for transmission to new hosts (e.g., cough, diarrhea). On the other hand, disease entails recruitment of diverse host defenses, loss of certain receptors and host cells, and occasionally death of the host. An organism that relies on a strategy that routinely produces disease is viewed as a "principal" pathogen—e.g., *N. gonorrheae*. Organisms that cause disease rarely or only in hosts with impaired defenses are viewed as opportunistic pathogens—e.g., *P. aeruginosa*. Bacteria that are better adapted to animals than they are to humans tend to be associated with severe disease when they infect the latter.

The steps taken by a bacterial pathogen upon entering a susceptible human host follow a common scheme. Figure 3.2 provides one version of this scheme as it pertains to *Bordetella pertussis* infection and the causation of whooping cough. The first step involves attachment to host cells and acquisition of an appropriate anatomic niche. Bacterial multiplication and colonization then ensue. A necessary next step involves bacterial avoidance or subversion of host immune defense mechanisms. As either part of or separate from this process, many bacteria intoxicate the host or release tissue-destructive molecules. At this point, some bacterial pathogens negotiate a more chronic phase of infection during which persistent organisms turn off one set of genes and turn on another. The final phase in pathogenesis concerns transmission of the pathogen to a new susceptible host. Little attention has been devoted to the identification of bacterial factors that are essential for this phase of the process.

### Regulation of virulence

Bacterial pathogens are particularly adept at evaluating their immediate environment and responding to it by turning on and off large numbers of genes in a coordinate manner. This would seem to make sense for several reasons: (*1*) from the time of entry into a host to the time of departure, a pathogen encounters changing growth conditions that differ radically from the external environment; (*2*) different host environments require entirely different bacterial responses, ranging from purposeful movement to toxin production to sporulation; and (*3*) a large and unnecessary metabolic burden is imposed by the synthesis of specialized virulence-associated gene products in situations where they are not needed. For these reasons, bacteria rely upon a variety of overlapping and interconnected regulatory schemes and mechanisms. Groups of coregulated genes are referred to as *regulons*.

One common theme among bacterial regulatory responses to the environment is the use of a "two-component" system, consisting of a *sensor* protein and a *response regulator* protein. Sensor proteins are usually anchored within the cytoplasmic membrane and detect environmental signals in the periplasm; signal input is transmitted to the response regulator protein, usually by transfer of high-energy phosphate groups. Response regulators often become more effective DNA-binding proteins upon activation, and cause upregulated transcription of target genes within the regulon. Families of sensor-response regulator proteins share sequence similarity, are widely dispersed among pathogenic bacteria, and regulate a variety of virulence-associated properties including exotoxin and adhesin production (e.g., AgrA/B in *S. aureus* and BvgA/S in *B. pertussis*; see Fig. 3.2).

Other regulatory mechanisms among pathogenic bacteria include the use of diffusible homoserine lactone derivatives (*autoinducers*) and autoinducer-dependent transcriptional regulators to monitor and respond to autologous bacterial population density; the use of repressor molecules, such as the Fur protein, that bind an environmental factor, such as iron, and subsequently turn off unneeded gene products, such as iron acquisition proteins, by binding to DNA transcription–control sequences; the use of alternative sigma factors (RNA polymerase subunits) to activate accessory groups of genes; and the use of changes in chromosomal topology to regulate gene transcription. Negative regulation and the repression of some gene products in vivo is a less well characterized but equally important feature in this story.

The environmental cues that are recognized by bacterial pathogens are as diverse as the conditions in which they find themselves. In the laboratory, signals such as temperature, pH, osmolarity, oxygen tension, amino acid, and calcium and iron concentrations cause defined responses; however, it is unclear which signals or combinations thereof are most relevant in vivo—e.g., on a mucosal surface or within an intracellular phagosomal vacuole. *Borrelia burgdorferi* synthesizes new outer surface proteins within the midgut of a tick immediately following the initiation of tick blood feeding. Thus, it is clear that bacterial pathogens respond in vivo to complex and perhaps unique environmental cues, and behave in a natural host in a very different fashion from that displayed in the laboratory.

## Adherence

Adherence between the bacterium and the host is one of the earliest steps in the pathogenetic process, and contributes substantially to defining the nature of the subsequent host–pathogen interaction. Adherence is the major determinant of cell and organ tropism by a bacterial pathogen; it provides a means for communication between pathogen and host and between pathogens; and it often dictates the fate of the pathogen in its interaction with any given host cell—e.g., whether internalization takes place. Bacterial attachment factors—i.e., *adhesins*—and host target binding molecules—i.e., receptors—may be either proteins, carbohydrates, or combinations and modifications thereof. Adhesin expression is often regulated by the bacterium in response to environmental signals, suggesting that at certain times or places adhesins may be disadvantageous to a pathogen. Because adherence is so critical for many bacterial pathogens, each organism usually expresses multiple adhesins, sometimes with overlapping function. Thus, single knock-out mutants may not demonstrate a defect in adherence, colonization, or virulence. The role of bacterial cooperation and communities in adherence—e.g., biofilms—is an important area of study as it pertains to pathogenesis.

One of the most prominent types of bacterial adhesins is a macromolecular hairlike appendage called a *pilus* or *fimbria*. They are most common to gram-negative bacteria. Pili are composed of one or more major structural subunits and often possess a tip protein (or proteins) that directly mediate binding to a host receptor. Members of different families of pili may be expressed by the same organism; each family—e.g., type 1, pyelonephritis-associated or P, bundle-forming, X, S, and type IV—may recognize different host receptors (e.g., molecules containing D-mannose, digalactosides, and sialic acid).

Nonfimbrial adhesins are diverse in structure and receptor recognition. Staphylococci and streptococci express a group of proteins anchored to their surface that mediate adherence to host extracellular matrix proteins and inhibit host defense mecha-

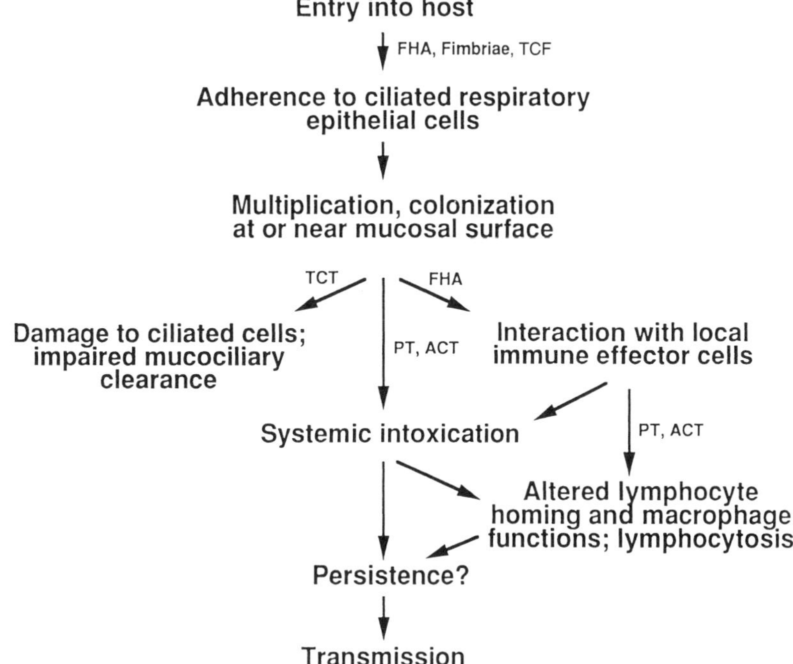


**Fig. 3.2** Schematic diagram of the steps and virulence factors involved in *B. pertussis* pathogenesis (see text). FHA, filamentous hemagglutinin; TCT, tracheal cytotoxin; PT, pertussis toxin; ACT, adenylate cyclase toxin; TCF, tracheal colonization factor. [Modified from Relman, 1995.]

**Table 3.1** Major bacterial pathogens by anatomic site

| Anatomic site | Bacterial pathogens | Pathogenic mechanisms | Host defense |
|---|---|---|---|
| Skin | *S. pyogenes*, *S. aureus* | Impetigo: exfoliative toxins<br>Erysipelas: streptococcal progenic exotoxin | Predisposing factors: trauma (especially for zoonotic infections), occluded follicles; impaired neutrophil function (pyogenic bacteria)<br>Dendritic cells may play important role in antigen presentation and cellular immune defense |
| | Mycobacteria, *B. burgdorferi* | Mycobacteria, *B. burgdorferi*: recruitment of T-lymphocytes, macrophages | |
| | *Bartonella henselae* | | |
| Eye | Cornea: *S. aureus*, P. *aeruginosa*, *N. gonorrheae*, *S. pneumoniae* | Proteolytic enzymes | Cornea, aqueous, vitreous are relatively avascular, sequestered sites<br>PMN response in cornea results in substantial local damage |
| | Diffuse: *S. aureus*, *S. epidermidis*, enteric Gram-negative bacilli, *Bacillus* spp., *M. tuberculosis* | Endophthalmitis: hematogenous route in setting of debility and immunosuppression; direct inoculation following eye surgery | Trauma, steroids, contact lens predispose to keratitis<br>Lysozyme degrades bacterial peptidoglycan |
| Ear | Middle: *S. pneumoniae*, *H. influenzae*, *B. catarrhalis* | Pathogens colonize nasopharynx; gain access to middle ear via eustacian tube | Eustachian tube dysfunction leads to middle-ear fluid accumulation<br>Local secretory IgA in middle ear |
| | External: *S. aureus* | Local skin commensals proliferate in external canal in setting of altered local defenses | Obstructed external canal or excessive moisture predispose to external otitis |
| | *P. aeruginosa* | *Pseudomonas* elastases, proteases, exotoxin A | Vascular insufficiency in osseous portion of canal leads to malignant otitis externa in diabetics |
| Respiratory tract | *S. pneumoniae* | Binding to immobilized fibronectin and other extracellular matrix proteins<br>Neutrophil response may cause substantial damage to host | Cilia and cough promote clearance<br>Respiratory-associated lymphoid tissue (e.g., tonsils) provide base for local immune responses |
| | *H. influenzae*, *Bordetella pertussis*, *Mycoplasma pneumoniae*<br>*Branhamella catarrhalis*<br>*Legionella pneumophila*<br>*M. tuberculosis* | Adhesins: pili, *B. pertussis* FHA, Mycoplasma P1 protein | Bronchoalveolar macrophages are major defense in lower tract, but also site for bacterial growth and persistence in some cases |
| Gastrointestinal tract: stomach | *Helicobacter pylori* | Vacuolating toxin causes epithelial cell injury; associated with ulcer formation<br>Urease as chemoattractant for inflammation, and produces ammonia with buffering capacity | Fucosylated blood-group antigens on gastric epithelial cells are targeted for *H. pylori* adherence. Individuals with blood group O phenotype are at elevated risk for developing ulcers<br>Low pH blocks many bacterial pathogens from infecting intestines<br>Mucus may block attachment, but can promote local colonization |

| | | | |
|---|---|---|---|
| Gastrointestinal tract | Enterotoxigenic *E. coli*, *V. cholerae*<br>*Shigella*<br>*Clostridium difficile*<br>Enteropathogenic *E. coli*<br>*Yersinia*<br>*Salmonella* | ADP-ribosylating exotoxins<br><br>Shiga toxin<br>*C. difficile* toxins A and B<br>Adherence: pili, intimin<br>Invasin, antiphagocytic toxins | M cells in the Peyer's patch are the targets for bacterial attachment, entry, and transgression of the mucosa<br>Secretory IgA is protective<br>Peristalsis and epithelial cell turnover clear bacteria and their products<br>Resident microflora in colon protects against colonization<br>Paneth cells produce antibacterial peptides: cryptdins |
| Urinary tract | Uropathogenic *E. coli*<br><br><br>*Proteus*<br>Enterococci<br>*S. saprophyticus* | Attachment: pili, afimbrial adhesin<br>Hemolysin<br>Siderophore: aerobactin<br>Urease: pH effect, calculus formation | Urine flow, bladder flushing<br>Anti-adherence effects of surface mucopolysaccharides<br>Antibodies may protect against upper tract disease |
| Genital tract | *C. trachomatis*<br>*N. gonorrheae*<br><br>*T. pallidum*<br>*Haemophilus ducreyi* | Antigenic mimicry<br>*N. gonorrheae*: pili, porins, antigenic variation, IgA protease (?) | Neutrophil response is prominent; macrophages and T lymphocyte response to *T. pallidum* |
| Central nervous system | *S. pneumoniae*; *N. meningitidis*;<br>*H. influenzae*, type b<br><br><br><br><br><br>*L. monocytogenes*<br>*B. burgdorferi* | Most pathogens colonize nasopharynx, then penetrate mucosa; fimbriae important adhesins for many<br>Capsule facilitates survival in bloodstream spread<br>LPS-induced leukocyte and cytokine responses lead to bloodbrain barrier breakdown | Opsonins are protective: specific antibody and complement<br>Bacterial cell wall components released during lysis lead to CSF leukocytosis, cerebral edema, vasculitis |
| Bones and joints | *S. aureus*<br><br><br>*B. burgdorferi*<br><br><br>*N. gonorrheae*<br>*S. pyogenes* | *S. aureus* binds to bone sialoprotein, as well as extracellular matrix at sites of damage<br>*B. burgdorferi* tropic for synovium, sheds antigenic membrane blebs into joint space | Preexisting arthritis or boney damage, trauma, poor perfusion, diabetes are predispositions<br>Poor vascular supply to affected area; host response sequesters infected site |
| Vascular compartment and endovascular surfaces | alpha-hemolytic Streptococci<br><br><br>Staphylococci<br><br><br>enteric gram-negative bacilli<br>Enterococci | Binding to immobilized fibronectin, fibrin, other extracellular matrix proteins, and platelets<br>Bacterial induction of platelet aggregation, cascade of host inflammatory pathways<br>Secretion of extracellular glycocalyx | Damaged endothelial surface leads to fibrin and platelet deposition<br>Hypercoagulability and turbulent flow increase risk of infection<br>Defenses: complement-mediated bacterial killing and reticuloendothelial system |

nisms. These proteins include protein A (immunoglobulin-binding protein), fibronectin-binding proteins, collagen-binding protein, and the fibrinogen-binding protein (clumping factor). Streptococcal lipoteichoic acid and M protein also act as adhesins. Staphylococcal adhesins are negatively regulated with respect to the group of secreted staphylococcal enzymes and toxins—i.e., when one group is repressed, the other is expressed.

Two other well-characterized adhesins are *B. pertussis* filamentous hemagglutinin (FHA) and enteropathogenic *E. coli* (EPEC) EaeA (intimin). *B. pertussis* FHA is a 220 kD surface protein and is the dominant adhesin for this organism. Multiple adherence domains mimic host adherence mechanisms, including at least two domains that are recognized by host integrin receptors. This family of receptors mediates cell–cell communication, migration, and differentiation, as well as binding of extracellular matrix. Integrin binding is a theme that is common to a number of bacterial pathogens; some express their own integrin ligand—e.g., FHA—and others borrow a host ligand—e.g., *T. pallidum* coats itself with fibronectin. Bacterial adherence to an integrin stimulates host cell signaling and may lead to host cell cytoskeletal rearrangements, bacterial internalization (see below, Under "Entry and Multiplication Within Host Cells"), or a more efficient means of mucosal colonization or toxin delivery. Other host cell receptor families also recognize bacterial ligands and lead to host cell responses. Enteropathogenic *E. coli* cause diarrhea after establishing an intimate form of adhesion to the small intestinal epithelium; EPEC EaeA and EaeB trigger calcium and inositol phosphate flux, protein tyrosine phophorylation, and actin polymerization, with formation of a host cell pedestal-like structure at the point of bacterial attachment. One of the phosphorylated proteins is an EPEC product that is secreted into host cells. In its phosphorylated state it becomes localized to the host cell membrane and serves as the EPEC attachment receptor. Virulent pneumococci may be recognized by platelet-activating factor receptors on activated host cells with a number of subsequent receptor-mediated events. Bacterial stimulation of host cell surface rearrangements and host receptor-mediated signaling are emerging themes in bacterial pathogenesis.

## Acquisition of nutrients

Bacteria compete with both the host and with each other for a variety of essential nutrients once they have arrived at their preferred niche. Iron is a critical nutrient whose availability to bacteria is restricted by high-affinity host iron-storage proteins, such as hemin, ferritin, transferrin, and lactoferrin. As a result, bacterial pathogens have developed sophisticated mechanisms for iron acquisition within the host. Bacterial strategies for iron acquisition include (*1*) removal of iron from host proteins by secreted bacterial iron chelators known as siderophores (e.g., *E. coli* aerobactin, *B. pertussis* alcaligin, *S. aureus* staphyloferrin, *Pseudomonas* pyoverdin) with subsequent bacterial receptor-mediated uptake of iron-siderophore complexes; (*2*) direct uptake of host iron complexes by specific bacterial receptors for complexed transferrin or lactoferrin (e.g., *Neisseria* and *Haemophilus* transferrin-binding proteins Tbp1 and Tbp2); and (*3*) secretion of hemolysins that can release iron from heme. Low iron concentration is often a regulatory signal for bacterial expression of these mechanisms as well as expression of other virulence factors (see above, under "Regulation of Virulence"). Clinical situations associated with increased iron availability, such as hemochromatosis, chronic liver disease, transfusion therapy, as well as deferoxamine therapy for these conditions, are associated with an elevated risk of *Yersinia enterocolitica*, *Vibrio vulnificus*, and *E. coli* bacteremia. As with other critical virulence-associated attributes, bacteria rely on multiple redundant systems for essential nutrient acquisition; thus, some but not all mutant strains with single defects in iron acquisition are avirulent. Iron is but one example of a critical nutrient for which there are diverse bacterial acquisition mechanisms; cyanocobalamin is another example.

## Exotoxins: ADP-ribosyltransferases

A number of bacterial pathogens secrete enzymes that share a common biochemical activity and structural organization, and are closely associated with virulence. This family of enzyme toxins, the bacterial ADP-ribosylating exotoxins (bAREs), is one of the most well-characterized groups of microbial virulence factors. It includes diphtheria toxin (DT), *Pseudomonas* exotoxin A (ETA), cholera toxin (CT), pertussis toxin (PT), and enterotoxigenic *E. coli* heat-labile toxin (LT). They are arranged as A:B proenzymes, where A is the ADP-ribosyltransferase and B is the binding and transmembrane delivery domain. A and B may be part of the same polypeptide, or separate but linked proteins. Enzymatic activity depends on a conserved active site with a glutamic acid residue that binds NAD and catalyzes transfer of the ADP-ribose portion to a eukaryotic target molecule, inactivating the latter. Targets include elongation factor II (for DT, ETA), heterotrimeric GTP-binding proteins (for CT, LT, PT), small-molecular-weight GTP-binding proteins, and actin. bAREs play important roles in pathogenesis; some bAREs alone reproduce disease in animal models, and null mutants for these toxins are usually attenuated for virulence. However, there is increasing appreciation of the roles played by accessory molecules in bARE expression, secretion, and delivery to target cells, as well as the importance of alternative toxins that act synergistically or in concert with bAREs.

## Pore-forming proteins and other toxins

A variety of bacterial pathogens secrete one or more cytolytic toxins (cytolysins) that belong to the "RTX" (Repeats in ToXin) family. These proteins share sequence similarity as well as tandem-nine residue repeats that are involved in calcium-dependent toxin binding to target cells; accessory bacterial gene products activate these cytolysins by covalent modification. The RTX toxins form pores in the plasma membrane of eukaryotic cells, leading to lysis. Toxins vary in their host species and cell-type specificity. Many of them are active against erythrocytes—hence their designation as hemolysins; however, the primary target cells for these toxins are believed to be leukocytes. *E. coli* $\alpha$-hemolysin (HlyA) is expressed by a larger proportion of urinary tract isolates than intestinal isolates. Mutant strains lacking this molecule are less virulent in a number of animal models. Other RTX toxins include the hemolysins of *Proteus*, *Serratia*, *Actinobacillus*, and *Pasteurella*. *B. pertussis* expresses a bifunctional molecule composed of a C-terminal hemolysin domain with sequence similarity to HlyA, and an N-terminal adenylate cyclase enzymatic domain. This adenylate cyclase toxin (ACT) penetrates host cells, presumably through a hemolysin-induced membrane pore and then catalyzes intracellular production of cAMP, leading to host cell (leukocyte) dysfunction. The ACT requires calmodulin, an exclusively eukaryotic product, for its activity; as well as post-translational palmitoylation by the *B. pertussis* CyaC gene product. In addition, ACT contributes to *B. pertussis* colonization of the lower respiratory tract and overall virulence in animals.

Gram-positive bacteria rely upon members of a family of thiol-activated hemolysins for disrupting host cell membranes. *Listeria* listeriolysin O is a well-characterized example that is required for escape of intracellular *Listeria* from the endocytic vacuole into the host cell cytoplasm (see below, under "Entry and Multiplication Within Host Cells"). Escape is essential for replication and spread of organisms, and hence virulence. *S. pyogenes*, *S. pneumoniae*, and *C. perfringens* express similar toxins, presumably for different purposes. *Listeria* may be aided in its vacuolar escape by a specific phospholipase. *C. perfringens* also expresses a phospholipase, which in this case is capable of directly inhibiting myocardial contractility and causing vascular shock. The molecular basis for the action of the clostridial neurotoxins, tetanus and botulinum toxins, hinges on their activity as zinc-dependent metalloendopeptidases. The substrates for both toxins are synaptobrevins, vesicle-associated peptides that are essential for neurotransmitter exocytosis. Cleavage of synaptobrevin blocks neurotransmitter release. The different effects of the two toxins lies in their tropism. Ingested botulinum toxin is absorbed and binds specifically to peripheral nerve cells, where internalized toxin prevents release of acetylcholine and leads to flaccid paralysis. On the other hand, tetanus toxin, absorbed from a wound infection, acts primarily on central nervous system (CNS) neurons, where it blocks release of inhibitory neurotransmitters and leads to spastic paralysis.

Other families of bacterial toxins include cell wall–derived muramyl peptides, bacterial superantigens, and endotoxins. *B. pertussis* tracheal cytotoxin (TCT) is an example of the first group; TCT is a disaccharide-tetrapeptide released by the organism during logarithmic growth. TCT induces IL-1 and nitric oxide production by ciliated respiratory epithelial cells and causes their subsequent death. *N. gonorrheae* may release a similar compound. Various *S. aureus* proteins, such as toxic shock syndrome toxin and enterotoxins A and B, and *S. pyogenes* toxins, such as erythrogenic toxin, act as superantigens. As such, they induce high levels of helper T-cell proliferation, prompt IL-2 and TNF-$\alpha$ release, and cause a shock syndrome. Sepsis and septic shock syndromes are classically associated with gram-negative endotoxin, and reflect activation of cytokine and complement cascades. The active moiety of endotoxin is lipid A (see Chapter 50). Gram-positive bacteria contain endotoxinlike cell wall components that have similar biological end results.

## Secretion and macromolecular assembly

Secretory and organelle assembly mechanisms are critical for bacterial growth and maintenance of viability. They are also critical for virulence, although alternative mechanisms are often involved in this setting. *Yersinia* outer proteins (Yops) are exported by a nontraditional process known as the type III secretion system; this system does not involve N-terminal processing of a signal sequence. The *Yersinia* Ysc proteins required for this export process share sequence similarity with proteins of similar function found in *Pseudomonas*, *Salmonella*, *Shigella*, *Bacillus*, and other bacteria. *Yersinia* Ysc mutant strains grow normally in nonrestrictive conditions, but they do not regulate Yop secretion properly, and are defective in virulence-associated traits. Some of the Ysc-related proteins mediate contact-dependent polarized transfer of virulence-associated products into host cells; others control assembly of flagella. A different bacterial export and assembly mechanism involves two groups of proteins, *chaperones* and *ushers*, which escort proteins across the gram-negative cell wall and mediate, for example, the assembly of pili.

## Entry and multiplication within host cells

Bacterial pathogens sometimes seek a niche within host cells. Moreover, entry into a host cell is essential for bacteria that can replicate only within host cells—i.e., obligate intracellular pathogens like *Rickettsia* and *Chlamydia*. Other bacterial pathogens survive or replicate within host cells as one facet of their pathogenic strategy, such as *Shigella*, *Salmonella*, and *Listeria*. Internalization affords an organism a means of escape from immune defenses as well as access to host nutrients and energy sources. Entry into one cell type—e.g., M cells of the small intestinal mucosa—may provide access to other cell types within deeper tissues and then blood or lymph-borne dissemination. Entry into a host cell can of course be detrimental to the bacterium, as well as the host cell. Given the diverse and profound consequences for the bacterium, it is not surprising that pathogens have evolved sophisticated and cunning mechanisms for entry and intracellular survival.

*Salmonella* expresses a number of invasion genes that are clustered in one region of its chromosome (see above, under "Bacterial Structure, Taxonomy, and Pathogenicity") and secretes their products into host cells by means of a type III system (see under "Secretion and Macromolecular Assembly"). *Salmonella* attachment to host epithelial cells induces membrane ruffling and formation of a "splash" effect. Resultant endocytic events engulf *Salmonella* within a vacuole that becomes rapidly modified by the bacterium for its own purposes. This "spacious phagosome" is partially blocked for acidification and provides the organism with nutrients and signals for subsequent replication. *Legionella*, *Coxiella*, and *Mycobacterium* also reside and replicate within phagocytic vacuoles, and in some cases block lysosomal fusion. Other intracellular pathogens, such as *Listeria*, *Shigella*, and *Rickettsia* require access to the cytoplasm for replication. *Listeria* expresses an adhesin, internalin, with features common to other cell wall-anchored proteins in gram-positive bacteria; it is recognized by members of the host cell cadherin receptor family and mediates internalization. Pore-forming hemolysins and phospholipases enable *Listeria* and other bacteria to leave the endocytic vacuole and enter the host cell cytoplasm. Once in the cytoplasm, some of these organisms catalyze actin polymerization at one bacterial pole, leading to "rocket"-like intra- and intercellular motility. The choice of host cell receptor may determine whether entry takes place, and the nature of the intracellular compartment. Pioneering studies of the *Yersinia* invasin protein demonstrated that a high binding affinity for $\beta$1-integrin receptors can trigger bacterial internalization. Bacterial coating with complement 3 fragments can lead to CR3 integrin-mediated internalization, with subsequent survival for only certain bacteria, such as *Legionella*.

## Avoidance of host immune defenses

Bacteria have evolved mechanisms for evading host immune defenses that are as diverse and complex as the defenses themselves. Bacterial capsule is composed of polysaccharide polymers and blocks complement deposition on the bacterial surface, either by preventing binding of protein B or by enhancing binding of protein H (which degrades complement C3b). Many capsules are nonimmunogenic, and mask the organism from eliciting antibody formation. LPS structure may also prevent activated complement complexes from damaging the bacterium. As mentioned above, some bacteria coat themselves with host proteins or enter modified intracellular niches, thereby avoiding the host immune response. Antigenic variation of immunogenic surface structures is one strategy for avoiding host humoral immune defenses. Gonococcal pilin variation is a classical example. Finally, certain bacterial-secreted proteins act as inhibitors of phagocytosis or phagocytic killing. *Yersinia* YopH, a tyrosine phosphatase, and YopE, a cytolysin, both possess this activity. *B. pertussis* adenylate cyclase toxin modulates neutrophil and macrophage antibacterial functions.

## Summary

Bacterial virulence should not be viewed as a deliberate attempt by a pathogen to damage or to incapacitate the host, but rather as a predictable outcome of certain bacterial strategies for replication within and spread between hosts. Microbial virulence is usually the consequence of a complex, dynamic interactive process between host and pathogen, and may reflect changing host behavior with subsequent microbial adaptation. The subtlety of this process and its dependence on fundamental host biological mechanisms have catalyzed the integration of previously separate scientific disciplines, such as bacterial pathogenesis, human cell biology, and immunology. Insights in one field often spawn insights in another. As the field of bacterial pathogenesis matures, an increasing amount of attention and study should become focused on more chronic, less dramatic host–pathogen relationships. And with this evolution will come a more refined definition of bacterial virulence.

### ANNOTATED BIBLIOGRAPHY

Cotter PA, Miller JF. *In vivo* and *ex vivo* regulation of bacterial virulence gene expression. Curr Opin Microbiol 1998; 1:17–26.
*Excellent review of regulatory mechanisms and schemes utilized by bacteria for regulation of virulence-associated genes.*

Finlay BB, Falkow S. Common themes in microbial pathogenicity revisited. Microbiol Mol Biol Rev 1997; 61(2):136–169.
*A review of key steps and mechanisms involved in microbial pathogenesis.*

Fleischmann RD, Adams MD, White O et al. Whole-genome random sequencing and assembly of Haemophilus influenzae Rd [see comments]. Science 1995; 269:496–512.
*A milestone in a technology-driven approach to the understanding of bacterial behavior and function. The complete 1,820,137 bp nucleotide sequence of* H. influenzae *is revealed, and preliminary functions are assigned to its 1743 proposed genes.*

Hultgren SJ, Abraham S, Caparon M, Falk P, St. Geme JW III, Normark S. Pilus and nonpilus bacterial adhesins: assembly and function in cell recognition. Cell 1993; 73:887–901.
*A review of bacterial adherence that emphasizes pilus structure, assembly and function, the role of adherence in bacterial tropism, and some of the consequences of bacterial adherence for host cells.*

Isberg RR. Discrimination between intracellular uptake and surface adhesion of bacterial pathogens. Science 1991; 252:934–938.
*A discussion of the factors that determine whether adherence or internalization results from intimate contact between bacteria and host cells. Focuses upon the* Yersinia *invasin protein paradigm.*

Kenny B, DeVinney R, Stein M, Reinscheid DJ, Frey EA, Finlay BB. Enteropathogenic *E. coli* (EPEC) transfers its receptor for intimate adherence into mammalian cells. Cell 1997; 91(4):511–520.
*A surprising story of choreographed attachment to a host cell by a bacterial pathogen.*

Krueger KM, Barbieri JT. The family of bacterial ADP-ribosylating exotoxins. Clin Microbiol Rev 1995; 8:34–47.
*A thorough discussion that emphasizes the common structure–function relationships of this prominent class of bacterial toxins.*

Mekalanos JJ. Environmental signals controlling expression of virulence determinants in bacteria. J Bacteriol 1992; 174:1–7.
*Discusses the individual environmental cues that play a role in virulence gene regulation. Most of the available data derive from in vitro studies.*

Olsen GJ, Woese CR, Overbeek R. The winds of (evolutionary) change: breathing new life into microbiology. J Bacteriol 1994; 176:1–6.
*An overview of the impact of the molecular phylogeny on the fields of microbiology and bacterial systematics.*

Relman DA. *Bordetella pertussis*: determinants of virulence. In: Handbook of Natural Toxins. Moss J, Iglewski B, Vaughan M, Tu AT, eds. Marcel Dekker, New York, pp 367–405, 1995.
*Review of pertussis pathogenesis, as a model for toxin-secreting, non-invasive bacterial pathogens.*

Relman DA, Falkow S. A molecular perspective of microbial pathogenicity. In: Principles and Practice of Infectious Diseases, 4th ed. Mandell GL, Douglas RG, Bennett JE, eds. Churchill Livingstone, New York, pp 19–29, 1995.
*Reviews key aspects of microbial pathogenesis with selected examples. Provides an overview with reference to clinical issues.*

Waldor MK, Mekalanos JJ. Lysogenic conversion by a filamentous phage encoding cholera toxin. Science 1996; 272:1910–1914.
*A surprising discovery of horizontal virulence gene transfer: A* Vibrio cholerae *pilus serves as the receptor for a phage that carries the cholera toxin gene cassette; and both, pilus receptor and toxin genes, are coregulated by the same environmental sensing protein.*

# 4

# Pathophysiology of Viruses and Viral Diseases

DAVID M. KOELLE AND LAWRENCE COREY

Medical virology seeks to understand the pathogenesis and therapy of viral agents infectious for humans. Molecular detection systems, serology, electron microscopy, cell culture, and animal models have revealed an amazing diversity and specificity in the pathogenesis of viral infections. Every virus-host relationship has new lessons to teach us, and generalizations are becoming less and less possible as our analytic tools improve. However, certain broad themes have stood the test of time. This chapter will present a general overview of viral pathogenesis at the cell and organism level, introducing concepts developed in detail in discussions of individual agents and clinical syndromes.

Viruses challenge our definition of life. They were first characterized in the nineteenth century as *filterable agents* since they pass through porcelain filters, and electron microscopy shows they are much smaller than bacteria (typically less than 200 Å in diameter). Viruses are obligate intracellular organisms containing a nucleic acid genome, either DNA or RNA (but not both), and a protein capsid protecting the genome. The genome encodes at least one capsid protein, and in almost every case a nucleic acid polymerase involved in copying itself. Viruses lack organelles and are metabolically inert outside of cells. *Viroids* and *virusoids* are self-replicating RNAs infecting plants which are not known to encode protein, while the subacute spongiform encephalopathies such as Creutzfeldt-Jakob disease appear not to require the transmission of nucleic acids. A complete listing of viruses pathogenic for humans might include viruses causing agriculturally important plant and animal diseases as well as viruses that directly infect humans. In addition, some viruses that infect bacteria (bacteriophages) cause disease indirectly by encoding proteins such as diphtheria toxin. Both bacteria (*C. diptheriae*) and virus are thus central to the pathogenesis of diptheria.

For their survival, viruses must be transmitted from host to host. Because they use ribosomes for protein synthesis, the cell must remain at least partially intact during the early phase of viral infection. The host organism must also live long enough to spread progeny virus—for example, by respiratory droplet or gastrointestinal routes. Production of rapid or severe dysfunction at the cell or organism level may thus be detrimental to viral spread. Viruses causing severe disease or death in a large proportion of infected persons, such as rabies, are distinctly rare and are frequently less pathogenic in their usual animal host species. Some viruses, such as influenza, measles, and smallpox, produce disease in most infected individuals; most viruses cause inapparent or mild disease, and a few, such as human spumavirus, have yet to be linked to any disease at all.

Viral infections may be temporary or lifelong (Fig. 4.1). Some self-limited infections such as hepatitis A lead to protective immunity, while others, such as respiratory syncytial virus, do not. Permanent infection may be persistent, with constant viral replication and destruction of host cells, or marked by alternating periods of viral latency and replication. Latency is highly cell type–specific; examples include latency of herpes simplex in neurons, varicella zoster in glia, and Epstein-Barr (EBV) in B lymphocytes. During latency, viral transcription and translation are limited to certain regions of the viral genome. Occasionally, viruses that usually cause acute, self-limited infection can persist and cause chronic disease. Subacute sclerosing panencephalitis (SSPE), caused by persistent measles virus infection of the central nervous system, is an example of this pattern.

*Cancer* is yet another consequence of viral infection. Hepatocellular carcinoma (hepatitis B), nasopharyngeal carcinoma in South Asia, many lymphomas (Epstein-Barr virus), and cervical cancer (papillomavirus) are malignancies of major public health importance that are linked to viral infections. While viral genomes are detectable in the malignant tissues of virus-related cancers, productive viral infection is unusual in these tumors. Proposed mechanisms of viral oncogenesis include antagonism of tumor-suppressor proteins, translocation of cellular oncogenes to chromosomal locations where they are upregulated by strong host promoter sequences, dysregulation of host growth factors, and inhibition of apoptosis of host cells. Recently, a herpesvirus related to Epstein-Barr virus has been detected in Kaposi's sarcoma tissue. This agent, termed *Kaposi's sarcoma–associated herpesvirus* (KSHV) or *human herpesvirus 8* (HHV-8), is also associated with rare B-cell lymphomas arising within body cavities. Several possible mechanisms of tumorogenesis, including production of virally encoded cytokine homologs, evasion of cell-cycle checkpoints, and inhibition of apoptosis, have already been described for KSHV.

The pathogenicity of a virus for a specific host may depend on both virus and host characteristics. Genetic virulence and resistance factors have been extensively investigated by infecting cells and animals with genetically altered viruses, and by introducing or deleting key nucleic acid sequences in the host. Passage of a virus through cells or animals may also "condition" its behavior without altering its genetic structure. Some viruses with large genomes, such as herpesviruses, contain many genes that can be deleted without effect on viral growth in cell culture. These same genes, however, can have profound effects on virulence in animals, thus limiting the medical applicability of cell culture studies. Identification of virulence factors is important for the creation of attenuated viral strains for use as live vaccines.

Host factors affecting virulence can be specific to anatomic regions, as exemplified by the increased growth of rhinoviruses at the cool temperatures found in the nasal mucosa, or they can be cell-specific, due to interaction with receptors or transcription factors. Genetic host factors are typified by the polymorphism in the human population at the erythrocyte P antigen locus. This

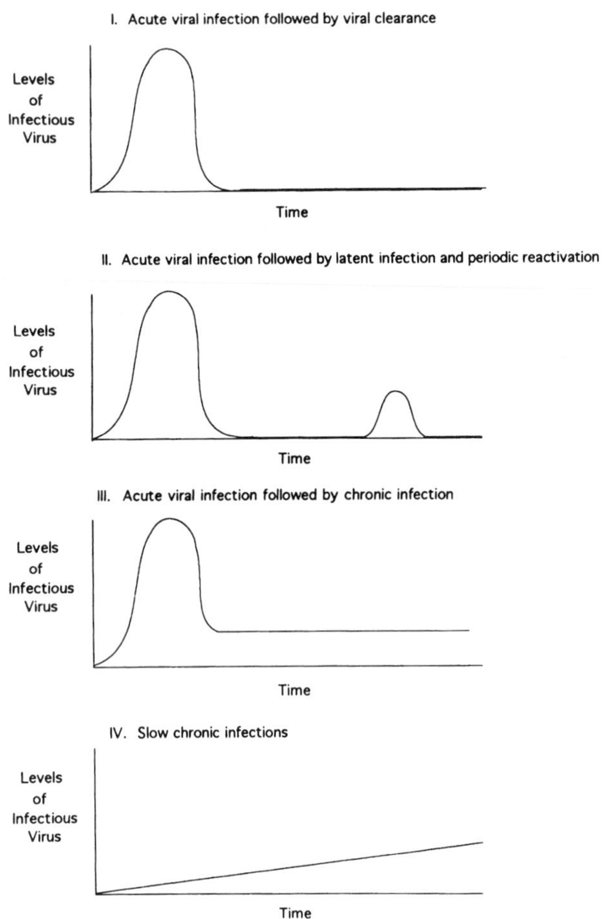


**Fig. 4.1** Temporal patterns of viral infection. [From Ahmed et al., Persistence of Viruses, p.221, in: *Fields Virology*, Third Edition, ed. Fields et al, Lippincott-Raven Publishers, Philadelphia, 1996, with permission]

protein serves as a receptor for parvovirus B19. Acquired host factors are also important, as demonstrated by the extreme virulence of measles in malnourished children. For most medically important viral infections, the status of the cellular immune system is a critically important host factor. Interventions aimed to improve the host immune response may be as appropriate and effective as direct antiviral chemotherapy.

## Taxonomy and Structure

Viral taxonomy is based primarily on genomic characteristics, replication strategy, and structure, and not on host species, tissue or cell tropism, or mode of transmission. For example, the Rhabdoviridae include both rabies virus and plant pathogens. The frequently used term "arbovirus" is not a taxonomic reference but refers to viruses spread through insect vectors. Arboviruses share pathogenetic properties such as the development of viremia in humans, productive infection within the gastrointestinal tract of insect vectors, and, frequently, a maintenance transmission cycle between nonhuman animal and insect hosts. The respiratory and enteric virus designations, referring to predominant organ system involvement, label agents that may share cell tropism despite disparate genetic and structural features. The defining traits of some virus families and representative human pathogens are listed in Table 4.1.

Taxonomic assignment is gaining medical relavence with advances in antiviral chemotherapy and vaccines, since antiviral strategies and even specific compounds may have cross-reactive activity against related agents. For example, most viruses with a reverse transcription step from RNA to DNA cause chronic infection, because the double-stranded DNA intermediate is able to integrate into the host genome. Inhibitors of reverse transcriptase would not be predicted to be active against most other RNA viruses, which do not include an RNA-to-DNA step in their replicative cycles, but are active, as predicted, against hepatitis B virus, a DNA virus with a reverse transcription step in its life cycle. Most retroviruses, such as HIV, utilize a highly error-prone reverse transcriptase. The resultant high rate of mutation leads to antigenic changes and alterations in the binding sites of antiviral agents, considerably increasing the challenges of making a universal vaccine and providing persistently effective antiviral chemotherapy.

Structural properties implied by taxonomic group include size, shape, presence or absence of envelope, and capsid structure (Fig. 4.2). Enveloped viruses are typically fragile and sensitive to detergents and organic solvents, while non-enveloped viruses are capable of withstanding harsher environmental conditions. Specific envelope and capsid proteins on the outside of enveloped and nonenveloped viruses, respectively, bind to specific receptors on susceptible cells.

## Viral Pathogenesis at the Organism Level

The envelope, if present, and the capsid enable the virus to survive long enough to reach the next host. Viruses must then gain entry into the host (Fig. 4.3). After entry into a cell, primary replication occurs at the site of inoculation. Some viruses then spread via blood or neural routes, and others remain localized. After seeding distant organs, a secondary viremia may occur after an additional cycle of viral growth. Finally, the virus must exit the body in a vehicle or vector suitable for transmission (Fig. 4.4).

Viruses gain entry through a variety of routes. Abrasion of the stratum corneum promotes infection by papillomavirus and herpes simplex virus, because only basal keratinocytes are metabolically active enough to support viral replication. These viruses cross the dermal–epidermal junction very poorly. Capillaries are rare in the epidermis, and thus viremia, while detectable by PCR (polymerase chain reaction), does not lead to seeding of distant organs and is of limited clinical importance. Sensory axons do, however, richly supply the epidermal–dermal junction, and thus retrograde axonal transport is possible for herpes simplex virus. Virus introduced into the dermis by insect (dengue) or human bite (hepatitis B) may spread via blood and lymphatics. Rabies also appears to require deep inoculation. Oral and genital mucosal surfaces are also susceptible to direct infection (herpes simplex), or provide viral access to mobile dendritic-lineage cells, which carry virus to local lymphoid tissue (human immunodeficiency virus).

Large airborne droplets are trapped in the nose to deliver "cold" agents such as rhinoviruses, coronaviruses, and adenoviruses. Small ($<5\ \mu$) airborne droplets gain access to the lower respiratory tract to deliver respiratory agents such as influenza. Varicella zoster and measles viruses are not typically associated with severe lower respiratory symptoms but are thought to use this route to enter the body. While influenza replication is lim-

**Table 4.1** Characteristics of medically important virus families

| Virus family | Common names of representative human pathogens | Nucleic acid | Envelope |
|---|---|---|---|
| Picornaviridae<br>Caliciviridae<br>Astroviridae | Polio<br>Norwalk agent<br>Astrovirus | RNA, single-stranded, positive sense, nonsegemented | No |
| Flaviviridae<br>Togaviridae | Dengue<br>St. Louis encephalitis virus | RNA, single-stranded, positive sense, nonsegemented | Yes |
| Coronaviridae | Coronavirus | RNA, single-stranded, positive sense, nonsegemented, nested transcription | Yes |
| Paramyxoviridae<br>Rhabdoviridae<br>Filoviridae | Measles<br>Rabies<br>Ebola | RNA, single-stranded, negative sense, nonsegmented | Yes |
| Orthomyxoviridae<br>Bunyaviridae<br>Arenaviridae | Influenza<br>Hantavirus<br>Lassa | RNA, single-stranded, negative sense, segmented | Yes |
| Reoviridae | Rotavirus | RNA, double-stranded, segmented | No |
| Hepadnaviridae | Hepatitis B | double/single-stranded DNA; reverse transcription | Yes |
| Retroviridae | Human immunodeficiency virus | RNA, single-stranded, positive sense; reverse transcription | Yes |
| Parvoviridae | Parvovirus B19 | DNA, single-stranded | No |
| Papovaviridae<br>Adenoviridae | Papillomavirus<br>Adenovirus | DNA, double-stranded | No |
| Herpesviridae<br>Poxviridae | Herpes simplex<br>Smallpox | DNA, double-stranded | Yes |

ited to the respiratory epithelium, varicella zoster and measles become widely disseminated to the skin after local respiratory replication leads to viremia. Viruses entering the stomach encounter acid, proteases, and bile salts. Enveloped viruses uncommonly initiate infection via the GI tract because bile salts denature lipid membranes. Rotavirus infectivity is actually enhanced by proteases present in the GI tract. In some instances, proteases are required to reveal active sites on viral attachment proteins mediating binding to target cells. Specialized M cells in the intestinal epithelium may mediate uptake of picornaviruses such as polio. Rarely, the conjunctiva may serve as the portal of viral entry. Blood-borne transmission by transfusion or injection drug use is of increasing medical importance, bypassing the stage of local replication typical of natural viral infection.

The pattern of viral spread (local or systemic) may be influenced by localization of progeny virus formation and budding in polarized epithelial cells. These phenomenon can now be studied in vitro with epithelial cell cultures that retain asymmetric surfaces and specialized intracellular junctions. If progeny virus is released from the basolateral membrane of an epithelium, locally invasive and ultimately systemic spread may occur. Examples of such viruses include vaccinia and vesicular stomatitis virus. If virus is released from the apical or lumenal surface, spread may be limited to adjacent epithelial cells. Influenza and parainfluenza are examples of such viruses.

Viremia may occur after spread of infection to local lymph nodes and transfer of virus to the blood by way of efferent lymphatics. Some viruses circulate as free infectious units, such as hepatitis B, while others, such as cytomegalovirus, appear to circulate primarily in association with cellular elements. Viruses that replicate in leukocytes, such as HIV, secrete infectious virus into the plasma. Viremia reflects a dynamic balance between production and clearance, which may be influenced by the development of opsonizing antibodies. Macrophage-derived cells of the reticuloendothelial system, rather than neutrophils, are the predominant mediators of clearance of antibody-coated virus. Some viruses, such as HIV, replicate within macrophages and may use such cells to deliver virus to other tissues, such as brain. Virus-specific immune-globulin preparations may attenuate infection by binding to circulating free virus and limiting viremic

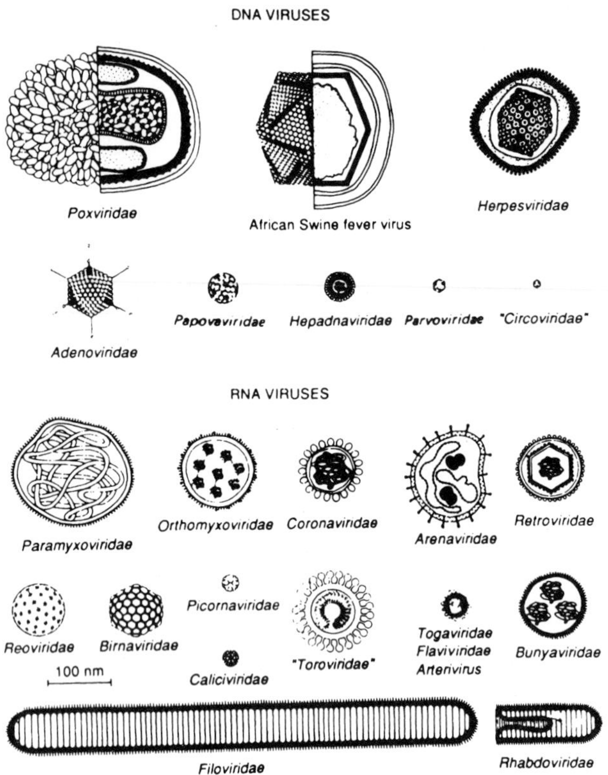


**Fig. 4.2** Morphology of some medically important virus families, to scale. [From Fenner FJ et al, *Veterinary Virology*, Second Edition, Academic Press, 1993, p. 21, with permission]

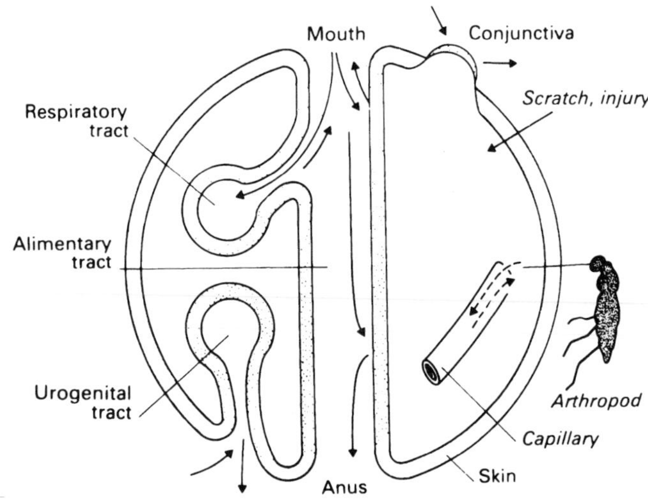


**Fig. 4.3** Routes of entry of viruses into a stylized host. [From Mims CA et al, *Viral Pathogenesis and Immunology*, Blackwell Scientific, Oxford, 1984. In: *Fields Virology*, Third Edition, ed. Fields et al, Lippincott-Raven Publishers, Philadelphia, 1996, with permission]

spread. Increasingly, qualitative and quantitative measures of cell-associated or plasma viremia are being used to diagnose viral infections and monitor the response to antiviral therapy.

Infection of the central nervous system is common among medically important viruses. Initial entry into the nervous system can take place through peripheral nerves or via tissue invasion from the blood or cerebrospinal fluid. Herpes simplex, rabies, and polio viruses usually access peripheral nerves after local replication and progress to the central nervous system (CNS) via afferent pathways. Once in the CNS, some viruses traverse synaptic spaces and infect secondary neurons with enough specificity that neuroanatomic pathways can be traced in this fashion. The blood–brain barrier limits direct neural invasion during viremia. Some viruses traverse, with or without infecting, brain capillary endothelial cells, to gain access to brain, while others gain access to the cerebrospinal fluid via the choroid plexus, which contains fenestrated endoethalial cells. Cytomegalovirus (CMV) uses this pathway to infect ependymal cells, followed by infection of subjacent brain tissue. Measles, mumps, and HIV may gain access to the brain by traveling within leukocytes that traverse capillaries. Some cases of herpes simplex encephalitis appear to occur after reactivation of virus from the trigeminal ganglia to the dura mater, which carries sensory enervation from the trigeminal nerve, followed by local spread to adjacent brain tissue.

After replication within the host, progeny virus is shed or transmitted to an intermediate vector (Fig. 4.4). Virus shedding responsible for transmission most frequently occurs from the genitourinary, respiratory, or gastrointestinal tract. Infection via semen is probably important for HIV, CMV, and hepatitis B virus

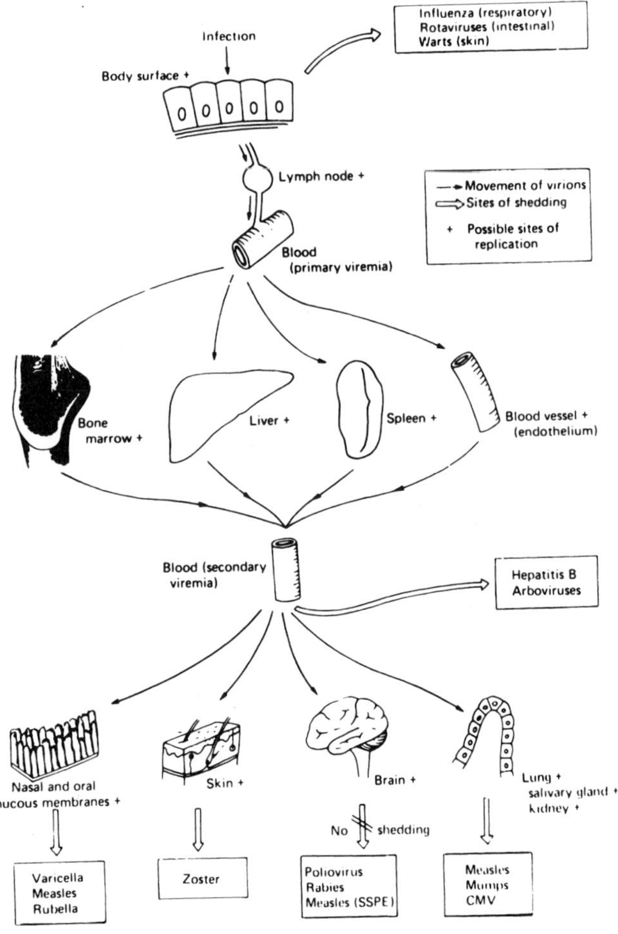


**Fig. 4.4** Routes of viral speed throughout the body, and sites of virus shedding with examples. [From Mims CA et al., *Viral Pathogenesis and Immunology*, Blackwell Scientific, Oxford, 1984, p. 52, with permission]

(HBV). Generation of respiratory droplets and direct inoculation of respiratory secretions by hand contact may both contribute to the spread of respiratory viruses. Hepatitis A, other picornaviruses, and rotaviruses are examples of agents spread via stool; transmission is facilitated by poor hygeine or contamination of water supplies.

Less frequently, shedding from intact skin or skin lesions may result in transmission, as for herpes simplex, papillomavirus, and some cases of varicella-zoster virus (most transmission of varicella zoster virus [VZV] is probably via respiratory droplet spread from patients with primary infection). Salivary transmission is important for the spread of EBV, CMV, and mumps. While many other viruses, including HBV, HIV, and human herpesvirus 6 (HHV-6) are frequently present in saliva, limitations on experimental inoculation studies have prevented full assessment of the role of salivary transmission of these agents. Transmission via infected blood is both a "natural" mode of transmission for many arboviruses and a human-dependent mechanism for some other infections characterized by prolonged, high-grade viremia, such as HIV, HBV, and CMV. Rarely, infections with transitory viremia, such as hepatitis A, are spread by blood exposure. Transmission by aerosolization of urine may be important for spread of the Sin Nombre hantavirus and lymphocytic choriomeningitis virus from rodents to humans, but it has rarely been implicated in human-to-human transmission. Milk may transmit several viruses, including human T-lymphotropic virus 1 (HTLV-1), HIV, and CMV.

## Cellular Events in Viral Pathogenesis

Despite variations in genome, structure, and replicative cycles at the organism level, the events of viral reproduction within the cell are constant enough to be summarized as a series of discrete steps. The replicative cycle leading to production of progeny virus and cell death is considered in detail here. Typically, complete viral replication leads to lysis and death of the infected cell. Some cells are thought to undergo abortive replication owing to virus or host cell factors preventing the complete viral life cycle. Viral antigens are detected, but progeny virus is not. Latent infection is the result of specialized, but poorly understood, genetic programs played out in specific virus/cell pairs. Latent infection is thus detailed in chapters on specific agents.

Viral replication begins with attachment, internalization, uncoating of the genome, and translocation of the genome to its site of replication. Host cell metabolism is specifically altered to favor viral replication. Following replication of the genome, the structural proteins required for capsid formation are synthesized. Formation of genome-capsid particles is facilitated by self-assembly properties of the capsid proteins. Egress of assembled virions is coupled, for some viruses, with acquisition of the envelope as the virus buds through the nuclear (herpes virus), Golgi (poxvirus), or cytoplasmic (retrovirus) membrane. Because uptake of virus is highly efficient and production of progeny virus takes time, an "eclipse" interval is noted in vitro in which little virus is present in the medium, ranging from 6 to 8 hours (picornaviruses) to 18 to 30 hours (herpesviruses). A single infected cell may give rise to up to hundreds of thousands of infectious progeny virus particles. The pace and efficiency of viral replication in vivo has not been as thoroughly studied.

Virus binding to cells typically does not require energy and is due to a strong, noncovalent interaction between specific viral attachment proteins and one or more host cell membrane receptor structures. Viral attachment proteins are typically located at the apices of capsomers of non-enveloped viruses and distally on membrane proteins of enveloped viruses. Host receptors are structurally diverse and include charged carbohydrate residues, glycosoaminoglycans, glycoproteins, glycolipids, and phospholipids (Table 4.2).

In some instances, the cell tropism of a virus can be understood from the limited distribution of its receptor or receptors. EBV, for example, binds to B-cells via CD21 and HLA class II, membrane proteins of limited distribution that are present on B-cells. HIV uses both CD4, present on some T-cells and monocytes, and specific chemokine receptors enriched on T-cells or monocytes. Detailed investigation now commonly reveals that more than one cellular component may contribute to virus binding. Prevention of infection by interference with viral binding remains an attractive target for antiviral chemotherapy and has been pursued extensively in the case of rhinovirus binding to intra-

**Table 4.2** Examples of receptors implicated in viral binding or internalization

| Virus | Cell type | Receptor class | Receptor |
|---|---|---|---|
| Adenovirus | Many | Integrin | $\alpha_v\beta_3$ |
| Human immunodeficiency virus | Lymphocyte, monocyte | Leukocyte HLA ligand | CD4 |
| Human immunodeficiency virus | $CD4^+$ lymphocyte | $\beta$chemokine receptor | CXCR4 |
| Human immunodeficiency virus | Monocyte | $\beta$chemokine receptor | CCR5 |
| Epstein-Barr virus | B lymphocyte, epithelial cell | Complement receptor (B lymphocytes, epithelial cells) | C3d receptor (CR2, CD21) |
| Epstein-Barr virus | B lymphocyte | HLA class II (B lymphocytes) | HLA DR |
| Vaccinia virus | Epidermal cell | Growth factor receptor | EGF receptor |
| Rhinovirus | Nasal epithelial cell | Adhesion molecule | ICAM-1 |

cellular adhesion molecule 1 (ICAM-1). Some neutralizing antibodies may operate by blocking virus binding.

## Viral Infection of Cells

After viral binding, the active, energy-requiring process of internalization takes place. The viral and host domains mediating binding and internalization are usually different. The entry of non-enveloped viruses is poorly understood and may occur in low-pH endosomes or by direct injection of nucleocapsids into the cytoplasm. For enveloped viruses, fusion between the viral envelope and a cellular membrane occurs, followed by uncoating of the nucleocapsid. Some enveloped viruses, such as HIV, fuse directly with the plasma membrane. Viral envelope proteins may contain two fusogenic domains, hydrophobic stretches of amino acids that may be revealed only after conformational changes after virus binding. Insertion of these hydrophobic domains into both envelope and host cell membrane may lead to the actual fusion event. Neutralizing antibodies exert some of their antiviral effect through binding to the fusion domains of proteins on the surface of enveloped viruses.

Other enveloped viruses, such as influenza virus, localize to clathrin-coated pits and are phagocytosed into coated vesicles. Fusion of phagosomes with lysosomes and acidification is required to produce a pH-dependent change in the conformation of the influenza hemagglutinin. A fusogenic domain is exposed, leading to fusion of the viral envelope with the phagolysosome membrane and release of viral genome/coat protein complexes into the cytoplasm. The influenza M2 protein may assist in acidification of phagolysosomes by acting as a hydrogen ion pore. Amantadine and rimantidine, drugs with activity against influenza A, bind specifically to M2 protein and limit acidification of phagolysosomes. Mutations in the M2 protein restore acidification and lead to resistance to these drugs.

Before host transcription or translational machinery can gain access to the viral genome, exposure of the genome is required. Disintegration of the capsid is only partial for reoviruses, and replication takes place within remnant capsids. Host proteins are required for disintegration of poxvirus capsids. The nucleocapsid may (herpesviruses, adenovirus, papovavirus, influenza virus) or may not (poxviruses) require transport to the nucleus prior to disintegration. After proper localization and exposure of the genome, viral protein synthesis requires the presence of mRNA. This arrives preformed in the case of positive single-stranded RNA viruses, but requires synthesis of new nucleic acid polymers from a viral template in the case of other types of virus. Either host or viral nucleic acid polymerases may be involved in the synthesis of viral mRNA.

The spatial and temporal pattern of viral gene transcription is tightly regulated. Transcriptional controls that are specific for specialized cells or tissues may contribute to viral tropism. For example, JC contains enhancer sequences that respond specifically to transcription factors present in glial cells, and JC virus infection appears limited to glia in vivo. Cell-specific enhancer sequences are also involved in papillomavirus infection of keratinocytes, Epstein-Barr virus infection of B lymphocytes, and hepatitis B virus infection of hepatocytes. Temporal control of transcription is initially provided in herpes simplex virus by the delivery, with the virion, of the transactivator protein VP16, which complexes with Oct-1 and other nuclear factors to activate transcription of immediate early viral genes. Other herpes simplex virion proteins immediately begin the process of shutting down host protein synthesis. The proteins encoded by immediate early genes in turn activate the transcription of early genes, which include genes required for genome replication, genes required to downregulate transcription of the first two sets of genes, and genes required to upregulate expression of late genes encoding structural genes required for assembly of new virions. Transcriptional regulation is not limited to DNA viruses and is also utilized by negative-stranded RNA viruses such as influenza, in which noncoding regions are thought to regulate transcription of critical virulence genes.

Because positive stranded RNA viruses serve directly as mRNA, regulation of gene expression occurs primarily at the level of translation rather than of transcription. For example, the 5′ noncoding region of picornaviruses contains conserved regions that function to promote ribosome binding to mRNA. Alterations in this region attenuating virus growth are present in the Sabin vaccine strain of polio.

Genome replication typically uses a virally encoded nucleic acid polymerase, either delivered preformed in the virion or synthesized in the infected cell. Several antiviral compounds are inhibitors of nucleic acid polymerases and show specificity for viral as compared to host enzymes. Mutations in the enzymes required to activate the prodrugs of the active compounds, or in the nucleic acid polymerases themselves, frequently give rise to viral resistance to this class of antiviral agents.

Retroviruses have a particularly complex replicative cycle. Preformed RNA-dependent DNA polymerase (reverse transcriptase) forms single-stranded DNA from viral single-stranded RNA, then catalyzes the formation of second complementary DNA strand to yield double-stranded DNA. The viral integrase, also delivered preformed in the virion, then inserts this DNA in the host genome. The viral DNA is then transcribed into a full-length mRNA. Translation may occur in more than one open reading frame, an example of the economy of viral genomes. The translation product of the dominant open reading frame contains the capsid/polymerase fusion protein and a protease region, which autocatalytically cleaves the polyprotein into shorter polypeptides. Inhibition of this protease activity is the basis for a class of anti-HIV drugs (see Chapter 98). Some HIV mRNAs are also derived from spliced pre-mRNAs containing exons. Transcription of HIV RNAs is highly dependent upon binding of cellular transcription factors such as NF$\kappa$B to specific regulatory DNA sequences. Translation of HIV RNA is dependent on binding of the HIV Tat protein directly to the TAR RNA sequence immediately upstream of the translation start. After synthesis of capsid, polymerase, and envelope proteins, two copies of full-length single-stranded RNA are incorporated into progeny virus, and the virus buds through the plasma membrane.

It is critical for viral survival that complete viral replication occur prior to host cell death. Cells infected with certain mutant adenoviruses undergo alterations in nuclear and membrane structure characteristic of programmed cell death or apoptosis at an accelerated rate compared to cells infected with wild-type virus. The product of the wild-type adenovirus gene E1B 19K is believed to inhibit apoptosis. The mechanism by which E1B 19K inhibits cell death appears similar to that used by bcl-2, an anti-apoptotic cellular protein activated in certain malignant cells. EBV has developed two strategies to combat apoptosis in B lymphocytes. Latently infected cells are protected from apoptosis by an increased level of cellular bcl-2, while lytically infected cells synthesize a viral homolog of bcl-2. Inhibition of apoptosis may also be important in evasion of immune cell–mediated killing of virally infected cells, since CTL and NK cells may kill virally infected host cells through induction of apoptosis (see below, under "Virus Interactions with the Immune System").

After replication of the genome and synthesis of new virion proteins, viral assembly occurs. Some viruses are self-assembling, while others require the participation of cellular chaperone proteins. Viruses containing single-stranded genomes preferentially include the proper nucleic acid strand. Nonenveloped viruses depend on disintegration of the host cell, caused by disruption of host cell metabolism, for release, while enveloped viruses bud through a cellular membrane. Herpesviruses first bud through the inner lamella of the nuclear membrane. The enveloped virus then accumulates between the inner and outer lamella, which is continuous with the lumen of the endoplasmic reticulum. Vesicles are budded off the endoplasmic reticulum which travel to and fuse with the cytoplasmic membrane, protecting the enveloped particle from the cytoplasm during transport. Finally, virus is shed from the body, a process that may be promoted by local tissue damage caused by viral replication and cell death.

## Virus Interactions with the Immune System

Both innate and acquired immunity contribute to the host response to viral infection. Innate immune mechanisms, lacking the memory and fine specificity of acquired cellular (T-lymphocyte) and humoral (antibody) responses, include the class I interferon proteins (alpha and beta) with broad antiviral activity, and natural killer lymphocytes capable of killing virally infected cells (see Chapter 10). The effector cells of the acquired immune response display virus-specific cell-surface receptors (T-cell receptors for T lymphocytes, immunoglobulin for B lymphocytes) capable of enormous diversity and fine specificity. Receptor diversity is generated in each case by very similar mechanisms of DNA rearrangement and somatic mutation. A diverse set of naive cells awaits stimulation and amplification by interaction with specific viral molecular determinants, converting them to virus-specific memory and effector cells. Some viruses undergo frequent antigenic change and present a moving target to the acquired immune system. Since reverse transcriptase has a higher error rate than DNA-dependent DNA polymerase, retroviruses are particularly adept at this form of immune evasion. The association of major influenza outbreaks with viral strains bearing new antigenic determinants on their hemagglutinin and neuraminidase proteins, acquired by reassortment of the segmented RNA genome, is probably explained by lack of preexisting host immunity to the new pandemic strain.

The distinction between innate and acquired immunity is not absolute, since antiviral cytokines may be secreted by effector cells from both systems, and the mechanisms used by cytotoxic effector cells to kill virally infected cells may also be common to both branches. In addition, the evolution of multiple closely related genes for innate host defense proteins, such as the class I interferons and granzymes, may indicate a primitive degree of specificity for "innate" responses. The use of genetic knock-out animals has revealed a great deal of redundancy within host defense systems; frequently, several compensatory mechanisms are capable of controlling viral infections. However, the discovery of many virally encoded inhibitors of both innate and acquired host defense mechanisms does imply a functional role for host defense mechanisms, including interferon and other cytokines, cytotoxic T lymphocytes, immunoglobulin, and other effector systems. Some viruses with large genomes, such as adenoviridae, poxviridae, and herpesviridae, devote a considerably a[illegible] of their nucleic acid to such immune evasion functions.

Class I interferons (interferons alpha and beta) are a fam[illegible] cytokines produced by many cell types upon interaction wi[illegible] a variety of viruses. Interferons interact with specific cell-surface receptors and mediate diverse antiviral effects on penetration, uncoating, transcription, translation, assembly, and release. Viruses must evade these effects long enough to replicate. Adenovirus, EBV, and hepatitis B virus each inhibit signal transduction through interferon receptors. Some of the effects of interferons are mediated by a protein kinase, PKR, which phosphorylates the initiation factor eIF2, limiting protein synthesis and thus viral replication. Of note, bacterial eIF may also be the target of antibacterial agents. Several viruses, including adenovirus, EBV, vaccinia, HIV, influenza, polio, and reovirus, encode proteins inhibiting the function of PKR. Viruses may also utilize side effects of interferon to their own advantage. Many of the symptoms of rhinovirus upper respiratory infection, such as nasal hypersecretion, may be due to local effects of interferon and other cytokines (see Chapter 11). It has been hypothesized that the virus takes advantage of this host response to spread to uninfected individuals.

Many DNA viruses in the adenoviridae, poxviridae, and herpesviridae families contain genes encoding for proteins homologous to other cytokines or their receptors, or inhibitors of cytokine action. EBV contains an IL-10 homolog gene that promotes the growth and transformation of B cells, while KSHV encodes an IL-6-like protein that may promote the growth of cells in KS tumors. Myxoma virus encodes a protein homologous to interferon-gamma receptor that neutralizes interferon-gamma activity, as well as soluble receptors for TNF and IL-1. Other poxviruses encode an inhibitor of IL-1$\beta$ converting enzyme (ICE). These genes, apparently captured from their hosts during viral evolution, may confer advantages that are difficult to discern in cell culture and animal model systems.

The acquired cellular immune response includes T lymphocytes with cytotoxic (cell-killing) potential (see Chapter 00). Within virally infected cells, cytoplasmic viral antigens are processed by a complex process of proteolytic cleavage and loaded onto class I histocompatibility antigens (termed HLA in humans), which are then translocated to the plasma membrane for monitoring by the host immune system. In contrast, exogenous viral antigens are phagocytosed, processed by proteolytic cleavage in acid lysosome compartments, and then translocated to the plasma membrane together with HLA class II antigens (Fig. 4.5). When the T-cell receptor of a highly specific cytotoxic T lymphocyte (CTL) interacts with a cell presenting viral antigen, it delivers a lethal signal to the virally infected cells, effectively shutting down viral replication. CTL bearing the CD8 molecule recognize HLA class I plus antigen, while CTL bearing the CD4 molecule recognize HLA class II plus viral antigen. A functional role for CTL has been proven in several animal systems. The importance of the $CD8^+$ subset of CTL in antiviral host defense may also be inferred from the consistency with which viruses in diverse taxonomic groups have devised mechanisms to subvert the presentation of viral antigens to this arm of the immune system.

Herpes simplex virus (HSV) provides an example of viral inhibition of antigen processing. When fibroblasts and keratinocytes, representative of cells infected with HSV during recurrent infection at peripheral sites, are infected with HSV they become resistant to the killing activity of $CD8^+$ T cells. This resistance correlates with downregulation of mature HLA class I

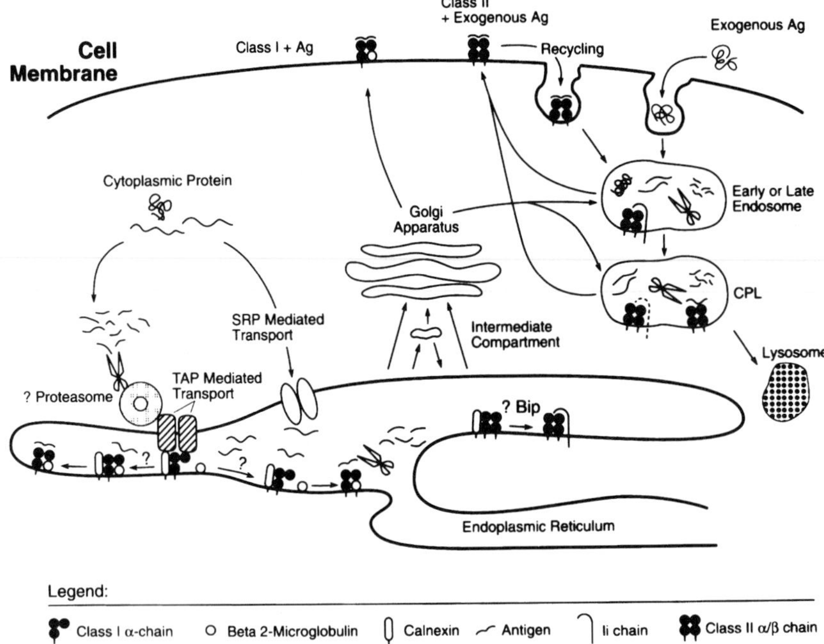


**Fig. 4.5** Endogenous (cytoplasmic) and exogenous pathways of antigen processing. Viral proteins that are synthesized in the infected cell, or delivered to the cytoplasm (left) are degraded by proteosomes (scissors) to peptides which are transported by TAP to the endoplasmic reticulum to associate with HLA class I. HLA class I-peptide complexes are transported to the plasma membrane, where they are recognized by CD8+ T-cells. Exogenous viral proteins are phagocytosed (upper left) and processed by proteolytic enzymes in endosomes: resultant peptides associate with HLA class II. HLA class II-peptide complexes are also transported to the plasma membrane where they are presented to CD4+ T-cells. [From Restifo NP, et al, Essentials of Immunology, p. 48, In: *Cancer: Principles & Practice of Oncology*, Fifth Edition, ed. Devita VT et al, Lippincott-Raven Publishers, Philadelphia, 1997, with permission]

peptide complexes at the cell surface. One viral protein responsible for this effect is ICP47, a cytosolic protein that inhibits the TAP1/TAP2 complex necessary for translocation of peptides into the endoplasmic reticulum for loading onto newly synthesized HLA class I. Despite this phenomenon, $CD8^+$ CTL specific for HSV are readily detectable in the blood of HSV-seropositive individuals. Thus, ICP47 may modify the timing or repertoire of proteins recognized by $CD8^+$ T-cells in such a way as to promote viral replication. Since NK cells have cytotoxic activity toward cells deficient in HLA class I, interference with $CD8^+$ T-cell recognition may allow a reciprocal increase in NK cell recognition of infected cells.

Adenovirus also interferes with the assembly of new HLA class I through the binding of the viral protein gp19K to newly synthesized HLA class I heavy-chain protein. EBV expresses a limited set of proteins during latency, and the recognition of one of these, EBNA 1, by HLA class I–restricted T cells is selectively downregulated by the presence of certain inhibitory amino acid regions within the viral polypeptide. CMV has several mechanisms for downregulation of assembly of new HLA class I molecules, limiting the display of viral epitopes on the cell surface. Since recognition of virally infected cells by $CD8^+$ T cells is highly sequence-specific, the high mutation rate of retroviruses such as HIV may allow escape from immune surveillance and contribute to viral persistence within the host.

Natural killer cells and CTLs trigger death in virally infected cells by several mechanisms, including exocytosis of toxic preformed granule contents such as perforin, secretion of cytokines such as TNF, and receptor–ligand interactions between proteins on the surfaces of killer and target cells, such as fas and fas ligand. These mechanisms kill cells by inducing apoptosis, or programmed cell death, in the virally infected cell. Viral genes, as discussed above, may allow cellular survival for long enough to permit production of progeny virus. Viruses also kill cells by induction of apoptosis. For example, gp160 of HIV may be sufficient to induce apoptotic cell death in susceptible cells such as neurons. HIV also primes T cells for the induction of apoptosis after activation through CD3 and presumably through physiologic stimulation by antigen. Thus, viruses manipulate cellular programs such as antigen processing and apoptosis in diverse ways that we are only beginning to understand.

In contrast to cellular immunity, impaired antibody responses, as well as granulocyte and complement deficiencies, are infrequently associated with severe viral infections. One exception is severe or chronic echovirus infections associated with immunoglobulin deficiency. Antibodies do appear to be important for protective immunity against some viruses after immunization or natural infection; prophylactic administration of specific immune-globulin products can prevent or ameliorate infection with HBV, VZV, and other viruses. If one accepts the premise that viral genomes are efficiently utilized, the presence of functional virally encoded Fc and complement component receptor homologs in herpes simplex and other viruses does argue that perturbation of these defense mechanisms is somehow advantageous to the virus. Herpes simplex viruses with alterations in their Fc receptors are, in fact, less virulent in certain model systems.

An immune response to viral infection may have deleterious effects. An example of this is dengue hemorrhagic fever, a severe form of acute dengue virus infection seen more frequently in patients with preexisting immunity to heterologous strains of dengue. Cross-reactive antibodies bind to the virus, enhancing viral entry via Fc receptors and triggering complement activation after the formation of immune complexes. Viruses are suspected, although not proven, to trigger a variety of inflammatory and autoimmune diseases. Herpetic keratitis is a frequent cause of anterior blindness, and is often associated with a leukocytic corneal infiltrate and little evidence of active viral infection. Juvenile-onset diabetes is associated with both certain HLA alleles and infection with enteroviruses. Molecular mimicry between viral and self antigens recognized by host HLA class II molecules may be responsible for these effects. Alternatively, viral infection may expose sequestered antigens in a local inflammatory microenvironment, which promotes the breaking of immunologic tolerance to self-antigens leading to autoimmune disease.

## Summary

Viruses have extraordinarily intricate and diverse relationships with their hosts at the cell, organism, and population levels. Generally, the signs and symptoms of viral infections are due to direct cytopathic effects of viral infection on host cells in specific tissues and organs, although host responses may lead to inflammatory tissue damage and may be involved in virus transmission. Many medically important viruses are persistent within the individual host, and accomplish this by a variety of mechanisms, including antigenic change, evasion of the cellular immune response through downregulation of antigen processing or apoptosis, and the establishment of episomal latent infections or integration into the host genome. The viral life cycle is so closely interwoven with the metabolism of host cells that additional selective chemotherapy has been very difficult to achieve. A detailed understanding of the specific events of binding, entry, and replication of diverse viral pathogens will hopefully lead to the development of selective antiviral agents, and should also lead to medically significant insights in the fields of cell biology, cancer, and immunology.

## ANNOTATED BIBLIOGRAPHY

Brown KE, Anderson SM, Young NS. Erythrocyte P antigen: cellular receptor for B19 parvovirus. Science 1993; 262:114–117.
*Example of virus dependence on a human allelic polymorphism highlights importance of binding in pathogenesis.*

Dragic T, Litwin V, Allaway GP et al. HIV-1 entry into $CD4^+$ cells is mediated by the chemokine receptor CC-CKR-5. Nature 1996; 381:647–648.
*An example of use of dual receptors for viral entry.*

Spriggs MK. One step ahead of the game: viral immunomodulatory molecules. Annu Rev Immunol 1996; 14:101–130.
*Emphasizes mimicry and evasion of host immune responses.*

Tyler KL, Fields BN. Pathogenesis of viral infections. In: Fields Virology, Third Edition, Fields BN, Knipe DM, Howley PM et al, ed. Lippincott-Raven Publishers, Philadelphia 1996, pp 173–218.
*Detailed review of key steps in viral pathogenesis.*

Vousden K. Interactions of human papillomavirus transforming proteins with the products of tumor suppressor genes. FASEB J 1993; 7:872–879.
*Summarizes tumorigenic mechanisms for this cancer-associated virus.*

# 5

# Parasitic Protozoa and Helminths

ADEL A. F. MAHMOUD

Parasitic protozoa and helminths constitute two of the larger groups of infectious agents that cause human morbidity and mortality (Table 5.1). In spite of the major biological, epidemiological, and clinical differences between these two groups of infectious agents, they have been traditionally identified as parasites. The acceptable definition of the phenomenon of parasitism, however, is a specialized, dependent, and obligatory mode of life. It, therefore, applies to all infectious agents and not particularly to any specific group whether it is viruses or helminths. The rationale for grouping protozoa and helminths together is therefore unclear except that both belong to the animal kingdom.

More important from the clinical point of view is the recognition of differences between protozoa and helminths. Protozoa are unicellular organisms; they are mainly microscopic in size and are, in general, capable of multiplying within their definitive mammalian host. Helminths, on the other hand, are multicellular; they vary in size from 1 mm to 10 m and are in general incapable of multiplication within the definitive mammalian host. There are, however, a few clinically relevant exceptions to this rule—e.g., strongyloidiasis and echinococcosis. Furthermore, helminth infections that migrate in host tissues are characteristically associated with tissue, as well as peripheral blood eosinophilia. Appreciation of these differences is essential in understanding host–parasite interaction and its pathologic sequelae.

## Classification

### Protozoa

The vast majority of protozoa are free-living. The parasitic species share the common features of the phylum. Structurally, all protozoa are unicellular and as other eukaryotes they possess well-defined nuclei. The cytosplasm of most protozoa contain one or more types of vacuoles and other inclusions, such as ribosomes, mitochondria, and Golgi complex. Protozoa exist as trophozoites or vegetative forms, but many are capable of encystation. Cysts of parasitic protozoa are essential for protection against environmental factors as well as for multiplication and transmission of the organisms between hosts.

Parasitic protozoa are classified into:

- Sarcomastiygophora, which possess pseudopodia or flagella as locomotor organelle during one or more stages of their life cycle.
- Apicomplexa, characterized by the presence of apical complexes
- Ciliophora, characterized by the presence of cilia or compound ciliary organelles.

The most recent classification of protozoa and examples of organisms is summarized in Table 2.

### Helminths

Parasitic helminths or worms are characteristically larger organisms when compared with protozoa. The smallest size of an adult worm is approximately 1 cm in length (*Entrobius vermicularis* or pinworms) and the largest is approximately 10 meters (*Diphyllobothrium latum* or fish tape worm). Infection with any of these large parasitic organisms is initiated through either ingestion of their eggs, by penetration of intact human skin by their larval stages (100–400 $\mu$m), or is carried into the host via the bite of an insect vector (e.g., mosquitoes transmit larvae of *Wuchereria bancrofti*). The body structure of parasitic worms is well developed and differentiated into organ systems. Most prominent is the outer structure, which protects the organism against host protective mechanisms. Examples of these structures include chitinous material and syncytium limited by a heptalaminate plasma membrane. Inside this protective coating exists several physiologic systems, such as digestive, neurologic, and reproductive organs. Significantly, the life cycle of parasitic helminths has evolved to secure several forms; each is capable of parasitizing a separate host. The life cycle in many parasitic worms may, therefore, alternate between the mammalian or definitive host and one or more intermediate hosts such as snails or fish.

Parasitic worms are generally divided into Nematodes (roundworms), Platyhelminths (flatworms), and Cestodes (segmented worms). The classification of the clinically significant members of each group is outlined in Tables 5.3, 5.4, and 5.5.

## Organ-specific infections

In most parasitic protozoan and helminthic infections a target organ in the human host can be identified. Disease associated with these infected organs may serve as an aid in establishing the correct diagnosis, but it also helps in understanding the pathological sequelae of host–parasite interaction. It has to be emphasized that many of these organisms are capable of producing disease in a primary site of infection that can spread to other sites in the body.

The subject of organ-specific infection will be approached in a system-by-system basis. In Table 5.6, infections of the gastrointestinal tract are summarized. The most characteristic manifestations are diarrhea in its different forms: frequent stools, malabsorption, and dysentery with passage of blood and mucus. In other circumstances, GI manifestations may be obstructive, as in infection with large numbers of *Ascaris* or when single worms migrate into the ampulla of Vater. Several infections may cause disease unrelated directly to the GI system—e.g., anemia in hookworm infection or $B_{12}$ deficiency in fish tapeworm infection.

Primary disease in the liver may be caused by several parasitic protozoa or helminth. These are summarized in Table 5.7.

**Table 5.1** Approximate quantification of the global burden of illness due to selective parasitic protozoan and helminthic infections

| Infection | Global prevalence (in millions) | Estimated burden of illness | |
|---|---|---|---|
| | | Morbidity | Mortality |
| PROTOZOA | | | |
| Malaria | 800 | +++ | ++++ |
| Amebiasis | 400 | + | ++ |
| Trypanosomiasis, American | 12 | ++ | ++ |
| Trypanosomiasis, African | 50 | ++ | ++ |
| HELMINTHS | | | |
| Schistosomiasis | 300 | ++ | + |
| Ascariasis | 1000 | + | − |
| Filariasis | 200 | ++ | − |
| Onchocerciasis | 50 | ++ | − |

**Table 5.2** Classification of parasitic protozoa

Phylum Sarcomastigophora: Flagella, pseudopodia, or both types of locomotor organelles
- Subphylum Mastigophora: One or more flagella typically present in trophozoites
  - Class Zoomastigophorea
    - Order Kinetoplastida
      - Suborder Trypanosomatina
        - *Leishmania, Trypanosoma*
    - Order Diplomonadida
      - Suborder Diplomonadina
        - *Giardia*
    - Order Trichomonadida
      - *Dientamoeba, Trichomonas*
- Subphylum Sarcodina: Pseudopodia or locomotive protoplasmic flow without discrete pseudopodia
  - Superclass Rhizopoda
    - Class Lobosea
      - Subclass Gymnamoebia
        - Order Amoebida
          - Suborder Tubulina
            - *Entamoeba*
          - Suborder Acanthopodina
            - *Acanthamoeba*
        - Order Schizopyrenida
          - *Naegleria*

Phylum Apicomplexa: Apical complex, generally consisting of polar ring(s), rhoptries, micronemes; conoid and subpellicular microtubules present at some stage
- Class Sporozoasida
  - Subclass Coccidiasina
    - Order Coccidiasina
      - Suborder Eimeriorina
        - *Isospora, Toxoplasma, Cryptosporidium*
      - Suborder Haemospororina
        - *Plasmodium*
  - Subclass Piroplasmasina
    - *Babesia*

Phylum Ciliophora: Simple cilia or compound ciliary organelles typical in at least one stage of life cycle; two types of nuclei; sexuality involving conjugation, autogamy, and cytogamy
- Class Litosomatea
  - Subclass Trichostomatia
    - Order Vestubuliferida
      - *Balantidium*

Source: Adapted from Warren KS, Mahmoud AAF. Tropical and Geographical Medicine, 2nd ed. McGraw-Hill, New York, 1990, p. 245.

The major disease manifestation is hepatomegaly, which usually does not help in establishing a definitive diagnosis. The associated symptoms and signs and the careful assessment of history of present illness may be helpful in differentiating the etiologic agents.

Infection with protozoans and helminths that parasitize human blood and the lymphatic system may be caused by several organisms (Table 5.8). The disease syndromes that are characteristic of these infections may be related to blood—e.g., anemia in malaria or obstruction of lymphatics in lymphatic filariasis—but also can manifest in other organs—e.g., liver in schistosomiasis or the central nervous system in African trypanosomiasis. Most of these infections are associated with peripheral blood eosinophilia.

Parasitization of other sites in the body occurs less frequently, but when it happens it is a major diagnostic challenge to the practicing physician. Tables 5.9 and 5.10, respectively, summarize the major parasitic protozoan and helminthic infections that may produce disease in the lungs or central nervous system.

The known spectrum of disease due to parasitic protozoan and helminthic infections has changed drastically over the past two decades. The introduction of steroids and other immunosuppressive regimens, the prolongation of the life span of many individuals with different malignant syndromes, and the occurrence of AIDS have increased the proportion of the population who are suffering from varying degrees of immunosuppression. New infections and new manifestations of known pathogens are now becoming a permanent feature of the treatment of infectious diseases. Table 5.11 summarizes the most common protozoan and helminthic infections in the immunocompromised.

## Pathogenesis

Disease due to parasitic protozoan and helminthic infections is one outcome of the host–parasite interaction. In certain circumstances the presence of the pathogens and the mechanical or nutritional sequelae may directly lead to pathological changes. Examples of this pathogenetic mechanism include anemia in hookworm disease and liver cysts in echinococcosis. Disease may also result from toxins produced by the invading organisms, such as *Entamoeba histolytica*. The other major pathological process seen in many protozoan and helminthic infections is an outcome of the host immunological reactions. While these may be important in limiting the extent of parasitization of the host or help in the development of acquired resistance, a by-product is pathological changes. The immune com-

**Table 5.3** Classification of parasitic nematodes

| Parasite | Infective stage | Mode of transmission |
|---|---|---|
| GUT ROUNDWORMS | | |
| *Ascaris lumbricoides* | Mature eggs | Ingestion |
| *Necator americanus* | Mature larvae | Penetration of skin |
| *Ancylostoma duodenale* | Mature larvae | Penetration of skin |
| *Strongyloides stercoralis* | Filariform larvae | Penetration of skin or gut |
| *Entrobius vermicularis* | Mature eggs | Ingestion |
| *Trichuris trichuria* | Mature eggs | Ingestion |
| TISSUE ROUNDWORMS | | |
| *Wuchureria bancrofti* | $L_3$ larvae | Bite of mosquito |
| *Brugia Malayi* | $L_3$ larvae | Bite of mosquito |
| *Onchocerca volvulus* | $L_3$ larvae | Bite of simulium |
| *Loa loa* | $L_3$ larvae | Bite of chrysops |

**Table 5.4** Classification of parasitic platyhelminth (flukes)

| | Infective stage | Mode of transmission |
|---|---|---|
| BLOOD FLUKES | | |
| *Schistosoma haematobium* | Cercaria | Penetration of skin |
| *S. mansoni* | Cercaria | Penetration of skin |
| *S. japonicum* | Cercaria | Penetration of skin |
| *S. intercalatum* | Cercaria | Penetration of skin |
| *S. mekongi* | Cercaria | Penetration of skin |
| LIVER FLUKES | | |
| *Fasciola hepatica* | Encysted metacercaria | Ingestion of aquatic plants |
| *Fasciola gigantica* | Encysted metacercaria | Ingestion of aquatic plants |
| *Clonorchis sinensis* | Encysted metacercaria | Ingestion of carp |
| LUNG FLUKES | | |
| *Paragonimus westermanni* | Encysted metacercaria | Ingestion of crabs and crayfish |
| INTESTINAL FLUKES | | |
| *Fasciolopsis buski* | Encysted metacercaria | Ingestion of acquatic plants |

**Table 5.5** Classification of parasitic cestodes (segmented worms)

| Helminth | Infective stage | Mode of transmission |
|---|---|---|
| *Cyclophyllidea* | | |
| *Taenia saginata* | Cysticercus | Ingestion of beef |
| *Taenia solium* | Cysticercus | Ingestion of pork |
| *T. solium* cysticercosis | Eggs | Auto-infection or ingestion of eggs |
| *Echinococcus granulosus* | Eggs | Ingestion (geohelminth) |
| *Pseudophyllidea* | | |
| *Diphyllobothrium latum* | Plerocercoid | Ingestion of raw fish |

**Table 5.6** Parasitic protozoan and helminthic infections of the gastrointestinal tract

| Site | Infection | Major disease manifestations |
|---|---|---|
| Small intestine | *Giardia lamblia* | Diarrhea, malabsorption |
| | Cryptosporidium | Watery diarrhea |
| | *Ascaris lumbricoides* | Nutritional defects, obstruction |
| | Hookworms | Anemia |
| | *Strongyloides stercoralis* (in immunocompetent host) | Abdominal pain, diarrhea, malabsorption |
| | *Taenia solium* | Nonspecific |
| | *Taenia saginata* | Nonspecific |
| | *Diphyllobothrium latum* | $B_{12}$ deficiency |
| Large intestine | *Entamoeba histolytica* | Dysentery, ameboma |
| | *Balantidium coli* | Bloody diarrhea |
| | *Trypanosoma cruzi* | Megacolon |
| | *Enterobius vermicularis* | Perianal irritation |
| | *Trichuris trichura* | Abdominal pain, malnutrition |

**Table 5.7** Parasitic protozoan and helminthic infection of the liver and biliary system

| Infection | Major disease manifestation |
|---|---|
| Amebiasis | Liver abscess: fever, tender hepatomegaly |
| Visceral leishmaniasis | Hepatomegaly, splenomegaly, fever, pancylopenia |
| Malaria | Hepatomegaly, splenomegaly |
| Fascioliasis | Abdominal pain, hepatomegaly |
| Clonorchiasis | Hepatomegaly |
| Toxocariasis | Abdominal pain, hepatomegaly |
| Schistosomiasis | Hepatomegaly, portal hypertension |
| Echinococcosis | Hepatomegaly, cyst in liver |

**Table 5.8** Parasitic protozoan and helminthic infection of blood, lymphatics or abdominal viscera

| Site | Infection | Major disease manifestation |
|---|---|---|
| Peripheral blood | Malaria | Fever, anemia, thrombocytopenia |
| | Babesiosis | Fever, anemia |
| | Trypanosomiasis, African | Fever, rash, sleeping sickness |
| Portal system | Schistosomiasis | Crampy abdominal pain, hepatosplenomegaly, portal hypertension |
| Vesical urinary system | Schistosomiasis haematobium | Hematuria, frequency of urination, hydroureter and hydronephrosis |
| Lymphatic | Lymphatic filariasis | Lymphangitis, lymphadenitis, elephantiasis |

**Table 5.9** Parasitic protozoan and helminthic infections of the lungs

| Infection | Major disease manifestations |
|---|---|
| Amebiasis | Lung abscess (rare) |
| *Pneumocystis carinii* | Cough, dyspnea, hypoxia |
| Ascariasis, hookworms, and strongyloidiasis | Loeffler's-like syndromes |
| Toxocariasis | Pulmonary infiltrate with eosinophilia |
| Schistosomiasis | Cor pulmonale |
| Echinococcosis | Lung cyst |
| Paragonimiasis | Lung infiltrate, abscess |

**Table 5.10** Parasitic protozoan and helminthic infections of the central nervous system

| Infection | Major disease manifestations |
|---|---|
| African trypanosomiasis | Altered mentation, coma |
| Malaria | Coma |
| Amebiasis | Space-occupying lesion |
| Primary amebic meningoencephalitis | Meningitis, encephalitis, or brain abcess |
| Schistosomiasis japonica | Grand mal epilepsy |
| Schistosomiasis mansoni or hematobium | Transverse myelitis |
| Cysticerosis solium | Space-occupying lesion |
| Echinococcosis | Space-occupying lesion |
| Angiostrongyliasis | Meningitis, eosinophilic |

plex–induced nephro-tic syndrome associated with *Plasmodium malariae* infection is a consequence of chronic antigenic stimulation and the corresponding host antibody response. Another well-studied disease mechanism is the host immunopathological granulomatous response to schistosome eggs.

The other significant aspect of the host–parasite relationship is the ability of most of these organisms to evade the protective responses of the host. These evasion mechanisms are well developed in many protozoan and helminthic organisms, thus ensuring survival of the pathogens for weeks or years in the host. Finally, protozoan and helminthic infections in humans may induce resistance against subsequent infection. For reasons that are still unclear, most of these infections induce, however, little or no demonstrable resistance in the infected hosts. In a few examples—e.g., cutaneous leishmaniasis—solid immunity against challenge infection may be demonstrated. The subject of vaccines for protozoan and helminthic infections is being pursued vigorously, and several candidate preparations have undergone clinical trials.

**Table 5.11** Parasitic protozoan and helminthic infections that are more prevalent in the immunocompromised host

| Protozoan | Helminthic |
|---|---|
| Toxoplasmosis | Strongyloidiasis |
| Cryptosporidium | |
| Isospora | |
| Leishmaniasis | |
| Pneumocystosis | |
| Giardiasis | |
| Amebiasis | |

## Approach to Diagnosis and Management

A history and physical examination are essential elements in approaching an individual with parasitic protozoan or helminthic infection. Traditionally, the question "Where have you been?" was considered central in examining the history of the present illness. This may not be enough. Geographic locations vary and the extent of other social, dietary, and recreational activities experienced by the traveler need to be assessed, as well as the duration of possible exposure and the time lapse between exposure and clinical presentation. Similarly, physical examination and initial workup plans should include particular attention from the practicing physician and collaboration with the laboratory personnel. Eosinophilia is a significant finding that may point toward tissue-migrating helminths (see Chapter 102). Interpreting a diagnostic test requires knowledge of the life cycle of the

**Table 5.12** Samples examined for definitive diagnosis of parasitic protozoan and helminthic infection*

| Sample or tissue | Stage of protozoa or helminth |
|---|---|
| Stools | Trophozoites or cysts: ameba, *Giardia*, *Cryptosporidium*, *Balantidium*<br>Eggs: *Ascaris*, hookworms, liver, intestinal and lung flukes, entrobiasis, trichiuriasis, schistosomiasis, *T. solium*, *D. latum*<br>Segments: taeniasis, diphyllobothriasis<br>Larvae: strongyloidiasis |
| Urine | Eggs: *Schistosoma haematobium* |
| Blood | Intraerythrocytic: malaria, babesiosis<br>Extraerythrocytic: African trypanosomiasis<br>Intraphagocytic: Leishmania |
| Rectal biopsy | Schistosomes |
| Muscle biopsy | Trichinosis |
| Brain biopsy | Toxoplasmosis, amebiasis |
| Liver biopsy | Schistosomes |

*See Chapter 19 for details.

pathogen, the specific stage to be searched for, and the correct handling of the clinical samples. In Table 5.12, the tissues to be examined and suspected agents are summarized. In addition, serological tests, which are available for most of these infections, may be of considerable help (see Chapter 19). Information about specific tests and their availability can be gotten from the state laboratories or from the Centers for Disease Control and Prevention in Atlanta, Georgia. Once the correct diagnosis is made, a therapeutic plan should be constructed to include cost-benefit analysis and possible outcome. Therapy of parasitic protozoan and helminthic infection is summarized in Chapter 40.

## ANNOTATED BIBLIOGRAPHY

Anderson RM, May RM. Infectious Diseases of Humans, Dynamics and Control. Oxford University Press, New York, p 757, 1991.
*A major source for the theory and application of epidemiological and mathematical modeling of infectious diseases as they occur in populations.*

Mahmoud AAF. Parasitic Protozoa and Helminths: Biological and Immunological Challenges. Science 1989; 246:1015.
*Examination of the immunological and molecular aspects of host–parasite relationships in select protozoa and helminths.*

Mahmoud AAF. (ed) Tropical and Geographical Medicine Companion Handbook, 2nd ed., McGraw-Hill, New York, p 468, 1993.
*A summary of the salient clinical, diagnostic and therapeutic approaches to protozoan and helminthic infections.*

Warren KS, ed. Immunology and Molecular Biology of Parasitic Infections, 3rd ed., Boston, Blackwell Scientific Publications, p 610, 1993.
*A detailed examination of the immunological and molecular aspects of protozoan and helminthic infections.*

Warren KS, Mahmoud AAF, eds. Tropical and Geographical Medicine, 2nd ed., McGraw-Hill, New York, p 1159, 1990.
*A comprehensive, textbook examination of the clinical, epidemiological, and scientific basis of host and parasite interactions in protozoan and helminthic infections.*

Wilson M, Schantz P. Nonmorphologic diagnosis of parasitic infections. In: Manual of Clinical Microbiology, 5th ed. Balows A, ed., American Society of Microbiology, Washington, 1991.
*A comprehensive source for diagnostic tests.*

# 6

# Fungi and Fungal Diseases

JOHN E. EDWARDS, JR. AND PETER G. PAPPAS

This chapter is divided into two main sections, "Opportunistic Mycoses" and "Endemic Mycoses." Because of the evolution of the fungal pathogens, this division has become imperfect in contemporary times. Many fungal pathogens that were previously classified as endemic have become opportunistic in severely immunocompromised hosts. For instance, *Histoplasma* frequently infects patients with the acquired immunodeficiency syndrome (AIDS). Furthermore, all of the fungal pathogens classified as opportunistic have occurred in individuals with no known immunocompromise. For example, rarely zygomycosis (mucormycosis) occurs in patients without diabetes, cancer, or renal failure. For convenience, this discussion will conform to the traditional classification. Instances where the classification becomes inappropriate will be pointed out within the description of each specific pathogen.

The evolution of the opportunistic fungal pathogens in the ever-growing population of severely immunocompromised patients has become increasingly important. *Candida* organisms have become the fourth most common organisms recovered from blood cultures in hospitalized patients. These organisms are now among the most common nosocomial pathogens in general. Cryptococcosis has become a relatively common infection in patients having AIDS. The number of cases of aspergillosis continues to increase in the cancer and bone marrow transplant populations. As the total number of patients with cancer, AIDS, immunosuppression following organ transplantation, prosthetic material implants, and protracted postoperative courses continues to grow, it is highly likely that the prevalence of serious fungal infections will increase substantially. Coupled with this increased prevalence of infections is the problem of the difficulty of treating fungal diseases. The organisms are eukaryotic and have cell structures that more closely resemble human cells than they do bacteria. Therefore, developing antifungal drugs that do not have toxicity against human cells is difficult and is an area requiring intense investigation.

## Opportunistic Mycoses

### Candidiasis

Of the deep fungal diseases, those caused by candidal organisms are the most common. The organisms are highly successful commensals that are part of the normal human flora. Additionally, they are found frequently in animals and in the environment. There are numerous species of these organisms (over 150). However, only a few have been reported to infect humans. Included in the most frequently recovered from man are *Candida albicans*, *C. tropicalis*, *C. glabrata* (*Torulopsis glabrata* is the term preferred by some mycologists), *C. parapsilosis*, *C. stellatoidea*, *C. pseudotropicalis*, *C. krusei*, and *C. guilliermondii*. *C. albicans* is traditionally considered the most pathogenic of these species, but all are capable of causing serious infections in the deep organs, and all are capable of causing mucocutaneous disease. Of recent importance regarding these species is the higher minimal inhibitory concentrations (MICs) that some species have to fluconazole. While the significance of these higher MICs is not known at this time, there is concern among clinical mycologists that they represent a relative resistance to this important azole. *C. krusei* predictably has higher MICs, and the MICs for *C. glabrata* tend to be variable. Importantly, *C. glabrata* is being recovered with higher frequency in the gastrointestinal tract in hospitalized patients. Because of differences in the pathology, epidemiology, and sensitivity to antifungal agents, careful speciation of candidal isolates is recommended as a routine procedure.

#### Pathogenesis

The reason for the emergence of candidal organisms as frequent and important nosocomial pathogens is probably related to their ability to heavily colonize individuals who are treated with multiple antibiotics. It is thought that *Candida* compete with bacteria for an ecological niche. When antibiotics suppress the normal bacterial flora, candidal organisms can proliferate and then disseminate to the deep organs. As advances have been made in antibacterial agents, candidal infections have increased dramatically. However, a number of additional factors are also important. They include the use of immunosuppressive therapy for treatment of cancer and management of organ transplantation, use of hyperalimentation fluids that support candidal growth, use of intravascular cannulation with plastic materials to which *Candida* adhere avidly, use of indwelling urinary tract catheters, steroid use, and implantation of prosthetic materials (such as artificial heart valves) that also serve as a focus for adherence of the organisms. Postoperative patients, usually without cancer, also constitute an important population susceptible to candidal infections.

Once a patient has become susceptible to candidal infections by being subjected to the predisposing factors, the candidal flora, particularly of the mucous membranes, becomes more dominant and the capability for entrance into the bloodstream increases. This scenario has led to the increasing recovery of candidal organisms from the blood of hospitalized patients. Once the organism enters the intravascular compartment, it can disseminate to virtually any organ and establish extensive infection. Those organs most commonly infected include the kidney, brain, heart, and eye. However, bones, skeletal muscle, liver and spleen (hepatosplenic candidiasis), gallbladder, endocrine glands, pancreas, peritoneum, heart valves, and virtually any organ may become severely infected. Establishment of the definitive diagnosis requires biopsy proof of the organisms invading a tissue, accompanied by confirmation by culture.

### Candidemia

One of the most difficult and controversial issues related to nosocomial candidal infection centers on the management of the candidemic patient. Undoubtedly, some patients subjected to these predisposing factors develop candidemia that they clear without any recognizable deep-organ infections or complications. No acceptable serodiagnostic tests have yet been developed for differentiating patients who have candidemia without deep-organ infection from those who develop deep-organ infection. During the period when amphotericin B was the only therapeutic agent available for the treatment of deep candidal infections, efforts were made to categorize candidemic patients according to likelihood of having deep infection. Those patients who were determined to have low likelihood of deep-organ infection were managed by removal of indwelling intravascular catheters only, and were not subjected to the serious toxicities accompanying the use of amphotericin B. However, two events have changed that approach, resulting in a consensus among clinical mycologists that all candidemic patients should receive some antifungal therapy. One has been the recognition from retrospective studies that the error rate in assuming candidemic patients did not have deep infection was approximately 30%. Also, the attributable mortality rate of candidemia is very high (38%). The other event has been the introduction of less toxic antifungals into widespread clinical use. The risk-benefit ratio now favors treating candidemic patients. It is likely that this consensus will remain strong, until a useful serodiagnostic test for deep-tissue invasion is developed. However, the probability that such a test will come into widespread clinical use during the next five to ten years is very low. Whether it is necessary to remove the indwelling lines in candidemic patients remains controversial. A consensus has developed that if it is logistically simple to remove the lines, they should be taken out. This consensus is stronger for the nonsurgically implanted lines. The expense and logistical complications of removal and reimplantation of surgically inserted lines is well recognized. Additional studies are critically needed in the area of line management (see Chapters 67, 85).

### Mucocutaneous candidiasis

Mucocutaneous candidal infection remains a frequent problem in immunocompromised patients. Since candidal infections are the most frequent infections complicating AIDS, the appearance of thrush in an individual, without other predisposing factors (such as recent use of antibiotics), should lead to evaluation for AIDS. Both severe thrush and candidal esophagitis occur in patients on chemotherapy for cancer and in patients with AIDS. There is a general consensus that if esophagitis is suspected in patients in either of these categories, a trial of antifungal therapy, usually an azole, is necessary. If there is no response, a definitive diagnosis with esophagoscopy is indicated, since both herpesvirus and cytomegalovirus are important causes of esophageal infection in these patients and require different therapy.

### Prevention

Currently there are ongoing studies on the prophylaxis of candidal infections in susceptible populations and on empiric therapy. These studies are critically important, since unless a prevention strategy is developed, it is highly likely that the prevalence of candidal infections will increase dramatically. Resistance to antifungal agents will eventually become prevalent also.

## Cryptococcosis

Organisms of the genus *Cryptococcus* are ubiquitous and have a worldwide distribution. With rare exception, *C. neoformans* is the infecting species.

### Pathogenesis

The usual route of infection with cryptococci is inhalation of the organisms, which then invade the pulmonary parenchyma. Entrance to the vasculature may occur from the respiratory tract, and hematogenous dissemination may result. The brain is the most common organ infected by the hematogenous route, but almost any organ may be involved. Cryptococcal meningitis has emerged as an important complication of AIDS and occurs in approximately 10% of patients with AIDS (recent studies are showing decreasing rates). Prior to the AIDS epidemic, approximately half the cases of cryptococcal meningitis were seen in patients receiving immunosuppressive therapy for either treatment of cancer or the management of organ transplantation. The other half occurred in patients who were seemingly normal and had no evidence of immunocompromise. Normal host defense mechanisms for cryptococcosis include predominant monocyte-derived macrophages, natural killer cells, and T lymphocytes. Both complement and antibodies assist these cells in defense. The dense polysaccharide capsule of *Cryptococcus* is considered an important virulence factor, since it is antiphagocytic. Patients having AIDS become particularly susceptible to infection when their $CD4^+$ lymphocyte counts fall below the 200 level.

### Diagnosis

Cryptococcal organisms can be seen readily in body fluids or secretions with the simple India ink preparation. This preparation is made by addition of a drop of India ink to approximately an equal volume of the clinical specimen. The yeast and its large capsule are clearly defined by the India ink. The definitive diagnosis of cryptococcosis requires biopsy-proven evidence of tissue invasion, with confirmation by culture. However, detection of the cryptococcal capsular antigen by latex agglutination is a reliable test that is both sensitive and specific. Despite the reliability of this test, confirmation by culture and tissue evidence of invasion is necessary for definitive diagnosis.

### Clinical manifestations

There is a broad spectrum of cryptococcal pulmonary infection, ranging from asymptomatic carriage in certain normal individuals to necrotizing pneumonia. The latter condition occurs more frequently in severely immunocompromised patients receiving cytotoxic chemotherapy. Not infrequently, asymptomatic individuals develop a solitary pulmonary nodule suggestive of a neoplasm. On biopsy or excision, cryptococcal infection is found. Of importance is the recognition that cryptococcal pulmonary infection may present with a clinical and radiographic picture indistinguishable from *Pneumocystis carinii* infection. This presentation has occurred predominantly in patients with AIDS. Culture, India ink preparation, and pulmonary biopsy assist in making this important differentiation.

Several aspects of cryptococcal central nervous system infection have been recognized in recent years and deserve comment. Fever is not always associated with cryptococcal meningitis. In such patients the diagnostic evaluation is usually directed more toward central nervous system neoplasm. If evaluation is terminated after radiographic studies, which may be normal, the diagnosis of cryptococcal meningitis may be missed. Sampling the cerebrospinal fluid and performing antigen detection, cultures, and India ink preparation would prevent a delayed diagnosis in such patients. With the advent of magnetic resonance imaging (MRI) and computerized tomography (CT) scans, cryptococcal mass lesions have been found with higher frequency than before. These lesions may increase the intracranial pressure and cause herniation of the brain. Therefore, in patients suspected of having cryptococcal meningitis, care should be taken to assure safety in performing a spinal tap. Some patients with AIDS have presented with no symptoms referable to the central nervous system. Nevertheless, they have had extensive cryptococcal meningitis. Usually the diagnosis has been made from a spinal tap performed in the course of evaluation for a fever of unknown etiology. Unfortunately, the spinal tap has generally been performed late in the diagnostic evaluation. The prognosis for cryptococcal meningoencephalitis depends on the underlying immunocompromise to some extent. Rough approximations for fatality rates range from 15% in nonimmunocompromised individuals to as high as 60% in certain patients with AIDS. High recurrence rates in patients with AIDS is thought to be due to their high prevalence of prostatic cryptococcal infections.

A number of tissues besides the brain, meninges, and lungs can be infected by *Cryptococcus*. They include predominantly the skin (by hematogenous dissemination), bones and joints, kidneys, and prostate. However, virtually any organ may be infected. The hematogenous skin lesions are nonspecific in appearance, and usually present as subcutaneous nodules that are clinically indistinguishable from similar lesions caused by *Candida* or *Mucor*. They are important to recognize on physical examination, since biopsy of the lesions will disclose the organisms. Finding such a lesion can be an especially helpful sign of widespread hematogenous dissemination.

### Treatment

Currently, extensive clinical trails are under way to define the most efficacious and appropriate therapy for cryptococcal meningoencephalitis. There is no clear consensus for patients with AIDS. The most attractive strategy at present is initial treatment with amphotericin B with or without 5-fluorocytosine followed by fluconozole. Most clinical mycologists are continuing to use amphotericin B as initial treatment in patients who do not have AIDS (see Chapter 42).

## Aspergillosis

Of all the fungal organisms, those in the species *Aspergillus* are among the most ubiquitous. They are found in an extremely diverse distribution of environmental sources, and are a component of the normal flora of man. Importantly, they are found throughout hospitals and frequently colonize hospital air-conditioning systems. Many outbreaks of aspergillosis have been traced to hospital environmental sources. The two most common species of *Aspergillus* infecting man are *A. niger* and *A. fumigatus*. Because of their ubiquitous distribution in hospitals, these organisms can easily contaminate specimens, both at the time of their collection from patients and during processing in the microbiology laboratory. Therefore, with *Aspergillus* infections, it is particularly important for making a definitive diagnosis to demonstrate invasion of tissues on histopathology as well as to have confirmation by culture. Additionally, it is not possible to distinguish *Aspergillus* from other filamentous fungi on histopathology. Therefore, confirmation by culture is imperative. In tissue, the organism appears as thin septated hyphae with dichotomous branching. Occasionally, the characteristic fruiting bodies may be seen. The cells important in defense are predominantly neutrophils, monocytes, and macrophages. Complement is considered to be important for optimal defense. Of particular importance is that *Aspergillus* organisms are angiotropic and have a tendency to invade blood vessel walls. Distal infarction is common following the vascular invasion.

### Clinical manifestation

The spectrum of types of infections with *Aspergillus* organisms is wide. The most common infection in nonimmunocompromised hosts is the formation of a fungus ball in a pulmonary cavity, usually caused by tuberculosis. These fungus balls generally do not require treatment unless they become invasive or are associated with frequent bleeding. An entity termed *allergic bronchopulmonary aspergillosis* occurs in patients who are not immunocompromised. Asthma, resolving pulmonary infiltrates, eosinophilia, elevated IgE levels, cutaneous hypersensitivity to *Aspergillus* antigens, and high IgG and IgE antibody titers to *Aspergillus* antigens are the hallmarks of this form of aspergillosis. Bronchiectasis and late-stage fibrosis are complications of the process. Systemic steroids have been helpful in management. Other forms of aspergillosis in nonimmunocompromised individuals include endobronchial colonization and chronic sinus infection.

Invasive aspergillosis in the immunocompromised patient is the most problematic infection caused by fungal organisms. The disease has a high fatality rate, at least 50%, the therapeutic options are very limited, and the diagnosis is very difficult to establish and usually made late into the patient's course. The delay in diagnosis usually occurs because blood cultures are rarely positive in disseminated aspergillosis, and there are no serodiagnostic tests for this disease that are currently available on a widespread commercial basis. Diagnosis depends on biopsy, with confirmation by culture. Patients who have been treated with cytotoxic chemotherapy and/or steroids are the most susceptible to invasive aspergillosis. In these patients, necrotizing pneumonia and/or hematogenous dissemination are the most common forms of the disease. Brain infection is very common when hematogenous dissemination occurs. Mass lesions usually occur, rather than diffuse meningitis. Sinus infection is also a prominent form of aspergillosis in neutropenic patients. Invasion into the orbit may occur, resulting in a syndrome clinically indistinguishable from rhinocerebral mucormycosis.

Other forms of aspergillosis are numerous, and include post-traumatic or postoperative keratomycosis, gastrointestinal invasion including *Aspergillus* esophagitis and infection of the intestinal mucosa, hematogenous or primary inoculation infection of the skin, and *Aspergillus* endocarditis.

Of particular importance is consideration of the possibility of aspergillosis in immunocompromised patients, especially those who are neutropenic, when there is unexplained infarction of deep organs, including lung, brain, and liver. Proof that these infarctions are caused by *Aspergillus* can be definitively obtained only through biopsy and confirmation by culture.

### Treatment

Successful management of immunocompromised hosts with aspergillosis requires a high index of suspicion coupled with aggressive diagnostic procedures directed at the sites of suspected infection. Care is necessary to assure that positive cultures do not represent contamination of clinical specimens from environmental sources. Rapid institution of amphotericin B, especially if the patient is neutropenic, is critical. While some success has been reported with azoles, especially itraconazole, their role in acute management remains secondary to amphotericin B. The role of lipid complex formulations of amphotericin B is currently under evaluation (see Chapter 42).

## Zygomycosis (mucormycosis)

Infections with organisms of the fungi subclass Zygomycetes have traditionally been referred to as mucormycosis. The term *mucormycosis* implies infection with organisms in the genus *Mucor*. However, the term actually encompasses infections caused by organisms in four genera: *Rhizopus*, *Absidia*, *Mucor*, and *Cunninghamella*. Therefore, certain mycologists prefer the term "zygomycosis," which is the term that will be used in this discussion. These filamentous fungi are ubiquitous and can be found as constituents of the normal flora of humans on occasion. In nature, they are usually found on decaying organic materials.

### Pathogenesis

The usual route of infection is by inhalation of spores. Infection in the sinuses, lungs, or widespread hematogenous dissemination may then occur. Alternatively, some patients are infected from environmental sources directly into surgical wounds, burn wounds, biopsy or injection sites, insect bites, and at sites of the application of adhesive tape. When the organisms infect tissue, the filamentous broad, nonseptate hyphae can be seen within the inflammatory reaction. The hyphae branch at right angles. Despite these morphological characteristics, culture is needed for differentiation from other filamentous fungi. Macrophages, neutrophils, and activation of the alternative complement pathway are considered the most important defense mechanisms against these organisms. Like *Aspergillus*, organisms causing zygomycosis are angiotropic and travel across tissue planes through invasion of blood vessels. A characteristic of infections is infarction. Also, because of the indolent nature of the infections, considerable necrotic debris is produced, forming a characteristic black material within the pus.

### Clinical manifestations and treatment

The forms of zygomycosis are divided into three areas for this discussion: *(1)* rhinocerebral in patients with diabetes and ketoacidosis, *(2)* pulmonary in patients rendered immunocompromised through cytotoxic chemotherapy, and *(3)* primary cutaneous. This division is imperfect and for convenience only, since all forms of zygomycosis can overlap within the categories of normal hosts, diabetics, and patients subjected to cytotoxic chemotherapy.

The classical presentation of *rhinocerebral zygomycosis* is the development of unilateral proptosis associated with pain, and mild to severe compromise in vision in a patient with diabetes and ketoacidosis. Sudden development of proptosis in a diabetic patient, particularly with acidosis, should initiate an aggressive evaluation for rhinocerebral zygomycosis, since the condition is frequently fatal and frequently results in permanent visual loss or loss of the entire eye. An extensive evaluation for intracerebral zygomycosis should also be considered in any diabetic acidotic patient in coma who does not have resolution of the coma with correction of acidosis, electrolyte abnormalities, and osmotic gradients owing to the hyperglycemia. Experimental evidence in animals coupled with clinical observations suggests that the acidosis contributes strongly to the pathogenesis and is more important than the hyperglycemia. Spores, which may be quiescent and harbored in the sinuses of the patient, develop the capability of invading the sinus tissue. The usual route of invasion is through the thin wall of the ethmoid sinus into the retroorbital space. Involvement of the extraocular muscles and retroorbital tissues causes the characteristic proptosis. Direct invasion of the optic nerve in the retroorbital space may severely compromise vision early in the process (see Chapter 77). Extension is usually retrograde, through the sinuses draining the orbit, into the frontal lobes of the brain. Extension may also occur into the maxillary sinus and inferiorly through the hard palate. Hematogenous dissemination may occur from this orbital infection, invading virtually any organ. This sequence of events may also occur in renal failure patients who are chronically acidotic. In recent years, zygomycosis has been linked to the use of deferoxamine as a chelation agent in renal failure patients on hemodialysis.

Once the consideration of rhinocerebral zygomycosis is entertained, mobilization of a large number of consultative services is required for adequate evaluation. Commonly, these disciplines include ophthalmology; ear, nose and throat (ENT); neurology; neuroradiology; infectious diseases; neurosurgery; and pathology. The most common finding on computerized tomography (CT) scan of the orbit is thickening of the medial rectus muscle associated with proptosis. Despite extensive infection in the retroorbital space, an organized retroorbital mass is rarely seen. Concluding that a patient does not have rhinocerebral zygomycosis because there is no retroorbital mass on CT scan has resulted in a delay of diagnosis. Surgery combined with antifungal therapy is the strategy for treatment. The organisms causing zygomycosis vary from very sensitive to very resistant to antifungal drugs. Therefore, if a patient is infected with an organism that is relatively resistant to amphotericin B, and is placed on that drug while the diagnosis is being explored, the patient may be virtually untreated during the time of the diagnostic evaluation. Hence the need for rapid mobilization of all appropriate resources to establish the diagnosis as quickly as possible and to add surgical debridement to the therapeutic strategy once the diagnosis is confirmed.

In recent years it has been established that the ocular muscles may appear normal or only slightly swollen on orbital exploration. However, when they have been biopsied and examined by histopathology, extensive invasion has been identified. Previously, most patients who were diagnosed with rhinocerebral zygomycosis underwent orbital exenteration. In recent years, patients have been managed successfully with early diagnosis, leading to early institution of amphotericin B and selective orbital and sinus debridement. This approach may avoid the cosmetically destructive orbital exenteration and loss of the entire ocular globe.

*Pulmonary zygomycosis* is seen most commonly in patients immunocompromised with cytotoxic chemotherapy for the treatment of cancer. It can occur either as a primary infection from inhalation of spores, or as a superinfection of a bacterial pneumonia. It may also result from septic pulmonary emboli. The infective process is indolent and results in extensive tissue necrosis. Radiographic appearances include bronchopneumonic infiltrates with or without cavitation and consolidation. If cavitation occurs, fungus ball formation may result. Pleural effusions may also occur. Because of the angiotrophic nature of the organisms, pulmonary infarction may be a complication. Definitive diagnosis requires biopsy proof of tissue invasion, with confirmation by culture.

*Cutaneous zygomycosis* may occur either by direct inoculation or by hematogenous seeding to the skin. Nonspecific subcutaneous nodules occur, as well as lesions similar to ecthyma gangrenosum. The organisms can be demonstrated on biopsy of the lesions. Cutaneous zygomycosis has occurred by direct inoculation of burn wounds, routine postoperative wounds, biopsies, spider bite, intravenous access sites, and injection sites for medicines. Additionally, periorbital skin may become involved from direct extension of rhinocerebral zygomycosis.

There are numcrous additional forms of zygomycosis. Widespread dissemination may occur in rhinocerebral disease, in patients with chronic renal failure, or in patients immunocompromised with cytotoxic chemotherapy. Virtually any organ may be infected. Gastrointestinal zygomycosis has occurred associated with gastric ulcers, trauma from indwelling intraluminal devices, and broad-spectrum antibiotics. It has also complicated other primary gastrointestinal diseases such as gastrointestinal *Salmonella* infection, amebic colitis, pellegra, and kwashiorkor. Intestinal zygomycosis may be complicated by perforation. Additional forms of infection are infection of the bladder, uterus, kidney, ear, venous grafts, bone, heart valves, prosthetic breast implants, and coronary arteries. In recent years zygomycosis has been linked to the use of iron chelation in patients undergoing chronic renal dialysis.

## Emerging opportunistic fungal pathogens

In recent years, infections caused by previously unreported fungal pathogens have been described with increasing regularity. Most authors have classified these emerging pathogens into four groups: *(1)* non-albicans species of *Candida*, *(2)* noncandidal yeasts, *(3)* organisms causing hyalohyphomycosis, and *(4)* organisms causing phaeohyphomycosis.

### *Candida species*

The non-albicans species of *Candida* of most importance are *C. tropicalis*, *C. parapsilosis*, *C. krusei*, *C.* (*Torulopsis*) *glabrata*, and *C. lusitaniae*. Others, occurring with lesser importance, are *C. guillermondii*, *C. stellatoidea*, *C. lipolytica*, *C. rugose*, *C. zeylanoides*, and *C. pseudotropicalis*.

*C. tropicalis* has become more prevalent, for reasons that are not clear. In some institutions, the organism constitutes over 30% of the species of *Candida* isolated from blood. The organism is capable of causing widespread hematogenous dissemination, similar to *C. albicans*. However, both experimental data and clinical experience suggest that the ocular infection rates are lower with all the non-albicans species of *Candida*. Increasing evidence of colonization as identified by surveillance cultures has been associated with an increase in frequency of dissemination. *C. parapsilosis* is important for its relationship to line sepsis, for reasons that are not clear. *C. glabrata* is being recovered with increasing frequency; it is becoming a frequent colonizer of the gastrointestinal tract in adults. Its major importance lies in its variable susceptibility to azoles, with some strains falling outside of what is considered to be the sensitive range. *C. krusei* recovery rates varies within individual institutions. However, with the exception of only a few institutions where the recovery rate has been very high, most centers have only an occasional blood isolate of this species. Its major significance is its intrinsic resistance to fluconazole.

*C. lusitaniae* has been recovered with increasing frequency, again for reasons that are not clear. Its significance is that some strains may be resistant to amphotericin B and poor outcome has been found to be related to this resistance. In general, each of these species should be viewed as having the potential to cause widespread hematogenous dissemination with fatal outcome.

### Other yeast species

Of the non-albicans yeast organisms, *Trichosporon* and *Malassezia* species require special emphasis. Others are *Rhodotorula* species and *Saccharomyces* species. The most important *Trichosporon* species are *T. asahii*, *T. asteroides*, *T. cutaneum*, *T. inkin*, *T. mucoides*, *T. ovoides*, and *T. capitatum*. The latter species has been renamed *Geotrichum capitatum* (*Blastoschizomyces capitatus*). There are now over 120 cases of hematogenously disseminated *Trichosporon* species infections reported in the literature, predominant in patients with bone marrow transplants and/or acute leukemia. Both the predisposing factors and clinical syndrome of extensive hematogenously disseminated disease resemble those of *Candida*, with the exceptions of hemochromatosis as a predisposing disease and the necrotic skin lesions seen in *Trichosporon* infections. Blood cultures are frequently positive. The infection may be rapidly fatal. Of significance is the variable sensitivities of these organisms to amphotericin B, flucytosine, and the azoles.

*Malassezia furfur* has been reported as a rare cause of deep infection in severely immunocompromised hosts who have received hyperalimentation with lipid-containing solution. *M. furfur*, as opposed to *M. pachydermitis*, requires fatty acid supplementation for growth. Discontinuation of the lipid-containing nutrients and removal of the lines is important in management. When deep infection is suspected, either amphotericin B or azoles should be used.

### Phaeohyphomycosis

Phaeohyphomycosis is a term used for infection by predominately *Alternaria*, *Bipolaris*, *Curvularia*, and *Exserohilum* species. *Chromomycosis* and *phaeosporotrichosis* are older terms used for these infections. These organisms have been traditionally described as the darkly pigmented or dematiaceous fungi found predominantly in soil. They cause a wide variety of cutaneous and sinus infections. Occasionally they disseminate to deep organs in normal hosts. In recent years they have caused serious infections in immunocompromised hosts, particularly those who have received cytotoxic chemotherapy for the treatment of cancer. A wide variety of infections has been reported with *Curvularia* species, including catheter infection, skin and subcutaneous tissue, sinus, lower respiratory tract, bone, and even cardiac valve. Treatment with either amphotericin B or the azoles, especially itraconazole, has been advocated. Surgery, in combination with antifungal treatment, is advised when feasible. Organisms of the genera *Bipolaris* and *Exserohilum* cause necrotizing pulmonary infection and/or widespread hematogenous dissemination to a variety of organs. Brain and sinus infection also occur. *Alternaria* species cause infection of the sinuses, skin,

**Table 6.1** Opportunistic mycoses

| Mycosis | Disease | Organism | Epidemiology | Pathogenic mechanisms | Manifestations | Diagnosis | Comments |
|---|---|---|---|---|---|---|---|
| *Candida* | Candidiasis | Candida species: *C. albicans*, *C. tropicalis*, *C. glabrata*, *C. krusei*, etc. | Ubiquitous human commensals | Colonizes mucous membranes, especially GI tract. Also skin. Becomes invasive when host defenses are compromised. | Thrush, esophagitis, vaginitis. Candidemia. Endophthalmitis. Candiduria. Deep-organ infection. | Typical white plaques that bleed when scraped and contain organisms. Blood culture for candidemia. Endopthalmitis—white lesions in chorioretina. Deep organs—micro- and small macro-abscesses. | There are no widely accepted serodiag-nostic tests. Azole resistance may occur in AIDS. All candidemics should be treated. Urinary tract may be a source for dissemination |
| *Cryptococcus neoformans* | Cryptococcosis | *C. neoformans* var neoformans var gattii | Ubiquitous in nature. Lives in soil contami-nated with pigeon droppings and on Eucalyptus trees. | Organism are inhaled into the lungs and disseminate hematogenously. | Pneumonia. Meningitis. Hematogenous dissemination to other organs. GU infection in AIDS | Cryptococcal antigen detection in serum and CSF. Culture from blood, urine, and tissue speicmens. | Meningitis has increased extensively since AIDS. Serodiagnostic test for antigen is very valuable for diagnosis. |
| *Aspergillus* | Aspergillosis | *Aspergillus fumagatis*, *A. flavus*, *A. niger* | Extremely ubiquitous organism throughout nature | Usually inhaled into the lungs and disseminates hematogenously. May contaminate burns or wounds. | Pneumonia. Central nervous system. Hematogenous dissemination to multiple organs. Burn wound infection. | Visualization of organisms in biopsy specimens. Interpretation of cultures difficult, since contamination may occur. Blood cultures are usually negative | Hallmark of infection is infarction. The organisms are angiotropic and invade blood vessel walls. No widely available serodiag-nostic tests. |
| Zygomycetes | Mucormycosis, Zygomycosis, Phycomycosis | *Rhizopus*, *Absidia*, *Rhizomucor*, *Mucor*, *Apophysomyces* | Ubiquitous in nature | Organisms colonize the nasal sinuses and occasionally the bronchi. | Rhinocerebral infection in diabetic ketoacidotics. Pulmonary infection in neutropenics. Wound infections on occasion. May hematogenously disseminate to multiple organs. Organisms are angiotropic and cause infection in deep organs. | Necrotizing sinus infection extending to retroorbital area in diabetics. May extend to the brain. Usually causes proptosis. Necrotizing pneumonia in neutropenics. | Should be suspected in any diabetic with ketoacidosis and proptosis. Black necrotic material may be seen draining from nose or eye. Surgery as well as amphotericin is critical for successful treatment. |
| *Fusarium* | Fusariosis Fusarium infection | *Fusarium solani*, *F. oxsporum*, *F. moniliforme*, and other species. | Ubiquitous soil saprophytes | Direct inoculation of skin. Infection of the sinuses, hematogenous dissemination to multiple organs. | Catheter-associated infection in neutropenics. Direct inoculation into the skin. Extensive sinus infection. | Cutaneous infection with ecthyma gangrenosa type lesions. Severe sinus infection. Widespread hematogenous dissemination. | Diagnosis is by culture. There are no widely accepted serodiagnostic tests. Organisms invade vessel walls. Dichomatous branch-ing hyphae with papallel orientation. |
| *Trichophyton* | Trichosporonosis | *T. asahii*, *T. asteroides*, *T. cutaneum*, *T. inkin*, *T. mucoides*, *T. ovoides* | Superficial skin saprophyte | Portal of entry is gastrointestinal tract, lung, or skin | Widespread dissemination. Necrotic skin lesions. | Biopsy. Blood cultures are frequently positive. | Susceptibility to antifungals is variable |
| *Melassezia furfur* infection | Catheter-associated. *M furfur* fungemia | *M. furfur* | Superficial skin saprophyte | Portal of entry is skin. | Pulmonary infiltrate | Cultured from blood | Associated with the use of intravenous intralipid |

**Table 6.2** Endemic mycoses

| Mycosis | Disease | Organism | Epidemiology | Pathogenic mechanisms | Manifestations | Diagnosis | Comments |
|---|---|---|---|---|---|---|---|
| *Coccidioides* | Coccidioidomycosis | *Coccidioides immitis* | Southwest U.S., Mexico, and Central America | Inhalation of arthrospores | Pulmonary. meningitis. Bone (hematogenous). Skin and joints (hematogenous). | Culture Complement-fixation serology | Increased incidence in pregnancy. Becoming important in AIDS patients. |
| *Histoplasma* | Histoplasmosis | *H. capsulatum* | Eastern U.S. and southeastern U.S., Latin America, and South America | Inhalation | Pulmonary. Wide-spread dissemination. Bone marrow. Oral. | Culture. Visualization of organisms in macrophages. Complement-fixation serology | Becoming very important in AIDS patients. |
| Blastomycetes | Blastomycosis | *Blastomyces dermatitidis* | Predominantly Ohio and Mississippi river valleys. Also Africa, Western Europe, and Canada. | Predominantly inhalation. Occasionally from skin innoculation. | Pulmonary. Cutaneous dissemination. Wide-spread hematogenous dissemination. Osteoarticular. Genitourinary tract. | Culture. Visualization in tissue sections. | Several cases have been reported in AIDS patients. |
| *Paracoccidioides* | South American blastomycosis | *Paracoccidioides brasiliensis* | Latin America | Inhalation | Pulmonary. Oral-pharyngeal. Wide-spread hematogenous dissemination. Gastrointestinal. Osseous. | Culture. Visualization in tissue sections. | Oral-pharyngeal form is very common. May not become clinically apparent for years after leaving endemic area. |
| Sporotrichosis | Sporotrichosis | *Sporothrix shenckii* | Worldwide | Inoculation through skin or inhalation | Cutaneous lesions along lymphatic drainage distribution | Culture and visualization in tissue sections. | May disseminate hematogenously |

lung, cornea, and peritoneum. Surgery is also helpful for these infections.

#### Hyalophyphomycosis

Hyalophyphomycosis refers to infection caused by molds that appear in tissue as light-colored and have no cell wall pigment. The most important organisms are *Fusarium* species, *Pseudoallescheria boydii*, *Scedosporium prolificans*, *Scopulariopsis* species, and *Penicillium* species. Of these, the most important in the immunocompromised hosts are the *Fusarium* species. The number of reports of infections with these organisms continues to increase, especially in those individuals who are immunocompromised from cytotoxic chemotherapy. The infections resembles aspergillosis and may involve the sinuses, lungs, and brain, as well as disseminate widely. However, characteristic nodular lesions with central necrosis have been more frequent with *Fusarium* infections, as well as a higher incidence of positive blood cultures. Additional skin lesions have included ecthymalike lesions and subcutaneous nodules. Infections from organisms of the *Scedosporium* genus are usually caused by *Pseudoallescheria boydii* and *Scedosporium inflatum*. Sinus and pulmonary involvement are common, but widespread infection of a large number of organs has occurred. Since these organisms are resistant to amphotericin B, miconazole, itraconazole or fluconazole may be useful. Infections with organisms of the genus *Scopulariopsis* are less common. The organisms have been resistant to antifungal therapy. *Penicillium marneffei* has infected patients with cancer and AIDS. However, apparently the organism is limited in distribution to Southeast Asia. It is usually sensitive to amphotericin B.

## The Endemic Mycoses

### Coccidioidomycosis

The organism causing coccidioidomycosis, *Coccidioides immitis*, is geographically limited to the lower Sonoran life zone of the Western Hemisphere. The regions are California, Texas, Arizona, Nevada, New Mexico, Mexico, Guatemala, Honduras, Paraguay, and Argentina. Since approximately 10% of Americans now live in California, and the population of the southwest United States is growing rapidly, an ever-increasing number of individuals are exposed to soil containing this organism and are at risk for infection. This organism has also been a cause of infection in immunocompromised patients who have had cytotoxic chemotherapy and infects patients with AIDS.

#### Pathogenesis

The organism lives in soil where rain induces germination and formation of the infectious form of the organism, the arthrospore. These spores infect man when wind, construction, or earthquakes create dust particles that facilitate delivery of arthrospores into the bronchi. The vast majority of patients develop a flulike illness or are asymptomatic. Some may develop erythema nodosum. The development of fever, cough, and the nodular lesions of erythema nodosum constitute the syndrome termed "valley fever." This form of the illness is self-limited. In certain circumstances there is a susceptibility to chronic pulmonary disease or hematogenous dissemination of the organism with development of meningitis, endophthalmitis, bone infection, joint infection, skin infection, or, less commonly, infection of other organs. Individuals susceptible to more serious forms of infection include African Americans, Filipinos, patients with diabetes, patients with AIDS, organ-transplant patients on immunosuppressive chemotherapy, and patients with cancer treated with cytotoxic chemotherapy. Additionally, pregnant women are susceptible to dissemination.

#### Diagnosis

Definitive diagnosis of coccidioidomycosis requires biopsy proof of the presence of spherules in infected tissue (once arthrospores infect, they develop into the characteristic thick-walled spherules). The complement-fixation test is a reliable and specific serodiagnostic test. Titers of 1:8 or 1:16 occur commonly in pulmonary infection. Titers of 1:32 or greater suggest dissemination. Any positive titer in the cerebrospinal fluid associated with a pleocytosis is highly suggestive of *Coccidioides* meningitis. Many patients who have become immunocompromised from cytotoxic chemotherapy, or who have AIDS, may have false negative CF titers.

Of particular importance is the recognition of the possibility that a patient with AIDS may have coccidioidomycosis simultaneously with other opportunistic infections. Commonly, this organism has been found to be present simultaneously with pneumocystis. Careful examination of sputum specimens should be done in patients who have been diagnosed as having pneumocystis and have not responded to appropriate therapy.

### Histoplasmosis

Histoplasmosis is caused by the organism *Histoplasma capsulatum*, which is endemic to the Mississippi and Ohio river valleys in the United States, the St. Lawrence River in Canada, and selected areas of northern Mexico. Infection results from inhalation of conidia from the soil or the excreta of bats or birds. Of greatest importance regarding histoplasmosis is its emergence as an important pathogen in patients with AIDS and in patients treated with cytotoxic chemotherapy for cancer. Similar to *Coccidioides*, the organism usually causes a self-limited, flu-like illness. Only rarely does chronic pulmonary disease develop or does widespread hematogenous infection occur. When widespread hematogenous dissemination does occur, the organism characteristically infects the bone marrow, mediastinum, liver, spleen, endocardium, adrenal gland, and, more rarely, central nervous system. Additionally, the eye may be infected by the hematogenous route.

The definitive diagnosis requires demonstration of the organism in tissue with confirmation by culture. Urinary antigen detection by radioimmunoassay is reliable and relatively specific. Complement fixation tests for antibody are also useful for diagnosis of deep-tissue infection. The organism may be seen in circulating monocytes or in bone marrow macrophages.

### Blastomycosis

*Blastomyces dermatitades*, the causative agent of blastomycosis, is indigenous in approximately the same areas in the United States as *Histoplasma*. However, it is also found in South America, Asia, and Africa. Acquisition of the infecting organism is presumably from soil. Patients are infected by aspiration of the conidia, which then establish a pulmonary focus. The disease process is similar to that of coccidioidomycosis and histoplasmosis in that the vast majority of patients are either asymptomatic or develop a mild flulike illness. They recover without sequelae. In a small percentage of patients, a chronic pulmonary form may develop or the organisms may disseminate hematogenously to infect skin, bones, the genitourinary tract, and meninges. The most common site for dissemination is the skin, where subcutaneous nodules are formed that ulcerate and form a verrucous border around the crater. The crater has darkly pigmented crusted material within it. The lesions may be on the extremities or the face. Central nervous system infection is rare. Because of the genitourinary tract involvement, sexual transmission has occurred.

The definitive diagnosis of blastomycosis requires demonstration of the organism invading tissue on histopathology, with confirmation by culture. Serodiagnostic tests are helpful for suggesting the diagnosis but are not conclusive. The enzyme immunoassay is the most sensitive serodiagnostic test.

An increasing number of AIDS patients with blastomycosis is being reported.

## Paracoccidioidomycosis

This infection is commonly referred to as "South American blastomycosis." It is caused by the organism *Paracoccidioides brasiliensis*. The endemic area spans from Mexico to Argentina. The organism lives in soil and infection is by inhalation of conidia. Two forms, juvenile and adult, have been described. In the juvenile form, usually seen in patients under the age of 30, the organism infects the reticuloendothelial system predominantly, causing hepatosplenomegaly. In the adult form, chronic pulmonary infection may occur with hematogenous spread to the skin and lymph nodes. Verrucous ulcers form in the skin and the lymph nodes may drain. Characteristic oral-pharyngeal ulcers are commonly seen. Hematogenous dissemination to the adrenals has also been noted frequently.

## Sporotrichosis

*Sporothrix shenckii*, the causative agent of sporotrichosis, is a saprophyte found on decaying vegetation throughout the world. It is usually acquired through direct inoculation into the skin. However, inhalation of the organism may cause a pulmonary infection as well. When inoculated into the skin, characteristic subcutaneous nodules form along the distribution of the lymphatics. These nodules may ulcerate and drain. They are usually not surrounded by erythema unless they become infected with bacteria. Cutaneous leishmaniasis is frequently considered in the differential diagnosis. Widespread hematogenous dissemination may occur, especially in immunocompromised hosts. The organisms may be seen in biopsy of the lesion, appearing as cigar-shaped yeasts. There are no useful serodiagnostic tests. Confirmation by culture is necessary for a definitive diagnosis.

*Acknowledgments*—This work was supported in part by the NIAID Mycoses Study Group contract NO1 AI 15082 and grants PO1-AI 37184 and RO1 AI 19990.

## ANNOTATED BIBLIOGRAPHY

Abi-said D, Anaissie EJ. New emerging fungal pathogens. In: Bailliere's Clinical Infectious Diseases, International Practice and Research. F. Meunier, ed. Billiere Tindall, London, pp 71–87, 1995.
*Excellent, comprehensive review of nearly all reported emerging fungal pathogens.*

Currie BP, Casadevall A. Estimation of the prevalence of cryptococcal infection among patients infected with the human immunodeficiency virus in New York City. Clin Infect Dis 1994; 19:1029–1033.
*A survey of New York City.*

Denning DW, Stevens DA. Antifungal and surgical treatment of invasive aspergillosis: review of 2,121 published cases. Rev Infect Dis 1991; 13:345.
*One of, if not the most, comprehensive review of the topic.*

Edwards JE Jr, Bodey GP, Bowden RA, Buchner T, de Pauw BE, Filler SG, Ghannoum MA, Glauser M, Herbrecht R, Kauffman CA, et al. International Conference for the Development of a Consensus on the Management and Prevention of Severe Candidal Infections [see comments]. Clin Infec Dis 1997, 25(1):43–59.
*In international consensus conference on management of a variety of forms of candidal infections.*

Fish DG, Ampel NH, Galgiani JN, Dols CL, Kelly PC, Johnson CH, Pappagianis D, Edwards JE, Wasserman RB, Clark JR et al. Coccidioidomycosis during human immunodeficiency infection: a review of 77 patients. Medicine 1990; 69:384–391.
*A comprehensive review.*

Galgiani JN. Coccidioidomycosis. Curr Clin Top in Infect Dis 1997, 17:188–204.
*Excellent and comprehensive review.*

Herbrecht R, Koenig H, Walker J et al. Trichosporon infections: clinical manifestations and treatment. J Mycol Med 1993; 3:129–136.
*An excellent review.*

Kauffman CA, Hedderwick S. Opportunistic fungal infections: filamentous fungi and cryptococcosis. Geriatrics 1997, 52(10):40–2, 47–49.
*Excellent current review.*

Kwon-Chung KJ, Bennett JE. Medical Mycology. Lea & Febiger, Philadelphia, 1992.
*A comprehensive, encyclopedic description of both the clinical and microbiological aspects of fungal diseases.*

Pfaller MA. Epidemiology and control of fungal infections. Clin Infec Dis 1994, 19 Suppl 1:S8–13.
*Comprehensive discussion of the topic.*

Powderly WG. Recent advances in the management of cryptococcal meningitis in patients with AIDS. Clin Infect Dis 1996; 22 Suppl 2:S119–123.
*Very up-to-date discussion of the topic.*

Vlasveld LT, Sweder van Asbeck B. Treatment with deferoxamine: a real risk factor for mucormycosis? Nephron 1991; 57:487–489.
*Excellent description of the association of deferoxamine and mucormycosis.*

Walsh TJ, Melcher GP, Lee JW, Pizzo PA. Infections due to Trichosporon species: new concepts in mycology, pathogenesis, diagnosis, and treatment. Curr Top Med Mycol 1993; 5:79–113.
*The authors have had an extensive clinical experience with Trichosporon infections.*

Wey SB, Mori M, Pfaller MA, Woolson RF, Wenzel RP. Hospital-acquired candidemia. The attributable mortality and excess length of stay. Arch Intern Med 1988; 148:2642–2645.
*A case-controlled epidemiology study to determine the attributable mortality of candidemia.*

Wheat J. Endemic mycosis in AIDS: A clinical review. Clin Microbiol Rev 1995; 8:146–159.
*A comprehensive review.*

Wright WL, Wenzel RP. Nosocomial Candida. Epidemiology, transmission, and prevention. Infect Dis Clin North Am 1997, 11(2):411–425. Pub type: Journal Article; Review; Review, Tutorial. Type D 11 AB to see abstract. (UI: 97331622)
*Excellent comprehensive review.*

# 7

# Epidemiology in Clinical Infectious Diseases

RICHARD A. GOODMAN AND JAMES M. HUGHES

The role of clinically based health care providers in diagnosing and treating their patients' problems uniquely positions clinicians to recognize new infectious agents and outbreaks. The detection of new disease agents and the recognition of outbreaks usually have broad implications for the public's health. Even though this book emphasizes clinical aspects of infectious diseases, the astute clinician can, by combining clinical skills with basic principles of epidemiology, simultaneously maximize the treatment of the individual patient and facilitate the proper public health response to an infectious-disease problem involving the community.

Infectious diseases are the leading cause of death worldwide. Based on an estimate by the World Health Organization (WHO), in 1997 approximately 17 million (33%) of the 52 million deaths worldwide were caused by microbial agents. In the United States, infectious diseases are the third-leading cause of death, and among persons aged 25–44 years, infection with human immunodeficiency (HIV) virus is now a leading cause of death.

This chapter provides an epidemiologic framework for clinicians who treat patients with infectious diseases; this framework encompasses the principles of epidemiology and public health in the diagnosis, treatment, and prevention of infectious-disease problems. Specifically, the chapter summarizes key concepts and principles underlying the public health approach to established and emerging infectious diseases, outlines the process of infectious-disease surveillance in the United States, and describes the role of and opportunities for clinicians in recognizing, responding to, and preventing the occurrence of transmissible infectious diseases.

## Concepts and Principles

### Definitions

Epidemiology is the study of the distribution and determinants of diseases of infectious origin and other etiologies, injuries, and other health states in populations, and the use of this information to prevent or control health problems and to improve health. The methods of epidemiology are used to solve epidemics, endemic problems, and pandemics. An epidemic can be defined as the occurrence of cases of disease in excess of what usually is expected for a given period of time; the term *epidemic* can be used interchangably with the term *outbreak*. Epidemics may be short in duration (e.g., manifestations of staphylococcal infection associated with a food-borne outbreak may last from 12 to 24 hours), or persist for years (e.g., the ongoing epidemic of acquired immunodeficiency syndrome [AIDS] and HIV infection). In contrast to epidemics, *endemic* problems are those that occur at high background levels, often as the result of multiple or continuous chains of transmission. The term *pandemic* is closely related to *epidemic*, but usually indicates a problem of global dimensions, as illustrated by the influenza pandemic of 1918–1919.

Understanding the domain of infectious-disease epidemiology requires an understanding of the interaction among three factors—infectious agents, susceptible hosts, and environmental conditions—that permit host exposure to the agent. Knowledge of how these factors interact is crucial for selecting the proper approach for preventing or controlling further spread of specific infectious diseases. The importance of this agent–host–environment relationship is illustrated by the problem of epidemic influenza. In this example, the agent—influenza A or B virus—is highly infectious, and the susceptible host is someone who never before has been infected by the strain and therefore lacks specific protective antibodies. When the environment is a closed setting, such as a nursing home, there may be enhanced efficiency of transmission of the virus from a source case of infection to a susceptible host.

### Modes and patterns of transmission

Infectious agents include bacteria, viruses, chlamydia, rickettsia, fungi, protozoa, and parasites; these agents persist in nature only if they are able to pass from one host to another member of the same or a different species. Epidemics can occur when large numbers of susceptibles are exposed to these agents under conditions conducive to the spread of the agent. The spread of an infectious disease occurs through a "chain of transmission," which comprises the agent, a source for the agent, a route of exit from the reservoir or source host (e.g., the respiratory or gastrointestinal tracts), a suitable mode from the source to the new susceptible host, and a route of entry into the new susceptible host.

Modes of infectious-disease transmission are characterized as being *vertical* or *horizontal*. Vertical transmission occurs from mother to fetus or newborn prior to or during delivery. For example, some viruses may be transmitted vertically from mother to fetus, either via the placenta, via passage through the birth canal, or via the integration of viral DNA directly into the DNA of the fertilized egg. Vertical transmission of an infectious agent may be associated with congenital disease (e.g., cytomegalovirus, herpes simplex virus type 2, parvovirus B19, rubella, *Treponema pallidum*, *Toxoplasma gondii*, and HIV).

Most transmission of infectious diseases occurs through the horizontal mode, involving spread between individuals within the population at risk. Routes of horizontal transmission of infectious agents can be characterized as *contact*, *common vehicle*, *airborne*, or *vectorborne*. Some infectious agents are transmitted exclusively by one route, while others spread through a combination of pathways. Contact transmission can be further subdivided into *direct* and *indirect* modes. Direct contact transmission involves physical contact (e.g., through shaking of hands, kissing, or sexual intercourse) between the infected host and the susceptible. Indirect contact transmission may involve contaminated vehicles (fomites), such as shared eating utensils, toys in a child care facility, or improperly sterilized surgical equipment or nondisposable needles and syringes. Certain respiratory infections are transmitted by direct and indirect contact (e.g., rhinovirus infections), while others are transmitted through exposure to contaminated large droplets emitted during coughing and sneezing (e.g., meningococcal infections).

Common vehicle transmission may involve contaminated food and water (e.g., shigellosis, hepatitis A, giardiasis, cryptosporidiosis), meats or vegetables cooked inadequately prior to consumption (e.g., salmonellosis, listeriosis, *E. coli* 0157:H7 disease), blood or blood products (e.g., hepatitis B and C), and intravenous solutions (e.g., some gram-negative bacteria). Although common vehicle transmission is often associated with epidemic disease, exposure to contaminated food vehicles also may cause endemic disease in which the role of food is difficult to recognize. Air-borne transmission, which typically results in epidemic disease, involves very small droplets that evaporate before settling and produce infectious droplet nuclei (less than 5 $\mu$m in diameter); such droplets may originate from infected persons (e.g., *M. tuberculosis*) or environmental sources (e.g., *L. pneumophila*), remain airborne for long periods, and travel substantial distances before being inhaled by a susceptible person. Vector-borne transmission involves exposure of susceptibles to arthropod vectors (e.g., mosquito-borne malaria and encephalitis viruses, and tick-borne Lyme disease, babesiosis, ehrlichiosis, and Colorado tick fever).

Epidemiologic patterns of occurrence and transmission of infectious diseases in the United States have evolved as a reflection of changes in demographic, social, and environmental factors. For example, the transmission of many infectious agents has been enhanced in recent decades as a consequence of demographic changes in relation to institutional settings, including day care facilities for children (Table 7.1) and long-term-care facilities for the elderly. Many of these patterns and changes have important ramifications for clinical providers in relevant specialties, including family medicine, pediatrics, and adult primary care. Other examples of the effects of the changing epidemiology of infectious diseases include the risks of transmission in some occupational settings (Table 7.2), in competitive sports (Table 7.3), and among persons who travel internationally (Table 7.4). The importance of obtaining a travel history in persons with an infectious disease cannot be overemphasized, since the frequency and efficiency of international travel continue to increase.

**Table 7.1** Selected examples of syndromes and agents acquired in child care settings

| Syndrome | Agents |
|---|---|
| Diarrhea | *Escherichia coli* 0157:H7<br>*Shigella* spp.[a]<br>Rotavirus |
| Otitis media | *Streptococcus pneumoniae*[a]<br>Nontypable *H. influenzae* |
| Hepatitis | Hepatitis A |
| Meningitis | *Neisseria meningitidis*[a] |
| Acute respiratory infection | Influenza<br>Respiratory syncytial virus |

[a]Drug-resistant organisms may be involved.

**Table 7.2** Selected examples of syndromes and agents acquired in selected occupational settings

| Syndrome | Agents |
|---|---|
| HEALTHCARE WORKERS | |
| Hepatitis | HAV<br>HBV<br>HCV |
| Fever and rash | Rubella<br>Rubeola<br>Varicella |
| Mononucleosis | CMV<br>HIV |
| Acute respiratory infections | *Bordetella pertussis*<br>Influenza<br>Respiratory syncytial virus<br>Parainfluenza<br>Adenovirus |
| Acute diarrhea | *Salmonella* spp.<br>Norwalk-like viruses<br>*Cryptosporidium* |
| Chronic respiratory infections | *Mycobacterium tuberculosis* |
| Hemorrhagic fever | Ebola, Marburg, Lassa |
| ANIMAL HANDLERS* | |
| Meningoencephalitis | Rabies<br>Herpes B |
| Hepatitis | *Coxiella burnetti* |
| Fever and myalgia | *Brucella* spp. |

*Including veterinarians and abbatoir workers.

## Basic strategies of infectious-disease control and prevention

The basic strategies for controlling and preventing the further transmission of infectious diseases are related directly to the principles of the agent–host–environment relationships, and to the opportunities presented by the links in the chain of transmission of infectious agents. Four of these strategies, of fundamental im-

**Table 7.3** Selected examples of syndromes and agents acquired through competitive sports

| Syndrome | Agents |
|---|---|
| Skin lesions | Herpes simplex<br>Group A streptococci<br>*Staphylococcus aureus*<br>*Trichophyton* spp.<br>Molluscum contagiosum (pox virus) |
| Fever and rash | Measles |
| Aseptic meningitis | Enteroviruses |
| Hepatitis | Hepatitis B |
| Acute respiratory infection | Influenza<br>Parainfluenza<br>Adenoviruses |

**Table 7.4** Selected examples of syndromes and agents acquired during travel

| Syndrome | Agent |
|---|---|
| Fever | *Plasmodium* spp.<br>*Salmonella typhi* |
| Acute respiratory infection | Influenza<br>*Legionella pneumophila* |
| Acute diarrhea | *Escherichia coli*<br>*Vibrio cholerae*<br>*Shigella* spp.<br>*Giardia lamblia*<br>*Entamoeba* spp. |
| Meningoencephalitis/encephalomyelitis | Rabies<br>*Trypanosoma brucei* |

portance for clinical providers, are (*1*) treating the source of the infection and/or eliminating the source from the environment (e.g., suspending from work a food handler infected with an enteric pathogen until the food handler has been appropriately treated); (*2*) cohorting infected patients in institutional settings (e.g., grouping infected patients together for dedicated care in hospitals, child day care facilities, and nursing homes); (*3*) preventing subsequent transmission through behavior modification or other interventions (e.g., facilitating reductions in high-risk behaviors associated with transmission of HIV infection); and (*4*) protecting the persons at risk (e.g., appropriate vaccination of persons and groups at increased risk for vaccine-preventable diseases).

## Infectious-Disease Surveillance and Reporting

### Notifiable conditions

In the United States, infectious diseases diagnosed by clinicians and other health care providers are monitored through the National Notifiable Diseases Surveillance System (NNDSS). As of January 1, 1997, a total of 52 infectious diseases had been designated by the Council of State and Territorial Epidemiologists (CSTE) as "notifiable" at the national level and as reportable to CDC (Table 7.5). A notifiable disease is one for which regular, frequent, and timely information on individual cases is considered necessary for the prevention and control of the disease. Of these diseases, 8 (15%) have been added to the list since January 1995. The NNDSS is an example of passive surveillance—that is, the system is dependent primarily on the voluntary reporting of notifiable conditions by clinical providers, health care facilities, diagnostic laboratories, and other sources. However, these reports are critical in ensuring prompt detection of and response to outbreaks, as well as long-term assessment of trends in the occurrence of infectious-disease problems.

The basis for infectious-disease surveillance in the United States can be traced to 1878, when Congress authorized the U.S. Marine Hospital Service (the forerunner to the Public Health Service [PHS]) to collect and report information on cases of cholera, smallpox, plague, and yellow fever from U.S. consuls; this information was to be used to assist in preventing the introduction and spread of these conditions into the United States. In 1893, Congress expanded the authority for weekly reporting to include data from states and municipal authorities. The scope of

**Table 7.5** Nationally notifiable infectious diseases (United States)

| | |
|---|---|
| Acquired immunodeficiency syndrome (AIDS) | Legionellosis |
| Anthrax | Lyme disease |
| Botulism | Malaria |
| Brucellosis | Measles |
| Chancroid | Meningococcal disease |
| *Chlamydia trachomatis*, genital infections | Mumps |
| Cholera | Pertussis |
| Coccidioidomycosis[a] | Plague |
| Congenital rubella syndrome | Poliomyelitis, paralytic |
| Congenital syphilis | Psittacosis |
| Cryptosporidiosis[a] | Rabies, animal |
| Diphtheria | Rabies, human |
| Encephalitis, California[b] | Rocky Mountain spotted fever |
| Encephalitis, Eastern equine[b] | Rubella |
| Encephalitis, St. Louis[b] | Salmonellosis |
| Encephalitis, Western equine[b] | Shigellosis |
| *Escherichia coli* 0157:H7 | Streptococcal disease, invasive, group A[a] |
| Gonorrhea | *Streptococcus pneumoniae*, drug-resistant[a] |
| *Haemophilus influenzae*, invasive disease | Streptococcal toxic-shock syndrome[a] |
| Hansen disease (leprosy) | Syphilis |
| Hantavirus pulmonary syndrome[a] | Tetanus |
| Hemolytic-uremic syndrome, post-diarrheal[a] | Toxic-shock syndrome |
| Hepatitis A | Trichinosis |
| Hepatitis B | Tuberculosis |
| Hepatitis, C/non-A, non B | Typhoid fever |
| HIV infection, pediatric (i.e., in persons ages <13 years)[a] | Yellow fever |

[a]Condition added to notifiable disease list since January 7, 1995.

[b]Primary encephalitis deleted and replaced with these.

surveillance continued to evolve, and by 1928 all states were participating in national reporting of nearly 30 specified conditions. In 1950, the State and Territorial Health Officers authorized a conference of state and territorial epidemiologists to determine which diseases should be reported to PHS, and in 1961 the Centers for Disease Control and Prevention (CDC) assumed responsibility for the collection and publication of data on nationally notifiable diseases.

The list of nationally notifiable infectious diseases is revised periodically by public health officials at state health departments (CSTE) with input from CDC; some diseases may be deleted as their incidence declines and others may be added to the list as new pathogens emerge. Reporting of nationally notifiable diseases to CDC by the states is voluntary. Because reporting is mandated at the state level only (by legislation or regulation), the list of diseases that are considered notifiable varies slightly by state. Reported cases of notifiable diseases are published each week in CDC's *Morbidity and Mortality Weekly Report* (*MMWR*).

Infectious-diseases data reported by physicians and other clinical providers to health departments and *MMWR* must be interpreted in light of reporting practices. Some diseases that cause severe clinical illness (e.g., plague or rabies), if diagnosed by a clinician, are likely to be reported accurately. However, persons with cases of diseases that are usually clinically mild and infrequently associated with serious consequences when they affect immunologically competent individuals (e.g., salmonellosis) may not even seek medical care from a clinical health care provider and, even if these less severe diseases are diagnosed, they are less likely to be reported. Other factors influencing the completeness of reporting include the availability of diagnostic facilities; presence and effectiveness of control measures; and the interests, resources, and priorities of state and local health officials responsible for disease control and surveillance.

### Most commonly reported infectious diseases in the United States

Among the nationally notifiable diseases, sexually transmitted diseases (STDs) have accounted for the most commonly reported infectious-disease conditions in the United States. For example, during 1995, the ten most frequently reported nationally notifiable infectious diseases were, in descending order, chlamydia, gonorrhea, acquired immunodeficiency syndrome (AIDS), salmonellosis, hepatitis A, shigellosis, tuberculosis, primary and secondary syphilis, Lyme disease, and hepatitis B. The STDs of chlamydia, gonorrhea, AIDS, primary and secondary syphilis, and hepatitis B accounted for 87% of cases reported for these ten diseases. Although 1995 was the first year genital infections with *Chlamydia trachomatis* were nationally notifiable, this condition was the most commonly reported disease for 1995.

The most commonly reported infectious diseases varied by age group. Among younger children (aged <5 years), salmonellosis and shigellosis were the most commonly reported conditions, while among those aged 5–14 years, gonorrhea and shigellosis were the most frequent. Gonorrhea also was the most commonly reported disease among persons aged 15–24 years. Gonorrhea and AIDS were common among adults aged 25–64 years, while among the elderly (aged >65 years), TB was the most commonly reported notifiable disease.

## Emerging Infectious Diseases

### Concepts in emerging infectious diseases

In 1992, a committee of the National Academy of Science's Institute of Medicine (IOM) issued a report titled *Emerging Infections: Microbial Threats to Health in the United States.* In this report, the committee defined emerging infections as those that have increased in incidence in the past 20 years or threaten to increase in the near future. The report described the threats posed by microbial agents, identified the factors that contribute to disease emergence and reemergence, and stressed the need to heighten vigilance and strengthen response capacity.

The six factors that contribute to the emergence of infectious diseases identified by the IOM committee are (*1*) changes in human demographics and behavior, (*2*) advances in technology and industry, (*3*) economic development and changes in land use, (*4*) dramatic increases in travel and commerce, (*5*) microbial adaptation and change in response to selective pressures, and (*6*) deterioration of the public health system at the local, state, national, and international levels because of financial and human resource constraints. These factors help to explain the emergence and reemergence of a number of diseases currently posing challenges to clinicians, microbiologists, and public health officials.

As a result of improvements in sanitation and overall living conditions during the early part of the twentieth century and the subsequent introduction of many vaccines and antibiotics, considerable complacency has developed regarding infectious diseases that many regard as either preventable by immunization or treatable by antibiotics. The 1970s and early 1980s produced the beginning of a series of what, in retrospect, heralded the sustained domestic and global challenges of infectious diseases, including, for example, rotavirus gastroenteritis, Lyme disease, Legionnaires' disease, and toxic shock syndrome. The most dramatic example of an emerging infectious disease, AIDS, was recognized in 1981, and hemorrhagic colitis caused by *Escherichia coli* 0157:H7 was identified in 1982. The end of the 1980s was marked by the reemergence of measles and tuberculosis in the United States and the emergence of multiple drug resistance in *Mycobacterium tuberculosis* strains causing disease predominantly in persons infected with HIV. Experiences with these and other emerging and reemerging diseases should have alerted physicians, microbiologists, researchers, public health officials, policy makers, and the public to the critical importance of ensuring the capacity to detect, respond to, and control these infections.

### Public health response to emerging infectious diseases

In 1994, CDC, in consultation with outside experts in clinical infectious diseases, microbiology, and public health, developed a strategy for addressing emerging infectious diseases. The strategy contains four goals, which focus on strengthening surveillance and response capability, addressing research priorities, improving prevention and control strategies, and strengthening the public health infrastructure at the local, state, and federal levels.

Implementation of the CDC plan requires effective partnerships with other federal, state, and local public health agencies, clinicians, clinical microbiologists, academic institutions, industry, the World Health Organization (WHO), and other international organizations and agencies. CDC has begun implementing this strategy by establishing Emerging Infections Programs (EIPs) based in seven state health departments, initiating publication of the journal *Emerging Infectious Diseases*, which is distributed electronically to provide timely peer-reviewed information on emerging diseases, and organizing a laboratory training fellowship program in collaboration with the Association of State and Territorial Public Health Laboratory Directors.

Strengthening surveillance is critical to the successful implementation of this strategy. Use of uniform case definitions that include laboratory components is essential. The flow of information in an infectious-disease surveillance system is critically important. One of the approaches to strengthening surveillance and response capacity has involved establishment of EIPs in California, Connecticut, Georgia, Maryland, Minnesota, New York, and Oregon. These programs involve partnerships between state and local health departments, academic institutions, and health maintenance organizations. Each program is conducting core projects that focus on invasive bacterial diseases, the etiology of unexplained deaths in persons between the ages of 1 and 49 years, and food-borne disease. In addition, each state has included two or three additional projects of high priority in their geographic area. The EIPs also have played important roles in assessing the occurrence (e.g., a new variant of Creutzfeldt-Jakob disease) and the magnitude and geographic extent of disease (e.g., *Cyclospora* cases associated with raspberries imported from Guatemala) in the United States.

Minnesota identified an outbreak caused by *Salmonella* serotype Enteriditis in the fall of 1994 when the state laboratory noted an increase in the expected number of isolates submitted to the state public health laboratory. Prompt epidemiologic investigation identified the vehicle as a contaminated ice-cream product produced in Minnesota and distributed to 48 states. The product was removed from distribution; follow-up investigation identified culture-confirmed cases in 41 states and approximately 250,000 cases of illness nationwide.

Oregon identified an increase of the incidence of meningococcal disease in the state between 1992 and 1994 associated with the emergence of the ET-5 clone of group B meningococci, which has caused epidemic disease in other countries. Cases have more recently been identified in the adjacent state of Washington, raising concerns about epidemic disease in the Pacific Northwest.

### Addressing antimicrobial resistance

Antimicrobial-resistant organisms also have posed major challenges in both hospital and community settings since publication of the IOM report. Antimicrobials are the second most commonly prescribed class of drugs in the United States. The National Foundation for Infectious Diseases has estimated the annual cost of infection caused by drug-resistant organisms to be over $4 billion.

Surveillance data on drug resistance in bacterial pathogens causing hospital-acquired infections are reported to CDC by the nearly 250 hospitals that voluntarily participate in the National Nosocomial Infections Surveillance (NNIS) system. These data have documented a dramatic increase in the frequency of vancomycin resistance in enterococci since 1989. Many of these infections are not treatable by any available antibiotics. The possibility exists for the transfer of the gene mediating resistance to vancomycin to *Staphylococcus aureus*, which would result in severe untreatable infections and has caused concerns regarding the advent of a "post-antibiotic era." Surveillance has been intensified in hospitals in the United States in an effort to ensure prompt recognition of and response to vancomycin-resistant staphylococcal infections.

Surveillance of drug resistance in community-acquired infections in the United States is limited primarily to infections caused by *M. tuberculosis*, *Neisseria gonorrhoeae*, and *Streptococcus pneumoniae*. The frequency of high-level penicillin resistance in sterile site isolates of pneumococci from patients in 13 hospitals in 12 states increased more than 60-fold, from 0.02% in 1987 to 1.3% in 1991 and subsequently to 3.2% in 1993–94. The frequency of high-level resistance is even higher in some geographic areas (e.g., 7.1% in metropolitan Atlanta in 1994).

The increasing incidence of antimicrobial resistance has important implications for clinical management of patients, surveillance, laboratory diagnosis, infection-control practices, professional and public education strategies, and drug and vaccine development priorities. Clinicians, microbiologists, and public health personnel must work together effectively to address this problem. Programs to improve antimicrobial usage must be implemented to help preserve the effectiveness of these valuable drugs, since few new antimicrobial agents are currently being introduced.

## Practitioner's Role in the Control and Prevention of Infectious Diseases

### Recognition of outbreaks and emerging problems

Routine surveillance for infectious disease in the United States is especially dependent on the timely and accurate reporting of cases by physicians and other clinical practioners. In addition, however, thoughtful observations and reporting by clinical practitioners can be critical in the recognition of outbreaks of established infectious diseases, and in the discovery or characterization of new and emerging agents. For example, primary care providers, specialists, and others have been responsible for initially recognizing and reporting to health departments problems that have run the gamut from a focal outbreak of toxoplasmosis, to multistate outbreaks of hantavirus pulmonary syndrome and of *E. coli* O157:H7–associated bloody diarrhea and hemolytic uremic syndrome from hamburgers, to the global pandemic of AIDS. This role for practitioners is not restricted to infectious diseases, as illustrated by the actions of physicians in New Mexico and Minnesota who, in 1989, initially detected and reported the outbreak of eosinophilia-myalgia syndrome associated with ingestion of contaminated L-tryptophan.

### Clinical assessment

When evaluating or treating patients with conditions of known or likely infectious etiology, clinical practitioners should address basic factors related to the potential for identifying the source of the problem and/or preventing secondary spread or recurrence (Table 7.6). In addition to asking specific questions that may lead to identification of the source of the problem and provide guidance for stemming further transmission, the provider should at the same time consider the possible relation to patterns of infectious diseases in his/her community (for example, see Tables 7.1 to 7.4). Finally, specific clinical indicators (signs/symptoms)

**Table 7.6** Essential questions for the clinician when assessing a patient with a possible infectious disease of public health importance

| |
|---|
| Is this condition a transmissible infectious disease? |
| What is/was the source (e.g., common, other)? |
| Where has the patient traveled recently? |
| What laboratory studies are indicated if an infectious disease of public health importance is strongly suspected? |
| How can additional cases be prevented? |
| Are there secondary cases associated with the patient (e.g., in the family/household, child day care, co-workers, social contacts, or friends)? |
| Who needs to be contacted (e.g., local and/or state health department)? |
| What measures are indicated to prevent other cases from occurring among other patients (e.g., vaccination)? |

should be used as a guide for both rapid diagnosis and reporting to public health officials (Table 7.7).

## Relationship to other key partners/organizations

Infection-control practitioners (ICPs) have an important role to play in the surveillance of infectious diseases. ICPs may be considered to be an extension of local public health agencies, as they are on the front lines in the proper management of hospitalized persons with infectious diseases. These individuals can play an important liaison role with local and state health departments and represent important partners in the detection and response to emerging infectious diseases.

The challenges posed by emerging infectious diseases will continue to demand a multidisciplinary approach and a supply of trained clinicians, microbiologists, pathologists, rodent and vector biologists, ecologists, behavioral scientists, and public health officials. The ability to address these emerging and reemerging microbial threats requires adequate surveillance and response capacity, ongoing research programs, strengthened prevention and control programs, and repair of the public health system locally, at the state and national levels, and internationally. The discipline of pathology has played an important role in recognition and characterization of the hantavirus pulmonary syndrome outbreak, diagnosis and subsequent prospective surveillance of Ebola hemorrhagic fever in Central Africa, identification of the etiologic agent in the leptospirosis outbreak in Nicaragua, and characterization of the variant form of Creutzfeldt-Jakob disease in the United Kingdom. Pathologists have also made vital contributions to recognition of opportunistic infections in HIV-infected and other immunocompromised patients.

**Table 7.7** Selected clinical syndromes and infectious agents with potential public health implications

| Syndrome condition | Common infectious agents |
|---|---|
| Febrile diarrhea | *Salmonella* spp., *E. coli* 0157:H7 |
| Meningitis | *N. meningitidis* |
| Encephalitis | Rabies |
| Pneumonia | *Legionella pneumophila*, Sin Nombre virus, *Yersinia pestis* |
| Febrile URI | Influenza |

## Conclusions

Infectious diseases are important, evolving, complex public health problems. Their prevention and control will increasingly require sophisticated epidemiologic, molecular biologic, statistical, and behavioral approaches and technologies and the integration of epidemiologic and laboratory sciences. Ensuring information exchange and technology transfer through intercountry networks is critical if future emerging infectious-disease threats are to be recognized in time to implement cost-effective control measures. As the authors of the IOM report noted, "Pathogenic microbes can be resistant, dangerous foes. Although it is impossible to predict their individual emergence in time and place, we can be confident that new microbial diseases will emerge."

Future challenges are difficult to predict but certainly include more problems with antimicrobial-resistant infections, the threat of another influenza pandemic, and the likelihood of increasing problems of dengue hemorrhagic fever and the risk of urban yellow fever in the Western Hemisphere. The global HIV epidemic will put large numbers of people at risk for currently recognized and new opportunistic infections. The role of hepatitis B and C viruses in chronic liver disease and hepatocellular carcinoma, human papillomavirus in cervical cancer, and *Helicobacter pylori* infection in peptic ulcer disease and gastric cancer are now well established. Additional chronic diseases are likely to be found to have an infectious etiology. Physicians and other clinical providers clearly will have an important role in the future in surveillance, diagnosis, and response to emerging and reemerging infections.

Clinicians and clinical laboratories today are under pressure to control health care costs. However, definitive diagnosis of most infectious diseases is critically dependent on the microbiology laboratory. Decreases in stool cultures will increase the likelihood that common-source food-borne and water-borne disease outbreaks will be detected late or missed entirely. Decreases in the frequency of bacteriologic studies will also compromise the ability of clinicians and public health professionals to acquire data on and monitor trends in local patterns of antimicrobial resistance. At the same time, many state public health laboratories face profound resource constraints, as part of the deterioration of support for the infectious-disease public health infrastructure. Public health laboratories in some states even face the threat of privatization. The critical functions of public health laboratories in recognition, monitoring, and molecular characterization of emerging and reemerging infectious diseases must be preserved and strengthened if we are to be prepared to confront these threats.

## ANNOTATED BIBLIOGRAPHY


Bell BP, Goldoft M, Griffin PM et al. A multistate outbreak of *Escherichia coli* O157:H7-associated bloody diarrhea and hemolytic uremic syndrome from hamburgers. JAMA 272:1349–1353, 1994.
*Summary of investigation of large interstate* E. coli *O157:H7 outbreak traced to fast-food restaurant chain.*

Berkelman RL, Pinner RW, Hughes JM. Addressing emerging microbial threats in the United States. JAMA 275:315–317, 1996.
*Summary of progress in implementing the CDC Emerging Infections Plan.*

Centers for Disease Control and Prevention. Addressing emerging infectious disease threats: A prevention strategy for the United States. U.S. Department of Health and Human Services, Public Health Service, Atlanta, Georgia, 1994.
*CDC Strategic Plan for responding to emerging infectious diseases at the local, state, national, and international level.*

Cox NJ, Brammer TL, Regnery HL. Influenza: Global surveillance for epidemic and pandemic variants. Eur J Epidemiol 10:467–470, 1994.
*Description of the global influenza surveillance system.*

Dowdle WR. The future of the public health laboratory. Annu Rev Public Health 14:649–664, 1993.
*A thoughtful discussion of the unique roles and responsibilities of public health laboratories.*

*Emerging Infectious Diseases.* published by the Centers for Disease Control and Prevention. Access by: http://www.cdc.gov
*Quarterly peer-reviewed journal addressing emerging infections issues.*

Garrett L. The coming plague: Newly emerging diseases in a world out of balance. Farrar, Straus and Giroux, New York, 1994.
*A comprehensive, thoroughly documented assessment of challenges posed by emerging pathogens over the past 35 years.*

Goodman RA, Solomon SL. Transmission of infectious diseases in outpatient health care settings. JAMA 265:2377–2381, 1991.
*Review of the literature focused on microbial agents transmitted in outpatient settings and risk factors for transmission.*

Goodman RA, Thacker SB, Solomon SL, Osterholm MT, Hughes JM. Infectious diseases in competitive sports. JAMA 271:862–867, 1994.
*Review of the literature focused on microbial agents transmitted during competitive sporting events and risk factors for transmission.*

Gregg MB. Conducting a field investigation. In: Field Epidemiology, Gregg MB, Dicker RC, Goodman RA, eds. Oxford University Press, New York, 1996.
*Description of practical approach to outbreak investigation.*

Hennessy TW, Hedberg CW, Slutsker L et al. A national outbreak of *Salmonella enteritidis* infections from ice cream. N Engl J Med 334:1281–1286, 1996.
*Summary of epidemiologic and laboratory investigation of a very large interstate food-borne disease outbreak.*

Hertzman PA, Blevins WL, Mayer J et al. Association of the eosinophilia-myalgia syndrome with the ingestion of tryptophan. N Engl J Med 322:869–873, 1990.
*Description of national outbreak of illness linked to a dietary supplement.*

Lederberg J. Infectious disease—A threat to global health and security. JAMA 276:417–419, 1996.
*Discussion of national security implications of emerging infectious diseases.*

Lederberg J, Shope RE, Oaks SC. Emerging infections: Microbial threats to health in the United States. National Academy Press, Institute of Medicine, Washington, D.C.: 1992.
*A landmark IOM report that defines emerging infectious diseases, identifies the factors associated with disease emergence, and recommends approaches required to address challenges posed by emerging microbes.*

LeDuc J. World Health Organization strategy for emerging infectious diseases. JAMA 275:318–320, 1996.
*Summary of WHO strategy for confronting emerging infections globally.*

*Morbidity and Mortality Weekly Report (MMWR)* Series: published by the Centers for Disease Control and Prevention. Access by: http://www.cdc.gov
*Weekly publication providing timely summaries of investigations of problems of public health importance.*

Osterholm MT. Infectious disease in child day care: an overview. Pediatrics 94(Suppl):987–990, 1994.
*An overview of infectious diseases of public health importance affecting children, family members, and staff in child day care settings.*

Pinner RW, Teutsch SM, Simonsen L et al. Trends in infectious diseases mortality in the United States. JAMA 275:189–193, 1996.
*Analysis of national mortality data between 1980 and 1992 showing increasing importance of infectious diseases that ranked third behind heart disease and cancer in 1992.*

Sepkowitz KA. Occupationally acquired infections in health care workers: parts I and II. Ann Intern Med 1996, 125:826–834 and 917–928.
*Comprehensive review of infectious diseases acquired in health-care settings and risk factors for transmission.*

Stroup NE, Zack MM, Wharton M. Sources of routinely collected data for surveillance. In: Teutsch SM, Churchill RE (ed): Principles and Practice of Public Health Surveillance. Oxford University Press, New York, pp 31–85, 1994.
*Thoughtful discussion of potential sources of data useful for public health surveillance.*

# 8

# Epidemiology and Control of Infectious Diseases in Health Care Facilities

HUAN J. CHANG AND WILLIAM R. JARVIS

Nosocomial infections are a major cause of morbidity and mortality in the United States, annually affecting over 2 million patients at an estimated cost of $4.5 billion in 1992 dollars. Health care facilities present a unique set of conditions for interaction of pathogens with patients, for at least four reasons. First, many hospitalized patients already are uniquely susceptible to infection owing to their underlying medical conditions or therapeutic maneuvers. Second, hospital settings support the development of antimicrobial-resistant microorganisms. Third, even within a hospital, the type and frequency of infections vary by the case mix, the service the patient is on, the severity of patient illness, and device use. Fourth, the increasing use of outpatient facilities and home therapy present unique challenges for infection-control personnel. For all these reasons, it is important to understand the special relationships among infecting organism, host, and health care environment that foster transmission of nosocomial infections.

In 1975–1982, the Study of the Efficacy of Nosocomial Infection Control (SENIC) programs documented that infection-control programs were cost-effective. The presence of a physician with special interest in infection control (e.g., hospital epidemiologist) and at least one infection-control practitioner per 250 beds were critical elements of effective infection-control programs. Additional studies documented that about 1/3 of all nosocomial infections were preventable, and many of those that were potentially preventable were not being prevented. With the implementation of prospective payment by insurance companies based on diagnostic-related groups, nosocomial infections became more costly to hospitals.

Overall, nosocomial infections are defined as those infections that develop during hospitalization but are neither present nor incubating upon the patient's admission to the hospital. The definitions of specific nosocomial infections have been modified over the past 25 years. The current definitions in the United States were developed by the Hospital Infections Program, Centers for Disease Control and Prevention (CDC), to facilitate surveillance of nosocomial infections. Most infections manifest during hospitalization; however, with shorter patient stays and more frequent use of outpatient and home therapy, more infections are manifesting after patient discharge.

Use of accepted definitions has been critical to studying the epidemiology of nosocomial infections and to comparing intra- and interinstitutional infection rates.

## Epidemiology of Nosocomial Infections

The epidemiology of nosocomial infections is constantly evolving. Influencing factors include the following: new medical technology, device use, severity of patient illness, case mix, managed care, health care reimbursement, outpatient care, and home care. In order to most effectively prioritize prevention and control efforts and maximize cost-containment efforts, it is essential to understand the sources, modes of transmission, and risk factors for nosocomial infection.

### Transmission of nosocomial infections

There are four major modes of transmission of infectious pathogens. The most common is *contact* transmission, which results from direct (between patients or between patients and health care workers [HCWs]) or indirect (between persons and contaminated inanimate objects—i.e., fomites) contact. The second most common mode of transmission is via *common sources* such as contaminated medications, devices, food, or blood products. The third most common cause is *air-borne* transmission of infectious agents; *Mycobacterium tuberculosis*, *Legionella* sp., influenza, and varicella virus are among the agents transmitted this way. Finally, *vector-borne* transmission is rare in hospital settings in the United States but can be an important consideration in developing countries.

Both intrinsic and extrinsic risk factors predispose patients to nosocomial infections. Intrinsic factors include patient characteristics such as age, sex, underlying disease, severity of illness, and immune status. Knowledge of these factors is useful in identifying high-risk patients for which special precautions may be provided. Extrinsic risk factors include surgical or other invasive procedures, diagnostic or therapeutic interventions, and personnel exposures.

Invasive devices, in particular, place patients at increased risk for infection. In some studies, ≥90% of infections are associated with invasive devices. Such devices bypass the normal defense mechanisms (e.g., skin or mucous membranes) and provide foci where pathogens can proliferate protected from the patient's immune defenses. These devices also facilitate transfer of pathogens from one part of the patient's body to another or from one patient to another via HCW hands. Reduction of infection risk associated with such devices requires careful attention to established guidelines for their insertion, manipulation, and maintenance.

## Surveillance

Surveillance, or "the systematic, active, ongoing observation of the occurrence and distribution of disease within a population and of the events or conditions that increase or decrease the risk of such disease occurrence," is a critical component of every hospital infection-control program. For surveillance to be effective, appropriate surveillance methods must be used, appropriate numerator and denominator data collected, the data regularly analyzed, and results disseminated to the individuals who need to know them in order to take appropriate actions. The purpose of surveillance should be to prevent infections by monitoring trends in infection rates, detecting outbreaks, collecting data that will assist in identifying areas where interventions should be instituted, and enabling evaluation of the effectiveness of introduced prevention measures. Many experts also believe that the direct contact and interaction between infection control practitioners conducting surveillance and hospital personnel heightens awareness of hospital-infection control activities and practices.

Although the concept of using surveillance methods to control nosocomial infections dates back at least to Dr. Semmelweiss's work in Vienna, Austria, in the 1840s, it was not until 1958 that the American Hospital Association (AHA) recommended that surveillance for nosocomial infections be conducted in hospitals as part of their nosocomial infection-prevention and control programs. While many hospitals originally practiced hospital-wide surveillance, increasing severity of illness of patients, insufficient personnel resources, and assessment of where infection risk was greatest led many infection control personnel to change to focused surveillance in the mid 1980s. In focused surveillance, only high-risk populations, services, or sites of infection associated with the greatest morbidity or mortality are surveyed. In many facilities, this method is more time and personnel efficient.

Presently the National Nosocomial Infections Surveillance (NNIS) System is the only source of national surveillance data on nosocomial infections in the United States. Begun in 1970, its main objectives are to monitor nosocomial infection trends in the United States and to provide data for inter- and intrainstitutional comparison. In the NNIS system, standardized surveillance methods and definitions are used. Results from the NNIS system have become the source for benchmark infection rates that many hospitals use for comparison with their own rates.

## Distribution of Nosocomial Infections by Site and Pathogen

Overall, *Staphylococcus aureus* is the most common pathogen among patients at participating NNIS hospitals performing hospital-wide surveillance. It was followed closely by *Escherichia coli*, coagulase-negative staphylococcus, *Enterococcus* spp., and *Pseudomonas aeruginosa.* Pathogen distributions vary by site and by intensive care or nonintensive care area (Table 8.1).

Nosocomial pathogens have changed markedly since the 1970s. The trends reflect, in part, the continued emergence of antimicrobial-resistant strains. Rates of *S. aureus*, coagulase- negative staphylococcus, enterococcus, *Candida* sp., methicillin-resistant *S. aureus* (MRSA), vancomycin-resistant enterococcus (VRE), and other antimicrobial-resistant pathogens have increased, whereas *E. coli* and *P. aeruginosa* infections have decreased.

**Table 8.1** Distribution of most common nosocomial pathogens for hospital-wide and ICU patients by site of infection, NNIS, October 1986–December 1990

| Hospital-wide component | | ICU component | |
|---|---|---|---|
| Blood | Percent | Blood | Percent |
| COAGULASE-NEGATIVE STAPHYLOCOCCI | 27.9 | COAGULASE-NEGATIVE STAPHYLOCOCCI | 28.2 |
| *S. aureus* | 16.5 | *S. aureus* | 16.1 |
| Enterococci | 8.3 | Enterococci | 12.0 |
| *Candida* spp. | 7.8 | *Candida* spp. | 10.25 |
| *E. coli* | 5.6 | *Enterobacter* spp. | 5.3 |
| SURGICAL WOUND | | SURGICAL WOUND | |
| *S. aureus* | 17.1 | Enterococci | 15.8 |
| Enterococci | 13.3 | Coagulase-negative staphylococci | 13.8 |
| Coagulase-negative staphylococci | 12.6 | *S. aureus* | 11.7 |
| *E. coli* | 9.4 | *Enterobacter* spp. | 10.3 |
| *P. aeruginosa* | 8.2 | *P. aeruginosa* | 9.5 |
| RESPIRATORY TRACT | | RESPIRATORY TRACT | |
| *P. aeruginosa* | 16.9 | *P. aeruginosa* | 20.8 |
| *S. aureus* | 16.1 | *S. aureus* | 17.1 |
| *Enterobacter* spp. | 10.5 | *Enterobacter* spp. | 11.1 |
| *S. pneumoniae* | 6.5 | *Acinetobacter* spp. | 6.4 |
| *H. influenzae* | 6.3 | *K. pneumoniae* | 5.6 |
| URINARY TRACT | | URINARY TRACT | |
| *E. coli* | 25.8 | *Candida* spp. | 25.0 |
| Enterococci | 15.9 | *E. coli* | 17.5 |
| *P. aeruginosa* | 12.0 | Enterococci | 13.0 |
| *Candida* spp. | 9.4 | *P. aeruginosa* | 11.3 |
| *K. pneumoniae* | 6.4 | *Enterobacter* spp. | 6.1 |

Source: Jarvis WR, Martone WJ. Predominant pathogens in hospital infections. J Antimicrob Chemother 1992; 29(Suppl A):19–24.

## Common pathogens

Approximately 80% of all nosocomial infections occur at four sites: the urinary tract, surgical wounds, bloodstream, and respiratory tract. The distribution of prominent pathogens varies by site. In addition, the risk factors associated with each site vary (see Fig. 8.1).

Patients hospitalized in intensive care units (ICUs) are at a higher risk of acquiring a nosocomial infection than are non-ICU hospitalized patients. This probably is partially due both to the severity of the patients' underlying illness and to their exposures to lifesaving invasive procedures. For instance, in the NNIS system, the risk of acquiring nosocomial pneumonia, bloodstream infection, or urinary tract infection (UTI) were significantly associated with device exposures.

## Nosocomial Urinary Tract Infections

UTIs are the most frequently diagnosed nosocomial infection, accounting for approximately 36% of the 2 million nosocomial infections that occur each year. Most UTIs are acquired endemically from strains of gram-negative organisms colonizing the gastrointestinal tract of catheterized patients. In the NNIS hospital-wide component, the most common nosocomial pathogens causing UTIs are *E. coli* (25.8%), enterococcus (15.9%), and *P. aeruginosa* (12%) (Table 8.1).

The gastrointestinal tract is an important reservoir of *E. coli* and enterococcus, but is rarely colonized by *P. aeruginosa*. Reservoirs for *P. aeruginosa* are usually contaminated inanimate objects or other infected patients.

### Risk factors

Approximately 80% of all nosocomial UTIs occur in patients with indwelling urinary catheters, and nearly 20% occur after other types of transient urologic instrumentation. Other extrinsic risk factors include the length of catheterization, catheterization insertion and maintenance practices, and antimicrobial therapy. Intrinsic risk factors are especially important for females; the risk of women acquiring nosocomial bacteriuria is approximately two

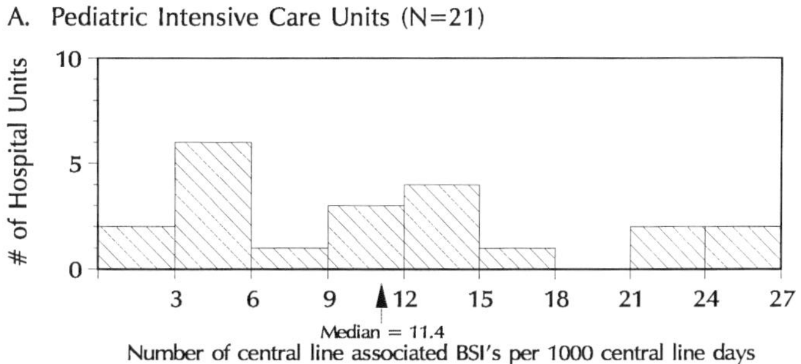


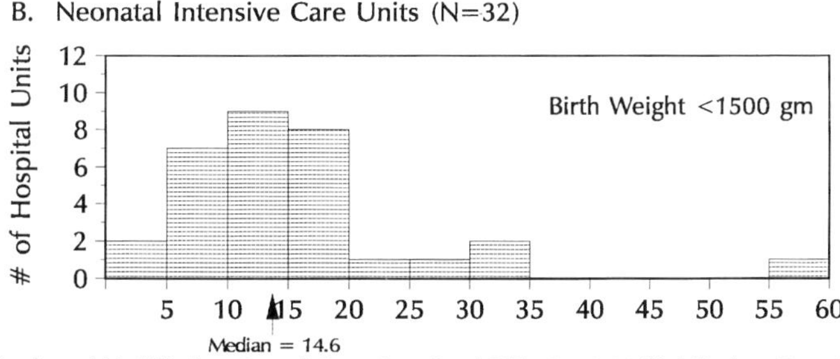


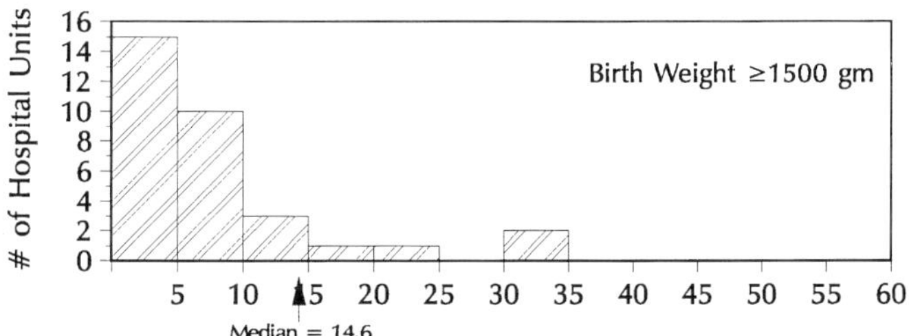


**Fig. 8.1** Distribution of nosocomial bloodstream infections per 1000 catheter days for pediatric or neonatal intensive care unit patients, NNIS, 1986–1990. [From Jarvis et al. Am J Med 1991; 91(Suppl 3B):3B–185S; Gaynes et al. Am J Med 1991; 91 (Suppl 3B):67–71.]

times that of men. Other intrinsic risk factors include older age, severe underlying illness, and meatal colonization with gram-negative bacilli (Table 8.2).

### Pathogenesis

Infecting microorganisms may enter the catheterized urinary tract by one of two routes. In women, infections most commonly arise by the periurethral route; namely, microorganisms from the bowel flora or elsewhere colonize the periurethral area and ascend into the bladder in the mucous sheath between the urethral meatus and external catheter surface. Microorganisms may also enter the bladder via the intraluminal route; such organisms gain access to the catheter lumen via the disconnected catheter collection tube junction after contamination of the collecting bag. This appears to be the predominant route of entry in men. While UTI most commonly follows catheterization, other factors such as presence of stones, anatomic defects, and prostatic infection may lead to persistence of colonization and invasive symptomatic disease. Some diseases, such as diabetes mellitus, greatly increase the risk of UTI by altering metabolic and neurogenic factors. Any conditions, such as vesicoureteral reflux, that interfere with normal urinary flow and bladder emptying also predispose to UTI.

**Table 8.2** Risk factor for nosocomial infection at major sites

| Site | Risk factors |
|---|---|
| Urinary tract | Advanced age<br>Female sex<br>Breaks in closed system<br>Failure of personnel to wash hands<br>Severity of illness |
| Lung (Pneumonia) | Underlying disease<br>  Altered mental status<br>  Diabetes<br>  Alcoholism<br>Intubation<br>Mechanical ventilation<br>Respiratory therapy equipment<br>Tracheostomy<br>Malnutrition<br>Thoracoabdominal surgery<br>Histamine II blockers, antacids<br>Severity of illness |
| Bloodstream (primary) | Extremes of age<br>Underlying disease<br>  Immunosuppression<br>  Burns<br>Intravascular devices<br>Severity of illness |
| Surgical wound | Advanced age<br>Malnutrition<br>Wound classification<br>Prosthesis<br>Type of procedure<br>Preoperative shaving<br>Severity of illness |

Source: Beck-Sague CM, Jarvis WR. The epidemiology and prevention of nosocomial infections. In: Disinfection, Sterilization, and Preservation, 4th ed. Block SS, ed. Lea & Febiger, Philadelphia, 1991, pp 663–675.

### Prevention

CDC has published guidelines for prevention of catheter-associated urinary tract infections. Prevention of catheter-associated UTI depends on (*1*) restriction of catheterization to those for whom it is essential, (*2*) appropriate preparation of the insertion site and aseptic catheter insertion, and (*3*) maintenance of a closed urinary drainage system. Some investigators suggest that intermittent catheterization with bladder emptying reduces the incidence of bacteriuria and subsequent UTI in patients requiring long-term catheterization. When an indwelling catheter is necessary, aseptic cleaning of the meatus and aseptic insertion and maintenance of a closed system with prompt removal of the catheter reduce the risk of UTI.

## Surgical Site Infections (SSIs)

In NNIS hospitals conducting hospital-wide surveillance, nearly 17% of nosocomial infections were due to SSIs. However, in institutions that focused on surgical patients, SSIs were the most common nosocomial infection site (37%); 24% of SSIs were incisional and 13% were organ/space. These data showed that nearly 9% of nosocomial infections occurred in surgical patients who subsequently died. Of those infections that were related to the patient's death, SSIs accounted for 21%.

Since 1964, SSIs have been classified by the level of contamination present at the time of surgery; the different levels of contamination include *clean* (class I), *clean-contaminated* (class II), *contaminated* (class III), and *dirty* (class IV) procedures. Rates of infection increase as the classification of surgery progresses from clean to dirty. Recently, studies have shown that a risk index is a better measure of SSI risk, since risk indexes control for confounders such as type and duration of procedure, wound class, and severity of illness. Such risk indexes are better predictors of SSI risk than is use of the wound class alone.

At NNIS hospitals, *S. aureus* is the most common pathogen associated with SSIs, followed by enterococcus and coagulase-negative staphylococcus (Table 8.1).

### Risk factors

The SENIC and NNIS studies have each developed simple indexes for predicting risk of SSI. The SENIC index includes an operation involving the abdomen, an operation lasting >2 hours, an operation classified as either contaminated or dirty, and a patient having ≥3 discharge diagnoses. The NNIS index includes a measure of severity of disease, the American Society for Anesthesia (ASA) score, the length of the procedure, and the wound class. In both of these indices, important confounding risk factors are included, which are not accounted for in the wound classification system alone.

Extrinsic risk factors predisposing patients to SSIs are multiple and are related to every aspect of the procedure, from preoperative skin preparation to wound closure. These include age, sex, type of surgery, skin preparation, surgical technique, and aseptic preparation of the patient. A number of factors associated with preoperative skin preparation have been associated with increased infection risk. Shaving patients' skin before surgery, particularly more than several hours before surgery, increases the risk of SSI, possibly by causing multiple microscopic nicks where bacterial growth can occur inaccessible to skin antisepsis; clipping the hair or shaving immediately before surgery decreases infection risk. The hands of surgical staff also can serve as reservoirs for organisms that can cause SSIs. A given patient's skin may be heavily colonized with a wide variety of potential pathogens, particularly if the patient has been hospitalized for a long time before surgery.

### Pathogenesis

Surgical infections are usually bacterial in origin, due to intraoperative seeding of exogenous bacteria or dissemination of endogenous bacteria to the operative site. Bacterial inoculation causing infection of a closed wound is thought to be uncommon. Less frequently, SSIs can result from postoperative manipulation, such as postoperative inoculation of cardiac surgery sites with *Legionella* sp. through the use of tap water to clean the area around the surgical site.

### Prevention

CDC guidelines for the prevention of SSIs include measures for prevention in the pre-, intra-, and postoperative periods. In general, prevention of SSIs depends on (*1*) reducing the amount and type of microbial contamination of the wound, (*2*) using techniques that protect the condition of the wound during the operation, and (*3*) enhancing the patient's ability to withstand microbial contamination. Preoperative measures include treating any known infection, minimizing the preoperative stay, preoperative bathing with an FDA-approved antiseptic, avoiding shaving, and correcting known nutritional deficiencies if possible. Intraoperative measures include appropriate preparation of the operative site with an FDA-approved antiseptic; adequate scrubbing of surgical personnel's hands and use of sterile gloves; good operative aseptic technique, including careful handling of tissue; and appropriate and judicious use of prophylactic antimicrobials.

## Nosocomial Bloodstream Infections (BSIs)

Nosocomial BSIs currently account for 13.9% of all nosocomial infections. Patients admitted to ICUs have the highest incidence of all nosocomial infections, but especially BSIs. In ICU settings, approximately 1.3% of patients acquire a BSI, and BSIs comprise 15.8% of nosocomial infections. Coagulase-negative staphylococci are the most common pathogens, accounting for 27.9% of all BSIs; *S. aureus* (16.5%) and enterococcus (8.3%) are the next most common pathogens (Table 8.1).

### Risk factors

The major extrinsic risk factor for nosocomial BSI is use of an intravascular catheter. Over 80% of BSIs occur among patients with intravenous (IV) lines. In NNIS ICU patients, the central venous catheter (CVL) BSI rate was 8.6 per 1000 line-days, compared with 0.02 per 1000 patient-days among patients without IV lines.

Intrinsic risk factors for BSI include extremes in age and severity of underlying disease. Extremes in age also affect host immune responses, with rates of infection highest among low-birthweight infants and the elderly. Patients with fatal underlying diseases are at greatest risk for BSI. In these patients, infections at other sites may not adequately be contained or pathogens either gain access to the bloodstream or small numbers of microorganisms may disseminate, causing secondary BSIs. Often these infections are not clearly related to the presence of intravascular catheters.

### Pathogenesis

The increasing incidence of BSIs appears to be related in part to the increasing use of prolonged central and peripheral IV cannulation. Most catheter-related infections are caused by skin microorganisms that invade the cutaneous tract during catheter insertion or during the course of IV therapy. Concomitantly, an important step in the pathogenesis of catheter-related infections is the formation of a fibrin sheath around a cannula inserted into a vessel. The sheath then becomes colonized with the entering cutaneous microbes, and the bacteria replicate and are released into the bloodstream. Loose connections between intravascular and extension tubing, and stopcock or hub contamination by skin organisms, also have been recognized as important causes of BSI.

Contamination of infusates is a less frequent cause of endemic BSI; however, it is one of the most common causes of epidemic BSI and can be classified as either intrinsic or extrinsic. Intrinsic contamination is caused by inadvertent introduction of microorganisms during manufacture into substances intended for infusion. This includes contamination of caps or containers of intravenous fluids (IVF). Since the 1971 nationwide outbreak of intrinsically contaminated IVF, no other epidemic of intrinsic IVF contamination has occurred in the United States, although such outbreaks still occur outside the United States.

Extrinsic contamination of infusates is more common than intrinsic contamination. It is caused by introduction of pathogens after manufacture, usually during use in a health care setting; this continues to be the most common cause of recognized epidemic BSI. *Enterobacter cloacae, P. aeruginosis,* and *Candida parapsilosis* are so prevalent in epidemics of extrinsic contamination, particularly where total parenteral nutrition is involved, that when they are recovered from blood cultures a high index of suspicion of extrinsic IVF contamination should exist and a prompt search for such contamination should be undertaken.

### Prevention

CDC has published guidelines for the prevention of nosocomial intravascular catheter-related infections. Strict adherence to both handwashing and aseptic technique remains the cornerstone of prevention of catheter-related infections. Other measures, however, may confer additional protection and must be considered when formulating prevention strategies. These measures include selection of an appropriate site for catheter insertion and type of catheter material, use of barrier precautions during catheter insertion, change of catheters and administration sets at appropriate intervals, catheter-site care, and the use of filters, flush solutions, prophylactic antimicrobials, and newer intravascular devices.

## Nosocomial Pneumonia

Although its incidence in hospitals has decreased significantly over the past few years, pneumonia remains one of the most frequent types of nosocomial infection, accounting for nearly 13%

of all nosocomial infections. These infections are especially important since nosocomial pneumonia causes the greatest morbidity and mortality of all nosocomial infections. Most nosocomial pneumonias occur in patients who are intubated and/or hospitalized for longer than 7 days. The three most common pathogens causing nosocomial pneumonia are *P. aeruginosa* (16.9%), *S. aureus* (16.1%), and *Enterobacter* sp. (10.5%).

### Risk factors

Intrinsic risk factors for nosocomial pneumonia include advanced age, underlying chronic cardiopulmonary disease, and immunosuppression of the host. Immunocompromised patients are susceptible to a wider range of organisms than are nonimmunocompromised patients, and pneumonias caused by fungi, mycobacteria, and viruses often are seen in addition to the more common organisms.

Extrinsic risk factors include thoracic or abdominal surgery, intubation, or hospitalization in an ICU. Among extrinsic risk factors, surgery is especially important, since half of all nosocomial pneumonias occur postoperatively. Factors strongly associated with pneumonia in thoracic or abdominal surgery patients include preoperative markers of underlying disease severity, such as low serum albumin or greater severity of illness; length of preoperative stay; duration of surgery; and thoracic or upper abdominal surgical sites. Mortality due to nosocomial pneumonia varies by patient characteristics and type of organism but may often be high. For instance, gram-negative pneumonia in hospitalized patients is associated with mortality rates approaching 70%.

### Pathogenesis

Most nosocomial pneumonias occur after the oropharynx or the stomach or both become colonized with pathogenic organisms. Both these potential reservoirs routinely spill small amounts of their contents into the trachea. Colonized patients are much more susceptible to nosocomial pneumonia.

Colonization of the oropharynx is facilitated by a number of factors, including underlying disease; persons with medical conditions such as alcoholism, diabetes mellitus, or viral pharyngitis have higher colonization rates of gram-negative organisms. Age, history of respiratory disease, and activity level also affect colonization rates.

Intubation and mechanical ventilation are very important factors associated with nosocomial pneumonia. These procedures bypass the natural nasopharyngeal mechanical barrier and expose the respiratory tract to oropharyngeal flora. Intubation and tracheotomy increase the incidence of infection by approximately 20% and 25%, respectively. Respiratory therapy equipment also can serve as reservoirs for organisms associated with nosocomial pneumonia, especially if tap water is used or the equipment is not properly disinfected or sterilized.

### Prevention

The prevention of nosocomial pneumonias largely depends on (*1*) restricting invasive techniques, such as intubation or mechanical ventilation, to clinically indicated uses, (*2*) avoiding specific devices associated with high risk of infection, such as nebulizers that create droplets to humidify air, and (*3*) improving postoperative respiratory care via specific preoperative patient preparation, including patient instruction designed to prevent pulmonary complications.

Administration of antacids or H-2 blockers for prevention of stress bleeding in critically ill patients has been associated with gastric bacterial overgrowth. In contrast, sucralfate, a cytoprotective agent, has little effect on gastric pH, may have antibacterial properties, and has been suggested as a potential substitute for antacids and H-2 blockers. Studies of the risk of nosocomial pneumonia in patients receiving sucralfate versus H-2 blockers and/or antacids have had variable results. Most ICU patients on mechanical ventilation and antacids with or without H-2 blockers have had increased gastric pH, bacterial counts, and pneumonia rates compared to those receiving sucralfate.

## Transmission in Special Settings

### Pediatric

The distribution of nosocomial infections in pediatric patients differs from that seen in adults. In infants and children, cutaneous infections, BSIs, and lower respiratory tract infections account for slightly over 50% of reported infections; SSIs and UTIs each account for <10% of infections. In contrast, in adults, UTIs account for >40% of infections, and SSIs and lower respiratory tract infections account for 19% and 16%, respectively; BSIs and cutaneous infections each account for approximately 6%.

The pathogens that cause nosocomial infections also differ between pediatric and adult patients. Gram-negative and gram-positive aerobes each account for approximately 40% of the nosocomial infections in infants and children, while gram-negative aerobes account for nearly 60% of nosocomial infections in adults. *S. aureus* is the most frequently reported pathogen causing infections in infants and children, whereas *E. coli* is the most frequently reported pathogen in adults. Coagulase-negative staphylococci and group B streptococcus are reported more frequently from pediatric patients, while enterococci, *P. aeruginosa*, and *Enterobacter* spp. are reported more frequently from adults. Viruses also are an important cause of nosocomial infections in pediatric patients. In the NNIS system, pediatric patients were five times more likely to develop a nosocomial viral infection than were adult patients. In one study, viruses were reported to account for >25% of the pediatric nosocomial infections; rotavirus, respiratory syncytial virus, parainfluenza virus, and adenovirus were all associated frequently with nosocomial infections.

### Neonatal intensive care units (NICUs)

The predominant sites of infection in neonates in NICUs differ from those in older infants and children or the overall pediatric population. Skin or surface infections are most frequently reported, followed by pneumonias and BSIs. Among neonates, SSIs and UTIs account for a smaller percentage of infections, and central nervous system and upper respiratory tract infections account for a larger percentage of the infections than in older children.

*S. aureus* and *E. coli* are the predominant pathogens causing infections in NICU patients. Coagulase-negative staphylococci and *Candida* spp. are emerging as other important nosocomial pathogens. *Candida* sp. infections have increased in very-low-birthweight infants (<1500 g), perhaps as a result of prolonged vascular cannulation, antimicrobial therapy, and the increasing use of steroids.

Numerous risk factors for developing a nosocomial infection have been identified among NICU patients. In addition to those identified for all pediatric patients, these factors include birthweight and the number, type, and duration of invasive procedures (Fig. 8.1). Neonates admitted to NICUs do not acquire "normal" aerobic gastrointestinal flora but instead become colonized with the prevalent NICU environmental organisms; the probability of such colonization is dependent on the duration of NICU stay. Birthweight is a particularly important determinant of infection risk. Hemming and co-workers found an inverse relationship between birthweight and the risk for nosocomial infection; 9% of infants weighing ≥2500 g contracted an infection, versus 46% of infants weighing <1000 g. The risk of acquiring a nosocomial infection has been estimated at 3% for every 500 g decrement of birthweight.

Most nosocomial infections in NICU patients result from person-to-person transmission via the hands of medical personnel. Although intrinsic or extrinsic product or device (e.g., intravenous fluids, intralipid, cannulae) contamination can lead to nosocomial infections, such episodes result in only a small proportion of all NICU nosocomial infections.

### Pediatric intensive care units (PICUs)

Among the pediatric population, those admitted to PICUs are second only to NICU patients in the risk of acquiring nosocomial infections. Infection rates from such units range from 6.2 to 24.1 infections per 100 patients discharged (mean, 13.5 infections per 100 patients discharged). The reported infection rate in PICU patients is higher at children's hospitals (range, 11–24.1; mean, 13) than at general hospitals (range, 6.2–21.6; mean, 9.6); this may reflect differences in severity of illness or case mix. Factors influencing the infection rate are similar to those found for pediatric patients in general and include the subspecialty service, length of stay, and severity of illness.

The distribution of infections by site and pathogen varies considerably among the reported PICU studies. In general, pulmonary infections are most frequently reported, followed by UTIs and SSIs; cutaneous infections account for <15% of infections. These results differ from those reported from adult ICUs. The predominant pathogens have differed in various studies published to date. In a study performed in two PICUs, *Candida* spp. and *S. aureus* predominated in one PICU while *Pseudomonas* spp., *Candida* spp., and *Klebsiella* spp. predominated at the other. The mean severity of patients' illnesses differed markedly between the two PICUs, and the severity of illness as measured by physiologic abnormalities or therapeutic interventions correlated with both mortality and risk of acquiring a nosocomial infection.

### Long-term care

As the U.S. population ages, the proportion of elderly hospitalized patients will increase. In addition, as the elderly population increases, the proportion receiving care in long-term-care facilities will increase. This will pose a challenge to HCWs, since the elderly are more prone to nosocomial infection and epidemiologically have a slightly different distribution of nosocomial infections than does the general population. Among the elderly, risk factors for nosocomial infection include exposure to certain high-risk medical devices. NNIS data suggest that the risk of dying from a nosocomial infection is related more to the site of infection and complication than to the age of the patient.

Often, ongoing surveillance for infections in long-term-care facility residents does not exist. For surveillance in this population, either modified acute-care-facility nosocomial infection definitions or specific infection definitions for the elderly in long-term care can be used. A better understanding of the characteristics of nosocomial infections in elderly patients and their associated risk factors will assist in the development of the most beneficial and cost-effective infection-control measures.

### Home health care (HHC)

Recent trends in health care have emphasized increased patient care in home settings. However, no surveillance system exists for HHC-associated infection, and often these infections are not detected because they do not occur in the hospital and the HHC company may not employ infection-control personnel. Although limited data are available regarding infection in HHC patients, such patients probably are at lower risk of contracting infections from multiply resistant bacteria and other typically "hospital-acquired" pathogens while they receive care at home. Thus, the home environment may lower the risk of infection for some patients.

Currently, there are no standardized definitions of infection or guidelines for infection-control practices in HHC settings. Recently, several outbreak investigations of BSIs in HHC patients identified needleless devices and infection-control practices associated with these devices as risk factors for BSIs in this population. Because of the growing importance of HHC, studies have begun to address infection-control parameters in HHC. Surveillance systems, nosocomial infection definitions, and guidelines for HHC practice will be needed for this area.

## Recent Developments in Epidemiology and Control of Hospital-Acquired Infections

### Antimicrobial resistance

Nosocomial infections due to multidrug-resistant microorganisms are increasingly common and of concern to health care professionals. MRSA emerged in the early 1980s and has become prevalent at many United States hospitals. More recently, VRE has emerged and is spreading throughout United States hospitals. NNIS data show an increased percentage of MRSA from 2.4% among all hospitals in 1975 to over 30% by the early 1990s. Similarly, the incidence of VRE has risen from 0.3 to 7.9% between 1989 and 1993. The emergence of VRE has presented a serious treatment challenge, because these organisms often have high-level resistance to penicillins and aminoglycosides and no effective therapy is available. An increased risk of VRE infection and colonization has been associated with severe underlying disease, immunosuppression, previous treatment with multiple antimicrobials or vancomycin, and intraabdominal surgery. The simultaneous occurrence of MRSA and VRE in selected populations increases the risk of transmission of the vancomycin resistance gene to MRSA; vancomycin-resistant MRSA would be a public health emergency.

Different methods are being used to prevent selection for and further nosocomial transmission of multidrug-resistant organisms. In many hospitals, infection-control specialists and epidemiologists are aggressively limiting the use of broad-spectrum antimicrobials to those situations that specifically warrant them. These actions, in addition to specific isolation precautions recommended by the Hospital Infection Control Practices Advisory Committee (HICPAC), are being adopted by increasing numbers of health care facilities in hopes of controlling spread of antimicrobial-resistant organisms.

## Nosocomial tuberculosis

Nosocomial transmission of *Mycobacterium tuberculosis* (TB), both drug-sensitive and multidrug-resistant strains, has increased concurrent with the overall rise of TB in the United States. Both HCWs and patients are at risk of contracting TB infection in the hospital. Maloney et al. (1995) showed that failure to apply CDC-recommended control measures, including (*1*) prompt isolation and treatment of patients with TB; (*2*) rapid diagnostic techniques for processing TB specimens; (*3*) negative-pressure isolation rooms; and (*4*) appropriate HCW respiratory protection contributed to nosocomial transmission of multidrug-resistant *M. tuberculosis*. Implementation of the CDC-recommended control measures interrupted patient-to-patient transmission within the hospital. CDC has recently published new guidelines for preventing transmission of TB in health care facilities. The recent approval of N-95 respirators, which cost about the same as dust-mist respirators, should reduce the cost of respirators and protect HCWs from air-borne droplet nuclei.

## Bloodborne pathogens

Occupational exposures of HCWs to blood-borne pathogens include percutaneous, mucous membrane, or cutaneous exposure to blood or other potentially infectious materials. Organisms of concern include hepatitis B and C, and human immunodeficiency virus (HIV). Risk of transmission following percutaneous injury by contaminated needles or other sharp objects has been estimated at 2%–40% for hepatitis B and 3%–10% for hepatitis C. The risk of HIV infection depends on several factors, including the prevalence of HIV in the patient population, the nature and frequency of occupational blood contact, and the risk of HIV transmission after a single contact with blood. Based on prospective surveillance of more than 3000 exposed HCWs, the risk of seroconversion after a single percutaneous exposure to HIV-infected blood is approximately 0.3%.

Risk reduction can be accomplished most effectively by reducing the frequency of blood exposures among HCWs. In 1987, CDC introduced its "Universal Precautions" to prevent contact with blood, certain other body fluids, and tissues of *all* patients. These recommendations, coupled with the Occupational Safety and Health Administration's (OSHA) blood-borne pathogen standard in 1991, have become an important component in the overall strategy to prevent occupational blood contact. In 1995, new patient-isolation precautions have been published. The revised guidelines contain two tiers of precautions. The newly introduced "standard precautions" synthesize the major features of "Universal Precautions" and "Body Substance Isolation" and are intended to prevent transmission of many non-blood-borne and blood-borne pathogens. Standard precautions apply to blood, all body fluids, secretions and excretions (except sweat), nonintact skin, and mucous membranes. "Transmission-Based Precautions," the second tier, are for patients documented or suspected to be infected with highly transmissible or epidemiologically important pathogens for which additional precautions beyond standard precautions are needed to interrupt transmission in hospitals. There are three types of transmission-based precautions: airborne precautions, droplet precautions, and contact precautions. Transmission-based precautions are to be used in addition to standard precautions.

Personal protective equipment also is important in reducing blood exposure among HCWs. Studies have found that besides decreasing the incidence of blood–hand contact, use of double gloves also may reduce the volume of blood associated with percutaneous injury. Selection of gowns, masks, and protective eyewear should be guided by knowledge about the nature and frequency of blood contact; the type, duration, and estimated blood loss associated with a procedure; the occupation/role of the HCW during a surgical procedure; the worker's training and experience; cost; and acceptability to the worker. New devices with features intended to reduce the likelihood of percutaneous injury by hollow and solid-bore needles and scalpels increasingly are available.

Detailed recommendations for management of exposures to blood and blood-borne pathogens have been published. These include prompt reporting of the exposure to receive necessary counseling and management, evaluation of the need for postexposure prophylaxis, testing of the patient with consent for hepatitis B surface antigen, HIV antibodies, and serologic follow-up of the HCW. Postexposure testing of HCWs exposed to hepatitis C can also be considered to detect hepatitis C antibodies and evidence of hepatitis. The confidentiality of the source patient and the HCW should be maintained.

Although failures of postexposure zidovudine (ZDV) to prevent HIV infection in HCWs have been documented, a recent case-control study found that the use of ZDV following percutaneous exposure to HIV-infected blood may reduce the risk of subsequent HIV infection. Serious toxicity associated with short-course ZDV therapy appears to be rare; nausea, vomiting, headache, malaise, and fatigue are the most commonly reported side effects. Because of limited data regarding its efficacy and toxicity, the Public Health Service, in an earlier statement, did not recommend for or against the use of ZDV after exposure. The PHS is currently evaluating the possible need for revision of these earlier recommendations regarding the postexposure use of ZDV and other antiretroviral agents.

## Role of HCWs

HCWs play a major role in transmission of nosocomial pathogens. They can transmit an illness to, and contract an illness from, a patient they care for. In addition, HCWs can inadvertently serve as vectors for disease transmission between patients. Diseases such as chickenpox or measles have a high risk of transmission either to or from HCWs, while other diseases, such as HIV, have a low risk of transmission. CDC has published guidelines for infection-control activities intended to protect both the hospitalized patient and the HCW.

Breaks in HCW sterile technique or recommended handwashing practices have resulted in numerous documented outbreaks of disease. In addition, although difficult to document, failure to follow recommended handwashing procedures is probably a major factor contributing to transmission of endemic nosocomial infections. Maintenance of a clean environment is crucial to controlling spread of nosocomial infection, but handwashing before and between all patient contacts is the single most important procedure for preventing nosocomial infections. In many VRE outbreaks, environmental contamination has been documented. Patients in high-risk units, such as ICUs, are more often infected or colonized with virulent or multidrug-resistant organisms and are more susceptible to infection than are other patients, making HCW handwashing even more critical in these units.

It is important to remember that hands must be washed after patient care even if gloves were worn during care, since small holes in gloves may allow microorganisms to contaminate hands. Numerous studies have shown that both physicians and nurses often do not wash their hands as recommended; often, <50% wash hands appropriately. As more multidrug-resistant microorganisms evolve, the use of standard precautions becomes especially important in order to prevent HCWs from becoming inadvertent vectors of infection.

## Conclusion

Nosocomial infections cause substantial morbidity and mortality. Reducing nosocomial infections requires active surveillance and infection-control programs. Use of standardized definitions of infection and surveillance methods facilitates both identification of areas where preventive interventions are necessary and inter- and intrahospital comparison of infection rates. Control measures include education of HCWs about nosocomial infection control, full implementation of infection-prevention guidelines, and careful and judicious use of antimicrobial therapy and invasive devices and procedures. By fully implementing these measures, hospital personnel can maximally reduce the risk of nosocomial infection in their patients.

### ANNOTATED BIBLIOGRAPHY


Centers for Disease Control and Prevention. Case-control study of HIV seroconversion in health-care workers after percutaneous exposure to HIV-infected blood—France, United Kingdom and United States, January 1988–August 1994. MMWR 1995; 44:929–933.*

*A retrospective case-control study assessing potential risk factors influencing seroconversion after percutaneous exposure to HIV-infected blood which found that risk was increased if the exposure was associated with specific risk factors.*

CDC National Nosocomial Infection Surveillance. Nosocomial infection rates for interhospital comparison: limitations and possible solutions. Infect Control Hosp Epidemiol 1991; 12:609–621.

*Discussion of the importance of nosocomial infection surveillance data that can be used for interhospital comparison and describes several new infection rates, including device-associated, device day rates, and a NNIS surgical wound infection risk index.*

Cullen DJ, Civetta JM, Briggs BA et al. Therapeutic intervention scoring system: A method for quantitative comparison of patient care. Crit Care Med 1974; 2:57–60.

Garner JS, Jarvis WR, Emori TG, Horan TC, Hughes JM. CDC definitions for nosocomial infections, 1988. Am J Infect Control 1988; 16:128–140.

*Definitions of nosocomial infections; the article provides algorithms that combine specific clinical findings and laboratory results.*

Gaynes RP, Martone WJ, Culver DH et al. Comparison of rates of nosocomial infections in neonatal intensive care units in the United States. Am J Med 1991; 91(Suppl 3B):67–71.

*Shows the value of device-specific and birthweight-stratified nosocomial infection rates among NICUs for interhospital comparisons.*

Haley RW, Culver DH, White JW et al. The efficacy of infection surveillance and control programs in preventing nosocomial infections in U.S. hospitals. Am J Epidemiol 1985; 121:182–205

*Documented intensive infection surveillance and control programs decreased rates of the four most common nosocomial infections.*

Jarvis WR, Edwards JR, Culver DH et al. Nosocomial infection rates in adult and pediatric intensive care units in the United States. Am J Med 1991; 91(Suppl 3B):3B–185S.

*Introduces the concept of and describes the effectiveness of using ICU-specific and device-specific days as the denominator for inter- and intrahospital comparison when analyzing nosocomial infection rates in adult and pediatric ICUs.*

Maloney SA, Pearson ML, Gorson MT et al. Efficacy of control measures in preventing nosocomial transmission of multidrug-resistant tuberculosis to patients and health care workers. Ann Intern Med 1995; 122:90–95.

Shay DK, Maloney SA, Motecalvo M et al. Epidemiology and mortality risk of vancomycin-resistant enterococci bloodstream infections. J Infect Dis 1995; 172:993–1000.

*Study to determine risk factors for vancomycin-resistant enterococcal bloodstream infection at a tertiary care hospital.*

Yeh TS, Pollack MM, Ruttimann UE et al. Validation of a physiologic stability index for use in critically ill infants and children. Pediatr Res 1984; 18:445–451.

*Descriptions of the first severity of illness scoring systems for pediatrics, based on therapeutic intervention and physiologic measurements.*


### RECOMMENDED READING

#### Surveillance


Haley RW, Culver DH, White JW, Morgan WM, Emori TG, Munn VP, Hooton TM. The efficacy of infection surveillance and control programs in preventing nosocomial infections in U.S. hospitals. Am J Epidemiol 1985; 121:182–204.

Hughes JM, Jarvis WR. Epidemiology of nosocomial infections. In: Manual of Clinical Microbiology, 4th ed. Lennette EH, Balows A, Hausler WJ, Jr., Shadomy HJ, eds. American Society of Microbiology, Washington, DC, 1985, pp 99–104.

Beck-Sague CM, Jarvis WR. The epidemiology and prevention of nosocomial infections. In: Disinfection, Sterilization, and Preservation, 4th ed. Block SS, ed. Lea & Febiger, Philadelphia, PA, 1991, pp 663–675.

Jarvis WR, Martone WJ. Predominant pathogens in hospital infections. J Antimicrob Chemother 1992; 29(Suppl A):19–24.

Emori TG, Gaynes RP. An overview of nosocomial infections, including the role of the microbiology laboratory. Clin Microbiol Rev 1993; 6:428–442.

LaForce FM. Lower respiratory tract infections. In: Hospital Infections, 3rd ed. Bennett JV, Brachman PS, eds. Little Brown and Company, Boston, MA, 1992, pp 611–639.

Wollschlager CM, Conrad AR, Khan FA. Common complications in critically ill patients. DM 1988; 34:221–293.

Brachman PS. Epidemiology of nosocomial infections. In: Hospital Infections, 1st ed. Bennett JV, Brachman PS, eds. Little, Brown and Company, Boston, MA, 1979, p 9.

Haley RW, Gaynes RP, Aber RC, Bennett JV. Surveillance of nosocomial infections. In: Hospital Infections, 3rd ed. Bennett JV, Brachman PS, eds. Little, Brown and Company, Boston, MA, 1992, pp 79–108.

Haley RW, Culver DH, Morgan WM, White JW, Emori TG, Hooton TM. Increased recognition of infectious diseases in U.S. hospitals through increased use of diagnostic tests, 1970–1976. Am J Epidemiol 1985; 121:168–181.


#### Urinary tract infections


Garibaldi RA. Hospital acquired urinary tract infection. In: Wenzel RP, ed., CRC Handbook of Hospital Acquired Infections. CRC Press, Boca Raton, FL, 1981, pp 371–512.

Stamm WE. Nosocomial urinary tract infections. In: Hospital Infections, 3rd ed. Bennett JV, Brachman PS, eds. Little, Brown and Company, Boston, MA, 1992, pp 597–610.


#### Surgical site infections


Horan TC, Culver DH, Gaynes RP, Jarvis WR, Edwards JR, Reid CR, the National Nosocomial Infections Surveillance (NNIS) System. Nosocomial infections in surgical patients in the United States, January 1986–June 1992. Infect Control Hosp Epidemiol 1993; 14:73–80.

Cruse PJE, Ford R. The epidemiology of wound infections: A ten-year prospective study of 62,939 wounds. Surg Clin North Am 1980; 60:27–40.


#### Bloodstream infections


Maki DG. Epidemic nosocomial bacteremias. In: CRC Handbook of Hospital Acquired Infections. Wenzel RP, ed. CRC Press, Boca Raton, FL, 1981, pp 371–512.


*Copies may be purchased from National technical Information Service, U.S. Department of commerce, 5285 Port Royal Road, Springfield, VA 22161. Tel: (703) 487–4650.

Maki DG, Rhame FS, Mackel DC et al. Nationwide epidemics of septicemia caused by contaminated intravenous products: I. Epidemiologic and clinical features. Am J Med 1976; 60:471–485.

Hamory BH. Nosocomial bloodstream and intravascular device-related infections. In: Prevention and Control of Nosocomial Infections. Wenzel RP, ed. Williams & Wilkins, Baltimore, MD, 1993, pp 283–319.

### Nosocomial pneumonia

Beck-Sague, Sinkowitz, Chinn et al. Risk factors for ventilator-associated pneumonia in surgical intensive care unit. Infect Control Hosp Epidemiol 1996; 17:374–376.

Garibaldi RA, Britt MR, Coleman ML et al. Risk factors for postoperative pneumonia. Am J Med 1981:70:677–680.

### Pediatric

Hemming VG, Overall JC Jr, Britt MR. Nosocomial infections in a newborn intensive-care unit. N Engl J Med 1976; 294:1310–1316.

Welliver RC, McLaughlin S. Unique epidemiology of nosocomial infection in a children's hospital. Am J Dis Child 1984; 138:131–135.

### Long-term Care

Emori TG, Banerjee SN, Culver DH et al. Nosocomial infections in elderly patients in the United States, 1986–1990. Am J Med 1991; 91(Suppl 3B):289S–293S.

McGeer A, Campbell B, Emori TG et al. Definitions of infection for surveillance in long-term care facilities. Am J Infect Control 1991; 19:1–7.

### Home health care

Simmons B, Trusler M, Roccaforte J, Smith P, Smith R. Infection control in home health care settings. Infect Control Hosp Epidemiol 1990; 11:362–370.

American Association for Respiratory Care. Guidelines for disinfection of respiratory care equipment used in the home. Respir Care 1988; 33:801–808.

Valenti WM. Infection control, human immunodeficiency virus, and home health care: 1. Infection risk to the patient. Am J Infect Control 1994;22:371–2.

Danzig LE, Short LJ, Collins K et al. Bloodstream infections associated with a needleless intravenous system in patients receiving home infusion therapy. JAMA 1995; 273:1862–1864.

### Antimicrobial resistance

Panlilio AL, Culver DH, Gaynes RP et. al. Methicillin-resistant *Staphylococcus aureus* in U.S. hospitals, 1975–1991. Infect Control Hosp Epidemiol 1992; 13:582–586.

Shay DK, Goldmann DA, Jarvis WR. Reducing the spread of antimicrobial-resistant microorganisms. Pediatr Clin North Am 1995; 42:703–716.

### Nosocomial tuberculosis

Quebbeman EJ, Short LJ. How to select and evaluate new products on the market. Surg Clin North Am 1995; 75:1159–1165.

Dooley SN, Villarino ME, Lawrence M et. al. Nosocomial transmission of tuberculosis in a hospital unit for HIV-infected patients. JAMA 1992; 267:2632–2634.

Beck-Sague C, Dooley SW, Hutton MD et al. Hospital outbreak of multidrug-resistant *Mycobacterium tuberculosis* infections. JAMA; 268:1280–1286.

Frieden TR, Fujiwara PI, Washko RM et al. Tuberculosis in New York City—turning the tide. N Engl J Med 1995; 333:229–233.

### Bloodborne pathogens

Mast ST, Woolwine JD, Gerberding JL. Efficacy of gloves in reducing blood volumes transferred during simulated needlestick injury. J Infect Dis 1993; 168(6):1589–1592.

Fry DE, Telford GL, Fecteau DL et al. Prevention of blood exposure. Body and facial protection. Surg Clin North Am 1995; 75:1141–1157.

Gerberding JL. Management of occupational exposures to blood-borne viruses. N Engl J Med 1995; 332:444–451.

Tokars JI, Marcus R, Culver DH et al. Surveillance of HIV infection and zidovudine use among health care workers after occupational exposure to HIV-infected blood. Ann Intern Med 1993; 118:913–919.

### Outbreaks

Lowry PW, Blankenship RJ, Gridley W, Troup NJ, Tompkins LS. A cluster of *Legionella* sternal-wound infections due to postoperative topical exposure to contaminated tap water. N Engl J Med 1991; 324:109–113.

Richet HM, Craven PC, Brown JM et al. A cluster of *Rhodococcus (Gordona) bronchialis* sternal-wound infections after coronary- artery bypass surgery. N Engl J Med 1991; 324:104–109.

Mastro TD, Farley TA, Elliott JA et al. An outbreak of surgical-wound infections due to group A streptococcus carried on the scalp. N Engl J Med 1990; 323:968–72.

Welbel SF, McNeil MM, Pramanik A et al. Nosocomial *Malassezia pachydermatis* bloodstream infections in a neonatal intensive care unit. Pediatr Infect Dis J 1994; 13:104–108.

### Guidelines and recommendations**

Centers for Disease Control and Prevention. Guideline for Handwashing and Hospital Environmental Control. Am J Infect Control 1986; 14:110–129.

Centers for Disease Control and Prevention. Guideline for Prevention of Catheter-associated Urinary Tract Infections. Am J Infect Control 1983; 11:28–33.

Centers for Disease Control and Prevention. Guideline for Prevention of Surgical Wound Infections. Infect Control 1986; 7:193–200.

Centers for Disease Control and Prevention. CDC Definitions of Nosocomial Surgical Site Infections, 1992: A modification of CDC Definitions of Surgical Wound Infections. Am J Infect Control 1992; 20:271–274.

Centers for Disease Control and Prevention. Guideline for Prevention of Intravascular Device-Related Infections. Draft: Fed Reg 9/27/95;60(187): 49978–50006.

Centers for Disease Control and Prevention. Guideline for Prevention of Nosocomial Pneumonias. Infect Control Hosp Epidemiol 1994; 15:587–627.

Centers for Disease Control and Prevention. Guideline for Infection Control in Hospital Personnel. Infect Control 1983; 4:326–349.

Centers for Disease Control and Prevention. Guidelines for preventing the transmission of *Mycobacterium tuberculosis* in health-care facilities, 1994. MMWR 1994; 43:i–132.

Centers for Disease Control. Update: Universal precautions for prevention of transmission of human immunodeficiency virus, hepatitis B virus, and other bloodborne pathogens in health-care settings. MMWR 1988; 37:377–382.

Centers for Disease Control and Prevention. Public health service statement on management of occupational exposure to human immunodeficiency virus, including considerations regarding zidovudine Postexposure use. MMWR 1990; 39(RR-1).

Centers for Disease Control and Prevention. Caring for someone with AIDS—information for friends, relatives, household members, and others who care for a person with AIDS at home.

Garner J, Jarvis WR, Emon G, Horan TC, Hughes JM. The Centers for Disease Control. CDC Definitions for Nosocomial Infections, 1988. Am J Infect Control 1988; 16:128–140.

Hospital Infection Control Practices Advisory Committee. Guideline for Isolation Precautions in Hospitals. Infect Control Hosp Epidemiol 1996; 17:53–80.

Hospital Infection Control Practices Advisory Committee (HICPAC). Recommendations for preventing the spread of vancomycin resistance. Infect Control Hosp Epidemiol 1995; 16:105–113.

# 9

# Host Responses to Infection: Fever, Hyperthermia, and Hypothermia

RICHARD K. ROOT

Fever has been recognized as a cardinal manifestation of disease since ancient times. The first reliable measurements of body temperature were made in the mid 19th century, and since then its documentation has been a major aspect of the evaluation and management of a large variety of illnesses and diseases (Table 9.1). The majority of acute infectious diseases are accompanied by fever, and its occurrence accounts for a large percentage of visits to physicians and other health care givers worldwide. In evaluating patients with elevated body temperature it is important to distinguish between disorders that lead to *hyperthermia* as opposed to *fever*. Hyperthermia is the elevation of body temperature above the level established by a central set point in the hypothalamus, owing to an imbalance between heat-generating and -dissipating mechanisms. Fever is the controlled elevation of body temperature above the normal range in response to a set point change. The change in set point that initiates the febrile response is mediated by endogenous cytokines termed *pyrogens*.

For fever to occur, not only does a change in the set point need to take place, but heat-generating and -conserving mechanisms must be intact. Some patients, in particular neonates and the very elderly, may not be capable of generating febrile responses to infection, and paradoxically very severe infection or "sepsis" may sometimes be accompanied by a fall in temperature owing to a failure of heat-conservation mechanisms. The treatment of fever may assume an importance in patient management independent of the primary disease process, and this has spawned controversy since evidence exists that fever might be a beneficial component of the host immune response. On the other hand, the resolution of fever is usually perceived as a welcome clinical sign by patients and their caregivers.

This chapter will review the mechanisms involved in the pathogenesis of fever and distinguish these from conditions causing hyperthermia. Conditions that might blunt the febrile response or cause hypothermia will be described. Finally, the role of fever in host defense and the treatment of fever, hyperthermia, and hypothermia will be discussed.

## Thermoregulation

In 1868, following one million recordings in 25,000 healthy subjects, Wunderlich reported that the average body temperature was 37.0°C (98.6°F). For years this was held to be the standard, which the body's heat-generating and -dissipating mechanisms strove to maintain despite wide swings in ambient temperatures and activity. However, recent studies on a large group of healthy adults aged 18 to 40 years with modern thermometric methods have established that the average normal basal temperature is 36.8° ± 0.4°C (98.2° ± 0.7°F), with females exhibiting slightly higher mean values (36.9°C [98.4°F]) than males (36.7°C [98.4°F] $p <$ .001). For 99% of the population, the range of normal temperatures varies between 36.0°C (96.8°F) and 37.7°C (99.9°F) and follows a circadian rhythm, a phenomenon first demonstrated by Wunderlich and his colleagues. The lowest temperatures are routinely recorded in the early morning (4 A.M.) and the peak at 4 to 6 P.M. The average daily oscillation is about 0.55°C (1.00°F), but in some may be as broad as 1.0°C (1.8°F). Fever (or hyperthermia) can be said to be present if the oral, basal body temperature exceeds 37.2°C (99.0°F) in the morning or 37.8°C (100.0°F) in the late afternoon or early evening. Rectal temperatures generally average about 0.5°C (0.9°F) higher than oral.

Basal metabolic processes, in particular these governed by the action of thyroid hormones, generate 55–75 kcal/h in healthy adults and are responsible for the normal resting body temperature. Thermogenesis may be increased by fivefold with moderate activity or following ingestion of a large meal; and transient rises in temperature are usually recorded until activation of heat-dissipating mechanisms return the temperature to baseline. Shivering can increase thermogenesis by two- to fivefold. Hyperthyroidism can increase and hypothyroidism decrease basal thermogenesis by as much as 80% and 50%, respectively. The actions of catecholamines and growth hormone can also increase thermogenesis. Age over 65 is associated with a moderate decrease in basal metabolism, and a lower body temperature (0.5°C on average) and the elderly may have blunted responses to catechols and thyroid hormone.

Exogenous heat may be gained from the environment by radiation, conduction or convection if the ambient temperature exceeds that of the body. Conversely, radiation accounts for about half of body heat loss and is modified by the ambient temperature, subcutaneous fat, peripheral blood flow, and clothing. Other mechanisms of heat loss involve conduction, convection, and vaporization. Vaporization in the lungs and from the skin (*insensible loss*) accounts for about 30% of body heat loss at rest. Heat loss by radiation and convection increases with vasodilation at ambient temperatures below that of the body. At high environmental temperatures, evaporation of sweat is the principal mechanism of heat loss and together with pulmonary water vaporization accounts for all heat loss at ambient dry temperatures greater than 36°C (96.8°F). Young adults may sweat up to 1.5–2.0 liters/h depending on training and acclimatization, thereby dissipating up to 900 kcal/h; elderly individuals can sweat at about one-half this rate. The cardiovascular system participates critically in heat dissipation through increases in cardiac output and cutanous vasodilation. Impairments in sweating or cardiovascular function can markedly reduce heat loss at high

**Table 9.1** Diseases causing fever

| |
|---|
| Infections |
| Inflammatory disorders |
| Immune disorders |
| Granulomatous disorders |
| Neoplastic disorders |
| Vascular disorders |
| Trauma or tissue infarction |
| Metabolic disorders |

ambient temperatures and can be factors leading to hyperthermia.

The central orchestration of heat-generating or heat-loss responses takes place in the hypothalamus, specifically in the anterior, preoptic area. This region contains temperature-sensitive neurons the firing rate of which controls heat-generating and -conserving responses (cold-sensitive neurons) or heat-dissipating responses (heat-sensitive neurons), respectively. Heat and cold receptors located in the skin, abdominal viscera, great veins, and spinal cord send impulses to the anterior preoptic region of the hypothalmus, thereby triggering heat-generating or -dissipating responses. This region is also sensitive to the temperature of blood that is bathing it. Coordination and integration of the thermoregulatory responses is achieved in the hypothalamus at a set point level that functions like a thermostat and determines the relative discharge rates of the cold- and heat-sensitive neurons. When heat-sensitive neuronal discharges predominate, cutaneous vasodilation and sweating occur, as well as behavioral changes to reduce activity and to seek a cooler environment. When the firing rates of the cold-sensitive neurons predominate, heat generation is increased through shivering and heat loss is reduced by diversion of cutaneous blood to core regions, piloerection ("goose pimples"), and behavioral attempts to seek a warmer environment or to add clothes or blankets. The hypothalamic set point varies over an average 0.55° (1.0°F) range during the day and is responsible for the circadian variation in temperature.

## Pathogenesis of Fever

### Physiologic events

The major manifestation of fever is an elevation of body temperature. Basal oral temperatures in excess of 37.2°C (99.0°F) in the morning and 37.8°C (100.0°F) in the evening should be considered as elevated. Temperature elevation is initiated by the upregulation of the hypothalamic set point in response to pyrogenic stimuli. Upregulation leads to an increase in the firing rate of cold-sensitive neurons, thereby activating the heat-conserving and -generating mechanisms discussed above. During the rising phase of fever, cutaneous blood flow is diverted to deep beds, sweating is decreased, the blood pressure and pulse rate all increase, reflecting increased sympathetic nerve system activity, which with shivering leads to an abrupt rise in the body temperature. There is often a sense of being cold ("chills") and a corresponding search for warmth under bedclothes and blankets. Other accompaniments of fever, listed in Table 9.2, can include malaise, somnolence, and anorexia; arthralgias and myalgias may also occur. A number of endocrine and metabolic events also take place during fever, as noted. When the new set point is reached, the equilibrium between heat generation and loss is reestablished at the higher body temperature. The patient may then be flushed and warm to the touch, and shivering ceases. Tachycardia remains and vasodilation replaces vasoconstriction.

If the thermoregulatory mechanisms are operating normally, the peak temperatures achieved in most fevers rarely exceed 41°C (105.8°F) (values above this are termed *hyperpyrexia*) and with many febrile conditions may be elevated to only 1.0° to 1.5°C (1.8°–2.7°F) above the baseline. The highest daily temperatures often occur at the peak of the baseline circadian rhythm—i.e., in the late afternoon or early evenings. Some febrile states are associated with a loss of the circadian temperature rhythm, and the circadian fluctuation of temperature during fever may also be obscured by the use of antipyretics.

During defervescence the hypothalamic set point falls toward normal, thereby triggering heat-loss mechanisms, principally sweating and a search for a cooler environment. Antipyretics do not lower baseline normal body temperatures, but serve to lower the elevated set point (Fig. 9.1). When they are used, the central responses to pyrogenic cytokines are blocked and heat-loss responses in the febrile patient predominate, with a fall in temperature toward normal values. If the pyrogenic stimulus remains when the antipyretic effect wears off, heat-generating and -conservation mechanisms will predominate, with return of all of the manifestations of fever. Intermittent use of antipyretics can induce a state of recurring chills, rigors, and fever interspersed with soaking sweats and defervescence, which may make some patients quite uncomfortable.

## Pyrogens

A list of known pyrogens involved in the pathogenesis of fever in humans and lower mammals is provided in Table 9.3. Also shown are endogenous substances that may serve to limit responses to pyrogens; they have been termed "cryogens" by some investigators, but since they do not lower basal temperatures, "antipyrogen" seems like a better term.

**Table 9.2** Components of the febrile state

| |
|---|
| AUTONOMIC |
| Shift in blood flow from cutaneous to deep beds |
| Increased pulse and blood pressure |
| Decreased sweating |
| BEHAVIORAL |
| Shivering (rigors) |
| Search for warmth (chills) |
| Anorexia |
| Somnolence |
| Malaise |
| ENDOCRINE AND METABOLIC |
| Increased production of glucocorticoids |
| Increased secretion of growth hormone |
| Increased secretion of aldosterone |
| Decreased secretion of vasopressin |
| Hypoferremia |
| Increased synthesis and secretion of acute-phase proteins |

Source: Adapted with permission from Saper CB, Breder CD. The interrelationship between systemic inflammatory response syndrome (SIRS), sepsis and infection. N Engl J Med 1994; 330:1880–1886.

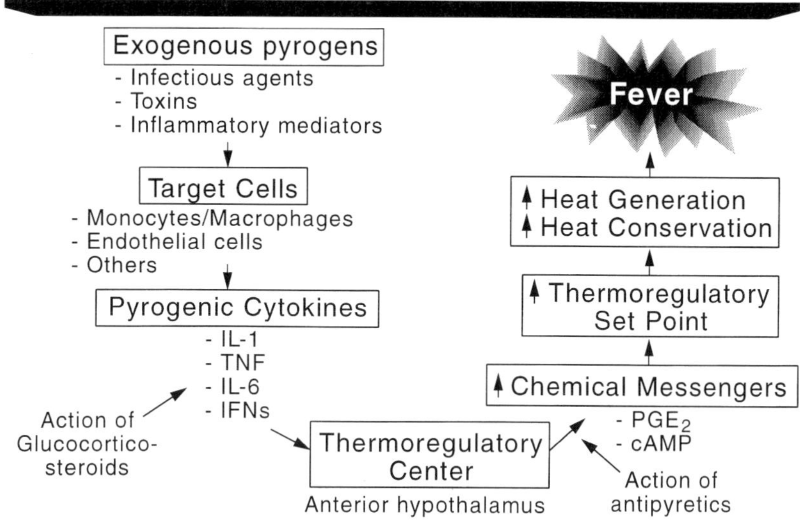


**Fig. 9.1** Sequences in fever induction.

### Exogenous pyrogens

These are substances which when administered intravenously or intramuscularly in sufficient dosage will predictably induce fever in the recipient. Microbes, in particular bacteria and viruses, or certain microbial products were the first exogenous pyrogens described. The lipopolysaccharide outer envelope (LPS or *endotoxin*) found universally in Gram-negative bacteria is one of the best-defined pyrogens with respect to structure–function relationships and mechanisms of action. The lipid A component of endotoxin is responsible for virtually all of the acute systemic responses to its administration, including fever, leukocytosis, coagulopathy, shock, and death. Neutralization of lipid A with antibodies or the antibiotic polymyxin B will abolish these effects (see Chapter 50). Good evidence exists that most of the systemic responses to endotoxin or lipid A are actually produced by secondary mediators released from host cells. Formation and release of these mediators are initiated when lipid A binds to responding host cells by a specific LPS-binding receptor, CD14.

Other microbial pyrogens that appear to act by analogous mechanisms include the pyrogenic exotoxins of *Staphylococcus aureus* and group A streptococci. These exotoxins can trigger pyrogenic cytokine release from the macrophages. In addition, in some patients these exotoxins bind directly to V beta portions of the antigen receptor on T cells (T3) and thus establish a link with the MHC locus of macrophages and other antigen-presenting cells. This linkage allows the exotoxins to function as so-called *superantigens*, triggering massive cytokine release and causing fever and shock (see Chapters 11 and 50). Bacterial cell wall peptidoglycans and mannans from the cell walls of fungi can also serve as pyrogenic stimuli; the precise mechanisms involved remain to be elucidated but also appear to involve cytokine intermediates.

Other substances that have been shown to be pyrogenic are components of immunological and inflammatory reactions, including antigen–antibody complexes and the C5a fragment of the complement system. Inflammatory bile acids, certain androgenic steroid metabolites, and crude products of necrotic tissue are also pyrogenic. While these substances may be endogenously derived, they differ from true *endogenous pyrogens* in their site and mechanisms of actions—i.e., all are pyrogenic through inducing secondary mediators of the febrile response.

**Table 9.3** Pyrogens and "antipyrogens" in the pathogenesis of fever

| |
|---|
| EXOGENOUS PYROGENS |
| Microbes |
| Microbial products |
| Lipopolysaccharide (endotoxin) |
| Pyrogenic exotoxins |
| Host-derived substances |
| Antigen–antibody complexes |
| Complement components |
| Inflammatory bile acids |
| Androgenic steroid metabolites |
| Products of tissue necrosis |
| ENDOGENOUS PYROGENS |
| Interleukin 1 |
| Tumor-necrosis factor alpha |
| Interferons |
| Interleukin 6 |
| Prostaglandins |
| ENDOGENOUS "ANTIPYROGENS" |
| Arginine vasopressin |
| Melanocyte-stimulating hormone |
| Cytokine inhibitors |
| IL 1 receptor antagonist |
| Soluble TNF receptors |
| Others? |

### Endogenous pyrogens

The stereotypic nature of febrile responses regardless of the stimulus used led to early speculation that an endogenous mediator or mediators were produced that actually triggered the resulting fever. Subsequently, a large body of work has demonstrated the role of endogenous mediators, including various cytokines, and arachidonate metabolites in the pathogenesis of both fever and other manifestations known collectively as the *acute phase response* (see Chapter 10).

Interleukin (IL-1) was the first endogenous pyrogen described and is one of the best-characterized pyrogenic cytokines. IL-1 is formed by a large variety of host cells, including such diverse types as leukocytes (predominantly macrophages), endothelial cells, renal mesangial cells, astrocytes, and keratinocytes. Two molecular forms have been defined: IL-1 alpha, which is minimally secreted, and IL-1 beta, which is secreted from appropriately stimulated cells and may be found in the circulation of febrile subjects given endotoxin or suffering from sepsis. Despite having a different primary structure, both forms of IL-1 can bind to specific IL-1 receptors, which are widely distributed among different cell types. Binding induces the acute phase and immunologic responses discussed in Chapters 10 and 11 as well as other responses, such as stimulation of fibroblast growth and activation of osteoclastic activity.

The availability of recombinant forms of IL-1 has permitted both the confirmation of its multiple biological effects as well as a clarification of its role in participating with other cytokines, specifically *tumor necrosis factor alpha* (TNF$\alpha$), *interleukin 6* (IL-6), and *interferon gamma* (IFN$\gamma$) in mediating the acute-phase response and fever. Intravenous injection of recombinant TNF, IL-6, or any of the interferons will produce fevers that are very similar in form and duration to those induced by IL-1. When the plasma of rabbits or man made febrile by injections of LPS is analyzed for the presence of these cytokines, they appear in a characteristic sequence: first TNF (within minutes), followed by IL-1 $\beta$ (within a half hour), then IFN$\gamma$ (after one hour). It is of interest that TNF can induce endothelial and other cells to release IL-1 and both IL-1 and TNF can induce lymphocytes to form and release IFN$\gamma$. Finally, IFN$\gamma$ can induce the expression of TNF receptors on a variety of cell types, thereby augmenting the activities of this inflammatory cytokine.

The pyrogenic cytokines appear to act by a common mechanism, involving the induction of prostaglandin synthesis—in particular, $PGE_2$ by responding cells. This prostanoid is found in increased amounts in the CSF of animals made febrile by injection of pyrogenic cytokines. Administration of cyclooxygenase inhibitors will block febrile responses to LPS or any of the recombinant cytokines by inhibiting $PGE_2$ synthesis. Application of pyrogenic cytokines to hypothalamic minces will induce $PGE_2$ formation, and intracisternal administration of $PGE_2$ induces a brisk febrile response in rabbits. Finally, a number of the other peripheral responses to the pyrogenic cytokines also appear to be mediated through $PGE_2$ production. Current evidence suggests that endothelial cells in the *organum vasculosum* adjacent to the preoptic area of the hypothalamus may be the principal source of $PGE_2$ that triggers the temperature set point change.

A number of regulatory steps for the production and action of pyrogenic cytokines have been defined. Both promoters (stimuli such as LPS or the cytokines themselves) and inhibitors of IL-1 and TNF formation (e.g., glucocorticoids) have been shown to act at the level of transcription of RNA in responding cells. As noted, inhibitors of cyclooxygenase (aspirin, NSAIDs) block pyrogenic cytokine action by preventing formation of $PGE_2$. Conversely, $PGE_2$ itself has been shown to inhibit IL-1 and TNF synthesis, thereby exerting a negative feedback regulation. Other factors induced by cytokine action may bind to IL-1 or TNF (*IL-1 receptor antagonist protein*, IL-1 RAP, and *soluble TNF receptors*, sTNFR, respectively), and block access to their cellular targets. IL-1 RAP was originally isolated from the urine of febrile subjects; sTNFR is found in the circulation of septic animals and patients. Pituitary hormones secreted during fever (ACTH and MSH) can also inhibit responses to pyrogens. ACTH acts through stimulating glucocorticoid release; MSH appears to act centrally, although a precise mechanism for its action remains to be defined. Finally, arginine vasopressin (AVP) has also been demonstrated to inhibit responses to both exogenous and endogenous pyrogens, presumably through a central mechanism. AVP levels decrease during the rising phase of fever. The existence and operation of so many regulating factors for inflammatory cytokine production and action emphasize the highly orchestrated nature of fever as just one component of the acute-phase and immunologic responses to infection.

## Effects of Fever on Host–Microbe Interactions

Fever as a response to infection is exhibited by invertebrates and poikilothermic vertebrates as well as all endothermic animals, and forms of IL-1 and TNF have been isolated from all animal species. This suggests that fever and its responsible cytokines evolved phylogenetically hundreds of millions of years ago as a means of enhancing host defenses against infection. In poikilotherms infection leads to heat-seeking behavior, which if prevented results in a generalized inhibition of the inflammatory response and increased mortality. Pharmacologic suppression of fever may result in increased mortality to viral or bacterial infections in some mammalian species. In man the failure to develop fever during severe bacterial infection has been associated with higher morbidity and mortality in some clinical studies. These observations suggest that temperature elevation per se may have favorable effects on host–microbe interactions beyond the actions of cytokines.

Febrile temperatures could alter microbial viability or susceptibility to host defense mechanisms or enhance host defenses. Evidence for all three effects has been obtained in a variety of in vitro studies (Table 9.4). Multiplication of some pathogens (e.g., *Streptococcus pneumoniae* and *Treponema pallidum*) is inhibited at febrile temperatures. Others may become more sus-

**Table 9.4** Effects of febrile temperatures on host–microbe interactions

| |
|---|
| ANTIMICROBIAL EFFECTS[a] |
| Inhibition of replication (some organisms) |
| Enhancement of complement-mediated lysis |
| Enhancement of susceptibility to some antibiotics |
| Enhancement of hypoferremic effect on growth inhibition |
| EFFECTS ON HOST DEFENSE |
| Enhanced survival from infection (some species) |
| Augmented lymphocyte responses[a] |
|   Mitogenesis |
|   Production of IL-2 |
|   Antibody production by B cells |
| Augmented neutrophil responses |
|   Entry into inflammatory sites |
|   Motility in vitro[a] |
|   Bactericidal activity[a] |
| Augmented macrophage responses[a] |
|   Oxidative metabolism |
| Production and actions of the interferons[a] |

[a]Effects demonstrated in vitro only.

ceptible to lysis by complement or antimicrobials. Proliferation of some microbes is impaired by hypoferremia, an action in vivo of the pyrogenic cytokines; this impairment is more pronounced at higher temperatures and can be related to reduced microbial synthesis of iron-chelating proteins. Human neutrophil function in vitro is enhanced at 40°C (104.0°F) and reduced at hypothermic temperatures. Macrophage oxidative metabolism is increased at 40°C (104.0°F). These enhancements are lost at higher temperatures, and in fact exposure to temperatures above 42°C (107.6°F) is eventually cytotoxic. The antiviral and antitumor actions of interferons as well as their production are increased at febrile temperatures. Finally, elements of the specific immune response may be augmented at febrile temperatures, including IL-1–induced T-cell activation and IL-2 production as well as T-cell help for production of immunoglobulins by B cells.

The investigations with various animal models in vivo and human immune and inflammatory cells in vitro support a beneficial role for fever during acute infection and in stimulating the immune response. It is more difficult however, to translate this into benefit for man during most established infections, or conversely into a clear conclusion that inhibition of fever by antipyretic measures may be deleterious.

## Hyperthermia

Hyperthermia is elevation of body temperature above that established by the hypothalamic set point and occurs when heat-generating and -conserving responses exceed the effects of heat dissipation. Hyperthermia can be caused by excessive heat production, diminished heat dissipation, or loss of regulatory function by the hypothalamus (Table 9.5). Neither the height nor pattern of temperature elevation can clearly distinguish fever from hyperthermia; however, the clinical situation will usually provide a diagnostic clue. Any temperature in excess of 41.1°C (106.0°F), regardless of the cause, usually implies disordered thermoregulatory mechanisms.

**Table 9.5** Causes of hyperthermia

| |
|---|
| DISORDERS OF EXCESSIVE HEAT PRODUCTION |
| Exertional hyperthermia |
| Exertional heatstroke[a] |
| Malignant hyperthermia of anesthesia |
| Neuroleptic malignant syndrome[a] |
| Lethal catatonia |
| Thyrotoxicosis |
| Pheochromocytoma |
| Salicylate intoxication |
| Drug abuse (e.g., cocaine and amphetamines) |
| Delirium tremens |
| Status epilepticus |
| Generalized tetanus |
| DISORDERS OF DIMINISHED HEAT DISSIPATION |
| Classic heatstroke[a] |
| Extensive use of occlusive dressings |
| Dehydration |
| Autonomic dysfunction |
| Use of anticholinergic agents |
| Neuroleptic malignant syndrome[a] |
| DISORDERS OF HYPOTHALAMIC FUNCTION |
| Neuroleptic malignant syndrome[a] |
| Cerebrovascular accidents |
| Encephalitis |
| Sarcoidosis and granulomatous infections |
| Trauma |

[a]Mixed pathogenesis.

Source: Adapted with permission from Simon HB. Hyperthermia. New Engl J Med 1993; 329:483–487.

### Exertional hyperthermia

This is the most common condition that gives rise to hyperthermia. During vigorous exercise skeletal muscles can increase their energy consumption by as much as 20-fold, about 75% of which may be converted to heat produced from cleavage of ATP. Heat dissipation by cutanous vasodilation (radiation) and sweating are impaired by high ambient temperatures and humidity. Vasodilation may also be impaired by volume depletion. Hyperthermia is an almost universal occurrence with intense prolonged exercise in a warm, humid environment; for example, temperatures of marathoners commonly reach 39° and 40°C (102.2° to 104.0°F) rectally by the conclusion of a race.

The clinical consequences of exertional hyperthermia can include *heat exhaustion* and *heatstroke*. Heat exhaustion results from fluid and electrolyte depletion with profuse sweating and is usually characterized by extreme fatigue, dizziness or lightheadedness, near syncope, nausea, and muscle cramps. It will usually respond promptly to rest in a cool environment and administration of cool fluids orally. Exertional heatstroke results from a failure of heat loss mechanisms after prolonged vigorous exercise in very warm, humid weather. While the use of anticholinergic or beta-blocking drugs may predispose to this complication by interfering with heat loss during exercise, most of the victims are young and healthy. Lack of acclimatization, poor cardiovascular conditioning, excessively warm clothes, and fluid depletion are predisposing factors in the warm environment. Heatstroke is characterized by its acute onset, extremely high temperatures, usually in excess of 40°C (104.0°F), absence of sweating, tachycardia, hypotension, hyperventilation, and altered mental status. Laboratory studies may reveal hemoconcentration, leukocytosis, proteinuria, hematuria and azotemia, elevated muscle enzymes, coagulopathy, and respiratory alkalosis or metabolic acidosis. (Many of these are manifestations of the *systemic inflammatory response syndrome* (SIRS), which is discussed in Chapter 50.) The recognition and proper management of heatstroke constitute a medical emergency; otherwise, development of fatal *multiple organ failure* can result.

### Classic heatstroke

While exertional heat syndromes are relatively easy to recognize and treat, other conditions that give rise to hyperthermia may not be easily differentiated from those causing true fever. For example, *classic heatstroke* usually affects the sedentary elderly or the very young who are unable to care for themselves. These are often the same individuals who are prone to severe infections and sepsis. Besides a warm environment, predisposing factors include neurological disorders with impaired consciousness, cardiovascular diseases, and the use of medication with anticholinergic (e.g., tricyclic antidepressants, phenothiazines, antihistamines) beta-blocking or diuretic effects. The clinical and laboratory manifestations are often difficult to differentiate from SIRS caused by infection (*sepsis* or *septic shock*; see Chapter 50). Besides measures to replace volume and to cool the patient, systemic antibiotic administration after obtaining appropriate cultures is usually indicated. Despite appropriate therapy, the mortality rate from heatstroke remains high, often exceeding 10%.

### Hyperthermia caused by drug intoxication or withdrawal

Other common medical conditions that can give rise to acute hyperthermia and may be difficult to distinguish from sepsis include drug withdrawal, in particular delirium tremens, and cocaine or amphetamine intoxication. In each case, heat generation is excessive and heat dissipation diminished through overstimulation of the sympathetic nervous system. Eliciting the history of drug or alcohol use as well as using toxicological screening are key to making the correct diagnosis.

### Endocrine disorders and hyperthermia

Thyroid storm and pheochromocytoma are rare but distinctive endocrinological causes of acute hyperthermia. Both conditions increase the basal metabolic rate, and in the case of pheochromocytoma, intense vasoconstriction impairs heat loss. Hyperthyroid storm is usually precipitated by stress (e.g., surgery or infection) and accompanied by other manifestations of hyperthyroidism (e.g., exopthalmos or weight loss or supraventricular tachycardias). Besides occasionally causing hyperthermia, marked hypertension is characteristic of the discharge of catecholamines from a pheochromocytoma.

### Neuroleptic malignant syndrome and malignant hyperthermia

Conditions in which repetitive or sustained muscle contraction give rise to hyperthermia include grand mal seizures, particularly status epilepticus, generalized tetanus or catatonia, and two unique disorders, the *neuroleptic malignant syndrome* (NMS) and *malignant hyperthermia* (MH). In addition to persistent muscle contraction that generates increased heat, hypothalamic dysfunction and vasoconstriction from sympathetic discharge may contribute to the hyperthermia. NMS is so named because it is an idiosyncratic response to the administration of neuroleptics. More than 25 drugs have been found to have the potential to cause NMS, with the most frequently reported being butyrophenones (e.g., Haldol), phenothiazines, and thioxanthines (e.g., Navane). Lithium administration and, rarely, withdrawal of dopaminergic agents in Parkinson's disease may also precipitate NMS. The mechanism for development of NMS involves dopaminergic blockade at several sites: centrally in the striatum, which leads to muscle rigidity, and in the hypothalamus, which alters thermoregulatory responses; and peripherally, by interfering with dopamine-induced muscle relaxation.

NMS occurs more frequently in men (2:1), in patients starting therapy at high dosages or with depot neuroleptic drugs, and in those who are dehydrated, agitated, or confused. In many patients the onset of symptoms is delayed until 4 to 5 days into treatment with escalating drug dosages. Besides the febrile psychiatric patient, other clinical settings for NMS can include the patient with preoperative or postoperative fever, given neuroleptics as premedication or sedation, the postoperative combative patient, or the patient using phenothiazine antiemetics. Typical features include hyperthermia, with temperatures sometimes exceeding 41°C (105.8°F), and increased muscle tone, manifest as rigidity, cogwheeling, or, less commonly, as akinesia or dyskinesia. Dysautonomic signs include pallor, diaphoresis, tachycardias, or dysrhythmias (80%–90%), and blood pressure fluctuations (55% to 80%). Mental status changes, including coma, confusion, and agitation, occur in more than 50% of affected patients. Sustained muscle contraction can lead to rhabdomyolysis; elevation of creatine kinase levels is common. Other laboratory abnormalities include leukocytosis and left shift (70% to 80%), abnormal liver function tests, coagulopathies, hypophosphatemia, increased creatinine and urea nitrogen, and myoglobinuria. Elevated CSF protein without pleiocytosis is characteristic. These abnormalities may be similar to those seen in sepsis or heatstroke; the clinical circumstances and the muscle rigidity provide the diagnostic cue.

The treatment of NMS involves recognition of the syndrome, excluding sepsis or other diagnoses, stopping the neuroleptic(s), providing general fluid and cardiovascular support as needed, administering antipyretics, providing physical cooling for temperatures in excess of 41°C (105.8°F), and reversing muscle rigidity and dysautonomia pharmacologically. Centrally acting dopamine agonists that have been successfully employed to treat NMS include bromocriptine (2.5 to 10 mg orally three times per day), Carbidopa-levodopa (25/250 mg orally three to four times per day), and amantadine (100–200 mg orally two times per day). Muscle relaxation can be achieved by administering dantrolene, 2–3 mg/kg per day, orally, in divided doses or intravenously. Dantrolene acts at the level of the sarcoplasmic reticulum by inhibiting calcium release. Muscle relaxation and resolution of other extrapyramidal symptoms is usually achieved within the first 24 hours; defervescence may take several days.

*Malignant hyperthermia* (MH) is an acute hypermetabolic syndrome characterized by muscle rigidity and high fever in patients administered either potent inhalation anesthetics, depolarizing muscle relaxants (e.g., succinyl choline), or both. The cause of the syndrome is excessive release of calcium from the sarcoplasmic reticulum, which initiates both muscular contraction and mitochondrial hypermetabolism and leads to muscle rigidity, increased heat production, ATP depletion, metabolic acidosis, and eventually "energy crisis." Susceptibility to MH is inherited as an autosomal-dominant trait, and a positive family history for similar episodes is often elicited. Some patients have a defect in the ryanodine receptor of the major calcium-release channel of the sarcoplasmic reticulum, while others have altered muscle phospholipase A2 activity, indicating the multifactorial nature of the mechanisms that control calcium release. Musculoskeletal abnormalities are seen in up to two-thirds of all patients with MH, and patients with some neuromuscular disorders (e.g., myotonic and other forms of dystrophy) appear to have a high frequency of MH-like events following anesthetic administration.

While almost all anesthetics have been implicated in triggering the syndrome in susceptible patients, halothanes with or without the use of succinyl choline predominate. MH typically begins shortly after administration of the agent, but in some cases the onset may be delayed for up to 11 hours. Up to half of the patients may have had previous general anesthesia without developing MH. Patients may fail to relax upon the administration of succinyl choline or develop progressive rigidity during general anesthesia. Many patients develop arrhythmias and hypertension. Fever develops in only about a third of patients with MH, but when it occurs it is often extreme, with temperatures of as high as 45°C (113.0°F) having been reported. Laboratory abnormalities include lactic acidosis, hyperkalemia, hyperphosphatemia, elevations of CK, renal failure, and myoglobinuria (all due to rhabdomyolysis). Leukocytosis and left shift are common, as is disseminated intravascular coagulation.

Left untreated, the mortality rate from MH may reach 70%; its recognition and prompt therapy constitute a medical emergency. General treatment consists of prompt discontinuation of the anesthesia, correction of the hypoxia and metabolic disorders, and cardiovascular support. In hyperthermic patients physical cooling with ice packs or evaporative methods until the temperature falls below 39°C (102.2°F) is recommended. The use of antipyretics to treat MH is controversial and not likely to be of significant benefit. The cornerstone of therapy for MH is the administration of dantrolene at an initial dosage of 2.5 mg/kg intravenously, with repeat dosing of 2.5 mg/kg at 6 hour intervals up to a total dose of 10 mg/kg until muscle relaxation and resolution of the syndrome is achieved. Given appropriate treatment, the mortality of MH is less than 7%.

Identification of MH-susceptible individuals is possible by a functional assay on biopsied skeletal muscle or in about 50% of cases by documentation of elevated serum CK values. Individuals who have a family history of anesthetic deaths or high fevers, and those with neuromuscular disorders, are candidates for evaluations, as are those who have had anesthetic complications that might suggest MH. In the MH-susceptible patient who must undergo surgery, nontriggering agents should be used for anesthesia (barbiturates, narcotics, nitrous oxide, pancuronium or vecuronium.)

## Hypothermia

Not all patients with acute or chronic infections develop fever, and paradoxically some patients with sepsis or septic shock will be hypothermic. Both neonates and the very elderly appear to be less likely to develop fever with bacteremias. For example, in a study of 187 episodes of pneumococcal bacteremia in adults, 29% of the elderly were afebrile. In another study of bacteremias complicating pneumonia, urinary tract infection, peritonitis, cholangitis, or cellulitis in which all the patients were afebrile, most were over the age of 65. Multiple mechanisms could explain the apparently decreased febrile responses in elderly patients. As noted in Table 9.6, hypothermia (or absent febrile responses) could be the consequence of pathologic conditions causing decreased heat production, increased heat loss, or impaired thermoregulation. In addition, elderly (or neonatal) patients could have diminished responses to exogenous pyrogens at the level of generation of pyrogenic cytokines or hypothalamic responses to their action. More data are needed to clarify the precise mechanisms responsible for the clinical observations, but they point out the need to rely on signs other than fever to indicate infection in patients who are at the extremes of age.

In patients who exhibit poor febrile responses to major infections, it is also important to consider the possibility of the existence of a medical condition or conditions that may inhibit pyrogenic responses, as noted in Table 9.6. This is particularly true for patients with hypothyroidism, hypopituitarism, or hypoadrenalism, in whom severe infection is often the precipitating stress for critical acute endocrinological failure. Other patients who are notorious for not developing significant fevers or becoming hypothermic when infected are those with protein-caloric malnutrition, burned patients, those with diffuse erythrodermas, or those with uremia. Very ill patients in the acute stages of severe trauma are often hypothermic for a multiplicity of reasons; they are at high risk for infections complicating their in-

**Table 9.6** Factors predisposing to hypothermia

| |
|---|
| DECREASED HEAT PRODUCTION |
| *ENDOCRINOLOGIC FAILURE* |
| Hypothyroidism |
| Hypopituitarism |
| Hypoadrenalism |
| *INSUFFICIENT FUEL* |
| Hypoglycemia |
| Protein calorie malnutrition |
| Marathon exertion |
| Toxicologic |
| *NEUROMUSCULAR INEFFICIENCY* |
| Impaired shivering |
| Inactivity |
| Toxicologic |
| INCREASED HEAT LOSS |
| *ENVIRONMENTAL* |
| Immersion |
| Nonimmersion |
| *INDUCED VASODILATATION* |
| Pharmacologic |
| Toxicologic |
| *SKIN DISORDERS* |
| Burns |
| Diffuse erythroderms |
| Ichthyosis |
| Iatrogenic |
| IMPAIRED THERMOREGULATION |
| *PERIPHERAL FAILURE* |
| Neuropathies |
| Acute spinal cord transection |
| *METABOLIC* |
| Diabetes |
| Anorexia nervosa |
| Toxicologic |
| *CENTRAL FAILURE* |
| CNS trauma |
| Cardiovascular accident |
| Subarachnoid hemorrhage |
| Hypothalamic dysfunction |
| Neoplasm |
| Granulomatous lesion |
| Multiple sclerosis |
| Parkinsonism |
| MULTIPLE MECHANISMS |
| *SYSTEMIC INFLAMMATORY RESPONSE SYNDROME* |
| Sepsis |
| Hemorrhagic pancreatitis |
| Massive trauma |
| Shock |
| *CARDIOVASCULAR DISEASE* |
| Carcinomatosis |
| Uremia |

Source: Adapted with permission from Harchelroad F. Acute thermoregulatory disorders. Clin Geriatric Med 1993; 9:621–39.

juries or management, a fact that may be obscured by the lack of a febrile response (see Chapter 84).

Finally, another group of patients in whom severe infection is often coupled with hypothermia are those found in an obtunded or comatose state either outside or in an unheated dwelling. Neurological impairments of many types, including cranial trauma, intracranial bleeds or strokes, and drug or carbon monoxide intoxication, can all disrupt thermoregulatory mechanisms and impair shivering responses to falling body temperatures. In addition, alcohol intoxication may be a complicating factor that can accelerate heat loss through vasodilation. In one study at a general city hospital, 50% of patients admitted with exposure-induced hypothermia had severe infections, predominantly sepsis or pneumonia. In such patients, complete evaluation for systemic infection and empirical broad-spectrum antimicrobial treatment are indicated as part of the initial management.

## Treatment of Fever and Hyperthermia

Proper treatment of fever should be focused on specific therapy for its cause whenever available. Resolution of fever as a manifestation of the therapeutic effect of an antibiotic is one of the more reassuring aspects of managing infections. Since fever per se is rarely dangerous to the patient and may in fact be beneficial to the balance between an invading microbe and host defense mechanisms, antipyretic therapy for infections should not be initiated automatically. Consideration should be directed toward the need to reduce fever versus its value as a marker of the therapeutic response to specific antimicrobial therapy. A further potential drawback of vigorous antipyretic therapy is that it may obscure complications or delay a needed antimicrobial change in patients not responding to treatment. In contrast to infectious causes of fever, the primary therapy of inflammatory conditions that give rise to fever often requires the use of agents that have both anti-inflammatory and antipyretic properties. Resolution of fever in these cases often coincides with diminishing inflammation and provides evidence that the condition is responding to treatment.

General management of febrile patients involves rest and the administration of hypotonic fluids. Insensible losses of water increase by as much as 1000 ml/day in adults for each 2°C (3.6°F) temperature elevation, due to increased metabolic rates. With sweating there will be further losses of hypotonic fluid containing small amounts of sodium. If the febrile patient is also losing fluids from the gastrointestinal tract, then these losses should also be estimated and replaced with fluids containing sodium and potassium. Maintenance of a replete plasma volume assists normal thermoregulatory mechanisms, in addition to its role in cardiovascular support.

### Selection of patients for antipyretic therapy

With the exception of hyperpyrexia or hyperthermia causing very high body temperatures, there are few absolute indications for using antipyretics or physical means to lower temperature. Patients with neurological disorders or complications, or those with cardiovascular disease, and perhaps pregnant women are exceptions (Table 9.7). Delirium, obtundation, and, rarely, seizures may be seen in patients with fever. If the fever is very high (>41.1°C [106.0°F]), concern can be raised about brain injury or damage. While encephalopathy can develop as a consequence of sustained hyperthermia, the likelihood of its occurrence is quite low and most specific neurologic abnormalities seen during fever are due either to the causative disease or to exacerbation of underlying defects. Some children may experience self-limited seizures, typically during the early phases of temperature elevation with a fever. In the vast majority of these patients there is no evidence of organic brain disease or sequelae, and in many these episodes do not recur. Early administration of antipyretics does not prevent recurrences, and while anticonvulsants may prevent subsequent episodes the lack of serious consequences from febrile seizures militates against their use for long-term treatment. Other patients with organic brain disease may exhibit obtundation or worsening of their neurological defects during fever. While it is not clear that it is the temperature elevation per se that causes this phenomenon as opposed to a central action of some of the pyrogenic cytokines, these patients appear to benefit from pharmacological antipyresis.

Patients who have cardiovascular disease, in particular coronary disease, may not tolerate the hypermetabolic state that accompanies fever. Besides developing tachycardia in response to increased sympathetic nervous system stimuli, cardiac work has been estimated to increase by 15%–20% with each 1°C (1.8°F) elevation in temperature during fever, particularly during the rising or stable phases of temperature elevation. Pharmacologic antipyresis is indicated in this patient population, particularly if they become more symptomatic with temperature elevation. Unless they are hyperthermic or hyperpyrexic, physical cooling should be generally avoided in this group, because they may provoke shivering and vasoconstriction, thereby increasing cardiac work

**Table 9.7** Treatment of fever and hyperthermia

| |
|---|
| INDICATIONS FOR THERAPY |
| Hyperpyrexia (Temperature >41°C, 106°F) |
| Central nervous system disorder |
| Cardiovascular disease |
| Pregnancy |
| Comfort? |
| GENERAL SUPPORT |
| Fluids |
| Rest |
| PHARMACOLOGIC ANTYPYRESIS |
| Aspirin (325–650 mg q4–6h PO up to 4 g/day)[a] |
| Acetaminophen (Paracetamol) (325–650 mg q4–6h PO up to 4 g day)[a] |
| NSAIDs |
| Ibuprofen (200–400 mg q4–6h PO up to 3600 mg g/day)[a] |
| Indomethacin (25–50 mg q6–8h PO up to 200 mg/day)[a] |
| Naproxen (250 mg q6–8h PO up to 1250 mg/day)[a] |
| Glucocorticosteroids |
| Hydrocortisone (25–50 mg IM or IVq4–6h up to 250 mg/day)[b] |
| Inhibition of shivering |
| Meperidine (25–50 mg IM, IV or SC q4–6h as needed)[a] |
| Morphine sulfate (2.5–5 mg q4h IV, IM, or SC as needed)[a] |
| PHYSICAL COOLING |
| Contact |
| Cooling blanket or mattress |
| Ice packs |
| Immersion |
| Evaporation |
| Core cooling |

[a]Adult dosages.

[b]Not generally recommended as an antipyretic (see text).

and the potential for further complications. Fetal malformations or spontaneous abortions have been ascribed to fever occurring in the mother. In retrospective human studies it has been difficult to separate effects due to fever from those due to causative infections, and in at least one prospective study no excess in fetal malformations was seen in women reporting high fever during the first trimester.

The most common reason for treating fever is patient "comfort." In many patients the discomfort of a febrile illness is greatest during the rising phase of fever, when the patient is experiencing chills and rigors. Patients with stable temperature elevations may not experience much discomfort. The common practice of administering antipyretics only after the temperature has risen beyond a certain value will occasionally precipitate abrupt defervescence with profuse sweating and rarely hypotension. This may create more discomfort than before, particularly after the antipyretic effect wears off and the patient redevelops fever with chills and rigors. The malaise and myalgias that occur during febrile illnesses have been ascribed to the action of proteases that are active in mobilizing amino acids from muscle, a cyclooxygenase-dependent process. In experimental studies in subjects administered endotoxin, blockade of these symptoms occurred only if aspirin, NSAIDs, or glucocorticoids were administered before the endotoxin. Thus, administration of antipyretics may give broad symptomatic relief, which should be most noticeable if administered *before* marked temperature elevation. For an optimal effect, antipyretics should be continued on a regular basis until other manifestations of the illness have resolved or improved, at which point antipyretic therapy can be discontinued.

## Antipyretic drugs

Most antipyretics have as a major locus of their action the hypothalamus, where they promote a resetting of the "thermostat," presumably by inhibiting synthesis of prostaglandins (Fig. 9.1). Inhibition of prostaglandin synthesis peripherally also makes most of these drugs effective analgesics and, to a variable degree, antiinflammatory agents. An exception to this rule are the glucocorticosteroids, which have generally minor effects on inhibiting central prostaglandin synthesis but act peripherally to block production of TNF and IL-1, as well as the entrance of neutrophils into inflammatory sites. The glucocorticosteroids also have the most potent antiinflammatory actions of the antipyretics and are used extensively to treat a variety of inflammatory and immune disorders. Because of their broad immunosuppressive and antiinflammatory properties, a major complication of high-dose glucocorticoid therapy is secondary infection with opportunistic organisms (see Chapter 87). Glucocorticoids are therefore not generally used as antipyretics.

Aspirin and acetaminophen have been used as antipyretics and analgesics for over 100 years; more recently, a proliferating array of NSAIDs have been marketed for this purpose. Aspirin and the NSAIDs are potent inhibitors of cyclooxygenase peripherally and centrally; acetaminophen (paracetamol) may be more selective in inhibiting brain cyclooxygenase. All of these agents can block the development of fever to various pyrogenic stimuli or cause defervescence in a wide variety of species. While ibuprofen and other NSAIDS are more potent antipyretics than aspirin or acetaminophen on a weight basis, all appear to be about equally potent in their antipyretic actions in humans with standard dosages. Thus, the selection of a particular antipyretic is usually based on its potential for causing adverse effects.

With the exception of the glucocorticosteroids, none of the antipyretic drugs have been convincingly shown to have an adverse effect on infection outcome. However, there have been case reports of the sudden development of fulminant soft-tissue infections in patients taking NSAIDs. Aspirin and the NSAIDs at standard dosages have predictable activities against platelet cyclooxygenase, which can inhibit aggregation and may promote excessive bleeding with trauma. Aspirin in high doses can inhibit prothrombin formation, thereby further disrupting normal coagulation mechanisms. Both aspirin and the NSAIDs can have adverse effects on the gastrointestinal tract: aspirin can be directly cytotoxic to gastric cells; NSAIDs can inhibit gastric and duodenal cytoprotective mechanisms and increase the likelihood of gastritis or peptic ulcer disease. The use of both aspirin and the NSAIDs should be avoided in patients at high risk for upper gastrointestinal bleeding or ulceration. NSAIDs can variably inhibit renal blood flow, another prostaglandin-regulated function, and reduce renal function as well as cause sodium and fluid retention. Edema formation and precipitating or worsening congestive heart or renal failure may occur. Unless there are strong specific indications for their antiinflammatory properties, NSAIDs should not be used routinely for antipyresis in patients with these medical conditions. For similar reasons, they should also be used with caution in elderly patients. NSAIDs have become preferred drugs for the relief of mild to moderate inflammatory conditions, including gouty arthritis, in which fever might be a manifestation. They may also be more effective than other antipyretics in relieving the myalgias that can accompany fever.

The development of Reye's syndrome following influenza, varicella, or other viral infections in children has been attributed to aspirin. This has led to the widespread use of acetaminophen for fever and analgesia by most pediatricians and many who care for adult patients. The major negative effect of acetaminophen is its potential for causing severe hepatotoxicity in overdosage. Patients who have liver disease, who are heavy imbibers of alcohol, or who are taking other hepatotoxic drugs should avoid acetaminophen for antipyresis and analgesia.

Besides the administration of antipyretics to reduce fever, it may be desirable at times to inhibit shivering and its effects on heat generation. Administration of meperedine or morphine sulfate in low to moderate dosages (Table 9.7) is effective for this purpose. Patients given these compounds should be monitored for hypotension.

## Physical antipyresis

Physical methods of lowering body temperatures should generally be reserved for those patients who have life-threatening temperature elevation or for treating fever at high ambient temperatures. The patient who develops fever is already reacting as if the environmental temperature is too low, and placing such patients on cooling blankets will greatly exacerbate chills, rigors, and the feeling of discomfort. Several studies have shown that sponging children with tepid water after the administration of antipyretics did not speed defervescence and only added to their discomfort.

When it is necessary to rapidly reduce body temperature, as in the treatment of heatstroke or hyperpyrexia (temperatures in excess of 41.1°C [106.0° F]), physical cooling is the treatment of choice rather than antipyretics. In these patients, monitoring of core temperatures should be continuous, aiming for a cooling rate of >0.1°C (0.18°F)/min and cooling measures should be continued until a target temperature of 38.5°C is achieved.

Drastic and impractical methods such as plunging the patient into an ice bath, while capable of promoting cooling at the desired rate, have largely been replaced by those that promote evaporation and convection. Evaporation of 1 g of water consumes seven times as much heat as the melting of 1 g of ice. Under proper conditions, shivering and vasoconstriction can be eliminated and patient temperatures may drop at a rate of 0.31°C/min. In the absence of special units to promote evaporative cooling, simple methods that employ tepid water and a fan would appear to be preferable to ice applications or even cooling blankets. Other methods of inducing rapid cooling are either too cumbersome and impractical (e.g., iced peritoneal lavage or cardiopulmonary bypass) or have not been shown to be as effective (iced gastric lavage, cold intravenous fluids, iced enemas, cold humidified oxygen) as evaporative techniques.

Additional management of patients with heatstroke or hyperpyrexia includes judicious monitoring of fluid administration. Many of these patients may be hypotensive when initially seen; hypotension is often the consequence of vasodilation and high-output cardiac failure. The primary management of this complication is cooling; alpha-agonistic drugs should be avoided, because they will interfere with the cooling process by causing vasoconstriction. With redistribution of fluid from the periphery during cooling, volume overload may occur if the administration of fluids has been undertaken too aggressively.

## Treatment of Hypothermia

Patients with accidental hypothermia may have complicating infection, and conversely sepsis may trigger a hypothermic response (<36°C [95.0°F]) in some individuals. Thus, evaluation of hypothermic patients for infection as well as combined management of infection and hypothermia are often necessary. Appropriate radiologic procedures and culturing of blood, urine, and other sites must be done on hypothermic patients. If the patient has been lying or sitting in one position for a long period of time, the development of skin necrosis or compartment syndromes and aspiration pneumonia should be considered. Administration of broad-spectrum antibiotics (modified as needed for a suspected site of infection) should be part of the initial management of almost all hypothermic patients, particularly if they have other manifestations of sepsis or are victims of prolonged exposure to cool ambient temperatures. Initial management should focus on airway control using endotracheal intubation in any obtunded patient, cardiac monitoring for atrial or ventricular arrhythmias (common below temperatures of 32°C [89.6°F]), and intravenous isotonic fluids (not lactated Ringer's solution because of impaired hepatic lactate clearance). Pressors should generally be avoided because of their arrhythmic potential and marked prolongation of half-life in the hypothermic liver. Most atrial arrhythmias will revert spontaneously upon warming the patient; ventricular arrhythmias are treated sparingly with electroshock and CPR, as needed, below core temperatures of 30°C (86.0°F), while instituting active rewarming. Procainamide should be avoided as an antiarrhythmic agent in the hypothermic patient; the preferred agent for treating ventricular arrhythmias is bretylium or magnesium sulfate.

Rewarming the hypothermic patient is an essential part of management. Rewarming techniques can be either passive or active, depending on the degree of the hypothermia. For most adults with body temperatures over 32°C (89.6°F) who are capable of generating sufficient heat through basal metabolism, passive rewarming is sufficient. This should include placement of the patient at an ambient temperature of >21°C (69.8°F), ideally in a high-humidity environment, and covering with blankets to prevent further heat loss. These measures will allow gradual rewarming at a rate of 0.5°–2.0°C (0.9°–3.6°F)/hr in appropriately selected patients. In older or malnourished patients this rate may be reduced due to glycogen depletion, volume depletion, or cardiovascular disease. Other patients who fail to respond to these simple measures may have thyroid, adrenal, or pituitary insufficiency.

Active rewarming involves the direct transfer of heat to the patient and may require either external or internal methods. These methods should be reserved for patients who have moderate to severe hypothermia (body temperatures <32°C [89.6°F]), who have cardiovascular or endocrine disorders leading to hypothermia, who do not respond to initial rewarming methods, or who have traumatic or toxicologic hypothermia. Active rewarming may be accomplished by the external application of heat sources or core-rewarming methods. If external heating is applied, it should be centered on the thorax while allowing vasoconstriction of the extremities to conserve body heat.

External rewarming is not nearly as effective as core rewarming using heated (up to 42°C [107.6°F]), humidified oxygen, usually delivered by ventilator after intubating the patient. As water vapor condenses and cools to the current core temperature, heat is yielded; the amount delivered can be increased by increasing the ventilation rate. Administration of heated intravenous fluids is not effective in rewarming and should be avoided. Warm peritoneal lavage can transfer up to 2°–3°C° (3.6°–5.4°F)/hr using a dialysate at 40°–45°C (104°–113°F). Other methods for rapid core rewarming include cardiopulmonary bypass, hemodialysis, and continuous arteriovenous rewarming using femoral arterial and venous catheters connected to a countercurrent fluid warmer. These approaches should generally be reserved for the most serious cases in whom simpler methods have failed or who have severe electrolyte disturbances from rhabdomyolysis. The complications of rapid rewarming from severe hypothermia can include pulmonary edema, hemolysis, DIC, and acute tubular necrosis; the outcome is usually related to the degree of hypothermia and the presence of underlying medical conditions.

## ANNOTATED BIBLIOGRAPHY

Dinarello CA, Cannon JG, Wolff SM. New concepts in the pathogenesis of fever. Rev Infect Dis 1988; 10:168–189.

*An excellent review of the state of knowledge through 1987 stressing the role of cytokines and prostaglandins and the mechanisms of their action in producing fever.*

Harchelroad F. Acute thermoregulatory disorders. Clin Geriatr Med 1993; 9:621–639.

*An up-to-date review that focuses on hyperthermic and hypothermic syndromes and their recognition, pathogenetic mechanisms, and management in elderly patients.*

Heiman-Patterson TD. Neuroleptic malignant syndrome and malignant hyperthermia. Important issues for the medical consultant. Med Clin North Am 1993; 77:477–492.

*An excellent, thorough, and practical review of these two conditions stressing clinical recognition, differential diagnosis, mechanisms and management with dopaminergic agents, and inhibitors of unregulated ionized calcium release in the sarcoplasm of skeletal muscles.*

Kluger MJ. Fever: role of pyrogens and cryogens. Physiol Rev 1991; 71:93–127.

*A detailed review of the comparative biology and physiology of fever, covering the potential adaptive functions of fever, the role of cytokines and other mediators in fever, and host defense as well as antipyrogenic hor-*

*mones ("cryogens"), which can inhibit febrile responses in different species.*

Mackowiak PA, ed. Fever: Basic Mechanisms and Management. Raven Press, New York, 1991.

*An excellent monograph with 23 contributors covering various aspects of fever, including basic thermoregulatory mechanisms, exogenous and endogenous pyrogens, cardiovascular changes during fever syndromes, and management of fever, hyperthermia, and hypothermia.*

Mackowiak PA, Wasserman SS, Levine MM. A critical reappraisal of 98.6°F, the upper limit of the normal body temperature, and other legacies of Carl Reinhold August Wunderlich. JAMA, 1992; 268:1578–1580.

*A detailed study using modern thermometric methods to assess the normal body temperatures of 148 healthy men and women aged 18 through 40 years.*

Norman DC, Santiago DT. Infections in elderly persons. An altered clinical presentation. Clin Geriatr Med 1992; 8:713–719.

*A discussion centering on the occurrence and significance of reduced inflammatory and febrile responses in elderly patients with infection.*

Saper CB, Breder CD. The neurologic basis of fever. N Engl J Med 1994; 330:1880–1886.

*An up-to-date review of pathogenetic mechanisms in fever, stressing the role of specialized centers in the brain, the activities of specialized cells which constitute the blood–brain barrier, and the possible dual functions of cytokines and prostaglandins as both signaling agents and central neurotransmitters in fever and other acute-phase responses to infection.*

Simon HB. Hyperthermia. N Engl J Med 1993; 329:483–487.

*A practical review of the mechanisms and management of hyperthermia that distinguishes this condition from fever.*

Styrt B, Sugarman B. Antipyresis and fever. Arch Intern Med 1990; 150:1589–1597.

*A detailed and thorough review of the role, potential harm, and benefits of fever as a response to infection and other inflammatory stimuli and the indications and approaches for suppression of fever as part of patient management.*

# 10

## The Acute Inflammatory Response

JAN VERHOEF

When microbes breach local defense barriers, the host defenses of the body utilize two major mechanisms to contain and eliminate them. The first of these is the *acute inflammatory response*, which is nonspecific in nature and can be activated within minutes to hours. The second is the *specific immune response*, which takes days to weeks to become expressed. The elements of the acute inflammatory response are cellular—i.e., phagocytes including polymorphonuclear leukocytes, monocytes, and tissue macrophages—and humoral. Of the humoral mechanisms, the complement system plays a critical role of interfacing between phagocytes and microbes acutely, and when specific antibodies are produced, between the immune system, microbes, and phagocytes. This chapter will review the major elements and features of the acute inflammatory response and how it functions in host defense against infection.

### Inflammation

Inflammation is the reaction of the tissues to injury. In principle the local inflammatory reaction, with its cardinal signs—calor, rubor, dolor, and tumor—is aimed at elimination of the irritant (e.g., microbe) and subsequent repair of the damage done by the intruders. However, evidence accumulates that inflammation can also be promoted by the defense reactions themselves and the resulting tissue injury can in turn continue to promote the inflammatory reaction.

The hallmarks of the pathology of inflammation are vascular changes with arteriolar dilatation, increased capillary permeability, emigration of leukocytes, and escape of plasma into the tissues, leading to cellular exudate and tissue changes. Developing within hours after the breach of local barriers, the local inflammatory response acts to prevent the dissemination of infection before the advent of a specific immune response. Phagocytes and opsonins (complement factors and specific antibodies) play an important role in containing the infection. Some bacteria (e.g., staphylococci) appear to be easily contained, while others (e.g., $\beta$ hemolytic staphylococci) may spread before the inflammatory reaction manifests itself.

A failure to contain bacteria by the acute inflammatory response can be a major factor in their invasiveness. Invasion may lead to a generalized state of inflammation, often accompanied by an acute-phase response (see Chapter 14). The clinical signs of a generalized inflammatory reaction are fever, hypotension, tachycardia, and tachypnea—i.e., the *systemic inflammatory response syndrome* (SIRS) (see Chapter 50). Sometimes bacteria remain localized but bacterial products (e.g., endotoxins and exotoxins) disseminate, and these products contribute to a generalized inflammatory reaction. During the systemic inflammatory response many organ systems may malfunction, leading to the syndrome of multiorgan failure. As part of the process cells can be activated, including polymorphonuclear leukocytes, a variety of monocytes, macrophages, lymphocytes, platelets, endothelial cells, fibroblasts, and bone marrow cells. Many molecules play a role in mediating activation of these cells: complement factors, cytokines, coagulation factors, arachidonic acid metabolites (prostaglandins and leukotrienes), endorphins, nitric oxide, and acute-phase proteins. When the activation process becomes excessive and poorly regulated, the end result can be *septic shock*, *multiorgan failure*, and death. These processes are discussed in more detail in Chapter 50.

### The Complement System

The complement system plays a crucial role in host defense against invading microorganisms, even before its activities are harnessed and directed by the specific immune response. Some microorganisms are killed and lysed directly by complement; others are opsonized through complement, then bind to receptors on phagocytic cells and are subsequently phagocytized and killed.

The complement system is composed of more than 30 components that can be activated in a cascadelike fashion (Fig. 10.1). Activation of the complement system can occur via two routes: *the classical* and *the alternative pathway*. The most abundant and central component of the complement cascade is the third complement component, C3, and its activation and cleavage leads to most of the biologic activities of the complement system in host defense.

The complement system can be activated via the *classical pathway* when antigen and antibody complexes combined with a subcomponent of $C_1$, $C_{1q}$. During infection this pathway does not predominate until antibodies, in particular those of the IgM class, are developed against microbial antigens. C1 is then converted to an esterase, which splits off a small peptide from both C4 and C2, leading to the formation of the $C_{4b\ 2b}$ complex. The $C_{4b\ 2b}$ complex has enzymatic activities as a C3 "convertase" that proteolytically cleaves C3 into two components: $C_{3b}$, which remains bound to $C_{14b\ 2b}$, and a soluble peptide, $C3_q$.

C3 convertase activity can also be generated by the alternative pathway in a process that is kinetically slower than that by the classical pathway but which is the principal one utilized before antibodies are formed. Certain microbial molecules such as endotoxin (lipopolysaccharide [LPS]) cell wall peptidoglycan and capsular polysaccharides can trigger the alternative cascade by binding with properdin factors B and D. The resulting complex leads to the development of C3 convertase activity when it combines with $C_{3b}$. In normal plasma there is always some $C_{3b}$ present owing to spontaneous activation of C3. This $C_{3b}$ is able to complex with factor B, producing $C_{3b}B_b$ in the presence of the plasma enzyme factor

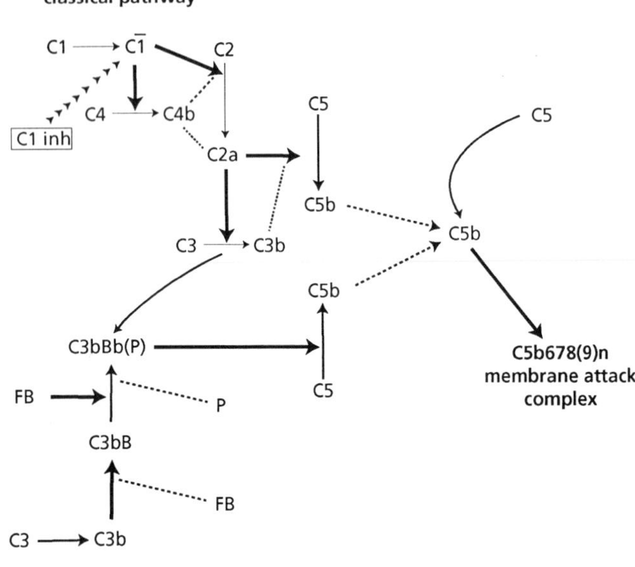


**Fig. 10.1** The complement system: activation and effector pathways. [From Host defense against infection by Jan Verhoef. In: Crossley KB, Archer GL (eds.) *The Staphylococci in Human Disease*. Churchill Livingstone Inc.; New York 1997.]

D. Like $C_{14b\ 2b}$, $C_{3b\ Bb}$ convertase is stabilized against breakdown, thereby accelerating the activity of the alternative pathway.

$C_{3a}$ and a second cleavage product of $C_3$, $C_{3b}$, bound to the microbial surface serve as opsonins, recognized by specific receptors ($CR_1$ and $CR_3$) on phagocytes. Soluble $C_{3a}$ acts as an "anaphylatoxin," promoting vasodilation and increasing capillary permeability as part of the inflammatory response.

In a continuation of activation of the complement cascade the fifth complement factor ($C_5$) is cleaved by $C_{3b}$, $B_bD$, or $C1_{423b}$ to produce $C_{5b}$, which is also able to bind to bacterial cell walls. This subsequently binds C6, C7, and C8, which form a complex capable of inducing a critical conformational change in the terminal component $C_9$. In gram-negative organisms and certain other cells the unfolded $C_9$ molecules become inserted into the lipid bilayer of the cell membrane and polymerize to form an annular "membrane attack complex." This behaves as a transmembrane channel that is fully permeable to electrolytes and water and that eventually leads to lysis of susceptible microorganisms. Only a minority of pathogenic bacteria are susceptible to lysis by the complement system; gram-positive organisms are generally resistant because their thick peptidoglycan cell wall denies access of the membrane attack complex to the plasma membrane.

## Cytokines

The functions of both early and late inflammation and immunity are regulated by the actions of glycoproteins secreted by many different cells. These glycoproteins are signal molecules responsible for communication between cells of the immune and inflammatory systems. They are responsible for the fine-tuning of the function of different cells involved in the fight against intruders. Under special circumstances the coordination of the network of cytokines is disturbed and a systemic inflammatory response syndrome (SIRS) may occur, where cells and cell systems react out of control (see Chapter 50).

As soon as monocytes and macrophages encounter microorganisms, TNF$\alpha$ is released from these mononuclear cells, shortly followed by interleukin-1$\alpha/\beta$ (IL-1$\alpha/\beta$), IL-6, IL-8, IL-10, IL-12, IFN-$\alpha$, granulocyte-macrophage derived colony-stimulating factors (GM-CSF), G-CSF, and M-CSF. Most of these cytokines can also be produced by other cells: endothelial cells, macrophages, fibroblasts, lymphocytes, and bone marrow stromal cells. Indeed, fibroblasts, macrophages, and stromal cells are also important sources for colony-stimulating factors (CSFs), IL-1, and IL-6. Upon stimulation, B lymphocytes produce IL-1, IL-10, and IL-12; T lymphocytes release TNF-$\alpha$, IL-6, and IL-10; and natural killer (NK) cells are important producers of TNF-$\alpha$ (see Chapter 46). Stimulation of monocytes leads to activation of factors needed for transcription of specific cytokine genes in the genome of the monocytes. This is followed by translation of mRNA into proteins and extracellular secretion of these cytokines. Important transcription factors are NF-$\kappa$B (see Chapter 11).

TNF-$\alpha$ and IL-1$\alpha/\beta$ induce an increase in the expression of adhesion molecules on endothelial cells and promote egress of neutrophils into the tissues invaded by microbes. At about the same time IL-8, IL-10, and IL-12 are produced by the mononuclear cells and possibly also by neutrophils. IL-8 changes the shape of the neutrophil and induces the cell to migrate (chemotaxis) through the endothelial cell layer into the tissues. IL-8 also activates the neutrophil (i.e., enhances the respiratory burst) so that the cell is better equipped to kill bacteria. Interestingly, IL-10 downregulates IL-8 and may play an important role in the resolution of an inflammatory response. IL-12 upregulates the production of IFN-$\gamma$ by NK cells. IFN-$\gamma$ produced by NK cells can then activate the mononuclear cells to produce more inflammatory cytokines as well as increase oxidative metabolism.

Neutrophils are further recruited and activated by colony-stimulating factors (CSFs). These factors are responsible for the observed leukocytosis during infection and for upregulation of receptors of the neutrophil plasma membranes needed for optimal phagocytosis. During inflammation, not only are cytokines released but also membrane receptors are shed from many cells. These receptors include those for $C_{3b}$ (Cri) and $C_{3i}$ (CR3), TNFR, IL-1R, and the LPS-binding receptor, CD14. At the same time, antagonists of these receptors are also produced and released (e.g., IL-1R antagonist). The soluble receptors are able to bind and inactivate specific cytokines before they bind to their target cells. The interactions of cells with cytokines, cytokine receptors, and receptor antagonists creates an enormously complex regulatory network for the inflammatory response that enables cells to communicate. The resulting interaction not only determines the outcome of encounters between microbes and host defense systems at the local level but also gives rise to many of the systemic manifestations of infection, such as fever (see Chapter 9). If infection or tissue injury (as in trauma or burns) is not contained or is poorly regulated, massive cytokine expression or inactivation may play an important role in some of the systemic deleterious effects of inflammation, as discussed in Chapter 50.

## The Acute-Phase Response

Collectively the metabolic and cellular events that accompany the acute inflammatory changes early in infection are known as "the acute-phase response." In the acute-phase reaction the number and function of the phagocytic cells is increased. Inflammatory cells and humoral factors are delivered to the site of infection, fever often develops, and its accompanying metabolic changes assist the host in defending against the invading microorganisms (see Chapter 9). Production of a number of plasma proteins by hepatocytes increases in response to the inflammatory cytokines, in particular IL-1, TNF, and IL-6. Acute-phase proteins that dramatically rise in plasma concentrations include C-reactive protein (CRP), mannose-binding proteins (MBP), $\alpha$1-acid glycoprotein, serum amyloid A protein (SAA), fibronectin, fibrinogen, and C3. A precise role for each of these proteins in host defense is still being defined, but some can function as antimicrobial opsonins (CRP, MBP, C3) in the absence of specific antibodies.

Other events that characterize the acute-phase response include the mobilization of amino acids from muscle through the action of TNF and IL-1 to activate proteases, and mobilization of lipids presumably to supply energy from adipose stores by activation of lipoprotein lipase. While hepatocyte production of acute-phase proteins is enhanced, that of albumin is diminishcd; this and thc increased utilization of albumin as an energy supply results in hypoalbuminemia, which can be an early and dramatic finding in acute infection.

During acute infection inflammatory cytokine-induced stimulation of a number of hormones occurs, including insulin and glucagon release from the pancreas, growth hormone and ACTH release from the pituitary, and glucorticoids and catecholamines from the adrenals (see Chapter 14). As a result glycogenolysis occurs, and glucose is released from the liver and utilized in the periphery. Depending on the adequacy of glycogen stores, tissue demands, and the counteracting actions of insulin and the other regulatory hormones, the results may be hyper- or hypoglycemia. For example, in patients with limited hepatic glycogen stores (e.g., cirrhotics, neonates) infection may trigger hypoglycemia. In those with diabetes and impaired insulin production, infection is a notorious cause of insulin resistance, which may culminate in hyperglycemia, hyperosmolar states, and/or ketoacidosis.

Finally, when acute infections become chronic many of the acute-phase responses remain active. The wasting, hyperlipidemia, and hypoalbuminemia that characterize chronic intracellular infections (or malignancy) can be ascribed to the continued actions of TNF$\alpha$, IL-1, and IL-6. Elevation of the erythrocyte sedimentation rate, and in rare cases amyloidosis complicating chronic infection, can be ascribed to elevations of fibrinogen and deposition of serum amyloid A protein, respectively. Leukemoid reactions complicating acute or chronic infections are the result of excessive activation and stimulation of myelopoesis by G-CSF and other colony-stimulating factors.

## Phagocytes in Host Defense

Once the barriers of the skin and mucous membranes have been breached by invading microbes, the host's health depends acutely on the actions of neutrophilic polymorphonuclear leukocytes (PMN), monocytes, and macrophages coupled with those of other host resistance factors to limit the spread of microbes and their products (see Fig. 10.2).

## Polymorphonuclear leukocytes

### Kinetics

Under the influence of CSFs, PMN originate in the bone marrow and are continuously discharged in vast numbers into the bloodstream. The average time spent in the blood is about 12 hours before exiting the circulation and entering tissues. This time may be shortened to just several hours when the demand for these cells is increased during acute infection. Normally, adults produce about $10^{10}$ PMN/day, a number that is matched by the senescence and clearance of these cells in tissues and in the GI tract. Approximately 50% of the PMNs in the bloodstream that are freely circulating can be measured by counting them in peripheral venous or capillary blood. The remainder of the cells are in a marginated state in the spleen, the lungs, or in the microvasculature preparing to exit the circulation into the tissues.

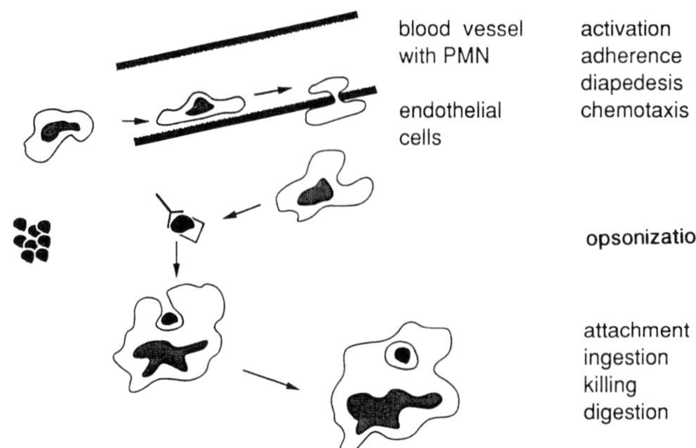


**Fig. 10.2** Processes involved in phagocytosis of bacteria by polymorphonuclear leukocytes. [With permission from Verhoef & Visser: Neutrophil phagocytosis and killing. In: Abramson JS, Wheeler JG (eds.) *The Neutrophil*; Oxford University Press Inc.; Oxford, New York 1993.]

Leukocytosis occurs acutely when stored maturing PMN are released from the bone marrow maturation pool (about 50% of the PMN precursors in the bone marrow). Neutrophilia is maintained chronically during infection when myeloid cell production is increased up to tenfold under the influence of CSFs, in particular G-CSF. Leukocytosis can also be seen when the ability of circulating PMN to exit the vasculature is impaired, as by the action of glucocorticoids or in rare disorders involving the lack of production of key PMN adhesion proteins (see below, under "Diapedesis and Chemotaxis"). Prolonged high-dose glucocorticoid therapy may lead to an increased incidence of bacterial infections through this influence on the acute PMN inflammatory response.

Neutropenia may be seen during infection if PMN production and maturation are impaired. Production may be impaired by cytokines such as gamma interferon, produced in excess during chronic infections or more often by alcohol, drugs, or nutritional or other factors. Neutropenia can also be seen when the margination of cells is increased or demand for PMN in tissues increases and the marrow is unable to keep with this increased demand. During active bacterial infection, myelopoesis may be increased by tenfold within 24 to 48 hours in normal individuals; if utilization in the periphery exceeds production, neutropenia can result.

### Diapedesis and chemotaxis

As soon as microbes invade the tissues, circulating PMN are activated, adhere to activated endothelial cells, leave the bloodstream (diapedesis), and move through the endothelial barrier to the site of the infection. This process of migration is called chemotaxis and is defined as cell movement in one direction in response to an agent that signals and induces the cell to move.

Neutrophil chemotaxis requires binding of chemoattractants to specific membrane receptors. Chemoattractants can be bacterial products (e.g., LPS and formylated peptides), activated complement factors (C5a), arachidonic acid metabolites (LTB4), IL-1, platelet-activating factor (PAF), or degraded tissue proteins. Chemoattractant receptors bind to G proteins in order to transmit signals to the interior of the cell. These signals alter cell polarity, stimulate a change in the gel-sol state of intracellular contraction proteins (actin), and promote forward movement.

When viewed microscopically, the first event in the microvasculature at an inflammatory site is the slowing or margination of the circulating leukocytes within postcapillary venules. Rather than free linear flow, the PMN become loosely tethered to the vessel wall and roll along the surface of the endothelium. After rolling, many neutrophils firmly adhere to the endothelial cell surface and become activated, changing from a spherical configuration to a flattened shape. This is followed by diapedesis, in which the adherent PMN exit the postcapillary venules by squeezing between adjacent endothelial cells.

Recently the mechanisms involved in leukocyte rolling, sticking, and diapedesis have been defined (Fig. 10.3). During tethering, a family of three lectinlike carbohydrate-binding molecules found either on PMN or endothelial cells and called "selectins" are expressed on the cell surfaces. Each of these selectins promotes leukocyte rolling. These selectins are named L-selectin, E-selectin, and P-selectin, according to the cell type on which they were first described: lymphocyte, endothelium, and platelets. L-selectins are expressed on most leukocytes; the E- and P-selectins are synthesized and expressed by endothelial cells. E-selectins or P-selectins recognize specific carbohydrate sequences on leukocytes (L-selectin) and thereby mediate tethering of leukocytes to the endothelium. The selectins mediate a degree of intercellular adhesion that is strong enough to induce rolling of PMN along the vessel wall but not so strong as to stop them completely. Strong adhesion of leukocytes to endothelium is mediated by a second set of intercellular adhesion molecules called *integrins*. After activation, specific integrins promote strong adhesion that can fix the rolling leukocyte to the endothelial cell and then induce diapedesis.

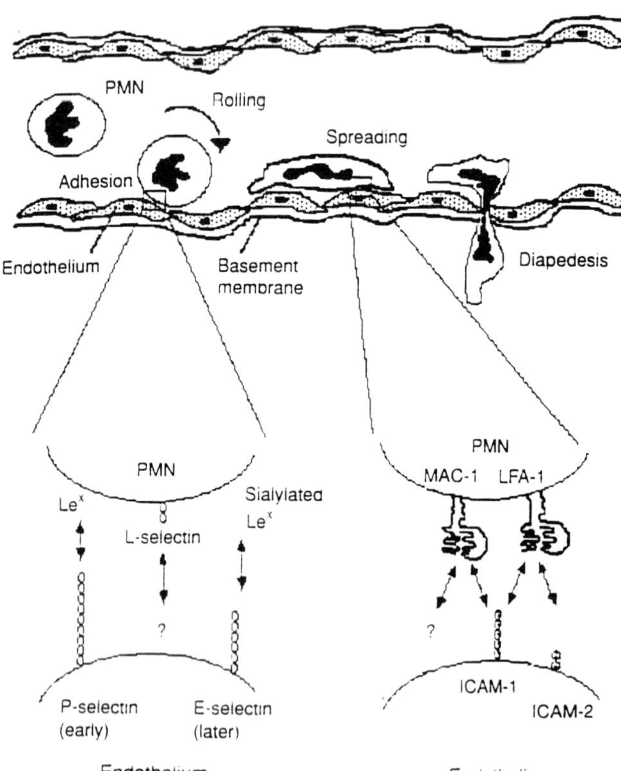


**Fig. 10.3** Processes involved in the diapedesis of polymorphic nuclear leukocytes. [With permission from Rosales & Brown: Neutrophil receptors and modulation of the immune response. In: Abramson JS, Wheeler JG (eds.) *The Neutrophil*. Oxford University Press Inc.; Oxford, New York 1993.]

Integrins are a family of membrane glycoproteins found on almost all cells and responsible for cell–cell or intracellular cell-matrix adherence. Each integrin consists of an $\alpha$ and $\beta$ subunit. Based on the structure of their $\beta$ subunit, integrins can be grouped into subfamilies. The most important of these subfamilies for leukocytes are: the $\beta 1$ integrins—also known as the VLA proteins—which have a common $\beta$ chain (CD29) paired with different $\alpha$ subunits (CD49a-CD49f), and the $\beta 2$ integrins—also known as leukocyte cell-adhesion molecules—which share the $\beta$ chain CD18 paired with CD11a (LFA-1), CD11b (Mac-1), or CD11c $\alpha$ chains.

An important activator of selectin and integrin expression is the chemotactic cytokine IL-8. Other activators of neutrophil and monocyte selection and integrin expression are platelet-activating factor, a phospholipid that is produced rapidly by endothelial cells after stimulation with leukotrienes, TNF$\alpha$, IL-4, etc., bacterial cell wall components (endotoxin), and complement products. Many of the cytokines that trigger strong adhesion may also act as chemotactic factors. Thus, IL-8 induces chemotaxis of neutrophils as well as triggering their adhesion.

Many of the activators responsible for chemotaxis and adhesion of PMN and endothelial cells are produced by the endothelial cells themselves, the monocytes, or the bacteria. There is growing evidence that the neutrophil is also able to produce its own chemotactic factors and activators.

## Opsonization

Opsonization refers to the process by which microbial surfaces are altered by humoral factors to permit their binding and ingestion by phagocytes. The major opsonins are antibody and complement factors. PMN have receptors specifically designed to bind to the Fc fragment of the IgG molecule present on the surface of the opsonized bacteria and other receptors (CR1 and CR3) designed to bind to the activated complement factors.

Opsonization through activation of complement is primarily a function of C3b and iC3b. The PMN receptor that recognizes C3b is CR1, while the receptor that recognizes iC3b is CR3. Ingestion is also facilitated by opsonic antibodies that are of the IgG isotype. Antibodies bind to specific antigens on the cell wall of bacteria, and bind to PMNs, monocytes, or macrophages by specific IgG Fc receptors. Receptors for the Fc portion of the IgG are present on the phagocytic cell membrane: FcRII and FcRIII. FcRII can bind to antigen–antibody complexes of IgGI and IgG3 equally well, and better than IgG2 and IgG4. FcRIII binds only monomeric IgG.

Many bacteria have developed a defense against opsonophagocytosis and are thus able to escape phagocytosis by PMN. The most prominent antiphagocytic defense of bacteria is the presence of an enveloping capsule. These capsules protect the microbes against PMN by interfering with opsonization. For example, *Hemophilus influenzae*, *Neisseria meningitidis*, *Escherichia coli*, *Streptococcus pneumoniae*, *Klebsiella pneumoniae*, and group B streptococci have polysaccharide capsules on their surface. Non-encapsulated derivatives of these organisms are readily phagocytized and are less virulent. Some other cell wall components that help microbes evade the phagocytic defense of the host are protein A (*Staphylococcus aureus*), which binds opsonic IgG by the Fc portion, thereby preventing linkage with Fc receptors and protein M (group A streptococci).

### Phagocytosis in the absence of antibody and complement

Some bacteria are able to adhere to PMN in the absence of antibodies and/or complement. *E. coli* adhesins, for example, are important components that may mediate adherence of *E. coli* directly to PMN without antibodies and complement. These adhesins can be divided into two groups: one where D-mannosides inhibit their adherence and one where they do not. The mannose-sensitive (MS) adhesins recognize the mannose residues of three different membrane glycoproteins in the PMN—gp150, gp70–80, and gp100—and this interaction leads to phagocytosis and killing by PMNs.

A serum factor other than complement or antibody that can function as an opsonin against gram-negative organisms is the *lipopolysaccharide-binding protein* (*LBP*). LBP is an acute-phase reactant that binds bacterial LPS. LBP binds to the LPS rich outer envelope of some gram-negative bacilli and in turn strongly enhances attachment of the organisms to the CD14 molecule in the cell membrane of phagocytic cells. This leads to enhanced phagocytosis.

In plasma there is a high-molecular-weight glycoprotein, *fibronectin*, that aids the reticuloendothelial system in removing microorganisms from the bloodstream and helps maintain vascular stability. Several bacteria—for example, *S. aureus* and groups A, B, C, and G streptococci—have receptors for fibronectin. Because PMN can also bind fibronectin, it is possible that this glycoprotein acts as a bridge between PMN and the bacteria and therefore facilitates phagocytosis in the absence of specific opsonins.

### Microbial resistance of opsonization

Many microorganisms can escape from opsonization by varying their surface antigenic structure. Some bacteria are master chameleons. For example, *N. gonorrhoeae* possess at least two mechanisms for altering surface antigens:

1. They can change PII proteins. Most *N. gonorrhoeae* express several different PII proteins at any given time, and a given strain can potentially express up to seven different PII proteins. The genetic control of each PII gene appears unrelated to other PII genes, which results in many different combinations.
2. They can change pilins. There are usually many silent pilin gene sequences. The gonococcus can undergo gene conversion by placing one of these incomplete sequences into the expression site, thus synthesizing a new antigenically distinct pilin molecule. Antigenic variation occurs in many other bacteria as well—e.g., group B streptococci, *H. influenzae*, *P. aeruginosa*, *Salmonella*, *Borrelia*, etc.

### Effect of antibodies on opsonization

Exposure of bacteria to specific antibiotics below the minimal inhibition concentration (MIC) may increase their susceptibility to the antimicrobial action of normal human PMN and monocytes. Low concentrations of antibiotics influence cell wall composition. Clindamycin, for example, has an inhibitory effect on the expression of M protein of streptococci and protein A of *S. aureus* and thereby facilitates phagocytosis. Antibiotics may also interfere with capsular (K antigen) synthesis and LPS assembly in *E. coli*, allowing the organisms to be more readily opsonized and subsequently phagocytized. Thus, during infections antibiotics may act in different ways: they may either kill the microbe directly or change the cell wall composition in such a way that opsonophagocytosis is enhanced.

### Phagocytosis

During phagocytosis, PMN take up opsonized microorganisms into phagosomes that fuse with secretory granules (lysosomes) to form phagolysosomes. Killing and digestion of microorganisms take place within these phagolysosomes.

### Normal phagocytosis

Phagocytosis is the process that describes ingestion of particles by phagocytic cells. It involves both particle attachment to membrane receptors and subsequent engulfment. Phagocytosis starts with receptor-ligand binding between PMN and the microbe. The receptor–ligand interaction activates the contractile protein complex actin, myosin, and actin-binding proteins. At the site of particle attachment actin microfilaments in the cytoplasm are polymerized. This polymerization leads to puckering of the plasma membrane at the site of contact, because the microfilaments attach to the membrane. The plasma membrane then extends around the particle, and the formation of a pseudopod and new particle-membrane contacts results. As the particle becomes surrounded by pseudopodia a phagocytic vacuole (phagosome) is created. As this is happening, granules in the cytoplasma fuse with the phagosome membrane, producing a phagolysosome (Fig. 10.2).

### Microbial evasion of phagocytosis

Some bacteria are able to inhibit the fusion of the granules with the phagosome and thereby escape killing by PMN. By inhibition of degranulation these microorganisms become intracellular pathogens. For example, *Mycobacterium tuberculosis* is an obligate intracellular bacterium that survives by interfering with lysosome–phagosome fusion. When viable *M. tuberculosis* organisms are ingested, the azurophilic granules remain intact and do not fuse with the phagosomes containing *M. tuberculosis*. In contrast, lysosomes do fuse with phagosomes containing nonviable *M. tuberculosis*. Viable *M. tuberculosis* produce strongly acidic sulfatides that accumulate in azurophilic granules and prevent lysome-phagosome fusion. Surface components of *M. leprae* and *M. tuberculosis* are also responsible for the inhibition of fusion. For example, the cord factor, a cell wall glycolipid of mycobacteria, inhibits fusion between phospholipid vesicles in general and between phagosomes and lysosomes in particular. Abnormalities in lysosome–phagosome fusion have also been demonstrated in neutrophils and macrophages that have phagocytized other bacteria (such as *Salmonella* and gonococci), fungi (such as *Histoplasma capsulatum*), and live *Toxoplasma gondii*. This suggests that certain fungal and protozoal species also secrete factors that inhibit the disruption of lysosomes.

Virulent gonococci attach to PMN and stimulate an oxidative metabolic response. The azurophilic granules, however, do not release their contents into phagocytic vacuoles and the intracellular gonococci remain viable. Virulent gonococci possess the major outer membrane protein, protein I. Protein I is a porin, one of a class of specialized proteins used by bacteria to permit the passage of ions and nutrients through their otherwise impermeable outer membrane (see Chapter 3). Protein I has the unusual ability to translocate from the gonococci into human cells, including into the phagolysosome membrane, where it remains in an open and functional state. This allows an influx of anions into the phagosome. As the potential difference increases, the porin closes. Closure and cessation of ion flow inhibits degranulation but does not affect superoxide anion ($O_2^-$) generation. Some virulent gonococci may survive in phagocytes as a result.

Opsonization itself may alter the capacity of microorganisms to inhibit phagosome–lysosome fusion. For example, live *Chlamydia* organisms are readily phagocytized but little degranulation occurs and the organisms replicate within the phagosomes. However, when antibody-coated *Chlamydiae* are phagocytized, prompt lysosome–phagosome fusion is observed.

## Killing of Microorganisms

PMN are able to kill microorganisms by two distinct systems. One antimicrobial system is oxygen-dependent, while the other can kill bacteria in the absence of oxygen.

### Oxygen-dependent events

The oxygen-dependent antimicrobial mechanisms are set in motion when PMN undergo a "respiratory burst." NADPH oxidase in the phagolysosome membrane is activated and reduces $O_2$ to superoxide ($\cdot O_2^-$). $O_2$ reduction is the first step in a series of reactions that produce toxic oxygen species. For example, $\cdot O_2^-$ dismutates to $H_2O_2$ and the azurophil granule enzyme MPO catalyzes the oxidation of $Cl^-$ by $H_2O_2$ to yield HOCl. $H_2O_2$ is a powerful oxidant; however, it reacts sluggishly with biological materials. In addition, most microorganisms contain enzymes that detoxify $H_2O_2$, such as catalase and/or NADH or sulfhydryl peroxidase, and therefore are highly resistant to killing by $H_2O_2$.

$H_2O_2$ and $\cdot O_2^-$ can give rise to more potent oxidants in the presence of ferric ion or $Fe^{3+}$ chelates such as transferrin or lactoferrin. $O_2^-$ reduces $Fe^{3+}$ or $Fe^{3+}$ chelates to $Fe^{2+}$. The subsequent reaction of $H_2O_2$ with $Fe^{2+}$ chelates yields iron–oxygen complexes that react directly with microbial components or that release hydroxyl radicals ($\cdot OH\cdot$, HaberWeiss reaction). OH· reacts rapidly with chemical bonds of all kinds and can cause damage near the site where it is produced. However, its high reactivity within phagosomes suggests that most of the OH· is likely to be consumed in the oxidation of microbial surface components that are not essential to viability and an enormous amount would be required for killing. Recent studies, therefore, cast doubt on the significance of ·OH· as a critical antimicrobial reactive oxygen species of PMN.

HOCl is a potent microbicidal agent. However, it is unlikely that HOCl acts directly as the microbial substance in phagolysosomes. HOCL reacts rapidly with ammonia ($NH_4^+$) to yield monochloramine ($NH_2CL$) and with amines to yield mono- and dichloramines (RNHCL and $RNCL_2$). Since the concentration of donor nitrogen compounds is very high within phagosomes, evidence supports the concepts that the toxicity of the MPO/ $H_2O_2/Cl^-$ system is mediated by chloramines.

### Microbial evasion of oxygen-dependent killing

Microorganisms differ greatly in their susceptibility to killing by oxidants. These differences are due in part to differing levels of intracellular protective enzymes produced by certain bacteria, such as superoxide dismutase (SOD), catalase, various reductases, and peroxidases. However, it is not known whether any microorganism has sufficiently high levels of such antioxidant enzymes to escape killing by PMN oxidants in vivo. For example, *E. coli*, *Salmonella typhimurium*, and *Bacillus subtilis* exposed to sublethal concentrations of $H_2O_2$ adapt in such a way that they can survive subsequent exposures to considerably higher concentrations of this oxidant. Adaptation has been linked to the induction of antioxidant enzymes, enhanced DNA repair, and the synthesis of a variety of stress proteins. These proteins, resulting from oxidant stress, are similar to heat-shock proteins.

For example, *S. typhimurium* becomes resistant to killing by $H_2O_2$ when pretreated with nonlethal levels of this oxidant. This adaptation results in the transient accumulation of a distinct group of proteins. Most of these proteins are under the control of the so-called OXY R gene product. The expression of the kat G (catalase) gene also appears to be regulated by OXY R at the level of mRNA. *Candida albicans*, a leading cause of opportunistic mycosis (see Chapter 6), undergoes genetically programmed reversible high-frequency phenotypic switching. The resulting changes in properties of surface proteins of blastoconidia and pseudohyphae lead to differences in colony morphology (white and opaque phenotypes). Blastoconidia of the opaque phenotypes are more susceptible than are those of the white phenotype to killing by neutrophilis or cell-free oxidants, such as $H_2O_2$ or the MPO-$H_2O_2$-$CL^-$ system. When ingested, opaque blastocondidia are also more potent stimuli of neutrophil superoxide formation than are the white blastocomidia. Both neutrophils and oxidants (rcagent $II_2O_2$ or NOCl, as well as the MPO-$H_2O_2$-$CL^-$ systeni) can induce unidirectional increases in the spontaneous rates of switching from white to opaque phenotypes. Differences in expression of *C. albicans* phenotypes, therefore, may determine the relative susceptibility to neutrophil fungicidal mechanisms, and the neutrophils themselves appear capable of selectively augmenting the switching process.

*Listeria monocytogenes*, the causative agent of listeriosis, is also able to avoid the lethal effects of oxygen metabolites. Interestingly, this resistance appears to be related to the growth phase of the bacteria. In vitro *Listeria* in the logarithmic phase of multiplication are more resistant to toxic oxygen species than are Listeria in the resting stage. This is because of a higher production of catalase during the logarithmic phase of growth.

Exposure of gonococci to sublethal concentrations of superoxide and $H_2O_2$ also promotes resistance to oxidant stress. This adaptation requires new protein synthesis but is not specifically related to increased production of SOD or catalase. It appears that gonococci bound to human PMN use PMN-derived lactate as an energy source. This leads to an increase in oxygen consumption and the creation of an anaerobic environment for the gonococcus. The resulting anaerobiasis shuts down the PMN $O_2$-generating system. It is possible that other facultatively anaerobic organisms utilize a similar mechanism to escape killing by phagocytes.

*Legionella pneumophila* replicates intracellularly in macrophages and fibroblasts, behaving like an obligate intracellular organism. Since *L. pneumophila* does not replicate extracellularly in vivo, some aspect of the macrophage metabolism would appear to contribute to the bacterial replication. Viable *L. pneu-*

*mophila* can produce a toxin that inhibits the oxidative response of macrophages during phagocytosis. Both virulent and avirulent strains are susceptible to products of the oxidative reaction of phagocytes; survival and replication of these organisms within macrohages are thus enhanced by inhibition of host cell oxidative metabolism.

Resting conidia of *Aspergillus* are resistant to killing. Despite their susceptibility to phagocytosis, these conidia only marginally stimulate production of superoxide anion, hydrogen peroxide, and hypochlorous acid (HOCl) and induce less MPO-dependent iodination by PMN than do metabolically active conidia. Metabolically active conidia are more readily killed by PMN than are resting conidia. PMN of patients with chronic granulomatous disease (CGD) (unable to form $O2^-$ and $H_2O_2$) do not kill *Aspergillus* conidiae, indicating the importance of toxic oxygen species in this process.

Certain group B streptococci are also readily ingested but not killed, presumably owing to inhibition of the PMN respiratory burst by the bacteria. Evidence suggests that this may be because of the presence of C protein in the cell wall of these bacteria.

### Oxygen-independent events

PMN cytoplasmic granules contain additional antimicrobial agents that are released into phagolysosomes and do not require the production of oxidants for activity. These agents include proteases, hydrolytic enzymes such as phospholipases, glycosidases, and lysozymes, and proteins and peptides that disrupt microbial functions or structural components. All of these agents must bind to the microbial cell surface to exert antimicrobial activity, and the activity of each agent is limited to certain classes and species of microorganisms. Three well-characterized granule components, known as bactericidal/permeability-increasing protein (B/PI), CLCP (chymotrypsinlike cationic protein), cathepsin G, and defensins, have microbicidal activity in vitro.

#### B/PI

This 58 kD protein is found in the primary (azurophil) granules and may contribute to the ability of neutrophils to kill gram-negative bacteria. Within 15 seconds after exposure to B/PI *E. coli* no longer form colonies. Loss of viability is caused by an increase in outer-membrane permeability to hydrophobic molecules and by activation of enzymes that are able to degrade peptidoglycan and outer-membrane phospholipids. The specificity of B/PI for gram-negative bacteria is due to the interactions between B/PI and LPS. The interactions between cationic B/PI molecules and anionic phosphate or 2-keto-3deoxy-D-mannooctulonic acid (KDO) residues disrupt the LPS layer. Binding of B/PI to the outer membrane of gram-negative bacilli also leads to displacement of KDO- and phosphate-bound divalent cations that stabilize the outer membrane. The displaced calcium ions then activate bacterial phospholipases.

#### CLCP

Azurophil granules of human PMN contain three immunologically cross-reactive cationic proteins that have both antibacterial and chymotrypsinlike neutral protease activity in vitro. Exposure of *S. aureus* or *E. coli* to CLCP inhibits multiplication by suppressing macromolecular (protein, RNA, and DNA) synthesis. The microbicidal activity of CLCP persists when protease activity is abolished by heat or by active-site inhibitors. Therefore, the microbicidal activity of CLCP does not depend on a primary proteolytic activity. CLCP has also been shown to sensitize gram-negative bacteria *Acinobacter* 199A to lysozyme and to act synergistically with PMN elastase against *E. coli* and *S. aureus*.

#### Defensins

The azurophilic (primary) cytoplasmic granules of PMN contain a variety of antimicrobial cationic proteins with potent antimicrobial activity. Three structurally and functionally homologous peptides, called defensins, exist in human PMN. The peptides are small (3.5 kD), cysteine rich, only moderately cationic, and identical except at their amino-terminal residues. They are also remarkably abundant, up to 5%–7% of the total protein of human PMN and 30%–50% of the total protein of the primary granules. These peptides have a broad spectrum of activity in vitro against gram-positive and gram-negative bacteria, fungi (including *Candida* species and *Cryptococcus neoformans*), and certain enveloped viruses. Human PMN defensins kill only metabolically active bacteria and induce loss of outer- and inner-membrane integrity.

Other granular agents that contribute to the bactericidal activity of the PMN are elastase and lactoferrin. Lactoferrin binds iron and produces an iron-free milieu in the PMN. It is bacteriostatic because most bacteria do not multiply in the absence of iron. Lactoferrin also alters the cell wall of bacteria so that it becomes more accessible to lysozyme. Thus, lactoferrin and lysozyme act synergistically.

## Intracellular Digestion of Microbes

Most microorganisms are digested after being killed and bacterial components are rapidly degraded by the numerous granule-associated hydrolytic enzymes. Intracellular killing of ingested bacteria usually takes place during the first minutes of phagocytosis. The degree of subsequent digestion of engulfed bacteria depends on the structure of the bacterial cell envelope and on the presence of digestive enzymes in the phagosome. For example, PMN can rapidly and extensively degrade macromolecules such as proteins, RNA, and peptidoglycan of unencapsulated *E. coli*. In contrast to the rapid killing and extensive breakdown of unencapsulated *E. coli* strains, strains with capsular K antigen are more resistant to killing and resist degradation by PMN.

## Role of PMN in Regulation of the Inflammatory Response

The phagocytic cell is the cornerstone in acute host defense against bacteria. Without adequate numbers of properly functioning PMN, patients suffer from bacterial and opportunistic fungal infections (see Chapter 86). The PMN has long been regarded as a terminally differentiated cell, incapable of protein synthesis, and fulfilling only a "passive" effector role in inflammation via phagocytosis and the release of performed enzymes and cytotoxic compounds. However, it is now clear that mature PMNs retain the capacity to synthesize a restricted, but significant, range of mRNAs and proteins. For example, PMN have been shown to synthesize and release several important mediators, including alpha interferon (IFN-$\alpha$), platelet-activating factor (PAF), and leukotriene $B_4$, IL-$\alpha$ and $\beta$, and TNF.

Negative regulators of inflammation may also be produced by PMNs during phagocytosis or in response to LPS, including IL-1 RAP and soluble TNF receptors. As IL-1 RAP blocks IL-1 activity both in vitro and in vivo, PMN possess the capacity to inhibit an IL-1–mediated inflammatory response.

Neutrophils play an important role in localizing the infection. However, when the invading microorganisms overwhelm the host, a generalized inflammatory reaction occurs—i.e., SIRS (Chapter 50). In this process the monocyte/macrophage plays a crucial role as the prime producers of inflammatory mediators when they become activated. Therefore, these cells are at the center stage when the acute-phase reaction turns into a general inflammatory response.

## ANNOTATED BIBLIOGRAPHY


Abramson J, Wheeler JG, eds. The Neutrophil. IRL Press at Oxford University Press, Oxford, New York, Tokyo, 1993.
*This book is an excellent source of information on leukocytes.*

Adams DH, Shaw S. Leucocyte-endothelial interactions and regulation of leucocyte migration. The Lancet 1994; 343:831–836.
*A very good overview.*

Baumann H, Gauldie J. The acute phase response. Immunol Today 1994; 15:74–80.
*A clearly written overview.*

Bone RC. Sepsis and its complications: The clinical problem. Crit Care Med 1994; 22:S8–S11.
*Good example of the definition of interaction, clinical picture, and pathogenesis.*

Dale DC. Potential role of colony-stimulating factors in the prevention and treatment of infectious diseases. Clin Infect Dis 1994; 18(Suppl 2):S180–S188.

Davies MG, Hagen PO. Systemic inflammatory response syndrome. Br J Surg 1997; 84:920–935.

Densen P, Mandell GL. Granulocytic phagocytes. In: Principles and Practice of Infectious Diseases, 3rd ed., Mandell SL, Douglas RG, Bennet JE, eds. Churchill Livingstone Inc., New York; 1990, pp 81–101.
*Practical and good reference book.*

Johnston RB Jr. The complement system in host defense and inflammation: The cutting edges of a double edged sword. Pediatr Infect Dis J 1993; 12:933–941.
*Ins and outs of complement. Well written.*

Jones TC. The effect of granulocyte-macrophage colony stimulating factor (rGM-CSF) on macrophage function in microbial disease. Med Oncol 1996; 13:141–147.

MacMicking J, Xie QW, Nathan C. Nitric oxide and macrophage function. Annu Rev Immunol 1997; 15:323–350.

Morgan RW, Christman MF, Jacobson FS, Storz G, Ames BN. Hydrogen peroxide-inducible proteins in *Salmonella typhimurium* overlap with heat shock and other stress proteins. Proc Natl Acad Sci USA 1986; 83:8059–8063.
*Very interesting article.*

Proost P, Wuyts A, van-Damme J. The role of chemokines in inflammation. Int J Clin Lab Res 1996; 26:211–223.

Silver GM, Fink MP. Possible roles for anti- or pro-inflammatory therapies in the management of sepsis. Surg Clin North Am 1994; 74:711–723.

Simms HH, D'Amico R. Studies on polymorphonuclear leukocyte bactericidal function: II. The role of oxidative stress. Shock 1997; 7:339–344.

Thomas, LT, Lehrer RI. Human neutrophil antimicrobial activity. Rev Infect Dis 1988; Suppl 2:S450–S456.
*Good update.*

Verhoef J, Visser MR. Neutrophil phagocytosis and killing: Normal function and microbial evasion. *In*: The Neutrophil, Abramson J, Wheeler JG, eds. IRL Press at Oxford University Press. Oxford, New York, Tokyo; 1993, pp 109–137.

Wardle EN. Cytokines: An overview. Eur J Med 1993;2:417–423.

# 11

## The Specific Immune Response

JOHN M. DWYER

The specific immune response mounted by higher species is necessarily complicated. But the logic associated with the broadening of our immunological repertoire under evolutionary pressure to produce this complexity is likely to be readily appreciated by those interested in infectious diseases. While most of the microbes we encounter are harmless, so many are not that the survival pressures on "selfish genes" throughout the eons has seen both the immune system and the pathogens with which it must struggle become increasingly sophisticated. Rare congenital and increasingly frequent acquired immune deficiency states demonstrate that we humans cannot live without our immune system.

Unlike those ancient useful but nonspecific mechanisms that can induce an inflammatory response, specific immunity involves three quite extraordinary biological developments. First, cells of the immune system recognize "foreignness" and "self" and appreciate the difference; this recognition occurs at the level of the individual cell. Second, an encounter with foreignness leads to an expansion of the cellular entities capable of recognizing that particular example of "nonself." Third, an encounter with foreignness is usually associated with a long-lived immunological memory of the event so that a more rapid and more efficient response is made to a second encounter. The human brain is the only other biological system capable of recognizing, distinguishing, and remembering (learning) and therefore adapting to second encounters. It is indeed fascinating that hormonal and neuronal links exist that allow specific immune and neurological functions to influence each other.

Before looking at the trees in the immunological forest it is sensible to stand back and look at the forest that is specific immune function. In so doing one notes that:

1. Nonspecific immune responses that produce inflammation by activating the alternate pathway of complement, polymorphonuclear cells (granulocytes), monocytes, basophils, mast cells, and eosinophils were available to developing species before a specific immune response developed. However, specific immune responses are designed to harness these factors and cells in a more measured fashion.

2. The specific immune response features two major cooperating but different defensive mechanisms: cellular and humoral immunity. In general, cellular immunity requires *cell contact* with the peptide determinants that provoked the response for destruction and elimination to occur. Humoral immunity requires soluble *circulating* or mucosa-bound proteins (immunoglobulins) to interact with targets during the attack phase. Last century, invisible soluble factors whose effects were clearly demonstrable, though invisible, were referred to as the "humors." Cellular immunity developed during the evolution of specific immunity before humoral immunity, and this may be a major reason why cellular immune mechanisms control humoral immune events.

3. The major challenge for any specific immune system involves the development of fail-safe mechanisms which ensure that foreignness, not self, is attacked. To date, security systems have not been perfected and self peptides occasionally induce and sustain an immune response that results in an autoimmune disease.

Strictly speaking, the term *antigen* refers to a small molecule (almost always a peptide sequence) that is recognized by the immune system. Recognition, however, is not always followed by the generation of an inflammatory or other attack response. Thus, we constantly recognize self antigens and respond with immunological indifference. An *immunogen* is an antigen that so excites specific immunological cells that attempts at killing or elimination follow. Most texts, however, equate antigens and immunogens using the former rather than the latter to denote foreignness and immunogenicity. To avoid confusion, that terminology will be employed in this discussion.

4. In any first encounter with microbial antigens, experiments of nature tell us clearly that we are dependant on the integrity of our *cellular immune response* if we are to handle satisfactorily viruses, fungi, parasites, and intracellular bacteria such as *Listeria monocytogenes* and *Mycobacterium tuberculosis*. On the other hand, the challenge associated with infection by rapidly dividing extracellular bacteria, especially those wrapped in a polysaccharide coat, requires an effective *humoral* response. Thus, patients with an antibody deficiency state can die of overwhelming bacterial infection but not be troubled by an attack of measles. Conversely patients, such as those with AIDS, who have severely damaged or absent cellular immune responses cannot respond satisfactorily to cytomegalovirus. Indeed, the very existence of the two major divisions of labor within the immune system can be thought of in adaptive terms. Humoral immune mechanisms, by which we produce a series of antigen-specific immunoglobulins, were an essential addition to our defensive repertoire if we were to handle bacterial infection.

5. The cells of the immune system don't "see" whole viruses or bacteria. They can only recognize antigenic determinants—that is, digestion fragments of antigen usually containing no more than 15–17 amino acids. Hence it is absolutely essential for antigen to be engulfed and digested by specialized cells and then be re-presented as "bite size" determinants. "Fractured foreignness" is presented to the cells of our specific immune system for inspection. Monocytes (which are precursors of macrophages) are the major antigen-presenting cells in the body, but specialized cells in the skin (Langerhans' cells) and intestinal tract (M cells), as well as certain lymphocytes, can also perform this task satisfactorily.

6. The many trees in the immunological forest (lymphoid cells) are, in fact, constantly patrolling around the body in a routine and not entirely random fashion. They circulate in the blood and lymphatic fluid and must be summoned and then guided from their circulation pathways into a tissue that is infected. A continuity of cellular signposts and chemoattractants, activated only after an antigen enters a tissue, accomplishes this extraordinary task.

7. As hinted at above, immune responses are tightly controlled and positive (deliberate) interactions may result in signals that "upregulate" or "downregulate" the inflammatory potential of the immune response. In a manner analogous to the way in which our autonomic nervous system is designed, an immune response at any given moment represents the net result of simultaneously active stop and go signals. With time, immune responses are actively terminated. Thus, the family of cells that supplies us with a specific immune response are referred to as either immunoregulatory or effector cells.

8. Many microorganisms have developed tactics that allow them to

subvert our immune response. The ultimate (we hope) example of this is the destruction by the human immune deficiency virus (HIV) of critical cells within the immune system. Apart from HIV, however, many examples of less dramatic but nonetheless important perturbations of immunological performance can be induced by certain microbes to their own survival advantage. Similar protective mechanisms are generated by some tumor cells.

Ironically, many infectious agents are harmless in that they would produce little or no damage in a tissue or cell in which they had taken up residence. It is the potent immune response they provoke that may cause the disease process (for example, hepatitis B).

We can now look at how lymphocytes recognize antigens, how they interact with macrophages and other cells that prepare antigen for recognition, and then follow the events that ensue in the generation of a specific immune response.

## The Cellular Elements of the Specific Immune System

### Thymus-derived lymphocytes—"T cells"

The thymus is a bilobed gland that sits astride the grest vessels leaving the heart. It develops early in human embryonic life and ten weeks into gestation it begins to function. The gland has three major functions:

1. It secretes a chemoattractant that recruits primitive stem cells, initially from the fetal liver and later from the bone marrow, for "education" within the gland.
2. It educates those recruits by activating genes within the now intrathymic cells that program the production of membrane receptors to "recognize" the one antigenic determinant that will have a best-fit status within this receptor molecule. This "T" cell receptor (TCR) is positioned on the surface of the cell so that its binding site projects out into the microenvironment (see Fig. 11.1).

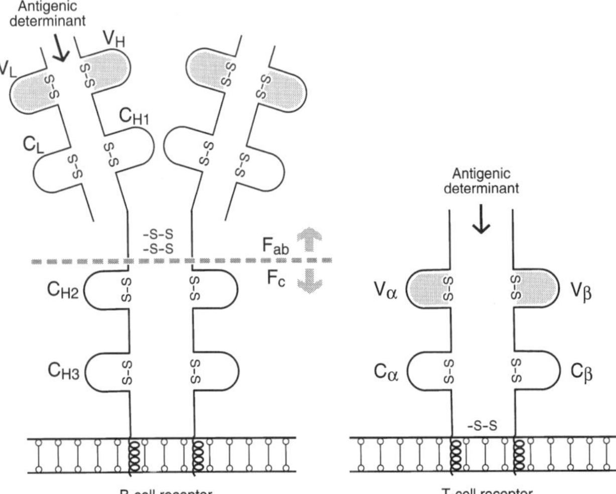


**Fig. 11.1** Both B and T lymphocytes have surface-membrane receptors for antigenic determinants. All binding sites for antigen on any one cell are identical. T cells have receptors for antigen that are constructed from two chains of amino acids—$\alpha$ and $\beta$ (a small subset have variations known as gamma and delta chains), each of which has a constant and variable domain. B-cell receptors for antigen are immunoglobulin molecules. They have a valency of two, three constant domains, and a variable terminal domain whose three-dimensional shape allows one antigenic determinant best-fit status.

Four morphologically identical but functionally distinct T-cell subtypes have been identified:

- Cells that must be activated by an encounter with antigen to initiate the chain of events that leads to a *cellular* immune response (TH1 cells).
- Cells that must be activated by an encounter with antigen to initiate the chain of events that leads to a *humoral* immune response (TH2 cells).

Both of these cells have clustered on their outer membranes a protein that allows their function to be differentiated from that of other T-cell subsets. This "cluster of differentiation" (CD) protein is referred to by the number 4. The cells are referred to as CD4 T lymphocytes or in biological shorthand, "T4" cells. In descriptions of their function they are usually referred to as inducer or helper lymphocytes, but as the former term is more accurate it is used throughout this text.

- The thymus educates a class of T cells that has the capacity to lyse (kill) infected cells and some tumor cells, but only after receiving specific instruction from CD4 lymphocytes. These cells are referred to as cytotoxic or "killer" T lymphocytes.
- Finally, a class of T cells produced by the thymus gland plays a vital role in the regulation of specific immune functions. As most interactions between these cells and the effector cells of the immune apparatus result in a downregulation of effector function, these T cells are often referred to as "suppressor" T lymphocytes. However, these cells may occasionally upregulate effector function and thus are better referred to as *immunoregulatory* T lymphocytes.

Both cytotoxic and immunoregulatory T cells have a cluster of differentiation protein on their surface, referred to as CD8. Complicated flow cytometric analysis in research laboratories can distinguish cytotoxic from immunoregulatory CD8 cells, but these differentiating techniques are not yet available in clinical laboratories.

There is inconclusive but certainly suggestive evidence for a further subset of T lymphocytes that regulate CD8 immunoregulatory cells. These cells are referred to as contrasuppressor cells, and it is more likely than not that further research will solidify their place in the functional family of human T lymphocytes.

3. The third function of the thymus gland is perhaps the most complicated. The generation of T-cell receptors for antigenic determinants is accomplished by randomized genetic permutations and combinations. We thus generate receptors for peptide sequences of both foreignness and self. Mechanisms for eliminating or controlling T cells that are naturally programmed to recognize self are essential.

We have evolved such mechanisms, but they are not perfect. We all live with T cells in our body that have the potential for autoimmune activity. It is true, however, that millions of T cells generated in the thymus die an intrathymic death because they have receptors for certain self antigens. The mechanisms responsible will be discussed later in the chapter. The process is known as *negative selection*. The thymus, however, may destroy many of the cells it has created in a process known as *positive selection*. These selection mechanisms can be best understood after describing the events involved in antigen presentation.

### Immunogenetics and antigen presentation

Receptors on T cells for antigenic determinants consists of two chains of amino acids, the terminal portion of which has a three-dimensional shape in space that allows one and only one antigenic determinant to have "best fit" status within that receptor. However, the lock into which the antigenic key must fit is more complicated than that. An antigenic determinant is presented to a T cell packaged with a "presenting" molecule. Both antigenic determinant and presenting molecule come clustered together on the surface of the antigen-presenting cell. Imagine that you extend your index finger from a clenched fist. The finger is the antigenic determinant being presented to the T cell. The T-cell receptor that will accept that finger, however, is structured to allow both finger and fist to fit snugly into the T-cell receptor. Indeed, antigen will be recognized and therefore provoke a response only if the presenting molecule is embraced just as intimately as is the antigen in question. Why?

Immunological "mortal sin" involves the generation of an attack on self. Since evolution has not succeeded in eliminating T cells that could respond to self antigens, a secondary fail-safe mechanism demands that we actively present antigenic determinants for inspection. If we don't "present" self antigens appropriately, then a casual encounter between T-cell receptors and self antigens, even if that encounter involves a degree of binding, will not stimulate a response. T cells are activated only if they recognize antigen in the context of a presenting molecule. Using an explanatory style that personifies immunological reactions, lets look at this concept of "decision making."

Nature has found it necessary to separate inducer (CD4) and effector (CD8) lymphocytes so that a crucial decision-making step is possible. Effector lymphocytes, even if they recognize antigenic determinants presented appropriately, are not functional unless they receive a series of activating signals from CD4 lymphocytes and some other cells. For this reason, the molecules that present antigens to CD4 inducer T cells are different from those that present antigen to effector cells.

With the exception of red blood cells, every cell in our body can present antigens to effector lymphocytes. This is essential because at least theoretically every cell in our body could become infected or malignant. In such circumstances an immunological response against the cell would be appropriate. However, the majority of the time the presenting molecules that pepper the surface of all cells bind *self antigens*. After all, we are in a constant state of breakdown and repair, and the self determinants released may be trapped by the presenting molecules. It would be disastrous if these self antigen-presenting molecule complexes provoked an immune response; there is no shortage of T cells that can recognize this combination. Hence the crucial CD4 decision-making role.

Cells that present antigens to CD4 lymphocytes are highly specialized. They present only antigens that they have endocytosed or pinocytosed from the surrounding environment. They do not present soluble proteins. Hence CD4 lymphocytes are most likely to be presented with foreignness. CD8 cells will be presented constantly with foreignness and self. Being dependent on CD4 signals to attack, CD8 cells will in most circumstances not get the signal that would allow them to attack self, because self, unlike foreignness, will not have been presented to CD4 lymphocytes by their antigen-presenting cells. Some of the molecular details are described later in this chapter.

In looking at the nature of antigen presentation for the activation of cellular immune responses, another teleological concept seems reasonable. Immune responses involve the release of potent inflammation-inducing molecules. Battles with foreignness should therefore be intensely local affairs. By and large they are, and while we may experience fever and myalgia as a result of the *systemic* effects of the chemicals released, the *local* intensity of the reaction is far more extreme. Hence, having effector cells and antigen-presenting cells that have been infected by a virus physically bound together by presenting molecules, allows the killing to proceed with a minimum of bystander damage.

### The major histocompatibility loci

In immunology, terminology often obstructs ease of understanding. Historical appellations are not easily changed. For example, the genetic loci on the short arm of human chromosome 6 responsible for the production of antigen-presenting molecules should by rights be called "antigen-presenting loci." But they are not; they are referred to as "major histocompatibility loci."

This unfortunate state of affairs developed this way. With the first attempts at transplanting organs, cells, or tissue between nonidentical twins (or in a laboratory, non-inbred animals) the uniqueness of an individual's organ-associated antigens became clear. Nothing provokes a stronger immune response than cells or tissue from a genetically nonidentical individual. We now know that it is the presence of antigen-presenting molecules on the surface of nonidentical cells that provokes the strongest attempts at rejection. Within the human genetic pool there are hundreds of allelic arrangements that can occupy the loci responsible for the coding of these very immunogenic molecules. Despite this heterogeneity it is possible to find in the community individuals that have, by chance, the same combination of antigen-presenting molecules that we display and to which, because they represent self, we are tolerant. The closer the match, the less violent is the attempt to reject transplanted tissue. These antigen-presenting molecules were therefore referred to as "histocompatability antigens" and the loci that coded for them the "major histocompatability loci." Tissue typing, in which allelic expressions of antigen-presenting molecules on the cells of donor and potential recipient are matched, became available before we knew the function of the proteins whose structures were being compared.

The polymorphism that generates so many different antigen-presenting molecules was not an evolutionary development intended to make transplantation difficult. Some alleles code for presenting molecules that present certain microbial antigens better than others. For the sake of the species this heterogeneity is an advantage, but it matters little to the individual. The phenomenom does, however, explain why it is that the antigen-presenting molecules one produces are linked to disease susceptibility as well as the variability in response to an identical organism that is made by different individuals. These susceptibility (and protection) linkages are further strengthened because very close to those genetic loci on chromosome 6 that code for antigen-presenting molecules are genes involved in coding for the performance of immunoregulatory phenomena. Regulatory and antigen-presenting alleles are likely to coincide through many generations because of their proximity to each other on the one chromosome.

With that explanation we can approach the terminology involved. On each arm of chromosome 6 there are four loci where the genes present code for the production of antigen-presenting molecules. Genes inherited from both mother and father are fully expressed. Again the terminology is unfortunate; these gene products are present on the surface of all cells are most commonly referred to as human leukocyte associated antigens (HLA antigens) because they were first discovered on human leukocytes. HLA antigens are, in fact, antigen-presenting molecules, although of course there are thousands of other antigens on the surface of leukocytes that have nothing to do with antigen presentation (Fig. 11.2).

HLA antigens are coded for at four loci (A, B, C, or D) on chromosome 6. The antigen-presenting molecules on the surface of all cells except red cells are coded for at the A, B, and C loci,

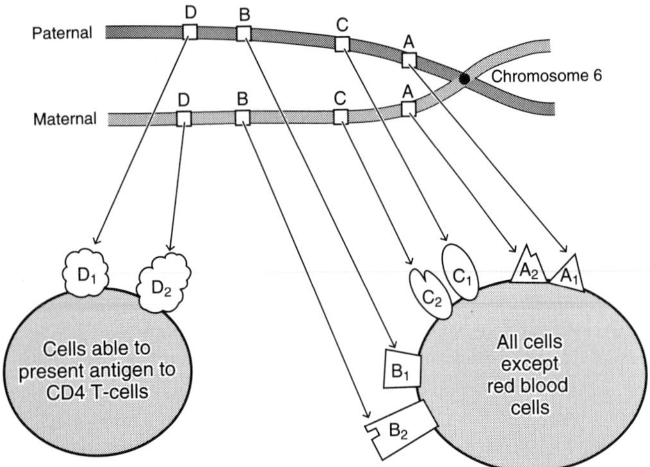


**Fig. 11.2** Antigen-presenting molecules are present on the surface of all but red blood cells. They are coded for by alleles that occupy loci on the short arm of chromosome 6. Inherited maternal and paternal alleles are fully expressed. Products coded for at A, B, and C loci (class I molecules) can present self and foreignness to CD8 T cells and B lymphocytes. Products coded for at D loci are expressed on the surface of a restricted number of cells and can present antigen to inducer CD4 T cells.

and these are collectively referred to as class I antigens. These are the molecules that present foreignness and self to CD8 lymphocytes. D locus class II antigens are present only on specific cells: macrophages, Langerhan's cells in the skin, dendritic cells in lymph nodes, certain mucosal cells, the lymphocytes that are responsible for antibody production (B cells) and in humans, activated T cells themselves. All of these cells can present processed exogenous peptides to CD4 lymphocytes. Since T cells must interact with class II antigen-presenting molecules before a response is made to antigen bound to class I molecules, it's a pity the numbers are not reversed.

## Selection in the thymus

Understanding antigen presentation mechanisms is a prerequisite to further discussion of the all-important subject of T-cell selection in the thymus. As T cells mature in the thymus, they eventually display their receptor for antigen (TCR). In the thymus are antigen-presenting cells displaying their A, B, C, and D loci–induced molecules. Undoubtedly there are many other self antigens present as well. The random process that produces TCR means that cells will be created that recognize an individual's A, B, C, and D loci products as antigens. Those T cells that recognize and bind such antigens need to be eliminated prior to release from the thymus. The majority of such cells, as well as other cells that see self antigens in the thymus, are destroyed on binding to antigen. Programmed cell death (apoptosis) is activated following such a happening intrathymically. This is called *clonal abortion*, as the "family" of T cells that could attack our own tissues displaying the antigens seen in the thymus are destroyed.

As mentioned earlier, the process is not perfect. Not all self-recognizing cells are destroyed. Some survive but are rendered tolerant (clonal anergy) by mechanisms that are still poorly understood. Perhaps of more importance is the obvious imperfection in this *negative selection* process. During their time of intrathymic development, T cells with TCR for tissue- and organ-specific antigens will not encounter those antigens that do not enter the thymic milieu; hence the need for additional safeguards to prevent reactivity to self at the time of antigen presentation.

An additional selection process is now known to be operative in the thymus. TCR are produced randomly and, as described earlier, consist of three-dimensional shapes that recognize antigen and presenting molecules simultaneously. An individual inherits a specific allelic pattern of presenting molecules. T cells that can recognize only foreignness in the context of other arrangements of antigen-presenting molecules are useless to us. Such cells are also destroyed in the thymus (*positive selection*). The result of all this intrathymic destruction is that only about 5% of the stem cells that enter the thymus leave the gland to provide us with a specific immune system (Fig. 11.3).

## T-cell maturation

The human thymus develops from the third and fourth pharyngeal pouches; as these are paired the thymus develops as a bilobed structure. Each thymic lobe is encapsulated by a membrane that migrates into the gland to form inner partitions (septa) and divide the gland into lobules. Each lobule consists of two distinct regions: an inner medulla and an outer cortex.

Other structures developed from the third and, more specifically, the fourth pharyngeal pouches include the parathyroid glands and the great vessels that come out of the heart. Embryonic disaster affecting the third and fourth pharyngeal pouches presents as DiGeorge's syndrome. Neonates with the syndrome are recognized because of hypocalcemia (tetany) and abnormalities affecting the great vessels coming from the heart. The thymic shadow normally seen on chest X ray will be absent. In such children normal cell-mediated immunity cannot develop.

Stem cells that carry a differentiation antigen known as Thy-I preferentially enter the thymus and progressively mature as they move from the cortex to the medulla. It is in the medulla that antigen-presenting molecules are well displayed and much of the selection process starts. Necessarily, much of the intimate maturation detail we have discovered comes from studies on laboratory mice, but we have good evidence to suggest that the essentials are similar in humans.

In the cortex, cells display initially one of the two chains of their TCR (the beta chain), with the alpha chain developing sometime later. With the development of the two chains the cells begin to display a universal T-cell cluster of differentiation protein, CD3, which is an intimate associate of the TCR. Soon after the expression of the alpha and beta chain of the T-cell receptor on the surface of a maturing T cell, CD4 and CD8 proteins appear simultaneously on the surface of the still-developing T cell. These CD4 and CD8 cells move into the medulla of the thymus, where positive and negative selection occurs as the cells finally differentiate into either CD4- or CD8-positive cells. Those cells that survive in this demanding microenvironment leave the thymus via the medulla.

## The secondary lymphoid organs

The thymus is the major primary lymphoid organ. Lymph nodes (including the spleen) are secondary lymphoid organs designed to facilitate the presentation of antigen to specific receptors on the surface of lymphocytes. At any given moment, most lymphocytes would be found resident in these secondary organs, though 1% of the total lymphocyte pool recirculates each hour. As there are approximately $10^{12}$ lymphocytes in the adult human

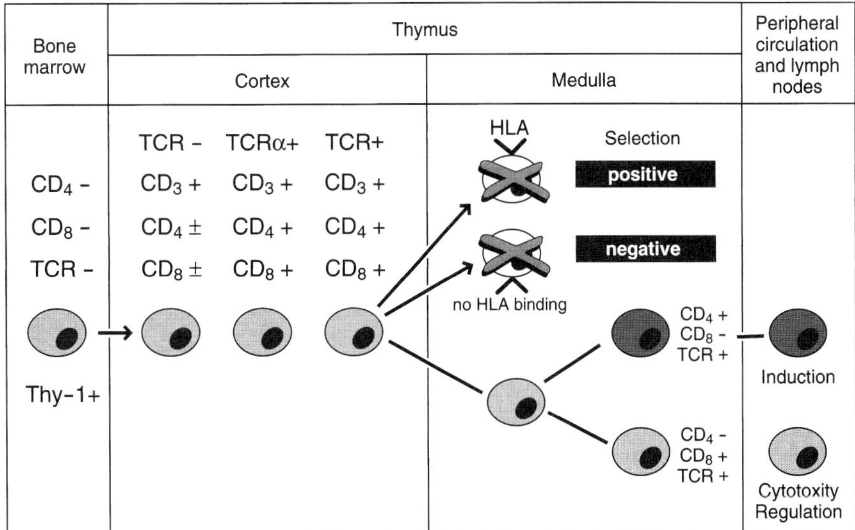


**Fig. 11.3** Would-be T cells are attracted into the cortex of the thymus from bone marrow. As they mature there they display their T-cell receptor and become both CD4- and CD8-positive. In the medulla they differentiate to become inducer CD4 cells or cytotoxic or regulatory cells expressing CD8. T cells that recognize self A, B, C, or D locus antigens are largely eliminated (positive selection), as are T cells that cannot recognize antigen in the context of self antigen-presenting molecules (negative selection).

body, many lymphocytes are found in blood and lymphatic vessels, where they circulate in lymph. Circulation pathways involve cells migrating from blood to lymphoid tissue, then on into lymphatic vessels, which run parallel to blood vessels, and back again into the bloodstream via the thoracic duct. In the circulation pathway, migration through the bone marrow is a regular event. The circulation pathway for many cells involves entrance into the specialized lymphoid areas found in association with our bowel, (gut-associated lymphoid tissue, or GALT) and the bronchial tree.

These migratory patterns are not as random as they might first appear. Certain lymphocytes tend to home repeatedly to a specific lymphoid organ such as the spleen- or the mucosa-associated lymph nodes of the GALT system. Lymphocytes leave the bloodstream to enter lymphoid tissue via postcapillary high endothelial venules (HEV). On the cuboidal HEV cells of vessels entering lymphoid organs are distinctive homing proteins that bind subsets of lymphocytes that have receptor molecules complimentary to these particular structures. This ensures that certain cells migrate preferentially to certain lymphoid organs. Once in the lymph node or spleen, cells cluster in anatomically distinct portions of the organ. For example, in lymph nodes, T cells congregate in the cortex of the node while the B cells (to be discussed below) gather into dense round lymphocytic follicles that are surrounded by CD4 and CD8 T cells. Lymphatic fluid, which often contains antigen, circulates through tiny lymphatic tributaries within the T- and B-cell areas of the organ to maximize the chance that antigen will be taken up from the lymph by antigen-presenting cells present in both T- and B-cell areas.

## T-cell migration into tissues

Just as T cells can be lured from blood vessels into specific lymphoid organs via interaction with homing receptors, lymphocytes can be summoned into tissues when a potentially dangerous invader is present. In this way the full repertoire of antigen-reactive lymphocytes has access to different body tissues.

Local, non-antigen-specific mechanisms result in the release of chemicals that upregulate the expression of homing molecules in the local vasculature. In this way cells circulating through such tissue are induced to migrate into the surrounding tissues, where a chemoattractant gradient guides lymphocytes to the very source of the alarm signal.

When a T cell arrives at a site of invasion, adhesion molecules on antigen-presenting cells (non-antigen-specific) bind to complimentary receptors on T cells and provide an opportunity for locally processed antigen to be introduced to the T cells' TCR. Unless an antigen in combination with an antigen-presenting molecule is recognized, the T cell is released and allowed to go on its way and the next T cell that migrates by is hooked for inspection of the antigen. Thus it is that the primary encounter between a T cell and an antigen on the surface of an antigen-presenting cell can occur in either a tissue or a secondary lymphoid organ.

## A cellular immune cascade

We are now in a position where we can look at the chain of events that links all of the mechanisms discussed above into a smooth, powerful, but controlled continuum.

When foreign antigens encounter specific antigen-presenting cells they will be in the form of either exogenous proteins or particulate material. Exogenous proteins are internalized by antigen-presenting cells and taken up intracellularly by *endosomes*. Therein enzymatic processing reduces the proteins to small peptides. Particulate antigen is *phagocytosed* into the antigen-presenting cell only to be taken up into *phagolysosomes*. Here also, proteolytic cleavage results in the production of small peptides. While this activity is proceeding, class II antigen-presenting mol-

**Table 11.1** Immunological responses to bacterial infection associated with the clearance of the organism

| | | Humoral response | | | | Cellular response | |
|---|---|---|---|---|---|---|---|
| Bacteria | Disease | Class | Antitoxin | Opsonisation[a] | Complement | DTH[b] | CD8 Killing |
| *S. aureus* | Boils | M,G | – | + | +++ | – | – |
| *S. pyogenes* | Tonsillitis | M,G | – | + | +++ | – | – |
| *S. pneumoniae* | Pneumonia | M,G | – | +++ | +++ | – | – |
| *N. gonorrheae* | Gonorrhea | G,A | – | ++ | + | – | – |
| *C. diphtheriae* | Diphtheria | G | +++ | + | + | – | – |
| *C. tetani* | Tetanus | G | +++ | + | + | – | – |
| *T. pallidum* | Syphilis | G,E | – | + | ++ | + | – |
| *B. burgdoferi* | Lyme disease | G,E | – | + | ++ | + | ++ |
| *L. pneumophila* | Legionnaires' disease | G | – | + | +++ | +++ | – |
| *R. prowazeki* | Typhus | – | – | – | – | +++ | ++ |
| *C. trachomatis* | Trachoma | – | – | – | – | ++ | ++ |
| Mycobacteria | TB, leprosy | – | – | – | – | ++++ | ++ |

[a]Promotes not only phagocytosis but NK cell killing.
[b]CD4 T cells and macrophages.

ecules are being assembled on the cell's endocytoplasmic reticulum. These molecules are composed of two polymorphic chains, alpha and beta, of molecular weight 33 and 29 kd, respectively. Two domains containing intrachain disulphide bonds are present on each chain. Inside the antigen-presenting cell newly assembled alpha and beta chains of the class II molecule are linked to a third "invariant" chain that transports the molecule into the lysosomes and endosomes where the newly formed peptides are placed in a groovelike structure in the class II molecule. X-ray crystallography suggests that the take-up of antigen and its display resembles cargo (antigen) in the open bay of the space shuttle capsule (antigen-presenting molecule) (Fig. 11.4).

Once antigenic determinants and presenting molecules are displayed on the surface of the specialized presenting cell, it remains for one of the attracting mechanisms discussed above to bring the appropriate T cells onto the scene. Localized CD4 lymphocytes randomly interact with loaded antigen-presenting cells and the two players in the immunological drama bind to each other in a manner that ensures that what is being carried in the class II molecular groove is inserted into a CD4 TCR to see if a best fit is achieved.

On the side of the class II molecule is a specific protein sequence that CD4 molecules bind to. In addition on the CD4 cell surface is a homing antigen (leukocyte function antigen 1, or LFA-1) that interacts with a complimentary protein on the surface of the antigen-presenting cell: intracellular adhesion molecule 1, or ICAM-1. These adhesion molecules that hold antigen-presenting and T cells together are essential for the triggering of a normal response (Fig. 11.5).

LFA-1 belongs to a family of adhesion molecules known as

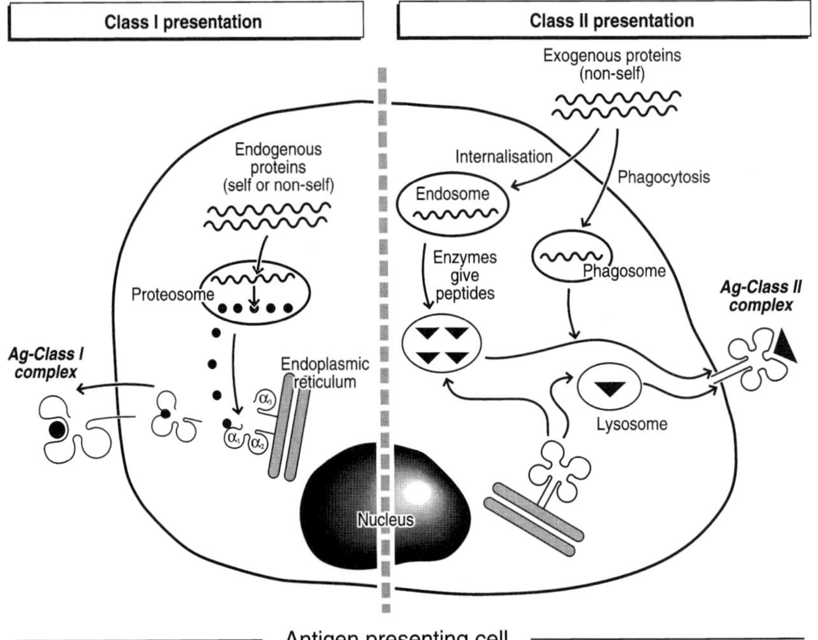


**Fig. 11.4** Endogenous proteins (usually self) are processed in proteosomes and the peptide fragments formed displayed to CD8 cells by class I presenting molecules. Exogenous proteins are digested and displayed to CD4 cells by class II molecules.

**Table 11.2** Immunological responses to nonbacterial infection associated with the clearance of the organism

| | | Humoral response | | | | Cellular response | |
|---|---|---|---|---|---|---|---|
| Organism | Disease | Class | Antitoxin | Opsonization[a] | Complement | DTH[b] | CD8 Killing |
| VIRUSES | | | | | | | |
| Variola | Smallpox | – | – | – | – | + | +++ |
| Varicella zoster | Chickenpox | M,G | – | + | + | – | ++ |
| Epstein-Barr | Mononucleosis | G | – | ++ | ++ | – | +++ |
| Influenza | Influenza | G,A | – | ++ | ++ | – | + |
| Mumps | Mumps | G | – | +++ | ++ | – | + |
| Polio | Poliomylitis | G | – | + | – | – | +++ |
| HIV | AIDS | – | – | – | – | – | + |
| FUNGI | | | | | | | |
| *Candida albicans* | Candidiasis | G,A | – | ++ | + | +++ | – |
| PROTOZOA | | | | | | | |
| Plasmodium | Malaria | G | – | ++ | ++ | ++ | – |
| *Toxoplasma gondii* | Toxoplasmosis | G | – | ++ | ++ | ++ | – |
| *Trypanasoma* spp. | Trypanosomiasis | G | – | ++ | ++ | ++ | – |
| *Leishmania* spp. | Leishmaniasis | – | – | – | – | ++++ | – |
| WORMS | | | | | | | |
| Schistosome | Schistosomiasis | – | – | – | – | ++++ | – |

[a]Promotes not only phagocytosis but NK cell killing.
[b]CD4 T cells and macrophages.

integrins. It is composed of alpha- and beta-chain dimers. A recessively inherited deficiency of the beta chain results in "leukocyte adhesion deficiency disease." Patients so deprived are susceptible to very severe infections (see Chapter 86).

As an example of how the system works, imagine that a viral peptide has been introduced appropriately to a TCR programmed to recognize that particular peptide. The chain reaction that follows will lead to an effective antiviral response involving many cells activated by chemicals or "cytokines" released by the cellular players. Two of the most important cytokines produced and released by CD4 cells are interleukin-2 (IL-2) and interferon gamma (IFN-$\gamma$).

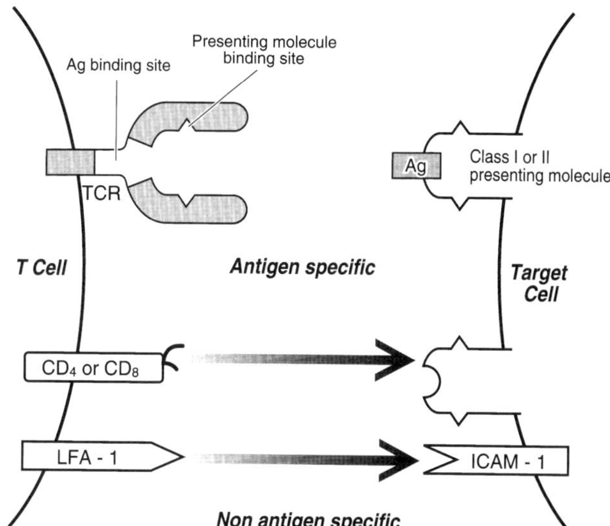


**Fig. 11.5** T cells bind to an antigen-presenting cell using antigen-specific and -nonspecific mechanisms. Presenting molecules holding an antigenic peptide will bind to a TCR. Adhesion molecules hold cells together while TCR and antigen attempt to interact.

## Cytokines

Over the last ten years, molecular biology has identified a series of chemicals released by specific cells that affect others that express on their surface membrane a receptor for one or more of these cytokines. The molecules in question are essential for cell growth, differentiation, proliferation, and the activation of specific functions (see Chapter 46).

Cytokines are produced by cells of the lymphoid system, and at this writing more than a dozen have been purified to homogeneity. Many are being used in clinical trials (see Chapter 46). Cytokines produced by both lymphocytes and macrophages are involved in the specific immune response. Rather than discussing them individually, we will examine them in the context of the evolving response to the viral peptides described above.

## The response to antigen recognition

Our antigen-presenting cell has just successfully introduced a viral peptide to a CD4 TCR that recognized its amino acid sequence. The antigen-presenting cell, usually a macrophage, will now release a cytokine known as interleukin-1 (IL-1). In specific immunity, the major function of this molecule (which induces a protean array of responses) (see Chapter 46) appears to be the stimulation of the primed CD4 lymphocyte to secrete interleukin-2 (IL-2).

Besides induction of IL-2, IL-1 is responsible for the fevers that so frequently accompany an infection and is in fact the same chemical as endogenous pyrogen (see Chapter 9). IL-1 is also responsible for the release into the circulation of acute phase reactants. In most infections, there is a dramatic rise in circulating levels of C-reactive protein, SAA (serum amyloid anticedent), and fibrinogen, the latter leading to an increase in the erythrocyte sedimentation rate (see Chapters 10 and 11).

At the beginning of the chapter we noted that CD4 inducer cells are functionally defined as TH1 and TH2 cells. TH1 cells specifically help CD8 lymphocytes to become activated and cytotoxic. TH2 cells, as we will see, help B cells begin the production cycle that will result in antibody formation.

A TH1 CD4 cell responding to a challenge from a viral peptide and spurred on by IL-1, for which it has a cell-surface receptor, secretes two interleukins, IL-2 and IL-12. These two can act independently but usually cooperate synergistically in that IL-12 augments IL-2 production.

IL-2 was at first known as "T-cell growth factor." Its discovery and use was instrumental in the culture of the human retroviruses responsible for T-cell leukemia and AIDS. IL-2 was first found in the supernatant of CD4 cells stimulated in vitro with the mitogen phytohemagglutinin (PHA). IL-2 is a 15 kd molecule that activates cells which have a receptor for IL-2 (IL-2R) on their surface. Resting CD8 cytotoxic cells do not display IL-2R, but antigenically primed CD8 cells do. If, and only if, these receptors bind IL-2 does cytotoxicity commence. IL-2 also stimulates some lymphocytes to secrete IFN-$\gamma$, which has potent antiviral and antiproliferative effects, and also activates macrophage functions.

IL-2 has the capacity to turn resting T cells into promiscuous tumor cell killers. These lymphokine-activated killer cells (LAK cells) don't respond to MHC restriction rules and kill both autologous and allogeneic tumor cells. Much is yet to be learned about the molecular mechanisms involved. Unfortunately, the administration of IL-2 to humans results in severe toxicity. Nevertheless, trials of IL-2 infusions in patients infected with HIV have produced encouraging results. (Chapter 46). There is good evidence to suggest that with time TH1, CD4 lymphocytes are preferentially killed by HIV and, as a result, CD8 cells are deprived of the IL-2 necessary for them to maintain their antiviral activity (Chapter 96). IL-12 stimulates T cells in a manner that is very similar to that of IL-2 and it also induces IFN-$\gamma$ production.

## The killing of virus-infected cells

While CD4 positive cells are activated by a peptide-class II presentation, CD8$^+$ cells can be readied for a cytotoxic attack on virus-infected cells. The virus, of course, has its own mechanism for getting inside a target cell, where it becomes an endogenous protein. Any internal endogenous protein (including self protein) can be processed in a proteosome and subsequently expressed on the surface of the cell in association with class I molecules.

Class I molecules are composed of a polymorphic alpha chain that noncovalently pairs with a nonpolymorphic molecule called beta 2 microglobulin ($\beta$2M). This latter molecule is encoded outside of the antigen-presenting loci on chromosome 6. Three regions of the class I molecule contain intrachain disulphide bridges and are designated as domains. Antigenic peptides are displayed in a groove within the molecular configuration of the class I molecule (Fig. 11.6).

CD8 potentially cytotoxic cells recognize these peptides after a similarly close inspection to the one carried out by CD4 cells seeing antigen attached to class II molecules. The same LFA-1 and ICAM interactions draw the virus-infected and CD8 T cells together, and indeed CD8 molecules can bind to class I molecules. TCR recognition of the peptide being presented leads to the upregulation in the expression on the surface of the CD8 lymphocytes of receptors for IL-2 and IL-12. The cell then awaits CD4 activation for attack in the form of IL-2 and IL-12 signals (Fig. 11.7).

Interestingly, the release of IFN-$\gamma$ upregulates the expression of class I antigens on virus-infected cells, making the target that much easier to recognize. With IL-2 and IL-12 binding to the surface of the CD8-positive cytotoxic cell, the killing commences. Death results from damage to the cell membrane and its permeability barrier. Even before membrane damage is evident, fragmentation of chromosomal DNA and loss of nuclear integrity can be detected. The biochemical mechanisms involved are both magnesium and calcium dependent. Perforin, a calcium-dependent pore-forming protein located in cytoplasmic granules within cytotoxic lymphocytes, is an important participant in the killing of an infected cell, as is the release from CD8 T cells of tumor-

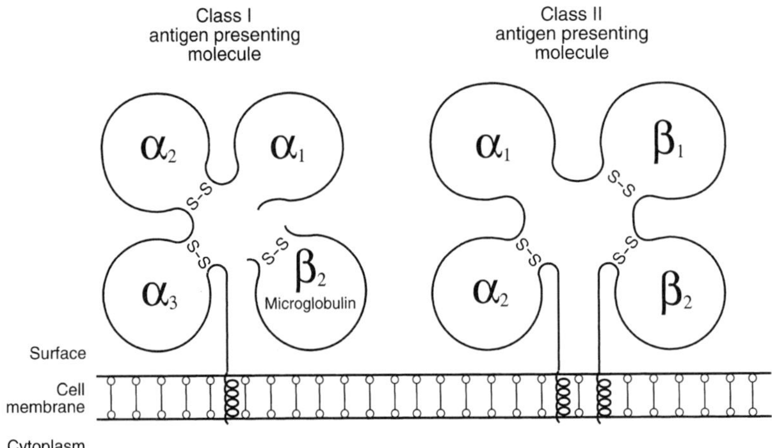


**Fig. 11.6** Class I and class II molecules are quite distinctive. $B_2$ microglobulin, produced separately from the class I $\alpha$ chain, completes the molecule. Class II molecules have $\alpha$ and $\beta$ chains and domains defined by disulphide bridges.

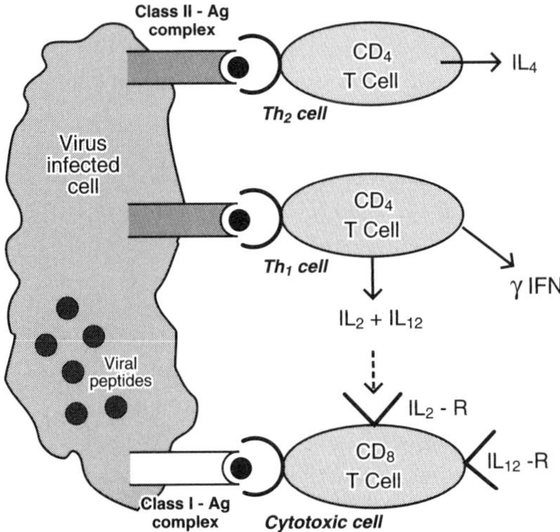


**Fig. 11.7** A virus-infected cell the displays class II as well as class I antigen-presenting molecules can activate CD4 and CD8 lymphocytes. If the cell cannot display class II molecules, a specialized antigen-presenting cell must do so to present viral peptides to a CD4 cell before the virus-infected target cell is attacked. TH2 cells stimulate antibody formation. TH1 cells give CD8 cells "permission" in the form of IL-2 and IL-12.

necrosis factor, a powerful cytokine that is toxic to infected cells and many tumor cells.

## Delayed-type hypersensitivity

T-cell effector responses are not restricted to cytotoxicity. Phylogenetically macrophagelike cells were phagocytosing and killing invaders before T cells became so sophisticated. At some point the evolutionary process selected for T cells that could harness macrophage properties, thus having them contribute to an antigen-specific response. Thus, when we discuss cell-mediated effector responses we must include delayed-type hypersensitivity (DTH) as well as the CD8 cytotoxic response.

Certain CD4 T cells have the capacity to migrate rapidly through tissues along the signed immunological biways as they respond to chemoattractants. The reactions are antigen specific, and local factors that are still poorly understood call these cells to action. Mast cells, basophils, and macrophages are involved early in the delayed hypersensitivity reaction, but macrophage recruitment and activation is markedly increased after the arrival on the scene of these CD4 T cells.

Whether these cells are typical TH1 cells or other specialized T cells is unknown. The collection of an appropriate mass of activated T cells (only some of which are specific for the antigen that has provoked the inflammatory melee) takes about 48 hours in humans in an already sensitized individual; visible DTH is a *secondary* immune response. Readily demonstrable is the role of regulatory cells in shutting down the inflammatory response, which features much edema and all of the cells mentioned above.

In older texts, DTH is known as type IV hypersensitivity. The best-known example in clinical medicine is the DTH reaction to tuberculin, which is provoked in a "positive Mantoux" test (see Chapter 57). DTH-like mechanisms may be stimulated by systemic infections once they have localized, but it seems that the rapid entry of antigen into local lymphatic vessels is necessary for the most vigorous response. This is why intradermal injections of antigen, which results in rapid lymphatic uptake, produces such strong reactions in the sensitized individual.

The inability to mount DTH reactions (anergy) occurs with cellular immune deficiency states but also in situations where the migration of T cells into the skin is interfered with. Interferon is a cytokine that can block DTH, and thus anergy is common in states where intense but poorly regulated immune responses are occurring. Many diseases that feature granuloma formation as part of their pathology are associated with anergy.

## Humoral Immunity

CD4 lymphocytes are essential for the production of the antibody repertoire, and the rules for antigen presentation are virtually identical in both humoral and cellular immune systems.

## Bone marrow–derived B lymphocytes

In birds, B lymphocytes that will be responsible for antibody production differentiate in a primary lymphoid organ that arises from the cloaca known as the bursa of Fabricius. It is a fortunate linguistic coincidence that the primary lymphoid organ responsible for the production of B lymphocytes in humans is the bone marrow.

B lymphocytes produce and secrete an array of immunoglobulin products as they mature following an encounter with antigen. Diversity in terms of antigen recognition is generated in the bone marrow in a manner similar to that used in the thymus to create antigen-specific T cells. B cells possess a receptor for antigen (BCR) that projects out into the microenvironment from the cell's surface. It allows any one B cell to bind a specific three-dimensional shape into the terminal portion of its BCR.

The fundamental difference between cellular and humoral immunity, and one that explains the unique design features of the latter system, is best understood in terms of local versus systemic influence. T cells kill and eliminate in their immediate environment; B cells secrete products that are effective remote from the factories that produce them. This fact appears to meet design demands for a system that must cope with rapidly dividing and disseminating extracellular bacteria, some of which are capable of secreting toxins that will be active systemically and must be neutralized.

Given the above, it is logical for B cells to use as a receptor for antigen the products that the activated cell will secrete. If antigen-trapping receptor molecules can bind antigen on the surface of a B cell, they will bind antigen once released into the circulation. Thus, B cell receptors are themselves immunoglobulin molecules.

Immunoglobulin molecules are composed of four polypeptides: two identical "heavy" chains of 50 kd each and two identical "light" chains of 25 kd each. The chains are held together by disulphide bridges. Their N-terminal region is referred to as the variable portion of the molecule. The C-terminal end of the molecule, which on the surface of the B cell is buried in its outer membrane, is relatively constant. It is the amino acid sequence within the variable region that determines which particular peptide can enter into an antigen–antibody reaction (Fig. 11.8). Fundamentally, an appropriately primed B lymphocyte encountering "its" antigen divides, matures, and secretes the molecule that trapped antigen on its surface in the first place.

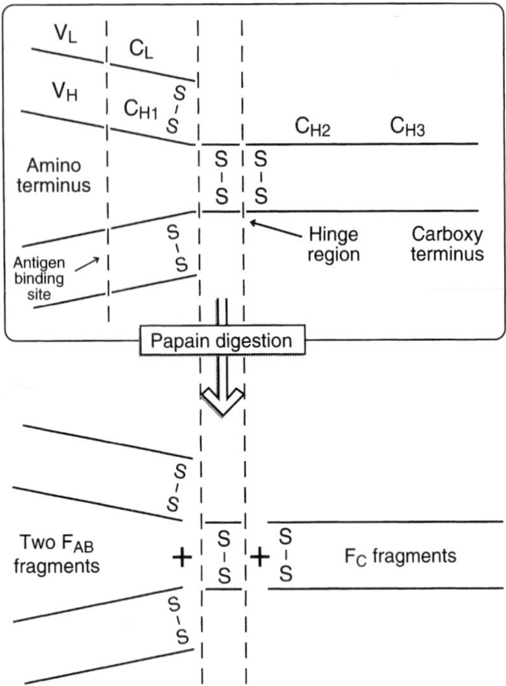


**Fig. 11.8** Immunoglobulin (antibody) molecules are composed of heavy and light chains. Digestion fragments reveal that the antigen-binding capacity of an immunoglobulin molecule is associated with the amino terminus–variable regions. Complement activation and binding of immunoglobulins to mast cells, phagocytic cells, and NK cells is mediated by amino acid segments in the Fc portion of the molecule.

## Immunoglobulins

It is necessary to look at the product of B cells before we review the generation and action of the cells themselves. In humans, B cells produce five major isotypes (classes) of immunoglobulin (antibody), and they are referred to as Ig (for immunoglobulin) types M, D, E, G, and A. Three classes of immunoglobulin—IgM, IgG, and IgA—are further subdivided into subclasses, variations on a theme that add to the diversity of function needed by our humoral immune system.

While the once-popular concept that ontogeny recapitulates phylogeny may have been discredited by a number of biologists as a generally applicable principle of evolution, there is no doubt that it is true with respect to antibody production. Looking at surviving species with immune systems less well developed than our own, the phylogenetic addition of immunoglobulin classes to the humoral immune repertoire is obvious and appropriate. As this evolutionary layering is recapitulated during fetal and postfetal life, developmental arrest can occur for various reasons, depriving us of some immunological classes and subclasses.

IgM was nature's first production model for an immunoglobulin, and B cells as they leave the bone marrow and migrate to the B cell areas (lymphocytic follicles) of the lymphoid organs are covered with five hundred thousand or so receptors for an antigenic determinant. All of these receptors are IgM in nature.

The differentiation of B cells occurs in two stages; the first is antigen independent, while the second follows an antigenic encounter. During the early stages of its differentiation, an individual precursor B cell rearranges the genes that code for the variable regions of the heavy and light chains of immunoglobulins and in so doing randomly selects a particular BCR. This random rearrangement occurring throughout the B-cell population is responsible for diversity in terms of antigen recognition. Again the system begins to mature very early in fetal life, and it is thought that by 16 weeks of gestation B cells recognize more than a million different antigenic determinants.

Pre–B cells contain only the heavy chain of IgM ($\mu$ chains) in their cytoplasm. As this pre–B cell matures it produces light chains and assembles a complete IgM molecule. The molecule is then fixed to its outer cell membrane. At this point it is referred to as an immature B cell. During its development to this point the B cell has also acquired other surface markers: the D locus class II antigens and three clusters of differentiation antigens: CD19, CD20, and CD21. B cells are destined to be able to present antigen to CD4-positive T cells (Fig. 11.9).

Without an encounter with antigen, immature B cells begin to produce intracytoplasmic IgD molecules, the variable regions of which are identical to those of the IgM already on the cell's surface. This specificity in the variable region is also referred to as *idiotypic specificity*. With the coexpression of IgM and IgD on the surface of an individual B cell, it has reached the end of its antigen-independent maturation.

## Antigen presentation and the activation of B cells

From the earliest experiments involved in the removal of the thymus from neonatal mice it was obvious that a lack of T cells was associated with a dramatic reduction in antibody production. T-cell help is indeed essential for normal humoral immune function. It is interesting to speculate that the preservation of many aspects of humoral immune function in patients with advanced HIV infection is associated with the preservation of TH2 rather than TH1 helper cells, which may be preferentially destroyed by HIV.

A mature B cell binds an antigenic determinant to its IgM class receptor, and this triggers numerous changes to the cell that prepare it for antibody secretion if "permission" is received from a TH2 CD4 T cell. The activated B cell upregulates, on its surface, receptors for IL-2, IL-4, and IL-6, all products of TH2 cells. It also displays more prominently an antigen known as CD40. The TH2 cell in its vicinity must see the appropriate antigenic determinant in the context of a class II antigen, and in a primary immune response this usually involves the presentation of antigen to B cells by macrophages.

A B cell could theoretically present the antigen it has bound to its BCR to the TH2 CD4 cell in its vicinity if the B cell processed that antigen and re-presented it in the groove of its class II molecules. The two processes are, however, quite independent of each other. Thus, the antigen present in the groove of a class II antigen on the surface of an unprimed B cell will not necessarily be related to the antigenic determinants that have been bound to that cell's antigen-specific BCR.

In a secondary immune response, however, B cells are much more likely to present to TH2 CD4 lymphocytes antigen that is bound to the cell's BCR, as with the maturation of the immune response the affinity of the receptors for antigen on a given B cell will increase and result in an abundance of trapped antigen being rapidly taken into the cytoplasm of the cell. After antigen binds to a BCR there is movement of the receptor/antigen complex to one pole of the cell, followed by phagocytosis of these

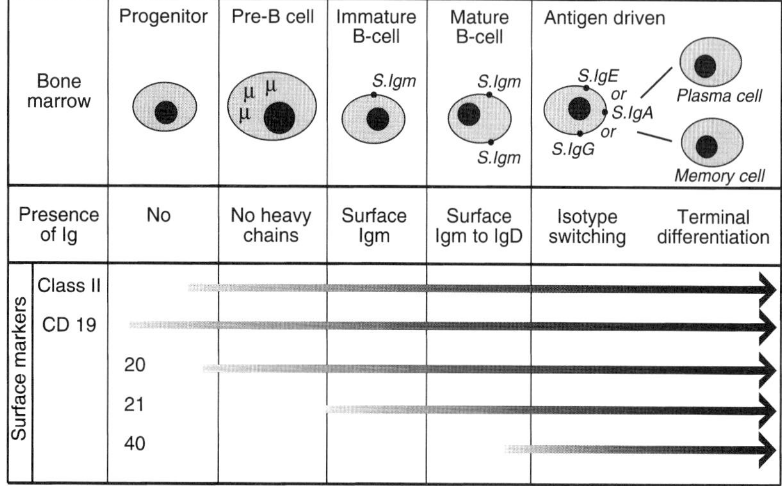


**Fig. 11.9** B cells mature in the bone marrow independent of the presence of antigen until that point in their differentiation when they express both surface IgM and IgD. In the presence of antigen that binds to the B cell's receptor, the cells switch the surface isotype they display and secrete different forms of immunoglobulin as they mature to plasma cells. A portion of the stimulated cells become "memory" B cells ready for the rapid secretion of IgG on a second encounter with antigen.

"capped" complexes. Thus, in a secondary immune response it's very much more likely that antigen displayed on the surface of the B cell in conjunction with a class II antigen will be the same antigen trapped in the immunoglobulin receptors on the surface of that cell.

Once the TH2 cell was recognized antigen appropriately presented, it displays on its surface a 33 kd protein that binds to the CD40 molecule now present on the activated B cells. This interaction holds the cell in place in a manner analogous to the way in which LAF-1 and ICAM molecules interact. Thus, B cell and TH2 cell are held in place while the B cell receives signals via the interleukins secreted by the now-activated T cell.

Interleukin-4 is a product of activated TH2 cells that was first given the name "B cell growth factor" (BCGF). It allows for the specific expansion of B cells responding to antigen. In a nice example of synergistic facilitation, IL-4 also stimulates the growth of CD4 TH2 cells themselves. It is involved in the switch of the B-cell immunoglobulin factory from IgM to IgE and IgG production.

Interleukin-5 is also a product of activated T cells and upregulates the expression of IL-2R on B cells, thus facilitating and promoting B cell division. Interleukin-6 (IL-6) is a product of monocytes and T cells that enhances the secretory phase of immunoglobulin production by B cells. Interleukin-7 (IL-7) is a recently identified molecule produced by thymic and bone marrow cells that induces the proliferation of pre–B cells.

A B cell's response to an antigenic encounter, and the help with which it is swamped, ensures that blast formation and proliferation of the stimulated B cells will occur rapidly to increase the number of antigen-specific B cells. The differentiation of this progeny into mature plasma cells that can secrete 2000 molecules of immunoglobulin per second follows rapidly. During all this TH2-dependent activity, plasma cells first secrete the IgM isotype. Interleukins, and perhaps yet-to-be-discovered factors, induce in time an isotype "switch" in which the factory rearranges the genes it is using for antibody production to produce IgE, IgG, and finally IgA. The specificity of all these molecules for the initiating antigen remains constant (Fig. 11.10).

Plasma cell formation represents terminal differentiation, and these antibody production factories are short-lived. Hence not all the progeny of activated B cells differentiate into plasma cells. Many mature, in that their membrane receptors for antigen display IgG receptors rather than IgM receptors, and reside as "memory" B cells in the follicular areas of the lymph node. This phenomenon explains the basis of the common serological characteristic of primary and secondary humoral immune responses. The presence in serum of IgM indicates a recent primary infection. Secondary infection will immediately activate IgG production from memory B cells that mature into IgG-secreting plasma cells. Memory B cells also have receptors on their surface for some components of the complement system and for the Fc por-

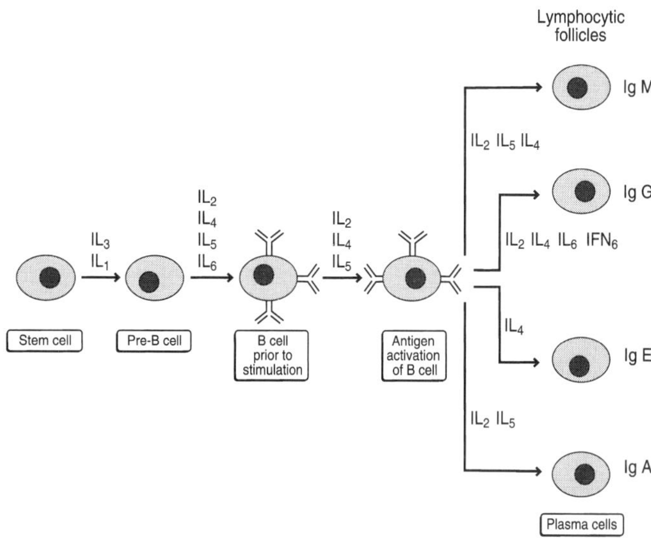


**Fig. 11.10** B cells mature under the influence of numerous cytokines and usually respond to antigen, terminally differentiating and secreting IgG, in the lymphocytic follicles of lymph nodes.

tion of immunoglobulins themselves. The significance of both these facts will be obvious when we examine antibody function.

## The functions of immunoglobulin molecules

What can immunoglobulins do for us? The rapid secretion of IgM following bacterial infection clearly offers some protection, but as this molecule in secreted form (as opposed to its B cell membrane form) clusters as a pentameric molecule, it cannot leave the bloodstream to provide tissue protection. Hence the primary immune response to extracellular bacteria takes time to be maximally effective, and during that time we are vulnerable to the pathogenic potential of these organisms.

The primary humoral response is of little use in coping with a new viral infection. Viral entry into target cells will occur more rapidly than will the production of neutralizing antibodies. Such antibodies are of course useful in second and later encounters with a virus, an important principle in vaccine immunology.

Antibodies can be likened to the laser beam in your compact disc player. They recognize that all those digital signals are representing the notes of Beethoven's fifth symphony, but their recognition of this fact is of no use to us without an amplification process. With the exception of IgA, which acts uniquely, immunoglobulins bind specifically and then harness nonspecific inflammatory "amplification" mechanisms to eliminate what they have bound.

When an antibody molecule is subjected to digestion by papain in the presence of cysteine as a reducing agent, the molecule is split into two functionally distinct units. N-terminal portions of the molecule retain their antigen-binding properties, and so these fragments are referred to as the *Fab* portion of the molecule (fragments with *antibody activity*). The remaining fragment, which does not bind antigen, *crystallizes* easily and is relatively *constant*, and it is referred to as the *Fc* portion of the antibody molecule. In general, the amplification mechanisms promoted by immunoglobulins involve the Fc portion of the molecule, the idiotypic Fab determinant being confined to assuring that the actions are antigen-specific.

A total of five antigenically distinct immunoglobulin heavy chains have been demonstrated. These are designated mu, delta, epsilon, gamma, and alpha to match the terminology given to the intact molecule (IgM, IgD, IgE, IgG, and IgA, respectively). Only two antigenically distinct light chains have been found: kappa and lambda.

### IgM

IgM is a pentamer whose monomers are linked by a J chain and disulphide bridges. There are five Fc portions available to activate and fix components of the complement cascade. IgM is very active, therefore, in promoting the cytolytic activity of complement, but only in the intravascular space, to which it is confined. The activation by an antigen antibody complex of the classical complement cascade results in (*1*) vasodilatation that facilitates the extravascular accumulation of cells and serum factors, (*2*) the production of chemoattractants for polymorphonuclear cells, (*3*) the activation of their phagocytic mechanisms, and (*4*) the activation of those terminal sequences in the complement cascade that can produce cell lysis by inducing pores in cell membranes.

In general, therefore, it is these proinflammatory mechanisms that represent the amplification strategy used by IgM and IgG. Because of its size, IgM is easily broken down into fragments that are useless. Its effective half-life in the serum is only 2 to 3 days. Individuals whose B-cell maturation is arrested at the IgM-secreting stage cannot survive without immunoglobulin therapy. There are two subclasses of IgM, but any functional distinction associated with these differences is as yet unknown. In an adult, IgM plasma concentration is normally 100–175 mg/dl.

### IgD

Any function of secreted IgD is yet to be defined, and indeed secretion of IgD by B cells is minimal. Thus, the concentration of IgD in adult serum is only 3–5 mg/dl. Membrane-bound IgD may well be involved in mechanisms associated with a switch in isotype production, but the role of the molecule remains far from clear. It is not present on the surface of B cells involved in the production of immunoglobulins other than IgM.

### IgE

This class of immunoglobulin may have arisen under the evolutionary pressure associated with the problem of parasitic infestation. The molecule is produced in relatively large quantities in response to the presence of antigenic determinants associated with many forms of parasites. On mast cells and basophils there are receptors for the Fc portion of IgE, and in the gastrointestinal tract the release of chemicals from these cells following the binding of an antigen–antibody complex to an Fc receptor increases bowel peristalsis, helping to eliminate parasites.

IgE in small amounts is a useful "immunological gatekeeper," and in this capacity plays a universal role in humoral immunity. Numerous vasoactive substances released from basophils in the blood and mast cells in the tissues dilate blood vessels locally and promote changes that enhance cellular trafficking into an area where antigen resides. The normal serum concentration of IgE is less than 30 $\mu$g/dl. It has a very short half-life of only 2 to 3 days. As the vasoactive potency of IgE is so powerful, production of the molecule is closely and actively regulated. Individuals who produce inappropriate amounts of IgE may suffer the clinical consequences that follow the release of excessive quantities of mast cell products—namely, vasodilatation and bronchial smooth-muscle cell contraction. The systemic effects can occur almost instantly, a phenomenon known as *immediate hypersensitivity*.

### IgG

This immunoglobulin plays a major role in defense against a large variety of microorganisms. The normal serum concentration of IgG is 1000–1500 mg/dl, and it has a serum half-life of 23–30 days. In general, it is capable of fixing and therefore activating complement, and it can diffuse readily into tissues. IgG is the predominant "opsonin" in serum (from the Greek word for "to prepare for a meal"), and particles coated with IgG are very likely to be phagocytosed by polymorphonuclear cells and to a lesser extent monocytes. On the surface of the phagocytes are receptors for both the Fc portion of IgG and complement components that may be bound to an antigen-antibody complex.

Over the evolutionary eons, B cells have been selected to produce four functionally distinct variations on the IgG theme. The clinical significance of these subclasses is only now being appreciated, and much is still to be learned. $IgG_1$ is the major immunoglobulin in serum and can activate complement. It has a half-life of 25 days. Together with $IgG_3$ it provides the major antibody response to protein antigens.

$IgG_2$ is essential for an adequate response to polysaccharide antigens and therefore to encapsulated bacteria. Selective deficiency of $IgG_2$ is well recognized, and the clinical consequences are predictably repeated severe infections with pneumococci and *Hemophilus influenzae*. The concentration of $IgG_2$ in human serum is 220–300 mg/dl and it also has a half-life of about 25 days.

$IgG_3$ has a half-life of only 9 days, because it has many more disulphide bridges holding its heavy and light chains together than do other IgG subclasses. This makes it easier for functional degradation to occur by proteolytic mechanisms. $IgG_3$ seems to be particularly important in the neutralization of viruses in a secondary immune response.

$IgG_4$ in serum represents only 4% of total IgG. It is unique among IgG subclasses in that there are receptors for the Fc portion of this molecule on mast cells and basophils. It has a half-life of 25 days and is generated, albeit in small quantities, in response to polysaccharide antigens. Selective deficiency often features severe bacterial infections in the lower respiratory tract (such as bronchiectasis), sinusitis, and abnormally high levels of IgE, suggesting that $IgG_4$ may play an important role in the defense of the lower respiratory tract. Frequently congenital deficiencies in subclass formation present with $IgG_1$ and $IgG_3$ deficiencies occurring simultaneously or $IgG_2$ and $IgG_4$ deficiencies present at the same time.

### IgA

Mucosal immunity is a huge and fascinating topic well worthy of detailed study. For one thing, more and more candidate vaccines for organisms that gain entry via mucous membranes are being prepared to take advantage of the mucosa's specialized immunological capacity.

Delicate mucous membranes, often richly supplied with nerves, are not sites where the inflammatory response is comfortably endured even if it were to eradicate a dangerous organism. Hence, mucosal humoral immune mechanisms involving the "silent antibody," IgA, have been evolved.

IgA is produced in the lymph nodes in the submucosal region by B lymphocytes obeying all the pertinent rules we have discussed above. The molecule is secreted in the form of a dimer (four antigen-binding sites) joined at the C-terminal end by a J chain, just as in the case of secreted IgM. The molecule, once secreted, must be transported to the mucosal membrane nearby, and a product of the local epithelial cells known as secretory component binds to the linked Fc portion of IgA molecules and transports the dimer to the mucosal surface by marching it through layer after layer of epithelial cells. Once it has reached the mucous membrane, electrostatic forces associated with the mucus that covers these membranes align the dimer so that its V-shaped chain-linked C-terminal region is buried in the mucus itself, with the antigen-binding regions available to interact with antigenic determinants passing by. Recognition in this setting is effective but undramatic, with local antigen-antibody complexes and mucus all being constantly shed. IgA does not bind components of the classical pathway of complement and cannot amplify the inflammatory responses through this pathway.

There are two subclasses of IgA, and although functional differences cannot be ascribed to the structural differences, one such class, $IgA_2$, is predominant in secretions, while $IgA_1$ is predominant in serum where it is almost exclusively monomeric (Fig. 11.11).

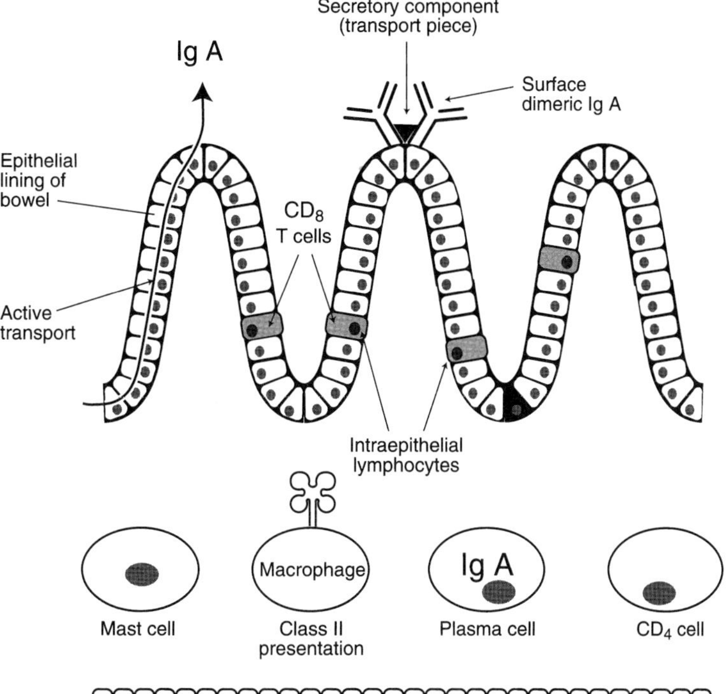


**Fig. 11.11** IgA is secreted by plasma cells of the lamina propria. The immunoglobulin is secreted as a dimer joined at its carboxy end by a J chain. Secretery component (transport piece) actively transports the dimer through bowel epithelial cells to align the molecule on the mucosal membrane.

### Humoral immunity and the newborn period

Neonates have few B lymphocytes that have encountered antigen, and therefore the first major meeting with bacteria and other potential pathogens in the birth canal represents a rude immunological awakening to the hostile microbial environment awaiting. B cells in the neonate must make IgM before they can make IgG. IgA production occurs later still, and the entire system is not satisfactorily mature until early in the second year of life.

Maternal IgG crosses the placenta in the last few weeks before birth and provides the neonate with passively acquired IgG that represents a library of maternal immunological experiences. If the baby encounters only those antigenic determinants present in the mother's community, all is well. An encounter with a hospital-acquired infection that mother has not herself previously encountered may place an infant at risk of overwhelming infection.

Maternal IgG gradually disappears from an infant's circulation during the first year of life. Apart from protection, there are two clinical consequences of this phenomenon. The presence of IgG antibody does not necessarily mean that a baby is infected with the provoking antigen (for example, HIV), and some vaccines will not be effective until levels of maternal neutralizing immunoglobulin fall satisfactorily (for example, measles).

Breast milk is rich in maternal IgA and contains useful amounts of IgG as well. Gut epithelial cells can selectively absorb IgG (transcytosis), and the maternal IgA will protect a baby's mucous membranes with the same limitations that apply to IgG in the circulation.

For reasons that are unknown, neonates are particularly inept at producing $IgG_2$ and hence do not respond adequately to conventionally delivered polysaccharide-encapsulated bacteria (for example, pneumococci and group B streptococci) until the second year of life. Indeed, care must be taken, since polysaccharide antigens introduced in the first few months of life can promote a long-lived tolerance that is detrimental to the infant.

## Regulation of the Immune Response

The key word in any analysis of immunoregulation is "appropriateness." As an enormous arsenal of destructive mechanisms is at the disposal of the various immunological components described, it is essential that control be extended to maximize efficiency and minimize bystander damage. Regulation of the immune response can be subdivided into three distinct but cooperating mechanisms:

1. The secretion of cytokines that modulate immune responses and terminate certain actions.
2. The regulation by idiotypic network interactions that occurs when an immune response is generated against the unique antigen-recognizing structure on the surface of T or B cells or the idiotypic regions of antibody.
3. The activation of a specialized group of immunoregulatory T cells.

To the three regulatory mechanisms described can be added three fundamentally important concepts. First, in the majority of cases, the symptoms and signs of infection are produced not by the presence of foreign antigenic epitopes per se but rather by the *response* to those determinants. Clinical experience with the administration of interferon and the interleukins highlights this fact. While knowledge that inadequate regulation of the production of IgE can produce a humoral immune allergic (*allos*, altered, *ergos*, anergy) response is decades old, only recently have we realized that a number of disease processes, from contact sensitivity to adult respiratory distress syndrome (ARDS) and Kawasaki syndrome, can be produced by T-cell allergies.

The most extreme example of clinically significant overstimulation of the cell-mediated immune system is supplied by confrontation with "superantigens," so called because they lead to cellular responses that are far more intense and far more systemic than those occurring after stimulation with normal antigens. Some individuals have allelic variations in the more constant portions of the beta chains of their T-cell receptors that will interact (bind) in a non-antigen-specific way with a microbial product—i.e., superantigen. As the TCR component binding the superantigen is not positioned in the unique idiotypic region found in the variable portion of TCR, a much larger percentage of T cells can bind and be activated by the product in question. The results are often disastrous. Superantigens are produced by many different pathogens, including bacteria such as staphylococci and streptococci, mycoplasma, and viruses. They combine directly to antigen-presenting molecules without being processed; indeed, fragmentation of superantigen molecules destroys their biological activity. Superantigens tend to bind to the lateral surface of both class II presenting molecules and the variable region of the beta chain of the T-cell receptor. Each superantigen can bind to one of the different beta-region sequences within the TCR found on an individual T cells. Not all T cells express the same variable-region sequences; indeed, there are some 20 to 50 variations in this part of the T-cell receptor known to occur on human T cells. So it is that in general a superantigen is able to stimulate 2% to 20% of all T cells.

The result of such binding is a massive production and release of cytokines, mainly by CD4 T cells. Not only can these cytokines produce systemic toxicity, but some are capable of suppressing adaptive immune responses, and the dual effect is responsible for the pathogenicity. Among the bacterial superantigens are the staphylococcal enterotoxins (SE) that so commonly cause food poisoning and the toxic shock syndrome toxin (TSST). Viral superantigens have been found in mice, particularly associated with the murine mammary tumor virus, and viral superantigens will probably be found to trouble humans as well.

Second, immunoregulation involves constant, harmless—indeed, necessary—reactions to self. These reactions, however, actually make it less likely that more sophisticated immune mechanisms will be activated that would damage the self antigens activating these primary immunoregulatory responses. For example, we all make IgM antibody in small quantities to self antigens, but that antibody prevents us from making IgG antibody to those same antigens. Were we to make IgG, as we know from clinical experience, we would be likely to experience autoimmune disease. The limitation of these responses involves the production of regulatory antibodies that block clinically significant autoimmune responses to determinants that are shared by a number of tissues. For example, one regulatory antibody can block autoreactivity to self antigens as varied as thyroid, factor VIII, and intrinsic factor determinants.

Third, while immunoregulation in its broadest sense must include intrathymic death and the induction of tolerance and anergy among T cells leaving the thymus (negative immunoregulation), the evolutionary state of the immune system of higher species for this millennium overwhelmingly involves positive immunoregulation in which T cells secrete modulatory cytokines.

## Cytokine modulation of the immune response

One way in which immune regulation is accomplished involves the differential production of lymphokines by immunological effector cells during an immune response to antigen. For example, the secretion of IL-4 by CD4 helper T cells activates B cells to express class II MHC molecules and to proliferate and secrete immunoglobulin. Interaction of IL-4 with macrophages, however, downregulates class II molecules and inhibits their biological activity. The secretion of IFN-$\gamma$ by inflammatory-producing T cells can activate macrophages to upregulate the expression of class II MHC molecules and so enhance their biological functions, whereas IFN-$\gamma$ inhibits the expression of class II MHC molecules and the production of immunoglobulin by B cells. This reciprocal regulation of cellular versus humoral immunity is under genetic influences that have been well characterized in mice and seem likely to apply to humans responding to different organisms.

Interleukin-10 is a relatively recently discovered lymphokine, the gene for which has been cloned in both mice and humans. It is produced largely by activated TH2 cells. IL-10 is an inhibitory factor suppressing the production of interferon $\gamma$ by TH1 cells. This function of IL-10 has a potential significance in various clinical situations, since it can inhibit at least some effector functions of TH1 cells. As TH1 cells mediate delayed-type hypersensitivity responses, IL-10 could, theoretically at least, be used to specifically suppress DTH responses without effecting antibody production. It is of interest that IL-10 has been found to have a 70% amino acid sequence homologous with an as yet unidentified gene product of the Epstein-Barr virus. It appears that the cellular gene encoding IL-10 has been picked up by the Epstein-Barr virus sometime during the evolutionary process and conserved, because it allows the virus to suppress the immune response in an infected host.

## Idiotypic networks

Antigen-specific receptors on T and B cells possess combining sites that recognize antigenic epitopes. As we have seen, the antigen specificity of these receptors is determined by unique variable regions. Receptors on different cells are composed of structures that are unique to that particular receptor, and this uniqueness provides the specificity and affinity of binding that the receptor has for its antigen (*epitope*). The unique antigenic structure of the variable regions of lymphocyte antigen receptors are called *idiotypes*.

When these arrangements for recognizing antigenic determinants were clarified it was soon postulated that the cells of the immune system would be capable of recognizing not only foreign antigen, but also the unique determinants on self receptors or idiotypes expressed or secreted by immune cells. According to this theory, we would not only produce antibodies to an antigenic determinant, but following the production of such an antibody (Ab1), other cells of our immune system would recognize Ab1 in an *antigenic* sense and produce Ab2. Ab2, which would share some of the antigenic properties of the antigenic determinant that stimulated the production of Ab1, would be capable of binding to receptors for that antigen. Binding would block the sites available to bind further antigen without stimulating further antibody production. After the demonstration that such theoretical happenings did in fact occur, the classical network-regulation theory was refined.

As the concentration of antigen begins to rise in the body, antibodies to that antigen (Ab1) are produced. As the level of Ab1 increases, two events occur. Ab1 binds to and clears antigen and the level of antigen begins to fall, but while that is happening, Ab1 is inducing the production of Ab2. As the level of Ab2 rises, the Ab2 binds to cells inducing Ab1 and inhibits further production. This leads to a drop in the amount of Ab1 and induces the production of Ab3. Ab3 then inhibits Ab2 production, leading to a drop in the amount of Ab2, and induces the production of Ab4, and so on. Just as when a stone is thrown into the middle of a pond, this ripple effect continues until the levels of antiidiotypic antibodies produced are sufficient to eliminate idiotypic-bearing antibodies but not sufficient to induce the production of anti-antiidiotypic antibodies, at which point the cascade ends (Fig. 11.12).

## Regulation by immunoregulatory T cells

In addition to regulation by idiotypic network interactions, immunological appropriateness is fine-tuned by specialized cells within the immune system that usually function to downregulate the activity of immune inducer and effector cells during an immunological response. Regulatory T cells play a role in determining the appropriateness of immune responses to a wide variety of antigens in a large number of different experimental situations, including immunological tolerance, humoral immune responses, inflammatory immune responses, immune responses to tumors, hypersensitivity responses, autoimmune diseases, and in genetically determined "low responder" animal strains or individuals. It is also clear that some antiidiotypic antibodies can actually activate regulatory T cells. The activity of regulatory T cells may be either specific for the immunizing antigen or nonspecific, suggesting that several different mechanisms exist for the generation and functional activity of these cells. The majority of immune-suppressive activity does appear to be mediated by specific regulatory T cells (Fig. 11.13).

There are two cells involved in the generation of suppressor T-cell activity, (1) a suppressor inducer CD4 T cell that activates the regulatory function of (2) the T cell directly responsible for suppression. The cells doing the regulating are CD8 positive and secrete unique T suppressor cell factors that are unlike any cytokine yet described and await detailed molecular characterization. Suppressor cytokines, however, have the following biological properties:

1. They bind to and are specific for native antigen or idiotype.
2. They exhibit genetic restrictions in their interactions with their target cells.
3. They express determinants linked to the major histocompatibility loci on chromosome 6.
4. They do not express serological determinants found on immunoglobulins or any known cytokine.
5. Like the cells that secrete them, they are functionally unique within the regulatory circuit, with some factors including the activity of suppressor cells and other factors released by those cells actually carrying out the suppression on susceptible target cells.

Regulatory (suppressor) T cells can exert inhibitory activities on macrophages, helper T cells, cytotoxic T cells, B cells, polymorphoneutrophilic leukocytes, and even other regulatory T cells. The effects of regulatory cytokines on macrophages include inhibition of IL-1 secretion and inhibition of tumoricidal activity and the inhibition of the capacity to prepare and present antigens to CD4 lymphocytes. Regulatory T cells can affect inducer and cytotoxic T cells by inhibiting their proliferation and secretion of lymphokines, while immune suppression of B cells re-

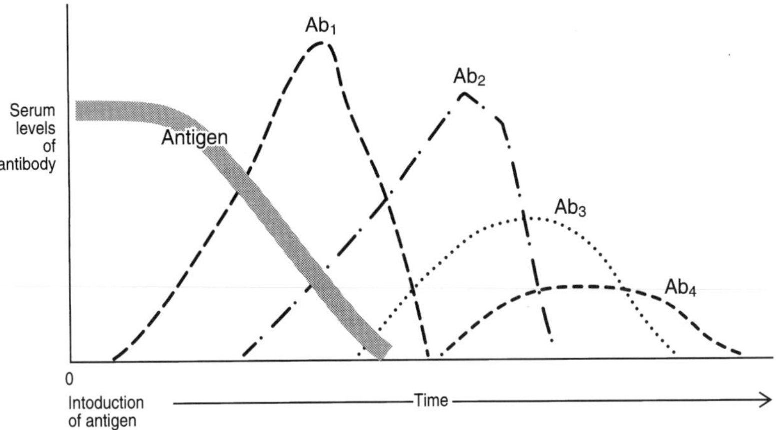


**Fig. 11.12** As the concentration of antigen begins to rise, antibodies to that antigen (Ab1) are produced. As the level of Ab1 increases, that immunoglobulin binds to and clears antigen. Ab1 then induces the production of Ab2. As the level of Ab2 rises, the Ab2 binds to cells producing Ab1 and inhibits further production. This leads to a fall in the amount of Ab1 secreted and induces the production of Ab3. Ab3 then inhibits Ab2 production, leading to a drop in the amount of Ab2 and induces the production of Ab4, etc. The cascade continues until the levels of antiidiotypic antibodies produced are sufficient to eliminate idiotype-bearing antibodies but not sufficient to induce to production of anti-antiidiotypic antibodies.

sults in their inability to produce immunoglobulin heavy chains. Inhibition of cell motility, homing, and even cell-surface phenotypic expression have been described. The point, of course, is that effector mechanisms for suppression are broad and significant.

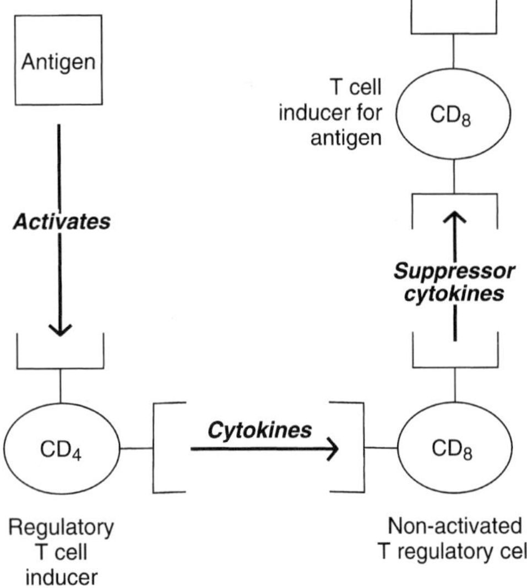


**Fig. 11.13** Antigen activates CD4 cells that will secrete IL-2 or IL-4 and activate CD8 and B effector cells. However, antigen also activates CD4 regulatory cell inducers that secrete cytokines and activate CD8 regulatory T cells. These cells, in turn, downregulate the activity of TH1 and TH2, CD4 inducer cells.

## Other Interleukins

Interleukin-3 is one of several glycoproteins that cause proliferation of bone marrow progenitor cells. IL-3 is capable of stimulating the growth of erythroid cells, granulocytes, monocytes, eosinophils, and megakaryocytes in human bone marrow and cord blood. Interleukin-8 is made by macrophages after stimulation by lipopolysaccharide, IL-1, TNF, IL-3, and GM-CSF. IL-8 affects neutrophils in much the same way as does the chemotactic protein produced during the complement cascade (C5a). It is more selective than C5a, however, because it has little effect on eosinophils or basophils and no effect on platelets, macrophages, or monocytes. It is of particular interest because it has been found in excessive amounts in the skin of patients with psoriasis and could be part of the pathogenesis of the inflammation seen in the skin and joints of these patients.

Interleukin-9 is a newly discovered lymphokine that can support the growth of TH2 cells in the absence of IL-2 or IL-4. It can enhance the proliferative effect of IL-3 on mast cells. IL-11 is a bone marrow stromal cell–derived cytokine involved in maturation of immature lymphocytes, red blood cells, and megakaryocytes. It appears to play a major role in platelet production. It can increase the number of antibody-forming B cells, but there is still much to be learned about this molecule.

## Variations on the Theme

The description of the immune response given in this chapter is somewhat didactic, and in fairness it is important to emphasize that there are some areas in which variations on the theme add to the complexity. Thus, some CD4 lymphocytes are inherently cytotoxic, while some antigens are capable of interacting with B cells and making them produce antibody without any CD4 lymphocyte involvement at all. Long-chain polysaccharide antigens are particularly good examples of this. While 90% of T cells carry receptors for antigenic determinants that are made up of alpha and beta chain, there is a very distinct subset of cells that instead use gamma- and delta-chain variants as part of their T-cell receptor. The function of these cells is unknown.

## Natural Killer Cells

Significant time is required for the induction of an antigen-specific CD8 cytotoxic response. Thus, there is need for an immediate reaction while antigen-specific cells are responding. This is supplied by cells that can be isolated from blood, spleen, and other lymphoid organs that kill various tumor lines without induction by immunization. A cytotoxic response requiring no induction by antigen is termed *natural cytotoxicity*, and the cells involved are known as *natural killer* or *NK*, cells. The cells probably have a T-cell lineage and can be described morphologically as large granular, lymphocyte-like cells filled with azurophilic granules.

Killing by NK cells is somewhat similar to killing by cytotoxic T cells. The cells will attack many transformed lines and normal cell types but show preference for killing less differentiated cells, especially in the hematopoietic linage, and may serve to limit the expansion of these cells. Natural killer cells seem to participate in resistance to tumors and also to viral infection.

Cytotoxic cells expressing surface receptors for various classes of immunoglobulin can bind cells coated with antibody molecules and kill them. Thus, even cells with no antigen-specific receptors can utilize the specificity of antibody in the production of "antibody-dependent cellular cytotoxicity" (ADCC). The majority of large granular lymphocytes referred to above do have Fc receptors for IgG and are capable of producing ADCC. While a number of textbooks have attributed ADCC to a unique population of blood cells called K cells, it now seems more likely that

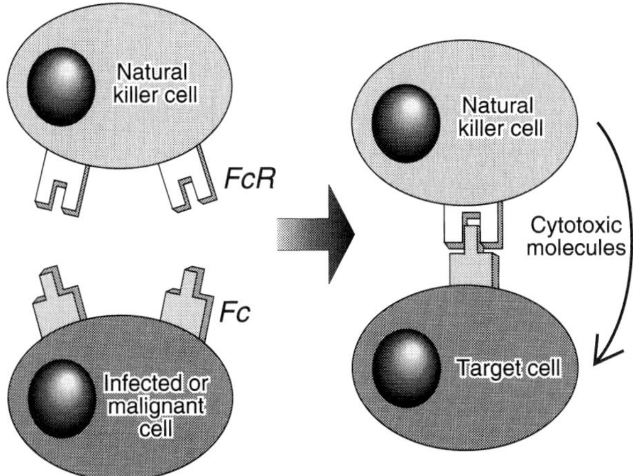


**Fig. 11.14** Natural killer cells under the influence of cytokines can kill virus-infected and malignant cells without the assistance of antigen-presenting cells. They do this even more efficiently if the target cell is coated with immunoglobulin. Natural killer cells have receptors on their surface membrane for the Fc portion of immunoglobulin. Binding of antibody molecules to Fc receptors ensures that target cells are brought into close proximity to effector cells.

ADCC activity and NK activity reside in related, if not identical, cells (Fig. 11.14).

Given the complexity described in these pages, it is not surprising that there are more than 60 distinct immune deficiency diseases resulting from the imperfect development or application of one or more elements. In general, immune deficiency diseases are characterized as isolated defects in antibody production, cell-mediated immune capacity, or a combination of both (see Chapter 90). Immune deficiency diseases, however, can be associated with a lack of NK cell activity, and an extraordinary array of molecular defects may be responsible. These experiments of nature clearly show the importance of each element in the immunological chain reaction in preserving our health. Increasingly, acquired immune deficiency states are being induced as a result of aggressive chemotherapy to treat cancer and make organ transplantation possible. The interested reader should seek more information on all these topics. It is particularly interesting to review the mechanisms by which individual drugs known to produce immunosuppression interfere with the elements of the immune system that we have detailed.

There is much yet to be learned about the immune system, and undoubtedly we will improve our capacity to harness its remarkable properties. There are many examples of genetic variations within families of bacteria and viruses that have provided them with survival advantages by allowing them to minimize the effectiveness of one or more elements of the immune response. On the other hand, there is no doubt that no strategy developed by modern medicine has done as much to minimize suffering and death as has the application of our knowledge of the immune system to provide protection against infectious diseases. The battle between formidable foes continues.

### ANNOTATED BIBLIOGRAPHY

Alt FW, Blackwell TK, Yancopoulos GD. Development of the primary antibody repertoire. Science 1987; 238:1079–1087.
*An approachable overview of how B cells respond to antigens to produce specific antibody.*

Anderson G, Moore NC, Owen JJT, Jenkinson EJ. Cellular interactions in thymocyte development. Ann. Rev. Immunol. 1996; 14:73–99.
*An excellent overview of the role of the thymus in T cell maturation.*

Ashwell JD, Klausner RD. Genetic and mutational analysis of the T cell receptor. Annu Rev Immunol 1990; 8:139.
*An excellent review of how the T-cell repertoire develops by intrathymic programming of T-cell receptor formation.*

Bevilacqua MP, Stengelin S, Gimbrone MA, Seed B. Endothelial leukocyte adhesion molecule 1: An inducible receptor for neutrophils related to complement regulatory proteins and lectins. Science 1989; 243:1160–1165.
*This paper provides additional information on adhesion molecules and emphasizes the importance of such in antigen-specific mechanisms.*

Biron CA. Cytokines in the generation of immune responses to, and resolution of, virus infection. Curr. Opin. Immunol. 1994; 6:530–538.
*The role of interferon in viral replication and host-defense response is explored in a clinically relevant manner.*

Borden EC, Sandel PM. Lymphokines and cytokines as cancer treatment: Immunotherapy realized. Cancer 1990; 65:800–814.
*An excellent review of the potential of immunotherapy in the control of malignancy.*

Chan AC, Irving BA, Weiss A. New insights into T cell antigen receptor structure and signal transduction. Curr Opin Immunol 1992; 4:246.
*An approachable overview of the structure of T-cell receptors and the reasons why superantigens are so potent.*

Clark EA, Lane PJL. Regulation of human B cell activation and adhesion. Annu Rev Immunol 1991; 9:97–108.
*A comprehensive review of how B cell function is regulated and how these cells bind to antigen presenting cells.*

Fremont DH, Hendrickson WA, Marrack P, Kappler J. Structures of an MHC class II molecule with covalently bound single peptides. Science 1996; 272:1001–1004.

*The distinctive subunit structures of MHC molecules are examined in a way that makes the spacial arrangements readily understandable.*

Janeway CA. The T cell receptor as a multicomponent signalling machine: CD4/CD8 co-receptors and CD45 in T cell activation. Annu Rev Immunol 1992; 10:645.

*A fascinating review of the molecular details associated with the activation of T-cell receptors.*

Kosco MH, Tew JG. Microanatomy of lymphoid tissue during humoral immune responses: Structure function relationship. Ann Rev Immunol 1989; 7:91–109.

*An approachable overview of the functional anatomy of lymphoid tissue.*

Moller G, ed. Lymphocyte homing. Immunol Rev 1989; 108 (special issue).

*An excellent review of lymphoid trafficking from blood vessels to antigens present in tissues.*

Moller G, ed. The T cell repertoire. Immunol Rev 1988; 101 (special issue).

*Basic review of the different functions of specific T cells.*

Rajewsky K, von Boehmer H, eds. Lymphocyte development. Curr Opin Immunol 1992; 4:131–166.

*An overview of the intrathymic and bone marrow phases of lymphocyte development.*

Ravetch JV, Kinet JP. Fc receptors. Annu Rev Immunol 1991; 9:457–492.

*A review of the way in which phagocytic cells are able to attack antibody-coated (opsonized) targets.*

Song R, Harding CV. Roles of proteasomes, transporter for antigen presentation (TAP), and $\beta_2$-microglobulin in the processing of bacterial or particulate antigens via an alternate class I MHC processing pathway. J. Immunol. 1996; 156:4182–4190.

*Explores the major reason for all the complexity associated with antigen presentation.*

Strober W, Brown WR. The mucosal immune system. In: Immunological Diseases, Samter M, Talmage DW, Frank MM, Austen KF, Claman HN, eds. Little, Brown, Boston, pp. 79–139, 1988.

*An excellent review of the arrangement and functional organization of mucosal and submucosal immunity.*

Strober W, James SP. The immunologic basis of inflammatory bowel disease. J Clin Immunol 1986; 6:415–432.

*An excellent discussion of the basic mechanisms by which immune responses can damage normal body structures.*

Wardlaw AJ, Moqbel R, Kay AB. Eosinophils: biology and role in disease. Adv. Immunol. 1995; 60:151–266.

*A clinically relevant review of a major character in immediate hypersensitivity.*

# II

# DIAGNOSTIC METHODS IN INFECTIOUS DISEASE

# 12

## Modern Imaging Techniques in Infectious Disease

ERIC J. STERN, HANH V. NGHIEM, JOHN F. HIEHLE, JR., AND DAVID H. LEWIS

This chapter provides a regional and organ-system overview of the role of radiologic procedures in diagnosing infectious diseases. Emphasis is placed on the newer, more advanced imaging techniques, such as computed tomography (CT) and magnetic resonance imaging (MRI), and their most appropriate uses and indications. For each organ system, the relative advantages and limitations of these new, advanced imaging modalities is specifically discussed, including their relationship to older, more traditional imaging techniques. Specific nuclear imaging techniques in diagnosing infectious diseases is discussed.

### Central Nervous System

Any discussion of imaging of the central nervous system (CNS) would be incomplete without a comparison of the relative merits of the two major tomographic imaging modalities used in the head and spine, MRI and CT. CT is less time-consuming and less expensive than MRI in most instances, and generally more available. Unless there is a history of contrast allergy or atopy, there is no particular patient preparation for CT scanning. The benefits of CT imaging far outweigh the small radiation-exposure risk. CT imaging is limited to axial and sometimes coronal scan planes. Severe streak artifacts can occur that are caused by metallic foreign objects, such as dental amalgam, and CT is notoriously poor at visualizing structures in the posterior fossa. MRI, on the other hand, is better for the posterior fossa and offers superb soft-tissue contrast and essentially unlimited multiplanar imaging capability. MRI is an extremely safe test, as long as care is taken to screen for those patients with contraindications. MRI should never be performed in patients with pacemakers, non-MRI-compatible vascular clips, or intraorbital metallic foreign bodies; there are no known direct health risks from exposure to the magnetic field and radio waves. Unlike iodinated contrast agents for CT or angiography, allergic reactions to MRI contrast agents are extremely rare. Many patients feel claustrophobic in the small magnet bore during an MRI examination. Adequate explanation of the nature of the examination, possibly supplemented with an oral sedative to take upon arrival at the MRI center, may significantly improve the successful outcome of the study. Patients with severe claustrophobia may not tolerate the exam even after sedation. MRI is much more sensitive to motion than CT, so uncooperative patients are more appropriately imaged with CT.

There are a wide variety of MRI pulse sequences and imaging planes that can be used. Standard spin echo images, commonly referred to as *T1-weighted*, *proton density–weighted*, and *T2-weighted images*, can be obtained with or without intravenous contrast enhancement. Gradient echo images permit high-resolution images without sacrificing time and image contrast. A wide variety of MRI angiography techniques may be helpful in evaluation of vascular anatomy and pathology. Inversion recovery images are helpful in eliminating high signal from fat and accentuating soft-tissue edema. All of these techniques may be used with an essentially unlimited range of resolution parameters and image planes. Unfortunately, owing to cost and time constraints, only a few pulse sequences can be obtained on each patient. Although a "routine" MRI will often answer the clinical question, in the absence of a thorough clinical history it becomes impossible to exploit the extreme flexibility of MRI to tailor the exam to the specific clinical history and questions. Therefore, the advantage of MRI is not fully realized unless there is good communication between the referring physician and the radiologist.

Intraaxial CNS infection may manifest as a demyelinating process, a cerebritis or encephalitis, or as an abscess (Fig. 12.1). In addition to leptomeningeal inflammation, meningitis may or may not cause inflammatory or ischemic change in subjacent brain parenchyma. Extraaxial CNS infections usually involve the subdural space, and less commonly the epidural space. Osteomyelitis of the skull base or cranial vault may complicate infections arising in the soft tissues around the skull. For almost all CNS indications, the multiplanar capabilities and excellent image contrast of MRI make it an imaging modality superior to CT. The exception to this rule is in the evaluation of bone and calcification; improved bone visualization may be important in the evaluation of osteomyelitis or secondary intracranial extension of complicated sinusitis or mastoiditis. Identification of calcifications may be helpful when granulomatous disease, specifically CNS cysticercosis, is included in the differential diagnosis.

Other neuroradiological tests play a comparatively minor role in evaluation of infection. Cerebral angiography may be useful in the patient with known or strongly suspected septic emboli to evaluate for mycotic aneurysms, which typically occur along the distal branches of the cerebral arteries, or in the evaluation of postinfectious vasculitis, such as herpes ophthalmica.

Immunocompromised patients, including those with acquired immune deficiency syndrome (AIDS), have increased susceptibility to CNS infections. Human immunodeficiency virus (HIV) infection of the white matter is endemic, but specific imaging findings usually lag behind clinical symptoms; therefore, treatment is not based on imaging findings. In general, CT is not as efficacious as MRI in the detection of white matter diseases, including HIV, cytomegalovirus, and progressive multifocal leukoencephalopathy, none of which typically enhance following administration of an intravenous contrast agent.

Detection of cerebral toxoplasmosis is clinically imperative so that an appropriate treatment course may be initiated. MRI is the favored imaging technique in the evaluation of these patients and may reveal multiple lesions when only single lesions are detected by CT. Cerebral non-Hodgkin's lymphoma may have an appear-

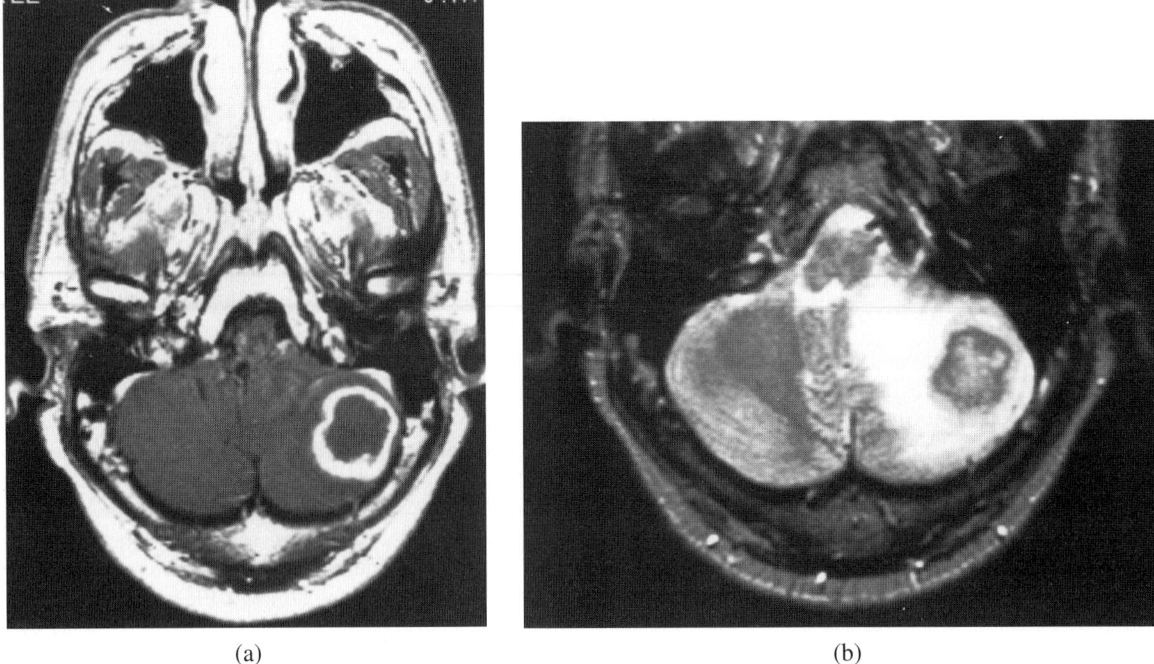

(a) (b)

**Fig. 12.1** T2-weighted (*a*) and post-gadolinium T1-weighted (*b*) MR images of the cerebellum show a ring-enhancing mass with surrounding vasogenic edema and mass effect causing rightward shift of the fourth ventricle and downward herniation of the left cerebellar tonsil. Surgical evacuation of abscess cavity demonstrated acid-fast organisms consistent with mycobacterium tuberculosis.

ance similar to that of cerebral toxoplasmosis, including multiple, ring-enhancing masses. It may not be possible to distinguish between toxoplasmosis and lymphoma on imaging criteria alone until a trial treatment course has been attempted. Improvement in toxoplasmosis lesions is usually evident within two to four weeks (see Chapter 80).

Because the diagnosis of meningitis is usually made clinically, imaging plays a secondary role in the workup and management of these patients. Depending on the patient's presentation, however, imaging may be indicated to rule out the presence of mass effect that might obviate a lumbar puncture. For that application, unenhanced CT is sufficiently sensitive. Imaging findings in early, acute meningitis are usually normal, although secondary signs, including distention of the subarachnoid space, diffuse cerebral swelling, and communicating hydrocephalus, may be seen. The major applications of imaging in the evaluation of meningitis are in the assessment of complications or the discovery of parameningeal foci that may have contributed to the meningitis. Some of the many complications potentially encountered include subdural effusions or empyemas, encephalitis, parenchymal abscess, ventriculitis, vasculitis, or infarction. These complications are all shown best by MRI, with the exception of vasculitis, which is best imaged with catheter angiography. Rarely, contrast cisternography may be helpful in the patient with recurrent meningitis and suspected CSF fistula to the paranasal sinuses or mastoid air cells.

## Head and Neck

Evaluation of the head and neck is one area in which CT has not been supplanted by MRI. The combination of respiratory motion and vascular pulsation may cause significant degradation of MRI image quality caudal to the hard palate. On the other hand, soft-tissue contrast of CT is augmented in the neck by the presence of multiple normal fat planes. Intravenous contrast is essential in CT evaluation of the neck, not just to elucidate the enhancement pattern of tumors or infections, but to assist in differentiation of vascular structures from other, potentially important soft-tissue densities, particularly cervical adenopathy. It is important to be aware that infections in the retropharyngeal space can extend along fascial planes into the mediastinum along the cervico-thoracic continuum (see Chapter 84). To evaluate infectious involvement of the spinal column, MR is the preferred modality (see below, under SPINE).

## Sinuses

In the past, screening for sinusitis has generally been done with plain radiographs. Unfortunately, plain radiographs are notoriously inaccurate in evaluation of mucoperiosteal changes and offer essentially no information on the status of the ostiomeatal complex, the main therapeutic target of flexible endoscopic sinus surgery. Therefore, routine plain radiographs have been essentially replaced by CT. Probably the only current indication for plain sinus films is in the evaluation of a patient who cannot be transported to CT, such as an unstable ICU patient being evaluated for fever of unknown origin. Many institutions offer a "screening sinus CT" that will render a much more accurate view of inflammatory sinus disease for the same cost as a plain radiographic sinus series. If surgical intervention is contemplated, the otorhinolaryngologist will request a more detailed CT examination, including high-resolution coronal images of the sinuses to accurately visualize the ostiomeatal units or drainage pathways of the sinuses and plan functional endoscopic sinus surgery. CT is optimal since it allows visualization of the small bony structures that form the drainage channels of the sinuses. Key issues in CT of uncomplicated sinusitis include delineation of normal and anomalous bony anatomy, mucosal thickening, and sinus opacification. Intravenous contrast is not generally useful for imaging in simple sinusitis, but becomes so in complicated sinusitis when there is extension into the orbit or frontal lobe. Similarly, MRI is not indicated in the workup of routine inflammatory sinus disease, but may be helpful if secondary complications are suspected, such as intracranial abscess or empyema or periorbital infection. Additionally, if there is a question of sinus neoplasm, MRI can help to distinguish tumor from inflammatory change.

## Spine

Infections in the spine are usually the result of hematogenous spread and classically involve the intervertebral disk and/or epidural space. The pathogen lodges at the vertebral end plate and destroys both the disk and adjacent bone. Gadolinium-enhanced MRI is the most sensitive imaging modality in the detection of discitis and associated osteomyelitis (Fig. 12.2), although plain radiographs and/or CT may be helpful in the evaluation of associated bony erosion and sclerosis. In postoperative patients, it may be difficult to distinguish normal MRI postoperative enhancement of the disk space from infection. End-plate erosion and enhancement of adjacent vertebral bodies then become important secondary clues. Pott's disease, or tuberculous infection of the spine, may be indistinguishable from bacterial discitis, but typically involves the lower thoracic spine, may skip vertebra, and late in the disease may paradoxically preserve the disk space (see Chapter 78).

Isolated spinal epidural abscess becomes a serious clinical consideration in the immunocompromised patient or intravenous drug user with back pain and progressive neurologic impairment. Once again, MRI is the ideal imaging modality because of its multiplanar capability and superb soft-tissue image contrast. The dorsal epidural space is most commonly involved owing to the close approximation of the ventral dura to the posterior longitudinal ligament.

In summary, MR is the imaging modality of choice for the majority of patients with brain and spine infections. The radiologist equipped with a prior awareness of appropriate clinical history and specific questions to be addressed by the exam is best able to exploit the flexibility of MRI. CT is preferable in the evaluation of uncomplicated sinusitis and soft-tissue neck infections, and is a reasonable alternative for screening a patient with suspected uncomplicated meningitis.

## Musculoskeleton

Diagnostic imaging modalities that can be used for evaluating musculoskeletal infections include plain radiographs, radionuclide imaging (see below, under NUCLEAR IMAGING), CT, and MRI. Each method has its own indications and inherent limitations. MRI has become an important imaging technique for the evaluation of musculoskeletal infections owing to its excellent soft-tissue contrast, multiplanar capability, and improved assessment of bone marrow involvement. Changes within the bone marrow space of the earliest stages of acute osteomyelitis can be clearly defined by MRI, which shows decreased signal intensity of bone marrow on T1-

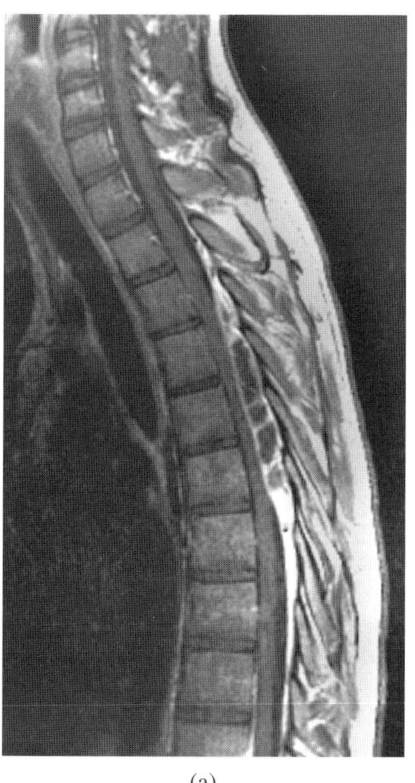

(a)

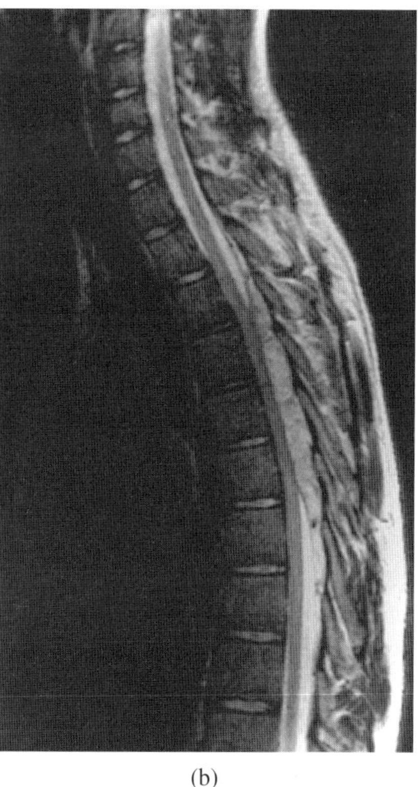

(b)

**Fig. 12.2** T2-weighted (*a*) and post-gadolinium-weighted (*b*) images of the upper thoracic spine show a dorsal epidural abscess in this 18-year-old male college student presenting with several days of fever, neck stiffness, and progressive myelopathy. After surgical evacuation, culture were positive for *S. aureus*.

weighted images and increased signal intensity on T2-weighted images. MRI can also define the extent of soft-tissue infection and identify soft-tissue abscess. (Fig. 12.3).

## Chest

Newer imaging techniques for pulmonary infections revolve predominantly around CT of the chest, particularly in the evaluation of the immunocompromised host.

CT, including high-resolution CT (HRCT), is the best noninvasive imaging technique for the evaluation of the lung and airways. CT accurately determines the extent and distribution of pulmonary abnormalities and can be used to determine the most appropriate lung biopsy technique, such as open lung biopsy, transbronchial biopsy/bronchoalveolar lavage, or transthoracic fine needle aspiration biopsy, and to then guide the lung biopsy procedure to the most appropriate region(s) of lung.

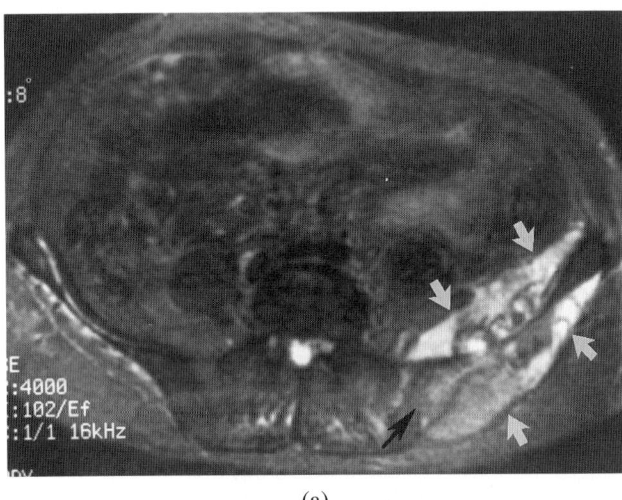


(a)

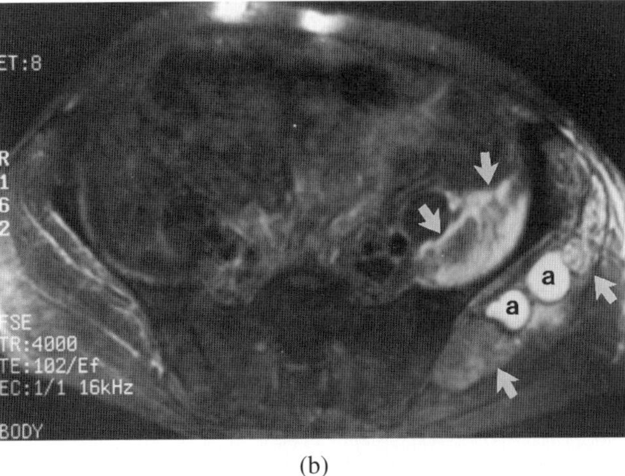


(b)

**Fig. 12.3** Axial T2-weighted images through the pelvis in a patient with acute osteomyelitis of the left ilium. *a.* Abnormal high signal intensity is seen in the marrow of the left iliac bone (*black arrow*). There is an extensive area of high signal intensity involving the adjacent soft tissue and muscles, representing associated soft-tissue infection and edema (*white arrows*). *b.* Level slightly inferior to A. Two well-demarcated high-signal-intensity fluid collections are seen in the gluteal muscle, representing soft-tissue abscesses (*a*). Again, an extensive area of high signal intensity involving the adjacent soft tissue and muscle is seen (*arrows*).

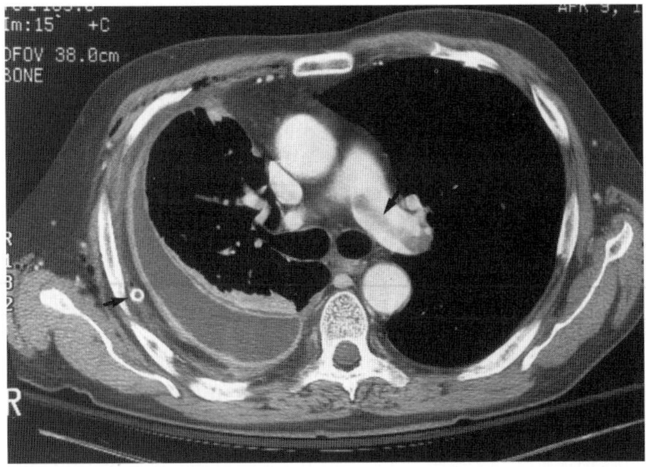


**Fig. 12.4** Contrast-enhanced chest CT in a patient with pleuritic chest pain, fevers, and a nonfunctioning chest tube shows a large right pleural fluid collection surrounded by enhancing thickened pleura consistent with an empyema. There is no significant adjacent parenchymal disease. Note that the thoracostomy tube (*left arrow*) is extrapleural. Incidentally, there is a large clot in the left pulmonary artery (*right arrow*).

MRI has little role in the workup of patients with infectious pulmonary disease; with current imaging sequences, the magnetic imaging properties of the lung parenchyma preclude a diagnostic quality MRI examination. However, in selected cases, the multiplanar imaging capabilities of MRI permit sagittal or coronal imaging of mediastinal and chest wall abnormalities.

### Infectious-disease indications for CT scanning of the chest

CT of the chest is not used routinely in the evaluation of uncomplicated intrathoracic infections in the immunocompetent host. However, CT may be very helpful in detecting unsuspected complications in immunocompetent patients with abnormal but stable chest radiographs that are not responding as expected to medical and/or surgical therapy. For instance, CT scanning of the chest is particularly useful to define loculated empyemas, large-vessel pulmonary emboli, or necrotizing pneumonias or lung abscesses (Fig. 12.4). In other patients, CT also identifies unsuspected adenopathy, fluid collections in the mediastinum, and chest wall involvement by an underlying pleural or parenchymal process. Parietal pleural thickening seen with contrast-enhanced CT is strongly indicative of an exudative pleural effusion, while a pleural effusion in the absence of pleural thickening occurs most often in patients with a malignant or uncomplicated parapneumonic effusion. CT allows the clinician to follow the efficacy of medical or interventional therapy—for example, the adequacy of empyema drainage or urokinase therapy for loculated pleural fluid collections. Finally, in patients with radiographic features of a prior pulmonary granulomatous infection and clinical symptoms of active disease, CT scanning of the chest is useful in distinguishing active infection from fibronodular scarring (Fig. 12.5).

### The immunocompromised host

#### Non-AIDS

CT scanning of the chest is an important tool for evaluating the lungs in the immunocompromised host prone to malignancies

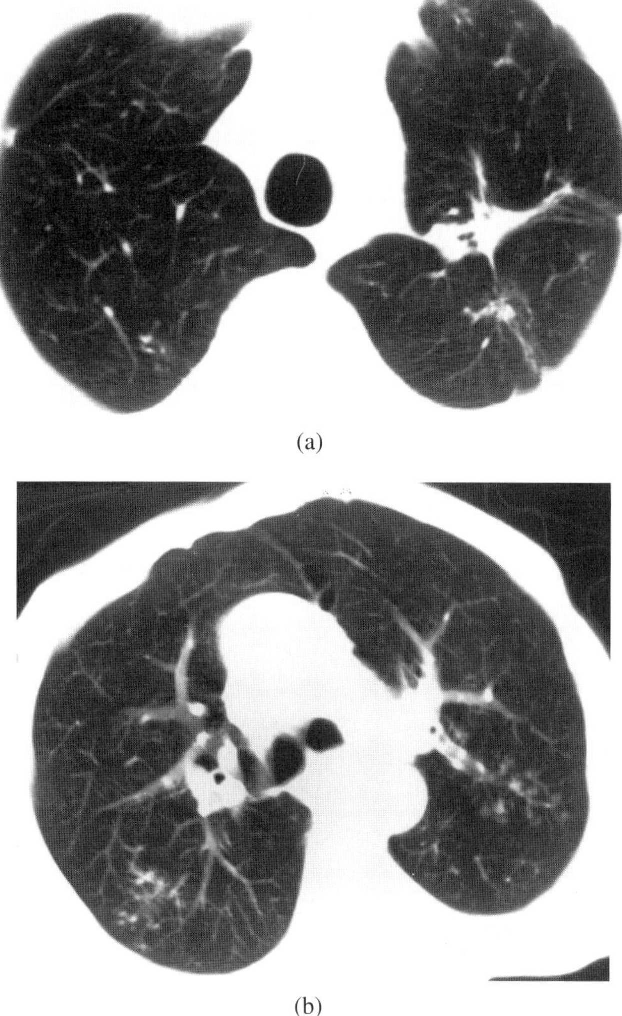


**Fig. 12.5** Chest CT from two patients with tuberculosis. *a.* CT scan shows typical fibronodular scarring in the left lung apex consistent with a prior tuberculous infection. There is no evidence of activity. *b.* CT scan in a patient with sputum-positive tuberculosis shows ill-defined nodules distributed along the bronchovascular bundles at both lung bases. This nodular appearance is nonspecific, but in the appropriate clinical setting is highly suggestive of an active granulomatous process such as tuberculosis and distinguishes active infection from healed or dormant tuberculosis.

and atypical infections with opportunistic organisms, as well as unusual manifestations of each of these processes. In symptomatic immunocompromised patients, chest radiographs are often normal, and when abnormal, usually nonspecific. CT can better characterize the underlying disease process, often directing specific medical or surgical intervention.

Common CT findings of acute pulmonary infections in the immunocompromised host include nodules (with or without cavitation), patchy or diffuse "ground-glass" attenuation (hazy infiltrate that does not obscure bronchovascular structures—a nonspecific finding that may indicate interstitial or airspace inflammation or fibrosis), and consolidation (a more opaque infiltrate than ground glass fills the airspaces, often with air bronchograms).

In an immunocompromised host, nodules frequently define fungal infection, but may also represent bronchiolitis obliterans organizing pneumonia (BOOP) or lymphoma. Nodules that have a lucent parenchymal zone or "halo" suggest invasive pulmonary aspergillosis. The halo corresponds to a rim of coagulative necrosis and hemorrhage. The CT halo sign is nonspecific, however, and may also be seen with other infections, such as candidiasis, cytomegalovirus, and herpes simplex viral infections, as well as noninfectious conditions such as Wegener's granulomatosis, Kaposi's sarcoma, and, rarely, metastatic angiosarcoma.

CT is much more sensitive in detecting ground-glass attenuation than chest radiography. Ground-glass attenuation is a strong indicator of an abnormality; however, it is a nonspecific finding. In the immunocompromised host, CT scans showing ground-glass attenuation suggests an interstitial inflammatory process such as *Pneumocystis carinii* pneumonia (PCP), but may also represent BOOP, other infectious pneumonias, or even lymphoma or cytotoxic drug reaction. When ground-glass attenuation is focal or patchy, CT can direct the bronchoscopist or surgeon to the most appropriate lavage or biopsy site, greatly improving diagnostic yield.

Consolidation is also a nonspecific finding at CT scanning, and in addition to pyogenic infections, may also represent atelectasis, BOOP, pulmonary infarction due to fungal infection, and pulmonary hemorrhage.

### AIDS

The chest radiographic appearance of PCP typically shows a fine interstitial infiltrate with a perihilar distribution. AIDS patients with PCP may also have a normal or near-normal chest radiograph, typically with an early infection. In these patients, CT scans are almost always abnormal. The most common CT scan pattern of disease is a fine ground-glass patchwork pattern. However, atypical CT appearances of PCP can occur and include nodules, cavities, peripheral infiltrates only, upper or lower lung zone predominance to infiltrates, unilateral infiltrate, and cystic lung destruction. Nodules and cavities, however, when seen in addition to the fine ground-glass patchwork pattern, should suggest the possibility of a superimposed infection or neoplasm. Associated, though uncommon, CT findings with PCP include pneumothorax, adenopathy, and pleural effusions.

In summary, while chest radiographs remain the best radiographic screening tool for intrathoracic infections, CT is the advanced imaging modality of choice for the majority of immunocompetent and immunocompromised patients. Chest radiographs are often normal or nonspecific, and CT can better characterize the underlying disease process and often direct specific medical or surgical intervention.

## Abdomen

Contrast-enhanced CT and sonography have proven to be of significant clinical value in the assessment of patients with intraabdominal and pelvic infections. The role of MRI remains limited owing to limited spatial resolution, artifacts resulting from respiration and peristalsis, and lack of an effective oral and rectal contrast agent.

## Solid organ abscess

Solid organ abscesses (hepatic, splenic, pancreatic, renal) are best demonstrated by iodinated contrast-enhanced CT, and sometimes ultrasonography exams. On CT exam, abscesses are seen as single or multiple areas of low attenuation either without contrast enhancement or with an enhancing peripheral rim of edematous

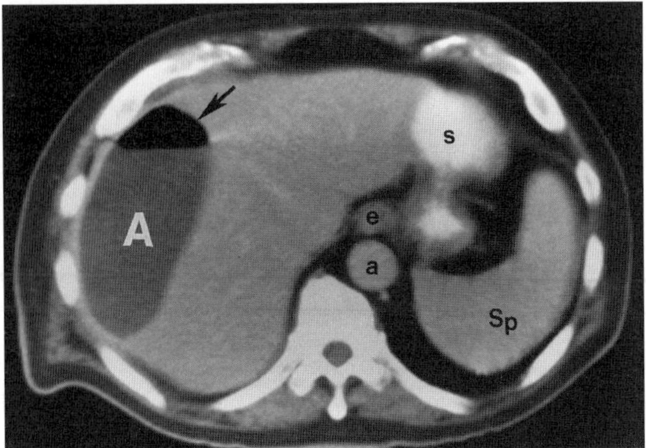


**Fig. 12.6** CT of a pyogenic abscess in the right lobe of the liver. The abscess (*A*) is large and contains fluid and air (*arrow*). L, liver; Sp, spleen; s, stomach; a, aorta; e, esophagus.

and inflamed parenchymal tissue (Figs. 12.6, 12.7). The presence of gas within an abscess, seen more readily on CT than sonography, increases the diagnostic specificity.

On ultrasound, abscesses are seen as irregular, poorly defined anechoic or hypoechoic areas. A "wheels within wheels" or "target sign" appearance has been described in patients with fungal infection of the liver and spleen, particularly candidiasis (Fig. 12.8).

When the radiographic appearance is nonspecific and the diagnosis of abscess is uncertain, CT or ultrasound-guided percutaneous aspiration can confirm the diagnosis.

## Peritoneal abscess

CT is the preferred radiologic study for detection of peritoneal abscess. Sonography is limited by the patient's body habitus and the presence of overlying bowel gas. Peritoneal abscesses typically are seen in patients after abdominal or pelvic surgery. In patients who have not undergone a surgical procedure, common causes of peritoneal abscesses include appendicitis, diverticulitis,

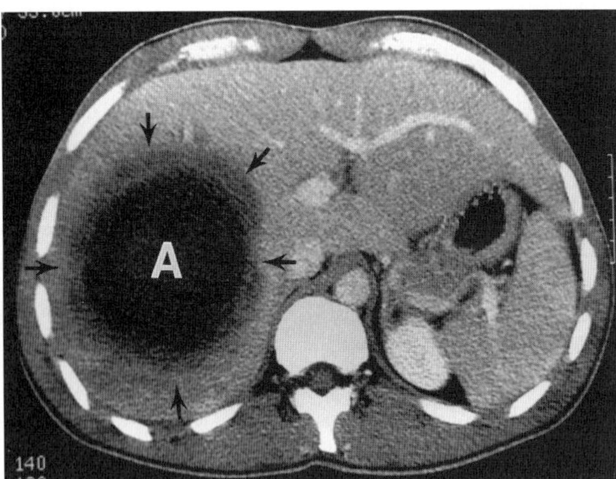


**Fig. 12.7** CT of an amebic abscess in the right lobe of the liver. The low-attenuation abscess (*A*) has a peripheral rim of decreased attenuation, representing edematous liver tissue (*arrows*).

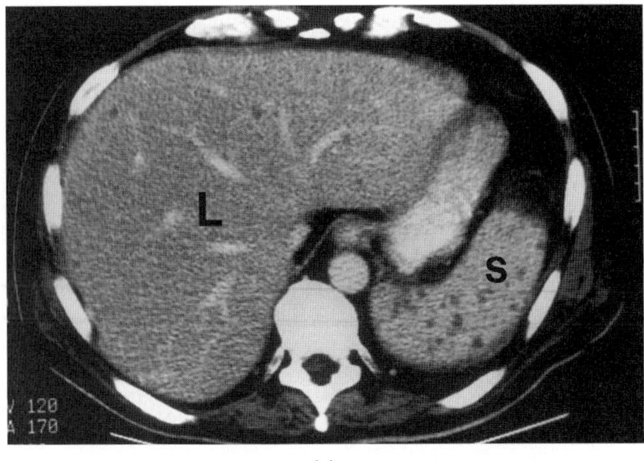


(a)

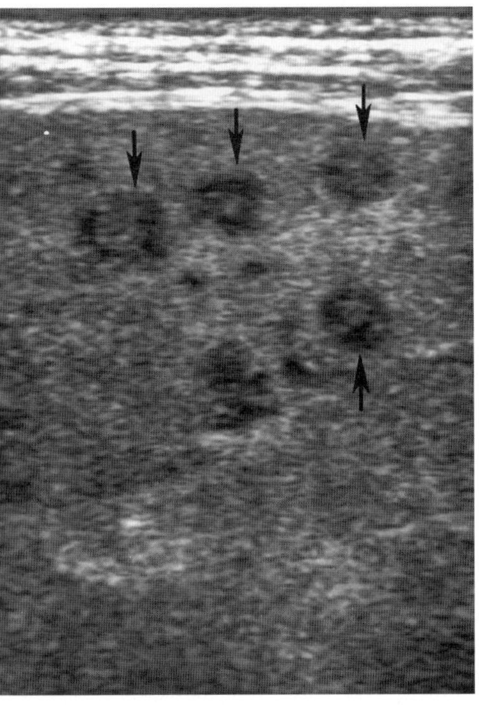

(b)

**Fig. 12.8** *Candida* abscess in an immunocompromised patient. *a.* CT image demonstrates multiple small low-attenuation lesions in both liver (*L*) and spleen (*S*), representing *Candida* abscess. *b.* Ultrasound image of the spleen in the same patient shows the target sign appearance of *Candida* abscess (*arrows*).

perforated carcinoma, cholecystitis, and inflammatory bowel disease. A well-circumscribed fluid attenuation with an enhancing rim are distinctive CT features and enable a confident diagnosis in most cases (Fig. 12.9). CT also can demonstrate the presence of gas within an abscess, which increases diagnostic specificity.

## Enteritis and colitis

A barium study is the most effective radiographic technique for the evaluation of mucosal disease of most forms of enteritis and colitis. However, CT has recently made significant contributions in the assessment of the bowel wall and of extraluminal abnormalities in various types of infectious and inflammatory conditions of the small bowel and colon. CT can define the extent of bowel involvement and evaluate complications, such as fistulae or abscess. The bowel wall in colitis and enteritis is usually thickened, and the usual sharp definition of the serosal surface is obscured by adjacent inflammation. Common conditions that exhibit these striking CT features are Crohn's disease, pseudomembranous colitis, and cytomegalovirus colitis in patients with AIDS (Figs. 12.9, 12.10). Neutropenic colitis is a localized form of colitis that is seen in patients with leukemia, usually after receiving chemotherapy (Fig. 12.11). CT usually shows bowel wall thickening and inflammatory infiltration of the pericolonic fat localized to the cecum and the right colon.

## Imaging of the gastrointestinal tract in patients with HIV infection

Double-contrast barium study is still the preferred method for evaluating the GI tract in patients with HIV infection, since pathology is usually limited to the mucosal surface. However, CT is an important adjunctive imaging modality for detection of adenopathy, associated malignancy, hepatic and splenic abnormalities, and other extra-intestinal masses. The role of sonography is limited predominantly to the evaluation of the gallbladder and the biliary system.

## Appendicitis

Graded-compression sonography has proven to be of significant clinical value in the assessment of patients with right lower quadrant pain and possible appendicitis. The sonographic diagnosis of acute appendicitis can be established with confidence if a noncompressible, blind-ended tubular structure arising from the cecal tip measuring 7 mm or greater in anteroposterior dimension is visualized. Appendicoliths can be detected sonographically as bright echogenic foci with acoustical shadowing. Graded-compression sonography is now the preferred initial study in patients with clinical symptoms suggestive of acute appendicitis in centers where the sonographic study can be properly performed. Limitations of sonography include obesity and lack of cooperation in patients who are extremely distressed or restless. CT exam is more helpful in patients with a septic presentation (see Chapter 65).

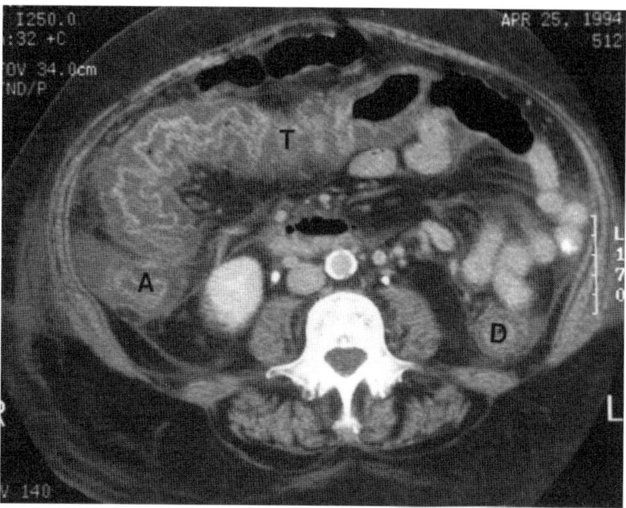


**Fig. 12.10** CT of pseudomembranous colitis shows severe edematous and thickened bowel wall of the ascending (*A*), transverse (*T*), and descending (*D*) colon.

## Acute cholecystitis

Sonography and biliary scintigraphy are of proven clinical value in diagnosing acute cholecystitis. In general, the sensitivity of both studies exceeds 90%. However, sonography is less expensive and can be performed more rapidly. It can also elucidate other causes of right upper quadrant pain and fever, such as abscess. Typical sonographic findings in uncomplicated acute calculous cholecystitis include gallstones, focal gallbladder tenderness (sonographic Murphy's sign), and gallbladder wall thickening from subserosal edema.

In summary, CT is the imaging modality of choice for the majority of patients with infraabdominal infections. However, given a particular clinical situation, the radiologist is best able to recommend the most appropriate imaging technique. CT is preferable in the evaluation of solid organ abscesses (hepatic, splenic, pancreatic, renal), peritoneal abscesses, and associated malig-

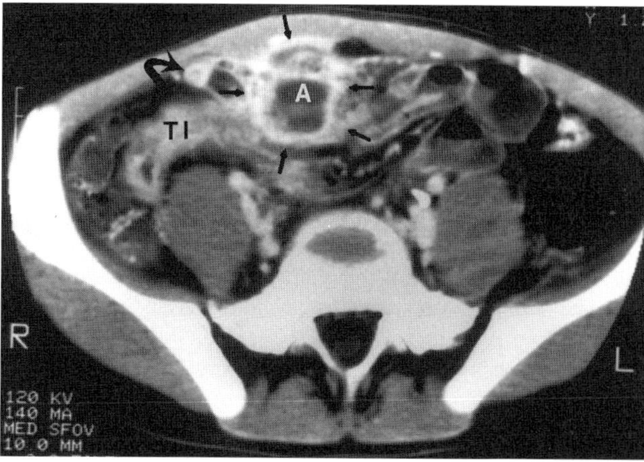


**Fig. 12.9** CT of peritoneal abscess in a patient with Crohn's disease involving the terminal ileum and appendix. The abscess (*A*) is seen as a fluid collection with an enhancing rim (*straight arrows*). The adjacent terminal ileum (*TI*) and appendix (*curved arrow*) have abnormally thickened wall.

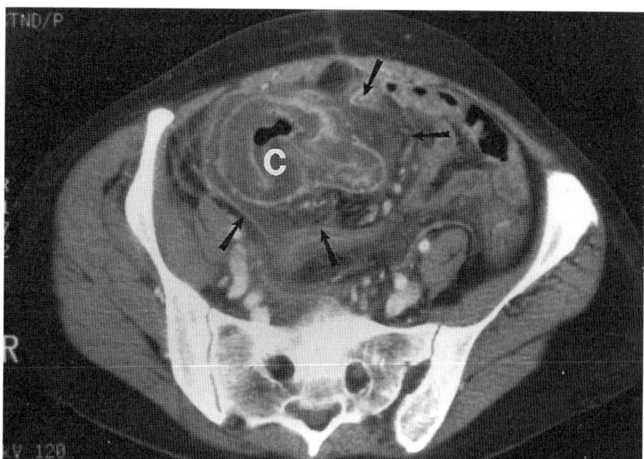


**Fig. 12.11** CT of neutropenic right-sided colitis in a patient undergoing chemotherapy for leukemia. The bowel wall of the cecum (*C*) is markedly thickened, and there is considerable pericolonic inflammation (*arrows*).

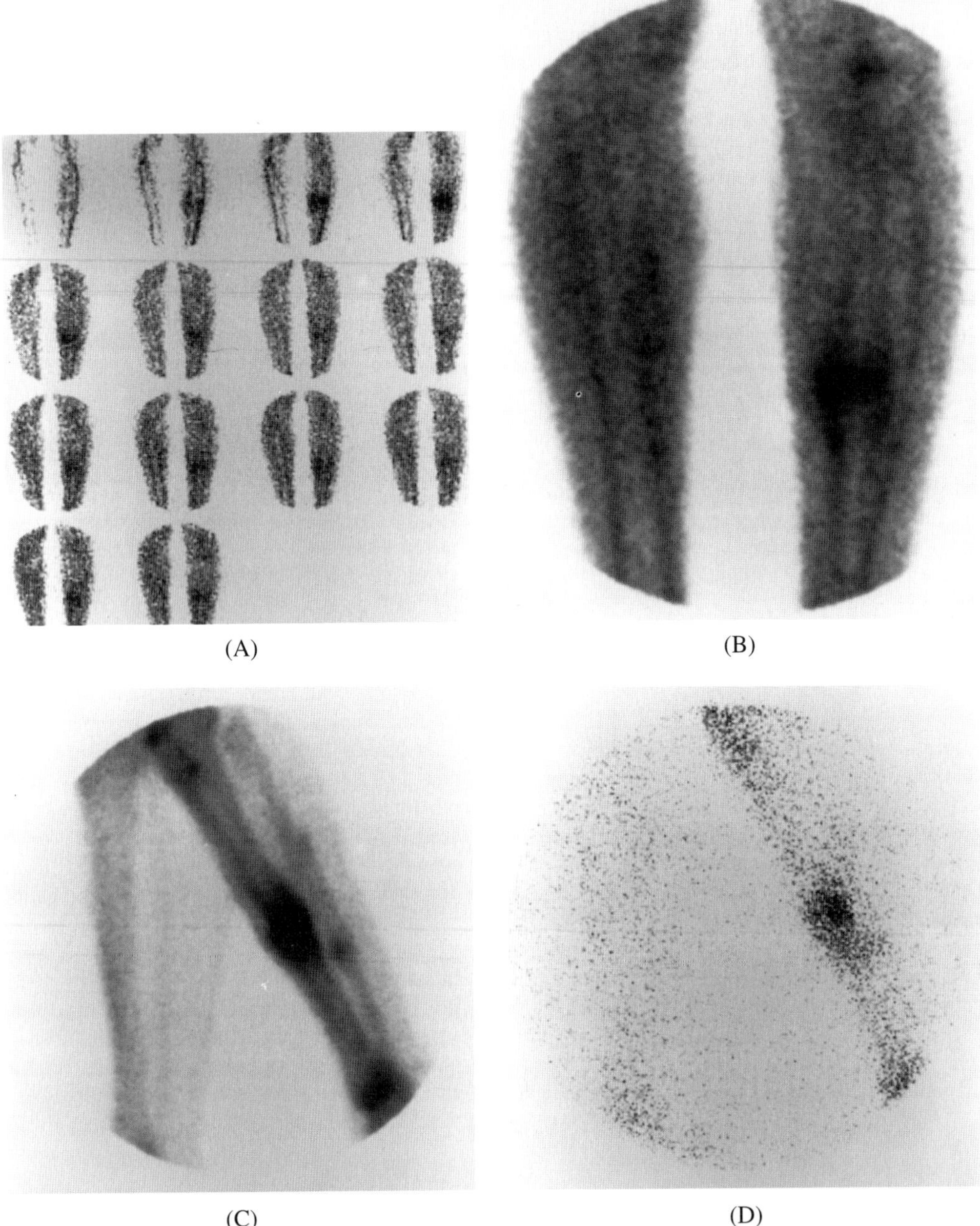

**Fig. 12.12** *A.* Blood flow. *B.* Blood pool. *C.* Three-hour delayed Tc-99m methylene diphosphonate bone image. *D.* In-111 WBC image. Images show left tibial osteomyelitis in a patient s/p fracture and intramedullary rod fixation.

nancies or adenopathy. CT is an important adjunctive imaging modality in the assessment of the bowel wall and extraluminal abnormalities. Sonography is used primarily in the evaluation of the gallbladder, biliary system, pelvic infections including the appendix, and prostatitis.

## Nuclear Imaging

Radionuclide techniques for the imaging of infection rely on the physiologic principles of the infection's inflammatory response for localization of specific tracers. The phenomena of increased blood flow, increased capillary permeability, and active recruitment of white blood cells to sites of infection underlie the nuclear medicine strategy for imaging. Often, when focal infection is suspected, imaging studies such as CT or ultrasound will be used to clarify findings on physical exam. However, when these studies are nonspecific or unrevealing, or when there is no reliable direction for an imaging search from the physical exam, a nuclear medicine exam, such as a whole-body bone scan, white blood cell (WBC) scan, or gallium scan can aid in the detection of sites of "occult" infection by screening the entire skeleton, white blood cell distribution, or whole-body gallium distribution, respectively. Therefore, specific indications for nuclear imaging include: (*1*) abscess/phlegmon detection when there is lack of localization or specificity on physical exam and other imaging studies; (*2*) simple or complicated osteomyelitis that may be hematogenously spread or occurring in bone with antecedent pathology, such as trauma or fixation; (*3*) persistent fevers despite apparently appropriate antibiotic choice because occult abscess or untreated infection may be present; (*4*) fever of unknown origin (FUO) in which infection, inflammatory disease, and/or malignancy is suspected; (*5*) contrast-agent allergies in which intravenous iodinated contrast material is necessary for diagnosis (adverse reactions to radiopharmaceuticals are extremely rare even in "iodinated contrast allergic" patients).

In this short review of infection imaging with nuclear medicine, the areas for specific applications of methods are divided into osseous and nonosseous imaging.

## Osseous infection

The three- or four-phase bone scan, using technetium-99m diphosphonate (Tc-99m), is the most commonly used nuclear medicine procedure for the identification of osteomyelitis. The phases consist of: (*1*) blood flow, (*2*) blood pool, (*3*) delayed 3- to 5-hour static images, and (*4*) 24-hour delayed images. Osteomyelitis is characterized by increased flow, pooling, and progressively increasing skeletal-to-background activity on the delayed images. Caveats include previous bone injury, which may cause a similar pattern of uptake, and photopenic or "cold" defects, which can occur because of high pressure in the infectious mass actually disrupting the arterial input and reducing the bony uptake. In the former case, the addition of a WBC image or gallium-67 (Ga-67) scan can improve the specificity in structurally abnormal bone (Fig. 12.12). In the latter case, astute recognition of the significance of photopenia is essential because a bone abscess may be present.

Particular problems arise in dealing with diabetic pedal osteomyelitis, because other pathologic states of bone, such as diabetic osteoarthropathy as well as soft-tissue infections, may complicate the diagnosis. In these cases, combined use of bone scans and indium-111 (In-111) WBC scans in a dual-isotope, simultaneous acquisition have been helpful. The bone scans provide a structural and localizing background for the WBC image, as the latter has poorer spatial resolution but higher specificity for infection.

In hematogenously disseminated infection, bone scans are sensitive for bone and joint involvement. Alternatively, whole-body Tc-99m or In-111 labeled white blood cell scans or Ga-67 scans can also evaluate for focal uptake in bone at the same time that soft-tissue and organ involvement may be addressed. In the spine and other areas with significant marrow components, WBC scans can show "cold" spots in areas of abscess formation. Other space-occupying or marrow-destructive processes can result in similar findings; thus the finding of photopenia is nonspecific but must be always considered suspicious for infection. Ga-67 scans have less incidence of the photopenic phenomenon and may be preferred for evaluation of the spine. In the setting of chronic osteomyelitis, Ga-67 also may be indicated over WBC imaging. The cells for WBC imaging are labeled in proportion to the differential blood count, and therefore polymorphonuclear cells are the predominant cell type. In chronic osteomyelitis, the predominant cell type in the infection is often mononuclear. As such, WBC scans may be falsely negative in chronic osteomyelitis, whereas the Ga-67 scan is more sensitive. Another imaging technique, such as MRI or CT, may be employed for focal osseous infection. Yet these techniques are impractical for rendering a skeletal or whole-body survey.

## Nonosseous infection

WBC scans with either In-111 or Tc-99m labeling are the preferred imaging methods for whole-body screening for localization of infection. In-111 scans are ideal for abdominal infections, as are Tc-99m scans, but the latter only when imaged within the first 4 hours after administration of the agent. Tc-99m WBCs have some impurities that are due to a lower tagging efficiency and that result in some gut excretion after 4 hours. The impurities, though problematic for interpretation, do not cause any adverse reactions in patients. White blood cell scans have been shown to have utility in the evaluation of vascular graft infections. Ga-67 scans are preferred in certain subpopulations of patients, such as AIDS, neutropenic, and FUO patients. Because of physiologic gut excretion of Ga-67, these scans are poor for evaluating intraabdominal infections.

The technique of cellular labeling requires handling of blood products and in vitro tagging. Stringent precautions are taken to avoid misadministration of the labeled cells to the wrong patient. Newer, "safer" radiopharmaceuticals for use in imaging the whole body for infection are under investigation. They include In-111 polyclonal IgG, Tc-99m labeled IgG, Tc-99m antigranulocyte monoclonal antibodies, and chemotactic peptides.

In summary, the whole-body screening capability of these nuclear medicine tests can provide unique and highly diagnostic images of suspected and occult infection. When taken in concert with the clinical scenario and other imaging studies, a detailed definition of a patient's infection is possible. No imaging study is truly inexpensive, but a well-considered imaging plan arrived at through consultation with nuclear medicine specialists and radiologists can result in cost containment and wise use of resources.

## ANNOTATED BIBLIOGRAPHY


Brown ML, Collier BD Jr., Fogelman I. Bone scintigraphy: Part 1. Oncology and Infection. J Nucl Med 1993; 34:2236–2240.

*Excellent, well-referenced review article on applications of bone scintigraphy in skeletal metastatic disease and osteomyelitis.*

Callen P. Computed tomographic evaluation of abdominal and pelvic abscesses. Radiology 1979; 131:171.

*Well-referenced article that describes CT characteristics of abdominal and pelvic abscesses and discusses the specificity of these characteristics.*

Goodman, P. C. Mycobacterial disease in AIDS. J Thorac Imaging 1991. 6:22–27

*This is a good, well-referenced review article describing the radiologic manifestations of mycobacterial disease in AIDS.*

Grossman RI, Yousem DM. Neuroradiology: The Requisites. Mosby, Philadelphia, 1994.

*A general neuroradiology text targeted primarily at radiology residents and fellows. The authors include a concise, yet remarkably complete chapter on brain infections, as well as other chapters on temporal bone, sinonasal, and head and neck inflammatory processes.*

Hesselink JR, ed. Neuroimaging Clinics of North America: Infectious and Inflammatory Diseases, vol 1. WB Saunders, Philadelphia. 1991.

*A thorough, up-to-date review of current radiographic evaluation of CNS infections, including the brain and spine.*

Imaging of CNS Infection, Topics in Magnetic Resonance Imaging. Raven Press, New York, 1994.

*Another thorough review of the modern radiologic approach to CNS infections.*

Jeffrey R, Laing F, Townsend R. Acute appendicitis: High resolution real time US findings. Radiology 1988; 167:327–329.

*Excellent article that describes sonographic criteria for the diagnosis of acute appendicitis in a large series with surgical correlation. Key references on ultrasound of acute appendicitis are included.*

Kuhlman JE, Kavuru M, Fishman EK, Siegelman SS. *Pneumocystis carinii* pneumonia: spectrum of parenchymal CT findings. Radiology 1990; 175:711–714.

*This article describes the spectrum and frequency of CT manifestations of* Pneumocystis carinii *pneumonia (PCP) in 39 patients.*

McAfee JG, Gagne G, Subramanian G, Schneider RF. The localization of Indium-111-leukocytes, Gallium-67, Polyclonal IgG and other radioactive agents in acute focal inflammatory lesions. J Nucl Med 1991; 32:2126–2131.

*Experimental study of* E. coli *abscess formation in rabbits and uptake of various radiopharmaceuticals in the lesions. The highest target-to-background uptake was shown with In-111 white blood cells.*

Moskovic E, Miller R, Pearson M. High resolution computed tomography of *Pneumocystis carinii* pneumonia in AIDS. Clin Radiol 1990; 42:239–243.
*This article describes the wide variety of CT appearances of* Pneumocystis carinii *pneumonia (PCP), with emphasis on early PCP infection in the face of a normal chest radiograph.*

vanSonnenberg E, D'Angostino H, Casola G, Halasz N, Sanchez R, Goodacre B. Percutaneous abscess drainage: Current concepts. Radiology 1991; 181:617.
*Excellent review of current and future concepts of percutaneous abscess drainage with a large number of pertinent references. The article reviews the indications, imaging modalities, and techniques for management of a variety of abscesses.*

# 13

# Hematologic Alterations in Infectious Disease Patients

PHOTIS BERIS AND FRANCIS A. WALDVOGEL

Defense of the host against infectious agents covers a large spectrum of mechanisms, which include: acute inflammatory reactions, activation of complement, activation of macrophages, activation of granulocytes, polyclonal activation of some T-cell subsets, and T cell–dependent or T cell–independent polyclonal B cell activation. Cellular and humoral blood elements are involved in protection against infection and, when this is not possible, in its eradication or control. Hematologic alterations in infectious diseases vary, and may be characterized by an increased proliferation of lymphohematopoietic tissue, an increased destruction of blood elements in the periphery, resulting in cytopenia(s), and an insult to stem cells, progenitors, or the microenvironment, leading to different forms of bone marrow aplasia. Infectious diseases may also interfere with coagulation, leading to thrombohemorrhagic phenomena by a direct or indirect effect on platelets or by activation of coagulation factors.

In the past, infectious diseases were thought to cause only benign or "polyclonal" hematologic alterations. However, molecular biology techniques and increasing understanding of the pathogenesis of malignancies have now provided evidence that some infections, particularly viral, can induce monoclonal hematologic malignancies. In this chapter, we systematically describe hematologic manifestations of infectious diseases.

## Erythrocytes and Infections

### Inflammatory anemia

Inflammatory anemia is defined as the anemia occurring in chronic infections and in inflammatory or neoplastic disorders. This anemia is mild to moderate (Hb is rarely lower than 9 g/dl) and is normochromic/normocytic or normochromic/microcytic It is characterized by decreased serum iron and total iron-binding capacity with normal or increased iron stores demonstrated by serum ferritin levels or by Prussian blue stain for marrow iron. Reticulocytes are not increased in proportion to the degree of anemia.

Inflammatory anemia or anemia of chronic disease (ACD) is the anemia most frequently diagnosed in general hospitals in western countries. Advances in research on cytokines and mediators in inflammation, as well as improved understanding of erythropoiesis, have greatly enhanced our appreciation of the pathogenesis of ACD.

#### Pathogenesis

Tumor-necrosis factor (TNF) and interleukin-1 (IL-1) directly or indirectly (mediated by interferon-$\beta$ (IFN-$\beta$) and interferon-$\gamma$ (IFN-$\gamma$), respectively) inhibit erythropoiesis. TNF and IL-1 have been observed to be increased particularly in patients with parasitic and bacterial infections. In addition, IFN-$\gamma$ is produced mainly by T lymphocytes in response to IL-1, and IFN-$\beta$ is produced by marrow stromal cells in response to TNF. Both mediators have been found to be elevated in patients with infectious diseases, thus suggesting their pathogenetic role in ACD.

Besides the negative effects on erythroid progenitors, IL-1 and TNF contribute to the development of ACD by inhibiting erythropoietin (EPO) production and by altering iron metabolism. In fact, studies on the role of cytokines in inflammatory anemia have demonstrated a blocking of the release of reticuloendothelial iron, leading to the well-known hypoferremia and to a decreased iron incorporation in red blood cells (RBCs). Furthermore, IL-1 increases ferritin production, suggesting that this additional ferritin could act as a trap for iron otherwise available for erythropoiesis. A schematic diagram of the contribution of some cytokines to the development of inflammatory anemia is shown in Figure 13.1. Resolution of infection leads to decrease of inflammatory cytokines and correction of anemia.

### Iron-deficiency anemia

Gastrointestinal bleeding represents the main cause of iron-deficiency anemia. Although a benign or malignant anatomic lesion must be excluded in such patients, in tropical areas an important source of gastrointestinal blood loss is parasitic infection. Hookworm (*Necator americanus* or *Ancylostoma duodenale*) affects some 20% of the world population. It is endemic in a zone extending from the southern United States to northern Argentina, as well as in Mediterranean countries, South Asia, and Africa (see Chapter 5). The worms attach to the proximal small intestine and suck blood from the host. The amount of blood lost is proportional to the number of worms harbored, which in turn can be estimated by the fecal excretion of hookworm eggs. With *Necator* infections, each worm accounts for the loss of about 0.05 ml blood per day. Women harboring more than 100 worms (= 5 ml/day blood loss) and men harboring more than 250 worms (12.5 ml/day blood loss) tend to become anemic. The daily blood loss may be as great as 250 ml. Even larger amounts are lost in *Ancylostoma* infection.

This anemia possesses all the characteristics of iron deficiency (microcytosis, hypochromia) and can be corrected by iron therapy, whether the worms are eliminated or not. Conversely, elimination of worms with an effective antihelminthic agent does not correct the anemia unless iron stores are replenished.

Schistosomiasis and trichinosis are other parasitic infections associated with iron deficiency. With *Schistosoma mansoni*, blood loss is from the intestine, whereas with *Schistosoma hematobium*, it is from the urinary tract.

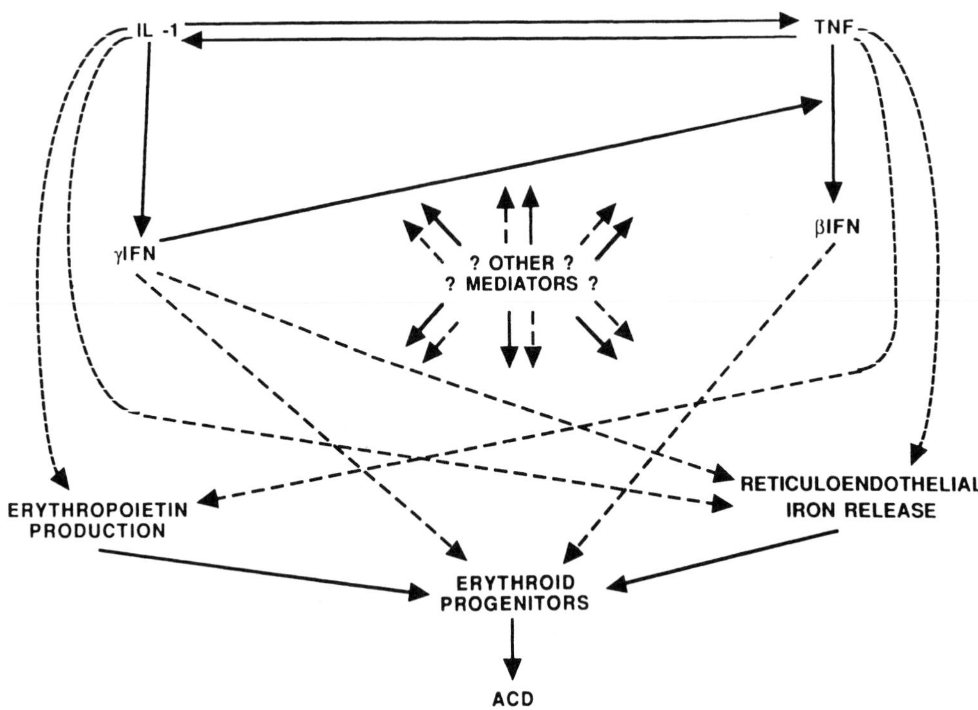


**Fig. 13.1** Schematic diagram representing the effects of inflammatory cytokines on processes involved in the impairment of erythropoiesis in ACD. Positive regulatory effects are indicated by solid lines and negative effects by broken lines. [From Means RT et al. Progress in understanding the pathogenesis of the anemia of chronic disease. Blood 1992; 80:1639–1647, with permission.]

## Megaloblastic anemia

Another parasite-creating anemia is the fish tapeworm *Diphyllobothrium latum. D. latum*, a common parasite of freshwater fish, in particular salmon, is distributed widely in the lakes of many parts of Europe as well as those of the northern part of central North America. Human infestation results from ingestion of inadequately cooked fish. Carriers of *D. latum* develop megaloblastic anemia because the tapeworm competes with the host for dietary $B_{12}$ and is able to take up and firmly bind the vitamin. Little, if any, improvement in absorption is observed when the vitamin is given with intrinsic factor. Schilling's urinary excretion test gives results similar to those seen in nontropical sprue. The anemia responds to expulsion of the worms, but the response is often suboptimal if no vitamin $B_{12}$ is given. Parenterally administered vitamin $B_{12}$ is effective even when the worms are not expelled.

## Pure red cell aplasia

Parvoviruses are the smallest DNA-containing viruses (*parvum* in Latin means "small") infecting human cells. Because of their limited genetic capacity, parvoviruses are absolutely dependent for their replication on actively cycling cells. Consequently, animal parvoviruses cause diseases by infecting rapidly proliferating tissues such as hematopoietic tissue.

In normal humans, parvovirus B19 causes "fifth disease" in children, and an acute febrile illness characterized by polyarthralgia rather than rash in adults (see Chapter 79). Hematologic disease secondary to B19 parvovirus is seen mainly in patients with chronic hemolytic anemias and is characterized by a transient aplastic crisis. B19 parvovirus can induce transient pure red cell aplasia in patients with sickle-cell disease, hereditary spherocytosis, thalassemias, erythrocyte enzyme deficiency, autoimmune hemolytic anemia, and, possibly, in patients with hemorrhage-induced erythropoietic stress. In addition to complicating the course of a patient with known chronic hemolytic anemia, transient aplastic crisis may precipitate anemia in patients with compensated hemolysis.

Pure red cell aplasia is characterized by the abrupt onset of severe anemia with an absence of reticulocytes in the peripheral blood and a paucity of erythroid precursor cells in the bone marrow. Giant pronormoblasts are seen in the bone marrow with prominent nucleoli or nuclear inclusion bodies. Anemia dominates the clinical presentation of transient aplastic crisis, but both neutropenia and thrombocytopenia have also been observed. Platelet counts as low as 15,000/mm$^3$ and neutrophil numbers as low as 600/mm$^3$ have been reported. Although recovery usually occurs after 1 to 2 weeks with sequential appearance of peripheral blood normoblasts, reticulocytes, and a rising hemoglobin, transfusion is usually required and may be lifesaving.

### Pathogenesis

Experimental data in colony assays as well as molecular biology studies of B19 parvovirus give evidence of the specificity of the virus for erythroid cells. Inhibition of granulopoiesis is probably mediated by a noncapsid protein transcription product of the viral genome. The disappearance of erythroid cells is the result of cell death rather than blocked differentiation. Cytopathic effects in isolated, infected erythroid progenitors visualized by electron microscopy include pseudopod formation, cytoplasmic vacuolization, and mitochondrial swelling.

Chronic bone marrow failure due to persistent B19 parvovirus infection with hypoplastic bone marrow has been noted in patients with congenital (Nezelof's syndrome) or acquired immunodeficiency syndromes (AIDS). In these cases, clinical improvement is correlated with disappearance of the virus from the blood and can be induced by IV high-dose immunoglobulin administration (see Chapter 44).

## Hemolytic anemia

Infectious diseases can cause hemolytic anemia either by an *immune* or by a *nonimmune* mechanism. Immune hemolysis may be mediated by warm or cold reactive antibodies. *Warm-reactive autoantibodies* with specificity for red cell antigens have been described in association with viral and some protozoan infections. In particular, autoimmune hemolytic anemia (AIHA) has been observed following hepatitis, cytomegalovirus infections, Epstein-Barr virus (EBV) and rubella. In children with AIHA, infection is a common triggering factor, more so than in affected adults. In parasitic diseases, AIHA may be found in malaria, visceral leishmaniasis, and trypanosomiasis.

Autoimmune hemolytic anemia may be explosive in onset and life-threatening in patients with acute viral infections. In contrast, hemolysis in patients with protozoan infections is often of mixed origin (hypersplenism, toxic effects of the parasites, and immune origin), and although the direct antiglobulin (Coombs') test may be quite strongly positive, immunoglobulin affinity and avidity for erythrocytic antigens is weak and immune erythrocytic destruction very low.

*Cold-reactive antibodies* react most effectively with red cell antigens at temperatures below 32°C. This reaction may give rise to one of two clinical syndromes, depending on the functional properties of the anti–red cell antibodies involved: the *cold agglutinin syndrome* and *paroxysmal cold hemoglobinuria*. Infections have been associated with both.

Cold agglutinins may be polyclonal or monoclonal. Infections usually generate the former, while malignant lymphocytic proliferation generates the latter. The most frequent causes of cold agglutinins are summarized in Table 13.1.

### Pathogenesis

Most cold agglutinins are specific for one of the I antigens (anti-I or anti-i). Some agglutinins that react equally with cord (i) and adult (I) cells have been named Pr. On occasion, examples of cold-reactive autoantibodies with anti-A, anti-B, anti-H, anti-M, anti-P, and anti-N specificity have been reported.

Generally, cold agglutinins are of the IgM class, although cold agglutinins of the IgG class have been observed in patients with infectious mononucleosis. The amount of lysis effected by cold agglutinins is related most directly to the ability of a given antibody to initiate complement activation. This property is, in turn, related to the thermal amplitude of the antibody. When thermal amplitude (i.e., the highest temperature at which the antibody binds to red cells) is near core body temperature, cold agglutinins are manifested clinically by intravascular hemolysis (Coombs' C3b is positive, high serum lacticodehydrogenase (LDH), low haptoglobin level). If thermal amplitude is low, cold agglutinins are hematologically asymptomatic. Finally, since cells other than erythrocytes possess Ii or Ii-like surface antigens (e.g., B and T lymphocytes, polymorphonuclear leukocytes, monocytes, macrophages, and platelets), all formed blood elements may be affected by anti-Ii cold agglutinins.

Fortunately, hemolytic disease caused by cold agglutinins is rare. When it occurs, the hemolysis is of rather abrupt onset and is occasionally severe. The process is self-limited, however, and the cold agglutinin titre usually drops to normal levels within 3–4 weeks. HIV-infected individuals with symptoms and signs of AIDS may present with persistent cold agglutinins.

Patients with cold agglutinins secondary to infections need no specific therapy, and the most important principle besides specific treatment of the infectious disease is the maintenance of an ambient temperature above the maximal temperature at which the antibody reacts. If transfused, blood should be warmed to 37°C. Furthermore, the use of washed red cells and the slow infusion of the blood into a large vein are recommended. Finally, plasmapheresis may be of benefit for acutely ill patients.

*Paroxysmal cold hemoglobinuria (PCH)* is characterized by the sudden passage of hemoglobin into the urine after local or general exposure to cold. This syndrome is due to the presence of cold hemolysins of the Donath-Landsteiner type that are specific for the Pp blood group. This antibody was classically described in patients with tertiary or congenital syphilis. Classic PCH is now a rare disease and most cases of hemolysis associated with Donath-Landsteiner antibodies are acute transient episodes in children who had previously contracted an acute viral infection of the respiratory tract. Other patients have had measles, mumps, or infectious mononucleosis.

**Table 13.1** Diseases in which cold agglutinins may occur

| INFECTIOUS DISEASES | NONINFECTIOUS DISEASES |
|---|---|
| *POLYCLONAL* | *POLYCLONAL* |
| *Mycoplasma pneumoniae* | Collagen vascular and immune complex diseases |
| Infectious mononucleosis | Angioimmunoblastic lymphoadenopathy |
| Cytomegalovirus | *MONOCLONAL* |
| Mumps | Idiopathic chronic cold agglutinin disease |
| Listeriosis | Waldenström's macroglobulinemia |
| Subacute bacterial endocarditis | Lymphomas |
| Syphilis | Chronic lymphocytic leukemia |
| Trypanosomiasis | Myeloma |
| Malaria | |
| HIV (persistent) | |
| *MONOCLONAL* | |
| *Mycoplasma pneumoniae* (exceptional) | |
| Kaposi's sarcoma | |

*Nonimmune-mediated hemolysis* induced by infection may be due either to a corpuscular defect of erythrocytes or to direct toxic damage of red blood cells by the infectious agent. In the former group—i.e., hemolysis occurring in patients suffering from a hereditary corpuscular defect of erythrocytes, infections can act as a triggering factor and sometimes precipitate life-threatening hemolytic episodes: G-6-PD deficiency, unstable hemoglobins, and sickle-cell disease represent the main diseases.

In the latter group are malaria (particularly *P. falciparum*), babesia (in asplenic individuals), African trypanosomiasis, and bartonellosis (particularly in Peru). Other instances of nonimmune–mediated hemolytic anemia have been encountered in association with severe bacterial infections: *Clostridium welchii* septicemia, *Borrelia recurrentis*, and leptospirosis. The hemolysis caused by these agents is probably the result of toxins or, in the case of leptospirae, direct attack of the erythrocytic membrane by the microorganism. Table 13.2 is a summary of forms of anemia and associated infectious diseases.

## Leukocytes and Infection

### Granulocytes

Infection with pyogenic bacteria usually elicits a neutrophilic response, the magnitude of which depends on many factors, such as the virulence of the organism, the extent of the infection (localized or widespread), and the bone marrow's ability to respond to the process.

When the infection is mild, slight neutrophilia is seen, while in some patients with serious infection, a leukocyte count greater than $50 \times 10^9$ cells/L with the presence of immature cells in the peripheral blood (leukemoid reaction) can be observed. Successive detailed blood analyses are of considerable prognostic value in the event of serious infection: a low or falling count and a shift to the left with the appearance of metamyelocytes and myelocytes in the blood suggests exhaustion of marrow neutrophil reserves and a poor outcome. Mechanisms of granulocytosis during infection and changes in granulocyte kinetics are discussed in Chapter 10.

#### Morphology

In a pyogenic infection, the following morphologic alterations can be seen:

1. Toxic granules may be seen in mature or immature neutrophils (Fig. 13.2a). Electron microscopic (EM) findings and histochemical studies indicate that "toxic" granules are peroxidase-positive azurophilic (primary) granules that are more readily stained than the granules in normal cells. They are more visible because they are present in greater proportion to the pink specific granules than normal owing to accelerated myelopoiesis and decreased cellular divisions after the promyelocyte stage. These granules, as well as the increase in leukocyte alkaline phosphatase activity, are seen in association with infection and indicate that myelopoiesis is accelerated in response to inflammatory stimuli.

2. Another neutrophilic alteration associated with severe infection is the presence of Döhle's bodies. These are morphologically discrete, round or oval areas seen in the peripheral portions of the cytoplasm of neutrophils. They stain sky blue with Romanovsky's dyes and have been identified by EM as lamellar aggregates of rough endoplasmic reticulum. Like toxic granulation, they are indicative of accelerated myelopoiesis and reduced maturation. They are seen not only during infection, but also in patients with burns and after exposure to cytotoxic agents. They are similar to and must be differentiated from May-Hegglin bodies (Fig. 13.2b).

3. Cytoplasmic vacuoles in neutrophils may be seen. They represent phagosomes or autophagocytic vacuoles and are indicative of cellular activation by inflammatory stimuli while still in the vasculature. A variety of microbial products, complement factors, and cytokines (TNF, IL-1, IFN-$\gamma$) are capable of inducing vacuolation (see Chapter 10). There is some specificity between the appearance of vacuoles and the presence of bacteria in blood cultures.

Toxic granulations, cytoplasmic vacuoles, diffuse cytoplasmic basophilia, pyknotic areas in the nucleus, and Döhle's bodies may all occur during severe infection and have grave prognostic implications. The presence of one or more of these changes suggests the development of septicemia or bacteremia and points to the possibility of generalized infection as opposed to a localized process (see Chapter 53). The degenerative index is a means of quantitating these changes. An index greater than 50% (>50% neutrophils exhibiting toxic granulation) suggests severe infection and a poor prognosis. Serial indices are more informative than changes in leukocyte number or a left shift in the differential count. Finally, the presence of cytoplasmic vacuoles in blood neutrophils is found to correlate well with the presence of bacteremia and impaired granulocyte function.

**Table 13.2** Anemia and infectious disease

| Form of anemia | Associated diseases |
|---|---|
| Inflammatory anemia | Many infections |
| Iron-deficiency anemia | Hookworm, schistosomiasis |
| Megaloblastic anemia | *Diphyllobothrium latum* |
| Red cell aplasia | PV B19 |
| Hemolytic anemia characterized by | |
| Immune warm antibodies | Viral and protozoan infections |
| Immune cold antibodies | Mycoplasma, EBV, CMV, Listeria, syphilis |
| Nonimmune | In normal subjects, malaria, babesia, bartonellosis |
| | Any infectious agent in patients suffering from a hereditary erythrocyte defect |

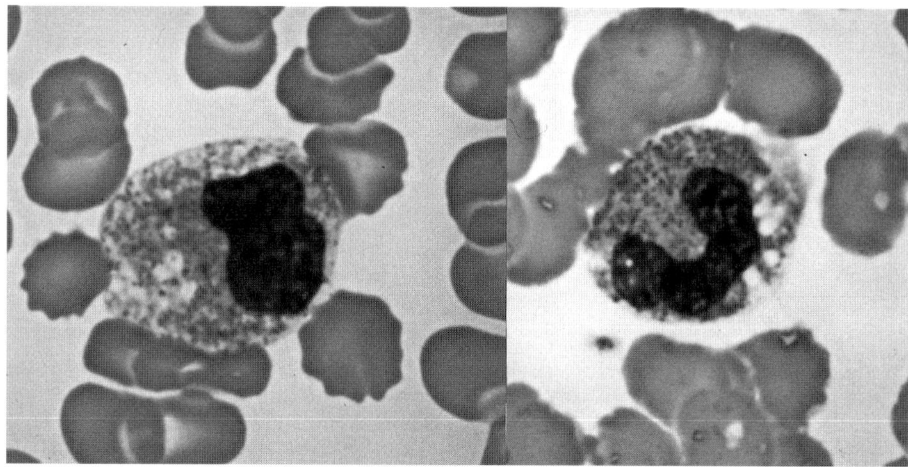

**Fig. 13.2a** Toxic granulation, cytoplasmic vacuoles, Döhle bodies. Peripheral blood from a patient with pneumococcal pneumonia. Wright staining, ×1000.

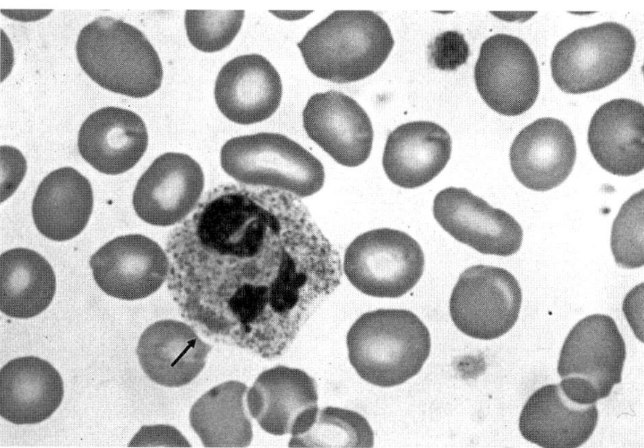

**Fig. 13.2b** May-Hegglin anomaly. Note presence of "pseudo"–Döhle bodies. Peripheral blood. Wright staining, ×1000.

In contrast to the pyogenic infections, leukopenia and neutropenia are commonly associated with some bacterial and viral infections (see below) and do not necessarily have a poor outcome.

## Lymphocytes

With most acute nonviral infections (e.g., pneumonia, active tuberculosis, malaria), lymphocytopenia occurs, the only exception being pertussis where lymphocytosis (lymphocyte count $> 4.0 \times 10^9$ cells/L) is seen. Glucocorticoids found in the blood in increased amounts during the stress of severe infection reduce lymphocyte numbers by their action on $CD4^+$ helper cells, which is to direct them out of the circulation into the periphery.

Conversely, reactive (polyclonal) lymphocytosis may occur, usually as the result of viral infection. Most of the lymphocytes can be shown to be $CD8^+$ cells, and an inversion in the CD4/CD8 ratio (normally ~2:1) is common during acute viral infection.

Infectious mononucleosis is usually characterized by marked lymphocytosis. In contrast to pertussis and infectious lymphocytosis, in EBV infection lymphocytes are atypically large with basophilic cytoplasm and fine chromatin. In the classic mononucleosis syndrome, lymphomonocytosis comprises at least 50% peripheral leukocytes with 10% or more atypical stimulated large lymphocytes (also known as Pfeiffer's cells) (Fig. 13.3). Flow cytometric analysis of the peripheral blood cells revealed that 90% of atypical lymphocytes were $CD3^+$ T cells, 80% were CD8 T cells, and 9% were CD4 T cells. The CD8 cells expressed the T-cell receptor $\alpha$ and $\beta$ chains, the activation-associated antigens Human leucocytic antigen (HLA)-DR and CD45 RO, an antigen associated with memory T cells, as well as other T cell–related antigens, confirming the normal phenotype of mature activated CD8 T cells. The mononucleosis syndrome may also be seen in cytomegalovirus (CMV) infection, infectious hepatitis, and human immunodeficiency virus (HIV) seroconversion.

In children, acute infectious lymphocytosis, a disease with as yet no definite etiologic agent, is mainly characterized by lymphocytosis (average peak value $34 \times 10^9$/L) persisting for 3–7 weeks.

Although lymphocytosis is mainly seen in viral infections, persistent high lymphocyte numbers may also suggest certain chronic bacterial infections such as brucellosis, tuberculosis, secondary and congenital syphilis, or a parasitic infection, toxoplasmosis.

## Eosinophils

*Protozoan* infections (pneumocystis, toxoplasmosis, amebiasis, and malaria) are rarely associated with eosinophilia, and when it

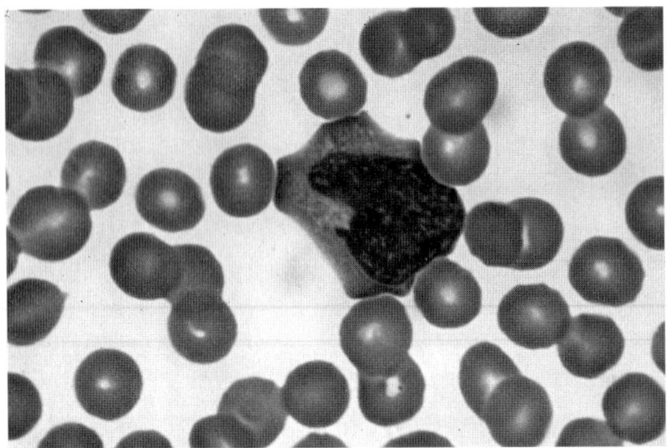

**Fig. 13.3** Atypical and large lymphocytes in a case of infectious mononucleosis (Pfeiffer's cells). Peripheral blood smear. Wright staining, ×1000.

does occur, the eosinophilia is always mild. Conversely, *metazoan* infections (nematodes, hematodes, cestodes, and arthropods) can create reactive hypereosinophilic syndromes with persistent blood eosinophilia (>1.5 × $10^9$/L) and eosinophilic infiltration of tissues.

It is not possible to distinguish morphologically between eosinophils associated with parasites and primary or malignant eosinophilia, since hypodense activated eosinophils with intracytoplasmic vacuoles are seen in both conditions. For this reason, the finding of a hypereosinophilic condition should always be a reason to look for a possible parasitic infection as well as bronchopulmonary aspergillosis where eosinophilia is the result of an acute allergic-inflammatory response (see Chapter 55). Successful treatment of parasites leads to normalization of the high eosinophil count.

Eosinopenia (counts <50/ml) is a feature of most acute bacterial infections. This is most likely due to the action of glucocorticoids released in increased amounts during an acute infectious episode and can be seen with other similarly stressful disorders (e.g., pancreatitis, myocardial infarction).

## Mononuclear phagocytes

It has long been recognized that there are certain microorganisms that can enter, resist killing, and replicate within the mononuclear phagocyte. For the hematologist, the most important human pathogens that can replicate within macrophages are: *Mycobacteria* sp., *Histoplasma capsulatum*, *Toxoplasma gondii*, and *Leishmania* sp. At an early stage, these organisms provoke monocytosis or lymphomonocytosis, which may be followed by other hematologic complications, including immune-mediated and hemophagocytic syndrome with pancytopenia (see below, under Pancytopenia Secondary to Infection) or hypersplenism. Monocytosis may also be seen with chronic intravascular infections, in particular subacute bacterial endocarditis.

In vitro studies have shown that fresh, unstimulated circulating blood monocytes can kill and digest almost all intracellular (amastigote) forms of *L. donovani* or the trophozoite forms of *T. gondii*. In contrast, the human monocyte-derived macrophage fails to exert any activity against these intracellular pathogens and readily supports their replication. Incubation of the macrophages with crude T-cell lymphokines, or in particular with immune (gamma) interferon (IFN-γ), restores their microbicidal activity as a manifestation of macrophage activation (see Chapter 11). These experimental data explain why, in T cell–deficient immunosuppressed patients, intracellular pathogens are almost always seen in bone marrow macrophages.

The role of the hematologist in the case of suspected infection with these slowly replicating intracellular pathogens is to offer a rapid diagnosis through detection of pathogens in bone marrow aspirates (Plate 1 and Fig. 13.4) or histologic sections (Plate 2). Histoplasmosis must be differentiated from leishmaniasis by PAS staining: negative for leishmaniasis, positive for histoplasmosis. Fungal infections in bone marrow histologic preparations are best seen upon Grocott staining and mycobacteria upon Ziehl-Neelsen staining. In cases of disseminated toxoplasmosis, cysts can be seen in simple bone marrow aspirates stained upon Wright's staining (Fig. 13.4). Bone marrow examination is the simplest and most rapid method for diagnosis and monitoring of treatment in visceral or systemic leishmaniasis.

Table 13.3 summarizes leucocyte disorders and associated infectious diseases.

## Coagulation Disorders and Infection

Infectious diseases can alter hemostasis through (*1*) vascular injury, (*2*) abnormal blood coagulation, (*3*) enhanced plasma proteolysis, and/or (*4*) disorders of platelets. Table 13.4 lists the most frequent patterns of thrombohemorrhagic manifestations secondary to infection:

*Thrombocytopenia* of immune origin is classically produced by the lymphotropic viruses, e.g., EBV, CMV, etc., and is usually self-limited. It has also been described as a manifestation of HIV infection and may be a persistent defect in some HIV-infected patients before the advent of AIDS-defining illnesses (see Chapter 100). Autoimmune thrombocytopenia may be a secondary immune reaction following some other viral infections and most often persists for some time after the infectious process has subsided. Finally, a wide range of infectious agents can cause thrombocytopenia in the absence of disseminated intravascular coagulation by a direct effect on platelets (varicella, rubella, lep-

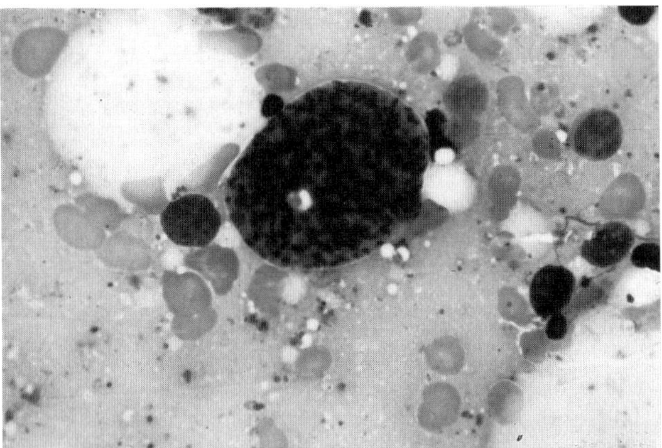

**Fig. 13.4** *Toxoplasma gondii*. Single cyst in bone marrow smear of a patient who received aggressive immunosuppressive therapy for severe acute GVHD after unrelated HLA-compatible bone marrow transplantation for acute myeloid leukemia M4 type. Wright staining, ×1000. [From Soulier-Lauper M et al. Disseminated toxoplasmosis in a severely immmunodeficient patient: Demonstration of cysts in bone marrow smears. Am J Hematol 38: 324–326, 1991, with permission].

**Table 13.3** Leukocytes and infection

| Leucocyte disorders | Associated source of infection |
|---|---|
| Leukemoid blood picture | Pyogenic bacteria |
| Leukopenia | Exhaustion of marrow neutrophil reserve in case of pyogenic infection |
| | Gram-negative bacteria, disseminated fungal disease, disseminated tuberculosis |
| Lymphocytosis | Viral infections |
| Monocytosis | Chronic infections (Tbc, endocarditis) |
| Eosinophilia | Metazoan infections |
| Eosinopenia and lymphopenia | Most acute bacterial infections |

tospirosis), by damage to the vessel wall (*Yersinia*, dengue), or by a direct effect on megakaryocytes (HIV).

Reactive or secondary *thrombocytosis* is seen in any inflammatory disorder (neoplasia, infection, tissue necrosis). However, in active pulmonary tuberculosis secondary thrombocytosis is particularly pronounced and its correction parallels clinical improvement on antituberculosis therapy.

*Disseminated intravascular coagulation (DIC)* can be a striking complication of acute bacteremia with the development of the sepsis syndrome (see Chapter 50). Factors that can trigger DIC during sepsis include endothelial injury and direct effects of microbial mediators, such as gram-negative endotoxin, peptidoglycans, and techoic acids from gram-positive bacteria, and direct endothelial injury by certain viruses (e.g., varicella, zoster, CMV, or hemorrhagic fever viruses) on platelets and coagulation proteins. Cellular mediators are released when endothelial cells are activated and/or shed, exposing the subendothelial surfaces. This exposure is another source of activation of the coagulation cascade and of the fibrinolytic system. Circulating platelets adhere to both the exposed subendothelium and damaged endothelial cells. Increased levels of circulating cytokines, in particular TNF, also promote intravascular coagulation by upregulating the expression of thrombospondin on endothelial cells. Activated macrophages may release thromboplastin and thus contribute to DIC. Even minimal hemolysis may provide negatively charged phospholipids that, together with activated platelets, help to sustain activation of serine proteases of the coagulation system. Activation of the complement system (C3a, C5a) and release of elastase from polymorphonuclear cells further increase the leakiness of the microcirculation, amplifying tissue injury via arterial blood pressure decrease. At the stage of further decompensation, significant amounts of thrombin may be produced locally or generally in the blood circulation and cause multiple secondary alterations, particularly thrombus formation, severe thrombocytopenia and a decrease of fibrinogen and other clotting factors. The detection of DIC is summarized in Table 13.5.

**Table 13.4** Thrombohemorrhagic manifestations secondary to infection

| |
|---|
| Thrombocytopenic purpura |
| Thrombocytosis |
| Disseminated intravascular coagulation |
| Hemolytic uremic syndrome (HUS)/thrombotic thrombocytopenic purpura (TTP) |
| Purpura fulminans |
| Specific organ bleeding<br>pulmonary hemorrhage<br>intracerebral hemorrhage<br>gastrointestinal hemorrhage |

The *hemolytic uremic syndrome* (HUS) is probably closely related to *thrombotic thrombocytopenic purpura* (TTP). A common feature is an early involvement of the microcirculation, mainly affecting the kidney (in HUS), but also any other organ. Both HUS and TTP are characterized by hemolytic anemia (high reticulocyte count), the presence of helmet cells in peripheral blood, and a low platelet count, all features of a *"microangiopathic" disorder* (Fig. 13.5). Cerebral damage is responsible for neurologic manifestations in TTP. Although the pathogenesis of microangiopathic syndromes is still unknown in the majority of cases, some infectious agents have been implicated in causing, or participating in the pathogenesis of, HUS or TTP: *Shigella*, *Escherichia coli* D1:H157, and HIV infections in HUS; *Campylobacter* and *Corynebacterium diphtheria* in TTP. Proposed therapeutic regimens in such cases include plasma exchange using frozen plasma, antiaggregants, and above all, the elimination of the infectious agent.

Summarized in Table 13.5 are the most helpful hematologic laboratory tests for patients with suspected coagulation disorders associated with infectious disease.

Finally, abnormal bleeding or any abnormal coagulation test in a febrile patient may not be the consequence of an infectious

**Table 13.5** Hematologic evaluation of coagulation disorders associated with infectious disease

| |
|---|
| Platelet count. In the case of an isolated decreased count, a viral infection, especially HIV or EBV, should be looked for. DIC should be looked for if bacteremia is suspected. Finally, if severe anemia coexists, (the possibility of) a microangiopathic syndrome should be excluded. |
| Red blood cell, reticulocyte count, red blood cell morphology, and hemolysis tests (bilirubin, LDH). |
| Fibrinogen concentration. Normally, infection produces a high fibrinogen concentration (acute phase protein). A normal or low fibrinogen level is indicative either of a production deficit or hyperconsumption of coagulation factors. |
| Prothrombin time and activated partial thromboplastin time. |
| Concentration of cofactors V, VII, VIII, and X: Factor VIII determination is of particular interest, as it is involved in DIC but not in hepatic pathology. |
| Concentration of fibrinogen-degradation products. |

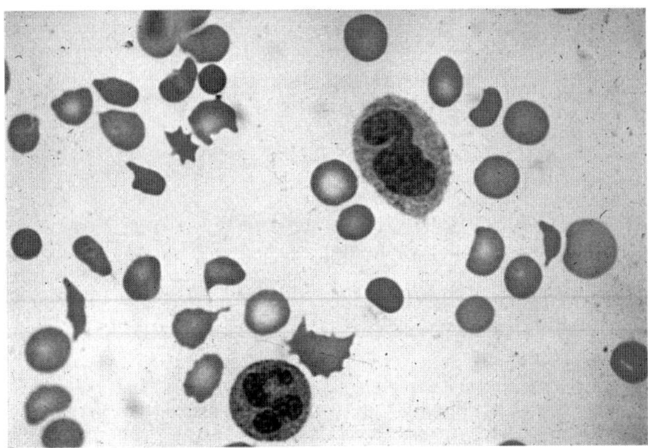

**Fig. 13.5** HUS in a case of AIDS. Peripheral blood smear (×1000).

episode. The possibilities of preexistent hematologic or liver disease or side effects of drugs used to treat either the infection or an underlying disease must be considered. Table 13.6 summarizes coagulation disorders and associated infections.

## Pancytopenia Secondary to Infection

Pancytopenia may be a complication of many diseases, including nutritional disorders (folate or $B_{12}$ deficiency), primary myelopoietic disorders, immune disorders (e.g., systemic lupus erythematosus), hypersplenism, marrow infiltrative disease (e.g., metastatic cancer), and certain infectious diseases. It may be of peripheral or central origin. *Peripheral* pancytopenia secondary to infection is seen in patients with malaria and kala-azar. In such cases, pancytopenia is the result of hypersplenism plus immune-mediated destruction of blood elements. Disseminated tuberculosis and disseminated fungal disease can cause pancytopenia, mainly through accelerated hemophagocytosis by the activated and hyperplastic histiomonocytes of bone marrow and the spleen.

Pancytopenia of *central* origin is known as aplastic anemia. Some viruses have been reported to cause aplastic anemia—e.g., hepatitis A and, less frequently, hepatitis B, rubella virus, EBV, HIV, and parvovirus B19 (in AIDS patients). The precise mechanisms by which infection with these viruses causes aplasia is not known. It is possible that the virus directly attacks stem cells. Alternatively, virus-induced immunologic disorders may damage either stem cells or the bone marrow microenvironment leading to bone marrow failure. An increase in the production of gamma-interferon by chronic infection may play a major role in inhibiting hematopoiesis.

Pancytopenia of central origin is of insidious onset and the degree of severity may vary. Aplastic anemia following an attack of infectious hepatitis is generally severe, and without treatment, the mortality in adults is extremely high. Laboratory features classically show a macrocytic anemia with a decreased absolute number of reticulocytes, absolute granulocytopenia, and moderate to severe thrombocytopenia. The presence of nucleated red cells on the blood film or immature myeloid precursors is an unusual finding and suggests marrow dysfunction rather than bone marrow aplasia. A typical finding is an increased serum iron concentration with almost complete saturation of iron-binding capacity. The diagnosis can be confirmed by bone marrow aspiration and biopsy that reveals fatty material with diffuse sparse accumulation of lymphocytes, phagocytizing macrophages, conspicuous mast cells, and plasma cells. Normal hematopoietic precursors are scarce and often greatly dispersed.

Without aggressive treatment (bone marrow transplantation or IV immunosuppression with antithymocyte globulin), the prognosis is poor. One exception is aplastic anemia secondary to parvovirus B19, which generally responds to high-dose IV administration of immunoglobulin (see above, under "Pure Red Cell Aplasia"), which presumably contains sufficient neutralizing antibody against the offending virus.

Although bone marrow suppression is not usually a feature of CMV infection in immunocompetent hosts, pancytopenia has been observed in immunocompromised individuals with generalized CMV infection. Hematologic evaluation can reveal infiltration of the bone marrow and lymph nodes (and other tissues) with lymphocytes and macrophages. The macrophages exhibit hemophagocytosis (see below, under "Virus-Associated Hemophagocytic Syndrome"). Alternatively, other CMV-positive allogeneic marrow graft recipients who develop progressive pancytopenia post-transplant may show hypocellular bone marrow biopsies without evidence of disease recurrence. CMV can usually be identified in the blood and urine. Many of these patients will respond to anti-CMV treatment with ganciclovir with improvement in the hematologic parameters.

### Virus-associated hemaphagocytic syndrome

EBV, CMV, *herpes simplex*, and adenovirus have been the most commonly implicated infectious agents in the genesis of virus-associated hemophagocytic syndrome (VAHS). Other intracellular infections that can trigger the syndrome are tuberculosis, histoplasmosis, cryptococcosis, babesiasis, ehrlichiosis, and AIDS. This disorder is characterized by a benign generalized histiocytic proliferation with marked hemophagocytosis. Clinically, the patients present with fever, generalized constitutional symptoms, myalgias, malaise, and wasting. On physical examination, hepatosplenomegaly and lymphadenopathy are common.

Hematologic manifestations in VAHS include coagulopathy and pancytopenia. Early in the disease, the bone marrow is hypercellular with infiltrating histiocytes showing pronounced hemophagocytosis (Plate 3). Later, the bone marrow is hypocellular

**Table 13.6** Coagulation disorders and infection

| | |
|---|---|
| Thrombocytopenia | Lymphotropic viruses (EBV, CMV, etc.)<br>Malaria |
| Thrombocytosis | Active pulmonary tuberculosis |
| Disseminated intravascular coagulation (DIC) | Sepsis syndrome |
| Microangiopathic disorders | *Shigella*, *E. coli*, HIV, *Campylobacter* |

and histiocytes become the main feature. At this stage, differential diagnosis between malignant histiocytosis and VAHS may be difficult.

VAHS has been most frequently observed in individuals with underlying immunosuppression (allograft recipients, patients receiving high-dose corticosteroids), which probably plays a role in its pathogenesis; EBV and CMV are potent stimulators of the immune system. Because of the underlying immunoregulatory disturbances allowing an inappropriate antiviral defense, cytokines (e.g., IFN-$\gamma$) secreted by activated T lymphocytes probably elicit the proliferation and activation of histiocytes. Table 13.7 gives causes of pancytopenia and associated infectious diseases.

## Hematologic Malignancies Secondary to Infection

It has long been a common belief that some cases of malignant lymphocytic proliferation could be secondary to viral infections. Molecular biology techniques and recently acquired knowledge of the pathogenesis of malignancies has provided evidence of the primordial role of some viruses of the herpes simplex family (EBV, CMV) and of retroviruses in the genesis of hematological malignancies, especially B-cell lymphoma, chronic lymphocytic leukemia (CLL), T-cell lymphoma, and leukemia. In addition, one has to consider that certain viruses can induce "prognostically malignant" polyclonal proliferation in some immunocompromised patients.

### EBV-associated neoplasms

*Fatal infectious mononucleosis*, in which the B-cell proliferation of acute mononucleosis fails to resolve and persists, resulting in fatal proliferation, has been described in boys carrying the genetically controlled immunodeficiency XLP (= X-linked lymphoproliferative syndrome or Duncan syndrome). EBV-infected B cells from these individuals are resistant to killing by T cells. Patients with the XLP syndrome have elevated white blood cell counts and marked atypical lymphocytosis. Because of fulminant liver failure, a bleeding diathesis secondary to coagulopathy is frequently seen. Fifteen percent of these patients develop lymphoma, while in those males surviving EBV infection, an uncontrolled anomalous T cell–mediated immune response results in B-cell aplasia with a picture of common variable immunodeficiency.

*Burkitt's lymphoma (BL)* (see Fig. 13.6) was the first hematologic malignancy found to be directly related to an infectious agent. In fact, based on epidemiologic studies, EBV was found to be responsible for most (96%) Burkitt's lymphomas occurring in Africa.

Molecular analysis has revealed that the specific chromosomal translocation found in EBV-associated Burkitt's lymphoma results in the juxtaposition of c-myc oncogene (chromosome 8) with immunoglobulin heavy chain gene (chromosome 14), while in sporadic Burkitt's lymphoma the juxtaposition of the c-myc oncogene is with the lambda light-chain gene (chromosome 22) or with the kappa light-chain gene (chromosome 2). To explain the role of EBV in BL genesis, the following scenario has been proposed:

The translocation of c-myc into the immunoglobulin gene occurs at a regular but low frequency when B cells are actively rearranging their immunoglobulin genes during differentiation. Chronic malaria is a potent polyclonal activator of B cells, an activation that results in an increase in the pool of B cells available for the rare translocation event. If EBV infects such a cell, it then provides the complementary signal for proliferation. In sporadic BL (lymphomas that lack any detectable viral DNA, RNA, or proteins), another genetic event replaces the EBV signal for immortalization.

*Lymphomas related to EBV infection* can develop in allograft recipients (renal, liver, cardiac, and bone marrow transplantation). In such cases it appears that impaired immune response and chronic antigen stimulation from the graft allow the malignant transformation and growth of EBV-infected B lymphocytes. The majority of these post-transplant lymphomas are diffuse large-cell lymphomas with immunoblastic features. Ig heavy- and light-chain genes are rearranged but no specific cytogenetic abnormality is described.

Human herpes virus 8 (HHV-8) has recently been found to be the causal agent of Kaposi's sarcoma in HIV-infected patients. This virus is closely related to the transforming EBV and can also be detected in body-cavity-based lymphomas. Its relation to multiple myeloma is still hypothetical.

### HIV infections and lymphomas

AIDS patients are at increased risk for developing *malignant lymphomas*. In HIV-seropositive patients, HIV proteins, as well as the wide range of infections from which they suffer, are acting as polyclonal B-cell stimulators predisposing to subsequent malignant chromosomal translocation. Furthermore, HIV-infected adults frequently demonstrate evidence of past EBV infection. Because of chronic destruction and loss of the T helper/inducer lymphocyte populations, the expanded pool of latently infected B lymphocytes will continue to grow and proliferate, and if the c-myc into immunoglobulin gene translocation occurs, an oligoclonal or monoclonal Burkitt's lymphoma will result. In BL in patients who are HIV-positive or who have AIDS, EBV genomes occur in 25%–40% of cases where the typical t(8;14) translocation is found.

Patients with advanced AIDS develop tumors that resemble those found in immunosuppressed transplant patients (large-cell lymphomas with immunoblastic features). Using molecular biology techniques, EBV genomes are demonstrated in the majority of biopsy specimens taken from these patients.

Besides malignant lymphoma, and in rare cases CLL, patients

**Table 13.7** Pancytopenia secondary to infection

| | |
|---|---|
| Peripheral origin | Malaria, kala-azar |
| Central origin (immunocompetent host) | Hepatitis A and B, rubella, EBV |
| Central origin (immunocompromised individuals) | CMV, parvovirus B19 |
| Pancytopenia with histiocytic proliferation (hemophagocytic syndrome) | Virus (EBV, CMV, HS) and other intracellular infections (Tbc, histoplasmosis, cryptococcosis, etc.) |

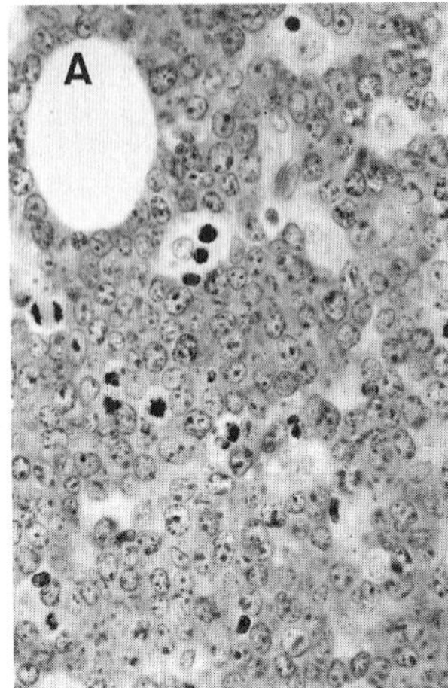


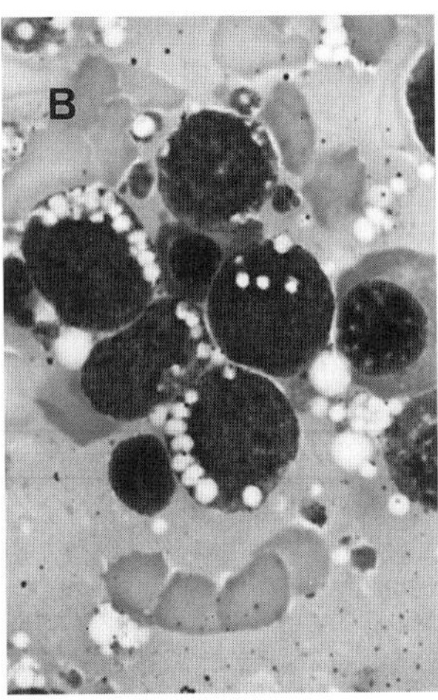


**Fig. 13.6** Burkitt's lymphoma (*panel A*: E&H, ×200) with bone marrow involvement (*panel B*: Wright staining, ×1000).

with HIV infection in advanced AIDS may develop pancytopenia with cellular dysplastic bone marrow features. Myelodysplasia in such cases is the result of HIV or other infectious injury to the bone marrow microenvironment or hematopoietic progenitors rather than of a mutation at the stem-cell level leading to a monoclonal dysplastic hematopoiesis.

## HTLV-I-associated malignancies

A spectrum of hematologic complications following infection with HTLV-I has been described. The vast majority of HTLV-I infected individuals are carriers of the virus and do not manifest any overt signs or symptoms. Some of them, however (approximately 0.4%), will develop the preleukemic phase of adult T-cell leukemia (pre-ATL). These patients will present with a modest leukocytosis and abnormal lymphocytes. DNA extracted from the peripheral blood lymphocytes of pre-ATL patients contain oligoclonally integrated HTLV-I. Approximately one-half of pre-ATL patients evolve to a more aggressive stage of the disease (acute ATL), while the remainder appear to regress into a carrier state. Features of acute ATL include leukocytosis, abnormal lymphocytes in peripheral blood that have characteristic lobulated or flower-shaped nuclei, mild to moderate lymphadenopathy, hepatosplenomegaly, and leukemic infiltration of the skin and bone.

Some ATL patients have been described in whom the presentation is predominantly that of a T-cell lymphoma rather than a leukemia. These lymphomas vary in histology and can involve any organ. Leukemic cells as well as lymph node biopsy specimens from these ATL patients contain oligoclonally integrated HTLV-I as determined by Southern hybridization.

Diagnosis can be established if the following criteria are met: positive HTLV-I serology, elevated serum $Ca^{++}$ and LDH, negative TdT staining in proliferating lymphocytes, specific immunophenotyping of ATL cells expressing CD4 and Tac antigens, and prcscncc of monoclonally integrated HTLV-I in the malignant T-cell clone.

Between 300 and 500 cases of ATL are diagnosed yearly in Japan, and the incidence of ATL has been estimated at less than one in 600 HTLV-I–infected carriers. Potential cofactors affecting the course of HTLV infection include parasitic infections such as strongyloides stercoralis, filariasis (in Japan), and malaria (in Africa).

## HTLV-II–associated hairy cell leukemia

HTLV-II virus has been reported in a patient with a T-cell lymphoproliferative disorder and concomitant B-cell hairy cell leukemia. In that patient, HTLV-II was detected in the expanded T-cell clone only. Table 13.8 summarizes hematological malignancies and associated infectious agents.

## Conclusion

Hematologic alterations in infectious diseases may be either specific or (in the majority of cases) nonspecific for the invading microorganism. Study of peripheral blood and—when indicated—of the bone marrow can be of great help in the establishment or orientation of a diagnosis. Furthermore, successive detailed blood analyses are of considerable prognostic value and quite often give an early indication of cure—or success of antiinfectious therapy. Almost any blood dyscrasia seen in a febrile patient may be secondary to infection; however, one must keep in mind the possibility of preexisting abnormalities of peripheral blood or the possibility of side effects of drugs used.

Finally, certain monoclonal lymphoproliferative disorders may be secondary to viral—most often retroviral—infections. Studies of these cases at a molecular level may provide invaluable information on oncogenesis.

*Acknowledgments*—We thank Dr. Christophe Girardet of the Department of Pathology, Geneva University Hospital, for providing us with the preparations shown in Figures 13.6 and 13.9. We are grateful to Ms. Jean Ringrose for excellent secretarial assistance.

**Table 13.8** Hematological malignancies secondary to infection

| | |
|---|---|
| Fatal B-cell polyclonal proliferation | EBV infection in patients with XLP syndrome |
| Burkitt's lymphoma | EBV |
| High-grade malignant lymphoma | HIV + EBV |
| Adult T-cell leukemia | HTLV-I |
| Hairy cell leukemia | HTLV-II? |
| Kaposi's sarcoma, mm(?) | HHV-8 |

## ANNOTATED BIBILIOGRAPHY


Beck EA, Dejana E. Thrombohemorrhagic phenomena associated with infectious diseases. Semin Hematol 1988; 25:91–100.

*An excellent review of the thrombohemorrhagic phenomena associated with infectious diseases, with particular emphasis on pathophysiological mechanisms.*

Bilgrami S, Almeida GD, Quinn JJ, Tuck D, Bergstrom S, Dainiak N, Poliquin C, Ascensao JL. Pancytopenia in allogeneic marrow transplant recipients: role of cytomegalovirus. Br J Haematol 1994; 87:357–362.

*A recent excellent article on the role of cytomegalovirus as a causative agent of aplastic anemia in allogeneic marrow transplant recipients. An excellent example of a disease in humans caused by a new therapeutic method.*

Cheeseman SH. Infectious mononucleosis. Semin Hematol 1988; 25:261–268.

*This excellent paper gives a complete description of the classic clinical syndrome of infectious mononucleosis. Unfortunately, it lacks figures and would have been greatly improved by the inclusion of plates illustrating the evolution of specific antibodies to EBV and the presence of stimulated lymphocytes in peripheral blood.*

Fleming AF. Iron deficiency in the tropics. Clin Hematol 1982; 11:365–388.

*Although written in the early 1980s, this paper remains a classic with regard to iron-deficiency states. The relationship between helminthic infections and iron-deficiency anemia is particularly well developed. Furthermore, the reader has the opportunity to review diagnostic problems and treatment of iron deficiency.*

Grierson H, Purtilo DT. Epstein-Barr virus infections in males with the X-linked lymphoproliferative syndrome. Ann Intern Med 1987; 106:538–545.

*This is the classic description of EBV infection in male patients with the X-linked lymphoproliferative syndrome. It contains an excellent discussion of the three main clinical phenotypes: fatal or chronic infectious mononucleosis, acquired hypo- or agammaglobulinemia, and high-grade malignant B-cell lymphoma.*

Hamilton-Dutoit SJ, Pallesen G, Franzmann MB, Karkov J, Black F, Skinhoj P, Pedersen C. AIDS-related lymphoma. Histopathology, immunophenotype, and association with Epstein-Barr virus as demonstrated by in situ nucleic acid hybridization. Am J Pathol 1991; 138:149–163.

*This excellent paper suggests the existence of two main groups, each with a different pathogenesis, of AIDS-related lymphoma. First, there are immunoblast-rich lesions, which are usually associated with EBV and morphologically resemble lymphomas described in immunosuppressed organ-transplant patients. Second, there are Burkitt-type tumors in which EBV sequences are less common and which may be pathogenetically analogous to sporadic Burkitt's lymphoma.*

Hanto DW. Classification of Epstein-Barr virus-associated posttransplant lymphoproliferative diseases: implications for understanding their pathogenesis and developing rational treatment strategies. Annu Rev Med 1995; 46:381–394.

*The Epstein-Barr virus (EBV) is associated with a spectrum of B-cell lymphoproliferative diseases (LPD) that develop following organ transplantation. In this very recent review, a classification scheme for these disorders has been developed based on the clinical, histologic, immunologic cell-typing, cytogenetic, immunoglobulin gene-rearrangement, and virologic characteristics of these LPD. This classification has furthered our understanding of the pathogenesis of these diverse LPD and has allowed the development of rational treatment protocols.*

Kurtzman G, Frickhofen N, Kimball J, Jenkins DW, Nienhuis AW, Young NS. Pure red-cell aplasia of 10-year duration due to persistent parvovirus B19 infection and its cure with immunoglobulin therapy. N Engl J Med 1989; 321:519–523.

*In the Cheeseman and Fleming studies cited above, the spectrum of B19 parvovirus diseases, with particular emphasis on the hematological manifestions, is comprehensively described. Specific diagnostic procedures and therapeutic approaches for the immunocompromised host suffering from B19 parvovirus infection are discussed.*

Means RT, Krantz SB. Progress in understanding the pathogenesis of the anemia of chronic disease. Blood 1992; 80:1639–1647.

*This is an excellent review of the pathophysiology of anemia of chronic disease (ACD). The role of specific cytokines such as TNFα, IL-1, and IFN-γ in the inhibition of erythropoiesis and in altered iron metabolism in ACD is very elegantly discussed.*

Nydegger UE, Kazatchkine MD, Miescher PA. Immunopathologic and clinical features of hemolytic anemia due to cold agglutinins. Semin Hematol 1991; 28:66–77.

*In this relatively recent review of cold agglutinins in humans, the mechanisms of anemia and the laboratory findings in cold agglutinin disease are successfully developed.*

Pelicci PG, Knowles DM, Magrath I, Dalla-Favera R. Chromosomal breakpoints and structural alterations of the c-myc locus differ in endemic and sporadic forms of Burkitt lymphoma. Proc Natl Acad Sci USA 1986; 83:2984–2988.

*This paper describes the molecular pathology of endemic and sporadic forms of Burkitt's lymphoma. Different genetic mechanisms are involved in chromosomal translocation/c-myc activation in endemic and sporadic forms of BL.*

Reiner AP, Spivak JL. Hematophagic histiocytosis. Medicine 1988; 67:369–388.

*An excellent and exhaustive review of hematophagic histiocytosis. Excellent plates and figures complete the description of this syndrome, which, in the majority of cases, is secondary to an infectious episode.*

Rosenblatt JD, Chen ISY, Wachsman W. Infection with HTLV-I and HTLV-II: evolving concepts. Semin Hematol 1988; 25:230–246.

*See Yamaguchi et al for annotation.*

Straus DJ. HIV-associated lymphomas. Curr Opin Oncol 1997; 9(5):450–454.

*The pathologic and clinical features of the HIV-associated lymphomas and treatment approaches and results are the subjects of this review. Unusual types of NHL and manifestations of Hodgkin's disease in HIV-infected individuals are also discussed.*

Tosato G, Taga K, Angiolillo AL, Sgadari C. Epstein-Barr virus as an agent of haematological disease. Baillieres Clin Haematol 1995; 8(1):165–199.

*In this review article, the relationship between EBV infection and hematologic manifestations is described didactically and successfully. In particular, the pathophysiological basis of EBV-related lymphomas is discussed exhaustively.*

Wicki J, Samii K, Cassinotti P, Voegeli J, Rochat T, Beris P. Parvovirus B19-induced red cell aplasia in solid-organ transplant recipients. Two case reports and review of the literature. Hematol Cell Ther 1997; 39(4):199–204.

*Excellent review of the parvovirus B19-induced red cell aplasia in solid-organ transplant recipients with pathognomonic microphotograph of an infected proerythroblast. Very good discussion concerning diagnostic procedures by molecular biology techniques.*

Yamaguchi K, Yoshioka R, Kiyokawa T. Lymphoma type adult T-cell leukemia—a clinicopathologic study of HTLV related T-cell type malignant lymphoma. Hematol Oncol 1986; 4:59–65.

*This and the Rosenblatt et al. reference both give an excellent review of human malignant lymphoproliferative diseases associated with HTLV-I and HTLV-II, including the epidemiology and molecular biology of these two retroviruses.*

Zon Li, Groopman JE. Hematologic manifestations of the human immune deficiency virus (HIV). Semin Hematol 1988; 25:208–218.

*A very elegant description of the variety of hematological abnormalities affecting circulating blood cell populations, bone marrow progenitors, and the coagulation system in association with HIV infection.*

# 14

# Metabolic and Endocrine Alterations in Infectious Disease Patients

FRANCIS A. WALDVOGEL

Any infectious disease, as a confrontation and interaction between microorganisms and its host, elicits by different mechanisms a variety of metabolic changes that often result in characteristic and sometimes impressive clinical pictures. Thus, the cerebrospinal fluid (CSF) acidosis of bacterial meningitis promotes the hyperventilation syndrome associated with the disease, the cytotoxic T-cell response to hepatitis B antigens expressed on the surface of hepatocytes leads to massive increase in Aspartate and Alanine Transaminases (AST/ALT) and hyperbilirubinemia, and the brisk inflammatory response induced by bacterial pneumonia leads to an abrupt change in liver metabolism, resulting in the synthesis of increased amounts of acute-phase proteins and a marked concomitant decrease in albumin synthesis. Schematically, these changes, which are the essence of the host's response to infectious diseases, can be subdivided into two groups:

1. *Nonspecific general changes in the host*, occurring in any infectious disease and encompassing (*1*) metabolic alterations, (*2*) neuroendocrine changes, (*3*) systemic inflammatory reactions, and (*4*) autonomic and behavioral responses to infection (e.g., shivering, fever, tachycardia, sweating, thirst, search for a warm environment, etc.) These are covered in Chapters 9 and 10.
2. *Specific organ involvement* by the infectious process leads to target organ dysfunction with its own metabolic consequences, such as liver failure in hepatitis, renal failure in papillary necrosis, or electrolyte disturbances in cholera. This chapter will concentrate on the alterations described under (*1*), and the reader is referred to the relevant chapters for the alterations summarized under (*2*).

Generally, although not invariably, bacterial diseases are more likely to produce more profound inflammatory, endocrine and metabolic alterations than are viral diseases: this results clinically in a more dramatic or "toxic" (septic) presentation, as observed, for instance, in bacterial versus viral meningitis, or bacterial versus viral pneumonia. Viruses, on the other hand, when infecting an organ, usually invade and disrupt functional cells; bacterial diseases cause a more generalized inflammation of an organ. Viral infection, therefore, often results in more profound changes in organ-specific tests: thus, alterations of liver-function tests or transient hyperthyroidism are characteristic of viral hepatitis or thyroiditis, whereas bacterial involvement of these two organs (liver or thyroid abscess) usually causes little functional change. Bacterial pneumonia tends to be localized and confined to bronchioles and alveoli, whereas viral pneumonia is usually bilateral and diffuse, and can directly involve pneumocytes. Finally, the generalized response of the host to infection, the systemic inflammatory reaction syndrome (SIRS) (see Chapter 50), which encompasses an inflammatory reaction owing to the action of cytokines and other biological products, is more severe in bacterial infections. Bacterial products alter more profoundly the host's metabolism and endocrine system, leading, among other responses, to lactic acidosis, diabetic decompensation, etc.

## Metabolic Alterations in Infectious Diseases

### Glucose metabolism

Alterations in glucose metabolism are frequently seen during infectious diseases, leading sometimes to the unmasking of a hitherto unknown diabetic state or in known diabetics to hyperosmolar or ketoacidotic decompensation. These complications are attributable to the fact that the production and secretion of glucagon, growth hormone, cortisol, and catecholamines are increased under infectious conditions. Conversely, hypoglycemia has been described particularly in the setting of major systemic infectious diseases, such as overwhelming meningococcal and pneumococcal sepsis or disseminated varicella, or in patients with starvation, alcoholism, cirrhosis or active hepatitis. In these situations, hyperinsulinemia caused by the action of interleukin-1 (IL-1) and tumor-necrosis factor (TNF) may be a contributing factor. Decreased hepatic glycogen stores and impaired gluconeogenesis, as well as a shift to anaerobic hepatic metabolism, are additional major responsible mechanisms of infection-induced hypoglycemia.

### Acid–base disturbances

Sepsis produced by infection leads to *lactic acidosis*, defined as a metabolic acidosis with an increased anion gap (>17 mM/L) and the presence of >5 mM/L of lactic acid. Systemic lactic acidosis may occur as a result of increased production of lactate owing to tissue hypoxia (type A) or to decreased catabolism (type B) in liver failure or sepsis. Lactic acidosis should not be confused with other causes of increased anion gap, such as uremia, ketosis, salicylate or ethylene glycol intoxication, or even severe hypoalbuminemia. Lactic acidosis is frequently observed in intensive care patients as part of multiple organ dysfunction syndrome (MODS) and is associated with a poor prognosis. In a recent prospective multicenter study encompassing 126 patients, all patients had mixed-type (A and B) lactic acidosis, which could be clearly related to a septic episode in 58% of the patients. Despite modern therapeutic strategies, the death rate in patients with lactic acidosis was high, with a survival rate of only 17% at 30 days.

### Electrolyte disturbances

A second cause of metabolic acidosis in patients with infectious diarrhea can be due to excessive gastrointestinal loss of bicarbonate. This is a nonanion gap–type acidosis, usually with hyperchloremia, and is a particularly striking feature of patients with secretory diarrheas, such as cholera. In addition, multiple electrolyte disturbances may occur during an active infectious disease: for example, *hyponatremia* due to inappropriate secretion of antidiuretic hormone (ADH) can be observed in meningitis due to *M. tuberculosis* or fungi, in other central nervous system (CNS) infections (encephalitis) and occasionally in pulmonary infections (pneumonia or tuberculosis). It is characterized by a hypoosmolar state with normal renal function, and urine hyperosmolarity with Na loss. Hyponatremia may also be a consequence of hypovolemia (vomiting or diarrhea), or adrenal insufficiency. Hypernatremia can occasionally be observed after prolonged sweating and poor rehydration. This is often a prominent finding in elderly patients disabled by strokes or other diseases that make it difficult or impossible to voluntarily increase their water intake.

#### Hyperkalemia

*Hyperkalemia* is occasionally observed, and is usually secondary to extracellular efflux induced by lactic acidosis. Other diagnoses to be considered include hemolysis, rhabdomyolysis (often with marked hyperkalemia), and renal or adrenal insufficiency. Hypokalemia is a common finding: it may be due to excessive losses from prolonged vomiting or diarrhea, and is part of the picture observed with concomitant metabolic acidosis in cholera. Urinary K levels are conspicuously low under these circumstances. Hypokalemia may also be induced by the action of catecholamines (intracellular shift) or glucocorticosteroids (increased renal losses) produced during sepsis.

True hypocalcemia is often observed in severe infections, for reasons that are still unknown. Hypophosphatemia can be a hallmark of sepsis due to insulin action, and it may be aggravated by glucose infusions, because insulin acts to promote intracellular entry of phosphate from its extracellular location. Severe hypophosphatemia may lead to hemolysis and a Guillain-Barré–like syndrome with respiratory muscle insufficiency. Chronic hypophosphatemia favors the loss of Mg, which in turn will stimulate further renal phosphate and K loss. All these alterations can occur even in noncritically ill patients with a septic process, and alcoholic patients are at particular risk because of chronic phosphate depletion.

All four major *acid–base disturbances* have been described during bacterial, viral, or parasitic infection. Two conditions, however, should be stressed, because they may help in the early identification of infection: they include respiratory alkalosis and, independently or associated with it, metabolic acidosis. For instance, hyperventilation and respiratory alkalosis can be the heralding sign of gram-negative sepsis in an elderly patient. Persistent metabolic acidosis with lactacidemia in an intensive care patient can be an early sign of an intraabdominal septic process in a postoperative patient.

*General protein and lipid metabolism* is shifted in severely infected patients toward catabolism. This subject is reviewed in detail in Chapter XX. Catecholamines, IL-1, and TNF—possibly by IL-6 induction—and other mediators are responsible for these effects, resulting in a three- to fivefold increase in catabolism ("septic cannibalism"). Great attention should be given to the restoration of protein calories in an infected patient to avoid severe comorbidity from malnutrition. Furthermore, both TNF and IL-1 are promoters of lipoprotein lipase activity, which leads to mobilization of triglycerides from adipose tissue stores. Hyperlipidemia may therefore be a prominent feature of sepsis.

## Endocrine Abnormalities and Infectious Diseases

Endocrine abnormalities during infectious diseases can be subdivided into three groups: (*1*) those due to local invasion of an endocrine organ by pathogenic organism; (*2*) specific changes that are associated with certain infectious diseases; and (*3*) endocrine abnormalities occurring nonspecifically during an infectious process. Finally, the special relationship between HIV infections and endocrine disorders will be discussed separately (see also Chapter 100).

### Invasion of endocrine organs

Although rare, organ invasion by pathogens may be associated with severe metabolic perturbations; thus, *M. tuberculosis* or fungal meningitis may lead to inappropriate ADH secretion or, in exceptional cases, to the opposite condition of diabetes insipidus. Both types of meningitis and occasionally viral encephalitis can directly involve the pituitary stark and lead to pituitary insufficiency, provided that more than 50% of the gland is destroyed. Sheehan's syndrome (pituitary apoplexy) has been described after septic shock. Addison's disease has been classically reported with *M. tuberculosis* and with fungal infection (e.g., histoplasmosis): under these conditions, the adrenals are enlarged and contain calcifications on computed tomography (CT) scan; the latter finding, however, is nonspecific and has also been described with adrenal hemorrhage and adrenal cancer. Finally, adrenal insufficiency is a well-known complication of fulminant meningococcemia and can occasionally be seen in other patients with septic shock. More recently, it has also been described in disseminated cytomegalovirus (CMV) infection in HIV-positive patients and in patients who have undergone bone marrow transplantation. Infections of the thyroid can be focal as observed in suppurative thyroiditis—which is due to pyogenic organisms in more than two thirds of cases—other agents including *M. tuberculosis*, *Actinomyces* species, and, rarely, *Pneumocystis carinii*. The gland shows local signs of inflammation and occasionally frank abscess formation. Thyroid tests are normal under these circumstances. Subacute thyroiditis, on the other hand, which is probably of viral origin, presents with a diffusely enlarged, tender gland and transient signs of hyperthyroidism; full recovery is expected after a few days, and thyroid-function tests return rapidly to normal values in these cases.

### Infectious diseases complicating endocrine disorders

Many hormonal dysfunctions have been either associated with or shown to promote various infectious diseases. Thus, Cushing's syndrome—whether pituitary, adrenal, or ectopic—leading to increased cortisol levels, favors the risk of *M. tuberculosis* or fungal infections: in one series, 43% of patients with Cushing's syndrome had either superficial or deep fungal infections, and there was a correlation between the severity of the endocrine disorder and the specific infection rate. Chronic mucocutaneous candidiasis is a T-cell disorder associated with various endocrinopathies of autoimmune nature, as well as with thymoma, myasthenia gravis, pernicious anemia, chronic hepatitis, and dental dysplasia. It is characterized by repeated superficial fungal infections. Hypothyroidism poses the problem of the recognition of a simultaneous infectious process, since fever may be absent and pleural and pericardial effusions are part of the clinical picture. Bacterial infections in these patients may precipitate myxoedematous coma. Very high thyroid-stimulating hormone (TSH) levels and low T3 and T4 values are the biological hallmarks of the disease.

### Nonspecific endocrine alterations associated with infection

Many severe infectious diseases may be accompanied by, or responsible for, transient endocrine abnormalities. These abnormalities are not an exclusive consequence of the infectious process, since they have also been described after trauma, febrile illnesses of noninfectious causes, and severe malnutrition. They are therefore observed with increased frequency in intensive care patients. Recent and extensive studies have concentrated on thyroid dysfunctions. A low T3 state has been described, this decrease being related to the severity of the infection. It has been explained by a decreased peripheral conversion rate of T4 to T3; conversely, rT3 is usually elevated under these circumstances. This condition does not require any therapy, as evidenced by TSH levels that remain normal at all times.

A low T3/T4 state has also been observed. This condition has been correlated with the APACHE score and appears in intensive care patients after several days or weeks of infection, representing, in fact, a continuum with the isolated low T3 state. More elaborate investigations have shown that, in fact, T4 production is normal under these conditions; thyroxin-binding globulin (TBG) is decreased, leading to low total T4, whereas free T4 measured by ultrafiltration or dialysis is normal. In case of a low T3/T4 state, TSH may be normal, low, or high: substitution therapy should be considered only with markedly elevated TSH levels.

All other endocrine organ systems may occasionally show abnormalities, which are summarized in Table 14.1. As a general rule, only major deviations from normal values should be considered for treatment, since most of the minor dysfunctions will return to normal with the control of the infectious process.

### HIV-positive patients

Recently, many endocrine abnormalities with advancing disease have been described, due either to opportunistic infections or to the consequences of the HIV infection itself. *M. tuberculosis* and fungal infections may lead to pituitary or adrenal insufficiency; the latter condition has been recently reported several times to be also due to disseminated CMV infection. Thyroid involvement with *Pneumocystis carinii* is a new, although rare disease. The situation is less clear regarding involvement of the adrenal glands by HIV infection. Most patients have a normal basal and adrenocorticotropic hormone (ACTH)-stimulated cortisol levels; other patients show either an abnormal immediate response to ACTH or a blunted response to a 3-day stimulation test, pointing toward an insufficient adrenal reserve. Some patients have elevated basal and subnormal stimulation tests, implying a stressed state due to the infection. Finally, the euthyroid sick syndrome, as described above, with either low T3 only, or low T3/low T4, is frequently observed. This condition does not require any therapy, as long as TSH is within normal values.

## Acute-Phase Reactions Associated with Infectious Diseases

It has become axiomatic that an acute infectious process will elicit first a local and thereafter a generalized swift inflammatory response, mediated by various cytokines, anaphylatoxins, and glucosteroids: the *acute-phase reaction* refers to this wide range of physiological changes that are initiated immediately after the onset of infection, but also after trauma, burns, and even violent exercise, and which lead to striking changes in the serum protein profile. Since these cytotokine-induced mechanisms are discussed in detail in Chapter 50 on sepsis only those modifications pertaining to the daily clinical monitoring of a patient and implying the so-called *acute-phase reactants* will be discussed: clinically, the most important ones are the C-reactive protein (CRP), serum amyloid A protein (SAA), and $\alpha_1$-antitrypsin. One should keep in mind, however, that the acute-phase reaction encompasses more than 30 proteins, including complement and coagulation proteins, specific proteinase inhibitors, metal-binding proteins, other carriers, etc., which are probably of utmost importance in generating the mechanism of the host response, but which cannot be measured on a routine basis.

**Table 14.1** Major endocrine changes during infection

HYPOTHALAMUS/NEURAL CONTROL

CRF stimulates release of ACTH
ADH: increased production and release
Epinephrine: increased secretion from adrenal medulla
Norepinephrine: increased secretion from sympathetic terminals

PITUITARY

ACTH: increased
Growth hormone: increased
Prolactin: increased
TSH: normal or decreased

ADRENAL GLAND

Cortisol: normal, increased, blunted response
Aldosterone: increased secretion
Catecholamines: increased secretion

THYROID GLAND

T4: normal or moderately decreased
T3: decreased

PANCREAS

Glucagon: increased
Insulin: blunted response

RENIN-ANGIOTENSIN SYSTEM

Activation

*C-reactive protein* (CRP) belongs to the family of the pentraxins, a group of proteins with a cyclic pentameric structure. During infection serum levels increase from 1 $\mu$g/ml by 100 to 1000 times within hours, this rapid increase owing to a specific induction of hepatic synthesis. The CRP gene is situated on chromosome 1. Under its polymeric form, CRP precipitates with C carbohydrate from *Streptococcus pneumoniae*; hence its name. The physiological role of CRP, however, is still not completely clear: CRP binds to human nuclear material and chromatin and increases their clearance, thereby avoiding possibly an inappropriate autoimmune response to host nuclear material during necrosis. CRP also promotes opsonization of bacteria, activates complement, and binds to immune complexes. Increases of serum CRP to 100 times the normal value during acute infections are often observed: they usually precede the increase in sedimentation rate, and the same but inversed sequence is observed at the end of an infection. Bacterial infections traditionally lead to the most dramatic increases in CRP, and its measurement in a febrile patient may be a useful screen for bacterial infection.

*Serum amyloid A protein* (SAA) is a collective name given to a group of polypeptides that increase rapidly in the circulation during infection and associate with high-density lipoproteins (HDL3). They sometimes exceed apolipoprotein A in quantity. Although not measured routinely, evidence suggests that SAA may be an important control factor of the inflammatory response—i.e., a feedback molecule to control fever, a compound codeposited in truncated form in AA amyloidosis, and a factor leading to abnormal cholesterol metabolism in chronic infection.

*Other important acute-phase reactants* include $\alpha_1$-antitrysin—a strong inhibitor of elastase -, fibrinogen, some complement components, in particular C3, C4, and factor B. Total complement hemolytic activity is therefore frequently elevated in major infections.

This chapter would not be complete without some comments regarding *erythrocyte sedimentation rate* (ESR), a time-honored, venerable test. Paradoxically, the test has escaped the scrutiny of well-planned prospective studies to demonstrate its diagnostic value; when analyzed as a screening test, it has been shown to be of poor predictive help. Few studies, however, have investigated its possible utility as a long-term monitoring test to follow infections of various types during therapy.

The mechanisms of erythrocyte sedimentation are poorly understood. Basically, since many of the acute-phase plasma proteins are positively charged, they should increase the ESR by neutralizing the negatively charged erythrocyte surfaces, leading to a loss of coercive suspension forces and increasing the gravitational effect on erythrocytes. Indeed, on a scale of 10, fibrinogen scores 10, $\beta$-globulin 5, $\alpha$-globulin 2, gamma globulin 1, whereas CRP—at normal concentration—has no effect on ESR.

In a patient without localizing symptoms, and because of the complexity of the mechanisms subtending the ESR, only frank abnormalities should be considered, and even then, the test should be repeated before embarking on costly investigations. Very high values in the range of 100 mm/hr should, however, be investigated: infection is usually the first diagnosis, followed by malignancy and by connective tissue disorders, among which giant-cell arteritis is the most common.

Finally, the skilled clinician will use the ESR, despite its shortcomings, to follow a benign infection that apparently does not require antibiotics, or an infection that requires a prolonged antibacterial treatment such as endocarditis, osteomyelitis, or an intraabdominal or pulmonary abscess, in order to confirm his clinical intuition of the therapeutic response.

## ANNOTATED BIBLIOGRAPHY

Dluhy RG. Editorial. The growing spectrum of HIV-related endocrine abnormalities. J Clin Endocrinol Metab 70 1990; 563–65.

*An editorial that reviews the endocrine abnormalities, most of them nonspecific, observed in severe HIV infections.*

Dowton SB, Colten HR. Acute phase reactants in inflammation and infection. Semin Hematol 1986; 25:84–90.

*A scholarly review on acute phase reactants, with emphasis on those that can be easily measured in the clinical laboratory.*

Merenich JA et al. Evidence of endocrine involvement early in the course of human immunodeficiency virus infection. J Clin Endocrinol Metab 1990; 70:566–70.

*A review of the many often subtle, endocrine abnormalities observed in HIV-positive patients without infections, tumors, or specific antiviral therapy.*

Nicoloff JT et al. Nonthyroidal illness. In: The Thyroid, 6th ed. Braverman LE, Utiger RD, eds. Lippincot, New York and London, pp 357–368, 1991.

*A great variety of acute and chronic infectious diseases can alter reversibly thyroid function. This review summarizes the major changes, and makes conclusively the point that most often, careful follow-up is better than aggressive therapy.*

Preuss HG et al. Evaluation of renal function and water, electrolyte, and acid-base balance. In: Clinical Diagnosis and Management by Laboratory Methods, 18th ed. Henry JB, ed. WB Saunders, Philadelphia, pp 128–139.

*Infectious diseases can alter water balance and electrolyte balance in many ways, and nonspecifically. These changes are summarized in a concise way in this review.*

Sox HC, Liang MH. The erythrocyte sedimentation rate. Guidelines for rational use. Ann Int Med 1986; 104:515–23.

*A state-of-the-art article on the clinical use of the sedimentative rate. If its role as a screening test is disputed, no information is given, however, on its role as a follow-up test to guide therapy, or the absence thereof.*

Stacpoole PW. Lactic acidosis. Endocrinol Metab Clin North Am 22:221–245.

*A landmark study to follow the clinical course of lactic acidosis and to establish its role as a predictive survival test.*

Tuazon CU, Labriola AM. Infectious diseases causing hormonal or metabolic disorders. In: Principles and Practice of Endocrinology and Metabolism, 2nd ed. Becken KL, ed. chap. 214: Infectious Diseases and Endocrinology, pp 1571–1577 and p 1622.

*Infectious diseases of many kinds can cause hormonal and metabolic disorders; conversely, many endocrine disorders can predispose to certain infectious diseases. This review summarizes both aspects in a synthetic manner.*

Imura H. Endocrine and metabolic manifestations associated with infectious and inflammatory diseases. FEMS Immunol Med Microbiol (Netherlands), 1997, 18(4):221–226.

*An excellent review of the relationship between infection and metabolism.*

Beisel WR. Herman Award Lecture: infection-induced malnutrition—from cholera to cytokines. Am J Clin Nutr (United States), 1995, 62(4):813–819

*Why do people lose weight during infection: a global, useful account.*

# 15

## Specimen Management and Rapid Detection of Infectious Agents

FRED C. TENOVER

The microbiology laboratory plays a central role in the diagnosis of infectious illnesses by detecting microorganisms, or their products, in clinical samples. A variety of techniques, including direct staining, antigen and antibody tests, nucleic acid–based assays, and culture are often performed. The host's immune response to a microorganism also provides clues to acute, chronic, and past infections, and tests to measure those responses are useful for diagnosis. Today, there is increased emphasis in the laboratory on rapid identification of pathogens through the use of immunologic and nucleic acid–based techniques. Rapid recognition of an infectious agent can help guide therapy early in the course of an illness, can indicate when isolation precautions may or may not be necessary, and may decrease the number of invasive diagnostic procedures that are required for definitive diagnosis. The exhaustive identification of multiple organisms present in a sample is usually unwarranted and is now a rare event. Rather, the identification of key pathogens pertinent to the site of infection is routinely performed. Ultimately, the goal of the clinical microbiology laboratory is to provide rapid, accurate, and clinically relevant information to the physician regarding the presence of microorganisms in clinical samples, in the most cost-effective manner. While rapid methods play an important role in diagnosis of disease and can, in some cases, provide definitive identification of infectious agents, the low sensitivity of a number of the commercially available antigen and DNA probe methods often precludes the abandonment of culture techniques. The recovery of organisms in pure culture is still advantageous, because it allows ancillary tests, such as antimicrobial susceptibility tests and strain typing, to be undertaken. Susceptibility testing, particularly in an age of increasing resistance to antimicrobial agents, remains an important activity of the laboratory.

### Specimen Collection

Accurate and timely microbiology tests require appropriately selected and properly collected specimens of sufficient quality and quantity. Table 15.1 lists some common specimens submitted for microbiologic analysis, the preferred methods of collection, and a guide to the types of culture media that should be used for recovery of pathogenic bacteria and fungi. Given the critical nature of specimen collection, it is ironic how often this task is left to untrained personnel who do not appreciate the need for adequate site preparation and prompt transport of specimens to the laboratory. Site preparation is particularly critical for collection of blood cultures, cerebrospinal fluid, and other specimens obtained by aspiration from normally sterile sites where the presence of normal skin flora in the sample can produce confusing or misleading culture results. Given the number of indwelling lines and intravascular devices used in modern medicine, it is often difficult to ascertain the clinical significance of organisms, such as *Staphylococcus epidermidis,* from sterile sites, particularly in immunocompromised hosts. Thus, the relatively small amount of additional time required for proper site preparation prior to collection of specimens by venipuncture or aspiration can reduce the time spent in ascertaining the significance of skin flora that are recovered from such cultures.

The collection and transportation of surgical samples for microbiologic studies present two recurring problems for clinical microbiologists. First, many of the bacteria responsible for infection of sites such as the abdomen and pelvis are anaerobic and exquisitely sensitive to oxygen. While it is preferable to send purulent aspirates to the laboratory in the syringes in which they are collected, all too frequently a small amount of material is expressed onto a swab, which is then placed in an anaerobic transport tube and dispatched to the laboratory. Thus, instead of receiving 5–10 ml of purulent fluid for staining and culture, the microbiology laboratory receives a sample of 0.1 ml or less that has been exposed to oxygen. Purulent material, because of its low pH, is an excellent transport medium for most pathogenic microorganisms; a filled syringe can be sent to the laboratory once the needle has been appropriately removed and the syringe sealed. Likewise, tissue removed during surgery should be placed in sterile cups and transported immediately to the microbiology laboratory, where sections can be removed and prepared for culture, and the remaining material sent to cytology. All too often, large tissue samples are placed directly in formaldehyde and sent for cytologic examination without consideration for microbiologic culture. Manuals describing (*1*) procedures for collection and transport of specimens, (*2*) safety precautions for specimen handling, (*3*) critical volumes of specimens, (*4*) policies for specimen rejection, and (*5*) storage instructions for delayed transport of specimens, should be available on each hospital ward and updated periodically. In addition, frequent in-service training for personnel responsible for specimen collection should be advocated. Subsequent chapters provide detail on collection of specimens for bacteriological (Chapter 16), virological (Chapter 17), mycological (Chapter 18), and parasitological (Chapter 19) studies. Direct staining can allow rapid identification of the nature of the infecting organisms as well as relate this to the character of the inflammatory response. Appropriate staining techniques and their interpretation are described in the individual sections.

### Direct Tests for Specific Identification of Microorganisms

A number of methods are available in the clinical microbiology laboratory for the rapid detection of pathogenic microorganisms directly in clinical specimens. A summary of the more commonly

**Table 15.1** Collection procedures and primary agar and broth media for isolation of infectious agents

| Source | Indication | Specimen | Growth media[a] |
|---|---|---|---|
| Nasopharyngeal | Pertussis | Calcium alginate swab | Regan-Lowe, Bordet-Gengou |
| Throat | Streptococci | Swab | BA+SXT |
| Throat | Diphtheria | Swab | BA, Tinsdale |
| Sputum | Bacteria | Expectorated | BA, CA, Mac, CNA, BCYE[b] |
| Sputum | Mycobacteria | Expectorated, BAL | LJ, M-7H11, M-7H12 broth (BACTEC) |
| Urine | Bacteria and fungi | Clean catch, in/out catheter | BA, Mac |
| CSF | Bacteria and fungi | Sterile tube | BA, CA |
| Cervical/Urethra | Gonorrhoea | Calcium alginate swab | CA, ML |
| Deep wound infection, abscess | Bacteria and fungi | Aspirate in syringe | BA, ABA, CA, Mac, CNA, thio broth |
| Lung biopsy | Bacteria and fungi | Tissue | BA, ABA, CA, Mac, BCYE[b] |
| Superficial wound | Bacteria | Swab, aspirate | BA, CA, Mac, Tins[c] |
| Skin | Fungi | Scrapings | BHI+, SDA |
| Blood | Bacteria and fungi | Venipuncture | Broth, aerobic and anaerobic |
| Pleural, synovial, pericardial and other body fluids | Bacteria and fungi | Aspirate in syringe | BA, ABA, CA, Mac, CNA, thio broth |

[a]Abbreviations: BA, blood agar; SXT, sulfa-trimethoprim; CA, chocolate agar; Mac, MacConkey agar; CNA, Columbia nalidixic acid agar; BCYE, buffered charcoal yeast extract agar; BAL, bronchoalveolar lavage; LJ, Lowenstein Jensen agar; M-7H11, Middlebrook 7H11 agar; ABA, anaerobic blood agar; ML, Martin-Lewis agar; Tins, Tinsdale agar; BHI+, brain heart infusion agar plus antimicrobial agents; SDA, Saboraud's dextrose agar.

[b]For detection of *Legionella* species on request (not routine).

[c]For detection of *C. diphtheriae*.

**Table 15.2** Rapid tests for respiratory pathogens[a]

| Organism | Gram stain | Acid-fast stain | KOH prep | DFA | Latex | EIA | DNA probe | PCR | TMA |
|---|---|---|---|---|---|---|---|---|---|
| UPPER RESPIRATORY | | | | | | | | | |
| *Streptococcus pyogenes* | | | | x | x | x | x | | |
| *Bordetella pertussis* | | | | x | | | | | |
| *Corynebacterium diphtheriae* | | | | x | | | | | |
| LOWER RESPIRATORY | | | | | | | | | |
| Bacteria | x | | | | | | | | |
| Legionella | | | | x | | | x | | |
| Mycobacteria | | x | | | | | | x | x |
| Mycoplasma | | | | x | | x | | | |
| Nocardia | x | x | | | | | | | |
| Fungi | | | x | | | | | | |

[a]Abbreviations: KOH, potassium hydroxide mount; DFA, direct fluorescent antibody test; Latex, latex agglutination assay; EIA, enzyme immunoassay; PCR, polymerase chain reaction; TMA, transcription-mediated amplification.

**Table 15.3** Rapid tests for genital pathogens[a]

| Organism | Gram stain | Darkfield | DFA | EIA | DNA probe | LCR | PCR |
|---|---|---|---|---|---|---|---|
| *Neisseria gonorrhoeae* | x | | x | | x | x | x |
| *Chlamydia trachomatis* | | | x | x | x | x | x |
| *Treponema pallidum* | | x | x | | | | |
| *Haemophilus ducreyii* | x | | x | | | | |

[a]Abbreviations: DFA, direct fluorescent antibody test; EIA, enzyme immunoassay; PCR, polymerase chain reaction; LCR, ligase chain reaction.

used tests for bacterial and fungal respiratory pathogens is given in Table 15.2, for genital pathogens in Table 15.3, for enteric pathogens in Table 15.4, and for pathogens in cerebrospinal fluid in Table 15.5.

### Latex agglutination tests

Latex agglutination tests, while highly specific and easy to use, often have lower sensitivity than many enzyme immunoassay methods for direct detection of bacterial antigens. Latex tests are useful screening tests for Group A $\beta$-hemolytic streptococci from throat samples, and are helpful for detecting bacterial infection in cerebrospinal fluid (CSF), especially in patients who received antimicrobial therapy prior to the time the specimens were collected. The sensitivity of latex tests for detecting bacteria in CSF, however, is only comparable to that of the Gram stain.

### Enzyme immunoassay

Enzyme immunoassay tests are available for a wide variety of microbial pathogens, including bacteria, fungi, viruses, and parasites. They are more expensive than latex agglutination tests, but frequently have higher sensitivity and often are at least semiquantitative. Endpoints for many tests are determined visually, while others require instrumentation. Many commercially prepared kits allow determination of both IgM and IgG antibody responses, which is often helpful in distinguishing between acute and resolving infections.

### Direct fluorescent antibody tests

The detection of bacteria in tissues, aspirates, or material from swab specimens using fluorescein-labeled antibodies to specific antigens is a key diagnostic tool for the recognition of *Chlamydia trachomatis*, *Cryptosporidium* species, *Bordetella pertussis*, *Giardia* species, *Legionella* species, *Streptococcus pyogenes*, *Pneumocystis carinii*, and several other organisms. Direct fluorescent antibody tests require from 0.5 to 3 hours to perform and often incorporate monoclonal antibodies to improve specificity. Because of relatively low sensitivity of the reagents for *Legionella* species and *B. pertussis*, culture procedures are still recommended to maximize the sensitivity of detection of these organisms.

## Nucleic Acid–Based Methods

### DNA probes

DNA probes are small pieces of nucleic acid that bind in a predictable way to complementary nucleic acid sequences during hybridization reactions. Hybridization can occur between two complementary strands of DNA, two strands of RNA, or between DNA and RNA strands to form a stable hybrid. The degree of mismatch between the two strands that can be tolerated and still allow the strands to remain together is a function of the temperature and ionic strength of the buffer used in the hybridization reaction, and is referred to as "stringency." The development of

**Table 15.4** Rapid tests for enteric pathogens

| Organism | Latex | EIA[a] | Rapid urease | Calcofluor | Iodine prep |
|---|---|---|---|---|---|
| *Clostridium difficile* | x | x | | | |
| *Helicobacter pylori* | | | x | | |
| Rotavirus | x | x | | | |
| Amoeba | | x[b] | | | x |
| Giardia | x | x | | | x |
| Cryptosporidia/ Microsporidia | | x | | x | x |

[a]EIA, enzyme immunoassay.

[b]For extraintestinal infections only.

**Table 15.5** Rapid tests for organisms in cerebrospinal fluid

| Organism group | Gram stain[a] | Latex | DFA[b] | India ink | Acid-fast stain | Wet mount |
|---|---|---|---|---|---|---|
| Bacteria | x | x | x | | | |
| Mycobacteria | | | | | x | |
| Fungi-Cryptococcus | | x | | x | | |
| Amoeba | | | | | | x |

[a]Sensitivity is enhanced by cytocentrifugation of CSF prior to staining.

[b]DFA, direct fluorescent antibody test.

extraction protocols that release nucleic acids from organisms contained in blood, sputum, tissue, and stool samples has made the use of hybridization-based tests, which include DNA probes and nucleic acid amplification methods, feasible in clinical microbiology laboratories.

When used as diagnostic tools, DNA probes are usually labeled with a substrate such as biotin, or a chemiluminescent moiety, that allows easy detection of the double-stranded molecules after a hybridization reaction. The most commonly used DNA probe tests in clinical laboratories are those in which all of the reaction steps take place in a single tube; they are referred to as homogeneous assays. DNA probe tests serve two functions: identification of organisms grown in pure culture on agar or in a liquid culture medium (culture confirmation), and direct detection of organisms in clinical specimens. A list of commercially prepared DNA probe tests for culture confirmation assays for bacteria and fungi is given in Table 15.6.

Commercial DNA probe tests have gained widespread acceptance in clinical laboratories for the culture confirmation of mycobacteria, including *M. tuberculosis*, *M. avium*, *M. intracellulare*, *M. kansasii*, and *M. gordonii,* particularly when acid-fast growth is detected in BACTEC vials (Becton Dickinson Microbiology Systems, Cockeysville, Md) that contain a liquid medium designed to support the growth of mycobacteria. Other

**Table 15.6** DNA probes available for culture confirmation of bacterial and fungal isolates

| Organism | Sensitivity[a] | Specificity[a] | Remarks |
|---|---|---|---|
| Campylobacters | 100 | 100 | Thermophilic species only |
| Enterococci | 100 | 100 | |
| *Haemophilus influenzae* | 98.4 | 100 | |
| *Listeria monocytogenes* | 100 | 100 | |
| *Mycobacterium avium* | 100 | 100 | Can use with BACTEC pellet[b] |
| *Mycobacterium avium* complex | 100 | 100 | Can use with BACTEC pellet[b] |
| *Mycobacterium gordonii* | 98.7 | 98.4 | Can use with BACTEC pellet[b] |
| *Mycobacterium intracellulare* | 97.5–100 | 100 | Can use with BACTEC pellet[b] |
| *Mycobacterium kansasii* | 100 | 100 | Can use with BACTEC pellet[b] |
| *Mycobacterium tuberculosis* complex | 93.4–100 | 96.6–100 | Can use with BACTEC pellet[b] |
| *Neisseria gonorrhoeae* | 100 | 100 | |
| *Streptococcus agalactiae* | 100 | 100 | Group B streptococcus |
| *Streptococcus pneumoniae* | 100 | 100 | |
| *Blastomyces dermatitidis* | 100 | 100 | Hyphal growth |
| *Coccidioides immitis* | 100 | 100 | Hyphal growth |
| *Cryptococcus neoformans* | 100 | 100 | Hyphal growth |
| *Histoplasma capsulatum* | 100 | 100 | Hyphal growth |

[a]Data taken from published studies.

[b]DNA probes not yet approved for use with other commercial liquid mycobacterial growth systems.

**Table 15.7** Characteristics of direct DNA probe and nucleic acid amplification assays for genital pathogens

| | DNA probe | | PCR | | LCR | |
|---|---|---|---|---|---|---|
| Organism | Sensitivity | Specificity | Sensitivity | Specificity | Sensitivity | Specificity |
| *Neisseria gonorrhoeae* | 88.9% | 100% | 92.4% | 100% | 94.6% | 99.6%–100% |
| *Chlamydia trachomatis*[a] | 84%–95% | 98%–100% | 60%–97% | 98%–99.2% | 87.5%–96% | 100% |

[a]Data from published studies; sensitivity varies significantly with patient population studied.

liquid culture systems specifically designed for mycobacteria may also be used in conjunction with probe tests. Probes frequently decrease the time to recognition and identification of *M. tuberculosis* in specimens from weeks to days. The mycobacterial DNA probes cannot be used for direct detection of organisms in clinical samples, since they lack sensitivity. Rather, biological amplification through culture or nucleic acid amplification (see below, under "Amplification Methods") is mandatory.

DNA probes for the culture confirmation of a variety of other bacterial and fungal pathogens are also available (Table 15.6). One novel application of probes is their use on organisms obtained from blood culture vials for rapid identification of pneumococci, enterococci, and staphylococci. In the current regulatory environment, however, such nonlabel use of these reagents requires in-house studies to document the validity of this approach.

The development of probes to the dimorphic fungal pathogens *Histoplasma capsulatum, Blastomyces dermatitidis,* and *Coccidioides immitis* has played an important role in allowing laboratories that do not have trained mycologists to recognize these pathogens with high accuracy. They can be used on mycelial phase growth before spores or other diagnostic morphologic structures are present in slide cultures.

## DNA probes for direct detection of organisms in clinical samples

DNA probes are also used for the direct detection and identification of organisms in clinical samples. For example, two commonly used commercial probes are those for detection of the sexually transmitted pathogens *Neisseria gonorrhoeae* and *Chlamydia trachomatis* (Table 15.7). These tests are highly specific and have sensitivities approximating and in some cases exceeding that of culture. The lower range of sensitivity in Table 15.7 reflects studies conducted among asymptomatic women attending an outpatient clinic. One commercially available test kit allows the detection of both *N. gonorrhoeae* and *C. trachomatis* from a single cervical swab. These tests have found widespread use in public health laboratories where large numbers of specimens are processed, and the specimens often are delayed in reaching the laboratory due to long transit times from remote clinics and hospitals. With DNA probe tests, the organisms do not need to be viable to be identified accurately. A note of caution, however: the use of nucleic acid–based tests, with or without amplification, has not yet been accepted in a court of law in the United States as valid evidence in cases of rape or child abuse. (The same is true of antigen-detection methods.) In such cases, culture techniques should continue to be used for detection of these pathogens.

Probe tests for detection of *Streptococcus pyogenes* in throat samples are also available. These tests can be completed in less than 2 hours and compare favorably with culture.

## Amplification methods

The newest diagnostic methods in clinical microbiology are the nucleic acid–amplification and signal-amplification technologies (Table 15.8). Nucleic acid–amplification methods can be divided into two types: target amplification and probe amplification. Target-amplification technologies include the polymerase chain reaction (PCR); the self-sustaining sequence-replication reaction (3SR) and the related technologies, nucleic acid sequence–based amplification (NASBA) and transcription-mediated amplification (TMA); and strand-displacement amplification (SDA). Ligase chain reaction (LCR) and the Q$\beta$ replicase system are examples of probe amplification methods. Branched DNA (bDNA) is currently the most prominent signal-amplification method. While specific nucleic acid sequences can be identified and amplified from virtually any microorganism by one of the amplification strategies, at present the clinical relevance of using amplification technology for early detection of many microorganisms has yet to be established. Furthermore, many in-house amplification assays (the "home-brewed assays") suffer from false-positive and false-negative results and should be used with caution. Particular attention to the use of both positive and negative controls, including internal controls to monitor for the presence of inhibitory substances present in clinical samples, can improve the accuracy and reliability of noncommercially prepared assays. Commercial amplification methods at present focus on *M. tuberculosis*, *C. trachomatis*, *N. gonorrhoeae*, hepatitis C virus, and human immunodeficiency virus (HIV). The *C. trachomatis* amplification tests, including PCR and LCR, suggest that they are comparable or better in sensitivity than the culture methods used in many laboratories. However, inhibitory substances present primarily in female urine samples has placed some restrictions on the use of these technologies as screening tests. Nonetheless, one cost-benefit analysis has recommended use of amplification methods over culture, enzyme immunoassay, and direct fluorescent antibody methods, in populations with a prevalence of >6%. The specificity of both the PCR and LCR tests for *C. trachomatis* is very high.

Evaluations of the PCR, TMA, SDA, and NASBA assays for *M. tuberculosis* suggest that while they are highly sensitive and specific for detection of tubercle bacilli in acid fast smear-positive samples, the sensitivity of these assays in smear-negative samples where the organism load is small dips to 60–70%. Thus, the algorithm defining how these assays will be used in various

**Table 15.8** Characteristics of amplification methods

| Test | Amplification assay type | Target | Enzymes used | Thermal cycling required | Commercial applications |
|---|---|---|---|---|---|
| PCR | Target | DNA (RNA)[a] | Thermostable DNA polymerase | Yes | Mtb, Ct, Ng, HCV, HIV[b] |
| TAS | Target | DNA/RNA | Reverse transcriptase + RNA polymerase | Yes | — |
| TMA | Target | RNA (DNA)[c] | Reverse transcriptase + RNA polymerase + RNase H | No | Mtb, Ct |
| SDA | Target | DNA[c] | *Hinc*II + DNA polymerase I | No | Mtb |
| NASBA | Target | RNA (DNA)[c] | Reverse transcriptase + RNA polymerase + RNase H | No | Mtb, HIV |
| Q$\beta$ | Probe | DNA/RNA | Q-$\beta$ replicase | No | Ct |
| LCR | Probe | DNA | Thermostable DNA ligase | Yes | Ct, Ng |
| bDNA | Signal | DNA/RNA | Alkaline phosphatase | No | HCV, Mtb, HIV |

[a]Requires reverse transcriptase to prepare RNA from DNA template.

[b]Mtb; *M. tuberculosis*; Ct, *C. trachomatis*; HIV, human immunodeficiency virus; HCV, hepatitis C virus.

[c]DNA must be denatured prior to amplification.

clinical laboratories (e.g., only on acid-fast smear-positive samples, or only on samples from HIV-infected patients) may depend on the patient population served and other factors. The sensitivity of commercial amplification methods for detecting *M. tuberculosis* outside of the respiratory tract, such as in cerebrospinal fluid, is approximately the same as in smear-negative respiratory samples, although the data are few. The role of amplification tests for mycobacteria other than *M. tuberculosis* has yet to be established.

Another emerging use of amplification technology is for monitoring the viral load in patients on antiviral therapy. Commercial PCR, NASBA, and bDNA assays are available to monitor the plasma viral load, and thus presumably disease progression, of patients with human immunodeficiency virus infections who are being treated with nucleoside analogues and protease inhibitors. This assay is now performed routinely in many large medical centers. Similarly, the viral loads of patients with hepatitis C virus infections who are being treated with interferon can also be monitored using quantitative amplification methods.

The most novel application of amplification technology is for the detection of uncultureable agents, such as the bacterium of Whipple's disease, *Tropherema whippelii*, using universal primers that recognize rDNA sequences common to all bacteria. By performing DNA sequence analysis of the amplified products of the rRNA genes, a genus and species determination can be made. This technology can also be used to identify the presence of microorganisms that are difficult to culture from clinical samples, or in specimens from patients who have received antimicrobial chemotherapy prior to the time cultures were obtained. Advances in DNA sequencing methods, including oligonucleotide probe arrays, have made this technology more accessible to clinical microbiology laboratories. These advances promise to make this type of analysis even faster and more affordable for clinical use.

### Detection of antimicrobial resistance genes

Amplification tests can also be used to detect antimicrobial resistance genes in organisms directly in clinical samples to predict therapeutic responses. For example, detection of mutations in the *rpoB* locus in *M. tuberculosis*, which indicates probable rifampin resistance, can serve as a surrogate marker for multidrug-resistant *M. tuberculosis* and guide therapy early in the course of mycobacterial illness. Other tests, such as for the *mecA* gene in *Staphylococcus aureus* (which mediates methicillin resistance), could be used to analyze organisms directly in blood cultures to aid the physician in selecting therapy for nosocomial bacteremia.

Oligonucleotide arrays have made detection of point mutations in the HIV genome associated with resistance to protease inhibitors and nucleoside analogues accessible to the clinical laboratory.

## Antibody Tests

The detection of antibodies in serum and cerebrospinal fluid remains an important diagnostic tool, both for initial diagnosis of infectious illnesses and, in some instances, for following the effects of therapy. Table 15.9 lists a number of commonly used

**Table 15.9** Serologic tests for bacterial and fungal diseases

| Organism | Method[a] | Test results |
|---|---|---|
| Anthrax | Immunoblot | Any titer |
| *Blastomyces dermatitidis* | CF, EIA | >1:8 (CF); ≥32 (EIA) |
| *Brucella* spp. | Agglutination | ≥1:80 positive |
| *Bartonella henselae* (cat scratch disease) | IFA | 4× rise |
| *Chlamydia pneumoniae* | CF, IFA | 4× rise, IgG ≥512 |
| *C. psittici* | CF | 4× rise |
| *Coccidioides immitis* | Tube precipitins; EIA; skin test | 4× rise (Tp or EIA); positive reaction |
| *Cryptococcus spp.* | Latex agglutination | Any titer |
| *Francisella tularensis* | Agglutination | ≥1:40 |
| *Histoplasma capsulatum* | CF; skin test | 4× rise or IgG ≥32; positive reaction |
| Legionella | Immunofluorescence | ≥1:128 positive |
| Leptospirosis | Agglutination, EIA | ≥1:128 positive |
| Lyme disease | IFA | 4× rise |
| Mycoplasma | CF, EIA | 4× rise |
| Plague | Passive hemagglutination | 4×rise |
| Q fever | EIA, CF | 4× rise |
| Rickettsia | Immunofluorescence | ≥1:128 positive |
| *Streptococcus pyogenes* | ASO | 4× rise |
| *Treponema pallidum* | RPR (nonspecific) | agglutination = positive |
| *T. pallidum* | MHA-TP; FTA-ABS | agglutination = positive; fluorescence |

[a]Abbreviations: ASO, antistreptolysin O titer; CF, complement fixation; FTA-ABS, fluorescent treponemal antibody test—absorbed; IFA, indirect immunofluorescent assay; EIA, enzyme immunoassay; RPR, rapid plasma reagin test; Immunoblot, Western blot assay; MHA-TP, microhemagglutination test for *Treponema pallidum*; FTA-ABS, fluorescent treponemal antibody adsorption.

serologic tests. While serologic tests are important for diagnosing many viral and parasitic illnesses, the role of serology in the diagnosis of bacterial diseases is rather limited. Rickettsial, leptospiral, and treponemal disease, together with legionellosis and the zoonotic infections—Lyme disease, brucellosis, and tularemia—constitute the major bacterial illnesses for which serologic studies are undertaken. While serologic diagnosis of helicobacter infections is undertaken with increasing frequency, alternate testing methods, including the urea breath test, are gaining acceptance for detecting infections caused by this pathogen.

## Culture

Culture of microorganisms on agar, in liquid media, or in cell culture remains the gold standard for the laboratory diagnosis of most bacterial, fungal, and viral infections, and is helpful for several parasitic diseases. The appropriate culture techniques for various species are discussed in Chapters 16–19.

## BIBLIOGRAPHY


Baron EJ, Murray P, Tenover FC, Pfaller MA, Yolken RA, eds. Manual of Clinical Microbiology, 6th ed. American Society for Microbiology, Washington, D.C., 1995.

Centers for Disease Control and Prevention. Recommendations for the Prevention and Management of *Chlamydia trachomatis* Infections, Morbidity Mortality Weekly Report Recommendations and Reports 1993; 42(12):1–20.

Davis GL, Lau JY-N, Urdea MS et al. Quantitative detection of hepatitis C virus RNA with a solid phase signal amplification method: definition of optimal conditions for specimen collection and clinical application in interferon-treated patients. Hepatology 1994; 19:1337–1341.

Ehlers S, Ignatius R, Regnath T, Hahn H. Diagnosis of extrapulmonary tuberculosis by Gen-Probe amplified Mycobacterium tuberculosis direct test. J Clin Microbiol 1996; 34:2275–2279.

Genç M, Mårdh P-A. A cost-effectiveness analysis of screening and treatment for *Chlamydia trachomatis* infection in asymptomatic women. Ann Int Med 1996; 124:1–7.

Hamed KA, Dormitzer PR, Su CK, Relman DA. *Haemophilus parainfluenzae* endocarditis: application of a molecular approach for identification of pathogenic bacterial species. Clin Infect Dis 1994; 19:677–683.

Isenberg HD, ed. Clinical Microbiology Procedures Handbook. American Society for Microbiology, Washington, D.C., 1993.

Jaschek G, Gaydos CA, Welsh LE, Quinn TC. Direct detection of *Chlamydia trachomatis* in urine specimens from symptomatic and asymptomatic men by using a rapid polymerase chain reaction assay. J Clin Microbiol 1993; 31:1209–1212.

Kozal MJ, Shah N, Shen N et al. Extensive polymorphisms observed in HIV-1 clade B protease gene using high density oligonucleotide arrays. Nature Medicine 1996; 2:753–759.

Limberger RJ, Biega R, Evancoe A et al. Evaluation of culture and the Gen-Probe PACE-2 assay for detection of *Neisseria gonorrhoeae* and *Chlamydia trachomatis* in endocervical specimens transported to a state health laboratory. J Clin Microbiol 1992; 30:1162–1166.

Miller N, Hernandez SG, Cleary TJ. Evaluation of Gen-Probe Amplified Mycobacterium tuberculosis direct test and PCR for direct detection of *Mycobacterium tuberculosis* in clinical specimens. J Clin Microbiol 1994; 32:393–397.

National Committee for Clinical Laboratory Standards. Microbiology Diagnostic Methods for Infectious Diseases; Approved Guideline MM3-A, vol. 15, no. 22. National Committee for Clinical Laboratory Standards, Wayne, PA, 1995.

Noordhoek GT, van Embden JDA, Kolk AHJ. Reliability of nucleic acid amplification for detection of *Mycobacterium tuberculosis*: an international collaborative quality control study among 30 laboratories. J Clin Microbiol 1996; 34:2522–2525.

Pease AC. Light-directed oligonucleotide arrays for rapid DNA sequence analysis. Proc Natl Acad Sci USA 1994; 91:5022–5026.

Persing DH. In vitro nucleic acid amplification techniques. In: Diagnostic Molecular Microbiology. Persing DH, Smith T, Tenover FC, White TH, eds. American Society for Microbiology, Washington, D.C. pp. 51–87, 1993.

Pokorski SJ, Vetter EA, Wollan PC, Cockerill FR, III. Comparison of Gen-Probe Group A Streptococcus direct test with culturing for diagnosing streptococcal pharyngitis. J Clin Microbiol 1994; 32:1440–1443.

Relman DA, Schmidt TM, MacDermott RP, Falkow S. Identification of the uncultured bacillus of Whipple's disease. N Engl J Med 1992; 327:293–301.

Revets H, Marissens D, De Wit S et al. Comparative evaluation of NASBA HIV-1 RNA QT, AMPLICOR-HIV Monitor, and QUANTIPLEX HIV RNA assay, three methods for quantification of human immunodeficiency virus type 1 RNA in plasma. J Clin Microbiol 1996; 34:1058–1064.

Scembri MA, Lin SK, Lambert R. Comparison of commercial diagnostic tests for *Helicobacter pylori* antibodies. J Clin Microbiol 1993; 31:2621–2624.

Schacter J, Stamm E, Quinn TC et al. Ligase chain reaction to detect *Chlamydia trachomatis* infection of the cervix. J Clin Microbiol 1994; 32:2540–2543.

Telenti A, Imboden P, Marchesi F et al. Direct, automated detection of rifampin-resistant *Mycobacterium tuberculosis* by polymerase chain reaction and singe-strand confirmation polymorphism analysis. Antimicrob Agents Chemother 1993; 37:2054–2058.

Tenover FC, Popovich T, Olsvik Ø. Genetic methods for detecting antibacterial resistance genes. In: Manual of Clinical Microbiology, 6th ed. Baron EJ, Murray P, Tenover FC, Pfaller MA, Yolken RA, eds. American Society for Microbiology, Washington, D.C. pp. 1368–1378, 1995.

Tenover FC, Unger ER. Nucleic acid probes for detection and identification of infectious agents. In: Diagnostic Molecular Microbiology. Principles and Applications. DH Persing, T Smith, FC Tenover, T White, eds. American Society for Microbiology. Washington, D.C. pp. 3–25, 1993.

Wolcott M. Advances in nucleic acid-based detection methods. Clin Microbiol Rev 1992; 5:370–386.

Yang LI, Panke ES, Leist PA et al. Detection of *Chlamydia trachomatis* endocervical infection in asymptomatic and symptomatic women; comparison of deoxyribonucleic acid probe test with tissue culture. Obstet Gynecol 1991; 165:1444–1453.

# 16

## Clinical Bacteriology

JAMES J. PLORDE

The definitive diagnosis of bacterial infections is most commonly accomplished by the cultural recovery of the causative agent(s) from body surfaces, fluids, tissues or excreta of the affected patient. The reliability of this approach is dependent on *(1)* the collection of clinical specimens free of colonizing, but potentially pathogenic, bacteria, and *(2)* the transportation of these specimens to the laboratory in a manner that ensures the survival of fastidious pathogens.

### Specimen Collection and Transportation

#### Specimen categories

The extent to which specimens can be collected free of resident bacteria is linked to the anatomic characteristics of the sampling site. The most advantageous areas are the *deep, closed body sites* such as the vascular system, subarachnoid space, pleural cavity, peritoneal cavity, and joints. Specimens obtained from such normally sterile areas by needle aspiration through an intact and appropriately disinfected skin surface are seldom contaminated with resident flora. Cultural recovery of bacteria in such circumstances is prima facie evidence of infection. Less satisfactory sampling locations are the *deep communicating body sites.* Examples include lung, bladder, uterus, and fistulated tissue. Although these sites are also normally sterile, the pathways by which they communicate with the external world (e.g., oropharynx, urethra, endocervix, fistula) are invariably colonized with a wide variety of bacterial flora. Specimens collected following transit through these pathways are invariably contaminated. The level of contamination can be diminished by disinfecting the pathway's orifice and flushing its lumen prior to specimen collection (e.g., clean-voided, midstream urine specimens); aspirating the specimen through a sterile catheter placed deep into the pathway (e.g., endobronchial, endocervical, and fistula aspirates); or by direct, percutaneous needle aspiration through intact skin, thus bypassing the communicating pathway (e.g., suprapubic or transthoracic aspirates). With the exception of the latter approach, contamination is never totally eliminated. Its continuing presence is suggested by the isolation of multiple bacterial species. Except for anaerobic infections, most infected sites harbor a single organism, or occasionally two. Additionally, quantitative bacteriology permits reasonable differentiation of clinically significant and insignificant bacterial growth in certain specimens (e.g. urine, bronchoalveolar lavage fluid). The least satisfactory sampling locations are *superficial body sites* such as the skin, mucous membranes, open ulcers, and the gastrointestinal tract. These sites are so heavily contaminated with resident flora that culture is seldom of value unless a specific bacterial pathogen is being sought, such as *Streptococcus pyogenes* from the throat, *Neisseria gonorrhoeae* from the genital tract, or *Salmonella* and *Shigella* from the stool.

#### Specimen transport

Transportation times greater than 60 minutes may result in the death of fastidious organisms through desiccation, oxygenation, or metabolic competition with more hardy pathogens and contaminants. This risk is particularly high for specimens less than 1 $cm^3$ in volume. Such fluids and tissues are best transported in special sealed, anaerobic vials or tubes. Swab specimens should be transported in one of the several commercially available transport media; the use of swabs is strongly discouraged if the recovery of anaerobic organisms is anticipated. Large-volume respiratory, tissue, urine and body fluid specimens are safely transported in any sterile, leakproof plastic container. Syringes used in the collection of large-volume aspirates may be used to transport the specimen to the laboratory provided all air is expressed and the syringe is adequately sealed.

#### Percutaneous needle aspirates

The aspiration site should be cleansed with 70%–95% isopropyl or ethyl alcohol and then disinfected by applying a 2% tincture of iodine or an iodophor in concentric circles around the intended aspiration site. Although tincture of iodine is a more effective bactericidal agent, iodophors are generally preferred as they induce skin sensitization less frequently. As it takes approximately 1–2 minutes to achieve maximum killing of the skin flora, the iodine-preparation area should be allowed to dry before proceeding. It should not be touched with the finger unless clad with a sterile glove. Following aspiration, the residual iodine is removed with alcohol; this is particularly important if tincture of iodine was used.

#### Blood specimens

Cultures should be obtained from febrile and hypothermic patients who manifest rigors, hypotension, prostration, altered sensorium, or a cardiac murmur, or who are immunosuppressed. If a viral, mycobacterial, fungal, or fastidious bacterial infection is suspected, the laboratory should be contacted for special instructions. In adults, blood culture yield is dramatically influenced by specimen volume, increasing approximately 2% for each additional milliliter of blood drawn between 5 and 30 ml. The timing of specimen collection is less critical. In patients with endovascular infections, overwhelming sepsis, and salmonellosis, bacteremia is generally constant. While often intermittent in other circumstances, the scheduling of blood draws is generally dictated by the patient's clinical condition and urgency of antimicrobial therapy. Generally, two or three cultures of 20 to 30 ml taken at intervals of no less that 60 minutes are adequate to document adult bacteremia. In critical situations, two cultures taken from different anatomic sites is generally sufficient. If the patient has received antimicrobial therapy within the previous two weeks, if the clinical probability of bacteremia is high, or if the expected pathogen is a member of resident skin flora, a second series of cultures should be obtained the following day. In patients who are currently receiving antimicrobial agents, blood specimens should be collected immediately prior to the next scheduled antimicrobial dose, and the laboratory should be notified to ensure they employ techniques to minimize in vitro bacterial killing. Specimens are best collected by percutaneous venipuncture as described in the preceding section. Collections from the femoral vein should be avoided, as the concentration of organisms in the venous drainage of the lower extremities is less than that found in arm veins. The hirsute nature of the groin also renders skin disinfection procedures less effective. Blood culture specimens drawn through intravascular catheters are no more productive than percutaneously drawn specimens and are more frequently contaminated. This is probably related to the frequency with which the interiors of the catheter hubs become colonized with organisms found on the surrounding skin. It has been suggested that disinfection of the hub interior with an ethanol-soaked swab prior to the collection of the specimen may serve to decrease the contamination rate.

### Cerebrospinal fluid specimens

The rapidly lethal nature of untreated bacterial meningitis demands a prompt etiologic diagnosis. In adults, the new onset of fever and confusion, even in the absence of headache, vomiting, nuchal rigidity, and hyperreflexia, warrant a lumbar puncture. The site should be prepared in the manner described as above for percutaneous aspirates. If possible, at least 2 ml of CSF is collected in one or more sterile screw-cap tubes with leakproof caps. When only a single tube is used, it should be dispatched to the microbiology laboratory. Here an aliquot will be aseptically removed and the remainder sent to the chemistry laboratory. If multiple tubes are collected, a tube other than the first should be sent for microbiologic studies; the remaining tubes may be routed to chemistry for cell count, glucose, and protein determinations. The laboratory should be notified if the specimen was collected from an abscess within the central nervous system to ensure that it is cultured anaerobically as well as aerobically. Similarly, the laboratory needs to know if a viral, fungal, mycobacterial, or parasitic etiology is being considered. To prevent die-off of temperature-sensitive organisms such as *Neisseria meningitidis* during transport, it is desirable to immediately dispatch the specimen to the laboratory in the care of a responsible individual. Commercial antigen-detection procedures are available for the diagnosis of the common bacterial causes of childhood meningitis, *Haemophilus influenzae, N. meningitidis, Streptococcus agalactiae,* and *Streptococcus pneumoniae*. With sensitivities roughly equivalent to that of Gram-stained smears, they are most useful in children with suspected meningitis who have already been started on antimicrobial therapy and have a negative CSF smear. The value of antigen-detection tests for the diagnosis of adult bacterial meningitis is doubtful. Only a small fraction of adult cases are now caused by one of the four organisms mentioned above. As a result, false-positive results may outnumber true-positives despite generally excellent specificities. Moreover, false-negative results may inappropriately result in antimicrobial withdrawal.

### Other body fluids and exudates

Pericardial, pleural, peritoneal, and synovial fluids as well as pus from closed abscesses are best collected and transported as described in the preceding sections. Large fluid volumes may accumulate in these normally sterile cavities, producing low bacterial concentrations; thus, large-volume collections are advised. The risk of clot formation may be decreased by prior rinsing of the syringe with heparin. The use of cultural techniques that result in the leukocyte lysis appears to improve organism recovery from peritoneal dialysis patients experiencing clinical evidence of peritonitis, possibly by releasing entrapped organisms prior to intracellular killing. The same may be true of patients with pleural effusions. The collection and/or transportation of specimens on swabs is ill advised. The small sample size exposes the limited number of retained organisms to the twin dangers of desiccation and oxidation. The difficulty of collecting specimens from deep suppurative lesions communicating with the body surface through a fistula or sinus has been described above (deep, communicating body sites). The level of specimen contamination with a fistula's bacterial flora can be diminished somewhat by aspirating the specimen through a sterile catheter placed deep in the fistula after careful disinfection of the orifice. Bacteriologic diagnosis is better served with culture of currettings or biopsy.

### Lower respiratory tract specimens

While sputum culture remains the single most frequently used technique for establishing the etiologic diagnosis of lower respiratory tract infections, its value has been repeatedly challenged. Studies of patients with bacteremic pneumonia have shown the causative agent to be absent from the sputum in as many as 50% of cases. Moreover, careless collection procedures or inability of the patient to cooperate adequately result in the submission of specimens heavily contaminated with oropharyngeal organisms, including bacterial species commonly associated with pulmonary infection. Some of the attendant confusion can be avoided by examining a Gram-stained smear prepared at the time of culture plating. If fewer than ten squamous epithelial cells (SEC) are found per low-power field, the culture is more likely to yield a pure or near-pure growth of a known respiratory pathogen. Only in this situation can the isolate be confidently assumed to represent the etiologic agent. Expectorated specimens, either induced or spontaneous, are most useful when used to establish the presence of an infection produced by organisms absent from the oropharynx, such as mycobacteria and *Legionella* spp. The culture of three fresh, early-morning expectorated specimens is almost always adequate to establish the diagnosis of pulmonary mycobacterial disease.

For patients unable to expectorate, respiratory secretions may be collected by nasotracheal or endotracheal suction. These specimens are contaminated with oropharyngeal flora carried to the lower respiratory tract during the passage of the aspirating instrument; accordingly, they share many of the limitations of expectorated sputum collections. Contamination can be avoided if a protected bronchial brush catheter is utilized. Material obtained in this fashion is also suitable for anaerobic culture. Brush yields of $\geq$1000 colony-forming units (CFUs) of a specific organism indicate that the isolate is likely of etiologic significance. More recently, quantitative bronchoalveolar lavage has proven popular for the diagnosis of lower respiratory tract infections, particularly in immunocompromised hosts and patients with ventilator-associated pneumonia. Growth of $\geq$100,000 CFU of a specific organism per ml of lavage fluid is considered clinically significant.

Techniques that totally bypass the oropharnx are occasionally required to establish an etiologic diagnosis. Radiographically monitored needle aspiration of pulmonary infiltrates has largely supplanted transtracheal aspiration. The former provides more accurate results and a higher yield, albeit at a somewhat higher morbidity.

## Urinary tract specimens

Voided urine is invariably contaminated with the resident flora of the urethra and external genitalia (mainly staphylococci, diphtheroids, lactobacilli, and streptococci). When the periurethral area is carefully disinfected and the urethra flushed with the initial portion of the urine stream prior to the collection of a mid- to late-stream specimen, contamination with these organisms is usually minimal. Quantitative culture techniques and speciation are used to distinguish such low-level bacterial contamination from true bacteriuria. Colony counts generally display a bimodal distribution, with concentrations of <1000 and ≥100,000 CFU/ml separating the former and latter conditions. These breakpoints are modified in certain clinical situations. Thus, counts of ≥100 CFU/ml of a uropathogen such as *E. coli* in young, acutely dysuric women and ≥1000 CFU in symptomatic men may reflect the presence of infection. Low numbers of organisms may also be significant in clean-voided specimens from patients receiving antimicrobial agents, and in specimens obtained by ureteral or urethral catheterization or suprapubic aspiration.

Under certain circumstances, contaminating bacteria may be present in numbers exceeding 100,000 CFU/ml, resulting in false-positive culture results. This is most frequently the consequence of inadequate instruction in, or execution of, the clean-catch midstream urine-collection procedure. As urine is a good culture medium, it may also occur when voided urine specimens are allowed to sit at room temperature for prolonged periods of time prior to plating. Accordingly, urine culture specimens should be plated within 1 hour or refrigerated at 4°C until appropriate transportation can be arranged. The latter can be held for up to 6 hours without an appreciable increase in colony count. If neither is possible, transport kits with preservatives designed to temporarily inhibit bacterial growth at room temperatures should be employed. Such specimens must be plated within 24 hours. Contaminants can also multiply to high concentrations in stagnant urine present in the collection tubes and bags of patients with indwelling urethral catheters, making these locations inappropriate collection sites. More suitably, specimens should be aspirated directly from the catheter with a sterile syringe and needle following disinfection of the catheter's exterior surface or sampling port. Finally, as most urinary tract infections are caused by one or, at the most, two bacterial species, the isolation of three or more species suggests contamination, even when the colony count is high. True polymicrobial bacteriuria is commonly seen only in patients with nephrostomy tubes or chronic indwelling urinary catheters.

Culture-suitable specimens can be obtained from incontinent males by cleansing the glans penis with an iodophor, applying a new, unsterile condom catheter and drainage system, and collecting the first void from the urine bag. When adequate specimens cannot be obtained by other means or when anaerobic cultures are desired, suprapubic aspiration may be employed. As such specimens are unlikely to be contaminated, any growth may be significant. For the reasons outlined above, information on the clinical diagnosis, method of specimen collection, time obtained, and antimicrobial therapy should accompany the specimen to the laboratory.

A number of screening tests for bacteriuria have been developed. Among the most widely used are Gram-stained smears of uncentrifuged urine and leukocyte esterase–bacteria nitrate kits. Positive screening tests reliably detect the presence of ≥100,000 CFU/ml; they are significantly less sensitive in detecting true bacteriuria at lower colony counts.

## Fecal specimens

Fecal cultures are used for determining the etiologic agent(s) of acute diarrheal illness and in detecting carrier states. In either situation, recovery of the responsible agent is complicated by the enormous number and diversity of the normal fecal flora ($10^{12}$ CFU/g feces). Moreover, in this "haystack" of organisms one is not simply mounting a search for a single "needle" but for an ever-growing list of potential enteropathogens, many of which require unique cultural procedures for their isolation Most laboratories routinely culture for *Salmonella, Shigella, Campylobacter,* and *Clostridium difficile*. Reference laboratories routinely, and smaller laboratories on special request, may employ procedures capable of detecting *Vibrio parahaemolyticus, V. cholerae, Yersinia enterocolitica, E. coli* O157:H7, enterotoxigenic and verotoxigenic *E. coli*, *Aeromonas,* and *Plesiomonas*. The diagnosis of *Bacillus cereus, Clostridium perfringens,* and *Staphylococcus aureus* food poisoning usually falls within the province of the public health laboratory.

To appropriately focus the laboratory effort, it is essential that the clinician provide relevant epidemiologic and clinical data. Knowledge of the patient's age, history of contact with other diarrheal patients, duration of illness, recent antimicrobic use, hospital stay, dietary adventures, or other epidemiological exposures can narrow the list of potential pathogens. Similarly, knowledge of the frequency and nature of stools (e.g., "rice water," watery, bloody), and presence of other gastrointestinal manifestations (e.g., vomiting, flatulence, lower abdominal pain), may significantly shorten the time required to diagnosis.

Ideally, liquid stool should be collected during the acute disease; formed stools procured late in the course of the disease are less likely to yield the causative agent. Rectal swab specimens are usually adequate for the diagnosis of acute bacterial diarrhea, but are less satisfactory for the detection of carrier states. If used, the swab must be inserted through the anal sphincter into the rectal cavity. The withdrawn swab should show obvious fecal soiling, and be sent to the laboratory in an appropriate transport medium. Swabs of rectal or colonic lesions visualized through an endoscope are more productive than those collected blindly. Whole stool should be collected free of urine, placed in a clean, waxed cardboard carton, and promptly sent to the laboratory. If delivery cannot be made within 1 hour, it should be placed in Cary-Blair transport medium. The submission of a second, and occasionally a third, specimen may be productive, particularly when seeking a carrier. It is seldom necessary to submit more than three consecutive daily specimens.

## Genital tract specimens

Genital specimens are collected primarily for the diagnosis of venereal disease, several of which are caused by bacterial agents. These include *Neisseria gonorrhoeae, Chlamydia trachomatis, Haemophilus ducreyi,* and *Treponema pallidum*. Of these, the first three are routinely identified by culture, the latter by dark-field or fluorescent-antibody microscopy. When gonorrhea is suspected in a woman, medical personnel should collect swab specimens from the cervical os and, if possible, the rectum. In males specimens are taken from the urethral orifice and, if the patient is known to be homosexual, the pharynx and rectum. The swabs are placed into modified Stuart's medium and immediately transported to the clinical laboratory. Directions for the collection of specimens for the remaining agents should be sought in the chapters dealing with sexually transmitted diseases (Chapters 70–72).

In addition to the venereal pathogens, a number of organisms may infect the endometrium, tubovarian tissues, and vagina. In patients with postpartum endometritis, specimens are best collected with a double-lumen vacuum catheter inserted through a decontaminated cervical os. When intrauterine-device actinomycosis is suspected, the entire device and associated exudate should be collected. Both of these endometrial specimen types should be dispatched immediately to the clinical laboratory or placed in a gassed-out environment to ensure recovery of anaerobic organisms. In patients with suspected vaginitis, swab specimens are collected from the vaginal fornix under direct visualization. KOH wet mounts and Gram-stain smears are then prepared and examined for the characteristic "clue cells" of bacterial vaginosis (see Chapter 72) and for motile trichomonads budding yeast, or pseudohyphae.

## Vascular catheters

Local infection and bacteremia are major infectious complications of intravascular catheters (see Chapter 67). It has been estimated that 50,000 to 120,000 patients in the United States develop nosocomial infusion-related bacteremia annually. The preponderance of evidence suggests that the majority of these result from the contamination of external surface of the catheter during insertion and subsequent manipulation. Organisms may penetrate the insertion site and then colonize the intravascular segment of the catheter. Microbiologic techniques for demonstrating bacterial colonization have focused on the removal and subsequent quantitative culture of the catheter's exterior surface. The skin around the insertion site is first cleansed with alcohol and allowed to dry. The cannula is then withdrawn, taking care to avoid contact with the skin. Using sterile technique, a segment of the catheter is aseptically excised and placed in a sterile container for transport to the clinical laboratory. For short devices, the entire catheter should be amputated just below the old skin–catheter junction. For catheters ≥8 inches in length, two 5 cm segments are cultured, one taken from the tip and the other from the intracutaneous portion of the catheter. The growth of ≥15 CFU of a single organism per catheter denotes a *local* catheter-related infection. In the presence of clinical evidence of sepsis or thrombophlebitis, it is presumptive evidence of the isolate's etiologic role. Recent studies have suggested that catheters in place for periods of several weeks may be more commonly infected with organisms that initially colonize the interior of the catheter hub and subsequently track along the interior wall to the vascular space. Proposals have been made that catheter-related infections could be reliably detected by culture of the hub interior. Other investigators have advocated defining catheter-related sepsis on the basis of quantitative cultures performed on blood specimens collected simultaneously by catheter and percutaneous draws. Bacterial concentrations in catheter-drawn blood that exceeded that of percutaneously drawn blood by five- to tenfold were thought to define catheter-related sepsis. The clinical utility of these two approaches has not yet been adequately defined.

## Direct microscopic examination

In this era of molecular microbiology, the direct microscopic examination of a specimen is still, as it has been for a century, the single best technique for the rapid diagnosis of bacterial infection. The power of the technique is dramatically enhanced with the use of stains that provide contrast between microbial agents and their surrounding environment. The Gram, acridine orange, acid-fast, and immunofluorescent stains are discussed below. Most require the sequential application of a stain directed at a target organism, a mordant that fixes that stain to the target, a decolorizing agent that removes unfixed stain, and a counterstain to provide contrast and/or color to the background and to untargeted organisms. In addition to the skill and diligence of the microscopist, the sensitivity and specificity of the stained smears reflect *(1)* the number of pathogenic microorganisms at the inflammatory site, *(2)* the degree to which the specimen-collection process circumvented contamination with resident flora, *(3)* the use and efficiency of bacterial concentration procedures, *(4)* the quality of smear preparation, *(5)* the level of contrast provided by the stain, and *(6)* the resolving power of the microscope. As the microscopic visualization of bacteria occurs at the very limits of optical capacity, the resolving power of the microscope must be fully optimized if small microbes are to be detected. Most critical to this is the adjustment of the condenser to focus its transmitted light on the plane of the specimen. This can be accomplished quickly, and fairly accurately, on most bright-light microscopes, by raising the condenser to its highest station and then lowering it slightly by turning the adjustment knob one-eighth of a revolution in the opposite direction. Neglecting this step may result in the failure to detect small, gram-negative organisms.

## Gram stain

The Gram-stain procedure utilizes crystal violet to color all bacterial and host cells a deep blue; application of iodine selectively fixes this stain to gram-positive organisms. Following removal of the unfixed crystal violet with a decolorizing agent, gram-negative bacteria, host cells, and exudate are counterstained reddish-pink with safranin, or, occasionally, with the more intensely red carbol-fuchsin. With the notable exception of upper respiratory tract samples, most clinical specimens submitted for bacterial culture are candidates for Gram's stain examination. Body fluids (excluding urine) and BAL specimens are concentrated by centrifugation prior to smear preparation and staining. The completed stain is screened under low magnification (100×) for the presence of neutrophils and squamous epithelial cells (SEC). An abundance of the latter suggests the specimen was contaminated during collection and is not suitable for further processing. In the absence of such cells, the smear is carefully scanned under the oil immersion lens (1000× magnification) for bacteria.

The sensitivity of optimally prepared and examined Gram-stained smears is approximately 25%, 60%, and 95% at bacterial concentrations of $<10^3$, $10^3$–$10^4$, and $\geq 10^5$ CFU/ml, respectively. As concentrations often vary by specimen types, so do the sensitivities of the Gram-stained smear. Typical sensitivities for culture-positive voided urine, CSF, expectorated sputum specimens, and peritoneal fluids are 95%, 75%, 50%, and 30%, respectively. The color and morphology of the visualized organ-

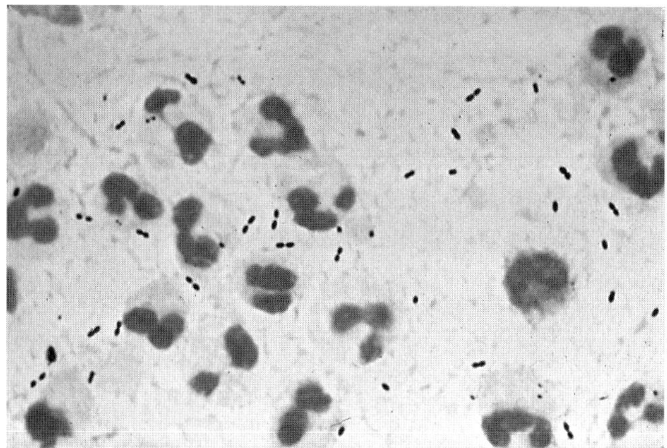

**Fig. 16.1** Pneumococci—CSF.

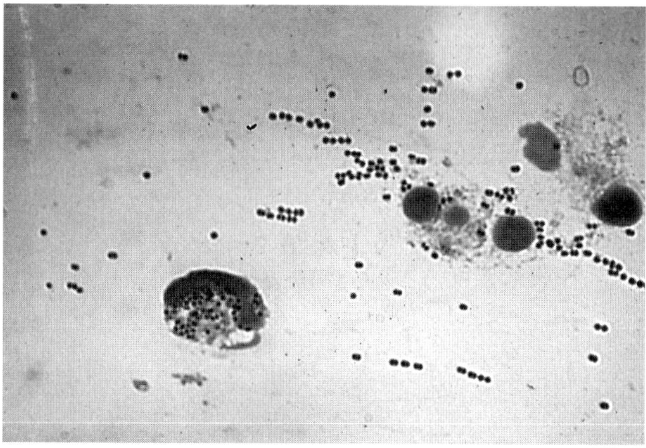

**Fig. 16.3** Gonococci—urethral exudate.

isms is often sufficiently unique to permit a presumptive identification of the genus, and occasionally the species, of the organism in question. Staphylococci, streptococci, pneumococci, clostridia, *Nocardia,* Coryneforms, *Neisseria,* coliforms, pseudomonads, and *Hemophilus influenzae* can be identified with considerable accuracy (see Figs. 16.1–16.6 and Plates 4 and 5). The failure to recover organisms in culture that are prominent on the Gram-stained smear suggests that antimicrobial agents are present in the specimen and/or that cultural procedures need to be optimized for the visualized organisms.

## Acridine orange stain

Acridine orange (AO) is a fluorochrome stain that intercalates into nucleic acid, making it valuable for the detection of host inflammatory cells and all classifications of microorganisms. When examined under UV light, bacteria and yeast stain bright red-orange and leukocytes stain pale green. It is capable of detecting organisms at a concentration of $\geq 10^4$ CFU/ml, one log less than that regularly detected by the Gram's stain. It is also said to be more sensitive than the Gram's stain in specimens obtained from patients recently started on antimicrobial therapy. This increased sensitivity results from the striking contrast between the bright, fluorescent organisms and the dark background. This contrast permits rapid examination of most smears under 400× magnification. AO stains have been particularly helpful in screening CSF and peritoneal fluid specimens for the presence of microbes. It is also useful for staining slow-growing microorganisms in broth culture. AO-positive smears must subsequently be Gram-stained to verify the presence of bacteria and to determine their gram-reaction. Fortunately, AO smears can be overstained with Gram reagents without prior decolorization of the acridine orange. The major disadvantage of this stain is the need for a fluorescence microscope.

## Acid-fast stains

Mycobacteria, and to a lesser degree the actinomycetes, stain poorly with routine bacterial stains owing to the high lipid content of their cell walls. Heat and/or detergents will enhance stain uptake. Once the stain is fixed to the target cells, they are highly resistant to decolorization, even when combinations of strong organic acids and alcohol are employed. The two most widely used stains for the visualization of mycobacteria are the Ziehl-Neelsen and Kinyoun. Both employ carbol fuchsin as the primary stain, a mixture of hydrochloric acid and ethanol as decolorizing agents, and methylene blue as a counterstain. The major difference between the two techniques lies in their use of mordants; heat is employed in the former and phenol in the latter. In smears stained by either method, mycobacteria appear as red bacilli ("red snappers") against a blue background. As actinomycetes cannot resist the harsh decolorization procedures utilized in the standard

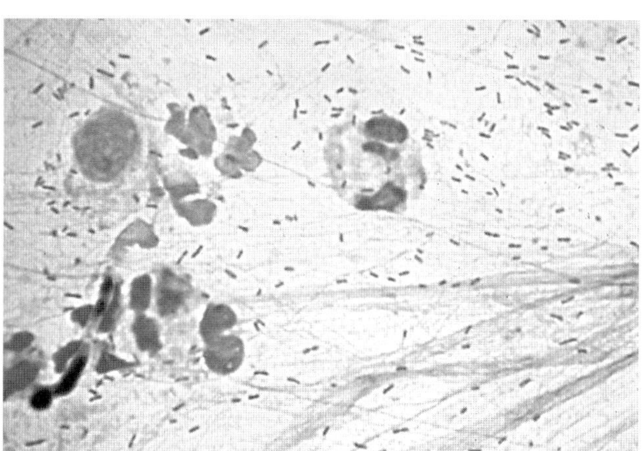

**Fig. 16.2** *H. influenzae*—sputum.

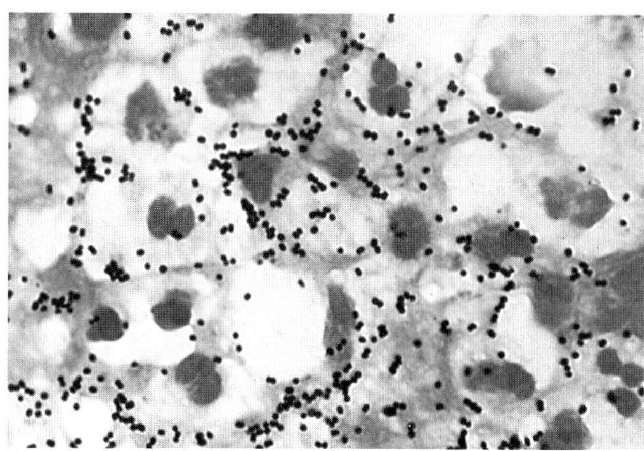

**Fig. 16.4** Staphylococci—sputum.

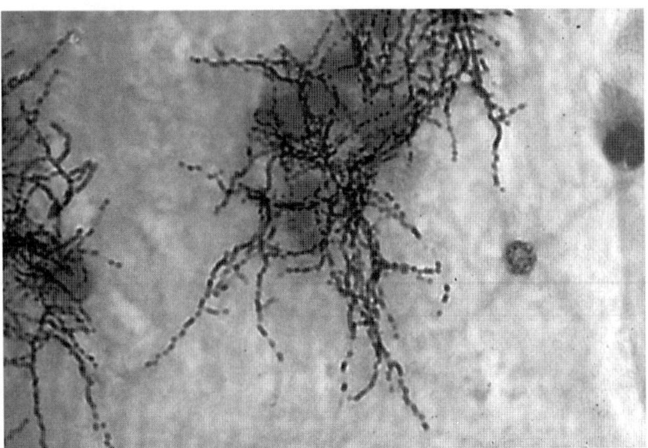

**Fig. 16.5** Nocardia—exudate.

Ziehl-Neelsen and Kinyoun techniques, a "Modified Kinyoun" stain employing gentler decolorization is used to distinguish the weakly acid-fast *Nocardia* group from other actinomycetes.

In many medical centers, the Ziehl-Neelsen and Kinyoun strains have been supplanted by the more sensitive auramine-"rhodamine fluorochrome procedure. As in the case of the acridine orange stain, enhanced sensitivity results from the striking contrast between the bright green, fluorescent organisms against a dark background, permitting the microscopist to scan the entire smear at relatively low magnification. The overall sensitivity of the acid-fast stains is approximately 40%–50%. It is higher in patients with *M. tuberculosis* infections than in those with illness caused by other mycobacterial species, and higher in respiratory than tissue or body fluid specimens. In all cases, sensitivity appears directly related to the number of colonies recovered in culture, reaching a low of 13% when $\leq$10 colonies are seen and a high of more than 90% when >100 colonies are isolated. In our institution, 65% of respiratory specimens that are culture-positive for *M. tuberculosis* have positive direct smears. If more than one respiratory tract specimen is submitted, 96% of patients with pulmonary tuberculosis will have at least one positive direct stain. Reported specificities have usually ranged from 80% to 90%. The majority of false-positive smear results occur in patients on antimycobacterial therapy. False-positive smear results in this setting have been attributed to the staining of dead mycobacteria by the auramine-rhodamine stain.

### Immunofluorescent stains

Direct immunofluorescent stains combine the speed of direct microscopy with the specificity of immunologic procedures. In this technique, smears thought to contain certain bacterial pathogens are stained with specific antibody preparations labeled with fluorescent compounds and examined with a fluorescence microscope. In the bacteriology laboratory this technique is widely used for the detection of *Legionella* spp. in expectorated sputum and *Bordetella pertussis* in nasopharyngeal cells. Commercial polyvalent fluorescein isothiocyanate-conjugated monoclonal antibodies will detect the majority of legionella serotypes implicated in human disease. The sensitivity of such preparations are limited (~60%); specificity depends on the experience of the testing laboratory. Sensitivities and specificities of 60% and 90% have been reported for the *Bordetella* immunofluorescent stain.

### Nucleic acid–detection techniques

These are rapid sensitive and specific for a variety of bacterial species and are discussed in detail in Chapter 15.

## Culture Techniques

Cultivation and subsequent identification of the infecting microorganism is usually the most sensitive and specific method for establishing an etiologic diagnosis of a bacterial infection. While almost all important bacterial pathogens can be readily grown on artificial media, the selection of *media, conditions of incubation*, and *detection procedures* vary greatly with the specimen type submitted and the microorganisms sought.

### Media composition

The principal ingredients of bacterial media are protein digests—generally poorly defined slurries of polypeptides, amino acids, enzymes, and trace metals. To these mixes are added various supplements, including salts, carbohydrates, vitamins, reducing substances, and/or blood products to provide specific bacterial pathogens with the nutritional substrates they require for optimal growth.

When specimens are collected from sites heavily colonized with resident flora, *selective media* are employed. These either contain enrichments designed to enhance the growth of the pathogen or inhibitors that selectively suppress growth of the resident flora. Among the latter are antibiotic-containing media used for the recovery of *Neisseria gonorrhoeae* from the urethra and uterine cervix, and several species of *Campylobacter* from the stool. Unfortunately, the selectivity of such media is never total; resident flora resistant to the selecting agent are often present, and the organisms sought may be occasionally inhibited. For this reason, selective media are generally used in combination with nonselective preparations.

If the specimen to be cultured potentially contains a wide variety of pathogenic organisms, *differential media* are more useful. These contain supplements that permit the recognition of certain organism groups sharing common metabolic capacities or protein products. Carbohydrates and pH indicators are commonly used differential agents. Organisms capable of fermenting the carbohydrate become visually apparent when the acid metabolites of sugar fermentation force a shift in the color of the pH

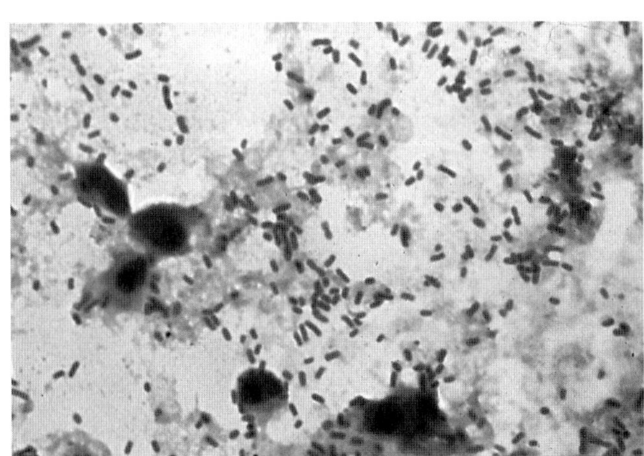

**Fig. 16.6** *E. coli*—peritoneal exudate.

**Table 16.1** Characteristics of common bacterial pathogens

| Organism group | Stain appearance | Special culture conditions | Colonial characteristics | | | Rapid tests | | Comment |
|---|---|---|---|---|---|---|---|---|
| | | | Morphology | Hemolysis | Other | One | Two | |
| GRAM-POSITIVE COCCI | | | | | | | | |
| *STAPHYLOCOCCI* | | | | | | | | |
| *Staphylococcus aureus* | Clusters | None | Opaque, cream | $\beta$ (70%) | | Catalase + | Coagulase + | |
| *S. epidermidis* | Clusters | None | Opaque, white | None | | Catalase + | Coagulase − | |
| *S. saphrophyticus* | Clusters | None | Opaque, white | None | | Catalase + | Coagulase − | Urinary pathogen |
| *LANCEFIELD STREPTOCOCCI* | | | | | | | | |
| *Streptococcus pyogenes* | Chains | None | Translucent | $\beta$ | Push Test + | Catalase − | Gp A, PYR + | |
| Strep equi & Grp G | Chains | None | Translucent | $\beta$ | Push Test + | Catalase − | Gps C, G | |
| *S. agalactiae* | Chains, pairs | None | Transl., orange | $\beta$ | Push Test − | Catalase − | Gp B | |
| *S. anginosus* (milleri) | Chains | $CO_2$ | Transl., minute | $\beta$, $\alpha$ | Lactic acid odor | Catalase − | Gp F ± | Abscesses |
| S. bovis | Chains | None | Translucent | None | | Catalase − | Gp D | Colonic CA |
| *GREENING STREPTOCOCCI* | | | | | | | | |
| *S. pneumoniae* | Lancet-shaped diplococci | None | Transl., umbilicate | $\alpha$ | | Catalase − | Bile soluble | Autolytic enzymes |
| *S. sanguis* | Chains | None | Transl., convex | $\alpha$ (None) | | Catalase − | Bile insoluble | Caries, endocarditis |
| *S. mutans* | Coccobacillary pairs | $CO_2$ | Transl., convex | $\alpha$ (None) | Pits agar | Catalase − | | Caries, endocarditis |
| *ENTEROCOCCI* | | | | | | | | |
| *S. faecalis* | Chains, pairs | None | Transl., gray-green | None ($\alpha$) | | Catalase − | Gp D +, PYR + | |
| *S. faecium* | Chains, pairs | None | Transl., gray-green | $\alpha$, (None) | | Catalase − | Gp D +, PYR + | |
| *S. durans* | Chains, pairs | None | Transl., gray-green | None | | Catalase − | Gp D +, PYR + | |
| GRAM-POSITIVE RODS | | | | | | | | |
| *CORYNEFORMS* | | | | | | | | |
| *Corynebacterium diphtheriae* | Clubbed pleomorphic coccobacilli | Special media | Opaque, white | $\beta$ (10%) | Black colonies & brown halos on Tinsdale medium | Catalase + | Nonmotile | |
| *Listeria monocytogenes* | As above | None | Transl., gray | $\beta$ (Narrow) | | Catalase + | Motile-tumbling | Grows at 4°C |
| *ACTINOMYCETES* | | | | | | | | |
| *Nocardia* spp. | Branching, beaded | Slow-growing | Rough, white-pink | None | Adherent colonies | Catalase + | Acid-fast +(wk) | Aerial hyphae |
| *Actinomyces israelii* | Branching, beaded sulfur granules | Anaerobic | Molar-tooth colonies | None | Spider colonies | Catalase − | Acid-fast − | DFA stain |
| *CLOSTRIDIA* | | | | | | | | |
| *C. perfringens* | Big, square ends | Anaerobic | Smooth, transl. erose border | $\beta$-double zone | | Lecithinase + | Nonmotile | Spores uncommon |
| *C. difficile* | Big, square ends | Anaerobic Special media | Watery, gray erose border | None | Chartreuse fluorescence | | Motile | Horse-barn odor |

*(continued)*

**Table 16.1** Characteristics of common bacterial pathogens (*Continued*)

| Organism group | Stain appearance | Special culture conditions | Colonial characteristics | | | Rapid tests | | Comment |
|---|---|---|---|---|---|---|---|---|
| | | | Morphology | Hemolysis | Other | One | Two | |
| GRAM-NEGATIVE COCCI | | | | | | | | |
| *Neisseria gonorrhoeae* | Intracellular diplococci | Special media | Opaque, gray domed | None | | Oxidase + | Rapid glucose + Rapid maltose − | Rapid enzyme ID |
| *N. meningitidis* | Intracellular diplococci | Special media | Opaque, yellow-gray | None | | Oxidase + | Rapid glucose + Rapid maltose + | Rapid enzyme ID |
| *Moraxella catarrhalis* | Diplococci | None | Raised, opaque yellow | None | | Oxidase + | Rapid glucose − | DNAse + |
| GRAM-NEGATIVE RODS | | | | | | | | |
| *LACTOSE-FERMENTING ENTEROBACTERIACEAE* | | | | | | | | |
| *Escherichia coli* | Short-plump | None | Gray, translucent flat, irreg. edge | $\beta$ (70%) | LF | Indole + | Motile | |
| *Klebsiella* spp. | Short-plump | None | Gray, translucent domed, smooth edge often mucoid | None | LF | Indole −(+) | Nonmotile | |
| *Enterobacter* spp. | Short-plump | None | Gray, translucent domed, smooth edge often mucoid | None | LF | Indole − | Motile | |
| *NON-LACTOSE-FERMENTING ENTEROBACTERIACEAE* | | | | | | | | |
| *Proteus mirabilis* | Medium-plump pleomorphic | None | Gray, translucent Swarms on BA | None | NLF, Browns BA | Indole − | Urease +, motile | Chocolate odor |
| *Providencia* spp. | Medium-plump pleomorphic | None | Gray, translucent | None | NLF, Browns BA | Indole + | Urease −, motile | |
| *Morganella morganii* | Medium-plump pleomorphic | None | Gray, translucent | None | NLF, Browns BA | Indole + | Urease +, motile | |
| *Serratia marcescens* | Long, plump | None | Gray, translucent | None | NLF, red pigment (20%) | Indole − | DNAse + | |
| *Citrobacter* spp. | Long-plump | None | Gray, translucent flat, irregular edge | None | NLF (50% LF) | | | |
| *Salmonella* spp. | Long-plump | Special media | Gray, translucent | None | NLF | H2S + | Motile, Agglut + | |
| *Shigella* spp. | Long-plump | Special media | Gray, translucent flat, irregular edge | None | NLF | | Nonmotile, Agglut + | |
| OTHER AEROBIC GRAM-NEGATIVE RODS | | | | | | | | |
| *Pseudomonas aeruginosa* | Long, thin | None | Gray, translucent flat, irregular edge metallic sheen | $\beta$ (70%) | NLF, green pigment | Oxidase + | Motile | Grape odor |
| *Xanthomonas maltophilia* | Long, thin | None | Gray, translucent pale yellow | None | NLF | Oxidase − DNAse + | Motile | |
| *Acinetobacter baumanii* | Large coccobacillary pairs | None | Transl., convex | None | NLF | Oxidase − | Nonmotile | |
| *Haemophilus influenzae* | Tiny coccobacilli | Special media | Transl., convex | None | | XV requirement | Nonmotile | Musty odor |

| | | | | | | | | |
|---|---|---|---|---|---|---|---|---|
| *Campylobacter jejuni* | Curved, seagull | Special media microaerophilic | Transl., convex | None | | Catalase + | Hippurate + | Darting motility |
| *Legionella* spp. | Coccobacilli | Special media $CO_2$ | Transl., convex opalescent | | | DFA | | DNA probe |
| ANAEROBIC GRAM-NEGATIVE RODS | | | | | | | | |
| *Bacteroides fragilis* group | Pale, pleomorphic, irregular staining | Special media | Gray-white, convex | None | Black colony on BBE agar | Bile + | Resistant Kan, Van, Colistin | |
| Prevotella melaninogenica | Coccobacillary | Special media | Tan, convex | None | Brick-red | Bile − | Resistant K & V Sens colistin | |
| *Fusobacterium nucleatum* | Pointed ends, thin | Special media | Opaque, speckled breadcrumb, smooth | None | Chartreuse | Bile + | Indole + | |

| | |
|---|---|
| $CO_2$ | Requires increased concentrations of this gas for optimal growth. |
| $\beta$ | Colony demonstrates beta hemolysis on blood agar. |
| $\beta$-double zone | Colony has inner zone of complete and outer zone of partial hemolysis. |
| $\alpha$ | Colony demonstrates alpha hemolysis (greening) on blood agar. |
| Push test | Colony can be pushed intact across the surface of the agar plate. |
| Gp A, B, C, D, F | Lancefield group antigen A, B, C, D, or F demonstrated in cell wall. |
| PYR | Pyrrolidonyl arylamidase test. |
| Bile solubility | Organisms are lysed in the presence of bile. |
| LF | Lactose-fermenting organism. |
| NLF | Nonlactose-fermenting organism. |
| Tinsdale | Selective media for isolation of *C. diphtheriae*. |
| Browns BA | Colony turns blood agar a reddish-brown color. |
| Lecithinase | A phospholipase C that hydrolyzes lecithin and sphingomyelin. |
| Indole + | Organism is able to produce indole, a benzopyrrole, from tryptophan. |
| Urease + | Organism is able to hydrolyze urea to ammonia with an increase in pH of maltos C. |
| Rapid glucose/maltose | A rapid procedure for detecting the ability of an organism to break down carbohydrates. |
| Rapid enzyme | Procedures for identifying organisms by detecting presence of constituative enzymes. |
| DNase + | Organism has ability to hydrolyze DNA present in media. |
| Swarming | Growth swarms over the surface of agar plates. |
| BBE agar | Blood-bile esculin medium for grouping anaerobic gram-negative rods. |
| $H_2S$ + | Organism is able to produce hydrogen sulfide. |
| XV requirement | Determines the organism's need for hemin (X) and/or NAD (V) for growth. |
| DFA | Direct fluorescent antibody test. |
| Agglutination+ | Organism agglutinates in the presence of specific antiserum. |
| Hippurate + | Organism is able to hydrolyze sodium hippurate. |

**Table 16.2** Characteristis of other bacterial pathogens

| Organism group | Microscopic appearance | Special culture conditions | Colonial characteristics | | | Rapid tests | | Comment |
|---|---|---|---|---|---|---|---|---|
| | | | Morphology | Hemolysis | Other | One | Two | |
| MYCOBACTERIA | | | | | | | | |
| *M. tuberculosis* | AFB: deep red, thin, beaded cording | Special media, $CO_2$, BACTEC TB Slow growth (wks) | Rough, buff | NA | No pigment | NAP + | Niacin + | DNA probe available |
| *M. avium-intracellulare* | AFB: uniform stain, coccobacillary | As above, blood culture in AIDS | Thin, translucent to opaque | NA | No pigment | NAP − | Biochemically unreactive | DNA probe available |
| *M. haemophilum* | AFB: deep red, short, curved, uniform stain | Hemin required 10% $CO_2$, 28°–32°C + blood cultures | Smooth–rough | NA | No pigment | PZA + | Biochemically unreactive | Seen in AIDS patients |
| *M. genavense* | AFB: clumps, coccobacilli | BACTEC13A broth 2–10 weeks | Pinpoint | NA | Difficult to grow on solid media Requires mycobactin | Catalase + | PZA & urea + | Bacteremic AIDS patients |
| SPIROCHETES | | | | | | | | |
| *Treponema pallidum* | Tight, regular spirals 5–15 $\mu$ | Grown in cell culture, not subcultured | NA | NA | NA | Darkfield microscopy | DFA | Syphilis |
| *Borrelia* | | | | | | | | |
| *B. recurrentis* | Irregular spirals 10–30 $\mu$ gram-negative | Special media requires long-chain fatty acids | NA | NA | NA | Wright's stain of blood smear | | Tick- and louse-borne, relapsing fever |
| *B. burgdorferi* | As above | Grows poorly in artificial media | NA | NA | NA | Western blot serology | PCR (?) | Lyme disease |
| *Leptospira* spp. | Tight, regular semispirals 5–15 $\mu$ | Enriched, semisolid medium | NA | NA | NA | Bacteria seen with darkfield | Serology | |
| MYCOPLASMA | | | | | | | | |
| *M. pneumoniae* | Pleomorphic—cocci, filaments Does not stain | Mycoplasma agar | Pinpoint, 3–20 d, fried-egg appearance | $\beta$ | NA | Urea-, glucose+ | CF serology | |
| *Ureaplasma urealyticum* | As above | Urea-enriched agar pH $< 7.0$ | Pinpoint, 1–4 d | NA | Grows into media | Urea+, glucose− | | Present as normal flora |

| | | | | | | | | |
|---|---|---|---|---|---|---|---|---|
| CHLAMYDIA | | | | | | | | |
| *C. trachomatis* | Small, round bodies on DFA | Cell culture | Intracytoplasmic inclusions on DFA | NA | NA | DFA | Ligase chain reaction, PCR | |
| *C. pneumoniae* | | | | | | Dx established serologically | | Walking pneumonia and pharyngitis |
| BARTONELLA GROUP | | | | | | | | |
| *B. quintana* | Tiny GNR, often clumped | Blood culture media; detected c acridine stain | Tiny, transl., tan punctate on CA in several days | NA | Gummy | DFA | Biochemical ID | Trench fever, cat scratch |
| *B. henselae* | Tiny curved rod, c silver stain, weakly GN | Lysis centrifugation blood culture subed to chocolate | As above | NA | Passed on heart infusion rabbit blood agar | | PCR, IFA | Bacillary angiomatosis, cat scratch disease, bacillary peliosis |
| *Afipia felis* | Tiny, pleomorphic c silver stains weakly GN and intracellular | Cell culture and biphasic brain-heart browth | As above | NA | | Oxidase + | PCR, IFA | Cat scratch ?? |
| WHIPPLE'S BACILLUS | | | | | | | | |
| *Tropheryma whippelii* | Tiny GPR seen c PAS, silver and EM | Not recovered in culture | NA | NA | NA | Tissue bx | PCR | An actinomycete |

$\beta$ Colony demonstrates beta hemolysis.
NAP + P-Nitro-$\alpha$-acetylamino-$\beta$-hydrozxypropiophenone, an analogue of chloramphenicol, inhibits *M. tuberculosis*, but not other mycobacteria.
Niacin + Almost all strains of *M. tuberculosis* accumulates niacin and excretes it into the culture medium; few other mycobacteria do.
PZA + Test for the enzyme pyrazinamidase. Most commonly used to differentiate *M. marinum* from *M. kansasii* and *M. bovis* from *M. tuberculosis*.
DFA Direct fluorescent antibody test.
IFA Indirect fluorescent antibody test.
PCR Polymerase chain reaction.
LCR Ligase chain reaction is a recently developed molecular amplification procedure that can serve as an alternate to the PCR.

indicator in the immediate vicinity of the bacterial colony. The inclusion of blood in the media allows the detection hemolysins produced by organism groups such as the $\beta$ hemolytic streptococci. Other media are designed to enhance the pigment production of organisms such as *Pseudomonas aeruginosa.* MacConkey's agar is an example of a medium that has both selective and differential properties. The presence of crystal violet and bile inhibits the growth of gram-positive organisms, while lactose and a pH indicator permits the visual differentiation of lactose-fermenting and nonlactose-fermenting gram-negative bacilli.

## Liquid and solid media

All media are initially prepared in liquid form. Agar, a polysaccharide derivative of seaweed, can be added later, allowing the production of agar plates or slants (tubes). Both liquid and solid media are used in the clinical microbiology laboratory; each have their own unique advantages and disadvantages. Agar plates and slants have a limited absorptive capacity, making them unsuitable for inocula significantly in excess of 0.05 ml. In contrast, a broth media can accommodate huge inoculum volumes, rendering them more suitable for culturing specimens likely to contain small concentrations of pathogens (e.g., blood, body fluids, exudates, and other specimens unlikely to be contaminated by normal flora). As a result of the oxygen gradient between the top and bottom of a stagnant column of fluid, broth media is able to simultaneously support the growth of obligate aerobes and anaerobes. To achieve the same result with solid media, duplicate plates must be inoculated for incubation in aerobic and anaerobic atmospheres. Finally, broth culture specimens may be maintained under incubation conditions for prolonged periods of time.

Plate media, with their shallow depth and large surface area, suffer large evaporative water losses daily. Unless special measures are taken to control these losses, agar plates lose their capacity to support bacterial growth within a few days. If a solid medium is appropriately inoculated, bacteria will grow in separate, distinct colony-forming units. The advantage to this is twofold. First, the colonies of many bacterial species and/or genera have distinct morphologic characteristics, allowing an early, preliminary identification to be made. This early information is often of significant assistance in the timely selection of antimicrobial agents. Second, the presence of distinct colonies facilitates the preparation of pure subcultures, a requisite for definitive bacterial identification and susceptibility testing.

## Conditions of incubation

Most cultures are incubated in dry air at 35° to 37°C. More humid environments are required for the optimal growth of some pathogens. Higher and lower temperatures can be used to selectively favor the growth of *Campylobacter jejuni* and *Listeria monocytogenes*, respectively. A number of aerobic or facultative organisms, including *C. jejuni* and *M. tuberculosis*, grow either more luxuriantly or obligately, at concentrations of $CO_2$ higher than that found in the atmosphere. The growth of aerobes in broth is accelerated by the enhanced oxygenation that accompanies agitation of the culture media. Cultural recovery of strict anaerobes generally requires both the use of highly reduced medium, such as thioglycollate, and an atmosphere devoid of oxygen.

## Detection times and procedures

Incubation periods vary by specimen type and the nature of the organisms sought. Given the concentration and nature of pathogens typically isolated from throat, sputum, and urine specimens, bacterial growth is generally detected within 18–48 hours of media inoculation. Incubation periods of 3 to 7 days are more typical for body fluids, tissues, and deep wounds, as the microbes found in them are often present in small numbers and are more fastidious in nature (e.g., anaerobes). When certain slow-growing bacteria such as mycobacteria or actinomycetes are sought, incubation periods can reach several weeks.

Growth on solid media is detected visually as distinct colonies or, more rarely, as confluent bacterial lawns. Unfortunately, bacterial growth in broth media is not visually apparent until organism concentrations of $10^6$ organisms/ml or more are reached. Until recently, early detection required the collection of "blind" aliquots from the broth for Gram stain and subculture to solid media. There are now a number of automated or semiautomated instruments that detect early growth indirectly by monitoring increases in $CO_2$ concentrations or pressure changes in the head space gas. These instruments have become the de facto standard against which other methodologies for the culture of blood and mycobacteria must be measured.

## Identifying characteristics of common bacterial pathogens

In Tables 16.1 and 16.2 are abbreviated lists of identifying characteristics of common and recently described bacterial pathogens. The information is intended to provide the clinician with the capacity to make tentative bacterial identifications based on preliminary microbiologic data.

### REFERENCES


Bryant JK, Strand CL. Reliability of blood cultures collected from intravascular catheter versus venipuncture. Am J Clin Pathol 1987;88:113–116.
*Blood culture contamination with coagulase-negative staphylococci were found to be more frequent in specimens collected from intravascular catheters.*

Goldman DA, Pier GB. Pathogenesis of infections related to intravascular catheterization. Clin Microbiol Rev 1993;6:176–192.
*An excellent review of this increasing threat to hospitalized patients.*

Gray LD, Fedorko DP. Laboratory diagnosis of bacterial meningitis. Clin Microbiol Rev 1992;5:130–145.
*A comprehensive review of appropriate techniques for the diagnosis of bacterial meningitis, including discussions of CSF concentration procedures and utilization of antigen-detection procedures.*

Li J, Plorde JJ, Carlson LG. Effects of volume and periodicity on blood cultures. J Clin Microbiol 1994;32:2829–2831.
*Study confirms the linear relationship between blood volume and culture positivity rates, and establishes that the collection of specimens at 30- to 60-minute intervals does not increase yield vis-à-vis simultaneously drawn specimens.*

Lipsky BA. Urinary tract infections in men: epidemiology, pathophysiology, diagnosis and treatment. Ann Intern Med 1989;110:138–150.
*Most studies of urinary tract infections have been done in predominantly female populations. This study establishes several unique characteristics of this common infection in males.*

Lipsky BA, Gates J, Tenover FC, Plorde JJ. Factors affecting the clinical value for acid-fast bacilli. Rev Infect Dis 1984;6:214–222.
*Discusses the factors affecting the clinical value of direct acid-fast stains and confirms their high sensitivity and specificity, when properly performed, for the diagnosis of pulmonary tuberculosis.*

Maki DG, Weise CE, Sarafin HW. A semiquantitative culture method for identifying intravenous-catheter-related infection. N Engl J Med 1977;296: 1305–1309.

*The original description of the most widely used procedure for the laboratory diagnosis of intravenous-catheter-relation infections. A golden oldie.*

Morris AJ, Wilson ML, Mirrett S, Reller LB. Rationale for selective use of anaerobic blood cultures. J Clin Microbiol 1993;31:2110–2113.

*The authors' data suggest that anaerobic bacteremias occur in predictable clinical settings, and that it may be cost-effective to limit the use of anaerobic blood cultures to these settings.*

Morris AJ, Wilson SJ, Marx CE, Wilson MI, Mirrett S, Reller LB. Clinical impact of bacteria and fungi recovered only from broth cultures. J Clin Microbiol 1995;33:161–165.

*It is common to culture tissues and body fluids, excluding blood and urine, on both solid and liquid media. The authors point out that microorganisms isolated exclusively from a liquid medium are frequently contaminants.*

Pezzlo M. Detection of urinary tract infection by rapid methods. Clin Microbiol Rev 1988;1:268-280.

*A good review of a very commonly misused diagnostic technique.*

Raad II, Bodey GP. Infectious complications of indwelling vascular catheters. Clin Infect Dis 1992;15:197–210.

*A "state-of-the-art" clinical article.*

Salzman MB, Isenberg HD, Rubin LG. Use of disinfectants to reduce microbial contamination of hubs of vascular catheters. J Clin Microbiol 1993;31:475–479.

*Colonization of vascular catheter hubs is an increasing antecedent of both catheter-induced bacteremia and the source of contamination of blood culture specimens. The authors address procedures to control such colonization.*

Siegman-Igra Y, Anglim AM, Shapiro DE, Adal KA, Strain BA, Farr BM. Diagnosis of vascular catheter-related bloodstream infection: a meta-analysis. J Clin Microbiol 1997;35:928–936.

Strand CL, Wajsbort RR, Sturmann K. Effect of iodophor vs iodine tincture skin preparation on blood culture contamination rate. JAMA 1993;269:1004–1006.

*Preparation of the skin with iodine tincture decreases blood culture contamination rate, vis-à-vis iodophor preparation.*

Torres A et al. Specificity of endotracheal aspiration, protected specimen brush, and bronchoalveolar lavage in mechanically ventilated patients. Am Rev Respir Dis 1993;147:952–957.

*A good review.*

Von Graevenitz A, Amsterdam D. Microbiologic aspects of peritonitis associated with continuous ambulatory peritoneal dialysis. Clin Microbiol Rev 1992;5:36–48.

*Peritoneal fluid cultures are frequently negative in patients with bacterial peritonitis. This review discusses factors that contribute to this situation and microbiologic techniques for improving bacterial culture yield.*

# 17

# Clinical Virology

RHODA L. ASHLEY

Laboratory tests for viral diagnosis include cell culture methods for viral isolation, rapid assays that detect viral macromolecules, molecular techniques such as polymerase chain reaction (PCR) that amplify and identify viral nucleic acids, and serologic tests that detect serum antibody responses to viral infections (Fig. 17.1). With the advent of molecular techniques and availability of reagents to detect viral antigens and nucleic acids, the spectrum of tests offered and the complexity of specimen requirements has increased dramatically. Communication between health care providers and the laboratory is essential to assure that the most effective tests are used for each situation.

## Specimen Collection

Specimens for viral detection should be collected early in the illness from the most appropriate site(s) as determined by clinical presentation. In general, methods that result in collection of cells rather than exudate provide the highest yield (Table 17.1).

### Respiratory tract specimens

Swabs, washes, and aspirates are the most common specimens. Swabs should not be moistened prior to sampling. Washes and aspirates should not be diluted.

#### Throat swab (TS)

A dry cotton swab is rubbed firmly over the posterior pharynx or both tonsils and over any lesions. The openings of Stensen's ducts are swabbed when mumps is suspected.

#### Nasopharyngeal (NP) swab

An NP swab with flexible wire shaft and small cotton or Dacron tip is gently inserted through the nostril to the nasopharynx, then gently rotated before removal. TS and NP specimens may be combined in a single vial.

#### Nasal wash

This method is preferred to swab collection for respiratory syncytial virus (RSV). Sterile buffered saline (5 ml) is drawn into a sterile bulb syringe and, with the patient lying on his or her side, the solution is instilled into the nose and quickly aspirated back into the bulb. The sample is placed into a sterile container.

#### Tracheal aspirates

Transtracheal or transbronchial aspirates are preferred to sputum for lower respiratory tract pathogen recovery because of the risk of contamination of sputum with oral secretions. These are sent undiluted.

#### Bronchoalveolar lavage

The affected area is identified by bronchoscopy, then washed with 5–10 ml sterile saline. The sample is aspirated and a minimum of 5 ml is placed in a sterile vial for transport.

### Gastrointestinal specimens

Rectal swabs and stool are the most common specimens. Gastric lavage and biopsy material from the gastrointestinal tract can also be processed for viral detection. Rectal swabs from patients with aseptic meningitis or motor neuron diseases may be sent for enterovirus isolation when molecular tests are unavailable. Stool or rectal swabs may be used for diagnosis of gastroenteritis syndromes caused by Norwalk agent, rotavirus, astrovirus, and adenovirus.

#### Rectal swab (RS)

A swab is gently inserted far enough into the rectum to dirty it, then is placed immediately into transport medium.

#### Stool

Collect 5–10 grams in a sterile container for transport.

### Urine

First-voided morning urine is sent, undiluted, for isolation of cytomegalovirus (CMV), adenovirus, and herpes simplex virus (HSV) and is the best specimen for isolation of mumps virus after shedding from respiratory sites has ceased. Papillomaviruses and polyomaviruses (JC and BK) are also shed in urine. Molecular techniques are required to detect these viruses; therefore, the laboratory should be apprised if these pathogens are suspected.

### Mucocutaneous lesions

Varicella zoster virus (VZV), HSV, and some Coxsackie viruses can be isolated from vesicular or ulcerative lesions. Macular lesions rarely yield viable virus. Cotton, Dacron, rayon, and polyester swabs are all acceptable for viral culture. Calcium alginate swabs inhibit HSV growth and should not be used. Vesicles are opened and firmly swabbed with a cotton or Dacron swab. Vigorous swabbing is necessary to collect cells both for culture and for direct antigen or nucleic acid detection. Vesicle fluid may also contain cultivable virus and may be collected via aspiration with a 20-gauge needle or by wicking the fluid onto a swab once the vesicle is opened. In collecting from mucous membranes of the mouth or genital tract, a dry cotton swab should be used to

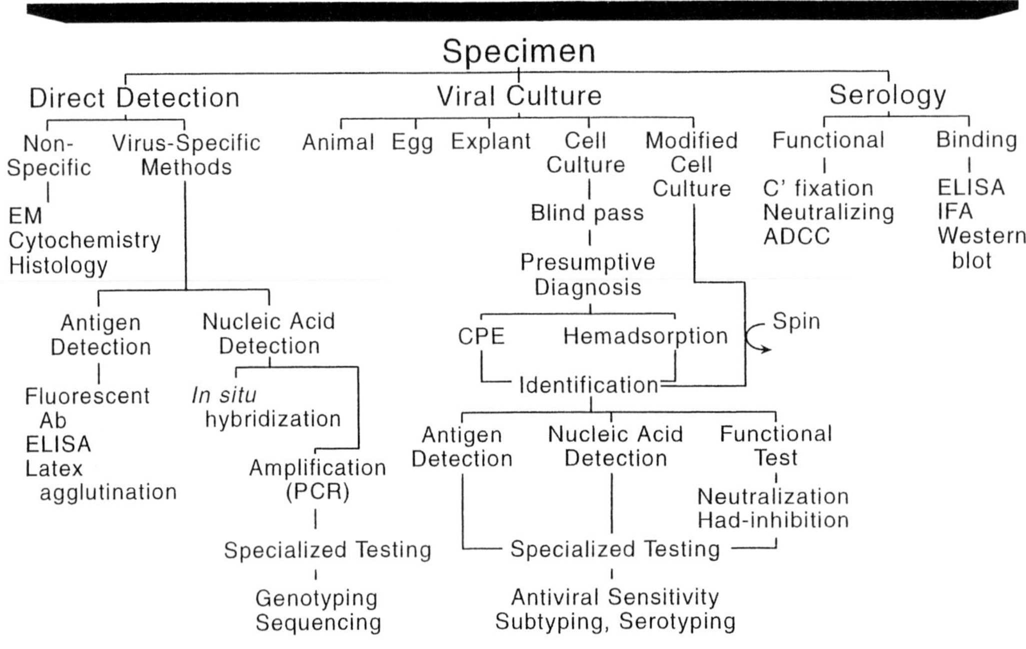


**Fig. 17.1** Strategies for viral diagnosis.

**Table 17.1** Collection and transport of viral specimens

| Specimen for culture or direct FA | Collection method | VTM | Transport (T) |
|---|---|---|---|
| Aspirates and lavages | Collect in sterile container 5 ml minimum. | None | Cold pack or −70°C |
| Body fluids | Sterile container; 5 ml minimum. | None | Cold pack or −70°C |
| Bone marrow | Collect in heparinized syringe or transfer into heparinized blood tube. | None | Room temperature |
| Buffy coat | Draw into 10 ml green or lavender top tube (3–5 ml for pediatric patients). | None | Room temperature |
| Cerebrospinal fluid | Sterile container; 1 ml minimum. | None | Cold pack or −70°C |
| Cervical swab | Clean secretions with cotton swab. | 2 ml | Cold pack or −70°C |
| | Using new swab, rub exocervix. Avoid vaginal contamination. | | |
| Conjunctiva swab; separate swabs for each eye; may be pooled. | Rub the lower conjunctiva with swab moistened in sterile PBS. | 2 ml | Cold pack or −70°C |
| Lesion swab | Vigorously rub base of lesion after clearing pus or necrotic debris. | 2 ml | Cold pack or −70°C |
| | Unroof vesicles and collect fluid plus basal cells. | | |
| Nasal wash | With patient lying on side, instil 3–5 ml of PBS with bulb syringe into nostril; suction back immediately. | None | Cold pack or −70°C |
| Nasopharyngeal swab (NP) | Insert dry swab on flexible wire through nostril to posterior nasopharynx. Rotate and withdraw. | 2 ml | Cold pack or −70°C |
| Rectal swab (RS), do *not* pool with NP or TS | Insert dry swab, rotate then withdraw; RS should be soiled. | 2 ml | Cold pack or −70°C |
| Stool | Collect 5–10 g in clean container. | None | Cold pack |
| Throat swab (TS); can pool with NP | Rub dry swab over posterior pharynx or tonsillar fossae and over any lesions. | 2 ml | Cold pack or −70°C |

gently remove secretions or exudate from lesion sites before sampling.

### Cerebrospinal fluid (CSF) and body fluids

Cerebrospinal fluid (CSF) can yield HSV, enteroviruses, human immunodeficiency virus type 1 (HIV-1), human herpes virus 6 (HHV-6), and, less commonly, VZV, CMV, measles, mumps, and adenoviruses from individuals with central nervous system (CNS) disease. A minimum of 1.0 ml should be collected aseptically and sent in a separate, sterile container. Other body fluids obtained aseptically from pericardium or peritoneum are sent without dilution in sterile containers.

### Blood

Blood for CMV or HIV culture is collected in green or lavender top tubes and transported at room temperature. Bone marrow is collected in a heparinized syringe and transported at room temperature.

### Specimen collection for molecular virology tests

Specimens to be submitted for detection of viral nucleic acid after amplification of either the target molecule or other test components must be collected under aseptic conditions that minimize the risk of contamination with exogenous nucleic acids. The collection site should be isolated with sterile drapes and gloves, masks, and caps should be worn during the sampling procedure. Mucocutaneous sites and lesions are sampled using Culturettes.™ Tissues are sent without additional fluid added. A minimum of 0.5 ml of CSF, urine, or plasma is sent in sterile collection vials. To avoid handling and possible contamination in the laboratory, specimens should be dedicated for molecular tests; if other tests are required, additional specimens should be collected.

## Specimen Transport

### Processing specimens for cell culture before transport

Swabs and tissues being submitted for viral isolation or for tests requiring intact cells are placed in viral transport medium (VTM) to maintain cell integrity and prevent proteolytic breakdown of infectious virus. VTM is composed of a buffered protein solution with antibacterial and antifungal agents. Because of these added elements, swabs should not be moistened with VTM before sampling. Leak-free vials are used for all specimens; those with snap caps or internally threaded caps are unacceptable. With the exception of blood and bone marrow, which are sent at room temperature, specimens for viral culture are sent to the laboratory on wet ice or cold packs unless transport requires more than 2 days, in which case, specimens are frozen immediately at −70°C and shipped on dry ice (Table 17.1). Freezing at −20°C reduces viability of most viruses.

### Processing specimens for antigen detection

Specimens being submitted for in situ tests such as immunofluorescence require intact cells and, therefore, should be handled in the same way as specimens being submitted for cell culture. If collected properly, most specimens contain enough infected cells to be divided for both cell culture and antigen-detection tests.

Specimens for solution-based tests for viral antigen or nucleic acid do not require intact, infected cells. Specimens for these tests should be sent in the sample buffer compatible with the particular test. As these solutions vary with manufacturer and with the test, the laboratory should be consulted before sampling. Most transport solutions for antigen or DNA detection serve to disrupt infected cells and will destroy viral infectivity as well. Therefore, if both viral isolation and antigen detection are desired, *separate specimens* must be obtained.

### Processing for viral serology

Blood collected for viral serology must be processed before transport. Blood is allowed to clot and the serum is removed to a sterile, leakproof vial for transport with cold packs or, for prolonged transit, on dry ice.

### Packaging for transport

All specimens must be placed in a leakproof container with the requisition form in a separate plastic bag for transport. Shipment of biological specimens by commercial carriers must adhere to federal regulations, which require that the specimen be wrapped in sufficient material to absorb the entire specimen should a leak occur. The wrapped specimen and the separately wrapped requisition form are then placed in a crushproof and leakproof container, which is then enclosed, with insulation, cold packs, or dry ice, in a labeled shipping container.

## Viral Culture Techniques

### Animal and explant systems

Because cell culture systems have been developed for most human viral pathogens, use of animals, organ or tissue explant cultures, and eggs is generally limited to reference or research laboratories. The most readily available animal system, the newborn suckling mouse, is used for Coxsackie virus A and for togavirus isolation. Explants of human organs or tissues are used for fastidious viruses such as rotovirus (intestine explants), coronavirus (embryonic trachea), or polyoma viruses (glial explants).

### Cell culture

Conventional culture continues to be a major tool in the diagnostic lab. A broad spectrum of viral isolates can be amplified and detected in cell culture, providing a clear advantage over other virus-detection methods. The limitations of cell culture include the variable nature of cell lines and the resulting need for comprehensive quality-control programs and the need for highly trained personnel to recognize the different patterns of cell pathology caused by individual viruses. A further difficulty with cell culture systems, particularly nonhuman primate cells, is the possibility that endogenous viruses in the cell culture will either inhibit replication of viruses from the specimen or produce misleading cytopathology in inoculated cells.

Three types of cell cultures—primary, semicontinuous, and continuous—are used in combination to accommodate the variation in host range and growth characteristics of different viruses. The laboratory is guided in its selection of cells to inoculate by

**Table 17.2** Identifying characteristics of human viruses in culture

| Virus | Permissive cell system | Time to CPE | Comments |
|---|---|---|---|
| Adenovirus 1–39 | Hep 2, 293 | 2–7 days | Freeze/thaw passage to increase titer. May also grow in HDF. Grapelike clusters of infected cells. |
| Adenovirus 40, 41 | 293 | 2–14 days | Fastidious; difficult to grow. |
| Coxsackie A7,9,16 | HDF | 1–7 days | Other serotypes require animal inoculation. |
| Coxsackie B | Hep-2, PMK, BGM | 1–7 days | Poor growth in HDF. Uniform cell rounding or teardrop-shaped cells—degeneration of monolayer. |
| Cytomegalovirus | HDF only | 1–25 days | Trypsin passage to increase titer. Slow-growing. Scattered, focal patches of rounded cells. |
| EBV | Cord blood or B-cell transformation | 4–6 weeks | Time-consuming, impractical for normal use. |
| Echovirus | HDF; also PMK | 1–7 days | Poor growth in heteroploid cells. Uniform cell rounding. Degeneration of monolayer. |
| Enteroviruses | HDF, PMK, also BGM | 1–7 days | Combination of culture systems is desirable. |
| HHV-6,7 | T-cell lines or co-cultivation with cord blood cells or PBMC | 7–14 days | Cultivation difficult. |
| HIV-1 | Human PBMC cocultivation | 2–4 weeks | T-cell lines also available. |
| HSV-1,2 | HDF, ML, PRK | 1–7 days | Focal refractive, granular cells. Degeneration of monolayers at edges. |
| HTLV-1, II | Human PBMC cocultivation | 2–4 weeks | |
| Influenza | PMK, MDCK | 2–14 days | Large granular or vacuolated cells. Hemadsorption with guinea pig cells. |
| Measles | PMK | 5–8 days | Syncytia, giant cells. |
| Mumps | PMK, Hep-2 | 6–14 days | Syncytia and vacuolation. Hemadsorption with guinea pig cells important. |
| Parainfluenza | PMK; also Hep-2, HDF | 1–14 days | Irregular syncytia mainly with para 2. Hemadsorption with guinea pig cells. |
| Parvovirus B19 | Human bone marrow cells | 2–3 weeks | Not widely available. |
| Poliovirus | PMK, Hep-2, HDF | | Uniform small rounded cells. Monolayer degeneration usually rapid. |
| Polyomaviruses | Primary human fetal kidney or glial cells | 4–8 weeks | Not widely available. Vacuolaton and degeneration. |
| Rhinovirus | HDF; also BGM | 1–14 days | Round, refractile cells. Acid labile. |
| RSV | Hep 2; also PMK | 2–5 days | Syncytia |
| Rubella | AGMK, LLC | 14–21 days | Interferes with infection by second "signal virus." |
| VZV | HDF only | 3–21 days | Requires actively growing cells. Trypsin pass to increase titer. Slow-growing. |

specimen site, syndrome, and the virus suspected (Table 17.2). Communication with the laboratory is, therefore, a key factor in the effective use of cell culture isolation systems for viral diagnosis.

Primary cell cultures have been freshly prepared from animal tissue and can be maintained in culture for only one or two generations or "passages" before undergoing genetic changes that alter permissiveness for viral infection. Primary cultures contain a number of different cell types, including differentiated cells, which are predominantly diploid and are characterized by contact inhibition in culture. Monkey kidney (PMK) or rabbit kidney (PRK) provide commonly used primary cultures for virus isolation. Suspension cultures of human peripheral blood mononuclear cells (PBMC) are used in limited passage numbers for human retrovirus isolation. Primary culture of human embryonic tissue is extremely sensitive for many viruses but is not widely available.

Semicontinuous lines are derived from primary cell cultures and are characterized by maintenance of diploid chromosomes, and by the selection of a single type of cell, most often fibroblasts. These lines remain stable for a longer period of time in culture than do primary cell cultures but will eventually either die or undergo a selection process for cells that differ substantially in character from the original line. The most useful lines include human diploid fibroblasts (HDF) derived from primary cultures of human foreskin or human embryonic tissues.

Continuous cell lines are derived from those cells that survive the "crisis" observed in long-term semicontinuous cultures. These lines are characterized by heteroploidy and their lack of contact inhibition and can be maintained in culture indefinitely. Widely used continuous lines such as HeLa, Hep-2, or A549 lines are derived from human neoplasms. Cell lines such as 293 have been altered by viral elements for continuous culture but do not express the virus used for transformation. Lines derived from nonhuman primates (BGM, Vero, AGMK, LLC) and other mammalian cells such as canine kidney (MDCK) or mink lung (ML) are selectively used in addition to human diploid and heteroploid cells to isolate specific viruses (Table 17.2).

## Presumptive diagnosis of viruses in culture

Once inoculated, cultures are placed in rotating roller drums and observed daily for 7 days, then every 2 days for an additional 7–21 days. Cytopathic effect (CPE) is readily observed by light microscopy for many viruses (Table 17.2). The speed with which CPE appears, the rate of spread of the CPE, the cell lines affected, and the appearance of the infected cells all help make a presumptive diagnosis (Fig. 17.1).

Other viruses may not cause distinctive or rapid CPE but, rather, cause cell changes that can be detected with an additional step. For example, influenza, parainfluenza, and mumps viruses code for hemagglutinin proteins that are inserted into the infected cell membrane. As a result, adsorption of guinea pig red blood cells are used to detect infection. This hemadsorption step is performed blindly 2–5 days and 10–14 days after inoculation and in cell cultures of respiratory specimens showing CPE consistent with one of the hemadsorbing viruses.

Other viruses require special conditions to detect in culture. For example, rubella does not induce visible CPE but can be detected by its ability to interfere with replication of a second "signal" virus. When rubella is suspected, LLC or AGMK cells are inoculated, incubated for 10–14 days, then challenged with echovirus 7. After an additional 2–4 days, failure of the signal virus to cause typical CPE is taken as presumptive evidence for rubella. If rubella is suspected, the laboratory must be notified so that it can initiate this specialized culture.

## Blind passage of putative isolates

When CPE is absent or atypical, cells are subcultured or "passed" to new cells to amplify the titer of virus. This technique also helps identify nonspecific cytotoxicity commonly caused by semen, urine, rectal, and genital tract specimens. Toxic elements in the original culture are diluted out after passage so that cytotoxic effects are reduced or eliminated. To amplify most suspected viruses by passage, cells are scraped from the culture tube or dislodged by shaking with sterile glass beads and the resulting slurry is added to fresh cells. If adenovirus is suspected, the cells are frozen and thawed before passing to new cells. For highly cell-associated viruses such as CMV and VZV, the infected cells are disrupted with trypsin before passage. Blind passage adds to the sensitivity of culture but requires an additional 1 to 2 weeks to complete.

## Definitive identification of viral isolates

The combination of cytopathic effect patterns, the rate of CPE progression, and the cells permissive for infection can provide a presumptive diagnosis. Putative virus isolates are definitively identified by biologic methods or by antigen or genome detection. Rhinovirus isolates are confirmed by their inability to infect cells after pretreatment with medium at pH 3.0. Neutralization of virus infectivity and resulting inhibition of CPE or hemadsorption can be performed using virus-specific antibodies or intersecting antibody pools for viruses, such as enteroviruses, which have many serotypes. Solid-phase or soluble-antigen detection using virus-specific antibodies and colorimetric or fluorescing signals is a more rapid and cost-effective method than neutralization to identify viral isolates with limited serotypes or group-specific antigens. These tests allow the confirmation step to be combined with a subtyping or serotyping step by using type-specific antisera.

## Modified cell culture methods

Conventional culture systems provide the ability to detect the broadest possible spectrum of viruses—occasionally, more than one in a single specimen. However, the isolation and identification process can take days to weeks (Table 17.2). To increase the speed of virus diagnosis, several modified culture systems are now widely used. Centrifugation of the inoculum onto cell monolayers speeds detection, possibly by increasing the contact between virus and cell membrane or by altering the cell membrane to enhance viral entry. In a further modification, the spin amplification step is performed using cell monolayers grown on circular coverslips and incubated in shell vials. The coverslips are removed after 16–48 hours and reacted with virus-specific antisera to detect viral antigen before CPE is apparent. For detection of HSV and CMV, antisera directed against early antigens that are expressed in advance of structural proteins provide the basis for rapid staining after overnight culture. Shell vial assays have been adapted to 24- or 48-well plates, which allows simultaneous setup of multiple specimens. While convenient for the laboratory, this method increases the risk of contaminating the culture of one specimen with detectable levels of virus from an unrelated specimen in a neighboring well.

While the combination of culture amplification and identification steps can provide rapid results, low-titer viruses may not be sufficiently amplified to be detected. The sensitivity of shell vial or spin amplification tests versus conventional culture varies widely with the cells used, the virus, the antibody reagent(s), and the length of time the shell vials and conventional cultures are incubated. While shell vial sensitivity can approach that of culture in studies in which the conventional cultures are incubated 7 days, comparisons after longer culture times reduce the relative sensitivity of shell vial tests. Shell vial–type tests are limited to the virus to which the antibody reagent is directed. Moreover, viral isolates cannot be harvested for further analyses, such as those to determine sensitivity to antiviral agents. For optimal diagnosis and flexibility, conventional culture on an appropriate variety of cell lines should be performed in parallel.

Transgenic reporter systems are being developed to rapidly detect virus. For example the enzyme-linked virus inducible system (ELVIS™) is comprised of BHK cells genetically engineered to contain a reporter $\beta$-galactosidase gene under the control of a promoter for HSV. Transactivation of the HSV promoter by the incoming viral structural protein VP16 results in expression of the reporter gene. This gene product is detected within 6–24 hours by addition of the enzyme's substrate, which, in turn, results in color change. The tests are specific and very sensitive.

## Direct Detection Methods

The most rapid viral diagnostic methods detect virions, viral macromolecules, or infected cells in the specimen without culture amplification (Fig. 17.1). Electron microscopy or immune electron microscopy are effective for viruses with distinctive ultrastructure and may be useful for special cases. For routine use, these methods have been replaced in most laboratories by virus-specific direct detection methods. Similarly, cytochemical stains of smears or cytospin preparations can be performed to detect cells altered in appearance by viral infection. However, these methods are less sensitive and less specific than stains based on detecting viral macromolecules in specimens.

With the exception of labile viruses such as RSV or VZV, immunostaining methods are less sensitive than culture or modified culture techniques. However, the tests are completed within hours of specimen receipt and do not require infectious virus. As with shell vial tests, the diagnosis is limited to those viruses sought. Thus, for optimal diagnostic power, conventional culture should be requested along with direct detection tests.

### Immunostains for antigen detection

Immunostaining methods use virus-specific antibodies and a variety of signals. Immunofluorescence (IF) and "fluorescent antibody" (FA) tests use fluors such as fluoroscene or rhodamine, while immunoperoxidase (IP) methods use the enzyme horseradish peroxidase to detect viral antigen in intact cells. Enzyme-linked immunosorbent assays (ELISA) use other enzymes in in situ formats.

Most immunostains, regardless of signal, use an indirect format that entails a two-step binding procedure to, first, bind a specific, unlabeled antivirus antibody and, second, to add an enzyme- or fluor-conjugated secondary antibody that is directed against the species-specific epitopes of the primary antibody. Because the secondary antibody can bind to many sites on the primary antibody, indirect immunostaining assays are about tenfold more sensitive than assays using a conjugated primary antibody. This strategy also allows the use of a number of primary antibodies against different viruses in a specimen while a single secondary system is used to detect the binding of virus-specific antibody. In this type of multiplex test, cells are dripped onto slides with multiple rings to separate tests or cells are dispended into microwells. Tests are performed on samples with sufficient intact cells to provide 20 cells per low-power field per test. In situ immunostaining tests allow a measure of specificity; most viruses have a typical distribution of antigen in infected cells that can be readily distinguished from nonspecific binding of reagents.

### Solid-phase immunodetection tests

Cells are not the only substrate for antigen detection. Capture antibodies specific for a number of viruses have been bound to polystyrene plates, latex beads, or polystyrene beads. The specimen is treated with detergent to solubilize the viral antigen and the treated specimen is added to the capture system. Bound antigen is then incubated with a primary, antivirus antiserum and, if necessary, an enzyme-conjugated secondary antiserum. These tests have the advantage of not requiring intact cells; the specimen preparation is usually easier and, often, is accomplished as the specimen is transported or stored. Further, these tests can be automated for high throughput and rapid results. The disadvantage of these tests is the arbitrary cutoff values assigned to distinguish a positive test from background or nonspecific reactivity. On occasion, a true positive will be obscured by background binding or a true negative will be mistakenly interpreted as positive due to nonspecific binding.

### Direct detection of viral nucleic acid

In situ hybridization of virus-specific DNA or RNA probes can be performed to detect viral genome or mRNA within cells. While this technique offers some of the same advantages as immunostaining or solid-phase antigen-detection tests, acceptable sensitivity has been difficult to achieve. Most nucleic acid–detection tests are performed after target amplification.

## Molecular Detection Methods

### Target amplification

A number of protocols have been published for amplification of viral DNA and RNA. The most widely used technique is the polymerase chain reaction (PCR), which amplifies DNA or cDNA generated from viral RNA. Other methods are rapidly becoming routine for RNA amplification as well.

#### PCR

This technique uses oligonucleotide primer sets complementary to virus target sequences 50–1500 nucleotides apart on opposite strands of the DNA. The sample DNA is denatured at high temperature to allow primer annealing, then primers are extended by a temperature-stable DNA polymerase to yield two copies per DNA molecule of target sequence. The process is repeated ("thermocycling") to allow exponential amplification of the target sequence. Nested primers internal to the first set of primers may be used after conventional PCR to dilute out the effects of inhibitors in the sample or to increase sensitivity. Viral RNA can be detected by conversion to DNA using reverse transcriptase and subsequent PCR amplification.

#### Transcription-based amplification system (TAS)

Transcription-based amplification systems, including nucleic acid sequence–based amplification (NASBA) and an isothermal self-sustaining sequence replication ("3SR") method, are examples of systems that amplify RNA. Both methods use T7 phage RNA polymerase promoter on primer ends in concert with reverse transcriptase and RNAse H to generate multiple target RNA molecules via a double-stranded DNA intermediate and antisense RNA copies of the target. TAS methods are rapid, sensitive, and highly selective for viral RNA molecules, which can be useful to detect RNA viruses. TAS can also be used to distinguish active DNA virus infection from quiescent or latent infections by detecting RNA transcripts.

#### Ligation-activated transcription

This method uses DNA ligase, reverse transcriptase, RNA polymerase, and RNAse H in a single isothermic reaction to generate amplified RNA transcripts from DNA target molecule that has been ligated to a partially double-stranded hairpin primer containing the T7 RNA polymerase. The method is rapid and self-sustaining and can be used to amplify either RNA, through a reverse transcription step, or DNA.

### Strand-displacement amplification (SDA)

SDA is another isothermal reaction system that uses a primer with a Hinc II restriction site that is annealed to target DNA and extended. Hinc II is used to nick the recognition site, displacing the downstream strand. The polymerization-nicking-displacement cycle continues as a nickable Hinc II site is regenerated.

## Probe amplification

These methods include ligase chain reaction and the Q-$\beta$ replicase system and serve to amplify a probe that, in contrast to PCR primers, covers all or most of the target sequence.

## Detection systems

The final step in these amplification systems is the identification of the amplified sequences by binding of a target-specific probe. These probes may be isotopically labeled (Southern blot), but recent tests incorporate enzymatic or chemiluminescent signals to detect bound probe. Protocols and reagents are also available to detect low levels of viral nucleic acids by amplification of the signal in addition to or rather than the target molecule. These "Christmas tree" methods use multiple enzymes, multiple probes, or a combination of multiple probes and multiple enzymes (branched-chain detection) spaced to amplify the signal. Signal amplification by branched chain allows binding of as many as 300 enzyme signal molecules per target molecule.

Amplified target sequences can also be detected by hybrid capture, a method that uses antibodies to duplex DNA. Bound target is detected by a second enzyme-labeled antibody that catalyzes a color change.

A recent advance allows direct detection of amplified sequences via the endonucleolytic activity of the *Thermus aquaticus* (Taq) polymerase. A fluorogenic reporter dye is released upon completion of each PCR cycle and cleavage of the reporter probe. Fluorescence cannot be released in the absence of the viral sequence being sought. Because extra steps are not necessary to identify the amplified sequences, the resulting test is rapid as well as specific and sensitive.

The advantages of PCR and other amplification methods include speed of detection and a high level of sensitivity, allowing diagnosis from low-volume specimens or those with low viral titer. In some cases, such as HIV-1 infection, diagnosis by PCR can precede that possible by seroconversion by days to weeks. Nucleic acid amplification is particularly valuable for viruses that are difficult to culture in the laboratory (Table 17.3). Further, infectivity of the virion is not required; thus, archival samples can be tested. Specimens from acute infections of class 4 agents, including arenaviruses (Lassa, Junin, Machupo) and filoviruses (Marburg, Ebola), can be subjected to molecular diagnostic methods in order to avoid culture amplification of infectious virus.

The disadvantages of these approaches include the high cost of the special facilities and training required to perform these tests accurately and of unique reagents that may not be subject to market pressure. In many areas, reimbursement for molecular diagnostic tests is limited. In addition, as with direct antigen-detection tests, the test diagnosis is limited to the virus-specific reagents selected; the broad spectrum of findings possible with culture techniques have not been achieved with current nucleic acid–amplification tests. Multiplex PCR tests incorporating several primer sets in one test are designed to overcome this problem. Finally, the exquisite sensitivity of PCR coupled with the need for only fragments of viral nucleic acid for a positive result require that caution be applied when interpreting test results, since finding a specific viral genome segment does not guarantee its etiology in the disease under study.

As summarized in Table 17.3, reagents are available and protocols have been published for molecular detection of most human viral pathogens. Due to the higher cost of nucleic acid–amplification methods, the decision to seek a diagnosis by one of these methods should take into account the need for rapid and sensitive testing as well as the nature and availability of alternative tests. In some cases, such as monitoring antiviral therapy of HIV and hepatitis C infections, molecular testing is the only available alternative.

## Viral Serologies

Testing for serum antibody to a viral pathogen is the principal diagnostic test to determine the immune status of an individual. In particular, seroconversion, as determined by rising antibody titers between samples drawn during acute illness and 4–8 weeks later, is diagnostic. Serology provides an alternative method when sampling or transport conditions for virus culture cannot be met, for viruses that are difficult to culture, or in cases where molecular testing is not feasible. Detection of antibodies can also be diagnostic in infections, such as hepatitis A, in which viral shedding has ceased when symptoms develop. Finally, with the recent development of virus-specific vaccines, serology provides a means of determining immune status when vaccination is considered and may also be used to track vaccine recipients for waning protective immunity. The use of serology for diagnosing central nervous system disease by demonstrating antibodies in CSF or to diagnose fetal or neonatal infections is rapidly being supplanted by molecular diagnostic tests. In general, with the exception of determining immune status to guide vaccination decisions or to detect silent carriers of chronic viruses such as hepatitis B or HSV-2, diagnostic methods should emphasize the demonstation of virus or viral macromolecules.

Methods for detecting antiviral antibodies fall into two categories: functional tests and binding tests. Functional assays include neutralization of virus infectivity, inhibition of hemadsorption, and complement fixation. These tests have been largely supplanted by binding assays, which are, in general, more sensitive and more amenable to quality control and automation. Binding assays include immunoassay formats in which the viral target antigen is bound to a solid surface such as a microwell plate, paper strip, or bead, or to a capture antibody on such a substrate. Serum is added and the bound antibodies detected with a secondary antibody directed against human immunoglobulin. The secondary antibody is conjugated to a signal molecule, including a variety of fluors (immunofluorescence assays) or enzymes (enzyme immunoassays, or EIAs). EIAs use color-changing substrates or light-emitting chemicals as signals. Latex agglutination assays use antigen-coated latex particles which agglutinate to a visible endpoint when crosslinked by specific antibodies. These tests are rapid and effective for serologic screening but lack the sensitivity to provide reproducible quantitative end points.

More-specialized binding tests include Western blot methods,

**Table 17.3** System-specific molecular diagnostic tests

| System | Specimens used | Diagnostic application | Alternative test |
|---|---|---|---|
| EYE | | | |
| CMV | Aqueous, subretinal fluid; retinal biopsies | Retinitis | Culture |
| EBV | Corneal scrapings | | Test of choice |
| Enterovirus | Conjuntival scapings | Conjunctivitis | Culture |
| HSV | Corneal, conjunctival scrapings | Dendritic keratitis, particularly stromal keratitis | Culture |
| VZV | Vitreous fluid | Acute necrotizing retinitis | Culture |
| GI TRACT AND LIVER | | | |
| Adenovirus 40,41 | Stool | Gastroenteritis | Culture |
| Hepatitis A | Stool | Hepatitis (active) | Serology |
| Hepatitis B | Serum | Hepatitis; monitor antiviral therapy Hepatocellular carcinoma | Test of choice |
| Hepatitis C | Serum | Hepatitis; genotype, monitor antiviral therapy | |
| Hepatitis G | Serum | Non A-E hepatitis | |
| Rotavirus | Stool | Diarrhea; identifying groups A, B, C | Antigen detection |
| STDS | | | |
| HIV | Blood | Detection; monitor antiviral therapy | |
| | | Condyloma, genital tract dysplasia | DNA detection |
| HPV | Biopsy | Atypical lesions | Culture |
| HSV | Lesion scrapings CSF | Recurrent meningitis | Test of choice |
| CONGENITAL, NEONATAL | | | |
| CMV | Urine | Neonatal diagnosis | Culture |
| HIV-1 | Blood | Neonatal diagnosis | Test of choice |
| HSV | CSF | Neonatal diagnosis | Test of choice |
| Parvo B19 | Blood | Fetal infection | Test of choice |
| Rubella | Blood, brain, fetal tissue | Congenital rubella syndrome | Test of choice |
| RESPIRATORY TRACT | | | |
| HPV | Biopsy | Laryngeal papilloma | *In situ* DNA detection |
| Influenza or Parainfluenza | Respiratory secretions, cell culture fluids | Pneumonia; typing and subtyping of isolates | Culture, antigen detection |
| Hantavirus | Serum | Hantavirus pulmonary syndrome | Test of choice |
| CENTRAL NERVOUS SYSTEM | | | |
| Bunyaviruses | CSF | Encephalitis | Culture |
| Enterovirus | CSF | Meningitis | Culture |
| Flaviviruses | CSF | Encephalitis | Serology |
| HHV-6, 7 | CSF | Febrile seizures | Test of choice |
| HIV-1 | CSF | Meningitis, myelitis, AIDS dementia | Culture |
| HSV | CSF | Encephalitis | Culture |
| HTLV | CSF, blood | Tropical spastic paraparesis | |
| JC | Brain biopsy | PML | Antigen detection |
| Measles | CSF | Encephalitis | Culture |
| Mumps | CSF | Encephalitis | Culture |
| VZV | CSF | Encephalitis | Test of choice |
| HEMORRHAGIC FEVER | | | |
| Ebola, Lassa | Serum, CSF | Class 4 agents | Serology |

which use denatured, electrophoretically separated mixtures of viral proteins as the bound phase for enzyme immunoassay. This technique allows a detection of antibodies to multiple viral proteins while discriminating between true antibody binding and nonspecific binding by the location of reacting bands. This added specificity is exploited in most confirmatory tests for HIV-1 EIA-positive samples. It has also allowed the successful differentiation of antibodies to HSV-1 and HSV-2 in patient samples.

## ANNOTATED BIBLIOGRAPHY

Hsiung GD, Fong CKY, Landry ML, eds. Diagnostic Virology, 4th ed. Yale University Press, New Haven, CT, 1994.

*A lavishly illustrated book featuring electron micrographs and color plates of direct antigen detection and cell culture for viral diagnosis. Supplementary reading lists with each chapter provide a well-balanced glimpse of primary sources describing most aspects of viral diagnosis.*

Lennette EH, Lennette DA, Lennette ET, eds. Diagnostic Procedures for Viral, Rickettsial, and Chlamydial Infections, 7th ed. American Public Health Association, 1995.

*Excellent overall text with numerous protocols for diagnostic tests. While this text is of greatest value to the laboratorian, its comprehensive nature makes it a valuable reference for clinicians.*

Specter S, Lancz G, eds. Clinical Virology Manual, 2nd ed., Elsevier, New York, 1992.

*Detailed reference text that extends the lab protocols it provides with sources for test kits and reagents for most human viruses. Most important for clinicians, this book contains unique chapters that (1) list State Public Health laboratories, (2) list, by state, laboratories that offer viral diagnostic services, and (3) outlines viral testing and consulting services at the Centers for Disease Control and Prevention, along with contact numbers for these services.*

Wiedbrauk DL, Farkas DH, eds. Molecular Methods for Virus Detection. Academic Press, New York, 1995.

*A comprehensive text that goes beyond PCR to describe in depth state-of-the-art molecular testing for viral diagnosis. Laboratory protocols and descriptions of highly technical methods are presented in a clear and organized manner. Citation lists give useful references to original descriptions of methods.*

# 18

# Clinical Mycology

MICHAEL A. PFALLER

The spectrum of fungal infection runs the gamut from superficial mucosal and cutaneous mycoses to locally destructive and highly invasive infections due to both classic systemic and opportunistic pathogens. The frequency of fungal disease, particularly that due to the systemic and opportunistic pathogens, has increased substantially during the past two decades. This increase is due in large part to expanding patient populations with high risk of developing opportunistic life-threatening fungal infections, including individuals with AIDS or neoplastic disease, and those undergoing organ transplantation and aggressive surgery. These opportunistic infections are clearly important causes of morbidity and mortality and are due to an ever-increasing array of pathogens. In addition to the well-known pathogenic fungi such as *Candida albicans*, *Cryptococcus neoformans*, and *Aspergillus* spp., serious infections are being reported due to yeasts such as *Trichosporon beigelii* and species of *Candida* other than *C. albicans*, hyaline hyphomycetes including *Fusarium* and *Penicillium* spp., and a wide variety of dematiaceous fungi. In many ways, modern medical mycology has become the study of infections due to opportunistic fungi.

Due to the complexity of the patient population involved and the increasing variety of potential fungal pathogens, the opportunistic mycoses pose the greatest diagnostic challenge to clinicians and microbiologists alike. It is absolutely essential that institutions caring for high-risk immunocompromised patients place a high priority on maximizing their diagnostic capabilities for the early detection of opportunistic fungal infections. The successful diagnosis and treatment of such infections in the compromised patient is highly dependent on a team approach involving clinicians, microbiologists, and pathologists. This chapter summarizes the major issues to be considered in the laboratory diagnosis of systemic and opportunistic fungal infections. The general aspects of specimen collection, microscopic examination, culture, serodiagnosis, and identification of the major systemic and opportunistic fungal pathogens will be presented. The interested reader is directed to several excellent reference texts for more detailed information.

## Clinical Recognition of Fungal Infection

With the increased frequency of invasive mycoses has come an enhanced index of clinical suspicion and a greater appreciation and recognition of the major risk factors that predispose patients to fungal infections. The current diagnostic approach consists of clinical suspicion; thorough history and physical examination, including evaluation for skin or mucosal lesions; inspection of all intravascular devices; and a careful ophthalmologic examination, diagnostic imaging of appropriate organ systems, and, finally, procurement of appropriate specimens for laboratory diagnosis. Unfortunately, although specific fungal pathogens may be associated with specific case scenarios, such as sinus infection due to zygomycetes in a diabetic patient with ketoacidosis or fungemia due to *C. tropicalis* in a neutropenic patient with sudden onset of myalgias and myositis, clinical signs and symptoms are frequently not helpful in distinguishing between bacterial and fungal infections. Because the clinical symptoms and radiographic findings in fungal infections are not specific, diagnosis usually depends on three basic laboratory approaches: (*1*) microbiologic, (*2*) immunologic, and (*3*) histopathologic (Table 18.1). More recently, the application of nucleic acid-based detection and identification methods offers promise as an additional rapid approach for diagnosis of fungal infection. Despite these investigations, the clinician frequently cannot wait, and the decision to treat often has to be made on the basis of the clinical information at hand and the physician's subjective assessment.

## Laboratory Diagnosis

### Specimen collection and processing

Successful laboratory diagnosis of fungal infection is directly dependent on the proper collection of appropriate clinical specimens and the rapid transport of the specimens to the clinical laboratory. Selection of appropriate specimens for culture and microscopic examination should be based on clinical and radiographic examination and consideration of the most likely fungal pathogen (Table 18.2). Specimens should be collected under aseptic conditions or after appropriate cleaning and decontamination of the site. It must be stressed that an adequate amount of suitable clinical material be submitted. Unfortunately, many specimens submitted to the laboratory are of insufficient amount or are not appropriate to make a diagnosis. Whenever possible, specimens should be submitted in a sterile, leakproof container and should be accompanied by a relevant clinical history. Clinical information is very important in directing laboratories' efforts in processing and interpreting the results of fungal cultures. This is particularly important when dealing with specimens from nonsterile sites, such as sputum, bronchial washings, and skin. Furthermore, it is the only way of alerting the laboratory that they may be dealing with a potential laboratory hazard such as *Histoplasma capsulatum* or *Coccidioides immitis*.

Transportation of specimens to the laboratory should be rapid; however, delayed processing of specimens for fungal culture is not as detrimental as with specimens for virologic, parasitologic, or bacteriologic examination. Fungi may be recovered from specimens submitted in most bacteriologic transport media, although direct microscopic examination of such material is not recommended. In general, if processing is delayed, specimens for fungal culture may be safely stored at 4°C.

**Table 18.1** Approaches to the laboratory diagnosis of fungal infections*

| |
|---|
| MICROBIOLOGIC APPROACH |
| Direct microscopic examination of clinical material |
| Isolation of etiologic agents in culture |
| Identification of isolates by morphologic, physiologic, immunologic, and molecular criteria |
| IMMUNOLOGIC APPROACH |
| Tests for antibodies (serum and cerebrospinal fluid): agglutination, complement fixation, immunodiffusion, enzyme immunoassay, and immunofluorescence |
| Tests for antigens (serum, cerebrospinal fluid and urine): enzyme immunoassay, latex agglutination, and radioimmunoassay |
| MOLECULAR APPROACH |
| Tests for direct detection and identification from clinical material: polymerase chain reaction (PCR) and other amplification-based methods |
| Tests for identification of isolates from culture: nucleic acid probes |
| HISTOPATHOLOGIC APPROACH |
| Conventional microscopic examination using routine and special stains |
| Direct immunofluorescence of deparaffinized sections of formalin-fixed tissue |

*Adapted from Chandler and Watts (1987).

As with specimens for bacteriologic examination, there are specimens that are more and those that are less optimal for diagnosis of fungal infections (Table 18.2). Certainly cultures of blood and other normally sterile body fluids should be obtained if clinical signs and symptoms are suggestive of involvement of these sites. Diagnosis of oral or vaginal mucosal infections may be better established by clinical characteristics and direct microscopic examination of secretions or mucosal scrapings, as cultures may be positive in a significant percentage of asymptomatic individuals. Likewise, diagnosis of many fungal infections of the gastrointestinal tract are better established by biopsy and histopathologic examination of involved tissue. Care should be taken in collecting lower respiratory and urine specimens in order to minimize contamination with normal oral and periurethral

**Table 18.2** Selection of clinical specimens for recovery of opportunistic fungal pathogens[a]

| | Clinical specimen source[b] | | | | | | | | |
|---|---|---|---|---|---|---|---|---|---|
| Suspected pathogen | Blood | Bone marrow | Brain and CSF | Joint fluid | Eye | Urine | Respiratory | Skin and mucous membranes | Multiple systemic sites |
| YEASTS | | | | | | | | | |
| *Candida* spp. | ++++ | + | + | + | + | +++ | + | +++ | +++ |
| *C. neoformans* | +++ | + | ++++ | | + | ++ | +++ | + | ++ |
| *T. beigelii* | ++++ | | | | | ++ | +++ | ++ | +++ |
| MOULDS | | | | | | | | | |
| *Aspergillus* spp. | | | + | | + | + | ++++ | ++ | +++ |
| Zygomycetes | | | + | | + | | ++++ | ++ | +++ |
| *Fusarium* spp. | +++ | | | + | + | | ++ | ++++ | +++ |
| *P. boydii* | ++ | | + | | + | | ++ | +++ | ++ |
| Dematiaceous fungi | | | +++ | | + | | +++ | ++ | ++ |
| DIMORPHIC | | | | | | | | | |
| *H. capsulatum* | +++ | ++ | + | + | + | + | ++++ | ++ | ++ |
| *B. dermatitidis* | | | + | + | | ++ | ++++ | +++ | ++ |
| *C. immitis* | ++ | + | + | + | + | + | ++++ | +++ | +++ |
| *S. schenckii* | + | | + | + | | | +++ | ++++ | + |
| OTHER | | | | | | | | | |
| *P. carinii* | | + | | | | | ++++ | | + |

[a]Adapted from Muslal et al. (1988).

[b]Predominant sites for recovery are ranked in order of importance and frequency (++++ most important or most frequent, + less important or less frequent), based on the most common clinical presentation.

flora. Twenty-four-hour collections of sputum or urine are inappropriate for mycologic examination, as they will become overgrown with both bacterial and fungal contaminants.

## Stains and direct examination

Direct microscopic examination of tissue sections and other clinical material is perhaps the most rapid, useful, and cost-effective means of diagnosing fungal infection. Detection of fungal elements microscopically may provide a diagnosis in less than an hour, whereas culture results are not available for days or weeks. In some cases, infections are caused by organisms that can be identified specifically on direct microscopy because they are morphologically distinct. For example, if typical organisms are observed microscopically an etiologic diagnosis can be made of infections due to *Histoplasma capsulatum*, *Blastomyces dermatitidis*, *Coccidioides immitis*, and *Pneumocystis carinii*. In other infections, such as aspergillosis, candidiasis, and trichosporonosis, the morphologic appearance may allow a diagnosis to the genus, but not the species, level. Detection of fungi in tissue or on direct examination of other clinical material may also be helpful in determining the significance of culture results. This is especially true when the fungi isolated in culture are part of the normal human flora or the environment. Finally, detection of specific fungal elements on microscopy may assist the laboratory in selecting the most appropriate means by which to culture the clinical specimen.

Although direct examination may be extremely valuable in diagnosing fungal infections, one must keep in mind that both false-negative and false-positive results may occur. As in other areas of microbiology, direct examinations are less sensitive than culture and a negative direct examination does not rule out fungal infection.

A number of different stains and procedures may be used to demonstrate fungi on direct examination of clinical material (Table 18.3). Most commonly, microscopy as performed in the clinical microbiology laboratory consists of examination of wet mounts in 10% KOH stained with the fluorescent reagent Calcofluor white and staining of smears or touch preparations with Gram, Giemsa, and/or periodic acid–schiff (PAS) stain. The Calcofluor white reagent stains all fungi in KOH wet mounts or in tissue and causes them to fluoresce, allowing for easier and faster detection. The Gram stain is useful for detection of yeasts such as *Candida* and *Cryptococcus* and also stains hyphal elements of filamentous fungi such as *Aspergillus* and *Fusarium*. The Giemsa stain is particularly useful for detection of *H. capsulatum* in bone marrow, peripheral blood smears, or touch preparations of lymph nodes or other tissues.

The laboratory diagnosis of *Pneumocystis carinii* infection is also commonly made in the clinical microbiology laboratory by direct examination of induced sputum and specimens collected by bronchoscopy. In addition to more general stains, such as Gomori's methenamine–silver stain (GMS), Giemsa, and toluidine blue, the recent development of fluorescent monoclonal antibody stains has enhanced the detection of *P. carinii*.

Specific cytologic and histologic stains, including the Papanicolaou, hematoxylin-eosin (H&E), GMS, and PAS stains, are used for detection of fungi in cytologic preparations, tissues, body fluids, and exudates. The Papanicolaou stain is usually performed in the cytopathology laboratory and may detect fungi such as *B. dermatitidis*, *C. neoformans*, *C. immitis*, and the hyphae of zygomycetes (*Rhizopus*, *Mucor*, etc.) and *Aspergillus* spp. When present in sufficient numbers, most fungi can be detected in tissue stained with H&E; however, *Candida* and *Aspergillus* may be missed in H&E–stained sections, and special stains such as GMS and PAS are essential for detecting small numbers of organisms and for characterizing their morphology in detail. Although not widely available, specific immunofluorescent stains may be extremely helpful in confirming a presumptive histologic identification of certain fungi. The microscopic morphologic features of several of the more common etiologic agents are presented in Table 18.4, and Figures 18.1 to 18.12.

## Culture

The isolation of fungi on culture media is the most sensitive means of diagnosing infection and in most instances is necessary to allow the identification of the specific etiologic agent. Optimal recovery of fungi from clinical material is dependent on multiple factors. Because no single medium alone is sufficient to recover all medically important fungi, a battery of fungal culture media should be employed. In general, at least two types of culture media, nonselective and selective, are essential for primary recovery of fungi from clinical specimens. The nonselective media should permit the growth of both rapidly growing yeasts and molds as well as the more fastidious or slower-growing fungi. Examples of acceptable nonselective media include brain-heart infusion (BHIA) agar, inhibitory mold agar, and Sabhi agar. Sabouraud dextrose agar is generally considered inferior to these media for primary isolation and should not be used except when infections with dermatophytes are suspected. Most fungi will grow on routine bacteriologic media such as blood agar; however, growth is often slow and may not be visible in the time usually allowed for bacterial cultures. In addition to the nonselective primary isolation media, a blood-containing medium (e.g., BHIA with 5%–10% sheep blood) is helpful in recovery of fastidious dimorphic fungi. The addition of cycloheximide to this medium will also enhance the recovery of the slower-growing dimorphic fungi by inhibiting rapidly growing yeasts and molds that may contaminate the specimen. Specimens that may be contaminated with bacteria should also be cultured on selective media such as inhibitory mold agar, Sabhi, or BHIA plus gentamicin, chloramphenicol, penicillin plus streptomycin, norfloxacin, or ciprofloxacin. The recent introduction of CHROMagar Candida (Hardy Diagnostics Inc., Santa Maria, CA) provides an excellent selective, chromogenic medium for isolation and presumptive identification of *Candida* spp., including *C. albicans*, *C. tropicalis*, and *C. krusei*. CHROMagar has proven particularly useful in detecting mixed infections with more than one species of *Candida* and formulations incorporating fluconazole into the agar have allowed investigators to simultaneously screen for infections due to *Candida* and to detect potential fluconazole resistance. Finally, specialized media for recovery of specific fungi, such as media containing or overlaid with olive oil or another source of long-chain fatty acids for recovery of *Malassezia furfur* or caffeic acid–containing media for detection of *C. neoformans* by its phenol oxidase activity, may be used.

The detection of fungi in blood is a very important means of diagnosing invasive fungal infection. There have been numerous advances in blood culture methodology over the past 10 to 15 years that undoubtedly have contributed to improved detection of fungemia. Presently, the lysis/centrifugation method provides a very flexible and sensitive method for detection of fungemia due to yeasts, molds, and dimorphic pathogens. Recent advances

**Table 18.3** Methods and stains available for direct detection of fungi in clinical specimens by microscopic examination[a]

| Method | Use | Time required (min) | Comments |
|---|---|---|---|
| Gram stain | Detection of bacteria and fungi | 3 | Rapid; commonly performed on clinical specimens. Will stain most yeast and hyphal elements. *Cryptococcus* may stain weakly. |
| KOH | Clearing of specimen to make fungal elements more visible | 5–15 | Rapid; some specimens difficult to clear. May produce artifacts that are confusing. Most useful in combination with Calcofluor white stain. |
| Calcofluor white | Detection of all fungi and *Pneumocystis carinii* | 1–2 | Rapid; detects fungi due to bright fluorescence. Useful in combination with KOH. Requires fluorescent microscope and special filters. Background fluorescence may make examination of some specimens difficult. |
| India ink | Detection of encapsulated yeasts | 1 | Rapid; insensitive (40%) means of detecting *C. neoformans* in spinal fluid. |
| Wright's stain | Examination of bone marrow, peripheral smears, and touch preparations | 5–10 | Useful for diagnosis of histoplasmosis. |
| Giemsa stain | Examination of bone marrow, peripheral smears, touch preparations, and respiratory specimens | 5–10 | Useful for diagnosis of histoplasmosis and *Pneumocystis carinii* pneumonia (induced sputum). |
| Toluidine blue | Examination of respiratory specimens | 5–10 | Useful for diagnosis of *P. carinii* pneumonia. |
| Methenamine silver stain | Detection of fungi in histologic section and *P. carinii* in respiratory specimens | 5–60 | Staining of tissue may require up to 1 h. Respiratory specimens more rapid (5–10 min). Best stain to detect fungi. Yeast cells and *P. carinii* may appear similar. |
| Papanicolaou stain | Cytologic stain used primarily to detect malignant cells | 30 | Stains most fungal elements. Hyphae may stain weakly. Allows cytologist to detect fungal elements. |
| Periodic acid–Schiff stain | Detection of fungi | 20–25 | Stains both yeasts and hyphae well. Artifacts may be confused with yeast cells. |
| Mucicarmine stain | Stains mucin | 60 | Used to demonstrate mucoid capsule of *C. neoformans* and differentiate it from other yeasts. May also stain cell walls of *Blastomyces dermatitidis* and *Rhinosporidium seeberi*. |
| Fontana-Masson | Melanin stain | 60 | Confirms the presence of melanin in lightly pigmented cells of dematiaceous fungi. Useful for staining the cell wall of *C. neoformans*. |
| Hematoxylin-eosin (H&E) | General purpose histologic stain | 30–60 | Best stain to demonstrate host tissue reaction. Stains most fungi. Useful in demonstrating natural pigment in dematiaceous fungi. |

[a]Adapted from Chandler and Watts (1987), Musial et al. (1988), and Woods and Gutierrez (1993).

**Table 18.4** Summary of characteristic features of selected opportunistic and pathogenic fungi[a]

| Fungus | Cultural characteristics | Microscopic morphologic features in Culture | Microscopic morphologic features in Tissue | Additional tests for identification |
|---|---|---|---|---|
| *Candida* spp. | Colonies vary in morphology but are usually pasty, white to tan, and opaque. May have smooth, wrinkled, or fuzzy topography. Some colonies produce fringes of pseudohyphae at periphery. | Most species produce blastoconidia, pseudohyphae or true hyphae. *C. albicans* (all) and *C. tropicalis* (some) may produce chlamydospores. See Figure 18.1. | Oval, budding yeasts 2–6 $\mu$m in diameter and pseudohyphae or hyphae may be present. | Germ tube production by *C. albicans*. Carbohydrate utilization. |
| *C. neoformans* | Colonies are typically shiny, mucoid, dome-shaped, and cream to tan in color. | Cells are variable in size, spherical, and encapsulated. Cells may have multiple, narrow-based buds. See Figure 18.2. | Spherical, budding yeasts of variable size, 2–15 $\mu$g. Evidence of encapsulation may be present. | Tests for urease (+) phenoloxidase (+), and nitrate reductase (−) production. Latex agglutination test for polysaccharide antigen. Carbohydrate utilization. Mucicarmine and melanin stains in tissue. |
| *T. beigelii* | Colonies are smooth, shiny to membranous, dry, and cerebriform. | Hyphae and pseudohyphae; blastoconidia, and arthroconidia; no chlamydospores. | Hyaline arthroconidia and blastoconidia 2–4 by 8 $\mu$m. | Carbohydrate utilization. May produce cross-reaction with cryptococcal latex test. |
| *Aspergillus* spp. | Varies with species. Colonies of *A. fumigatus* usually blue-green to gray-green, *A. flavus* yellow-green, *A. niger* black, other species wide variety. | Varies with species. *A. fumigatus*: uniserate heads with phialides covering upper half of 2/3 of vesicle. See Figure 18.3.<br>*A. flavus*: uniserate or biserate or both with phialides covering entire surface of vesicle.<br>*A. niger*: biserate with phialides over entire surface of vesicle. Conidia are black.<br>*A. terreus*: biserate with phialides covering the surface of a hemispherical vesicle. | Septate, dichotomously branched hyphae of uniform width (3–6 $\mu$m); conidial heads rarely seen in cavitary lesion. See Figure 18.4. | Identification based on microscopic and colonial morphology. |
| Zygomycetes | Colonies are rapid growing, woolly, and gray to brown to gray-black in color. | *Rhizopus* spp.: rhizoids at the base of a sporangiaphore. See Figure 18.5.<br>*Mucor* spp.: no rhizoids produced. | Broad, thin-walled, infrequently septate hyphae, 6–25 $\mu$m wide, with nonparallel sides and random branches. Hyphae stain poorly with methenamine silver stain. See Figure 18.6. | Identification based on microscopic morphologic features. |
| *Fusarium* spp. | Colonies are purple, lavender, or rose-red with occasional yellow variants; cottony or woolly in appearance. | Both macroconidia and microconidia may be seen; Macroconidia are cylindrical, multicelled, andsickle-shaped; Microconidia are arranged in clusters on top of short delicate phialides. See Figure 18.7. | Septate hyphae that are uniform in width (3–8 $\mu$m) and branch at right angles. Angioinvasion is common. Hyphae may be indistinguishable from those of *Aspergillus* spp. See Figure 18.8. | Identification based on microscopic and colonial morphology. |
| *P. boydii* (*S. apiospermum*) | Colonies are woolly and mousy gray with dark brown or brown-black reverse. | Single-celled brownish conidia are produced singly or in groups at the tips of single conidiophores (*Scedosporium apiospermum*); cleistothecia containing ascospores may be produced (*P. boydii*) | Septate, randomly branched hyphae, 2–5 $\mu$m wide; angioinvasion common; conidia of *Scedosporium* type may be formed in cavitary lesions. | Identification based on microscopic and colonial morphology. |

(*continued*)

**Table 18.4** Summary of characteristic features of selected opportunistic and pathogenic fungi[a]—*Continued*

| Fungus | Cultural characteristics | Microscopic morphologic features in: Culture | Microscopic morphologic features in: Tissue | Additional tests for identification |
|---|---|---|---|---|
| Dematiaceous fungi (*Alternaria*, *Cladosporium*, *Curvularia*, etc.) | Colonies are generally rapidly growing, woolly, and gray, olive, black, or brown in color. | *Alternaria* spp: Conidiophores usually solitary and simple or branched; Conidia develop in branching chains and are dematiaceous, muriform, smooth, or rough and taper toward the distal end. See Figure 18.9.<br>*Cladosporium* spp: Conidiophores arise from hyphae and are dematiaceous, tall, and branching; conidia may be shield shaped, smooth or rough, one to several-celled and form in branching chains at apex of conidiophore.<br>*Curvularia* spp: Conidiophores are dematiaceous, solitary or in groups, septate, sympodial, and geniculate; conidia are dematiaceous, two to several celled and curved. | Pigmented (brown) hyphae, 2–6 $\mu$m wide, may be branched or unbranched and are often constricted at their frequent and prominent septations. | Identification based on microscopic and colonial morphology. |
| *H. capsulatum* | Colonies slow-growing, white or buff-brown, suedelike to cottony with pale yellow-brown reverse (25°C). Yeast-phase colonies are smooth, white, pasty (37°C). | Thin, branching, septate hyphae that produce tuberculate macroconidia and microconidia (25°C) small round to oval budding yeast-like cells produced at 37°C. See Figure 18.10. | Small, narrow-based budding yeasts (2–4 $\mu$m); often clustered due to growth within mononuclear phagocytes. See Figure 18.11. | Conversion from mold to yeast phase; exoantigen test; nucleic acid probe test. |
| *C. immitis* | Colonies initially moist and glabrous, rapidly becoming suedelike to downy, grayish white with a tan to brown reverse. | Single-celled, hyaline, rectangular to barrel-shaped, alternate arthroconidia, 2–4 × 3–6 $\mu$m, separated by disjunctor cell. | Spherical, thick-walled, endosporulating spherules, 20–200 $\mu$m; mature spherules contain small, 2–5 $\mu$m endospores; arthroconidia and hyphae may form in cavitary lesions. | Exoantigen and nucleic acid probe tests. |
| *B. dermatitidis* | Colonies may grow rapidly with fluffy white mycelium or slowly as glabrous, tan, nonsporulating colonies (25°C). Yeast phase colonies are wrinkled, folded, and glabrous (37°C). | Hyaline, ovoid to pyriform, one-celled, smooth conidia, borne on short lateral or terminal hyphal branches (25°C). Large (8–15 $\mu$m), thick-walled, budding yeast (37°C). | Spherical, multinucleated yeasts, 8–15 $\mu$m, with thick walls and single, broad-based buds. See Figure 18.12. | Conversion from mold to yeast; exoantigen and nucleic acid probe tests. |

[a]*Source*: Adapted from Chandler and Watts (1987), Musial et al. (1988), and Woods and Gutierrez (1993).

in broth and biphasic (broth/agar) culture methods by agitation and lysis have improved the ability of these systems to recover *Candida* spp.; however, they remain inadequate for detection of *C. neoformans*, *H. capsulatum*, and filamentous fungi such as *Fusarium* spp. Despite the merits of any individual blood culture system, analysis of the available data clearly indicates that maximum detection of fungemia is achieved when more than one blood culture system is employed. Thus, the approach to the diagnosis of invasive mycoses should include the collection of adequate volumes of blood and the use of both a broth- (vented, agitated) and an agar-based (lysis/centrifugation) blood culture method for optimal detection of fungemia.

Once inoculated, fungal cultures must be incubated at proper incubation temperature and for sufficient duration to optimize the recovery of fungi from clinical specimens. A temperature of 30°C is near the optimal temperature for growth of many fungi, although incubation at room temperature (~25°C) will suffice. Although culture dishes are preferred, test tubes may be used for

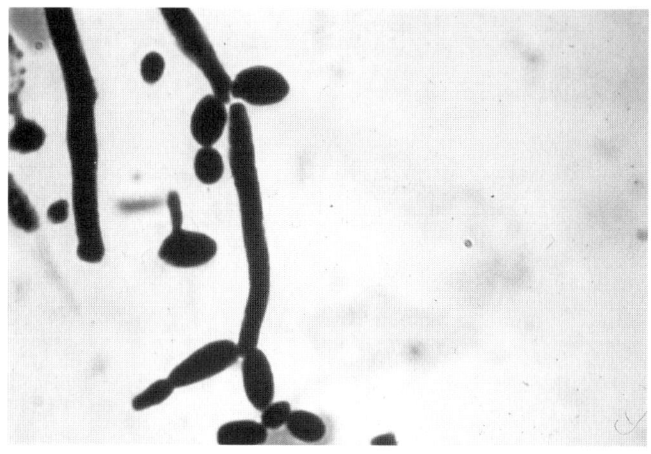

**Fig. 18.1** Gram stain of *Candida albicans* demonstrating blastoconidia, germ tube and pseudohyphae.

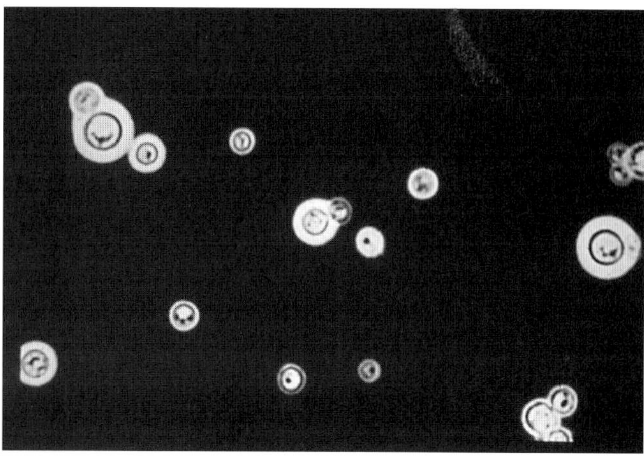

**Fig. 18.2** India ink preparation demonstrating the capsule of *Cryptococcus neoformans.*

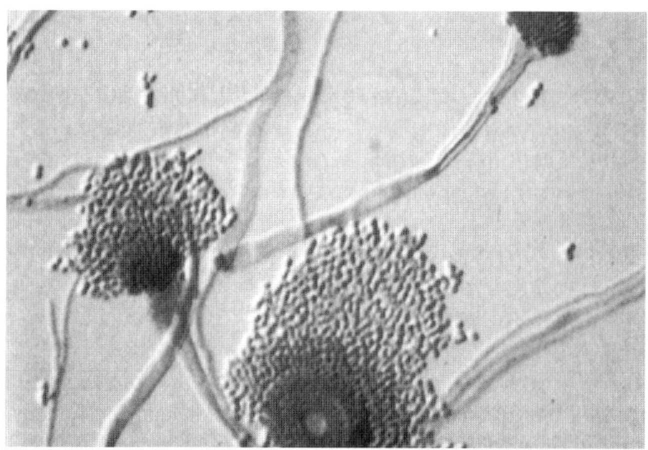

**Fig. 18.3** Microscopic appearance of *Aspergillus fumigatus*. [Reprinted with permission (McClatchey KD. *Clinical Laboratory Medicine,* Williams & Wilkins, Baltimore, MD, 1994.)]

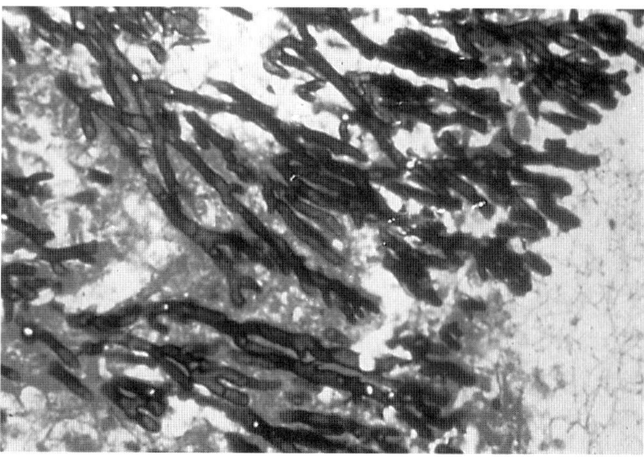

**Fig. 18.4** Tissue section from an individual with invasive aspergillosis demonstrating characteristic septae and 45°-angle branching.

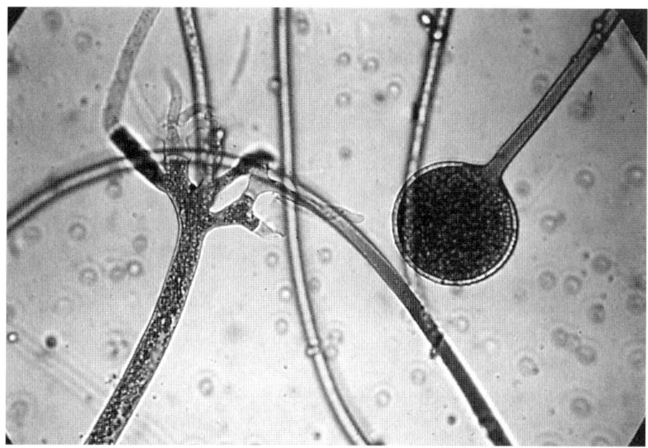

**Fig. 18.5** Microscopic appearance of *Rhizopus* spp.

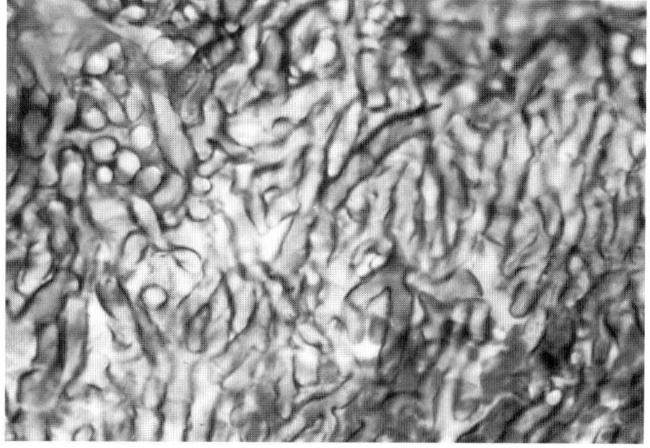

**Fig. 18.6** Tissue section from an individual with zygomycosis demonstrating nonseptate hyphae with characteristic pleomorphic ribbon appearance.

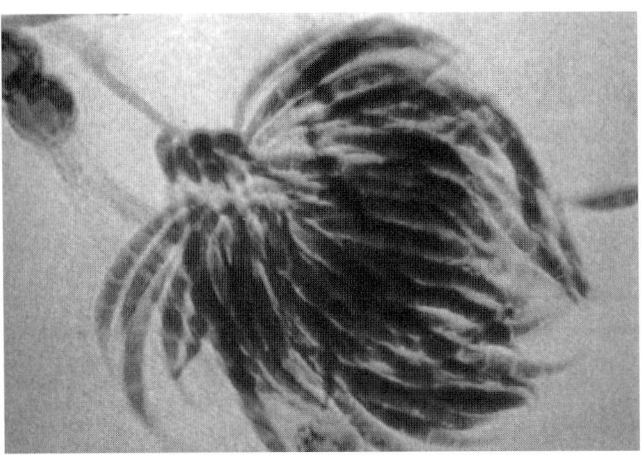

**Fig. 18.7** Microscopic appearance of *Fusarium* spp. demonstrating sickle-shaped macroconidia [Reprinted with permission (McClatchey KD. *Clinical Laboratory Medicine,* Williams & Wilkins, Baltimore, MD, 1994.)]

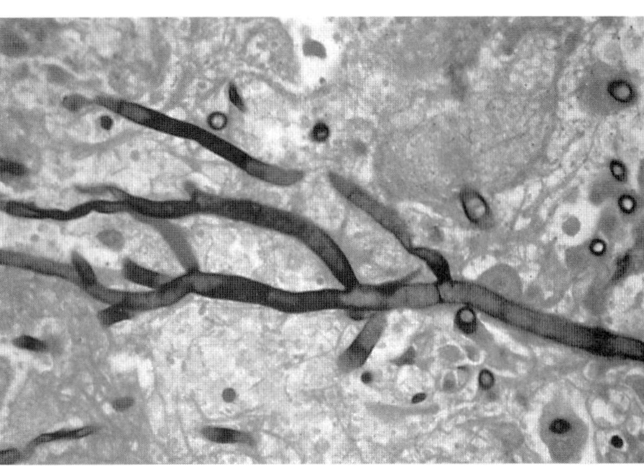

**Fig. 18.8** Tissue section from individual with invasive fusariosis. [From Chandler and Watts, *Pathologic Diagnosis of Fungal Infections*, ASCP Press, Chicago, 1987, with permission.]

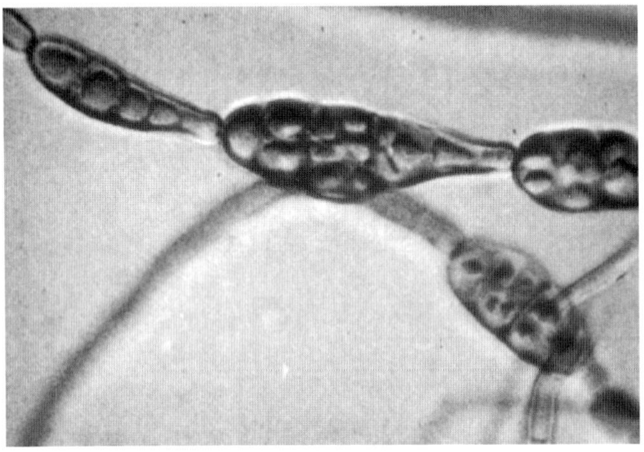

**Fig. 18.9** Microscopic appearance of *Alternaria alternata* [Reprinted with permission (McClatchey KD. *Clinical Laboratory Medicine,* Williams & Wilkins, Baltimore, MD, 1994.)]

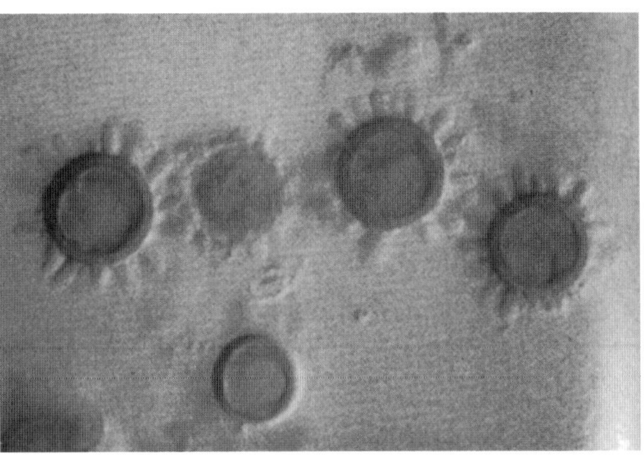

**Fig. 18.10** Microscopic appearance of the mold phase of *Histoplasma capsulatum* demonstrating tuberculate macroconidia. [Reprinted with permission (McClatchey KD. *Clinical Laboratory Medicine,* Williams & Wilkins, Baltimore, MD, 1994.)]

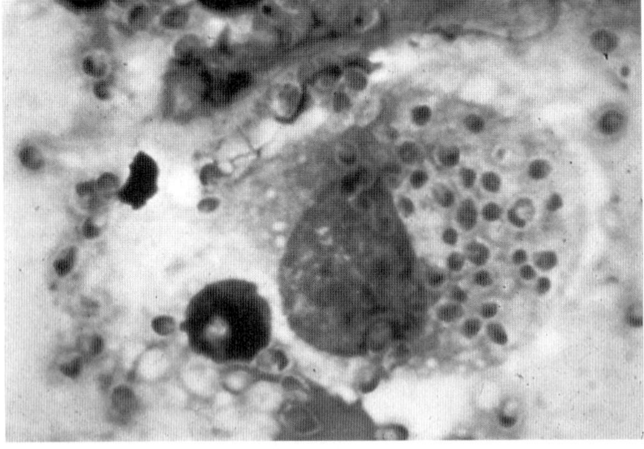

**Fig. 18.11** Touch preparation of a lymph node demonstrating intracellular yeast forms of *H. capsulatum.*

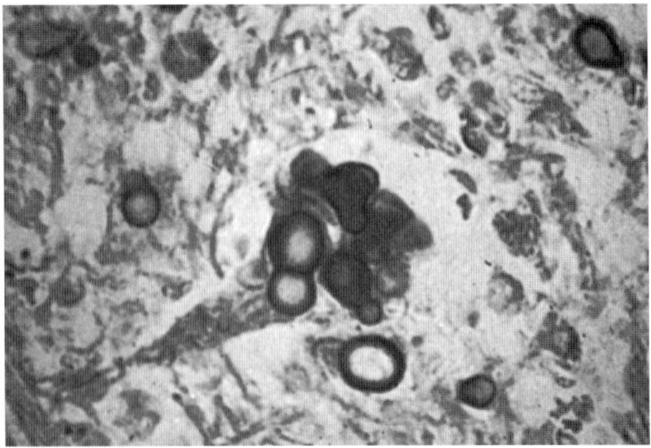

**Fig. 18.12** Microscopic appearance of the tissue phase of *Blastomyces dermatitidis* demonstrating a large, broad-base budding yeast [Reprinted with permission (McClatchey KD. *Clinical Laboratory Medicine,* Williams & Wilkins, Baltimore, MD, 1994.)]

culture; however, care must be taken to leave all screw caps loosened to allow for proper aeration. All specimens should be incubated for 4–6 weeks and examined regularly for growth. As a rule, the laboratory should report the isolation of any fungus. Determination of the clinical significance of a fungal isolate must be made on consultation with the responsible clinician in the context of the clinical setting of the patient.

## Serologic and Nucleic Acid–Based Methods of Diagnosis and Identification

Although culture and histopathology remain the primary means of diagnosing fungal infections, there continues to be a need for more rapid, nonculture methods for diagnosis. Tests for detection of antibodies, rapid detection of specific fungal antigens, metabolic by-products, and fungal species–specific RNA and/or DNA sequences have the potential to yield rapid diagnostic information and can guide the early and appropriate use of antifungal therapy. Some progress has been made in these areas; however, with few exceptions, these tests have yet to make a significant impact on the diagnosis of fungal infections.

Serologic tests can provide a rapid means of diagnosing fungal infections and may also be used to monitor the progression of disease and the response to therapy by serial determinations of antibody and/or antigen titers. Most serologic tests in current use are based on detection of antibodies to specific fungal antigens. Perhaps the most reliable and widely used serodiagnostic tests in mycology are the tests for histoplasmosis and coccidioidomycosis. Both complement fixation and immunodiffusion tests have been found useful for diagnosis of these infections. Complement-fixation titers of >1:32 may be diagnostically significant, whereas lower titers may represent early infection, a cross-reaction, or residual antibodies from a previous infection. Immunodiffusion tests are generally less sensitive than complement-fixation tests but may be useful in identifying cross-reactions. In contrast to serologic tests for other fungal diseases, these tests employ well-standardized commercially available reagents.

The serodiagnostic tests for the opportunistic mycoses lack both sensitivity and specificity, are poorly standardized, and are not widely available. Antibody tests for *Candida* and *Aspergillus* may be performed; however, these tests are frequently unable to distinguish between active and past infection on the one hand and colonization or transient fungemia on the other. In addition, a negative serologic test does not rule out infection with one of these fungi, because immunocompromised patients, and some individuals with disseminated infection, may not mount an antibody response to the infecting organism.

Tests designed to detect fungal antigens or metabolic by-products in serum or other body fluids seem to represent the most direct means of providing an improved method for serodiagnosis of invasive fungal infection. Significant advances have been made in recent years; however, for most fungal infections an acceptable method is not widely available. Most methods for rapid detection of fungal antigens are available in research laboratories only. The exception to this statement are the latex and enzyme immunoassay (EIA) tests for the polysaccharide antigen of *Cryptococcus neoformans*. The tests for cryptococcal antigen are available and detect >95% of cryptococcal meningitis and approximately 67% of disseminated cryptococcal infection. The antigen tests for cryptococcal infection are well-standardized and widely available and have supplanted the India ink test (sensitivity of <40%) for the diagnosis of cryptococcal meningitis. Another useful antigen test that is available from a reference laboratory (Histoplasmosis Reference Laboratory, Indianapolis, IN) is the test for *Histoplasma* antigen. The antigen test for histoplasmosis has been shown to be rapid (<24 hr), sensitive (50%–99%), specific (>98%), and reproducible. This test employs a radioimmunoassay (RIA) or enzyme immunoassay (EIA) format and allows detection of *Histoplasma* polysaccharide antigen in body fluids. Urine and serum are the most common specimens tested for *Histoplasma* antigen; however, antigen may be detected in the spinal fluid of 42%–67% of patients with *Histoplasma* meningitis and in alveolar lavage fluid of 70% of patients with AIDS and severe pulmonary histoplasmosis. Unfortunately, the availability of the test is limited to a single laboratory; however, results are available within one working day, providing rapid turnaround for specimens shipped by overnight mail.

In contrast to the antigen tests for cryptococcosis and histoplasmosis, immunoassays for antigens of *Candida* and *Aspergillus* have been disappointing. Although efforts to develop commercial assays to detect *Candida* mannan and enolase antigens have been encouraging, problems in achieving optimal sensitivity and specificity remain and these tests are not currently available. Likewise, both EIA and latex assays detecting *Aspergillus* galactomannan antigens have shown promise but are not widely available. Further work is needed in this area both to establish which antigens are diagnostically relevant and to determine the most appropriate format for performing these assays in the clinical laboratory.

Similar to antigen detection, the detection of candidal metabolites is another potential method for rapid diagnosis of invasive candidiasis. The detection of arabinitol in serum appears to be an indicator of hematogenously disseminated candidiasis. The diagnostic specificity of arabinitol detection may be improved by correcting for renal function (arabinitol:creatinine ratio) and/or by detection of specific isomers (D-arabinitol). The reported sensitivity and specificity of arabinitol determinations for diagnosis of candidiasis is quite variable and appears to be method dependent. Thus, the diagnostic utility of metabolite detection remains uncertain.

As in other areas of microbiology, the application of molecular biology, specifically the polymerase chain reaction (PCR), offers great promise for the rapid diagnosis of fungal infections. Presently, most of the work has been focused on the diagnosis of invasive candidiasis; however, PCR has also been applied to the diagnosis of aspergillosis and other fungal infections.

PCR-amplified *Candida*-specific DNA has been recovered from blood and other body fluids in a small number of patients. Amplification targets include the lanosterol demethylase gene, mitochondrial DNA, 18S rRNA, the actin gene, and the chitin synthetase gene. Detection of as few as 2–10 cells per ml have been reported, although most assays do not approach this level of detection in clinical samples. The true diagnostic sensitivity of this approach is unknown, but sensitivities of 76%–96% have been reported. Current PCR-based approaches to the diagnosis of fungal infection must be considered cumbersome yet promising prototypes.

Immunologic and molecular approaches have also been applied to the identification of fungi once isolated in culture. Both exoantigen- and nucleic acid probe–based methods have proven to be quite useful for identification of the systemic dimorphic pathogens *H. capsulatum*, *B. dermatitidis*, and *C. immitis*. A nucleic acid probe for the identification of *C. neoformans* is also available.

In the exoantigen test, antigens are extracted from culture material and reacted against specific antibodies for each dimorphic fungus in an immunodiffusion test. These tests may be completed within 24–72 h and have an accuracy of 98%–100% when compared to classical mycologic techniques. In the nucleic acid probe tests, nucleic acids are extracted from culture material and reacted against a chemiluminescent-labeled probe specific for *H. capsulatum*, *B. dermatitidis*, *C. immitis*, or *C. neoformans* rRNA. These tests may be completed within 2 h and have an accuracy of 99%–100%.

## Identifying Characteristics of Different Fungi

There are several reasons for identifying fungi to genus and/or species level. In many instances their clinical presentations are indistinguishable yet determination of the specific etiologic agent may have direct bearing on therapeutic considerations and prognosis. It is becoming increasingly clear that a single therapeutic approach (amphotericin B) is inadequate for many fungal infections and that appropriate classification of the various etiologic agents is necessary. Additionally, the identification of fungal pathogens may have further diagnostic and epidemiologic implications and may provide access to the literature regarding the clinical course of infection and response to therapy for the more unusual opportunistic mycoses.

Of course, the first level of identification is to distinguish infection with a yeast versus a mould. Visual examination of a colony growing on agar usually distinguishes yeasts, which produce pasty opaque colonies, from moulds, that form larger filamentous colonies of varied texture, color, and topography. Microscopic examination further delineates these two large groups. Further identification to genus and species requires more detailed microscopic examination coupled with specific biochemical and physiologic tests supplemented by immunologic and molecular characterization (Table 18.4).

Yeasts may be identified morphologically as single-celled fungi that reproduce by simple budding to form blastoconidia. To varying degrees, certain yeasts may form true hyphae or pseudohyphae and some may be encapsulated. Colonies are usually moist or mucoid, cream-colored in appearance, and grow on most agar media within a few (2–5) days. Because *C. albicans* accounts for approximately 75% of all yeasts recovered from clinical specimens, a rapid simple test that distinguishes it from other yeasts should be performed on all yeasts isolated from clinical specimens. This may be accomplished by performing a germ tube test or a rapid colorimetric test based on the detection of *C. albicans*–specific enzymes (L-proline aminopeptidase and $\beta$-galactosaminidase). A positive germ tube or colorimetric test is generally considered diagnostic for *C. albicans* and further identification is not indicated.

More than 100 species of *Candida* have been identified; however, only a few have been isolated from humans. *C. albicans* and *C. tropicalis* are the two species most commonly isolated from clinical material. Recent reports suggest that shifts have occurred in the distribution of infections caused by specific species. Although *C. albicans* remains the most frequent cause of fungemia and hematogenously disseminated candidiasis, there has been an increase in infections caused by *Candida* (*Torulopsis*) *glabrata*, *C. tropicals*, *C. parapsilosis*, *C. krusei*, and *C. lusitaniae*. For these reasons, further identification of all germ tube– or colorimetric test–negative yeasts should be performed on those isolates obtained from blood and other normally sterile body fluids or tissues. All encapsulated yeasts from any site should be identified, because *C. neoformans* from any site may be clinically significant. Rapid screening tests for the presumptive identification of *C. neoformans* include the urease test (positive), nitrate test (negative), and production of phenol oxidase (positive).

The identification of germ tube–negative yeasts to species is based on the biochemical and physiologic profile and on the cellular structure of the organism on cornmeal agar. Carbohydrate utilization profiles may be performed using one of several commercially available identification systems. These systems are standardized and provide a reasonably accurate identification of most clinical yeast isolates in 24–96 h. The microscopic appearance of many yeasts on cornmeal agar is characteristic and may allow differentiation of yeasts with similar biochemical characteristics. The characteristic features of several of the commonly isolated yeasts are provided in Table 18.4.

The identification of molds is based on growth rate, gross colony appearance, and microscopic morphology. Colonies of the zygomycetes, most hyaline (light-colored hyphae and conidia), and some dematiaceous (dark-colored hyphae and conidia) fungi often grow within 1–5 days, whereas the dimorphic fungi grow more slowly, often requiring 2–4 weeks of incubation. Additionally, the dimorphic fungi are not inhibited by cycloheximide, a compound that inhibits the growth of most rapidly growing molds.

The macroscopic appearance of filamentous fungi may be useful; however, it cannot be used as the sole criterion for identification owing to both natural and medium-dependent variation. Useful characteristics include surface texture, topography and pigment, reverse pigment, and growth at 37°C. For identification purposes, potato dextrose agar and cornmeal agar are two of the most suitable media and exposure to light is recommended to maximize color development.

The definitive identification of a mould is based on its microscopic morphology. The important features include the shape, method of production, and arrangement of conidia or spores, and the size and appearance of the hyphae. The preparation of material for microscopic examination must be done in a way that produces minimal disruption of the precise arrangement of the conidiophores and the way in which the conidia are produced. This may best be obtained by cellophane-tape preparations or (preferably) slide cultures. Determination of the presence (dematiaceous) or absence (hyaline) of hyphal and conidial pigmentation and thermal-regulated dimorphism (yeast at 37°C and mold at 25°–30°C) are also important characteristics. As noted previously, the systemic dimorphic pathogens may also be identified by immunologic- or nucleic acid probe–based methods, in addition to the demonstration of classic thermal dimorphism. The characteristic features of several of the commonly isolated filamentous and dimorphic pathogens are listed in Table 18.4.

## Antifungal Susceptibility Testing

The field of antifungal susceptibility testing has progressed considerably over the past 10–15 years. Presently, the state of the art for susceptibility testing of yeasts is comparable to that of bacteria. Standardized methods for performing antifungal susceptibility testing are reproducible, accurate, and available for use in clinical laboratories. The development of quality control guidelines and interpretive criteria for a limited number of antifungal agents (Table 18.5) provides a basis for limited application of this testing in the clinical laboratory (Table 18.6).

**Table 18.5** Interpretive guidelines for in vitro susceptibility testing of yeast isolates to fluconazole, itraconazole, and flucytosine using National Committee for Clinical Laboratory Standards approved methods[a]

| Antifungal agent | MIC ($\mu$g/ml) | Interpretation | Clinical outcome (% success)[b] |
|---|---|---|---|
| Fluconazole | ≤8.0 | Susceptible | 97 |
| | 16–32 | Susceptible-dose dependent | 82 |
| | ≥64 | Resistant | 60 |
| Itraconazole | ≤0.12 | Susceptible | 90 |
| | 0.25–0.5 | Susceptible-dose dependent | 63 |
| | ≥1.0 | Resistant | 53 |
| Flucytosine | ≤4.0 | Susceptible | NA[c] |
| | 8.0–16 | Intermediate | NA |
| | ≥32 | Resistant | NA |

[a]Macrodilution and microdilution broth methods as described by Pfaller et al. (1997) and Rex et al. (1997).

[b]Clinical outcome data for treatment of oropharyngeal candidiasis in AIDS patients as described by Rex et al. (1997).

[c]Clinical data not available.

Although establishing a correlation between *in vitro* susceptibility tests and clinical outcome has been difficult, it is now clear that antifungal susceptibility testing can predict outcome in several clinical situations, the most notable of which is fluconazole and itraconazole treatment of oropharyngeal candidiasis in AIDS patients. The establishment of interpretive breakpoints for *in vitro* susceptibility of yeasts to these antifungal agents has now been accomplished (Table 18.5). Efforts are now underway to develop reference methods for testing of filamentous fungi as well.

Despite this progress, it remains to be seen how useful antifungal susceptibility testing will be in guiding therapeutic decision making. Guidelines for the use of susceptibility testing in the clinical laboratory have been developed (Table 18.6) and include routine identification of fungi to species level and only selective application of in vitro susceptibility testing. Future efforts must be directed towards establishing and validating interpretive breakpoints for currently available antifungals as well as those new antifungals now under development. In addition, procedures must be optimized for testing non*Candida* yeasts (e.g., *Cryptococcus neoformans*) and moulds.

## Summary

Our understanding of the clinical importance of fungal infections has improved considerably over the past decade. By weight of sheer numbers, we have the best understanding of candidal infections; however, there is little doubt that newer fungi previously considered as "nonpathogens" have now emerged as significant human pathogens. Recognition of these emerging fungal pathogens has resulted in improved understanding of their clinical presentation and of the laboratory techniques necessary to aid in the diagnosis. Clearly we have an increasing number of laboratory aids for the diagnosis of many fungal infections, in-

**Table 18.6** Recommendations for studies of fungal isolates in the clinical laboratory[a]

| Setting | Recommendation |
|---|---|
| Routine | 1. Species level identification of all *Candida* isolates from deep sites.<br>2. Genus level identification of moulds. Identification to species desirable but not necessary.<br>3. Routine antifungal susceptibility testing not recommended. |
| Epidemiological survey | 1. Periodic batch susceptibility testing of *Candida* species.<br>2. Establish antibiogram for an institution.<br>3. Relevant drugs: Fluconazole, itraconazole, flucytosine. |
| AIDS and oropharyngeal candidiasis | 1. Routine antifungal susceptibility testing not required.<br>2. Susceptibility testing may be useful for patients unresponsive to azole therapy.<br>3. Relevant drugs: Fluconazole, itraconazole. |
| Invasive candidiasis | 1. Isolates of *Candida* species (especially non-*albicans*) from deep sites.<br>2. Susceptibility testing offered on request for selected patients.<br>3. Relevant drugs: Fluconazole, itraconazole, flucytosine. |
| Cryptococcosis | 1. Testing not recommended.<br>2. Interpretive guidelines have not been established. |
| Mould infections | 1. Testing not recommended.<br>2. Interpretive guidelines have not been established. |

[a]Adapted from Pfaller et al. (1997).

cluding improved microscopic, culture and serologic techniques. In addition, the exciting new tools of molecular biology offer great promise. However, as our understanding of fungal infections increases, it is obvious that no single diagnostic test is completely adequate. Optimal diagnostic sensitivity and specificity will require a heightened index of suspicion clinically, collection of appropriate specimens, and the application of both culture and nonculture methods.

## ANNOTATED BIBLIOGRAPHY


Chandler FW, Watts JC. Pathologic Diagnosis of Fungal Infections. ASCP Press, Chicago, 1987.
*Excellent discussion and illustration of the use of histopathologic examination in the diagnosis of fungal infections.*

Chanock SJ, Walsh TJ. Molecular diagnosis of *Candida* infection in the immunocompromised host: Current status and future prospects. In: Int J Infect Dis 1(Suppl 1): pp. S20–S24. 1997.
*Recent review of technical issues and potential applications of PCR-based methods for detection of Candida in clinical specimens.*

Connor DH, Chandler FW, Schwartz DA. Pathology of Infectious Diseases. Appleton and Lange, Stanford, CT, 1997.
*Outstanding text and atlas discussing all aspects of infectious diseases with excellent photomicrographs of common and uncommon mycoses.*

Einsele H, Hebart H, Roller G, Löffler J, Rothenhöfer I, Müller CA, Bowden RA, van Burik JA, Engelhand D, Kanz L, Schumacher U. Detection and identification of fungal pathogens in blood by using molecular probes. In: J Clin Microbiol 35: pp. 1353–1360, 1997.
*Description of a PCR assay with high sensitivity and specificity for detection and identification of fungal pathogens in vivo.*

Fridkin SK, Jarvis WR. Epidemiology of nosocomial fungal infections, In: Clin Microbiol Rev 9: pp. 499–511, 1996.
*Comprehensive review of fungal epidemiology with discussion of diagnosis and antifungal susceptibility.*

Hajjeh RA, Brandt ME, Pinner RW. Emergence of cryptococcal disease: Epidemiologic perspectives 100 years after its discovery, In: Epidemiologic Rev 17: pp. 303–320, 1995.
*Excellent and comprehensive review of cryptococcal disease. Includes diagnosis and therapy.*

Hazen KC. New and emerging yeast pathogens, In: Clin Microbiol Rev 8: pp. 462–478, 1995.
*Very useful discussion of Candida and other species of yeast pathogens that may be encountered in the clinical setting.*

Kaufman L, Reiss E. Serodiagnosis of fungal diseases. In: Manual of Clinical Laboratory Immunology, 4th ed. Rose NR, DeMacario EC, Fahey JL, Friedman H, Penn GM, eds. American Society for Microbiology, Washington D.C., pp. 506–528, 1992.
*Comprehensive reference for immunologic tests used in the diagnosis of fungal diseases.*

Kaufman L, Standard PG, Jalbert M, Kraft DE. Immunohistologic identification of *Aspergillus* spp. and other hyaline fungi by using polyclonal fluorescent antibodies, In: J Clin Microbiol 35: pp. 2206–2209, 1997.
*Contemporary demonstration of the value of immunohistochemistry in identifying hyaline moulds in formalin-fixed tissue sections.*

Kwon-Chung KJ, Bennett JE. Medical Mycology. Lea & Febiger, Philadelphia, 1992. Up-to-date reference text on all aspects of clinical mycology.

Liu K, Howell DN, Perfect JR, Schell WA. Morphologic criteria for the preliminary identification of *Fusarium*, *Paecilomyces*, and *Acremonium* species by histopathology, In: Am J Clin Patholog 109: pp. 45–54, 1998.
*Very provocative discussion of several subtle morphologic features exhibited by fungi that may allow the pathologist to distinguish them from Aspergillus.*

McGinnis MR. Mycology, In: Clinical Microbiology Procedures Handbook. Isenberg HD, ed. American Society for Microbiology, Washington, D.C., 1992.
*Detailed how-to procedures in medical mycology.*

McGough DA, Fothergill AW, Rinaldi MG, Pfaller MA. Fungi and fungal infections, In: Clinical Laboratory Medicine. McClatchey KD, ed. Williams and Wilkins, Baltimore, MD, pp 1169–1196, 1994.
*Recent review of contemporary mycology.*

Musial CE, Cockerill EF III, Roberts GD. Fungal infections in the immunocompromised host: clinical and laboratory aspects. Clin Microbiol Rev 1988; 1:349–364.
*Very useful review of the laboratory diagnosis of opportunistic fungal infections.*

Nelson PE, Dignani MC, Anaissie EJ. Taxonomy, biology, and clinical aspects of *Fusarium* species, In: Clin Microbiol Rev 7: pp. 479–504, 1994.
*Complete review of the biology and clinical aspects of Fusarium infection.*

Odds FC, Bernaerts R. CHROMagar Candida, a new differential isolation medium for presumptive identification of clinically important *Candida* species, In: J Clin Microbiol 32: pp. 1923–1929, 1994.
*Initial description of CHROMagar with outstanding color photos.*

Pfaller MA. Laboratory aids in the diagnosis of invasive candidiasis. Mycopathologia 1992; 120:65–72.
*Recent update on culture and nonculture methods for diagnosis of candidiasis.*

Pfaller MA. Nosocomial candidiasis: Emerging species, reservoirs and modes of transmission, In: Clin Infect Dis 22(Suppl 2): pp. S89–S94, 1996.
*Discussion of the clinical importance of species of Candida other than C. albicans.*

Pfaller MA, Rex JH, Rinaldi MG. Antifungal susceptibility testing: Technical advances and potential clinical applications, In: Clin Infect Dis 24: pp. 776–784, 1997.
*Review of the state of the art of antifungal susceptibility testing.*

Reiss E, Morrison CJ. Nonculture methods for diagnosis of disseminated candidiasis. Clin Microbiol Rev 1993; 6:311–323.
*Excellent critical review of antigen, metabolite, and nucleic acid–based methods for diagnosis of candidiasis.*

Rex JH, Pfaller MA, Galgiani JN, Bartlett MS, Espinel-Ingroff A, Ghannoum MA, Lancaster M, Odds FC, Rinaldi MG, Walsh TJ, Barry AL. Development of interpretive breakpoints for antifungal susceptibility testing: Conceptual framework and analysis of in vitro - in vivo correlation data for fluconazole, itraconazole, and *Candida* infections, In: Clin Infect Dis 24: pp. 235–247, 1997.
*The first description of the development of in vivo correlates for antifungal susceptibility tests. A useful review of the limitations of all antimicrobial susceptibility tests.*

Sandhu GS, Kline BC, Stockman L, Roberts GD. Molecular probes for diagnosis of fungal infections, In: J Clin Microbiol 33: pp. 2913–2919, 1995.
*Description of a universal fungal detection and identification protocol utilizing a panel of oligonucleotide probes.*

Schell WA. New aspects of emerging fungal pathogens, In: Clin lab Med 15: pp. 365–386, 1995.
*Excellent review and new insights into emerging fungal pathogens.*

Stockman L, Clark K, Hunt JM, Roberts G. Evaluation of commercially available acridinium ester-labeled chemiluminescent DNA probes for the culture identification of *Blastomyces dermatitidis*, *Coccidioides immitis*, *Cryptococcus neoformans*, and *Histoplasma capsulatum*. J Clin Microbiol 1993; 31:845–850.
*Comparative evaluation of new molecular identification methods for dimorphic pathogens and C. neoformans.*

Tanner DC, Weinstein MP, Fedorciw B, Joho KL, Thorpe JJ, Reller LB. Comparison of commercial kits for detection of cryptococcal antigen. J Clin Microbiol 1994; 32:1680–1684.
*Critical evaluation of five commercially available kits for detection of cryptococcal antigen. Evaluation includes both latex and enzyme immunoassay kits as applied to CSF and serum.*

Walsh TJ, Chanock SJ. Laboratory diagnosis of invasive candidiasis: A rationale for complementary use of culture- and nonculture-based detection systems, In: Int J Infect Dis 1(Suppl 1): pp. S11–S19, 1997.
*Recent update on culture- and nonculture-based methods for diagnosis of candidiasis.*

Wheat J. Endemic mycoses in AIDS: A clinical review, In: Clin Microbiol Rev 8: pp. 146–159, 1995.
*Excellent review of clinical and laboratory aspects of endemic mycoses including a discussion of the use of antigen detection for diagnosis of histoplasmosis.*

Wheat J, Wheat H, Connolly P, Kleiman M, Supparatpinyo K, Nelson K, Bradsher R, Restrepo A. Cross-reactivity in *Histoplasma capsulatum* variety *Capsulatum* antigen assays of urine samples from patients with endemic mycoses, In: Clin Infect Dis 24: pp. 1169–1171, 1997.
*Demonstration of cross-reactivity in samples from patients with blastomycosis and disseminated Penicillium marneffii infection.*

Woods Gl, Gutierrez Y. Diagnostic Pathology of Infectious Diseases. Lea & Febiger, Philadelphia, 1993.
*Excellent general reference text for clinical mycology and microbiology.*

# 19

# Clinical Parasitology

JAMES J. PLORDE

The majority of parasitic infections are diagnosed by the recovery and morphologic identification of the etiologic agent in the excreta, blood, body fluids, or tissues of the host (see Table 19.1, Figs. 19.1, 19.2, 19.3, 19.4, 19.5, 19.6). In intestinal infections, this is accomplished by examining wet amounts and/or stained smears of fecal material. Wet mounts and smears of peripheral blood are employed for the diagnosis of malaria, leishmaniasis, trypanosomiasis, and filariasis, while examination of sputum or urine can yield the diagnosis of paragonimiasis and schistosomiasis haematobium, respectively. Tissue sections taken from skin or muscle can be productively examined for *Onchocerca volvulus* or *Trichinella spiralis*. Morphologic identification of the recovered parasite is often facilitated by the use of special stains, especially for protozoans.

## Specimen Collection and Transportation

A summary of the specimen-collection procedures used in our laboratory is presented in Table 19.1

### Gastrointestinal specimens

#### Normally passed stool

With the exception of a few helminths (*Ascaris, Trichuris,* hookworm), most intestinal parasites are passed into the stool intermittently or in fluctuating numbers. For this reason, a single aliquot of a fresh, normally passed stool from an infected patient will yield the diagnosis for 30% to 50% of the time, depending on the parasite. Generally, three specimens collected at intervals of 2–3 days will substantially improve the yield, particularly in protozoan infection; daily collection is less preferable but may be employed to avoid prolongation of hospitalization. In suspected cases of giardiasis, three additional specimens taken at weekly intervals should be collected if the original series is negative. Post-treatment specimens should be collected in the same manner, beginning two weeks after completion of therapy for helminthic infections, four weeks for protozoan infections, and six weeks for *Taenia* infections. Follow-up specimens may be checked at three and six months, if desired.

Certain drugs and compounds, including purgatives, antidiarrheal agents, antacids, antibiotics and contrast agents, interfere with the detection of stool parasites. Barium, magnesium, kaolin, and bismuth compounds produce crystalline or particulate debris that can obscure parasites and alter the appearance of trophozoites. Oil globules from castor or mineral oil interfere with microscopic examination. Antibiotics and cathartics temporarily decrease the protozoan population to a level where organisms may not be detected. Specimens should be obtained before these compounds are used, or their collection delayed until their effects are passed. Collection should be delayed for seven to ten days following barium, bismuth, kaolin, magnesia, castor oil, or mineral oil administration, and three weeks following antibiotics or after gallbladder dye has been given.

Whole fecal specimens should be collected to allow an adequate sample for the gross and microscopic examination; rectal swabs are unacceptable. Fecal specimens should be obtained in a manner that precludes contamination with urine, water, dirt, or soil. Urine and water will destroy trophozoites that may be present, and dirt interferes with the examination. Further, soil may contain free-living larvae or other organisms that can be confused with human pathogens. Collection of the specimen in a clean, dry bedpan, or directly into a plastic specimen cup with a threaded, leakproof lid, is preferable. Ideally, specimens should be immediately transported to the laboratory. If a delay of 1–2 hours is anticipated, the specimen should be refrigerated at 5°C. Greater delay requires use of stool preservative kits, each containing one vial of 10% formalin and one of polyvinyl alcohol (PVA).

#### Purged stool and sigmoidoscopic aspirates

One purged stool will result in the recovery of more protozoan species (90%) than the cumulative total from three normally passed stools. This is presumably due to the evacuation of the cecal area, where many protozoa are concentrated. However, there are a number of disadvantages to purged specimens: (*1*) trophozoites predominate in purged specimens and are more difficult to identify than cysts; (*2*) the cathartic may affect the appearance and behavior of the organism; and (*3*) protozoan parasites frequently cannot be demonstrated in stool for up to a week after purgation. Purging should be avoided in patients with diarrhea or significant abdominal pain; sodium-containing cathartics should not be used in patients with congestive heart failure, or a magnesium one in those with renal failure. Purging is generally employed only when there is strong clinical evidence of an *Entamoeba histolytica* infection and the routine stool examinations have proved negative.

Sigmoidoscopic aspirates are a convenient alternative to purged stool specimens. For either specimen type, the clinical laboratory should be contacted for specific instructions of the collection and transportation of the specimen.

#### Anal swabs

Cellophane tape anal swabs are the best means of detecting infections with *Enterobius vermicularis* and *T. saginata. Enterobius* eggs are deposited directly on the perianal skin by the nocturnally migrating female. In the case of *Taenia* infections, the eggs

**Table 19.1** Diagnosis of parasitic diseases

| Disease | Etiologic agent | Clinical indication | Specimen | Test | Diagnostic form/test |
|---|---|---|---|---|---|
| Amebiasis | *Entamoeba histolytica* | Compatible history or PE | Stool series (3 specimens) | Wet mount, concentration, stained smear | Cysts/trophozoite |
| | | Negative stool smear; asymptomatic | Purged stool | Wet mount, stained smear | Trophozoites |
| | | Negative stool smear; symptomatic | Sigmoidoscopic aspirate | Wet mounts, stained smear | Trophozoites |
| | | Therapeutic liver aspiration | Terminal (bloody) portion of aspirate | Wet mount, culture | Trophozoites |
| | | Chronic colitis or liver abscess | Blood | Serology | IHA EIA |
| Amebic keratitis | *Acanthamoeba* | Chronic corneal lesion | Corneal scraping | Wet mount, culture | Cysts/trophozoites |
| Amebic meningoencephalitis | *Naegleria* or *Acanthamoeba* | Meningoencephalitis after swimming | CSF | Wet mount, culture | Trophozoites |
| Ascariasis | *Ascaris lumbricoides* | Compatible history | Stool series | Wet mount, concentration | Egg |
| Cryptosporidiosis | *Cryptosporidium* | Compatible history | Stool | Acid fast stain | Oocyst (Plate 6) |
| | | Compatible history | Stool | Serology | EIA, DFA |
| Cutaneous larva migrans (Creeping eruption) | Several helminthic agents | Skin rash | Blood | Serology | IFAT |
| Cysticercosis | *Taenia solium* | Compatible history or PE | Soft tissues of patient | X ray | Calcified cysticerci |
| | | | Blood | Serology | IHA, EIA, IB |
| Dracunculiasis | *Dracunculus medinensis* | Compatible PE | Ulcer washings | Wet mount | Larvae |
| Echinococciasis | *Echinococcus granulosus*, *Echinococcus multilocularis* | Compatible history or PE | Liver | X ray | Hepatic calcification |
| | | | | Radioisotope scan | Cold spot |
| | | | Lung | X ray | Opaque irregular mass |
| | | | Blood | Serology | IHA, DD, EIA, IB |
| Enterobiasis (pinworm infection) | *Enterobius vermicularis* | Compatible history or PE | Perianal swab q.d. ×3 (early A.M. or late P.M.) | Scotch-tape slide | Eggs, adult female |
| Filiariasis (Bancroftian filariasis) | *Wuchereria bancrofti*, *Brugia malayi*, *Brugia timori* | Compatible history or PE | Blood (day & night) and/or ascites fluid | Wet mounts, thin and thick films, and concentration | Microfilariae |
| | | Negative blood or ascites preparation | Blood 1 hour after 100 mg of diethylcarbamizine | Wet mount, thick film, concentration | Microfilariae |
| | | Negative blood | Blood | Serology | IHA, BF, Nucleopore filtration |
| (Loiasis) | *Loa loa* | Compatible history or PE | Blood (day) or Calabar swelling aspirate | Wet mounts, thin and thick films, concentrates | Microfilariae |
| | | Visible adult worm | Extracted worm | Macroscopic exam | Adult worm |
| | | Negative exams for microfilariae and adults | Blood | Serology | IHA, BF, Nucleopore filtration |
| (Onchocerciasis) | *Onchocerca volvulus* | Compatible history or PE | Skin snip | Wet mount | Microfilariae |
| | | | Node excision | Histologic section | Adult worm |

| | | | | | |
|---|---|---|---|---|---|
| Giardiasis | *Giardia lamblia* | Compatible history | Stool series (3 specimens) | Wet mount, concentrate, smear | Cysts/trophozoites (Fig. 19.4) |
| | | Negative stool series | Stool (3 specimens per week) | Wet mount, concentrate, smear | Cysts/trophozoites |
| | | | String Test (Entero-test) | Wet mount, smear | Trophozoites |
| | | | Stool | Culture | Trophozoites |
| | | | Stool | Serology | EIA |
| Hookworm disease | *Ancylostoma duodenale*<br>*Necator americanus* | Compatible history or PE | See Ascariasis | | |
| Intestinal flukes | *Fasciolopsis buski*<br>*Nanophyetus salmincola* | Compatible history or PE | See Ascariasis | | |
| Intestinal nematodes | See Ascariasis, Enterobiasis, or Stronglyoidiasis | | | | |
| Leishmaniasis (kala-azar) | *Leishmania donovani* | Compatible history or PE | Blood, bone marrow | Giemsa smear | Intracellular amastigote form (Fig. 19.2) |
| | | | Blood | Culture | Promastigote form (Isoenzyme electrophoresis) |
| | | | Blood | Serology | IF, IHA, direct agglut. |
| (Oriental sore) | *Leishmania tropica* | Compatible history or PE | Biopsy or aspirate | Giemsa smear | Intracellular amastigote form |
| | | | As above | DNA probe | + blot |
| | | | Blood | Serology | IHA, direct agglut. |
| (Espundia) | *Leishmania braziliensis* | Compatible history or PE | As above | As above | As above |
| (Chiclero ulcer) | *Leishmania mexicana* | Compatible history or PE | As above | As above | As above |
| Liver Flukes | *Fasciola hepatica,*<br>*Clonorchis sinensis*<br>*Opisthorchis* sp. | Compatible history or PE | Stool series and/or biliary drainage | Wet mounts and concentration | Eggs and adult worms |
| Microsporidiosis | *Enterocytozoon bienusi*<br>*Encephalitozoon cuniculi*<br>*Encephalitozoon hellem*<br>*Villaforma corneum*<br>*Encephalitozoon intestinalis*<br>*Pleistophora* sp. | Compatible history | Stool, urine sediment, nasal smears, corneal scraping, biopsy | *Calcofluor* stain<br>Weber's Trichrome<br>Electron microscopy | Spores |

*(continued)*

**Table 19.1** Diagnosis of parasitic diseases (*Continued*)

| Disease | Etiologic agent | Clinical indication | Specimen | Test | Diagnostic form/test |
|---|---|---|---|---|---|
| Malaria | *P. vivax*, *P. ovale*, *P. malariae*, *P. falciparum* | Compatible history or PE | Finger prick blood Q 6–8 h × 3 days | Thin and thick Giemsa smear | *P. falciparum*: rings and gametocytes (Fig. 19.3) |
| | | Evenings, weekends | Venous blood (EDTA) q 6–8 h | Thin Wright-Giemsa smear | *P. vivax, P. ovale, P. malariae:* rings, mature trophozoites, schizonts, gametocytes |
| | | History, chronic relapsing fever, negative smears | Blood | Serology | IFAT, IHA |
| Paragonimiasis | *Paragonimus* spp. | Compatible history or PE | Stool and sputum series | Wet mount and concentration | Eggs |
| | | | Blood | Serology | CF, IB (Fig. 19.4) |
| Pneumocystosis | *Pneumocystis carinii* | Compatible history and CXR | Endobronchial brush, open lung biopsy, BAL, bronchial wash | Processing done in Pathology | Cysts |
| | | Productive sputum | Induced sputum smear | As above | Cysts |
| Schistosomiasis | *Schistosoma mansoni*, *Schistosoma japonicum*, *Schistosoma mekongi* | Compatible history or PE | Stool series | Wet mount, concentration, hatching test | Eggs, miracidia (Fig. 19.5) |
| | | | Rectal biopsy | Wet mount | Eggs |
| | | | Blood | Serology | CF, BF, IF, EIA, IB |
| | *Schistosoma haematobium* | Compatible history or PE | Terminal portion of noon urine ×3 | Wet mount and concentration | Eggs |
| | | | Blood | Serology | CF, BF, IF, EIA |
| Strongyloidiasis | *Strongyloides stercoralis* | Compatible history | Stool series | Wet mount, concentration | Rhabditiform larvae |
| | | Negative stool series | String test (Enterotest) | Wet mount | Rhabditiform larvae |
| | | Negative stool and string test | Stool | Culture | Filariform larvae |
| | | Negative stool and string test | Blood | Serology | IHA, IFAT, EIA |
| Taeniasis | *Taenia saginata* *Taenia solium* | Compatible history or PE | Stool | Wet mount | Proglottids, eggs |
| | | | Vaspar swab ×3 | Scotch-tape slide | Eggs |

| | | | | | |
|---|---|---|---|---|---|
| Tapeworm (See also Cysticercosis, Echinococciasis Taeniasis) | *Diphyllobothrium* spp. | Compatible history or PE | Stool series | Wet mount and concentration | Eggs |
| | *Hymenolepis nana* | As above | As above | Wet mount and concentration | Eggs |
| | *Hymenolepis diminuta* | As above | As above | Wet mount and concentration | Eggs |
| Toxocariasis (Visceral larva migrans) | Toxocara canis<br>Toxocara cati | Compatible history and PE | Blood | Serology | EIA |
| Toxoplasmosis | *Toxoplasma gondii* | Compatible history or PE | Blood | Serology | IHA, IFAT, EIA |
| | | | Lymph node/aspirate | Giemsa stain | Tachyzoite |
| | | | Brain biopsy | Giemsa stain | Cyst |
| Trichinosis | *Trichinella spiralis* | Compatible history and PE | Blood | Serology | EIA, IFAT, BFT |
| | | | Muscle tissue 3rd week | Wet mount, histologic section (H&E), press prep | Larvae |
| Trichuriasis | *Trichuris trichuria* | Compatible history and PE | Stool series | Wet mount, concentration | Egg |
| Trypanosomiasis (Chagas' Disease) | *Trypanosoma cruzi* | Compatible history or PE | Blood | Wet mount, thin and thick smears | *Trypomastigote* |
| | | | Bone marrow aspirate | Stained smears | Amastigote |
| | | | Blood | Culture | Trypomastigote |
| | | | Blood | Serology | CF, IHA (Fig. 19.6) |
| Trypanosomiasis (Sleeping Sickness) | *Trypanosoma brucei* complex | Compatible history or PE | Blood | Wet mount, thin and thick smears | Trypomastigote |
| | | | Lymph node aspirate | Thin and thick smears | Trypomastigote |
| | | | CSF | Smear | Trypomastigote |

Abbreviations: PE, physical examination; CSF, cerebrospinal fluid; IHA, indirect hemagglutination assay; DFA, direct fluorescent antibody test; IFAT, indirect fluorescent antibody test; IF, immunofluorescent antibody test; EIA, enzyme immunoassay; BF, bentonite flocculation; DD, immunodiffusion; CF, complement fixation; IB, immunoblot.

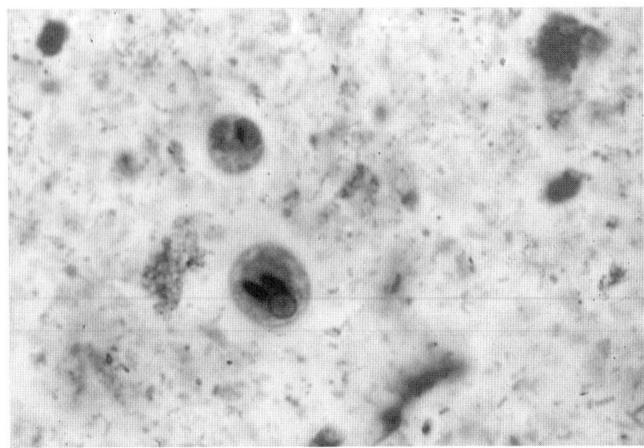

**Fig. 19.1** *E. histolytica* stool cysts—iron hematoxylin.

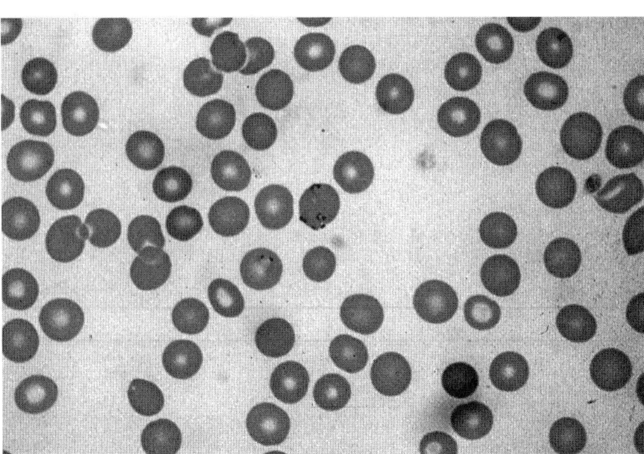

**Fig. 19.3** *P. falciparum*—multiple trophs.

reach this area as a result of proglottid rupture during passage through the anal canal. Three to six consecutive daily collections are required to detect all pinworm infections. They should be obtained between 9 P.M. and midnight or early in the morning before defecation or bathing. Instructions and materials can be obtained from the clinical laboratory. After collection, the cellophane tape is placed sticky side down on a glass slide and stored in a sealed container at refrigerator temperature until all specimens have been collected.

### Duodenal drainage (Enterotest®)

Duodenal specimens may be useful for the diagnosis of giardiasis and strongyloidiasis when the examination of stool specimens has not been fruitful. The Enterotest or "string test" is a convenient technique for collecting such specimens. Patients are asked to swallow a weighted string after firmly fixing the proximal end of the string to the patient's cheek. The string is withdrawn 4–6 hours later, placed in a sealed plastic container, and sent immediately to the laboratory.

## Genitourinary specimens

*Trichomonas vaginalis* is frequently recovered from the urine sediment of both men and women who are infected. In addition, urine is the most common pathway for the excretion of *Schistosoma haematobium* eggs. More rarely, *Entamoeba histolytica* may be found in the urine of patients with amebic ulceration of their genitalia and microfilaria in the urine of patients who are chyluric with Bancroft's filariasis. *Dioctophyma renale,* a rare parasite of man, and *Strongyloides stercoralis* may also be rarely seen.

### Trichomonas vaginalis

Women should be instructed not to douche for 3–4 days prior to the collection of vaginal or urethral specimens. If possible, an unlubricated or lightly lubricated speculum should be used during collection to avoid microscopic artifacts. The specimen is obtained with a sterile swab that is then placed in a tube containing a small amount of saline; a second swab may be inoculated into a *Trichomonas* culture tube. Urethral and prostatic secretions from men are managed in a similar fashion. The first portion of voided urine, procured without preceding cleansing, may be profitably examined for *Trichomonas vaginalis* if urethral, vaginal, or prostatic secretion specimens cannot be obtained. All specimens should be sent immediately to the microbiology laboratory for preparation and examination of a wet mount. Old specimens are unsatisfactory, since the flagellates may be immobile.

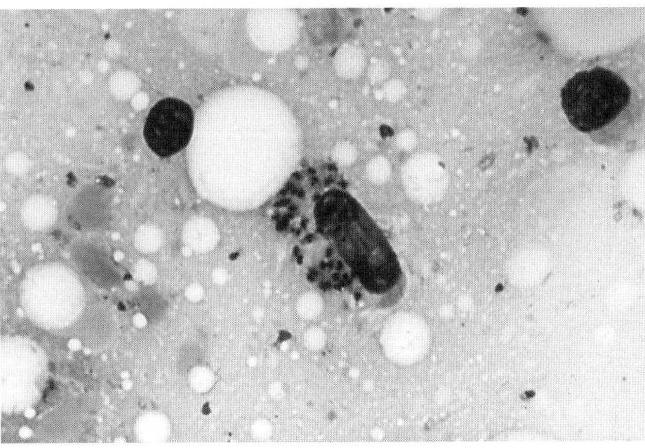

**Fig. 19.2** Leishmania—bone marrow Giemsa.

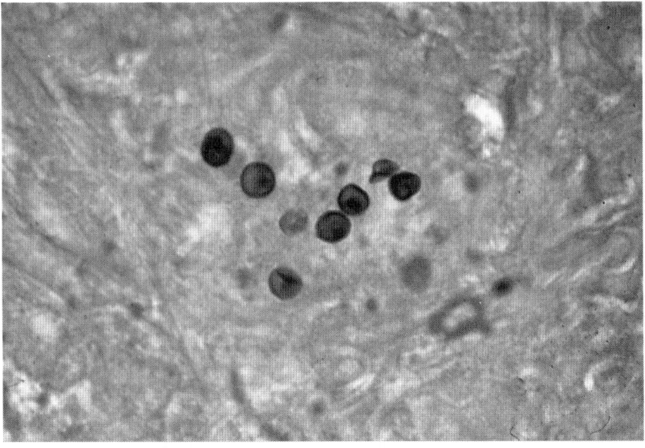

**Fig. 19.4** *P. carinii*—Wright-Giemsa.

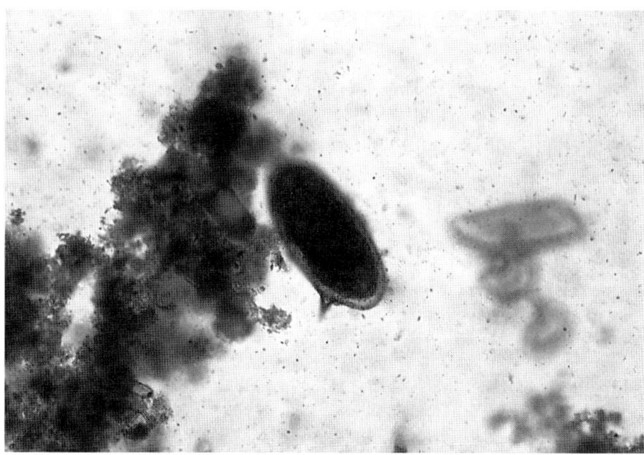

**Fig. 19.5** *Shistosoma mansoni*—iodine prep stain.

### Schistosoma haematobium

Since the passage of schistosome eggs in the urine fluctuates, it is often necessary to collect three consecutive daily specimens. Eggs are most likely to be found in the urine passed between noon and 2:00 P.M., particularly if blood or pus are present. Since eggs are concentrated in the last few drops of urine, collect only the last third of the void. It should be placed in a sterile plastic jar, tightly sealed, and sent immediately to the laboratory.

## Respiratory specimens

In human lung fluke infections, the eggs of *Paragonimus* spp. are usually discharged in the sputum, although some are swallowed and later appear in the stool. For this reason, both sputum and fecal specimens should be obtained. Pulmonary amebic abscesses may rupture into a bronchus, resulting in the expectoration of blood, mucus, necrotic tissue, and trophozoites of *E. histolytica.* Similarly, hydatid cysts may discharge fragments of the cyst wall and many free protoscolices of *Echinococcus granulosus.* Larvae of *Ascaris lumbricoides, Strongyloides stercoralis,* and the hookworms may also be found in the sputum during their phase of pulmonary migration. Expectorated sputum specimens are collected as for bacterial cultures (Chapter 16).

In cases of suspected amebiasis, the specimen should be immediately hand-delivered to the laboratory for a wet-mount examination. If this is not possible, mix the specimen 1:3 with PVA fixative. For all other specimens, deliver to the laboratory within an hour of collection or preserve 1:3 in 5% formalin. The laboratory should be contacted for instruction on the collection of endobronchial specimens.

## Blood and bone marrow specimens

Blood specimens may be submitted for serologic examination, culture, or, more commonly, direct examination for the presence of parasitic organisms. The collection techniques for serologic and cultural examination are the same as for other microbial diseases. Direct examination of blood is useful for the detection of malaria parasites, microfilariae, leishmania, and trypanosomes. Preferably, fresh capillary blood is used to prepare wet mounts as well as thin and thick smears. Alternatively, fresh venous specimens may be collected. A laboratory technologist should collect the fresh specimen and prepare wet mounts (trypanosomes, microfilariae) and/or thin and thick smears at the bedside using precleaned slides. The presence of soda lime or potash on new uncleaned slides will alter the pH of the stain, making recognition of parasites more difficult. If experienced technologists are not available, venous bloods should be collected in an EDTA vacutainer and sent to the laboratory.

### Filariasis

The only definitive method of diagnosing Bancroft's filariasis is the demonstration of microfilariae in the circulating blood. Unfortunately, they can be seen only in the intermediate stages of the disease, being absent both very early (first 6–12 months) and very late in the disease. When present, many display nocturnal periodicity (see Table 19.1), requiring blood collection after 10:00 P.M. Alternatively, one can administer diethylcarbamazine (DEC) to the patient to provoke a transitory emergence of the microfilariae into the peripheral circulation during the day in numbers approximating one-third of the nocturnal level. If *Wuchereria bancrofti* or *Brugia malayi* infections are suspected, blood should be drawn between 10 P.M. and 2 A.M. For *Loa Loa* and *Mansonella* infections, collect the specimen between 11:00 A.M. and 2:00 P.M. If nocturnal collections are not feasible, a 100 mg oral dose of DEC may be administered and blood collected one hour later. DEC should not be given to patients who might have loiasis or onchocerciasis, as it can provoke a severe clinical reaction. If a wet mount and direct smear is negative, one or more specimens should be collected for concentration.

### Leishmaniasis

Definitive diagnosis of systemic leishmaniasis (kala-azar) depends on the demonstration of *L. donovani* group organisms in stained smears of the bone marrow, spleen, lymphatic gland fluid, or buffy coat, and by culture of blood or other tissue. Blood smears are usually negative except in Indian kala-azar. Thin smears should be prepared from bone marrow aspirate and submitted to the laboratory. When ordering buffy coat smears, draw 2–3 ml of venous blood into a citrate vacutainer tube and dispatch to the laboratory.

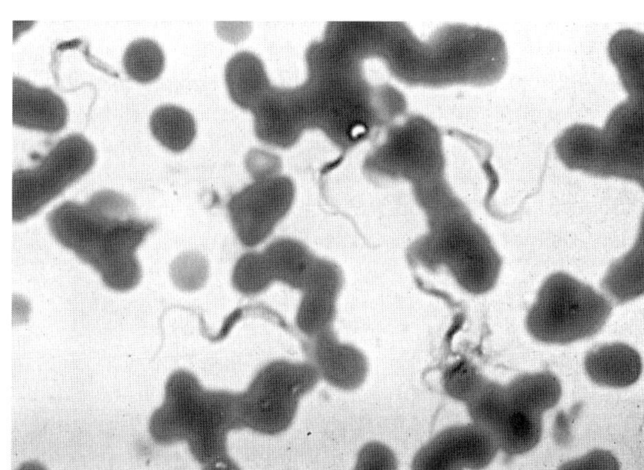

**Fig. 19.6** *Trypanosomes bruseii*—Giemsa blood.

### Malaria

Specimens should be collected every six hours for three days. The best diagnostic forms are found 12 hours after the chill. A microbiology technologist should collect and prepare thin and thick smears as outlined above. If a technologist is unavailable, draw the blood specimen into an EDTA vacutainer tube and send to Hematology for a differential white count. The resultant Wright-Giemsa–stained thin smear is scanned for malaria parasites.

### Trypanosomiasis

Trypanosome forms are frequently rare and difficult to find in the peripheral blood. Nevertheless, they can sometimes be seen, especially in sleeping sickness, where they actually multiply in the blood. Routine specimens are collected as described for malaria. In addition, blood should be drawn into three citrate or EDTA tubes and sent to the laboratory for concentration.

## Aspirates

Parasites can often be recovered from aspirates when conventional methods have failed. Duodenal and sigmoidoscopic aspirates are dealt with under gastrointestinal specimens. Aspirates of liver, lymph nodes, bone marrow, spinal fluid, and cutaneous ulcers are discussed below. A microbiologist should be present at the time of aspiration to accept the specimen. If this is not possible, the aspirate should be immediately hand-carried to the laboratory in a sterile container or sealed syringe and examined as soon as possible.

### Liver

The most frequent material submitted for the diagnosis of extraintestinal amebiasis is aspirate taken from a liver abscess. This material harbors only trophozoites, and since these forms rapidly deteriorate in the external environment, immediate examination is mandatory. Even under optimal conditions, however, it is difficult to demonstrate organisms, for two reasons: (*1*) most of the organisms are in the peripheral area of the abscess; relatively few are free in the abscess contents; (*2*) the organisms may be partially immobilized by coagulum. The yield is increased if the terminal (brownish-red or bloody) portion of the aspirate is treated with proteolytic enzymes to free the organism. Prior notification of the laboratory will permit them to prepare the enzymes. The initial part of aspirate should be sent to the laboratory for bacterial cultures. The reddish-brown or bloody portion of the terminal aspirate is then collected with a new syringe. A drop of this aspiration is placed on a clean slide and mixed with 2 or 3 drops of PVA fixative. The syringe with the remainder of the specimen is sealed and sent together with the PVA slide to the laboratory.

### Lymph nodes, spleen, bone marrow, and spinal fluid

Aspirates of these tissues are often obtained from patients suspected of having African trypanosomiasis, leishmaniasis, or Chagas' disease. Notify the laboratory when an aspiration will be performed; send the specimen immediately to the laboratory in a sterile container or sealed syringe.

### Cutaneous ulcers

The diagnosis of cutaneous leishmaniasis is established by demonstrating the presence of intracellular organisms in the suspected ulcer. Material should be obtained from below the ulcer bed through uninvolved skin, not from the surface of the ulcer. Introduce a few drops of saline with a 25-gauge needle and syringe. Aspirate the material back into the syringe, seal the syringe, and send it to the laboratory.

## Biopsy material

### Skin

Skin biopsies are helpful in the diagnosis of onchocerciasis, cutaneous amebiasis, and leishmaniasis. The presence of onchocerciasis is confirmed by finding microfilariae in skin snips taken from areas of involved skin. In the absence of detectable lesions, snips are taken from the thighs, buttocks, and iliac crests in African cases and from the scapulae, buttocks, and face regions in American cases. Provide the laboratory with prior notice that an onchocerciasis biopsy is to be submitted. The skin should then be disinfected with 70% alcohol or an iodophor and allowed to dry. A sterile 25-gauge needle point is then slipped under the epidermis and raised, and a small piece of skin (2–3 mm in diameter) is sliced off with a safety razor blade or scalpel. The snip should be so thin that significant bleeding does not occur, just a slight oozing of fluid. The skin snip is placed in a small amount of saline and delivered immediately to the laboratory. Amebiasis and leishmaniasis specimens are collected and processed for tissue sectioning and culture.

### Lymph nodes

Tissue specimens for the diagnosis of trypanosomiasis, leishmaniasis, Chagas' disease, and toxoplasmosis should be submitted to the Pathology service for impression smears and tissue sections. Smears are processed as thin smears and stained with Giemsa stain.

### Muscle biopsies

Muscle biopsy can be used to diagnose both trichinosis and cysticercosis. Biopsy of the deltoid, biceps, pectoralis major, or gastrocnemius muscle during the third to fourth week of trichinosis will often reveal larvae or cysts of that parasite. Because of the extreme rarity of cysticercosis in this country, muscle biopsy for this disease is seldom indicated. A small piece of muscle should be delivered to the Microbiology laboratory for a compression slide and digestion procedures; the remainder is dispatched to Pathology for tissue sectioning.

### Rectal or bladder biopsies

Rectal and bladder biopsies frequently reveal the presence of schistosome eggs in patients with chronic or light infections of *S. mansoni*, *S. japonicum* (rectal), and *S. haematobium* (bladder) when they cannot be found in the stool or urine.

Rectal biopsies should be taken from the level of the dorsal fold (Houston valve) with tracheal forceps. The greatest concentrations of eggs are found 9 cm from the anus. No special preparation of the patient is required. Bladder biopsies are similarly obtained from the area of the trigone. Both should be submitted to the Microbiology Laboratory for compression slides.

## Mature worms and proglottides

Worms and proglottides should be placed in a sterile bottle half filled with saline and delivered immediately to the Microbiology laboratory. If delay is expected, the bottle should be refrigerated until delivery is made.

## Stains

Some of the more commonly used stains for identification of parasites in excreta, blood, body fluids, and tissues are described below.

## Stool wet mounts

Lugol's iodine solution is routinely employed in stool wet mounts examined for the presence of protozoa. The yellow-brown stain makes *cysts* visually obvious and the characteristics of their nuclei more distinct than they appear in unstained wet mounts. Unfortunately, iodine distorts *trophozoites*, making it unsuitable for the visualization of this parasite stage. Two supravital stains, Quensel's and buffered methylene blue, can be used for staining *Entamoeba histolytica* trophozoites, producing levels of nuclear detail comparable to that achieved with permanently stained preparations. Merthiolate-iodine-formaldehyde (MIF), a solution used as a preservative for protozoa and helminths, stains both protozoan trophozoites and cysts in wet-mount preparations.

**Table 19.2** Immunologic tests performed at the Centers for Disease Control

| Disease | Test[a] | Diagnostic endpoint | Sensitivity[b] | Specificity[b] | Comment |
|---|---|---|---|---|---|
| Amebiasis | IHA | ≥1:256 | 70[1], 95[2] | 90[1] | 1. Active intestinal infection<br>2. Extraintestinal infection<br>3. Titers may persist for years |
| Cysticercosis | IB[1] | + or − | 70[2], 82[3], 98[4] | 100[4] | 1. Seven major bands<br>2. Single, enhancing CSF cyst<br>3. Multiple calcified CSF cyst<br>4. Serum >> CSF results |
| Echinococcosis | IHA | ≥1:256 | 60[1], 90[2] | 90–95[3,4] | 1. Lung or calcified cyst<br>2. Liver or peritoneal<br>3. Cysticercosis cross-reacts<br>4. Titer may persist for years |
| | IB[5] | + or − | 91[2] | 100[3,6] | 5. 8 kDa antigen<br>6. *E. multilocularis* cross-reacts |
| Paragonimiasis | IB[1] | + or − | 96 | 99 | 1. 8 kDa protein, Chaffee agn |
| Schistosomiasis | FAST-ELISA[1] | ≥ 8 U/μl | 99[2], 50[3] | 99 | 1. *S. mansoni* adultmicrosomal antigen<br>2. *S. mansoni* infections<br>3. *S. japonicum* infections |
| | IB[1] | + or − | High | High | 1. Separate Sm, Sh, SJ antigens |
| Strongyloidiasis | EIA | ≥1:8 | 84–92[1] | 80[2,3] | 1. *S. stercoralis* larval antigen<br>2. No absolute reference<br>3. Cross-reacts with filariasis, ascariasis |
| Toxocariasis | | | | | |
| Visceral | EIA[1] | ≥1:32 | 78 | 92[2] | 1. TES antigen<br>2. In children |
| Ocular | EIA | ≥1:8<br>≥1:32 | 90<br>73 | 91[1]<br>95 | 3. Patients with ocular disease |
| Toxoplasmosis | Capture EIA-IgM | ≥1:4 | High[1,3,4] | High[1,3] | 1. No absolute reference stnd<br>2. Antibodies persist for years<br>3. Antibodies persist for months<br>4. May be (−) in immunocompromised host |
| Trichinosis | BFT | ≥1:5 | 97[1] | 90[2] | 1. Detected after 3rd week of illness<br>2. Titers may persist for years |

[a]Abbreviations: IHA = Indirection hemagglutination; IB = immunoblot assay; ELISA = enzyme-linked immunosorbent assay; EIA = enzyme immunoassay; IFA = indirect fluorescent assay; BFT = bentonite flocculation.

[b]Superscript numbers refer to comments in far right column.

**Table 19.3** Key to malaria parasites found on thin film smear of blood

| | |
|---|---|
| INFECTED ERYTHROCYTE ENLARGED | |
| Many fimbriated erythrocytes:<br>Parasite fills 1/3 or more of cell<br>Schuffner's Dots seen in Giemsa-stained smears<br>Rings, schizonts & gametocytes present | *Plasmodium ovale* |
| No fimbriated erythrocytes:<br>Parasite fills 1/3 or more of cell<br>Schuffner's Dots seen in Giemsa-stained smears<br>Rings, schizonts, & gametocytes present | *Plasmodium vivax* |
| INFECTED ERYTHROCYTE NOT ENLARGED | |
| Ring forms are delicate, often with double chromatin dot<br>Only ring forms and banana-shaped gametocytes present<br>May have more than 1 parasite per cell<br>Parasite fills less than 1/3 of cell | *Plasmodium falciparum* (Fig. 19.3) |
| Rings form small with thick, bold staining cytoplasm<br>Rings, mature trophozoites, schizonts present<br>Mature trophozoites take band form<br>Parasite fills less than 1/3 of cell | *Plasmodium malariae* |

**Table 19.4** Key to microfilaria found in blood

| | |
|---|---|
| MICROFILARIAE ARE SHEATHED | |
| 275–325 μm in length, graceful curves, transparent sheath, discrete nuclei that do not reach tip | *Wuchereria bancrofti* |
| 300 μm in length, sheath visualized only with Delafield's stain, nuclei extend in continuous row to tip | *Loa loa* |
| 225–275 μm in length, kinky curves, nuclei overlapping and smudged, not continuous, two nuclei in tail | *Brugia malayi* |
| MICROFILARIAE ARE UNSHEATHED | |
| 200 μm in length, blunt tail large nucleus in tail | *Mansonella perstans* |
| 220 μm in length, clear cephalic space, sharp tail without nuclei | *Mansonella ozzardi* |

## Stool smears

In addition to the microscopic examination of saline and iodine wet mounts of direct and concentrated stool specimens, parasitologists recommend the use of stained smear microscopy. Since this significantly extends the time required to complete a parasitologic workup, many laboratories choose to restrict their workup to wet mounts. Nevertheless, examination of a stained concentrate significantly extends the sensitivity of microscopic examination (particularly for trophozoites and small cysts), increases the reliability of organism identification, permits later referral to consultants, and provides a permanent record of the organisms detected.

### Routine stains

The premier stain, Heidenhain's iron-hematoxylin technique, provides superb detail and can be used with either fresh or pre-

**Table 19.5.** Characteristics of protozoan cysts in the stool

| Parasite | Shape | Size (mm) | Number nuclei | Nuclear karyosome | Chromatoidal bodies | Comments |
|---|---|---|---|---|---|---|
| *Entamoeba histolytica* | Spherical | 10–15 | 14 | Small, central | Cigar-shaped | Glycogen mass in young cysts (Fig. 19.1) |
| *Giardia lamblia* | Ovoid | 8–12 × 6–10 | 4 | Tiny, central | None | Nuclei at anterior poles<br>Longitudinal fibers<br>Cytoplasm retracts from wall (Fig. 19.7) |
| *Isospora belli* | Ovoid | Oocyst 12 × 30 | NA | NA | NA | 2 sporozoites (9 × 11 μm) in oocyst wall; acid-fast |
| *Cryptosporidium parvum* | Spherical | Oocyst 5–6 | NA | NA | NA | 1–6 dark large granules and several small granules on phase microscopy; acid-fast |
| *Cyclospora cayetanensis* | Wrinkled spheres | Oocyst 8–10 | NA | NA | NA | 2 sporocysts per oocyst fluoresce under UV light; acid-fast |
| Microspora (several species) | Ovoid | Spore 1 × 2 | NA | NA | NA | Banded staining with Weber's stains. Fluoresce with the fluorochrome, Calcofluor White |

*Invasive and non-invasive (E. dispar) strains of Entamoeba histolytica cannot be differentiated by microscopy.

served specimens. Protozoan organisms appear blue-gray with black nuclear structures and inclusions. Unfortunately, the staining process is prolonged, cumbersome, and requires critical attention to detail. For routine laboratory work, the simpler and more rapid trichrome stain of Wheatley is usually employed. Like the iron-hematoxylin stain, it may be used with both fresh and preserved specimens. Protozoan cytoplasm is blue-green. The nuclear chromatin, chromatoid bodies, and ingested red cells and bacterial stain red. Eggs and larvae stain red, providing strong contrast with the green background.

### Supplemental stains

A number of coccidian protozoa, including *Cryptosporidium parvum, Isospora belli,* and *Cyclospora cayetanensis* have been recently recognized as important diarrheal agents, particularly of immunocompromised individuals. The small size and irregular staining characteristics of the coccidia have led to the introduction of a number of additional staining protocols for diarrheal stools. The stool oocysts of *Cryptosporidium, Isospora,* and *Cyclospora* can be readily visualized, and usually identified, with a number of acid-fast staining techniques. The Ziehl-Neelsen and Kinyoun stains can be viewed with a standard light microscope and provide good morphologic detail, permitting definitive parasite identification. The technically simpler Kinyoun stain is usually preferred to the Ziehl-Neelsen. The bright contrast provided by the auramine-rhodamine fluorescent stain makes it more convenient to scan large numbers of slides, and more sensitive in detecting small numbers of oocysts. The lack of morphologic detail afford by this stain, however, requires confirmation of the parasite's identification with a second procedure. A direct immunofluorescent stain is also available for the detection of *Cryptosporidium* oocysts in stool; a second direct immunofluorescent stain detects both giardia and cryptosporidia. Both are more expensive and time-consuming to

**Table 19.6** Key to helminth ova in stool

| | |
|---|---|
| OPERCULUM PRESENT | |
| *LARGE, OVER 50 MM* | |
| 140 × 80 μm: Ellipsoidal, rounded at poles, thin shell small indistinct operculum | *Fasciola hepatica* |
| 95 × 55 μm: Ellipsoidal, thick shell, flat distinct operculum (common in sputum, less frequent in stool) | *Paragonimus* species |
| 70 × 45 μm: Oval, small, slightly domed operculum, abopercular knob | *Diphyllobothrium* species |
| *SMALL, UNDER 50 MM* | |
| 29 × 16 μm: Ovum widened at nonoperculated pole, giving appearance of electric lightbulb | *Clonorchis sinensis* |
| 29 × 16μm: No widening at nonoperculated pole | *Opisthorchis* species<br>*Heterophyes heterophyes* |
| OPERCULUM ABSENT | |
| *WALL SMOOTH* | |
| Wall opaque | |
| Ovum elongated, wall thin with spines: | |
| 140 × 65 μm: terminal spine (present in urine, rare in feces) | *Schistosoma haematobium* |
| 150 × 65 μm: lateral spine | *Schistosoma mansoni* (Fig. 19.5) |
| 85 × 60 μm: minute lateral knob | *Schistosoma japonicum* |
| 57 × 37 μm: minute lateral knob | *Schistosoma mekongi* |
| Ovum round, wall thick with radial striae, hexacanth embryo with hooklets, 30–40 μm | *Taenia saginata*<br>*Taenia solium* |
| Wall transparent | |
| Wall thick | |
| 52 × 23 μm: Barrel-shaped with polar plugs | *Trichuris trichiuria* |
| 52 × 35 μm: Globular, bipolar filaments on inner shell, hexacanth embryo with hooklets | *Hymenolepsis nana* |
| Wall thin | |
| 60–70 × 38–40 μm: Ovoid with bluntly rounded ends, partially embryonated | *Ancylostoma duodenale*<br>*Necator americanus* |
| 55 × 26 μm: Asymmetrical, one side convex and other flattened, usually fully embryonated with rhabditiform larva | *Enterobius vermicularis* |
| *WALL ORNAMENTED* | |
| 60 × 45 μm: Ovoidal with brown outer mammillated covering, thick outer shell. | *Ascaris lunbricoides* |

**Table 19.7.** Key to cestode proglottids found in stool

| | |
|---|---|
| UTERUS FORMS A CENTRAL ROSETTE | *Diphyllobothrium* species |
| UTERUS DOES NOT FORM CENTRAL ROSETTE | |
| *UTERUS HAS CENTRAL STEM RUNNING LENGTH OF PROGLOTTID:* | |
| Central stem has 7–13 main lateral branches | *Taenia solium* |
| Central stem has 15–20 main lateral branches | *Taenia saginata* |
| *UTERUS WITHOUT A CENTRAL STEM:* | |
| Proglottid wider than long | *Hymenolepsis* species |
| Proglottid longer than wide | *Dipylidium caninum* |

use than the nonimmunologic stains. As *Cyclospora* oocysts are intensively autofluorescent, they can be recognized by their blue color under ultraviolet light.

Until recently, the diagnosis of human intestinal microsporidiosis required the recognition of the these tiny obligate intracellular protozoa in tissues submitted for light and electron microscopy. Now the availability of two simple staining procedures allow their spores to be identified directly from stool. The Weber modification of the trichrome stain permits a skilled and patient microscopist to find the distinctive, 1–2 $\mu$ red-stained, coccobacillary-shaped spores with central unstained bands amid the fecal debris. Although it requires the use of a fluorescence microscope, calcofluor white, a commonly used fungal stain, permits the more rapid and sensitive detection of fecal microsporidia. This, however, is not specific for microsporida.

## Blood smears

Direct examination of stained blood smears is useful for the detection of malaria parasites, leishmania, trypanosomes, and microfilaria. Fresh capillary or, less satisfactorily, venous blood is collected for the preparation of thin and thick smears. Precleaned glass slides must be used, as traces of soda lime and other contaminants may alter the pH of the stain, making identification of the parasites more difficult. Giemsa is the preferred stain for all blood parasites. Field's stain, widely used in malarious areas because of its simplicity of preparation, stability during storage, and speed of staining (3–4 seconds), is an appropriate alternative for the identification of malaria parasites. Wright's or Wright's-Giemsa stains are commonly substituted for Giemsa in nonendemic areas. However, they are not suitable for the staining of thick smears, and do not demonstrate Schüffner's granules characteristically seen in *Plasmodium vivax*– and *P. ovale*–infected erythrocytes. Delafield's hematoxylin stain is often substituted for Giemsa when staining blood obtained from patients suspected or known to have lymphatic filariasis. Delafield's stain better demonstrates the presence or absence of microfilarial sheaths, a morphologic feature important in the speciation of filarial pathogens.

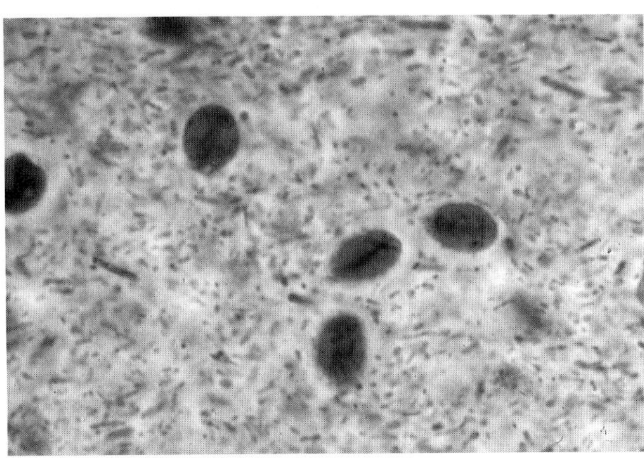

**Fig. 19.7** Giardia cysts.

## Serologies

Immunodiagnostic tests can be useful when it is difficult to recover the parasite or its progeny from the infected patient. Although such tests have been available for decades, their diagnostic value has been limited by low specificity and sensitivity. The recent availability of purified homologous antigens and highly reactive test systems has improved both of these parameters. At present, clinically useful tests are available for amebiasis, babesiosis, Chagas' disease, cysticercosis, echinococcosis, filariasis, leishmaniasis, paragonimiasis, schistosomiasis, toxocariasis, toxoplasmosis, and trichinosis (Table 19.2). Tests of marginal usefulness have been described for several others. The detection of specific antibodies to one of the diseases in the former group provides compelling evidence of infection, past or present. As antibody levels persist for periods of months to years, they cannot, with notable exceptions, differentiate past from current infections or be used to monitor the success of chemotherapy. Over the past decade, commercial firms have marketed antibody-detection kits for several parasitic diseases mentioned above. Due to the lack of standard methods for expressing test results, however, it is difficult to compare results obtained with kits from different companies.

Soluble antigens of several parasites have been demonstrated in body fluids, tissues, and excreta of infected patients. Commercial test kits are currently available for the detection of *Entamoeba histolytica, Giardia lamblia,* and *Cryptosporidium parvum* antigens in stool specimens and *Trichomonas vaginalis* in genitourinary tract specimens. A commercial stool antigen test capable of differentiating invasive from non-invasive (Eidispar) strains of *E. histolytica* is now available. Molecular diagnostic tests have been developed for most parasitic infections. At present, none are available commercially in the United States and few are suitable for routine diagnostic parasitology.

## Identifying Characteristics

Pertinent identifying characteristics of common pathogenic parasites are listed in Tables 19.3 to 19.7 (Fig. 19.7).

### REFERENCES

Alicna AD, Fadell EI. Advantage of purgation in recovery of intestinal parasites or their eggs. Am J Clin Pathol 1959; 31:139–142.

*Frequently recommended, but seldom employed, purgation remains useful for the diagnosis of organisms concentrated in the cecum, most notably* E. histolytica.

Bruckner DA. Amebiasis. Clin Microbiol Rev 1992; 5:356–369.

*A review of amebiasis with an emphasis on diagnostic approaches.*

Current WL, Garcia LS. Cryptosporidiosis. Clin Microbiol Rev 1991; 4:325–358.

Gottstein B. Molecular and immunological diagnosis of echinococcosis. Clin Microbiol Rev 1992; 5:248–261.
*A still-current, in-depth review of recent approaches to the diagnosis echinococcosis in United States.*

Maddison Shirley E, 1991 Serodiagnosis of Parasitic Diseases. Clin Microbiol Rev 1991; 4:457–469.
*The most comprehensive, recent review of parasitic serologies.*

Morris AJ, Wilson ML, Reller LB. Application of rejection criteria for stool ovum and parasite examinations. J Clin Microbiol 1992; 30:3213–3216.
*The majority of stool specimens submitted to the clinical laboratory are unsuitable for the diagnosis of intestinal parasitosis.*

Nanduri J, Kazura JW. Clinical and laboratory aspects of filariasis. Clin Microbiol Rev 1989; 2:39–50.
*A good review of a confusing—and frequently confused—diagnostic area.*

Spencer FM, Monroe LS. The Color Atlas of Intestinal Parasites. Charles C. Thomas, 1961.
*Still a classic.*

Sun T. Current topics in protozoal Diseases. Am J Clin Pathol 1994; 102:16–28.
*The author provides concise, current reviews of cryptosporidiosis, cyclosporiasis, isosporiasis, microsporidiosis, pneumocystosis, and toxoplasmosis as they appear in patients with AIDS.*

Tanowitz HB, Kirchhoff LV, Simon D, Morris SA, Weiss LM, Wittner M. Chagas' disease. Clin Microbiol Rev 1992; 5:400–419.

Weber R, Bryan RT, Schwartz DA, Owen RL. Human microsporidial infections. Clin Microbiol Rev 1994; 7:426–461.
*Microsporidiosis is increasingly recognized in patients with AIDS. This article provides an exhaustive review of this disease complex.*

Weiss JB. DNA probes and PCR for diagnosis of parasitic infections. Clin Microbiol Rev 1995; 8:113–130.
*Molecular diagnostic procedures are, at last, finding their way into the armamentarium of parasitologists, providing highly sensitive and specific alternatives to morphologic diagnosis.*

Wilcox A. Manual for the Microscopical Diagnosis of Malaria in Man. U.S. Public Health Service Publication N796, 1960.
*Still the best after 35 years.*

Wilson M, Schantz P, Pleniasek N. Diagnosis of parasitic infections: immunologic and molecular methods, In: Manual of Clinical Microbiology, 6th ed. Murray PR, Baron EJ, Pfaller MA, Tenover FC, Yolken RH, eds. American Society for Microbiology, Washington, D.C., pp. 1159–1170, 1995.
*The most recent review of the immunologic and molecular techniques currently employed for the diagnosis of parasitic diseases.*

Wolf MS. Giardiasis. Clin Microbiol Rev 1992; 5:93–100.

# 20

## Rickettsia and Chlamydia

W. CONRAD LILES AND WALTER E. STAMM

### Rickettsial and Related Diseases

The agents causing human rickettsial disease comprise a diverse group of bacteria, considered similar because of both their characteristic ability to defy cultivation on artificial media and their tendency to be associated with transmission by arthropod vectors. The order Rickettsiales includes four genera—*Rickettsia, Coxiella, Ehrlichia*, and *Bartonella*—with members capable of causing human disease. In general, rickettsial diseases are characterized by nonspecific systemic clinical manifestations, including fever, malaise, myalgias, and headache early in the course of illness, rendering specific diagnosis difficult at this stage. Nevertheless, it is often imperative that the clinician initiate appropriate empiric therapy against rickettsiae based on clinical suspicion alone, with subsequent confirmation of the diagnosis serologically. Such empiric therapy is necessary early in the disease course to avoid excessive morbidity and possible mortality associated with delayed treatment.

### Rickettsia (see Tables 20.1 and 20.2)

Human infections due to members of the genus *Rickettsia* are generally divided into three groups: the spotted fever group, the typhus group, and the scrub typhus group. The epidemiologic and clinical features of these diseases are summarized in Tables 20.1 and 20.2, respectively. Although most rickettsiae can be successfully cultivated with appropriate reagents, routine attempts to culture rickettsiae from clinical samples are discouraged because of the attendant risk of transmission to laboratory personnel. Serologic testing remains the cornerstone of routine clinical laboratory diagnosis of rickettsial diseases. However, the clinician should bear in mind that an antibody response rarely occurs with any of the rickettsioses before the end of the first week of illness. At present, serologic testing consists of (*1*) the Weil-Felix agglutination reaction (nonspecific), which is generally available in hospital laboratories as part of commercial "febrile agglutinin" packages, and (*2*) species-specific serologic tests, which are generally available at state health departments, the Rickettsial Laboratory at the CDC (Atlanta, GA), and the WHO reference laboratories.

The Weil-Felix agglutination reaction is based on common expression of unique polysaccharide antigens on certain *Proteus* strains and some rickettsiae. This relatively simple, but nonspecific, test is performed with suspensions of rough *Proteus* OX-2, OX-19, and OX-K strains. Typical Weil-Felix results are summarized in Table 20.3. Although utilized extensively in the past for the diagnosis of clinical rickettsial disease, the Weil-Felix reaction has now been largely supplanted by more definitive, specific serologic studies (see relevant sections in this chapter).

Of the specific serologic tests, the indirect fluorescent antibody (IFA) test is currently the most widely used method for diagnostic and epidemiologic purposes. The IFA test can be made group-specific or species-specific. Agglutination and complement-fixation (CF) tests are generally less sensitive and specific than comparable IFA tests. Ideally, both acute and convalescent sera should be obtained for simultaneous serologic testing. A fourfold or greater rise in specific antibody titer between acute and convalescent sera confirms the diagnosis of rickettsial disease. A single elevated titer suggests acute or recent infection. Enzyme-linked immunosorbent assays (ELISA), which offer high sensitivity, are currently under development or evaluation for the diagnosis of several rickettsial diseases. Polymerase chain reaction (PCR) technology also offers promise for rapid diagnostic testing in the future.

### Rocky Mountain spotted fever (RMSF)

The diagnosis of RMSF should be considered in any patient from an endemic region (especially the southeastern and lower midwestern United States) who presents with a history of potential tick exposure and fever, myalgias, and headache with or without a rash during the months of May through September.

#### Culture

Attempts to culture *R. rickettsii* require laboratory facilities with biohazard class 3 certification. *R. rickettsii* can be isolated from human blood or tissue biopsy specimens by cultivation in Vero cells, L cells, primary chicken embryo fibroblasts and other cell lines, or by intraperitoneal inoculation of adult male guinea pigs.

#### Serology

In general, serologic studies will not become positive until day 7–10 of clinical illness. Early appropriate therapy may partially blunt or delay the antibody response, and antibodies generally fall to nondiagnostic titers in approximately 2 months. The Weil-Felix agglutination reaction is typically positive for OX-19 and OX-2 late in the course of illness. Currently available RMSF-specific serologic tests include IFA, indirect hemagglutination assay (IHA), and latex agglutination. Whereas IFA, which is highly sensitive and specific, is the preferred serologic test, the latex agglutination test offers the advantages of simplicity and speed. Commercial reagents for IFA and latex agglutination are available from Integrated Diagnostics, Inc., Baltimore, MD. A fourfold or greater rise in antibody titer between acute and convalescent sera measured by any of these serologic tests confirms the diagnosis of RMSF. Moreover, a single titer ≥1:64 by IFA or ≥1:16 by CF is considered diagnostic of acute or recent infection, while a single titer ≥1:128 by IHA or latex agglutination strongly suggests RMSF.

### Histology

Demonstration of *R. rickettsii* in vascular endothelium and smooth muscle from biopsy specimens of the RMSF rash by immunofluorescence or immunoperoxidase methods provides early definitive diagnosis of RMSF. The CDC can be contacted to provide reagents for a highly specific direct immunofluorescence (DFA) test (sensitivity 70%). Optimal results with DFA are obtained when the test is performed on a 3 mm punch biopsy of a classic petechial lesion located on an erythematous base. An immunoperoxidase method has also been described for the detection of *R. rickettsii* in biopsy samples.

### PCR

DNA of *R. rickettsii* has been detected following PCR amplification in blood samples from patients with severe RMSF. Currently, this method is not available in clinical laboratories for the rapid diagnosis of RMSF.

## Boutonneuse fever (Mediterranean spotted fever)

### Culture

*Rickettsia conorii* can be isolated from blood samples in tissue culture using Vero cells, L cells, primary chicken embryo fibroblasts and other cell lines, or by intraperitoneal inoculation of adult male guinea pigs.

### Serology

IFA is most commonly employed to confirm the diagnosis. However, this test is only spotted fever group–specific in most circumstances. As in RMSF, the Weil-Felix agglutination reaction is typically positive late in the course of illness.

### Histology

Early diagnosis is possible by identification of *R. conorii* in biopsy specimens of the inoculation site or rash with specific fluorescein- or peroxidase-labeled antibody.

**Table 20.1** Epidemiologic features of selected human rickettsial diseases

| Disease | Organism | Arthropod vector | Mammalian host | Usual mode of transmission to man | Risk factors | Geographic distribution |
|---|---|---|---|---|---|---|
| TYPHUS GROUP | | | | | | |
| Murine typhus | *Rickettsia mooseri* (*R. typhi*) | Flea | Rodents | Cutaneous contact with infected flea feces, or aerosolized contact with mucous membranes | Rat-infested environments (e.g., old grain silos, warehouses, etc.) | Scattered foci woldwide |
| Epidemic typhus | *R. prowazekii* | Body louse | Man | Cutaneous contact with crushed lice or feces, or aerosolized contact with mucous membranes | Lice-infested human population | Scattered foci worldwide (esp. East Africa) |
| Brill-Zinsser disease | *R. prowazekii* | Body louse | Man | Relapse of louse-borne typhus months to years after primary illness | Lice-infested human population | Scattered foci worldwide |
| SPOTTED FEVER GROUP | | | | | | |
| Rocky Mountain spotted fever | *R. rickettsii* | Dermacentor ticks | Small mammals | Bite of infected tick | Tick-infested environments, dogs | Western hemisphere (esp., North America) |
| Boutonneuse fever (Mediterranean spotted fever) | *R. conorii* | Ixodid ticks | Rodents, dogs | Bite of infected tick | Tick-infested environments, dogs | Mediterranean basin, sub-Saharan Africa |
| Rickettsialpox | *R. akari* | Mouse mite | Mice | Infected mouse mite bite | Mouse-infested environments (both urban and rural) | United States, former USSR, Korea |
| SCRUB TYPHUS GROUP | | | | | | |
| Tsutsugamushi disease | *R. tsutsugamushi* | Chigger | Rodents | Infected chigger bite | Chigger-infested terrain, such as scrublands and grasslands | Asia, Australia, New Guinea, Pacific islands |

**Table 20.2** Clinical features of selected human rickettsial diseases

| Disease | Incubation period (days) | Skin manifestions | Duration of illness (days) | Usual severity of illness | Duration of fever following initiation of effective treatment (hours) |
|---|---|---|---|---|---|
| TYPHUS GROUP | | | | | |
| Murine typhus | 8–16 | Macular or macuolopapular rash of trunk and extremities | 8–16 | Moderate | 48–72 |
| Epidemic typhus | 10–14 | Macular, maculopapular, or petechial rash of trunk and extremities | 10–18 | Severe | 48–72 |
| Brill-Zinsser disease | — | Macular rash of trunk and extremities | 7–11 | Mild | 48–72 |
| SPOTTED FEVER GROUP | | | | | |
| Rocky Mountain spotted fever | 3–12 | Macular, maculopapular, or petechial rash of extremities, trunk, and face | 10–20 | Severe | 24–72 |
| Boutonneuse fever (Meditteranean spotted fever) | 5–7 | Eschar often present (tache noire); macular, maculopapular, or petechial rash of entire body surface | 7–14 | Moderate | — |
| Rickettsialpox | 9–17 | Eschar often present; papulovesicular rash of trunk, face, and buccal mucosa | 7 | Mild | — |
| SCRUB TYPHUS GROUP | | | | | |
| Tsutsugamushi disease | 9–18 | Eschar often present; macular or maculopapular rash of trunk and extremities | 10–20 | Mild to severe | 24–36 |

## Rickettsialpox

This disease is usually diagnosed on clinical grounds. The clinical presentation of rickettsialpox is relatively distinctive but can be confused with primary varicella. Typically, the rash of rickettsialpox consists of vesicuopapules, which appear in one crop. Often, an eschar is present at the site of the causative mite bite.

### Culture

Isolation of the agent is not recommended.

### Serology

Confirmation of rickettsialpox infection is usually based on serologic testing available through state health departments. The Weil-Felix agglutination reaction is negative in rickettsialpox.

## Other spotted fever diseases

Serologic tests are usually employed to confirm the diagnosis of other spotted fever rickettsial diseases, including North Asian tick-borne rickettsiosis and Queensland tick typhus. Typically, these diseases are associated with a positive Weil-Felix agglutination reaction for OX-19 and OX-2. The Rickettsial Laboratory at the CDC or WHO reference laboratories should be contacted about the availability of reagents for specific serologic studies.

## Murine typhus

### Culture

*Rickettsia typhi* can be cultivated, but this is not performed by most clinical laboratories.

**Table 20.3** Typical Weil-Felix agglutination test results

| Rickettsial disease | OX-19 | OX-2 | OX-K |
|---|---|---|---|
| Typhus group | +++ | + | Negative |
| Brill-Zinsser disease | Variable; often negative | Variable; often negative | Negative |
| Spotted fever group | + to +++ | + to +++ | Negative |
| Rickettsialpox | Negative | Negative | Negative |
| Scrub typhus group | Negative | Negative | Negative to +++[a] |
| Q fever | Negative | Negative | Negative |

[a]Usually positive in primary infection; unlikely to be positive in subsequent reinfections with different serotypes.

### Serology

Laboratory confirmation of murine typhus is usually achieved by specific serologic testing. Available serologic tests include IFA, latex agglutination, and solid-phase immunoasssay. Antibodies directed against *R. typhi* are almost always detectable by day 15 of illness.

### Histology

Immunohistology has been used to demonstrate *R. typhi* in infected tissues. However, this technique is not readily available in most laboratories.

### PCR

A PCR-based assay to detect DNA from *R. typhi* has been developed but is not widely available at the present time.

## Epidemic typhus

### Culture

Although not generally performed in most clinical laboratories, *Rickettsii prowazekii* can be isolated from blood or infected tissues by inoculation of guinea pigs or tissue culture.

### Serology

Definitive diagnosis of epidemic typhus is usually made by demonstrating a ≥fourfold rise in antibody titer using one of a variety of serologic tests. The IFA test demonstrates a predominant IgM response in primary typhus, while an IgG response is detected in relapsed typhus (Brill-Zinsser disease). Complement-fixation (CF) and toxin-neutralization tests are also available. The Weil-Felix agglutination reaction may be positive for OX-19 and OX-2. Antibodies against *R. prowazekii* persist for years following primary infection.

### PCR

A PCR-based assay to detect DNA from *R. prowazekii* in blood specimens has been developed. However, the current availability of this test is limited.

## Scrub typhus (tsutsugamushi disease)

### Culture

Although not routinely recommended, *Rickettsia tsutsugamushi* can be isolated by inoculation of infected blood or tissue homogenates intraperitoneally into white mice.

### Serology

Laboratory confirmation of the diagnosis of scrub typhus is almost excusively based on serologic studies at the present time. Antibodies directed against *Proteus* OX-K (Weil-Felix agglutination reaction) are present in approximately 50% of cases during the second week of illness. A single titer ≥1:320 or a fourfold rise in titer is considered diagnostic. Both an IFA test and an immunoperoxidase test, with similar sensitivity and specificity, have been developed and are available for use in clinical laboratories.

### PCR

PCR-based methodology has been developed to detect acute scrub typhus infection but is not widely available.

## Coxiella (see Tables 20.4 and 20.5)

## Q fever

### Culture

*Coxiella burnetti* can be isolated from blood, tissues, and valvular vegetations following inoculation into guinea pigs, mice, and embryonated eggs. Because of the associated risk of laboratory transmission, attempts to cultivate and isolate *C. burnetii* are generally not recommended.

### Serology

Serology remains the mainstay for the diagnosis of Q fever in the clinical setting. Highly specific microagglutination, IFA, ELISA, and CF tests have been used for diagnosis; the CF test is the most commonly used. A fourfold or greater rise in titer between acute and convalescent sera is diagnostic of Q fever. In acute uncomplicated disease, phase II complement-fixing antibodies appear approximately 7 days into the course of illness, peak in 3–4 weeks, and gradually decline over the ensuing 24–36 months. Phase I antibodies are usually not significantly elevated. Elevated phase I antibodies (i.e., ≥1:200) suggest chronic infections, such as endocarditis or hepatitis. Antibody titers decline slowly with effective antimicrobial treatment.

### Histology

Organisms have been demonstrated in tissues (granulomas) and valvular vegetations using fluorescein-labeled anti–*C. burnetti* immune serum. This methodology is not generally available in most clinical laboratories.

**Table 20.4** Epidemiologic features of human rickettsial-like diseases

| Disease | Organism | Arthropod vector | Mammalian host | Usual mode of transmission to man | Risk factors | Geographic distribution |
|---|---|---|---|---|---|---|
| Q fever | *Coxiella burnetii* | ?Ticks | Mammals (esp., livestock and cats) | Inhalation of dried airborne infective material | Exposure to parturient domestic livestock or cats; ?tick bite | Worldwide (esp. Australia) |
| Trench fever | *Bartonella quintana* | Body louse | Man | Cutaneous contact with infected crushed lice or feces | Lice-infested human population; urban homeless street population | Africa, Mexico, United States |
| Cat scratch disease | *B. henselae* (major etiology) *Afipia felis* (minor etiology) | None known | Cats | Bite or lick from a cat, especially a kitten | Exposure to cats | Worldwide |
| Bacillary angiomatosis | *B. henselae* (major) *B. quintana* (minor) | None known | ?Cats | ?Exposure to cats | HIV disease | Worldwide |
| Bartonellosis | *Bartonella bacilliformis* | Phlebotomine sandflies | Man | Bite of infected sandfly | Residence in valleys 800–2500 meters above sea level in Peru, Ecuador, and Columbia | Specific highland valleys in Peru, Ecuador, and Columbia |
| Ehrlichiosis | *Ehrlichia chaffeensis* | Ticks | Unknown; possibly small mammals | Bite of infected tick | Outdoor activity during warm weather months in tick-infested areas | United States |
| Sennetsu fever | *Ehrlichia sennetsu* | ?Ticks | Probably small mammals | ?Bite of infected tick | ?Outdoor activity in endemic regions during summer and fall months | Japan (esp., western coastal regions) and Malaysia |

#### PCR

DNA of *C. burnetti* in clinical specimens has been detected following PCR amplification. Currently, PCR-based tests for Q fever are not routinely available in clinical laboratories.

## *Ehrlichia* (see Tables 20.4 and 20.5)

### Ehrlichiosis

The diagnosis of ehrlichiosis should be considered in patients presenting with fever, leukopenia, thrombocytopenia, elevated serum transaminases, and a history of recent tick bite in endemic regions (southeastern and lower midwestern United States) from May through August.

#### Culture

Cultivation of *Ehrlichia chaffeensis* is possible but laborious, and thus is not recommended for routine clinical diagnosis at the present time.

#### Serology

At present, definitive diagnosis of ehrlichiosis depends chiefly on serologic studies utilizing an IFA test available at the CDC. Diagnosis is based on demonstration of a ≥fourfold rise or fall in antibody titer, with a minimal peak titer of ≥1:80.

#### Histology

Ehrlichial morulae can be detected in human tissue by immunohistochemistry. However, this technique is relatively insensitive.

#### PCR

A PCR-based method to detect DNA from *E. chaffeensis* has been developed but is not widely available.

**Table 20.5** Clinical features of human rickettsial-like diseases

| Disease | Incubation period (days) | Skin manifestions | Duration of illness (days) | Usual severity of illness | Duration of fever following initiation of effective treatment (hours) |
|---|---|---|---|---|---|
| Q fever | 10–26 | None | 2–21 (acute) Months to years (chronic) | Mild to moderate | 48–120 |
| Trench fever | 14–35 | Possible macular rash | 3–5, with possible relapses | Mild to moderate | — |
| Cat scratch disease | 3–10 | Vesiculopapular lesion at inoculation site; erythema over involved lymphadenopathy | 10–120 | Mild | — |
| Bacillary angiomatosis | Unknown | Diffuse vascular papules, nodules, and plaques | Chronic; relapses following treatment are common in immunocompromised patients | Mild to moderate | Variable |
| Bartonellosis | 7–100 | Verrucous skin lesions of extremities, trunk, and face during chronic phase of disease (verruga peruana) | 10–28 (acute phase) | Mild to severe | 8–12 |
| Ehrlichiosis | 1–21 | Maculopapular or petechial rash in <25% of patients | 7–21 | Mild to moderate | 12–48 |
| Sennetsu fever | Unknown | Skin rashes are unusual | 10–21 | Mild | 12–48 |

## Bartonella (including *Rochalimaea*) (see Tables 20.3 and 20.4)

### Trench fever

#### Culture

*Bartonella quintana* can be grown from blood on blood agar incubated for 10–14 days at 33°C in a 10% $CO_2$–90% air atmosphere. At the present time, the Isolator lysis-centrifugation system (Wampole Laboratories, Cranbury, NJ) is preferred for the detection of non-*bacilliformis Bartonella* spp. Isolator-processed blood should be plated on blood or chocolate agar and incubated in a humid $CO_2$-enriched atmosphere at 35°–37°C for 5–30 days. Recently, it has been shown that *B. quintana* can be detected by acridine orange staining of routine broth blood cultures (BACTEC nonradiometric aerobic resin blood cultures) from patients with bacteremia. Xenodiagnosis can also be achieved with clean lice.

#### Serology

IFA, CF, microagglutination, and ELISA tests have all been described but are not routinely available.

### Cat scratch disease

*Bartonella henselae* is the etiologic agent in the majority of cases of cat scratch disease (CSD). Infection with *Afipia felis* is responsible for relatively few cases of CSD. Most cases of CSD are presumptively diagnosed based on the clinical presentation and history of exposure to cats.

#### Culture

Lysis-centrifugation blood cultures can be used to isolate non-*bacilliformis Bartonella* spp., including *B. henselae*, from bacteremic patients. However, most CSD patients are not bacteremic. Direct plating of homogenized tissue has yielded rare isolates. Gas-liquid chromatography can be used as a confirmatory method once the organisms have grown in culture.

#### Serology

In most cases, serologic confirmation of CSD is not required. When clinically warranted, serum samples can be sent to the CDC for IFA testing for *B. henselae.* ELISA tests to detect IgG antibodies against *B. henselae* and *A. felis* are now commercially available (Specialty Laboratories, Santa Monica, CA). Serologic tests have essentially replaced use of the cat scratch skin test.

#### Histology

Histologic examination of lymph node tissue may be clinically indicated in atypical CSD. The diagnosis of CSD can be confirmed by demonstrating small, pleomorphic bacilli in Warthin-Starry– or Brown-Hopps–stained sections of biopsy specimens obtained from involved lymph nodes, skin, or conjunctiva. It should be noted, however, that interpretation of these stains is often difficult in inexperienced hands.

#### PCR

PCR-based technology has been employed to detect DNA from *B. henselae* in clinical specimens. This technique is currently a research tool and is not routinely used for diagnosis of clinical CSD.

### Bacillary angiomatosis

Recent studies indicate that disseminated infection with *Bartonella henselae* is responsible for the majority of cases of bacillary angiomatosis (BA). Infection with *Bartonella quintana* appears to account for most of the remaining cases.

#### Culture

Lysis-centrifugation blood cultures can be used to isolate *B. henselae* and *B. quintana* from the blood of patients with BA (see "Trench Fever," earlier in this chapter). *B. henselae* has also been isolated after direct plating of tissue from involved lymph nodes and spleen.

#### Serology

Serum samples from patients with suspected BA can be sent to the CDC for IFA testing for both *B. henselae* and *B. quintana.* An ELISA test to detect IgG antibodies against *B. henselae* is commercially available (Specialty Laboratories, Santa Monica, CA).

#### Histology

Biopsy of skin lesions is usually necessary to distinguish BA from Kaposi's sarcoma definitively. Examination by light microscopy is the most commonly used method to confirm the diagnosis. BA lesions show characteristic lobular vascular proliferations composed of plump "epithelioid" endothelial cells. Neutrophils are usually scattered in varying densities throughout the lesion, especially around eosinophilic aggregations, which prove to be collections of bacteria when viewed by light microscopy or following Warthin-Starry staining.

#### PCR

See "Cat Scratch Disease," earlier in this chapter.

### Bartonellosis

A presumptive diagnosis of acute bartonellosis is based upon the clinical presentation of fever, progressive hemolytic anemia, and generalized lympadenopathy in an individual with nocturnal exposure to sandfly bites in an endemic area (specific highland valleys of Peru, Ecuador, and Columbia at altitudes btween 800 and 2500 meters above sea level).

#### Culture

Definitive diagnosis of acute bartonellosis is based on the isolation of *Bartonella bacilliformis* from blood cultures. The organism can be cultivated on Columbia agar with 5% defibrinated human blood or semisolid nutrient agar with 10% fresh rabbit hemoglobin under aerobic conditions at 28°C. Colonies usually are apparent following 7–10 days of growth.

#### Serology

IFA, IHA, and ELISA tests have been developed in research laboratories but are not widely available.

#### Histology

Rapid confirmation of suspected acute bartonellosis can be obtained by demonstration of intraerythrocytic bacilli in a Giemsa-stained thin blood smear. Diagnosis of chronic bartonellosis (verruga peruana) can be made by identification of characteristic Giemsa-stained bacilli in a biopsy specimen of a representative skin lesion.

## Chlamydiae and Related Diseases

The genus chlamydiae contains three species that produce human disease: *Chlamydia trachomatis*, *Chlamydia pneumoniae*, and *Chlamydia psittaci*. *Chlamydia trachomatis* derives its name from its role as the causative agent in trachoma, a highly prevalent blinding infection of the eye found principally in arid, underdeveloped parts of the world. In both developed and underdeveloped countries, *Chlamydia trachomatis* is a major cause of sexually transmitted disease syndromes, including urethritis, cervicitis, pelvic inflammatory disease, epididymitis, proctitis and the other conditions shown on Tables 20.6 and 20.7. Cervical infection in the mother may be transferred vertically to newborn infants, producing conjunctivitis, rhinitis, and pneumonitis. Selected strains of *Chlamydia trachomatis* (serovars L1, L2, L3) produce the syndrome lymphogranuloma venereum, which is associated with genital ulceration and inguinal lymphadenopathy. Transmission of *Chlamydia trachomatis* occurs during sexual intercourse, during the birth of a newborn to a mother with cervical infection, or in the case of trachoma, from person to person via transfer of infected secretions through close personal contact in crowded conditions. No animal reservoirs are known, and man is the sole host.

In contrast, *C. psittaci* infects many species of birds and mammals. Man is infected accidentally, usually after exposure to infected birds, and is only an accidental host. The illness in man usually presents as an atypical pneumonia, but the infection is generally systemic, frequently involving the liver, spleen, meninges, and other sites. Infective endocarditis may also result. *Chlamydia psittaci* is not transmitted from man to man; the organism, however, is highly infectious in the laboratory and care must be taken to prevent laboratory-acquired infections. For this reason, culture is generally not utilized to make the diagnosis.

The third species of chlamydia infecting man is *Chlamydia pneumoniae*, which was recently discovered in the late 1980s. Although this species was originally considered to be a variant of *C. psittaci*, it is now clearly identified as a separate species. Like *C. psittaci*, *C. pneumoniae* primarily infects the respiratory tract, producing rhinitis, sinusitis, pharyngitis, and pneumonitis. Unlike *C. psittaci*, however, there appears to be no animal reservoir. To date, *Chlamydia pneumoniae* infections have been identified only in man, and transmission occurs from person to person via respiratory secretions much like mycoplasmal or viral infections of the respiratory tract (Table 20.1).

### Microbiological characteristics of chlamydiae

All chlamydia are obligate intracellular parasites and can multiply only in living eucaryotic cells. They produce characteristic intracytoplasmic inclusions in these cells and have unique life

**Table 20.6** Diagnosis of *C. trachomatis* infections in men

| Disease | Clinical criteria | Laboratory criteria | |
|---|---|---|---|
| | | Presumptive | Diagnostic |
| Nongonococcal urethritis (NGU) | Discharge, dysuria; urethral discharge on exam | Urethral GS with greater than or equal to 5 PMN/ 1000× field: pyuria on FVU | Positive culture or nonculture test (urethra) |
| Acute epididymitis | Fever, epididymal/testicular pain, evidence of NGU, epididymal tenderness/mass on exam | As for NGU | As for NGU; positive culture on epididymal aspirate |
| Acute proctitis (nonlymphogranuloma venereum strain) | Rectal pain, discharge; abnormal anoscopy (mucopurulent discharge, pain, spontaneous or induced bleeding) | Rectal GS with greater than or equal to 1 PMN/ 1000× field | Positive culture or nonculture test (rectal) |
| Acute proctocolitis (lymphogranuloma venereum strain) | Severe rectal pain, discharge, hematochezia, markedly abnormal anoscopy with lesions extending into colon; fever, lymphadenopathy | Rectal GS with greater than or equal to 1 PMN/ 1000× field | Positive culture or nonculture test (rectal); complement fixation antibody titer greater than or equal to 1/64 |

Abbreviations: GS, Gram stain; PMN, polymorphonuclear leukocyte; NGU, nongonococcal urethritis; FA, fluorescent antibody; FVU, first-void urine.

cycles in which an extracellular transmissible form (the elementary body) facilitates transmission from one cell to another or from one host to another, while an intracellular form of the organism (the reticulate body) is adapted to intracellular survival and multiplication. The three species all share a genus-specific lipopolysaccharide antigen, which is the basis of the complement-fixation antibody test. Each species, however, has major outer-membrane protein antigens that are unique and species-specific. Eighteen serovars of *Chlamydia trachomatis* have been identified to date. In contrast, all strains of *C. pneumoniae* appear to be serologically homogenous. The chlamydial species can be clearly differentiated on the basis of DNA hybridization tests, which indicate that each of the three is unique since less than 10% hybridization occurs with DNA from other species. Selected microbiologic and morphologic features also serve to differentiate the three species in the laboratory (Table 20.8).

Since all chlamydia are obligate intracellular pathogens, they must be isolated in cell culture systems. Cell culture systems have been effectively used in the clinical setting for isolation of *C. trachomatis* for years, but are largely available only in referral centers. Additionally, transport of specimens from clinics to the reference laboratory must be rapid and under refrigerated conditions to ensure viability of the organisms. Recent studies with more sensitive diagnostic tests, such as polymerase chain reaction, indicates that many chlamydia culture systems only detect 50%–60% of true infections, most likely due to poorly collected samples or nonviability after transport. Since chlamydia are intracellular parasites, collection of specimens that contain epithelial cells is critical for successful isolation of the organism. Specimens containing purulent discharge frequently will not grow the organism. *Chlamydia psittaci* can also be grown in various cell culture systems, but this is not widely practiced owing to the associated hazard of infecting laboratory workers. *Chlamydia pneumoniae* can be grown in HeLa cells, HL cells, and other cell lines, but it is fastidious and cell culture is not generally available for clinical purposes owing to lack of sensitivity.

Given these difficulties in utilizing cell culture for chlamydia diagnosis, much recent effort has been directed toward the development of nonculture tests for chlamydial infection. Considerable progress has been made in this regard with *C. trachomatis*. Nonculture tests that detect chlamydial antigen either by enzyme immunoassay or by direct visualization of chlamydial elementary bodies in smears utilizing fluorescein-conjugated monoclonal antibodies are widely available commercially. Studies indicate that these tests are highly specific but that their sensitivity compared with high-quality cell culture systems ranges from 60% to 85%. The recent development of DNA-amplification assays utilizing polymerase chain reaction and ligase chain reaction procedures has resulted in diagnostic tests that exceed culture in terms of sensitivity and are equal to culture in specificity. These tests are just now becoming commercially available and will probably become the tests of choice for diagnosis of most *C. trachomatis* infections. Of interest, these amplification tests appear to be sufficiently sensitive so that one can utilize a voided urine specimen in both males and females to diagnose chlamydial genital infection with sensitivity exceeding that of urethral and cervical swabs in men and women, respectively.

Unfortunately, nonculture tests have not been developed for the other chlamydial species. Although EIA, DFA, and PCR have all been studied for *Chlamydia pneumoniae*, commercially available tests that are sensitive and specific for this infection have not been forthcoming as yet. The same can be said for *C. psittaci*. For this reason, both *C. pneumoniae* and *C. psittaci* remain largely serologic diagnoses.

### *Chlamydia trachomatis* infections

*Chlamydia trachomatis* causes a variety of syndromes in infected men, women, and infants (Tables 20.6 and 20.7). In most instances, a presumptive diagnosis can be established based on clinical findings and evidence of inflammation on Gram stain or

**Table 20.7** Diagnosis of *C. trachomatis* infections in women

| Disease | Clinical criteria | Laboratory criteria: Presumptive | Laboratory criteria: Diagnostic |
|---|---|---|---|
| Mucopurulent cervicitis | Mucopurulent cervical discharge, cervical ectopy and edema, spontaneous or easily induced cervical bleeding | Cervical GS with greater than 20 PMN/100× field in nonmenstruating women; PMNS (often in strands of cervical mucus); positive swab test | Positive culture or nonculture test (cervix) |
| "Dysuria-pyuria" (urethritis) | Dysuria-frequency in young, sexually active women; recent new sexual partner; often more than 7 days of symptoms | Pyuria, no bacteriuria | Positive culture or nonculture test (cervix and/or urethra) |
| Pelvic inflammatory disease (PID) | Lower abdominal pain; adnexal tenderness on pelvic exam; evidence of MPC often present on exam | As for MPC; cervical GS positive for gonorrhea; endometritis on endometrial biopsy | Positive culture or nonculture test (cervix, endometrium, tubal) |
| Perihepatitis | Right upper quadrant pain, nausea, vomiting, fever; young, sexually active women; evidence of PID | As for mucopurulent cervicitis and PID | High-titer IgM or IgG antibody to *C. trachomatis* |

Abbreviations: GS, Gram stain, PMN, polymorphonuclear leukocyte; PID, pelvic inflammatory disease; MPC, mucopurulent cervicitis; FA, fluorescent antibody; FVU, first-void urine.

biopsy at the site of infection (Tables 20.6 and 20.7). A specific diagnosis can be established by utilizing culture, a nonculture diagnostic test, or serology. Tables 20.6 and 20.7 outline which of these tests is most appropriate for each clinical circumstance.

### Cultures

Chlamydia can be readily cultured in a variety of cell culture systems. Most laboratories utilize HeLa, McCoy, or BHK cells. Specimens for culture are generally collected with swabs or, in the case of cervical specimens in women, a cytobrush. Care should be taken to remove purulent discharge and sample epithelial cell scrapings for optimal results. Specimens must be placed in an appropriate transport medium and refrigerated during transport to the laboratory. Inoculation on the cell culture monolayer must be accomplished within 48 hours or the specimen should be frozen at −70°C until it can be inoculated. Cultures can be performed in monolayers grown in 96-well microtiter plates or on cover slips in glass vials. Seventy-two hours after inoculation, chlamydial inclusions are identified utilizing fluorescein-conjugated monoclonal antibodies. Cultures for chlamydia are technically difficult, reasonably expensive, and in

**Table 20.8** Comparison of *Chlamydia* spp. causing human disease

| | Principal diseases | | |
|---|---|---|---|
| | *C. pneumoniae* pneumonia, bronchitis pharyngitis, sinusitis | *C. psittaci* pneumonia, FUO | *C. trachomatis* STD, trachoma, LGV |
| Natural host | Human | Birds, mammals | Human |
| Serovars | 1 | Unknown | 18 |
| Sulfa sensitive | No | No | Yes |
| Tetracycline-sensitive | Yes | Yes | Yes |
| Elementary body morphology | Pear-shaped, periplasmic space | Round, no periplasmic space | Round, no periplasmic space |
| Iodine-staining inclusions | No | No | Yes |
| LPS complement-fixing antigen | Yes | Yes | Yes |

many circumstances probably have sensitivity only in the range of 50%–60%. Further, the relatively restrictive transport conditions limit the availability of cultures. It is likely that DNA amplification–based tests (PCR and LCR) will largely replace culture in the next few years.

### Nonculture diagnostic tests

Given the shortcomings of culture, considerable effort has been expended toward the development of nonculture tests for chlamydia. The first such tests utilized fluorescein-conjugated monoclonal antibodies, which could be used to demonstrate the presence of chlamydia elementary bodies in smears of infected discharge from the cervix, urethra, or eye. While technically laborious, this technique, when well performed, is highly specific and reasonable sensitive. However, the test cannot be used to process large numbers of specimens, owing to the lengthy periods of microscopy required. Antigen-detection tests utilizing enzyme immunoassays have also been developed. These tests, which now generally incorporate a confirmatory assay as well, are quite specific but considerably less sensitive than culture. More recently, two tests utilizing DNA amplification have been developed—namely, the PCR and LCR assays. Both assays appear to be highly sensitive and specific when applied to genital specimens. It also appears that the assays are sensitive enough to be able to utilize urine specimens rather than urethral and cervical swabs. The ability to use voided urine specimens obviously has great potential advantage from the perspective of patient convenience and has tremendous implications for the development of chlamydia screening programs. Depending on the site of infection being tested, these amplification assays appear to be 10%–30% more sensitive than the best culture systems. Pending further experience with these tests in a wider variety of patient populations and laboratories, it is likely that they will become the most widely used diagnostic approaches to most genital and ocular chlamydial infections.

### Staining procedures

Chlamydia inclusions can be identified by direct staining in some infected discharges, especially those obtained from ocular infections. However, the classical use of Giemsa staining to demonstrate chlamydial inclusions in smears has been largely replaced by the new diagnostic tests outlined above. The use of fluorescein-conjugated monoclonal antibodies to demonstrate elementary bodies rather than inclusions in infected discharges has greatly improved the sensitivity of staining techniques. However, in most cases, these tests are less sensitive and not much faster than the newer amplification tests described above. Hence, it is not likely that they will have a major place in patient management in the future.

### Serology

Two serological assays are available for *Chlamydia trachomatis* infections: the complement-fixation test available in many laboratories and health departments, and the microimmunofluorescence serologic test, which remains largely a research tool. The complement-fixation test measures antibody directed against the genus-specific lipopolysaccharide antigen of the organism. Thus, all three chlamydial species can induce antibody rises in the complement-fixation test. Most *C. trachomatis* infections are superficial mucosal infections that do not engender a dramatic immune response utilizing this test. Additionally, many chlamydial infections have been present for weeks or months at the time of initial serological evaluation, and thus it is often difficult to differentiate acute infection (characterized by the presence of IgM antibody or by titer rises or falls in IgG antibody) from chronic infection. For these reasons, the complement-fixation assay is not recommended for diagnosis of most *C. trachomatis* infections. It may be useful in patients with suspected LGV, in whom a titer of ≥1:64 is considered diagnostic.

The microimmunofluorescense test measures antibody directed against the *C. trachomatis* major outer-membrane protein and thus is species-specific. Additionally, it may be possible to identify the specific infecting serovar utilizing this test. The test has been most valuable as a diagnostic tool in infants with suspected chlamydial pneumonia, in patients with LGV infection, in patients with pelvic inflammatory disease and perihepatitis, and in selected other circumstances. However, the test is largely limited to research laboratories and hence is not widely available.

## *Chlamydia pneumoniae*

*Chlamydia pneumoniae* is one of many organisms that should be suspected in patients with upper or lower respiratory tract infections. Clinically, the syndromes produced by *Chlamydia pneumoniae* cannot be readily differentiated from other respiratory pathogens such as mycoplasma, streptococci, pneumococci, haemophilus, and respiratory viruses. In many instances, given the relative lack of severity and self-limited nature of the infection, it is not necessary to make a specific etiologic diagnosis. In cases of pneumonia or other more serious infections, however, specific diagnostic tests are often useful. Unfortunately, diagnostic tests for *C. pneumoniae* are presently limited. While the organism can be grown in cell culture and passaged in the laboratory, primary isolation from respiratory secretions or other respiratory specimens has been disappointingly insensitive. At present, antigen-detection tests that can identify *C. pneumoniae* infections with reasonable sensitivity and specificity are not available. PCR methodologies have been utilized and are being developed but are not yet available to clinicians. Thus, the only available diagnostic method in most patients is serologic testing, which has the limitations as outlined below.

### Culture

*C. pneumoniae* can be isolated in HeLa cells, McCoy cells, and other commonly used cell lines but appears to grow best on HL cells or HEPA cells. Attempts to isolate the organism from primary patient specimens have been disappointing, and more sensitive cell culture systems would be of great value.

### Nonculture diagnostic tests

As yet, there are no nonculture tests or DNA amplification tests that are commercially available for the diagnosis of *C. pneumoniae*. Efforts are under way to develop such tests.

### Serology

The greatest published experience with serologic tests for diagnosis of *C. pneumoniae* derives from a few centers utilizing the microimmunofluoresence test. Unfortunately, this test is not widely available to most clinicians and is technically difficult to perform. Utilizing the test, an IgM antibody ≥1:8, a fourfold rise or fall in IgG titer, or a single IgG titer ≥1:512 is considered indicative of current or recent infection. Other titers probably indicate preexisting or chronic infection. In recurrent infections, IgM antibody is frequently absent and IgG titer rises are less dramatic. *Chlamydia pneumoniae* infection also produces antibody rises utilizing the complement-fixation test. In the setting of respiratory infection, this test does not differentiate *C. pneumoniae* from *C. psittaci* infection. *C. pneumoniae* infection produces complement-fixation antibody titers ≥1:16 in most individuals with primary infection. In recurrent infections, complement-fixing antibody is frequently not seen. At present, although inadequate, the best diagnostic test for *C. pneumoniae* in patients with pneumonia is usually measurement of acute and convalescent antibody titers utilizing the microimmunofluoresence test in an appropriate reference laboratory.

## *Chlamydia psittaci*

Given the serious nature of many *C. psittaci* infections, a precise etiologic diagnosis and specific therapy is quite important. Either culture of the organism or serologic studies are most commonly utilized to confirm the diagnosis in patients with suspected psittacosis.

### Culture

*C. psittaci* can be isolated from respiratory secretions in HeLa, McCoy, or other cell lines. Given the potential laboratory hazard, laboratory personnel should be notified when such isolation is undertaken. Given the paucity of published clinical experience with the use of culture for diagnosis, the optimal sampling sites and methods and the true sensitivity of this approach are unknown.

### Nonculture diagnostic tests

Antigen detection, DNA hybridization, or DNA-amplification tests for *Chlamydia psittaci* have not been developed. Some of the enzyme immunoassays that have been developed for *Chlamydia trachomatis* infection and utilize genus-specific antigens should theoretically be positive in *C. psittaci* infections as well, but actual experience with this approach is limited.

### Serology

*Chlamydia psittaci* is usually diagnosed on the basis of titer rises observed in the complement-fixation assay. In most laboratories, a fourfold rise or fall in antibody titer in acute and convalescent sera confirms the diagnosis. A single titer ≥1:64 may also be indicative of acute or recent infection.

## ANNOTATED BIBLIOGRAPHY

### Rickettsial diseases


Dumler SJ, Walker DH. Diagnostic tests for Rocky Mountain spotted fever and other rickettsial diseases. Dermatol Clin 1994; 12:25–36.
*An excellent overview of the tests available for the diagnosis of human rickettsial diseases, with an emphasis on diagnosis during the acute phase of illness.*

Jones D, Anderson B, Olson J, Greene C. Enzyme-linked immonosorbent assay for detection of human immunoglobulin G to lipopolysaccharide of spotted fever group rickettsiae. J Clin Microbiol 1993; 31:138–141.
*Description of an ELISA assay for diagnosis of human rickettsial disease.*

McDade JE. Diagnosis of rickettsial diseases: a perspective. Eur J Epidemiol 1991; 7:270–275.
*A useful discussion of the available dignostic studies for rickettsial diseases from a respected authority in the field.*

Sexton DJ, Kanj SA, Wilson K et al. The use of a polymerase chain reaction as a diagnostic test for Rocky Mountain spotted fever. Am J Trop Med Hyg 1994; 50:59–63.

Sugita Y, Yamakawa Y, Takahashi K et al. A polymerase chain reaction system for rapid diagnosis of scrub typhus within six hours. Am J Trop Med Hyg 1993; 49:636–640.
*Use of the polymerase chain reaction of blood specimens to detect rickettsial infection.*

Spach DH, Liles WC, Campbell GL et al. Tick-borne diseases in the United States. N Engl J Med 1993; 329:936–947.
*A comprehensive review of the major tick-borne diseases in the United States, including Rocky Mountain spotted fever and ehrlichiosis.*

Walker DH, Cain BG, Olmstead PM. Laboratory diagnosis of Rocky Mountain spotted fever by immunofluorescent demonstration of *Rickettsia rickettsii* in cutaneous lesions. Am J Clin Pathol 1978; 69:619–623.

Woodward TE, Pederson CE, Oster CN et al. Prompt confirmation of Rocky Mountain spotted fever: Identification of rickettsiae in skin tissues. J Infect Dis 1976; 134:297–301.
These two papers describe an immunofluorescent technique to identify *R. rickettsii* in skin lesions from patients with acute Rocky Mountain spotted fever.

Weber DJ, Walker DH. Rocky Mountain spotted fever. Infect Dis Clin North Am 1991; 5:19–35.
*A thorough and useful discussion of the clinical and laboratory manifestations of Rocky Mountain spotted fever.*


### Ehrlichiosis


Anderson BE, Dawson JE, Jones DC, Wilson KH. *Ehrlichia chaffeensis,* a new species associated with human ehrlichiosis. J Clin Microbiol 1991; 29:2838–2842.
*Original identification of Ehrlichia chaffeensis as the causative agent of human ehrlichiosis.*

Anderson BE, Sumner JW, Dawson JE et al. Detection of the etiologic agent of human ehrlichiosis by polymerase chain reaction. J Clin Microbiol 1992; 30:775–780.
*Description of polymerase chain reaction technology to detect* Ehrlichia chaffeensis *infection from clinical blood samples.*

Bakken JS, Dumler SJ, Chen S-M et al. Human granulocytic ehrlichiosis in the upper midwest United States: a new species emerging? JAMA 1994; 272: 212–218.

Chen S-M, Dumler SJ, Bakken JS, Walker DH. Identification of a granulocytotropic *Ehrlichia* species as the etiologic agent of human disease. J Clin Microbiol 1994; 32:589–595.
*Clinical and microbiologic descriptions of a newly recognized form of human ehrlichiosis.*

Eng TR, Harkess JR, Fishbein DB et al. Epidemiologic, clinical, and laboratory findings of human ehrlichiosis in the United States, 1988. JAMA 1990; 264:2251–2258.

Fishbein DB, Dawson JE, Robinson LE. Human ehrlichiosis in the United States, 1985–1990. Ann Intern Med 1994; 120:736–743.

Harkess JR. Ehrlichiosis. Infect Dis Clin North Am 1991; 5:37–51.

McDade JE. Ehrlichiosis—a disease of animals and humans. J Infect Dis 1990; 161:609–617.
*These four papers provide a comprehensive, detailed summary of the clinical and laboratory features of human ehrlichiosis.*

Yu X, Brouqui P, Dumler JS, Raoult D. Detection of *Ehrlichia chaffeensis* in human tissue by using a species-specific monoclonal antibody. J Clin Microbiol 1993; 31:3284–3288.
*Description of methodology to detect Ehrlichia chaffeensis using an immunohistologic stain in tissues from infected patients.*


### Bartonella infections


Adal KA, Cockerell CJ, Petri WA. Cat scratch disease, bacillary angiomatosis, and other infections due to Rochalimaea. N Engl J Med 1994; 330:1509–1515.
*A recent review of the epidemiology, clinical manifestations, and diagnosis of infections due to Bartonella (formerly Rochalimaea) henselae and B. quintana.*

Anderson B, Sims K, Regnery R et al. Detection of *Rochalimaea henselae*

DNA in specimens from cat scratch disease patients by PCR. J Clin Microbiol 1994; 32:942–948.
*Use of polymerase chain reaction technology to detect Bartonella henselae infection in lymph node specimens from patients with cat scratch disease.*

Cotell SL, Noskin GA. Bacillary angiomatosis: clinical and histologic features, diagnosis, and treatment. Arch Intern Med 1994; 154:524–528.
*A recent discussion of the clinical presentation, diagnosis, and current approach to treatment of cat scratch disease.*

Knobloch J, Solano L, Alvarez D, Delgado E. Antibodies to *Bartonella bacilliformis* as determined by fluorescent antibody test, indirect hemagglutination and ELISA. Trop Med Parasitol 1985; 36:183–185.
*A comparison of serologic tests to diagnose bartonellosis in patients from an endemic area.*

Larson AM, Dougherty MJ, Nowowiejsli DJ et al. Detection of *Bartonella (Rochalimaea) quintana* by routine acridine orange staining of broth blood cultures. J Clin Microbiol 1994; 32:1492–1496.
*Method to detect* B. quintana *bacteremia by conventional blood culture.*

## Chlamydial infections

Grayston JT. Infections caused by *Chlamydia pneumoniae* strain TWAR. Clin Infect Dis 15:757–761, 1992.
*An excellent review summarizing all aspects of the microbiology, immunology, and clinical diagnosis and treatment of* C. pneumoniae *infections.*

Grayston JT, Campbell LA, Juo CC, Mordhorst CH, Saikku P, Thom DH et al. A new respiratory tract pathogen: *Chlamydia pneumoniae* strain TWAR. J Infect Dis 161:618–625, 1990.
*Description of the microbiologic and serologic characteristics of C. pneumoniae strain TWAR, as well the DNA of hybridization properties distinguishing it from both* C. trachomatis *and* C. pneumoniae.

Grayston JT, Kuo CC, Wong SP, Altman J. A new *Chlamydia psittaci* strain, TWAR, isolated in acute respiratory tract infections. N Engl J Med 314:161–168, 1986.
*The original article describing* Chlamydia pneumoniae *(which was first considered a* Chlamydia psittaci *strain) as a cause of respiratory illness, including sinusitis, pharyngitis, and pneumonitis.*

Orfial J, Byrne GI, Chersesky MA, Grayston JT, Jones RB, Ridgway GL, Saikku P, Schachter J, Stamm WE, Stephens RS, eds. Chlamydial Infections. Proceedings of the Eighth International Symposium on Human Chlamydial Infections. Societa Editrice Esculapio, Bologna, Italy, 1994.
*Proceedings of international symposium on chlamydial infections, with excellent reviews of key topics as well as research papers.*

Weinstock H, Dean D, Bolan G. *Chlamydia trachomatis* infections. Med Clin North Am 8:797–815, 1994.
*Well-written and complete overview of the epidemiology, diagnosis, and treatment of sexually transmitted chlamydial infection.*

Marrazzo JM, Stamm WE. New approaches to the diagnosis, treatment, and prevention of chlamydial infection. In Current Clinical Topics in Infectious Diseases vol. 18. J Remington, ed. in press.
*An excellent overview of recent developments in the clinical management and prevention of sexually transmitted chlamydial infections.*

Kuo CC, Jackson LA, Campbell LE, Grayston JT. *Chlamydia pneumoniae* (TWAR). Clin Micro Rev 8:451–461, 1995.
*Excellent overview of the microbiology, epidemiology, clinical manifestations, diagnosis, treatment, and pathogenesis of* C. pneumoniae *infections.*

# III

# ANTIMICROBIAL DRUGS: PRINCIPLES AND USAGE

# 21

# Mechanisms of Antimicrobial Action and Resistance

GEORGE A. JACOBY

Antimicrobial agents possess selective toxicity because, as predicted by Paul Ehrlich a century ago, there are targets in a microbe that are missing or significantly different from those in humans.

## General Principles of Antimicrobial Action

The bacterial targets (Table 21.1) include the following:

1. Cell wall peptidoglycan, which is a structural polymer composed of alternating units of *N*-acetylglucosamine and *N*-acetylmuramic acid stabilized by cross-linking bridges of D- and L-amino acids,
2. The machinery of protein synthesis and especially the prokaryotic ribosome, which differs in both protein and RNA components from its eukaryotic counterpart,
3. The outer cell membrane, which differs in chemical composition from those in humans;
4. Enzymes of bacterial nucleic acid metabolism, specifically DNA gyrase and DNA-dependent RNA polymerase,
5. Enzymes involved in folic acid synthesis, a pathway absent in humans.

### Cell wall active agents

Peptidoglycan synthesis can be divided into three stages. In the first stage, UDP-*N*-acetylglucosamine and UDP-*N*-acetylmuramic acid pentapeptide are assembled in the cytoplasm. In the second stage, these two compounds are transferred to a lipid carrier in the inner cell membrane, joined together, and added to the end of a growing peptidoglycan chain. In the final stage, the nascent glycan chain is cross-linked to pre-existing cell wall by transpeptidation.

D-cycloserine and fosfomycin interfere with steps in stage one. D-cycloserine blocks formation of the D-alanine-D-alanine terminus of the pentapeptide side chain by inhibition of alanine racemase and D-Ala:D-Ala synthetase. Fosfomycin inhibits pyruvate-UDP-*N*-acetylglucosamine transferase, which is required for UDP-*N*-acetylmuramic acid synthesis.

Bacitracin inhibits the conversion of phospholipid pyrophosphate to phospholipid and thus prevents the regeneration of the lipid carrier involved in the second stage of peptidoglycan synthesis.

$\beta$-lactam and glycopeptide antibiotics act at the third stage of cell wall synthesis. Vancomycin, and other glycopeptide antibiotics such as teicoplanin, bind directly to D-Ala-D-Ala at the end of a pentapeptide chain in a growing subunit prior to cross-linking. Peptidoglycan polymerization (transglycosylation) and transpeptidation are thus inhibited.

Penicillin and related $\beta$-lactam antibiotics interact with bacterial proteins on the cytoplasmic membrane, known as *penicillin-binding proteins* (*PBPs*). Bacteria have 4 to 8 PBPs varying in size from 35 to 120 kDa. Some are DD-carboxypeptidases or transpeptidases that are essential for peptidoglycan cross-linking. $\beta$-lactam antibiotics block this latter step by mimicking the structure of the acyl D-Ala-D-Ala end of a nascent peptide cross-link, forming a stable covalent bond with serine at the active site of peptidoglycan transpeptidase, thus inactivating it. Other PBPs have no demonstrable enzymatic activity but play important roles in cell shape or septation.

### Agents acting on the ribosome and other aspects of protein synthesis

The bacterial ribosome is a 70S particle made up of 50S and 30S subunits containing three kinds of ribosomal RNA, 52 ribosomal proteins, and a variety of enzymes and elongation factors. The two subunits together with mRNA contain what are termed the *A* and *P* sites. The cycle of protein elongation begins with polypeptidyl-tRNA in the P site and an empty A site. In the presence of elongation factor EF-Tu and GTP, aminoacyl-tRNAs are tested for complementarity to the A site codon. The match is checked for accuracy by a process termed *proofreading*, and if all is well, the peptidyl-tRNA in the P site is transferred to the new aminoacyl-tRNA bound at the A site. In the presence of elongation factor EF-G and GTP, the growing chain is translocated from the A site to the P site, and mRNA is moved by three nucleotides to expose a new codon at the A site so that the cycle can be repeated. A third, or *E* site, has also been proposed on the ribosome for the deacylated tRNA.

Antibiotics can block ribosomal function at several steps in the process of protein synthesis. Erythromycin, clindamycin, chloramphenicol, and streptogramin A or B primarily effect 50S ribosomal functions and compete with each other for binding to this subunit, while aminoglycosides and tetracycline target the 30S component. Tetracycline blocks binding of aminoacyl-tRNA to the A site in the presence of EF-Tu and GTP. Aminoglycosides such as amikacin, gentamicin, kanamycin, streptomycin, and tobramycin have multiple effects on ribosomal function, but they are noteworthy for their ability to promote misreading by a reduction in the accuracy of proofreading at the A site. Spectinomycin, an aminocyclitol, blocks protein synthesis without producing misreading. Macrolides, clindamycin, and chloramphenicol are all peptidyltransferase inhibitors and block transfer of peptidyl-t-RNA in the P site to the amino group of aminoacyl-tRNA in the A site. Finally, fusidic acid blocks the translocation step by binding to EF-G and locking it to the ribosome.

The topical antibiotic mupirocin also blocks protein synthesis but it does so by specifically inhibiting isoleucyl-tRNA synthetase, probably by competing with isoleucine for the active site of the enzyme.

**Table 21.1** Mechanisms of action of antimicrobial agents

| Target | Antimicrobial agent |
|---|---|
| CELL WALL PEPTIDOGLYCAN | |
| Synthesis of UDP-*N*-acetyl-glucosamine and UDP-*N*-acetylmuramic acid | D-cycloserine, fosfomycin |
| Transfer across cell membrane and polymerization | Bacitracin |
| Transpeptidation | Vancomycin, teicoplanin, penicillins, cephalosporins, monobactams, carbapenems, and other $\beta$-lactam antibiotics |
| PROTEIN SYNTHESIS | |
| 30S ribosome | Chloramphenicol, clindamycin, erythromycin and related macrolides; streptogramin A and B |
| 50 S ribosome | Aminoglycosides, aminocyclitols, tetracycline, fusidic acid |
| t-RNA charging | Mupirocin |
| OUTER CELL MEMBRANE | Colistin, polymyxin B, cationic peptides |
| NUCLEIC ACID METABOLISM | |
| RNA polymerase | Rifampin, rifabutin |
| DNA gyrase | Nalidixic acid, fluoroquinolones, novobiocin |
| DNA replication | Metronidazole |
| FOLIC ACID BIOSYNTHESIS | |
| Dihydropteroate synthase | Sulfonamides |
| Dihydrofolate reductase | Trimethoprim |

## Cell membranes

The cyclic polypeptides polymyxin B and colistin (which is polymyxin E) act like cationic detergents. They bind to anionic sites, especially phospholipids, in membranes of gram-negative organisms and enhance permeability so that the membranes become leaky.

There are many other antimicrobial peptides that upset membrane permeability, including linear magainins from frog skin and cecropins from insects as well as disulfide-containing defensins from mammalian phagocytes. These 3000 to 5000 molecular weight cationic molecules form pores in bacterial cell membranes, depolarizing and increasing the permeability of the membrane, and bringing about cell lysis.

## Enzymes of nucleic acid synthesis

Rifampin binds to the $\beta$-subunit of DNA-dependent RNA polymerase to block synthesis of all forms of RNA. Rifabutin has a similar site of action.

Nalidixic acid, oxolinic acid, and new fluoroquinolones such as norfloxacin, ciprofloxacin, levofloxacin, trovafloxacin, and others have as their targets the essential bacterial enzymes DNA gyrase and DNA topoisomerase IV. Gyrase controls DNA supercoiling, while topoisomerase IV decatenates interlinked daughter chromosomes following DNA replication. Both are tetramers composed of two subunits. In gram-negative bacteria, gyrase is usually the more important quinolone target, whereas in gram-positive organisms, topoisomerase IV predominates, but which target is more important also depends on the particular quinolone tested. Quinolones not only block gyrase and topoisomerase function but also trap the enzymes on DNA and cause lethal double-strand DNA breakage. Novobiocin also blocks DNA gyrase, but its target is the B subunit of the enzyme.

When the nitro group of metronidazole is reduced to produce the active form of the drug, it causes breaks and mutations in DNA, thus stopping DNA replication.

## Folic acid synthesis

Sulfonamides and trimethoprim block enzymes involved in the synthesis of tetrahydrofolic acid. Sulfonamides (and sulfones) compete with the native substrate p-aminobenzoic acid for dihydropteroate synthase, while trimethoprim inhibits dihydrofolate reductase. Tetrahydrofolic acid is an essential carrier of one-carbon units in the synthesis of purines, pyrimidine, and amino acids such as methionine. Starvation for thymidine seems to be particularly important since a minute supplement disrupts antibacterial activity.

# Resistance to Antimicrobial Agents

Bacteria may be naturally resistant to a particular agent or resistance may develop either by mutation or the acquisition of exogenous genetic information, such as that carried by a plasmid or transposon. There are four major mechanisms for resistance (Table 21.2):

1. A change in the drug target so that affinity for the agent is diminished, either by a reduction in receptor affinity or the substitution of an alternate pathway,
2. Production of an enzyme that modifies or inactivates the agent,
3. Reduced accumulation of the agent either by a permeability barrier limiting uptake or an active efflux system promoting export of the drug.
4. Loss of a pathway involved in drug activation.

Often resistant clinical isolates employ several resistance mechanisms that act synergistically. For example, diminished accumulation can augment resistance from either an altered target or enzymatic detoxification.

## Target alterations

### Cell wall biosynthesis

Penicillin-binding proteins are altered in most penicillin-resistant *Neisseria meningitidis*, some $\beta$-lactam-resistant *Neisseria gonorrhoeae* and *Haemophilus influenzae*, and all penicillin-resistant *Streptococcus pneumoniae*. In these pathogens, low-affinity hybrid PBPs have arisen by replacement of parts of one or more *pbp* genes with DNA from related organisms: from commensal species of *Neisseria* for meningococci and gonococci and from other streptococci for pneumococci. In *S. pneumoniae* with high-level (MIC $\geq 1$ $\mu$g/ml) resistance to penicillin, at least three of the five high-molecular-weight PBPs are altered and susceptibility to other $\beta$-lactam antibiotics is diminished as well. Recently, pneumococci with clinically significant resistance to ceftriaxone and cefotaxime have been responsible for failure of the these drugs in treating meningitis. Mosaic *pbp* genes have

**Table 21.2** Major mechanisms of resistance to antimicrobial agents

| Mechanism | Agents affected |
|---|---|
| ALTERED TARGET | |
| *CELL WALL BIOSYNTHESIS* | |
| Modified PBPs | β-lactams |
| Modified acyl D-Ala-D-Ala | Glycopeptides |
| *PROTEIN SYNTHESIS* | |
| Modified 30S ribosome | Streptomycin, spectinomycin, tetracycline |
| Modified 50S ribosome | Clindamycin, macrolides |
| *CELL MEMBRANE* | |
| Lipopolysaccharide | Polymyxin B |
| *NUCLEIC ACID METABOLISM* | |
| DNA gyrase | Fluoroquinolones, nalidixic acid, novobiocin |
| Topoisomerase IV | Fluoroquinolones |
| RNA polymerase | Rifampin |
| ENZYMATIC MODIFICATION | |
| *AMINOGLYCOSIDE* | |
| Acetyltransferase | Amikacin, gentamicin, kanamycin, tobramycin |
| Nucleotidyltransferase | Amikacin, gentamicin, kanamycin, spectinomycin, streptomycin, tobramycin |
| Phosphotransferase | Amikacin, kanamycin, streptomycin |
| β-Lactamase | Carbapenems, cephalosporins, monobactams, penicillins, and other β-lactams |
| Chloramphenicol acetyl-transferase | Chloramphenicol, fusidic acid |
| Fosfomycin glutathione-*S* transferase | Fosfomycin |
| DECREASED OUTER MEMBRANE PERMEABILITY | |
| OprD channel loss | Carbapenem |
| ACTIVE EFFLUX | |
| Fluoroquinolone efflux | Fluoroquinolones, nalidixic acid |
| Tetracycline efflux | Tetracycline, minocycline |
| LOSS OF ACTIVATION | |
| KatG catalase-peroxidase | Isoniazid |
| Nitroreductase | Metronidazole |
| Pyrazinamidase | Pyrazinamide |

presumably arisen in these organisms because these species can accept DNA by transformation. They can also donate resistance to related organisms, for example, between different serotypes of pneumococci or from *S. pneumoniae* to other viridans streptococci such as *Streptococcus sanguis* or *Streptococcus oralis*.

PBP-mediated resistance is also found in staphylococci and in enterococci which are not naturally transformable, but in these cases, a single, novel low-affinity PBP is involved. Methicillin-resistant *Staphylococcus aureus* (MRSA) has its normal complement of PBPs plus a new one, PBP 2′ or 2a, with reduced affinity for all β-lactam antibiotics. PBP 2′ is encoded by the *mecA* gene which is part of a 30–40 kilobase segment of DNA, including other resistance genes, which has integrated at a specific site in the staphylococcal chromosome. Expression of methicillin resistance is complex. Most MRSA populations are heterogeneous with only a few organisms expressing high-level resistance. At least five genes besides *mecA* influence the level of methicillin resistance. The mechanism of methicillin resistance in coagulase negative staphylococci is similar. In enterococci high-level resistance to penicillin is associated with PBP 5 having reduced affinity for β-lactam antibiotics.

Resistance to vancomycin is the result of a set of enzymes that modifies the D-Ala-D-Ala target to which the antibiotic binds in susceptible organisms. Genes for these enzymes are located on a transposon together with two genes that make the system inducible. VanH is a dehydrogenase that makes D-lactate from pyru-

**Table 21.3** Glycopeptide resistance phenotypes

| Phenotype | Genotype | MIC (μg/ml) | | Expression | Transfer by conjugation | Pentapeptide terminus | Bacterial species |
|---|---|---|---|---|---|---|---|
| | | Vancomycin | Teicoplanin | | | | |
| VanA | *vanA* | 64–>1000 | 16–512 | Inducible | + | D-Ala-D-Lac | *E. faecium*<br>*E. faecalis*<br>other enterococcal species |
| VanB | *vanB* | 4–1000 | 0.5–1 | Inducible | + | D-Ala-D-Lac | *E. faecium*<br>*E. faecalis* |
| VanC | *vanC-1* | 2–32 | 0.5–1 | Constitutive | − | D-Ala-D-Ser | *E. gallinarum* |
| | *vanC-2* | 1–8 | 0.25–1 | Constitutive | − | | *E. casseliflavus* |
| | *vanC-3* | 8 | 0.5–1 | Constitutive | − | | *E. flavescens* |
| VanD | *vanD* | 64 | 4 | Constitutive | − | D-Ala-D-Lac | *E. faecium* |

vate. VanA ligates D-Lac to D-Ala to produce a depsipeptide that can substitute for D-Ala-D-Ala at the end of the pentapeptide side chain to allow normal peptidoglycan polymerization and transpeptidation in the presence of vancomycin. VanX is a dipeptidase that hydrolyzes D-Ala-D-Ala produced by the host ligase, while VanY is a carboxypeptidase that prevents translocation of D-Ala-D-Ala containg precursors to the cell surface.

Four types of vancomycin resistance have been described in enterococci (Table 21.3). The VanA phenotype is inducible, usually plasmid mediated, and also causes resistance to the glycopeptide teicoplanin. VanB is inducible, usually encoded on the chromosome, and vancomycin specific. Both occur in *Enterococcus faecalis* and *Enterococcus faecium*. VanC is constitutive, low level, and confined to the infrequent clinical isolates *Enterococcus gallinarum*, *Enterococcus casseliflavus*, and *Enterococcus flavescens*. A fourth variety, VanD, has been described with a ligase having 69% amino acid identity to ligases from VanA and VanB and 43% homology to VanC. In the laboratory vancomycin resistance has been transferred on a plasmid to *S. aureus*, where it was fully expressed. Such high-level vancomycin resistance has not yet appeared in clinical isolates, but low-level vancomycin resistance (MIC 8 μg/ml) has recently been found in MRSA in Japan and the United States.

In *Mycobacterium tuberculosis* and related organisms, resistance to ethambutol results from amino acid substitutions in the *embB* gene, which is involved in the transfer of arabinogalactan into mycobacterial cell wall.

### Alterations in ribosomes and other machinery of protein synthesis

Resistance to agents blocking protein synthesis arises by changes in both ribosomal protein and rRNA. High-level resistance to streptomycin results from amino acid substitutions at particular sites in protein S12 of the 30S subunit, and changes in protein S5 produce resistance to spectinomycin. However, alteration at specific sites in 16S RNA also cause resistance to streptomycin or spectinomycin, and several altered residues in 23S RNA confer resistance to chloramphenicol or erythromycin.

In gram-positive organisms resistance to the macrolide-lincosamide-streptogramin B (MLS) group of antibiotics is produced by inducible plasmid-mediated enzymes that mono- or dimethylate adenine residue 2058 in 23S rRNA. Erythromycin is often the best inducer, thus an organism may appear clindamycin susceptible but have the potential for resistance by mutating to constitutive expression of the methylase. Erythromycin-resistant organisms are also resistant to azithromycin and clarithromycin.

Some tetracycline-resistant bacteria circumvent the ability of the antibiotic to block aminoacyl-tRNA binding to the ribosomal A site. Exactly how this is accomplished is not yet clear, but the protein involved has GTPase activity and considerable homology with EF-Tu and may function as an analog of this factor.

High-level mupirocin-resistant *S. aureus* isolates contain a new species of isoleucyl-tRNA that is plasmid mediated and resistant to mupirocin inhibition. In intermediate-level mupirocin-resistant strains, the chromosomal enzyme appears to have become less sensitive to inhibition.

### Cell membrane

Changes in both outer membrane proteins and lipopolysaccharides have been associated with acquired resistance to polymyxin B and to cationic antibacterial peptides. Naturally polymyxin-resistant organisms, such as *Proteus mirabilis*, have substitutions on lipopolysaccharide phosphates that lower the negative surface charge and peptide binding.

## Nucleic acid metabolism

Target-mediated quinolone resistance can occur by amino acid substitutions in either the A or B subunits of DNA gyrase in gram-negative bacteria or the ParC and ParE subunits of DNA topoisomerase IV in such gram-positive organisms as *S. aureus*. In *E. coli* and other gram-negative bacilli, high-level resistance has been associated with double substitutions in GyrA or combination of a *gyrA* mutation with one in *parC* or *parE*. Resistance to rifampin results from amino acid substitutions or small insertions and deletions at several sites in the β-subunit of RNA polymerase. Resistance can emerge so rapidly that rifampin should be combined in treatment with other agents.

### Folic acid metabolism

Resistance to sulfonamides and trimethoprim results from inhibitor-resistant dihydropteroate synthases and dihydrofolate reductases. The resistant enzymes are often carried by plasmids or transposons. At least 16 different plasmid-borne dihydrofolate reductases are known, but only two types of dihydropteroate synthase have been discovered.

## Detoxifying enzymes

### Aminoglycoside-modifying enzymes

Aminoglycosides are inactivated by acetyltransferases (AACs), nucleotidyl- (or adenylyl-) transferases (ANTs), and phosphotransferases (APHs) that attack particular amino or hydroxyl groups on these antibiotics. Different enzymes acetylate the 3-, 2′-, or 6′-amino group of the gentamicin or kanamycin families of aminoglycosides. Phosphorylation of the 3′-hydroxyl and adenylylation of the 2′-hydroxyl is common, whereas adenylylation at the 4′-hydroxyl is rare. Furthermore, a particular site may be modified by a number of enzymes. For example, AAC(3)-I attacks gentamicin. AAC(3)-II, and -IV attack tobramycin and netilmicin in addition to gentamicin, whereas AAC(3)-III modifies kanamycin and neomycin as well as gentamicin and tobramycin. These differences in substrate range are not the result of a few amino acid alterations since distinct AAC(3) enzymes vary in amino acid composition by as much as 50%.

Many resistant staphylococci and enterococci have an unusual aminoglycoside-modifying enzyme with both AAC(6′) and APH(2″) activity in separate protein domains. The bifunctional enzyme provides resistance to amikacin, gentamicin, netilmicin, and tobramycin. Its increasing prevalence in enterococci has compromised synergistic $\beta$-lactam/aminoglycoside therapy.

### $\beta$-lactamases

The major mechanism for bacterial resistance to penicillins, cephalosporins, monobactams, carbapenems, and related $\beta$-lactam antibiotics is production of enzymes that catalyze hydrolytic attack on the $\beta$-lactam ring, thus inactivating these drugs. In gram-positive bacteria, $\beta$-lactamase is an extracellular enzyme; in gram-negative bacteria, it is located in the periplasmic space. *bla* genes are found on plasmids, transposons, and the bacterial chromosome. Hundreds of $\beta$-lactamases have been distinguished by substrate and inhibitor spectra, molecular size, isoelectric point, and other properties, but all can be categorized into one of four structural classes based on amino acid homology (Table 21.4). $\beta$-lactamases of classes A, B, and C are the most important clinically. Class A $\beta$-lactamases are responsible for the resistance of *S. aureus* to penicillin and the resistance of *Escherichia coli* and other gram-negative pathogens to ampicillin, carbenicillin, and cephalothin. Class C $\beta$-lactamases are usually encoded on the chromosome and are mainly active against cephalosporins. Class B enzymes are metallo-$\beta$-lactamases that can hydrolyze carbapenems as well as penicillins and cephalosporins. Class A, C, and D $\beta$-lactamases have serine at their active site and are members of the family of penicilloyl serine transferases that includes PBPs.

$\beta$-lactamases have evolved in response to the continuing development of $\beta$-lactam antibiotics that have often been designed to be $\beta$-lactamase resistant. Since oxyimino-$\beta$-lactams such as cefotaxime, ceftazidime, ceftriaxone, and aztreonam were introduced, extended-spectrum $\beta$-lactamases have appeared, especially in isolates of *Klebsiella pneumoniae*, that are able to hydrolyze these agents. The molecular basis of resistance is the substitution of one, two, or three amino acids near the active site of TEM-1, TEM-2, SHV-1, or OXA-type $\beta$-lactamases that increases the catalytic efficiency of the enzymes toward these compounds. *Enterobacter, Citrobacter, Proteus, Pseudomonas*, and *Serratia* species have another way to overcome newer $\beta$-lactams. In these genera, the class C chromosomal $\beta$-lactamase, although very limited in its ability to attack oxyimino-$\beta$-lactams, is inducible, and mutations in the induction system allow it to be ex-

**Table 21.4** $\beta$-lactamase structural classes

| Class | Preferred substrates | Genetic location[a] | Examples |
|---|---|---|---|
| A | Penicillins, cephalosporins | C, P, T | Penicillinase of *S. aureus*, TEM- and SHV-type $\beta$-lactamases[b] |
| B | Most $\beta$-lactams, including carbapenems | C, P | L1 $\beta$-lactamase of *S. maltophilia*, IMP-1 $\beta$-lactamase |
| C | Cephalosporins | C, P | AmpC $\beta$-lactamase of *E. cloacae* and other gram-negative bacilli; MIR-1 $\beta$-lactamase |
| D | Penicillins, oxacillin | P, C, T | OXA-type $\beta$-lactamases |

[a]C, chromosomal; P, plasmid; T, transposon.

[b]$\beta$-lactamase nomenclature is bewildering and inconsistent at best. Most plasmid-mediated enzymes (and some encoded on the chromosome) have a three- or four-letter abbreviation. Some were named for biochemical properties, such as OXA for activity against oxacillin and SHV for activity which is variably affected by sulfhydryl reagents. AmpC $\beta$-lactamase alludes to resistance conferred to ampicillin, although the enzyme is more efficient hydrolyzing cephalosporins than penicillins. MIR-1 got its name from the Miriam Hospital, where it was discovered. TEM $\beta$-lactamase was named after a patient (Temoniera) and now comprises a family of over sixty varieties with amino acid substitutions at critical sites that alter the substrate spectrum, inhibitor response, and isoelectric point of the enzymes.

pressed at such high levels that resistance is produced to oxyimino-$\beta$-lactams and also to $\alpha$-methoxy-compounds such as cefoxitin or cefotetan. The same phenotype has been achieved in some *E. coli* or *K. pneumoniae* isolates by acquisition of class C chromosomal-type enzymes on transmissible plasmids. Presently, only a few organisms, such as *Xanthomonas maltophilia*, are predictably resistant to imipenem and other carbapenems. Most produce class B metallo-$\beta$-lactamases, although a few class A enzymes able to hydrolyze imipenem have appeared. A class B $\beta$-lactamase (IMP-1) has also been found on transmissible plasmids in carbapenem-resistant clinical isolates of *Pseudomonas aeruginosa*, *K. pneumoniae*, *Serratia marcescens*, and other genera but so far, such strains have been found only in Japan.

#### Other antibiotic modifying enzymes

Chloramphenicol is inactivated by acetyltransferases to produce inactive mono- and diacetyl derivatives. At least a dozen varieties of chloramphenicol acetyltransferase are known. One type binds fusidic acid and confers resistance to this structurally unrelated steroidal agent.

Fosfomycin can be inactivated by a plasmid-mediated glutathione-*S*-transferase. Clindamycin or lincomycin can be modified by *O*-nucleotidylation, and erythromycin by *O*-phosphorylation or hydrolysis of the lactone ring, although these are minor mechanisms of resistance to these drugs, compared with target site alteration. Target alterations are also the main mechanism for rifampin resistance, but glycosylation, phosphorylation, and ribosylation of rifampin have been found in some resistant *Nocardia* and *Mycobacterium* species.

### Reduced accumulation

Many antibiotics traverse the outer membrane of gram-negative bacteria via porin channels that allow hydrophilic molecules to penetrate the lipid bilayer. Where a specific and nonessential channel is used, loss of this pathway can produce significant resistance, such as loss of the OprD channel of *P. aeruginosa* associated with resistance to imipenem. Loss of a transport system is also one mechanism for mutational resistance to fosfomycin. Reduction in other, less specific, porin channels can augment resistance to chemically unrelated antimicrobial agents but often not to a clinically significant degree unless the permeability defect works in concert with another resistance mechanism, such as an enzyme that can better inactivate a slower flow of substrate.

Active efflux is a more effective resistance strategy. A major mechanism of tetracycline resistance in both gram-negative and gram-positive pathogens is the energy-dependent export of the drug mediated by cytoplasmic membrane proteins whose formation is induced by tetracycline. At least eight classes of tetracycline efflux genes are known. Some provide resistance to minocycline as well as to tetracycline. Active efflux transporters for chloramphenicol or erythromycin have also been described, and a major mechanism for fluoroquinolone resistance in addition to alterations in DNA gyrase involves active efflux. *E. coli* and other enteric gram-negative organisms also have a chromosomal locus termed *mar* (for multiple antibiotic resistance) that regulates susceptibility to unrelated antimicrobial agents and environmental stresses by a combination of active efflux and diminished production of the OmpF porin channel.

### Loss of an activating step

One mechanism for isoniazid resistance in tubercle bacilli is loss or mutation in the *katG* gene that encodes a catalase-peroxidase enzyme essential for isoniazid activation. Similarly, loss of pyrazinamidase that converts pyrazinamide to pyrazinoic acid in *M. tuberculosis* and diminished activity of the nitroreducatase that activates metronidazole in *Bacteroides* species have been associated with resistance to these agents.

### Multiresistance

Organisms resistant to one antimicrobial agent are more likely to be resistant to others. Sometimes a single resistance gene is responsible, but more often multiresistance results from the linkage of different resistance genes. When these are located on a conjugative plasmid or transposon, resistance can spread between unrelated organisms as well as by dissemination of a resistant clone. Plasmids present in bacteria stored away before the antibiotic era lacked resistance genes. Our success in using antibiotics has been all too closely paralleled by the success of bacterial adversaries in accumulating resistant determinants—to the point now where some organisms have become virtually untreatable.

### Circumventing resistance

Knowledge of resistance mechanisms has allowed rational development of new agents more resistant to bacterial modifying enzymes. Successive generations of cephalosporins have been developed with increasing resistance to existing $\beta$-lactamases. Amikacin is kanamycin acylated with amino-hydroxybutyric acid in such a way that many bacterial enzymes active on the parent compound are blocked. Fluorinated analogs of chloramphenicol with reduced substrate activity for chloramphenicol acetyltransferase have been produced. Unfortunately, $\beta$-lactamases have evolved to hydrolyze new cephalosporins, enzymes attacking amikacin have appeared, and chloramphenicol resistance due to active efflux can deal with the fluorinated derivatives.

A related approach is to develop a specific enzyme inhibitor. Clavulanate, sulbactam, and tazobactam are $\beta$-lactamase inhibitors used in combination with $\beta$-lactamase susceptible agents to increase their spectrum of action. Bacteria have counterattacked by porin loss to diminish inhibitor access, increased $\beta$-lactamase production to overcome inhibition, and, most recently, by amino acid substitutions in TEM and SHV $\beta$-lactamases that reduce inhibitor affinity.

Antimicrobial agents with novel targets or activity against resistant organisms are still being sought, but other, more traditional, strategies deserve continued attention. Since usage selects for resistance, antimicrobial agents need to be utilized optimally, both in and outside the hospital. In the hospital, better systems for concurrent monitoring of resistance need to be employed so that barrier precautions, hand washing, and other accepted methods of infection control can be instituted in a timely manner.

## ANNOTATED BIBLIOGRAPHY

Davies J. Inactivation of antibiotics and the dissemination of resistance genes. Science 1994; 264:375–382.
*A stimulating account.*

Drlica K, Zhao X. DNA gyrase, topoisomerase IV, and the 4-quinolones. Microbiol Mol Biol Rev 1997; 61:377–392.
*An up-to-date discussion of quinolone action and quinolone resistance.*

Gale EF, Cundliffe E, Reynolds PE, Richmond MH, Waring MJ. The Molecular Basis of Antibiotic Action. London, John Wiley & Sons, 1981.

*An entire book on how antibiotics work.*

Jacoby GA, Archer GL. New mechanisms of bacterial resistance to antimicrobial agents. N Engl J Med 1991; 324:601–612.

*A summary of what is known about antimicrobial resistance with emphasis on new and emerging mechanisms.*

Livermore DM. β-Lactamases in laboratory and clinical resistance. Clin Microbiol Rev 1995; 8:557–584.

*An informative and practical summary.*

Neu HC. The crisis in antibiotic resistance. Science 1992; 257:1064–1073.

*The bad news and some things to do about it.*

Nikaido H. Prevention of drug access to bacterial targets: permeability barriers and active efflux. Science 1994; 264:382–388.

*An expert summary of a major mechanism of resistance.*

Spratt BG. Resistance to antibiotics mediated by target alterations. Science 1994; 264:388–393.

*Another masterful account of a leading resistance mechanism.*

Woodford N, Johnson AP, Morrison D, Speller DCE. Current perspectives on glycopeptide resistance. Clin Microbiol Rev 1995; 8:585–615.

*A comprehensive review of a rapidly moving field.*

# 22

# Pharmacology of Antimicrobials

SANDRA L. PRESTON AND GEORGE L. DRUSANO

Pharmacokinetics can be defined as the time course and quantitation of a drug and its metabolites in the body. Pharmacokinetic principles are important in relation to anti-infective pharmacotherapy in that they (along with pharmacodynamic principles) can be utilized to guide decision-making for dosing regimens aimed at maximizing efficacy and minimizing development of toxicity.

In this chapter, we will provide an overview of the general principles of pharmacokinetics and their application to anti-infective pharmacotherapy with particular emphasis on treatment of central nervous system (CNS) infection in relation to drug penetration. Appropriate dosing of anti-infectives in renal or hepatic failure will also be discussed.

## General Principles

After administration of a drug, there are three basic pharmacokinetic processes that take place: absorption, distribution, and elimination. Elimination can be further subdivided into metabolism and excretion. Each of these processes will be discussed in more detail.

## Absorption

Absorption may be defined as the process by which a drug proceeds from the site of administration to the site of measurement within the body. The most common routes of administration include intravenous (IV), intramuscular (IM), subcutaneous, and oral. Drugs can also be administered regionally such as intraperitoneally or intrathecally. The IV route delivers drug directly into the site of measurement, therefore absorption is assumed to be 100%.

Absorption from other routes is more variable and often incomplete. Both physiochemical properties of the drug and physiologic properties of the patient can affect absorption. Drug properties affecting absorption can include formulation of the product. Differences in dissolution between various formulations (e.g., capsule, tablet, etc.) can affect the rate and sometimes, the extent of absorption. Use of the sodium salt of the drug or the acid form can also influence dissolution. Generally, use of a salt form results in faster dissolution. Physiologic properties of the patient that can affect absorption include blood flow through the site of administration (IM and subcutaneous), with increased blood flow in these regions hastening absorption. Decreased absorption may occur in low blood flow states, such as shock. This will have adverse effects on the absorption of any antibacterial agent administered by the IM route. Consequently, all routes of drug administration except IV are relatively contraindicated in this circumstance.

Absorption of orally administered drugs can be impaired by a number of different factors. Most drug absorption occurs in the proximal jejunum and in the ileum. Patients lacking those parts of the gastrointestinal system can have marked impairment in absorption of orally administered drugs. In such patients, alternative routes of administration may be prudent. Absorption of many drugs (most notably ketoconazole and itraconazole) can be affected by pH. These drugs need an acidic environment in order to be absorbed, therefore concurrent administration of antacids or $H_2$-antagonist drugs can impair their absorption. Drug absorption can be increased in such circumstances by administering with acidic beverages, such as Coca-Cola.

Drug absorption can also be impaired by competing reactions in the gastrointestinal tract. Antibacterials such as the tetracyclines and the quinolones can form complexes with polyvalent cations such as magnesium, aluminum, calcium, zinc, and iron. These insoluble complexes render the drug unabsorbable, potentially leading to a decrease in efficacy. Concurrent administration of a quinolone with sucralfate or didanosine (ddI preparation containing antacid) can also lead to complex formation and inactivity of the quinolone. Penicillin G's absorption can be decreased by acid hydrolysis, leaving the product inactive. Because of this, oral penicillin G is infrequently used clinically, and acid stable penicillins (e.g., penicillin VK) have been derived.

In some circumstances, lack of absorption is a desired effect. Examples include oral neomycin and oral vancomycin. These drugs have difficulty passing through the gastrointestinal mucosa (neomycin is a polar compound and vancomycin has a large molecular weight), yet they maintain their antibacterial activity. Neomycin is thus used in bowel decontamination regimens for its activity against gram-negative aerobes and vancomycin is used for the treatment of pseudomembranous colitis due to *Clostridium difficile*.

## Distribution

Distribution is the reversible transfer of drug to and from the site of measurement. Drug distribution can approximate total body water (e.g., gentamicin with a volume of distribution [$V_d$] of 0.2 L/kg). Alternatively, some drugs are more widely distributed into tissues leading to a very large apparent $V_d$ (e.g., 4 L/kg for amphotericin B, 25 L/kg for pentamidine). This apparent $V_d$ represents the proportionality of drug plasma concentrations to the total amount of drug in the body. Drugs with a very high apparent $V_d$ demonstrate significant binding to tissues and/or plasma proteins or penetration into cells. Knowledge of apparent $V_d$ is important when a loading dose of a drug needs to be calculated in order to achieve a desired plasma concentration. A rough approximation of the dose needed to achieve a drug concentration goal can be calculated employing the relationship of dose/$V_d$ = desired plasma concentration.

Factors affecting distribution include *tissue perfusion by blood*, *tissue permeability*, and *plasma protein binding*. In poorly perfused tissue (e.g., bone or fat), distribution into the tissue can take longer. Likewise, loss of drug from the tissue can also be prolonged. Tissue membrane permeability is an important factor affecting drug distribution, particularly with regard to sites where the capillary endothelium has tight junctions, such as the CNS and the eye. The prostate also represents a "specialized site" for drug penetration. Drug penetration into the CNS will be discussed in greater detail later.

Plasma protein binding can occur to a great extent with some drugs (e.g., some human immunodeficiency virus [HIV] protease inhibitors, sulfonamides) and can affect drug distribution. Acidic and neutral drugs commonly bind to albumin whereas basic drugs often bind to $\alpha$-1 acid glycoprotein. It is expected that only the fraction of unbound drug is available to exert a pharmacological effect because the drug–protein complex is unable to traverse capillary membranes on account of its size. In instances where protein binding is altered, an increased or decreased effect can occur. Ceftriaxone demonstrates a somewhat unusual concentration-dependent plasma protein–binding effect. As the drug concentration in the plasma increases from 0.5 $\mu$g/ml to 300 $\mu$g/ml, the number of free binding sites decreases and the free fraction of drug increases from 4% to 17%. The clinical significance of this finding, however, is most likely minimal because achievable serum concentrations clinically range from 150–300 $\mu$g/ml after a 1–2 g dose.

Clinically, certain patient populations are known to have higher $V_d$s as compared with that of a "normal" patient. Patients with cystic fibrosis, critically ill patients, and those with hematologic malignancies tend to have higher $V_d$s. This can be important when dosing antimicrobials. An example would be a patient in the intensive care unit who is receiving an aminoglycoside. Because of an increased $V_d$, peak serum concentrations would be lower than anticipated if dosing was based on a "normal" $V_d$. These patients would likely need higher doses to achieve desired serum concentrations. $V_d$ and plasma clearance are the physiologically linked variables and are related to each other through the following equation: clearance = ($V_d$)(ke). Ke is the elimination rate constant and is a derived term determined by the ratio of clearance and $V_d$. This rate constant is related to the half-life of the drug as follows: half-life = ln2/ke. Therefore, for any plasma clearance of drug, an increasing $V_d$ must give a smaller ke and hence, a longer half-life. Although the peak concentration of drug will be lower with the increased $V_d$, the area under the plasma concentration versus time curve (AUC) will be unchanged, because AUC equals dose/clearance.

## Metabolism

Unlike distribution, which is a reversible process, metabolism is the irreversible conversion of a drug from one form to another. Metabolism usually occurs in the liver, although other organs (kidneys, lungs, etc.) can also play a role in drug metabolism.

The liver microsomal drug oxidation/reduction system (cytochrome P450, CYP) is an enzyme complex located in the endoplasmic reticulum of hepatocytes and is responsible for metabolism of many drugs. These enzymes can be grouped into families and subfamilies (e.g., CYP3A). A cytochrome P450 family or subfamily can be induced (increased in activity) or inhibited (decreased in activity) in the presence of certain drugs, leading to a number of clinically significant drug interactions with other drugs metabolized via the same enzyme subfamily.

Drugs known to be enzyme inducers can cause a reduction of serum concentrations of other drugs metabolized by the same system. This effect tends to be gradual over a period of 1–2 weeks. One anti-infective known to be an enzyme inducer is rifampin. It is the most potent inducer of CYP3A in clinical use; however, it can also induce other enzyme families. Concurrent administration of rifampin with drugs such as oral contraceptives or warfarin can result in failure of the oral contraceptives and suboptimal anticoagulation. Phenytoin serum concentrations can also be decreased. Drug concentrations of HIV protease inhibitors can decline by 40%–50%.

A number of different anti-infectives are known to be enzyme inhibitors. Ciprofloxacin, erythromycin, clarithromycin, the azole antifungals (fluconazole, itraconazole, ketoconazole), and isoniazid can increase serum concentrations of certain drugs. Such enzyme inhibition is usually rapid and can occur within the first few doses of the inhibitor. Ciprofloxacin is metabolized through CYP1A2 and is known to increase serum concentrations of theophylline, potentially leading to theophylline toxicity. Erythromycin and terfenadine, an antihistamine, are metabolized through CYP3A. Concurrent administration of erythromycin and terfenadine has resulted in fatal cardiac arrhythmias due to the inhibition of metabolism of terfenadine to its metabolite. A similar interaction has been reported between ketoconazole and terfenadine. In instances in which known interacting drugs need to be prescribed together, it may be prudent to use a different agent, particularly in circumstances when the interaction can be life-threatening. Alternatively, one could monitor serum concentrations of the drug if available (e.g., theophylline), or monitor other markers of drug activity (e.g., international normalized ratio for warfarin) in order to adjust drug doses appropriately.

Hepatic clearance is dependent upon intrinsic hepatocellular activity. In patients with hepatic failure (e.g., cirrhosis), impairment of metabolism of hepatically cleared drugs may occur. This may warrant dosage adjustments of drugs primarily cleared by the liver. Unfortunately, liver function tests (ALT, AST, GGT, serum albumin, prothrombin time) can be relatively nonspecific and increases may not correlate with metabolic functional impairment. In other words, they do not consistently provide an indication of the liver's metabolic capacity. Because of this, it is difficult to provide precise recommendations for dosage adjustments of hepatically metabolized drugs. Anti-infective drugs that may need a dosing adjustment in hepatic failure are listed in Table 22.1. Clinical judgement should be used to assess the individual's degree of hepatic failure and when necessary, the drug in question should have serum concentrations determined. Extension of the dosing interval or decrease in dose should be made accordingly.

## Excretion

Excretion is the irreversible loss of chemically unchanged drug. The primary organ of excretion is the kidney, although other routes are rarely possible, such as the lung for drugs with a low vapor pressure. Drugs can be excreted by glomerular filtration or by active tubular secretion. Renal clearance of a drug can be altered by a patient's changing renal function or, less commonly, by drug interaction.

Impairment of a patient's renal function can markedly decrease clearance of drugs that are primarily eliminated by this route. Serum concentrations of the drug can be increased and prolonged. Because of this, patients may be at increased risk of drug-induced toxicity. Dose and/or dosing intervals should therefore be altered

**Table 22.1** Anti-infective agents in need of dosing adjustment in severe hepatic disease

| |
|---|
| Ampicillin |
| Cefoperazone |
| Chloramphenicol |
| Clindamycin |
| Erythromycin |
| Mezlocillin |
| Metronidazole |
| Nafcillin |
| Penicillin G |
| Rifampin |

in such patients in order to achieve appropriate serum concentrations. One must evaluate the patient's renal function, usually by assessing serum creatinine concentrations and calculated creatinine clearances (CrCL), in order to avoid toxicity associated with increased serum concentrations of drug. One must also be sure that enough drug is given on an appropriate schedule so that efficacy is maintained, incorporating known pharmacodynamic principles of particular drugs, such as (*1*) peak to minimum inhibitory concentration (MIC) ratio (peak/MIC), (*2*) AUC to MIC ratio (AUC/MIC), and (*3*) time that concentrations exceed the MIC (time > MIC). Briefly, these principles take into account measures of drug exposure, such as peak concentration and AUC, and they relate these variables to a measure of drug potency for the infecting organism (MIC). A summary of dosage modifications for patients with renal impairment for selected antimicrobials is provided in Table 22.2.

While it is well known that aminoglycoside dosing needs to be adjusted in patients with renal impairment to avoid the associated problems of nephro- and ototoxicity, it is also important to adjust doses of agents less likely to be associated with significant toxicity, such as the $\beta$-lactam antibiotics. In such cases, it is unnecessary to give patients more drug than needed and, indeed, toxicities can occur. Imipenem-cilastatin, for example is a $\beta$-lactam agent that is associated with development of seizures at high serum concentrations. It is important in this instance to pay attention to dosage adjustment so that unnecessary patient toxicity can be avoided.

Another mechanism of altering renal clearance of drug is by drug interaction. Probenecid is an acidic drug that is renally se-

**Table 22.2** Dosage modifications for selected agents for renally impaired patients

| Drug | CrCL[a] (mL/min) | Dosing recommendation |
|---|---|---|
| Acyclovir | >50 | 5–10 mg/kg q8h |
| | 25–50 | 5–10 mg/kg q12h |
| | 10–25 | 5–10 mg/kg q24h |
| | 0–10 | 2.5–5 mg/kg q24h |
| Amikacin[b] | | Loading dose 7.5 mg/kg, select maintenance dose and adjust to desired serum concentrations |
| Ampicillin/sulbactam | >29 | 1.5–3 g q6h |
| | 15–29 | 1.5–3 g q8–12h |
| | 5–14 | 1.5–3 g q24h |
| Aztreonam | >30 | 1–2 g q8h |
| | 10–30 | 1–2 g q12h |
| | <10 | 1–2 g q24h |
| Cefazolin | >50 | 1–2 g q8h |
| | 10–50 | 1–2 g q12h |
| | <10 | 500 mg–1 g q24h |
| Cefotaxime | ≥20 | 1–2 g q6h |
| | <20 | 500 mg–1 g q6h |
| Cefotetan | >30 | 1–2 g q12h |
| | 10–30 | 1–2 g q24h |
| | <10 | 1–2 g q48h |
| Cefoxitin | >50 | 1–2 g q8h |
| | 10–50 | 1–2 g q12h |
| | <10 | 1–2 g q24h |
| Ceftazidime | >50 | 1–2 g q8h |
| | 30–50 | 1–2 g q12h |
| | 10–30 | 1–2 g q24h |
| | <10 | 0.5–1 g q24h |
| Ceftizoxime | >50 | 1–2 g q8h |
| | 20–50 | 1–2 g q12h |
| | <20 | 1–2 g q24h |
| Cefuroxime | >20 | 0.75 g q8h |
| | 10–20 | 0.75 g q12h |
| | <10 | 0.75 g q24h |

(*continued*)

**Table 22.2** Dosage modifications for selected agents for renally impaired patients—*Continued*

| Drug | CrCL[a] (mL/min) | Dosing recommendation |
|---|---|---|
| Ciprofloxacin IV | ≥20 | 400 mg q12h |
| | <20 | 400 mg q24h |
| PO | >50 | 500–750 mg q12h |
| | 30–50 | 500 mg q12h |
| | <30 | 250–500 mg q24h |
| Fluconazole IV/PO | >50 | 100% of usual dose[c] |
| | 20–50 | 50% of usual dose |
| | <20 | 25% of usual dose |
| Ganciclovir IV (induction) | ≥80 | 5 mg/kg q12h |
| | 50–79 | 2.5 mg/kg q12h |
| | 25–45 | 2.5 mg/kg q24h |
| | <20 | 1.25 mg/kg q24h |
| Gentamicin[b] | | Loading dose 2 mg/kg, then select maintenance dose and adjust to desired serum concentrations |
| Imipenem-cilastatin | >50 | 0.5–1 g q6h |
| | 20–50 | 0.5–1 g q8h |
| | <20 | 0.5–1 g q12h |
| Piperacillin | >50 | 3 g q4h |
| | 20–50 | 3 g q6h |
| | 10–20 | 3 g q8h |
| | <10 | 3 g q12h |
| Tobramycin[b] | | Loading dose 2 mg/kg, then select maintenance dose and adjust to desired serum concentrations |
| Vancomycin[d] | >50 | 1 g q12h |
| | 10–50 | 1 g q1–4d |
| | <10 | 1 g q4–7d |

[a]Calculated creatinine clearance.

[b]Aminoglycoside dosing should be determined on a case-by-case basis, taking into account present dose and dosing interval, patient renal function, actual serum concentrations obtained at steady state, and desired peak and trough serum concentrations based often on site of infection.

[c]Usual dose varies with indication.

[d]Dosage should be individualized for desired serum concentrations (peak < 40 mcg/ml, trough 8–12 mcg/ml).

creted by an anionic transport system and reabsorbed. When used in combination with penicillin (also secreted by an anionic transport system), probenecid competitively inhibits the renal secretion of penicillin and therefore its clearance. Increased serum concentrations of penicillin result. Because of the availability of alternative antimicrobials with the ability to produce more sustained serum concentrations than penicillin, probenecid is rarely used today for this indication.

## Pharmacodynamic Principles

Knowledge of the pharmacokinetics of a drug is important in that it allows description of its disposition. This has practical importance only if some measure of drug exposure can be linked to clinical outcome and/or toxicity. Measures of drug exposure that are to be linked to outcome must also be viewed relative to some measure of the potency of the agent against the pathogen in question, such as the MIC. Consequently, attempts to link outcome to measures of drug exposure should examine peak/MIC ratio, AUC/MIC ratio, and the time >MIC. These evaluations may be made using plasma drug concentrations or at drug concentrations at primary infection sites.

A determinant of which of these measures of drug exposure is most closely linked to outcome is the manner in which the drug kills target pathogens. If the pathogen cell kill is relatively concentration independent, as is the case for the $\beta$-lactam class of antibiotics, then time > MIC is the measure that is usually linked to outcome. For drugs that are concentration dependent in kill rate, such as the aminoglycoside and fluoroquinolone classes of antimicrobials, the AUC/MIC ratio is more likely to be linked to outcome. Peak/MIC ratio can also be linked to outcome, usually occurring through suppression of emergence of resistant variants with agents which are concentration dependent in cell kill. This can occur when the peak concentration is quite high (usually >10/1, peak/MIC ratio) and suppresses not only the parent strain, but the mutant organism as well. This occurs when the mutation increases the MIC by a relatively small multiple, such as four- to eightfold. The fluoroquinolone antimicrobials are a case in point, where parent strain MICs usually increase with gyrA mutation by four- to eightfold. Animal model data in neutropenic rats of Drusano and colleagues have shown that an increase in MIC of a strain of *Pseudomonas aeruginosa* from 1 $\mu$g/ml to 8 $\mu$g/ml changed the survivorship after administration of 80 mg/kg/day of lomefloxacin from circa 70%–75% to 0%. In this same study, it was shown that once-daily administration of the

80 mg/kg dose was highly significantly superior to administration of the same dose on a more fractionated schedule. This implies that the peak/MIC ratio is the dynamically linked variable in this circumstance. However, with a lower total daily dose in which the once-daily schedule did not produce peak/MIC ratios of >10/1, AUC/MIC ratio was the best dynamic variable. This outcome was most likely due to the relatively higher lomefloxacin peak/MIC ratios being able to suppress gyrA or transport mutants pre-existent in the challenge population. Clinical trials support these findings as Forrest et al. (1993) found that AUC/MIC was linked to outcome in their retrospective evaluation of ciprofloxacin therapy. Approximately 50% of these patients had peak/MIC ratios of ≤10/1. These investigators did find that a low peak/MIC ratio was significantly associated with emergence of resistance. Prospectively generated data of Preston et al. in which >80% of patients had peak/MIC ratios of >10/1 indicate that the peak/MIC ratio was the variable most closely linked to outcome.

Like fluoroquinolones, aminoglycosides are drugs that are concentration dependent in bactericidal rate. Indeed, in an *in vitro* evaluation (Blaser et al., 1987), the dynamics of drug action with an aminoglycoside followed exactly the same principles as with fluoroquinolones. Consequently, it is not a surprise that the peak/MIC ratio and AUC/MIC ratio are variables most closely linked to outcome for aminoglycosides.

β-lactams are a drug class that is relatively concentration independent in bactericidal rates. Because of this, the time that drug concentrations remain in excess of the pathogen's MIC is the primary determinant of the outcome of the infection. This has been demonstrated in animal model systems (Craig 1995), and in a clinical trial (Schentag 1984).

Another pharmacodynamic principle that can be considered when dosing antimicrobial agents is the postantibiotic effect (PAE). The PAE is a period of time for which there is continued suppression of bacterial growth after a limited period of drug exposure, despite the fact that antimicrobial concentrations in the body have fallen to undetectable levels. The PAE is variable, depending upon the infecting organism and the antimicrobial agent used. The mechanism is believed to result from nonlethal damage caused when the antimicrobial agent was taken up by the bacteria. This principle is considered to be one rationale for single-daily dosing of aminoglycosides. In giving one large daily dose of the aminoglycoside, concentration-dependent bactericidal activity can be maximized, and when drug concentrations fall below the organism MIC, the PAE may provide prolonged suppression of bacterial growth. Table 22.3 lists drugs exerting a PAE. The postantibiotic sub-MIC effect (PASME) has also been examined. This effect examines bacterial regrowth when drug concentrations of one-quarter the MIC are present, as opposed to the traditional PAE where drug concentrations are negligible. The regrowth is much slower in this instance. This scenario may actually be more clinically relevant, as such low concentrations (less than the MIC, but not zero) may be found in patients and may indicate that PAE values are conservative estimates of time to organism regrowth.

## Drug Penetration into the Central Nervous System

Infections of the central nervous system (CNS) are serious and life threatening. Expeditious, appropriate treatment with an anti-infective agent upon diagnosis is therefore essential. The goal of therapy is to deliver sufficient concentrations of anti-infective to the site of infection in the brain and cerebrospinal fluid (CSF). Because normal host defense mechanisms (including leukocytes, immunoglobulin, and complement) are limited in the CNS and CSF, concentrations of drug should be bactericidal. In fact, studies from a variety of animal models suggest that CSF drug concentrations should be 10–20 times above the minimum bactericidal concentration in order to achieve rapid bacterial killing. A number of natural barriers limit the ability of drug to enter the CSF from the systemic circulation.

### Barriers to drug entry into the CNS

The blood-to-brain barrier can limit the exchange of drug between the systemic circulation (capillary blood) and the CNS. This barrier in the brain tissue is composed of capillary endothelial cells joined tightly together. In order to penetrate the barrier, the drug must be able to pass directly through the capillary endothelial cell by passive diffusion and then penetrate the glial cells that envelop capillaries of the brain. Based upon animal and some human studies, many antibiotics achieve CSF concentrations of less than 5% of simultaneous serum concentrations because of the function of this barrier in the absence of inflammation.

The blood-to-CSF barrier controls the passage of drugs between the brain and CSF and is made up of ependymal cells of the choroid plexus. These cells utilize an active transport mechanism in a manner similar to that of renal tubular epithelial cells and can effectively pump certain organic acids such as many β-lactam agents out of the CSF. The function of these cells can be inhibited by probenecid and can also be impaired in the presence of inflammation. Thus, anti-infective agents may achieve higher CSF concentrations when probenecid is used or in the setting of meningitis.

**Table 22.3** Drugs exerting a significant postantibiotic effect (PAE)

| Drug class | Gram-positive organisms | Gram-negative organisms |
|---|---|---|
| Penicillins | +/++ | 0 |
| Cephalosporins | +/++ | 0 |
| Carbapenems | +/++ | +/++ |
| Aminoglycosides | 0 | ++ |
| Fluoroquinolones | +/++ | ++/+++ |
| Vancomycin | +/++ | 0 |

0 = no PAE; + = minimal PAE; ++ = moderate PAE; +++ = extensive PAE.

**Table 22.4** Anti-infective penetration into the CNS

| | |
|---|---|
| Therapeutic CSF concentrations achieved | Rifampin<br>Chloramphenicol<br>Trimethoprim<br>Sulfamethoxazole |
| Therapeutic CSF concentrations achieved only with inflamed meninges | Penicillin G<br>Ampicillin<br>Cefotaxime<br>Ceftriaxone<br>Ceftazidime<br>Imipenem/cilastatin<br>Meropenem |
| Therapeutic CSF concentrations unlikely to be achieved | Amikacin<br>Gentamicin<br>Tobramycin<br>Cefazolin<br>Ketoconazole<br>Vancomyin |

## Factors affecting CSF anti-infective penetration

There are several factors that influence the transfer of drug from the blood into the CNS. As stated previously, increased meningeal inflammation promotes increased drug penetration. Some drugs normally unable to penetrate can attain therapeutic concentrations in the CSF with inflammation. Specific drugs and their ability to penetrate are listed in Table 22.4.

Small-molecular-weight compounds are more capable of penetrating biological barriers by passive diffusion than are large-molecular-weight compounds. Ionized drugs, on account of their increased affinity to plasma water, penetrate CNS barriers poorly because of poor transport across cellular membranes. Drugs that are unionized at physiologic or pathologic pH penetrate more effectively. Drugs that are highly lipid soluble cross cell membrane barriers well and are likely to penetrate into the CSF even in the absence of inflammation. Low plasma protein binding of drugs allows for an increased free fraction capable of passing into the CNS.

### Factors affecting anti-infective bactericidal activity within the CNS

The pH of the CSF is generally decreased in acute bacterial meningitis because of the elevation of CSF lactate. Drugs that are less effective in an acidic environment, such as the aminoglycosides, may therefore be less effective for treatment of bacterial meningitis.

### Effect of corticosteroid therapy on subsequent anti-infective drug penetration

The use of steroids (usually dexamethasone) as adjunctive treatment is efficacious in children with *Haemophilus influenzae* meningitis by decreasing inflammation and subsequent neurologic sequelae. Use of dexamethasone in children with other organisms causing meningitis and in adults remains controversial because of lack of data proving efficacy. One area of concern regarding dexamethasone use in meningitis patients is that the drug's anti-inflammatory effect may decrease drug penetration into the CNS. There is indeed some evidence from rabbit pneumococcal meningitis studies indicating that dexamethasone decreases the CSF penetration of ceftriaxone and vancomycin, thereby delaying CSF sterilization. Penetration of rifampin, however, is not affected. Clinically, dexamethasone use has been associated with prolongation of positive CSF cultures in patients with *Streptococcus pneumoniae* meningitis when compared with nondexamethasone-treated patients. More data are needed to determine the exact role of corticosteroids as adjunctive therapy in treatment of meningitis.

Because of the problems associated with passage of drug into the CNS when administered by the IV route, direct administration into the CNS may increase drug CSF concentrations. Lumbar intrathecal administration is limited by the caudal unidirectional flow of the CSF, therefore distribution throughout the CNS may not occur. Intraventricular administration usually requires surgical placement of a reservoir (Ommaya or Rickham) for repeated dosing. Drug can be administered into the ventricle and will then be distributed throughout the intracerebral and extracerebral CSF. As stated previously, probenecid can increase the CSF concentration of penicillin and some cephalosporins because the active transport system is inhibited in the choroid plexus. The clinical utility of this approach, however, is unclear.

## Monitoring Serum Concentrations of Antimicrobials

Therapy with some antimicrobial agents, including aminoglycosides and vancomycin, can be monitored by obtaining serum concentrations. Dosages can be then be adjusted on the basis of this information. Aminoglycoside monitoring is desirable because increased exposure can increase the chance of developing nephrotoxicity and ototoxicity. Desired peak serum concentrations for aminoglycosides vary, depending on the site of infection. Generally, peak concentrations for gentamicin and tobramycin of 7–8 $\mu$g/ml are desirable for treatment of a pneumonia. For other sites of infection, levels of 5–6 $\mu$g/ml are generally acceptable. Lower levels (4 $\mu$g/ml) are acceptable for treatment of urinary tract infection because the drug concentrates in the urine, achieving high concentrations at the site of infection. Trough concentrations of less than 2 $\mu$g/ml are desirable. Ranges of concentration goals for efficacy are for empiric use only. When pathogens are identified, it is important to realize that the 7 $\mu$g/ml peak concentration of aminoglycosides is quite adequate for a patient with a *Klebsiella pneumoniae* pneumonia with an MIC of 0.25 $\mu$g/ml, but it is inadequate for the patient whose pneumonia is caused by *P. aeruginosa*, where that MIC is 4 $\mu$g/ml.

Once-daily dosing of aminoglycosides is a treatment strategy that incorporates pharmacodynamic variables of concentration-dependent bactericidal activity and PAE to theoretically maximize efficacy. One large daily dose of drug can potentially maximize bacterial killing early in the dosing interval and the PAE can sustain antimicrobial effect even after the drug concentration falls below the organism MIC. In clinical trials, differences in efficacy between once- and multiple-daily dosing regimens has not clearly been demonstrated; however, this type of dosing may be used to prolong the time to development of nephrotoxicity that can be associated with aminoglycoside use.

Vancomycin serum concentration monitoring is often conducted to avoid any potential toxicity, particularly ototoxicity. For vancomycin, there are few convincing data linking drug exposure to either infection outcome or occurrence of toxicity. Consequently, plasma concentration monitoring is often overused. For the patient not responding adequately to standard, CrCL-adjusted doses of vancomycin, plasma concentration monitoring is prudent. Patients of this type should have their trough vancomycin concentrations adjusted to achieve about four times the MIC of the infecting pathogen (the drug is 50% protein bound and a one tube dilution error in the MIC is possible).

## Summary

Pharmacokinetic principles can help to guide clinical decision-making with regard to appropriate dosing regimens for anti-infective agents. These principles, however, must be individualized, as variability exists from patient to patient.

### ANNOTATED BIBLIOGRAPHY


Blaser JB, Stone BB, Groner MC, Zinner SH. Comparative study with enoxacin and netilmicin in a pharmacodynamic model to determine importance of ratio of antibiotic peak concentration to MIC for bactericidal activity and emergence of resistance. Antimicrob Agents Chemother 1987; 31:1054–1060.
*This study demonstrated peak/MIC ratio as a primary determinant for efficacy.*

Craig WA. Interrelationship between pharmacokientics and pharmacodynamics in determining dosage regimens for broad-spectrum cephalosporins. Diagn Microbiol Infect Dis 1995; 22:89–96.
*This animal model demonstrated a significant correlation between decreased amount of bacteria in the tissue and increasing time above the MIC.*

Drusano GL, Johnson DE, Rosen M, Standiford HC. Pharmacodynamics of a fluoroquinolone antimicrobial agent in a neutropenic rat model of *Pseudomonas* sepsis. Antimicrob Agents Chemother 1993; 37:483–490.
*This study demonstrated that peak/MIC ratio of lomefloxacin was linked to survivorship when ratios of >10/1 were achieved and AUC/MIC ratio was most strongly linked to outcome when peak/MIC ratios of <10/1 were achieved. The authors stated that a potential reason for this finding was that higher peak/MIC ratios can suppress resistant mutant organisms.*

Forrest A, Nix DE, Ballow CH, et al. Phamacodynamic of intravenous ciprofloxacin in seriously ill patients. Antimicrob Agents Chemother 1993; 37:1073–1081.
*This study retrospectively linked AUC/MIC ratio of ciprofloxacin to bacteriologic and clinical response in seriously ill patients. The authors provided guidelines for targeting dosing regimens to achieve an AUC/MIC ratio that would increase the probability of a positive outcome.*

Gerber AU, Feller-Segessenmann C. In-vivo assessment of in-vitro killing patterns of Pseudomonas aeruginosa. J Antimicrob Chemother 1985; 15(Suppl A):201–206.
*This animal model study linked a single daily gentamicin dose with increased bactericidal activity versus intermittent dosing. This finding linked peak to outcome.*

Moore RD, Lietman PS, Smith CR. Clinical response to aminoglycoside therapy: Importance of peak concentration to minimum inhibitory concentration. J Infect Dis 1987; 155:93–99.

Moore RD, Smith CR, Lietman PS. Association of aminoglycoside plasma levels with therapeutic outcome in gram-negative pneumonia. Am J Med 1984; 77:657–662.
*These two studies associated peak concentration of aminoglycosides to patient outcome. They are an important basis for therapeutic drug monitoring for aminoglycosides.*

Paris MM, Hickey SM, Uscher MI, Shelton S, Olsen KD, McCracken GH. Effect of dexamethasone on therapy of experimental penicillin and cephalosporin-resistant pneumococcal meningitis. Antimicrob Agents Chemother 1994; 38:1320–1324.
*This study demonstrated that in this animal model, penetration of certain antibiotics into the CSF may be substantially reduced when dexamethasone therapy is given.*

Powell SH, Thompson WL, Luthe MA, et al. Once-daily versus continuous aminoglycoside dosing: efficacy and toxicity in animal and clinical studies of gentamicin, netilmicin, and tobramycin. J Infect Dis 1983; 14:918–932.
*In cystic fibrosis patients, no difference in efficacy or toxicity was found between groups. This was one of the first clinical studies examining single-dose aminoglycosides.*

Preston SL, Drusano GL, Berman AL, et al. Prospective development of phamacodynamic relationships between measures of levofloxacin exposure and measures of patient outcome: a new paradigm for early clinical trials. JAMA 1998; 279:125–129.
*A prospective relationship between levofloxacin peak/MIC ratio was developed for clinical and microbiological outcome. A peak/MIC ratio of ≥12 was found to be the breakpoint for increased probability of successful outcome.*

Roosendaal R, Bakker-Woudenberg IA, van den Berg JC, et al. Therapeutic efficacy of continuous versus intermittent administration of ceftazidime in an experimental *Klebsiella pneumoniae* model. J Infect Dis 1985; 152:373–378.
*This animal model study demonstrated that continuous infusion β-lactam was significantly better in prevention of mortality versus intermittent infusion.*

Schaad UB, Kaplan SL, McCracken GH. Steroid therapy for bacterial meningitis. Clin Infect Dis 1995; 20:685–690.
*An excellent review of this topic.*

Schentag JJ, Smith IL, Swanson DJ, et al. Role for dual individualization with cefmenoxime. Am J Med 1984; 77(Suppl 6a):43–50.
*These clinical data have suggested a link between time > MIC and positive outcome for the β-lactam, cefmenoxime. This was a retrospective study that linked increased time > MIC to number of days to bacterial eradication.*

Vogelman B, Gudmundsson S, Legget J, et al. Correlation of antimicrobial pharmacokinetic parameters with therapeutic efficacy in an animal model. J Infect Dis 1988; 158:831–847.
*Again, in this animal model study, time > MIC was most strongly linked to bacterial killing versus other parameters such as peak/MIC ratio or AUC/MIC ratio.*

Zinner ZH, Dudley MN, Gilbert D, et al. Effect of dose and schedule on cefoperazone pharmacodynamics in an in-vitro model of infection in a neutropenic host. Am J Med 1988; 85(Suppl 1A):56–58.
*This in vitro experiment demonstrated that time > MIC was the most important variable in determining bacterial growth, with the regimens having the greater time > MIC having significantly less bacterial regrowth.*

# 23

# Antimicrobial Toxicities and Drug Interactions

JAMES E. LEGGETT AND SUSAN R. RABER

"Above all, do no harm," states the Hippocratic oath. Yet, antibiotics have been shown to cause over 10% of all drug-related emergency department visits. Use of any antimicrobial agent can lead to adverse effects ranging from mild to life threatening. Several factors impact upon the frequency and severity of adverse effects, including the patient's genetic background, physiologic age, and underlying disease, as well as the antimicrobial regimen, duration of therapy, and presence of other drugs. The mechanism of most adverse effects is incompletely understood, although progress is being made in elucidating genetic predisposition and precise biochemical pathways for many antibacterial-induced toxicities. On the other hand, the incidence of clinically significant drug interactions involving antibiotics appears to be increasing as new classes of drugs are employed and polypharmacy proliferates. This chapter will deal with the most common and serious adverse events associated with antibacterial agents.

## Allergic–Hypersensitivity Reactions

Allergic–hypersensitivity reactions may occur with any drug. These reactions rarely cause death but are responsible for morbidity in about 1%–5% of patients treated with penicillins or sulfonamides, as shown in Table 23.1. There is little difference among specific penicillins with regard to potential for inducing such effects. Anaphylactic reactions, which are the most serious because they may cause sudden death, occur in about 0.01% of those treated with a parenteral penicillin. Death due to such reactions is estimated to occur in 0.002%–0.015% of penicillin-treated patients. Hypersensitivity reactions are caused by antibodies directed against the so-called major and minor determinants of penicillin. Ninety-five percent of the penicillin that undergoes protein coupling forms the major penicilloyl structure, while the remaining 5% that becomes immunogenic forms the minor determinants penicilloate, the intact molecule itself, and other breakdown products. Immediate allergic reactions are mediated by immunoglobulin E (IgE) antibodies to the minor determinants, whereas accelerated and late urticarial reactions result from major determinant-specific antibodies measured in commercially available skin tests. Maculopapular cutaneous reactions may be due to immune complexes involving IgM antibodies. They are not predicted by skin tests.

One large retrospective study of approximately 16,000 patients reported that 8% of patients with a history of penicillin allergy also reacted to cephalosporins whereas only 2% of patients without such a history developed a cutaneous reaction. Anaphylactic or accelerated cross-reactions to cephalosporins occur in less than 5% of penicillin-allergic patients. Aztreonam shows no cross-allergenicity with penicillin, but may do so with ceftazidime. Imipenem may produce hypersensitivity reactions in penicillin-allergic patients.

Drug-induced cutaneous reactions may lead to minor or life-threatening consequences. The most common clinical manifestations include maculopapular rashes, urticaria, pruritus, fixed drug eruptions, erythema nodosum, erythema multiforme, toxic epidermal necrolysis, contact dermatitis, and photosensitivity. Overall, amoxicillin, trimethoprim-sulfamethoxazole, and ampicillin appear to produce the highest reaction rates. Ampicillin also very frequently causes a nonallergic skin reaction in patients with infectious mononucleosis or acute lymphocytic leukemia, and in those treated with allopurinol. Phototoxicity is seen most often with tetracyclines and quinolones. Rapid infusion of vancomycin has been associated with a histamine-induced erythematous reaction, which may be attenuated by antihistamine administration.

Fever may be the only sign of an allergic reaction. While it has been reported for every class of antibacterial drugs, β-lactams and sulfonamides account for most cases. Certain drugs appear to be associated with relatively high frequencies of drug fever, such as penicillin G, cephapirin, cephalothin, azlocillin, mezlocillin, and piperacillin when used in high doses for long durations.

## Gastrointestinal Reactions

Gastrointestinal side effects may accompany use of any antimicrobial agent. The frequency of diarrhea depends upon the amount of active drug that reaches the intestinal tract and its antibacterial spectrum. The biliary excretion of cephalosporins possessing a methylthiotetrazole side chain or a similar structure—as in the case of ceftriaxone—results in a higher frequency of diarrhea than renally excreted cephalosporins. The addition of clavulanate to amoxicillin significantly increases the frequency of loose stools. Alteration of gastrointestinal flora may play an integral role in this process. This enigmatic, relatively benign side effect accounts for approximately 80% of antibiotic-associated diarrhea. In contrast, *Clostridium difficile* toxin-associated enterocolitis, which accounts for 20% of antibiotic-associated diarrhea, may be life threatening. Although the risk of developing *C. difficile* colitis is highest with clindamycin, the majority of cases are seen after use of penicillins and cephalosporins, on account of their much wider use. Many drugs may produce nausea, including trimethoprim-sulfamethoxazole, tetracyclines, rifampin, metronidazole, imipenem, and fluoroquinolones.

Although the liver is particularly exposed to antibacterials and their metabolites, adverse hepatic events are far less frequent than other gastrointestinal side effects. The liver may sustain hepatocellular or cholestatic injury and may progress to steatosis, chronic active hepatitis, or cirrhosis. In addition, certain drugs such as sulfonamides, ceftriaxone, and cefoperazone may displace bilirubin to cause encephalopathy in some neonates.

Subclinical two- to threefold elevations of transaminases have been seen in up to 20% of those treated with prolonged high doses of carbenicillin or acylureidopenicillins such as mezlocillin, azlocillin, and piperacillin. Oxacillin and ampicillin are also commonly responsible for mild elevations. Rarely are these

**Table 23.1** Adverse reactions to antibacterial drugs—*Continued*

| Reaction | Occurrence: Frequent | Occurrence: Infrequent | Comments |
|---|---|---|---|
| ALLERGIC-HYPERSENSITIVITY | | | |
| Anaphylaxis | | β-lactams, tetracyclines | About 1:10,000 |
| Cutaneous reactions | β-lactams, clindamycin sulfonamides | Vancomycin | 1%–5% overall |
| Fever | β-lactams, sulfonamides | Any drug | 1%–5% |
| Histamine reactions | Vancomycin | | With rapid infusion |
| Phototoxicity | Tetracyclines | Quinolones | 2% with lomefloxacin |
| Serum sickness | | β-lactams, sulfonamides | <1:1000 overall, children > adults (cefaclor) |
| SLE-like reactions | | Nitrofurantoin | Rare |
| ELECTROLYTE ABNORMALITIES | | | |
| Hypokalemia | Carbenicillin, ticarcillin | | 5 mEq $Na^+$/g ticarcillin |
| Hypomagnesemia | Aminoglycosides | | |
| GASTROINTESTINAL | | | |
| Diarrhea | Amoxicillin-clavulanate, ampicillin, cefixime, clindamycin | Any drug | 7%–15% with some drugs, *C. difficile* related in many cases |
| Esophagitis | | Tetracyclines | Rare, related to acidic pH of drugs such as doxycycline |
| Nausea, vomiting, cramps | Macrolides | Oral β-lactams, imipenem, metronidazole, quinolones, tetracyclines | 1%–3% β-lactams, 10%–25% with macrolides |
| Pancreatitis | | Metronidazole, nitrofurantoin, sulfonamides | Case reports |
| HEMATOPOIETIC | | | |
| *BLEEDING* | | | |
| Hypoprothrombinemia | | Cefamandole, cefmetazole, cefoperazone, cefotetan, ceftriaxone | Conflicting data about increased risk of methyl-tetrathiazole side chain |
| Platelet dysfunction | Penicillin G, ticarcillin | Extended-spectrum penicillins, | Dose-related, increased with renal failure |
| Thrombocytopenia | | β-lactams, rifampin, sulfonamides, trimethoprim | Rare |
| *HEMOLYSIS* | | | |
| G6PD associated | Chloramphenicol, nitrofurantoin sulfonamides | | Rare |
| Immune | | β-lactams, rifampin, sulfonamides | Very rare with β-lactams |
| Coombs reaction | Cephalosporins, penicillins | | 3% with high-dose penicillin G, 4%–6% for cephalosporins |
| Eosinophilia | β-lactams | Any drug | <1%–11% for β-lactams |
| Neutropenia | Sulfonamides, trimethoprim | β-lactams, clindamycin, metronidazole vancomycin | >10% with nafcillin ≥21 days, 6% piperacillin in 1 study, 2% with vancomycin |
| Pancytopenia | Chloramphenicol | β-lactams, clindamycin, sulfonamides | Decreased RBC in 1/3, aplastic anemia in 1:60,000 courses of chloramphenicol |
| HEPATIC | | | |
| Cholestasis | Erythromycin estolate | Amoxicillin-clavulanate | 1:1000 risk with erythromycin estolate 1:100,000 risk with amox-clav, asymptomatic gallbladder sludge 9% with ceftriaxone |
| Hepatitis (overt) | | Nitrofurantoin, oxacillin, rifampin, sulfonamides | Rare |
| Transaminase elevation rifampin | Ampicillin, oxacillin, | β-lactams, clindamycin, quinolones | 6% with ampicillin, 15% with oxacillin >6 g/d, transient 10% with rifampin |

**Table 23.1** Adverse reactions to antibacterial drugs—*Continued*

| Reaction | Occurrence: Frequent | Occurrence: Infrequent | Comments |
|---|---|---|---|
| NEUROLOGIC | | | |
| Central | | | |
| Encephalopathy | Quinolones | Metronidazole | <1%–4% insomnia, headache, dizziness with quinolones |
| Optic neuritis | | Chloramphenicol, quinolones | Very rare |
| *OTOTOXICITY* | | | |
| Cochlear | Aminoglycosides | Macrolides, vancomycin | Subjective <1%, 1%–5% audiometric toxicity with aminoglycosides, very rare with vancomycin |
| Vestibular | Minocycline | Aminoglycosides, β-lactams, vancomycin | <1% with aminoglycosides, up to 30%–90% for minocycline |
| Seizures | Imipenem, penicillins | Metronidazole, quinolones | ~20% with 4 g/day imipenem (0.2% with 2 g/day) |
| *PERIPHERAL* | | | |
| Muscular blockade | | Aminoglycosides, clindamycin | Use with caution in patients with myasthenia gravis, Parkinsonism, botulism |
| Neuropathy | | Metronidazole, nitrofurantoin, tetracyclines | Very rare |
| PHLEBITIS | β-lactams, erythromycin, tetracyclines, vancomycin | | Cephalothin and nafcillin 17%–50%, others 1%–13% |
| PULMONARY | | | |
| Bronchospasm | | β-lactams | Generally single case reports |
| Interstitial pneumonitis | | Nitrofurantoin | Rare |
| Nodular infiltrates | | TMP/SMX | Rare |
| RENAL | | | |
| Crystal deposition | Sulfadiazine | Quinolones | Crystalluria with large doses |
| *NEPHRITIS* | | | |
| Hypersensitivity | | Sulfonamides | Rare |
| Interstitial | | β-lactams, minocycline, quinolones, rifampin | Very rare with β-lactams |
| *TUBULAR TOXICITY* | | | |
| Distal | | Tetracyclines | Rare |
| Proximal | Aminoglycosides | | ~1%–5% in most recent studies |

drugs, the first generation cephalosporins, or rifampin associated with overt hepatitis. Cholestatic and mixed injuries have been reported in up to 0.6% of sulfonamide-treated patients, although subclinical transaminase elevations have been reported in up to 10% of recipients. Erythromycin estolate appears to be the derivative most frequently responsible for erythromycin-induced hepatitis. This hepatitis often resembles cholangitis, with moderately increased transaminases (less than 10 times normal), mildly elevated alkaline phosphatase, and serum eosinophilia in one-half of cases. A similar picture has recently been described with amoxicillin-clavulanate and rarely with quinolones.

## Hematopoietic Reactions

Hematopoietic side effects appear to result from a number of different mechanisms, including immune reactions and dose-related pharmacologic effects. Some hematologic reactions, such as thrombocytosis and many cases of eosinophilia, may actually represent manifestations of the inflammatory response to the underlying infection itself.

Although rare, neutropenia has been reported following exposure to most antimicrobials. β-lactams given at high doses for prolonged periods may alter the bone marrow's ability to promote maturation of granulocytes. In general, onset of neutropenia is late (10–30 days) and values return to normal within 7 days of cessation of the drug. Drugs particularly implicated include penicillinase-resistant penicillins and piperacillin. Folate inhibitors such as trimethoprim and sulfonamides given at high doses can produce leukopenia despite their low affinity for human dihydrofolate reductase, particularly in AIDS patients.

Thrombocytopenia may also involve several mechanisms. Folate antagonists may produce thrombocytopenia via biochemical inhibition of synthesis. β-lactams, sulfonamides, and rifampin may rarely cause immune-mediated platelet destruction in the spleen. Some penicillins may bind to the adenosine diphosphate receptor in sufficient quantity to prevent aggregation. While this is a property of nearly all penicillins, those antipseudomonal penicillins given in gram quantities are the most commonly implicated agents, especially in the postoperative patient who may also have received aspirin, has renal failure, or has other coagulation problems.

Folate antagonists may induce a megaloblastic anemia because of their inhibition of dihydrofolate reductase. Hemolysis has been reported rarely with several β-lactams, and is probably caused by IgG antibodies to erythrocytes. Hemolytic anemia can also occur in genetically predisposed individuals with glucose-6-phosphate dehydrogenase deficiency who are treated with sulfonamides, nitrofurans, and chloramphenicol. On the other hand, a high frequency of false-positive direct Coomb's tests without hemolysis has been reported with cephalosporins (innocent bystander hemolysis).

Pancytopenia and aplastic anemia are most often associated with chloramphenicol. A dose-related maturation arrest of erythroid and other precursors occurs at prolonged serum levels above 25 mcg/ml (or doses greater than 4 g/day). An idiosyncratic aplastic anemia that occurs with about 1 in 60,000 treatment courses may have a genetic predisposition. The gray baby syndrome results from diminished conjugation of chloramphenicol by immature hepatic glucuronyl transferase in neonates, coupled with decreased renal function producing toxic serum levels that lead to cardiovascular collapse.

The incidence of hypoprothrombinemia in patients treated with cephalosporins has varied from 4% to 68%. In addition to the presumed microbiologically induced suppression of intestinal vitamin K synthesis that results from their use, cephalosporins may impair the biosynthesis of vitamin K–dependent clotting factors in the liver. The N-methyltetrathiazole (NMTT) side chain inhibits vitamin K epoxide reductase and thus interferes with vitamin K synthesis. Other studies have suggested instead that only cephalosporins with a free sulfhydryl group can interfere with such synthesis. Predisposing factors such as malnutrition and renal or hepatic insufficiency are undoubtedly involved.

## Neurologic Reactions

Neurotoxicity may accompany the use of several antibiotics. Nonspecific manifestations such as headache, agitation, or insomnia have been reported for many agents. More severe encephalopathy appears to occur in up to 1–4% of patients treated with fluoroquinolones, which are known to inhibit the binding of γ-aminobutyric acid (GABA) to synaptic receptors. Interference with the normal inhibitory activity of GABA has been correlated with the epileptogenic potential of β-lactams. Imipenem in particular has caused a high rate of seizures when given at high doses or in the presence of renal impairment. All aminoglycosides cause ototoxicity. It is frequently irreversible, may occur after discontinuing the drug, may be cumulative with repeated courses, and may be genetically controlled by one or more loci on mitochondrial DNA. Both vestibular and cochlear toxicity are clinically apparent in less than 1% of patients treated with aminoglycosides, although high-frequency auditory damage is more prevalent. In contrast, as many as 30%–90% of patients treated with minocycline develop self-limited vestibular toxi-cities. High doses of macrolides may also produce temporary deafness, but hearing usually returns to normal following discontinuation of the drug. Peripheral neuropathy has developed rarely following treatment with metronidazole, nitrofurantoin, and tetracyclines. Aminoglycosides and clindamycin may rarely cause neuromuscular paralysis by preventing the release of acetylcholine, especially in the presence of presynaptic impairment by medications or illness.

## Renal Reactions

Renal damage affecting the glomeruli or the collecting tubules follows exposure to many antimicrobials. Crystal deposition leading to obstructive nephropathy is observed with large doses of sulfadiazine, which is poorly soluble at acid pH. Quinolones may form crystals at alkaline pH, but only at higher doses than are currently administered.

Hypersensitivity nephritis is typically an interstitial process manifested by renal impairment accompanied by fever, eo-sinophilia and eosinophiluria, and rash. Although methicillin is the prototypical offending agent, many β-lactams have been implicated rarely. Aminoglycoside nephrotoxicity has received much attention over the years, as it has been the limiting factor to the broader use of these agents. An historical incidence of 5% to 25% has recently been lowered to 1%–5% with most regimens, including those with dosing intervals prolonged to 24 hr or more. Since renal toxicity is usually reversible, alteration of dose with rising serum creatinine is effective in allaying toxicity. Electrolyte abnormalities such as hypokalemia or hypomagnesemia may result from aminoglycoside-

**Table 23.2** Adverse reactions associated with childhood

| Factor | Drug | Toxicity |
|---|---|---|
| AGE-RELATED | | |
| Altered pharmacokinetics | β-lactams, aminoglycosides | Volume of distribution and elimination half-life may require dosage adjustment to avoid subtherapeutic or excessive concentrations |
| Immature hepatic function | Chloramphenicol | Decreased conjugation may lead to excessive concentrations that result in cardiovascular collapse (gray baby syndrome) |
| Bilirubin displacement | Cefoperazone, ceftriaxone | Displaced free bilirubin may cause encephalopathy in some neonates |
| DISEASE-RELATED | | |
| Cystic fibrosis | β-lactams, aminoglycosides | Altered hepatic and other functions may require dosage adjustment to avoid subtherapeutic or excessive concentrations |
| UNIQUE | Quinolones | Cartilage toxicity in young animals |
| | Tetracyclines | Tooth and bone abnormalities in children <8 yr of age |

**Table 23.3** Adverse drug reactions more common in the elderly

| Reaction | Drug | Comment |
|---|---|---|
| Anaphylaxis | β-lactams | Greater potential for prior exposure, ambiguous history |
| Antibiotic-associated colitis | β-lactams, clindamycin | Increased relapse frequency as well |
| HEMATOPOIETIC | | |
| Bone marrow suppression | Chloramphenicol, TMP/SMX | Higher concentrations due to decreased elimination |
| Hemorrhage | Cephalosporins with NMTT side chain | |
| Nephrotoxicity | Aminoglycosides | Higher concentrations due to decreased elimination |
| Ototoxicity | Aminoglycosides, vancomycin | Higher concentrations due to decreased elimination |
| Seizures | Imipenem | Higher concentrations due to decreased elimination |

induced damage. Large doses of disodium salts such as ticarcillin deliver a large load of nonreabsorbable anion to the distal tubule and alter hydrogen ion exchange, causing hypokalemia without actually causing renal damage.

## Special Populations

The clinical pharmacology of antibacterial agents varies with age. Physiologic characteristics unique to the fetus, the child, and the elderly adult may lead to differences in the frequency and severity of adverse events, as shown in Tables 23.2 and 23.3. Gestational and chronologic-age-related pharmacokinetics for β-lactams and aminoglycosides may vary significantly. The high affinity of ceftriaxone or cefoperazone for albumin binding sites may lead to bilirubin encephalopathy in the newborn. Unique adverse effects of tetracyclines in the fetus and in children include discoloration and hypoplasia of the teeth and depressed skeletal growth, while quinolones may cause cartilage damage. Advanced age is associated with many physiologic changes that alter the pharmacokinetics of antimicrobials. Many of the adverse effects seen more commonly in the elderly reflect the greater effective doses that these patients may be administered.

The use of antibiotics in pregnancy is a frequent cause for concern. Table 23.4 shows some of the known prenatal risks of an-

**Table 23.4** Safety of antibacterial drugs in pregnancy

| Drug | FDA category[a] | Fetal toxicity | Safest trimester | Comments |
|---|---|---|---|---|
| Aminoglycoside | C–D | Ototoxicity | Third | Risk of ototoxicity increases in 2nd trimester; use with caution |
| β-lactams | B | None known | All | Probably safe |
| Chloramphenicol | C | "Gray baby" | First, second | Use with caution, especially at term |
| Clindamycin | B | None known | All | Probably safe |
| Macrolides | B–C | None known | All | Avoid erythromycin estolate. Clarithromycin has shown fetal toxicity in primates |
| Metronidazole | B | Perhaps teratogenic in humans | | |
| Nitrofurantoin | B | Hemolysis (G6PD) | All | Contraindicated at term |
| Quinolones | C | Arthropathy in animals | Avoid | Contraindicated |
| Rifampin | C | Teratogenic in animals, neonatal bleeding | Second, third | Avoid in early pregnancy. Use with caution |
| Sulfonamides | B | Folate antagonism, hemolysis (G6PD) kernicterus | Second | Contraindicated at term |
| Tetracyclines | D | Skeletal, tooth abnormalities, cataracts | Avoid | Contraindicated |
| Trimethoprim | C | Folate antagonism | First, third | Use with caution |
| Vancomycin | C | None known | | Probably safe |

[a]FDA pregnancy categories: A, adequate studies in pregnant women show no risk; B, animal studies show no risk but human studies inadequate or animal toxicity but human studies show no risk; C, toxicity in animal studies, inadequate human studies, but benefit may exceed risk; D, evidence of human risk, but benefit may exceed risk.

tibacterials, but the teratogenic potential of many drugs is unclear. Antibacterial choice should balance the seriousness of the infection with the drug's safety at any given point in fetal development.

## Antibacterial Drug Interactions

Nearly all antibacterial agents have the potential to interact with other drugs. While many of these interactions may not result in clinically significant effects, those that are associated with substantial morbidity are more likely to occur in patients on long-term maintenance therapy with medications for other underlying diseases such as diabetes, asthma, or seizure disorders. To avoid unnecessary toxicity or hospital visits, it is essential for clinicians to be familiar with interactions among antibacterials and the other drugs a patient may be taking before deciding on an antibacterial regimen.

Pharmacokinetic drug interactions, those resulting when one drug alters the absorption, distribution, metabolism, or excretion of another drug, account for the majority of antibacterial interactions. Of these, induction or inhibition of metabolism of the

**Table 23.5** Antibacterial drug interactions

| Antibacterial agent | Interacting drug | Effect |
|---|---|---|
| CAUSING ALTERED ABSORPTION | | |
| Clindamycin | Kaolin-pectin containing anti-diarrheals | Q clindamycin absorption |
| Fluoroquinolones | Antacids<br>Didanosine (ddI)<br>Ferrous sulfate<br>Sucralfate<br>Zinc | Q fluoroquinolone concentration due to chelation with di- and trivalent cations |
| Tetracyclines | Antacids<br>Bismuth subsalicylate<br>Didanosine (ddI)<br>Ferrous sulfate | Q tetracycline concentration due to chelation |
| CAUSING ALTERED METABOLISM | | |
| Chloramphenicol | Oral sulfonylureas | q sulfonylurea concentration; hypoglycemia |
| | Phenytoin | q phenytoin concentration |
| | Rifampin | Q chloramphenicol concentration |
| | Warfarin | q anticoagulation effect and q PT |
| Clarithromycin | Carbamazepine | q carbamazepine concentration |
| | Cisapride | q cisapride concentration with risk of life-threatening arrhythmias |
| | Cyclosporine | q cyclosporine concentration |
| | Nonsedating histamines: astemizole, terfenadine | q antihistamine concentration with risk of life-threatening arrhythmias |
| | rifabutin | q rifabutin concentration, risk of uveitis |
| | theophylline | q theophylline concentration |
| Doxycycline | Barbiturates | Q doxycycline concentration |
| | Carbamazepine | Q doxycycline concentration |
| | Phenytoin | Q doxycycline concentration |
| Erythromycin/ troleandomycin (TAO) | Carbamazepine | q carbamazepine concentration |
| | Cisapride | q cisapride concentration with risk of life-threatening arrhythmias |
| | Cyclosporin | q cyclosporin concentration |
| | Methylprednisolone | q steroid concentration |
| | Nonsedating histamines: astemizole, terfenadine | q antihistamine concentration with risk of life-threatening arrhythmias |
| | rifabutin | q rifabutin concentration; q risk of uveitis |
| | Theophylline | q theophylline concentration |
| | Warfarin | q anticoagulation effect |
| Fluoroquinolones (ciprofloxacin, enoxacin, grepafloxacin) | Caffeine | q caffeine concentration |
| | Cimetidine | q fluoroquinolone concentration |
| | Theophylline | q theophylline concentration/toxicity |
| | Warfarin | q anticoagulation effect |

(continued)

**Table 23.5** Antibacterial drug interactions—*Continued*

| Antibacterial agent | Interacting drug | Effect |
|---|---|---|
| Metronidazole | Barbiturates | Q metronidazole concentration |
| | Warfarin | q anticoagulation effect |
| Rifampin | Antiarrhythmics | Q antiarrhythmic concentrations |
| | Azole antifungals | Q azole concentration/effectiveness |
| | Calcium channel blockers | Q concentration of diltiazem, nifedipine, and verapamil |
| | Chloramphenicol | Q chloramphenicol concentration |
| | Corticosteroids | Q steroid concentration |
| | Cyclosporine | Q cyclosporine concentration |
| | Dapsone | Q dapsone concentration |
| | Diazepam | Q diazepam concentration |
| | Methadone | Q methadone concentration |
| | Oral contraceptives | Q estrogen concentration/effectiveness |
| | Phenytoin | Q phenytoin concentration |
| | Protease inhibitors | Q protease inhibitor concentration |
| | Sulfonylureas | Q sulfonylurea concentration |
| | Theophylline | Q theophylline concentration |
| | Warfarin | Q anticoagulation effect |
| Sulfonamides | Sulfonylureas | q sulfonylurea concentration/ hypoglycemia |
| | Warfarin | q anticoagulation effect and q PT |
| Trimethoprim | Phenytoin | q phenytoin concentration |
| CAUSING ALTERED EXCRETION | | |
| $\beta$-lactams | Probenecid | Q tubular secretion of renally-eliminated $\beta$-lactams |
| Ciprofloxacin | Probenecid | Q ciprofloxacin clearance |
| Trimethoprim | Dapsone | q concentrations of both dapsone and trimethoprim |
| MISCELLANEOUS | | |
| Aminoglycosides | Neuromuscular blocking agents | Enhanced muscular blockade; respiratory depression or apnea |
| $\beta$-lactams: cefoperazone, cefotetan, cefamandole, cefmetazole, moxalactam | Ethanol | Disulfuram-like reaction; CNS toxicity |
| Clindamycin | Nondepolarizing neuromuscular blocking agents | Enhanced muscular blockade; respiratory depression or apnea |
| Erythromycin, clarithromycin | Digoxin | q digoxin bioavailability due to suppression of *Eubacterium lentum* in the gut |
| Metronidazole | Disulfuram<br>Ethanol | CNS toxicity, disulfuram-like reaction |

interacting drug or the antibacterial itself is by far the most frequently encountered, as shown in Table 23.5. These metabolic interactions are secondary to effects on the cytochrome P (CYP) 450 enzyme system responsible for oxidative (phase I) metabolism of drugs in the liver and in the gut. Knowledge and identification of the CYP-450 isoenzymes has expanded significantly over the past decade. Those involved the most with drug metabolism, and therefore drug interactions, are the CYP3A4, CYP2D6, CYP1A2, and CYP2C isoenzymes. The list of drug–drug interactions involving the CYP-450 isoenzymes has grown beyond that which can be committed to memory. Recognition of the drugs that act as substrates, inhibitors, or inducers of the CYP-450 isoenzymes can assist clinicians in predicting potentially significant drug–drug interactions. However, the clinical outcome of these interactions, as with other types of drug interactions, are highly situational and have high interpatient variability.

Fluoroquinolones and macrolides tend to inhibit CYP-450 enzymes, but generalization among the entire class of agents is problematic since interaction potential is not uniform among members of the classes. Within the macrolide class, troleandomycin (TAO) and erythromycin are the most potent inhibitors of CYP3A4, followed by clarithromycin. Azithromycin and dirithromycin each have low affinity for CYP-450 with minimal to no inhibitory effects. Significant prolongation of the QT interval and life-threatening arrhythmias can occur in patients prescribed macrolide therapy in combination with either terfenadine, astemizole, or cisapride, all of which undergo significant metabolism via CYP3A4. Similarly, theophylline serum concentrations may be elevated in the presence of macrolides or some fluoroquinolones, manifesting as tachycardia, arrhythmias, nausea/vomiting, and headache. These symptoms may be confused with those of an infectious process. Within the fluoroquinolone class, enoxacin, ciprofloxacin, and grepafloxacin are the most potent inhibitors of CYP1A2, while the other members of the class appear to have a lesser inhibitory effect.

Not all of the significant metabolic antibacterial interactions result in toxicity. Rifampin, and to a lesser extent rifabutin, exhibit potent induction of the CYP-450 enzymes, which can lead to increases in the clearance of many drugs including antiarrhythmics, oral sulfonylureas, antiepileptics, and other antimicrobials. These interactions may lead to treatment failure or exacerbation of an underlying condition.

Many drug–drug interactions involving CYP-450 isoenzymes have the potential to occur during HIV therapy with highly active antiretroviral regimens including protease inhibitors and/or non-nucleoside reverse transcriptase inhibitors. Please refer to Chapter 101, Antiretroviral Therapy.

Antibacterial treatment failure may occur for a number of reasons. One avoidable scenario is inadequate serum antibacterial concentrations as a result of decreased absorption. Tetracyclines and fluoroquinolones are chelated by magnesium, calcium, iron, and other ions found in antacids, foods and other drugs. Chelation prevents absorption and results in minimal or undetectable serum concentrations. Concurrent use of agents of chelating potential with tetracyclines or fluoroquinolones should be avoided if possible. If the combination is unavoidable, at least a 2 hr interval is recommended between the times of their administration.

Recognition of potential antibacterial drug interactions with appropriate clinical intervention is essential to providing the best possible treatment of infectious diseases. Whether the interaction leads to therapeutic failure or to toxic adverse effects, it can be detrimental to the patient. Careful selection of antibacterial regimens, appropriate adjustment of doses, and close monitoring can prevent unnecessary morbidity and mortality in patients being treated for infectious diseases.

## ANNOTATED BIBLIOGRAPHY


Bartlett JG. Antibiotic-associated diarrhea. Clin Infect Dis 1992; 15:573–581.
*A state-of-the-art clinical review of enigmatic and* C. difficile*–associated diarrhea. It provides good management guidelines for patients.*

Bigby M, Jick S, Jick H, Arndt K. Drug-induced cutaneous reactions. JAMA 1986; 256:3358–3363.
*A 7-year review of 15,438 hospitalized patients that provides drug-specific reaction rates. Amoxicillin, ampicillin, and trimethoprim-sulfamethoxazole had the highest reaction rates.*

Cooper K, Bennett WM. Nephrotoxicity of common drugs used in clinical practice. Arch Intern Med 1987; 147:1213–1218.
*A succinct review of the pathophysiology and clinical spectrum of antibiotic-induced nephrotoxicity.*

Doucet J, Chassagne P, Trivalle C, Landrin I, Pauty MD, Kadri N, Menard JF, Bercoff E. Drug–drug interactions related to hospital admissions in older adults: a prospective study of 1000 patients. J Am Geriatr Soc 1996; 44:944–948.
*Drug interaction may be a more common cause of hospitalization in an elderly population subjected to polypharmacy.*

Gillum JG, Israel DS, Polk RE. Pharmacokinetic drug interactions with antimicrobial agents. Clin Pharmacokinet 1993; 25:450–482.
*A compilation of the most relevant drug interactions, describing their mechanisms and the increasing scope of these interactions.*

Hedstrom S, Martens MG. Antibiotics in pregnancy. Clin Obstet Gynecol 1993; 36:886–892.
*A brief overview of antibiotics deemed safe or hazardous during pregnancy. It emphasizes the varying potential toxicities of antibiotics according to the physiologic changes in the fetus during pregnancy.*

Michalets EL. Update: clinically significant cytochrome P-450 drug interactions. Pharmacotherapy 1998; 18:84–112.
*A detailed review of an increasingly complex subject.*

Norrby SR. Problems in evaluation of adverse reactions to $\beta$-lactam antibiotics. Rev Infect Dis 1986; 8(Suppl 3):358–370.
*An extensive review of $\beta$-lactam-associated adverse reactions and of the marked differences in their reported frequencies among studies. The author reasons that the lack of strict uniform definitions of adverse events accounts for much of this observed variability.*

Roujeau JC, Stern RS. Medical progress: severe adverse cutaneous reactions to drugs. N Engl J Med 1994; 331:1272–1285.
*An excellent review of the clinical recognition, epidemiology, pathophysiology, and treatment of severe cutaneous drug reactions, accompanied by representative figures.*

Sanford JP, Gilbert DN, Moellering RC, Sande MA. The Sanford Guide to Antimicrobial Therapy 27th ed. Antimicrobial Inc., Dallas, TX, 1997.
*An exhaustive tabulation of antimicrobial interactions and toxicities, updated yearly.*

Westphal JF, Vetter D, Brogard JM. Hepatic side effects of antibiotics. J Antimicrob Chemother 1994; 33:387–401.
*A detailed review of idiosyncratic and dose-related hepatotoxicity including hypoprothrombinemia.*

# 24

## Selection of Antimicrobials for Treatment

JAY P. SANFORD AND RICHARD K. ROOT

Antimicrobial therapy is either empirical, based upon clinical symptoms, signs, laboratory findings, and epidemiologic information or definitive, based upon the results of microbiologic tests and where appropriate, in vitro antimicrobial susceptibility testing. The two approaches should not be considered mutually exclusive. In many cases, it may be appropriate to initiate an empirical regimen, then change to definitive therapy. In some circumstances, initiation of therapy can be deferred until the results of cultures and susceptibilities are available. Finally, in certain circumstances, empirical therapy alone may be adequate. The decision as to which approach to take should be based upon clinical evaluation of the patient as well as knowledge of antimicrobial susceptibilities and the pharmacological properties of the agents selected. Mechanisms of antimicrobial resistance, the pharmacology of different agents, adverse effects, and drug interactions are discussed in Chapters 21 to 23.

Decision making in clinical practice has evolved away from the focus on determining the most likely diagnosis or etiology to the questions of what might the patient have, and what drugs will cover most, if not all, of the possibilities. As a result, many patients expect that physicians will empirically prescribe antimicrobial agents for virtually all febrile illnesses, with the exception of the common cold (the approach of "take this for a few days and if you aren't better I'll see you again"). But even the most empirical approach should include considerations of host and microbial factors.

In deciding to use empirical therapy, a logical decision tree should be followed. Clinically, the site of infection should be localized. This can usually be based on the patient's history and physical examination: we shall take here the clinical situation of a patient with a sore throat, fever, and erythematous tonsils with an exudate. Next, environmental or host factors that might modify the likely causative organisms should be considered—i.e., is the patient in his teens, is there associated generalized lymphadenopathy or splenomegaly, does the peripheral blood smear show atypical lymphocytes? Based on such information, what are the likely organisms? Will a Gram's stain, rapid antigen detection tests, or other procedures narrow the possibilities? Occasionally, imaging studies may be required. If a microbial etiology is likely, to what antimicrobial agents are these organisms likely to be susceptible? In the example given, major considerations include group A streptococci, *Arcanobacterium hemolyticum*, *Corynebacterium diptheriae*, infectious mononucleosis (EB virus), herpes simplex (HSV-1 or HSV-2) and herpangina. A rapid group A streptococcal antigen test, if positive, has a high degree of specificity but less sensitivity. For example, group A streptococci are isolated from throat cultures in 3%–33% of cases of infectious mononucleosis. Although group A streptococci are susceptible to all $\beta$-lactam antibiotics, benzathine penicillin G (IM) or penicillin V (PO) remain the drugs of choice. In some cases, second generation cephalosporins may be more effective. When infectious mononucleosis is suspected, aminobenzyl penicillins (ampicillin, amoxicillin) should be avoided because of the high frequency (50%–80%) of skin rashes.

In summary, the physician should assess whether to treat or wait. If treatment is chosen, site, modifying circumstances, likely organisms, likely susceptibilities, then dosage, adverse effects, and duration should be considered.

### Antimicrobial Susceptibility Testing

Antimicrobial susceptibility testing is one of the keystones to the selection of optimal therapy. The information used in the decision process is at three levels: broad, focused, or specific. At the broad level, knowledge of the inherent in vitro susceptibility of the likely infecting organism(s) is used; for example, *Pseudomonas aeruginosa* are susceptible to ceftazidime but are resistant to amoxicillin. At the more focused level, knowledge of the in vitro susceptibility patterns in the patient's community or in the hospital is used; for example, 35% of *Haemophilus influenzae* strains produce $\beta$-lactamase and are resistant to amoxicillin. Finally, the specific in vitro susceptibility of the organisms isolated from the individual patient—for example, a methicillin-resistant *Staphylococcus aureus* from a blood culture—is of most value.

In vitro susceptibility tests measure the concentrations of antimicrobial agents required to inhibit or kill organisms in vitro compared with the expected concentration of the drug achieved in the blood or urine with usual dosages of the drug in healthy volunteer subjects or in moderately ill patients. Such tests essentially ignore all host factors and conditions. The results of broth dilution and diffusion (disc sensitivity tests such as the Kirby Bauer procedure or the more recent E test) susceptibility tests are greatly influenced by the reagents and conditions under which the tests are run. Inoculum density, phase of growth, incubation time and temperature, pH, incubation atmosphere, and ionic content of the media may influence end points.

The *disc diffusion test* has been most widely used. Its major advantage is the ease of setting up individual tests to evaluate a large number of antimicrobial agents. Diffusion tests are influenced by the depth, type, and concentration of the agar used. Only with standardization of methods and use of reference organisms can reproducibility be achieved. The innoculum tested should be derived from several colonies and be reasonably heavy, to increase the chance of detecting resistant mutants or heteroresistant strains. Diffusion tests are qualitative tests; although organisms are reported as susceptible, intermediate, or resistant, only inhibition of growth in vitro is measured and the concentrations of antibiotic necessary to accomplish this are not measured. Further, neither bactericidal activity nor factors that modify action at the site of infection are evaluated. Other deficiencies include lack of applicability to slowly growing organisms or anaerobes and inability to use agents, such as the polymyxins, that diffuse poorly. The E test, a recently developed method based on diffusion of a continuous concentration gradient of an antimicrobial from a plastic strip, provides quantitative results comparable to standardized dilution tests.

*Dilution tests* provide the most quantitative method for susceptibility testing. Either agar or broth dilution techniques are used. Commercially available semi-automated microdilution devices have made dilution tests practical and economical. Knowledge of the concentration of antibiotic causing growth inhibition may influence not only choice of a specific agent but its dosage and route of administration. Dilution tests also enable determination of bactericidal activity. Results of individual susceptibility tests are reported as minimum inhibitory concentrations (MIC) or minimum bactericidal concentrations (MBC). In some infections it is critical to achieve bactericidal concentrations of a drug; e.g., in meningitis, concentrations of the drug in vivo must be at least eight- to tenfold above the MBC for optimal results (see Chapter 73).

When susceptibility results are compiled, they are usually reported as the $MIC_{50}$, $MIC_{90}$, or MBC for a given bacterial species. The $MIC_{50}$ is the median antibiotic concentration at which one-half of strains are more sensitive, while one-half are more resistant. The $MIC_{90}$ is the concentration that inhibits 90% of the isolates. Knowledge of $MIC_{90}$ or MBC values is more useful than the $MIC_{50}$ value in the initial empirical selection of an antibiotic.

## Host Factors

The adequacy of multiple host factors should be considered in the decision to initiate empirical or definitive therapy and in the selection of specific agents. Such factors include the physiological responses of the individual to the infection, the patient's age, the presence of underlying disease, the presence or absence of prosthetic materials, pregnancy, and the adequacy of the patients inflammatory and immune responses. The importance of assessing the physiological responses to infection can be illustrated by considering the decision to hospitalize patients with community-acquired pneumonia. Physiologic determinants indicative of severity and higher risk of poor outcome include temperature $>101°$ F, respiratory rate $>30$ per minute, blood pressure $<90/60$ mm Hg, peripheral leukocyte count $<4000$ or $>30{,}000/mm^3$, hematocrit $<30\%$, $PaO_2$ $<60$ mm Hg, $PaCO_2$ $>50$ mmHg, serum creatinine $>1.2$ mg/dl or requirement for mechanical ventilation (see Chapter 56).

*Age*, at either extreme, is a surrogate marker for a number of anatomic, immunologic, hormonal and other as yet unidentified changes which affect susceptibility to infection as well as organisms to which an individual is exposed or colonized. For example, the most common cause of neonatal sepsis is the group B streptococcus acquired from the mother's vaginal flora during delivery. A risk factor for pharyngeal colonization with aerobic gram-negative bacilli is advanced age. The increased frequency of recurrent urinary tract infections in postmenopausal women appears to be related to vaginal estrogen deficiency. Both cellular and humoral defenses diminish with advancing age. This is apparent when analyzing the frequency with which groups of individuals respond to an antigen such as hepatitis B vaccine where response rates decrease from 97% in the $<30$ age-group to 58% in the $>60$ age-group. Herpes zoster, a manifestation of diminished cell-mediated immunity against childhood varicella-zoster virus infection occurs with increasing frequency with advancing age. Age also influences drug absorption, metabolism, and excretion.

During pregnancy, selection of drugs must include considerations of potential embryopathy and fetal toxicity as well as altered metabolism leading to maternal toxicity such as occurs with tetracycline. Underlying or concomitant diseases may predispose to infection with specific organisms. Examples include overwhelming pneumococcal or *H. influenzae* sepsis in patients with asplenia (sickle cell disease or splenectomy), meningococcal or gonococcal sepsis in individuals with complement deficiencies, sepsis due to *Vibrio vulnificus* after ingestion of raw shellfish by individuals with underlying liver disease, postinfluenzal pneumococcal or staphylococcal pneumonia or the association of *Streptococcus bovis* endocarditis with carcinoma of the colon.

Underlying disease may also alter the pharmacology of antimicrobial drugs. There is broad awareness of the importance of assessing renal function in the dosing of most antimicrobials (see Chapter 22). A common error in dosing patients with advanced renal disease, however, is lack of appreciation that the initial or loading dose should seldom be decreased. The dosage should be decreased or the interval between doses extended with subsequent administration. In the patient with cystic fibrosis, renal clearance of $\beta$-lactam and aminoglycoside drugs is significantly increased so that higher-than-usual doses are required to achieve and maintain expected serum levels.

## Microbial Factors

Microbial factors must also be considered in the decision to initiate and choose specific antimicrobial therapy. It is also important to consider the natural history of the probable infection(s). The list of infections that can be rapidly fatal is long, including bacteremia with shock, meningitis, many pneumonias, bacterial peritonitis, the streptococcal and staphylococcal toxic shock syndrome, and infections in the profoundly neutropenic patient. In other infections, progression may not be rapid, however, specific microbial data are virtually essential for management. These include most cases of infective endocarditis, or patients with chronic osteomyelitis.

The likelihood of obtaining meaningful microbiologic results in a timely manner can also affect antibiotic choice. For example, in the patient with suspected ventilator-associated pneumonia, data do not exist to support specific antimicrobial choices based on invasive methods to determine infecting agents and their antimicrobial susceptibilities over empiric therapy. In the patient suspected of having tuberculosis, a positive acid-fast smear may be obtained promptly, but measurement of antimicrobial susceptibility often takes weeks. Thus, the selection of an antimicrobial regimen is based upon factors such as the patient's place of residence—e.g., recent immigration from Latin America or Asia or residence in an area of increased prevalence of resistant *Mycobacterium tuberculosis*, or risk of exposure to multiply resistant *M. tuberculosis* (see Chapter 37).

## Site of Infection

In vitro susceptibility testing is keyed to serum (or urinary) concentrations and does not take into account host factors or conditions that alter antimicrobial access. There are sites of infection in which host defense mechanisms are absent or impaired. In the subarachnoid space (meningitis) the ability of neutrophilic leukocytes to phagocytize is impaired. Therefore, for effective treatment of bacterial meningitis, it is necessary to achieve cerebrospinal fluid (CSF) antimicrobial levels that are bactericidal at a dilution of 1:8 or 1:10. The milieu of the kidney, particularly the medulla, is inhibitory for many host defense mechanisms.

The site of infection and nature of the pathological process can affect antimicrobial contact with pathogens as well as antibiotic activity. This should be considered when choosing an antimicrobial, as well as the dosage, duration, and adjunctive approaches to therapy. Only a limited number of antimicrobial agents diffuse well into CSF or into the eye; as a result, high dosages of most agents are usually required. It is often not appreciated that as the inflammatory response subsides, entry of most drugs, particularly the $\beta$-lactam antibiotics, into the CSF decreases. Hence, as a patient is recovering, the dosage of a drug such as ampicillin in a child with meningitis (initially 200 mg/kg/day) should not be decreased. Although intrathecal therapy may be required in some circumstances, prospective studies in neonatal meningitis have not demonstrated a survival advantage. With endopththalmitis, intravitreal administration is the standard therapy for creating adequate antibiotic concentrations (see Chapter 77).

*Abscesses* represent a pathological process that will subvert the antibacterial activity of many antimicrobials. In addition to the large bacterial inoculum contained in abscesses, aminoglycosidic antibiotics diffuse poorly across the abscess wall which acts as a semipermeable membrane. Aminoglycosidic antibiotics have decreased antibacterial activity at acid pH levels and in the presence of nucleoproteins derived from dead leukocytes, and they are inactive at decreased levels of oxygen tension—all of which are characteristics of abscess cavities. With $\beta$-lactamase-susceptible drugs such as ampicillin, the $\beta$-lactamases released from killed organisms and retained within the abscess may be sufficient to inactivate later doses of ampicillin. Finally, there are a number of organisms that are intracellular pathogens. Since $\beta$-lactam and the aminoglycosidic antibiotics are not delivered well nor active intracellularly, intracellular organisms are usually protected from the antibacterial effects. They are exposed only when released into the extracellular milieu. A current therapeutic enigma is the evaluation of in vitro susceptibility testing with a drug such as azithromycin, which quickly diffuses from the intravascular pool into tissues and intracellularly where azithromycin concentrations may be 20-fold higher than serum concentrations.

## Route of Administration

Antimicrobial agents can be administered by several routes: enterally (oral or rectal), parenterally (intravenous, intramuscular, intraperitoneal), small particle (less than 5 $\mu$m) aerosol, intrathecally, intravitreally, or topically (skin or mucous membranes). Except for specialized circumstances such as endophthalmitis, coccidiodal meningitis, or peritoneal dialysis infections, most antimicrobial agents are administered orally, intravenously, or intramuscularly. The route of administration is determined in many instances by characteristics of the drug. Drugs to be given orally must be inherently resistant to degradation by gastric acid or coated to protect them until they enter the duodenum. Drugs such as the antiretroviral didanosine must be given with a buffer. Other drugs such as ketoconazole require gastric acidity for absorption. Among the oral cephalosporins, the absorption of some drugs, e.g., cefuroxime axetil, is increased with food. In contrast, food has no effect on absorption of cefixime and it is recommended that the oral carbacephem loracarbef be administered 1 h before or 2 h after meals. There are clinical circumstances in which proximal gastrointestinal (GI) absorption may be too good; amoxicillin is less active in shigellosis than is ampicillin, presumably because amoxicillin is better absorbed with lower intraluminal concentrations in the colon.

In the United States and many other countries, most parenteral antibiotic administration is intravenous (IV). The limiting factor for IV use is the drug's aqueous solubility. In other parts of the world, the intramuscular (IM) route is more widely used. Disadvantages to the IM route include local pain, local tissue damage, and dependence on adequate local tissue perfusion. In shock, drugs administered intramuscularly may not be absorbed.

A subject of intense current interest is the appropriate time to switch from parenteral to oral therapy as a means of decreasing hospital cost and duration of stay. The subject is not new. In the 1960s, children with *H. influenzae* meningitis treated with chloramphenicol were divided into a group that had oral therapy after the second day compared with a group with IV chloramphenicol for the full course. The outcomes were equivalent in both groups. More recently, studies have compared switching from parenteral to oral ciprofloxacin after 72 h of parenteral therapy, again with comparable results between regimens. In switching patients to oral therapy it is important to be certain that the patient's condition permits reliable intake and GI absorption and that the levels of drug achieved in the blood after oral administration are adequate to treat the infection. Furthermore, in selecting any patient for oral therapy, the ability and willingness of the patient to comply with the prescribed treatment must be considered.

## Requirement for Bactericidal as Compared with Bacteristatic Agents

There are several generalizations that apply in the selection of an antimicrobial regimen. As with generalizations, there are exceptions. The first generalization is that the $\beta$-lactam and aminoglycoside antibiotics are potentially bactericidal agents, whereas chloramphenicol, the tetracyclines, the macrolides, and lincosamides are bacteriostatic (Table 24.1). The second generalization is that one has to consider specific organisms. It has been clearly shown that chloramphenicol is bactericidal for *H. influenzae*, *Streptococcus pneumoniae*, and *Nesseria meningitidis*, hence its value in treating bacterial meningitis caused by these organisms. Similarly, ampicillin by itself is bactericidal against *Enterococcus faecalis*. Although there are exceptions and differences in antimicrobial susceptibilities and pharmacology, the selection of a bactericidal agent is usually preferable to treat most serious infections. This is especially true with infections in which host defenses are lacking or impaired, such as in meningitis, endocarditis, or the immunocompromised, neutropenic patient. In these patients, failure to select bactericidal agents for treatment is associated with an unacceptably high failure or relapse rate.

## Combination Therapy

There are three reasons to consider use of combinations of antimicrobials, to treat infections: broad spectrum coverage, synergistic activity, or prevention of resistance. The major reason

**Table 24.1** Categorization of bacteriocidal and bacteriostatic agents*

BACTERIOCIDAL AGENTS

*β-LACTAM DRUGS*

Penicillins
- Natural: penicillin G, V
- Penicillinase-resistant: methicillin, nafcillin, oxacillin, cloxacillin, dicloxacillin, flucoxacillin
- Aminobenzyl penicillins: Ampicillin, amoxicillin, bacampicillin
- Antipseudomonal (caboxy and ureidopenicillins): carbenicillin, ticarcillin, mezlocillin, piperacillin, azlocillin

Cephalosporins
- First generation: cephalothin, cefazolin, cephradine, cephalexin, cefadroxil
- Second generation: cefaclor, cefamandole, cefoxitin, cefuroxime, cefonicid, cefmatozole, cefotetan, cefprozil, loracarbef, ceftibuten
- Third generation: cefetamet pivoxil, cefoperazone, cefotaxime, ceftizoxime, ceftriaxone, cefixime, cefpodoxime proxetil
- Fourth generation: cefpirome, cefepime

Carbapenems: imipenem, meropenem

Monobactams: aztreonam

*AMINOGLYCOSIDES*

Amikacin, gentamicin, kanamycin, neomycin, netilmicin, streptomycin, tobramycin

*FLUOROQUINOLOLONES*

Ciprofloxacin, ofloxacin, norfloxacin, enoxacin, lomefloxacin, pefloxacin, rufloxacin

*PEPTIDES*

Bacitracin

Polymixin: polymyxin B, colistin

Glycopeptides: vancomycin, teicoplanin

*NITROIMIDAZOLES*

Metronidazole,[a] ornidazole, tinidazole, albendazole

BACTERIOSTATIC AGENTS

Macrolides/azalides: erythromycin,[b] azithromycin, clarithromycin, roxithromycin

Chloramphenicol[c]

Tetracyclines: tetracycline, doxycycline, minocycline

Lincosamides: lincomycin, clindamycin

Rifamycins: rifampin, rifabutin

Sulfonamides/trimethoprim

*Some agents are bacteriostatic against some organisms and bacteriocidal against others. Some are bacteriostatic at lower concentrations and bacteriocidal at higher concentrations.

[a]Metronidazole: bacteriocidal against *T. vaginalis*, *E. histolytica*.

[b]Erythromycin: predominantly bacteriostatic, but slowly bacteriocidal at higher concentrations.

[c]Chloramphenicol: bacteriostatic against almost all bacterial species but bacteriocidal at 2–4 times the MIC against *S. pneumoniae*, *H. influenzae*, *N. meningitidis*.

that combination therapy is used in most patients is to provide a broad spectrum of action to "cover the possibilities." The infection itself may be polymicrobial, or more likely, the possible causes include multiple organisms against which there is no single effective drug. For example, even imipenem, a β-lactam with very broad activity is not effective against methicillin-resistant staphylococci, *Legionella* spp., chlamydia, mycoplasma, mycobacteria, or fungi. Although it is common to use multiple drugs with an overlapping activity spectrum in the febrile neutropenic patient, a number of recent comparative studies have demonstrated the efficacy of monotherapy (see Chapter 86).

The second and more sound reason for combination therapy is to take advantage of synergism between two agents. The classical example is the synergistic action of streptomycin or gentamicin (not amikacin) plus ampicillin or penicillin G against *E. faecalis* in vitro or in patients with enterococcal endocarditis. Use of these combinations in enterococcal endocarditis leads to a higher cure rate and lesser relapses than with penicillin ampicillin alone (see Chapter 66).

The third reason for utilizing combination therapy has been to decrease the likelihood of the emergence of resistant organisms. Treatment of tuberculosis with isoniazid plus rifampin has been shown to decrease the emergence of resistant strains when compared with the use of either drug alone. The rationale for the current empirical use of four drugs to treat tuberculosis is to increase the likelihood that organisms will be sensitive to at least two of the four and this has become common practice when resistant tuberculosis is a consideration (see Chapter 37). Evidence that combination therapy use has decreased the emergence of resistance by the more common pathogens is lacking.

A potential downside of combination therapy is antagonism between drugs. In the 1950s there was a large literature on antibiotic synergism and antagonism. It was shown in vitro that the combination of a bacteristatic agent such as tetracycline would negate the bactericidal action of penicillin against a susceptible organism such as *S. pneumoniae.* Antibacterial antagonism in the clinical setting was shown only in bacterial meningitis where the mortality associated with penicillin alone was 30% whereas that with penicillin plus chlortetracycline was 79%. Because of this experience, the general rule has evolved to avoid the combined use of bacteristatic and bactericidal antibiotics to treat infections caused by single organisms.

## Adjunctive Approaches in the Treatment of Infection

In the management of some infections, particularly those which are life threatening, antimicrobial therapy, even if prompt, appropriate, and adequate, may be insufficient to promote a good outcome without other adjunctive and supportive measures. It is essential to correct life-threatening physiological derangements. Shock, if present, requires volume replacement with crystalloid solutions; hypoxemia will require supplemental oxygen with or without ventilatory support; cardiac arrhythmias such as those associated with Lyme disease or diphtheria may require pharmacologic or electromechanical support. Even when all *S. pneumoniae* were exquisitely sensitive to penicillin G, comparison of survival curves in patients with pneumococcal bacteremia suggested that antimicrobial therapy had little or no effect upon the outcome of infection among those destined at the onset of illness to die within 5 days. The drainage of abscesses or other closed sites remains a cardinal principle. In management it is essential to eliminate or bypass obstruction to normal drainage (paranasal sinuses, gall bladder, kidneys, or bladder) and to drain loculated areas of infection (abscesses, empyema). If there are prosthetic materials in the patients, consideration must be given to removal where possible (see Chapter 85).

There are circumstances in which it may be advantageous to suppress the inflammatory response through the use of corticosteroids. Again, one cannot generalize. In bacterial meningitis, especially that from *H. influenzae* in children, pretreatment with dexamethasone 15–20 min before antibiotics significantly decreases mortality and morbidity Inversely, in patients with cerebral Falciparum malaria, use of dexamethasone increased the duration of coma in a controlled study. In patients with more chronic illnesses or co-morbid conditions, correction of caloric, protein, trace metal, and nutritional deficiencies will facilitate recovery. Assisted organ function may be life saving, especially in those diseases where dysfunction is relatively transient, such as in the Hantavirus pulmonary syndrome or the use of renal dialysis in leptospirosis or hemorrhagic fever with renal syndrome.

## Monitoring Responses to Therapy

In many instances, the monitoring of response to treatment is more of an art than a science and often, just as with art, it "is in the eye of the beholder." The clinical parameters followed include the temperature (fever), signs of inflammation (erythema, pain, and swelling), and organ function. The response of any of these parameters is seldom as rapid as we would wish. Even in young patients with community-acquired pneumococcal pneumonia, the duration of fever after initiation of appropriate therapy is 2 to 4 days. Because of this natural course of response to treatment, therapy should not be changed within the first 72 h unless there is marked clinical deterioration. The rate with which patients with pyelonephritis defervesce with appropriate antimicrobial therapy varies from 3 to 13 days, depending upon whether or not the patient has focal or diffuse mass-like lesions on CT scan (see Chapter 69). In patients treated for infective endocarditis caused by streptococcus viridons, one-half are afebrile within 3 days, three-fourths by 1 week, and 90% by 2 weeks. In other patients the rate of defervescence depends upon the infecting organism, the size of the vegetations, and the presence of complications (see Chapter 66).

Laboratory parameters usually followed include leukocyte counts both in the peripheral blood and where possible, in specific fluids such as cerebrospinal fluid or peritoneal fluid. In cirrhotic patients treated for spontaneous bacterial peritonitis, the finding of $\leq$250 neutrophils/mm$^3$ and a sterile culture after 48 h indicated that 5 days of treatment was adequate in one study. The decline in acute-phase reactants, such as the erythocyte sedimentation rate or C-reactive protein, may also provide supporting evidence of therapeutic efficacy, especially in conditions such as osteomyelitis.

Imaging studies, X ray, CT, or MRI may provide additional evidence of resolution, although radiologic resolution may be delayed compared with clinical improvement. For example, with community-acquired pneumococcal pneumonia in young nonsmokers, only 60% will have X-ray resolution by 4 weeks. In a study of amebic liver abscesses in U.S. Army personnel returned from Vietnam who were treated with emetine, chloroquine, diodoquin, and tetracycline or metronidazole, the average radiologic resolution time was 4.3 months, which is far beyond clinical resolution or the continued need for active therapy.

Microbiologic parameters to follow include repeat cultures. Repeat blood cultures, if originally positive and subsequently negative, are extremely helpful. In patients treated with nafcillin and gentamicin for *S. aureus* endocarditis, blood cultures are usually negative by 48 h. Likewise, repeat urine cultures are useful in selected patients with complicated urinary tract infections (see Chapter 69). In contrast, repeat cultures of the sputum or draining wound or sinus tract as a measurement of treatment seldom do more than confuse interpretation. As a general rule, there is a great tendency to anticipate that responses occur more rapidly than is usual, and to overinterpret random variations in temperatures, leukocyte counts, and meaningless cultures, resulting in an irrational antibiotic merry-go-round changing of drugs to "cover" bacterial isolates that have been selected by the preceding therapy.

## Duration of Therapy

For all the studies of the treatment of infections with various antimicrobial agents there have been almost none that have established the minimal duration of therapy for any infection. Early in the antibiotic era, in infective endocarditis caused by *Streptococcus viridans* the failure rate was 83% after a 5-day course, 50% after 10 days, and only 2% after 20 days. It was also shown that 6 weeks of treatment with penicillin and streptomycin was optimal for enterococcal endocarditis, while shorter courses could be used for viridans streptococci and tricuspid endocarditis from *Staphylococcus aureus* in addicts. Ten days of penicillin (IM or oral) of group A streptococcal pharyngitis was the required treatment for preventing development of acute rheumatic fever. One to three days of trimethoprim sulfamethoxazole is adequate treatment for curing an initial episode of cystitis and prevent relapse (see Chapter 69).

Beyond these examples, most treatment duration recommendations are based on anecdotal experiences either of success or often of an occasional failure or relapse. Short-course therapy is given for 3 to 14 days and includes most uncomplicated bacterial infections. Intermediate courses of about 4 to 6 weeks are given for more difficult-to-eradicate infections, such as endocarditis. Long courses of >6 months are reserved for organisms in intracellular loci, such as tuberculosis, and many of the endemic mycoses. This is an area in which well-designed prospective studies are needed.

## Pharmacoeconomics

With cost containment becoming a major goal in health care delivery, the specialty of pharmacoeconomics has arisen. In considering the cost of an illness, not only must medical expenditures (cost of a provider visit, cost of medications, cost of administration) be considered but also the lost productivity of the patient or parent. Given these considerations, the least costly way to manage many common infections, especially when the efficacy of antimicrobial agents is questionable and illnesses are episodic and self-limiting, is through self-care. Conversely, the administration of a less costly but ineffective drug, when clinically indicated, is the most costly; the patient is subjected to the hazards of the infection as well as the potential adverse effects of the drug.

Cost of a drug should be a tertiary consideration, after effectiveness and safety. If agents can be identified that are equally effective and safe, then cost (both of acquisition and administration) can be a determinant in drug selection. Table 24.2 illustrates the enigma one faces in drug selection. All of the drugs listed are approved by the FDA for treatment of adults with acute bacterial exacerbations of chronic bronchitis. Although FDA approved, the specific value of antimicrobial therapy is controversial. The major pathogens incriminated include *H. influenzae* (28% of isolates) and *Moraxella catarrhalis* (10% of isolates). Resistance to ampicillin is found in 35% of isolates

**Table 24.2** Antimicrobial costs: treatment of an adult with acute bacterial exacerbation of chronic bronchitis*

| Antimicrobial agent[a] | Dose/frequency | Dose: Cost ($) | Cost/course[b]($) |
|---|---|---|---|
| LOWER COST GROUP | | | |
| Amoxicillin | 500 mg tid | 250 mg: 0.09 | 5.40 |
| Doxycycline | 100 mg bid | 100 mg: 0.17 | 3.40 |
| Erythromycin ethyl succinate | 400 mg qid | 400 mg: 0.22 | 8.80 |
| Penicillin V | 500 mg qid | 500 mg: 1.08 | 3.20 |
| Trimethoprim/sulfamethoxazole | 1 DS tab bid | 1 ds tab: 0.11 | 2.20 |
| INTERMEDIATE COST GROUP | | | |
| Amoxicillin Clavulanate | 500 mg tid | 500 mg: 2.60 | 78.00 |
| Azithromycin | 500 mg, 250 qd × 4 days | 250 mg: 6.04 | 36.24 |
| Cefaclor | 250 mg tid | 250 mg: 2.08 | 62.40 |
| Cefadroxil | 1.0 g bid | 500 mg: 3.06 | 61.20 |
| Cefixime | 400 mg qd | 400 mg: 6.07 | 60.70 |
| Cefpodoxime | 200 mg bid | 200 mg: 3.15 | 63.00 |
| Cefuroxime axetil | 250 mg bid | 250 mg: 3.11 | 62.20 |
| Ciprofloxacin | 500 mg bid | 500 mg: 3.13 | 62.60 |
| Clarithromycin | 250 mg bid | 250 mg: 2.97 | 59.40 |
| Loracarbef | 400 mg bid | 400 mg: 3.78 | 75.60 |
| Ofloxacin | 400 mg bid | 400 mg: 3.66 | 73.20 |
| HIGHER COST GROUP | | | |
| Cefprozil | 500 mg bid | 500 mg: 5.33 | 106.60 |
| Cefuroxime axetil | 500 mg bid | 500 mg: 6.11 | 122.20 |

*Costs are based on average wholesale price (AWP) in U.S. dollars to pharmacist. *Drug Topics Red Book 1995.*

[a]Prices for lower cost group based on generic not name brand products; prices for intermediate and higher cost groups based on name brand products.

[b]Course of therapy 10 days, except for azithromycin which is 5 days.

of *H. influenzae*. Resistance to tetracycline and TMP/SMX occurs but is less common. Erythromycin is only marginally effective against *H. influenzae.* Amoxicillin clavulanate, second and third generation cephalosporins, azithromycin, and the quinolones are effective against almost all strains, although many feel that ciprofloxacin should not be used for this indication because of the potential for increasing resistance as well as marginal effectiveness against *S. pneumoniae.* Approximately 80% of strains of *M. catarrhalis* are resistant to ampicillin. The other comments regarding *H. influenzae* also hold for *M. catarrhalis*. Thus, 15%–20% of isolates would be anticipated to be resistant to lower-cost drugs. Does this justify the use of more costly agents? Some might ask, what is the drug of choice for a nonindication?

## ANNOTATED BIBLIOGRAPHY


American Thoracic Society. Guidelines for the initial management of adults with community-acquired pneumonia: diagnosis, assessment of severity and initial antimicrobial therapy. Am Rev Respir Dis 1993; 148: 1418–1426.

*Includes a concise summary of risk factors to be considered in deciding whether to hospitalize patients with pneumonia.*

Austrian R, Gold J. Pneumococcal bacteremia with special reference to bacteremic pneumococcal pneumonia. Ann Intern Med 1964; 60:759–776.

*The classic review of pneumococcal bacteremia in the antibiotic era. Antibiotic treatment was no better than serum or no therapy in changing mortality rates in the first 48 h.*

Baker CN, Stocker SA, Culver DH, Thornsberry C. Comparison of the E test to agar dilution, broth microdilution and agar diffusion susceptibility testing techniques by using a special challenge set of bacteria. J Clin Microbiol 1991; 29:533–538.

Cates JE, Christie RV. Subacute bacterial endocarditis. Q Intern Med 1951; 20(NS)L 93–130.

*An early study that documented treatment success rates with different durations of proper antimicrobial therapy.*

Chambers HT. Short-course combination and oral therapies of *Staphylococcus aureus* endocarditis. Infect Dis Clin North Am 1993; 7:69–80.

*In patients with tricuspid valve endocarditis due to S. aureus without other complications, 2 weeks of treatment usually suffice.*

Fong TL, Akriviadis EA, Runyon BA, Reynolds TB. Polymorphonuclear cell count response and duration of antibiotic therapy in spontaneous bacterial peritonitis. Hepatology 1989; 9:423–426.

*When PMN counts fell below 250/mm³ in the peritoneal fluid, cure was obtained. In most patients, only 5 days of treatment were needed.*

Huang JJ, Sung JM, Chen KW, et al. Acute bacterial nephritis: a clinicoradiologic correlation based on computed tomography. Am J Med 1992; 93:289–298.

*Patients with focal or mass-like lesions took longer to defervesce with appropriate antimicrobial treatment.*

Lederman MM, Sprague L, Wallis RS, Ellner JJ. Duration of fever during treatment of infective endocarditis. Medicine 1992; 71:52–57.

*A retrospective analysis of patients treated for proven endocarditis with appropriate antimicrobial therapy. Certain organisms (*S. aureus, P. aeruginosa*) were associated with the longest times to defervescence compared with* Streptococcus viridans. *Prolonged fever despite proper therapy was also associated with vegetation size >1 cm and myocardial abscesses.*

Lepper MH, Dowling HF. Treatment of pneumococcic meningitis with penicillin compared with penicillin and aureomycin. Arch Intern Med 1951; 88:489–494.

*A striking example of in vivo antagonism of penicillin by a tetracycline.*

MacFarlane JT, Miller AC, Roderick Smith WH, et al. Comparative radiographic features of community acquired legionnaires disease, pneumo-

coccal pneumonia, mycoplasma pneumonia and psittacosis. Thorax 1984; 39:28–33.
*Natural history of responses to treatment on chest X ray of pneumonias caused by different pathogens.*

McCraig LF, Hughes JM. Trends in antimicrobial drug prescribing among office-based physicians in the United States. JAMA 1995; 273:214–219.

McGowan JE JR, Chesney PJ, Crossley KB, LaForce FM. Guidelines for the use of systemic glucocorticosteroids in the management of selected infections. J Infect Dis 1992; 165:1–13.
*This is the consensus of the Antimicrobial Agents Committee of the Infectious Diseases Society of America. An excellent analysis.*

Neiderman MS, Torres A, Summer W. Invasive diagnostic testing is not needed routinely to manage ventilator-associated pneumonia. Am J Respir Crit Care Med 1994; 150:565–569.
*This view is not shared by others. See Chastre J, Fagon JV. Invasive diagnostic testing should be routinely used to manage ventilated patients with suspected pneumonia. Am J Respir Crit Care Med 1994; 150:570–574.*

Paladino JA, Sperry HE, Backes JM, et al. Clinical and economic evaluation of oral ciprofloxicin after an abbreviated course of intravenous antibiotics. Am J Med 1991; 91:462–470.
*When used after 3 days of IV antibiotics, oral ciprofloxicin was as effective and safe as full courses of IV antibiotics.*

Roome AJ, Walsh SJ, Cartter ML, Hadler JL. Hepatitis B vaccine responsiveness in Connecticut Public Safety Personnel. JAMA 1993; 270: 2931–2934.
*An excellent example of the influence of age on responsiveness to a vaccine.*

Saint S, Bent S, Vittinghoff E, Grady D. Antibiotics in chronic obstructive pulmonary disease exacerbations. JAMA 1995; 273:957–960.
*This meta-analysis suggests a small but statistically significant improvement due to antibiotic therapy. Other analyses are less clear; see Murphy TF, Sethi S. Bacterial infections in chronic obstructive pulmonary disease. Am Rev Respir Dis 1992; 146:1067–1083.*

Shulman ST, Gerber MA, Tanz RR, Markowitz M. Streptococcal pharyngitis: the case for penicillin therapy. Ped Infect Dis J 1994; 13:1–7.
*On the basis of a meta-analyses of cephalosporins as compared with penicillin V, the argument has been made that cephalosporin regimens result in higher bacteriological and clinical cure rates. This article argues for the traditional approach. This is an area where changing recommendations seem likely.*

# 25

## Outpatient Parenteral Therapy of Serious Infections

ALAN D. TICE

Hospitals have played an important role in the evaluation and management of serious infections. In fact, for many years, some institutions were devoted simply to the care of patients with infection. As therapies and our understanding of disease have improved, however, the sanitoria and leprosaria have been closed and the majority of the hospitals in the United States are now downsizing with the cost constraints of health care reform. This transition has been brought about by advances in available antibiotics and increasingly in the technology of delivery as well. Oral antibiotics, such as the quinolones, have been substituted for parenteral ones in the therapy of gram-negative bacteria. New intravenous (IV) antibiotics have been developed which need to be given only once a day. All this makes it difficult to justify hospitalization for antibiotic therapy alone. Increasingly safe and reliable vascular access has been developed for home care. A variety of pumps now automatically administer antibiotics at any intervals desired, and with a reliability and accuracy equal to that given in the hospital.

While the stimulus for outpatient intravenous therapies has come largely from cost savings, other benefits to the patient and family are increasingly recognized and appreciated. Many patients are able to return to work or school. People generally prefer life outside the hospital to that inside—for the quality of the food if nothing else. Patients receiving intravenous antibiotics are also more involved in the treatment process if they are sent home. With outpatient therapy, patients and their families must understand their disease better and may be able to administer their own intravenous medication. Participation of patients in therapy helps them understand their disease and contributes to compliance as well as cost savings.

Since the first report of its use to treat recurrent infections in children with cystic fibrosis in 1974, outpatient intravenous antibiotic therapy (OPAT) has developed rapidly in the United States. Now over 300,000 patients are treated each year (more than 1 in 1000 Americans) with expenditures in the billions of dollars. The meteoric rise of outpatient intravenous care has not only stimulated a new form of medicine but has spawned a new industry called "home infusion." Its growth has been fueled further by the AIDS epidemic as most HIV-infected people shun hospitalization and prefer to be treated and die at home, despite the potential safety and theoretical benefits of hospital care.

Outpatient parenteral antibiotic therapy offers a challenge to the physician with new technology, new ways to use antibiotics, and special considerations about patient care that are different from those in the hospital. Despite the lack of control over patient care outside the hospital, the physician is nevertheless responsible legally and ethically for the quality of that care. It is the ordering physician's obligation to assure that the quality of care of outpatient IV therapy is comparable to that of continued hospitalization. He or she is relied upon to provide the safety net of quality for the patient—with the only backup being the legal profession. It behooves the physician to take a leadership role with pharmacists and IV therapy nurses to coordinate an effective, safe program of care as modern medicine shifts more and more to an outpatient setting.

### Patient Selection

The general principles of home or outpatient care require knowledge of appropriate patient selection, choice of antibiotics, knowledge of administration systems, and plans for ongoing medical monitoring (Table 25.1). Patient selection must be individually adapted according to the programs, resources, and expertise available. The first consideration is whether the diagnosed infection and other related diseases are appropriate to treat as an outpatient. This would not be the case for patients who are toxic, unstable, or may have endocarditis, meningitis, or septic arthritis. Patients with heavy nursing needs such as wound care or dementia and those who need special hospital procedures such as debridement or close laboratory monitoring are often best left in the hospital. Before any decision about home intravenous antibiotic therapy is made, consideration must be given to an oral antibiotic regimen. If the infection appears appropriate for management in the outpatient setting and to require intravenous therapy, then patients should be evaluated for their willingness and ability to accept the responsibility of outpatient therapy. Without their interest and participation, safety and compliance issues favor hospitalization. If, however, the patient is interested in home therapy, the family and home situation should be further explored. It is most helpful and often essential that there be another person in the home to assist with therapy. A person should not be sent home unless they have a telephone and ready access to transportation in case they need prompt medical evaluation. Patients to be trained in self-administration should have not only a telephone but a refrigerator and running water in order to store their medication and prepare for their administration.

### Models for Outpatient Intravenous Therapy

The three basic models for providing outpatient therapy are those of the visiting nurse, the infusion center, and that of self-administration (Table 25.2). The visiting nurse model offers convenience for the patient as the nurse visits the home to give the medication and supervise the administration. This may pose a problem, however, if medications must be given more than once a day, as the cost of the nurse's visits may be prohibitive. The infusion center model can be located in a hospital clinic, doctor's office, or nursing home, or it may be free-standing. It offers the safety of complete medical equipment and backup should there be problems with a vascular line or a need to change med-

**Table 25.1** Patient selection criteria for outpatient infusion therapy

| |
|---|
| DISEASE CONSIDERATIONS |
| Clear diagnosis |
| Appropriate infection |
| Oral therapy not reasonable |
| Other diseases |
| Nursing needs |
| PATIENT CONSIDERATIONS |
| Clinically stable |
| Willing to try |
| Physically able |
| Mentally able |
| Substance abuse |
| HOME SITUATION |
| Transportation |
| Telephone |
| Family support |
| Refrigeration |
| Running water |

ication. It is less attractive to the patient who has to travel to the infusion facility. Furthermore, the cost of maintaining the infusion therapy center must also be considered. A select group of patients may also be considered for training in self-administration or for training a family member to administer the antibiotic at home for the patient. This approach works particularly well for willing patients with few other medical problems, with good family support, and who are able to go back to work or school. Children are often saved the stress of hospitalization if their parents can learn to administer the medication. Most programs that carefully select patients and families have had few problems with intravenous infusions done without direct medical supervision.

## Types of Infection

There appears to be no contraindication to outpatient intravenous antibiotics by type of infection. Some diseases, such as sepsis, endocarditis, meningitis, and septic arthritis, should clearly be hospitalized initially, but even these patients can often complete their course of therapy on an outpatient basis if the patient responds well to the initial therapy. The infections most suited to outpatient intravenous antibiotic therapy are those that require repeated or prolonged courses of intravenous therapy in patients who are otherwise relatively well. This is often the case with osteomyelitis, endocarditis, recurrent lung infections, and in selected opportunistic infections in immunocompromised hosts. HIV-infected patients, for example, are excellent candidates for outpatient therapy, particularly when lifelong treatments such as ganciclovir or foscarnet are necessary. Increasingly, however, there is interest in treating as an outpatient diseases that need a shorter course of antibiotic therapy. This is especially true if hospitalization can be avoided altogether. It is possible to treat patients with cellulitis and postoperative wound infections with empiric parenteral antibiotic therapy and then change to the most active and specific drug when the culture results become available. If close outpatient monitoring and ready access to medical resources can be provided, these patients can be treated entirely as outpatients. If they respond well within a few days of therapy, often they can be switched to oral medications to complete their course.

## Antibiotic Selection

It is increasingly clear that not only can any infection be treated on an outpatient basis but that any antibiotic can be used to do so. Published series of patients treated with outpatient therapy indicate that the primary antibiotics used are ceftriaxone, cefazolin, vancomycin, and penicillin. Generally, more toxic drugs such as amphotericin B and pentamidine are best administered in infusion clinics, but even these are sometimes given at home under the supervision of a nurse. Antibiotic selection factors to consider in outpatient therapy are different from those in the hospital. There are multiple reasons to select a drug that can be given once a day. Ceftriaxone has a particular advantage in this regard because of its half-life of 6 to 8 h. It has been well studied and proven effective with a single daily dose for most infections where it is indicated. The convenience of once-daily dosing has also stimulated interest in using other drugs once a day. It appears that the majority of people over 65 can be treated with vancomycin once a day as their renal function is slightly compromised. In the elderly, the half-life of vancomycin becomes equivalent to that of ceftriaxone, if not longer. In addition, our increasing knowledge of the pharmacodynamics of aminoglycosides has indicated that, because of their concentration-dependent killing and prolonged postantibiotic effect, these drugs are also effective when given only once a day. It appears they are also less toxic when given once a day and that their toxicity correlates with trough levels. Some of the new quinolones and azithromycin also have half-lives such that they can be given once a day. (Suggested drugs and regimens for specific infections are shown in Table 25.3).

For the drugs that do not have the pharmacologic parameters to justify once-a-day therapy, new and evolving vascular access devices and pumps have been developed. They make it possible

**Table 25.2** Models for delivery of outpatient IV antibiotic delivery

| Model | Advantages | Disadvantages |
|---|---|---|
| Visiting nurse | Home assessment<br>Supervised infusion | Nurse time<br>Travel costs<br>Privacy |
| Infusion center | Ease of monitoring<br>Medical equipment<br>Supervised infusion | Patient travel<br>Overhead costs |
| Self-administration | Low labor costs<br>Patient autonomy | Patient training<br>Unsupervised |

**Table 25.3** Common outpatient treatment regimens

| Antibiotic | Infections commonly treated | Dosing in adults[a] | Weekly monitoring[b] |
|---|---|---|---|
| Ceftriaxone | Osteomyelitis<br>Cellulitis<br>Lower respiratory<br>Meningitis<br>Endocarditis<br>Wound<br>Urinary | 1 or 2 g q24h | CBC twice<br>Renal once |
| Vancomycin | Wound infections<br>Methicillin-resistant staphylococci | 1 g q12h (q24h in elderly) | CBC once<br>Renal twice |
| Cefazolin | Cellulitis<br>Wound<br>Osteomyelitis<br>Urinary | 2 g q8h | CBC twice<br>Renal once |
| Penicillin | Endocarditis<br>Meningitis | 2–4 million units q4h or continuous infusion with a pump | CBC twice<br>Renal once |
| Gentamicin or | Urinary | 5–7 mg/kg | Renal twice |
| Tobramycin | Enterococci<br>Resistant gram-negative rods | q24h | CBC once |
| Oxacillin | Staphylococci<br>Osteomyelitis<br>Wound<br>Cellulitis | 2 gm q6h (with a pump) | CBC twice<br>Renal once<br>Liver once |
| Ceftazidime | Pseudomonas | 2 gm q8 or 12h | CBC twice<br>Renal once |
| Ganciclovir | Cytomegalovirus | Induction, then 6 mg/kg q24h | CBC once<br>Renal once |
| Foscarnet | Cytomegalovirus | Induction, then 90–120 mg/kg q24h | Renal, electrolytes, calcium, magnesium, liver function once<br>CBC once |

[a]If normal renal function.

[b]If laboratory parameters otherwise stable.

to reliably administer medications at any intervals desired, including by continuous infusion. The major limitation of this methodology is the stability of the antibiotics. Ampicillin, for example, is relatively unstable once it is put into a solution and must therefore be mixed fresh daily.

## Monitoring Therapy

One of the most important and often overlooked aspects of outpatient therapy is that of monitoring the clinical response and looking for signs of toxicity from the drugs. This is a growing concern as increasingly ill and complex patients are sent home to receive IV therapy. Problems with the treatment programs themselves must also be considered. Limited studies suggest a wide variation in complications depending on the quality of the organization and the population being treated. A good program should have rates of phlebitis, compliance, and adverse drug events comparable to the hospital, if not better.

To assure that the quality of care is comparable to that in the hospital, patients must be followed and monitored closely (Table 25.4). Physician visits are usually once or twice a week, although

**Table 25.4** Monitoring on outpatient intravenous antibiotic therapy

| | |
|---|---|
| Physician visits | As needed but usually once or twice weekly when stable |
| Hematology | White blood cell count at least weekly on penicillins, cephalosporins, and vancomycin<br>Hemoglobin/hematocrit weekly<br>Platelet count, coagulation studies if any bleeding problems, concomitant nutritional compromise, or with specific antibiotics such as moxalactam |
| Renal function | Blood urea nitrogen or creatinine weekly on penicillins or cephalosporins, twice weekly with aminoglycosides or vancomycin, and more often if unstable or with amphotericin B |
| Liver function | Liver enzyme levels weekly or every other week on nafcillin |

unstable patients may need to be seen every day and those that are stable on prolonged therapy with drugs such as ganciclovir may only need to be seen every few weeks. It is important to work closely with the IV therapy nurses seeing the patient and to monitor appropriate blood studies depending upon the antibiotic used. The white blood cell count, for example, may fall to dangerous levels with penicillins, cephalosporins, and vancomycin (see Chapter 23). It is important to note that leukopenia usually does not develop until 2 or 3 weeks into therapy. A reduction in dose may be sufficient to reverse the effect, but usually the antibiotic must be changed. Renal function should be checked periodically with all antibiotics and probably twice a week with patients receiving aminoglycosides and vancomycin. Serum concentrations of aminoglycosides and vancomycin are often monitored to assure therapeutic levels as well as to avoid toxicity. With the use of once-daily aminoglycosides and the low incidence of vancomycin toxicity, the need for routine monitoring of levels in patients with normal renal function has been questioned. Vestibular toxicity from aminoglycosides must also be watched for clinically as it may not correlate with antibiotic levels or renal function and may not occur until several weeks into the treatment course (see Chapter 23).

Other adverse events such as allergic reactions to the antibiotic must also be considered and actively monitored. Infections or complications related to medical therapy at home can also occur. The incidence of *Clostridium difficile* colitis, superinfections, and line infections appear to be less frequent with outpatient therapy than in the hospital. When secondary infections do arise, they are less likely to involve the multidrug-resistant organisms of the hospital.

The use of outpatient intravenous antibiotic therapy is growing rapidly but has not been well studied. How much it can or should be used is uncertain. It is essential that standards for monitoring and outcomes research be developed to understand how best to maximize its potential benefits and to understand its limitations and risks, especially since cost factors continue to challenge the quality of care.

In summary, outpatient therapy for serious infections is increasingly feasible and utilized. It offers a challenge to the physician to assemble an effective team to provide this form of therapy, to determine how best to use new antibiotics, and to most appropriately employ established drugs. With expertise, physicians can provide very cost effective and safe care for their patients.

## ANNOTATED BIBLIOGRAPHY


American Medical Association. Physician Guide to Home Health Care. Mineola, New York: Dover, American Medical Association, 1989, pp 19–28.
*Guidelines for home health care considerations for the physician, prepared by the American Medical Association.*

Balinsky W, Nesbitt S. Cost-effectiveness of outpatient parenteral antibiotics: a review of the literature. Am J Med 1989; 87:301–305.
*A review of cost factors related to savings of outpatient parenteral antibiotic therapy.*

Craig WA. Kinetics of antibiotics in relation to effective and convenient outpatient parenteral therapy. Int J Antimicrob Agents 1995; 5:19–22.
*Review of pharmacokinetics and pharmacodynamics of antibiotics with particular relevance to OPAT therapy.*

Hindes R, Winkler C, Kane P, Kunkel M. Outpatient intravenous antibiotic therapy in medicare patients: cost-savings analysis. Infect Dis Clin Pract 1995; 4:211–217.
*Detailed review of cost effectiveness issues and cooperative effort between hospital and physician for Medicare patients.*

Gilbert DN, Dworkin RJ, Raber SR, Leggett JE. Outpatient parenteral antimicrobal-drug therapy. N Engl J Med 1997; 337:829–838.
*Review of vascular access devices that may be particularly relevant to OPAT therapy.*

Poretz DM, Eron LJ, Goldenberg RI et al. Intravenous antibiotic therapy in an outpatient setting. 1982; JAMA 248:336–339.
*A basic early reference.*

Stivers HG, Telford GO, Mossey JM et al. Intravenous antibiotic therapy at home. Ann Intern Med 1978; 89:690–693.
*A basic early reference.*

Tice AD. An office model for outpatient parenteral antibiotic therapy. J Infect Dis 1991; 13(Suppl 2):S184–S188.
*Description of a physician-directed, clinic-based intravenous antibiotic therapy program and how it arose.*

Tice AD. Experience with a physician-directed, clinic-based program for outpatient parenteral antibiotic therapy in the USA. Eur J Clin Micro Inf Dis 1995; 14:23–29.
*Review of experiences with a private practice program with emphasis on patient selection and appropriate antibiotics.*

Tice AD. Handbook of Outpatient parenteral therapy. New York: Scientific American Medicine, 1997:1–122.
*Basic review of OPAT therapy with practical aspects of treatment.*

Tice AD, et al. Outpatient Parenteral Antimicrobial Therapy: Current Status. Proceedings of an OPAT Advisory Board Meeting. Chicago, Illinois, May 16–18, 1996. Scientific American Medicine (A special report). 1997; 5–83.
*Recent review of some practical aspects of OPAT therapy*

Tice AD (ed). Outpatient Parenteral Antibiotic Therapy: management of Serious Infections. Part I: Medical, Socioeconomic, and Legal Issues. 1993; Hosp Pract 28(Suppl 1).
*A supplement of nine chapters about practical management issues involved in providing outpatient parenteral antibiotic therapy..*

Tice AD (ed). Outpatient Parenteral Antibiotic Therapy: Management of Serious Infections. Part II: Amenable Infections and Models for Delivery. 1993; Hosp Pract 28(Suppl 2).
*A second supplement of twelve chapters discussing the primary infections treated with outpatient intravenous antibiotic therapy and the organization models used to treat them.*

U.S. Congress, Office of Technology Assessment, Home Drug Infusion Therapy Under Medicare, OTA-H-509 (U.S. Government Printing Office, Washington, DC; May 1992).
*A comprehensive report to Congress on the home infusion industry with a particular emphasis on reimbursement issues and their implications for the federal Medicare program.*

Williams D. Home intravenous antibiotic therapy (HIVAT): indications, patients and antimicrobial agents. Int J Antimicrob Agents 1995; 5:3–8.
*Review of experiences in a hospital-based OPAT program.*

Williams DN, Rehm SJ, Tice AD, Bradley JS, Kind AC, Craig WA. Practice guidelines for community-based parenteral anti-infective therapy. Clin Infect Dis 1997; 25:787–801.
*Infectious Diseases Society of America guidelines for evaluation and management of OPAT patients with criteria for program quality assurance.*

# 26

# Control of Antimicrobial Usage

PETER G. DAVEY

There is global concern about the need to control antibiotic usage. This stems from widespread evidence, mainly from hospitals, of misuse of antimicrobial drugs leading to escalating drug costs, increased burden of side effects, and the rapid spread of resistance. In contrast to irrational use of other drugs (e.g., anti-hypertensives), the latter problem is unique to antibiotic usage. Ideally, assessment of the benefits of controlling usage should be based on audits of mortality or morbidity from infection and should show that regulation limits the spread of resistance. In reality such comprehensive audit or research is beyond the scope of most hospitals and they must be content with implementation of processes that have been shown to control antibiotic use and to improve clinical outcome in other centers. Setting realistic objectives is a key component of audit.

## Where Should Control of Antibiotic Usage Be Implemented?

Most studies to date have addressed the problem of inappropriate usage of antibiotics from a hospital perspective. Indeed, guidelines for improving the use of antimicrobial agents in hospitals have long been established. Considering that most antibiotic usage occurs in the ambulatory setting and despite evidence that excessive use of certain antibiotics by general practitioners has led to increasing incidence of bacterial resistance in the community, attempts at control of antibiotic usage in this area have been sparse. A recent study from England and Scotland (Davey et al. 1996), which examined data from antibiotic prescriptions in general practice over a 13-year period, revealed consistent, linear growth in antibiotic prescriptions and also in cost per prescription. Alarmingly, growth has been most rapid for recently introduced drugs, such as the quinolones, which are relatively expensive and against which resistance may develop rapidly. There is no epidemiological justification for this steady rise, and failure to halt or reverse this trend will increase the prevalence of drug-resistant bacteria in primary care.

## Who Should Be Involved in Controlling Antibiotic Usage?

National guidelines exist in some countries regarding use of antibiotics in some conditions, for example, pneumonia. However, practical local guidelines are needed for the community or hospital physician. In hospitals, a multidisciplinary approach could incorporate the local infectious disease clinicians, microbiologists, clinical pharmacists, and, most importantly, the senior clinicians whose junior staff would be the principle users of the policy. Family practitioners are being exposed to an increasing number and variety of antibiotics that have no clear advantages over those already available. They are also being persuaded to use potent expensive drugs, such as quinolones, initially directed towards hospital use. These factors and the spread of resistance to some of these agents has been the stimulus for introducing antibiotic policies within individual or groups of family practices. The primary care teams have devised a policy in conjunction with the local microbiologists and infectious disease clinicians as well as the community pharmacists.

## What Are the Aims of the Key Control Measures?

The concerns outlined previously have led to the introduction of measures to control antibiotic usage. There is good evidence that these measures reduce unwanted clinical effects of antibiotics, allow their cost-effective use, and limit spread of resistance. The impact of the latter is a delay in clearing the infection and treatment with second-line agents that often have more side effects and are generally more expensive. Measures that reduce the number of cases in which second-line agents are necessary should at least ensure that resistance to these second-line agents is kept low.

The main tool to achieve these objectives have been the introduction of *antibiotic policies*. Each policy encompasses a number of measures and aims along with their desired impact or effect. These are summarized in Table 26.1.

## What Is the Level of Success of Various Key Methods Used to Implement Antibiotic Policies?

Once an antibiotic policy is agreed upon, the next step is to ensure that the staff using the guidelines are aware of them and the intentions of the policy. The four general intervention strategies for influencing prescribing habits are re-education, persuasive, facilitative, and power strategies. When comparing the impact of a range of strategies to rationalize antibiotic usage, superiority and benefit of one strategy over another has to be measured in prospective comparative clinical trials. One of the best examples is a multicenter trial of four strategies to reduce use of pre-operative chest X rays (Fowkes et al. 1986). Of the four strategies, the appointment of a multidsciplinary utilization review committee was the most successful. This trial reinforces the need to involve clinicians in setting standards and the importance of feeding information back to clinicians on a regular basis.

**Table 26.1** Summary of methods and effect of antibiotic policies

| Measures | Effect |
|---|---|
| Narrow range of familiar drugs | Promotes awareness of their effectiveness and potential side effects<br>Facilitates educational programs within hospital<br>Lessens the impact of aggressive pharmaceutical marketing<br>Encourages appropriate use of antibiotics |
| | PHARMACY BENEFITS<br>Reduces bulk orders<br>Reduces number of orders<br>Better stock control<br>Easier prescription review |
| | MICROBIOLOGY BENEFITS |
| Advise on "best guess" in empiric therapy | Rationalize sensitivity testing<br>Improve general familiarity with drugs<br>Identify patient's risk category<br>Intravenous vs. oral<br>Duration of therapy<br>Penicillin allergy |
| Make rational choice among "equivalent" drug(s) based on | Dose/frequency/route<br>Route of excretion<br>Drug formulations<br>Spectrum of activity<br>Cost |
| Aim for cost-effectiveness for the hospital | Contains costs for:<br>The pharmacy<br>Clinical staff<br>Microbiology staff |
| Promote good practice | Facilitates peer review<br>Reduces ineffective prescribing and bad practice<br>Provides a focus for education and training<br>Reduces use of nonformulary drugs |
| Reduce the emergence of resistant strains | Maximizes patient benefit from first-line drugs<br>Reduces use of costly second-line drugs<br>Reduces reliance on new drug development |

Many strategies have been used to control the use of antibiotics with varying degrees of success. Table 26.2 summarizes examples of some key strategies that have been successful in implementing policies concerned with control of antibiotics. Re-education and persuasive strategies tend to be noninteractive and rely on the user to make a decision based on the information or options provided. In general terms, these strategies only have a transient effect on prescribing habits. Power strategies are often felt to be rather restrictive and dictatorial. Strategies that appeal to the prescriber's desire to do better, for example, reducing the length of hospital stay or cutting cost of certain antibiotics, may be more appealing. Facililtative strategies encompass the principles of good audit, which are defining a goal, providing the information to assess the best method for achieving the goal, measuring the results, and feeding them back to the prescriber. One of the best examples of this is a study by Feely et al. (1990) who examined the impact of introduction of new drugs in a hospital formulary with an intensive prescribing feedback program over a 1-year period. Prescribing habits were monitored for a further year, but feedback was discontinued. In the year in which the intervention occurred, generic prescribing rose by 50%, inappropriate prescribing and the overall use of third generation cephalosporins fell, and drug costs remained static against a projected increase for that year. During the next year, when no form of feedback intervention took place, previous gains were eroded and drug costs rose.

## Economic Issues

There are several studies showing that antibiotic policies reduce hospital drug costs. In general, these savings are achieved by reduction in the use of new, expensive parenteral drugs. There are relatively few studies that quantify the cost of introduction and maintenance of control measures and compare these costs (mainly staff time) with the benefits achieved. Nonetheless, even elaborate and costly control measures can be shown to save resources. The key to success is to define a specific goal, estimate the financial savings or improvement in patient care that may be achieved, and estimate the resources required to make the change. It is vital that all concerned are convinced that the benefits of control measures are likely to justify the time and effort required to implement them.

**Table 26.2** Examples of key strategies used in controlling antibiotic usage

| Target | Strategy | Outcome/reference |
|---|---|---|
| RE-EDUCATION STRATEGIES | | |
| Reduces use of specific drug | Mailed information | Transient effect, unsuccessful Avorn and Soumerani, 1983 |
| Substitution of specific drugs | Drug bulletin | Successful Fendler et al., 1984 |
| Compliances with formulary | Issuing formulary without feedback | Unsuccessful Feely et al., 1990 |
| PERSUASIVE STRATEGIES | | |
| Reduction in costs of IV | Feedback of costs to individual antibiotics | Unsuccessful Parrino, 1989, with peer comparison |
| Promote use of cheaper alternative agents | Educational advertising poster campaigns | Successful Harvey et al., 1986 |
| Improve antibiotic dosing | Structured educational order form for parenteral antibiotics | Successful Avorn et al., 1988 |
| Reduction in IV antibiotic | Cost information added to microbiology form | Successful Rubenstein et al., 1988 |
| Reduction in IV antibiotic costs | Guidelines for IV vs. oral switch | Successful Quintiliani et al., 1987 |
| FACILITATIVE STRATEGIES | | |
| Substitution of specific drugs | Computerized feedback of potential cost savings | Successful Evans et al., 1986 |
| Reduce use of specific drugs | Mailed information and feedback at interview | Successful Fendler et al., 1984 |
| | Academic detailing | Successful Avorn and Soumerai, 1983 |
| Compliance with formulary | Regular feedback to individual prescribers | Successful Feely et al., 1990 |
| Reduce costs of surgical prophylaxis | Educational marketing | Successful Landgren et al., 1988 |
| Identification of educational needs for 10 most commonly prescribed drugs | Individual tailored instruction packets | Successful Manning et al., 1986 |
| POWER OR RESTRICTIVE STRATEGIES | | |
| Controlled use of "expensive," broad-spectrum parenteral agents | Automatic stop orders for specific high-cost agents | Successful Marr et al., 1988 |
| | Prior approval of infectious diseases specialist, microbiologist | Successful Marr et al., 1988 |
| | Required infectious diseases consultation prior to prescription | Successful Marr et al., 1988 |
| | Written justification by clinician | Transiently successful McGowan and Finland, 1974 |

## REFERENCES


Avorn J, Soumerai SB. Improving drug therapy decisions through educational outreach. A randomized controlled trial of academically based "detailing." N Engl J Med 1983; 308:1457–1463.

Avorn J, Soumerai SB, Taylor W, Wessels MR, Janousek RPh, Welner M. Reduction of incorrect antibiotic dosing through a structured educational order form. Arch Intern Med 1988; 148:1720–1724.

Davey PG, Bax RP, Newey J, Reeves D, Rutherford D, Slack R, Warren RE, Watt B, Wilson J. Growth in the use of antibiotics in the community in England and Scotland in 1980–1993. Br Med J 1996; 312(9 March): 613.

Davey P, Nathwani D. Antibiotic policies. In: Antibiotic and Chemotherapy. O'Grady F, Lambert H, Finch RG, Greenwood D, eds. Churchill Livingstone, London, 1997, pp 149–163.

*A comprehensive review of the literature and the evidence that antibiotic policies do influence patterns of prescribing, cost-effectiveness of prescribing, and the emergence of drug resistance.*

Evans RS, Larsen RA, Burke JP, Gardner RM, Meier FA, Jacobson JA, Conti MT, Jacobson JT, Hulse RK. Computer surveillance of hospital acquired infections and antibiotic use. JAMA 1986; 256:1007–1011.

Fowkes FGR, Evans KT, Hartley G, Nolan DJ, Roberts CJ, Davies ER, Green G, Hugh AE, Power AL, Rozdzinski E. Multicentre trial of four strategies to reduce use of a radiological test. Lancet 1986; i:367–369.

Feely J, Chan R, Cocoman L, Mulpeter K, O'Connor P. Hospital formularies: need for continuous intervention. BMJ 1990; 300:28–30.

Fendler KJ, Gumbhir AK, Sall K. The impact of drug bulletins on physician prescribing habits in a health maintenance organization. Drug Intel Clin Pharm 1984; 18:627–631.

Fowkes FGR, Evans KT, Hartley G, Nolan Dj, Roberts CJ, Davies ER, Green G, Hugh AE, Power AL, Rozdzinski E. Multicentre trial of four strategies to reduce use of a radiological test. Lancet 1986; i:367–369. *Although this study relates to reducing unnecessary pre-operative chest X-rays, the methodology is relevant to prescribing policies. The trial clearly showed that involvement of clinicians in writing standards produced the greatest initial change in practice and that continuous feedback of audit results to clinicians was necessary to maintain changes in practice.*

Harvey KJ, Stewart R, Hemming M, Nalsmith N, Moulds RFW. Educational antibiotic advertising. Med J Aust 1986; 145:28–32.

Landgren FT, Harvey KJ, Mashford L, Moulds RFW, Guthrie B, Hemming M. Changing antibiotic prescribing by educational marketing. Med J Aust 1988; 149:595–599.

Manning PR, Lee PV, Clintworth WA, Denson TA, Oppenheimer PR, Gilman NJ. Changing prescribing practices through individual continuing education. JAMA 1986; 256:230–232.

Marr JJ, Moffet HL, Kunin CM. Guidelines for improving the use of antimcobial agents in hospitals: a statement by the Infectious Diseases Society of America. J Infect Dis 1988; 157:869–876.

McGowan JE, Findland M. Usage of antibiotics in a general hospital: effect of requring justification. J Infect Dis 1974; 130:165.

Parrino TA. The nonvalue of retrospective peer comparision feedback in containing hospital antibiotic costs. Am J Med 1989; 86:442–448.

Quintiliani R, Cooper BW, Briceland LL, Nightingale CH. Economic impact of streamlining antibiotic administration. Am J Med 1987; 82(Suppl 4A):391.

Rubenstein E, Barzilai A, Segev S, Samra Y, Modan M, Dickerman O, Haklai C. Antibiotic cost reduction by providing cost information. Eur J Clin Pharmacol 1988; 35:269–272.

# 27

# Penicillins

CATHERINE M. CRETICOS AND JOHN N. SHEAGREN

The now famous discovery by Alexander Fleming in 1928 of a substance produced by a culture of *Penicillium notatum* that inhibited the growth of *Staphylococcus aureus* did not evolve into a therapeutic compound until over 10 years later. In 1939, Dr. Howard W. Florey and co-workers isolated the compound and determined its structure and properties. After sufficient quantities of penicillin were produced, testing in humans began in 1941 when a British policeman infected with both staphylococci and streptococci was treated with penicillin-G. Improvements in production techniques as well as greater yields of the compound utilizing *Penicillium chrysogenum*, a new production strain, combined with increased interest by the United States in the production of penicillin because of the war led to its general use in the United States by the end of the 1940s. Many penicillins have since been found or synthesized, making this family of antimicrobials one of the largest and most important.

Penicillin derivatives remain useful today because of their bactericidal activity, excellent therapeutic-to-toxic ratio, and generally good tissue penetration. Spawned by the emergence of resistant bacteria, the development of first the penicillinase resistant penicillins (1950s), followed by ampicillin, the carboxypenicillins and ureidopenicillins (1960s), and most recently, combinations with $\beta$-lactamase inhibitors (1980s) have permitted these agents to maintain their effectiveness and to expand their spectra of activity.

## Chemistry

The basic structure of penicillin (6-aminopenicillanic acid) has three components to the nucleus (see Fig. 27.1): a thiazolidine ring, a $\beta$-lactam ring, and a side chain. This nucleus results from a combination of the two amino acids alanine and cysteine. Changes made in the side chains account for differences in the antimicrobial spectrum or pharmacologic properties between the various penicillins. Alteration of the side chain may occur naturally, by the selection of the fermentation medium in which penicillin is grown, or by chemical attachment as in the semisynthetic penicillins.

## Mechanism of Action

Although the exact mechanism by which penicillins kill bacteria has still not been fully elucidated, it includes inhibition of bacterial cell wall synthesis, binding to bacterial targets located beneath the cell wall (called *penicillin-binding proteins* [PBPs]), and also, at least in some cases, activation of bacterial autolysis.

Interference with the final step of bacterial cell wall formation was one of the earliest mechanisms by which penicillins were found to kill bacteria. It is now known that cell wall synthesis in bacteria is a process that contains multiple steps and at least 30 enzymes. The peptidoglycan component of gram-positive bacteria is 50–100 molecules thick, compared with only one or two molecules thick for gram-negative bacteria; in both, it is important in maintaining the osmotic integrity of the bacterial cell. In addition, gram-negative bacteria have an outer lipopolysaccharide layer, which can interfere with delivery of penicillins to their target sites.

Formation of peptidoglycan cell wall is divided into three stages. First is the creation of the building blocks UDP-*N*-acetylmuramyl (NAM) pentapeptide and UDP-N-acetylglucosamine (NAG) from nucleic acid precursors. Next, these proteins are carried across the cytoplasmic membrane and transglycosylation occurs, transforming the NAM-pentapeptide and NAG into peptidoglycan polymers. Finally, the polysaccharide chains are cross-linked via peptide side chains. This transpeptidation reaction, which occurs at the surface of the cell membrane, is the primary step inhibited by penicillins via acylation of transpeptidase enzymes (Fig. 27.2). Specific transpeptidases may incorporate new peptidoglycan into old, cross-link specific structures, or build the cell wall septum.

Additional targets of penicillins at the level of the cell membrane are the penicillin-binding proteins (PBPs), first detected and described in 1972. The PBPs are numbered according to molecular weight, which may vary from 35,000 to 120,000, in order of decreasing size, and differ from one species of bacteria to another. No relationship exists between the PBPs of gram-positive and gram-negative bacteria. PBPs can vary in number (typically 7 to 10 for gram-negative bacilli compared to 3 to 5 for gram-positive cocci) and amount. Some PBPs are known to correspond to distinct cellular enzymes such as carboxypeptidases, transpeptidases, and endonucleases. Binding to some PBPs may induce cell death while binding to others may change cell morphology. For example, in *Escherichia coli*, the binding of the PBP-1 complex results in cell lysis, while the specific binding of PBP-2, as occurs with amdinocillin, is associated with loss of rod shape and the formation of ovoid cells which later lyse. Again, in *E. coli*, PBP-3 is important in cell division and binding results in filament formation without septa; PBPs 4 and 5 are less important since mutants lacking these PBPs grow and survive.

For some bacterial species, induction of autolysis may be an important killing mechanism for penicillin. Autolysis may be activated by interference with the normal inhibitors of the autolytic enzyme system (e.g., inhibition of peptidoglycan hydrolases). Penicillins exert a postantibiotic effect of several hours duration for gram-positive bacteria, but do not show a similar effect on gram-negative bacteria.

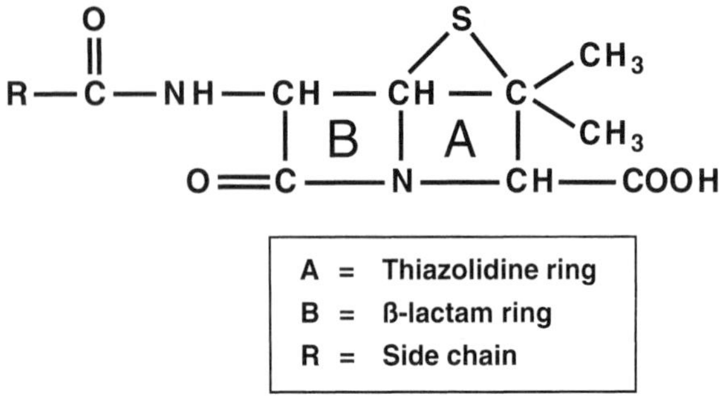

A = Thiazolidine ring
B = ß-lactam ring
R = Side chain

**Fig. 27.1** The basic structure of penicillins.

## Resistance

Bacteria have developed many important mechanisms of resistance to penicillin, the most significant of which is the ability to hydrolyse the $\beta$-lactam ring of penicillin by $\beta$-lactamases. The $\beta$-lactam ring must be intact for the antibacterial activity of a penicillin to be preserved. In gram-positive bacteria, $\beta$-lactamases are inducible and plasmid mediated, and they are excreted into the extracellular environment. Enzyme production may be in large amounts and with a high affinity for penicillin (Fig. 27.3A). Activity against staphylococci of methicillin and isoxazolyl penicillin is due to their $\beta$-lactamase stability.

In contrast, in gram-negative bacteria, $\beta$-lactamases may be either inducible or constitutive enzymes, plasmid or chromosomally mediated, with affinity for penicillins or cephalosporins or both. Also, $\beta$-lactamases are located in the periplasmic space between the lipopolysaccharide coat and the inner membrane (ideally located to protect the targets of penicillin) and may vary in amount of production (Fig. 27.3B). Probably all gram-negative bacteria produce at least small amounts of $\beta$-lactamases. To be effective, a penicillin must cross the periplasmic space of a gram-negative bacterium and reach its target site before being hydrolyzed by local $\beta$-lactamases. Changes in the side chains of penicillins to enhance permeability and increase affinity for penicillin target sites are generally more important in improving gram-negative activity than those to reduce the susceptibility to hydrolysis. $\beta$-lactamase stability may contribute somewhat to differences in gram-negative activity between some of the other penicillins, but bulky side chains that increase $\beta$-lactamase stability may also interfere with passage across the outer membrane of gram-negative bacteria.

Plasmid-mediated $\beta$-lactamases may spread between bacterial species, e.g., the spread of the TEM-1 among *Enterobacteriaceae* and to *Haemophilus influenza* and *Neisseria gonorrhoeae*, or the spread staphylococcal penicillinase to *Enterococcus faecalis*. Increased numbers of plasmid-mediated $\beta$-lactamases over the last several years, and the ability of some to also destroy cephalosporins have compounded the problem of resistance. Chromosomally mediated $\beta$-lactamase produced by stable derepressed genes is an important mechanism of penicillin resistance in *Pseudomonas aeruginosa* and *Enterobacter* species.

Another mechanism of resistance of increasing importance is alteration of the penicillin target site. Reduced affinity of PBPs for penicillin has been identified as the mechanism of resistance for streptococci, in particular, *Streptococcus pneumoniae*, and for non-$\beta$-lactamase-resistant *Neisseria* and *H. influenzae* strains, as well as for methicillin resistance in staphylococci.

Reduced permeability of the outer membrane of gram-negative bacteria may occur concomitantly with alteration in PBPs or $\beta$-lactamases and hinder approach to the penicillin target site. This mechanism of resistance is not important for gram-positive bacteria. Changes in the bacterial outer membrane component due to mutation may raise MICs to some penicillins by two to sixfold, but resistant clinical isolates are unlikely to owe their resistance solely to altered permeability.

Finally, one mechanism of resistance to killing by the penicillins seen in gram-positive bacteria is the phenomenon of tolerance that occurs when the concentration of penicillin required to kill the bacteria (the minimum bactericidal concentration or MBC) is much greater (usually more than 16-fold) than the concentration needed to inhibit bacterial growth (the minimum inhibitory concentration [MIC]). Suppression or reduction of penicillin triggered autolytic activity after exposure to penicillin is seen in tolerant organisms and can be observed in strains of staphylococci, streptococci, enterococci, and *Listeria monocytogenes*.

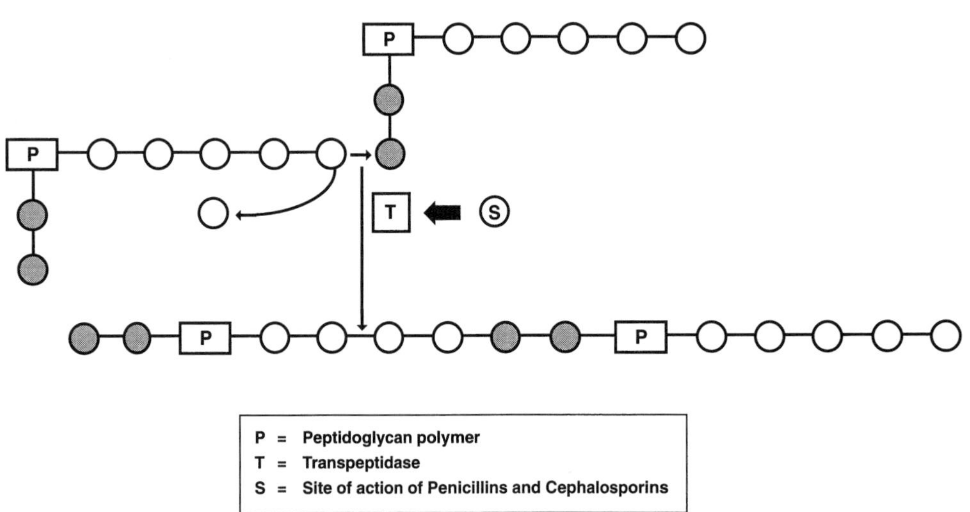


**Fig. 27.2** The transpeptidase step in gram-positive bacteria inhibited by penicillins and cephalosporins.

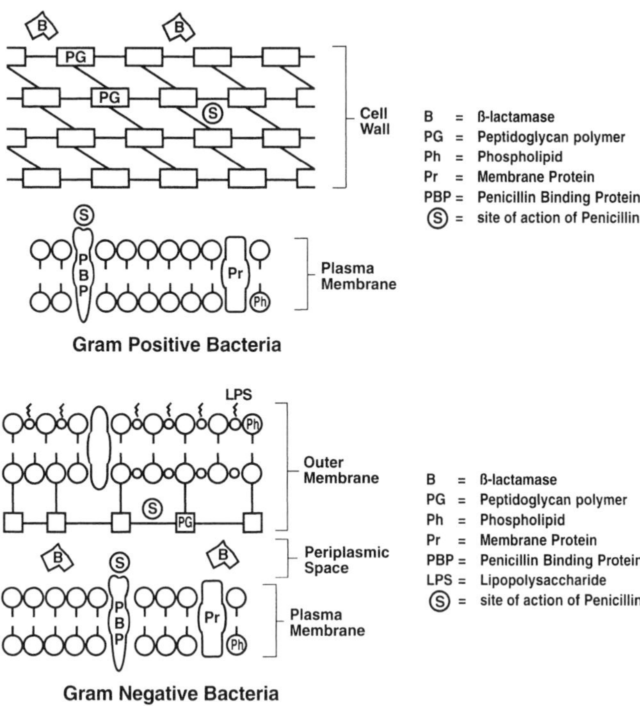


**Fig. 27.3** Comparison between gram-positive and gram-negative cell walls and sites of action of penicillins.

## Pharmacokinetics

The acidic environment of the stomach destroys a number of penicillins including penicillin G, methicillin, the carboxypenicillins, and the ureidopenicillins, making them unsuitable for oral use. Penicillins not affected by gastric acid are generally well absorbed in the duodenum, and peak serum levels after oral administration are attained in 1 to 2 h. Nafcillin has intermediate acid stability and variable absorption. Ampicillin has only 30% to 60% absorption, whereas amoxicillin and the carboxylester formulations are well absorbed. Food delays absorption of most penicillins (ampicillin esters show increased absorption) and thus may also lower peak serum levels.

Absorption of drug after intramuscular administration is rapid, and peak serum levels occur within 1 h. Exceptions are the procaine and benzathine salts of penicillin G which are relatively insoluble, and intramuscular injection of these salts generates slower absorption and lower but more sustained blood levels than after sodium penicillin G injection.

Penicillins bind largely to albumin, and the extent of protein binding can vary greatly, from 17% to 97%. Drug must be unbound to pass through cellular or bacterial channels and concentrate in tissues or exert bactericidal activity. Penicillins that are highly protein bound show lower tissue concentration; and in general, concentrations of drug in tissue correlate with serum levels of unbound drug. Concentrations of drug in tissues such as lung, liver, kidney, muscle, bone, and placenta are good, and penicillins penetrate adequately in the presence of inflammation into abscesses, middle ear, and pleural, peritoneal, and synovial fluids. The cerebrospinal fluid (CSF), eye, prostate, human milk, saliva, tears, and respiratory secretions have lower tissue levels. CSF levels in particular are also lowered by the presence of an active transport system that moves penicillins back to the serum from the CSF and the eye. Normally CSF drug levels are less than 3% of those in serum. In the presence of inflammation, penicillin levels in the CSF are adequate because of better penetration of the drug and interference with the export pump. Fetal serum and amniotic fluid levels of drug best correlate with the maternal serum level of unbound penicillin.

Penicillins are minimally metabolized and are renally excreted via tubular secretion. Protein binding does not significantly affect this mechanism. Excretion is rapid for most penicillins, with half-lives ranging from 30 to 75 min. Probenecid prolongs serum half-lives by blocking renal tubular secretion of penicillins. By competing with penicillin for binding sites on albumin, probenecid also releases more free drug. Furthermore, probenecid blocks the anion transport system in CSF, allowing for increased penicillin levels in CSF.

Changes in dosage regimens for most penicillins are not necessary if the creatinine clearance is greater than 10 ml/min; exceptions are carbenicillin, ticarcillin, and temocillin. Urinary concentrations of penicillins are high and exceed blood levels except when creatinine clearance drops below 10 ml/min, when levels may equal those in blood. When renal function further deteriorates and the creatinine clearance becomes less than 10 ml/min, adjustments should be made in daily dosages of most penicillins; exceptions here include oxacillin, nafcillin, cloxacillin, and dicloxacillin. In newborns, the tubular secretory functions are not fully developed and renal excretion of penicillins is considerably less, requiring significant dose reduction.

Biliary secretion occurs for most penicillins, yielding high levels in bile, ranging from 10 times those in serum for penicillin G, ampicillin, and amoxicillin, to 100 times the serum level for nafcillin. However, biliary levels are substantially lower in the presence of common duct obstruction, becoming equal to serum levels under that condition. Although penicillins are not significantly metabolized, breakdown products of penicillin are important in that such derivatives, including penicilloyl and penicillenic acid, and others, factor in hypersensitivity reactions.

## Spectrum of Activity and Clinical Applications

As a family, the penicillins exhibit a wide spectrum of activity and are indicated for the treatment of numerous infections, often being the primary agents of choice (Table 27.1). For many common pathogenic bacteria, the penicillins remain highly active and because of favorable safety and cost profiles are excellent therapeutic agents. The development of resistant pathogens over the last several years has prompted a change in some of the indications for the older penicillins. For example, because of increasing numbers of penicillin-resistant *N. gonorrhoeae* strains, penicillin G is no longer indicated for treatment of these infections without known susceptibilities. On the other hand, penicillin G is still the treatment of choice for treponemal infections.

### Natural penicillins

The natural penicillins were the first penicillins used clinically. Penicillin G, or benzylpenicillin, is the parent compound of this group and is available for use orally, parenterally, intrathecally, subcutaneously, or as a repository salt. An aqueous salt of crystalline penicillin G has been used via all these routes of administration, except in repository form. Although available in both sodium and potassium salts, the latter is most commonly used because the sodium form is more expensive. The sodium and potassium forms provide only 2.0 mEq of sodium or 1.7 mEq of potassium per one million units of drug, respectively. The amount of sodium or potassium administered with penicillin is rarely important clinically unless massive doses are employed in the setting of reduced cardiac or renal function.

Intravenously, the aqueous salt of crystalline penicillin G provides high serum concentrations rapidly and should be used for serious infections. Dosages for routine streptococcal infections vary from 0.5 to 1.0 million units every 6 h, but for endocarditis, meningitis, or other severe infections should be increased to 12 million to 24 million units per day. These dosages can be administered in a more cost-effective way as a continuous infusion of 20 to 24 million units over 24 h.

Penicillin G is acid-labile and destroyed by gastric acid unless taken 1 to 2 h before a meal. Intramuscular administration of an aqueous salt of crystalline penicillin G are more useful when these routes are preferred.

The repository forms of penicillin G include procaine penicillin (an equal molar mixture of procaine and penicillin) and benzathine penicillin (a mixture of one mole of penicillin and two moles of an ammonium base). These preparations can only be used intramuscularly. Administration of procaine penicillin is less painful than that of aqueous crystalline penicillin G and it is absorbed more slowly so that peak plasma concentrations occur 2 to 4 h after injection and are still detectable up to 24 h post-administration. Allergic reactions after administration of procaine penicillin intramuscularly are distinctly more common and neurologic reactions may occur if the procaine component is inadvertently injected into the bloodstream. Benzathine penicillin allows for very slow release of drug from the site of injection, producing low but sustained plasma levels. Depending on the initial dose, plasma levels are detectable 15 to 30 days later and are adequate for highly susceptible organisms.

The forms of penicillin G most resistant to gastric destruction are the phenoxymethyl- and phenoxyethyl-analogues. Penicillin VK is the potassium salt of phenoxymethyl penicillin (a sodium salt is also available), is most commonly used, and produces serum levels two or more times higher than oral penicillin G. These forms are indicated for mild infections due to susceptible organisms, usually in the throat, respiratory tract, or soft tissues.

Pneumococcal pneumonia responds equally well to treatment with procaine penicillin G 600,000 units q12h or penicillin G 20 million units a day. Treatment of gonorrhea with procaine penicillin G should be given only if susceptibility is assured because of the widespread occurrence of penicillin-resistant strains;

**Table 27.1** Therapeutic indications for commonly used penicillins

| Penicillins | Indications |
|---|---|
| Penicillin | Penicillin-susceptible pneumococcal infections; infections due to other streptococci; meningococcal disease; syphilis; actinomycosis; diphtheria; anthrax; clostridial infections; rat-bite fever; listeria infections; erysipeloid; infections in the mouth due to anaerobes and fusobacterium/spirochetes; prophylaxis for streptococcus pyogenes exposure and rheumatic fever; prophylaxis for procedures in patients with valvular heart disease |
| Ampicillin, amoxacillin | Upper respiratory infections; urinary tract infections due to susceptible organisms; meningitis (in combination with third generation cephalosporins) |
| Oxacillin, nafcillin, dicloxacillin | Skin and soft tissue infections due to staphylococci and streptococci (not methicillin-resistant staph. species) |
| Antipseudomonal penicillins (Ticarcillin, piperacillin, mezlocillin) | Serious infections due to gram-negative bacteria; empiric therapy for febrile immunocompromised patients; nosocomial gram-negative infections |
| $\beta$-Lactamase inhibitors | Mixed gram-positive, gram-negative, and anaerobic infections; ampicillin/sulbactam more active against enterococci, ticarcillin/clavulanate and piperacillin/tazobactam more active against gram-negative bacteria |

dosage is 4.8 million units divided between two sites intramuscularly and given with 1 g of probenecid orally. Benzathine penicillin G is indicated for the treatment of early and latent syphilis; aqueous crystalline penicillin G for tertiary syphilis. Concentrations in the CSF after administration of the repository forms of penicillin G are unreliable and may be inadequate to treat neurosyphilis. In HIV-positive individuals, CSF involvement must be ruled out before treatment of early or latent stages of syphilis; and even in the absence of central nervous system (CNS) involvement, failures and relapses in this patient population may occur (see Chapters 70, 100). Pharyngitis or skin infections due to group A $\beta$-hemolytic streptococci (*Staphylococcus pyogenes*) may be treated with benzathine penicillin G, and postrheumatic prophylaxis or prophylaxis against recurrent streptococcal cellulitis is commonly administered via this method. Penicillin VK is beneficial in early Lyme disease and parenteral penicillin G in late disease, but tetracycline and ceftriaxone respectively may be more effective agents. In addition, penicillin G is recommended for other fusospirochetal infections, as well as for actinomycosis, anthrax, rat-bite fever, fusospirochetal infections, erysipeloid, periodontal infections, and infections due to *Pasteurella multocida*. It may also be beneficial in cases of severe leptospirosis.

Indications for the use of penicillin G include streptococcal infections, especially those due to *Streptococcus pyogenes*, and for *S. viridans* endocarditis. Penicillin-resistant *Streptococcus pneumoniae* strains had been rare in the United States, but they are becoming increasingly clinically significant; in regions where these isolates have not yet been identified, penicillin G is still effective. Strains that are relatively resistant to penicillin G and exhibit MIC values of 0.1 to 1.0 mg/L require higher drug concentrations for successful therapy. Penicillin G remains effective for meningitis due to *Neisseria meningitides* since nearly all strains remain susceptible, but it is not useful in eradicating the carrier state. Penicillin G is used prophylactically to prevent recurrences of rheumatic fever, bacterial endocarditis in susceptible hosts, and to abort outbreaks of streptococcal infection due to *S. pyogenes*.

## Penicillinase-resistant penicillins

The emergence of penicillinase producing staphylococci in the 1950s led to the development of semi-synthetic penicillins possessing an acyl side chain which sterically inhibits the action of penicillinase enzymes, preserving the integrity of the $\beta$-lactam ring. These penicillinase-resistant penicillins include methicillin, the first developed; nafcillin, and the isoxazolyl penicillins. They have excellent activity against methicillin sensitive staphylococci and remain the agents of choice for these infections. The antibacterial activity of the penicillinase-resistant penicillins against streptococci is somewhat less than that of penicillin G, but remains adequate to treat infections due to streptococci except enterococcus. These agents lack activity against gram-negative bacteria and penicillin-resistant *S. pneumoniae*. The emergence of staphylococci resistant to these semisynthetic penicillins has become increasingly more important over the last decade. These bacteria have been referred to as methicillin-resistant staphylococci (MRSA), but are better termed $\beta$-lactam antibiotic-resistant staphylococci as they are resistant to the penicillins and all the cephalosporins as well. The mechanism of resistance is via altered penicillin-binding proteins. $\beta$-lactam resistance is highly prevalent among the coagulase-negative staphylococci. Much less prevalent but more frequent clinical pathogens are the $\beta$-lactam antibiotic-resistant strains of *Staphylococcus aureus* (i.e., MRSA).

Methicillin must be administered parenterally because it is rapidly destroyed by gastric acid. After intramuscular injection, absorption is rapid. It is not highly protein bound (38%), and is rapidly excreted by the kidneys. Toxicity due to interstitial nephritis, which may be more common with methicillin than with other agents in this class, has led to a decline in its use clinically, as equally effective, less toxic congeners are available in nafcillin and oxacillin.

Oxacillin and nafcillin are highly protein bound, and dose reduction in renal failure is unnecessary because they are primarily excreted via the liver. Absorption of nafcillin after an oral dose is erratic, and levels after intramuscular injection are low; hence intravenous administration is preferred. Oxacillin is an isoxazolyl penicillin and available as an oral drug, but it should be taken 1 to 2 h before food and shows the lowest serum levels after ingestion among the oral preparations of this class of agents.

The other isolazolyl penicillins include cloxacillin, dicloxacillin, and flucloxacillin (not available in the United States). Absorption of flucloxacillin is best, followed by dicloxacillin and cloxacillin. These drugs are indicated for the primary oral treatment of less serious staphylococcal infections and the longer-term, ambulatory follow-up of more serious, deep infections after an initial course of parenteral therapy. Osteomyelitis and septic arthritis due to *S. aureus* in children and adults have been successfully treated with these oral agents. Occasionally, they are also used as long-term suppressive agents for staphylococcal infections treated parenterally but not deemed curable. Due to hepatic excretion, as with the other penicillinase-resistant penicillins, dosage modifications are unnecessary in renal failure.

## Aminopenicillins

The clinical importance of gram-negative isolates not effectively treated by penicillin quickly prompted further modifications of the basic benzylpenicillin nucleus; first formed was ampicillin by the addition of an amino group. The other aminopenicillins include the following: amoxacillin, bacampicillin, betacillin, and cyclacillin. Not available in the United States, but used elsewhere are pivampicillin, talampicillin, and epicillin. These agents more effectively penetrate through the outer membrane of gram-negative bacteria and possess a higher affinity for PBPs as their primary mode of increased gram-negative activity. They are not resistant to the penicillinase produced by staphylocci, and many gram-negative organisms.

Ampicillin has better activity than penicillin G against enterococci and *Listeria monocytogenes*, and initially had activity against most strains of *E. coli*, *Proteus mirabilis*, *Salmonella*, *Shigella*, *H. influenzae*, and *N. gonorrhoeae*. Increasing gram-negative resistance due to $\beta$-lactamases has led to the development of ampicillin resistant strains and the use of ampicillin for infections due to these organisms has been supplanted by other agents. If $\beta$-lactamase-positive strains of *H. influenzae* are still uncommon in the area, initial therapy with ampicillin or amoxacillin for otitis media, acute sinusitis, or upper respiratory tract infections may be warranted on account of their low cost and good safety profile. Ampicillin is not useful for the treatment of infections due to most strains of *Klebsiella*, or to *Serratia*, *Enterobacter*, *Acinetobacter*, *Pseudomonas*, and *Bacteroides fragilis*. In combination with an aminoglycoside, ampicillin is indicated for the treatment of infections caused by the HACEK group of organisms; and the combination is also recommended for endocarditis prophylaxis for patients at high risk, including those undergoing genitourinary or gastrointestinal procedures.

Ampicillin is orally absorbed, and peak serum levels occur in 1–2 h; probenecid increases the height of serum levels and delays the disappearance of drug from the serum. Therapeutic levels are achieved in body fluids, including CSF, in the presence of inflammation. A close relative of ampicillin, amoxacillin, is its parahydroxyl derivative and is similar in antibacterial activity. Amoxacillin is significantly better absorbed orally than ampicillin, and peak blood levels are two to three times higher than those produced by a similar dose of ampicillin. More drug is absorbed and thus less drug acts locally in the gastrointestinal tract, making it less effective for the treatment of shigellosis. Diarrhea may be less common than with ampicillin. The consistency that amoxacillin provides in absorption and subsequent plasma concentrations has given it preference over ampicillin for the following uses: treatment of respiratory tract infections caused by susceptible bacteria, treatment of urinary tract infections and gonorrhea (when bacterial susceptibilities are known), treatment of pediatric infections due to susceptible organisms, and in the revised American Heart Association guidelines prevention of bacterial endocarditis (instead of penicillin VK).

Bacampicillin is an aminopenicillin that itself is inactive until after an oral dose, when the drug is completely hydrolyzed to free ampicillin. Although initially higher, after 2.5 h, serum levels are equivalent to those of amoxacillin and activity is similar to that of ampicillin. Cyclacillin also has similar activity and is the most rapidly absorbed aminopenicillin with excellent blood levels after ingestion, up to four times those achieved after ingestion of ampicillin. However, it is also rapidly cleared and offers no advantage over ampicillin. Hetacillin similarly shows no added benefit over ampicillin or amoxacillin. Pivampicillin and talampicillin are inactive agents that are rapidly hydrolyzed to ampicillin and are well absorbed; however, they are not available in the United States. Epicillin has a slightly different structure from the other aminopenicillins but offers no advantages beyond ampicillin and is not available in the United States.

## Carboxypenicillins

As more resistant gram-negative bacteria, including *Pseudomonas aeruginosa*, gained clinical importance as pathogens, penicillins with activity against these bacteria were developed. Carbenicillin was the first of these expanded-spectrum agents, formed by the substitution of a carboxyl group for the amino group on ampicillin. Further modifications produced ticarcillin, which is similar pharmacologically but is two to four times more active than carbenicillin against *P. aeruginosa*. In addition to pseudomonas, the antibacterial spectrum of both drugs includes enterobacter, morganella, indole-positive proteus, and providencia. However, klebsiella and some strains of serratia are not susceptible to these drugs and may cause bacterial superinfection during treatment. Activity of carbenicillin and ticarcillin against enterococci is less than that of ampicillin, and carbenicillin may also be less efficacious than ampicillin against *S. pyogenes* and *S. pneumoniae*. The remainder of the spectrum of activity is similar to that of ampicillin. Carbenicillin and ticarcillin act synergistically with the aminoglycosides against *P. aeruginosa*.

Both drugs can be administered intramuscularly or intravenously. Only carbenicillin is available in an oral form (indanyl carbenicillin), but adequate levels are only produced in the urinary tract and it is of limited therapeutic value. Intravenous therapy is preferable because of the drug's rapid clearance. Carbenicillin is a disodium salt and contains 4.7 mEq of sodium per gram; ticarcillin contains 5.2 mEq/g but lower total dosages of ticarcillin are required for the same antibacterial effect. The sodium load of the carboxypenicillins must be considered when instituting treatment since congestive heart failure may be precipitated. Hypokalemia may be significant because of potassium wasting in the distal tubule. Also, platelet function may be inhibited by the binding of drug to ADP receptor sites on platelets. The carboxypenicillins should not be physically mixed with the aminoglycosides, since they can form complexes and inactivate both drugs. Ticarcillin's better activity against *P. aeruginosa* and the lower dosages that can be used compared with those of carbenicillin, thus reducing the problems of salt load, hypokalemia, and platelet effects, give ticarcillin advantages over carbenicillin. Both drugs are efficacious in the treatment of various gram-negative infections and are indicated for the treatment of infections due to *P. aeruginosa* in particular. In the latter case, the addition of an aminoglycoside not only promotes synergistic killing but helps to prevent the emergence of resistant strains during treatment.

## Ureidopenicillins

Despite the development of the carboxypenicillins, there was still an additional need for agents with further activity against gram-negative bacteria, especially *P. aeruginosa*, and with fewer side effects. In response to this need, the acylureidopenicillins, mezlocillin and azlocillin, and a piperazine derivative, piperacillin, were developed. Mezlocillin has a similar antibacterial spectrum to carbenicillin and ticarcillin but has enhanced activity against *Klebsiella* species, *E. faecalis*, *Pseudomonas*, and *B. fragilis*. Mezlocillin's improved activity appears to be due to greater affinity for PBPs and better penetration into the periplasmic space of gram-negative bacteria. Piperacillin is fourfold more active and azlocillin is about twofold more active than mezlocillin against *P. aeruginosa*, but whereas piperacillin is active against klebsiella species, azlocillin is not as active. Although the acylureidopenicilins have greater in vitro activity against *P. aeruginosa* than ticarcillin, comparative clinical trials have not clearly demonstrated superiority of these drugs. Side effects seen with the carboxypenicillins can also be seen with these agents, but the frequency of hypokalemia and platelet effects is less than that with carbenicillin and the salt content is lower because they are monosodium salts.

Unlike the carboxypenicillins, the ureidopenicillins show nonlinear dose dependent kinetics. They have short serum half-lives that are increased only to 4 h in renal failure. Biliary excretion is substantial (20% to 30%) and high biliary levels are achieved. Penetration into tissues including the CSF under conditions of inflammation is excellent. These drugs are also synergistic with aminoglycosides against *P. aeruginosa* and should not be mixed directly with those agents because of inactivation of the latter. The development of bacterial resistance during therapy has been seen with the ureidopenicillins as with the carboxypenicillins when they are used as single agents. Because of their wide spectrum of activity and good distribution into tissue, the ureidopenicillins are efficacious in the treatment of many serious infections. These drugs are not orally absorbed and are only available in parenteral form.

## Amdinocillin

Amdinocillin, a 6-$\beta$-acylaminopenicillanic acid, is an extended spectrum penicillin with a unique affinity for PBP-2 in gram-negative bacteria. Thus the drug has poor activity against gram-positive bacteria. Because amdinocillin preferentially binds PBP-2 while other $\beta$-lactam drugs bind alternative PBPs, there may be synergism against some gram-negative bacteria when amdinocillin is combined with other $\beta$-lactams. This effect is not universal, however, and amdinocillin was not widely adopted after its introduction. It is no longer available in the United States.

## $\beta$-lactamase inhibitors

Another strategy to circumvent the problem of bacterial resistance was developed with the concept of combining $\beta$-lactamase inhibitors, which attack the most common mechanism of penicillin resistance, with a parent penicillin. The $\beta$-lactamase inhibitors bind irreversibly and with high affinity to many bacterial $\beta$-lactamases, preventing the hydrolytic action of the $\beta$-lactamase against the companion penicillin. Thus, the activity of the penicillin against $\beta$-lactamase-producing bacteria is greatly enhanced when combined with a $\beta$-lactamase inhibitor. The $\beta$-lactamase inhibitors provide no added benefit in situations where the bacteria are already susceptible to the penicillin, or when bacterial resistance is not $\beta$-lactamase mediated.

Clavulanic acid was the first $\beta$-lactamase inhibitor developed, followed by sulbactam and later tazobactam. All three have weak intrinsic antibacterial activity, but alone they are not useful therapeutic agents. There are differences among the three agents in the specific $\beta$-lactamases which are inhibited by each.

Amoxacillin-clavulanic acid was the first $\beta$-lactamase inhibitor–penicillin combination available. This combination expanded the antibacterial spectrum of amoxacillin to include $\beta$-lactamase-producing strains of *S. aureus*, *H. inflenzae*, *N. gonorrhoeae*, *E. coli*, and *Moxarella catarrhalis*, and *Proteus*, *Klebsiella*, and *Bacteroides* species. This fixed combination drug is broadly efficacious for the treatment of otitis media, sinusitis, bronchitis, skin and soft tissue infections, lower respiratory tract infections, and for infections from human and animal bites.

Next released was the first parenteral $\beta$-lactamase inhibitor–penicillin combination, ticarcillin-clavulanic acid. The antibacterial activity of ticarcillin-clavulanic acid includes that of ticarcillin and further extends its activity to $\beta$-lactamase-producing strains of *S. aureus*, *H. influenzae*, *M. catarrhalis*, and *N. gonorrhoeae*, as well as *Klebsiella*, *Proteus*, *Providencia*, and *Bacteroides* species. MRSA are resistant to ticarcillin-clavulanic acid, and indeed to all $\beta$-lactamase inhibitor–penicillin combinations, since the mechanism of resistance for these bacteria is not $\beta$-lactamase production. Ticarcillin-clavulanic acid is efficacious in many serious infections, and is particularly useful in polymicrobial or mixed aerobic and anaerobic infections.

The combination of ampicillin-sulbactam was the next available parenterally administered drug in this class. Again, the addition of the $\beta$-lactamase has extended the spectrum of the parent ampicillin to include $\beta$-lactamase-producing strains of *S. aureus*, *H. influenzae*, *N. Gonorrhoeae*, *M. catarrhalis*, and *E. coli*, *Klebsiella*, *Providencia*, *Proteus*, and *Bacteroides* species. Ampicillin-sulbactam has no activity against *P. aeruginosa* but retains excellent activity against enterococci. The combination drug is distributed well into tissues and is most useful in the treatment of polymicrobial or mixed infections especially when enterococci may be present; it should be used with an aminoglycoside if resistant gram-negative bacteria are suspected.

Piperacillin-tazobactam is the most recently released combination in this class of drugs. The addition of tazobactam to the parent compound piperacillin has, similar to ticarcillin-clavulanic acid, increased the activity of piperacillin against $\beta$-lactamase-producing strains of many organisms. Piperacillin-tazobactam has demonstrated efficacy in lower respiratory tract, gynecologic, skin and soft tissue, and intro-abdominal infections. This agent will probably be most useful in the management of polymicrobial or mixed infections. The side effects of the $\beta$-lactamase inhibitors generally follow those of the parent penicillin, and may ultimately play a role in the selection of the agent used clinically. The problem clinically is that when a patient receiving a combination of drugs develops a hypersensitivity reaction, it is extremely difficult to ascertain which drug induced the reaction, and both agents must be withheld in the future.

## Adverse Reactions

Overall, the penicillins are safe, but adverse reactions are not uncommon. Most common are hypersensitivity reactions, which can range from fever alone to a rash or (rarely) immediate anaphylaxis. Hypersensitivity reactions are least common when the penicillin is given orally, and occur most often when given intramuscularly; larger doses and longer duration of therapy may also increase the likelihood of allergic reactions. Hypersensitivity reactions are mediated by antibodies made to penicillin degradation products which become haptens when bound to proteins. Benzylpenicilloyl and penicillanic derivatives of penicillin are the major penicillin degradation products and are known as the *major determinants*; *minor determinants* include benzylpenicilloate and benzylpenicillin (Table 27.1). Both major and minor determinants are involved in anaphylaxis, but the minor determinants are more common in anaphylaxis while the major determinants are more common in urticarial reactions. Anaphylaxis occurs in 0.004% to 0.015% of cases; urticaria in 1% to 5%. Immunoglobulin E (IgE) antibodies are involved in both types of reactions. Nonurticarial, morbilliform rashes are produced by IgM and IgG antibodies and are much more common. The incidence of rash in patients who have infectious mononucleosis is high after receiving ampicillin. Patients allergic to one penicillin often are allergic to other penicillins, but allergenicity may wane over time. Premedication with antihistamines does not prevent allergic reactions to the penicillins. Skin testing may predict an immediate hypersensitive reaction, but a negative test does not exclude this possibility. If a penicillin drug must be administered to a patient with a known hypersensitivity reaction or a positive skin test, desensitization by an oral or parenteral protocol must be performed under supervision.

Serum sickness from the penicillins is uncommon today and results from immune complex deposition in tissues, causing fever, joint pains, urticaria, and angioneurotic edema. Exfoliative dermatitis and erythema multiforme types of reactions (including the Stevens-Johnson syndrome) occur rarely. A severe form of vasculitis with both cutaneous and visceral lesions has occurred but is very rare.

Hematologic toxicities of the penicillins include Coomb's positive hemolytic anemia and neutropenia, the latter being more common after high doses and/or prolonged administration.

Platelet dysfunction, especially from the carboxypenicillins can occur, but clinical bleeding is uncommon. Allergic interstitial nephritis may occur with any penicillin, but has most often been associated with methicillin. Clinical manifestations include fever, eosinophilia, proteinuria, eosinophiluria, hematuria, and rash. Initially there is nonoliguric renal failure with a decrease in creatinine clearance, which can progress to renal failure and anuria. However, the renal function usually normalizes upon discontinuation of the offending agent. Kidney biopsy will usually reveal an interstitial mononuclear and eosinophilic cellular infiltrate.

Hepatic toxicity has been seen during therapy with oxacillin and carbenicillin, is usually mild, and is reversible. Fluid overload and hypokalemia may occur with penicillins with high sodium content. High-dose intravenous therapy, especially in patients with renal insufficiency, may produce myoclonic jerks, seizures, hyperreflexia, or coma.

When administered orally, penicillins can cause gastrointestinal irritation and produce nausea, vomiting, or diarrhea. By altering the bacterial flora of the gut, penicillins can cause overgrowth with penicillin-resistant organisms such as gram-negative bacteria or candida. Also, all penicillins have on occasion produced enterocolitis due to toxigenic *Clostridium difficile*.

## Conclusion

Since 1941, the penicillin antibiotics have been important and efficacious as therapeutic agents. For the treatment of infections due to susceptible bacteria, these drugs remain the agents of choice, and expanded-spectrum penicillins are useful in managing infections caused by many of the bacteria resistant to the earlier penicillins. This family of antibiotics continues to be well distributed and well tolerated, and it consists of bactericidal agents that are clinically useful in a broad variety of situations.

### ANNOTATED BIBLIOGRAPHY

Dajani AS, Taubert KA, et al. Prevention of bacterial endocarditis: recommendations by the American Heart Association. JAMA 1997; 277: 1794–1801.
*Recommended guidelines for prophylaxis against bacterial endocarditis for patients undergoing surgical and dental procedures and instrumentations.*

Drusano GL, Schimpff SC, Hewitt WL. The acylampicillins: mezlocillin, piperacillin, and azlocillin. Rev Infect Dis 1984; 6:13–32.
*An excellent review of the in vitro spectrum of activity, therapeutic utility, and indications for use of these expanded-spectrum penicillins.*

Eliopoulos GM, Moellering RC. Azlocillin, mezlocillin, and piperacillin: new broad-spectrum penicillins. Ann Intern Med 1982; 97:755–760.
*A comparison and review of early clinical studies of these broad-spectrum antibiotics at the time of their introduction.*

Fass RJ, Copelan EA, et al. Platelet-mediated bleeding caused by broad-spectrum penicillins. J Infect Dis 1987; 155:1242–1248.
*A prospective study looking at the risks for bleeding complications from selected expanded-spectrum penicillins.*

Hackbarth CJ, Chambers HF. Methicillin-resistant staphylococci: genetics and mechanisms of resistance. Antimicrob Agents Chemother 1989; 33: 991–994.
*A concise review of mechanisms of resistance, and their genetic base, to methicillin of staphylococci.*

Lees L, Milson JA, Knirsch AK. Sulbactam plus ampicillin: interim review of efficacy and safety for therapeutic and prophylactic use. Rev Infect Dis 1986; 8(Suppl 5):S644–S650.
*A review of 39 therapeutic and 6 prophylactic studies on ampicillin/sulbactam.*

Moellering RC. β-lactamase inhibition: therapeutic implications in infectious diseases—an overview. Rev Infect Dis 1991; 13(Suppl 9):S723–S726.
*A brief overview of the development of β-lactamases, inhibitors to β-lactamase, and a summary of symposium discussions on their therapeutic uses.*

Neu HC. Antistaphylococcal penicillins. Med Clin North Am 1982: 66:51–60.
*A thorough review of this group of penicillins.*

Neu HC. Carbenicillin and ticarcillin. Med Clin North Am 1982; 66: 61–76.
*An extensive discussion of these first extended-spectrum penicillins.*

Saxon A. Immediate hypersensitivity reactions to β-lactam antibiotics. Rev Infect Dis 1983; 5(Suppl 2):S369–S379.
*A detailed discussion of hypersensitivity (primarily IgE-mediated) reactions to the penicillins and cephalosporins.*

Tomasz A. Penicillin-binding proteins and the antibacterial effectiveness of β-lactam antibiotics. Rev Infect Dis 1986; 8(Suppl 3):S260–S278.
*An in-depth look at penicillin-binding proteins and their role in the efficacy of β-lactam antibiotics against bacteria.*

Wright AJ, Wilkowske, CJ. The penicillins. Mayo Clin Proc 1991: 66:1047–1063.
*An excellent broad review of the penicillins as part of the Mayo Clinic symposium on antimicrobial agents.*

# 28

# Cephalosporins

JAMES B. MALOW AND JOHN N. SHEAGREN

The discovery of penicillin by Alexander Fleming in 1929 and the eventual clinical use of the purified product in the 1940s led to the search for other antibacterial agents produced by naturally occurring fungi. Giuseppi Brotzu was the first to isolate a cephalosporin from *Cephalosporium acremonium* in 1945. This substance was subsequently further fractionated and found to be made up of several active components. The most active, Cephalosporin C, became the parent compound for the first cephalosporin, used in clinical practice.

This new class of antibiotics was found to have a broader spectrum of antimicrobial activity than penicillins, as well as having an inherent resistance to $\beta$-lactamase degradation. These factors, as well as the lack of toxicity, have led to the development of multiple agents within the class of cephalosporins.

The classification of the cephalosporins is traditionally done by generations. This scheme at times is imprecise, and slight differences in classifications are found in standard texts. In general, the first generation agents tend to have a narrower spectrum of activity but are the most potent against gram-positive bacteria. The second generation drugs, including the cephamycins, cefoxitin, cefotetan, and cefmetazole, have extended gram-negative activity as well as anaerobic activity. The third generation drugs have an even broader spectrum and an enhanced in vitro activity against gram-negative bacilli; these advantages, however, are accompanied by a relative decrease in gram-positive activity. Additionally, unlike the older cephalosporins, most of these drugs reach therapeutic levels in the cerebrospinal fluid (CSF) and can be used in the therapy of meningitis.

## Chemistry and Nomenclature

The basic structure of the cephalosporins is similar to that of the penicillins. Both contain a $\beta$-lactam ring; however, the five-membered thiazolidine ring characteristic of the penicillins is replaced by a six-membered dihydrothiazine ring (Fig. 28.1). Acid treatment of Cephalosporin C produces 7-aminocephalosporonic acid which, when modified, creates the family of cephalosporin compounds.

Chemical modification can be made at the 3 and the 7 positions of the cephalosporin molecule. In general, modifications at position 3 alter metabolic and pharmacokinetic parameters, whereas changes at position 7 alter the antibacterial activity. The addition of methylthiotetrazole (MTT) at position 3 causes enhanced activity against gram-negative bacilli (cefamandole, cefotetan, moxalactam, cefoperozone, and cefmetazole). However, this change also causes disulfuram-like reactions and hypoprothrombinemia, at times, leading to serious bleeding problems.

Bulky side chains at position 3 lead to altered gastrointestinal (GI) absorption of compounds. Therefore, oral agents commonly have simple methyl groups or chlorine atoms at position 3 (cephalexin, cephradine, cefodroxil and cefaclor). Acidic substitutions at position 7 enhance activity against *Pseudomonas aeruginosa* (ceftazidime, moxalactam and cefsulodin). Addition of an aminothiazolyl group causes increased affinity for penicillin-binding proteins, as well as providing better penetration of gram-negative cell walls. The presence of a methoxy group at the 7 position leads to enhanced stability against cephalosporinases, especially those produced by *Bacteroides* species. This change, however, is accompanied by a relative decrease in gram-positive activity, including *Staphylococcus aureus*. Compounds with this substitution are called cephamycins but are commonly included with the cephalosporins (cefoxitin, cefotetan, moxalactam, and cefmetazole).

## Mechanisms of Action and Resistance

### Actions

Cephalosporins, like the penicillins, exert their antimicrobial activity by inhibiting peptidoglycan cross-linkage in the cell wall. The formation of the lattice structure of the peptidoglycan layer is catalyzed by transpeptidases, endopeptidases, and carboxypeptidases. These enzymes, otherwise known as *penicillin-binding proteins* (PBPs), are the target sites for all of the $\beta$-lactam antibiotics that bind to and inactivate them.

The penicillins and cephalosporins have different binding affinities for the PBPs. The PBP or combination of PBPs bound by a given antibiotic determines its subsequent effect. Binding of drugs to PBPs 1A, 1BS, 2, or 3 leads to cell death, whereas binding to PBPs 4, 5, or 6, which apparently are not as essential to the organism's survival, causes nonlethal changes. In some instances the action of a cephalosporin may lead to cell lysis. Organisms that contain autolysins may lose enzyme inhibitors to the autolysins when exposed to $\beta$-lactam antibiotics, which subsequently leads to lysis and death of the cell. Bacteria lacking autolysins may develop bizarre forms when exposed to $\beta$-lactam antibiotics and only show growth inhibition.

In summary, the cephalosporins require three steps in order to effect their antibacterial action: (*1*) penetration of the bacterial cell wall, (*2*) avoidance of hydrolysis by $\beta$-lactamases, and (*3*) binding to target sites on the cell membrane. Resistance to the effects of the cephalosporins can occur at any of these three essential steps.

### Resistance

Resistance to penetration of cephalosporins through the cell wall does not appear to be a problem in gram-positive organisms. The

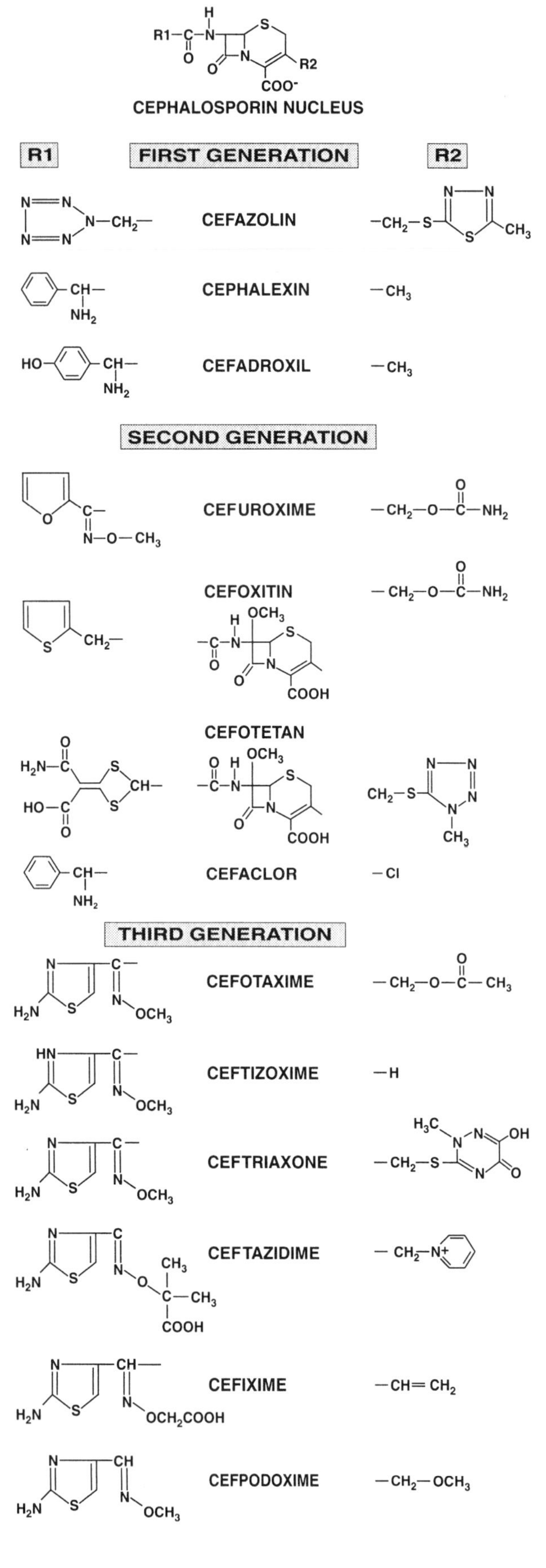

CEPHALOSPORIN NUCLEUS

R1 FIRST GENERATION R2

CEFAZOLIN

CEPHALEXIN

CEFADROXIL

SECOND GENERATION

CEFUROXIME

CEFOXITIN

CEFOTETAN

CEFACLOR

THIRD GENERATION

CEFOTAXIME

CEFTIZOXIME

CEFTRIAXONE

CEFTAZIDIME

CEFIXIME

CEFPODOXIME

**Fig. 28.1** Chemical structure of commonly used cephalosporins by class.

peptidoglycan structure in these bacteria readily permit the passage of cephalosporin-sized molecules. However, the outer membrane of gram-negative bacteria is much more complex, consisting of lipids, proteins, and polysaccharides, which, in some instances, represent a formidable barrier to entry of the cephalosporin. The outer membrane contains protein pores known as porins, which pass through the membrane. These channels appear to allow passage of substances slightly larger than the size of penicillins or cephalosporins into the periplasmic space where they can ultimately gain access to PBPs after subsequent passage through the thin cell wall. Passage through the porins is not only dependant on molecular size, but also on the lipophilicity or hydrophilicity of the compounds. Penetration resistance can be of clinical importance for some gram-negative bacilli, especially *P. aeruginosa* and *Enterobacter* species.

$\beta$-lactamases are enzymes produced by bacteria that inactivate penicillins and cephalosporins by hydrolyzing the cyclic amide bond of the $\beta$-lactam ring. In the case of gram-positive organisms, especially *S. aureus*, the $\beta$-lactamase is released into the surrounding environment. The cephalosporins, as a group, are relatively resistant to hydrolysis by these staphylococcal $\beta$-lactamases. In gram-negative organisms, the $\beta$-lactamases are released into the periplasmic space between the cell wall and outer membrane. This action appears to make the enzyme more effective as the cephalosporin traverses the periplasmic space to reach its target proteins. The production of gram-negative $\beta$-lactamases may be encoded chromosomally or extrachromosomally via transposons or plasmids. The enzymes can be constituitive or inducible. The susceptibility to $\beta$-lactamase hydrolysis is variable among the cephalosporins. Cefuroxime, cefoxitin, and the third generation cephalosporins are, as a rule, quite resistant to hydrolysis by gram-negative beta-lactamases. However, organisms producing inducible $\beta$-lactamases, including *Serratia* species, *Citrobacter* species, *Enterobacter* species, *Proteus vulgaris*, *P. aeruginosa*, and other nonfermenting gram-negative rods, may produce enzymes that fail to hydrolyze cephalosporins, but instead bind them, not allowing them to reach their target sites. This binding process may produce broad levels of resistance against all or most $\beta$-lactam drugs.

The last method of resistance to the cephalosporins involves alteration of the antibiotic binding site, decreasing the drug's affinity for its site of action. This process has been well characterized in methicillin-resistant *S. aureus* where the organism produces an altered PBP, mainly PBP 2′ or $PBP2_a$, which has markedly decreased affinity for penicillinase-resistant penicillins and cephalosporins. Similar altered PBPs have been seen with $\beta$-lactam-resistant *Streptococcus pneumoniae* and enterococci.

## Spectrum of Activity and Clinical Applications

### First generation cephalosporins

The antibacterial spectrum of the first generation cephalosporins includes most gram-positive bacteria. They are the most active cephalosporins against *Staphylococcus* species and streptococci. They are also quite active against gram-positive anaerobes and *Actinomyces* species. Exceptions include $\beta$-lactam antibiotic-resistant staphylococci, enterococci, penicillin-resistant pneumococci, and *Listeria* species. Their gram-negative spectrum includes *Escherichia coli*, *Proteus mirabilis*, and most *Klebsiella* species. They have limited activity against *Hemophilus influenzae* and little activity against other enterobacteriaceae and

*Bacteroides fragilis*. The antibacterial spectrum is virtually identical between the various first generation cephalosporins. Differences between agents include routes of administration and drug half-lives.

The parenteral agents include cephalothin, cefazolin, cephapirin, and cephradine. Cefazolin is presently the agent of choice because of its longer half-life and increased tolerability to intramuscular injection. These agents can be used in persons not anaphylactically allergic to the penicillins as penicillin alternatives for skin and soft tissue infections, as well as serious methicillin-sensitive staphylococcal infections. They are adequate agents for sensitive urinary tract infections but may not be cost-effective. The first generation agents should not be used to treat meningitis, as they fail to cross the blood-brain barrier in amounts adequate to provide bactericidal CSF concentrations. They are safe and cost-effective for orthopedic and cardiovascular surgical prophylaxis.

The oral first generation agents include cephalexin, cefodroxil, and cephradine. The short half-lives of cephalexin and cephradine require four-times-daily dosing. Cefodroxil has a prolonged half-life with increased serum and urinary levels and can therefore be dosed once or twice daily. These agents can be used as oral treatment for skin and soft tissue infections or pharyngitis due to streptococci and sensitive staphylococci. They are effective agents for urinary tract infections due to *E. coli*, *P. mirabilis*, and *Klebsiella* species.

## Second generation cephalosporins

The second generation cephalosporins consist of a heterogeneous group of drugs which, in general, have increased gram-negative and anaerobic activity and some decreased in vitro, antistaphylococcal activity. The parenteral agents include cefamandole, cefonicid, ceforanide, and cefuroxime, as well as the cephamycins, cefoxitin, cefotetan, and cefmetazole. Oral agents include cefuroxime axetil, cefaclor, and cefprozil. Unlike the first generation drugs, the antibacterial spectra of these agents are not interchangeable and individual in vitro testing is necessary.

Cefuroxime and cefamandole have very similar antibacterial activity. When compared with first generation agents, they are consistently more active against *H. influenzae*, *E. coli*, indole-positive *Proteus*, *Enterobacter*, and *Klebsiella* species. Their anaerobic activity is *not* enhanced. They retain good activity against *S. aureus* and *S. pneumoniae*. These drugs are especially useful in the treatment of community acquired pneumonias, but they have also been used successfully for bacteremia, soft tissue infections, and urinary tract infections caused by susceptible bacteria. Cefuroxime has become popular because it has a longer half-life with less frequent dosing, and it lacks the MTT side chain present on cefamandole, which may contribute to the occasionally seen coagulopathy and to an antabuse-like effect. Additionally, cefuroxime is the only second generation agent that crosses the blood-brain barrier and has been used successfully for the treatment of meningitis. However, the third generation cephalosporins have even better central nervous system (CNS) penetration.

Ceforanide and cefonicid are both similar to cefamandole: they have long half-lives and are dosed every 12 or 24 h, respectively. Clinically, they have failed to show significant advantages over existing drugs and are therefore seldom employed.

Cefoxitin, introduced in 1978, was the first of the cephamycins. It is active against most organisms susceptible to the first generation cephalosporins except for somewhat decreased activity against gram-positive cocci. In addition, it has enhanced activity against many first generation cephalosporin-resistant strains of *E. coli*, *Klebsiella*, *Proteus*, and *Serratia*. Cefoxitin is also active against *Neisseria gonorrhoeae* (penicillinase positive or negative), but has little or no activity against *H. influenzae* and *Enterobacter* species. The most notable characteristic of cefoxitin is its extended anaerobic coverage. It remains the most active cephalosporin against *B. fragilis*, demonstrating an approximately 80% rate of in vitro sensitivity. It also retains excellent activity against other gram-negative and gram-positive anaerobes.

The newer cephamycins, cefotetan and cefmetazole, share the resistance to $\beta$-lactamases of cefoxitin, therefore having an extended antibacterial spectrum when compared with the first generation cephalosporins. Both demonstrate enhanced anaerobic activity, except cefotetan is less active in vitro against non-fragilis *Bacteroides* species than cefoxitin. Cefotetan, however, is somewhat more active against aerobic gram-negative bacilli than cefoxitin; further, it has a prolonged half-life of 3.3 h, permitting it to be dosed twice daily. Thus, cefotetan is emerging as the second generation drug of choice because of all these positive characteristics.

Cefmetazole's spectrum is similar to that of cefoxitin; however, it is approximately two- to eightfold more active against most species of *E. coli*, *P. mirabilis*, *Klebsiella*, *S. aureus*, *H. influenzae*, and non-enterococcal streptococci.

Despite the differences in activity, clinical trials have failed to show any significant differences between the cephamycins. These agents appear to be quite useful in the treatment of polymicrobial infections such as diverticulitis, appendicitis, pelvic inflammatory disease, aspiration pneumonia, and diabetic foot infections. These agents have also been shown to be efficacious as prophylaxis for pelvic and intra-abdominal surgical procedures. The cephamycins should not be used for life-threatening infections where *Bacteroides* species are suspected of being the primary pathogen or for nosocomial intra-abdominal infections where more resistant gram-negative bacilli may play a significant role.

The second generation cephalosporins available for oral use include cefaclor, cefuroxime axetil, and cefprozil. Cefaclor has a spectrum of activity similar to the first generation cephalosporins except for enhanced activity against *H. influenzae*. Cefuroxime axetil shares the same spectrum with its parent compound, the injectable cefuroxime, but because of its enhanced lipid solubility it is well absorbed from the gastrointestinal tract. Cefprozil has a spectrum of activity very similar to cefuroxime axetil. All three drugs have been effective in the treatment of pharyngitis, bronchitis, otitis media, cellulitis, and impetigo in both adults and children. All these drugs can be administered twice daily; however, they are expensive alternatives to standard agents for most common infections.

## Third generation cephalosporins

The third generation cephalosporins as a group have enhanced resistance against hydrolysis by $\beta$-lactamases produced by many gram-negative bacilli, therefore giving them a very broad gram-negative antibacterial spectrum. They do not have enhanced gram-positive activity and may be inferior for covering gram-positive bacteria when compared with the first and second generation cephalosporins. Anaerobic activity varies from agent to agent, but none is more active than cefoxitin. None of the drugs in this class has activity against listeria, β-lactam antibiotic-resistant staphylococci, enterococci, or strains of pseudomonas other than *P. aeruginosa*. All of the third generation drugs cross the blood-brain barrier well and achieve therapeutic levels in the cerebrospinal fluid, making them useful agents in the treatment of meningitis due to susceptible bacteria. The parenteral third generation drugs include cefotaxime, ceftizoxime, ceftriaxone, moxalactam, cefoperazone, and ceftazidime. Cefixime and cefpodoxime are the only oral third generation drugs released for clinical use.

Cefotaxime, released in 1981, was the first of the third generation cephalosporins available in the United States and therefore is the drug for which there has been the most experience. Its half-life is 1 h and therefore it is dosed every 4 to 6 h. Ceftizoxime is quite similar in spectrum to cefotaxime, but it has a slightly more prolonged half-life of 1.7 h and can be safely dosed on an every 8 h basis. Both drugs have a broad gram-negative spectrum of activity, including most strains of *E. coli*, *Klebsiella*, *H. influenzae*, indole-positive and -negative proteus, *Salmonella*, *Neisseria meningitidis*, and *N. gonorrhoeae*. Many strains of otherwise resistant bacteria including *Enterobacter* species, *Citrobacter freundii*, *Morganella morganii*, and *Serratia* species may be sensitive. Neither drug is active against *P. aeruginosa*, nor do they have exceptional anaerobic activity. Of the third generation drugs, cefotaxime and ceftizoxime are the most active in vitro against staphylococci and streptococci.

These drugs have been effective primarily in the treatment of infections caused by resistant gram-negative bacilli. Because of their extremely broad spectrum, they are especially useful in the therapy of nosocomial infections. Narrower-spectrum and cheaper agents are preferable for most community-acquired infections. These drugs have been efficacious in the therapy of pneumonias, bacteremias, skin and soft tissue infections, urinary tract infections, and intra-abdominal infections. Cefotaxime has had the greatest usage in the therapy of meningitis and, it and ceftriaxone are listed as the third generation cephalosporins of choice by the Committee of Infectious Diseases of the American Academy of Pediatrics for the treatment of meningitis, based on extensive data on pediatric usage. Although the data is limited for ceftizoxime, it too is useful in the treatment of meningitis due to ampicillin-sensitive and -resistant *H. influenzae* type B, *N. meningitidis*, and for all but the highly penicillin-resistant strains of *S. pneumoniae*. For gram-negative meningitis caused by strains other than *P. aeruginosa*, these agents are quite active with cure rates of 80%–90%.

The spectrum of activity of ceftriaxone is comparable to that of cefotaxime and ceftizoxime; however, its long half-life of 8 h allows dosing intervals of 12 to 24 h, depending on the severity of infection. It remains useful in the therapy of multiple types of infectious processes as listed for cefotaxime and ceftizoxime. Its enhanced in vitro activity against penicillin-sensitive and -resistant *N. gonorrhoeae*, along with good tolerance of intramuscular injection has made ceftriaxone the drug of choice for all forms of gonorrhea, including ophthalmia neonatorum (see Chapters 73, 74). It also is an effective agent in the therapy of chancroid. It is the drug of choice for complicated Lyme disease including meningitis. Infrequent dosing has made this drug extremely attractive for home IV infusion in today's cost-conscious environment (see Chapter 25). Similarly, in-hospital savings in pharmacy preparation costs have led to the broad use of ceftriaxone as a first-line cephalosporin in many hospitals.

Moxalactam is mentioned for historical reasons only. Its structure is unique in that an oxygen is substituted for the sulfur atom in the six-membered ring of the cephalosporin nucleus. Its activity against gram-positive cocci is poor, but the drug is more active against gram-negative bacilli, including *P. aeruginosa* and *B. fragilis*, than cefotaxime, ceftizoxime, or ceftriazone. The methylthiotetrazole (MTT) side chain is present at the 3 position of the moxalactam nucleus and has been associated with enough episodes of clinically significant bleeding that the drug is no longer marketed in the United States.

Third generation cephalosporins with the best activity against *P. aeruginosa* include cefoperazone and ceftazidime. However, cefoperazone in vitro is less active against *P. aeruginosa* than ceftazidime and against other gram-negative bacilli when compared with all the other third generation drugs. Additionally, it has the MTT side chain at position 3 and has also been associated with prolonged prothrombin time and rare bleeding episodes.

Ceftazidime, therefore, is the most active third generation cephalosporin against *P. aeruginosa*. It also retains activity against other gram-negative bacilli equivalent to cefotaxime. These characteristics have made ceftazidime a popular choice in the treatment of the febrile neutropenic patient, usually but not necessarily in combination with an aminoglycoside (see Chapter 90). Although some data exist to support monotherapy in this setting, many clinicians still favor combination therapy for serious pseudomonas infections or gram-negative bacteremia. Ceftazidime is the drug of choice for *P. aeruginosa* meningitis with response rates of approximately 80% because of its excellent in vitro activity coupled with its ability to achieve therapeutic cerebrospinal fluid levels.

The oral third generation cephalosporins, cefixime and cefpodoxime, are highly active in vitro against group A streptococci, pneumococci, *N. gonorrhoeae*, *Moraxella catarrhalis* (including β-lactamase-producing strains), *H. influenzae*, and many enterobacteriaceae. Cefpodoxime, unlike cefixime, also exhibits some activity against β-lactam antibiotic-sensitive strains of *S. aureus*. Neither drug is active against species of *Enterobacter*, *Pseudomonas*, or *Enterococci*. Clinical trials have shown both drugs to be effective therapy for upper and lower respiratory infections, otitis media, sinusitis, and urinary tract infections. Cefixime is dosed once daily, and cefpodoxime twice daily. In most instances, however, cheaper alternatives provide adequate coverage. Both drugs show promise for single-dose, oral therapy of uncomplicated gonorrhea.

## Adverse Reactions

The safety profile of the cephalosporins is quite favorable when compared with other antibiotics. Life-threatening reactions are rare lending to their widespread usage.

Hypersensitivity reactions, as with the penicillins, are the most common side effects of the cephalosporins. Immediate type reactions with angioedema, bronchospasm, or anaphylaxis have been reported but are rare. More commonly one sees urticaria, pruritis, or nonspecific rashes. Drug fever with or without eosinophilia can also be seen.

Cross-allergenicity between the cephalosporins and penicillins has always been a controversy because they are similar in structure. Patients with a history of penicillin allergy have a higher incidence of reactions to cephalosporins (5%–16%) than patients

**Table 28.1** Therapeutic indications for commonly used cephalosporins

| Agent | Indication |
|---|---|
| FIRST GENERATION | |
| *Drugs in this class are interchangeable because they possess identical antibacterial spectra* | |
| Cefazolin | Skin and soft tissue infections, urinary tract infections. Effective alternative agent for serious staphylococcal infections. Inexpensive and effective drug for surgical prophylaxis |
| *ORAL AGENTS* | |
| Cephelexin | Skin and soft tissue infections, pharyngitis, and susceptible urinary tract infections |
| Cefodroxil | Same indications as cephelexin, but longer half-life allows once or twice daily dosing |
| SECOND GENERATION | |
| *Antibacterial spectra of individual agents not interchangeable. In general, increased gram-negative and anaerobic activity and decreased anti-staphylococcal activity* | |
| Cefuroxime | Community-acquired pneumonias, skin and soft tissue infection; bacteremias and urinary tract infections |
| Cefoxitin | Polymicrobial infections such as diverticulitis and other intra-abdominal infections, pelvic inflammatory disease; aspiration pneumonia; and diabetic foot infections. Prophylactic agent for intra-abdominal and pelvic surgical procedures |
| Cefotetan | Similar to cefoxitin, but longer half-life allows for less frequent dosing (twice daily) |
| *ORAL AGENTS* | |
| Cefaclor | Pharyngitis, bronchitis, otitis media, cellulitis, and impetigo |
| Cefuroxime axetil | Same indications as cefaclor but useful for continuation of therapy following parenteral cefuroxime, especially for community-acquired pneumonia |
| THIRD GENERATION | |
| *Antibacterial spectra of individual agents not interchangeable. As a group the gram-negative spectrum is markedly enhanced but the gram-positive activity is inferior when compared to first and second generation drugs* | |
| Cefotaxime | Pneumonia, bacteremias, skin and soft tissue infections, urinary tract infections, and meningitis |
| Ceftizoxime | Similar to cefotaxime, but longer half-life allows less frequent dosing (three times daily) |
| Ceftriaxone | Spectrum similar to cefotaxime and therefore useful for same indications. Additionally, useful for gonorrhea, chancroid, and complications of Lyme disease. Long half-life allows once or twice daily dosing |
| Ceftazidime | Same indications as cefotaxime; however, because of its increased Pseudomonal activity, ceftazidime is the only third-generation agent used in the febrile neutropenic host. "Drug of choice" for *Pseudomonas aeruginosa* meningitis |
| *ORAL AGENTS* | |
| Cefixime | Upper and lower respiratory infections, otitis media, sinusitis, urinary tract infections, and uncomplicated gonorrhea. No activity against *Enterobacter* sp., *Pseudomonas* sp., or enterococci. Once daily dosing, expensive |
| Cefpodoxime | Same indicators as cefixime but dosed twice daily and provides some activity against $\beta$-lactam antibiotic sensitive strains of *Staphylococcus aureus* |

with no penicillin allergy (1%–2.5%). Additionally, patients with a history of penicillin allergy have a rate of adverse drug reactions that is three times higher than that of nonallergic individuals even when the drugs are dissimilar immunologically. It has been estimated that the rate of cross-sensitivity is somewhere between 3% and 7%. In that there is no accurate way to predict cross-sensitivity between the two drug classes, most practioners recommend avoiding cephalosporins, if possible, in patients who have previously experienced IgE-mediated, anaphylactic-type reactions to penicillins. In patients with a history simply of skin rashes to penicillins, cephalosporins can be safely used, if needed.

All of the injectable forms have the potential for phlebitis, although no specific agent appears to have a higher frequency. Cefoxitin and cephalothin, however, cause pain with intramuscular injection more frequently than do the other cephalosporins.

Renal insufficiency was reported with cephaloridine, but this drug is no longer in clinical use. The combination of cephalothin and aminoglycosides has been implicated as causing synergistic nephrotoxicity. No other cephalosporins appear to share this trait. In general, the cephalosporins do not cause significant nephrotoxicity with the rare exception of interstitial nephritis which may occur as part of a hypersensitivity reaction.

Hepatic abnormalities may manifest themselves as elevated transaminases. These are rarely of clinical significance and can occur with any of the drugs within the class.

Drug-associated diarrhea can occur with any of the cephalosporins but is more common with oral agents owing to direct irritation of the intestinal tract along with alteration of the GI flora. Cefoperazone and ceftriaxone are reported as having a greater frequency of diarrhea on account of their hepatic metabolism and high biliary levels. *Clostridium difficile* colitis has been reported with all of the drugs in this group but at no greater frequency than seen with other antimicrobial agents. Ceftriaxone can cause the syndrome of pseudocholecystitis, which is more frequently seen in infants and children, secondary to formation of biliary sludge. This syndrome is reversible with discontinuation of the drug.

Hematologic side effects are reported in up to 3% of individuals, the most common of which is the development of a positive Coombs test. However, this event is rarely associated with the development of hemolysis. One may also see eosinophilia, thrombocytosis, and rarely, neutropenia.

Bleeding problems have been reported from hypoprothrombinemia, platelet aggregation defects, and thrombocytopenia. All broad-spectrum antibiotics may cause prolongation of the prothrombin time because of suppression of gut flora leading to decreased vitamin K synthesis. Additionally, cephalosporins with the MTT side chain at position 3 appear to inhibit competitively the formation of vitamin K–dependent clotting factors, as well as inhibiting the formation of vitamin K from its precursor. These effects can be reversed with administration of vitamin K or, in the presence of severe bleeding, by administering fresh frozen plasma. The MTT side chain is present on cefamandole, cefotetan, moxalactam, cefoperazone, and cefmetazole. Moxalactam is the only cephalosporin to cause a defect in platelet aggregation. Subsequently, because moxalactam has the greatest propensity to cause bleeding complications, it has been removed the U.S. market. The rest rarely cause any coagulation problems.

Cephalosporins with the MTT side chain or with similar substitutions (ceforanide and cefonicid) may also cause flushing, tachycardia, nausea, vomiting, and occasional hypotension and confusion when administered with alcohol. This antabuse-like effect can occur during or for a few days after the drug is given. This reaction is due to an accumulation of acetaldehyde from the inhibition of aldehyde dehydrogenase by a metabolite of methylthiotetrazole.

Lastly, because of their broad spectrum of antimicrobial activity, there is a risk of bacterial or fungal superinfection with prolonged usage of cephalosporins. Organisms encountered in this setting commonly include *Enterococcus*, *Pseudomonas*, *Enterobacter*, or *Candida* species. Thus, as with all antibiotics, usage should be brief, just enough to suppress or cure the primary infection, and no longer. Because superinfecting and colonizing microbes may become the cause of secondary (and often more serious) infections, appropriate adjustments of antimicrobial therapy may be necessary should these bacteria become clinically significant.

## ANNOTATED BIBLIOGRAPHY

Antimicrobial prophylaxis in surgery. Med Lett Drugs Ther 1992; 34:5–8.
*This article covers the choice and duration of antibiotic prophylaxis for a variety of surgical procedures.*

Cherubin CE, Eng RHK, et al. Penetration of newer cephalosporins into cerebrospinal fluid. Rev Infect Dis. 1989; 11:526–548.
*A review of the world literature on cerebrospinal fluid penetration of members of the various classes of cephalosporin antibiotics.*

Fong IW, Tompkins KB. Review of Pseudomonas aeruginosa meningitis with special emphasis on treatment with ceftazidime. Rev Infect Dis 1985; 7:604–612.
*Antimicrobial therapy of Pseudomonas aeruginosa meningitis with special emphasis on ceftazidime.*

Gustaferro CA, Steckelberg JM. Cephalosporin antimicrobial agents and related compounds. Mayo Clin Proc 1991; 66:1064–1073.
*An excellent comprehensive review of cephalosporins as part of the Mayo Clinic Antimicrobial Symposium.*

Le Saux N, Ronald AR. Role of ceftriaxone in sexually transmitted diseases. Rev Infect Dis 1989; 11:299–309.
*Experience with ceftriaxone treatment of gonococcal infections and chancroid.*

Morrow JD. The oral cephalosporins—a review. Am J Med Sci 1992; 303:35–39.
*A practical review contrasting the three generations of oral cephalosporins.*

Neu HC. Structure–activity relations of new β-lactam compounds and in-vitro activity against common bacteria. Rev Infect Dis 1983; 5(Suppl 2):S319–S337.
*A comprehensive review of the relationship between chemical structure modifications and the antimicrobial activity of β-lactam antibiotics.*

Norrby SR. Role of cephalosporins in the treatment of bacterial meningitis in adults: overview with special emphasis on ceftazidime. Am J Med 1985; 79(Suppl 2A):56–61.
*Treatment of meningitis with cephalosporins highlighting the efficacy of the third generation drugs.*

Pizzo, PA. Management of fever in patients with cancer and treatment induced neutropenia. N Engl J Med 1993; 328:1323–1332.
*An overview of the approach to the febrile neutropenic patient.*

Pizzo PA, Hathorn JW, Hiemenz J, et al. A randomized trial comparing ceftazidime alone with combination antibiotic therapy in cancer patients with fever and neutropenia. N Engl J Med 1986; 315:552–558.
*A classic study comparing monotherapy with ceftazidime with triple antibiotic therapy in the febrile neutropenic patient.*

Sanders CC, Sanders WE Jr. Emergence of resistance during therapy with the newer β-lactam antibiotics; role of inducible β-lactamases and implications for the future. Rev Infect Dis 1983; 5:639–648.
*A discussion of mechanisms of resistance of gram-negative bacteria with emphasis on inducible β-lactamases.*

Sattler FN, Weitekamp MR, Ballard JO. Potential for bleeding with the new β-lactam antibiotics. Ann Intern Med 1986; 105:924–930.
*Abnormal hemostasis associated with structural relationships of various β-lactam antibiotics.*

Saxon A, Beall GN, et al. Immediate hypersensitivity reactions to β-lactam antibiotics. Ann Intern Med 1987; 107:204–215.

*A comprehensive discussion of hypersensitivity reactions with all types of β-lactam antibiotics.*

Thornsberry C. Review of in-vitro activity of third generation cephalosporins and other newer β-lactam antibiotics against clinically important bacteria. *Am J Med 1985; 79(Suppl 2A):14–24.*

*In vitro susceptibility data for third generation cephalosporins, carbapenems, and monobactams is compared with first and second generation cephalosporins.*

Tomasz A. Penicillin-binding proteins and the antibacterial effectiveness of β-lactam antibiotics. Rev Infect Dis 1986; 8(Suppl 3):S260–S278.

*A review of the interractions between β-lactam antibiotics and penicillin-binding proteins and their effect on bacterial killing and resistance.*

# 29

# Other Beta-lactam Antibiotics: Penems, Carbapenems, and Monobactams

PIERRE TATTEVIN, GUILLAUME BRETON, AND CLAUDE CARBON

In the late 1970s, a new group of $\beta$-lactam antimicrobial agents was discovered: the carbapenems. Initially, these were olivanic acid (derived from *Streptomyces olivacus*) and thienamycin (derived from *Streptomyces catleya*). At about the same time, the first penem was synthesized by introducing a double bond into the thiazolin ring. The monobactam antibiotics, first synthesized in 1981, are monocyclic $\beta$-lactams.

## Penems and Carbapenems

The penems and carbapenems, new and very similar compounds, can be structurally considered as a combination of the two major classes of $\beta$-lactams: a penicillin $\beta$-lactam ring with a cephalosporin unsaturated C2–C3 bond (Fig. 29.1).

In the early development of the two compounds, two problems had to be solved: chemical instability, and the enzymatic degradation of most of these agents by the dehydropeptidase in the brush border of the renal tubuli. This led to the development of imipenem, which is stabilized by the crystallization of the N-formimidoyl derivative of thienamycin; and of cilastatin, a selective competitive antagonist of the dehydropeptidase 1. Their combination in the 1:1 ratio (Primaxin or Tienam) is the main compound of this group. It has been widely prescribed all over the world since 1981; the following data therefore mainly concern imipenem.

## Mechanisms of action

Although the fundamental mechanism of action of imipenem is similar to that of the classical $\beta$-lactams, three major differences (discussed below) may explain its specific antibacterial activity.

### Binding to different "penicillin-binding proteins" (PBP)

Imipenem mostly binds to PBP2, 1A, 1B, 4, and 5, and has a lower affinity to PBP3 compared with that of benzylpenicillin. In the presence of imipenem, gram-negative rods form small spherical or ellipsoidal cells ("lemon shape"), instead of the filamentous forms observed with penicillins and cephalosporins (probably because of their binding to PBP3). These lemon shapes are more easily phagocytized by polymorphonuclear leukocytes than the filaments. This could explain the postantibiotic effect (PAE) observed with imipenem on gram-negative rods. In contrast, penicillins and cephalosporins have a PAE on gram-positive organisms, which do not form filaments when exposed to $\beta$-lactams. This mechanism of action could also explain the lower endotoxin-liberating potential of imipenem than that of cephalosporins.

### High stability to most of the $\beta$-lactamases

This is probably due to the unusual *trans*-conformation of the hydroxyethyl side chain of imipenem as opposed to the *cis*-conformation of the acylamino-substituent on the $\beta$-lactam ring of the penicillins and cephalosporins.

### High diffusion rates through porin channels

These occur because of a more compact molecular structure. All these characteristics may explain the rare cross-resistance of imipenem with other $\beta$-lactams, its postantibiotic effect for most of the strains tested (including gram-negative rods), and its fast, dose-dependent bactericidal effect, independent of the inoculum size (except for some strains of *Bacteroides fragilis*).

## Mechanisms of resistance

It is worth noting that in spite of wide usage all over the world, the minimal inhibition concentrations (MICs) have not changed for most pathogens. Nevertheless, two mechanisms of resistance are well known.

### Enzymatic degradation

Imipenem has a very high degree of stability to $\beta$-lactamase action and is only hydrolyzed by zinc-containing enzymes, including other chromosomal $\beta$-lactamases produced by *Xanthomonas maltophilia*, some *Aeromonas* species and *Flavobacterium species*; or a carbapenemase produced by a few strains of *Enterobacter cloacae*, *Serratia marcescens*, *Aeromonas hydrophilia*, and *B. fragilis*. Although imipenem is a strong $\beta$-lactamase inducer, it remains active against most of the strains in which it has induced these enzymes.

### Loss of permeability

This is the major mechanism for treatment-induced resistance. It has mainly been described with *Pseudomonas aeruginosa*, especially in lower respiratory tract infections. In some studies, 50% of the initially sensitive strains may become resistant. A chromosomally coded alteration of outer membrane proteins (of 45–46 kd) that serve as porins makes the bacteria impermeable to carbapenem. The anti-Pseudomonas activity of other $\beta$-lactams is not impaired, since imipenem uses different porins (mainly protein D2) for its penetration through the outer membrane of *P. aeruginosa*. Thus, these imipenem-resistant strains may remain sensitive to ceftazidime and cefoperazone.

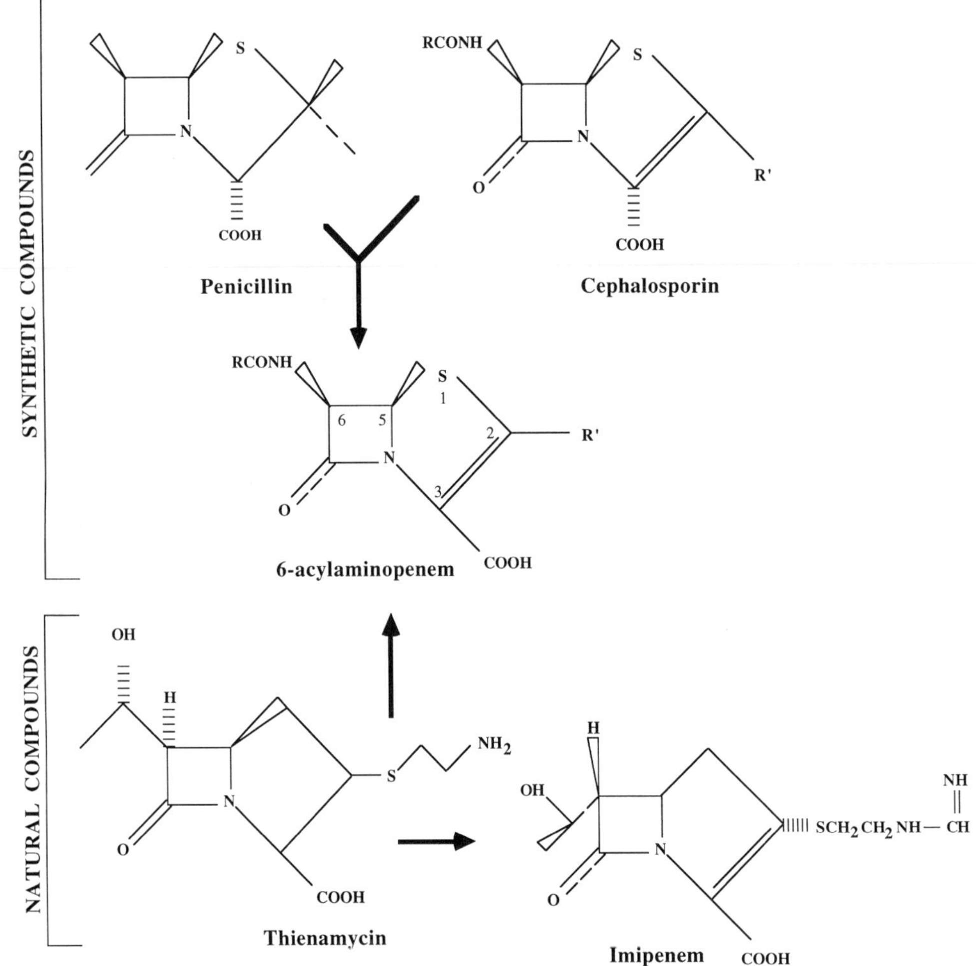


**Fig. 29.1** Chemical structure of some $\beta$-lactams.

### Efflux

Active efflux proteins have been shown to contribute significantly to multidrug resistance in *P. aeruginosa.* Some of them can confer resistance to carbapenems.

## Spectrum of action

Imipenem has a very broad antibacterial spectrum, thus it is easier to focus on the resistant strains rather than the sensitive ones.

### Gram-positive bacteria

Methicillin-resistant *Staphylococcus aureus* (MRSA) strains have minimum inhibitory concentrations (MICs) to imipenem of between 6 and 64 $\mu$g/ml when tested at 30°C. Despite lower MICs at 37°C, imipenem is ineffective for treatment of MRSA infections. Most strains of *Enterococcus faecalis* are readily inhibited by imipenem; (MICs $\leq$ 1.5 $\mu$g/ml), however, activity against *Enterococcus faecium* (MICs $\geq$ 8$\mu$g/ml) is poor. Moreover, ampicillin-resistant *faecium* or *faecalis* have MICs of 16–256 $\mu$g/ml). Among the gram-positive rods, only *Corynebacterium* JK is predictively resistant. *Listeria monocytogenes* will be discussed below.

### Gram-negative bacteria

Imipenem has excellent activity against almost all gram-negative bacteria. It is the only $\beta$-lactam with predictable activity against Gram-negative aerobes (e.g., *Enterobacter* sp., *Serratia* sp.) that express extended $\beta$-lactamase (TEM- or SHV-related $\beta$-lactamases) activity that inhibits ceftazidime and other third generation cephalosporins. *X. maltophila* is almost always resistant (MICs > 128 $\mu$g/ml), as are 50% of *Pseudomonas cepacia* strains, and most of *Flavobacterium* strains. The development of acquired resistance of *P. aeruginosa* during treatment with imipenem has been described above. Despite initial sensitivity of more than 80% of *P. aeruginosa* strains, clinical studies have proved that treatment failure is commonly due to the emergence of resistance. New carbapenems are being developed to circumvent this phenomenon.

### Intracellular pathogens

Despite good extracellular in vitro activity, imipenem should not be considered as a treatment for intracellular infections. *L. monocytogenes* has a high minimal bactericidal concentration (MBC) in spite of a MIC $\leq$0.06 mg/L. Treatment failures have been reported in animal models of *Legionella pneumophila* infection. These results appear to be due to the poor intracellular diffusion of imipenem in mammalian cells. On the other hand, imipenem is the most active β-lactam antibiotic against *Nocardia asteroides*, inhibiting 79% of 52 isolates at 4 μg/ml.

### Anaerobic bacteria

Almost all gram-negative anerobes are very susceptible (including most *B. fragilis* strains). Except for *Clostridium difficile*, Imipenem's activity is also high against gram-positive anaerobes. Imipenem is therefore selected by many clinicians as a treatment of choice in mixed polymicrobial infections with suspected presence of anaerobic pathogens.

### Mycobacteria

Imipenem binds to *Mycobacterium tuberculosis* PBPs at therapeutically achievable concentrations and is relatively stable to the mycobacterial β-lactamases. Further evaluation of this drug is warranted for the treatment of tuberculosis.

## Other carbapenems and penems

### Carbapenems

Meropenem (SM 7338) has been recently approved by the FDA. This carbapenem seems of particular interest in the treatment of imipenem-resistant *P. aeruginosa*. Compared with imipenem, it is more active against enterobacteriaceae (2–3 fold), slightly less active against most gram-positive cocci (and not active against *E. faecium*), and two- to fourfold more active against imipenem-resistant *P. aeruginosa.*

### Penems

None are actually available for clinical use. Their antibacterial activity is four to eightfold less than that of imipenem, but they are of interest mainly because of their resistance to renal dehydropeptidase and a significantly higher enteral absorption rate, which allows oral administration.

## General use

The broad antibacterial spectrum and high intrinsic bactericidal activity of imipenem places it among the most powerful antibiotics available to treat infections caused by mixed aerobic/anaerobic flora or by multiresistant hospital-acquired pathogens. Its efficacy has been widely confirmed in almost all organ infections.

### Lower respiratory tract infections

Acar has reviewed the worldwide experience with imipenem for lower respiratory tract infections. Of 204 assessable patients, 173 (85%) were cured or improved. The principal pathogens were *P. aeruginosa*, *Streptococcus pneumoniae*, *Klebsiella* spp., *Haemophilus influenzae*, *Escherichia coli*, and *S. aureus*. Because of the high rate of acquired resistance of *P. aeruginosa* to imipenem, it has been suggested that it should be combined with an aminoglycoside for treatment of pneumonia caused by this organism.

### Urinary tract infection

In preclinical studies, imipenem produced clinical improvement in patients with complicated urinary tract infection (including bacteremia), of which more than half were due to *P. aeruginosa*.

### Intra-abdominal infection

In clinical trials, imipenem as monotherapy has proved to be as effective as aminoglycosides combined with floroquinolones or clindamycin or third generation cephalosporins.

### Osteomyelitis

Gentry reviewed 33 patients who had been treated by one of the newer broad-spectrum β-lactams (imipenem, ceftazidime, cefotaxime, and ceftizoxime). There were no significant differences among the four antibiotics. In many hospitals, imipenem is reserved for the treatment of multiresistant hospital-acquired pathogens and is considered a second-line choice in other instances.

### Pelvic infection

Imipenem has a good activity against the mixed aerobic and anerobic bacteria that cause pelvic inflammatory disease (PID) or tuboovarian abscesses. It should be used in combination with a tetracycline such as doxycycline or a fluoroquinolone because of its poor activity against *Chlamydia* species.

### Meningitis, endocarditis, septicemia

Imipenem has proved effective against a wide range of pathogens. Many clinicians reserve its use for cases of clinical or bacteriological failure of the classical treatments, particularly when bacteria with extended-spectrum β-lactamase activity may be the responsible pathogens.

### Fever in neutropenic patients

Imipenem as monotherapy has been therapeutically equivalent to combination therapy with aminoglycosides plus ureidopenicillins or third generation cephalosporins or fluoroquinolones. In some situations, coverage of some Gram-positive cocci may be insufficient. Meropenem has been demonstrated to be efficacious in bacterial meningitis, febrile episodes in neutropenic patients, and complicated intraabdominal, lower respiratory, and urinary tract infections.

## Pharmacology

### Administration

The imipenem–cilastatin combination is administered by intermittent intravenous infusion or by intramuscular injection. Total daily doses may range from 1 to 4 g, depending on clinical indication, given as 250–500 mg every 6 or 8 h. Meropenem is given by intravenous infusion. The recommended doses are 20 mg/kg given every 8 h in children; 1 to 2 g every 8 h in adults.

### Blood and tissue levels

The intravenous infusion of a 500 mg dose immediately produces peak levels of 30 to 35 mg/L until 6 h after infusion. The intramuscular administration of a 500 mg dose produces peak levels at 2 h of 4 mg/L. The concentrations 8 h later are approximately 1 mg/L. Bioavailability by the intramuscular route is 60%. Drug accumulation occurs in healthy subjects despite repeated dosing.

The penetration of imipenem into body tissues and fluids is excellent (Table 29.1). High concentrations are obtained in urinary tract, lung, biliary tract, sinus, or bone. The diffusion into

**Table 29.1** Concentration of imipenem in various tissues or fluids

| Tissue or fluid | Dose IV (g) | Concentration (mg/kg or mg/L) | Time after infusion (min) |
|---|---|---|---|
| Renal parenchyma | 0.5 | 15–90 | 90 |
| Prostatic tissue | 0.5 | 5 | 90 |
| Prostatic fluid | 0.5 | 0.2 | 60 |
| Female genital tract | 0.5 | 3–15 | 60 |
| Pelvic dead space exudate | 0.5 | 13 | 120 |
| Biliary tract | 0.5 | 2 | 90 |
| Sputum | 0.5 | 1.5 | 60 |
| Sputum | 1.0 | 3.0 | 60 |
| Lung | 1.0 | 13 | 20 |
| Cerebrospinal fluid | 1.0 | 1–2 | 60 |

[From Clissold, 1987, with permission.]

cerebrospinal fluid is comparable to that of all $\beta$-lactams. The CSF concentration measured in patients with inflamed meninges is about 2 $\mu$g/ml following a 1 g dose.

Imipenem is 10% to 20% bound to human plasma proteins in vitro. The extent of serum protein binding for cilastatin is 35%. The combination of imipenem/cilastatin does not modify imipenem's protein binding. The serum half-life of imipenem is approximately 1 h in patient with normal renal function; that of cilastatin is slightly shorter. The plasma clearance is about 0.2 L/h/kg. Meropenem is widely dispersed into body tissues and fluids. Its terminal elimination half life is around 1 h.

### Excretion pathways

Imipenem is excreted almost entirely unchanged in the urine by glomerular filtration and tubular secretion. Administered alone, imipenem is hydrolyzed by dehydropeptidase I, an enzyme located in the brush border of the proximal tubule epithelium, which opens the $\beta$-lactam ring and produces an inactive metabolite. Under such circumstances, the urinary recovery of active imipenem is only 15% to 30%. The combination of imipenem with cilastatin, an inhibitor of the dehydropeptidase (DHP) increases the urinary recovery of active imipenem by 60%–75%. Seventy per cent of the administered dose of meropenem is excreted primarily unchanged through the kidneys. Meropenem is stable to human DHP, so it can be given as a single agent.

### Dose modifications in renal or hepatic failure

Reduced renal function increases the elimination half-life of imipenem, and dose adaptation is necessary (Table 29.2). For hemodialysis patients, the dose administered should be 0.5 g every 12 h. Dialysis removes 90% of imipenem; requiring replacement after the procedure. Imipenem does not undergo hepatic metabolism, so dose modifications in patients with liver disease are unnecessary. Similar dose modifications are needed with meropenem.

## Toxicities

Allergic manifestations occur in 2% to 3% of patients and usually include rash, fever, arthralgia, or neutropenia, similar to other $\beta$-lactam drugs. The cross-allergenicity rate with other $\beta$-lactams is about 50%.

Neurological toxicities are observed in 1% and consist mostly of convulsion or seizure. These incidents occur more frequently in patients with underlying neurological disease, renal failure (long-term treatment), or high dosage. In most cases, dose reduction is sufficient for neurologic symptoms to improve.

Nausea, vomiting, and diarrhea occur in 7% to 8%. Pseudomembranous colitis due to *C. difficile* has been reported. Liver enzyme abnormalities are frequent and moderate; neutropenia and anemia have been observed. No nephrotoxicity has been reported in humans; however, in animals, interstitial nephropathy occurs with high doses of imipenem. This toxicity decreases with concomittant administration of cilastatin.

Meropenem appears to have a safety profile similar to that of imipenem and other $\beta$-lactam antibiotics, and to be as safe in children as in adults. In keeping with animal data, meropenem is less likely to be epileptogenic than imipenem.

## Monobactams

Although a few new compounds are being studied, the first monobactam to be marketed, aztreonam, (a completely synthetic member) is still the only one available for clinical use. Its main characteristics include a well-defined antibacterial spectrum resembling that of the aminoglycosides against aerobic gram negative bacteria and weaker immunogenicity than other $\beta$-lactams. Compounds under study include S82291, which is orally absorbed.

**Table 29.2** Imipenem dose modification in case of renal failure

| Glomerular filtration rate (mL/min/1.73 m$^2$) | Daily dose (g/IV) |
|---|---|
| >70 mL | 2 |
| 70–31 | 1.5 |
| 30–11 | 1.0 |
| 10–5 | 0.5 |
| <5 | No use without hemodialysis |

[From Clissold, 1987, with permission.]

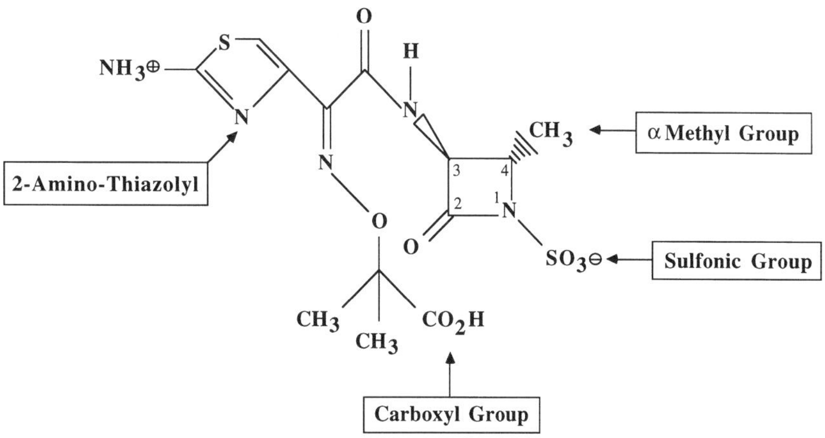

**Fig. 29.2** Aztreonam: structure–function relationships.

## Mechanism of action

Like heterocyclic $\beta$-lactams, monobactams bind to the penicillin-binding proteins of Gram-negative bacteria, leading to the production of filamentous forms and causing cell death. Aztreonam has a great affinity to PBP3, but none for the PBPs of anaerobic or gram-positive bacteria. Many of its structure–function relations have been described (Fig. 29.2): The sulfonic group ($SO^{3-}$) at C1 activates the $\beta$-lactam ring, directly leading to the acetylation of the PBP. The 2-amino-thiazolyl group at C3, similar to that of ceftazidime, increases its activity against *Pseudomonas*. The $\alpha$-methyl group at C4 gives aztreonam high stability to $\beta$-lactamases.

## Mechanism of resistance

Aztreonam is highly resistant to enzymatic hydrolysis by most of the $\beta$-lactamases because it has poor substrate affinity for these enzymes. Both chromosomal and plasmid $\beta$-lactamases, including TEM1, TEM2, SHV1, and those from *Staphylococcus* spp. and *B. fragilis*, are inactive against aztreonam. It is neutralized, however, by TEM3, TEM5, TEM7, and SHV2, the recently discovered plasmid-mediated $\beta$-lactamases. Other features of importance include a weak ability to induce chromosomally mediated $\beta$-lactamases. Permeability resistance in infecting organisms has occasionally occurred during treatment and if resistance is present to other $\beta$-lactam antibiotics, cross-resistance to aztreonam has been reported mainly in nonfermenting gram-negative bacteria.

## Spectrum of action

Almost all gram-negative aerobes are sensitive to monobactams. Enterobacteriaceae are killed at concentrations two to four times the MIC; the $MIC_{90}$ is less than 1 $\mu$g for most susceptible bacteria except for *Citrobacter freundii*, *Enterobacter*, and *S. marcescens* (MIC = 8, 4, and 2 $\mu$g/ml, respectively). The $MIC_{90}$ for *P. aeruginosa* is 8 $\mu$g/L, which is twofold that of ceftazidime. Aztreonam remains active against most aminoglycoside-resistant strains. It kills *P. aeruginosa* at concentrations four- to 16-fold above the MIC. Other *Pseudomonas* species such as *P. cepacia* must be considered as resistant, as are *X. maltophila*, *Acinetobacter* spp., *Achromobacter scylosascidans*, *Alcaligenes*, and *L. pneumophilia*. *Neisseria gonorrheae* and *H. influenzae* are usually susceptible with a $MIC_{90}$ of 0.25 $\mu$l/ml.

## General use

The antibacterial spectrum of aztreonam resembles that of the aminoglycosides, and it has been shown to be an effective therapy for gram-negative infections, especially when aminoglycoside-induced oto- or nephrotoxicity is likely to occur. Aztreonam has been effective as monotherapy in gram-negative aerobic septicemia, respiratory tract infections, urinary tract infections, osteomyelitis, arthritis, septic arthritis, cutaneous infections, and malignant otitis externa. It is also effective in treating *Salmonella* carriers and gonorrhea. Because of its low rate of allergenicity, even when previous reactions to $\beta$-lactams have been reported, it has been offered as safe and effective therapy in patients with a history of penicillin allergy. The lack of activity of aztreonam against gram-positive bacteria and anaerobes may be advantageous in reducing the potential for antibiotic-induced gastrointestinal disturbances. Thus, aztreonam has been proposed for selective reduction of bowel flora. Aztreonam in combination with other antibiotics has been suggested as treatment for intra-abdominal or gynecologic infections. Less toxic than aminoglycosides, aztreonam may also be more effective when local tissue conditions (low Ph, low $PO_2$) inhibit the activity of aminoglycosides. The compounds most frequently combined with aztreonam are clindamycin or metronidazole for mixed anerobic infections and glycopeptides or other $\beta$-lactams when mixed infections with gram-positive species are suspected. A synergistic effect has been described (in vitro only) with aminoglycosides which may be of little clinical relevance. Most of the other combinations have an additive effect. For empiric treatment of febrile granulocytopenia, the cure rates obtained with the combination of aztreonam and vancomycin are comparable to those reported for other frequently used combinations.

## Administration

Aztreonam may be administered intramuscularly or intravenously. The oral bioavailability is poor. Daily doses from 2 to 6g/24 h are usually given, administered as 500–2000 mg every 6 or 8 h.

## Pharmacology

The intravenous infusion of 1000 mg doses produces a peak serum level of 150 mg/L. The serum concentration falls to about 2 mg/L 8 h later. No accumulation is observed following repeated

**Table 29.3** Concentrations of aztreonam in tissues

| Tissue | IV dose (g) | Concentration (mg/kg or mg/L) | Time after injection (h) |
|---|---|---|---|
| Blister fluid | 1 | 20 | 1 |
| Bronchial secretion | 2 | 4–16 | 4 |
| Bile | 1 | 20–50 | 2 |
| Cerebrospinal fluid (inflamed meninges) | 2 | 3–18 | 1–4 |
| Pleural fluid | 2 | 40–60 | 1–3 |
| Endocardium | 2 | 22 | 0.9–1.6 |
| Synovial fluid | 2 | 70–95 | 1–2 |
| Muscle | 2 | 15 | 0.5–1 |
| Skin | 2 | 25 | 1 |
| Bone | 2 | 10–15 | 2 |
| Gall bladder | 2 | 20 | 4 |
| Kidney | 2 | 50–70 | 2–6 |
| Prostate | 1 | 9 | 1–3 |
| Endometrium | 2 | 9 | 1–2 |
| Liver | 2 | 40–50 | 1–2 |
| Lung | 2 | 20–25 | 1–2 |
| Urine | 2 | 500–3000 | 2–4 |

[From Neu, 1980, with permission.]

doses. The intramuscularly bioavailability is 100%. Aztreonam is widely distributed into the body tissues or fluids and high levels are obtained in bone, synovial fluid, kidneys, liver, and biliary tract (Table 29.3).

Aztreonam is 45% to 60% bound to serum proteins in vivo, and its elimination half-life is 1.6 h. About 60% to 70% of aztreonam is excreted unchanged in the urine by glomerular filtration and tubular secretion, only 1% being excreted in the feces or the biliary tract. Some is metabolized by a dehydropeptidase, the location of which is unknown.

## Dose modification in renal or hepatic failure

Because of its high percentage of renal excretion, aztreonam dosages have to be adapted to creatinine clearance. For a creatinine clearance between 80 and 30, 30 and 10, and 10 and 2 ml/min, the half-life is 3.5, 5.6, and 7.8 h, respectively. Daily doses must be modified by one-half, one-fourth, or one-eighth either by increasing the interval of administration or reducing the unitary dose. Aztreonam is removed by hemodialysis and has to be administered after dialysis. A 4-hour period of hemodialysis removes 25–30% of a dose. Patients with hepatic failure do not require dose modification.

## Toxicities

Aztreonam demonstrates few adverse effects (about 7% of patients). Allergic manifestations such as pruritis and rash are observed in 2% of patients and cross-reactions with other β-lactams occur in less than 1%. The most common adverse affects are local reaction at injection site, gastrointestinal side effects (diarrhea, nausea, vomiting), and slight elevations of ASAT and ALAT levels. There is no neurotoxicity and no nephrotoxicity; pseudomembranous colitis is rare (<1%).

## ANNOTATED BIBLIOGRAPHY


Acar JF. Therapy for lower respiratory tract infections with imipenem/cilastatin: A review of worldwide experience. Rev Infect Dis 1988; 7:573–577.
*A comprehensive review of the use of imipenem in lower respiratory tract infections.*

Adhinson NF. Immunogenicity and cross-allergenicity of aztreonam. Am J Med 1990; 88:12–15.
*A specific discussion on reduced allergic side effects of monobactams as compared with penicillins.*

Brewer NS, Hellinger WC. The monobactams. Mayo Clin Proc 1991; 66:1152–1157.
*A general article on this antibiotic class.*

Chambers HF, Moreau D, Yajko D, Miick C, Wagner C, Hackbarth C, Kocagoz S, Rosenber E, Hadley WK, Nikaido H. Can penicillins and other beta-lactam antibiotics be used to treat tuberculosis? Antimicrob Agents Chemother 1995; 39:2620.
*A very interesting in vitro approach of a potential antituberculosis effect of various β-lactams, including imipenem.*

Clissold SP. Imipenem/cilastatin: a review of its antibacterial activity, pharmacokinetic properties and therapeutic efficacy. Drugs 1987;33:193–241.
*Extensive review of the main properties and therapeutic use of imipenem.*

Finch RG, Bint AJ, White LO, Wood MJ. Meropenem: focus on clinical performance. J Antimicrob Chemother 1995; 30(Suppl A):1–22.

Hellinger WC, Brewer NS. Imipenem. Mayo Clin Proc 1991; 66:1074–1081.
*Practical clinical approach of imipenem.*

Igari J. Nationwide survey of antibacterial susceptibility of clinical isolates to imipenem in Japan, 1991. In: Recent Advances in Chemotherapy pp. 175–176, 1993.
*A paper on the relative stability of in vitro efficacy of imipenem.*

Masuda N, Sakagawa E, Ohya S. Outer membrane proteins responsible for multidrug resistance in *Pseudomonas aeruginosa*. Antimicrob Agents Chemother 1995; 39:2392.
*Description of three types of multidrug resistant mutants of P. aeruginosa, over expressing different types of outer membrane proteins.*

McClean KL, Sheehan GJ, Harding GKM. Intra-abdominal infection: a review. Clin Infect Dis 1994; 19:100–116.
*A review of the therapeutic impact of imipenem on polymicrobial difficult-to-treat infections.*

Neu HC. Aztreonam activity, pharmacology and clinical use. Am J Med 1990; 88:2–6.

*A comprehensive review of the main properties of aztreonam with practical perspectives.*

Norrby SR. Penems and carbapenems. In: The Antimicrobial Agents Annual, vol. 3. Peterson PK, Verhoef V, eds. Elsevier, Amsterdam, pp. 151–157, 1988.

*Good chapter on these agents, coming from a well-documented collection.*

Norrby SR, Newell PA, Faulkner KL, Lesky W. Safety profile of meropenem. J Antimicrob Chemother 1995; 30(Suppl A):207–223.

Priors JM, Van Agtmael MA, Kuijper EJ, Van Deventer SJ, Speelman P. Antibiotic induced endotoxin release in patients with gram-negative urosepsis: a double blind study comparing imipenem and ceftazidime. J Infect Dis 1995; 172:886.

*Evidence of a difference favoring imipenem. The clinical relevance remains to be established.*

Quinn JP. Emergence of resistance to imipenem during therapy for *P. aeruginosa* infections. J Infect Dis 1986; 154:289–294.

*One of the first descriptions of this specific risk with clinical relevance.*

Rolston KVI, et al. Aztreonam in the prevention and treatment of infection in neutropenic cancer patients. Am J Med 1990; 88:245–295.

*One of the first papers describing the potentials of aztreonam in these infections.*

Sirot D. Extended-spectrum plasmid-mediated beta-lactamases (ESBLs). J Antimicrob Chemother 1995; 36(Suppl. A):19.

*Valuable review of the different types of ESBLs clearly defining the resistance of imipenem and meropenem to the hydrolysis induced by these various enzymes.*

Spratt BG, Tobanputra V, Zimmerman W. Binding of thienamycin and clavulanic acid to the PBP of *E. coli* K12. Antimicrob Agents Chemother 1977; 12:406.

*Early assessment of the mechanism of action of imipenem.*

Wiseman LR, Wagstoff AJ, Brogden MN, Bryson HM. Meropenem: a review of its antibacterial activity, pharmacokinetic properties and clinical efficacy. Drugs 1995; 50:73.

*Extensive review of the main properties of meropenem with direct comparison with imipenem.*

# 30

# Aminoglycosides

DAVID N. GILBERT

The aminoglycoside antibiotics are a group of highly charged cationic molecules with rapid concentration-dependent bactericidal activity against the majority of aerobic gram-negative bacteria, some mycobacteria, and an occasional protozoan. The aminoglycosides are often combined with a $\beta$-lactam antibiotic for empiric or specific therapy of suspected or proven infection due to aerobic gram-negative bacilli. Aminoglycosides are rarely used for prophylaxis. Microbial resistance is at a low level, although occasional epidemic infection by resistant organisms is described. The aminoglycosides share the potential risk of renal injury, eighth nerve damage, and rarely, neuromuscular blockade. For years the aminoglycosides have been administered twice or three times per day. For reasons of equal efficacy, ease of administration, and reduced risk of toxicity, there is increasing use of once-a-day dosing.

## Aminoglycoside Family

The members of the aminoglycoside family are shown in Table 30.1. All have a necessary six-membered ring with amino-group substituents, hence the name aminocyclitol. The more common descriptor, aminoglycoside, derives from glycosidic bonds between the aminocyclitol and two or more sugars that may or may not have amino-group substituents. Spectinomycin is included because it does have an aminocyclitol ring but it lacks amino sugars or glycosidic bonds.

Aminoglycosides were discovered by screening soil bacteria for elaboration of antimicrobial substances. Aminoglycosides ending with the suffix "mycin" were derived from the Streptomyces whereas those ending in "micin" derive from Micromonospora. Kanamycin, neomycin, and gentamicin are products of fermentation with two or three chemical constituents. Netilmicin, amikacin, dibekacin, and isepamicin are semisynthetic derivatives of the fermentation product. Including spectinomycin, there are nine aminoglycosides marketed in the United States; in addition, sisomicin, dibekacin and isepamicin are in clinical use in Japan, Europe, and elsewhere.

## Antimicrobial Activity

### Mechanism

The bactericidal activity of aminoglycosides results from an initial passive ionic interaction between the cationic aminoglycoside and the anionic cell wall, subsequent energy-dependent internalization, and then binding to ribosomes. Subsequent to binding, there is a measurable decrease in protein synthesis and a concomitant increase in misreading of messenger RNA. Cell death may result from both alteration of the cell surface and ribosomal dysfunction.

The energy for the update phase of internalization is dependent on aerobic metabolism. Consequently, anaerobic organisms are resistant to aminoglycosides. Selected aerobic bacteria, some mycobacteria, and selected aerobic protozoa are susceptible to the antimicrobial influence of aminoglycosides.

### Spectrum of antimicrobial activity

#### Clinical microbiology

The aminoglycosides demonstrate concentration-dependent bactericidal activity in vitro against a wide spectrum of aerobic and facultative gram-negative bacilli (Table 30.2).

Of equal import are the microorganisms that consistently demonstrate no susceptibility to aminoglycosides—i.e., all anaerobic bacteria, fungi, *Mycoplasma* species, and viruses. Aminoglycosides have no predictable in vitro activity against *Streptococcus pneumoniae.*

Aminoglycosides demonstrate in vitro activity against some organisms known to cause intracellular infection, e.g., *Legionella* species. Despite documentation of low measurable intracellular aminoglycoside concentrations, gentamicin in vitro demonstrates cidal activity against intracellular *Escherichia coli* after incubation in solution with "therapeutic" concentrations of drug. Nonetheless, aminoglycosides are not used to treat *Legionella* species infection, but they are used successfully in the treatment of other intracellular pathogens, such as Brucellosis, tuberculosis, tularemia, and Yersiniosis. Aminoglycosides are not active against other intracellular pathogens such as chlamydiae or rickettsia.

The activity of the aminocyclitol spectinomycin is limited to *Neisseria gonorrhoeae.*

The in vitro activity of gentamicin, tobramycin, netilmicin, and amikacin against aerobic gram-negative bacteria is virtually identical with two exceptions. The minimum inhibitory concentration and minimum bactericidal concentration (MIC/MBC) of gentamicin against *Serratia* species is twofold lower than other aminoglycosides; the MIC/MBC of tobramycin against *Pseudomonas aeruginosa* is consistently twofold lower than that of other aminoglycosides.

#### MIC testing

The testing of the aminoglycosides is influenced by the cation content and the pH of the test media but is not influenced by the test inocula of organisms. In contrast, the MICs of the $\beta$-lactams are influenced by the test inoculum. Aminoglycosides exhibit concentration-dependent killing of susceptible bacteria; $\beta$-lactam

**Table 30.1** The aminoglycoside family

| Generic name | Proprietary name |
|---|---|
| Streptomycin | None |
| Neomycin | Mycifradin, neobiotic |
| Kanamycin | Kantrex |
| Paromomycin | Humatin |
| Gentamicin | Garamycin |
| Tobramycin | Nebcin |
| Amikacin | Amikin |
| Netilmicin | Netromycin |
| Spectinomycin | Trobicin |
| Sisomicin | Siseptin |
| Dibekacin | — |
| Isepamicin | [a] |

[a]Multiple names are used in Europe and Asia. Isepamicin is not marketed in the U.S.

antibiotics require concentrations above the MIC for killing, but increases to drug concentrations beyond 10–20 times the MIC do not enhance, and paradoxically may decrease, the rate of killing of bacteria. The aminoglycosides demonstrate an in vitro postantibiotic effect against aerobic gram-negative bacilli; the $\beta$-lactams do not demonstrate a postantibiotic effect against aerobic gram-negative bacilli.

### Synergy

In vitro antimicrobial synergy is defined as a magnitude of bacterial killing by two different drugs that exceeds the sum of the killing by each drug individually. Synergy was initially demonsterated with the combination of penicillin and streptomycin against strains of enterococci isolated from patients with endocarditis. Subsequently, in vitro synergy has been demonstrated with a variety of aminoglycosides combined with a $\beta$-lactam antibiotic or vancomycin against viridans streptococci, *Staphylococcus aureus*, *Staphylococcus epidermidis*, *Enterobacteriaceae*, *P. aeruginosa*, and other organisms.

**Table 30.2** Anticipated in vitro spectrum of aminoglycoside antimicrobial activity*

| Predictably active | Predictably inactive |
|---|---|
| Enterobacteriaceae: e.g., *E. coli*, *Proteus* sp., *Klebsiella* sp., *Morganella* sp., *Serratia* sp. | |
| *P. aeruginosa* | *Stenotrophomonas (Xanthomonas) maltophilia* |
| *H. influenzae* | |
| Methicillin-susceptible *S. aureus*[a] | Methicillin-resistant *S. aureus* |
| *Neisseria gonorrhoeae*[b] | |
| *Brucella* sp. | |
| *Yersinia pestis*[c] | *Burkholderia (Pseudomonas) cepacia* |
| *Francisella tularemia* | |
| *M. tuberculosis*[d] | |
| *M. avium intracellulare*[e] | |
| *Entamoeba histolytica*[f] | *Giardia lamblia* |
| *Cryptosporidium parvum*[f] | *Trichomonas vaginalis* |
| | *Legionella* sp. |
| | *Mycoplasma pneumoniae* |

*Refers to gentamicin, tobramycin, netilmicin, and amikacin, unless specified.

[a]May lose activity after 24–48 h.

[b]Spectinomycin.

[c]Streptomycin.

[d]Streptomycin.

[e]Amikacin.

[f]Paromomycin.

## Pharmacology

### Administration

Therapeutic serum concentrations of aminoglycosides are achieved by intravenous (IV), intramuscular (IM), or intraperitoneal (IP) route. Because a rapid increase in serum level to a high peak might precipitate neuromuscular blockade, IV infusions are extended over 15–60 min.

There is minimal absorption from the gastrointestinal (GI) tract. Rare instances of deafness have occurred after oral absorption of neomycin in patients with hepatic encephalopathy and impaired renal function. There is theoretic concern of absorption in patients with inflammatory bowel disease.

Aminoglycosides instilled into the peritoneal cavity are rapidly absorbed with subsequent serum concentrations proportionate to the concentration of drug instilled. For this reason, use of an aminoglycoside solution as abdominal irrigant in surgery is not recommended; rapid absorption and neuromuscular blockade has occurred. Smaller doses are instilled safely in the abdomen in patients with peritonitis complicating chronic ambulatory peritoneal dialysis.

Aminoglycosides are also applied topically to the skin, in ear drops, into the conjunctival sac, as an aerosol, as a bladder irrigant, and by direct instillation into the lumbar sac or lateral ventricles.

### Distribution

After parenteral administration, the aminoglycosides distribute throughout the vascular and interstitial spaces. Drug distribution characteristics are consistent with a high level of solubility in water and a low level of protein binding of approximately 10%. Intracellular penetration is poor, as is its ability to cross the blood-brain and blood-cerebrospinal fluid barriers. In contrast, synovial fluid concentrations are only slightly less than serum levels. Biliary levels are only 30% of concomitant blood concentrations. Penetration into vitreous humor of the eye is poor. Concentrations in bronchial secretions are low.

Overall, the volume of distribution ($V_D$) is 0.2–0.3 L/kg in the absence of disease or infection. The $V_D$ is less in obese individuals. There is a variable increase in the $V_D$ in patients with edema, ascites, burns, bacteremia, and any severe infection with "leaky" capillaries.

### Excretion

Of a given parenteral dose of aminoglycoside, 94% is excreted by the kidney. The remainder is eliminated in feces, saliva, and other body fluids. There is no evidence of in vivo metabolism of any aminoglycoside.

Virtually all of a given dose of aminoglycoside undergoes

glomerular filtration with minimal evidence of secretion by proximal tubular cells. Of filtered drug, approximately 5% is reabsorbed in the proximal tubule and the rest excreted. Urine concentrations exceed plasma levels by 25- to 100-fold within 1 h of parenteral administration. Drug reabsorbed in the proximal tubule cells is subsequently, but slowly, returned to the lumen of the nephron. After termination of administration of several doses of drug, the urine drug levels remain in the therapeutic range for days. The urine terminal half-life is between 48 and 200 h compared with a serum half-life of 1.5–3.0 h. Low levels of drug can be detected in urine for 20 days or longer after discontinuation of therapy.

## Pharmacokinetics

Although some aminoglycosides are administered three times a day, and others twice a day, all the aminoglycosides have similar kinetics. The initial distributive phase requires 15–30 min, hence the suggestion that peak serum levels be collected 30 min after the end of an IV infusion.

The elimination phase of kinetics is determined by the glomerular filtration rate. The half-life, $T_{1/2}$, of aminoglycosides in infants less than 1 week old or in low-birth-weight premature infants is 8–11 h; in neonates who weigh over 2 kg, roughly 5 h; in children and young to middle-aged adults, 1.5–3.0 h; and in older age-groups, somewhere beyond 3.5 h because of age-related decrement in renal function.

## Clinical Indications

### Empiric therapy

The aminoglycosides are employed for empiric therapy in the clinical setting of possible infection due to aerobic gram-negative bacilli. After collection of appropriate specimens for culture, an aminoglycoside is usually combined with one or more of other classes of antimicrobial drugs to increase the likelihood of activity against aerobic cocci and/or anaerobic bacteria. Empiric combination therapy has the added advantage of a possible synergistic or additive antibacterial effect. Examples of clinical settings wherein the empiric use of an aminoglycoside is appropriate is listed in Table 30.3. The list is not all-inclusive, and the companion drugs are meant as examples only.

For additive or synergistic effect against aerobic gram-negative bacilli, it is desirable to combine the aminoglycoside with an antimicrobial with a similar antimicrobial spectrum but a different site of action. Hence, the combination of a cell wall–active penicillin or cephalosporin with the aminoglycoside is frequently used. The fluorinated quinolones interfere with DNA gyrase and thus target a different site than the ribosomal dysfunction induced by aminoglycosides. The combination of ciprofloxacin or ofloxacin with an aminoglycoside is unpredictable with respect to an additive, synergistic, indifferent, or even antagonistic interaction. Imipenem is a $\beta$-lactam highly active against aerobic gram-negative bacilli as well as aerobic cocci and anaerobic organisms. There are no data, however, indicating the value of adding an aminoglycoside to empiric imipenem ther-

**Table 30.3** Examples of clinical settings with a high likelihood of infection with aerobic gram-negative bacilli and consideration of the empiric use of an aminoglycoside antibiotic

| Clinical setting | Other antimicrobial drug(s) considered for combination use |
|---|---|
| Fever without obvious source, possible bacteremia | PRSP, metronidazole, ampicillin, vancomycin, BL/BLI |
| Burn wound infection, possible/probable infective endocarditis | ESP, ESC, BL/BLI, penicillin, ampicillin, vancomycin |
| Intra-abdominal infection: appendicitis, diverticulitis, fecal-soilage peritonitis | Metronidazole, clindamycin, ampicillin, BL/BLI |
| Post-traumatic or postoperative meningitis | Vancomycin, ceftazidime |
| Neutropenia and fever following chemotherapy | ESP |
| Post-traumatic or postoperative septic arthritis or osteomyelitis | Vancomycin, BL/BLI |
| Malignant external otitis media in diabetic patient | ESP, ceftazidime |
| Respirator-associated pneumonia | ESP, ESC, BL/BLI |
| Severe pyelonephritis, | ESP |
| Foley catheter associated | |
| Hospitalized PID | Clindamycin |
| Febrile hospitalized diabetic patient with infected foot | Metronidazole, ampicillin |

Abbreviations: PRSP, penicillinase-resistant semisynthetic penicillins (e.g., nafcillin); BL/BLI, $\beta$-lactam $\beta$-lactamase inhibitor combination (e.g., ticarcillin-clavulanic acid); ESP, extended spectrum penicillin (e.g., ticarcillin, mezlocillin); ESC, extended spectrum cephalosporin (e.g., ceftriaxone, cefotaxime, ceftizoxime).

apy. An exception might be in institutions with *P. aeruginosa*, or other aerobic gram-negative bacilli known to be resistant to imipenem.

The other consideration in selecting companion empiric drug(s) is whether the infection under consideration might be due at least in part to an anaerobic organism, *S. aureus*, *S. pneumoniae*, or *Enterococcus* species. Aminoglycosides have in vitro activity against *S. aureus*, but small colony-resistant strains appear after 24 h of exposure unless a concomitant antistaphylococcal $\beta$-lactam or vancomycin is administered. Aminoglycosides are active against *Enterococcus* species only when combined with penicillin, ampicillin, an extended-spectrum penicillin, or vancomycin. Aminoglycosides have no intrinsic activity against anaerobic organisms or the pneumococcus.

For the above reasons, it is rare to administer an aminoglycoside alone. Aminoglycosides should never be used alone in the febrile neutropenic patient. Dual or triple therapy is often indicated until culture results are available and/or the clinical situation has clarified. The patient with pyelonephritis and visible gram-negative bacilli on a Gram stain of uncentrifuged urine is a reasonable indication for empiric therapy with only an aminoglycoside.

## Specific therapy

Regardless of empiric therapy or in the absence of any prior treatment, culture identification of a pathogen with concomitant in vitro susceptibility test results requires consideration of the wisdom of aminoglycoside therapy as opposed to other active drugs of a different antimicrobial class. As always, the choice of an anti-infective is first and foremost based on anticipated efficacy. Toxic potential, allergy history, convenience of administrations, and expense are other factors in the choice of drug. It may be reasonable to discontinue aminoglycoside therapy (if given empirically) and switch to an equally effective but less potentially toxic alternative. Alternatively, efficacy considerations may require continuing the aminoglycoside with an active $\beta$-lactam. In some instances, monotherapy with an aminoglycoside is indicated.

The specific indications for aminoglycoside therapy are summarized in Table 30.4. The clinical setting is the major determinant. In patients with plague or tularemia, gentamicin or streptomycin have established records of efficacy as monotherapy; in patients with brucellosis, the addition of doxycycline to gentamicin increases efficacy and lowers the rate of relapse.

In contrast, infections with Enterobacteriaceae or *P. aeruginosa*, especially if severe, often require combination therapy for one or two reasons. The prospects for efficacy may be enhanced by two active drugs of differing class or the infection may be polymicrobic and include enterococci or anaerobic gram-negative bacilli. Patients with peritonitis due to contamination by fecal flora may reasonably be given an aminoglycoside, metronidazole, and ampicillin in anticipation of the presence of enterococci and *Bacteroides fragilis*. Patients with respirator-associated pneumonia due to *P. aeruginosa* optimally receive tobramycin plus an active $\beta$-lactam in hope of an additive therapeutic effect; if due to *Serratia* species, gentamicin would be combined with an active $\beta$-lactam.

**Table 30.4** Specific indications for aminoglycoside or spectinomycin therapy

| Pathogens | Aminoglycoside/ aminocyclitol | Drug(s) used in combination |
|---|---|---|
| AEROBIC GRAM-NEGATIVE BACILLI | | |
| *Enterobacter aerogenes* | A, G, N, T | ESP, ESC |
| *Klebsiella* sp. | A, G, N, T | ESP, ESC |
| *Pseudomonas aeruginosa* | T | ESP, APC |
| *Serratia marcescens* | G | ESP, ESC |
| *Yersinia pestis* | G or St | None |
| *Francisella tularensis* | G or St | None |
| *Brucella* sp. | G or St | Doxycycline |
| AEROBIC GRAM-POSITIVE COCCI | | |
| *Enterococcus* sp. | G | Pen G, Ampicillin, ESP |
| *Staphylococcus aureus* | G | Nafcillin |
| *Staphylococcus epidermidis* | G | Vancomycin ± rifampin |
| *Streptococcus viridans* | G | Penicillin |
| MYCOBACTERIA | | |
| *Mycobacterium avium intracellulare* | A | Multiple |
| *Mycobacterium tuberculosis* | St | Multiple |
| PROTOZOA | | |
| *Cryptosporidium parvum* | P (oral only) | None |
| *Entamoeba histolytica* | P (oral only) | None |
| *Neisseria gonorrhoeae* | Sp | Doxycycline for concomitant *C. trachomatis* |

Abbreviations: A, amikacin; G, gentamicin; N, netilmicin; P, paromomycin; Sp, spectinomycin; St, streptomycin; T, tobramycin; ESP, extended-spectrum penicillin; ESC, extended-spectrum cephalosporin; APC, antipseudomonal cephalosporin

Endocarditis due to gram-positive cocci often results in aminoglycoside therapy but for differing reasons (see Chapter 69). Penicillin or ampicillin with concomitant gentamicin for 4–6 weeks is a necessity to ensure bactericidal activity in patients with enterococcal endocarditis. In patients with endocarditis due to *viridan streptococci*, the addition of an aminoglycoside to penicillin is a strategy to reduce the duration of therapy from the standard 4 weeks to 2 weeks. For patients with *Staphylococcus epidermidis* prosthetic valve endocarditis, gentamicin is combined with vancomycin and rifampin to increase efficacy for at least the first 2 weeks of combination therapy. For patients with *Staphylococcus aureus* endocarditis, adding gentamicin to standard nafcillin or oxacillin therapy shortens the duration of bacteremia by 1–2 days; there is no clear need to continue the gentamicin beyond 3–5 days.

In patients with disseminated *Mycobacterium avium intracellulare* infections, the only aminoglycoside that might be considered as part of combination therapy is amikacin. The availability of clarithromycin, rifabutin, ethambutol, and clofazamine has placed amikacin in the role of secondary therapy. Similarly, streptomycin is a second-line drug for *Mycobacterium tuberculosis* therapy. In areas with multidrug-resistant *M. tuberculosis*, streptomycin may be included in empiric and/or specific treatment regimens.

Paromomycin is the only drug, to date, that has shown some measure of efficacy against cryptosporidia infections in patients with AIDS. It is only given orally. Like neomycin, it is too toxic for parenteral therapy.

Spectinomycin is an aminocyclitol, given parenterally, for *N. gonorrhoeae*. Spectinomycin has no activity against concomitant *Chlamydia* infection.

## Prophylaxis

Aminoglycosides are recommended as prophylactic anti-infectives in two situations. Genitourinary and gastrointestinal surgical procedures may be associated with enterococcal bacteremia. Patients with valvular heart disease are at risk for endocarditis and prophylaxis with the combination of ampicillin and gentamicin is recommended. In the patient allergic to penicillin, vancomycin is substituted for the ampicillin.

In patients scheduled for elective colectomy, the combination of mechanical cleansing plus oral neomycin and erythromycin reduces the risk of surgical infection. One gram of each drug is given three times during the 18–24 h prior to surgery.

## Resistance

Microbial resistance is usually the result of bacterial enzymes adenylating, acetylating, or phosphorylating aminoglycosides with subsequent loss of antibacterial activity. Less often encountered mechanisms are alteration of the drug binding site on ribosomes or reduced uptake of drug because of decreased cell wall permeability.

Genes encoding enzymatic resistance are acquired via conjugative or nonconjugative plasmids. Resistance genes are associated with transposable genetic elements called transposons. Once acquired, gene transcription is constitutive. Less is known about the genetic basis of other mechanisms of resistance.

Enterococci resistant to the synergistic interaction of a penicillin plus an aminoglycoside are of particular import. Resistance can result from a $\beta$-lactamase that hydrolyzes the penicillin or an aminoglycoside-modifying enzyme or both. The aminoglycoside-modifying enzymes are encoded by plasmids or transposons. In patients with endocarditis due to enterococci, the patient's isolate should be tested for high-level (MIC above 2000 $\mu$g/ml) resistance to gentamicin; if present, there is a loss of the synergy with a cell wall–active penicillin.

Resistance of aerobic gram-negative bacilli to gentamicin, tobramycin, netilmicin, and amikacin varies with the magnitude of aminoglycoside use, the patient population, and the types of infections. In institutions with modest usage, overall rates of resistance vary from 0 to 5% among clinical isolates of *P. aeruginosa* and Enterobacteriaceae. Outbreaks of resistant organisms have occurred after intense use for prophylaxis in burn patients and in the intensive care unit setting. Exclusive use of one aminoglycoside tends to select, albeit slowly, for resistant organisms to that drug. In contrast to some $\beta$-lactams, resistance to aminoglycosides rarely emerges during therapy. The rare emergence of resistance occurs in situations requiring protracted treatment, such as cystic fibrosis, or where the inocula of bacteria is very large, e.g., in an infected burn wound.

## Toxicity

### General

With the exception of the aminocyclitol spectinomycin, all aminoglycosides are potentially toxic to the cells of the renal proximal tubule and the hair cells of the cochlea and the vestibular apparatus. Neuromuscular blockade occurs rarely in circumstances wherein a sudden increase to high serum concentrations occurs.

Estimates of the incidence of nephrotoxicity and ototoxicity vary widely as a result of differences in definition of toxicity and the sensitivity of measurement employed to detect toxicity. Nephrotoxicity is reported in 0–50% of patients, with most reports in the 5%–25% range. The incidence of cochlear toxicity is 3%–14% and vestibular injury is 4%–6%. Neuromuscular blockade is exceedingly rare.

Aminoglycosides are not associated with adverse effects often encountered with other classes of antimicrobial drugs. Thus, hypersensitivity reactions are uncommon; phlebitis at infusion sites is rare; IM injections do not become painful; instillation into the pleural space, abdominal cavity, or cerebrospinal fluid is free of irritation; and incorporation into methylmethacrylate prosthetic joint cement is well tolerated over long periods of time. The aminoglycosides are not hepatotoxic, do not induce photosensitivity, and have no known adverse influence on the coagulation cascade or hematopoiesis.

### Pathogenesis of nephrotoxicity

Aminoglycosides undergo glomerular filtration with subsequent binding to low-affinity high-capacity receptors on the brush border of proximal tubular cells. Only a small percentage of filtered drug binds. The bound drug is rapidly internalized by endocytosis, but the fate of internalized drug remains incompletely understood. There is a clear interaction with lysosomes. The result is generation of phospholipid-rich liposomal membranes in a whorl-like structure that resembles the myelin sheath; these structures are called myeloid bodies (or cytosegresomes by some authors). The myeloid bodies are found in the urine as a result of slow excretion by the cell or as a result of cell death. Myeloid bodies are not unique to aminoglycosides but occur after tubular cell exposure to a variety of other cationic amphiphilic drugs.

Dysfunction of a variety of other biochemical processes and cell organelles has been described. Aminoglycosides interfere with enzymes of the cell membrane phosphatidyinositol cascade. Functional abnormalities of mitochondria, ribosomes, and other cell membrane enzymes are well described. It is not clear whether there is a primary site of toxicity and then epiphenomena in injured or dying cells or whether there is simultaneous toxicity at multiple sites. Recent data hold the potential of explaining the intracellular trafficking of aminoglycosides. The endocytic receptor named megalin may be the means of delivering membrane bound gentamicin to endosomes. Regardless, death of the cell requires several days in the intact animal, which suggests the presence of an as-yet unidentified detoxifying mechanism(s). Clinically, the death of proximal tubule cells is reflected by a rise in the serum creatinine. Death or injury to the proximal tubule cells results initially in impairment of reabsorption of sodium and then in a decrease in glomerular filtration.

**Table 30.5** Risk factors for aminoglycoside nephrotoxicity

| Factors that increase risk of toxicity | Factors that decrease risk of toxicity |
|---|---|
| PATIENT FACTORS | |
| Older patients | Younger patients |
| Pre-existing renal disease | Normal renal function |
| Volume depletion, hypotension | Normotensive |
| Hepatic dysfunction | No hepatic dysfunction |
| AMINOGLYCOSIDE FACTORS | |
| Larger daily dose | Smaller daily dose |
| Treatment beyond 3 days | Treatment less than 3 days |
| Drug choice: e.g., gentamicin | Drug choice: e.g., tobramycin |
| Frequent dosing interval | Once-daily dosing |
| CONCOMITANT DRUGS | |
| Vancomycin | Carbenicillin |
| Amphotericin B | Ticarcillin |
| Furosemide | |
| IV radiocontrast | |

## Clinical nephrotoxicity

Aminoglycoside-induced renal injury is most often mild in severity. The most common manifestation is a nonoliguric fall in creatinine clearance. Progression to oliguric dialysis-dependent renal failure is uncommon. Furthermore, at least 3 days of drug exposure are usually required before the cell injury is of sufficient magnitude to be detected by a rising serum creatinine. Hence, the rapid onset of severe oliguric or anuric renal failure should prompt consideration of other potential etiologies of acute renal failure. Some patients have multiple risk factors for renal injury.

Risk factors for aminoglycoside nephrotoxicity can be divided into those that relate to the patient's underlying disease(s), the acute infectious disease that prompted aminoglycoside administration, frequency of aminoglycoside administration, and the concomitant administration of drugs known to alter the risk of renal injury (Table 30.5).

If the aminoglycoside is the nephrotoxic agent, the prognosis for recovery of renal function is excellent. Renal tubular cells can regenerate. In animal models and in patients, recovery from acute tubular necrosis occurs even if the aminoglycoside administration continues. The time to recovery varies from a few days to several weeks.

In models of nephrotoxicity in uninfected animals with no concomitant disease process, tobramycin is consistently less nephrotoxic than gentamicin. However, clinical trials in infected patients with a variety of underlying concomitant diseases have produced mixed results. One randomized prospective trial found a lower incidence of nephrotoxicity in tobramycin recipients, but other trials have produced mixed results.

The dosing interval was first shown to influence the risk of nephrotoxicity in animal models. When the total daily dose is held constant, the risk of nephrotoxicity increased with the frequency of dose administration. Similarly, many studies now show that patients receiving 80 mg three times a day are at greater risk than patients receiving 240 mg once a day.

Ill patients often require administration of a variety of different drugs. At least in adults, concomitant vancomycin increases the risk of renal injury. The mechanism is unclear in that modern preparations of vancomycin have virtually no nephrotoxic potential when administered alone.

In clinical trials that compared the combination of cephalothin plus an aminoglycoside with that of a penicillin plus an aminoglycoside, the risk of nephrotoxicity was greatest in the cephalothin–aminoglycoside combination. However, without an aminoglycoside-only group, it is not possible to separate an influence of the cephalosporin from the influence of the aminoglycoside.

Amphotericin B, foscarnet, and some IV radiocontrast agents have their own inherent toxicity. Furosemide may increase the toxic risk indirectly by reducing intravascular volume. Clindamycin was identified as a risk factor by statistical analysis of clinical trials. No mechanism is apparent. Two drugs, cyclosporin and *cis*-Platinum, have inherent nephrotoxic potential and amplify aminoglycoside toxicity in animals, but neither have been identified as risk factors for nephrotoxicity in clinical trials.

An aminoglycoside in combination with an extended spectrum penicillin is a standard empiric regimen for febrile neutropenic patients. The reported incidence of nephrotoxicity is only 2%–6% and suggests a protective effect of the penicillin. In animal studies, carbenicillin and ticarcillin have the greatest "protective effect"; one report described no protection by piperacillin.

A high trough serum level is often mentioned as a risk factor. The higher the trough serum level the longer the period of time drug is filtered and hence available for interaction with the cells of the proximal tubule. A high trough level results from dosage miscalculation or some impairment of glomerular filtration. With three-times-a-day dosing, low but detectable serum levels are desired just prior to the next dose; with once-daily dosing in patients with normal renal function, there is no detectable drug in serum for several hours at the end of a dosage interval. Hence, the trough serum level depends on the dosage regimen employed and the excretory ability of the kidney. The greater the dose of aminoglycoside, the higher the trough serum level and the greater the risk of toxicity. In a patient with a low trough serum level initially, a subsequent increase in the trough level is an indirect measurement of a reduced glomerular filtration rate.

## Cochlear toxicity

### Risk

Neurosensory hearing loss is a risk after administration of any of the aminoglycosides, but neomycin is the most dangerous and thus is not used systemically. Cochlear damage was recognized soon after the introduction of streptomycin into clinical practice. Modification of a simple streptomycin aldehyde group to an alcohol group produces dihydrostreptomycin; streptomycin is primarily vestibulotoxic whereas dihydrostreptomycin is primarily ototoxic.

The risk of cochlear damage is increased by concomitant vancomycin or "loop" diuretics. Loud ambient noise also heightens risk. There is a correlation between both dose and duration of therapy with risk of cochlear injury. In experimental animals, once-daily dosing reduced the risk.

It is of great interest that familial aminoglycoside-induced deafness has been described in several family pedigrees from the Far East and Middle East. A maternal inheritance pattern was observed and subsequently lead to identification of a mutation in the 12S rRNA mitochondrial gene.

### Pathogenesis

The toxic target of aminoglycosides is the outer hair cells of the basal turns of the organ of Corti. The nature of the interaction is unclear. Aminoglycosides can be detected in inner ear fluids but their concentration never exceeds serum levels. In experimental animals, inner ear tissues were saturated with gentamicin roughly 3 h after administration. However, cochlear damage, measured by brainstem-evoked potentials, was not detectable until after 3 weeks of daily injections.

The morbid anatomy is similar to kidney tubular cells. Lysosomal changes (myeloid bodies) are present with biochemical evidence of inhibition of phosphatidyl inositol metabolism.

### Detection

The hair cells of the basal turn of the organ of Corti detect high-frequency sounds to 20 kHz. Conversational speech is in the 0.3–3 kHz range. Even in the frequency range of normal conversation, a hearing threshold loss of 20–30 dB is necessary for patient awareness of the deficit. Hence, a great deal of hair cell damage occurs prior to patient recognition.

Clinical detection requires pure tone audiometry with an instrument designed to test high frequencies. In hospitalized febrile confused patients, meaningful bedside audiometry is rarely possible. If audiograms are done several days into aminoglycoside therapy, interpretation is difficult because elderly patients often have pre-existing high-frequency neurosensory hearing loss.

### Clinical

Cochlear injury is frustrating because of its unpredictability. Three or more days of therapy are a prerequisite. Some patients complain of tinnitus or a "fullness" in the ears. The hearing loss may be gradual with no associated symptoms, or it can occur rapidly without warning. It may be unilateral or bilateral. It can become apparent during drug therapy or within 1–2 weeks after the end of therapy. It is unusual to have associated vestibular or renal toxicity. Cochlear damage is traditionally described as irreversible. However, evidence of regeneration of cochlear cells has been demonstrated in animal models of ototoxicity.

### Prevention

Aminoglycosides are often given empirically. In many clinical circumstances it is desirable to substitute an effective non-aminoglycoside antimicrobial (a $\beta$-lactam or fluoroquinolone) when culture and sensitivity results become available. The necessary concomitant use of loop diuretics, vancomycin, or erythromycin may be reasons to avoid prolonged aminoglycoside use if other active agents are available.

In patients in whom weeks of aminoglycoside therapy is unavoidable (e.g., enterococcal endocarditis), it may be reasonable to perform serial audiometry.

## Vestibular toxicity

The site of aminoglycoside injury is the type 1 hair cell of the summit of the ampullar cristae. Less is known about vestibular toxicity in that animal studies are difficult and both animals and humans compensate for vestibular dysfunction by using visual and proprioceptive cues. Hence, patients can suffer substantial injury prior to overt symptoms or clinical findings.

The acute onset of vestibular injury is often manifest as nausea and vomiting secondary to vertigo. Nystagmus may be evident. If available, electronystagmography can confirm the diagnosis. Over time, symptoms abate. However, patients may have long-term symptoms in the dark or when eyes are closed or in other situations that block compensatory pathways.

Streptomycin is more likely to cause vestibular toxicity than the other commonly used aminoglycosides.

## Neuromuscular blockade

Neuromuscular blockade is a rare but life-threatening complication of aminoglycoside therapy. It has been described after exposure to all the aminoglycosides, but most frequently, neomycin. A rapid rise in serum drug levels usually precedes onset. Other risk factors include infant botulism, myasthenia gravis, paralysis with D-tubocurare or succinylcholine, hypomagnesemia, hypocalcemia, and perhaps calcium channel blockers.

Weakness of respiratory muscles leading to respiratory arrest is the most serious complication. Associated findings include flaccid paralysis, dilated pupils, and absent deep tendon reflexes.

The mechanism is inhibition of the presynaptic release of acetylcholine and blockade of the postsynaptic receptor sites for acetylcholine. The presynaptic release of acetylcholine requires calcium internalization; aminoglycosides block calcium internalization. The neuromuscular blockade is reversed rapidly by giving IV calcium gluconate.

The risk of neuromuscular blockade is lessened by avoidance of instillation of an aminoglycoside solution into a body cavity. Furthermore, the duration of IV infusions of aminoglycosides should extend over a minimum of 20–30 min.

## Administration of Aminoglycosides

The aminoglycosides are licensed for multiple administrations per day to patients with normal renal function—i.e., twice a day for streptomycin and amikacin and three times a day for gentamicin, tobramycin, and netilmicin. Currently, there is interest in once-daily aminoglycoside therapy. Each method is described for treatment of adults. Dosing methods in children and other special circumstances are described separately.

## Multiple daily dosing

### Loading dose

Aminoglycoside regimens are divided into an initial (loading) dose and subsequent maintenance doses. When the renal function is good (estimated endogenous creatinine clearance of 80 ml/min or higher), the loading and maintenance doses may be identical. With decrements in renal function, the maintenance dose is reduced.

Recommended loading doses for the aminoglycosides are summarized in Table 30.6. The purpose of a loading dose is to rapidly achieve a peak plasma concentration that exceeds the MIC/MBC for susceptible aerobic gram-negative bacilli. Important variables in the selection of a loading dose are body weight and anticipated volume of distribution. The loading dose calculation is independent of renal function.

Dosing weight in kilograms is calculated from formulae for ideal body weight as follows:

Female: 45 kg + 2.3 kg/inch of height over 5 ft

Male: 50 kg + 2.3 kg/inch of height over 5 ft

The dose is adjusted upward if there is more than a 30% difference between the actual and the ideal body weight (IBW) due to the altered volume of distribution to adipose tissue. The formula used is:

$$\text{Loading dose weight} = \text{IBW} + 0.4\,(\text{actual weight} - \text{IBW})$$

The results of clinical trials demonstrate a frequent failure of calculated loading doses to achieve targeted peak concentrations. The reason is probably failure to consider an altered volume of distribution ($V_D$) of drug. In uninfected healthy volunteers, the $V_D$ is 0.2–0.3 L/kg. The $V_D$ increases in patients with edematous states (ascites, congestive heart failure), in burn patients, and as a result of infection-induced "leaky" capillaries. At present, there is no way clinically to calculate the $V_D$. Because the peak serum level correlates with efficacy and because experience indicates frequent underdosing, it is suggested that the febrile critically ill patient have a loading dose that is at, or somewhat above, the calculated dose so as to account for a likely or possible increased $V_D$. Because of the obvious uncertainties, a peak serum level should be measured after either the loading dose or after the first maintenance dose.

### Maintenance dose

Excretion of aminoglycosides is primarily via the kidney. Hence, the maintenance dose requires an estimation of renal function. Calculation of the endogenous creatinine clearance (CrCL) is used to estimate the glomerular filtration rate. The equation of Cockcroft and Gault is used to calculate the estimated CrCL:

$$\text{CrCL} = \left[\frac{(140 - \text{age})(\text{ideal wt in kg})^*}{\text{Serum creatinine} \times 72}\right] = \text{CrCL in ml/min}$$

*For females, multiply answer by 0.85

The suggested maintenance doses for various levels of renal function are provided in Table 30.7. In critically ill patients, renal function often changes rapidly, and it is desirable to recalculate the maintenance dose frequently and to validate the results with measurements of peak and trough serum levels (discussed below).

If the estimated CrCL is below 80 ml/min, a reduced maintenance dose is necessary to avoid drug accumulation. Reduction can be accomplished by an extension of the dosage interval, reduction of the individual dose, or a combination of both. Table 30.7 provides dosage guidance for extension of the dosage interval. The advantages of this method are a maintenance of high peak serum levels for efficacy and convenience of dosage intervals that are some multiple of 12 with avoidance of every 36 h or every 60 h dosage.

The dose reduction method is not shown but is calculated easily as:

$$\text{New maintenance dose} = \frac{\text{CrCL}}{100} \times \begin{matrix}\text{maintenance dose for}\\ \text{CrCL over 80 ml/min}\end{matrix}$$

The calculated dose is given at the standard 8 or 12 h interval. A theoretic concern with this method is the fall in achieved peak serum levels that parallel the fall in renal function.

The aminoglycosides are removed by hemodialysis. It is necessary to administer a supplemental dose at the end of each hemodialysis (Table 30.7). The dosage suggested is based on an average clearance of approximately two-thirds of the circulating aminoglycoside. However, clearance in individual patients is unpredictable because of variable patient hemodynamics and other variables related to the specific dialyzer employed. Hence, in critical patients, it is mandatory to measure peak serum levels to en-

**Table 30.6** Multiple daily dosing: suggested loading doses, maintenance doses, and targeted serum concentrations of aminoglycosides in adult patients with an estimated creatinine clearance above 80 ml/min

| | | Daily maintenance dose | | Target serum concentrations ($\mu$g/ml) | |
|---|---|---|---|---|---|
| Drug[a] | Loading dose (mg/kg) | Total (mg/g) | Divided (mg/kg) | Peak | Trough |
| Gentamicin | 2 | 5.1 | 1.7 q8h | 4–10 | 1–2 |
| Tobramycin | 2 | 5.1 | 1.7 q8h | 4–10 | 1–2 |
| Netilmicin | 2 | 6 | 2 q8h | 4–10 | 1–2 |
| Amikacin | 7.5 | 15 | 7.5 q12h | 15–30 | 5–10 |
| Streptomycin[b] | 7.5 | 15 | 7.5 q12h | 15–30 | 5–10 |

[a]All drugs, including streptomycin can be given IM or IV.

[b]Maximum daily dose 2.0 g. Can administer 1.0 g IM (or IV) daily for tuberculosis.

**Table 30.7** Multiple daily dosing method: adjustment of dosage of aminoglycoside antibiotics in patients with variable degrees of impaired renal function using the method of prolongation of the dosage interval*

| Drug | Maintenance dose for normal renal function (mg/kg) | Estimated creatinine clearance (ml/min) | | | | Supplement after hemodialysis[a] (mg/kg) | Supplement during CAVH[a] mg/kg/day | Supplement during CAPD |
|---|---|---|---|---|---|---|---|---|
| | | 80–90 | 50–80 | 10–50 | <10 | | | |
| Gentamicin | 1.7 q8h | q12h | q12–24h | q24–48h | q48–72h | 1–2 | 2.5 | 3–4 mg lost/liter of dialysate/day[b] |
| Tobramycin | 1.7 q8h | q12h | q12–24h | q24–48h | q48–72h | 1–2 | 2.5 | 3–4 mg lost/liter[b] of dialysate/day |
| Netilmicin | 2 q8h | q12h | q12–24h | q24–48h | q48–72h | 2 | 2.5 | 3–4 mg lost/liter[b] of dialysate/day |
| Amikacin | 7.5 q12h | q12h | q12–24h | q24–48h | q48–72h | 5–7 | 4.0 | 15–20 mg lost per liter[c] of dialysate/day |

*Also shown are suggested doses of aminoglycoside for patients requiring hemodialysis, continuous arteriovenous hemofiltration (CAVH), and continuous ambulatory peritoneal dialysis (CAPD).

[a]Rate and absolute amount of drug removed influenced by a variety of host disease and dialysis-related factors. In critically ill patients, serum aminoglycoside levels should be monitored.

[b]Replace IV the 3–4 mg lost per liter of dialysate per day. Typically, 8 L/day × 4 mg/L = 32 mg.

[c]Replace IV 15–20 mg lost per liter of dialysate per day; e.g., 8 L × 20 mg/day = 160 mg.

sure therapeutic efficacy. The desired peak levels are those shown in Table 30.6.

Aminoglycosides given IV or IM are removed in the dialysate of patients undergoing continuous ambulatory peritoneal dialysis (CAPD). The standard procedure is to place 2 L of dialysis fluid in the abdomen, allow the fluid to "dwell" 6 h, and then repeat the process for a total of 8 L of dialysate in 24 h. The anticipated number of milligrams of aminoglycoside removed per liter of dialysate is summarized in Table 30.7 and allows calculation of the number of milligrams to be replaced over 24 h. Note that this is different from treating infection of the peritoneal fluid by addition of aminoglycosides to the dialysis fluid. The initial and maintenance doses of aminoglycosides for treatment of CAPD peritonitis are summarized in Table 30.8. In patients with severe CAPD peritonitis complicated by possible/documented bacteremia, initial therapy may include both parenteral and intraperitoneal therapy.

Continuous arteriovenous hemofiltration (CAVH) is employed with increasing frequency in the management of critically ill patients. The efficiency of CAVH depends on patient hemodynamics and the efficiency of individual filters. The result is kidney-like function at the equivalent of a creatinine clearance of between 10 and 50 ml/min. It is suggested that the "cleared" gentamicin be replaced via a dedicated IV access site in a once-daily dosage (Table 30.7). The achievement of the desired peak and trough concentration should be documented (see Table 30.6).

**Table 30.8** Intraperitoneal instillation of aminoglycosides to treat CAPD peritonitis

| Aminoglycoside | Dose (mg/2 L dialysis bag) | |
|---|---|---|
| | Initial | Maintenance |
| Gentamicin | 70–140 | 8–16 |
| Tobramycin | 70–140 | 8–16 |
| Netilmicin | 70–140 | 8–16 |
| Amikacin | 500 | 12–15 |

### Serum level measurements

Peak serum levels are needed to validate that the peak level is high enough to insure antibacterial efficacy. Peak levels are of particular import in patients with edematous states, bacteremia-induced leaky capillaries, or any other disease state with a likely altered volume of drug distribution. Trough serum levels are obtained to validate estimates of renal function. If the trough level is higher than predicted, it indicates renal functional impairment of greater magnitude than anticipated. After any necessary dosage adjustments, there is usually no need to repeat aminoglycoside serum levels unless there is a change in renal function. While administering aminoglycosides, it is reasonable to determine the serum creatinine concentration two times per week.

### Children

The suggested aminoglycoside regimen for neonates, infants, and children is summarized in Table 30.9. The dosages reflect altered pharmacokinetics because of the interplay of reduced renal clearance in a newborn combined with a larger $V_D$. Because the pharmacokinetics are unpredictable, peak and trough serum levels should be measured.

Kanamycin (because of the frequency of resistance among Enterobacteriaceae) and streptomycin (because of the risk of ototoxicity) should not be used in children and are not shown in Table 30.9.

### Cystic fibrosis

Owing to a combination of an altered volume of distribution, increased glomerular clearance, and a reduced serum half-life, the required dosage of parenteral aminoglycosides in patients with cystic fibrosis may be double the usual dose to achieve desired peak serum levels. Patients may require protracted parenteral therapy with a resultant high incidence of cochlear damage.

The risk of 8th nerve toxicity is reduced, without loss of antibacterial efficacy, by aerosol administration of drug. A well-studied regimen is 600 mg of tobramycin in saline, delivered three times daily by an ultrasonic nebulizer with specific speci-

**Table 30.9** Suggested aminoglycoside dosage regimens for neonates, infants, and children

| | Drug and dosage (mg/kg per day)[a] | | | |
|---|---|---|---|---|
| Age | Gentamicin | Tobramycin | Netilmicin | Amikacin |
| 0–7 days[b] | 5 | 4 | 5 | 15–20 |
| Infants | 5–7.5 | 5 | 7.5 | 20–30 |
| Children | 6–7.5 | 6–7.5 | 7.5 | 15 |

[a]Given in two or three divided doses.

[b]Assumes birth weight of 2000–2500 g or greater. Dose reduction necessary for neonates of lower weight.

fications. A commercial preparation of aerosolized tobromycin was recently approved by the FDA. The result of aerosolized tobromycin is therapeutic efficacy with reduced toxicity.

## Once-daily administration

### Premise

The motivation for administering aminoglycosides in a single daily infusion evolved from four separate but related experimental observations. First, experimental nephrotoxicity and ototoxicity were less severe in animals given a single daily dose as opposed to the same total milligrams given in divided doses daily. Rats administered a single daily dose accumulated less drug in the renal cortex. Similarly, patients scheduled for elective nephrectomy were randomized to standard q8h aminoglycoside or continuous infusion of drug for several days. The highest renal cortex drug concentrations were found in the patients given continuous infusions.

Second, aminoglycosides demonstrate a postantibiotic effect (PAE) against aerobic gram-negative bacilli both in vitro and in vivo. The higher the peak aminoglycoside concentrations, the longer the PAE. In neutropenic animals, the in vivo PAE is similar to the in vitro PAE of 1–3 h. In non-neutropenic animals, the in vivo PAE can extend to 12 h or longer. In vivo, the serum concentrations of drug can fall below the MIC of susceptible bacteria for several hours without loss of efficacy.

The third observation is that in in vitro systems, the rate of bacterial killing is proportional to the peak drug concentration.

Finally, once-daily dosing avoids the theoretical negative influence of adaptive resistance. Prolonged exposure of aerobic gram-negative bacilli to aminoglycosides results in an attenuation of their bactericidal activity. This adaptive resistance disappears within a few hours of the drug concentration falling below the MIC of the target organism.

Hence, a single daily, large bolus of drug results in a high peak serum concentration and, depending on renal function, an end of dosage interval period of several hours with no detectable drug in the bloodstream. The latter reduces the drug exposure time of kidney, cochlear, and vestibular sites of potential toxicity.

This premise has been tested in animal models of infection. Nephrotoxicity was reduced and antibacterial efficacy preserved

**Table 30.10** Suggested once-daily dosage regimens of gentamicin and tobramycin in patients with estimated creatinine clearnce (Est CrCl) between 20 and 100 mg/min; every other day regimens for creatinine clearance below 20 ml/min*

| Est CrCl (ml/min) | Dosage interval (h) | Dose (mg/kg) | $T_{1/2}$ (h) | Estimated serum level μg/ml at 1 h | 12 h | 18 h | 24 h |
|---|---|---|---|---|---|---|---|
| 100 | 24 | 5 | 2.5 | 20 | 1.0 | <1 | <1 |
| 90 | 24 | 5 | 3.1 | 20 | 2.0 | <1 | <1 |
| 80 | 24 | 5 | 3.4 | 20 | 2.5 | <1 | <1 |
| 70 | 24 | 4 | 3.9 | 16 | 2.0 | <1 | <1 |
| 60 | 24 | 4 | 4.5 | 16 | 3.0 | 1.5 | <1 |
| 50 | 24 | 3.5 | 5.3 | 14 | 3.5 | 1.0 | <1 |
| 40 | 24 | 2.5 | 6.5 | 10 | 3.0 | 1.5 | <1 |
| 30 | 24 | 2.5 | 8.4 | 10 | 4.0 | 2.5 | 1.5 |
| | | | | 1 h | 24 h | 36 h | 48 h |
| 20 | 48 | 4.0 | 11.9 | 16 | 4.0 | 2.0 | 1.0 |
| 10 | 48 | 3.0 | 20.4 | 12 | 5.0 | 3.0 | 2.0 |
| 0[a] (hemodialysis) | 48 | 2.0 | 69.3 | 8 | 7.0 | 6.0 | 5.0 |

*Predicted peak and trough serum levels are shown. Peak levels are calculated as follows:

$$\frac{\text{mg/kg administered} \times \text{kg body wt}}{V_D \text{ (L/Kg)} \times \text{kg body weight}}$$

Trough levels are calculated from peak concentration and published $T_{1/2}$ hours at varying levels of renal function.

[a]Example values for patient receiving hemodialysis every other day. Actual peak depends on efficiency of dialysis. Dose given postdialysis.

in both abscess and pneumonia models. In experimental *Pseudomonas aeruginosa* pneumonia in neutropenic guinea pigs, it was necessary to co-administer an active $\beta$-lactam to preserve antibacterial efficacy in the animals dosed once a day. It is important to note that once-a-day dosing has not proved efficacious in animal models of infective endocarditis.

### Clinical experience

The clinical experience with once-daily aminoglycosides now encompasses a wide range of patient groups, including critically ill and neutropenic patients. In most studies, and in all the trials including neutropenic patients, the aminoglycoside was administered with a concomitant $\beta$-lactam active against aerobic gram-negative bacilli. The various trials have employed gentamicin, tobramycin, netilmicin, or amikacin. There is no apparent difference between the drugs, and overall, there are no reports of failure or decrease in antibacterial efficacy. There is evidence of a reduction in the frequency, and prolongation of time to onset, of renal injury. No meaningful ototoxicity data are available.

The majority of clinical trials have compared the FDA-approved multiple daily dose regimen with the same dose as a single administration—e.g., gentamicin 1.7 mg/kg every 8 h vs. 5.1 mg/kg as a single infusion. One group has reported experience with over 2100 patients administered gentamicin or tobramycin in a dosage of 7 mg/kg per day. Toxicity rates were very low, with no evidence of decrease in efficacy.

### Dosing procedure

With once-daily administration, each dose is a loading dose. An estimated creatinine clearance is calculated using the patient's ideal body weight and the Cockcroft and Gault formula. Until more information is available, it is suggested that patients with an estimated creatinine clearance of 80 ml/min or greater receive gentamicin or tobramycin in a dosage of 5.1 mg/kg per day, netilmicin at 6 mg/kg per day, and amikacin at 15 mg/kg per day. For patients with an estimated creatinine clearance <80, the mg/kg dose is decreased with maintenance of a 24 h dosage interval (Tables 30.10 and 30.11). Note that as renal function declines, the serum half-life, $T_{1/2}$, lengthens progressively, the dosage decreases, the peak serum level decreases, and the period of time at the end of the dosage interval dependent on a PAE shortens progressively.

For an every-8-h or every-12-h dosage regimen, the usual infusion time is 15–30 min. With the larger dose of once-daily reg-

**Table 30.11** Suggested once-daily dosage regimens of netilmicin, amikacin, kanamycin, and streptomycin in patietns with estimated creatinine clearnce (Est CrCl) between 20 and 90 ml/min; every-other-day regimen for creatinine clearance below 20 mg/min*

| Est CrCl (ml/min) | Dosage interval (h) | Dose (mg/kg) | $T_{1/2}$ (h) | Estimated serum level μg/ml at | | | |
|---|---|---|---|---|---|---|---|
| | | | | 1 h | 12 h | 18 h | 24 h |
| NETILMICIN | | | | | | | |
| 90 | 24 | 6.5 | 3.1 | 26 | 2 | <1 | <1 |
| 70 | 24 | 5.0 | 3.9 | 20 | 2.5 | 1.0 | <1 |
| 50 | 24 | 4.0 | 5.3 | 16 | 4 | 1 | <1 |
| 30 | 24 | 2.0 | 8.4 | 8 | 3 | 2 | 1 |
| | | | | 1 h | 24 h | 36 h | 48 h |
| 20 | 48 | 3.0 | 11.9 | 13 | 3.0 | 1.5 | 0.75 |
| 10 | 48 | 2.5 | 20.4 | 10 | 4.0 | 3 | 2 |
| 0[a] (hemodialysis) | 48 | 2.0 | 69.3 | 8 | 7.0 | 6 | 5 |
| AMIKACIN, KANAMYCIN, STREPTOMYCIN | | | | 1 h | 12 h | 18 h | 24 h |
| 90 | 24 | 15 | 3.1 | 60 | 6.0 | <1 | <1 |
| 70 | 24 | 12 | 3.9 | 48 | 9.0 | 2.5 | <1 |
| 50 | 24 | 7.5 | 5.3 | 30 | 7.0 | 3.5 | 1.0 |
| 30 | 24 | 4.0 | 8.4 | 20 | 7.5 | 5.0 | 3.0 |
| | | | | 1 h | 24 h | 36 h | 48 h |
| 20 | 48 | 7.5 | 11.9 | 30 | 7.5 | 3.3 | 1.6 |
| 10 | 48 | 4.0 | 20.4 | 16 | 12 | 5.0 | 3.0 |
| 0[a] (hemodialysis) | 48 | 3.0 | 69.3 | 20 | 16 | 15 | 12 |

*Predicted peak and trough serum levels are shown. Peak levels are calculated as follows:

$$\frac{\text{mg/kg administered} \times \text{kg body wt}}{V_D\ (\text{L/kg}) \times \text{kg body weight}}$$

Trough levels are calculated from peak concentration and published $T_{1/2}$ hours at varying levels of renal function.

[a]Example values for patient receiving hemodialysis every other day. Actual peak depends on efficiency of dialysis. Dose given postdialysis.

imens, it is suggested that the infusion time be extended to 60 min as a precaution against possible neuromuscular blockade.

Peak serum levels are measured to ensure efficacy. With the large once-daily dosage, concern over failure to achieve the suggested targeted peak level (Tables 30.10, 30.11) arises in septic patients or other situations with a larger than usual $V_D$. In multiple clinical trials, the peak serum levels were often lower than anticipated because of the altered $V_D$. Hence, in critically ill patients, it is reasonable to obtain a peak serum level (10–15 min after the end of the infusion) after the first dose of drug.

In patients with a creatinine clearance over 80 mL/min who achieve targeted peak serum concentrations, the serum level should be undetectable 18 h later (Tables 30.10, 30.11). Serum levels above 1 $\mu$g/mL at 18 h suggest impairment of renal excretion; a repeat serum creatinine and recalculation of the estimated creatinine clearance and reassessment of the size of the daily dose are in order.

## ANNOTATED BIBLIOGRAPHY


Aronoff, GR. Drug Prescribing in Renal Failure, 4th ed. Philadelphia, American College of Physicians, 1998.

*Because the aminoglycosides are cleared almost exclusively by the renal route, dosage adjustment of aminoglycosides is necessary for any incremental fall in the glomerular filtration rate. This pocket monograph provides guidance for aminoglycosides and other commonly prescribed drugs.*

Brummett RE, Fox KE. Aminoglycoside-induced hearing loss in humans. Antimicrob Agents Chemother 1989; 33:797–800.

*A state-of-the-art review by career investigators in the field.*

Craig WA. Pharmacokinetic/pharmacodynamic Parameters: Rationale for antibacterial dosing of mice and men. Clin Infect Dis 1998; 26:1–12.

*The postantibiotic effect is necessary to understanding one of the principles underlying the once-daily dosing of aminoglycosides.*

Gilbert DN. Aminoglycosides. In: Principles and Practice of Infectious Diseases, 4th ed. Mandell GL, Bennett JE, Dolin R, eds. Churchill Livingstone, New York, pp 279–306, 1995.

*Encyclopedic review of all facets of the use of aminoglycosides. Greater emphasis on basic pharmacology than presented in this chapter.*

Gilbert DN. Once daily aminoglycoside therapy. Antimicrob Agents Chemother 1991; 35:339–405.

*A comprehensive review of the data that led to the current interest in the once-daily dosing of aminoglycosides.*

Gilbert DN, Bennett WM. Use of antimicrobial agents in renal failure. Infect Dis Clin North Am 1989; 3:517–531.

*Although all antimicrobials are reviewed, the emphasis is on the dosage calculations used, and on target peak and trough serum levels, in patients administered aminoglycosides in a once-daily regimen.*

Hutchin T, Cortopassi G. Proposed molecular and cellular mechanism for aminoglycoside ototoxicity. Antimicrob Agents Chemother 1994; 38: 2517–2520.

*Excellent summary of current knowledge on this most important adverse effct of aminoglycosides.*

Molitoris, BA. Cell biology of aminoglycoside nephrotoxicity: newer aspects. Current Opinion in Nephrology and Hypertension. 1997; 6:384–388.

*A concise update on the latest concepts of the pathophysiology of aminoglycoside nephrotoxicity.*

Nicolau DP, Freeman CD, Belliveau PP, et al. Experience with a once-daily aminoglycoside program administered to 2184 adult patients. Antimicrob Agents Chemother 1995; 39:650–655.

*The largest reported experience with once-daily dosing. No control group studied. Dosage was larger than that reported by other investigators.*

Ramsey BW, Dorkin HL, Eisenberg JD, et al. Efficacy of aerosolized tobramycin in patients with cystic fibrosis. N Engl J Med 1993; 328:1740–1746.

*Persistent and recurrent* Pseudomonas aeruginosa *bronchitis and pneumonia are common persistent infections in patients with advanced cystic fibrosis. Aerosol aminoglycoside, when properly administered, is as effective as systemic therapy without the risk of systemic drug toxicity.*

# 31

# Glycopeptides

ADEL S. SULAIMAN, ROBERT M. RAKITA, AND BARBARA E. MURRAY

Vancomycin is the only glycopeptide antibiotic licensed for clinical use in the United States. Another glycopeptide antibiotic, teicoplanin, is currently in clinical use in Europe, where, in addition, the glycopeptide avoparcin has been used in chicken and ruminant livestock feed as a growth promoter. Vancomycin was isolated in 1956 from *Streptomyces orientalis*. It was initially widely used for the treatment of staphylococcal infections, but, due to toxicity apparently related to impurities, its use declined dramatically after the discovery of anti-staphylococcal penicillins and cephalosporins. Because of the emergence of methicillin-resistant *Staphylococcus aureus* (MRSA), methicillin-resistant coagulase-negative staphylococci, multidrug-resistant enterococci, and more recently, penicillin-resistant streptococci (especially *Streptococcus pneumoniae*), the clinical use of vancomycin has once again become widespread. Current pure preparations of the antibiotic have made serious toxicity from this drug a relatively uncommon event.

Teicoplanin is derived from the fermentation products of *Actinoplanes teichomyceticus*. Although it shares a similar structure, mechanism of action, and antibacterial spectrum with vancomycin, it differs from vancomycin in having a longer half-life, and possibly a better safety profile (see Table 31.1). Studies of its clinical efficacy compared to that of vancomycin are still under way.

## Structure and Mechanism of Action of Glycopeptide Antibiotics

Glycopeptides are large, rigid, and complex molecules. Their structure is based on a central heptapeptide domain in which five of the seven amino acid residues are common to all glycopeptides, with sugars located on the outside of the molecules. In addition to having two different carbohydrate moieties and two different amino acid residues versus vancomycin, teicoplanin has a fatty acid substituent on the amino group of an aminosugar, with accordingly greater hydrophobicity.

The cell walls of gram-positive bacteria contain a relatively rigid layer of peptidoglycan. Studies indicate that the mode of action of vancomycin and other glycopeptides involves the inhibition of peptidoglycan synthesis. Vancomycin forms a stoichiometric 1:1 complex with the *N*-acetylmuramyl-pentapeptide component of the peptidoglycan precursor by forming hydrogen bonds with the terminal D-ala-D-ala of the pentapeptide (Fig. 31.1). This sterically interferes with the subsequent transfer of precursor disaccharide to the growing glycan polymer of the cell wall peptidoglycan. Since the terminal D-ala-D-ala of the pentapeptide is engulfed by the large glycopeptide molecule, the important transpeptidase reaction is inhibited as well. Although a report in 1959 described the inhibition of RNA synthesis as a mechanism of action of vancomycin, this has not been substantiated. Vancomycin and teicoplanin are bactericidal to most actively dividing susceptible bacteria, as are other cell wall–active agents, but are typically bacteriostatic against enterococci.

## Spectrum of Action

Both vancomycin and teicoplanin are active against *S. aureus* and coagulase-negative staphylococci, including strains resistant to methicillin. They are also active against streptococci, including *S. pyogenes*, *S. pneumoniae*, *S. agalactiae*, *S. bovis*, *S. milleri*, *S. mitis*, *S. sanguis*, viridans streptococci, and streptococci groups C, F, and G. Both antibiotics are active against gram-positive anaerobic bacteria including *Clostridium difficile*, *C. perfringens*, and *Propionibacterium* species. *Corynebacterium* species, including *Corynebacterium jeikeium*, are also susceptible to both antibiotics. Most gram-negative species are resistant to vancomycin and teicoplanin. While some *Neisseria gonorrhoeae* isolates may be susceptible to vancomycin and teicoplanin (and thus may be missed on screening with vancomycin-containing media, such as Thayer-Martin media), neither antibiotic should be used clinically for infections caused by this organism. Most enterococci (formerly classified as group D streptococci) display tolerance for the action of all cell wall–active agents, including vancomycin and teicoplanin. Synergy with an aminoglycoside (either gentamicin or streptomycin) is usually needed for bactericidal activity. The $MIC_{90}$ of teicoplanin for enterococci is generally lower than that of vancomycin (0.2–1.6 vs. 3.1–4.0 $\mu$g/ml), but the clinical significance of this awaits further study.

## Resistance to Glycopeptides

Resistance to glycopeptides is now known to occur in at least 7 genera of gram-positive organisms, including *Leuconostoc*, *Pediococcus*, *Lactobacillus*, *Erysipelothrix*, *Streptococcus*, *Enterococcus*, and *Staphylococcus*; the first four are thought to be intrinsically resistant. Glycopeptide resistance in staphylococci and enterococci is of great clinical importance. Recently strains of *S. aureus* with reduced susceptibility to vancomycin (MIC = 8 $\mu$g/ml, considered intermediately susceptible) have been isolated from several patients in different countries. These so-called VISA strains were all isolated from patients who had previously received prolonged treatment with vancomycin. Although clinical isolates have not yet demonstrated high-level resistance to vancomycin, this has been achieved in the laboratory by prolonged in vitro passage and by conjugative transfer of glycopeptide resistance genes from *Enterococcus faecalis* to

**Table 31.1** Comparative properties of vancomycin and teicoplanin

| | Vancomycin | Teicoplanin |
|---|---|---|
| Mechanism of action | Inhibits cell wall synthesis | Inhibits cell wall synthesis |
| General use | Gram-positive bacteria[a] | Gram-positive bacteria[a] |
| Administration | IV<br>1 g q12h infused over 30–60 min[b] | IV or IM<br>400 mg loading dose followed by 200–400 mg q24h[b,c] |
| Serum levels | Peak 20–50 $\mu$g/ml<br>Trough 5–10 $\mu$g/ml[d] | Peak 54–112 $\mu$g/ml<br>Trough 4 $\mu$g/ml[e] |
| Protein binding | 10%–55% | 90% |
| Excretion pathway | Renal excretion | Renal excretion |
| Dose modification | Dose adjustment needed in renal insufficiency | Dose adjustment needed in renal insufficiency |
| Removal by hemodialysis | No | No |
| Toxicity | "Red man" syndrome<br>Nephrotoxicity with aminoglycosides<br>Ototoxicity<br>Neutropenia<br>Drug fever | Hypersensitivity<br>Ototoxicity[f]<br>Nephrotoxicity[f]<br>Thrombocytopenia |

[a]See text for exceptions.

[b]For patients with normal renal function. Higher doses have been used to treat *S. aureus* endocarditis.

[c]In cases of serious infection, 400 mg every 12 h for 3 doses, followed by 400 mg/day.

[d]Utility of routine monitoring of levels recently questioned; see text.

[e]Peak levels after intravenous injections of 3 mg/kg and 6 mg/kg, respectively.

[f]Thought to occur less commonly than with vancomycin.

*S. aureus*. In addition, strains of coagulase negative staphylococci with vancomycin MICs of 10–20 $\mu$g/ml have been isolated from clinical specimens. In particular, nosocomial isolates of *S. haemolyticus* have been found to have relatively high MICs of vancomycin, with some showing a gradual increase in vancomycin MICs during the course of therapy.

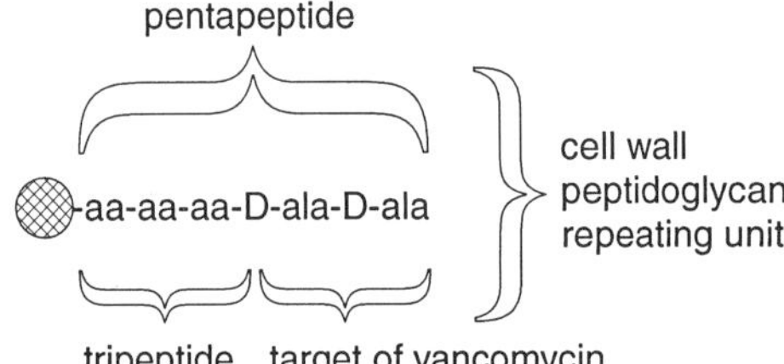


Binding of vancomycin to the pentapeptide-containing precursor prevents the precursor from being used for cell wall synthesis.

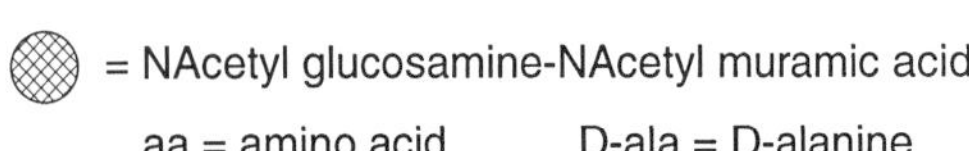


**Fig. 31.1** Site of action of vancomycin. Vancomycin binds to the terminal D-ala-D-ala dipeptide unit of the pentapeptide-containing cell wall precursor. This prevents the precursor from being used for cell wall synthesis. [From Murray, Antibiotic Resistance, in *Advances in Internal Medicine* Vol. 42, Mosby-Year Book Inc., Chicago, 1997, with permission.]

Glycopeptide resistance in enterococci has increased dramatically since it was first described in 1987. Almost 14% of enterococcal isolates from selected intensive care units in 1993 were vancomycin resistant, compared with only 0.4% of such isolates in 1989, and the proportion of centers in the United States isolating these organisms increased from 23% in 1992 to 61% in 1994. These organisms frequently exhibit concurrent resistance to multiple antibiotics, including $\beta$-lactams and aminoglycosides. The potential dissemination of resistance to other gram-positive organisms (such as *S. aureus*, as mentioned above) is an additional concern.

Four major phenotypes of glycopeptide resistance (VanA, VanB, VanC, and VanD) have been described in enterococci. The genetic basis of glycopeptide resistance in enterococci has been best characterized in VanA phenotype strains, which display high-level resistance to vancomycin and moderate-to-high resistance to teicoplanin. Nine proteins are encoded on a transposon (Tn*1546*) (Fig. 31.2) that mediates the VanA phenotype, including two involved in transposition and three, VanA, VanH, and VanX which are essential for glycopeptide resistance. VanS and VanR are involved in regulating expression of vancomycin resistance. VanH is a dehydrogenase that reduces pyruvate to lactate. VanA, a ligase produced when enterococci displaying the VanA phenotype are exposed to vancomycin or teicoplanin, preferentially catalyzes bond formation between D-alanine and D-2-hydroxy acids, especially D-lactate, forming the depsipeptide D-alanine-D-lactate; this is subsequently incorporated into the cell wall peptidoglycan precursor molecule, forming a pentadep-

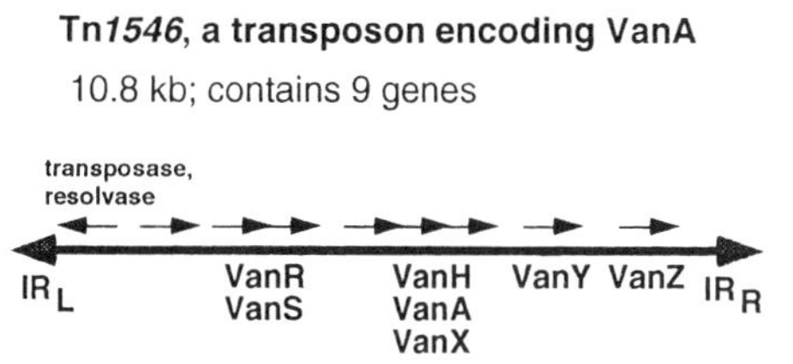

**Tn*1546*, a transposon encoding VanA**

10.8 kb; contains 9 genes

transposase, resolvase

IR L VanR VanS VanH VanA VanX VanY VanZ IR R

**Fig. 31.2** Schematic of Tn*1546* containing the vancomycin resistance gene cluster encoding the VanA phenotype. [Adapted from Arthur and Courvalin, 1993].

sipeptide (Fig. 31.3). This altered precursor does not form stable bonds with vancomycin and can, therefore, help render the organism resistant to the antibiotic. The protein VanX contributes to glycopeptide resistance by hydrolyzing D-ala-D-ala that is formed by the cell's normal D-ala-D-ala ligase, preventing the formation of normal pentapeptide precursors ending in this dipeptide. Should any normal pentapeptide precursors form, another protein, VanY (a carboxypeptidase), can cleave the terminal D-ala, resulting in a tetrapeptide terminal to which vancomycin does not bind. The function of VanZ is unknown. Enterococci producing the VanB ligase (and displaying the VanB phenotype) have a wide range of MICs of vancomycin. Although generally susceptible to teicoplanin, they become resistant if they are induced by vancomycin (but not teicoplanin). In addition, mutants constitutive for the production of VanB and resistant to teicoplanin can be selected on teicoplanin-containing agar. The VanB ligase is structurally related to the VanA ligase, displaying 75% identity. Strains with the VanC phenotype, which is constitutive, may have low-level resistance to vancomycin but are susceptible to teicoplanin. Strains with the VanD phenotype have moderate resistance to vancomycin and low-level resistance, or susceptibility, to teicoplanin, and the VanD ligase is also closely related to both VanA and VanB ligases, with 69% identity.

The VanA, VanB and VanD phenotypes represent acquired gene clusters not found in susceptible enterococci; these new genes have been found most often in vancomycin-resistant *E. faecium* and *E. faecalis*. Vancomycin resistance has also been found in a stool isolate of *Streptococcus bovis*. This strain contained a *vanB* gene 96% identical to that found in *E. faecalis*, demonstrating the potential for dissemination of vancomycin resistance among gram-positive bacteria. The VanC phenotype appears to be an inherent property of *E. gallinarum* and *E. casseliflavus*; the responsible genes, *vanC1* in *E. gallinarum* and *vanC2* in *E. casseliflavus*, appear to be normal and species-specific genes in these organisms. Because of the increasing prevalence of glycopeptide resistance in enterococci, these organisms are likely to continue to be very important pathogens in the future.

Vancomycin resistant enterococci, upon exposure to vancomycin, made a different cell wall peptidoglycan precursor:

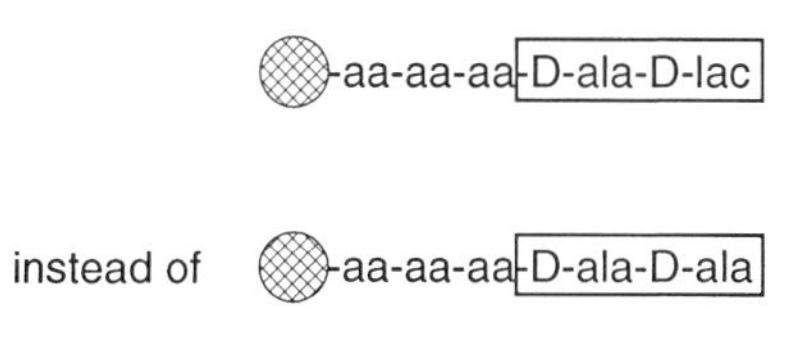


Vancomycin does not bind to -D-ala-D-lac and thus does not inhibit cell wall synthesis of these bacteria.

D-lac = D-lactate

**Fig. 31.3** Altered peptidoglycan precursor that is made by cells containing the *vanA* gene cluster after the cell is exposed to vancomycin. [From Murray, Antibiotic Resistance, in *Advances in Internal Medicine* Vol. 42, Mosby-Year Book Inc., Chicago, 1997, with permission.]

## Clinical Uses

Vancomycin, given intravenously, is the drug of choice for the treatment of most infections caused by methicillin-resistant staphylococci. It is also an appropriate alternative for the treatment of infections caused by streptococci and methicillin-susceptible staphylococci when the patient is allergic to penicillin and cephalosporins. Vancomycin has been used in combination with rifampin or a cephalosporin as initial therapy (pending identification and susceptibility testing) for the treatment of suspected *S. pneumoniae* infections in areas with a high prevalence of resistance to penicillin and cephalosporins. For treatment of prosthetic-valve endocarditis due to *S. epidermidis*, the addition of rifampin and/or gentamicin to vancomycin initially may improve clinical outcome. Serious infection due to *Corneybacterium* species have become more common, especially in the immunocompromised host. *C. jeikeium* are often resistant to multiple antibiotics while susceptible to vancomycin.

Enterococcal endocarditis is best treated with a combination of a cell wall–active agent and an aminoglycoside (gentamicin or streptomycin); when the organism is resistant to ampicillin, or when the patient is allergic to penicillin, vancomycin is the agent of choice for the cell wall–active component of treatment. Testing all enterococcal isolates causing serious infections (particularly endocarditis) for high-level gentamicin and streptomycin resistance is imperative when these aminoglycosides are used for synergy. In addition, patients receiving this combination should be monitored carefully for ototoxicity and nephrotoxicity.

Vancomycin is used for prophylaxis for bacterial endocarditis in patients undergoing dental, gastrointestinal (GI), or genitourinary (GU) procedures who are allergic to penicillin (see Chapter 66). Additionally, it can be used prophylactically in patients undergoing valve replacement surgery. Vancomycin can be used in the treatment of peritonitis caused by staphylococci in patients undergoing peritoneal dialysis, at times without removal of the peritoneal dialysis catheter. However, prolonged use for this indication should be avoided, as this may promote vancomycin resistance. Intrathecal vancomycin can be given as an adjunct to systemic therapy in complicated CNS infections caused by organisms susceptible to the antibiotic. For the empiric treatment of febrile neutropenic patients, vancomycin is often added when a high degree of suspicion exists for the presence of gram-positive infections. However, no survival advantage was found in several randomized studies when vancomycin was included initially to treat every neutropenic patient.

Oral vancomycin is effective for treatment of pseudomembraneous colitis caused by toxigenic strains of *Clostridium difficile*. Because of the vast cost differential, and concerns over emergence of vancomycin-resistant enterococci, oral vancomycin should generally be used only if therapy with metronidazole has failed.

Teicoplanin has been shown to be effective for the treatment of skin and soft tissue infections in hospitalized patients. It is also effective for the treatment of acute and chronic osteomyelitis and septic arthritis caused by susceptible organisms. It has been used successfully for the treatment of staphylococcal peritonitis in peritoneal dialysis patients. Teicoplanin seems to be as effective as vancomycin in the treatment of *C. difficile*–induced pseudomembranous colitis. Various infections caused by enterococci have been treated with teicoplanin, including endocarditis, septicemia, urinary tract infections (UTI), and soft tissue infections.

Early studies using teicoplanin for the treatment of gram-positive intravascular infections due to *S. aureus* showed a high failure rate. When higher doses of teicoplanin were used, however, better results were obtained. In serious gram-positive infections (including endocarditis), optimal dosing, comparative efficacy with vancomycin, and indications for combination therapy are factors that require clarification through additional clinical trials.

## Pharmacology and Dosing

When given intravenously, vancomycin should be mixed in 100–250 ml of 5% dextrose in water or normal saline, and infused over at least 60 min. Gastrointestinal absorption is poor. Ten to fifty percent of the drug is protein bound in the serum. Cerebrospinal fluid (CSF) penetration is poor, but it improves in cases of inflamed meninges, reaching 5%–19% of serum levels. As expected, excellent antibiotic levels are achieved in the urine following intravenous dosing, and adequate levels are seen in ascitic, pericardial, pleural, and synovial fluid.

Vancomycin is almost exclusively cleared by renal mechanisms, so dosage adjustment is mandatory in renal insufficiency. Removal of the antibiotic with hemodialysis is minimal.

The usual vancomycin dose for patients with normal renal function is 1 g every 12 h. While traditionally peak and trough ranges of 20–50 μg/ml and 5–10 μg/ml, respectively, were sought, and serum vancomycin levels were regularly determined, this practice has been questioned recently because of the lack of a clear correlation between vancomycin levels and either its clinical efficacy or toxicity. Monitoring vancomycin serum levels is indicated for (*1*) patients receiving concomitant nephrotoxic agents, such as aminoglycosides, (*2*) patients with renal insufficiency, rapidly changing renal function, or dialysis patients, and (*3*) patients receiving doses of vancomycin that are higher than usual, or patients with a volume of distribution predicted to be higher or lower than usual. For renal dialysis patients receiving intermittent dosing, levels should be maintained above 15 μg/ml.

When delivered via the intrathecal or intraventricular route for treatment of meningitis or ventriculitis, a dose of 10 mg/day can be given concomitantly with systemic therapy. Vancomycin can be added to the peritoneal dialysate at concentrations of 25 μg/ml to treat peritonitis in peritoneal dialysis patients as an adjunct to systemic therapy.

For penicillin-allergic patients who require prophylaxis to prevent endocarditis and are undergoing dental procedures, 1 g of vancomycin is given IV prior to the procedure. For similar patients undergoing GI or GU procedures, or for prosthetic valve surgery prophylaxis, vancomycin 1 g IV is given prior to the procedure, together with gentamicin 1.5 mg/kg. This may be repeated once 8–12 h later. The dose of oral vancomycin used to treat pseudomembranous colitis is 125 mg every 6 h.

Teicoplanin can be administered intravenously or intramuscularly, and, unlike vancomycin, it can be given rapidly. Gastrointestinal absorption of the antibiotic is poor. Plasma half-life with normal renal function is about 45–70 h and the drug is highly protein bound (90%). After teicoplanin dosing, adequate levels of the antibiotic are seen in bile, gallbladder, liver, pancreas, and bone. Lower concentrations are found in fat and the CNS, but urine levels are excellent. It is cleared by the kidneys, making dosage adjustment mandatory in renal failure. As with vancomycin, teicoplanin is not well removed by hemodialysis.

Teicoplanin dosage recommendations vary. In general, for soft tissue, skin, urine, and respiratory tract infections, a loading dose of 400 mg has been given on the first day, followed by a daily dose of 200 mg. For treatment of serious infections, including septicemia, endocarditis, osteomyelitis, and septic arthritis, patients have been given three loading doses of 400 mg every 12 h, followed by a daily dose of 400 mg/day. Doses of 12 mg/kg/day are standard for treatment of patients with *S. aureus* endocarditis, although doses up to 30 mg/kg/day may be needed. As an adjunct to systemic therapy, 20 mg of teicoplanin has been given intrathecally either daily or every other day for treatment of neurosurgical shunt infections. For intraperitoneal therapy, teicoplanin has been used at a concentration of 20 μg/ml in the dialysate. For treatment of *C. difficile* colitis, oral teicoplanin has been given at 100 mg twice daily for 10 days.

## Toxicity

The most common side effect of vancomycin is the "red-man" syndrome, manifested by erythema, flushing, and pruritus of the upper body, and occasionally angioedema and hypotension. It is mediated by histamine release and results from the rapid intravenous infusion of the antibiotic. This reaction can usually be alleviated by infusing the antibiotic more slowly (over 1 h or more) or by pretreatment with antihistamines. Muscle spasms of the chest and back may also result from rapid vancomycin infusion.

Nephrotoxicity is rare when vancomycin is used alone, but not uncommon when an aminoglycoside is used in combination. Ototoxicity may occur at high serum levels, and concomitant use of aminoglycosides appears to increase the risk for ototoxicity. Reversible neutropenia is the most common hematologic side effect of vancomycin. When this generally rare manifestation occurs, it usually does so after 14 days of therapy. Hypersensitivity, as manifested by drug fever and skin rash, can occur in up to 5% of patients receiving vancomycin.

The most common adverse reaction to teicoplanin is hypersensitivity (skin rash, drug fever), which rarely progresses to bronchospasm and anaphylaxis. Injection site intolerance is also seen, but is usually mild. Risks for ototoxicity and nephrotoxicity seem to be lower than those for vancomycin. Thrombocytopenia has been reported as an adverse effect of teicoplanin and is more common with higher doses.

## ANNOTATED BIBLIOGRAPHY

Campolli-Richards DM, Brogden RN, Faulds D. Teicoplanin: a review of its antibacterial activity, pharmacokinetic properties and therapeutic potential. Drugs 1990; 40:449–486.
*A very complete review of teicoplanin.*

Centers for Disease Control. Nosocomial enterococci resistant to vancomycin—United States, 1989–1993. MMWR 1993; 40:597–599.
*Summary of emergence and annual increase in vancomycin-resistant enterococci in the U.S. between 1989 and 1993.*

Centers for Disease Control. Recommendations for preventing the spread of vancomycin resistance. MMWR 1995; 44(Suppl. #RR12):1–13.
*CDC guidelines for prudent use of vancomycin and infection control measures for vancomycin-resistant enterococci.*

Centers for Disease Control. Update: *Staphylococcus aureus* with reduced susceptibility to vancomycin—United States, 1997. MMWR 1997; 46:813–815.
*Report of* S. aureus *clinical isolates with intermediate susceptibility to vancomycin.*

De Lalla F, Nicolin R, Rinaldi E, Scarpellini P, Rigoli R, Manfrin V, Tramarin A. Prospective study of oral teicoplanin versus oral vancomycin for therapy of pseudomembranous colitis and *Clostridium difficile*-associate diarrhea. Antimicrob Agents Chemother 1992; 36:2192–2196.
*Both are equally effective, but authors suggest that therapy should usually be initiated with metronidazole.*

Evers S, Reynolds PE, Courvalin P. Sequence of the *vanB* and *ddl* genes encoding D-alanine:D-lactate and D-alanine:D-alanine ligases in vancomycin-resistant *Enterococcus faecalis* V583. Gene 1994; 140:97–102.
*Comparison of the ligase gene of VanB-type resistance to the normal enterococcal ligase gene.*

Fekety R. Vancomycin and teicoplanin. In: Principles and Practice of Infectious Diseases, 4th ed. Mandell GL, Bennett JE, Dolin R, eds. Churchill Livingstone, New York, pp. 346–354, 1995.
*In-depth review of these two glycopeptides.*

Froggatt JW, Johnston JL, Galetto DW, Arthur GL. Antimicrobial resistance in nosocomial isolates of *Staphylococcus haemolyticus*. Antimicrob Agents Chemother 1989; 3:460–466.
*Describes multiresistance in S. haemolyticus including elevated MICs of vancomycin.*

Ingerman MJ, Santoro J. Vancomycin: a new old agent. Infect Dis Clin North Am 1989; 3:641–651.
*Succinct review of vancomycin.*

Johnson AP, Uttley AHC, Woodford N, George RC. Resistance to vancomycin and teicoplanin: an emerging clinical problem. Clin Microbiol Rev. 1990; 3:280–291.
*Excellent review published several years after VRE were discovered.*

Leclercq R, Courvalin P. Resistance to glycopeptides in enterococci. Clin Infect Dis 1997; 24:545–556.
*Excellent review of mechanisms, clinical experience, and therapeutic options.*

Moellering RC Jr. Editorial: Monitoring serum vancomycin levels: climbing the mountain because it is there? Clin Infect Dis 1994; 18:544–546.
*Recommendations regarding when vancomycin levels could be useful.*

Murray BE. Antibiotic resistance. In: Advances in Internal Medicine, vol 42. Fauci AS, ed. Mosby–Year Book, St. Louis, pp 339–367, 1997.
*Reviews the subject of antimicrobial resistance of enterococci with a special focus on vancomycin resistance.*

Nagarajan R. Antibacterial activities and modes of action of vancomycin and related glycopeptides. Antimicrob Agents Chemother 1991; 35:604–609.
*In-depth review of structure and mechanism of action of glycopeptides.*

Noble WC, Virani Z, Cree RGA. Co-transfer of vancomycin and other resistance genes from *Enterococcus faecalis* NCTC 12201 to *Staphylococcus aureus*. FEMS Microbiol Lett 1992; 93:195–198.
*This is the reference everyone refers to when expressing concern about transfer of vancomycin resistance to* S. aureus. *In a simple experiment involving mixing of VRE with* S. aureus *in the test tube and on the skin of a mouse, the authors were able to recover vancomycin-resistant* S. aureus.

Pizzo PA. Management of fever in patients with cancer and treatment-induced neutropenia. New Engl J Med 1993; 328:1323–1332.
*Extensive review and recommendations for management of febrile cancer and neutropenic patients.*

Poyart C, Pierre C, Quesne G, Pron B, Berche P, Trieu-Cuot P. Emergence of vancomycin resistance in the genus *Streptococcus*: characterization of a *vanB* transferable determinant in *Streptococcus bovis*. Antimicrob Agents Chemother 1997; 41:24–29.
*Isolation of a vancomycin resistant streptococcus from stools, demonstrating the potential for dissemination of these highly mobile vancomycin resistance determinants in gram-positive bacteria.*

Reynolds PE. Structure, biochemistry and mechanism of action of glycopeptide antibiotics. Eur J Clin Microbiol Infect Dis 1989; 8:943–950.
*Review of how glycopeptides inhibit bacteria by binding to the terminal 2 amino acids of a cell wall synthesis precursor, which then prevents this precursor from being added to the growing cell wall and thus subsequent steps of cell wall synthesis.*

Wilson APR, Gruneberg RN, Neu H. Dosage recommendations for teicoplanin. J Antimicrob Chemother 1993; 32:792–796.
*Discussion of conflicting outcomes associated with varying doses of teicoplanin.*

# 32

# Macrolides and Clindamycin

HOWARD S. GOLD AND ROBERT C. MOELLERING, JR.

Despite over 40 years of use, the macrolides continue to evolve in spectrum of activity and clinical application. Erythromycin is a natural compound secreted by *Streptomyces erythreus*. It is used most often to treat infections of the upper and lower respiratory tract, as well as the skin and soft tissues. Clindamycin is one of two clinically relevant lincosamide antibiotics, compounds composed of an amino acid linked to a sulfur-containing sugar. Lincomycin, the first described lincosamide, was isolated from a soil Streptomycete. It has been largely supplanted by its semisynthetic derivative, clindamycin, which is more active and better absorbed after oral administration.

## Macrolides

Macrolides are useful alternatives to $\beta$-lactams in patients with hypersensitivity to those agents. The spectrum of activity of the macrolides includes gram-positive cocci, gram-negative cocci, some gram-negative cocco-bacilli (e.g., *Moraxella catarrhalis* and *Bordetella pertussis*) and a number of intracellular pathogens. Newer macrolides, including clarithromycin, azithromycin, and roxithromycin, are semisynthetic derivatives of the original compounds with improved pharmacokinetics and antimicrobial activity.

### Structure and mechanism of action

The macrolides are compounds with a central 12- to 16-membered lactone ring to which one, two, or three neutral or basic sugars are linked. Macrolides with a 14-membered ring include erythromycin and its semisynthetic derivatives, including clarithromycin, roxithromycin, and dirithromycin. The sole 15-membered ring compound is azithromycin, which is also called an azalide because of its nitrogen-containing lactone ring. Sixteen-membered ring macrolides in current use include josamycin, midecamycin, and spiramycin, however, none of these is commercially available in the United States.

Macrolide antibiotics act by the inhibition of microbial protein synthesis. They bind to the 50S subunit of the bacterial ribosome and block protein elongation. The binding site for macrolides appears to overlap with the binding site of lincosamide (e.g., clindamycin) and streptogramin antibiotics, as well as that of chloramphenicol. Although macrolides are generally considered to be bacteriostatic, under certain conditions they appear to have bactericidal activity against *Streptococcus pneumoniae*, group A $\beta$-hemolytic streptococci, *S. mitis*, *Corynebacterium diphtheriae*, and *B. pertussis*.

### Mechanisms of resistance

Bacterial resistance to the activity of macrolides may be due to intrinsic factors or to one of a number of acquired mechanisms. The outer cell envelope of aerobic gram-negative bacilli acts as a permeability barrier, rendering them resistant to clinically achievable levels of most macrolides. An exception to this is azithromycin, which can penetrate the outer cell envelope of certain gram-negative bacilli and thus has improved activity against *Haemophilus influenzae* and some *Enterobacteriaceae*.

Acquired resistance to the macrolides may be due to target alteration, enzymatic inactivation, or active efflux. The macrolides' binding site on the bacterial ribosome may be altered by methylation of an adenine residue of the 23S ribosomal RNA. It is of interest to note that this modification is also present in the rRNA of the Streptomycetes that are the source of macrolide antibiotics. The methylating enzyme that produces macrolide resistance is encoded by one of a group of genes called *erm*, which are usually carried on a plasmid or transposon. Expression of this resistance determinant may be constitutive or inducible. When inducibly expressed in *Staphylococci*, macrolide resistance is considered "dissociated," as it is induced by 14- and 15-member ring macrolides, but not 16-member macrolides or the functionally related lincosamide and streptogramin antibiotics, which retain activity. Constitutive expression results in cross-resistance to all macrolides, lincosamides, and type B streptogramins, a phenotype called $MLS_B$. Macrolide-resistant streptococci bearing *erm* genes are often cross-resistant to lincosamides and type B streptogramins. $MLS_B$ is an important mechanism of resistance to macrolides, as it is found with significant frequency in clinically relevant organisms, including *Staphylococcus aureus*, *Streptococcus pyogenes*, *S. pneumoniae*, *Enterococcus faecalis*, *Clostridium* species, and *Bacteroides* species. A second form of target modification, alteration of the 50S ribosomal protein, has been postulated, but this has not been conclusively linked to resistance to macrolides.

Active efflux mechanisms for some macrolides have been described in *S. epidermidis* and more recently, in isolates of a number of streptococcal species with the M phenotype that are resistant to 14- and 15-member ring macrolides, but susceptible to 16-member ring macrolides, clindamycin, and streptogramin B drugs. This phenotype, which is mediated by the *mefA* and *mefE* genes, has been reported to be fairly common in *S. pyogenes*, *S. agalactiae*, and *S. pneumoniae*. Other acquired mechanisms of resistance are less prevalent in clinical isolates. Enzymatic modification of macrolides, mediated by erythromycin esterases and phosphotransferases, has been reported in *Escherichia coli* and *Pseudomonas aeruginosa*, as well as in *Lactobacillus* species. In some cases, more than one mechanism is present in an isolate, producing higher levels of resistance.

### Spectrum of antimicrobial activity

Macrolide antibiotics have a spectrum of activity that includes many common pathogens, as well as a number of more unusual ones. Most isolates of *S. pyogenes*, other $\beta$-hemolytic streptococci, viridans streptococci, and *S. pneumoniae* are highly susceptible to macrolides. However, resistant organisms of most species have been reported, particularly in geographic areas with heavy usage of these antibiotics. A particularly striking example of this problem was seen in Japan in the late 1970s when resistance to erythromycin among *S. pyogenes* peaked at over 83% of isolates, a figure that fell rapidly in subsequent years with more restrictive use of this agent. Multidrug-resistant pneumococci are a growing problem in many parts of the world, and a recent survey of >1000 clinical isolates of *S. pneumoniae* from the U.S. and Europe found that more than 20% were resistant to macrolides. In general, minimum inhibitory concentrations of clarithromycin for gram-positive organisms tend to be slightly lower than erythromycin and roxithromycin, whereas azithromycin is somewhat less active.

The in vitro susceptibility of *S. aureus* to macrolides often parallels methicillin susceptibility. Many isolates of methicillin-resistant *S. aureus* (MRSA) are impervious to multiple antibiotics, including macrolides. While more than 90% of MRSA may be resistant to macrolides, these agents do have activity against the majority of methicillin-susceptible isolates. This correlation between resistance to methicillin and macrolide resistance is also present in many coagulase-negative staphylococci. Less than 50% of isolates of *E. faecalis* are inhibited by macrolide antibiotics at concentrations below the recommended breakpoint and *E. faecium* are routinely more highly macrolide resistant than *E. faecalis*. Certain gram-positive bacilli, including *Corynebacterium diphtheriae*, *C. minutissimum*, *Listeria monocytogenes*, *Bacillus anthracis*, and *Erysipelothrix rhusiopathiae* are generally susceptible to macrolides. Macrolides have activity against *Actinomyces israelii* and related filamentous gram-positive organisms.

Gram-negative cocci and cocco-bacilli, including *Neisseria gonorrhoeae*, *N. meningitidis*, *Haemophilus ducreyi*, *Bordetella pertussis*, and *Moraxella catarrhalis*, are considered susceptible to macrolides. Azithromycin is the most active macrolide against this group of pathogens, followed by clarithromycin. Many isolates of *Haemophilus influenzae* are moderately resistant to erythromycin, but most are susceptible to azithromycin and clarithromycin. Some gram-negative enteric pathogens are inhibited by macrolides; for example, *Campylobacter jejuni* is routinely susceptible to erythromycin and azithromycin. Although azithromycin has activity against *Salmonella* and *Shigella* spp., macrolides are essentially inactive against most *Enterobacteriaceae* and all pseudomonads. Clarithromycin is highly active against *Helicobacter pylori*. Resistance to macrolides is common among many clinically important anaerobes, including *Bacteroides fragilis* and fusobacterium, however, the newer agents have somewhat better activity than erythromycin.

*Mycoplasma pneumoniae*, a common cause of community-acquired atypical pneumonia, is sensitive to all macrolides, while the uropathogen *Ureaplasma urealyticum* is most susceptible to clarithromycin. Macrolides have activity against a number of spirochetes, including *Treponema pallidum* and *Borrelia burgdorferi* (the agent of Lyme disease).

Several intracellular pathogens, such as *Legionella* species (including *L. pneumophila*) and *Chlamydia* species, are generally susceptible to macrolides. Macrolides have activity against *Rickettsiae* and the related genus *Bartonella*, including *B. henselae*, the cause of bacillary peliosus hepatis and bacillary angiomatosis in HIV-infected patients. Mycobacteria are another clinically important group of intracellular pathogens, and macrolides, particularly clarithromycin and azithromycin, have efficacy against the *Mycobacterium avium* complex, *M. fortuitum–chelonae* complex, and *M. leprae*. *M. tuberculosis* is generally not susceptible to macrolides. The spectrum of activity of the macrolides, particularly that of the newer agents, also includes a number of protozoan pathogens, including *Toxoplasma gondii*, *Plasmodium falciparum*, *Entamoeba histolytica*, *Giardia intestinalis*, and possibly several others.

## Pharmacokinetics

Macrolides are large, basic molecules, generally poorly soluble in water and unstable in gastric acid. Numerous strategies have been utilized to overcome these disadvantages, including the synthesis of salts and esters of erythromycin. Erythromycin base has been coated with a protective film or enteric coating for oral administration. Some macrolides, including azithromycin and roxithromycin, are more acid stable. Intravenous preparations of erythromycin utilize gluceptate or lactobionate salts. Erythromycin is not suitable for intramuscular administration because pain and sterile abscess develop at the injection site. A parenteral preparation of azithromycin dihydrate is available for intravenous infusion, however, it is not recommended for intramuscular injection. Parenteral clarithromycin is available in some European countries.

The various oral preparations of erythromycin produce peak serum levels ranging from 0.58 to 4.7 μg/ml after a single dose of 500 mg in a fasting subject. Erythromycin base, the stearate salt, and erythromycin ethylsuccinate are best absorbed in the fasting state, whereas absorption of enteric preparations of erythromycin base and the estolate form does not appear to be altered by food intake. Absorption of roxithromycin and azithromycin is significantly reduced by administration with food. Clarithromycin, the most bioavailable macrolide, is absorbed slightly better when taken with food.

Macrolides are highly lipid soluble and minimally ionized at physiologic pH, leading to distribution throughout the total body water and good penetration into most tissues. Protein binding, also a factor in tissue distribution, ranges from less than 50% to greater then 90%, depending on the compound. Tissue levels are generally good in the upper and lower respiratory tract; however, erythromycin diffuses slowly into the inner ear, achieving levels sufficient to treat only the most susceptible organisms. Clarithromycin achieves pulmonary parenchymal levels that are higher than those of erythromycin. Azithromycin produces sustained tissue levels in the lung, and although all macrolides concentrate in phagocytes and alveolar macrophages, azithromycin produces particularly high levels.

Macrolides produce good tissue levels in the skin but somewhat lesser levels in the fat, muscle, bone, and synovial fluid. In male and female urogenital tissues, azithromycin reaches sustained high tissue levels. Erythromycin crosses the placenta to a modest degree, and it produces significant levels in breast milk. In the gastrointestinal tract, macrolides are concentrated in the bile, where levels often exceed serum concentrations. Biliary excretion and nonabsorbed oral medication contribute to high fecal levels. Penetration into the central nervous system, cerebrospinal fluid, and aqueous humor is considered poor.

Although the peak serum concentration and elimination half-life of erythromycin may vary widely, depending on the preparation and test conditions, the half-life generally approximates 2 h. Several of the newer macrolides have more prolonged half-lives; for example, roxithromycin and azithromycin both have half-lives in excess of 10 h. Members of the macrolide family of antibiotics vary not only in their pharmacokinetics but also in their metabolism. Orally administered erythromycin base undergoes extensive hydrolysis by gastric acid. Erythromycin undergoes intramolecular cyclization, both in the stomach and after absorption, as well as rapid demethylation by the hepatic cytochrome P-450 system. Other macrolides are more resistant to gastric acid and may undergo varying degrees of modification by hepatic pathways. The major oxidative derivative of clarithromycin (14-hydroxy-clarithromycin) retains the antimicrobial activity of the parent compound; however, chemical modification of macrolides generally results in products with reduced antimicrobial potency. Macrolides and their metabolites are secreted in the bile, with urinary excretion playing a secondary role for most agents. As the macrolides have both hepatic and renal clearance, insufficiency of either system does not mandate dosage modification. Some authors, however, recommend dose reductions in patients with severe renal insufficiency. In the presence of *combined* liver and kidney failure, dose reduction is probably indicated. Neither hemodialysis nor peritoneal dialysis significantly alter levels of erythromycin.

## Toxicities and drug interactions

Adverse reactions to macrolide antibiotics, while not uncommon, are usually of a fairly mild nature. Gastrointestinal toxicity predominates, manifested by abdominal cramping, nausea, vomiting, and diarrhea. These symptoms, mediated by binding of the antibiotic to the receptor for motilin in gastroduodenal smooth muscle, may occur regardless of the mode of administration and are most pronounced after administration of 14-member ring macrolides, including erythromycin. Some of the newer macrolides, as well as 16-member ring macrolides, have been reported to cause less gastrointestinal toxicity. Hepatotoxicity resulting in cholestatic hepatitis is an uncommon event most often described in adult patients receiving erythromycin estolate and is most likely due to hypersensitivity to this particular form of the drug. Other allergic reactions are similarly unusual and may include skin rash, fever, and eosinophilia. Reports of anaphylaxis are rare. Ototoxicity, presenting as reversible sensorineural hearing loss and/or tinnitus has been seen, particularly in patients receiving large doses of macrolides in the presence of hepatic and/or renal dysfunction. Infusion of erythromycin into peripheral veins is often painful and may result in phlebitis, particularly if it is infused rapidly or in a concentrated solution. Drug interactions result from the effects of these antibiotics on the hepatic cytochrome P-450 system. Inhibition of this important metabolic pathway by erythromycin may result in elevated levels of a variety of other medications, including theophyllin, ergotderivatives, warfarin, cambamazepine, valproate, methylprednisolone, and cyclosporin. The combination of certain macrolides (erythromycin and clarithromycin) with the nonsedating antihistamines terfenadine and astemizole has been linked to cardiac arrhythmias, as has the combination of these macrolides and cisapride. Cardiotoxicity caused by erythromycin alone has been reported, but is rare. Uveitis was described in study subjects receiving clarithromycin and high-dose rifabutin. Rifampin, and to a lesser extent, rifabutin, decrease serum levels of clarithromycin. Certain 16-member ring macrolides (including spiramycin) and some of the newer agents (roxithromycin and azithromycin) produce fewer significant drug interactions by virtue of their more limited effect on the cytochrome P-450 system. Clarithromycin and erythromycin may interact with a number of antiretroviral drugs, e.g., coadministration of these drugs with several of the HIV protease inhibitors may result in elevated levels of both classes of drugs.

## Clinical use

The macrolides have proven themselves as effective and safe antimicrobials. As the family of macrolide antibiotics grows, the spectrum of activity and pharmacokinetics of these drugs continue to improve. Macrolides are very useful in the treatment of infections of the respiratory tract caused by streptococci, as well as lower respiratory infections caused by "atypical" agents including *Mycoplasma pneumoniae*, *Chlamydia pneumoniae*, and *Legionella pneumophila*. Intravenous erythromycin or azithromycin are used in patients hospitalized with community-acquired pneumonia. Azithromycin, with its improved activity against gram-negative bacteria, provides enhanced coverage of additional respiratory pathogens including *Haemophilus influenzae*, *Moraxella catarrhalis*, and *Bordetella pertussis*. In vitro, clarithromycin exhibits borderline activity against *H. influenza*, but in vivo it is metabolized to the 14-hydroxy derivative which is two- to fourfold more active against these organisms. Clarithromycin combined with the proton pump inhibitor, omeprazole, is an effective regimen for eradication of *H. pylori*, thought to be the causative agent of most peptic ulcer disease. Erythromycin is the drug of choice for treatment of diphtheria (as adjunctive therapy to antitoxin), as well as for chemoprophylaxis and elimination of the *Corynebacterium diphtheriae* carrier state.

Erythromycin is one of the drugs of choice to treat *Campylobacter jejuni* enteritis, while azithromycin is effective for the treatment of multidrug-resistant shigellosis. Because of improved activity and prolonged, high tissue levels, azithromycin has been approved for single-dose therapy for the treatment of nongonococcal urethritis and cervicitis caused by *Chlamydia trachomatis*. Macrolides are also useful in the treatment of other sexually transmitted diseases, including chancroid and granuloma inguinale (caused by *Haemophilus ducreyi* and *Calymmatobacterium granulomatosis*, respectively). Intravenous azithromycin has an indication for the treatment of pelvic inflammatory disease, administered with an appropriate drug to cover anaerobic bacteria. Macrolides fill an important role as an alternative therapy for $\beta$-lactam-allergic patients. Examples include the treatment of syphilis, prophylaxis against rheumatic fever, and prophylaxis of neonatal group B streptococcal disease. In the most recent American Heart Association guidelines for prophylaxis against infective endocarditis (in patients with underlying cardiac conditions who undergo dental or respiratory procedures), clarithromycin and azithromycin have replaced erythromycin for use in $\beta$-lactam-allergic patients. Clarithromycin and azithromycin are a cornerstone of multidrug therapy for infections caused by *Mycobacterium avium* complex (MAC). In patients infected with the human immunodeficiency virus (HIV), these agents are also effective primary prophylaxis against infections caused by MAC. Erythromycin is the drug of choice to treat bacillary angiomatosis and other infections caused by *Bartonella henselae* in HIV-infected individuals. Azithromycin may have activity against the difficult-to-treat enteric pathogen *Cryptosporidium parvum*, and this drug, as well as clarithromycin have been combined with pyramethamine/folinic acid to treat *Toxoplasma gondii* encephalitis in sulfa-allergic patients.

Spiramycin is sometimes used to treat pregnant women with toxoplasmosis. It is also used for prophylaxis against meningococcal disease for close contacts of infected patients. Macrolides are useful in the treatment of skin infections caused by susceptible organisms, especially streptococci and methicillin-susceptible *Staphylococcus aureus*. Erythromycin may be used to treat erythrasma. Topical erythromycin is effective therapy for acne vulgaris. Another effectual topical application for macrolides is the prophylaxis of neonatal chlamydial and gonococcal conjunctivitis with erythromycin ophthalmic ointment.

There are several important caveats in the use of macrolides.

Because their mechanism of action involves the inhibition of microbial protein synthesis, macrolides are primarily bacteriostatic agents. Although macrolides achieve excellent penetration into most tissues and fluids, they do not penetrate well into the central nervous system. Macrolide resistance is a growing problem among certain pathogens, most notably *S. pneumoniae*, *S. aureus*, and *Enterococcus* species. An interesting footnote is that the potentially unpleasant gastrointestinal side effects of erythromycin, mediated by motilin receptor agonist activity, are being exploited to synthesize promotility agents lacking antimicrobial activity.

### Administration

Please refer to Table 32.1 for recommended dosages of macrolide antibiotics.

## Clindamycin

With a spectrum of activity that includes aerobic gram-positive cocci and anaerobes, clindamycin is most often used to treat infections involving the abdomen, pelvis, skin, and soft tissues. Like the macrolides, clindamycin has been used to replace $\beta$-lactam antibiotics in hypersensitive patients.

### Mechanism of action

The lincosamides are functionally related to macrolides and streptogramins, as these agents share a similar mechanism of action. They bind to overlapping sites on the 50S subunit of the ribosome, specifically located on the 23S ribosomal RNA, and function by interfering with microbial protein synthesis. Like other antimicrobials with this mechanism of action, clindamycin and lincomycin are generally bacteriostatic, but they may be bactericidal under some conditions.

### Mechanisms of resistance

Resistance to lincosamides may occur because of insufficient access of the antimicrobial agent to its binding site, modification of that binding site, or enzymatic inactivation of the antibiotic. Facultative gram-negative bacilli, including *Enterobacteriaceae* and *Pseudomonas* species, are impervious to lincosamides, presumably because of poor penetration through the outer cell envelope. Other organisms with at least modest intrinsic resistance to clindamycin include *Haemophilus* species, *Neisseriaciae*, and enterococci. Bacteria may become resistant to lincosamides by acquiring one of the *erm* genes on a plasmid or transposon, encoding an ribosomal RNA-methylating enzyme. This enzyme alters the antibiotic binding site, and when expressed constitutively, produces cross-resistance to macrolides, lincosamides, and type B streptogramins (the $MLS_B$ phenotype). Although $MLS_B$ is the most clinically relevant form of acquired lincosamide resistance, some bacteria express the methylating enzyme only after induction. In some strains of staphylococci, 14- and 15-member ring macrolides induce resistance to all of the $MLS_B$ antibiotics. If induction has not occurred, clindamycin, streptogramins, and 16-member ring macrolides retain in vitro activity because they are poor inducers of the methylase; this phenomenon is called "dissociated resistance." It is noteworthy that staphylococci with this phenotype (erythromycin-resistant and clindamycin-susceptible) may develop cross-resistance to the latter agents with continued antibiotic exposure, both in vitro and in vivo. Enzymatic inactivation of lincomycin, and to a lesser degree, clindamycin, occurs in a minority of coagulase-negative staphylococci that bear genes of the *linA* group encoding a nucleotidyltransferase enzyme.

### Spectrum of antimicrobial activity

Clindamycin is active against many aerobic gram-positive cocci and a variety of anaerobes, as well as a few other pathogens. Most streptococci are susceptible to this antimicrobial; however, strains of *S. pneumoniae*, *S. pyogenes*, and others carrying the *ermAM* gene are constitutively or inducibly resistant to lincosamides as well as macrolides. Recent reports indicate that a sizable proportion of erythromycin-resistant streptococci are susceptible to clindamycin on account of specificity of an efflux mechanism, mediated by *mefA* and *mefE*, for the macrolide. While the majority of methicillin-resistant *S. aureus* are clindamycin resistant (>50%), clindamycin has activity against most methicillin-susceptible isolates (>85%). Many coagulase-negative staphylococci, particularly nosocomial isolates, are resistant to clindamycin. As noted previously, enterococci have intrinsic low-level resistance to lincosamides, and many strains also bear genes encoding high-level resistance. Although clindamycin is active against *Corynebacterium diptheriae*, *C. jeikeium* are resistant. Lincosamides have efficacy against other gram-positive organisms, including *Bacillus cereus*, lactobacilli, *Leuconostoc*, and *Actinomyces* species.

Lincosamides have, at best, modest activity against gram-negative cocci and cocco-bacilli, including *Neisseriaciae* and *Haemophilus influenzae*. These antimicrobials are completely ineffective against facultative gram-negative bacilli, but they are active against many anaerobic gram-negative and gram-positive bacteria. Most *Bacteroides fragilis* and other *Bacteroides* species are inhibited by clindamycin; however, resistance has occurred in as many as 20% of isolates in some series. Other anaerobes that are usually susceptible to clindamycin include *Fusobacterium* spp., peptococci, peptostreptococci, *Proprionobacterium acnes*, and *Clostridia perfringens*. *C. difficile* are resistant to clindamycin; in fact, this agent can cause antibiotic-associated colitis due to *C. difficile* overgrowth.

The spectrum of activity of clindamycin includes a few other, unrelated pathogens. This antimicrobial has fairly good activity against *Chlamydia trachomatis*. Unlike the macrolides, it lacks activity against *Ureaplasma* and *Mycoplasma* species. A number of protozoan pathogens, including *Toxoplasma gondii*, *Babesia microti*, *Plasmodium* spp., and *Pneumocystis carinii* are inhibited by clindamycin when it is used in combination with other antiprotozoal agents.

### Toxicity and drug interactions

The most significant adverse reactions caused by clindamycin involve the gastrointestinal system. Antibiotic-associated diarrhea may occur in up to 20% of patients receiving clindamycin, presumably because alterations in the bowel flora are caused by the compound's activity against anaerobic bacteria. A potentially more serious complication of this alteration of bowel flora is overgrowth of the colon by toxigenic *C. difficile*, resulting in antibiotic-associated colitis with pseudomembrane formation. Lincosamides are not the only cause of this syndrome, as $\beta$-lactam antibiotics produce a comparable relative risk per dose and are much more commonly used. The incidence of *C. difficile* colitis is lowest in outpatients and varies considerably by institution

**Table 32.1** Administration of macrolides

| Agent | Route of administration | Standard dosage for adults | Pediatric dosing | Comments |
|---|---|---|---|---|
| Erythromycin: | Oral | 250–500 mg qid (dose in erythromycin base equivalents) | 30–50 mg/kg/day divided into 3–4 doses | |
| Base | | | | Better absorbed in fasting state |
| Enteric coated | | | | Not affected by administration with food |
| Film coated | | | | Not affected by administration with food |
| Estolate | | | | Avoid use in adults, particularly pregnant women |
| Ethyl succinate | | | | Better absorbed in fasting state |
| Stearate | | | | Better absorbed in fasting state |
| Lactobionate | Intravenous | 250 mg–1 g q6hr | | |
| Gluceptate | | | | |
| Base | Topical | 0.5% ophthalmic ointment<br>2%–3% dermatologic gel or solution | | |
| Dirithromycin | Oral | 500 mg qd | | |
| Roxithromycin | Oral | 150 mg bid or 300 mg qd | 2.5 mg/kg q12hr | Better absorbed in fasting state |
| Clarithromycin | Oral | 500 mg bid | 15 mg/kg/day divided into 2 doses | Intravenous preparation available in some European countries |
| Azithromycin | Oral | 500 mg $\times$ 1 dose, then 250 mg qd | 10 mg/kg/day | Better absorbed in fasting state |
| | | (usually 5-day course) | | 1 g single-dose regimen for *C. trachomatis*. |
| | Intravenous | 500 mg qd | | |
| Spiramycin | Oral | 500–1000 mg bid or tid | 50–100 mg/kg/day divided into 2–4 doses | |
| | Intravenous | 500 mg q8hr | | |
| Josamycin | Oral | 500 mg tid or 1 g bid | 50–100 mg/kg/day divided into 2–4 doses | |
| Miokamycin | Oral | 600–900 mg bid or tid | 30–60 mg/kg/day divided into 2 doses | |

among inpatient populations. The spectrum of disease caused by *C. difficile* ranges from mild, self-limited diarrhea to fatal cases of toxic megacolon.

Other adverse effects of lincosamides include reversible elevation of hepatic enzymes, and rare cases of neutropenia and neuromuscular blockade, as well as manifestations of hypersensitivity, such as fever, rash, eosinophilia, and anaphylaxis. Cardiotoxicity and cardiopulmonary arrest, which had been reported after rapid infusion of lincomycin, are not known complications of clindamycin use. There are few important drug interactions involving lincosamides, but neuromuscular blocking agents may be potentiated by clindamycin.

## Clinical use

Clindamycin is an agent with several well-defined niches in antimicrobial chemotherapy. Infections containing anaerobic bacteria, particularly abdominal or pelvic abscesses, are amenable to treatment with clindamycin, usually in combination with an agent effective against Enterobacteriaceae. The combination of clindamycin with gentamicin is a reasonable alternative to $\beta$-lactam-doxycycline therapy for pelvic inflammatory disease. Clindamycin is probably superior to penicillin in the treatment of anaerobic infections of the lung, which may contain $\beta$-lactamase-producing *Bacteroides* species. Clindamycin may be used to treat odontogenic infections, or as an alternative drug for endocarditis prophylaxis in $\beta$-lactam-allergic patients undergoing dental or otorhinolaryngological procedures. Because of its good penetration into bone, clindamycin is sometimes used in the treatment of osteomyelitis caused by staphylococci or streptococci, or it may be combined with other agents for polymicrobial contiguous osteomyelitis, such as diabetic foot infections or decubitus ulcers. Skin infections caused by these organisms are often treatable with clindamycin. Because it inhibits ribosomal protein synthesis, some authors have advocated use of clindamycin-containing regimens (usually combined with a penicillin) in order to stop toxin production in patients with infections caused by clostridia, as well as toxin-producing streptococci and *S. aureus*. Clindamycin has additional advantages over $\beta$-lactams in that it is less affected by the large inoculum of organisms present in serious infections such as necrotizing fasciitis and may also have beneficial immunomodulatory effects.

Emerging uses of clindamycin take advantage of its activity against protozoan pathogens. Clindamycin combined with pyrimethamine has efficacy and toxicity comparable to pyrimethamine plus sulfadiazine in the treatment of central nervous system infection with *Toxoplasma gondii* in patients with AIDS. With the explosion of chloroquine resistance in *Plasmodium falciparum*, clindamycin combined with quinine (oral therapy) or quinidine gluconate (intravenous therapy), has proven useful. Clindamycin combined with quinine is the regimen of choice for infections due to *Babesia microti*.

There are several precautionary notes on the use of clindamycin. The mechanism of action of clindamycin is the inhibition of microbial protein synthesis, therefore it is usually only bacteriostatic. It does not penetrate the blood-brain barrier sufficiently to treat most bacterial infections of the central nervous system. Resistance to clindamycin is increasingly common among several important pathogens including methicillin-resistant *S. aureus*. While *C. difficile* colitis complicates a minority of therapeutic courses of clindamycin, the risk is not much greater than that caused by other antibiotics, particularly $\beta$-lactams.

## Administration

Clindamycin may be administered orally or parenterally. The standard oral preparation is clindamycin hydrochloride, which may be given in doses ranging from 150 to 450 mg every 6 h. Another oral preparation of clindamycin is a palmitate ester suspension. Oral preparations are absorbed rapidly and have approximately 90% bioavailability. Food may delay, but not decrease, the absorption of clindamycin. Peak serum levels of 3.6 $\mu$g/ml may be reached with a single 300 mg oral dose. For intravenous delivery, 600 to 900 mg of clindamycin phosphate is infused every 6 h to 8 h (higher doses have been used for treatment of toxoplasmic encephalitis) and peak serum levels of 14 $\mu$g/ml may be achieved with a single 900 mg dose. This preparation may also be administered intramuscularly in doses as high as 600 mg. Topical clindamycin, in a gel or solution, is available for dermatological (treatment of acne vulgaris) and gynecological (treatment of bacterial vaginosis) use.

Clindamycin has a serum half-life of between 2 and 3 h. It is highly protein bound with up to 90% serum protein binding in some studies. The esters of this drug (phosphate and palmitate) must be hydrolyzed in the blood to release active clindamycin. This agent penetrates into most tissues and fluids other than the cerebrospinal fluid. Animal model data indicate that clindamycin attains good levels in abdominal abscesses. Like the macrolides, it is concentrated in polymorphonuclear neutrophils and macrophages, but the clinical significance of this property is unclear. The metabolism of clindamycin occurs primarily in the liver, where the drug is converted to an *N*-demethyl metabolite with antimicrobial activity exceeding that of the parent compound, and a less-active sulfoxide metabolite. As these products are cleared through the urine and feces, significant dose reduction is recommended only for patients with severe hepatic failure *or* combined renal and hepatic dysfunction. Clindamycin levels are not reduced by either hemodialysis or peritoneal dialysis. Clindamycin crosses the placenta, and limited data have not revealed adverse effects on human fetal development.

### ANNOTATED BIBLIOGRAPHY

Bryskier AJ, Butzler JP, Neu HC, Tulkens PM. Macrolides. Arnette Blackwell, Paris, 1993.

*This is an encyclopedic reference text on the macrolides.*

Clancy J, Petitpas J, Dib-Hajj F, et al. Molecular cloning and functional analysis of a novel macrolide-resistance determinant, *mefA*, from *Streptococcus pyogenes*. Mol Microbiol 1996; 22:867–879.

*A report describing the gene encoding the M phenotype and its expression.*

Falagas ME, Gorbach SL. Clindamycin and metronidazole. Med Clin North Am 1995; 79:845–867.

*A review of clindamycin.*

Martin DH, Mroczkowski TF, Dalu ZA, et al. A controlled trial of a single dose of azithromycin for the treatment of chlamydial urethritis and cervicitis. N Engl J Med 1992; 327:921–925.

*A randomized comparative study of single-dose azithromycin versus one week of twice daily doxycycline for the treatment of chlamydial genital infection; Shows equivalent efficacy and adverse drug effects.*

Rodvold KA, Piscitelli SC. New oral macrolides and fluoroquinolone antibiotics: an overview of pharmacokinetics, interactions and safety. Clin Infect Dis 1993; 17(Suppl 1):S192–S199.

*Summary of current pharmacological data on clarithromycin and azithromycin. Extensive reference list provided.*

Shafran SD, Singer J, Zarowny DP, et al. A comparison of two regimens for the treatment of *Mycobacterium avium* complex bacteremia in AIDS: rifampin, ethambutol, and clarithromycin versus rifampin, ethambutol, clofazamine and ciprofloxacin. N Engl J Med 1996; 335:377–383.

Pierce M, Crampton S, Henry D, et al. A randomized trial of clarithromycin as prophylaxis against disseminated *Mycobacterium avium* complex infection in patients with advanced acquired immunodeficiency syndrome. N Engl J Med 1996; 335:384–391.

Havlir DV, Duké MP, Sattler FR, et al. Prophylaxis against disseminated *Mycobacterium avium* complex with weekly azithromycin, daily rifabutin, or both. N Engl J Med 1996; 335:392–398.

Horsburgh CR. Advances in the prevention and treatment of *Mycobacterium avium* disease. N Engl J Med 1996; 335:428–430.

*Three important trials involving prophylaxis and treatment of M. avium infections in persons with AIDS, along with the accompanying editorial supporting the use of clarithromycin and azithromycin for these indications.*

Schlossberg D. Azithromycin and clarithromycin. Med Clin North Am 1995; 79:803–815.

*A good general review of the newer macrolides.*

Stevens DL, Bryant AE, Hackett SP. Antibiotic effects on bacterial viability, toxin production and host response. Clin Infect Dis 1995; 20(Suppl 2):S254–S257.

*Results of this in vitro study comparing clindamycin with other agents supports the use of this agent in the treatment of infections caused by toxin-producing organisms.*

Sutcliff J, Tait-Kamradt A, Wondrack L. *Streptococcus pneumoniae* and *Streptococcus pyogenes* resistant to macrolides but sensitive to clindamyin: a common resistance pattern mediated by an efflux mechanism. Antimicrob Agents Chemother 1996; 40:1817–1824.

*Study detailing the M phenotype.*

# 33

# Tetracyclines and Chloramphenicol

THOMAS M. HOOTON

Tetracyclines, discovered in the late 1940s, were the first major group of antimicrobial agents for which the term "broad spectrum" was used. They are naturally occurring and synthetically derived antibiotics that constitute a very important class of drugs commonly used in clinical practice.

Chloramphenicol, a naturally occurring antibiotic, was also discovered in the late 1940s. Although it is a highly effective and inexpensive antibiotic, it should never be used for the treatment of minor infections because of concerns about its toxicity; effective and safer alternative agents are available. It is occasionally used, however, as an alternative agent for seriously ill patients when other alternatives are not feasible. Moreover, it continues to be used worldwide because of its broad spectrum, effectiveness, low cost, and ease of administration.

## Tetracyclines

Tetracyclines are generally bacteriostatic at therapeutic concentrations, but they may be bactericidal in certain situations. Tetracyclines inhibit protein synthesis by blocking the binding of aminoacyl-tRNA to the mRNA-ribosome complex through reversible binding, primarily to the 30S ribosomal subunit. The specificity of tetracyclines for bacteria depends both on their selectivity for bacterial ribosomes and on their requirement for an active, energy-dependent transport mechanism into the bacterial cell by a system not found in mammalian cell membranes.

### Pharmacology

Modifications of the tetracycline nucleus result in derivatives with different degrees of antibacterial activity, absorption, and protein binding. Although the antimicrobial spectrum of the different tetracyclines is similar, three groups can be distinguished by differences in their pharmacologic properties: the shorter-acting agents, tetracycline, oxytetracycline, and chlortetracycline, have a serum half-life of approximately 9 h; the intermediate-acting agents, demeclocycline and methacycline, have a serum half-life of approximately 13 h; and the longer-acting agents, doxycycline and minocycline, have a serum half-life of approximately 17 h. All but chlortetracycline and methacycline are commercially available for systemic use in the United States.

Doxycycline and minocycline are 95% to 100% absorbed from the gastrointestinal tract in fasting adults, compared with 60% to 80% absorption for the other commercially available agents. Concomitant administration of milk and food reduces the gastrointestinal absorption of tetracycline by 50% or more but that of doxycycline and minocycline only by 20%. The tetracyclines are secreted in the bile and undergo enterohepatic circulation with concentrations of drug in bile many times higher than serum concentrations. Peak serum concentrations occur approximately 2 h after oral dosing. Tetracyclines, some of which are up to 95% protein bound, are widely distributed throughout the body, readily cross the placenta, and are distributed into milk. However, cerebrospinal fluid levels are only 10% to 20% of those in serum. Tetracyclines are eliminated in urine and feces, and they are only minimally removed by hemodialysis or peritoneal dialysis.

The usual daily dose of tetracycline in adults is 1 to 2 g orally given at 6 h intervals. The maximum daily dose of tetracycline should not exceed 2 g. The usual oral dose of doxycycline is 100 mg twice daily or 200 mg on Day 1, followed by 100 mg once daily; for minocycline the dosage is 200 mg followed by 100 mg twice daily. Intravenous dosage of tetracycline, doxycycline, and minocycline is the same as oral dosage. Intramuscular injection of tetracyclines is painful and is not recommended. Tetracycline and doxycycline, but not minocycline, achieve therapeutic concentrations in the urine for those infections caused by susceptible uropathogens. The dosage of doxycycline needs little or no adjustment in renal failure and, as such, it is the tetracycline of choice in renal failure. However, it should not be used for urinary tract infections in patients with renal failure because of the low urine concentrations in such patients. The other tetracyclines should not be used in end-stage renal disease.

### Resistance

Resistance to tetracyclines is due to limitation of access to ribosomes through reduced uptake or energy-dependent efflux of antibiotic, ribosomal modification such that the antibiotic has decreased binding, and possibly through chemical inactivation of the antibiotic. The majority of tetracycline resistance determinants are located on plasmids or transposons. Plasmid-mediated resistance can be transferred between organisms of the same or different species and resistance to multiple antimicrobials may be tranferred on the same plasmid. Complete cross-resistance to the tetracyclines usually occurs, although some resistant strains remain susceptible to minocycline. The widespread use of tetracyclines in animal husbandry may be a factor resulting in increased resistance to this class of antibiotics through selective antibiotic pressure. In particular, increasing resistance to tetracyclines has been noted among *Neisseria gonorrhoeae*, staphylococci and streptococci, and several species of gram-negative bacilli.

### Clinical Indications

Tetracyclines exhibit a broad spectrum of activity against aerobic and anaerobic bacteria, spirochetes, *Mycoplasma* spp., *Chlamydia* spp., *Rickettsia* spp., and protozoans. However, tetracyclines have poor or no activity against many clinically important bacterial species, including enterococci, many strains of staphylococci, streptococci, *Escherichia coli* and other Enterobacteriaceae, and most strains of *Proteus* and *Pseudomonas aeruginosa*. Many strains of *N. gonorrhoeae*, especially those with chromosomally mediated resistance to penicillin, are resistant to tetracyclines. Although doxycycline is generally more active than tetracycline against anaerobic bacteria, including *Bacteroides fragilis*, other agents are usually preferred for treatment of infections caused by anaerobic bacteria. Tetracyclines are inactive against fungi and viruses.

Tetracyclines are widely used in a variety of infections and dermatologic conditions (see Tables 33.1 and 33.2). Tetracyclines also appear to have non-antimicrobial properties that are beneficial in the treatment of periodontal disease. The increased proportion of strains exhibiting resistance to the tetracyclines among pathogens causing common community-acquired infections, such as *S. pneumoniae*, *H. influenzae*, *N. gonorrhoeae*, and *E. coli*, along with the availability of effective alternative agents, has led to the decreased use of this class of antibiotics. Doxycycline and tetracycline are by far the most commonly used of the tetracycline analogs, and they can be used interchangeably for most infections. However, doxycycline is approximately two- to fourfold more active against many pathogens, can be administered twice rather than four times daily, and since becoming generic and less expensive, has become the most commonly used. Although minocycline tends to be the most active tetracycline against most susceptible organisms, side effects limit its usefulness (see below).

## Side Effects and Drug Interactions

The tetracyclines are generally very well tolerated. Gastrointestinal symptoms are the most common side effects and may be related to a direct irritant effect on the mucosa since tetracyclines can cause esophageal ulceration when they dissolve before entering the stomach. Photosensitivity reactions, considered to be a toxic rather than an allergic reaction, can be caused by all tetracyclines, but are most common with doxycycline. Other dermal reactions, including morbilliform rashes, urticaria, periorbital edema, hyperpigmentation of teeth, nails, and skin, and fixed drug eruptions are uncommon. Fatal hepatotoxicity may occur with administration of more than 2 g daily of tetracycline intravenously and at lower doses during pregnancy. Tetracyclines should be avoided in pregnancy because of the risk of hepatotoxicity and transplacental passage to the fetus leading to teeth and bone developmental abnormalities (see below). Pancreatitis is a rare complication of tetracycline therapy. Benign intracranial hypertension resulting in headache and blurred vision may occur with the use of tetracyclines. Minocycline is unique in causing vestibular symptoms (vertigo, ataxia, nausea, tinnitus) within 2 to 3 days of starting therapy. This adverse effect occurs in up to 70% of women and a smaller percentage of men; it is dose related and probably secondary to higher blood levels in women.

Tetracycline use in young children usually causes a permanent gray-brown to yellow discoloration of the teeth which may be associated with hypoplasia of the enamel and depression of skeletal growth in premature infants. The degree of enamel staining appears to be related to the cumulative dose of tetracyclines. Thus, tetracyclines should not be administered, unless there is no satisfactory alternative, to pregnant women or children up to the age of 8 years, which is the period when tooth enamel is being formed.

There are several significant drug interactions to be concerned about with tetracyclines. Divalent and trivalent cations, such as those found in antacids, dairy products, and iron preparations, can decrease the absorption of tetracyclines. Inducers of hepatic enzymes, such as phenytoin and barbiturates, may also decrease the levels of tetracyclines. On the other hand, tetracyclines have been shown to depress plasma prothrombin activity; patients on anticoagulants need close monitoring and possible dose adjust-

**Table 33.1** Conditions or pathogens for which tetracyclines are the therapeutic agents of choice*

| |
|---|
| Balantidiasis (*Balantidium coli*) (tetracycline) |
| Brucellosis (plus aminoglycoside or rifampin) |
| Chlamydial infections |
| *C. pneumoniae* |
| *C. psittaci* (psittacosis) |
| *C. trachomatis* (including cervicitis, epididymitis, inclusion conjunctivitis, lymphogranuloma venereum, pelvic inflammatory disease, proctitis, trachoma, and urethritis (usually in combination with an anti-gonococcal regimen) |
| Ehrlichiosis, monocytic (*Ehrlichia chaffeensis*) and granulocytic types |
| Glanders (*Burkholderia* (*Pseudomonas*) *mallei*) (plus streptomycin) |
| Granuloma inguinale (*Calymmatobacterium granulomatis*) |
| *Helicobacter pylori* (tetracycline plus bismuth and metronidazole) |
| Lyme disease, erythema chronicum migrans and arthritis (*Borrelia burgdorferi*) |
| Malaria (chloroquine-resistant *P. falciparum*) (plus quinine sulfate) |
| *Mycobacterium fortuitum* complex (plus amikacin) |
| Q fever (*coxiella burnetii*) (acute disease) |
| Relapsing fever (*Borrelia recurrentis*) |
| Rickettsial infections (Rocky Mountain spotted fever, Q fever (acute), endemic typhus, epidemic typhus, scrub typhus) |
| *Vibrio cholerae* (cholera) |
| *Vibrio parahemolyticus* |
| *Vibrio vulnificus* |

*Doxycycline unless otherwise noted.

**Table 33.2** Conditions or pathogens for which tetracyclines are effective alternative therapeutic agents

| |
|---|
| Acne, inflammatory |
| Acne rosacea |
| Actinomycosis (*Actinomyces israelii*) |
| Anthrax, cutaneous (*Bacillus anthracis*) |
| Bacillary angiomatosis (*Bartonella henselae*, *B. quintana*) |
| Bite (cat, rat) prophylaxis |
| Bronchitis (mild acute exacerbation of chronic bronchitis in smoker) |
| *Burkholderia* (*Pseudomonas*) *cepacia* (minocycline) |
| *Campylobacter jejuni* |
| *Clostridium perfringens* |
| *Clostridium tetani* |
| *Dientamoeba fragilis* |
| *Eikenella corrodens* |
| Leptospirosis (Leptospira) |
| Lyme disease—carditis (*Borrelia burgdorferi*) |
| Malaria (prophylaxis in areas of chloroquine-resistant strains) |
| *Moraxella (Branhamella) catarrhalis* |
| *Mycobacterium leprae* (leprosy) (minocycline) |
| *Mycobacterium marinum* (minocycline) |
| *Mycoplasma pneumoniae* |
| *Neisseria meningitidis*, prophylaxis of contacts (minocycline) |
| *Nocardia asteroides*, pulmonary (minocycline) |
| *Pasteurella multocida* |
| Plague (*Yersinia pestis*) |
| Pneumonia, mild community acquired |
| Melioidosis (*Burkholderia* (*Pseudomonas*) *pseudomallei*) (plus trimethoprim-sulfamethoxazole and chloramphenicol) |
| Rat-bite fever (*Spirillum minus*, *Streptobacillus moniliformis*) |
| Stenotrophomonas (*Xanthomonas*) *maltophilia* (minocycline) |
| Syphilis, all except neurosyphilis, pregnancy, congenital, HIV-associated (*Treponema pallidum)* |
| Yaws (*Treponema pertenue*) |
| Tularemia (*Francisella tularensis*) |
| *Ureaplasma urealyticum* |

ments. Tetracycline use can also decrease the efficacy of oral contraceptives, perhaps by altering bacterial hydrolysis of conjugated estrogen in the intestine. Women on these agents concomitantly should be advised to use additional contraception to prevent pregnancy. The anesthetic agent methoxyflurane has been reported to cause nephrotoxicity in patients receiving tetracyclines. Although clinical data are sparse, the bactericidal activity of other antibiotics may be decreased when used concomitantly with tetracyclines, which are bacteriostatic.

## Chloramphenicol

Chloramphenicol, although an excellent antimicrobial agent, is not the drug of choice for any infection in the United States because of the toxicity profile described below. Chloramphenicol should be used only for the treatment of serious infections caused by susceptible pathogens when other effective but less toxic regimens cannot be used.

Thiamphenicol is an analog of chloramphenicol in which the p-nitro group on the benzene ring is replaced by a methylsulfonyl group. Its antimicrobial spectrum is similar to that of chloramphenicol. Although thiamphenicol causes hemopoietic toxicity, it has not been reported to cause aplastic anemia, which suggests that the p-nitro moiety of chloramphenicol is the structural feature associated with the occurrence of aplastic anemia. Thiamphenicol is not available in the United States, but it is used extensively in Europe and Japan.

### Mechanism of action

Chloramphenicol inhibits protein synthesis by reversibly binding to the 50S subunit of the bacterial 70S ribosome, which prevents the attachment of the aminoacyl-tRNA to its binding region. Chloramphenicol is bacteriostatic against most susceptible pathogens, but it may be bactericidal when used in high doses or against highly susceptible pathogens. The major mechanism of resistance is drug inactivation by plasmid-mediated chloramphenicol acetyltransferase. Unrestricted use in some countries may be a factor resulting in increased resistance to this class of antibiotics through selective antibiotic pressure.

### Pharmacology

Chloramphenicol is highly bioavailable in the encapsulated form and results in peak serum levels after a 1 g oral dose of approximately 11 $\mu$g/ml of active antibiotic in 1 to 3 h, and approximately 18 $\mu$g/ml after several doses. Intravenous administration results in lower serum concentrations because of incomplete hydrolysis of the chloramphenicol sodium succinate to the biologically active chloramphenicol. The antibiotic diffuses well into many tissues and body fluids, including the aqueous and vitreous humor and cerebrospinal fluid, reflecting its high degree of lipid solubility and small molecular size. The concentration of chloramphenicol in cerebrospinal fluid is reported to be up to 50% of plasma concentrations in patients with uninflamed meninges and up to 89% of plasma concentrations in patients with inflamed meninges. Chloramphenicol crosses the placenta and is distributed into milk.

The plasma half-life of chloramphenicol in healthy adults is approximately 1.5 to 4 h. Chloramphenicol is metabolized primarily in the liver by glucuronyl transferase. Premature and newborn infants have immature mechanisms of glucuronide conjugation and renal excretion and the plasma half-life is increased to 24 h or longer. The usual oral and parenteral dose of chloramphenicol in adults and children is 50 (occasionally up to 100) mg/kg/day given at 6 h intervals, with a maximum daily dose not to exceed 4 g. The recommended dose in premature infants is 25 mg/kg/day. The dose of chloramphenicol should be adjusted in patients with hepatic failure because of the accumulation of chloramphenicol and subsequent toxicity. On the other hand, renal disease does not affect the half-life of biologically active chloramphenicol, therefore the dose does not need to be modified, even in the setting of peritoneal or hemodialysis. Because of the narrow therapeutic-to-toxic ratio, serum levels should be monitored, particularly in infants, in patients with hepatic disease, and when drugs that interact with chloramphenicol metabolism are used. Chloramphenicol levels should be maintained between 10 and 30 $\mu$g/ml in most cases. The course of therapy should be no longer than that required to produce a cure and minimize the risk of relapse, usually no longer than 10 to 14 days.

## Clinical Indications

Chloramphenicol is a very broad spectrum agent (Table 33.3). It demonstrates activity against many clinically important anaerobic bacterial species, including *Bacteroides fragilis* and *B. melaninogenicus* (*Prevotella melaninogenica*), *Clostridium* spp. (except *C. difficile*), and Fusobacterium. It also has activity against many important gram-positive aerobes, including *Streptococcus pyogenes* and *S. pneumoniae*, and many gram-negative aerobes, including *H. influenzae*, *N. gonorrhoeae*, and *N. meningitidis*. Chloramphenicol is also active against *Rickettsia* spp., *Chlamydia trachomatis*, and *Mycoplasma pneumoniae*.

Conditions for which chloramphenicol can be considered an alternative agent are listed in Table 33.3. It may occasionally have a role in the treatment of bacterial meningitis in the penicillin-allergic patient, for penicillin-resistant pneumococcal meningitis (although there are reports of high failure rates associated with chloramphenicol therapy), and as an oral agent when the use of parenteral therapy is impossible. Chloramphenicol is the drug of choice for rickettsial infections when tetracyclines cannot be used. It is generally considered the drug of choice for the treatment of rickettsial infection in young children and in pregnant women since tetracyclines are contraindicated in such patients, but the risk of serious side effects associated with chloramphenicol must be weighed against those associated with tetracycline therapy in such patients. Chloramphenicol may be useful when the differential diagnosis includes both meningococcemia and Rocky Mountain spotted fever, diseases that may be difficult to distinguish on clinical grounds, but other less toxic agents or combinations of agents can usually be used in these situations. It also has a role as an alternative agent in the treatment of typhoid fever, plague, and brucellosis.

## Side effects and drug interactions

### Hematologic toxicity

The most important toxicity associated with chloramphenicol can be divided into two types. The first is bone marrow suppression of all cell lines due to direct inhibition of mitochondrial protein synthesis. This type of toxicity is common at the maximal recommended doses of 4 g/day or in patients in whom serum levels are above 25 $\mu$g/ml, and is reversible when treatment with the antibiotic is discontinued. The second type of hematologic toxicity is a rare but usually fatal idiosyncratic reaction that is usually manifested as aplastic anemia. Although no prospective controlled trials have been performed, it has been estimated that aplastic anemia occurs once in 25,000 to 40,000 patients who are treated with chloramphenicol, a risk that is many times greater than that in the general population. Chloramphenicol was the single most commonly incriminated drug in cases of aplastic anemia. Aplastic anemia usually occurs weeks to months after completion of therapy and does not appear to be related to dose or duration of therapy. It may occur after a single dose of chloramphenicol. The mechanism of this toxicity is not known but may involve a genetic predispostition or preexisting marrow damage. Although it has been noted that aplastic anemia is much more common following oral administration of the drug, it may also follow its parenteral or topical ophthalmologic administration. Since marrow suppression may occur during the ad-

**Table 33.3** Conditions or pathogens for which chloramphenicol is an effective alternative agent alone or in combination with other agents

| Condition or pathogen | Agents of choice | Chloramphenicol |
|---|---|---|
| Bacterial meningitis (older infant/child)<br>*S. pneumoniae*<br>*N. meningitidis*<br>*H. influenzae* | Cefotaxime or ceftriaxone[a] | Plus vancomycin[b] |
| Bacterial meningitis (older child/adult)<br>*S. pneumoniae*<br>*N. meningitidis*<br>*Listeria monocytogenes* | Cefotaxime (or ceftriaxone)<br>+ ampicillin[a] | Plus TMP/SMX[b] |
| Brain abscess | Ceftriaxone (or penicillin G) + metronidazole | |
| Brucellosis | Doxycycline + (aminoglycoside or rifampin) | |
| *Burkholderia* (*Pseudomonas*) *cepacia* | TMP-SMX | |
| *Fusobacterium* sp. | Penicillin G | |
| Glanders (*Burkholderia* (*Pseudomonas*) *mallei*) | Doxycycline + streptomycin | Plus streptomycin |
| *H. influenzae*, life threatening | Cefotaxime or ceftriaxone | |
| Melioidosis (*Burkholderia* (*Pseudomonas*) *pseudomallei*) | Ceftazidime | Plus doxycycline and TMP/SMX |
| Plague (*Yersinia pestis*) | Aminoglycoside | |
| Psittacosis (*Chlamydia psittaci*) | Doxycycline | |
| Rickettsial infections | Doxycycline | |
| Tularemia (*Francisella tularensis*) | Aminoglycoside or doxycycline | |
| Typhoidal syndrome (*S. typhi*, *S. paratyphi*) | Fluoroquinolone or ceftriaxone | |
| *Vibrio vulnificus*, cellulitis, and/or sepsis | Doxycycline + ceftazidime | |

[a]Plus vancomycin if concern about high-level drug-resistant *S. pneumoniae*.

[b]If patient has a severe penicillin allergy.

ministration of the drug, complete blood counts should be obtained during drug administration (some recommend monitoring every 2 days), and the drug should be discontinued if significant hematologic toxicity is noted. However, such monitoring does not preclude the later development of the irreversible type of bone marrow depression.

Chloramphenicol use may also increase the risk of leukemia following aplastic anemia, leukemia not associated with aplastic anemia, paroxysmal nocturnal hemoglobinuria, and hemolytic anemia in patients with the Mediterranean form of glucose-6-phosphate dehydrogenase (G6PD) deficiency.

### Gray syndrome

The dose-related gray syndrome of premature and newborn infants, manifested by abdominal distension, vomiting, progressive pallid cyanosis, metabolic acidosis, circulatory collapse, and death, results from a diminshed ability of the newborn to conjugate chloramphenicol or excrete the unconjugated drug. Symptoms such as failure to feed or abdominal distention with or without vomiting usually develop several days after the start of chloramphenicol and, if recognized early enough and the drug is discontinued, the process may be reversible. The syndrome has also been reported in older children and after accidental overdose in adults in whom high levels have been noted.

### Other side effects

Optic neuritis resulting in decreased visual acuity to blindness has been reported in patients receiving prolonged high-dose therapy. Other neurologic sequelae such as peripheral neuritis, headache, depression, and mental confusion have been reported. Gastrointestinal symptoms, including nausea, vomiting and diarrhea, glossitis, and stomatitis may occur. Herxheimer-like reactions during therapy for typhoid fever have been reported. Hypersensitivity reactions are uncommon.

### Drug interactions

Chloramphenicol prolongs the serum half-life of tolbutamide, chlorpropamide, phenytoin, cyclophosphamide, and warfarin by inhibition of hepatic microsomal enzymes. It may also interfere with vitamin K production by intestinal bacteria and thus prolong the prothrombin time in patients receiving anticoagulant therapy. Dosages of such agents should be adjusted as necessary. Concomitant administration of chloramphenicol and phenobarbital or rifampin may result in decreased plasma concentrations of chloramphenicol. Chloramphenicol delays the reponse of anemias to iron, folic acid, and vitamin B12 therapy. Because of considerable in vitro data and conflicting in vivo data suggesting that chloramphenicol and $\beta$-lactams are antagonistic when used concurrently, it has been suggested that combined therapy with these agents should be avoided, particularly when bactericidal activity is desired.

## ANNOTATED BIBLIOGRAPHY


Abramowicz M, ed. Handbook of Antimicrobial Therapy. Med Lett 1996: 5–184.

*An excellent general review of antimicrobials with recommendations about appropriate use, dosing, and adverse effects.*

Chopra I, Hawkey PM, Hinton M. Review: tetracyclines, molecular and clinical aspects. J Antimicrob Chemother 1992; 29:245–277.

*A general review of the structure, mode of action, mechanisms of transport, mechanisms of resistance, and clinical uses of the tetracyclines.*

Egerman RS. The tetracyclines. Obstet Gynecol Clin North Am 1992; 19:551–561.

*A general review of the mechanism of action, pharmacokinetics, spectrum of activity, and side effects of the tetracyclines.*

Flegg P, Cheong I, Welsby PD. Chloramphenicol: are concerns about aplastic anaemia justified? Drug Safety 1992; 7:167–169.

*A review about the hematologic toxicities associated with chloramphenicol and a discussion about deciding when to use this compound.*

Friedland IR, Klugman KP. Failure of chloramphenicol therapy in penicillin-resistant pneumococcal meningitis. Lancet 1992; 339:405–408.

*A prospective study of children with pneumococcal meningitis demonstrating that chloramphenicol was associated with frequent treatment failures in those children with penicillin-resistant strains.*

Golub LM, Suomalainen K, Sorsa T. Host modulation with tetracyclines and their chemically modified analogues. Curr Sci Periodontol Res Dent 1992; 80–90.

*A review of the anticollagenase properties of the tetracyclines and the potential therapeutic roles of the tetracyclines in noninfectious disease conditions.*

Holt D, Harvey D, Hurley R. Chloramphenicol toxicity. Adverse Drug React Toxicol Rev 1993; 12:83–95.

*A general review of the adverse effects associated with chloramphenicol use.*

# 34

# Fluoroquinolones

RALF STAHLMANN AND HARTMUT LODE

Quinolones have been used therapeutically for more than 30 years, predominantly for treatment of urinary tract infections. As the antimicrobial and pharmacokinetic characteristics of the older quinolones, such as nalidixic acid or oxolinic acid, were far from optimal, they have been considered second-line therapeutics. The synthesis of a new series of drugs with a fluorine atom at position 6 of the molecule led to derivatives with markedly enhanced antibacterial activity. This group is referred to as fluoroquinolones.

These drugs represent a major advance in the chemotherapy of bacterial infections, but they also have a great potential for overuse and misuse, which in turn may result in the emergence of resistance. The future viability of the quinolones will depend on the ability of the medical community to use them wisely.

Table 34.1 provides an overview of those fluoroquinolones which are either on the market or at an advanced stage of their preclinical development. Since brand names differ in various countries, only the generic names are listed. Information on the range of doses usually recommended for treatment of bacterial infections with these drugs is also included.

## Structure–Activity Relationships and Mechanism of Action

A considerable amount of knowledge exists on the relationships between structure and antimicrobial activity of the fluoroquinolones (Fig. 34.1). The carboxy and carbonyl groups in positions 3 and 4 are essential for antibacterial activity because they mediate binding to the DNA–gyrase complex (probably via a magnesium ion). The fluorine at C6 is essential for high potency; it can provide 100-fold improvement of the antibacterial activity. A halogen (F or Cl) at the 8 position improves oral absorption and activity against anaerobes (e.g., lomefloxacin, fleroxacin, sparfloxacin). A cyclopropyl group at N1 (e.g., ciprofloxacin, sparfloxacin) and an amino substituent at C5 (e.g., sparfloxacin) improve overall antimicrobial potency.

Several potential side effects are also directly influenced by structural modification. For example, central nervous system (CNS) side effects and interactions with theophylline and nonsteroidal anti-inflammatory drugs (NSAIDs) are strongly influenced by the C7 substituent. Phototoxicity is determined by the nature of the 8-position substituent. A halogen atom in this position causes the greatest photoreaction whereas a hydrogen or a methoxy group show little light-induced toxicity. Some other side effects of the quinolones are class effects that probably cannot be modulated by molecular variation. These include the potential to induce gastrointestinal irritation or arthropathy in immature animals (Fig. 34.1).

The primary target of quinolones in the bacterial cell is the enzyme gyrase (also called topoisomerase II), which is found in bacteria only. Similar enzymes (topoisomerases III and IV) are found in mammalian cells. Gyrase introduces negative supertwists into the DNA double helix and separates interlocked DNA molecules. Quinolone concentrations that inhibit the DNA supercoiling and decatenating activities of purified DNA gyrase are often 10- to 100-fold higher than concentrations that inhibit bacterial growth. Thus other mechanisms for their antibacterial action may exist. Exposure of highly susceptible pathogens to fluoroquinolones results in rapid cell death. The exact details of the mechanisms of bacterial killing by quinolones still remain unclear.

## Resistance

Bacterial resistance to fluoroquinolones is an increasing problem. Laboratory observations have shown that serial passage of bacteria in increasing concentrations of fluoroquinolones can produce highly resistant strains of various bacteria.

Resistance to quinolones has been a problem primarily in two species, *Pseudomonas aeruginosa* and *Staphylococcus aureus*. Resistant strains of *P. aeruginosa* have been isolated from patients treated for urinary tract infections, cystic fibrosis, skin infections, or osteomyelitis. The incidence of resistance has been as high as 50%. In addition, in some countries, especially in Japan, the incidence of resistance against *Serratia marcescens* is significant. Among gram-positive bacteria the development of resistance in *S. aureus* is noteworthy. Ciprofloxacin-resistant methicillin-resistant *S. aureus* (MRSA) have been found in Europe, the United States, and other parts of the world.

Several mechanisms of resistance have been described. However, to date there is no evidence of a plasmid-mediated resistance to fluoroquinolones nor of destruction of these agents by bacterial enzymes. The mutants isolated so far show chromosomal mutations that alter the gyrase A or gyrase B subunit (the principle target of quinolone action) or the mutations affect the accumulation of quinolones in the cell. Accumulation of these agents in the bacterial cell involves several processes: in addition to passive diffusion, fluoroquinolones enter the bacterial cell via membrane protein porins (e.g., OmpF) and also by a "self-promoted" pathway. It has been suggested that quinolones disrupt bacterial lipopolysaccharides (LPS) through their chelating activity with magnesium—an ion which is essential for the LPS integrity—and thus facilitate their own uptake into the bacterial cell. In gram-negative and gram-positive bacteria, active efflux mechanisms exist for removing the quinolones from the cell. Alterations of transport into the cell or the efflux mechanism are possibilities for mutants to become resistant to quinolones.

**Table 34.1** Fluoroquinolones

| Name | Available as PO or IV formulation | Recommended daily doses |
|---|---|---|
| Norfloxacin | PO | 400 mg bid |
| Ciprofloxacin | PO | 250–750 mg bid |
| | IV | 200 mg q8–12h |
| Ofloxacin | PO | 200–400 mg bid |
| | IV | 200–600 mg bid |
| Enoxacin | PO | 400 mg bid |
| Lomefloxacin | PO | 400 mg qd |
| Fleroxacin | PO | 400 mg qd |
| | IV | 400 mg qd |
| Sparfloxacin | PO | 400 mg (1st day)<br>200 mg qd (subsequently) |
| Pefloxacin | PO | 400 mg bid<br>800 mg[a] |
| | IV | 400 mg bid |
| Grepafloxacin | PO | 400–600 mg qd |
| Levofloxacin | PO | 500 mg qd |
| | IV | 500 mg qd |
| Trovafloxacin | PO | 200 mg qd |
| | IV[b] | 300 mg qd |

[a]Single-dose therapy of uncomplicated cystitis.

[b]The intravenous formulation of trovafloxacin contains the prodrug alatrofloxacin.

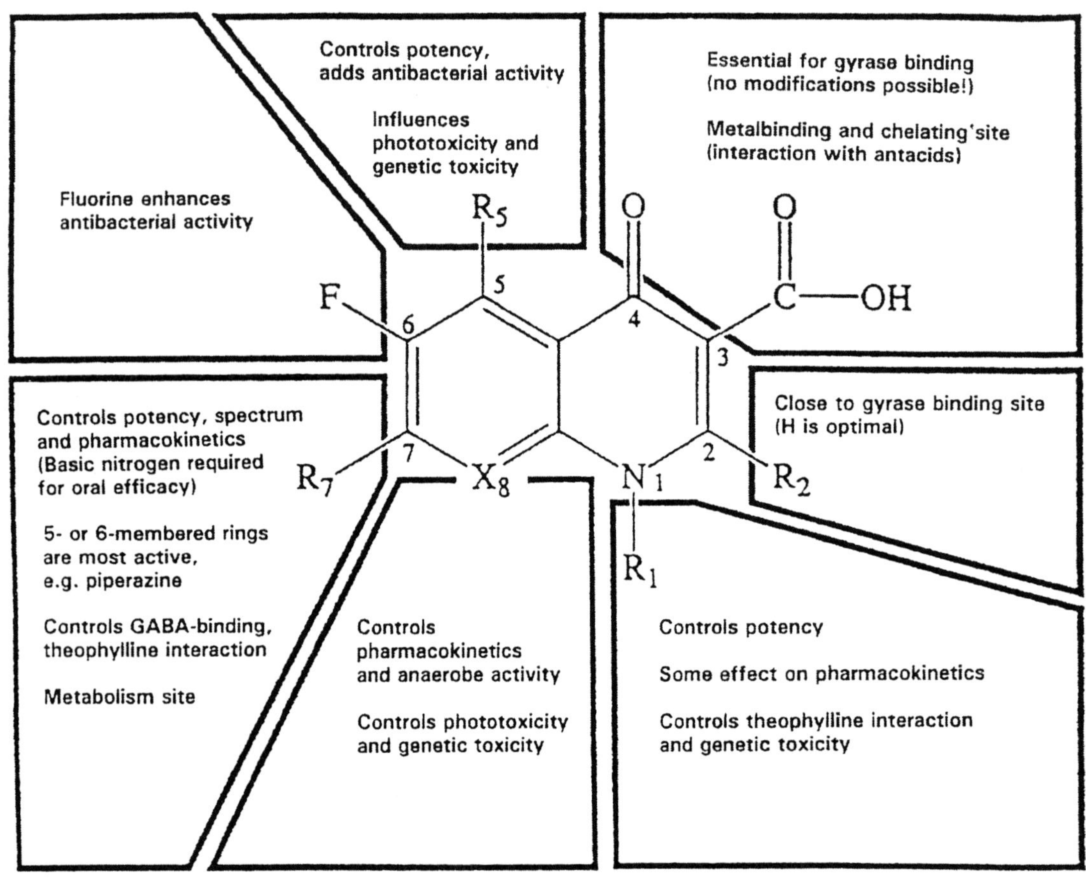


**Fig. 34.1** Summary of quinolone structure–activity relationships as derived from thousands of analogues. [Modified after Domagala, 1994.]

## Spectrum of Action

Quinolones have excellent activity against most Enterobacteriaceae and fastidious gram-negative pathogens such as *Haemophilus*, *Neisseria gonorrhoeae*, *Neisseria meningitidis*, and *Moraxella* (*Branhamella*) *catarrhalis*. Table 34.2 summarizes the antibacterial activity of the fluoroquinolones. Ciprofloxacin is the most potent fluoroquinolone against Enterobacteriaceae, inhibiting 90% of these bacteria at concentrations <0.5 mg/L. All enteric pathogens (e.g., enterotoxigenic *E. coli*, *Salmonella typhi*, and other *Salmonella* species, *Shigella* species, *Yersinia enterocolitica*, *Vibrio cholerae* and other *Vibrio* species, *Campylobacter jejuni*) are inhibited by fluoroquinolones at concentrations <2 mg/L.

The quinolones differ in activity against *P. aeruginosa* and other *Pseudomonas* species. Ciprofloxacin and tosufloxacin exhibit the highest activity against this pathogen.

Fluoroquinolones used today are less active against gram-positive bacteria. However, newer drugs, such as grepafloxacin, levofloxacin, trovafloxacin and sparfloxacin, exhibit increased activity against gram-positive organisms, inhibiting most of the staphylococci at concentrations <0.25 mg/L.

Important differences exist in the activities of fluoroquinolones against streptococci. Most of the derivatives have inadequate activity (e.g., enoxacin, fleroxacin, lomefloxacin). Ciprofloxacin and ofloxacin inhibit *Streptococcus pneumoniae* and the hemolytic streptococci of groups A, B, C, and G at concentrations <2 mg/L; however, a few strains have higher minimal inhibitory concentrations (MICs) and are resistant. Sparfloxacin and grepafloxacin, levofloxacin and trovafloxacin have increased activity against streptococci.

With a few exceptions (e.g., norfloxacin, enoxacin), most of the fluoroquinolones are active against *C. trachomatis*, *Ureaplasma urealyticum*, *Mycoplasma* species, and *Legionella* species. Ciprofloxacin, sparfloxacin, and ofloxacin are active against *Mycobacterium tuberculosis* and other mycobacteria. Quinolones also inhibit *Rickettsia* species and *Coxiella burnetii*, and they have some activity against *Plasmodium* species.

**Table 34.2** Antibacterial activity of fluoroquinolones ($MIC_{90}$)*

| Pathogen | Ciprofloxacin | Norfloxacin | Ofloxacin | Enoxacin | Lomefloxacin | Fleroxacin | Pefloxacin | Sparfloxacin |
|---|---|---|---|---|---|---|---|---|
| GRAM-POSITIVE COCCI | | | | | | | | |
| *Staphylococcus aureus* (methicillin-sens) | 0.5 | 1.0 | 0.5 | 2.0 | 4.0 | 2.0 | 0.5 | 0.25 |
| *Staphylococcus aureus* (methicillin-resi) | 32 | >16 | 16 | — | — | — | — | 8 |
| *Staphylococcus epidermidis* | 0.5 | 2.0 | 2.0 | 8.0 | 2.0 | 2.0 | 1.0 | 0.06 |
| *Streptococcus pyogenes* (group A) | 1.0 | 4.0 | 2.0 | 8.0 | 16.0 | 8.0 | 8.0 | 0.50 |
| *Streptococcus agalactiae* (group B) | 1.0 | 8.0 | 2.0 | 16.0 | 8.0 | 8.0 | 32 | 0.25 |
| *Streptococcus pneumoniae* | 2.0 | 8.0 | 2.0 | 16.0 | 16.0 | 16.0 | 12 | 0.5 |
| *Enterococcus faecalis* | 2.0 | 8.0 | 4.0 | 8.0 | 8.0 | 8.0 | 8.0 | 1.0 |
| ENTEROBACTERIACEA | | | | | | | | |
| *Escherichia coli* | 0.12 | 0.25 | 0.25 | 0.25 | 0.25 | 0.25 | 0.12 | 0.12 |
| *Klebsiella pneumoniae* | 0.12 | 0.5 | 0.25 | 0.25 | 0.50 | 0.50 | 2.0 | 0.25 |
| *Enterobacter* spp. | 0.12 | 1.0 | 0.25 | 0.50 | 0.50 | 0.50 | 0.5 | 0.25 |
| *Serratia marcescens* | 0.25 | 2.0 | 2.0 | 2.0 | 2.0 | 2.0 | 1.0 | 1.0 |
| *Proteus mirabilis* | 0.12 | 0.25 | 0.25 | 0.25 | 0.25 | 0.25 | 0.25 | 0.12 |
| *Proteus* (other) | 0.25 | 0.50 | 0.5 | 0.50 | 1.0 | 0.50 | 0.25 | 0.50 |
| *Providencia* spp. | 0.25 | 2.0 | 0.5 | 2.0 | 0.25 | 0.25 | 0.50 | 0.50 |
| *Shigella* spp. | 0.12 | 0.25 | 0.25 | 0.25 | 0.25 | 0.25 | 0.25 | 0.12 |
| OTHER BACTERIA | | | | | | | | |
| *Pseudomonas aeruginosa* | 0.5 | 8.0 | 4.0 | 2.0 | 4.0 | 2.0 | 2.0 | 2.0 |
| *Neisseria meningitidis* | <0.06 | <0.12 | <0.12 | <0.12 | 0.12 | 0.12 | <0.12 | <0.06 |
| Neisseria gonorrhoeae | <0.06 | <0.12 | <0.12 | <0.12 | 0.12 | 0.12 | <0.12 | <0.06 |
| *Haemophilus influenzae* | <0.06 | <0.12 | <0.12 | <0.12 | <0.12 | <0.12 | <0.12 | <0.06 |
| *Legionella* spp. | <0.12 | 0.5 | <0.06 | 0.2 | <0.06 | 0.06 | — | 0.06 |
| ANAEROBES | | | | | | | | |
| *Peptostreptococcus* | 4 | >32 | 2 | >32 | — | — | — | 2 |
| *Bacteroides fragilis* | 16 | >32 | 8 | >32 | 16 | 16 | 16 | 0.5 |
| OTHER PATHOGENS | | | | | | | | |
| *Mycobacterium tuberculosis* | 1.0 | 8.0 | 1.0 | >5.0 | 4.0 | 0.5 | 8.0 | 0.2 |
| *Mycoplasma pneumoniae* | 1.0 | 8.0 | 1.0 | 8.0 | 4.0 | 4.0 | 4.0 | 0.5 |
| *Chlamydia trachomatis* | 2.0 | 8.0 | 1.0 | 8.0 | 0.25 | 1.0 | — | 0.06 |
| *Ureaplasma* | 16 | 32 | 2.0 | 16.0 | 4 | 4.0 | — | 0.5 |

*MIC 90, minimal inhibitory concentration ( g/ml) that inhibits at least 90% of strains of a pathogen.

[Modified after Neu, 1992; Hooper, 1995.]

The older quinolones (e.g., ofloxacin, ciprofloxacin) do not inhibit anaerobic bacteria. Some newer derivatives (e.g. trovafloxacin) are active at clinically achievable concentrations. Sparfloxacin inhibits *Clostridium perfringens* and *Bacteroides fragilis.*

Quinolones have bactericidal action against most pathogens, with minimal bactericidal concentrations (MBCs) usually equal to or only twofold higher than the MICs. Urine reduces the antibacterial activity four- to 32-fold, but as the drug concentrations in urine are high, this effect is unlikely to be of clinical importance. The activity is also reduced by magnesium and at a low pH. Increasing the size of the inoculum has only minimal effect on the antimicrobial activity of fluoroquinolones.

Combinations of fluoroquinolones with other antibacterials have been investigated extensively. In most cases, neither a relevant synergy nor a clinically significant antagonism is found. When these drugs are combined with other antibiotics it is usually not for synergistic effects but rather to provide activity against bacteria inadequately inhibited by the fluoroquinolones.

## Pharmacokinetics

### Administration, absorption, elimination half-life

All commercially available fluoroquinolones as well as those under development are rapidly absorbed after oral administration. In addition, some drugs of this class (e.g., ciprofloxacin, ofloxacin) are available for intravenous infusion. The pharmacokinetics of these drugs after parenteral and oral administration are similar. Pharmacokinetic data compiled in Table 34.3 were calculated after oral administration of the drugs. Bioavailability is highest for ofloxacin and pefloxacin (>95%) and very low for norfloxacin. Mean peak plasma concentrations for most fluoroquinolones exceed 2.0 mg/L (exceptions: norfloxacin, sparfloxacin). Elimination half-lives of all compounds are long enough to allow a once- or twice-daily dose regimen. Ofloxacin has the longest half-life among the older drugs of this class (approximately 5 h); some of the newer derivatives have longer half-lifes (lomefloxacin, fleroxacin). Sparfloxacin is eliminated with a half-life of 18 h.

### Blood and tissue levels, protein binding

Fluoroquinolones reach high concentrations in many tissues and the total apparent volume of distribution ranges from 80 to >200 L, exceeding the total body water content. This indicates that these drugs reach significant intracellular concentrations, which is an important prerequisite for treating intracellular infections. This tissue accumulation differs from that of other antimicrobials, e.g., $\beta$-lactams or aminoglycosides; the volume of distribution of these antibiotics is approximately 20–25 L, corresponding to the extracellular volume.

The drugs achieve high concentrations in saliva, sputum, and bronchial mucosa. They are concentrated in phagocytes (polymorphonuclear leukocytes, alveolar macrophages) achieving concentrations in the range of 3 to 8 mg/L. The ability of fluoroquinolones to penetrate into cerebrospinal fluid is low. With the exception of ofloxacin, concentrations are below 50% of the corresponding serum concentrations.

Binding of fluoroquinolones to serum proteins is below 25% for most derivatives; protein binding of enoxacin is higher, but still at a level that would not be considered clinically significant.

### Clearance, excretion pathways

Fluoroquinolones are eliminated by different excretion pathways. Renal excretion, mainly by glomerular filtration, is the dominant route for ofloxacin and lomefloxacin, which are only minimally metabolized. Pefloxacin is metabolized (i.e., demethylated) almost completely in the liver to norfloxacin. For other drugs of this class, renal as well as hepatic elimination is of importance.

A piperazine ring in position 7 of the molecule is a common feature of most of the fluoroquinolones (Fig. 34.1). This basic ring structure is methylated in some compounds, with the methyl group either attached to the nitrogen or to one of the ring carbon atoms. This part of the molecule is one of the major targets for metabolizing enzymes that form oxometabolites. Glucuronidation is another important biotransformation for quinolones.

### Dose modifications in patients with renal or hepatic failure

Reduction of renal function prolongs the half-lives of norfloxacin, ciprofloxacin, enoxacin, and fleroxacin about twofold and the half-life of ofloxacin four- to fivefold. Doses of the re-

**Table 34.3** Pharmacokinetics of fluoroquinolones*

| Drug | Dose (mg) | $C_{max}$ $\mu$g/ml | $t_{1/2}$ (h) | Bioavailability (%) | AUC (mg × h/L) | Renal excretion (%)[a] | Metabolism (%) |
|---|---|---|---|---|---|---|---|
| Norfloxacin | 400 | 1.5 | 3.3 | (50) | 5.4 | 27 | 20 |
| Ciprofloxacin | 500 | 2.5 | 3.2 | 70 | 9.9 | 29 | 20 |
| Ofloxacin | 400 | 4.0 | 5.0 | >95 | 29.0 | 73 | 3 |
| Enoxacin | 400 | 2.3 | 4.9 | 88 | 16.0 | 44 | 20 |
| Pefloxacin | 400 | 3.2 | 10.5 | >95 | 55.0 | 11[b] | 90 |
| Lomefloxacin | 400 | 3.5 | 7.8 | >95 | 27.0 | 66 | 5 |
| Fleroxacin | 400 | 4.3 | 11.2 | 92 | 66.0 | 50[c] | 8 |
| Sparfloxacin | 400 | 1.6 | 17.6 | >60 | 32.0 | 35[d] | — |

*$C_{max}$, peak concentration; $t_{1/2}$, elimination halflife; AUC, area under the concentration time curve.

[a]Cumulative percentage of dose in urine after 24 h; [b]after 84 h; [c]after 72 h; [d]after 52 h.

[Modified after Hooper and Wolfson, 1991; Neu, 1993; Hooper, 1995.]

nally excreted compounds have to be adjusted in patients with severely impaired kidney function. Hepatic insufficiency is not known to have any major influence on the elimination of fluoroquinolones.

## Clinical Use

Fluoroquinolones find widespread use for the treatment of many bacterial infectious diseases. Fluoroquinolones are very beneficial drugs for use in severely ill, hospitalized patients as well as in outpatients, as these drugs can be taken orally. The proven and possible indications for these drugs have been listed in Table 34.4. These results are based on data from well-designed clinical trials.

### Urinary tract infections

Fluoroquinolones show excellent activity against almost all urinary tract pathogens, are excreted at high concentrations (most derivatives >200 $\mu$g/ml) in urine, and are therefore useful agents for the treatment of urinary tract infections, both uncomplicated and complicated (see Chapter 72). These drugs are highly effective in women with cystitis, with a 3-day regimen being more effective than single-dose therapy. However, if the pathogens are susceptible, fluoroquinolones are not more effective than trimethoprim-sulfamethoxazole. Because no clear-cut advantage of these antibacterials over older, less expensive drugs is recognizable in uncomplicated urinary tract infections, fluoroquinolones are not the first-choice drugs for treatment of such infections.

Fluoroquinolones are drugs of first choice in patients with complicated urinary tract infections. They may be particularly useful in replacing parenteral antibiotics and in reducing the need for hospitalization. In most studies of patients with nosocomial or complicated urinary tract infections, the fluoroquinolones have shown better efficacy than comparative drugs. Ciprofloxacin and other fluoroquinolones have been used successfully for treatment of *P. aeruginosa* infections. Development of bacterial resistance has been documented in about 10% of these patients, which is comparable to the effect of other antipseudomonal agents.

Bacterial prostatitis is a difficult-to-treat infection as only a few antibiotics penetrate sufficiently into prostatic fluid. Cure rates with fluoroquinolones have ranged from 65% to 90% after treatment periods of 4 to 6 weeks. These results are comparable or superior to the outcome with other antimicrobials.

### Sexually transmitted diseases

Single doses of fluoroquinolones are highly effective in curing uncomplicated gonococcal urethritis or cervicitis. Rectal infections have been cured in 99% of patients, but the therapeutic outcome in pharyngeal infections due to *N. gonorrhoeae* is lower (<90%). In infections with *C. trachomatis*, ofloxacin was as effective as doxycycline. Neither this drug nor any other quinolone tested so far is effective as single-dose therapy for *Chlamydia* infections.

Besides *C. trachomatis* and *N. gonorrhoeae*, Enterobacteriaceae and anaerobes are important pathogens in pelvic inflammatory disease (see Chapter 75). Combinations of quinolones with agents active against anaerobic bacteria (e.g., metronidazole, clindamycin) are currently being investigated. Fluoroquinolones have no activity against *Treponema pallidum*.

### Gastrointestinal infections

Fluoroquinolones show a high degree of activity against enteric pathogens and high levels of these drugs are achieved in feces (approximately 200 to 2000 mg/kg). Oral administration of fluoroquinolones eliminates major components of the gram-negative aerobic microflora without influencing the anaerobic flora. Another potential advantage of the quinolones in the treatment of gastrointestinal infections is the lack of plasmid-mediated resistance that could be transferred to other bacteria.

Several studies have documented that norfloxacin, ciprofloxacin, or other fluoroquinolones can reduce the duration of traveler's diarrhea from several days to approximately 1 day. *Salmonella*, *Shigella*, and pathogenic *E. coli* have been eliminated from the stool temporarily. Other pathogens (e.g., *Vibrio* species, *Plesiomonas shigelloides*, *Aeromonas* species) were eliminated by quinolones, but the effect on diarrhea has been minimal.

Quinolones can be used to treat typhoid fever. They rapidly eliminate *S. typhi* from the stool without development of a carrier state. Chronic fecal carriage of *Salmonella* has been eliminated with several fluoroquinolones, but late relapses occurred and the exact role of these drugs for this indication has not yet been defined. Fluoroquinolones have been useful against nontyphoidal salmonella infections in patients with HIV.

Although *Helicobacter pylori* is susceptible to quinolones in vitro, quinolone therapy has not eliminated this pathogen consistently, and emergence of resistance has been observed.

### Bone and joint infections

Fluoroquinolones offer several advantages over traditional compounds for treatment of osteomyelitis. They inhibit a broad spectrum of gram-negative and gram-positive bacteria, penetrate at sufficient concentrations into bone, and they can be administered orally. These are important features because osteomyelitis is caused by a variety of organisms and the treatment period is rather long (see Chapter 82). Ciprofloxacin at a dose of 750 mg bid has been used most widely for treatment of bacterial osteomyelitis. Cure rates for gram-negative organisms causing osteomyelitis have ranged from 60% to 80% for patients in whom the follow-up has been 6 months or longer.

### Skin and soft tissue infections

In a large double-blind study, oral ciprofloxacin was as effective as cefotaxime for treatment of patients with soft tissue infections (cellulitis, wounds, ischemic ulcers), with clinical cure rates of approximately 80%. Fluoroquinolones should not be used for skin infections caused by group A streptococci because of poor activity. Treatment of chronic ulcers with ciprofloxacin may lead to resistance of *P. aeruginosa* and staphylococci.

### Respiratory tract infections

Infections of the respiratory tract can be caused by a large variety of organisms (see Chapters 59–62), but not all of the possible pathogens are susceptible to fluoroquinolones. Most of the clinical experience reported is with compounds showing only poor activity against streptococci (e.g., ofloxacin, ciprofloxacin). Newer drugs such as sparfloxacin, grepafloxacin, levofloxacin, and trovafloxacin exhibit higher activity against gram-positive bacteria; they may be more useful for the treatment of respiratory tract infections.

**Table 34.4** Role of fluoroquinolones in the treatment of specific infections

| System affected<br>Disease | Possibly preferred agent | Alternative agent | Experimental agent[a] | Agent with little or no role |
|---|---|---|---|---|
| URINARY TRACT | | | | |
| Uncomplicated infections | | X | | |
| Complicated infections | X | | | |
| Prostatitis | X | | | |
| REPRODUCTIVE ORGANS | | | | |
| Uncomplicated gonorrhea | | X | | |
| Disseminated gonorrhea | | X | | |
| Chlamydial urethritis or cervicitis | | X[b] | | |
| Chancroid | | X | | |
| Pelvic inflammatory disease | | | X | |
| Syphilis | | | | X |
| GASTROINTESTINAL TRACT | | | | |
| Bacterial gastroenteritis | X[c] | | | |
| Chronic carriage of *Salmonella* | X | | | |
| Granulocytopenia (prophylaxis) | | X | | |
| Biliary tract infection | | | X | |
| RESPIRATORY TRACT | | | | |
| Acute exacerbation of | | | | |
| chronic bronchitis | | X[d] | | |
| cystic fibrosis | X | | | |
| Nosocomial pneumonia | X | | | |
| Community-acquired pneumonia | | X[d] | | |
| Aspiration pneumonia | | | | X |
| *Legionella* pneumonia | | X | | |
| *Mycoplasma* pneumonia | | X | | |
| Tuberculosis | | | X | |
| Meningococcal carriage | | X | | |
| Sinusitis or otitis media | | | X | |
| BONE AND JOINT | | | | |
| Osteomyelitis with gram-negative bacilli | X | | | |
| Staphylococcal infection | | X | | |
| Septic arthritis | | | X | |
| SKIN AND SOFT TISSUE INFECTIONS | | X | | |
| CENTRAL NERVOUS SYSTEM | | | | |
| Bacterial meningitis | | | X | |
| Invasive external otitis | X[e] | | | |
| BLOOD | | | | |
| Gram-negative enteric bacteremia | X | | | |
| *Pseudomonas* bacteremia | | | X | |
| Staphylococcal bacteremia | | | X | |
| Streptococcal or enterococcal bacteremia | | | | X |
| Anaerobic bacteremia | | | | X |
| Endocarditis | | | X | |

[a]Required additional study before routine use can be recommended.

[b]Ofloxacin appears to be promising; norfloxacin and ciprofloxacin are ineffective.

[c]Use should be limited to patients sufficiently ill that antimicrobial therapy would be considered on clinical grounds before a pathogen has been identified.

[d]Sparfloxacin, grepafloxacin, levofloxacin, and trovafloxacin may be the first fluoroquinolones with an indication for these infections.

[e]Results with ciprofloxacin are encouraging; drug may be considered for initial therapy.

[Modified after Hooper and Wolfson, 1991.]

At present, quinolones are not first-line therapy for respiratory tract infections caused by streptococci (e.g., pharyngitis, otitis media, sinusitis, acute exacerbations of chronic bronchitis, community-acquired pneumonia). If the infection is caused by *Haemophilus influenzae*, eradication and clinical cure rates are comparable or even superior to amoxicillin.

In nosocomial pneumonia, which is often caused by gram-negative pathogens including *P. aeruginosa*, fluoroquinolones may be first-choice antimicrobials. This also applies to patients with necrotizing external otitis due to *P. aeruginosa* (e.g., in diabetic patients).

Clinical experience with fluoroquinolones for treatment of *Mycoplasma* or *Legionella* infections of the respiratory tract is limited. They seem to be suitable drugs for these indications, but macrolides or rifampin remain the drugs of first choice.

## Adverse Effects and Toxicities

Fluoroquinolones are relatively safe and well tolerated. Under therapeutic conditions, there is no known predictable life-threatening organ toxicity that would essentially restrict their use. An exception is temafloxacin, which has caused a sometimes fatal syndrome of hemolysis, renal failure, thrombocytopenia, and hypoglycemia. A similar pattern of adverse effects has not been observed with other fluoroquinolones. The estimated reported incidence of the syndrome was 1 in 5000 prescriptions—an incidence too low to be detected reliably during clinical studies before marketing. As a result of this toxicity, the drug was rapidly withdrawn from the market. The mechanism of this rare side effect is still unknown.

The main target organs for common adverse effects of all fluoroquinolones are the gastrointestinal tract, the central nervous system, and the skin.

### Gastrointestinal tract

Nausea, diarrhea, vomiting, dyspepsia, and similar symptoms are among the side effects most often reported during therapy with quinolones. Reported frequencies of gastrointestinal tract disturbances range between 3% (ofloxacin) and 11% (temafloxacin). Antibiotic-associated colitis has been observed very rarely.

### Central nervous system

Mild neurotoxic reactions to fluoroquinolones include headache, dizziness, tiredness, or sleeplessness; abnormal vision, restlessness, bad dreams, etc., have also been reported in some instances. Severe neurotoxic side effects (psychotic reactions, hallucinations, depression, and grand mal convulsions) are rare (<0.5%).

### Skin (hypersensitivity, phototoxicity)

The incidences of cutaneous hypersensitivity reactions reported after fluoroquinolone treatment range between 0.4% and 1.1%; they include erythema, pruritus, urticaria, and rash. Phototoxic reactions have been described with nalidixic acid, therefore this risk has to be considered with the fluorinated derivatives as well. Patients taking fluoroquinolones should be advised to avoid prolonged sun exposure.

### Arthropathy (preclinical and clinical data)

All quinolones tested so far induce arthropathy in young dogs at rather low doses (15 to 50 mg/kg body weight). Articular cartilage damage is also inducible in several other animal species, such as rats, guinea pigs, rabbits, and nonhuman primates. On the basis of these data, pharmaceutical manufacturers and administrative authorities recommend that quinolones not be used in children. The exact mechanism of quinolone-induced arthropathy is still unknown. However, recent data indicate that the chelating properties of the quinolones for magnesium might play an important role because magnesium-deficient juvenile rats showed cartilage lesions that were identical to quinolone-induced lesions.

Fortunately, the chondrotoxic potential of quinolones in humans under therapeutic conditions is low. The vast majority of juvenile patients have shown no signs of arthropathy after treatment with these drugs. On the other hand, occasional reports of arthropathy in children and even adult patients have been published. The highest incidence of arthropathy reported so far has been observed after treatment with pefloxacin, reaching 14% in cystic fibrosis patients. Five patients who did develop arthralgia under treatment with pefloxacin did not show joint complications during treatment with ofloxacin. In a retrospective evaluation of 634 children and adolescents treated with ciprofloxacin on a compassionate basis, treatment-related arthralgia was reported in 8 (1.3%) children.

Many pediatricians have demanded that at least some of the newer quinolones be considered appropriate for use in children since the clinical data do not indicate a major risk. There is no doubt that the benefit of quinolone treatment in children with severe, life-threatening diseases will outweigh the risk of arthropathy. However, it is still unclear which compound is the most suitable one for quinolone therapy in children and whether lesions of articular cartilages are reversible and free of initiating secondary osteoarthritis.

## Drug Interactions

Bioavailability of fluoroquinolones is significantly reduced when co-administered with mineralic antacids, particularly those containing magnesium or aluminium; this drug interaction can result in therapeutic failure. Histamin ($H_2$) antagonists (e.g., ranitidine) have shown only little interference with the pharmacokinetics of quinolones. Ferrous sulfate administration sharply reduces the bioavailability of ciprofloxacin or ofloxacin.

Administration of quinolones with food may prolong absorption time and result in reduction of peak plasma concentrations. Total drug bioavailability in general, however, is not reduced.

Co-administration of some fluoroquinolones with theophylline has resulted in elevated theophylline plasma levels and adverse reactions. This interaction is most pronounced with enoxacin, but with high doses of some other fluoroquinolones, e.g., ciprofloxacin, the effect can also be observed. The mechanism of this interaction probably involves an inhibition of drug-metabolizing enzymes (CYP450 mono-oxygenases) by fluoroquinolones or by certain metabolites of these drugs.

## ANNOTATED BIBLIOGRAPHY

Andriole VT (ed). The Quinolones, 2nd ed. Academic Press, San Diego, 1998.
*All known aspects of quinolones as antimicrobial agents are discussed extensively in this book.*

Bauernfeind A. Comparison of the antibacterial activities of the quinolones Bay 12-8039, gatifloxacin (AM 1155), trovafloxacin, clinafloxacin, levofloxacin, and ciprofloxacin. J Antimicrob Chemother 1997; 40:639–651.
*The in-vitro activities of several fluoroquinolones against gram-positive and gram-negative bacteria are compared.*

Deppermann KM, Lode H. Fluoroquinolones: interaction profile during enteral absorption. Drugs 1993; 45(Suppl 3):65–72.

*Comprehensive review on the relevant interactions between fluoroquinolones and other drugs during enteral absorption.*

Domagala JM. Structure–activity and structure–side effect relationships for the quinolone antibacterials. J Antimicrob Chemother 1994; 33:685–706.
*This review describes the relationships of the quinolone structure to their antibacterial activity as well as their toxicities.*

Hooper DC. Quinolones. In: Principles and Practice of Infectious Diseases, 4th ed. Mandell GL, Bennet JE, Dolin R, eds. Churchill Livingstone, New York, pp 364–376, 1995.
*Book chapter on antimicrobial activity, pharmacokinetics, and clinical use of quinolones.*

Hooper DC, Wolfson JS. Fluoroquinolone antimicrobial agents. N Engl J Med 1991; 324:384–394.
*Review of the antimicrobial properties, pharmacokinetics, indications, and side effects of fluoroquinolones.*

Hooper DC, Wolfson JS, eds. Quinolone Antimicrobial Agents, 2nd ed. American Society for Microbiology, Washington, DC, 1993.
*All known aspects of quinolones as antimicrobial agents are discussed extensively in this book.*

Lode H. Pharmacokinetics and clinical results of parenterally administered new quinolones in humans. Rev Infect Dis 1989; 11(Suppl 5):S996–S1004.
*Review of the pharmacokinetics of parenterally administered fluoroquinolones and clinical results obtained by parenteral treatment with quinolones.*

Neu HC. Quinolone antimicrobial agents. Annu Rev Med 1992; 43:465–486.
*Review of the antimicrobial properties, pharmacokinetics, indications, and side effects of fluoroquinolones.*

Stahlmann R, Förster C, Shakibaei M, Vormann J, Günther T, Merker H-J Magnesium deficiency induces joint cartilage lesions in juvenile rats which are identical with quinolone-induced arthropathy. Antimicrob Agents Chemother 1995; 39:2013–2018.
*Results of this study indicate that in juvenile rats, a dietarily induced magnesium deficiency causes joint cartilage lesions identical to those seen after treatment with quinolones, indicating that quinolone-induced arthropathy is probably caused by a lack of functionally available magnesium in joint cartilage.*

Stahlmann R, Lode H. Concentration-effect relationship of the fluoroquinolones. In: Handbook of Experimental Pharmacology (vol. 127) Quinolone antibacterials. Kuhlmann J, Dalhoff A, Zeiler HJ, eds. Springer Verlag, Berlin-Heidelberg-New York, S. 407–420, 1997.
*This book chapter describes the pharmacodynamic properties of fluoroquinolones in comparison to those of β-lactams and aminoglycosides.*

# 35

# Sulfonamides and Trimethoprim

STEPHEN E. SANCHE AND ALLAN R. RONALD

Sulfonamide antibiotics are derivatives of sulfanilamide, the metabolite of a compound called prontosil that was developed by the German dye industry. Prontosil was reported to have antibacterial properties in 1932, and later in the same decade, sulfonamides were among the first antimicrobial agents to be used to treat infections in humans. Several synthetic derivatives with enhanced antimicrobial activity, improved pharmacokinetics, and more favorable side-effect profiles have subsequently been developed, allowing sulfonamides to maintain clinical usefulness six decades after the initial recognition of their anti-infective potential.

Trimethoprim (TMP) is one of the diaminopyridines, a group of antimicrobial compounds developed in the 1950s; TMP was first used in treatment of a human infection in 1962. The combination of TMP plus a sulfonamide was found to exhibit synergy in vitro, and it was introduced for clinical use in the form of TMP and sulfamethoxazole (SMX) in a fixed-dose combination formulation in Europe in 1968 and subsequently in the United States in 1973.

## Mechanisms of Action

Tetrahydrofolic acid (THF), a derivative of folic acid, is synthesized by bacteria and eukaryotic cells and is required for their production of purines, thymidine, and ultimately, DNA. Sulfonamides and TMP act at sequential steps in the same pathway to inhibit cellular THF synthesis.

Unlike humans, most bacteria are unable to use preformed folic acid and so must synthesize it from the precursors para-amino benzoic acid (PABA) and pteridine. The sulfonamides are structural analogues of PABA; they competitively block the production of the intermediate compound dihydropteroic acid by interacting with the enzyme dihydropteroic acid synthetase (Fig. 35.1).

Trimethoprim prevents the conversion of dihydrofolic acid to THF by inhibiting action of the responsible enzyme, dihydrofolate reductase (DHFR). Although humans also require DHFR for nucleic acid synthesis, the mammalian and bacterial enzymes are structurally different. Because TMP has several thousand-fold less affinity for the human DHFR than it has for the bacterial isoenzyme, it has minimal effect on human DNA synthesis. The DHFR of some eukaryotic species, in particular, *Pneumocystis carinii*, is also inhibited by TMP at clinically acheivable concentrations, in contrast to mammalian cells.

The sulfonamides and TMP are considered to be bacteriostatic agents in most situations. In vitro, the combination of TMP and SMX is synergistic and bactericidal against a variety of pathogens. The significance of synergy in clinical situations, however, is more difficult to demonstrate.

## Sulfonamides

### Pharmacology and preparations

With the exception of the TMP/SMX combination preparation, the sulfonamides currently employed for treatment of systemic infections are almost exclusively administered orally. The oral preparations currently used are short and intermediate-acting sulfonamides. This group of agents includes sulfamethizole (Thiosulfil), sulfadiazine (Microsulfon), sulfamethoxazole (Gantanol), sulfacytine (Renoquid), and sulfisoxazole (Gantrisin). These agents are all well absorbed from the gastrointestinal tract, reaching peak plasma concentrations 2–6 h after ingestion. Half-lives range from 4 to 12 h (Table 35.1).

Sulfonamides are variably acetylated and glucuronated in the liver; the resulting inactive metabolites as well as free drug are filtered through the glomerulus and actively secreted into the urine. Alkalinization of the urine increases renal excretion. Because inactive but toxic acetylated metabolites may accumulate in renal failure, sulfonamide dosage should be altered for creatinine clearances <50 ml/min. Plasma sulfonamide levels can be used as a dosing guide to avoid toxic effects but are unavailable in many clinical labs; peak sulfonamide levels should not exceed 120 mg/L. No dosage modification is required for patients with hepatic impairment.

Levels sufficient for activity have been documented in cerebrospinal fluid (CSF) (20%–80% of simultaneous serum levels) and in synovial, pleural, and peritoneal fluids. Sulfonamides cross the placenta and are detectable in breast milk.

Long-acting sulfonamides (with the exception of sulfadoxine as a component of Fansidar, see below) are no longer used on account of an unacceptably high incidence of severe cutaneous hypersensitivity reactions such as Stevens-Johnson syndrome. Poorly absorbed sulfonamide preparations were previously used for suppression of bowel flora prior to gastrointestinal tract surgery; this is no longer a common practice.

Several combination preparations are currently marketed. The most frequently used combination, TMP/SMX, is discussed separately below. Trisulfapyrimidines (Terfonyl) is a combination of equal amounts of sulfamethazine, sulfamerazine, and sulfadiazine. The combination of three structurally different sulfonamides allows a high total sulfonamide dose to be administered with a relatively low risk of crystalluria, but this preparation offers no advantage over more soluble sulfonamide preparations such as sulfisoxazole. The urinary analgesic phenazopyridine has been combined with each of the short-acting sulfonamides sulfisoxazole (Azo Gantrisin), sulfamethixole (Thiosulfil-A) and sulfamethoxazole (Azo Gantanol) specifically for urinary tract infection treatment. A preparation combining sulfisoxazole acetyl and erythromycin ethylsuccinate (Pediazole) is used primarily in treatment of pediatric respiratory tract infections. The long-act-

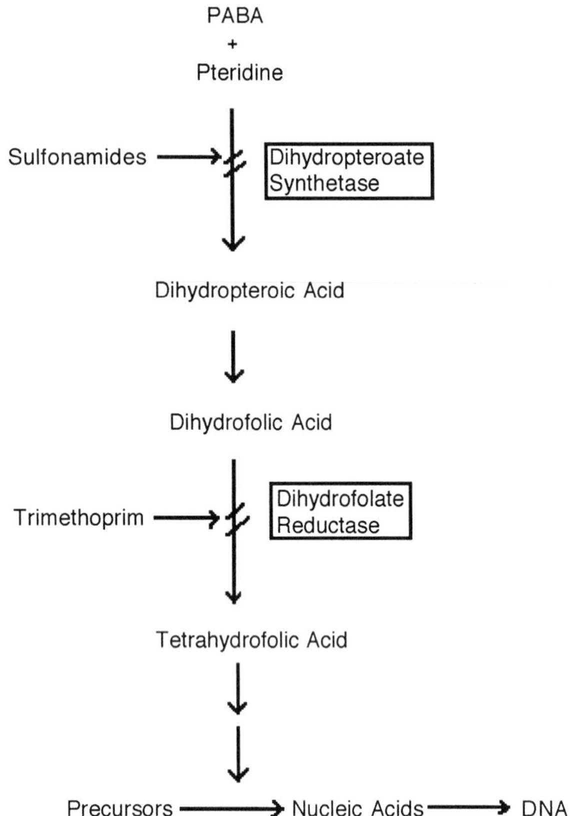


**Fig. 35.1** Trimethoprim and sulfonamides both act by inhibiting enzymes used in microbial synthesis of tetrahydrofolic acid, thus impacting nucleic acid synthesis.

ing sulfonamide sulfadoxine is available in combination with pyrimethamine (Fansidar) for prophylaxis and treatment of malaria.

Mafenide acetate (Sulfamylon) and silver sulfadiazine (Flamazine) creams have been used extensively in the topical treatment of burns. Sulfonamides are also employed in sulfacetamide ophthalmic solutions and ointments, and in a variety of vaginal suppositories and creams.

## Antimicrobial spectrum

Sulfonamides are active in vitro against a variety of gram-positive and gram-negative organisms. Community-acquired strains of *Escherichia coli* are intrinsically susceptible but may acquire plasmid-mediated resistance; *Klebsiella*, *Proteus*, and *Serratia* species are less predictably susceptible. *Streptococcus pneumoniae*, *Chlamydia trachomitis*, *Actinomyces* species, *Nocardia asteroides*, *Plasmodium falciparum*, and *Toxoplasma gondii* are also often susceptible. Anaerobes are generally resistant.

## Mechanisms of resistance

Three major mechanisms account for most of the currently recognized sulfonamide resistance. Restricted penetration of sulfonamides through the cell envelope can be responsible for either intrinsic or acquired resistance. Mutants that hyperproduce PABA are able to synthesize dihydropteroic acid even in the presence of competing sulfonamide. Several sulfonamide-resistant variants of the enzyme dihydropteroate synthetase have also been isolated. This latter mechanism can be plasmid mediated or on the basis of chromosomal mutation. Cross-resistance among the sulphonamides is usual.

## Clinical uses

The current major clinical use of the short- and intermediate-acting systemic sulfonamides is the treatment of uncomplicated urinary tract infections. Sulfonamides are also used for prophylaxis against recurrent attacks of rheumatic fever and erysipelas in penicillin-allergic patients as well as for treatment of nocardiosis and infections caused by *C. trachomatis*. Sulfonamides are used in combination with pyrimethamine for treatment of toxoplasmosis and for prophylaxis and treatment of malaria (see Chapter 40).

## Adverse reactions

Gastrointestinal disturbances, primarily nausea, vomiting, or diarrhea, are the most common adverse reactions, occurring in 3%–5% of patients. Liver enzyme abnormalities and pancreatitis are rare complications of sulfonamide therapy.

Hypersensitivity reactions usually present with an undifferentiated "drug rash," but more severe reactions such as erythema multiforme, Stevens-Johnson syndrome, toxic epidermal necrolysis, leukocytoclastic vasculitis, serum sickness-like reactions, and anaphylaxis can occur. Severe hypersensitivity reactions are more frequent with the long-acting agents such as sulfadimethoxine; for this reason, they are no longer used.

Hematologic toxicity can include aplastic anemia, leukopenia, thrombocytopenia, and hemolytic anemia, the last of which is more common in glucose-6-phosphate-dehydrogenase-deficient individuals.

Renal dysfunction due to tubular deposition of sulfonamide crystals is now rare. This was a relatively frequent complication

**Table 35.1** Pharmacokinetics of selected sulfonamides and trimethoprim

| Agent | Protein binding (%) | Peak blood level[a] ($\mu$g/ml) | Time to peak (h) | Plasma half-life (h) |
|---|---|---|---|---|
| Sulfisoxazole | 90 | 40–50 | 2–4 | 5–6 |
| Sulfadiazine | 45 | 30–60 | 3–6 | 17 |
| Sulfamethoxazole | 70 | 80–100 | 4–6 | 11 |
| Sulfadoxine | 85 | 50–75 | 3–6 | 100–230 |
| Trimethoprim | 45 | 2 | 1–4 | 10–12 |

[a]2 g doses of sulfonamide, 160 mg dose of TMP (adults).

of the older, less soluble preparations (e.g., sulfadiazine); it is preventable with proper attention to maintenance of urine volume. Interstitial nephritis and tubular necrosis are rarely associated with sulfonamide use.

Sulfonamides may displace bilirubin from binding sites on albumin and thus increase the risk of kernicterus in newborns. Adminstration of sulfonamides is therefore not recommended late in pregnancy, to nursing mothers or to neonates.

### Drug interactions

Displacement of oral anticoagulants and methotrexate from albumin binding sites may result in increased activity of the displaced drugs. The half-life of sulfonylureas can be prolonged, resulting in hypoglycemia. Sulfonamides themselves may be displaced from protein binding sites by indomethacin, salicylates, and probenecid.

## Trimethoprim

### Pharmacology

As a stand-alone agent, trimethoprim (TMP) is available only as oral tablets. Trimethoprim is rapidly absorbed from the gastrointestinal tract, with serum levels peaking at 1–4 h after ingestion. Eighty percent is excreted in the urine unchanged, a small amount is excreted in bile, and the remainder is found as inactive metabolites in the urine. Dosage must be adjusted in renal failure.

TMP is widely distributed in tissues: concentrations in kidney, lung, respiratory secretions and prostatic tissue and secretions are higher than those in plasma. Significant amounts are also found in breast milk, bile, and saliva, and CSF levels reach ~40% of simultaneous serum levels.

### Antimicrobial spectrum

Trimethoprim is active in vitro against many aerobic gram positive cocci including *Staphylococcus aureus* and most streptococci and against most common gram negative urinary tract pathogens. *Pseudomonas* species, *Neisseria* species, *Chlamydia* species, enterococci and most anaerobes are usually resistant.

### Mechanisms of resistance

The most important acquired mechanism of TMP resistance is the plasmid-mediated production of a resistant dihydrofolate reductase (DHFR) enzyme. Other reported mechanisms include cell wall impermeability, overproduction of unaltered DHFR enzyme, and chromosomally mediated production of resistant DHFR.

### Clinical uses

Trimethoprim is approved for use in acute uncomplicated urinary tract infections (UTI). Some experts prefer TMP alone to TMP/SMX, as efficacy is nearly equal and adverse effects are less common. Although there is theoretical concern that TMP resistance could develop more rapidly when it is used alone, this has not been observed in countries where TMP has been used as a single agent for many years. TMP is also used as an alternative to TMP/SMX for prophylaxis of recurrent UTIs in patients with sulfonamide allergy or intolerance. Because of its excellent penetration into prostatic tissue, TMP has been used with success as a single agent in treatment of chronic bacterial prostatitis. It has also been shown to be effective for prophylaxis and treatment of traveler's diarrhea, and (in combination with dapsone) for prophylaxis and treatment of *Pneumocystis carinii* pneumonia in patients intolerant to sulfonamides.

### Adverse reactions/drug interactions

Adverse reactions to TMP are less common than reactions to sulfonamides. Skin rashes have been reported in <3% of individuals. Decreases in any or all of the blood cell lines with associated megaloblastic marrow changes have been observed, particularly in individuals such as the elderly or alcoholics who are at risk for pre-existing folate deficiency. These marrow changes can be reversed through simultaneous administration of folinic acid, which does not reduce the antibacterial activity of TMP. Trimethoprim decreases the tubular secretion of creatinine, and therefore may increase serum creatinine levels in the absence of a true decrease in renal function. It has been shown to be teratogenic in rats and should therefore be avoided in pregnancy. Trimethoprim may predispose to phenytoin toxicity by increasing free levels of the latter drug.

## Trimethoprim/Sulfamethoxazole (TMP/SMX)

### Pharmacology

The combination TMP/SMX is available for both oral and intravenous administration as a fixed combination at a 1:5 weight ratio. Both drugs are well absorbed from the gastrointestinal tract. For oral administration, 80–400 mg (single strength [SS]) and 160–800 mg (double strength [DS]) tablets as well as 40 mg–200 mg/5 ml solution are used. The intravenous preparation contains 16 mg/ml TMP and 80 mg/ml SMX. The 1:5 ratio was chosen in order to achieve a 1:20 TMP:SMX plasma ratio, because in vitro synergy has been shown to be maximal at this ratio. The actual drug ratio at sites of infection, however, is usually quite different from 1:20, and the significance of synergy in vivo is therefore uncertain.

Both TMP and SMX are primarily excreted by the kidney and therefore dosage adjustments are recommended in advanced renal failure. One-half the usual dose is usually recommended for creatinine clearances of 15–30 ml/min; TMP/SMX is usually not recommended for use in patients with creatinine clearances <15 ml/min. Dosage adjustment is not necessary in hepatic failure.

### Antimicrobial spectrum

The combination TMP/SMX is active against a wide variety of organisms; it acts against *Staphylococcus aureus*, including many methicillin-resistant *Staphylococcus aureus* (MRSA) strains, *Staphylococcus epidermidis* and most streptococci. However, most penicillin-resistant *S. pneumoniae* isolates are also TMP/SMX resistant, and enterococci are variably sensitive combination even when susceptible in vitro. A wide spectrum of gram-negative organisms, including *Neisseria* species, *Moraxella catarrhalis*, *Pseudomonas cepacia* and *Stenotrophomonas (Xanthomonas) maltophilia* are usually susceptible, but anaerobes and *Pseudomonas aeruginosa* are typically resistant. This combination is also active in vitro against *Pneumocystis carinii*, *Listeria monocytogenes*, *Nocardia asteroides*, chlamydiae, and some atypical mycobacteria. Resistance among *Shigella* and *Salmonella* species is now widespread.

## Mechanisms of resistance

Resistance of the same organisms to both TMP and SMX could be attributable to any combination of the mechanisms discussed above for resistance to sulfonamides and TMP. Additionally, organisms can become resistant to both drugs by a mutation resulting in their conversion to "thymine auxotrophs." These mutant organisms lack the enzyme thymidine synthetase and are therefore dependent on exogenous thymine or thymidine for DNA synthesis. This mutation allows the organisms to bypass the single largest demand for tetrahydrofolate, which is thymidine synthesis. The effects of TMP and sulfonamides are therefore negated. This mechanism is likely to be less important clinically, however, because thymine auxotrophs are relatively avirulent.

Plasmid-mediated TMP and TMP/SMX resistance is becoming increasingly common, particularly among *E. coli*, *Salmonella*, and *Shigella* isolates. More than one-third of isolates of these organisms have been found to be resistant in recent studies in South America and Asia.

## Clinical uses

Because of increasing resistance, the number of infections for which TMP/SMX is recommended as the treatment of first choice is decreasing. It remains an excellent alternative in many clinical settings, however, especially if in vitro sensitivity can be established.

### Urinary tract infections (UTI)

The combination TMP/SMX has been shown to be effective treatment for acute uncomplicated urinary tract infections in women, and is considered the treatment of choice for these infections by many experts. A 3-day course of one DS tablet bid is as effective as 7- to 10-day therapy at the same dose. Single-dose treatment (two DS tablets) results in nearly the same rate of cure, but 3-day treatment seems to be preferred by most patients and practitioners because of reluctance to stop treatment before symptomatic improvement, and because the rate of relapse is slightly lower. TMP/SMX is also useful in management of acute uncomplicated pyelonephritis. Therapy can be initiated intravenously in moderately ill patients, or the entire course can be administered orally. Nightly or three times weekly TMP/SMX taken regularly or TMP/SMX postintercourse (SS or half SS tablets in both situations) are commonly used regimens for prophylaxis of recurrent UTI in women. Prolonged courses of TMP/SMX (12 weeks or more) are used in treatment of chronic bacterial prostatitis.

### Respiratory tract infections

The combination TMP/SMX is the preferred agent for *Pneumocystis carinii* pneumonia prophylaxis and treatment. The usual prophylactic regimens are one SS or one DS tablet daily or one DS tablet three times weekly. Treatment for severe infections is 20 mg/kg/day of the TMP component divided every 6 h intravenously, whereas milder episodes can be managed with eight DS tablets in four divided oral doses. Intolerance occurs among 40%–80% of AIDS patients, particularly at the higher treatment doses.

**Table 35.2** In vitro activity of TMP/SMX against selected organisms

| Organism | $MIC_{90}$[a] ($\mu$g/ml) | MIC range ($\mu$g/ml) |
|---|---|---|
| GRAM-POSITIVE | | |
| *Staphylococcus aureus* | 1/19 | 0.06/1.14–1.5/28.5 |
| *Staphylococcus epidermidis* | 4/76 | 0.06/1.14–8/152 |
| *Staphylococcus saprophyticus* | 1/19 | 1/19–16/304 |
| *Streptococcus pneumoniae* | 2/38 | 0.05/0.95–16/304 |
| *Streptococcus pyogenes* | 2/38 | 0.02/0.38–8/152 |
| *Enterococcus faecalis* | 1/19 | 0.02/0.38–>16/>304 |
| GRAM-NEGATIVE | | |
| *Escherichia coli* | 5/95 | 0.05/0.95–>16/>304 |
| *Klebsiella* sp. | 2/38 | 0.05/0.95–>16/>304 |
| *Proteus* sp. | 1/19 | 0.06/1.14–>16/>304 |
| *Salmonella* sp. | 2/38 | 0.05/0.95–16/304 |
| *Shigella* sp. | 2/38 | 0.02/0.38–>16/>304 |
| *Haemophilus influenzae* | 1/19 | 0.04/0.76–4/76 |
| *Moraxella catarrhalis* | 0.5/9.5 | 0.02/0.38–16/304 |
| *Pseudomonas aerugenosa* | >16/>304 | 4/76–>16/>304 |
| *Stenotrophomonas (Xanthomonas) maltophilia* | 1/19 | 1/19–>16/>304 |
| OTHER | | |
| *Nocardia asteroides* | 4/76 | 0.02/0.38–16/304 |

[a]Minimum concentration at which 90% of strains are inhibited.

TMP/SMX has been used with success for treatment of acute exacubations of chronic bronchitis and for pneumonia caused by sensitive gram-negative organisms. It is also useful for acute otitis media and sinusitis in patients with penicillin allergy or in regions with high proportions of $\beta$-lactamase producing *Haemophilus influenzae* or *Moraxella catarrhalis*.

### Gastrointestinal infections

The combination TMP/SMX is useful both in prophylaxis and in empiric treatment of traveler's diarrhea. However, resistance is now prevalent among *Shigella*, *Salmonella*, and *E. coli* isolates in many regions such as India and southeast Asia. For this reason, quinolones have become the preferred therapy for shigellosis, with TMP/SMX now an alternate. It is now also an alternate agent for treatment of *Salmonella* infections.

### Miscellaneous

The combination TMP/SMX is considered one of the preparations of choice for nocardiosis and for treatment of infections caused by *Moraxella catarrhalis*, *Yersinia enterocolitica*, *Aeromonas* species, *Pseudomonas cepacia*, and *Stenotrophomonas* (*Xanthomonas*) *maltophilia*. It has also been used successfully to treat meningitis, endocarditis, osteomyelitis, and other serious infections caused by gram-negative bacilli resistant or only moderately susceptible to $\beta$-lactam agents. The usual intravenous dosage ranges for such infections are 5–10 mg/kg/day in four divided doses. TMP/SMX may play an important role in combination treatment of MRSA infections, and in high oral doses it is an alternative to intramuscular ceftriaxone for pharyngeal gonococcal infection. TMP/SMX has also been shown to cause regression of the lesions of Wegener's granulomatosis.

## Adverse reactions

All adverse reactions decribed above for sulphonamides and trimethoprim have been reported with TMP/SMX. As with sulfonamides alone, the most frequent adverse reactions are mild drug rashes and gastrointestinal symptoms, both seen in 2%–5% of HIV-negative recipients. Severe skin reactions (e.g., Stevens-Johnson syndrome) are estimated to occur in between 1/10,000 and 3/100,000 patients. Megaloblastosis occurs rarely, generally in individuals predisposed to folate deficiency. Folinic acid supplements can be administered to these patients without impacting the effectiveness of antibacterial therapy. Isolated leukopenia, thrombocytopenia, and hemolytic anemia unassociated with megaloblastosis have also been reported. Fluid overload can be a sequela of the large fluid volumes required for intravenous administration. Other rare adverse effects of TMP/SMX include aseptic menigitis, hypoglycemia, hypothyroidism, hyperkalemia, cholestasis, hepatitis or hepatic necrosis, pseudomembranous colitis, and acute pancreatitis.

Adverse reactions are more frequently due to the sulfamethoxazole component of the combination, and thus trimethoprim alone can be substituted for TMP/SMX in clinically appropriate situations when the reaction is not life threatening. TMP/SMX is not recommended in pregnancy; in addition to data indicating that TMP is teratogenic in rats, a case–control study has shown an association between use of TMP/SMX in pregnancy and cleft lip and palate. Drug interactions are discussed separately above for TMP and the sulphonamides.

Adverse reactions to TMP/SMX are much more common among AIDS patients. Rash is observed in 40%–80% of individuals, and may be accompanied by fever, leukopenia, thrombocytopenia, and elevated hepatic transaminase levels. Several separate mechanisms likely contribute to this high rate of adverse effects in AIDS patients; toxicity of hydroxylamine metabolites of sulfamethoxazole is thought to be prominent among these mechanisms. Normally ~70% of sulfamethoxazole is acetylated in the liver while <10% is metabolized by the cytochrome p450 system to hydroxylamine metabolites. These metabolites are cytotoxic to peripheral blood mononuclear cells in vitro, and the degree of this cytotoxicity has been shown to be predictive of TMP/SMX hypersensitivity reactions in AIDS patients. This cytotoxicity can be inhibited by the addition of glutathione to the mononuclear cells of hypersensitive AIDS patients. Glutathione is thought to be key to detoxification of hydroxylamine groups in vivo, and is known to be deficient in some AIDS patients, perhaps predisposing them to hypersensitivity reactions. If this hypothesis is correct, "slow acetylators" would theoretically also be predisposed to hypersensitivity reactions because of production of larger-than-usual quantities of hydroxylamine metabolites. Because of the superiority of TMP/SMX in PCP prophylaxis, some physicians "treat through" mild rashes with antihistamines, and a 10-day "desensitization" regimen has recently been shown to be safe and effective in AIDS patients with a prior history of allergic reaction to TMP/SMX.

## ANNOTATED BIBLIOGRAPHY


Brumfitt W, Hamilton-Miller JMT. Limitations of and indications for the use of cotrimoxazole. J Chemother 1994; 6:3–11.
*The authors argue that treatment with trimethoprim alone would result in equal efficacy and less toxicity in several infections for which TMP/SMX is widely used, and discuss the limited clinical situations in which TMP/SMX has been shown to be superior.*

Cribb AE, Lee BL, Trepanier LA, Spielberg SP. Adverse reactions to sulphonamide and sulphonamide-trimethoprim antimicrobials: clinical syndromes and pathogenesis. Adverse Drug React Toxicol Rev 1996; 15(1):9–50.
*A review of sulphonamide-related adverse reactions and their postulated mechanisms.*

Cortese LM, Soucy DM, Endy TP. Trimethoprim/sulfamethoxazole desensitization. Ann Pharmacother 1996; 30(2):184–186.
*A brief review of TMP/SMX desensitization protocols for HIV patients.*

Harvey RJ. Synergism in the folate pathway. Rev Infect Dis 1982; 4:255–260.
*A theoretical discussion of interactions of inhibitors in metabolic pathways with specific reference to TMP and SMX. This and references # 5, 6, 8 and 9 are from a published symposium on on TMP and sulfonamides, which contains several other references of interest.*

Jick H. Adverse reactions to trimethoprim-sulfamethoxazole in hospitalized patients. Rev Infect Dis 1982; 4:426–428.
*The report of reactions in 1121 recipients of TMP/SMX in the Boston Collaborative Drug Surveillance Program.*

Koomans PP, van der Ven AJAM, Vree TB, van der Meer JWM. Pathogenesis of hypersensitivity reactions to drugs in patients with HIV infection: allergic or toxic? AIDS 1995; 9:217–222.
*This paper reviews recent theories regarding the causes of hypersensitivity reactions to sulfonamides (and other drugs) in AIDS patients.*

Ronald AR, Nicolle LE, Harding GK. Standards of therapy for urinary tract infections in adults. Infection 1992; 20 (Suppl 3):S164–S170.
*Current therapeutic standards for uncomplicated and complicated urinary tract infections in adults are discussed.*

Salter AJ. Trimethoprim-sulfamethoxazole: an assessment of more than 12 years of use. Rev Infect Dis 1982; 4:196–236.
*A comprehensive review of the TMP/SMX combination.*

Then RL. Mechanisms of resistance to trimethoprim, the sulfonamides, and trimethoprim-sulfamethoxazole. Rev Infect Dis 1982; 4:261–269.
*A review of the reported resistance mechanisms for the listed agents.*

# 36

# Miscellaneous Antibacterial Drugs

GORDON DOW AND ALLAN R. RONALD

## Urinary Anti-Infective Agents

Antimicrobial agents included in this category are not expected to achieve therapeutic concentrations outside the urinary tract. This unique drug disposition has advantages including reduced suppression of normal bacterial flora, decreased emergence of resistance, low rates of yeast overgrowth syndromes, and minimization of teratogenic risk and fetal toxicity. These agents are generally contraindicated for use in infections involving sites other then the urinary tract.

## Nitrofurantoin

Nitrothiazoles (niridazole), nitroimidazoles (metronidazole), and nitrofurans (nitrofurantoin) have all been developed through nitration of heterocyclic compounds. Several thousand nitrofurans have been evaluated as antimicrobial agents and of these, the hydantoin derivative, nitrofurantoin [(O-)5-nitrofurfurylidene-amino(-hydantoin)], has achieved widest clinical application. It has been in clinical use since 1953 in microcrystalline form and the macrocrystalline formulation has been available since 1967. Recently, a slow-release product has been developed, consisting of 75% nitrofurantoin monohydrate powder and 25% macrocrystalline nitrofurantoin.

### Physico-chemical properties

The structure of nitrofurantoin is shown in Figure 36.1. Nitrofurantoin has a molecular weight of 238 and consists of yellow, odorless crystals that will discolor upon exposure to light. It is a weak acid (pKa = 7.2) and its solubility in water improves dramatically with increasing pH.

### Mode of action

Nitrofurantoin is activated by flavoprotein enzyme systems that reduce it to a biologically inactive end product. Highly reactive intermediates produced during this degradative process inhibit bacterial enzyme systems. Nitrofurantoin intermediates also damage DNA directly, leading to strand breakage. These multiple toxic effects contribute to its spectrum or activity as well as reduced rates of bacterial resistance. Although nitrofurantoin is reduced to toxic intermediates within mammalian cells, oxygen scavengers prevent damage to host tissues.

### Pharmacokinetics

Nitrofurantoin is well absorbed from the gastrointestinal tract. Bioavailability increases when taken with food. Macrocrystalline formulations have comparable bioavailability but absorption is slower. The mean peak serum level is 0.72 $\mu$g/ml at 2 h after a dose of 100 mg of *micro-crystalline* nitrofurantoin. It is 90% protein bound.

Although widely distributed, rapid metabolic inactivation in the tissues and renal excretion result in a short half-life of 20 min. In the presence of normal renal function, therapeutic levels are only achieved in renal tissue and urine. The liver is the principle site of metabolic inactivation.

Approximately one-third of an oral dose is excreted unchanged in the urine, with peak urine levels varying from 50 to 250 $\mu$g/ml. Therapeutic urinary concentrations of drug are present for up to 6 h. Urinary excretion occurs primarily by glomerular filtration, with some tubular secretion. Tubular reabsorption provides therapeutic levels in renal medullary tissue. Although alkalinization of the urine reduces tubular reabsorption, resulting in increased urinary concentrations, the antibacterial activity of nitrofurantoin is significantly reduced above a urinary pH of 6.

Renal impairment increases host toxicity and decreases therapeutic efficacy. It also accumulates to toxic levels in newborns. Nitrofurantoin is contraindicated in patients with any renal insufficiency, children $<1$ month of age and women near delivery.

### Antimicrobial activity

Nitrofurantoin is active against a broad spectrum of gram-positive, gram-negative, and anerobic pathogens and is bactericidal at levels near the minimum inhibitory concentration (MIC). Bacteria with an MIC of 32 $\mu$g/ml or less are considered susceptible. Essentially 100% of urinary isolates of *Escherichia coli* and coagulase negative Staphylococci have remained susceptible to nitrofurantoin. Approximately 95% of Enterococci and 90% of *Staphylococcus aureus* are sensitive, while *Enterbacter* spp., *Proteus* spp., and *Klebsiella* spp. have an intrinsically higher MIC to nitrofurantoin with consequent lower susceptibility profiles. *Pseudomonas* spp. are usually resistant.

Resistant variants may be produced by passage in the presence of the drug, but this occurs slowly. Cross-resistance with other antibacterial agents is rare. Its broad mechanism of action, high oral bioavailability, and low concentrations at mucosal surfaces have ensured lack of development of resistance in normal flora during prolonged therapy. It is almost unprecedented for bacterial susceptibility to remain stable despite four decades of clinical use.

### Toxicity and side effects

Toxicity is due to the 5-nitrofuran ring and include cutaneous-allergic, pulmonary, hepatic, neurologic and hematologic adverse effects. The frequency of these drug reactions, based on over 120 million treatment courses, is presented in Table 36.1. The over-

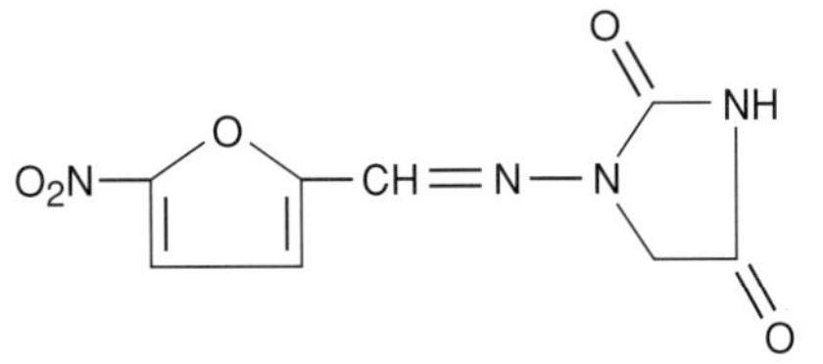

Fig. 36.1 Nitrofurantoin.

all estimated rate of serious adverse events is 28 per million treatment courses. All major adverse events are more common in the elderly.

Pulmonary reactions are the most frequently described severe toxicity, and may be acute, subacute, or chronic. Acute pulmonary reactions are characterized by fever, cough, dyspnea, and pleuritic chest pain with an interstitial-alveolar infiltrate on X ray. The onset is usually within 1 week of treatment and has features of a cell-mediated hypersensitivity pneumonitis. Peripheral eosinophilia is common. Recovery occurs rapidly upon discontinuation of the drug. Corticosteroids may be used in persons with a severe reaction. Subacute presentations are less likely to be associated with fever and eosinophilia and are slower to resolve. Chronic pulmonary reactions are rare and occur when the drug has been prescribed for >6 months. Patients present with the insidious progression of dyspnea and dry cough with an interstitial infiltrate on X ray; this likely represents a cumulative toxic drug effect. Chronic interstitial pneumonitis and fibrosis is evident histologically and the illness may not resolve when nitrofurantoin is stopped.

Hepatic reactions are rare and of two types. Acute cholestatic hepatitis presents with a prodrome of fever, rash, and eosinophilia followed by jaundice within a few days or weeks. This syndrome appears to be immunologically mediated, and as in acute pulmonary reactions, resolves with drug discontinuation and recurs with rechallenge. Prolonged therapy, usually for at least 6 months, is associated with the insidious onset of chronic active hepatitis. Recovery from chronic hepatitis occurs in about 80% of persons after discontinuation of nitrofurantoin.

The most common and serious neurologic toxicity of nitrofurantoin is an ascending sensory-motor polyneuropathy occurring in the presence of even modest renal impairment and in elderly persons who have had normal renal function. Sensory symptoms usually begin within 6 weeks of starting treatment, followed soon after by motor neuropathy. Total recovery occurs in one-third of cases and partial recovery in one-half. Prognosis correlates best with the severity of neuropathy at the time of drug discontinuation.

Nitrofurantoin may rarely be associated with hematologic abnormalities. Bone marrow depression has been described as well as hemolytic anemia in persons with glucose-6-phosphate dehydrogenase or enolase deficiencies. Hemolysis also occurs in infants <1 month of age in whom these red cell enzyme systems have not fully developed. Megaloblastic anemia may rarely occur, and is most likely related to hydantoin-induced folate deficiency.

Immunologically mediated cutaneous toxicities occur in approximately 1%–5% of patients, and subside rapidly with cessation of therapy. Other immunologic manifestations include drug fever, bronchospasm, arthralgia, and a lupus-like syndrome.

Anorexia, nausea, and vomiting are the most frequent adverse reactions reported with nitrofurantoin, occurring in 10%–20% of patients. However, these occur in a dose-related fashion, and are noted in only 1.6% of those taking recommended therapeutic doses of <4 mg/kg/day. Gastrointestinal side effects may also be related to the rate of drug absorption, since macrocrystals either alone or in combination with nitrofurantoin monohydrate powder appear to be better tolerated than the microcrystalline formulation.

Overall, most side effects occur at acceptably low levels when nitrofurantoin is prescribed at recommended doses. However, it is necessary to assess renal function, as an elevated creatinine contraindicates its use. Prolonged therapy requires periodic clinical assessment for pulmonary and neurologic toxicity as well as complete blood count and transaminase determinations and is rarely warranted in persons age 60 or greater.

### Interactions

Nitrofurantoin has been reported to reduce the bacteriostatic activity of quinolones. It may also reduce phenytoin levels in some patients.

## Therapeutic indications

Cure rates with nitrofurantoin for lower urinary tract infection (UTI) range from 70%–95%. Similar efficacy has been documented for patients with asymptomatic upper tract involvement and this may be related to the drug's ability to back diffuse into medullary tissue. However, nitrofurantoin should not be used for persons with complicated or symptomatic upper UTIs in which therapeutic levels of antibiotic may not be attained at the site of infection.

Three studies have assessed therapeutic efficacy by comparing conventional 7- to 10-day treatment regimens for UTI with either 3-day or single-dose therapy. Cure rates were similar and drug side effects were reduced in the patients receiving short-course therapy. Single-dose therapy with nitrofurantoin has not been directly compared with other regimens in randomized clinical trials. Current data suggests that 100 mg bid for 3 days is adequate for short course therapy.

Much of the clinical literature devoted to nitrofurantoin has described its low-dose, continuous use in the prophylaxis of recurrent UTI. Clinical efficacy is based on its local bactericidal activity in the bladder against reinfecting bacteria, as it does not influence vaginal or rectal colonization. Prophylaxis has been highly successful when given either as 50 or 100 mg once nightly. Postintercourse prophylaxis is also successful in women with

**Table 36.1** Nitrofurantoin and serious adverse events

| Reaction | Patients worldwide | Incidence (reactions/million treatment courses) |
|---|---|---|
| Acute pulmonary | 1138 | 9.4 |
| Subacute pulmonary | 22 | 0.2 |
| Chronic pulmonary | 281 | 2.3 |
| Miscellaneous pulmonary | 283 | 2.3 |
| Hepatic | 312 | 2.6 |
| Neurologic | 847 | 7.0 |
| Hematologic | 500 | 4.1 |
| Total | 3383 | 27.8 |

$n$ = 121.43 million courses of therapy

[From Drug Intelligence and Clinical Pharmacy 1985; 19:540–547.]

episodes of UTI that correlate temporally with sexual intercourse. Nitrofurantoin has been well tolerated when given long term for low-dose prophylaxis with efficacy comparable to trimethoprim and trimethoprim–sulfamethoxazole (TMP–SMX).

Antimicrobial regimens recommended for use in pregnancy have typically been restricted to $\beta$-lactams and nitrofurantoin. A meta-analysis of three studies of nitrofurantoin administration during the first trimester has shown no increase in teratogenic events nor fetal toxicity. Treatment of asymptomatic bacteruria in pregnancy with a single 200 mg dose of nitrofurantoin has a failure rate of 27%, which is equivalent to other single-dose failure rates. Although a 3- to 7-day course may have better efficacy, single-dose therapy has benefits of high compliance and low toxicity. Symptomatic bacteruria (acute cystitis) or relapse after single-dose therapy can be treated with 100 mg of nitrofurantoin twice daily for 3 to 7 days. Nitrofurantoin is appropriate for prophylaxis of recurrent UTI during pregnancy with postintercourse or nightly nitrofurantoin at a dose of 50 mg.

Two prospective studies in patients with spinal cord injury have demonstrated a significant reduction in UTI compared with placebo in patients utilizing intermittent self-catheterization.

## Methenamine

Methenamine (hexamethylenetetramine) was described by Butlerow in 1860 and it has been prescribed as an urinary antiseptic since 1895. This drug has advantages of economy, tolerability, minimal effect on gastrointestinal flora, and absence of bacterial resistance. Its niche has been largely supplanted by antibiotics, but the emergence of antimicrobial resistance has led to renewed interest. Methenamine is available as the pure base or in combination with organic acids to form the salts methenamine mandelate or methenamine hippurate. These formulations are available either in 0.5 or 1 g tablets.

### Physicochemical properties

Methenamine is a synthetic monoacidic base, formed by the condensation of ammonia and formaldehyde (Fig. 36.2). It occurs as clear crystals or as a white odorless powder that is freely soluble in water and alcohol. The pKa of methenamine is 4.8. One molecule of methenamine is hydrolyzed into four molecules of ammonia and six molecules of formaldehyde in an acid environment according to the following formula:

$$N_4(CH_2)_6 + 6H_2O + 4H^+ \ \mathrm{R}\ 4NH_{4+} + 6HCHO$$

### Mechanism of action

Methenamine lacks intrinsic bactericidal activity. Its anti-infective properties are due to the production of formaldehyde via acid hydrolysis in the bladder. Formaldehyde acts through protein denaturation and is bacteriostatic at a concentration of 10–15 $\mu$m/ml and bactericidal at concentrations >30 $\mu$m/ml. Mandelic and hippuric acids in the unionized state also possess bacteriostatic properties related to inhibition of bacterial oxidative metabolism. However, these organic acids must be given at a dose of approximately 12 g or more per day to render the urine inhibitory. Methenamine salts provide only 1–2 g/day of either organic acid with current formulations and there is little evidence that they reduce urinary pH enough to accelerate formaldehyde formation.

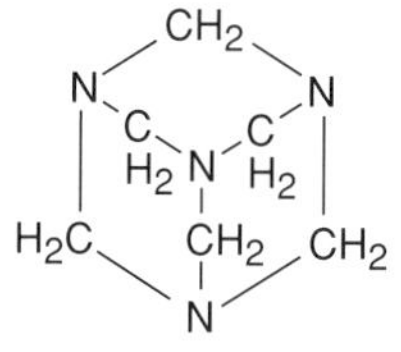

CH2
N N
C C
H2 N H2
H2C CH2 CH2
N

**Fig. 36.2** Methenamine.

### Pharmacokinetics

Pharmacokinetic studies of methenamine are inconsistent. Although hydrolysis in the stomach leads to some reduction in bioavailability, approximately 80% of an oral dose is recovered from the urine over a 24-h period. Enteric-coated methenamine mandelate may reduce gastric intolerance, but it may reduce bioavailability. Its volume of distribution closely approximates total body water. Methenamine has a half-life of 4 h and is rapidly excreted into the urine.

Accurate determination of free formaldehyde generation in the urine has only recently been possible, and ranges from 1 to 40 $\mu$m/ml at 2 h. This wide range varies with voiding pattern and urinary pH. The effect of pH on formaldehyde generation is logarithmic; over 5 h are required to produce a bactericidal formaldehyde concentration of >28 $\mu$m/ml in urine at a pH greater than 6.0. compared with 1.5 h at pH 5.6. Although adjunctive urinary acidification has been recommended, urine is acidic in most individuals, and acidifiers (vitamin C, methionine, ammonium chloride) are only effective at high doses over the short term. Fluid restriction is a more useful adjunctive measure as it acts to reduce voiding frequency, acidifies the urine, and increases bladder methenamine concentrations. Patients should be asked to reduce voiding frequency and restrict fluids to 1200–1500 ml per day so that the urine specific gravity is maintained at a level of 1.015 or greater.

### Antimicrobial activity

The antimicrobial action of methenamine is nonspecific and encompasses all bacteria and fungi causing urinary tract infections. Resistance has not been reported. Urea-splitting organisms such as *Proteus* spp., *Providencia* spp., and *Enterobacter* spp. can alkalinize the urine via production of ammonium hydroxide and thus block formaldehyde generation. The therapeutic activity of methenamine can be promoted in this setting by inhibiting bacterial urease with acetohydroxamic acid.

### Toxicity

Methenamine is well tolerated with adverse effects reported rarely. Most are related to excessive formaldehyde production. Gastrointestinal complaints include epigastric discomfort, anorexia, nausea, vomiting, and diarrhea. Bladder irritation may also occur, particularly at high doses resulting in dysuria, frequency, and hematuria. Cutaneous and pulmonary hypersensitivity reactions are rare.

Renal insufficiency does not contraindicate methenamine use, as it is nontoxic and urinary methenamine is readily converted to formaldehyde in the azotemic state. However, methenamine salts are contraindicated in renal failure where they may exacerbate acidosis or precipitate in the renal tubules. They also should be avoided in persons with gout.

Methenamine and its salts are contraindicated in severe hepatic impairment as ammonia release has the potential to induce or exacerbate hepatic encephalopathy.

The safety of methenamine and its salts in pregnancy has not been established by adequate studies. It has an excellent safety profile in children with adverse effects reported in approximately 1% of individuals.

### Drug interactions

Formaldehyde and some sulfa derivatives produce an inactive precipitate and should not be administered together. Formaldehyde can interfere with urinary hormonal assays, including false elevation of vanililmandelic acid, catecholamines, and 17-hydroxycorticosteroids. Discrepant low values for urine estriol and 5-hydroxyindoleacetic acid have also been reported.

## Clinical experience

While methenamine has been advocated for the treatment of acute bacterial cystitis, there are few modern studies which support this indication. It is contraindicated in persons with UTI involving the upper tract.

The primary role of methenamine and it salts has been for suppression and prophylaxis of UTI. Several prospective studies support this indication and its efficacy, although lower in some studies, has generally compared favorably with that of nitrofurantoin and trimethoprim-sulfamethoxazole. Failures with methenamine may be related to asymptomatic upper tract involvement, suboptimal dosing, and inadequate fluid restriction.

Methenamine has not proven efficacious for decreasing bacteriuria in persons with in-dwelling bladder catheters. This is expected on the basis of its mode of action, as urinary methenamine requires at least 2 h to produce adequate formaldehyde levels. Three comparative studies in spinal cord injured patients undergoing intermittent self-catheterization have demonstrated a significant reduction in UTI with methenamine salts. In one of these studies, ammonium chloride at a dose of 1 g given every 6 h was added to the prophylactic regimen.

For most indications, methenamine should be administered either as free base at a dose of 0.5 to 1 g qid, as methenamine mandelate at 1 g qid, or as methenamine hippurate at 1 g bid.

## Fosfomycin Trometamol

Fosfomycin is a unique substance that inhibits bacterial cell wall formulation by blocking the first phase of peptidoglycan synthesis. The trometamol salt is fully bioavailable and following single-dose administration orally achieves bactericidal activity in the urine against most urinary pathogens for 48 h or longer. No cross-resistance appears to occur with other antibacterial agents. A single-dose regimen of 3 g has been marketed in many countries in Europe and is currently being evaluated in the United States. Adverse effects are unusual and to date serious or life-threatening complications have not been reported. Single-dose regimens appear to be equivalent to other short-course treatment regimens used for acute cystitis. Further studies are necessary to determine its role in the overall management of urinary infection.

## Cranberry Juice

Cranberry juice has been widely promoted for the treatment and prophylaxis of UTI and four studies describe its use. While it may demonstrate some activity in acute UTI, efficacy rates appear to be significantly below those of other antibacterial agents. Its mechanism of action has been attributed to the inhibition of bacterial adherence, rather than the presence of vitamin C or hippuric acid, which are excreted in the urine following cranberry juice ingestion.

This postulated mode of action would support the use of cranberry juice for the prophylaxis of UTI rather than treatment. This has recently been demonstrated in elderly women, in whom prophylaxis with 300 ml of cranberry juice cocktail per day significantly reduced bacteruria with pyuria compared with those receiving placebo.

## Metronidazole

Metronidazole was introduced in 1959 for the treatment of *Trichomonas vaginalis* infections, which prior to that time, were treated topically with variable success. Its use as an anti-anaerobic agent was subsequently demonstrated in 1962.

## Physicochemical properties

Metronidazole (2-methyl-5-nitroimidazole-1-ethanol) occurs as a pale yellow crystalline powder which darkens on exposure to light (Fig. 36.3). It is a small molecule that is unionized at physiologic pH and only partly soluble in water and ethanol.

## Mode of action

Its mode of action appears to be identical to that of nitrofurantoin. The drug enters the cell and is reduced by accepting electrons from flavoprotein enzymes, producing highly reactive intermediates. These damage DNA and other macromolecules, eventually forming a stable end product. Inhibition of DNA synthesis appears to be immediate and thus the drug is rapidly bactericidal.

## Pharmacokinetics

Metronidazole is well absorbed from the gastrointestinal tract, with an oral bioavailability of 90%, which is delayed but not reduced by meals. Absorption is high after rectal administration and intravaginal administration achieves a bioavailability of 20%. Peak serum levels after a single 500 mg oral dose range from 1.0–16.0 $\mu$g/ml. The mean peak serum level with intravenous metronidazole 500 mg administered every 8 h is 26 $\mu$g/ml with a trough of 12 $\mu$g/ml. The elimination half-life is approximately 8 h.

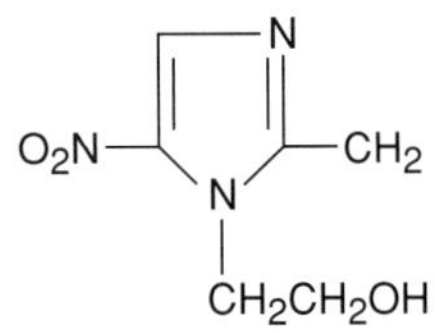

N
$O_2N$ — $CH_2$
N
$CH_2CH_2OH$

**Fig. 36.3** Metronidazole.

Metronidazole is poorly protein bound and has a high volume of distribution, approximating that of total body water. It is widely distributed, often with tissue levels comparable to serum levels. Therapeutic levels are also achieved in empyema fluid as well as in hepatic, cerebral, and pulmonary abscesses. Cerebrospinal fluid (CSF) concentrations are approximately 40% of serum and in alveolar bone this is reduced to 10%. Therapeutic concentrations are not achieved in the aqueous humor. Peak serum levels in the fetus approach maternal levels.

Metronidazole is extensively metabolized in the liver, where five major end products are formed, the most important of which is the hydroxy metabolite. This compound has significant anti-anaerobic activity.

Metronidazole and its derivatives are largely excreted by the kidney where 60%–80% may be recovered from the urine and 5%–15% in the feces. Parent compound may be almost undetectable in feces, except in circumstances where there is significant colonic mucosal inflammation, rapid gastrointestinal (GI) transit time, or high dosage. These low drug levels are likely related to its high bioavailability and extensive metabolic inactivation, which is carried out by both obligate and facultative anaerobic colonic flora.

Its pharmacokinetic profile is minimally influenced by renal failure, and metronidazole and its metabolites are completely removed by hemodialysis. Renal failure does not require a change in dosing. Plasma levels may become significantly elevated in the setting of hepatic failure, where once-daily dosing is warranted. There are no established clinical criteria as to when dosage reduction should be undertaken in this setting. Ideally, metronidazole levels are recommended to ensure that peak and trough levels do not exceed 25 and 18 μg/ml, respectively.

## Antimicrobial activity

Bacterial species with a MIC <16 μg/ml are considered susceptible. It is the drug of choice for infections with *Bacteroides fragilis*, and is active against most gram-negative obligate anaerobes. Whereas anaerobic gram-positive cocci are usually susceptible, most strains of gram-positive nonsporulating bacilli (*Actinomyces* sp., *Arachnia* sp., *Propionibacteria* sp.) and microaerophilic streptococci are resistant.

Gram-negative facultative anaerobes, including *E. coli*, *Klebsiella*, and *Proteus*, are also sensitive to metronidazole under strictly anaerobic conditions. This may explain why metronidazole has been successful in the treatment of mixed aerobic–anaerobic infections, but the clinical relevance of this observation is unclear. Colonic flora remain stable unless an agent is added that is active against facultative anaerobes, further supporting the fact that these bacteria can inactivate metronidazole.

Oral spirochetes, *Treponema pallidum*, *Helicobacter pylori*, and *Campylobacter fetus* are susceptible, as are the anaerobic protozoa *Trichomonas vaginalis*, *Entamoeba histolytica*, *Giardia lamblia*, and *Balantidium coli*. There has been one report of its successful use in *Fasciola hepatica* infection. It also expedites the removal of emerging worms in *Dracunculus medinencus* infection.

Plasmid and chromosomally mediated resistance to metronidazole have been described, but they appear rarely. Metronidazole resistance is seen in <1% of the *B. fragilis* group while increasing resistance has developed toward clindamycin (10%), ureidopenicillins (10%) and cephalosporins with anaerobic activity (5%–33%). Prevotella species have likewise remained susceptible to metronidazole. Resistant isolates of *T. vaginalis* have been reported.

Resistance is mediated by a decrease in nitroreductase activity, which also decreases metronidazole uptake by reducing the metronidazole concentration gradient.

## Toxicity and side effects

Metronidazole is usually well tolerated. The most frequently described side effects are gastrointestinal and include nausea, anorexia, and an unpleasant metallic taste. Pseudomembranous colitis has paradoxically been described in a few cases, sometimes with *C. difficile* sensitive to metronidazole. Pancreatitis has been described in one patient.

Transient reversible neutropenia has been noted in a few cases. Urine may become dark red-brown in color because of the presence of an azometabolite. Other minor adverse reactions include drowsiness, headache, and skin rash.

Its major toxicities are neurologic. Peripheral neuropathy has been reported in a number of patients receiving high doses for prolonged periods of time. Full recovery generally occurs with discontinuation or dose reduction. Seizures, encephalopathy, and cerebellar dysfunction have also been reported.

The greatest controversy associated with metronidazole toxicity has been related to the issue of mutagenic and carcinogenic potential. Reduction of the nitro group produces metabolites that react with deoxyribonucleic acid, therefore its antibacterial and mutagenic activity are inseparable. It is not surprising that urine from patients treated with metronidazole is mutagenic for *Salmonella tymphimurium* in the Ames test. This has not been shown in mammalian test systems. Prolonged treatment in patients with Crohn's disease has not been associated with an increase in chromosomal abnormalities.

Although an increase in lung tumors has been described in mice fed high doses of metronidazole over a prolonged period of time, this has not been reproducible in other species and may be related to an alteration in gut flora or the production of reactive intermediates in large amounts. Two large follow-up studies in humans have failed to reveal any excess cancer risk.

Animal models and follow-up of women given metronidazole at various stages of pregnancy have failed to show evidence of teratogenicity. However, it is prudent to avoid metronidazole during pregnancy except where no other alternative effective agents are available. Similarly, breast feeding should be discontinued during and for 48 h after treatment with metronidazole.

### Interactions

Metronidazole can produce a disulfiram reaction when ingested with alcohol by blocking the metabolism of acetaldehyde. It also inhibits metabolism of coumadin, requiring a dosage reduction, and may also elevate lithium levels. It can produce a spurius drop in SGOT (aspartate aminotransferase) when measured by some methods and can lead to a true decrease in cholesterol and triglycerides, the mechanism of which is unknown.

## Therapeutic indications

Metronidazole has been extensively reviewed in terms of its clinical efficacy in a wide range of anaerobic bacterial infections. Successful use has been demonstrated for intra-abdominal, obstetric-gynecologic, chest, head and neck, bone, and bacteremic infections. Its lack of efficacy for actinomycosis is a noteable exception. In many of these clinical settings, it has seldom been evaluated as monotherapy because of the mixed aerobic–anaerobic nature of these infections. Metronidazole should not be used as monotherapy for respiratory infection because of the presence of resistant microaerophilic streptococci.

Animal models of anaerobic osteomyelitis do not respond well to any antibiotic. However, anaerobic osteomyelitis in the setting of diabetic foot infection responds well to prolonged courses of appropriate antibacterial combinations that include metronidazole.

Oral and dental infections usually respond well to penicillin G. Metronidazole may be added if resistant *B. fragilis* group anaerobes are present.

Few comparative trials have been carried out to assess metronidazole in anerobic infection. However, intramuscular procaine penicillin compared with rectal/oral metronidazole for tetanus revealed a survival benefit in the latter group.

Although metronidazole is often given every 8 hours, its half-life is such that twice-daily dosing is adequate for most indications. For serious infections, 500 mg IV twice daily is recommended with an identical dosing regimen for oral therapy. Rectal metronidazole is an effective alternative to the oral route and can be administered as 1 g three times daily for 3 days followed by 1 g twice daily. Most dental and genital infections respond well to 250 mg orally three times daily.

Although primary resistance to metronidazole is seen in 20% to 40% of *Helicobacter pylori* isolates, triple therapy containing metronidazole has resulted in eradication rates of 60%–90%. For *Clostridium difficile* colitis, a dosage regimen of 250 mg of metronidazole given four times daily for 10–14 days is equivalent in efficacy to oral vancomycin. It has an efficacy rate approaching 90% for bacterial vaginosis when administered as 500 mg twice daily for 7 days, while success with a single 2 g dose is less than 50%. In contrast, the 2 g single dose provides effective treatment for both the patient with trichomonas and her consort. A dose of 500 mg twice daily for 5 days can also be used. Metronidazole is superior to quinacrine (no longer available in U.S.) for giardiasis, which may be treated with 250 mg twice daily for 7 days or 2 g daily for 3 days. Amoebiasis responds well to 750 mg three times daily for 7 days for dysenteric or hepatic disease, followed by iodoquinol.

High-dose metronidazole has been shown to have a beneficial effect in perineal Crohn's disease and possibly lessens diarrhea in the setting of active colitis. Prolonged use has been complicated by the development of neuropathy.

It is effective either orally or topically for acne rosacea, particularly for papules and pustules rather than the earlier erythema phase.

It has been shown to prevent intrahepatic cholestasis associated with total parenteral nutrition and hepatic steatosis associated with intestinal bypass, which suggests that both conditions may be related to intestinal overgrowth with anaerobic bacteria.

## Tinidazole

The usefulness of metronidazole has encouraged the development of numerous other nitroimidazoles, including tinidazole, nimorazole, ornidazole, carnidazole, and secnidazole. Tinidazole has received widest clinical application of these other cogeners.

Its antimicrobial spectrum is essentially identical to metronidazole but has been reported to have lower inhibitory concentrations for *B. fragilis*.

The pharmacokinetic profile of tinidazole is similar to that of metronidazole except that its half-life is longer (12 h) and its greater lipid solubility improves CSF levels and enhances in vitro activity.

Reported side effects have been comparable to those of metronidazole and it is also mutagenic using the Ames test.

Clinical use and indications are identical to those of metronidazole. Serious anaerobic infections are generally treated with 800 mg intravenously once daily. Oral treatment is given initially as 2 g followed by 1 g daily. It may have slightly better activity for Giardia than metronidazole and is given as a single 2 gm dose for this indication.

## Polymyxins

The polymyxins are cationic surface-active polypeptides that interact with the phospholipid component of the cytoplasmic membrane of susceptible bacteria and disrupt the osmotic integrity of the cell membrane. Polymyxin B and colistin (polymyxin E) have been used therapeutically in the past primarily to treat *Pseudomonas aeruginosa* infections. At one time, they were the only systemic therapeutic agents available for the treatment of *P. aeruginosa* infection. As no absorption occurs after oral administration, they must be administered parenterally. However, the polymyxins are currently rarely if ever prescribed for systemic use. They appear to be relatively ineffective for the treatment of deep tissue infections and have had limited efficacy for *Pseudomonas* infections outside the urinary tract. Dose-dependent nephrotoxicity and transient neurologic disturbances including neuromuscular blockage are also common and serious, although usually reversible.

Both polymyxin B and colistin sulphate are marketed topically in numerous products that are available as prescription drugs and over-the-counter preparations. Aerosolized polymyxin B has been used to treat *Pseudomonas* respiratory infections, particularly in patients with cystic fibrosis. It is prescribed as a bladder irrigant and topically for infections of the eye, ear, and skin. The evidence for the efficacy of all these regimens is equivocal; few controlled studies have been published on therapeutic efficacy for topical preparations of the polymyxins.

### ANNOTATED BIBLIOGRAPHY


Auger P, Bourgovin J, Bagot C. Intravenous metronidazole in the treatment of abdominal sepsis: once vs three times daily administration. Curr Ther Res 1988; 43(3):494–502.
*This study documents the efficacy of once daily metronidazole.*

Avorn J, Monane M, Gurwitz J, Glynn R, et al. Reduction of bacteriuria and pyuria after ingestion of cranberry juice. JAMA 1994; 271(10):751–754.
*A double-blind placebo controlled trial documenting the efficacy of cranberry juice as UTI prophylaxis in the elderly.*

Baily R, Roberts A, Gower P, De Wardener H. Prevention of urinary-tract infection with low-dose nitrofurantoin. Lancet 1971; 2:1112–1114.
*This describes the first trial using low dose nitrofurantoin to prevent urinary tract infection.*

Cunha B. Nitrofurantoin-current concepts. Urology 1988; 32:67–71.
*An excellent review of nitrofurantoin and its clinical utilization.*

Darcy P. Nitrofurantoin. Drug Intelligence and Clinical Pharmacy 1985; 19:540–547.
*A comprehensive review of adverse events associated with nitrofurantoin treatment as obtained through the Norwich Eaton data base.*

Gleckman R, Alvarez S, Joubert D, Mathews S. Drug therapy reviews: methenamine mandelate and methenamine hippurate. Am J Hosp Pharm 1979; 36:1509–1512.
*A good drug review of methenamine salts.*

Harding G, Ronald A. A controlled study of antimicrobial prophylaxis of recurrent urinary infection in women. N Engl J Med 1974; 291:597–601.
*This represents one of the original studies comparing the efficacy of methenamine as a urinary prophylactic agent with sulfamethoxazole, trimethoprim, co-trimoxazole and no drug therapy.*

Hooton T, Stamm W. Diagnosis and treatment of uncomplicated urinary tract infections. Infect Dis Clin North Am 1997 Sep; 11(3):551–581.

Roe F. Toxicologic evaluation of metronidazole with particular reference to carcinogenic, mutagenic and teratogenic potential. Surgery 1983; 93(1):158–164.
*A useful review of metronidazole associated toxicity.*

Stamm W, Counts G, Wagner K, Martin D, et al. Antimicrobial prophylaxis of recurrent urinary tract infections. Ann Intern Med 1980; 92;770–775.
*Utility of prophylaxis of UTI with nitrofurantoin is compared with co-trimoxazole, trimethoprim and placebo.*

Strom J, Jun H. Effect of urine pH and ascorbic acid on the rate of conversion of methenamine to formaldehyde. Biopharm Drug Dispos 1993; 14:61–69.
*The kinetics of conversion of methenamine to formaldehyde are described in terms of urinary pH and the presence of ascorbic acid.*

# 37

# Antimycobacterial Drugs

CHARLES A. PELOQUIN AND MICHAEL D. ISEMAN

Antimycobacterial agents embrace a wide array of drug classes and are used to treat a host of infections. These infections include tuberculosis, the disease caused by *Mycobacterium tuberculosis* (MTB); leprosy, the disease caused by *M. leprae*; and numerous infections due to mycobacteria other than tuberculosis (MOTT), such as *M. avium* complex, the most common nontuberculous mycobacterial pathogen in the United States. Among the nontuberculous mycobacteria (NTM), a major division exists between "slow growers," such as *M. avium* complex (MAC) and *M. kansasii*, and "rapid growers" such as *M. chelonae* and *M. fortuitum*. Aside from tuberculosis, well-designed prospective treatment studies are lacking for these conditions, so treatment recommendations vary from center to center and remain open to debate. With few exceptions, the treatment of mycobacterial diseases requires combination chemotherapy in order to prevent the emergence of drug resistance. Drug-resistant mutants are generally present among the population of organisms infecting the typical patient. Since most mutations are drug specific, it is unlikely that a spontaneously occurring mutant would be resistant to more than one drug. However, with careless prescribing or with patient noncompliance, the selection of drug-resistant isolates can occur readily. Therefore, it is important for each prescribing physician to be particularly diligent when employing the antimycobacterial drugs.

## Spectrum and Mechanism of Activity

Most of the antimycobacterial drugs are used only for mycobacterial infections. A few drugs, most notably rifampin, have a broader range of activity and may be employed in a variety of settings. Given the paucity of agents available for the world's most prevalent infectious killer, tuberculosis, it is desirable to reserve these drugs for mycobacterial infections whenever possible.

Limited pharmacological research on the antimycobacterial drugs has been performed over the past quarter century. Therefore, significant gaps remain in our knowledge about these agents. In addition, little is known about the mechanisms of action for several of the agents. This is due in part to the difficulty of studying mycobacteria in vitro. Therefore, the proposed mechanisms of action (Table 37.1) should be viewed with some level of caution.

The definitions of bacteriostatic and bactericidal as applied to the antimycobacterial drugs depart considerably from those used for other bacteria. Furthermore, these definitions depend upon whether an in vitro model or an animal model was used during the testing. Certain in vitro tests and many animal models use concentrations far above what can be achieved in humans, precluding any direct clinical correlation for the results. Therefore, considerable confusion exists in the medical literature as to which drugs are allegedly bacteriostatic (e.g., aminosalicylic acid and thiacetazone) and which are bactericidal (e.g., isoniazid and rifampin). Frequently, the term "bactericidal" is used to describe drugs that rapidly reduce the number of viable mycobacteria in sputum, regardless of their effect in vitro. Another term, "sterilizing activity," is used to describe drugs that eliminate "persisting" organisms in vivo (e.g., pyrazinamide and rifampin). These persisters are subpopulations of organisms believed to be either replicating very slowly or located in areas with limited blood supply. It is important to remember that these definitions were developed to describe the activity of drugs versus *M. tuberculosis*. Most of the anti-tuberculosis bactericidal agents are weakly bactericidal or only bacteriostatic against other mycobacteria, such as *M. avium* complex. A simpler, alternative nomenclature is to consider isoniazid and rifampin the two key drugs for MTB infection. The other drugs act as role players, shortening the duration of therapy or preventing the emergence of resistance to the key drugs. When isoniazid and rifampin are lost because of resistance or intractable toxicity, the treatment of tuberculosis becomes much more difficult. Critical drugs for the other mycobacterial infections are still being determined. For these NTM, macrolides such as clarithromycin and azithromycin will likely have more prominent roles than they do in treating tuberculosis.

An additional barrier to understanding how these drugs work is the distribution of rapidly growing, intermittently growing, and dormant mycobacterial organisms. Because it is impossible to know what portion of any patient's mycobacterial burden resides in any of these states, it is difficult to use this information clinically. These populations, should they truly exist in patients, further complicate the pharmacokinetic–pharmacodynamic modeling of drug action and the selection of optimal dosing strategies.

## Recommended Doses and Routes of Administration

The American Thoracic Society (ATS), the Centers for Disease Control and Prevention (CDC), and the American Academy of Pediatrics (AAP) have proposed dosing guidelines for the drugs intended for use in the treatment of tuberculosis (Table 37.2). The primary agents for drug-susceptible tuberculosis are isoniazid, rifampin, pyrazinamide, and frequently a fourth drug such as ethambutol or streptomycin. The other drugs are generally reserved for patients who cannot tolerate the primary agents, or patients infected with drug-resistant isolates. While similar drugs and doses are frequently employed when treating other mycobacterial infections, this practice clearly is without controlled documentation of efficacy. In particular, MAC is much more re-

**Table 37.1** Spectrum and mechanism of activity

| Drug name | Primary indications | Nonmycobacterial indications | General target | Specific target and mechanism of action | Resistance mechanism |
|---|---|---|---|---|---|
| Amikacin (AK) | MTB, MAC | Gram-negative infections | Target within mycobacteria | Ribosomal subunits inhibit translation | Altered target, ? Penetration and enzymatic modification |
| Aminosalicylic acid (PAS) | MTB | None | Target within mycobacteria | PABA antagonist ? Disrupt iron transport ? | ? Altered drug or target |
| Azithromycin (AZI) | MAC | Bacterial and atypical infections | Target within mycobacteria | 23 S rRNA inhibit initiation and translocation | Altered target |
| Capreomycin (CM) | MTB | None | Target within mycobacteria | Ribosomal subunits inhibit initiation and translocation | Altered target, ? penetration and enzymatic modification |
| Ciprofloxacin (CIP) | MAC, (MTB) | Gram-negative infections | Target within mycobacteria | DNA gyrase | Altered target |
| Clarithromycin (CLAR) | MAC | Bacterial and atypical infections | Target within mycobacteria | 23 S rRNA inhibit initiation and translocation | Altered target |
| Clofazimine (CFZ) | *M. leprae* MAC, (MTB) | Leprosy reactional states, pyoderma gangrenosum | Target within mycobacteria ? | Bind DNA ? | Not known |
| Cycloserine (CSN) | MTB (MAC) other NTM | Historically: Gram (+) and (−) UTI | Cell wall of mycobacteria | Block synthetase linkage of 2 D-alanine molecules | Altered target |
| Dapsone (DDS) | *M. leprae* | *Pneumocystis carinii* Plasmodium sp. | Target within mycobacteria | PABA antagonist ? | Not known |
| Ethambutol (EMB) | MTB, MAC other NTM | None | Cell wall of mycobacteria | Disrupt cell wall synthesis | Altered target |
| Ethionamide (ETA) | MTB (MAC) other NTM *M. leprae* | None | Cell wall of mycobacteria | Disrupt mycolic acid synthesis | Altered target |
| Isoniazid (INH) | MTB other NTM | None | Cell wall of mycobacteria | Disrupt mycolic acid synthesis | Altered target |
| Levofloxacin (LEVO) | MTB (MAC) | Gram-negative, other infections | Target within mycobacteria | DNA gyrase | Altered target |
| Kanamycin (KM) | MTB, MAC | Oral administration: bowel surgery preparation | Target within mycobacteria | Ribosomal subunits inhibit translation | Altered target, ? penetration and enzymatic modification |
| Pyrazinamide (PZA) | MTB | None | Target within mycobacteria | Unknown action via pyrazinoic acid | Not known |
| Rifabutin (RBN) | MAC, MTB (*M. leprae*) | None [active vs. gram (+)] | Target within mycobacteria | DNA-dependent-RNA polymerase: Prevent chain initiation | Altered $\beta$-subunit of RNA polymerase |
| Rifampin (RIF) | MTB, MAC other NTM *M. leprae* | Combination therapy: gram (+) infections *L. pneumophila* Meningitis prophylaxis: *H. influenzae* *N. meningitidis* | Target within mycobacteria | DNA-dependent-RNA polymerase: Prevent chain initiation | Altered $\beta$-subunit of RNA polymerase |
| Streptomycin (SM) | MTB, MAC other NTM | Brucella sp. *Yersinia pestis* Combination therapy: Enterococcal infections *Francisella tularenis* | Target within mycobacteria | 16 S rRNA inhibit translation | Altered target, ? penetration and enzymatic modification |
| Thiacetazone (Tb1) | MTB | None | Cell wall of mycobacteria | Disrupt mycolic acid synthesis | Altered target |

**Table 37.2** Recommended doses and routes of administration

| Drug name | Route and frequency | Adult daily | Adult 2× weekly | Adult 3× weekly | Pediatric daily | Pediatric 2× weekly | Pediatric 3× weekly |
|---|---|---|---|---|---|---|---|
| Amikacin (AK) | IV, IM QD | 12–15 mg/kg | 25–30 mg/kg[c] | 22–25 mg/kg[d] 25–30 mg/kg[c] | 12–15 mg/kg 20–40 mg/kg[c] | 25–30 mg/kg[c] | 25–30 mg/kg[c] |
| Aminosalicylic acid (PAS) | Oral, (IV[a]) BID or TID | 4 g/dose 8–12 g total | Not known | Not known | 150 mg/kg[c] divided TID | Not known | Not known |
| Azithromycin (AZI) | Oral QD | 250–300 mg pulmonary MAC | 1200 mg once weekly preventive tx | Not known | 5 mg/kg? (not studied) | Not known | Not known |
| Capreomycin (CM) | IM, IV QD | 12–15 mg/kg | Not known | Not known | 12–15 mg/kg 15–30 mg/kg[c] | Not known | Not known |
| Ciprofloxacin (CIP) | Oral, IV QD | 750–1250 mg | Not known | Not known | 10 mg/kg? (not studied) | Not known | Not known |
| Clarithromycin (CLAR) | Oral QD or BID | 500 mg | Not known | Not known | 7.5 mg/kg | Not known | Not known |
| Clofazimine[e] (CFZ) | Oral QD | 100–200 mg | Not known (MTB or MAC) | Not known (MTB or MAC) | Not known 2–3 mg/kg? | Not known (MTB or MAC) | Not known (MTB or MAC) |
| Cycloserine[f] (CSN) | Oral QD or BID | 250–500 mg/dose 750–1000 mg total | Not known | Not known | 15–20 mg/kg[c] | Not known | Not known |
| Dapsone (DDS) | Oral QD | 50–100 mg | Not known | Not known | 1.0–1.5 mg/kg (<5 yr: 25 mg; 6–14 yr: 50 mg) | Not known | Not known |
| Ethambutol (EMB) | Oral, [IV[a]] QD | 25 mg/kg (2 mo) then 15 mg/kg | 50 mg/kg | 25–35 mg/kg | 25 mg/kg (2 mo) then 15 mg/kg | 50 mg/kg | 25–35 mg/kg |
| Ethionamide[f] (ETA) | Oral QD or BID | 250–500 mg/dose 750–1000 mg total | Not known | Not known | 15–20 mg/kg | Not known | Not known |
| Isoniazid (INH) | Oral, IM, IV QD | 300 mg (5 mg/kg) | 15 mg/kg 900 mg max[c] | 15 mg/kg 900 mg max[c] | 10–20 mg/kg 300 mg max[c] | 20–40 mg/kg 900 mg max[c] | 20–40 mg/kg 600 mg max[c] |
| Levofloxacin (LEVO) | Oral, IV QD | 750–1000 mg | Not known | Not known | 10 mg/kg? (not studied) | Not known | Not known |
| Kanamycin (KM) | IM, IV QD | 12–15 mg/kg | 25–30 mg/kg[c] (like SM) | 22–25 mg/kg[d] | 12–15 mg/kg 15–30 mg/kg[c] | Not known | Not known |
| Pyrazinamide (PZA) | Oral QD or BID | 15–30 mg/kg 2 gram max[c] | 35–70 mg/kg 4 gram max[c] | 35–70 mg/kg 3 gram max[c] | 15–30 mg/kg 2 gram max[c] | 35–70 mg/kg 4 gram max[c] | 35–70 mg/kg 3 gram max[c] |
| Rifabutin (RBN) | Oral QD | 300 mg | Not known | Not known | 5–10 mg/kg proposed | Not known | Not known |
| Rifampin (RIF) | Oral, IV QD | 450–600 mg (10 mg/kg) | 450–600 mg (10 mg/kg) | 450–600 mg (10 mg/kg) | 10–20 mg/kg 600 mg max[c] | 10–20 mg/kg 600 mg max[c] | 10–20 mg/kg 600 mg max[c] |
| Streptomycin (SM) | IM, IV[b] QD | 12–15 mg/kg | 25–30 mg/kg[c] | 22–25 mg/kg[d] 25–30 mg/kg[c] | 12–15 mg/kg 20–40 mg/kg[c] | 25–30 mg/kg[c] | 25–30 mg/kg[c] |
| Thiacetazone (Tb1) | (Oral[a]) QD | 150 mg | Not known | Not known | 2–5 mg/kg proposed | Not known | Not known |

[a]Available outside of the United States; may be imported under IND.

[b]IV route of administration not FDA approved, but can be given IV like amikacin.

[c]ATS/CDC/AAP 1994 guidelines, which may differ from practice at National Jewish Medical and Research Center.

[d]Intermittent, high-dose, intravenous dosing protocol at National Jewish Medical and Research Center.

[e]Various intermittent clofazimine regimens have been proposed for leprosy, but not for MTB or MAC.

[f]Introduce gradually over several days.

sistant to the action of these drugs. Thus, a strong argument can be made for more aggressive dosing. Although this can be accomplished with certain agents, dose-limiting toxicities often prevent the universal implementation of such an approach. The drugs most frequently used for MAC infections include macrolides (clarithromycin, azithromycin), rifamycins (rifampin, rifabutin), ethambutol, clofazimine, aminoglycosides (streptomycin, kanamycin, amikacin) and ciprofloxacin. Well-designed, prospective clinical trials are needed to define the in vitro susceptibility breakpoints and the optimal doses and frequencies for these drugs versus MAC and other NTM. "Rapid growers" often respond to combinations of certain $\beta$-lactams (cefoxitin, imipenem) and some aminoglycosides (amikacin, streptomycin). Occasionally, certain tetracyclines, sulfonamides or macrolides may be used. Clarithromycin is more potent than erythromycin against the "rapid growers," and is emerging as an effective agent for such infections. While the suppression of the "rapid growers" is often achieved, true eradication has been much more difficult to accomplish.

Table 37.2 displays dosing regimens for selected agents. At our institution, starting doses are employed as described in Table 37.2. During the first 10 days of therapy, the serum concentrations for each drug in the regimen are determined. Doses are adjusted to achieve target serum concentration ranges (Table 37.3). Typically, these ranges are several multiples of the minimal inhibitory concentration (MIC) of most susceptible mycobacteria. While this approach requires additional prospective validation, it is consistent with that used for most infectious diseases. In particular, we prefer this approach for difficult infections, such as multidrug-resistant tuberculosis (MDR-TB), advanced pulmonary MAC infection, and tuberculosis or disseminated MAC infection in AIDS patients. Our clinical and research experience suggests that patients with AIDS are at particular risk of poor drug absorption.

## Therapeutic Drug Monitoring

Traditionally, therapeutic drug monitoring (TDM) has not been an integral part of antimycobacterial drug therapy. In patients with normal hepatic and renal function and fully drug-susceptible MTB infection, there is probably little to be gained by checking serum concentrations. However, patients with gastrointestinal, hepatic, or renal disease may be treated more safely and effectively by using serum concentrations to adjust doses. Malnourished patients and those with AIDS appear to have difficulty absorbing these drugs normally. In some patients, absorption may simply be delayed, but in others, the drugs never reach the systemic circulation. Therefore, the drugs will not be delivered to the sites of infection (other than along the gut wall itself). It is advisable to monitor therapy in such patients to verify the adequacy of the doses used. Failure to achieve adequate serum concentrations may be associated with bacteriological and clinical treatment failures. In the case of MTB infection, this can lead to the selection of further drug resistance, prolong the infectiousness of the patient, and prevent the timely and successful completion of therapy. All of these factors increase the cost of therapy far beyond the cost of the serum concentrations. When patients fail to respond to seemingly appropriate therapy and compliance with therapy is documented, serum concentrations should be obtained to verify the adequacy of the doses.

## Specific Drugs: Aminoglycosides, Polypeptides, Rifamycins, and Fluoroquinolones

Kanamycin, streptomycin, and amikacin show similar activity against both MTB and MAC. Capreomycin is less active against MAC than the other three drugs. Thus, the selection of an injectable agent should be based on in vitro activity against a given patient's isolate, and the cost and toxicity of the drug. While different doses and serum concentration ranges have been empirically proposed for capreomycin, kanamycin, streptomycin, and amikacin, there appears to be little rationale for this. The proposed differences in toxicity among these agents, while potentially real, appear largely to reflect substantial differences in the populations treated and the doses historically used. Therefore, with the exception of high-dose capreomycin, where less data has been accumulated, we dose capreomycin, kanamycin, streptomycin, and amikacin identically. Since these drugs appear to require high maximum concentration ($C_{max}$) to MIC ratios for optimal activity, some authorities have employed high-dose therapy ($C_{max}$ of 65–80 $\mu$g/ml three times per week). Toxicity with the high-dose regimens appears to be comparable to that seen with smaller daily doses ($C_{max}$ of 35–45 $\mu$g/ml five to seven times per week).

Capreomycin, streptomycin, kanamycin, and amikacin can be given intravenously. All can be infused in 100 ml of normal saline or 5% dextrose in water. Doses are typically 12–15 mg/kg five to seven times weekly, but with streptomycin, as high as 27 mg/kg three times weekly. Both peripheral and central catheters have been used successfully. It is advisable to use serum concentrations to adjust the doses. In addition, periodic monitoring (every 2–4 weeks) of the serum blood urea nitrogen, creatinine, calcium, potassium, and magnesium should be considered. Monthly audiograms, as well as symptomatic monitoring for vestibular effects, should also be employed if the drugs are to be used for extended periods.

Several new rifamycins may be introduced over the coming years. For the most part, these drugs are similar to rifampin in spectrum of activity and liability to resistance. The primary differences lie in their pharmacokinetics profiles. New, long-acting rifamycins may be advantageous for intermittent treatment of drug-susceptible MTB. Most rifamycins appear to exhibit cross-resistance with rifampin, so these drugs will likely have a minor role in the treatment of MDR-TB. Rifabutin appears to be a less potent hepatic enzyme inducer than rifampin, and may be slightly more active than rifampin against MAC when pharmacokinetics are considered. It does not appear to be superior to rifampin for the treatment of MTB, and generally cannot be relied upon for MDR-TB.

The fluoroquinolones appear to have a role in the treatment of MDR-TB and MAC. Detailed information regarding these drugs is provided in Chapter 34. Because of their relatively long serum half-lives and the slow doubling time of mycobacteria, we have adopted once-daily regimens of ciprofloxacin and levofloxacin in most adult patients; usual doses range from 750–1250 and 750–1000 mg, respectively. Using TDM, doses are adjusted to achieve target serum concentration ranges (4–6 $\mu$g/ml for ciprofloxacin; 8–12 $\mu$g/ml for ofloxacin) that exceed the MIC of most susceptible isolates. Our experience has shown these drugs to be well tolerated, even when treatment lasts for many months. They should never be used alone for the treatment of MTB or MAC.

## Pharmacokinetic Properties

The pharmacokinetic characteristics of the antimycobacterial drugs are shown in Tables 37.3 and 37.4. In many cases, the data are incomplete because thorough testing, in the modern sense, has never been performed. Genetic polymorphism (fast and slow acetylation) exists for isoniazid metabolism. Although the area under the serum concentration-versus-time curve (AUC) is lower for fast acetylators, clinical and bacteriological efficacy appears comparable for fast and slow acetylators when isoniazid is dosed two to seven times per week. Less frequent dosing of isoniazid may be less effective in fast acetylators. Mycobacteria may infect any part of the body, including the blood, lymphatics, vari-

**Table 37.3** Pharmacokinetic properties

| Drug name | Serum $C_{max}$ | Serum $T_{max}$ | Normal serum half-life | CSF penetration | Protein binding | Volume of distribution |
|---|---|---|---|---|---|---|
| Amikacin (AK) | 35–45 μg/ml<br>65–80 μg/ml[a] | 0.5–1.5 h (IM)<br>end infusion (IV) | 2–4 h | 20–40% est. | 0–60% est. | 0.2–0.3 L/kg |
| Aminosalicylic acid (PAS) | 20–60 μg/ml (granules) | 4–8 h (granules) | 0.5–2 h | 10%–50% | 50%–73% (15% in some reports) | 0.8–3.8 L/kg est. |
| Azithromycin (AZI) | 0.3–0.5 μg/ml | 2 h | 1–5 days | Not known | 50% | 25–100 L/kg |
| Capreomycin (CM) | 35–45 μg/ml | 1–2 h (IM)<br>end infusion (IV) | 2–4 h | 20%–40% est. | Not known<br>est. low | 0.2–0.3 L/kg |
| Ciprofloxacin (CIP) | 4–6 μg/ml targeted | 1–2 h | 3–5 h | 4%–10% | 20%–40% | 2.0–3.0 L/kg |
| Clarithromycin (CLAR) | 2–7 μg/ml | 2–3 h | 3–5 h<br>saturable elim. | Not known | 72% | 2.5–4.0 L/kg |
| Clofazimine (CFZ) | 0.5–2.0 μg/ml | 2–12 h | Biphasic:<br>a: 10 days<br>b: several weeks | Not known<br>est. poor | Not known | Not known<br>est. very large |
| Cycloserine (CSN) | 20–35 μg/ml | 2–4 h | 10–12 h | 50%–80% | Not known<br>0% est. | 0.2–0.35 L/kg est. |
| Dapsone (DDS) | 0.5–5.0 μg/ml | 2–8 h | 10–50 h | ? | 50%–90% | 1.5–2.5 L/kg est. |
| Ethambutol (EMB) | 2–6 μg/ml | 2–3 h | Biphasic:<br>a: 4–5 h<br>b: 10–15 h | 5%–65% est.<br>variable, inflammation | 6%–30% est.<br>also binds RBC | 1.6–3.8 L/kg |
| Ethionamide (ETA) | 1–5 μg/ml | 1–2.5 h | 2–4 h | 20%–100% est. | Not known<br>30% est. | 1.5–4.0 L/kg est. |
| Isoniazid (INH) | 3–6 μg/ml | 0.75–2 h | Polymorphic:<br>fast: 1.5–2 h<br>slow: 3.5–4 h | 20%–100% | 10% est. | 0.6–1.0 L/kg est. |
| Levofloxacin (LEVO) | 8–12 μg/ml targeted | 1–2 h | 5–8 h | 30%–90% | 8%–30% | 1.0–2.5 L/kg |
| Kanamycin (KM) | 35–45 μg/ml<br>65–80 μg/ml[a] | 0.5–1.5 h (IM)<br>End infusion (IV) | 2–4 h | 20%–40% est | 0%–60% est. | 0.2–0.3 L/kg |
| Pyrazinamide (PZA) | 20–60 μg/ml | 1–2 h | 9–11 h | 50%–100% | Not known | 0.6–0.7 L/kg est. |
| Rifabutin (RBN) | 0.3–0.9 μg/ml | 2–4 h | 20–25 h (steady state) | 30%–70% | 70%–90% | 8–9 L/kg |
| Rifampin (RIF) | 8–24 μg/ml | 2 h | 2–4 h | 5%–20% est.<br>variable, inflammation | 60%–80% est. | 0.6–1.0 L/kg est. |
| Streptomycin (SM) | 35–45 μg/ml<br>65–80 μg/ml† | 0.5–1.5 h (IM)<br>End infusion (IV) | 2–4 h | 20%–40% est. | 20%–57% est. | 0.2–0.3 L/kg |
| Thiacetazone (Tb1) | 0.9–2.4 μg/ml | 2–4 h | 12–20 h | Not known | Not known | 1–2 L/kg est. |

$C_{max}$, maximum concentration; $T_{max}$, time to maximum concentration; est., estimated

[a]Intermittent (2–3 times weekly) high-dose regimens.

ous tissues, and macrophages. Because portions of the mycobacterial burden reside intracellularly, the ability to penetrate *and act* within these cells is a desirable characteristic for any antimycobacterial drug. Drugs that are excluded from the macrophage, such as β-lactams and, to some degree, aminoglycosides, may still contribute to therapy. Early in the treatment of the infection, substantial portions of the mycobacterial burden may be in the blood or extracellular fluid, readily accessible to most drugs.

## Adverse Reactions and Drug Interactions

Adverse reactions are common with many of the antimycobacterial drugs (Table 37.5). Many authorities recommend monthly chemistry panels (for hepatic and renal function) and complete blood counts with platelets to help detect toxicities. Isoniazid, rifampin, and pyrazinamide may cause hepatotoxicity, which occurs with similar frequency in both fast and slow acetylators of isoniazid. It appears that although fast acetylators may generate

**Table 37.4** Routes of elimination and major adverse effects

| Drug name | % Renal excretion | % Hepatic clearance | Active metabolite | Metabolite excretion | Dose renal failure | Dose hepatic disease | Adverse effects[a] |
|---|---|---|---|---|---|---|---|
| Amikacin (AK) | >95 | 0 | None | None | 12–15 mg/kg 3× weekly | Unchanged | Ototoxicity, nephrotoxicity, cation wasting |
| Aminosalicylic acid (PAS) | 10 | 90 | None | Renal | Unknown avoid if possible | Not known | N, V, D, hypersensitivity, hypothyroidism |
| Azithromycin (AZI) | <10 | >90 nonrenal | None | Not known | Unchanged | Unchanged | N, V, D, ototoxicity |
| Capreomycin (CM) | >95 | 0 | None | None | 12–15 mg/kg 3× weekly | Unchanged | ototoxicity, nephrotoxicity, cation wasting |
| Ciprofloxacin (CIP) | 50–70 | 30–50 | None | Primarily renal | Unchanged unless severe | Unchanged unless severe | N, V, D, insomnia, restlessness |
| Clarithromycin (CLAR) | 20 | 80 saturable | 14-OH clari | Primarily renal | Unchanged | Unchanged | N, V, D, ototoxicity, hepatotoxicity |
| Clofazimine (CFZ) | <1 | yes (unknown) | None | Fecal | Unchanged | Unchanged | N, V, D, tissue discoloration, irritated skin and eyes |
| Cycloserine (CSN) | 70–100 | Not known | Not known | Not known | 250–500 mg 3× weekly | Unchanged | CNS: lethargy, depression, poor concentration |
| Dapsone (DDS) | 20 | 80 | None | Renal (70–85%) | Not known est. unchanged | Not known | Hemolytic anemia, methemoglobinemia, leprosy reactions |
| Ethambutol (EMB) | 80 | 20 | None | None | 15–25 mg/kg 3× weekly | Unchanged | Altered vision, retrobulbar neuritis, increased uric acid |
| Ethionamidc (ETA) | 5 | 95 | Yes: sulfoxide | Nonrenal | Unchanged | Not known | N, V, altered mood, hypothryoidism |
| Isoniazid (INH) | Polymorphic: fast: 10 slow: 30 | Polymorphic: fast: 90 slow: 70 | None | Renal (50–60%) and nonrenal | Unchanged or reduced to QOD 3 times/week | Unchanged in most patients | Hepatotoxicity, peripheral neuropathy |
| Levofloxacin (LEVO) | >90 | <10 | Not significant | Primarily renal | 750 mg 3× weekly | Unchanged | N, V, D, insomnia, restlessness |
| Kanamycin (KM) | >95 | 0 | None | None | 12–15 mg/Kg 3× weekly | Unchanged | Ototoxicity, nephrotoxicity, cation wasting |
| Pyrazinamide (PZA) | 5 | 95 | None | Renal | 15–30 mg/kg 3 times weekly | Not known | N, V, hepatotoxicity, increased uric acid |
| Rifabutin (RBN) | 10 | 90 | Yes: 25-O-deacetyl | Renal (35%) and nonrenal | Unchanged in most patients | Unchanged in most patients | N, V, uveitis, myalgia, anemia, neutropenia |
| Rifampin (RIF) | 10 | 90 | Yes: 25-deacetyl | Renal (20%) and nonrenal | Unchanged in most patients | Unchanged in most patients | N, V, hypersensitivity, flu syndrome, renal, hepatotoxicity |
| Streptomycin (SM) | >95 | 0 | None | None | 12–15 mg/kg 3 times weekly | Unchanged | Ototoxicity, nephrotoxicity, cation wasting |
| Thiazcetazone (Tb1) | <20 | >80 | Not known | Not known | Not known; avoid if possible | Not known; avoid if possible | Rashes, exfoliative dermatitis, anemia, hepatotoxicity |

[a]N, nausea; V, vomiting; D, diarrhea.

**Table 37.5** Drug interactions

| Drug name | Drug interaction | Clinical significance |
|---|---|---|
| Amikacin (AK) | May have additive nephrotoxicity with other drugs | Possibly significant |
| | May have additive ototoxicity with other drugs | Possibly significant |
| | May potentiate neuromuscular blocking agents | Possibly significant |
| Aminosalicylic acid (PAS) | May reduce absorption of digoxin | Possibly significant |
| | Slows metabolism of isoniazid | Not significant |
| | Probenecid slows renal clearance of PAS | Unlikely to be significant |
| Azithromycin (AZI) | Significant drug interactions have not yet been described | |
| Capreomycin (CM) | May have additive nephrotoxicity with other drugs | Possibly significant |
| | May have additive ototoxicity with other drugs | Possibly significant |
| | May potentiate neuromuscular blocking agents | Possibly significant |
| Ciprofloxacin (CIP) | Antacids, iron, cation supplements reduce ciprofloxacin absorption | Significant |
| | Ciprofloxacin can increase concentrations of theophylline and caffeine | Possibly significant |
| Clarithromycin (CLAR) | May slow the metabolism of other drugs directly or indirectly, including astemizole, carbamazepine, didanosine, digoxin, rifabutin, ritonavir, terfenadine, theophylline, zidovudine | Possibly significant |
| Clofazimine (CFZ) | May slow absorption and clearance of rifamycins | Possibly significant |
| Cycloserine (CSN) | May have additive CNS toxicity with other drugs | Possibly significant |
| Dapsone (DDS) | Antacids (including the DDI buffer) may reduce the absorption of dapsone | Possibly significant |
| | Dapsone may have additive hematological toxicity with other drugs | Possibly significant |
| | Rifampin may increase the metabolism of dapsone | Possibly significant |
| Ethambutol (EMB) | May have additive ocular toxicity with other drugs | Possibly significant |
| | Antacids reduce the absorption of ethambutol | |
| Ethionamide (ETA) | May have additive CNS toxicity with other drugs | Possibly significant |
| | May have additive gastrointestinal toxicity with other drugs | Possibly significant |
| Isoniazid (INH) | Antacids may reduce the absorption of isoniazid | Possibly significant |
| | Isoniazid may have additive CNS toxicity with other drugs | Possibly significant |
| | May slow metabolism of carbamazepine | Possibly significant |
| | May slow metabolism of phenytoin | Possibly significant |
| Levofloxacin (LEVO) | Antacids, iron, cation supplements reduce levofloxacin absorption | Significant |
| Kanamycin (KM) | May have additive nephrotoxicity with other drugs | Possibly significant |
| | May have additive ototoxicity with other drugs | Possibly significant |
| | May potentiate neuromuscular blocking agents | Possibly significant |
| Pyrazinamide (PZA) | May have additive gastrointestinal toxicity with other drugs | Possibly significant |
| Rifabutin (RBN) Rifampin (RIF) | Antacids may reduce the absorption of rifamycins | Possibly significant |
| | Clofazimine may slow absorption and clearance of rifamycins | Possibly significant |
| | Rifamycins may increase the rate of metabolism of many other drugs, including: chloramphenicol, clarithromycin, corticosteroids, cyclosporine, dapsone, digitalis derivatives, oral anticoagulants, oral antidiabetics, oral contraceptives, protease inhibitors, theophylline, verapamil, warfarin | Possibly significant |
| | Rifampin appears to be a more potent enzyme inducer than rifabutin | |
| Streptomycin (SM) | May have additive nephrotoxicity with other drugs | Possibly significant |
| | May have additive ototoxicity with other drugs | Possibly significant |
| | May potentiate neuromuscular blocking agents | Possibly significant |
| Thiacetazone (Tb1) | None well described | Not significant |

more potentially toxic metabolites, they appear to quickly detoxify them. Co-administration of isoniazid and rifampin does not appreciably increase the risk of hepatotoxicity beyond the risk found with either drug alone, and their combined efficacy more than compensates for this risk. Pyridoxine (vitamin B6, 10 mg daily) is generally given with isoniazid to reduce the risk of neuropathies. Ethambutol can cause ocular toxicity, which is generally reversible if detected early and the drug withdrawn. Ethambutol must be given less often in patients with renal insufficiency (e.g., three times per week instead of daily in end-

**Table 37.6** General treatment guidelines for MTB and MAC

| General treatment guidelines |
|---|
| *M. TUBERCULOSIS* |
| *PRIOR TO DRUG SUSCEPTIBILITY DATA, IN AN AREA WITH A LOW RATE OF DRUG RESISTANCE* |
| Isoniazid, rifampin, pyrazinamide and ethambutol or streptomycin until susceptibility known |
| *PRIOR TO DRUG SUSCEPTIBILITY DATA, IN AN AREA WITH A HIGH RATE OF DRUG RESISTANCE* |
| Isoniazid, rifampin, pyrazinamide, or up to three additional drugs, such as cycloserine, capreomycin, and either ciprofloxacin or ofloxacin until susceptibility known |
| Fully Drug-susceptible |
| Isoniazid, rifampin, pyrazinamide for 2 months, then |
| Isoniazid and rifampin for 4 months after consistent smear and culture negativity |
| *DRUG-RESISTANCE KNOWN* |
| Consult clinicians experienced with drug-resistant tuberculosis |
| Individualize therapy based on (*a*) prior use of TB drugs, and (*b*) current susceptibility data |
| Regimens will generally include an injectable agent plus several oral agents |
| *M. AVIUM* COMPLEX |
| *OBTAIN SUSCEPTIBILITY DATA USING RADIOMETRIC METHOD (NOT PROPORTION METHOD)* |
| Regimen should include multiple drugs (2 to 4), preferably to which isolate is susceptible |
| Number of drugs depends on extent of the disease and clinical goal ("cure" vs. palliation) |
| Clarithromycin currently is among the most active agents; azithromycin is a possible alternative |
| Rifampin (or rifabutin) and ethambutol frequently show in vitro synergy and may be used |
| *Note*: rifamycins increase the metabolism of clarithromycin; clinical significance not yet known |
| Aminoglycosides (streptomycin, kanamycin, or amikacin) may contribute to regimens |
| Role of ciprofloxacin or clofazimine debatable |

stage renal failure). Baseline opthamological exams are very helpful, along with periodic testing of visual acuity and red–green color discrimination during treatment. Other drugs, such as cycloserine and ethionamide, should be gradually introduced over several days to prevent overt central nervous system (CNS) or gastrointestinal (GI) toxicity, respectively. With cycloserine and ethionamide, most adults tolerate maximum daily doses of 750–1000 mg, which are generally divided into two daily doses (bid). Cycloserine dosing is greatly facilitated by serum concentration monitoring. Pyridoxine (50–100 mg daily for each 250 mg of cycloserine) is generally given with cycloserine to reduce the risk of CNS effects.

Clinicians must also be aware of potentially serious drug interactions, particularly with isoniazid, rifampin, and rifabutin. Among the more serious are interactions between isoniazid and certain anticonvulsants, and between rifamycins and oral contraceptives or oral anticoagulants. A newly identified interaction between rifamycins and macrolides such as clarithromycin has important clinical implications. Rifampin and rifabutin accelerate the clearance of clarithromycin via hepatic microsomal enzyme induction. Although the full clinical significance of this interaction is not yet known, it may require the removal of rifamycins from the treatment of MAC infections in order to preserve the efficacy of the more potent macrolides. Further research is needed to establish the proper roles of the rifamycins in the treatment of MAC infections. Interactions involving any of the antimycobacterial agents are particularly challenging in patients receiving numerous drugs, such as patients with AIDS. When the adequacy of antimycobacterial therapy is in doubt, clinicians should employ TDM to verify adequate bioavailability.

General treatment guidelines are provided for MTB and MAC in Table 37.6. Given the complexities of treating drug-resistant organisms such as MDR-TB and MAC, clinicians should identify consultants who are familiar with such infections and contact them prior to embarking on treatment regimens. This cautious approach should help stem the spread of drug-resistant mycobacteria.

## ANNOTATED BIBLIOGRAPHY

Baciewicz AM, Self TH. Isoniazid interactions. South Med J 1985; 78:714–18.
*Discussion of more important isoniazid–drug interactions.*

Baciewicz AM, Self TH, Bekemeyer WB. Update on rifampin drug interaction. Arch Intern Med 1987; 147:565–68.
*Discussion of more important rifampin–drug interactions.*

Bass JB Jr, Farer LA, Hopewell PC, O'Brien R, Jacobs RF, Ruben F, Snider DE Jr, Thornton G. Treatment of tuberculosis and tuberculosis infection in adults and children. Am J Respir Crit Care Med 1994; 149:1359–1374.
*Recent treatment recommendations from a nationally recognized panel of experts.*

Ellner JJ, Goldberger MJ, Parenti DM. *Mycobacterium avium* infection in AIDS: a therapeutic dilemma in rapid evolution. J Infect Dis 1991; 163:1326–1335.
*Clear review of the major features of disseminated MAC in patients with AIDS.*

Girling DJ. Adverse effects of antituberculosis drugs. Drugs 1982; 23:56–74.
Detailed review of side-effect profiles of the antituberculosis drugs.

Heifets LB, ed. Drug Susceptibility in the Chemotherapy of Mycobacterial Infections. CRC Press, Boca Raton, FL, pp 13–58; 89–146, 1991.
*The definitive textbook on the susceptibility testing of mycobacteria.*

Iseman MD. Treatment of multidrug-resistant tuberculosis. New Engl J Med 1993; 329:784–791.
*Complete review of the key issues for managing patients with TB in the era of multidrug resistance.*

Iwainsky, H. Mode of action, biotransformation and pharmacokinetics of antituberculosis drugs in animals and man. In: Antituberculosis Drugs. Bartmann K, ed. Springer-Verlag, Berlin, pp 399–553, 1988.
*Detailed textbook on the antituberculosis drugs, featuring translations of many non-English language references.*

Korvick JA, Benson CA. Mycobacterium avium-complex infection. Progress in research and treatment. Marcel Dekker, Inc., New York, 1996.

Peloquin CA, Antituberculosis drugs: pharmacokinetics. In: Drug Susceptibility in the Chemotherapy of Mycobacterial Infections. Heifets L, ed. CRC Press, Boca Raton, FL, pp 59–88, 1991.

*Complete review of the pharmacokinetics of the TB drugs, including their use in meningitis, renal failure, and pregnancy.*

Peloquin CA. Controversies in the management of *Mycobacterium avium* complex (MAC) infection. Ann Pharmacother 1993; 27:928–937.

*Detailed review regarding why so many different approaches are used for treating MAC, with recommendations for resolving these controversies.*

Peloquin CA. Pharmacology of the antimycobacterial drugs. Med Clin North Am 1993; 77:1253–1262.

*Focus on the practical use of TB drugs, particularly the "second-line" agents.*

Peloquin CA, Berning SE. Infections due to Mycobacterium tuberculosis. Ann Pharmacother 1994; 28:72–84.

*General review of TB, with focus on key treatment issues.*

Peloquin C, Nitta A, Burman W, Brudney K, McGuinness M, Miranda-Massari J, Gerena G. Incidence of low tuberculosis drug concentrations in AIDS patients. Abstract, 34th Interscience Conference on Antimicrobial Agents and Chemotherapy, Orlando, FL, October 4–7, 1994.

*Prospective study showing low drug concentrations in patients with AIDS and TB, especially rifampin and ethambutol.*

Tseng AL, Foisy MM. Management of drug interactions in patients with HIV. Ann Pharmacother 1997; 31:1040–1058.

Vareldzis BP, Grosset J, de Kantor I, Crofton J, Laszlo A, Felten M, Raviglione MC, Kochi A. Drug-resistant tuberculosis: laboratory issues. World Health Organization Recommendations. Tubercle and Lung Disease 1994; 75:1–7.

*Recent review of key laboratory issues that must be effectively addressed.*

Verbist L. Mode of action of antituberculosis drugs (parts I and II). Medicon Int. 1974; 3(1):11–23 and 3(2):3–17.

*Classic review of how antituberculosis drugs are thought to work.*

Winder, FG. Mode of action of the antimycobacterial agents and associated aspects of the molecular biology of the mycobacteria. In: The Biology of Mycobacteria, vol 1. Physiology, Identification, and Classification. Ratledge C, Stanford J, eds. Academic Press, London, pp 353–438, 1982.

*As above, a classic review of how antituberculosis drugs are thought to work, complementing the reference above.*

# 38

# Antimicrobial Therapy for Bacterial Diseases

DAVID H. SPACH AND W. CONRAD LILES

Antimicrobial therapy for bacterial diseases

| Organism/disease | First choice | Alternative choices | Comments |
|---|---|---|---|
| *Acinetobacter* spp. | Imipenem: 500 mg IV q6h × 10–14 days or<br>Meropenem: 500 mg IV q8h × 10–14 days | Ceftazidime<br>Amikacin (or tobramycin)<br>TMP-SMX | Combination therapy using $\beta$-lactam and aminoglycoside advised for serious infection |
| *Actinobacillus* spp.<br>Endocarditis | Penicillin G: 2–4 × $10^6$ units IV q4h × 4–6 weeks plus gentamicin (or tobramycin) 3–5 mg/kg/day IV × 4–6 weeks | Ampicillin<br>Cefazolin | Antimicrobial susceptibility testing recommended, but often difficult to rapidly obtain |
| Wound infection | Penicillin G: 1–2 × $10^6$ units IV q4–6h × 10–14 days | | |
| *Actinomyces* spp.<br>Actinomycosis | Penicillin G: 4 × $10^6$ units IV q4–6h × 2–6 weeks followed by penicillin V: 500–1000 mg PO qid × 6–12 months | Doxycycline<br>Clindamycin<br>Erythromycin | Generally resistant to metronidazole. Patients with less extensive involvement may require less intensive therapy |
| *Aeromonas hydrophilia*<br>Cellulitis/Wound infection | Ciprofloxacin: 200 mg IV bid (500 mg PO bid) × 10–14 days | TMP/SMX<br>Gentamicin (or tobramycin) | Bacteremia and sepsis usually involves immunocompromised patients |
| Bacteremia | Ceftriaxone: 2 g IV q24h × 10–14 days | | |
| Diarrhea | Norfloxacin: 400 mg PO bid × 5–7 days or<br>Ciprofloxacin: 500 mg PO bid × 5–7 days | | |
| *Alcaligenes* (*Achromobacter*) *xylosoxidans* | Imipenem: 500 mg IV q6h × 10–14 days or<br>Meropenem: 500 mg IV q8h × 10–14 days | Ceftazidime<br>TMP-SMX | Resistant to aminoglycosides and quinolones. Severe infections may require multiple drugs, but synergy has not been demonstrated. Duration of therapy depends on clinical response. |
| *Arcanobacterium haemolyticum*<br>Pharyngits (exudative) | Erythromycin: 250 mg PO qid × 10 days *or*<br>Penicillin VK: 500 mg PO qid × 10 days | Tetracyclines<br>Benzathine penicillin G | Resistant to TMP/SMX |
| *Bacillus anthracis*<br>Anthrax | Penicillin G: 4 × $10^6$ units IV q4–6h × 10 days | Erythromycin<br>Tetracyclines<br>Chloramphenicol | Corticosteroids often administered concomitantly for meningitis or disease complicated by malignant edema |
| *Bacillus cereus* | Vancomycin: 1 g IV q12h × 10–14 days | Clindamycin | Food poisoning does not require antimicrobial therapy. Topical therapy indicated for keratitis. Duration of therapy depends on clinical situation and response. |

(*continued*)

Antimicrobial therapy for bacterial diseases—*Continued*

| Organism/disease | First choice | Alternative choices | Comments |
|---|---|---|---|
| *Bacteroides* spp. (non-fragilis) | Metronidazole: 500 mg IV q6h × 7–14 days | Clindamycin<br>Cefoxitin (or cefotetan)<br>Imipenem<br>Meropenem<br>Ampicillin-sulbactam<br>Ticarcillin-clavulanic acid | Most laboratories do not routinely perform susceptibility testing, thus treatment is generally empiric. |
| *Bacteroides fragilis* group | Metronidazole: 500 mg IV q6h × 7–14 days | Clindamycin<br>Cefoxitin<br>Imipenem<br>Meropenem<br>Ampicillin-sulbactam<br>Ticarcillin-clavulanic acid | Cefotetan not active against "DOT" group. Duration of therapy depends on clinical situation and response. |
| *Bartonella henselae*<br>Cat-scratch disease | Erythromycin: 500 mg PO qid × 10 days | Doxycycline<br>Gentamicin<br>Ciprofloxacin<br>Azithromycin | Antimicrobial therapy may not be effective for HIV-negative patients. For HIV-infected patients with bacillary angiomatosis, longer courses are needed for involvement of liver, spleen, or heart. |
| Bacillary angiomatosis | Erythromycin: 500 mg PO qid × 2–3 months | Doxycycline<br>Rifampin<br>Azithromycin | |
| *Bartonella quintana*<br>Bacillary angiomatosis | Erythromycin: 500 mg PO qid × 2–3 months | Doxycycline<br>Rifampin | Longer courses are needed for involvement of liver, spleen, or heart. |
| Trench fever | Erythromycin: 500 mg IV (or PO) q6h × 21 days | Doxycycline | |
| *Bordetella pertussis*<br>Whooping cough | Erythromycin: 500 mg PO qid × 14 days | TMP/SMX | Close contacts of pertussis-infected persons should receive prophylactic 14-day course of erythromycin. |
| *Borrelia burgdorferi/*<br>Lyme disease | | | Success rates for treating Lyme disease generally higher earlier in the course of illness. Persistent symptoms following treatment usually not due to active infection. |
| Early (Erythema migrans) | Doxycyclinc: 100 mg PO bid × 14–21 days | Amoxicillin<br>Cefuroxime axetil | |
| Arthritis | Doxycycline: 100 mg PO bid × 30 days *or*<br>Ceftriaxone: 2g IV qd × 14–21 days | Amoxicillin<br>Penicillin G | |
| Cardiac | | | |
| Mild (AV block with PR ≤ 0.3 s) | Doxycyline: 100 mg PO bid × 21 days | Amoxicillin | |
| Serious | Ceftriaxone: 2g IV qd × 21 days | Penicillin G | |
| Neurologic | | | |
| Mild (facial palsy) | Doxycycline: 100 mg PO bid × 30 days | Amoxicillin | |
| Serious | Ceftriaxone: 2g IV qd × 14–21 days | Penicillin G | |
| *Borrelia* spp./relapsing fever | Doxycycline: 100 mg IV/PO bid × 10 days | Erythromycin | Jarisch-Herxheimer reaction common, especially with first dose of antimicrobial agent. |
| *Brucella* spp.<br>Brucellosis (acute, subacute, chronic) | Doxycycline: 100 mg IV/PO bid × 6 weeks *plus*<br>Rifampin: 300 mg IV/PO bid × 6 weeks | Doxycycline *plus* (TMP/SMX or gentamicin or streptomycin) | Chronic disease may require prolonged therapy (6–12 months). Gentamicin (or streptomycin) should be substituted for rifampin in patients with spondylitis. |
| *Burkholderia cepacia* | Ceftazidime: 1–2 g IV q8h × 10–14 days | Ciprofloxacin<br>TMP/SMX | Resistance to aminoglycosides, imipenem, and meropenem is common. |
| *Calymmatobacterium granulomatis*<br>Granuloma inguinale | Doxycycline: 100 mg PO bid × 3–4 weeks | Erythromycin<br>TMP/SMX | Continue therapy until lesion completely healed. Relapse occurs in 10%–20% of treated patients. |

*(continued)*

| Organism/disease | First choice | Alternative choices | Comments |
|---|---|---|---|
| *Campylobacter jejuni*<br>Diarrhea | Erythromycin 250 mg PO qid × 5–7 days *or*<br>Ciprofloxacin: 500 mg PO bid × 5–7 days | Clindamycin<br>Doxycycline | Most intestinal infections are self-limited and do not require antimicrobial therapy. Criteria for therapy include patients with high fever, bloody diarrhea, more than 8 stools per day, and symptoms for longer than 1 week. |
| *Campylobacter fetus*<br>Septicemia | Gentamicin: 3–5 mg/kg/day IV × 10–14 days | Ampicillin<br>Chloramphenicol<br>Imipenem | Treat with ampicillin if isolate susceptible to ampicillin. Endovascular infections with *C. fetus* require at least 4 weeks of therapy. |
| *Capnocytophaga ochracea* (DF-1) | Clindamycin: 300 mg IV/PO q6–8h × 7–10 days | Ampicillin-sulbactam<br>Ciprofloxacin<br>Imipenem<br>Amoxicillin-clavulanic acid | Duration of therapy often depends on patient's immune status and whether infection disseminated or localized to the mouth. |
| *Capnocytophaga canimorsus* (DF-2)<br>Septicemia | Penicillin G: 2–4 × $10^6$ units IV q4–6h × 14 days | Clindamycin<br>Imipenem<br>Ciprofloxacin<br>Amoxicillin-clavulanic acid | Infection often more severe in splenectomized patients. In vitro susceptibility testing difficult to perform. In most circumstances, duration of treatment is at least 14 days. |
| *Cardiobacterium hominis*<br>Endocarditis | Penicillin G: 2–4 × $10^6$ units IV q4h × 4–6 weeks *plus*<br>Gentamicin: 3–5 mg/kg/day × 4–6 weeks | Cefazolin<br>Chloramphenicol<br>Tetracycline | Ampicillin can be substituted for penicillin and tobramycin can be substituted for gentamicin. |
| *Chlamydia pneumoniae* (TWAR)<br>Pneumonia | Doxycycline: 100 mg IV/PO bid × 10–14 days | Erythromycin<br>Azithromycin<br>Clarithromycin<br>Fluoroquinolone | Treatment failures can occur (more often with erythromycin than with doxycycline). If treatment failure occurs, retreatment often successful. |
| *Chlamydia psittaci*<br>Psittacosis | Doxycycline: 100 mg PO bid × 14–21 days | Erythromycin | Patients with endocarditis generally require valve replacement and prolonged antimicrobial therapy. |
| *Chlamydia trachomatis*<br>Urethritis, cervicitis | Azithromycin: 1.0 g PO × 1<br>*or*<br>Doxycycline: 1.0 mg PO bid × 7 days | Ofloxacin<br>Erythromycin | Erythromycin drug of choice in pregnant women. For LGV, 21-day course with doxycycline recommended. |
| *Chromobacterium violaceum* | Gentamicin: 3–5 mg/kg/day IV × 14 days | Tetracycline<br>Chloramphenicol<br>TMP/SMX | Optimal therapy not known. Recommendation based on small number of patients. |
| *Citrobacter* spp. | Imipenem: 500 mg IV q6h × 10–14 days *or*<br>Meropenem: 500 mg IV q8h × 14 days | Ciprofloxacin<br>Gentamicin (or tobramycin) | Important to distinguish colonization from true clinical infection. |
| *Clostridium perfringens, C. septicum, C. tetani* | Penicillin G: 2–4 × $10^6$ units IV q4–6h × 10–14 days | Clindamycin<br>Metronidazole<br>Imipenem<br>Chloramphenicol | Some clostridial infections require prompt surgical intervention. Duration of therapy ≥14 days in severe cases. Unvaccinated patients with wounds at high risk for *C. tetani* infection should receive human tetanus immunoglobulin 500 IU IM (or infiltrated into wound), as soon as possible. Food poisoning from *C. perfringens* does not require therapy. |

(*continued*)

Antimicrobial therapy for bacterial diseases—*Continued*

| Organism/disease | First choice | Alternative choices | Comments |
|---|---|---|---|
| *Clostridium difficile*<br>Pseudomembranous colitis | Metronidazole: 500 mg PO tid × 10 days | Vancomycin | Cholestyramine may be beneficial in patients with severe diarrhea. Significant rate of relapse occurs following discontinuation of therapy. If vancomycin used, lower doses are adequate (125 mg PO qid). |
| *Corynebacterium jeikeium*<br>Catheter-associated bacteremia | Vancomycin: 1 g IV q12h × 14 days | Ciprofloxacin<br>Teichoplanin | Removal of infected catheter may be required for cure. |
| *Corynebacterium diphtheriae*<br>Diphtheria | Erythromycin: 500 mg PO/IV qid × 14 days | Penicillin G<br>Clindamycin<br>Rifampin | Diphtheria antitoxin should be administered to patients with laryngeal/pharyngeal disease. Contacts of patients with diphtheria should receive erythromycin ×7 days or benzathine penicillin: $1.2 \times 10^6$ units IM. |
| *Corynebacterium minutissimum*<br>Erythrasma | Erythromycin: 250 mg PO qid × 14 days | | Rare cases of bacteremia require intravenous therapy. |
| *Corynebacterium ulcerans*<br>Pharyngitis | Erythromycin: 250 mg PO qid × 14 days | | Diphtheria antitoxin should be given in presumed toxigenic cases. |
| *Coxiella burnetti* | | | |
| Pneumonia | Doxycycline: 100 mg PO bid × 14–21 days | Ciprofloxacin<br>Erythromycin *plus* rifampin | Duration of therapy for endocarditis has not been agreed upon; most recommend at least 1–2 years. |
| Hepatitis | Doxycycline: 100 mg PO bid × 14 days | | |
| Endocarditis | Doxycycline: 100 mg PO bid *plus* Rifampin: 600 mg PO qd | | |
| *Edwardsiella tarda*<br>Systemic infection | Ampicillin: 1–2 g IV q4–6h × 10–14 days | Cephalothin<br>Ciprofloxacin<br>Chloramphenicol | Treatment probably not indicated for uncomplicated gastroenteritis. |
| *Ehrlichia chaffeensis* | Doxycycline: 100 mg IV/PO bid × 7–10 days | Chloramphenicol | The same therapy is recommended for the recently described *Ehrlichia* species that causes human granulocytic ehrlichiosis. |
| *Eikenella corrodens* | | | |
| Endocarditis | Penicillin G: $2–4 \times 10^6$ units IV q4h × 4–6 weeks *plus* Gentamicin: 3–5 mg/kg/day × 4–6 weeks | Ampicillin<br>TMP-SMX | Patients with endocarditis should have aminoglycoside added and therapy should be continued for at least 6 weeks. |
| Soft tissue | Pencillin G: $2–4 \times 10^6$ units IV q6h × 10–14 days | Amoxicillin-clavulanic acid | |
| *Enterobacter* spp. | Imipenem: 500 mg IV q6h plus Gentamicin (or tobramycin): 3–5 mg/kg/day × 10–14 days | Meropenem<br>Mezlocillin<br>Piperacillin-tazobactam<br>Ticarcillin-clavulanic acid<br>Ciprofloxacin | Documented risk of rapid development of resistance to third-generation cephalosporins during therapy. |
| *Enterococcus* spp. | | | |
| Cystitis | Amoxicillin: 250–500 mg PO tid × 7 days | Ciprofloxacin<br>Ofloxacin<br>Nitrofurantoin | Bacteremia without endocarditis often effectively treated with ampicillin alone. |
| Endocarditis | Ampicillin: 3 g IV q4–6h *plus* Gentamicin: 3–5 mg/kg/day IV × 4–6 weeks | Vancomycin *plus* Gentamicin | |
| Other invasive infection | Ampicillin: 2 g IV q4–6 h × 14 days | Vancomycin | |

(*continued*)

| Organism/disease | First choice | Alternative choices | Comments |
|---|---|---|---|
| *Enterococcus* spp. ($\beta$-lactam resistant, high-level amino-glycoside resistant, vancomycin resistant) | | | No regimen of proven efficacy can currently be recommended. Most promising results have been with investigational drug quinupristin-dalfopristin |
| *Erysipelothrix rhusiopathiae*<br>Cellulitis, bacteremia | Penicillin G: 2–4 × $10^6$ units IV q4–6h × 10–14 days | Ceftriaxone | Resistant to vancomycin and aminoglycosides. A 4–6 week course of therapy is advised for endocarditis. |
| *Escherichia coli* | | | |
| Cystitis (uncomplicated) | TMP/SMX: 1 DS PO bid × 3 days | Norfloxacin<br>Ciprofloxacin<br>Nitrofurantoin | Parenteral therapy recommended for the treatment of pyelonephritis in a patient showing signs or symptoms of clinical toxicity. Conversion to oral therapy is recommended following resolution of fever and nausea. Ampicillin is preferred agent if isolate is ampicillin-susceptible |
| Pyelonephritis (uncomplicated) | TMP/SMX: 1 DS tab PO bid × 14 days | Norfloxacin<br>Ciprofloxacin<br>Ceftriaxone<br>Gentamicin<br>Aztreonam | |
| Gastroenteritis (traveler's diarrhea) | Norfloxacin: 400 mg PO bid × 3 days *or*<br>Ciprofloxacin: 500 mg PO bid × 3 days | TMP/SMX<br>Doxycycline | |
| Invasive infection (septicemia) | Cefazolin: 1–2 g IV q8h × 10–14 days *or*<br>other equivalent cephalosporin | Ampicillin-sulbactam<br>Ciprofloxacin<br>Ceftriaxone | |
| *Flavobacterium meningosepticum* | Vancomycin: 1 g IV q12h × 10–14 days | TMP/SMX<br>Ciprofloxacin | In vitro disk susceptibility testing often unreliable |
| *Francisella tularensis*<br>Tularemia | Streptomycin: 15 mg/kg IM q12h × 14 days *or*<br>Gentamicin: 3–5 mg/kg/day IV/IM × 14 days | Doxycycline<br>Chloramphenicol | Relapse is common if therapy is given for <14 days, especially if aminoglycoside not employed. |
| *Gardnerella vaginalis*<br>"Bacterial vaginosis" | Metronidazole: 500 mg PO bid × 7 days *or*<br>Metronidazole: 2 g PO × 1 | Clindamycin 2% vaginal cream<br>Metronidazole 0.75% vaginal gel | Some prefer intravaginal route because of fewer side effects. Metronidazole should be avoided in 1st trimester of pregnancy. Routine treatment of male sex partner not indicated. |
| *Haemophilus aphrophilus*<br>Endocarditis | Penicillin G: 2–4 × $10^6$ units IV q4h *plus*<br>Gentamicin: 3–5 mg/kg/day IV × 4–6 weeks | Cefazolin plus gentamicin<br>Ceftriaxone | Typically resistant to vancomycin, clindamycin, and methicillin. Ceftriaxone: 2 g IV qd × 4–6 weeks is a reasonable alternative regimen. |
| *Haemophilus ducreyi*<br>Chancroid | Azithromycin: 1 g PO × 1<br>*or*<br>Ceftriaxone: 250 mg IM × 1 | Erythromycin<br>Amoxicillin-clavulanic acid<br>Ciprofloxacin | Sexual contacts should be identified and treated for chancroid. |
| *Haemophilus influenzae* | | | |
| Meningitis/bacteremia/epiglottitis/ pneumonia | Ceftriaxone: 1–2 g IV q12h *or*<br>Cefotaxime: 2 g IV q4h × 10–14 days *or* | Cefuroxime<br>Chloramphenicol<br>Cefixime<br>Azithromycin | Ampicillin or amoxicillin can be employed if isolate is $\beta$-lactamase negative. Initial therapy with oral regimens not appropriate for serious infections. |
| Sinusitis | TMP/SMX: 1 DS tab PO bid × 14–21 days *or*<br>Amoxicillin-clavulanic acid: 875 mg PO bid × 14–21 days | | |
| *Haemophilus parainfluenzae*<br>Endocarditis/epiglottitis (supraglottitis) | Ceftriaxone: 2 g IV q24h | Cefotaxime<br>Ampicillin-sulbactam<br>TMP/SMX<br>Chloramphenicol | Ampicillin can be used if isolate is $\beta$-lactamase negative. Longer therapy (4–6 weeks) needed for endocariditis. |

(*continued*)

Antimicrobial therapy for bacterial diseases—*Continued*

| Organism/disease | First choice | Alternative choices | Comments |
|---|---|---|---|
| *Helicobacter pylori*<br>Type B gastritis/peptic ulcer disease | PeptoBismol: 1–2 tabs PO qid × 7 days *plus*<br>Metronidazole: 250 mg PO tid × 7 days *plus*<br>Tetracycline 500 mg PO qid × 7 days *plus*<br>Omeprazole: 20 mg PO qid × 7 days | Omeprazole *plus*<br>Clarithromycin | Amoxicillin can be substituted for tetracycline. Doxycycline less effective than tetracycline. |
| *Kingella kingii*<br>Endocarditis | Penicillin G: 2–4 × $10^6$ units IV q4h *plus*<br>Gentamicin: 3–5 mg/kg/day IV × 4–6 weeks | Ceftriaxone | Most reported cases have been treated with the combination of penicillin G (or ampicillin) and aminoglycoside. Ceftriaxone: 2 g IV qd × 4–6 weeks is a reasonable alternative regimen. |
| *Klebsiella pneumoniae, K. oxytoca* | Ceftriaxone: 1–2 g IV q 12–24h × 10–14 days *or*<br>Ciprofloxacin: 400 mg IV (or 500 mg PO) q12h × 10–14 days | Tobramycin (or gentamicin)<br>Piperacillin-tazobactam<br>Ticarcillin-clavulanic acid<br>Imipenem<br>Aztreonam | Imipenem recommended for isolates resistant to third generation cephalosporins. |
| *Klebsiella ozaenae, K. rhinoscleromatis*<br>Rhinoscleroma | Ciprofloxacin: 500 mg PO bid | TMP/SMX plus rifampin<br>Tetracycline<br>Chloramphenicol | Prolonged duration of therapy is required for treatment of clinical disease. |
| *Lactobacillus* spp.<br>Bacteremia | Clindamycin: 450–600 mg IV q8h × 10–14 days | Penicillin G<br>Erythromycin<br>Gentamicin (or tobramycin)<br>Imipenem | Isolates generally resistant to vancomycin |
| *Legionella* spp. | Erythromycin: 1 g IV q6h × 14 days *plus*<br>Rifampin: 300 mg IV/PO bid × 14 days | Fluoroquinolone<br>Azithromycin<br>Clarithromycin<br>TMP/SMX | Addition of rifampin not widely agreed upon. Risk of ototoxicity with erythromycin at 4 g/day. When patient becomes stable, they can be switched to oral erythromycin 500 mg qid. Longer therapy (21 days) recommended for immunocompromised patients. |
| *Leptospira* spp.<br>Leptospirosis | Penicillin G: 1.5 × $10^6$ units IV q6h × 7 days | Ampicillin<br>Doxycycline | Oral therapy for less severe cases |
| *Leptotrichia buccalis*<br>Bacteremia | Penicillin G: 2–4 × $10^6$ units IV q4–6h × 10–14 days | Doxycycline | |
| *Leuconostoc* spp.<br>Bacteremia | Penicillin G: 2–4 × $10^6$ units IV q4–6h × 10–14 days | Clindamycin<br>Erythromycin<br>Imipenem | Isolates resistant to vancomycin |
| *Listeria monocytogenes*<br>Bacteremia<br><br>Meningitis | Ampicillin: 2 g IV q6h × 14 days<br>Ampicillin: 3 g IV q6h × 14 days | Penicillin<br>TMP/SMX | Resistant to cephalosporins. Some recommend adding systemic and intrathecal gentamicin in patients with meningitis. Longer therapy (3–6 weeks) recommended for immunosuppressed patients. |
| *Moraxella catarrhalis* | Amoxicillin-clavulanic acid: 875 mg PO bid × 10–14 days *or*<br>TMP/SMX: 1 DS tab PO bid × 10–14 days | Cefuroxime<br>Cefixime<br>Azithromycin<br>Clarithromycin<br>Doxycycline | Amoxicillin can be employed for isolates that are $\beta$-lactamase negative. |
| *Morganella* spp. | Imipenem: 500 mg IV q6h × 10–14 days *or*<br>Ceftazidime: 1–2 g IV q8h × 10–14 days | Meropenem<br>Tobramycin (or gentamicin)<br>Ciprofloxacin<br>Aztreonam | Duration of therapy depends on clinical situation and response. |
| *Mycoplasma hominis*<br>Urethritis | Doxycycline: 100 mg PO/IV bid × 7 days | Clindamycin | Resistant to erythromycin and rifampin. Increasing resistance to tetracyclines. |

(*continued*)

Antimicrobial therapy for bacterial diseases—*Continued*

| Organism/disease | First choice | Alternative choices | Comments |
|---|---|---|---|
| *Mycoplasma pneumoniae*<br>Pneumonia | Erythromycin: 500 mg PO/IV q6h × 14 days *or*<br>Doxycycline: 100 mg PO/IV bid × 14d | Azithromycin<br>Roxithromycin<br>Clarithromycin<br>Fluoroquinolone | $\beta$-lactam antimicrobials not effective |
| *Neisseria gonorrhoeae* | | | |
| Cervicitis/urethritis/epididymitis | Ceftriaxone: 125–250 mg IM × 1 *or*<br>Cefixime: 400 mg PO × 1 | Ciprofloxacin<br>Ofloxacin<br>Trovafloxacin<br>Spectinomycin | Presumptive treatment of all recent (with the preceding 30 days) sexual partners is recommended. Patients should receive concomitant treatment for Chlamydia trachomatis. For patients with disseminated infection: following clinical improvement, reliable patients can complete the 7-day course of therapy with cefixime: 400 mg PO bid or ciprofloxacin: 500 mg PO bid. Patients should receive presumptive treatment for chlamydial infection. |
| Conjunctivitis | Ceftriaxone: 1 g IM × 1 | | |
| Arthritis/disseminated gonococcal infection | Ceftriaxone: 1 g IV/IM qd × 7 days | | |
| *Neisseria meningitidis* | Penicillin G: $4 \times 10^6$ units IV q4h × 10–14 days *or* Ampicillin: 2 g IV q4h × 10–14 days | Ceftriaxone<br>Cefotaxime<br>Ceftizoxime<br>Cefuroxime<br>Chloramphenicol | Prophylactic therapy is recommended for close contacts of patients with invasive disease. Regimens include rifampin: 600 mg PO bid × 2 days; Ceftriaxone: 250 mg IM × 1; or ciprofloxacin: 500 mg PO bid × 3 days. |
| *Nocardia asteroides*<br>Pulmonary infection | Sulfadiazine: 1.5 g PO qid *or* TMP/SMZ: 320 mg (TMP)/ 1600 mg (SMX) PO/IV tid | Minocycline<br>Amikacin<br>Imipenem | Prolonged course of treatment (months) is almost always required. |
| *Nocardia brasiliensis* | Sulfadiazine: 1.5 g PO qid *or* TMP/SMZ: 320 mg (TMP)/ 1600 mg (SMX) PO/IV tid | Ceftriaxone *plus* amikacin<br>Ampicillin-sulbactam | Resistant to imipenem. Duration of therapy depends on clinical situation and response. |
| *Pasteurella multocida*<br>Bite wounds | Amoxicillin-clavulanic acid: 875 mg PO bid × 14 days *or*<br>Penicillin VK: 500 mg PO qid × 14 days | Ampicillin-sulbactam<br>Tetracycline<br>Chloramphenicol<br>Ceftriaxone | Prolonged antimicrobial therapy recommended for patients with endocarditis or osteomyelitis. |
| Cellulitis/systemic disease | Penicillin G: $4 \times 10^6$ units IV q4–6h × 10–14 days | | |
| *Peptostreptococcus* spp. | Penicillin G: $1–2 \times 10^6$ units IV q4–6h × 10–14 days | Clindamycin<br>Doxycycline<br>Vancomycin | Antimicrobial susceptibility testing often not performed. Longer therapy (4–6 weeks) required for brain abscess. |
| *Plesiomonas shigelloides* | Doxycycline: 100 mg PO bid × 5 days | Ciprofloxacin | Often a self-limited diarrheal illness that does not require treatment. Intravenous therapy recommended in rare cases of disseminated disease. |
| *Propionibacterium acnes*<br>Acne | Doxycycline: 100 mg PO bid | Minocycline<br>Clindamycin (topical) | Prolonged therapy is generally required for successful treatment of acne. Most blood culture isolates represent contaminants. Unusual cases of serious infection require intravenous antimicrobial therapy. |
| *Proteus mirabilis* | Ampicillin: 500–1000 mg IV q6h × 10–14 days *or*<br>Amoxicillin: 500 mg qid × 10–14 days | TMP/SMX<br>Amikacin | In recent years, significant increase in resistance to many antimicrobials |

(*continued*)

Antimicrobial therapy for bacterial diseases—*Continued*

| Organism/disease | First choice | Alternative choices | Comments |
|---|---|---|---|
| *Proteus vulgaris* | Ceftriaxone: 1 g IV q24h × 10–14 days *or*<br>Ciprofloxacin: 400 mg IV q12h (or 500 mg PO bid) × 10–14 days | Amikacin<br>Imipenem<br>Aztreonam | |
| *Providencia* spp. | Ciprofloxacin: 400 mg IV q12h (or 500 mg PO bid) × 10–14 days *or*<br>Amikacin: 15 mg/kg/day IV × 10–14 days | Ceftriaxone<br>Ceftizoxime<br>Mezlocillin<br>Imipenem<br>TMP/SMX | Often resistant to gentamicin and tobramycin |
| *Pseudomonas aeruginosa* | | | |
| Urinary tract infection | Ciprofloxacin: 500 mg PO bid × 7–10 days | Piperacillin-tazobactam<br>Imipenem | Some clinical situations may require extended therapy (longer than 14 days) |
| Invasive disease | Ceftazidime: 1–2 g IV q8h × 10–14 days *plus*<br>Tobramycin: 3–5 mg/kg/day IV × 10–14 days | Meropenem<br>Aztreonam<br>Fluoroquinolone | |
| *Pseudomonas mallei*<br>Glanders | Sulfadiazine: 1.5–2.0 g PO q6h × 21 days | TMP/SMX | Clinical experience with agents other than sulfadiazine is limited. |
| *Pseudomonas pseudomallei*<br>Melioidosis | Ceftazidime: 1–2 g IV q8h ≥ 30 days *or*<br>Amoxicillin-clavulanic acid: 875 mg PO bid | Imipenem<br>TMP/SMX | Resistance to TMP/SMX is increasing in southeast Asia. Many authorities recommend combination therapy (ceftazidime plus TMP/SMX) for patients with septicemia. Prolonged therapy (6–12 months) recommended for suppurative extrapulmonary lesions. |
| *Rhodococcus equi* | Vancomycin: 1 g IV q12h | Erythromycin plus rifampin | Therapy should continue until patient stable and cultures are negative; this usually requires a minimum of 3–4 weeks. |
| *Rickettsia prowazekii*<br>Epidemic (louse-borne) typhus | Doxycycline: 100 mg IV (or PO) bid (continue 2–3 days after fever resolves) | Chloramphenicol | Recrudescent form (Brill-Zinsser) treated the same |
| *Rickettsia rickettsii*<br>Rocky Mountain spotted fever | Doxycycline: 100 mg IV (or PO) bid × 7–10 days | Chloramphenicol<br>Fluoroquinolone | Treatment often presumptive since rapid diagnostic test not widely available. |
| *Rickettsia tsutsugamushi*<br>Scrub typhus | Doxycycline: 100 mg IV (or PO) bid × 14 days | Chloramphenicol | Relapses can occur, especially if diagnosis delayed. |
| *Rickettsia typhi*<br>Endemic (murine) typhus | Doxycycline: 100 mg IV (or PO) bid; (continue 2–3 days after fever resolves) | Chloramphenicol | Relapses can rarely occur and require treatment. |
| *Salmonella* spp. | | | |
| Gastroenteritis (normal host) | No antimicrobial therapy | | Vascular involvement requires 6 weeks of IV therapy. AIDS patients should receive 2 weeks of IV therapy plus 4–6 weeks of oral ciprofloxacin. For eradication of the chronic carrier state, cholecystectomy may be required. |
| Gastroenteritis (immuno-compromised host) | Ciprofloxacin: 500 mg PO bid × 7 days | Amoxicillin<br>TMP/SMX<br>Ceftriaxone | |
| Bacteremia | Ceftriaxone: 2 g IV q24h × 14 days | Ampicillin<br>Ciprofloxacin<br>TMP/SMX | |
| Chronic carrier state | Ciprofloxacin: 500 mg PO bid × 4 weeks | Amoxicillin<br>TMP/SMX | |
| *Salmonella typhi* | Ciprofloxacin: 400 mg IV q12h (or 500 mg PO bid) × 10–14 days | Chloramphenicol<br>Ceftriaxone<br>TMP/SMX<br>Amoxicillin | Isolates demonstrating resistance to multiple drugs (i.e., chloramphenciol, ampicillin, TMP/SMX) are common in many developing countries. |

(*continued*)

Antimicrobial therapy for bacterial diseases—*Continued*

| Organism/disease | First choice | Alternative choices | Comments |
|---|---|---|---|
| *Serratia marcescens* | Ceftriaxone: 2 g IV q24h × 10–14 days | Amikacin<br>Ciprofloxacin<br>Imipenem<br>Meropenem<br>Aztreonam | Multiple resistance often seen. |
| *Shigella* spp. | Norfloxacin: 400 mg PO bid × 5–7 days *or* Ciprofloxacin: 500 mg PO bid × 5–7 days | TMP/SMX<br>Ampicillin | Resistance to TMP/SMX and ampicillin is common in Latin America and Middle East. Anti-diarrheal drugs not recommended. |
| *Spirillum minor*<br>Rat-bite fever | Amoxicillin-clavulanic acid: 875 mg PO bid × 10–14 days | Tetracycline<br>Streptomycin | Jarisch-Herxheimer reaction may complicate therapy. |
| *Staphylococcus aureus*, methicillin-sensitive | | | Cloxacillin can be substituted for nafcillin. Longer courses (6 weeks) favored with prosthetic valve endocarditis. Because of the rapid emergence of resistance during therapy, neither rifampin nor ciprofloxacin should be employed as single agents. Mupirocin is the preferred agent for eliminating nasopharyngeal carriage state. |
| Right-sided uncomplicated endocarditis secondary to intravenous drug use | Nafcillin: 2 g IV q4h × 4 weeks *or* Nafcillin: 2 g IV q4h × 14 days *plus* Tobramycin: 3–5 mg/kg/day IV × 14 days | Cefazolin<br>Vancomycin<br>Rifampin<br>Ciprofloxacin | |
| Left-sided endocarditis or complicated right-sided endocarditis | Nafcillin: 2 g IV q4h × 4–6 weeks *plus* Gentamicin: 3–5 mg/kg/d IV × 3–5 days | | |
| Bacteremia (no endocarditis) | Nafcillin: 2 g IV q4–6h × 14 days | | |
| *Staphylococcus aureus*, methicillin-resistant | Vancomycin: 1 g IV q12h × 10–14 days | Fluoroquinolone<br>TMP/SMX<br>Rifampin | Significant number of isolates are resistant to fluoroquinolone and TMP/SMX. Mupirocin can be employed to eradicate nasopharngeal carriage of organism, sometimes in combination with rifampin. |
| *Staphylococcus*, coagulase-negative<br>Bacteremia | Vancomycin: 1 g IV q12h × 10–14 days | Rifampin<br>TMP/SMX | Removal of infected prosthesis often required for cure. However, many cases of central venous line sepsis can be treated without removal of in-dwelling catheter. A 6-week regimen of vancomycin plus gentamicin plus rifampin is typically used to treat prosthetic valve endocarditis. |
| *Stenotrophomonas maltophilia* | TMP/SMX: (base on TMP component) 8–10 mg/kg/day divided q6h × 10–14 days | Ticarcillin-clavulanic acid<br>Fluoroquinolone | Usually resistant to imipenem and ceftazidime. |
| *Streptobacillus moniliformis*<br>Rat bite fever | Penicillin G: 1–2 × $10^6$ units IV q4–6h × 10–14 days | Doxycycline<br>Erythromycin<br>Clindamycin | With satisfactory clinical response, it is possible to convert from parenteral to oral therapy after 1 week. |
| *Streptococcus agalactiae* (group B) | | | |
| Bacteremia | Penicillin G: 2.0 × $10^6$ units IV q4h × 10–14 days | Vancomycin<br>Cefazolin | Regimens for neonates and infants are different from those listed here. |
| Meningitis | Penicillin G: 4.0 × $10^6$ units IV q4h × 14–21 days | | |
| Endocarditis | Penicillin G: 4 × $10^6$ units IV q4h × 4 weeks *plus* Gentamicin: 3–5 mg/kg/day IV × 4 weeks | | |

*(continued)*

Antimicrobial therapy for bacterial diseases—*Continued*

| Organism/disease | First choice | Alternative choices | Comments |
|---|---|---|---|
| *Streptococcus bovis*<br>Endocarditis | Penicillin G: 2–4 × $10^6$ units IV q4h × 4 weeks *or* Penicillin G: 2–4 × $10^6$ units IV q4h × 14 days *plus* Gentamicin: 3–5 mg/kg/day IV × 14 days | Vancomycin<br>Cephalosporins | The 4-week regimen generally recommended, especially for elderly patients and those with impaired renal function. Bacteremia without endocarditis can be treated with 2 weeks of IV penicillin. |
| *Streptococcus pneumoniae* | | | |
| Pulmonary disease | Penicillin G: 0.6–2.0 × $10^6$ units IV q4–6h × 10–14 days | Ampicillin<br>Cefazolin<br>Vancomycin | Older fluoroquinolones are unreliable in the treatment of pneumococcal disease. Newer quinolones are effective. Penicillin-resistant strains are increasing in North America. For isolates demonstrating MIC >2.0 (for penicillin), vancomycin is the antimicrobial agent of choice. |
| Meningitis | Penicillin G: 3–4 × $10^6$ units IV q4h × 10–14 days | Erythromycin | |
| Endocarditis | Penicillin G: 2–4 × $10^6$ units IV q4h × 4 weeks | | |
| Sinusitis | Amoxicillin: 500 mg PO tid × 10–14 days *or* TMP/SMX: 1 DS PO bid × 10–14 days | Grepafloxacin<br>Levofloxacin<br>Trovafloxacin | |
| *Streptococcus pyogenes* (group A) | | | |
| Pharyngitis | Penicillin V: 250–500 mg PO tid–qid × 10 days | Amoxicillin<br>Benzathine penicillin G<br>Erythromycin<br>Cephalexin | Treatment of pharyngitis important in preventing rheumatic fever. |
| Impetigo | Mupirocin ointment: apply bid × 10–14 days | Dicloxacillin<br>Cephalexin | Often co-infected with *Staphylococcus aureus*. Diffuse or severe cases will require systemic antimicrobial therapy. |
| Cellulitis | Penicillin G: 2 × $10^6$ units IV q4–6h × 7–14 days | Nafcillin (or cloxacillin)<br>Cefazolin<br>Vancomycin<br>Erythromycin | Oral antimicrobial therapy may be used in cases of mild cellulitis not involving the face. |
| Bacteremia | Penicillin G: 2 × $10^6$ units IV q4h × 10–14 days | Cefazolin<br>Vancomycin | Associated endocarditis is very rare. |
| *Streptococcus* (Viridans group)<br>Endocarditis | Penicillin G: 4 × $10^6$ units IV q4h × 14 days *plus* Gentamicin: 3–5 mg/kg/day IV × 14 days *or* Penicillin G: 4 × $10^6$ units IV q4h × 4 weeks | Vancomycin<br>Ceftriaxone | The 2-week regimen (penicillin G plus gentamicin) is limited to those cases with isolates having MIC ≤0.1 μg/ml. Moreover, the 4-week regimen is generally recommended for elderly patients and those with impaired renal function. A 6-week regimen is often recommended if the isolate has a MIC >0.5 μg/ml or the patient has a prosthetic valve. |
| *Treponema pallidum*/Syphilis | | | |
| Primary, secondary, early latent: not neurosyphilis | Benzathine penicillin: 2.4 × $10^6$ units IM × 1 | Doxycycline | Early latent defined as less than 1 year; many recommend that HIV-infected patients with any stage of syphilis should have evaluation for neurosyphilis. |
| Late latent, tertiary: not neurosyphilis | Benzathine penicillin: 2.4 × $10^6$ units IM q7 days × 3 | Doxycycline | |
| Neurosyphilis | Penicillin G: 2–4 × $10^6$ units IV q4h × 14 days | If allergic to penicillin, desensitize and give penicillin | |
| *Ureaplasma urealyticum*<br>Urethritis | Doxycycline: 100 mg PO bid × 7 days | Erythromycin | Erythromycin is drug of choice in pregnant women. |
| *Vibrio cholerae*<br>Cholera | Doxycycline: 100 mg PO q12h × 3–5 days | Fluoroquinolone<br>Furazolidone<br>TMP/SMZ | Rehydration therapy is critical. Furazolidone is recommended agent for treatment of children and pregnant females. |

(*continued*)

| Organism/disease | First choice | Alternative choices | Comments |
|---|---|---|---|
| *Vibrio parahemolyticus*<br>Gastroenteritis | Supportive therapy | Doxycycline<br>Furazolidone | Antimicrobial therapy has not been shown to shorten clinical course or duration of organism excretion. |
| *Vibrio vulnificus* | Doxycycline: 100 mg IV/PO q12h × 10–14 days *plus* Ceftazidime: 1–2 g IV q8h × 10–14 days | Chloramphenicol | Duration of therapy depends on clinical situation and response. |
| *Yersinia enterocolitica* | | | |
| Gastroenteritis | Norfloxacin: 400 mg PO bid × 10 days *or* Ciprofloxacin: 500 mg PO bid × 10 days | TMP/SMZ<br>Doxycycline<br>Fluoroquinolone | Value of antimicrobial therapy in uncomplicated gastroenteritis is not clear. |
| Septicemia | Gentamicin: 3–5 mg/kg/day IV × 10–14 days | | |
| *Yersinia pestis*<br>Plague | Streptomycin: 15 mg/kg IM bid × 10 days | Gentamicin<br>Chloramphenicol<br>Tetracycline | Patients with meningitis should be treated with chloramphenicol. Doxycycline therapy should be administered prophylactically to persons exposed to pneumonic plague patient or plague-infected animal. |
| *Yersinia pseudotuberculosis* | Ampicillin: 2g IV q4–6h × 10–14 days | Streptomycin<br>Tetracycline | Benefit of therapy for patients who have mesenteric adenitis remains unknown. |
| MYCOBACTERIA | | | |
| *Mycobacterium avium* complex | | | |
| HIV-negative | Clarithromycin: 500 mg PO bid × 6 months *plus* Ethambutol: 15 mg/kg PO qd × 6 months | | Disease among HIV-negative individuals is almost always pulmonary. Most studies have involved late-stage HIV-infected patients. Regimen for HIV infected individuals should include either clarithromycin or azithromycin and will be life-long. |
| HIV-infected | Clarithromycin: 500 mg PO bid *plus* Ethambutol: 15 mg/kg PO qd | Azithromycin<br>Ciprofloxacin<br>Rifabutin (or rifampin) | |
| *Mycobacterium chelonae* | Clarithromycin: 500 mg PO bid × 6 months | Amikacin<br>Cefoxitin | |
| *Mycobacterium fortuitum* | Amikacin: 15 mg/kg/day × 2–6 weeks *plus* Cefoxitin: 200 mg/kg/day × 2–6 weeks *plus* Probenecid: 500 mg PO qid × 2–6 weeks | TMP/SMX<br>Clarithromycin<br>Erythromycin | Patients should have surgical excision of infected areas. Following 2–6 weeks of intravenous therapy, if the organism is susceptible to oral antimicrobial, patient should be switched to oral therapy for 2–6 months. |
| *Mycobacterium kansasii* | Rifampin: 600 mg PO qd × 12–18 months *plus* Ethambutol: 20 mg/kg PO qd × 12–18 months | | |
| *Mycobacterium marinum* | Ethambutol 20 mg/kg PO qd × 6 months *plus* Rifampin: 600 mg PO qd × 6 months | Minocycline<br>Clarithromycin | No concensus on recommended duration of therapy. Recent review recommended minimum of 6 months. |
| *Mycobacterium leprae* | | | |
| Paucibacillary (tuberculoid or indeterminate) | Dapsone: 100 mg PO qd × 6 months (unsupervised) *plus* Rifampin: 600 mg PO once/month × 6 months (supervised) | Ethionamide may be substituted for clofazimine. | For multibacillary disease, therapy should be continued for a minimum of 2 years; preferably, one should document negative skin smears before stopping therapy. |

*(continued)*

Antimicrobial therapy for bacterial diseases—*Continued*

| Organism/disease | First choice | Alternative choices | Comments |
|---|---|---|---|
| Multibacillary (lepromatous) | Dapsone: 100 mg PO qd × 2 years (unsupervised) *plus* Clofazimine: 50 mg PO qd × 2 years (unsupervised) *plus* Rifampin: 600 mg PO once/month × 2 years (supervised) *plus* Clofazimine: 300 mg PO once/month × 2 years (supervised) | | |
| *Mycobacterium tuberculosis* | | | |
| Active disease | Isoniazid: 5 mg/kg PO qd (max 300 mg/d) × 6 months *plus* Rifampin: 10 mg/kg PO qd (max. 600 mg/d) × 6 months *plus* Pyrazinamide: 25 mg/kg PO qd (max. 2.0 g/days) × initial 2 months *plus* Ethambutol: 20 mg/kg/day (max. 2.5 gm/day) | Directly observed therapy given 2–3 times/week can be substituted for daily unsupervised therapy. Streptomycin can be substituted for ethambutol. | All isolates should be sent for susceptibility testing. If organism susceptible, then ethambutol can be discontinued. If organism resistant, then change therapy based on susceptibility testing. In areas where isoniazid resistance is documented to be less than 4%, ethambutol is not necessary to add to initial regimen. Therapy for HIV-infected patients should be continued for 9 months. |
| Drug-resistant | Consult expert | | |

## ANNOTATED BIBLIOGRAPHY

Amsden GW, Schentag JJ. Tables of antimicrobial agent pharmacology. In: Mandell, Douglas and Bennett's Principles and Practice of Infectious Diseases, 4th ed. Mandell GL, Bennett, Dolin R, eds. Churchill Livingstone, New York, pp 492–528, 1995.

*This chapter has elaborate and thorough tables of antimicrobial agents, including information on drug class, side effects, mechanism of action, and dosage adjustments.*

Donowitz GR, Mandell GL. Beta-lactam antibiotic (first of two parts). N Engl J Med 1988; 318:419–426.

Donowitz GR, Mandell GL. Beta-lactam antibiotics (second of two parts). N Engl J Med 1988; 318:490–500.

*This two part series is a classic—it provides an excellent overview of the differences between the major classes of β-lactams as well as discussing important differences within the individual classes. It is, however, limited because it obviously does not include a discussion of newer agents.*

Moellering RC. Principles of anti-infective therapy. In: Mandell, Douglas and Bennett's Principles and Practice of Infectious Diseases, 4th ed. Mandell GL, Bennett, Dolin R, eds. Churchill Livingstone, New York, pp. 199–212, 1995.

*This chapter provides an insightful look at the factors involved that lead to an appropriate choice of an anti-infective agent. In addition, the chapter discusses the indications for combination anti-infective therapy.*

Sanford JP, Gilbert DN, Mollering RC, Sande MA. The Sanford Guide to Antimicrobial Therapy, 27th ed. Antimicrobial Therapy, Inc. Dallas, 1997.

*This excellent pocket-sized manual remains the most commonly used antimicrobial reference by clinicians. The manual is thorough, up to date, and clearly organized. Information can be obtained specifically regarding an antimicrobial, as well as recommendations for treatment of specific organisms and syndromes.*

# 39

# Antiviral Drugs and Therapy

CATHERINE DIAMOND AND LAWRENCE COREY

Of the many drugs now available for the treatment of viral infections, several have only recently come into general clinical use. By clarifying the unique pharmacology of and indications for each antiviral drug, this chapter is intended as a guide to the appropriate use of these drugs. We will begin by reviewing drugs used for herpes simplex I (HSV-1) and II (HSV-2) and varicella zoster (VZV) viruses: acyclovir, valacyclovir, and famciclovir. We will then describe ganciclovir, foscarnet, and cidofovir, agents mainly employed in the treatment of cytomegalovirus. We will also cover two drugs used to treat influenza A, amantadine and rimantadine. We will conclude with a review of ribavirin and an outline of antiviral therapy with interferon. Antiviral drugs for HIV infection are discussed in Chapter 101.

## Drugs for Infection by Herpesviruses

### Acyclovir

Acyclovir (Zovirax, Glaxo-Wellcome; ACV) is the widely used standard drug for herpes simplex and varicella zoster infections.

#### Mechanism of action

Acyclovir is selectively phosphorylated intracellularly by HSV-1, HSV-2, and VZV thymidine kinase (TK) to acyclovir monophosphate. Cellular kinases then form acyclovir triphosphate (ACV-TP), which is a chain terminator and suicide inactivator of the HSV and VZV DNA polymerase.

#### Indications

Indications include HSV and VZV infections in immunocompetent and immunocompromised individuals, including neonatal HSV, genital HSV, varicella (chicken pox) and herpes zoster.

#### Pharmacokinetics

The kidney is the main route of drug elimination, so doses must be adjusted for renal insufficiency. Acyclovir peak concentration with 800 mg PO is 1–2 $\mu$g/ml and with 10 mg/kg IV therapy is approximately 20 $\mu$g/ml. Cerebrospinal fluid (CSF) ACV levels are about 50% of plasma levels. Acyclovir is removed by hemodialysis.

#### Clinical trials

Oral acyclovir is the drug of choice for the treatment of mucocutaneous HSV infections. Oral acyclovir shortens the duration of pain, viral shedding, and systemic symptoms in primary herpes simplex virus infection due to either HSV-1 or HSV-2. A dosage of 400 mg PO tid is as effective and more convenient than 200 mg PO 5 times per day. Oral ACV shortens the duration of viral shedding and lesions in patients with recurrent genital HSV. Acyclovir is also effective at 400 mg 5 times per day for first-episode HSV proctitis. Daily oral acyclovir is effective in reducing both clinical and subclinical reactivations of HSV-2 in immunocompetent persons. Suppressive therapy does not alter the long-term natural history of the disease. For persons with frequent outbreaks of oral labial HSV, 400 mg PO bid is also effective in suppressing frequently recurrent oral HSV, although the effectiveness (65%) is less than with genital disease (90%). Chronic suppressive therapy does not seem to induce resistance in immunocompetent hosts. When breakthrough recurrences occur, they are usually not due to ACV-resistant strains.

In the United States, 5% topical acyclovir in polyethylene glycol has little clinical utility. Topical therapy is effective in first-episode primary genital HSV; however, oral ACV is more effective and convenient. Two multicenter, placebo-controlled trials of treatment of recurrent genital HSV with topical ACV found no clinically significant effect on recurrent disease.

In Europe and Asia, topical acyclovir is distributed in modified aqueous cream base, which has greater cutaneous absorption. This topical formulation has been shown to be of modest benefit in speeding the healing of recurrent oral labial lesions in the normal host. It has recently become available as an over-the-counter (OTC) preparation in several European and Asian countries.

Acyclovir IV or oral is highly effective in the prevention, suppression, and treatment of HSV disease in immunosuppressed patients such as organ and bone marrow transplant recipients, patients undergoing chemotherapy, and AIDS patients. For instance, in a randomized, double-blind trial in 29 leukemic chemotherapy patients, culture-positive HSV infection occurred in 11 of 15 placebo recipients and none of the ACV recipients. Acyclovir has been shown to prevent cytomegalovirus (CMV) disease in bone marrow and renal transplant recipients. However, the advent of ganciclovir and foscarnet allows for more effective and directed CMV prophylaxis in the immunocompromised patient.

Intravenous acyclovir is the drug of choice for HSV encephalitis. In a randomized trial of ACV versus vidarabine in 69 patients who were diagnosed by brain biopsy with herpes encephalitis, the mortality in the vidarabine recipients was 54% versus 28% in the ACV recipients and the surviving ACV recipients had better functional outcomes than the surviving vidarabine recipients. High-dose acyclovir is also the gold standard in the treatment of neonatal HSV.

Acyclovir is also licensed for the therapy of varicella zoster infection and has been utilized extensively for varicella and VZV infections in immunocompetent and immunocompromised patients. However, valacyclovir, the L-valyl ester of acyclovir, is much better absorbed after oral administration, reaches higher blood levels, and provides a superior clinical response rate than acyclovir for VZV infections. As such, it is the preferred choice for oral therapy of VZV in the immunocompetent patient. Intravenous ACV halts progression of VZV in immunocompromised patients.

In 815 otherwise healthy children with varicella infection, acyclovir 20 mg/kg PO qid for 5 days decreased the number of pox, improved healing, and decreased the duration of fever and constitutional symptoms compared with placebo; there was no significant difference in VZV antibody titers between the two groups.

In a multicenter, randomized placebo-controlled, double-blind trial of ACV treatment of varicella in 62 otherwise healthy adolescents, ACV reduced cutaneous and constitutional illness. Varicella zoster antibody titers at 28 days were similar in the ACV and placebo group. In a double-blind, randomized trial in 148 adults with chicken pox, ACV 800 mg 5 times a day decreased fever duration, promoted cutaneous healing, and lessened symptoms when administered within 24 h of rash onset. Serious complications such as pneumonia and encephalitis were too rare to evaluate whether ACV influenced their incidence. The American Academy of Pediatrics recommends ACV for varicella in adolescents and secondary household cases.

### Dosage

Oral, intravenous, and topical therapy are available. Topical ACV is prepared as a 5% polyethylene glycol base or a 5% modified aqueous cream. Please refer to Table 39.1 for dosage information.

### Side effects

Acyclovir therapy is associated with reversible elevation of serum creatinine and renal dysfunction. Slow infusion and hydration decreases the risk of renal impairment. Neurotoxicity, including confusion, seizures, and agitation, has also been reported as an adverse effect. Headache and nausea are common minor side effects. Phlebitis may occur with IV ACV, and stinging and pruritus may occur with topical application.

### Precautions

Although ACV is not approved for use in pregnancy, treatment during pregnancy has not been associated with an increased risk of congenital abnormalities. A registry of pregnancy exposures is maintained by the manufacturer. Orally administered acyclovir is excreted in breast milk.

Probenecid reduces renal clearance of acyclovir by preventing tubular secretion of the drug.

### Resistance

Acyclovir resistance is defined as lack of inhibition of growth to >2 μg/ml in a plaque reduction assay. Thymidine kinase deficiency, TK alteration, and altered DNA polymerase can cause ACV resistance. Absence or deficiency of TK is the most common cause of resistance. ACV-resistant HSV may be seen in AIDS patients and marrow and organ transplant recipients on prolonged ACV therapy. ACV-resistant HSV-2 rarely occurs in immunocompetent patients. There are also case reports of acyclovir-resistant VZV in AIDS patients on prolonged ACV therapy. The clinical manifestations of ACV-resistant viruses are similar to those of sensitive strains. Because of time consumed during ineffectual ACV therapy and the immunosuppression of the host, the lesions may become large and ulcerated. ACV-resistant HSV and VZV infections usually respond to intravenous foscarnet therapy.

### Cost

All costs provided are average wholesale prices in U.S. dollars for 1997. The price of an oral acyclovir treatment course for acute genital herpes is $60. Chronic suppression costs about $125 per month. An oral treatment course for herpes zoster costs approximately $150–$200. Intravenous acyclovir for HSV encephalitis costs about $2400 for a 10-day course. A 15 g tube of 5% acyclovir ointment costs $40.

## Valacyclovir

Valacyclovir (Valtrex, Glaxo Wellcome) is a L-valyl ester of acyclovir that is well absorbed and converted to acyclovir.

### Mechanism of action

The mechanism of action is similar to that of acyclovir—phosphorylation by viral thymidine kinase with subsequent inhibition of viral DNA synthesis by inactivating the viral DNA polymerase enzyme.

### Indications

Valacyclovir demonstrates the same antiviral activity as acyclovir against HSV-1 and HSV-2 as well as VZV. The drug's advantage is higher absorption which allows greater serum levels of acyclovir. This is of clear benefit in the treatment of herpes zoster. Its advantages in HSV infection appear limited to dosing convenience.

### Pharmacokinetics

Valacyclovir is an ester of acyclovir that is cleaved by valacyclovir esterase, a novel enzyme in the small intestinal wall. This increases acyclovir absorption from approximately 20% to 80%, raising serum levels from 2 μg/ml with 800 mg of oral acyclovir to 5 μg/ml with 1 g of oral valacyclovir. Absorption is not altered by food.

### Clinical Trials

Two randomized, double-blind trials in immunocompetent patients with herpes zoster have been conducted. In patients under age 50, valacyclovir was compared with placebo; valacyclovir sped healing of lesions, but had no influence on postherpetic neuralgia. People under age 50 have a low frequency of postherpetic neuralgia. In patients over age 50, valacyclovir was compared with acyclovir; there was a decrease in the duration of zoster-associated pain in the valacyclovir arm. Optimal effectiveness was seen with a 7-day dosing regimen. Studies in immunocompromised patients are underway.

### Dosage

The recommended dosage for treatment of varicella zoster is 1 g (two 500-mg tablets) PO tid for 7 days. It is optimal to initiate therapy within 72 h of onset of rash. The dose is 1 g PO bid

**Table 39.1** Antiviral drugs

| Name | Mechanism of action | Indication | Pharmacology and interactions | Dosage | Side effects | Precautions |
|---|---|---|---|---|---|---|
| Acyclovir (ACV)<br>Zovirax<br>Glaxo-Wellcome | ACV is phosphorylated intracellularly by viral TK to then inhibit viral DNA polymerase | HSV-1 and -2 in immunocompromised host; initial genital HSV and suppression of >6 recurrences/yr; HSV encephalitis, neonatal HSV, VZV infections | Oral absorption is slow and incomplete; ACV cleared by kidney, so adjust dose for renal insufficiency; hydrate to avoid renal toxicity; probenecid reduces renal clearance; ACV is removed by hemodialysis; must be infused over at least 1 h | Primary genital HSV: 400 mg PO tid for 7–10 days<br>Recurrent genital HSV: 400 mg PO tid for 5 days. Suppression of genital HSV: ACV PO 400 mg PO bid<br>HSV encephalitis: 10 mg/k IV q8h for 10–21 days<br>Mucocutaneous disease in the immunocompromised host: 5 mg/kg or 250 mg/m$^2$ IV q8h or 400 mg PO tid for 7–14 days<br>Neonatal HSV: 45–60 mg/kg/day given intravenously q8h for 14–21 days<br>Varicella zoster: 800 mg PO 5 times a day for 7–10 days<br>Severe VZV in a compromised host: 10 mg/k IV q8h for 7–14 days<br>Adult with chicken pox: 800 mg 5 times a day for 7days | Neurotoxicity including seizures; increases creatine and causes renal dysfunction; headache, nausea, phlebitis | If therapy fails, consider resistance in immunocompromised host |
| Valacyclovir<br>Valtrex,<br>Glaxo-Wellcome | L-valyl ester of ACV; cleaved by enzyme in small intestine to ACV | Herpes zoster (preferred over acyclovir); recurrent genital herpes | Increases ACV bioavailablity three- to fivefold | VZV: 1 g tid for 7 days<br>Primary genital HSV: 1 gram bid for 7–10 days<br>Recurrent genital HSV: 500 mg bid for 5 days<br>Suppression of genital HSV: 500–1,000 mg once a day; if >10 outbreaks per year, use the higher dose | Headache, nausea, diarrhea, dizziness | TTP/HUS reported with chronic high doses, 8 g/day during therapy in immunocompromised patients |
| Famciclovir<br>Famvir<br>SmithKline Beacham | Prodrug of penciclovir, a guanosine analog that inhibits herpesvirus DNA synthesis; like ACV, it requires viral TK | Herpes zoster; recurrent genital herpes | Famciclovir is converted in the liver to penciclovir and excreted in the urine. Adjust dose for reduced renal function. Probenecid increases plasma drug concentration | VZV: 500 mg tid for 7 days<br>Primary genital HSV: 250 mg PO tid for 7–10 days<br>Recurrent genital HSV: 125 mg bid for 5 days<br>Suppression of genital HSV: 250 mg bid | Headache, nausea | Testicular toxicity and carcinogenesis in rats |

*(continued)*

**Table 39.1** Antiviral drugs—*Continued*

| Name | Mechanism of action | Indication | Pharmacology and interactions | Dosage | Side effects | Precautions |
|---|---|---|---|---|---|---|
| Ganciclovir (GCV) Cytovene Syntex | GCV must be converted to the corresponding triphosphate; GCV TP inhibits viral DNA synthesis through competitive inhibition and chain termination | CMV retinitis; clinically used in other AIDS-related CMV infections including esophagitis, colitis, and neurologic disease; oral GCV for maintenance treatment of non-sight-threatening retinitis with monthly ophthalmologic exams; GCV intravitreal implant. Prevention and treatment of CMV disease in bone and organ transplant recipients. Safety and efficacy have not been established for congenital/neonatal disease nor in immunocompetent host | The major elimination pathway for GCV is renal; adjust dose for renal dysfunction. Administer IV dose over 1 h. Bolus, IM, or SQ administration is toxic | CMV retinitis induction: 5 mg/kg IV q12 h for 14–21 days. Maintenance: 5 mg/kg IV qd or 6 mg/kg for 5 days every week; PO GCV: 1000 mg PO tid with food (four 250-mg caps) | Neutropenia, thrombocytopenia, and anemia. Neutropenia may be treated with GCSF; elevated creatinine; retinal detachment with implant | CMV retinitis in AIDS requires lifelong suppressive therapy. Progression may occur in time with the development of resistance or disease in the opposite eye or viscera with an implant. Combination therapy with foscarnet may work in cases that fail GCV alone. In animal studies, GCV was carcinogenic, teratogenic, and caused aspermatogenesis; safety has not been established in children. |
| Foscarnet Foscavir Astra | Pyrophosphate analog that inhibits the DNA polymerases of human herpes viruses | CMV retinitis; GCV-resistant CMV disease in the AIDS/transplant setting; ACV-resistant HSV and VZV | Renally eliminated; adjust dose for renal dysfunction; long-term bone deposition; concurrent use with IV pentamidine may exacerbate hypocalcemia | Induction: 60 mg/kg IV q8h over 1 h for 14–21 days. Maintenance: 90–120 mg/kg IV qd over 2 h; requires infusion pump. HSV and VZV: 40 mg/kg IV q8h for 14–21 days | Nephrotoxicity, which may be attenuated by prehydration with NS; genital ulcers; hypokalemia, hypocalcemia, increased Mg + $PO_4$; diabetes insipidus; must check electrolytes often; anemia; nausea, vomiting; seizures | Foscarnet has anti-HIV activity; in AIDS patients with CMV retinitis, foscarnet treatment is associated with improved survival over GCV treatment; lifelong suppressive therapy is needed for CMV retinitis in AIDS. Skeletal anomalies in offspring of laboratory animals treated with foscarnet |

| | | | | | | |
|---|---|---|---|---|---|---|
| Cidofovir Vistide, HPMPC Gilead Sciences | Nucleotide analogue that inhibits viral DNA polymerase. Contains a pre-existing phosphate group that enables it to bypass initial virus-dependent phosphorylation. Cellular enzymes convert cidofovir to the active diphosphate form in both infected and uninfected cells | AIDS-associated CMV retinitis | Long intracellular half-life. Avoid concurrent nephrotoxic drugs. Drug interactions with probenecid | 5 mg/kg weekly for 2 weeks as induction then every other week as maintenance | Nephrotoxic, proteinuria, glucosuria, Fanconi-like syndrome, increased serum creatinine. Serum creatinine and urine protein should be monitored prior to each dose. If serum creatinine increases 0.3–0.4 mg/dl, the cidofovir dose should be reduced from 5 mg/kg to 3 mg/kg. If serum creatinine increases >0.5 mg/dl or >3+ proteinuria develops, cidofovir should be discontinued. Also check neutrophils; neutropenia can occur. Also ocular hypotonia. Probenecid: nausea, vomiting, fever, hypersensitivity | Avoid use in pregnancy and nursing |
| Amantadine Symmetrel Dupont | Blocks uncoating of viral RNA within host cells | Influenza A prophylaxis and treatment | Excreted in urine unchanged; dosed weekly for HD patients; adjust dose for CrCl < 50 mL/min | Treatment and prophylaxis dosages are same, 100 mg PO bid for 3–5 days for treatment or for 2 weeks post-vaccination or until 1 week after the end of outbreak for prophylaxis; 100 mg PO qid for >65 years | Neurotoxicity, anxiety/light-headed/poor concentration, particularly in elderly; nausea, vomiting, anorexia | Seizures can occur with either amantadine or rimantadine in patients with a history of seizure disorder. Teratogenic in laboratory animals |
| Rimantadine Flumadine Forest Laboratories | Blocks uncoating of viral RNA within host cells | Influenza A prophylaxis and treatment | Metabolized by liver; decrease dose to 100 mg PO qd in patients with severe hepatic or renal dysfunction | Treatment and prophylaxis dosages are same 100 mg PO bid for 3–5 days for treatment or for 2 weeks post-vaccination or until 1 week after the end of outbreak for prophylaxis; decrease dosage to 100 mg PO qd in elderly NH patients | Fewer CNS side effects than amantadine; equal number of GI side effects | May decrease dosage to 100 mg PO qd in elderly who experience side effects. NB: the entire dose of 200 mg can be taken once a day without changing effectiveness or increasing side effects |

(*continued*)

**Table 39.1** Antiviral drugs—*Continued*

| Name | Mechanism of action | Indication | Pharmacology and interactions | Dosage | Side effects | Precautions |
|---|---|---|---|---|---|---|
| Ribavirin<br>Virazole<br>ICN | A synthetic nucleoside analogue that appears to interfere with the expression of mRNA and inhibit viral protein synthesis | Respiratory syncytial virus infections in hospitalized patients who are at risk for severe disease (CHD, AIDS, transplant, chemotherapy, etc.) or severely ill ($PaO_2 < 65$ mm HG, q $CO_2$), or mechanically ventilated; consider for infants at risk for severe disease at young age (<6 weeks) or underlying disease (congenital anomalies, cerebral palsy, neurologic dysfunction); hemorrhagic fevers | Aerosolized in oxygen hood/tent/mask; drug is concentrated in RBCs | 20 mg/ml aerosol for 12–20 h daily for 3–5 days for RSV; 2 g IV load then 1 g q6h for 4 days then 0.5 g q8h for 6 days for HF | Mucous membrane irritation conjunctivitis, rash, wheezing, arrthymia, anemia | Testicular lesions in rats and teratogenic in laboratory animals; pregnant women should avoid direct care of patients on ribavirin.<br>Deposition in the ventilator with subsequent malfunction can occur; only experienced staff should administer. IV ribavirin is unavailable in the U.S. |
| Interferon-$\alpha$<br>Intron A<br>Schering<br><br>Roferon-A<br>Roche | Induces cellular proteins that decrease viral expression | HBV; HCV; HPV | IM or SQ for intralesional (HPV) administration | HPV: 1 million units (.1 ml of a 10 million/ml vial) into lesion 3 times a week for 3 weeks, maximum 5 lesions<br>HBV: 5 million units/day SC/IM for 4 months<br>HCV: 3 million units SC or IM 3 times a week for 6–18 months | Flu-like syndrome fatigue, fever; myalgia; headache; anorexia; diarrhea; dizziness; rash; thyroid disease; Q WBC, Hgb, and platelets; depression. Flu symptoms decrease with premedication with acetaminophen | Interferon has been effective in HIV-related thrombocytopenia, HCV-related cryoglobulinemia, and HBV-related glomerulonephritis |

for 7–10 days for primary genital herpes and 500 mg PO bid for 5 days for recurrent genital herpes. For suppression of genital herpes, 500–1,000 mg daily can be utilized. Valacyclovir 500 mg once a day appears less effective than higher doses in patients who have more than 10 outbreaks per year. There is a dose adjustment for creatinine clearances <50 ml/min. A 4 h hemodialysis session removes about one-third of acyclovir in the body; thus, valacyclovir should be dosed after hemodialysis. Dose adjustment is not required for cirrhosis.

### Side Effects

Aside from occasional nausea and headache, the safety profile in immunocompetent hosts is favorable.

### Precautions

Thrombotic thrombocytopenic purpura/hemolytic uremic syndrome has been reported in AIDS patients and bone marrow and solid organ recipients in clinical trials of valacyclovir at high doses, 2 g qid for >6 months. Such high doses should not be used. Safety during breast feeding and pregnancy is unknown but generally should be regarded as similar to acyclovir.

### Resistance

Viruses resistant to acyclovir are resistant to valacyclovir as well.

### Cost

A 7-day course of valacyclovir for herpes zoster costs approximately $75. A course for recurrent genital herpes costs about $18.

## Famciclovir

Famciclovir (Famvir, SmithKline Beecham) is the oral prodrug of penciclovir. Famciclovir has been shown effective in the treatment of HSV-1, HSV-2, and VZV infections.

### Mechanism of action

Penciclovir triphosphate is a guanosine analog that inhibits herpes virus DNA synthesis by disrupting the action of viral DNA polymerase. Like acyclovir, penciclovir does not affect human DNA because viral rather than cellular thymidine kinase performs the first step in activating the drug, converting it to a monophosphate. Cellular kinases phosphorylate the monophosphate to penciclovir triphosphate which inhibits the viral DNA polymerase enzyme and thereby prevents viral replication.

### Indications

Famciclovir is indicated for oral treatment of acute uncomplicated herpes zoster in immunocompetent patients and in treatment of recurrent genital herpes. Studies of its effectiveness in the suppression of HSV infection in the normal host are ongoing. Topical penciclovir is being studied for the therapy of oral herpes labialis. The drug has not been studied in ophthalmic nor disseminated zoster nor in immunocompromised hosts. Famciclovir demonstrates in vitro activity against hepatitis B virus (HBV) as well as the expected activity against VZV and HSV-1 and HSV-2; a possible therapeutic use in HBV infection is being investigated. Both valaciclovir and famciclovir are more bioavailable than acyclovir and both are more convenient to administer.

### Pharmacokinetics

Famciclovir is quickly absorbed through the gastrointestinal (GI) tract and converted through deacetylation and oxidation in the liver to penciclovir. Famciclovir has greater oral bioavailability than acyclovir. Foods slows the absorption of famciclovir and rate of conversion to penciclovir but does not alter the final bioavailability of active drug. There is a decrease in the rate but not the extent of systemic availability of penciclovir in subjects with liver disease, so theoretically it should be unnecessary to alter famciclovir dosing in patients with compensated hepatic disease and normal kidney function. The serum half-life of penciclovir is 2.5 h but the intracellular half-life is longer. Penciclovir is excreted by the kidney. Dosage reduction is recommended for creatine clearances (CrCl) <60 ml/min.

### Clinical trials

In a placebo-controlled trial in 419 immunocompetent zoster patients, famciclovir accelerated lesion healing and reduced the duration but not the incidence of postherpetic neuralgia. A similarly designed large trial comparing famciclovir with acyclovir showed no difference in time to crusting, time to loss of acute pain, and duration of postherpetic neuralgia between the two drugs. Among persons with recurrent genital herpes, famciclovir 125 mg PO bid reduced the duration of viral shedding, pain, and itching, and sped healing of genital lesions. The relative reduction in each of these signs and symptoms was from two- to threefold.

### Dosage

The recommended dosage for herpes zoster is 500 mg PO every 8 h beginning within 72 h of rash onset and continued for 7 days. The dosage for primary genital herpes is 250 mg PO tid for 7–10 days and for recurrent genital herpes is 125 mg PO bid for 5 days. For suppression of genital herpes the dosage is 250 mg PO bid.

### Side effects

In four clinical studies, the most frequent adverse effects reported with famciclovir were headache, nausea, and diarrhea, which occurred with similar frequencies in the placebo arm. In animal studies, prolonged courses of high-dose famciclovir caused mammary adenocarcinoma in female rats and testicular changes and impaired fertility in male rats. However, men treated with oral famciclovir 250 mg bid for 18 weeks did not have altered spermatogenesis.

### Precautions

Safety in pregnancy and breast feeding is unknown.

### Resistance

Most acyclovir-resistant HSV and VZV clinical isolates are also resistant to famciclovir. Acyclovir resistance is usually due to absence of the viral thymidine kinase, and as such, cross-resistance is to be expected. Occasionally, acyclovir resistance is secondary to an altered TK; these viruses may be resistant to acyclovir and susceptible to famciclovir. However, because these strains are uncommon, empiric therapy with famciclovir for acyclovir-resistant viruses is not recommended without laboratory confirmation of a TK-altered phenotype.

### Cost

The price of a 7-day course of famciclovir for herpes zoster is similar to that of an equivalent course of oral acyclovir, $143. A course of famciclovir for recurrent genital herpes costs about $25.

## Ganciclovir

Ganciclovir (DHPG, Cytovene; GCV) is an acyclic nucleoside analog of guanosine that is licensed for the treatment of CMV infection.

### Mechanism of action

Ganciclovir is a prodrug that is phosphorylated intracellularly to its active triphosphate form, ganciclovir triphosphate, a competitive inhibitor of DNA polymerase. In cells infected with HSV or VZV, viral thymidine kinase phosphorylates the drug. In CMV-infected cells, the host cell performs this initial phosphorylation. The CMV virus specified gene UL97 then phosphorylates ganciclovir mono- and diphosphate to ganciclovir triphosphate. Ganciclovir owes its greater anti-CMV activity over acyclovir or famciclovir to the higher level of GCV-TP than ACV-TP or penciclovir-TP in CMV-infected cells.

### Indications

Ganciclovir has antiviral activity against HSV-1, HSV-2, VZV, and CMV. Since ganciclovir is far more toxic than the standard anti-herpes drug, acyclovir, its major clinical use is in the prevention and treatment of CMV rather than HSV disease. However, because of its anti-HSV activity, there is usually no reason to use acyclovir when intravenous ganciclovir is being administered.

GCV is indicated for use only in the treatment of CMV retinitis in immunocompromised individuals and in the prevention of CMV disease in transplant recipients. Ganciclovir and foscarnet appear to have equal efficacy in the treatment of CMV retinitis. However, foscarnet therapy for CMV retinitis has been shown to prolong survival in AIDS, presumably because of the agent's anti-retroviral activity. GCV is also used extensively in the treatment of CMV pneumonia, colitis, esophagitis, and nervous system disease in the immunocompromised, although its clinical effects in these conditions are more limited. Because of its hematologic toxicity, there is no definite indication for ganciclovir in the immunocompetent host.

### Pharmacokinetics

Oral, ocular implants, and intravenous ganciclovir are commercially available. Oral ganciclovir is poorly absorbed; bioavailability ranges from 2.6%–7.3%. A 1000 mg oral dose every 8 h produces a mean peak of 1.11 $\mu$g/ml and trough of 0.54 $\mu$g/ml. An intravenous dose of 5 mg/kg produces a peak of 5–10 $\mu$g/ml and trough of less than 2 $\mu$g/ml. Intravenous GCV is administered by slow infusion over 1 h. Concentration in the CNS is approximately 40% of plasma concentration. Intravitreal concentrations after intravenous administration may be subtherapeutic for many CMV isolates; this may explain disease progression despite intravenous therapy. Ocular levels with intravitreal implants are much higher. Ganciclovir is renally eliminated and requires dose adjustment for a creatinine clearance less than 80 ml/min. Approximately half the dose is eliminated by the end of a 4 h hemodialysis session. Thus, ganciclovir should be administered after the hemodialysis session.

### Clinical trials

Multiple studies have demonstrated the benefit of GCV in AIDS-associated CMV retinitis. Most patients respond to IV GCV therapy with stabilization or regression of disease. In 40 AIDS patients with CMV retinitis, 88% had a complete response to IV GCV. Reactivation occurred in 50% of patients on maintenance therapy for longer than 3 weeks. Lifelong suppressive therapy is required for AIDS-associated CMV retinitis. Despite suppressive therapy, most patients eventually relapse, requiring reinduction or the addition/substitution of foscarnet.

Ganciclovir has also been used in nonretinal CMV disease in the AIDS population. In a double-blind, placebo-controlled trial of 14 days of 5 mg/kg q12h GCV in 62 patients with AIDS-associated CMV colitis, GCV decreased CMV-positive colonic cultures, improved colonoscopy appearance, lowered the incidence of extracolonic CMV disease, and maintained body weight in treated subjects. It is unclear whether chronic suppression is necessary after treating AIDS-associated CMV colitis or esophagitis, but most clinicians attempt to stop therapy post-induction. There are scattered reports of GCV use in CMV neurological disease as well.

Ganciclovir and foscarnet have been shown to have synergistic inhibition of cytomegalovirus replication in vitro. Successful concurrent use of ganciclovir and foscarnet after failure of monotherapy has been reported. Alternating or concomitant use may have theoretical utility in reducing the emergence of GCV or foscarnet-resistant CMV. The rate of hematologic toxicity with combination therapy was higher than monotherapy, but 9 of 10 AIDS patients with progressive CMV disease responded to the combination.

Intraocular sustained-release GCV implants have been developed and are licensed for use in localized CMV retinitis. The implants are convenient and avoid systemic toxicity. In a randomized controlled trial of implants, 26 patients with previously untreated peripheral CMV retinitis were assigned to immediate or deferred treatment with the GCV implant. The median time to progression of retinitis was 15 days in the deferred group versus 226 days in the immediate treatment group. Intraocular GCV implants increase the risk of retinal detachment. An ocular implant will not prevent CMV disease in the other eye nor disseminated CMV disease.

The FDA has recently approved oral ganciclovir for maintenance therapy of CMV retinitis. An open-label randomized study compared the efficacy and safety of oral ganciclovir at a daily dose of 3000 mg with intravenous ganciclovir at 5 mg/kg/day as maintenance therapy for newly diagnosed AIDS-associated CMV retinitis in 115 patients. CMV disease was initially stabilized with intravenous ganciclovir. The mean time to progression of retinitis was 62 days in the intravenous group and 57 days in the oral group. Survival, alterations in visual acuity, incidence of viral shedding, and incidence of adverse GI side effects were similar in both groups. The intravenous ganciclovir group had more neutropenia, anemia, and catheter-related adverse events.

As serum and tissue levels of GCV are much less with oral than intravenous therapy, the use of oral GCV must be weighed againt the risk of relapse. Ideal candidates for oral maintenance therapy would include patients with stable disease or inactive peripheral retinitis. Patients suffering treatment failure or sight-threatening retinitis should receive intravenous therapy. Ophthalmological exam at the time of initiation of oral therapy, ideally with retinal photographs, is appropriate. Close ophthalmologic follow-up is mandatory. The efficacy of oral GCV in manifestations of CMV disease other than maintenance therapy in retinitis has not been established. Oral GCV may have some efficacy in prophylaxis against AIDS-associated CMV retinitis. However, the expense and incomplete protection offered make the benefit of oral GCV unclear. Further evaluation of this approach is needed.

Ganciclovir is frequently employed in the prophylaxis and treatment of CMV pneumonia in the bone marrow transplant (BMT) setting. In 40 allogeneic BMT patients with asymptomatic infection discovered on routine bronchoalveolar lavage, CMV pneumonia occurred in 5 (25%) of treated patients versus 14 (70%) of untreated patients. Ganciclovir combined with high-dose intravenous immune globulin (IVIG) improved the outcome of patients with CMV pneumonia after allogeneic BMT. Compared with 100% mortality in historical controls, seven of 10 patients receiving GCV and IVIG survived.

Prophylactic ganciclovir administered after engraftment suppresses CMV infection and disease. In 64 seropositive allogeneic BMT recipients randomized to either GCV or placebo after engraftment until day 100 post-BMT, 9 (29%) placebo recipients developed CMV disease in the first 100 days post-transplant compared with none of the GCV recipients; mortality between the two groups did not differ at 180 days. In a similar trial conducted in 85 seropositive allogeneic BMT recipients treated with placebo or prophylactic GCV pre-transplant continued until absolute neutrophil count (ANC) recovery, CMV disease occurred in 4 of 40 GCV patients (10%) versus 11 of 45 placebo patients (24%). Again, survival in both groups was equal.

Surveillance cultures may identify early CMV infection and therefore candidates for GCV therapy. In a double-blind trial, 72 seropositive or recipients of seropositive marrow patients were screened for CMV excretion by throat swabs, blood, urine, bronchoalveolar lavage (BAL) cultures, and excreters were assigned to either GCV or placebo. CMV disease occurred in 1 of 37 of the GCV arm (3%) versus 15 of 35 of the placebo arm (43%). In this trial, survival was significantly better in the GCV group. Late CMV disease (>100 days after BMT) may still occur after discontinuation of ganciclovir. Neutropenia, a risk factor for bacterial infection in the BMT population, is the major toxicity of ganciclovir.

Ganciclovir has been used to treat and prevent CMV disease in organ transplant recipients. In a randomized, placebo-controlled, double-blind, multicenter trial in heart transplant recipients, CMV illness occurred during the first 120 days after transplant in 26 of 56 (46%) seropositive patients given placebo compared with 5 of 56 (9%) seropositive patients treated with ganciclovir. Prophylactic GCV therapy is most effective when directed toward the patient most at risk and during the periods of greatest immunosuppression. Efficacy has not been established in congenital CMV disease.

#### Dosage

Retinitis induction requires 5 mg/kg IV q12h for 14–21 days; maintenance dosage is 6 mg/kg IV qd 5 days a week or 5 mg/kg/day 7 days a week.

Oral CMV retinitis maintenance dosage is 1 g PO tid with food (four 250-mg capsules three times daily).

CMV pneumonia in BMT requires 2.5 mg/kg IV q8h for 20 days then 5 mg/kg/day 3–5 times per week for 20 doses in combination with IVIG 500 mg/kg qod for 20 days then two times per week for eight doses.

Dosage for prophylaxis in transplant recipients is 5 mg/kg IV q12h for 14–21 days as induction followed by maintenance regimens similar to those used in retinitis (continued until day 100–120 in the BMT setting, depending on the degree of immunosuppression and risk of disease in the organ transplant setting).

#### Side effects

Neutropenia occurs in 25%–40% of patients during induction therapy but is reversible with withdrawal of the drug. Thrombocytopenia and anemia may also occur. Granulocyte cell–stimulating factor (GCSF) may reverse granulocytopenia. Hematologic toxicity may be exacerbated by drugs such as AZT and azathioprine. Phlebitis, GI disturbance, elevated serum creatinine, CNS side effects, and elevated liver function test can also occur. Bacterial endophthalmitis, conjunctival scarring, foreign body sensation, retinal detachment, scleral induration, and subconjunctival hemorrhage are adverse effects associated with ocular implants.

#### Precautions

In animal studies, GCV is teratogenic and carcinogenic, and has caused aspermatogenesis. Administration of high doses to nursing mice resulted in testicular hypoplasia in male offspring. Safety in childhood has not been established.

#### Resistance

Ganciclovir resistant isolates have in vitro inhibitory concentrations >3 $\mu$g/ml. Ganciclovir resistance in CMV is due to reduced intracellular phosphorylation or an altered viral DNA polymerase. In one prospective survey of 72 AIDS patients treated with ganciclovir, of 13 culture-positive patients treated for 3 months or more, 5 (38%) excreted virus resistant to ganciclovir. The resistant isolates are pathogenic. TK-negative, acyclovir-resistant HSV strains are also resistant to GCV.

#### Cost

Intravenous ganciclovir for CMV maintenance therapy costs over $1000 per month. The price of oral ganciclovir is approximately $1400 per month. Although oral therapy avoids the costs of administering intravenous GCV, it is still expensive to purchase and monitor appropriately.

### Foscarnet

Foscarnet (Foscavir, Astra USA, phosphonoformate) is a broad-spectrum intravenous antiviral used primarily in the treatment of CMV infections in immunosuppressed individuals.

### Mechanism of action

Foscarnet is a pyrophosphate analogue that inhibits the DNA polymerase of human herpesviruses (including HSV, CMV, VZV, EBV, and HHV-6) and the reverse transcriptase of HIV.

### Indications

The only approved indications for foscarnet are CMV retinitis and mucocutaneous acyclovir-resistant HSV infections in the immunocompromised. In light of improved survival in patients treated with foscarnet rather than ganciclovir, foscarnet may be the drug of choice in AIDS patients with CMV retinitis. Despite its limited approved indications, the drug has been used for acyclovir-resistant VZV and multiple manifestations of CMV disease in AIDS and bone marrow transplant patients. Uses include the previously mentioned CMV retinitis as well as esophagitis, colitis, and pneumonia, particularly for ganciclovir-resistant strains or in patients unable to tolerate ganciclovir.

### Pharmacokinetics

The drug is administered intravenously; plasma concentrations vary widely among individuals. The drug is minimally metabolized and renally eliminated. Sequestration in bone results in a long terminal half-life. Foscarnet penetrates the blood-brain barrier and thus may be useful in the treatment of CMV encephalitis.

### Clinical trials

Foscarnet is thought to be as effective as ganciclovir in AIDS patients with CMV retinitis; however, it is less convenient to administer and more toxic. In a randomized, controlled trial of foscarnet in 24 AIDS patients with CMV retinitis, the mean time to progression of retinitis was 3.2 weeks in the control group (delayed therapy) compared with 13.3 weeks in the treatment group. Two small, uncontrolled trials demonstrated stabilization or improvement in AIDS patients with CMV retinitis treated with foscarnet. Unfortunately, most patients eventually progress and require reinduction or change in therapy.

Foscarnet is also used in the treatment of acyclovir-resistant HSV. In a randomized trial comparing foscarnet with vidarabine for acyclovir-resistant mucocutaneous HSV in 14 AIDS patients, foscarnet demonstrated superior efficacy; the lesions of all 8 patients assigned to the foscarnet arm healed completely. In an uncontrolled trial of foscarnet therapy in 4 AIDS patients with severe ulcerative disease due to acyclovir-resistant, thymidine kinase negative HSV-2 infection, foscarnet resulted in dramatic clinical improvement.

Foscarnet has independent anti-HIV activity and intravenous foscarnet therapy decreases HIV p24 antigen in patients with CMV retinitis. This anti-HIV activity presumably is the cause of decreased mortality in patients with CMV retinitis treated with foscarnet compared with those treated with ganciclovir. In a multicenter, randomized trial in 234 AIDS patients with CMV retinitis, the median survival was 8.5 months in the ganciclovir group and 12.6 months in the foscarnet group. However, foscarnet's considerable toxicity and inconvenient administration limit the clinical utility of this improved survival data, particularly in patients with impaired kidney function.

### Dosage

Patients with a CrCl <1.6 ml/min/kg require dose adjustment. For CMV retinitis, induction therapy with 60 mg/kg q8h over 1 h for 14–21 days is reduced to maintenance dosing 90 to 120 mg/kg daily administered over 2 h. For HSV and VZV, 40 mg/kg IV q8h for 14–21 days is appropriate. The drug must be administered over 1 hour with an infusion pump to prevent toxicity induced by bolus injection. Thrombophlebitis occurs with administration through peripheral veins and if given peripherally, the drug must be diluted to prevent phlebitis. Foscarnet has been administered to hemodialysis patients with plasma level monitoring. The successful use of intravitreal foscarnet has been described.

### Side effects

Acute tubular necrosis, hypocalcemia, anemia, seizures, nausea, abnormal liver function tests, and penile ulcers are among the numerous adverse effects associated with foscarnet. When used with intravenous pentamidine, foscarnet may precipitate severe hypocalcemia. Up to two-thirds of foscarnet courses are complicated by renal toxicity. Administration with other nephrotoxic agents such as amphotericin B, cyclosporine, aminoglycosides, and pentamidine may exacerbate renal insufficiency. Prehydration with 500 ml to 1 L of normal saline appears to reduce foscarnet-associated nephrotoxicity. Anemia is also common, particularly when foscarnet is used in combination with AZT. Close monitoring of creatinine, electrolytes (calcium, phosphate, magnesium, potassium), and CBCs is necessary.

### Precautions

Rabbits and rats injected with foscarnet during gestation had an increased incidence of skeletal anomalies in their offspring. Lactating rats had high levels of foscarnet in their milk. Foscarnet is deposited in bone and may alter skeletal development with long-term use in children.

### Resistance

Both HSV- and CMV-resistant strains have occurred with prolonged foscarnet administration. Resistance is due to mutations in the viral DNA polymerase gene. These strains are pathogenic. Most strains will be sensitive to other antivirals. However, as foscarnet is frequently used for GCV- or ACV-resistant isolates that have already failed standard therapy with ganciclovir or acyclovir, respectively, foscarnet-resistant HSV and CMV may be difficult to manage. Strains resistant to both classes of drugs have also been described. Sensitivity testing is recommended if resistance is suspected clinically. Concurrent use of foscarnet and ganciclovir after failure of either alone may be successful.

### Cost

Foscarnet is expensive to purchase and incurs considerable cost in its administration and monitoring. Excluding the expense of prehydration and laboratory work, CMV maintenance therapy costs approximately $2200 a month.

## Cidofovir

Cidofovir (Vistide, HPMPC, Gilead Sciences) is a recently approved antiviral drug with activity against herpesviruses, including CMV, HSV, VZV, and EBV.

### Mechanism of action

Cidofovir is a monophosphate nucleotide analogue that inhibits viral DNA polymerase. In contrast to nucleoside analogues, such as ganciclovir and acyclovir, cidofovir contains a pre-existing phosphate group that enables it to bypass initial virus-dependent phosphorylation. Cellular enzymes convert cidofovir to the active diphosphate form in both infected and uninfected cells.

### Indications

Currently, the only indication for cidofovir is AIDS-associated CMV retinitis.

### Pharmacokinetics

Cidofovir has a long intracellular half-life and thus can be administered weekly during induction and every other week during maintenance therapy. Probenecid blocks active renal tubular secretion of cidofovir. There are minimal data on cidofovir pharmacokinetics in patients with renal insufficiency or requiring dialysis. Limited evidence shows that CSF concentrations of cidofovir are low.

### Clinical trials

In a randomized, controlled trial of 64 AIDS patients with previously untreated peripheral CMV retinitis, intravenous cidofovir slowed the progression of CMV retinitis. Median time to progression was 21 days in the group that received deferred therapy, 64 days in the low-dose (3 mg/kg) cidofovir group, and was not reached in the group that received high-dose (5 mg/kg) cidofovir. Of note, cidofovir did not substantially suppress CMV viremia. Another study was a randomized, controlled multi-center maintenance dose comparison trial conducted in 100 patients with relapsing CMV retinitis after extensive previous therapy with ganciclovir and/or foscarnet. There was a statistically significant difference in the median time to retinitis progression between the high-dose and lose-dose maintenance groups. Median time to retinitis progression for the 5 mg/kg maintenance group was 115 days and for the 3 mg/kg group was 49 days; unfortunately, few patients on the 5 mg/kg dose remained on therapy over time, limiting interpretation of these results.

### Dosage

The suggested dose is 5 mg/kg IV weekly for 2 weeks as induction, then the same dose every other week as maintenance. The drug is infused over 1 hour; compatibility with Ringer's solution or bacteriostatic infusion fluids has not been evaluated. Probenecid and hydration are required. Patients should receive 1 l of normal saline over 1–2 hours prior to receiving cidofovir. If extra fluid can be tolerated, patients should receive a second liter after the cidofovir infusion. Do not exceed the recommended dosage, frequency, or infusion rate. The probenecid dose is 2 g at 3 hours prior to the cidofovir dose and 1 g at 2 hours after the dose and 1 g at 8 hours, for a total of 4 g. The package insert provides a dosing schedule for renal insufficiency. Although there have been reports of intravitreal use, the manufacturer advises against intraocular injection.

### Side effects

Nephrotoxicity is the major side effect of cidofovir. This is manifested by proteinuria, glucosuria, a Fanconi-like syndrome (metabolic acidosis), and increased serum creatinine levels. Neutropenia may also occur, so neutrophil counts should be monitored. Serum creatinine and urine protein should be checked prior to each dose of cidofovir. If serum creatinine increases 0.3–0.4 mg/dl, the cidofovir dose should be reduced from 5 mg/kg to 3 mg/kg. If the serum creatinine increases >0.5 mg/dl or >3+ proteinuria develops, cidofovir should be discontinued. Administration of cidofovir with other nephrotoxic drugs should be avoided. Iritis and hypotonia can develop after intraocular injections. Ocular hypotonia may also occur with intravenous cidofovir.

Probenecid decreases nephrotoxicity but can cause side effects such as nausea, vomiting, fever, and hypersensitivity. Administration of probenecid with food and the use of antiemetics may decrease nausea and vomiting. While acetaminophen and antihistamines are suggested for minor hypersensitivity reactions, the use of probenecid and cidofovir is contraindicated in those with severe probenecid hypersensitivity. Probenecid has multiple drug interactions. On days of cidofovir infusion, HIV patients taking AZT may skip or half their dose because probenecid decreases AZT clearance.

### Precautions

Studies done in animals have reported an association between subcutaneous cidofovir and local neoplasms in female rats. Thus far, there have been no parallel findings in humans treated with cidofovir. Cidofovir inhibits spermatogenesis and is embryotoxic in animals and should not be given to pregnant women or nursing mothers. For these reasons, the National Institutes of Health recommends that preparation of cidofovir occur in a class II laminar flow biological safety cabinet by a gloved and gowned worker and that excess drug and soiled materials be disposed of safely.

### Resistance

Cidofovir resistance has developed in vitro; such cidofovir-resistant isolates were cross-resistant to ganciclovir but susceptible to foscarnet. The majority of ganciclovir-resistant CMV isolated from patients remain susceptible to cidofovir, but a minority are due to DNA polymerase mutations and are therefore resistant. Cidofovir is active against some foscarnet-resistant CMV isolates.

### Cost

The approximate price of a 5 mg/kg dose of cidofovir for a 70 kg patient is $750, not including the cost of hydration, equipment, nursing time, or laboratory tests.

## Drugs for Influenza A Virus

### Amantadine

Amantadine (Symmetrel, DuPont) is a symmetric tricyclic amine that is effective for the treatment and prophylaxis of influenza A infection.

#### Mechanism of action

Amantadine prevents viral uncoating upon cell entry so that viral RNA is not released into the cell; the drug alters the activity of the M2 protein found in the membrane of influenza A–infected cells.

#### Indications

Amantadine is used as prophylaxis against and treatment for influenza A. Prophylaxis with amantadine can reduce the morbidity from institutional outbreaks of influenza and protect high-risk individuals during epidemics. It can also be used for immunodeficient patients unable to adequately respond to vaccine and in those for whom influenza vaccine is contraindicated. When given for outbreak control, all residents of an affected institution should be prophylaxed, regardless of their vaccination status. Amantadine can be given with vaccination; neither amantadine nor rimantadine interferes with the efficacy of influenza vaccine or development of antibodies post-vaccination. Clinically amantadine is not effective against influenza B and parainfluenza virus.

#### Pharmacokinetics

Oral amantadine is well absorbed and available as capsules, tablets, or syrup. The drug is renally eliminated with minimal metabolism. Concentrations in CSF are about half those in plasma.

#### Clinical trials

When initiated before exposure to influenza A, amantadine is 70%–90% effective in preventing disease. In 450 volunteers in a placebo-controlled, double-blind, randomized trial of rimantadine and amantadine prophylaxis during an influenza outbreak, laboratory-documented influenza occurred in 21% of placebo recipients versus 2%–3% of treated subjects. When treatment is started within 48 h of onset of illness, it may reduce the duration of fever and symptoms. In 45 university students with proven influenza A infection treated with either amantadine, rimantadine, or placebo, the drug recipients had significantly less fever and greater improvement than the placebo recipients.

#### Dosage

A dosage of 200 mg/day for 3–5 days is the standard dose of amantadine in healthy adults. Amantadine can be given in one or two divided doses. The dosage should be adjusted to 100 mg daily orally in the elderly and decreased for renal impairment. Hemodialysis patients need only weekly dosing. The drug is safe for treatment and prophylaxis of children older than 1 year of age. Prophylaxis and treatment doses are the same. In outbreak situations, prophylaxis should be given for 2 weeks or until 1 week after the end of the outbreak. Children may require up to 6 weeks of prophylaxis after vaccination. There have been studies indicating that 100 mg daily may be an effective prophylaxis dose in healthy adults.

#### Side effects

Among healthy adults, 5%–10% suffer CNS side effects with amantadine use, including confusion, lightheadedness, anxiety, insomnia, seizures, and hallucinations. Elderly users are more likely to suffer untoward effects. About 40% of 79 treated retirement home patients had adverse reactions in one retrospective cohort study. The drug has anticholinergic-like side effects, such as dry mouth, blurred vision, constipation, and urinary retention. Five to ten percent of amantadine recipients report nausea. Side effects may diminish after the first week of therapy.

#### Precautions

CNS side effects are exacerbated by anticholinergic medications. Amantadine is teratogenic in animals and contraindicated in pregnancy and lactation. Children with epilepsy who receive amantadine have an increased incidence of seizures.

#### Resistance

In vitro resistance to amantadine develops easily through virus passage in the presence of drug. Studies have found amantadine-resistant strains of influenza A, particularly H3N2. Resistance may rapidly develop during treatment and transmission of amantadine-resistant strains among family members as well as among nursing home residents is well documented. This may result in failure of drug prophylaxis. Thus, it is advisable to separate treated patients and susceptible high-risk contacts. There is cross-resistance between amantadine and rimantadine. Resistant viruses cause typical influenzal illness. Because of the induction of resistance, treatment courses should be limited to 3–5 days or 24–48 h after illness resolution.

#### Cost

The drug is inexpensive, especially if a generic substitute is prescribed. A 5-day course costs about $6.

### Rimantadine

Rimantadine (Flumadine, Forest) is an analogue of amantadine that is effective for the therapy and prevention of influenza A.

#### Mechanism of action

The mechanism of action is the same as that of amantadine—the prevention of viral uncoating.

#### Indication

Rimantadine is indicated for the prophylaxis and treatment of influenza A in adults and prevention of influenza in children. Like amantadine, it is not active against influenza B.

### Pharmacokinetics

Like amantadine, rimantadine is well absorbed after oral administration. Unlike amantadine, the drug is extensively metabolized in the liver before being renally eliminated. This is beneficial in that dose adjustments are not needed unless the CrCl is <10 ml/min. The drug has a plasma half-life twice as long as amantadine.

### Clinical trials

In a randomized, double-blind, prophylaxis trial in 110 children, 31% of children in the placebo arm and 7% in the rimantadine arm developed influenza infection. In a randomized, double-blind treatment trial in 14 adults with uncomplicated influenza, rimantadine decreased viral shedding, fever, and symptoms compared with placebo.

### Dosage

The usual dose is 100 mg PO bid for 3–5 days. Pharmacokinetically, once-a-day dosing of 200 mg should be equally effective. The dosage of rimantadine should be reduced to 100 mg/day in elderly nursing home residents, patients with severe hepatic dysfunction, and recipients with a CrCl <10 ml/min. There are studies that indicate 100 mg/day may be adequate for prophylaxis in patients with normal metabolism as well.

### Side effects

The incidence of adverse experiences is similar to that in placebo recipients and less than with amantadine therapy. The risk of CNS side effects is much less with rimantadine than amantadine. However, the incidence of gastrointestinal side effects (such as nausea) is the same. There have been reports of seizures associated with rimantadine.

### Precautions

Rimantadine is FDA approved for prophylaxis but not for treatment of children. Like amantadine, rimantadine is contraindicated in pregnancy and breast feeding.

### Resistance

Resistance to rimantadine does occur clinically and may develop during treatment. The transmission of resistant viruses may present difficulties in the prophylaxis of family members. Viruses that are resistant to amantadine will be resistant to rimantadine and vice versa.

### Cost

Although rimantadine is more expensive than amantadine, a 3-day course of therapy still costs less than $10.

## Other Antiviral Drugs

## Ribavirin

Ribavirin (Virazole, ICN Pharmaceuticals) is a guanosine analog that inhibits the in vitro replication of a wide spectrum of viral pathogens including respiratory syncytial virus (RSV), influenza, paramyxo- and arena virus.

### Mechanism of action

The mechanism of action is not fully elucidated. As a synthetic nucleoside analog, ribavirin seems to interfere with the expression of messenger RNA and inhibit viral protein synthesis. Since the drug is active against a variety of viruses, it may employ several different mechanisms to inhibit viral replication.

### Indications

The American Academy of Pediatrics recommends aerosolized ribavirin for RSV in patients at risk for complications (congenital heart disease, cystic fibrosis, prematurity, immunodeficiency) and for those who are severely ill ($PaO_2 < 65$ mm Hg, increasing $PaCO_2$) or mechanically ventilated for RSV infection. Although it is acceptable to initiate empiric therapy, continuing therapy should be based on results of a rapid diagnostic method for RSV such as viral antigen detection by immunofluorescence. Aerosolized ribavirin has also been used in the treatment of parainfluenza and measles viral pneumonia. Anecdotal case reports suggest its utility in amantadine-resistant influenza A. However, controlled trials of these situations are not available.

Intravenous ribavirin decreases mortality in Lassa fever and hantavirus-induced hemorrhagic fever with renal syndrome (HFRS). Ribavirin has been used successfully for Congo-Crimean fever and Argentine hemorrhagic fever as well, but there are no controlled trials. Oral ribavirin has been suggested as a prophylactic agent for Lassa fever and Congo-Crimean fever contacts. Results of studies of its use in pulmonary hantavirus infections are pending.

Although ribavirin has beneficial effects on serum transaminases and liver histology in patients with chronic hepatitis C, these effects are not accompanied by decreased HCV RNA levels and regress when ribavirin is discontinued. As such, ribavirin as a single agent cannot be recommended for the treatment of HCV. Ribavirin is not an effective therapy for HIV infection.

### Pharmacokinetics

Ribavirin has complex pharmacokinetics and a long terminal half-life. The drug is concentrated in red blood cells and persists throughout the life of the cell. Only a third of a ribavirin dose is excreted by the kidneys. The drug is not removed by hemodialysis. Despite drug accumulation over time, peak plasma ribavirin concentrations following aerosolized therapy do not exceed 4 $\mu$g/ml. Respiratory secretion levels are about 1000 times higher than plasma levels.

### Clinical trials

Several trials have shown a modest benefit of aerosolized ribavirin in improving illness, lower respiratory tract signs, and arterial oxygen saturation and viral shedding in infants with pulmonary disease. In the late 1980s, a randomized double-blind, placebo-controlled trial in 28 infants on mechanical ventilation for RSV indicated that ribavirin decreased duration of mechanical ventilation, oxygen treatment, and hospital stay.

A trial in Sierra Leone compared untreated historical controls with Lassa fever with a group treated with IV or oral ribavirin demonstrated a survival benefit with oral and intravenous ribavirin in patients with severe illness as indicated by elevated aspartate aminotransferase and higher degrees of viremia. A prospective randomized double-blind, concurrent, placebo-controlled clinical trial of intravenous ribavirin was conducted in 242 patients with (HFRS) in the People's Republic of China; mortality was decreased sevenfold in the ribavirin arm.

### Dosage

Oral and intravenous ribavirin are not marketed in the United States. The aerosol is the only formulation licensed in the United States. In pediatric RSV infection, a small particle aerosol diluted to 20 mg/ml is delivered to the patient by oxygen hood, mask, or tent over 12–20 h/day for 3–5 days for RSV bronchiolitis or pneumonia. Higher doses given over shorter periods have been tried as a more easily administered alternative to standard therapy. A special nebulizer is provided by the manufacturer as the drug is relatively insoluble. An intravenous 2 g load then 1 g q6h for 4 days, then 0.5 g q8h for 6 days is the regimen used for Lassa fever.

### Side effects

Aerosolized ribavirin may cause rash, conjunctivitis, and wheezing. Acute deterioration of respiratory function in infants has occurred with initiation of aerosolized ribavirin; thus, close monitoring is required. Systemic ribavirin causes hemolysis with anemia, reticulocytosis, and hyperbilirubinemia, which is dose related and reversible.

### Precautions

Ribavirin is teratogenic and embryotoxic in animals and should not be used during pregnancy. While most institutions recommend that pregnant women not care for patients receiving ribavirin aerosol, health care workers absorb little of the aerosolized drug.

The aerosol tends to crystallize and obstruct mechanical ventilators. This can be prevented by inserting filters, modifying circuits, and frequent monitoring, but it requires that staff be familiar with this mode of drug administration.

Ribavirin has immunosuppressive effects in experimental animals and decreases the formation of RSV-specific neutralizing antibodies and nasopharyngeal RSV-specific IgE in treated children. The clinical consequences of this immunosuppression are unknown. Ribavirin causes seminiferous tubule atrophy and impaired spermatogenesis in rodents; the clinical implications of this finding are unclear.

### Resistance

Resistance to ribavirin has not been recognized clinically.

### Cost

Aerosolized ribavirin is expensive to purchase and administer. The price of a single dose is almost $1400 for the drug alone.

## Interferon $\alpha$

Interferon $\alpha$ (IFN-$\alpha$) is a protein induced by viral infections and double-stranded RNA, principally produced by peripheral blood leukocytes. Recombinant IFN-$\alpha$ products include $\alpha$-2a (Roferon-A, Roche) and $\alpha$-2b (Intron A, Schering).

### Mechanism of action

Interferon induces cellular proteins which, depending on the cell type and infecting virus, can inhibit viral protein synthesis and degrade viral components.

### Indications

Recombinant and natural IFN-$\alpha$ is approved in the United States for treatment of condyloma acuminatum and laryngeal papillomatosis, chronic HBV, chronic HCV, Kaposi's sarcoma in HIV-infected patients, and hairy cell leukemia. It has also been used for HIV-associated thrombocytopenia, HCV-associated cryoglobulinemia, and HBV-related glomerulonephritis. Although intramuscular or subcutaneous interferon has been tried for other illnesses including herpes zoster and intranasally for rhinovirus infection, there are better, less toxic treatments available for these disorders.

### Pharmacokinetics

Interferon is well absorbed after IM or subcutaneous administration. Levels peak 4–8 hours after IM injection. It is thought to be catabolized by the kidney. CNS penetration is poor.

### Clinical trials

There are multiple studies of both systemic and intralesional interferon for genital warts. In one randomized double-blind, placebo-controlled, multicenter study of 257 subjects, interferon used intralesionally 3 times weekly for 3 weeks significantly prevented wart progression and decreased wart area; 36% of interferon recipients had complete wart clearance. A similar trial in 158 patients using twice weekly IFN-$\alpha$ for up to 8 weeks eliminated warts in 62% of the treated patients compared with only 21% of the patients receiving placebo. Other studies have demonstrated a response rate closer to 50%. In one study using three different interferon preparations ($\alpha$-2b, $\alpha$-nl and $\beta$) $1 \times 10^6$ three times weekly, one-third of the interferon-injected warts recurred. In a double-blind, placebo-controlled trial employing 178 subjects, systemic interferon produced greater rates of condyloma resolution than placebo, but rates of complete response were low. The authors concluded that parenteral interferon might be useful as part of combination therapy. Intralesional interferon has been demonstrated to enhance the effect of topical podophyllin. Higher doses of interferon are associated with greater response, but the associated increased toxicity may be difficult for patients to tolerate.

The benefit of interferon therapy in chronic hepatitis B has been studied extensively. In a randomized controlled trial of IFN-$\alpha$-2b in 169 patients with chronic hepatitis B, five million units daily for 16 weeks resulted in the disappearance of HBeAg and

HBV DNA from serum in approximately 40% of patients. Decreased transaminases, disappearance of replicative forms of HBV DNA in the liver and improved histologic appearance are associated with response to therapy. Remissions in chronic HBV that are induced by interferon are long-lasting and may result in loss of HBsAg.

In about half of 14 patients with chronic hepatitis D treated with high doses of IFN-$\alpha$-2a for 48 weeks, HDV RNA became undetectable in serum, transaminases normalized, and there was histologic improvement. However, relapse was common once therapy was discontinued.

In chronic hepatitis C virus (HCV) infection, about 50% of those treated with interferon respond with decreased transaminases and improved liver histology. However, 50% of responders relapse after therapy is stopped. Long-term responders to IFN-$\alpha$ have eradication of HCV RNA in their serum and livers and significant improvement histologically. Patients with initially low HCV viremia are more likely to have a sustained response to interferon. Hepatitis C virus RNA persistence at the completion of interferon therapy predicts relapse. In chronic non-A non-B hepatitis patients randomized to 6 versus 18 months of three million units of IFN-$\alpha$-b three times weekly, patients treated longer had more sustained normalization of liver function tests (LFTs) and improved liver histology at 18 months. A subgroup treated with one million units did not show as much improvement in alanine aminotransferase values and liver histology as the three-million unit group. A lengthy course (18 rather than 6 months) at higher doses (three million rather than one million units) may produce more histological improvement and lower serum alanine aminotransferase values. A recent study of 90 patients with chronic active hepatitis C with cirrhosis indicated that interferon not only improved liver function but also decreased the incidence of hepatocellular carcinoma from 38% in the control arm to 4% in the interferon arm.

### Dosage

The dosing for genital warts is 1 million units per lesion up to a maximum of 5 lesions intralesionally 3 times weekly for 3 weeks. In chronic HBV, 5 million units SQ or IM daily for 4 months is recommended. In chronic HCV, the usual course is three million units SQ or IM 3 times per week for 6 to 18 months.

### Side effects

Interferon may cause a flu-like syndrome, particularly during the first week of IM or SQ therapy, with fever, chills, headache, myalgia, arthralgia, and nausea, vomiting, and diarrhea. These side effects can occur even after intralesional therapy. High-dose or chronic therapy may cause bone marrow suppression (particularly in combination with myelotoxic drugs such as AZT), fatigue, anorexia, psychiatric symptoms, hypo- or hyperthyroidism, elevated liver function tests, alopecia, autoantibody formation, and cardiotoxicity. Tenderness and erythema at injection site can occur as well. Premedication with acetaminophen is recommended.

### Precautions

High doses of interferon cause abortion in monkeys. The drug may impair fertility and alter estradiol and progesterone levels. Safety in human pregnancy is unknown and the drug is not recommended in pregnant nor nursing mothers.

Autoimmune chronic hepatitis is exacerbated by IFN-$\alpha$ therapy.

Interferon reduces the metabolism of certain drugs by the hepatic cytochrome P450 system; reduced theophylline clearance has been reported.

### Resistance

Although neutralizing antibodies may develop with interferon therapy, it is unclear whether such antibodies are associated with resistance.

### Cost

Interferon is expensive to purchase, administer, and monitor through laboratory work. A typical treatment course for HCV costs over $2200 for the medication alone. A meta-analysis of nine randomized controlled trials and cost-effectiveness analysis indicated that IFN therapy should lower costs for patients with chronic HBV who are HBeAg positive. However, this analysis may not apply to the HBeAg-negative HBV patients and HCV patients. A standard intralesional treatment course for genital warts costs about $360. Cryotherapy and podophyllin are generally much cheaper and adequate in the majority of patients with genital warts.

## ANNOTATED BIBLIOGRAPHY


Beutner KR, Friedman DJ, Forszpaniak C, et al. Valacyclovir compared with acyclovir for improved therapy for herpes zoster in immunocompetent adults. Antimicrob Agents Chemother 1995; 39:1546–1553.

*A randomized, double-blind, multicenter study demonstrating the safety and efficacy of oral valaciclovir for the treatment of herpes zoster; valaciclovir also accelerates the resolution of zoster-associated pain.*

Centers for Disease Control and Prevention. 1998 Guidelines for treatment of sexually transmitted disease. MMWR 1998; 47(No. RR-1):20–26.

Dolin R, Reichman RC, Madore HP, et al. A controlled trial of amantadine and rimantadine in the prophylaxis of influenza A infection. N Engl J Med 1982; 307:580–584.

*A large randomized, placebo-controlled, double-blind trial concluding that rimantadine is the drug of choice for the prophylaxis of influenza A.*

Drew WL, Ives D, Lalezari JP, et al. Oral ganciclovir as maintenance treatment for cytomegalovirus retinitis in patients with AIDS. N Engl J Med 1995; 333:615–620.

*An open-label randomized study demonstrating the safety, efficacy, and convenience of oral ganciclovir for maintenance therapy of cytomegalovirus retinitis in patients with AIDS.*

Emanuel D, Cunningham I, Jules-Elysee K, et al. Cytomegalovirus pneumonia after bone marrow transplantation successfully treated with the combination of ganciclovir and high-dose intravenous immune globulin. Ann Intern Med 1988; 109:777–782.

*Ganciclovir combined with high-dose intravenous immunoglobulin decreased mortality in a small number of bone marrow transplant recipients with CMV pneumonia as compared with historical controls.*

Eron LJ, Judson F, Tucker S, et al. Interferon therapy for condyloma acuminata. N Engl J Med 1986; 315:1059–1064.

*Describes a large randomized, double-blind trial of intralesional IFN-α-2b.*

Nishiguchi S, Kuroki T, Nakatani S, et al. Randomised trial of effects of interferon-$\alpha$ on incidence of hepatocellular carcinoma in chronic active hepatitis C with cirrhosis. Lancet 1995; 346:1051–1055.

*Interferon-α improved liver function in chronic active hepatitis C with cirrhosis and decreased the incidence of hepatocellular carcinoma.*

Perillo RP, Schiff ER, Davis GL, et al. Randomized controlled trial of interferon alfa-2b alone and after prednisone withdrawal for the treatment of chronic hepatitis B. N Engl J Med 1990; 323:295–301.

*In chronic hepatitis B, treatment with IFN-α-2b induced a biochemical and histologic remission in over a third of patients.*

Poynard T, Bedossa P, Chevallier M, et al. A comparison of three interferon alpha-2b regimens for the long-term treatment of chronic non-A, non-B hepatitis. N Engl J Med 1995; 332:1457–1462.

*Describes histologic and liver function test improvement with a regimen of 3 million units of IFN-α-2b given three times a week for 18 months.*

Safrin S, Crumpacker C, Chatis P, et al. A controlled trial comparing foscarnet with vidarabine for acyclovir-resistant mucocutaneous herpes simplex in the acquired immunodeficiency syndrome. N Engl J Med 1991; 325:551–555.

*A small study of successful foscarnet therapy in HIV-infected individuals with acyclovir-resistant HSV infections; relapse was common after treatment was discontinued.*

Smith DW, Frankel LR, Mathers LH, et al. A controlled trial of aerosolized ribavirin in infants receiving mechanical ventilation for severe respiratory syncytial virus infection. N Engl J Med 1991; 325:24–29.

*Supports the use of aerosolized ribavirin in infants requiring mechanical ventilation for RSV.*

Studies of Ocular Complications of AIDS Research Group, in collaboration with the AIDS Clinical Trials Group. Mortality in patients with the acquired immunodeficiency syndrome treated with either foscarnet or ganciclovir for cytomegalovirus retinitis. N Engl J Med 1992; 326:213–220.

*Foscarnet was associated with longer survival but greater toxicity than ganciclovir treatment for CMV retinitis in this multicenter randomized trial.*

Studies of Ocular Complications of AIDS Research Group, in collaboration with the AIDS Clinical Trials Group. Parenteral cidofovir for cytomegalovirus retinitis in patients with AIDS: the HPMC peripheral cytomegalovirus trial. Ann Intern Med 1997; 126:264–274.

*Intravenous cidofovir effectively slowed the progression of CMV retinitis but nephrotoxicity was a major side effect.*

Tyring S, Barbarash RA, Nahlik JE, et al. Famciclovir for the treatment of acute herpes zoster: effects on acute disease and postherpetic neuralgia. Ann Intern Med 1995; 123:89–96.

*A randomized, double-blind, placebo-controlled, multicenter trial showing decreased duration of postherpetic neuralgia with oral famciclovir therapy of herpes zoster.*

Van Voris LP, Betts RF, Hayden FG, et al. Successful treatment of naturally occurring influenza A/USSR/77H1N1. JAMA 1981; 245:1128–1131.

*A placebo-controlled demonstration of the benefits of antiviral therapy for influenza A in university students.*

Whitley RJ, Alford CA, Hirsch MS, et al. Vidarabine versus acyclovir therapy in herpes simplex encephalitis. N Engl J Med 1986; 314:144–149.

*Describes improved survival and decreased morbidity with acyclovir treatment of herpes simplex virus encephalitis.*

# 40

# Antiparasitic Drugs and Therapy

KEITH B. ARMITAGE

While therapy of many infections due to parasitic protozoa and helminths has improved in the past 10 years, many problems remain, including development of resistance to previously effective agents, toxic side effects of some of the currently recommended agents, and unavailability of certain drugs in the United States. In this chapter the mechanism of action, route of administration, major toxicities, and other pharmacological parameters of antiparasitic drugs are reviewed. Antiparasitic agents can be divided by the class of organism they primarily target (e.g., protozoa, or subgroups of helminths, e.g., nematodes, cestodes, and trematodes) or by whether they are systemic agents or primarily act locally. The indications and dosage for specific infections, as well as other treatment issues, are discussed following the pharmacologic information.

In Table 40.1, antiparasitic agents are listed in alphabetical order with indications, toxicity, and route of administration. Table 40.2 lists specific parasitic infections and the primary and alternative therapies. Additional information is provided in the text. Throughout the chapter and tables, the doses listed are for average-sized adults unless otherwise specified.

## Systemic Anti-protozoan Drugs

### Antimalarials

Antimalarials are used for both prophylaxis and treatment of infection due to *Plasmodium* species. The use of a specific therapy depends on the species involved and the geographic location.

#### Chloroquine phosphate

This is a 4-aminoquinolone used primarily for treatment and prophylaxis of *Plasmodium vivax*, *P. malaria*, *P. ovale*, and sensitive strains of *P. falciparum* (now limited to a few geographic areas). Chloroquine can be given orally with food or injected parenterally. Parenteral dosing may be associated with respiratory depression, hypotension, cardiac arrest, and seizures, particularly following rapid administration. Parenteral therapy should be used for patients unable to take oral medicine, and patients should be switched to the oral route as soon as possible.

Oral doses of chloroquine are greater than 90% absorbed, and intramuscular (IM) and subcutaneous (SQ) doses are also rapidly absorbed. Because of the large volume of distribution, a loading dose is required. The drug undergoes extensive metabolism, and approximately 50% is excreted by the kidney. In renal failure the therapeutic dose is not altered, but prophylactic doses should be reduced. The precise mechanism of action of chloroquine is unknown; it is known that chloroquine raises the pH of *Plasmodium* lysosomal vesicles and inhibits proteolysis of hemoglobin.

In therapy of malaria, chloroquine is very active against the asexual erythrocytic stages of sensitive strains and its administration leads to rapid clinical improvement. Chloroquine is indicated for the erythrocytic stage of sensitive strains of malaria species. In most areas of the world, *P. falciparum* is resistant; in addition, there have been isolated reports of *P. vivax* resistance in Papua New Guinea and Indonesia. Chloroquine has no exo-erythrocytic activity and therefore is of no use against tissue stages. When used to treat the erythrocytic stages of *P. vivax* and *P. ovale*, its use must be followed with an agent active against the tissue phase.

Chloroquine phosphate is supplied as 250 and 500 mg tablets and in the United States is sold under the trade name Aralen. Hydroxychloroquine sulfate (Plaquinil) is supplied in 200 mg tablets, and for dosing 400 mg of hydroxychloroquine sulfate is equal to 500 mg of chloroquine hydrochloride. Chloroquine hydrochloride for injection is supplied at a concentration of 50 mg/ml. For prophylaxis, 500 mg of chloroquine is given once a week. Therapy is started 2 weeks before exposure, and continued 8 weeks after. The dose in acute infection is 1 g, followed by 500 mg 6–8 h later, followed by 500 mg/day for 2 days for a total dose of 2.5 g. Parenteral dosing schedules are not as well established, but chloroquine can be given in a dose of 3.5 mg/kg q6h, for a total dose of 2.5 g. Children should not be given more than 10 mg/kg/day regardless of the route, and the usual dose is 5 mg/kg.

Common side effects of the dose of chloroquine used in acute attacks include gastrointestinal (GI) upset, pruritus, headache, and visual changes. As above, intravenous preparations are available, and should be used cautiously as rapid infusion can lead to cardiovascular collapse. The prophylactic dose is usually very well tolerated, although prolonged use can lead to skin eruptions and nail changes. Prolonged high daily doses have been associated with more serious side effects such as myopathy and neuropathy. Chloroquine is contraindicated in severe hepatic disease, psoriasis, and porphyrias. Chloroquine is an optional therapy in the treatment of extraintestinal amoebiasis, and because of its anti-inflammatory properties, chloroquine is used for the treatment of rheumatoid arthritis and some forms of lupus.

#### Mefloquine

This is a quinoline-carbinolamine compound active against chloroquine resistant *P. falciparum* in most parts of the world, and is used for prophylaxis and treatment of malaria where chloroquine resistance is likely. It is only available orally. Mefloquine has a very long half-life; the elimination time is 2–3 weeks. It is excreted in the feces and dosage adjustments do not need to be made in renal failure. The mechanism of action is unknown, but is probably similar to that for chloroquine. Like chloroquine, mefloquine is active only against the erythrocytic forms of the parasite. In the United States mefloquine is sold under the trade name Lariam and is supplied as 250 mg tablets.

**Table 40.1** Antiparasitic agents

| Agent | Indications | Route | Toxicity | Comments |
|---|---|---|---|---|
| Albendazole | Intestinal nematodes (including *Ascaris lumbricoides*, hookworm, *Trichuris trichiura*, *Enterobius vermicularis*, *Strongyloides stercoralis Capillaria philippinensis*,); cutaneous larva migrans, cysticercosis, hydatid cyst disease, *Trichostribgylus* sp., *Gnathostoma spinigerum* | PO | Common: diarrhea, abdominal pain<br>Rare: alopecia, leukopenia, increased hepatic transaminases | Some evidence for efficacy against *Enterocytozoon bieneusi* |
| Allopurinol | Leishmaniasis | PO | Rare: hypersensitivity reactions | Used in combination with antimonials; not FDA approved for this indication |
| Amphotericin B | Amoebic meningoencephalitis, leishmaniasis | | Common: nephrotoxicity immediate febrile reactions | Not FDA approved; for *Naegleria* infection, success reported with addition of rifampin and miconazole |
| Artemisinin | Therapy of chloroquine-resistant *P. falciparum* malaria | PO, IM, PR | Common: fever<br>Rare: transient heart block | Not FDA approved; artesunate and arteether have similar toxicity profiles; current use primarily limited to China and Vietnam |
| Atovaquone | PCP pneumonia, toxoplasmosis | PO | Common: rash, nausea, diarrhea | For PCP, oral alternative in patients unable to tolerate TMP/SMX; not FDA approved for toxoplasmosis |
| Azithromycin | Toxoplasmosis | PO, IV | Common: nausea | Pyrimethamine/sulfa is first choice; not FDA approved |
| Benznidazole | American trypanosomiasis | PO | Common: rash, GI upset, anxiety, dose-dependent neuropathy | Not FDA approved; not available in the U.S. |
| Bithionol | *Fasciola hepatica*<br>paragonimiasis | | Common: GI upset, abdominal pain, urticaria<br>Rare: leukopenia, hepatitis | Not FDA approved |
| Chloroquine | Prophylaxis and therapy of erythrocytic phase of *P. vivax*, *P. ovale*, and sensitive strains of *P. falciparum* malaria | PO, IV, IM | Occasional: GI upset, pruritus, myalgias, photophobia, dermatitis, alopecia<br>Rare: neuropathy, retinal injury heart block, myelosuppression, hemolysis | Toxicities dose related; parenteral > PO; toxicities more common with therapeutic dose than prophylactic dose |
| Clindamycin | Babesiosis, toxoplasmosis, PCP | PO, IV | Rare: antibiotic-associated diarrhea | Not approved by FDA for this indication |
| Dapsone | *Pneumocystis carinii* pneumonia | PO | Rare: GI upset, rash, hemolysis in G6PD deficiency, methemoglobinemia | Not approved by FDA for this indication |
| Diethylcarbamazine | *Wuchereria bancrofti*, *Brugia malayi*, *Mansonella ozzardi*, *Loa loa*, tropical eosinophilia, visceral larva migrans, *Onchocerca volvulus* | PO | Common: Mazzotti reaction (severe allergic reaction to dying microfilaria), GI upset<br>Rare: encephalopathy | |
| Diloxanide furoate | *Entamoeba histolytica* (asymptomatic), *Entamoeba polecki* luminal infection | PO | Common: GI upset, flatulence<br>Rare: diplopia, dizziness, pruritus, urticaria | Contraindicated in pregnancy; available from CDC; used for asymptomatic cyst passers and following therapy with metronidazole or other agent for system disease |

| | | | | |
|---|---|---|---|---|
| Doxycycline | Prophylaxis of resistant *P. falciparum* malaria | PO | Occasional: GI upset, rash from photosensitivity | Contraindicated in pregnancy, children <8 yr old; can be used therapeutically with quinine for chloroquine resistant *P. falciparum* malaria (see tetracycline) |
| Eflornithine (DFMO) | West African CNS trypanosomiasis | | Common: anemia, leukopenia, diarrhea<br>Rare: seizures, hearing loss | |
| Emetine | Amoebic liver abscess | IV, SQ | Common: GI upset, cardiac toxicity (EKG monitoring needed), muscle weakness, injection site pain<br>Rare: encephalopathy | Contraindicated in pregnancy; largely replaced by other agents in children <5 yr old, because of toxicity; EKG monitoring indicated while drug is being administered; dehydroemetine is similar to emetine, but is possibly less toxic |
| Furazolidone | Giardiasis | PO | Common: nausea, vomiting, headache rash, fever, allergic reaction including pulmonary infiltrates<br>Rare: hypotension, hemolytic anemia in G6PD deficiency, disulfiram reaction, polyneuritis, MAO-inhibitor reaction | Only drug available in liquid form for giardiasis; contraindicated in breast-feeding mothers and neonates |
| Halofantrine | Therapy of chloroquine resistant falciparum malaria | PO | Common: diarrhea, abdominal pain<br>Rare: prolongation of QT interval, pruritus | Not approved by FDA, experimental |
| Iodoquinol | Amoebiasis (asymptomatic), balantidiasis, *Dientamoeba fragilis* | PO | Occasional: GI upset, acne, rash, pruritus, slight enlargement of the thyroid gland<br>Rare: peripheral neuropathy after long-term use (months), optic neuritis, optic atrophy, loss of vision, iodine sensitivity | Contraindication: sensitivity to iodine; most toxicity is dose/duration dependent |
| Ivermectin | *Onchocerca volvulus*, *Strongyloides stercoralis* (alternative), *Wuchereria bancrofti*, *Brugia malayi* (alternative), broad range of nematodes and blood-sucking arthropods (use for these indications is investigational) | PO | Common: Mazzotti reaction (less than diethylcarbamazine)<br>Rare: hypotension | Contraindications: pregnancy, children <5 yr old; emerging agent for a variety of filarial and other helminthic infections |
| Ketoconazole | Leishmaniasis | PO | Rare: hepatitis | Drug interactions common; not FDA approved for this indication |
| Mebendazole | *Ascaris lumbricoides*, hookworm, *Trichuris trichiura*, *Enterobius vermicularis*, *Capillaria philippinensis*, *Gnathostoma spinigerum* (surgical removal is an alternative), *Mansonella perstans*, *Angiostrongylus cantonensis*, *Trichostrongylus* spp. (alternative), *Trichinella spiralis* (recommended by some; used with steroids), visceral larva migrans (alternative), *Echinococcus* spp. (alternative) | PO | Occasional: primarily GI upset<br>Rare: leukopenia, agranulocytosis, hypospermia | Minimal toxicity at usual doses; contraindicated in pregnancy |

(*continued*)

**Table 40.1** Antiparasitic agents—*Continued*

| Agent | Indications | Route | Toxicity | Comments |
|---|---|---|---|---|
| Mefloquine | Prophylaxis and therapy of chloroquine resistant *P. falciparum* malaria | PO | Occasional: GI upset, nightmares, visual disturbance, vertigo<br>Rare: seizures, confusion, psychosis, paresthesias, hypotension | Safety in pregnancy not established. Avoid use in patients with cardiac conduction abnormalities, or those taking beta-blockers for arrhythmias; toxicity more common with therapeutic dose; resistance is emerging in some areas, check with CDC for latest information |
| Meglumine antimonate | Leishmaniasis | IM, IV | Common: GI upset, rash, pruritus, nephrotoxicity | Not approved by FDA |
| Melarsoprol (arsenical) | African trypanosomiasis (CNS stage) | IV | Common: myocardial damage, proteinuria, hypertension, GI upset, peripheral neuropathy encephalopathy, local skin irritation<br>Rare: shock | Available from the CDC |
| Metronidazole | *Entamoeba histolytica* (invasive disease), giardiasis, trichomoniasis, *Blastocystis hominus*, *Entamoeba polecki*, *Balantidium coli* | PO, IV | Common: GI upset, headache, dry mouth, metallic taste, disulfiram-like effect with alcohol, vertigo, diarrhea, insomnia<br>Rare: seizures, encephalopathy, ataxia, peripheral neuropathy, pancreatitis, stomatitis | Not approved by FDA for giardiasis; avoid use in first trimester; more severe toxicities dose related; for amoebiasis, follow therapy with luminal agent |
| Niclosamide | *Diphylobothrium latum*, *Taenia solium*, *Taenia saginata*, *Dipylidium caninum*, *Hymenolepis nana* (alternative), *Fasciolopsis buski* | PO | Occasional: GI upset, pruritus<br>Rare: rash | Activity is limited to lumen of GI tract because of poor oral absorption; for treatment of *Taenia solium*, treatment is followed with a purge to reduce risk of autoinfection |
| Nifurtimox | American trypanosomiasis | PO | Common: insomnia, GI upset, polyneuritis, weight loss, memory loss, tremor, paresthesias<br>Rare: fever, pulmonary infiltrates seizures, psychological disturbances | Not approved by FDA; available from CDC |
| Ornidazole | Amoebiasis, giardiasis, trichomoniasis | PO | Common: dizziness, headache, GI upset<br>Rare: peripheral neuropathy | Similar to metronidazole; not available in the U.S.; some authors report less side effects than metronidazole |
| Oxamniquine | *Schistosoma mansoni* | PO | Occasional: headache, dizziness, GI upset<br>Rare: seizures, psychosis | |
| Paromomycin | Asymptomatic amoebiasis, cryptosporidiosis, *Dientamoeba fragilis* | PO | Common: GI upset<br>Rare: renal damage, eighth nerve damage | Efficacy in cryptosporidiosis not proven; also used for giardiasis in pregnancy |
| Pentamidine | *P. carinii* pneumonia, leishmaniasis, alternative for early stage of African trypanosomiasis | IV, IM | Common: abscesses at site of IM injection; fever, hypotension, hypoglycemia followed by diabetes mellitus, GI upset, hypocalcemia, nephrotoxicity<br>Rare: anaphylaxis, acute pancreatitis, hyperkalemia, liver damage, cardiotoxicity, rash, delirium | |
| Piperazine | Ascariasis | PO | Occasional: hypersensitivity, neurotoxicity<br>Rare: exacerbation of seizure disorder, visual disturbance, ataxia | Seizure disorder; not availble in the U.S.; used primarily when biliary or bowel obstruction from ascariasis |

| | | | | |
|---|---|---|---|---|
| Praziquantel | *Schistosoma* spp., *Clonorchis sinensis*, *Opisthorchis viverrini*, *Paragonimus westermani*, *Fasciolopsis buski*, *Heterophyes*, *Metagonimus yokogawai*, *Nanophyetus salmincola*, *Diphyllobothrium latum* (alternative), *Taenia solium* (adult worm and cysticercosis), *Taenia saginata* (alternative), *Dipylidium caninum* (alternative), *Hymenolepis nana* | PO | Occasional: GI upset, dizziness, hypersensitivity to dying cysticerci, malaise, sedation, eosinophilia, fatigue, fever<br>Rare: pruritus, rash | Contraindicated in ocular cysticercosis |
| Primaquine | Radical cure of exoerythrocytic stage of *P. vivax* and *P. ovale* malaria | PO | Common: hemolysis in G6PD deficiency, GI upset, neutropenia<br>Rare: CNS symptoms, arrhythmias, hypertension | Contraindicated in pregnancy |
| Propamidine | *Acanthamoeba* keratitis (topical application) | eye drops | | |
| Proguanil | With chloroquine, prophylaxis for *P. falciparum* in East Africa | PO | Rare: hematologic; higher doses, GI upset, hematuria, proteinuria | Not available in the U.S.; failures have been reported; must be taken daily |
| Pyrantel pamoate | Alternative for ascariasis, hookworms, enterobiasis, *Trichostrongylus* spp. | PO | Occasional: dizziness, GI upset<br>Rare: rash, fever | Contraindicated in pregnancy |
| Pyrimethamine | Presumptive therapy of chloroquine-resistant *P. falciparum* malaria; toxoplasmosis (use with clindamycin or sulfadiazine) | PO | Common: folic acid deficiency<br>Rare: fatal cutaneous reaction when combined with sulfadoxine (as Fansidar), rash, vomiting, convulsions, shock | Prophylactic use in malaria associated with fatal cutaneous reactions and is no longer recommended |
| Quinacrine HCL | Giardiasis | PO | Common: dizziness, headache, GI upset, yellow staining of skin,<br>Occasional: toxic psychosis, insomnia, bizarre dreams, blood dyscrasias, urticaria rash<br>Rare: seizures, fulminant hepatitis, severe dermatitis, retinal damage | Contraindicated in pregnancy and in patients with psoriasis; not available in the U.S. |
| Quinidine, quinine | Treatment of chloroquine resistant *P. falciparum* malaria, babesiosis | PO, IV<br>IM | Common: cinchonism (tinnitus, headache, nausea, abdominal pain, visual disturbance), photosensitivity, urticaria, GI upset;<br>Occasional: arrhythmias, drug fever hemolytic anemia, deafness, hypoglycemia,<br>Rare: with iv therapy: hypotension, heart block | For severe falciparum malaria: IV quinidine and exchange transfusion; parenteral toxicity > PO; EKG monitoring recommended during IV therapy; quinidine not FDA approved for this indication |
| Spiramycin | Cryptosporidiosis, toxoplasmosis | PO | Common: GI upset<br>Rare: allergic reaction | Used for toxoplasmosis in pregnancy; efficacy in cryptosporidiosis not proven, not available in the U.S. |
| Stibogluconate sodium (antimonial) | Leishmaniasis | IM, IV | Common: GI upset, pruritus, urticaria, paresthesias, photophobia, peripheral neuropathy<br>Rare: nephrotoxicity, EKG changes, shock, optic atrophy, blood dyscrasias | Not approved by FDA, available from the CDC |
| Sulfonamides | Malaria, toxoplasmosis, *P. carinii* pneumonia (treatment and prophylaxis when combined with pyrimethamine or trimethoprim) | PO | Common: allergic reactions<br>Rare: fever and severe dermatitis, serum sickness, crystalluria, neurotoxicity, and hepatotoxicity | Contraindicated in pregnancy, newborns |

(*continued*)

**Table 40.1** Antiparasitic agents—*Continued*

| Agent | Indications | Route | Toxicity | Comments |
|---|---|---|---|---|
| Suramin | African trypanosomiasis (hemolymphatic stage) | IV/IM | Common: nausea, vomiting, shock, fever, urticaria, rash, dermatitis, stomatitis, neuropathy, photophobia, renal dysfunction, diarrhea<br>Occasional: jaundice, hemolytic anemia, agranulocytosis | Available from the CDC |
| Tetracycline | Therapy of chloroquine-resistant *P. falciparum* malaria (with quinine), balantidiasis, *Dientamoeba fragilis* | PO | Occasional: GI upset, rash from photosensitivity | Contraindicated in pregnancy, children <8 yr old |
| Thiabendazole | Strongyloidiasis, trichinosis, toxocariasis, trichostrongyliasis, cutaneous larva migrans, visceral larva migrans, *Angiostrongylus costaricensis* (surgical intervention is the alternative), *Dracunculus medinensis* (alternative), *Capillaria philippensis* (alternative), *Trichinella spiralis* (alternative, used with steroids) | PO | Common: GI upset, vertigo<br>Occasional: leukopenia, crystalluria, hallucinations, erythema multiforma, olfactory disturbance, rash, pruritus, headache,<br>Rare: hypoglycemia, hypotension, seizures, cholestasis, tinnitus, angioneurotic edema, Stevens-Johnson syndrome | Contraindicated in pregnancy |
| Trimethoprim | (when combined with sulfamethoxazole) Prophylaxis and treatment of *P. carinii* pneumonia; *Isospora belli* | PO | Rare: allergic reactions: fever and severe dermatitis, serum sickness, crystalluria, neurotoxicity, and hepatotoxicity | Most toxicities due to sulfa component of trimethoprim/sulfa combinations |
| Trimetrexate | *P. carinii* pneumonia | IV | Occasional: rash, peripheral neuropathy, bone marrow depression | Antifolate; must be given with leucovorin to prevent hematoxicity; not approved by FDA |
| Tryparsamide (arsenical) | West African CNS trypanosomiasis (when combined with suramin) | IV, IM | Common: GI upset<br>Occasional: encephalopathy, local skin irritation | |

**Table 40.2** Parasitic diseases and their therapy

| Infection | Drug(s) of choice/dose[a] | Alternatives/dose[a] | Pediatric dose/comments |
|---|---|---|---|
| AMOEBIASIS | | | |
| (*Entamoeba histolytica*) Asymptomatic | Diloxanide furoate 500 mg tid × 10 days | Iodoquinol: 650 mg tid × 21 days *or* Paromomycin: 25–30 mg/kg/day in 3 doses × 7 days | Diloxanide 20 mg/kg/day in 3 doses × 10 days; follow metronidazole with luminal agent<br>Iodoquinol 30–40 mg/kg/day in 3 doses × 20 days |
| Intestinal disease | Metronidazole 750 mg tid × 10 days (followed by luminal agent) | Tinidazole: 1.0 g PO q12h × 3 days *or* Ornidazole: 500 mg PO q12h × 5 days (followed by luminal agent for both drugs) | Paromomycin 25–30 mg/kg/day in 3 doses × 7 days<br>Metronidazole 30–50 mg/kg/day in 3 doses × 10 days; tinidazole and ornidazole are similar to metronidazole but are not available in the U.S. |
| Hepatic abscess | Metronidazole 750 mg tid × 10 days *or* tinidazole 800 mg tid × 5 days (followed by luminal agent) | Dehydroemetine: 1–1.5 mg/kg/day (max. 90 mg/day) IM in 2 doses for up to 5 days followed by chloroquine phosphate 600 mg base (1 g)/day × 2 days, then 300 mg base (500 mg)/day × 2–3 weeks | Metronidazole 35–50 mg/kg/day in 3 doses × 10 days followed by diloxanide furoate 20 mg/kg/day in 3 doses × 10 days; emetine/dehydroemetine much more toxic than metronidazole; tinidazole available outside the U.S. |
| AMOEBIC MENINGOENCEPHALITIS, PRIMARY | | | |
| *Naegleria* | Amphotericin B 1 mg/kg/day IV, uncertain duration | Intraventricular amphotericin B via reservoir: 0.1–1.0 mg qod | Amphotericin: 1 mg/kg/day, uncertain duration<br>Amphotericin B: uncertain duration; success reported with addition of rifampin and miconazole |
| *Acanthamoeba* | No proven therapy | | Topical therapy for keratitis |
| *Ancylostoma duodenale*, see Hookworm | | | |
| *Anglostrongylus cantonensis* | Mebendazole: 100 mg bid × 5 days | | Mebendazole: 100 mg bid × 5 days; corticosteroids, analgesics and removal of CSF can help alleviate symptoms |
| *Angiolostrongylus costaricinsis* | Thiabendazole: 75 mg/kg/day in 3 doses × 3 days (max. 3 g/day) | | Thiabendazole: 75 mg/kg/day in 3 doses × 3 days (max. 3 g/day) |
| Anasakiasis (*Anasakis simplex*) | Surgical or endoscopic removal | Thiabendazole: 25 mg/kg × 3 days (max. 3g/day; not a proven therapy in humans) | Surgical or endoscopic removal |
| ASCARIASIS (*Ascaris lumbricoides*) | Mebendazole: 100 mg bid × 3 days | Pyrantel pamoate: 11 mg/kg once (max. 1 g) *or* Albendazole: 400 mg once | Mebendazole: 100 mg bid × 3 day *or* Pyrantel pamoate: 11 mg/kg once (max. 1 g *or* Albendazole: 400 mg once |

(*continued*)

**Table 40.2** Parasitic diseases and their therapy—*Continued*

| Infection | Drug(s) of choice/dose[a] | Alternatives/dose[a] | Pediatric dose/comments |
|---|---|---|---|
| BABESIOSIS (*Babesia microti*) | Clindamycin: 1.2 g bid parenteral or 600 mg tid oral × 7 days; plus quinine 650 mg tid oral × 7 days | Exchange transfusion in severe cases (greater than 10% parasitemia) | Clindamycin: 20–40 mg/kg/day in 3 doses × 7 day *plus*<br>Quinine: 25 mg/kg/day in 3 doses × 7 day. In Europe infection is due to *B. divergens*, *B. bovis*. |
| BALANTIDIASIS (*Balantidium coli*) | Tetracycline: 500 mg PO qid × 10 days | Iodoquinol: 650 mg PO tid × 21 days *or*<br>Metronidazole: 750 PO tid × 5 days | Tetracycline: 40 mg/kg/day in 4 doses × 10 days; max. 2 g/day; do not use in children <8 yr<br>Iodoquinol: 40 mg/kg/day in 3 doses × 21 days<br>Metronidazole: 35–50 mg/kg/day in 3 doses × 5 days |
| *BLASTOCYTIS HOMINIS* | Metronidazole: 750 mg tid × 10 days | Iodoquinol: 650 PO tid × 10 days | Treat only clinically apparent infection, role of *B. hominis* in human disease not proven, efficacy of therapy with metronidazole not proven.<br>Metronidazole: 35–50 mg/kg/day in 3 doses × 10 d *or*<br>Iodoquinol: 30–40 mg/kg/day in 3 doses × 20 days |
| CAPILLARIASIS (*Capillaria philippinensis*) *Clonorchis sinensis*, see Flukes | Mebendazole: 200 mg bid × 20 days | Albendazole: 200 mg bid × 10 days *or*<br>Thiabendazole: 25 mg/kg/day in 2 doses × 30 days | Mebendazole: 200 mg bid × 20 days<br>Albendazole: 200 mg bid × 10 days<br>Thiabendazole: 25 mg/kg/day in 2 doses × 30 days |
| CRYPTOSPORIDIOSIS (*Cryptosporidium parvum*) | No known effective therapy | Somatostatin analog octreotide used to decrease stools | Paromomycin: 500–750 mg PO qid reported to be effective in uncontrolled studies |
| CUTANEOUS LARVA | Thiabendazole: topically and/or 50 mg/kg/day in 2 doses (max. 3 g/day) × 2–5 days *or*<br>Albendazole: 200 mg bid × 3 days | | Thiabendazole: topically and/or 50 mg/kg/day in 2 doses (max. 3 g/day) in 2–5 days *or*<br>Albendazole: 200 mg bid × 3 days |
| MIGRANS (creeping eruption, dog and cat hookworm) Cysticercosis, see Tapeworms | | | |
| CYCLOSPORA | Trimethoprim/sulfamethoxazole: TMP 160 mg, SMX 800 mg bid × 3 days | | TMP: 5 mg/kg, SMX: 25 mg/kg bid × 3 days |

| | | | |
|---|---|---|---|
| *DIENTAMOEBA FRAGILIS* | Iodoquinol: 650 mg tid × 20 days | Paromomycin: 25–30 mg/kg/day in 3 doses × 7 days<br>Tetracycline: 500 mg qid × 10 days<br>Doxycycline: 100 mg PO bid × 10 days | Iodoquinol: 40 mg/kg/day in 3 doses × 20 days *or*<br>Tetracycline: 10 mg/kg qid × 10 days (max. 2 g/day) *or*<br>Paromomycin: 25–30 mg/kg/day in 3 doses × 7 days |
| *Diphyllobothrium latum*, see Tapeworms | | | |
| DRACUNCULUS *MEDINENSIS* (guinea worm) | Metronidazole: 250 mg tid × 10 days (adjunct to surgical removal; traditionally, emerging worm is wrapped on stick) | Thiabendazole: 50–75 mg/kg/day in 2 doses × 3 days (adjunct to surgical removal) | Metronidazole: 25 mg/kg/day (max. 750 mg/day) in 3 doses × 10 days<br>Thiabendazole: 50–75 mg/kg/day (max. 2 g/day) in 4 doses × 10 days |
| Echinococcus, see Tapeworms | | | |
| *Entamoeba histolytica*, see Amoebiasis | | | |
| ENTAMOEBA *POLECKI* | Metronidazole 750 mg PO tid × 10 days | | Metronidazole: 35–50 mg/kg/day in 3 doses × 10 days |
| ENTEROBIUS *VERMICULARIS* (pinworm) | Pyrantel pamoate 11 mg/kg once (max. 1 g); repeat after 2 weeks *or*<br>Mebendazole: single dose of 100 mg; repeat after 2 weeks | Albendazole: 400 mg once; repeat in 2 weeks | Pyrantel pamoate: 11 mg/kg once (max. 1 g); repeat after 2 weeks *or*<br>Mebendazole: single dose of 100 mg; repeat after 2 weeks *or*<br>Albendazole: 400 mg once, repeat in 2 weeks (albendazole not available in the U.S.); piperazine used when there is intestinal or biliary obstruction, 75 mg/kg PO qd × 2 doses; levamisole used for mass therapy |
| *Fasciola hepatica*, see Flukes | | | |
| FILARIASIS | | | |
| *Wuchereria bancrofti*, *Brugia malayi* | Diethylcarbamazine: Day 1: 50 mg, PO after meals, Day 2: 50 mg tid, Day 3: 100 mg tid, Days 4–21: 6 mg/kg/day in 3 doses | | Day 1: 1 mg/kg, oral, p.c.<br>Day 2: 1 mg/kg tid<br>Day 3: 1–2 mg/kg tid<br>Days 4–21: 6 mg/kg/day in 3 doses |
| *Loa loa* | Diethylcarbamazine: Day 1: 50 mg, PO after meals, Day 2: 50 mg tid, Day 3: 100 mg tid, Days 4–21: 9 mg/kg/day in 3 doses | | Day 1: 1 mg/kg, oral, p.c.<br>Day 2: 1 mg/kg tid<br>Day 3: 1–2 mg/kg tid<br>Days 4–21: 9 mg/kg/day in 3 doses; doxycycline may offer prophylactic benefit |
| *Mansonella ozzardi* | Ivermectin: 150 $\mu$g/day for 30 days | | Efficacy no proven; diethylcarbamazine has no effect |
| *Mansonella perstans* | Mebendazole: 100 mg bid × 30 days | | |
| *Onchocerca volvulus* | Ivermectin 150 $\mu$g/kg oral once, repeated every 6 to 12 months; if flukes in eye use prednisone 1 mg/kg/day, starting several days before therapy | | 150 $\mu$g/kg oral once, repeated every 6–12 months |
| *FLUKES, HERMAPHRODITIC* | | | |
| *Clonorchis sinensis* (Chinese liver fluke) | Praziquantel: 75 mg/kg/day in 3 doses × 1 day | | 75 mg/kg/day in 3 doses × 1 day |

(*continued*)

**Table 40.2** Parasitic diseases and their therapy—*Continued*

| Infection | Drug(s) of choice/dose[a] | Alternatives/dose[a] | Pediatric dose/comments |
|---|---|---|---|
| *Fasciola hepatica* (sheep liver fluke) | Bithionol: 30–50 mg/kg on alternate days × 10–15 doses | | 30–50 mg/kg on alternate days × 10–15 doses; praziquantel emerging as an alternative |
| *Fasciolopsis buski* (intestinal fluke) | Praziquantel: 75 mg/kg/day in 3 doses × 1 day | Niclosamide: single dose of 4 tablets (2 g), chewed thoroughly | Praziquantel: 75 mg/kg/day in 3 doses × 1 day *or*<br>Niclosamide: 11–34 kg: 2 tablets (1 g); >34 kg: 3 tablets (1.5 g) |
| *Heterophyes heterophyes* (intestinal fluke) | Praziquantel: 75 mg/kg/day in 3 doses × 1 day | | Praziquantel: 75 mg/kg/day in 3 doses × 1 day |
| *Metagonimus yokogawai* (intestinal fluke) | Praziquantel: 75 mg/kg/day in 3 doses × 1 day | | Praziquantel: 75 mg/kg/day in 3 doses × 1 day |
| *Nanophyetus salmincola* | Praziquantel: 60 mg/kg/day in 3 doses × 1 day | | 60 mg/kg/day in 3 doses × 1 day |
| *Opisthorchis viverrini* (liver fluke) | Praziquantel: 75 mg/kg/day in 3 doses × 1 day | | 75 mg/kg/day in 3 doses × 1 day |
| *Paragonimus westermani* (lung fluke) | Praziquantel: 75 mg/kg/day in 3 doses × 2 days | Bithionol: 30–50 mg/kg on alternate days × 10–15 doses | Praziquantel: 75 mg/kg/day in 3 doses × 2 days<br>Bithionol: 30–50 mg/kg on alternate days × 10–15 doses |
| Tropical pulmonary eosinophilia | Diethylcarbamazine: 6 mg/kg/day in 3 doses × 21 days | | 6 mg/kg/day in 3 doses × 21 days |
| GIARDIASIS (*Giardia lamblia*) | Metronidazole: 250 to 750 mg tid × 5 days | Quinacrine HCl: 100 mg tid p.c. × 5 days<br>Tinidazole: 2 g once<br>Furazolidone: 100 mg qid × 7–10 days<br>Paromomycin: 25–30 mg/kg/day in 3 doses × 7 days | Quinacrine: contraindicated in patients with a history of psychosis<br>Furazolidone: 1.25 mg/kg qid × 7–10 days<br>Metronidazole: 5 mg/kg tid<br>Quinacrine HCl: 2 mg/kg tid po × 5 days (max. 300 mg/day; not available in the U.S.); tinidazole available outside the U.S.; paromomycin used in pregnancy 500 mg PO qid × 7 days |
| GNATHOSTOMIASIS (*Gnathostoma spinigerum*) | Surgical removal plus albendazole: 400 mg qd × 21 days | | |
| HOOKWORM (*Ancylostoma duodenale*, *Necator americanus*) | Mebendazole: 100 mg bid × 3 days *or*<br>pyrantel pamoate: 11 mg/kg (max. 1 g) × 3 days *or*<br>albendazole: 400 mg once | | Mebendazole: 100 mg bid × 3 days *or*<br>Pyrantel pamoate: 11 mg/kg (max. 1 g) × 3 days *or*<br>*Albendazole: 400 mg once;*<br>albendazole not available in the U.S.; pyrantel not FDA approved for this indication |
| Hydatid cyst, see Tapeworms | | | |
| Hymenolepis nana, see Tapeworms | | | |
| ISOSPORIASIS (*Isospora belli*) | Trimethoprim/sulfamethoxazole: 160 mg TMP, 800 mg SMX qid × 10 days, then bid × 3 weeks | Pyrimethamine: 75 mg PO qd with folinic acid 10 mg/day, for 14 days | Trimethoprim-sulfamethoxazole: 10 mg/kg/day as TMP in 4 divided oral doses × 3 weeks; maintenance therapy required in AIDS patients |

| | | | |
|---|---|---|---|
| Leishmaniasis (*L. mexicana*, *L. braziliensis*, *L. donovani* (Kala azar) | Sodium stibogluconate: 20 mg Sb/kg/day IV or IM × 20–28 days *or*<br>meglumine antimonate: 20 mg Sb/kg/day × 20–28 days | Amphotericin B: 0.25–1 mg/kg by slow infusion daily or every 2 days for up to 8 weeks | Stibogluconate sodium: 20 mg/kg/day IM or IV (max. 800 mg/day) × 20 days;<br>Allopurinol: 5 mg/kg PO qid with probenecid 500 mg PO qid × 28 days, reported effective in *L. mexicana*<br>Pentamidine isethionate: 2–4 mg/kg daily or every 2 days IM for up to 15 doses alternative for *L. donovani*, allopurinol: 20 mg/kg/day used as adjunct. For *L. mexicana*, and *L. braziliensis*, ketoconazole: 600 mg/day for 28 days effective as pentamidine |
| *L. tropica*, *L. major* (Old World cutaneous) | Sodium stibogluconate: 20 mg antimony/kg/day × 20 days | Topical therapy: application of heat 39°–42°C directly to the lesions for 20–32 h over 10–12 days has been reported to be effective in *L. tropica* | Stibogluconate sodium: 10 mg/kg/day IM or IV (maximum 600 mg/day) × 6–10 days |
| *Loa loa*, see Filaria | | | |
| MALARIA<br>(*Plasmdoium falciparum*, *P. ovale*, *P. vivax*, and *P. malariae*) | | | |
| Therapy of chloroquine-resistant *P. falciparum* | *Oral*: Quinine sulfate: 650 mg q8h × 3–7 days *plus* Pyrimethamine-sulfadoxine: 3 tablets at once on last day of quinine *or plus*<br>Tetracycline: 250 mg qid × 7 days *or plus*<br>Doxycycline: 100 mg PO bid × 7 days *or* plus<br>Clindamycin: 900 mg tid × 3 days<br>*Parenteral*: Quinidine gluconate: 10 mg/kg loading dose 9 (max. 600 mg) in normal saline slowly over 1–2 h, followed by continuous infusion of 0.02 mg/kg/min until oral therapy can be started *or*<br>Quinine dihydrochloride: 20 mg salt/kg loading dose in 10 ml/kg 5% dextrose over 4 h, followed by 10 mg salt/kg over 2–4 h q8h (max. 1800 mg/day) until oral therapy can be started | Mefloquine: 1250 mg once<br>Halofantrine: 500 mg q6h × 3 doses; repeat in 1 week<br>Artemisinin (available for use in China and Vietnam, see text for doses) | Oral: Quinine sulfate: 25 mg/kg/day in 3 doses × 3 days *plus*<br>Pyrimethamine: <10 kg: 6.25 mg/day × 3 days<br>10–20 kg: 12.5 mg/day × 3 days<br>20–40 kg: 25 mg/day × 3 days *plus*<br>Sulfadiazine: 100–200 mg/kg/day in 4 doses × 5 days (max. 2 g/day) *or*<br>Quinine sulfate: 25 mg/kg/day in 3 doses × 3 days *plus*<br>Tetracycline: 5 mg/kg qid × 7 days; quinine has been used extensively in pregnancy; no teratogenicity, but hearing loss has occurred<br>Parenteral: Quinine dihydrochloride: 25 mg/kg/day in 3 doses × 3 days *or*<br>Quinidine: gluconate 10 mg/kg IV, then 0.02 mg/kg/min IV × 72 h |

*(continued)*

**Table 40.2** Parasitic diseases and their therapy—*Continued*

| Infection | Drug(s) of choice/dose[a] | Alternatives/dose[a] | Pediatric dose/comments |
|---|---|---|---|
| MALARIA All *Plasmodium* except chloroquine-resistant *P. falciparum* | *Oral*: Chloroquine phosphate: 600 mg base (1 g), then 300 mg base (500 mg) 6 h later, then 300 mg base (500 mg) at 24 and 48 h<br>*Parenteral*: Quinidine gluconate: same as above *or*<br>Quinine dihydrochloride: same as above | 6 h later, then 5 mg base/kg/day × 2 days<br>Chloroquine: optimal dosing not established, see text | *Oral*: Chloroquine phosphate: 10 mg base/kg (max. 600 mg base), then 5 mg base/kg<br>for *P. vivax* and *P. ovale*, follow treatment with primaquine—see below<br>*Parenteral*: Quinine dihydrochloride: 25 mg/kg/day; give 1/3 of daily dose over 2–4 h, repeat every 8 h until oral therapy can be started (max. 1800 mg/day IV) *or*<br>Quinidine gluconate: 10 mg/kg IV, then 0.02 mg/kg/min IV × 72 h<br>for *P. vivax* and *P. ovale*, follow treatment with primaquine—see below |
| MALARIA Prevention of relapses: *P. vivax* and *P. ovale* only | Primaquine phosphate: 15 mg base (26.3 mg)/day × 14 days or 45 mg base (79 mg)/week × 8 weeks | | Primaquine phosphate: 0.3 mg base/kg/day × 14 days |
| MALARIA Prophylaxis in chloroquine-sensitive areas | Chloroquine phosphate: 300 mg base (500 mg salt) orally, once a week | | Chloroquine phosphate: 5 mg/kg base (8.3 mg/kg salt) once per week, up to maximum adult dose of 300 mg base |
| MALARIA Prophylaxis in chloroquine-resistant areas | Mefloquine: 250 mg oral once a week *or*<br>Doxycycline: 100 mg daily | Chloroquine phosphate *plus* pyrimethamine-sulfadoxine for presumptive treatment (carry a single dose [3 tablets] for self-treatment of febrile illness when medical care is not immediately available) *or* plus proguanil 200 mg daily (in East Africa south of the Sahara) | Chloroquine phosphate: 5 mg/kg base (8.3 mg/kg salt) once per week, up to maximum adult dose of 300 mg base *plus*<br>Proguanil (in Africa, south of the Sahara): <2 yr: 50 mg daily; 2–6 yr: 100 mg daily; 7–10 yr: 150 mg daily 10 yr: 200 mg daily *plus*<br>Pyrimethamine-sulfadoxine (Fansidar) 2–11 months: 1/4 tablet; 1–3 yrs: 1/2 tablet; 4–8 yr: 1 tablet; 9–14 yrs: 2 tablets; >14 yr: 3 tablets<br>Take single dose of above for self-treatment of febrile illness when medical care is not immediately available *or*<br>Chloroquine phosphate (as above) *plus* doxycycline >8 yr of age: 2 mg/kg/day, up to adult dose of 100 mg/day<br>Resistance patterns change often; call CDC for latest information: 404-488-4046 days or 404-639-2888 nights/weekends |

| | | | |
|---|---|---|---|
| MICROSPORIDIOSIS | | | |
| *Naegleria* sp., see Amoebic | | Albendazole: 400 mg PO bid × 10–20 days reported to be effective for *Enterocytozoon bieneusi* | One case report of therapy with albendazole for infection with *Septata intestinalis*; role of various therapeutic agents in this class of organisms is still being defined |
| *Naegleria* sp., see Amoebic meningoencephalitis | | | |
| *Necator americanus*, see Hookworm | | | |
| *Onchocerca volvulus*, see Flukes | | | |
| *Opisthorchis viverrine*, see Flukes | | | |
| *Paragonimus westermani*, see Flukes | | | |
| Pinworm, see *Enterobius vermicularis* | | | |
| *PNEUMOCYSTIS CARINII* Pneumonia | Trimethoprim-sulfamethoxazole: TMP 15–20 mg/kg/day, SMX 75–100 mg/kg/day, oral or IV in 3 or 4 doses × 14–21 days *or*<br>Pentamidine: 3–4 mg/kg IV per day × 14–21 days | Trimethoprim: 5 mg/kg PO q6h × 21 days *plus*<br>Dapsone: 100 mg PO qd × 21 days<br>Atovaquone: 750 mg tid PO × 21 days<br>Primaquine: 15 mg base PO qd × 21 days *plus*<br>Clindamycin: 600 mg IV q6h × 21 days, or 300–450 mg PO q6h × 21 days<br>Trimetrexate: 45 mg/m$^2$ IV qd × 21 days *plus*<br>Folinic acid: 20 mg/m$^2$ PO or IV q6h × 21 days | Trimethoprim-sulfamethoxazole: TMP 20 mg/kg/day, SMX 100 mg/kg/day oral or IV in 4 doses × 14 days *or*<br>Pentamidine: 4 mg/kg/day IM or IV × 14 days<br>In severe cases of PCP ($pO_2$ <70) give steroids prednisone 40 mg bid × 5 days, 40 mg qd × 5 days, the 20 mg qd × 11 days; acute therapy must be followed by suppressive therapy |
| Primary and secondary prophylaxis | Trimethoprim-sulfamethoxazole: 1 DS tab PO qd or 3 times per week | Dapsone: 25–50 mg PO qd, or 100 mg PO 2 times per week;<br>aerosol pentamidine: 300 mg inhaled monthly via nebulizer | Aerosol pentamidine: use associated with increased failures and atypical presentation of PCP |
| SCHISTOSOMIASIS (*Bilharziasis*) | | | |
| *S. haematobium* | Praziquantel: 40 mg/kg/day in 2 doses × 1 day | Metrifonate: 10 mg/kg PO as a single dose (less expensive, less effective, also has activity against hookworm) | Praziquantel: 40 mg/kg/day in 2 doses × 1 day |
| *S. japonicum* | Praziquantel: 60 mg/kg/day in 3 doses × 1 day | | Praziquantel: 60 mg/kg/day in 3 doses × 1 day |
| *S. mansoni* | Praziquantel: 40 mg/kg/day in 2 doses × 1 day | Oxamniquine: 15 mg/kg once | Praziquantel: 40 mg/kg/day in 2 doses × 1 day<br>Oxamniquine: 20 mg/kg/day in 2 doses × 1 day (alternative) |
| *S. mekongi* | Praziquantel: 60 mg/kg/day in 3 doses × 1 day | | Praziquantel: 60 mg/kg/day in 3 doses × 1 day |
| KATAYAMA FEVER (acute toxic schistosomiasis) | Praziquantel: 25 mg/kg PO q4h with food for a total of 3 doses | | Control systemic symptoms, fever with steroids |
| SLEEPING SICKNESS, see Trypanosomiasis | | | |
| STRONGYLOIDIASIS (Strongyloides stercoralis) | Thiabendazole: 50 mg/kg/day in 2 doses (max. 3 g/day) × 2 day *or*<br>Ivermectin: 200 μg/kg/day × 1–2 days | Albendazole 400 mg po every day × 3 days | Thiabendazole: 50 mg/kg/day in 2 doses (max. 3 g) × 2 days; ivermectin becoming drug of choice;<br>in disseminated strongyloides, continue thiabendazole for a minimum of 5 days |

*(continued)*

**Table 40.2** Parasitic diseases and their therapy—*Continued*

| Infection | Drug(s) of choice/dose[a] | Alternatives/dose[a] | Pediatric dose/comments |
|---|---|---|---|
| TAPEWORM Adult (intestinal stage) *Diphyllobothrium latum* (fish), *Taenia saginata* (beef), *Taenia solium* (pork), *Dipylidium caninum* (dog) | Praziquantel: 5–10 mg/kg once | Niclosamide, single dose of 4 tablets (2 g), chewed thoroughly | Praziquantel: 5–10 mg/kg once *or* Niclosamide: 11–34 kg: single dose of 2 tablets (1 g); >34 kg: single dose of 3 tablets (1.5 g); for *T. solium*, therapy with niclosamide should be followed with a purge in 3–4 h. It causes disintegration of segments and release of viable eggs, and there is a theoretical risk of cysticercosis |
| *Hymenolepsis nana* (dwarf tapeworm) | Praziquantel: 25 mg/kg once | Niclosamide: single daily dose of 4 tablets (2 g), chewed thoroughly, then 2 tablets daily × 6 days | Praziquantel: 25 mg/kg once; alternative: niclosamide: 11–34 kg: single dose of 2 tablets (1 g) × 1 day, then 1 tablet (0.5 g)/day × 6 days; >34 kg: single dose of 3 tablets (1.5 g) × 1 day, then 2 tablets (1 g)/ day × 6 days |
| Larval (tissue stage) *Echinococcus granulosus* (hydatid cyst) | Albendazole: 400 mg PO bid with food × 28 days, repeated as necessary | | Albendazole: 15 mg/kg/day × 28 days, repeated as necessary; albendazole not available in the U.S.; albendazole therapy curative without surgery in 33 percent; mebendazole also has some efficacy (see text); drug therapy not effective with calcified cysts |
| *Echinococcus multilocularis* | Surgical excision | | Albendazole also may be effective |
| Neurocysticercosis (*Cysticercus cellulosae*) | Albendazole: 7.5 mg/kg/day in 2 doses × 8 days (not available in the U.S.) | Praziquantel: 20 mg/kg/day in 3 doses × 14 days | Albendazole: 15 mg/kg/day in 3 doses × 28 days, repeated as necessary *or* Praziquantel: 50 mg/kg/day in 3 doses × 15 days. Corticosteroids should be given 2–3 days before and during praziquantel therapy; surgery indicated for hydrocephalus, ventricular and spinal cysts; do not treat with drugs during acute phase; do not treat ocular disease with praziquantel |
| TOXOCARIASIS, see Visceral Larvae Milgrans | | | |
| TOXOPLASMOSIS (*toxoplasma gondii*) | Pyrimethamine: 25–100 mg/day × 3–4 weeks *plus* Sulfadiazine: 1–2 g qid × 3–4 weeks | Spiramycin: 3–4 g/day (safe in pregnancy) | Pyrimethamine: 2 mg/kg/day × 3 days, then 1 mg/kg/day (max. 25 mg/day) × 4 weeks *plus* Trisulfapyrimidines: 100 mg/kg/day × 3–4 weeks; corticosteroids should be used in ocular toxoplasmosis Spiramycin: 50–100 mg/kg/day × 3–4 weeks |

| | | | |
|---|---|---|---|
| TRICHINOSIS<br>*Trichinella spiralis* | Steroids (prednisone 40–60 mg PO qd for 5 days with taper) for severe symptoms plus mebendazole 200–400 mg tid × 3 days, then 400–500 mg tid × 10 days | | Mebendazole should not be given in the first trimester of pregnancy |
| *Trichomonas vaginalis* | Metronidazole 2 g once or 250 mg tid orally × 7 days *or*<br>Tinidazole: 2 g once | Outside the U.S., ornidazole and tinidazole have been used. | Metronidazole: 15 mg/kg/day orally in 3 doses × 7 days; avoid in first trimester; sexual partners should be treated simultaneously; resistance to metronidazole has been reported, higher doses are sometimes effective |
| TRICHOSTRONGYLUS | Pyrantel pamoate: 11 mg/kg once (max. 1 g)<br>Mebendazole: 100 mg bid × 3 days *or*<br>Albendazole: 400 mg once | | Pyrantel pamoate: 11 mg/kg once (max. 1g); alternative:<br>mebendazole: 100 mg bid × 3 days *or*<br>Albendazole: 400 mg once |
| TRICHURIASIS<br>*Trichuris trichiura* (whipworm) | Mebendazole: 100 mg/bid × 3 days *or*<br>Albendazole: 400 mg once | | Mebendazole: 100 mg BID × 3 days *or*<br>Albendazole: 400 mg once; albendazole not available in the U.S. |
| TRYPANOSOMIASIS<br>*T. cruzi* (South American, Chagas disease) | Nifurtimox: 8–10 mg/kg/day orally in 4 doses × 120 days | Benznidazole: 5–7 mg/kg/day × 30–120 days | Nifurtimox, 1–10 yr: 15–20 mg/kg/day in 4 divided doses × 90 days<br>Benznidazole, 11–16 yr: 12.5–15 mg/kg/day in 4 divided doses × 90 days.<br>Nifurtimox therapy associated with 70% parasitological cure, clinical benefit unclear, side effects 40%–70% |
| *T. brucei gambiense*;<br>*T.b. rhodesiense*<br>Hemolymphatic stage | Suramin: 100–200 mg (test dose) IV, then 1 g IV on Days 1, 3, 7, 14, and 21 *or*<br>Eflornithine: 400 mg/kg/day IV in 4 divided doses for 14 days, followed by oral 300 mg/kg/day for 3–4 weeks | Pentamidine isethionate 4 mg/kg/day IM × 10 days | Suramin: 20 mg/kg on Days 1, 3, 7, 14, and 21<br>Pentamidine: 4 mg/kg/day IM × 10 days |
| Late disease with CNS involvement | Melarsoprol: 2–3.6 mg/kg/day IV × 3 days; after 1 week 3.6 mg/kg per day IV × 3 days; repeat again after 10–21 days *or* eflornithine as for hemolymphatic stage | Tryparsamide: one injection of 30 mg/kg (max. 2 g) IV every 5 days to total of 12 injections; may be repeated after 1 month, *plus* suramin one injection of 10 mg/kg IV every 5 days to total of 12 injections; may be repeated after 1 month | Melarsoprol: 18–25 mg/kg total over 1 month initial dose of 0.36 mg/kg IV, increasing gradually to maximum 3.6 mg/kg at intervals of 1–5 days for total of 9–10 doses<br>Dose of tryparsamide and suramin unknown |
| VISCERAL LARVA MIGRANS | Diethylcarbamazine: 6 mg/kg/day in 3 doses × 7–10 days | Albendazole: 400 mg bid × 3–5 days<br>Mebendazole: 100–200 mg bid × 5 days | Diethylcarbamazine: 6 mg/kg/day in 3 doses × 7–10 days; alternative:<br>Albendazole: 400 mg bid × 3–5 days |
| Whipworm, see Trichuris | | | |
| *Wuchereria brancrofti*, see Filariasis | | | |

The most common prophylactic dosing schedule is mefloquine 250 mg/week, beginning one week before travel. The drug should be continued 4 weeks after the last exposure. A single dose of 1000 to 1500 mg is used for treatment of resistant falciparum malaria. Side effects are uncommon at doses of less than 1000 mg; nausea, vomiting, abdominal pain, and dizziness have been reported. Serious CNS side effects such as seizures, hallucinations, psychosis, and depression occur rarely at prophylactic doses (<0.5%). Use of mefloquine in patients with cardiac conduction abnormalities or those taking beta-blockers for anti-arrhythmic indications has rarely been associated with sudden death, and its use should be avoided in these circumstances. Mefloquine is teratogenic in animals, and data are not currently available regarding safety in pregnancy. The therapeutic dose for children is 25 mg/kg. Resistance to antimalarials may emerge rapidly, and the most recent information may be obtained from the Centers for Disease Control (CDC) Malaria Branch (404-488-4046). In 1997, mefloquine resistance has been most often reported in parts of Thailand, and has also been reported in West Africa.

### Quinine

This is an alkaloid extracted from the bark of the cinchona tree that is active against blood forms of malaria. Quinine is more toxic and less efficacious than chloroquine, and its primary use is therapy for resistant falciparum malaria. Quinine can be given by the oral, IV, or IM route; it is metabolized in the liver and excreted by the kidney. The exact mechanism of action is unknown. The most commonly used preparation is quinine sulfate; the oral dose is 650 mg tid after meals for 7–10 days; the duration can be decreased if other antimalarials are used. Parenteral quinine is more toxic and should be reserved for more severe cases; the dose is 20 mg of the salt/kg in 500 cc saline infused over the first 4 h, followed by a 10 mg/kg 4 h infusion every 10 h. Patients severely ill with falciparum malaria who have high levels of parasitemia (>5%–10%) or massive hemolysis should also be treated with exchange transfusion in combination with chemotherapy.

In the United States parenteral quinine is not available. Quinidine is a stereoisomer of quinine and can used in place of quinine in patients who need parenteral therapy. Quinidine is given by continuous IV infusion. The most commonly used dosage schedule is 10 mg of the salt/kg load, followed by 0.02 mg of salt/kg/min. Quinidine undergoes hepatic metabolism and is excreted in the urine. Blood levels should be followed in patients with hepatic and renal failure.

Intravenous quinine and quinidine can lead to hypotension and serious cardiac arrhythmias, particularly when given as boluses, and cardiac monitoring should be used. The fatal oral dose of quinine for adults is 2 to 8 g. Oral quinine is associated with a variety of side effects including nausea, vomiting, diarrhea, and hypoglycemia. Gastrointestinal side effects are decreased by dosing with meals. Dose-related side effects include tinnitus, headaches, visual changes, and vertigo. Tinnitus, optic neuritis and hypersensitivity reactions are contraindications.

### Pyrimethamine

This is a dihydrofolate reductase inhibitor which is highly active against the protozoan enzyme and is used in the prophylaxis and treatment of resistant falciparum malaria, as well as toxoplasmosis (see below). Pyrimethamine is well absorbed orally and has an extremely long tissue half-life (80–95 h). Pyrimethamine is particularly effective when used in combination with other folic acid antagonists, and combination therapy delays emergence of resistance. A common pyrimethamine/sulfa combination used for prophylaxis of malaria is Fansidar, which consists of pyrimethamine 25 mg and sulfadoxine 500 mg. Pyrimethamine, 12.5 mg, is also available in combination with dapsone, 100 mg, as Maloprim; it is not available in the United States.

Pyrimethamine in a single dose of 75 mg in combination with a sulfa drug is used for the treatment of acute attacks of falciparum malaria. Resistance to the pyrimethamine/sulfa combination among *P. falciparum* has been encountered in some areas. In therapy of acute malaria, quinine is frequently added as pyrimethamine is slow in clearing parasitemia. The pediatric therapeutic dose of pyrimethamine is one-quarter 25 mg tablet for children 2–11 months, one-half 25 mg tablet for children 1–3 years, one tablet for children 4–8, and two tablets for children 9–14.

Long-term prophylactic use of pyrimethamine/sulfa combinations has been associated with severe cutaneous skin reactions, and its use has largely been supplanted by mefloquine and doxycycline. Pyrimethamine/sulfa combinations have been used for individuals with prolonged exposure to resistant falciparum malaria and limited access to medical care who cannot tolerate mefloquine or doxycycline. The prophylactic dose is one Fansidar tablet weekly 1 week before and 6 weeks after exposure. The CDC now recommends that travelers not taking mefloquine or doxycycline who may be exposed to chloroquine-resistant malaria carry a therapeutic dose of pyrimethamine/sulfa which is to be taken if a febrile illness develops and medical care is not available. There have been no reports of fatal cutaneous reactions to Fansidar when used only for acute febrile episodes. High doses of pyrimethamine lead to megaloblastic anemia, which can be prevented with concurrent use of folinic acid (leucovorin).

### Proguanil (chloroguanide)

This is also an inhibitor of protozoan dihydrofolate reductase. The drug is well absorbed orally, readily excreted and does not accumulate in the body. To be effective for prophylaxis it must be taken daily. Proguanil is used in the prophylaxis of resistant falciparum malaria, particularly as an alternative to pyrimethamine/sulfa in East Africa. For reasons that are not clear, proguanil is less effective in West Africa. The prophylactic dose is 200 mg daily and is associated with few side effects (occasional mouth ulcers, nausea and diarrhea). In areas of *P. falciparum* resistant to chloroquine, the combination of daily proguanil and weekly chloroquine is only about 75% effective in preventing falciparum malaria, vs. >95% for mefloquine. In addition, the need for a daily dose (vs. weekly mefloquine) may lead to diminished compliance.

### Primaquine

This is an 8-aminoquinoline, and is the prototype tissue antimalarial. The drug is well absorbed orally and extensively metabolized. Primaquine interferes with mitochondrial function of *Plasmodium*. Primaquine is primarily used to treat the liver phase of malaria due to *P. vivax* and *P. ovale*; patients treated for the blood phase of *P. vivax* or *P. ovale* must receive therapy for the tissue phase to prevent relapse. Infection with *P. falciparum* is synchronous, and primaquine is not needed when the blood phase is successfully treated. However, patients who acquire *P. falciparum* malaria who are not taking chloroquine or other prophylaxis should be treated with primaquine, as co-infection with another species is common, and relapses occur without treatment of the liver phase. The dosage of primaquine is expressed in terms of the base. Primaquine is supplied in tablets containing 26.3 mg of the salt, equal to 15 mg of base. Primaquine 15 mg/day combined with chloroquine provides cure of sensitive strains of *P. vivax* malaria. For resistant strains, 45 mg of primaquine is given with chloroquine weekly for 7 weeks. Primaquine should always given with a schizonticidal agent (preferably chloroquine) in acute malaria to prevent the development of resistance.

Primaquine can cause GI distress at a higher dose; however, the major toxicity is related to the drug's redox potential. In high doses primaquine can cause methemoglobinemia. In G6PD-deficient individuals, primaquine provokes hemolysis at usual doses, and patients should be screened for G6PD deficiency prior to treatment. With higher doses or in susceptible patients the rbc count should be followed. Primaquine can rarely cause central nervous system (CNS) toxicity. Agranulocytosis has also been reported and primaquine is contraindicated with neutropenia. Primaquine should not be used during pregnancy.

### Artemisinin (qinghaosu)

This is a member of a group of compounds traditionally used in China to treat fever which has recently been found to have antimalarial activity. It is emerging as an alternative therapy for resistant falciparum malaria, and has been used extensively in China and Vietnam. Artemisinin and several related compounds (see below) are among the most rapidly schizonticidal drugs available. The mechanism of action is not well understood, but is thought to be mediated by free radical damage to parasitic membranes.

Artemisinin is commonly given orally or as a suppository. The oral dose is 50 mg/kg total dose given over 3 days, with the first dose greater than 10 mg/kg. Suppository administration of artemisinin is used extensively in cases of severe malaria where parenteral therapy is not available; usually 2800 mg is given over 3 days in 5–6 doses with the first dose greater than 10 mg/kg. Recent reports have suggested the use of artemisinin along with mefloquine for therapy of *P. falciparum* in areas where mefloquine resistance may be encountered. Two compounds very similar to artemisinin, artemether and artesunate, have also been used. Artemether is given intramuscularly in an initial dose of 3.2 mg/kg, followed by 1.6 mg/kg every 12–24 h for a total of six doses. Artesunate is given parenterally with a similar schedule. Severe toxicities to artemisinin and its related compounds are rare. Transient first-degree heart block, abdominal pain, diarrhea, fever, and cytopenias have been reported, but are uncommon, and artemisinin and the related compounds are generally well tolerated. Their safety in pregnancy has not been established.

### Halofantrine

This is a 9-phenathrenemethanol effective against chloroquine sensitive and chloroquine resistant falciparum malaria. The drug is only available in the oral form; absorption is best when taken with a fatty meal. Halofantrine is excreted in the feces. The mechanism of action is not known. Like chloroquine and mefloquine, it is active only against the intraerythrocytic stages of *Plasmodium* sp. Halofantrine is used in areas where there is resistance to chloroquine and mefloquine. There is some evidence of cross-resistance with mefloquine, which may limit the future usefulness of halofantrine. The dose is 500 mg given 3 times at 6 h intervals for adults and children over 40 kg, and 8 mg/kg at the same intervals for children under 40 kg. A second course after 7 days is recommended for patients not previously exposed to malaria. The most common side effects are headache, nausea, abdominal pain, diarrhea, and rash. The use of halofantrine is contraindicated in pregnancy and lactating women.

### Tetracyclines

Members of the tetracycline family can be used to treat multiply resistant falciparum malaria. They are slow to act and should be used with quinine. Tetracycline is given at a dose of 250 mg PO qid. Doxycycline at a dose of 100 mg/day can be used for short-term prophylaxis. Tetracyclines are associated with sun sensitization. They should not be used in children or during pregnancy.

### Prevention

At present, no drug treatment guarantees protection against malaria in all areas of the world. Travelers to countries with malaria should be advised to avoid mosquito bites by using insect repellents containing diethyltoluamide ("deet") and using mosquito netting when sleeping in exposed areas. The development of fever two to three weeks after visiting an area with malaria should prompt patients to seek medical attention.

## Therapy of Babesiosis

Infection with *Babesia* is sometimes confused with *P. falciparum* because of the similar appearance on smears of peripheral blood. Many patients with babesiosis have a mild illness and do not require specific treatment. Patients who are splenectomized, have underlying immunosuppression, and/or have a more severe presentation can be treated with the combination of clindamycin 300–600 mg given IM or IV, and oral quinine every 6–8 h for 7–10 days. The dose in children is clindamycin 20 mg/kg/day and quinine 25 mg/kg/day given in the same schedule as for adults. Chloroquine, sometimes given to patients with babesiosis mistakenly thought to have malaria, is not effective. Exchange transfusion can be used in combination with chemotherapy in patients with high levels of parasitemia, massive hemolysis or who are severely ill.

## Intestinal protozoa therapy

### Amebiasis

Agents used in the treatment of *Entamoeba histolytica* can be divided into those with activity limited to the lumen of the gut, those effective only in invasive systemic infection, and those effective in both settings.

*Metronidazole* (*Flagyl*) is a nitroidazole compound active against both luminal and invasive *E. histolytica*, and is also effective therapy for infections due to *Giardia lamblia* and *Trichomonas vaginalis* (see below). Metronidazole is metabolized in the liver, with some renal excretion of metabolites. It is completely and rapidly absorbed when given orally, and can also be given intravenously. Because of the extensive hepatic metabolism, lower doses should be used in patients with liver failure, but dosage adjustment is unnecessary in renal failure.

Metronidazole is selectively metabolized in anaerobic or hypoxic cells to a chemically reactive reduced form of the drug which is cytotoxic. The exact mechanism of action is unknown.

Metronidazole is the drug of choice for tissue amoebiasis including liver abscess, but is less effective in the treatment of asymptomatic cyst carriers. The dosage for systemic amoebiasis in adults is 750 mg tid IV or PO for 5–10 days. The dose in children is 35–50 mg/kg/day in three divided doses. Metronidazole is generally well tolerated, and side effects are usually not severe enough to lead to discontinuation. Headache, nausea, dry mouth, and a metallic taste may occur. Neurologic toxicities have included dizziness, vertigo and a sensory neuropathy. Metronidazole may cause a disulfiram like reaction. Metronidazole is contraindicated in the first trimester of pregnancy. Patients treated for amoebiasis with metronidazole or other agents should have follow-up stool examinations to insure eradication of intestinal infection. Many authorities recommend sequential treatment with an anti-luminal agent in all cases as some studies have found a failure rate of 5%–10% in eradicating cyst passage in metronidazole treated patients. Tinidazole and ornidazole are compounds related to metronidazole, with similar pharmacologic profiles and indications.

*Chloroquine*, discussed above, is efficacious in amoebic liver abscess, and is used when metronidazole is contraindicated. The dose is 1 g daily for 2 days, followed by 500 mg/day for 2 to 3 weeks. Chloroquine is not active against intestinal amoebae, and treatment with a luminal agent is recommended to prevent relapse.

*Emetine* (or its equivalent congener dehydroemetine) is a salt of an ipecac alkaloid effective in system amoebiasis, but has largely been replaced by the less toxic metronidazole. It is not absorbed when given orally. The mechanism of action is unclear, but emetine has a direct lethal action against *E. histolytica* trophozoites; it is much less effective against cysts. Its use is limited to cases of systemic amoebiasis in which metronidazole is ineffective or contraindicated. In addition, some authors recommend using emetine in combination with metronidazole for the first 2–3 days in patients who are severely ill or who have perforation of an amoebic liver abscess. Emetine can also be used in combination with chloroquine for therapy of systemic amoebiasis. The dose is 1–1.5 mg/kg/day up to 90 mg for 5 days. Among the disadvantages are the requirement for subcutaneous injection, which is associated with local reactions, and severe systemic reactions. Emetine is contraindicated in pregnancy, renal failure and in neuromuscular disease. In the United States, dehydroemetine is available from the CDC; emetine is not available.

*Diloxanide* is the drug of choice for asymptomatic cyst passers. The drug is well absorbed but is ineffective against systemic amoebiasis. It is excreted in the urine, and should be used cautiously in patients with renal failure. The mechanism of action is unknown, but the drug is very active in the lumen of the bowel against *E. hystolitica* cysts. The dose of diloxanide is 500 mg tid for 10 days. The pediatric dose is 20 mg/kg/day in three divided doses. Diloxanide is inexpensive and well tolerated; flatulence is a common side effect; vomiting, pruritus and urticaria occur rarely. Diloxanide and the other luminal agents are also used in combination with a systemic agent in patients with systemic amoebiasis. Diloxanide is available from the CDC.

*Iodoquinol and clioquinol* are luminal amoebicides which are alternatives to diloxanide. They are not well absorbed and in short-term use have little toxicity. The mechanism of action is not known. The dose is 650 mg tid with meals. Long term use has been associated with neurologic complications. Paromomycin, discussed below, is also effective for asymptomatic cyst passers at a dose of 500 mg PO qid.

### Giardiasis

Infection with *Giardia lamblia* is most commonly treated with metronidazole (see above) at a dose of 250 to 750 mg TID for 5–7 days; the lower dose is better tolerated but more often associated with treatment failures. *Quinacrine* is a yellow acridine dye which is an alternative agent for giardiasis, though its greater toxicity makes metronidazole the drug of choice, and quinacrine is not commonly used today and is not available in the United States. The precise mechanism of action is unknown. The dose is 100 mg TID for 5–7 days. For children the dose is 2 mg/kg tid up to 300 mg day. Toxicities include headache, dizziness, vomiting, blood dyscrasiia, dermatitis and ocular changes. Psoriasis, pregnancy, and a history of psychosis are contraindications. *Paromomycin*, discussed below, has been used for giardiasis in pregnancy at a dose of 500 mg PO qid.

*Furazolidone* is a nitrofuran derivative active against *Giardia*. The only drug used for giardiasis available as a liquid, furazolidone is often used for therapy in children. The drug is well absorbed and excreted in the urine. Its efficacy is equal to metronidazole. It is available as a suspension containing 25 mg/5 ml and as a 100 mg tablet. Side effects include nausea, vomiting, diarrhea, and fever, and the drug may cause darkening of the urine. Rare side effects include hypotension, urticaria, serum sickness, and hypersensitivity reactions. Furazolidone may cause mild hemolysis in patients with G6PD deficiency, and can cause a disulfiram like reaction. It should not be given to breast feeding mothers or to neonates.

### Other intestinal protozoans

Infection due to *Dientamoeba fragilis* is usually treated with iodoquinol (see above) at a dose of 650 mg tid for 20 days. Iodoquinol is also active against *Balantidium coli* and *B. hominis.* Tetracycline is an alternative for *D. fragilis* in a dose of 500 mg qid for 10 days. Tetracycline is also active against *B. coli.*

Trichomoniasis can be treated with metronidazole at a dose of 250 PO tid for 7 days, or a single dose of 2 g. The latter is preferred for first-episode or sporadic infections. If sexual partners are not treated, reinfection is likely.

Although the role of *Blastocystis hominis* as a cause of disease remains controversial, metronidazole is clinically active against *B. hominis* and is used at a dose of 750 mg PO tid for 10 days when infection is believed to be a cause of symptoms.

## Drugs used in opportunistic Protozoa in AIDS

### *Pneumocystis carinii* pneumonia

The combination of folate antagonist drugs *trimethoprim* and *sulfamethoxazole* (*TMP/SMX*) is the primary therapy for *Pneumocystis carinii* pneumonia (PCP) in AIDS. Trimethoprim is a dihydrofolate reductase inhibitor with increased activity against some bacterial and protozoan enzymes. Sulfamethoxazole is a folic acid antagonist with similar pharmacokinetics to trimethoprim. The combination TMP/SMX is very well absorbed orally and is excreted by the kidneys. The dose should be adjusted for renal insufficiency. Adverse reactions are increased in patients with AIDS and include rash, fever, nausea and vomiting, thrombocytopenia, leukopenia and hepatitis. The dosage for PCP is 20 mg/kg/day of trimethoprim and 100 mg/kg/day of sulfamethoxazole in 4 divided doses given orally or by the IV route for 14 to 21 days (the latter is recommended for patients with AIDS). If there is no clinical improvement in 5–7 days, alternative therapies should be considered (e.g., pentamidine). When tolerated, TMP/SMX is also the first choice for prophylaxis of PCP in immunocompromised patients in a dose of 5 mg/kg/day trimethoprim and 25 mg/kg/day sulfamethoxazole given three times per week. Desensitization to sulfamethoxazole has been used in patients with allergic reactions, particularly in patients with very low CD4 counts who fail other prophylactic regimens.

Adjunctive corticosteroids in patients with AIDS and PCP have been shown to improve survival, and should be considered for patients with moderate to severe disease (room air arterial oxygen tension <70 mm Hg). The usual dose is prednisone 40 mg bid for 5 days, followed by 40 mg/day for 5 days and then 20 mg/day for the duration of therapy.

*Trimethoprim* in combination with *dapsone*, a long-acting sulfone folic acid inhibitor, is also effective in PCP, although its use is usually reserved for patients with milder cases. Dapsone is well absorbed orally and is given 100 mg once a day, along with trimethoprim 20 mg/kg/day. This combination is better tolerated than TMP/SMX, although side effects such as nausea and vomiting, rash, hemolysis, methemoglobinemia, and granulocytopenia are not uncommon. Trimethoprim/dapsone and dapsone alone are also useful for prophylaxis but not as effective as TMP/SMX. Dapsone is contraindicated in patients with G6PD deficiency.

*Pentamidine* is an aromatic diamidine used to treat *P. carinii* pneumonia in immunocompromised patients, and is useful in leishmaniasis and trypanosomiasis (see below). The drug is given by the IV or IM routes. The mechanism of action is unclear. Pentamidine accumulates in tissues and little of the drug is eliminated via the kidneys. The drug should be used cautiously in patients with liver and kidney disease.

For PCP in AIDS patients, *pentamidine* is considered an alternative parenteral therapy for patients unable to tolerate trimethoprim/sulfamethoxazole (TMP/SMX). Patients are treated with 4 mg/kg/day for 14 days. The drug should be infused over at least one hour to avoid toxicities. Toxicities include sterile abscesses at the site of injections, hypotension following rapid IV infusion, pancreatitis, hypoglycemia, and, paradoxically, hyperglycemia in diabetics. The use of inhaled pentamidine in prophylaxis against PCP in AIDS patients is diminishing as recent trials have shown TMP/SMX regimens to be superior. For patients unable to tolerate TMP/SMX, monthly doses of aerosolized pentamidine given via nebulizer is effective in preventing PCP. Side effects of aerosolized pentamidine include a metallic taste, cough, and bronchospasm. Use of aerosolized pentamidine is associated with atypical X-ray presentations, upper lobe disease, and pneumothorax in patients who develop PCP. In addition, disseminated *P. carinii* has been reported in patients given PCP prophylaxis with pentamidine.

The antimalarial *primaquine* in combination with the lincosamide antibiotic *clindamycin* is an alternative therapy for mild-moderate PCP. Primaquine/clindamycin is most useful in patients intolerant of other therapies, or for whom oral therapy is desirable. The toxicities of primaquine are discussed above. The dose for PCP is primaquine 30 mg daily and clindamycin 900 mg tid for 14 to 21 days.

*Atovaquone* is a hydroxynaphthoquinone with activity against *T. gondii* and *P. carinii*. It is less effective than TMP/SMX or pentamidine in treating PCP in AIDS patients but is better tolerated. It is approved by the FDA for oral therapy of PCP in AIDS patients who are unable to tolerate TMP/SMX. The dose is 750 mg tid for 21 days. Atovaquone must be taken with a fatty meal for proper absorption. Reported side effects include rash, gastrointestinal upset, headache and insomnia.

*Trimetrexate* is a lipid soluble dihydrofolate reductase inhibitor which has been shown to be useful in treating PCP in patients intolerant or refractory to TMP/SMX. The drug is given by the IV route at a dose of 45 mg/m$^2$ over 60–90 min. qd for 21 days. Folinic acid (leucovorin) is administered concurrently at a dose of 20 mg/m$^2$ IV q6h for 24 days to prevent bone marrow suppression. Adverse reactions include leukopenia, fever, rash, nausea, vomiting, and peripheral neuropathy.

### Toxoplasmosis

*Pyrimethamine* (discussed above) in combination with *sulfadiazine* is the primary therapy for toxoplasmosis in immunocompromised patients. Pyrimethamine is given as a loading dose 200 mg on Day 1, followed by 50–75 mg/day with folinic acid 10 mg day along with sulfadiazine 4–8 g/day for 3–6 weeks. Adequate hydration is essential for patients receiving high doses of sulfa. Pyrimethamine in combination with *clindamycin* is an alternative for ocular toxoplasmosis or toxoplasma encephalitis, particularly in patients intolerant of sulfa. In this setting clindamycin is given 600 mg q6h IV or PO in addition to pyrimethamine. Acute therapy in AIDS patients with toxoplasmosis is followed by lifetime chronic suppression (pyrimethamine 50 mg PO qd with folinic acid 10 mg, with sulfadiazine 1.0 g PO bid or clindamycin 300 mg PO qid.

Pyrimethamine/sulfadiazine is also used for congenital toxoplasmosis and for acute toxoplasmosis in immunocompetent patients; the dose in these settings is 100 mg loading followed by 25 mg/day with sulfadiazine 4–6 g day PO for 4–5 weeks. The use of this combination in toxoplasmosis during pregnancy is problematic as pyrimethamine is contraindicated during the first trimester, and sulfonamides cannot be used near the time of delivery. The optimal therapy for toxoplasmosis in pregnancy is uncertain; the new macrolides such as clarithromycin and azithromycin may be useful in this setting.

The macrolide compounds spiramycin, azithromycin and roxithromycin have shown promise in therapy of toxoplasmosis. Azithromycin (1800 mg PO loading dose followed by 1200 mg/day) plus pyrimethamine had been used in patients intolerant of sulfa or who fail other therapy. There is preliminary evidence that atovaquone (discussed above) is useful in treating toxoplasmic encephalitis in AIDS patients who fail standard therapy.

### Therapy of intestinal protozoan in AIDS

Therapy of *Cryptosporidium* in immunocompetent patients is usually limited to supportive care. Many agents have been used in the treatment of cryptosporidium in immunocompromised patients, with little success. There is currently no agent that reliably produces a clinical response. Elimination of immunosuppression in non-HIV-infected immunosuppressed patients and efforts to increase CD4 counts in HIV patients may result in clearance of the parasite. In AIDS patients refractory to anti-parasitic treatment, hydration, nutritional support and octreotide, a somatostatin analog shown to decrease the volume of stools in some studies, are the mainstay of supportive care.

*Paromomycin* is an aminoglycoside used as a luminal agent in the therapy of several protozoa parasites which has been reported in uncontrolled studies to have some efficacy against cryptosporidiosis. It is not absorbed when given orally and activity is limited to the GI lumen. The mechanism of activity is similar to other aminoglycosides. The dose for cryptosporidiosis is 500 mg qid or 750 mg tid given for 2 to 3 weeks. Patients who respond are frequently treated with a lower maintenance dose, although there are no controlled studies. Side effects are largely limited to diarrhea and GI upset.

*Isospora belli* causes a similar illness to cryptosporidium in AIDS patients and responds to trimethoprim/sulfamethoxazole (see above) given qid for 10 days, then bid for 2 weeks.

The role of Microsporidium infection in immunocompromised patients is still being defined. Successful therapy with albendazole (see below) at a dose of 800 mg bid and metronidazole in patients with *Enterocytozoon bieneusi* has been reported, but this therapy remains to be proven in controlled trials.

Therapy of giardiasis is discussed above; AIDS patients usually respond to the normal doses, although the need for prolonged treatment and relapses have been reported

## Therapy of other systemic protozoan parasites

### Leishmaniasis

The therapy of *Leishmania* sp. varies with the clinical syndrome; visceral or disseminated, cutaneous and mucocutaneous leishmaniasis. *Pentavalent antimony* compounds are the primary therapy for disseminated leishmaniasis, and *sodium stibogluconate* remains the drug of choice for disseminated leishmaniasis and some forms of cutaneous leishmaniasis. In French speaking countries and parts of South America *meglumine antimonate* is used instead of sodium stibogluconate. Sodium stibogluconate acts by inhibiting oxidative energy producing processes of *Leishmania* amastigotes; other mechanisms may be involved. The drug is given by the IM or IV route and is excreted by the kidneys.

Pentavalent antimony compounds are much less toxic than the previously used trivalent antimony compounds. Toxicities include pain at the injection site, gastrointestinal symptoms, pancreatitis, headache, arthralgia, nephrotoxicity and reversible prolongation of the Q-T interval which may lead to cardiac arrhythmia. Electrocardiographic monitoring as well as monitoring of renal and hepatic function is recommended. In the United States the drug is available from the CDC. Treatment recommendations vary, but a standard dose is 20 mg/day for 20–40 days. This dose is also used for mucocutaneous leishmaniasis, when indicated (see below). The same mg/kg dose is used for children. The dose can be given every other day in debilitated patients who have difficulty tolerating daily doses. Response to therapy is measured on clinical grounds such as resolution of fever, regression of hepatosplenomegally and normalization of hematopoetic parameters. Pancreatitis, hepatitis and myocarditis are relative contraindications. *Interferon-*$\gamma$, in combination with pentavalent antimony compounds, has shown promise in refractory and relapsing cases.

An alternative therapy for patients with disseminated leishmaniasis who fail to respond (up to 15% in East Africa) is *pentamidine* (discussed above) 4 mg/kg/day for 12 to 15 days, or every other day for 24–30 days. Longer therapy may be required in more severe cases. Other alternatives include amphotericin B, ketoconazole and allopurinol. The specifics of amphotericin therapy are discussed elsewhere (Chapter 38); the mechanism of activity of amphotericin against leishmaniasis is uncertain. For leishmaniasis, a total amphotericin dose of 1 to 3 g is given. The purine analog *allopurinol* has been used in combination with antimonials in patients who failed monotherapy with antimonials. The dose is 21 mg/kg/day in three divided doses for 2–10 weeks. Allopurinol is cleared by the kidney and the dose should be adjusted in renal failure. *Ketoconazole* has been shown to be effective for infection due to *L. mexicana* and *L. panamensis*, but not *L. braziliensis*. Reports of the efficacy of ketoconazole in visceral leishmaniasis vary.

Cutaneous leishmaniasis in Africa, India and the Middle East frequently heals spontaneously and may not require therapy. Lesions that progress or are large at presentation can be treated similarly to visceral or mucocutaneous leishmaniasis. Cutaneous leishmaniasis in Latin America more frequently progress and may spread to mucosal sites, and should always be treated. Pentavalent antimony compounds are the first choice.

## Trypanosomiasis

The therapy of African trypanosomiasis varies with the stage of the disease and the species. The drug of choice for the early hemolymphatic stages of East African (*Trypanosoma brucei rhodesiense*) trypanosomiasis is *suramin*. The drug is active against West African (*Trypanosoma brucei gambiense*) trypanosomes but has been replaced by the less toxic agent *eflornithine* (see below). The primary mechanism of action of suramin is not known; the drug inhibits several trypanosomal enzymes and inhibition of energy metabolism has been shown. Suramin must be given parenterally. The drug has a half-life of 48 h and is primarily cleared by the kidney. Patients with renal insufficiency should be treated with extreme caution and the renal function followed closely. The drug is highly bound to plasma proteins, and small amounts persist in the circulation for up to 50 days. Suramin penetrates the CNS very poorly, consistent with its poor efficacy in trypanosomiasis once the CNS has been invaded. Suramin is usually administered via slow IV infusion in 10% aqueous solution. The normal dose for adults is 1 g given on days 1, 3, 7, 14, and 21, followed by weekly doses for 5 weeks. A test dose of 200 mg is usually given to detect sensitivity. It is advisable to wait until 24 h after diagnostic lumbar puncture, and suramin should be given cautiously to patients suspected of having onchocerciasis as severe systemic reactions may occur. The pediatric dose is 200 mg/kg, given in the same schedule.

Toxicities tend to be more severe in the more debilitated patients; immediate hypotension, seizures and obtundation occur in about 0.01% to 0.3%. Nausea, malaise, fever, chills, and fatigue occur more commonly. Skin rashes and neurologic complications such as headache, paresthesias, and peripheral neuropathy are also not uncommon and occur later. Abdominal pain and edema have also been noted. Patients with AIDS treated with suramin have been noted to develop adrenal insufficiency and vortex keratopathy.

In addition to therapy for hemolymphatic trypanosomiasis, suramin has been used for prophylaxis. It is not recommended for travelers with limited exposure due to its toxicity. The dose is 1 g weekly for 5 to 6 weeks. Suramin is not active against American trypanosomiasis. In the United States suramin is available from the CDC.

*Pentamidine*, discussed above, is effective for the early stages of West African (gambiense) but not East African (rhodesiense) trypanosomiasis. The dose is 4 mg/kg per day for 10 days.

The arsenical compound *melarsoprol* is the drug of choice for the later meningeoencephalitic stages of East African trypanosomiasis (rhodesiense), and is also used for patients with West African trypanosomiasis (gambiense). Melarsoprol can be used in the early stage of trypanosomiasis in patients who cannot tolerate suramin or pentamidine, or who fail therapy with less toxic drugs. Its toxicities preclude use as a first line agent in this setting. Melarsoprol is concentrated in susceptible trypanosomes and exerts a severe oxidative stress on the organism, inhibiting many enzymatic reactions. The drug must by given by the IV route and great care must be taken as it is very irritative to veins and extravisation may lead to severe skin reactions. Melarsoprol penetrates the CNS, accounting for its success in treating later stages of African trypanosomiasis and the propensity for severe CNS side effects. The dose is 3.6 mg/kg on 3–4 successive days, repeated once or twice, with a 1-week interval between each course. Children and debilitated patients should be treated with lower doses. Cures are achieved in about 80%–90% of patients. The prognosis is poor in the nonresponders.

Melarsoprol is toxic and should be given under hospital supervision. A severe reactive encephalopathy occurs in about 5% of patients, and is fatal in 50% to 70%. Other toxicities include hypersensitivity reactions, hypotension, proteinuria, hepatitis, nausea and vomiting. Hemolytic anemia occurs in patients with G6PD deficiency. In the United States the drug is available from the CDC.

For patients with West African (gambiense) trypanosomiasis who are intolerant of melarsoprol, another arsenical, *tryparsamide*, combined with suramin, is an alternative therapy. The doses are tryparsamide 30 mg/kg/day and suramin 10 mg/kg/day every 5 days for a total of 12 doses. Tryparsamide has a mechanism and side effect profile similar to melarsoprol. Tryparsamide is not reliably active against East African (rhodesiense) trypanosomiasis.

*Eflornithine* is a less toxic alternative for early and late stage West African trypanosomiasis, and has been approved by the FDA for this indication. Many strains of East African trypanosomiasis are resistant to eflornithine. The drug is an inhibitor of ornithine decarboxylase and prevents trypanosomal nucleic acid synthesis. Eflornithine penetrates the CNS well; the ratio of CSF to serum concentrations range from 0.09 to 0.45, and the higher concentrations are found in patients with the most severe CNS involvement. The drug is administered intravenously at a dose of 400 mg/kg in four divided doses for 2 weeks, followed by oral therapy at the same dose. Eighty percent of the drug is excreted unchanged in the urine. Eflornithine does not cause the severe systemic reactions seen with the arsenicals, but may cause cytopenias, and cell counts should be followed biweekly. Nausea, vomiting, diarrhea and ototoxicity also occur.

There are no reliable agents for the treatment of chronic American trypanosomiasis (Chagas' disease), and the drugs used for acute Chagas' diseases may not prevent chronic sequelae. *Nifurtimox* is a nitrofuran derivative that is used to treat Chagas' disease. The mechanism of action is mediated through the production of toxic oxygen radicals. The drug is well absorbed after oral administration. The dosage is 8–10 mg/kg/day PO divided into four doses for 90–120 days. For children 15–20 mg/kg/day in four doses are given for 90 days. The reported response rate for acute Chagas' is 90%. The efficacy for chronic Chagas' is questionable, and there is some geographic variability within South America. Drug-related side effects include hypersensitivity reactions, GI upset and weakness. Central and peripheral nervous system side effects also occur. In the United States nifurtimox is available from the CDC.

An alternative agent available only in South America is *benzimidazole*, which is used widely in Brazil. The recommended dose is 5 mg/kg orally bid for 30–120 days. Toxicities include dermatitis, GI upset, myelosuppression and peripheral neuropathy.

### Therapy of infection from free living amoebae

Optimal therapy of primary amoebic encephalitis due to *Naegleria fowleri* is poorly defined. The mortality in this condition is >95%, and there are only four patients with documented infection who survived. *Amphotericin B* was used systemically and intrathecally in these patients, and at least one patient received therapy with several other agents (miconazole, rifampin and sulfasoxizole). The specifics of amphotericin B therapy are discussed in Chapter 38.

Optimal treatment of granulomatous encephalitis due to *Acanthamoeba* species is also unclear. Most cases are diagnosed postmortem, and drug susceptibility testing has varied among different species and strains of the same species. Diamidine derivatives, including *pentamidine* and *propamidine*, have the greatest activity, and *miconazole*, *ketoconazole*, *neomycin*, and to lesser extent *amphotericin B* also have activity.

Treatment of *Acanthamoeba* keratitis with topical therapy, when combined with debridement, has been successful. Several topical anti-amoebics are used together, including 1% *miconazole nitrate*, neosporin, and 0.1% *propamidine isethionate*. Propamidine is a diamidine derivative with anti-protozoan activity similar to pentamidine. Most authorities recommend dosing topical propamidine at least 9 times per day. Therapy should be continued for at least 3–4 weeks. Topical propamidine has produced a reversible epithelial keratopathy after prolonged treatment and can be confused with a relapse of amoebic keratitis.

## Anti-Helminthic Agents

### Agents used primarily for intestinal nematodes

*Mebendazole* (Vermox), *thiabendazole* (Mintezol) and *albendazole* are benzimidazole derivatives that are broad spectrum antihelminthics which act by inhibiting microtubule synthesis and glucose uptake. They are used primarily for intestinal nematodes.

*Mebendazole* is highly effective in ascariasis, enterobiasis, trichuriasis, whipworm, and hookworm. It is active against both larval and adult forms of these worms, and is ovicidal for ascaris and trichuris. Mebendazole is poorly absorbed and undergoes extensive first pass metabolism, so plasma concentrations are low. Systemic toxicity is rare. Gastrointestinal distress is seen in some patients with heavy worm burdens. High doses used for hydatid disease (see below) are sometimes associated with allergic reactions, alopecia and neutropenia. The drug is contraindicated in pregnancy and in children less than 2 years of age.

Mebendazole is supplied as 100 mg tablets. The doses are the same for adults and children greater than 2 years of age. For enterobiasis, a single 100 mg tablet is given, with the dose repeated in 2 weeks. Ascariasis, trichuriasis and hookworm are treated with 100 mg bid for 3 days. A second course is given if evidence of persistent infection is present after 3 weeks. Mebendazole is particularly useful for patients with multiple roundworm infections. *Capillaria philippinensis* requires higher doses; 200 mg bid for 20 or more days. Mebendazole is also used for infection due to *Angiostrongylus cantonensis*. Mebendazole is also used in therapy for *Trichinella spiralis*; most authors recommend concomitant therapy with mebendazole (300 mg PO tid for 3 days, then 500 mg PO tid for 10 days) and corticosteroids (prednisone 40–60 mg PO qd for 3–5 days, followed by taper) in patients ill with trichinosis. Mebendazole and albendazole have been used for cystic hydatid disease, although surgery is usually required. The dose of mebendazole is 400 to 600 mg tid for 3 weeks or longer. Albendazole is the first choice in this setting.

Albendazole was approved for use by the FDA in 1997. The drug is active against a variety of helminths includ-ing *Ascaris*, *Trichuris*, *Enterobius*, *Capillaria*, hookworm, *Clonorchis*, and with prolonged therapy, *Strongyloides*. Albendazole is successful in treating hydatid disease due to *Echinococcus* sp. without surgery in about one-third of cases. Albendazole has also been used as adjunctive therapy with percutaneous drainage procedures in the therapy of echinococcal liver abscess. The drug is also used in the treatment of neurocysticercosis.

Albendazole is supplied as 400 mg tablets. It is poorly water soluble and should be taken with a fatty meal. The drug undergoes first pass metabolism and is primarily excreted in the bile. The mechanism of action is similar to mebendazole. The 400 mg dose used for intestinal nematodes is well tolerated; diarrhea and abdominal discomfort are the most common side effects. Higher doses have been associated with bone marrow suppression, transaminase elevation and alopecia. Albendazole is contraindicated during pregnancy.

*Thiabendazole* is more toxic than mebendazole and is generally not more efficacious, with the specific exceptions noted below. Thiabendazole is well absorbed after oral dosing and is excreted in the urine. The drug is available as 500 mg tablets and as a suspension. It should be given after meals. The use of thiabendazole is limited by toxicities which include pruritus, gastrointestinal upset, fatigue, hypoglycemia, anorexia, and confusion. Fever, rash, hallucinations, angioneurotic edema, and leukopenia are less common. The drug should not be given to patients whose activity requires alertness and its use should be avoided in liver failure. Thiabendazole is contraindicated in pregnancy.

Although active against many roundworms, toxicities have limited the use of thiabendazole primarily to strongyloidiasis. The dose in strongyloides is 25 mg/kg by mouth bid for 2–3 days. Symptoms of strongyloidiasis resolve in >90% of patients; a repeat course is indicated for nonresponders. Disseminated strongyloidiasis should be treated with the same daily dose for 1 to 3 weeks. Thiabendazole is efficacious in cutaneous larva migrans (5 days of therapy) and toxocara visceral larva migrans (1 to 3 weeks). There is evidence that thiabendazole is effective against *Trichinella spiralis*, and appears to reduce symptoms and eosinophilia early in the infection. It is not clear if there is any effect on larvae that have migrated to muscle. Some authors consider mebendazole to be a better, less toxic alternative. Thiabendazole is also used for infection due to *Angiostrongylus costaricensis*.

*Pyrantel pamoate* is a broad spectrum anti-helminthic, active against hookworm, enterobiasis and ascariasis, but not whipworm (trichuris). Pyrantel pamoate is a depolarizing neuromuscular blocking agent that induces spastic paralysis of the worms. Only 15% of a dose is absorbed and excreted in the urine; the remainder is excreted in the feces. Transient gastrointestinal upset is common, while headache, fever, dizziness and rash occur rarely. The dose is 11 mg/kg, up to 1 g, given orally once. Patients with pinworm should be retreated in 2 weeks. The drug should not be used during pregnancy or in children less than 2 years of age. Pyrantel pamoate and piperazine are antagonistic and should not be used together.

*Piperazine* is active against several roundworms, but is more toxic and less effective than other agents, and is used primarily for treating ascariasis when intestinal or biliary obstruction is present. Piperazine causes flaccid paralysis of the worms leading to expulsion from normal intestinal peristalsis. Piperazine is absorbed after an oral dose and excreted in the urine. Renal insufficiency is associated with increased toxicity, and alternative agents should be used. Piperazine is available in 250 mg tablets and in suspension. For ascariasis, 75 mg/kg in a single dose (up to 3.5 g) is given once a day for two days. Children are given the same dose. In patients with intestinal obstruction due to ascariasis, the drug can be given by nasogastric tube in an attempt to expel the worms and avoid surgery. The drug is also active against pinworm, and can be used when dual infection with *Ascaris* and *Enterobius* is present. Piperazine is usually well tolerated, but gastrointestinal upset, hypersensitivity reactions and neurotoxicity can occur. The drug is contraindicated in patients with seizures.

## Drugs active against tissue nematodes

*Diethylcarbamizine* is a piperazine derivative active against *Wucheria bancrofti*, *Brugia malayi*, *Loa loa*, *Mansonella* sp., and microfilaria of *Onchocerca volvulus*. The drug acts by decreasing muscular activity and immobilizing the parasites, and by altering microfilarial surface markers, increasing the susceptibility to host defenses. The drug kills adult worms of *Loa loa*, *W. bancrofti*, and *B. malayi*, but not *Onchocerca volvulus*. Diethylcarbamizine is given orally and is well absorbed and excreted by the kidney. The dose should be reduced in renal failure. Side effects are common but are usually mild and include headache, anorexia, nausea, and at high doses, vomiting. Fever and hypotension can also occur. The major adverse effects come indirectly or directly from the destruction of the microfilaria, and can be severe in patients with heavy infections. In patients suspected of having a heavy infection, therapy should be initiated with lower doses, or pretreatment with steroids should be considered. In patients with onchocerciasis a reaction (known as a Mazzotti reaction) frequently occurs a few hours following therapy characterized by itching, rashes, tachycardia, headache, fever, arthralgia, and enlargement and tenderness of the lymph nodes.

For reducing levels of microfilaria in infections due to of *W. bancrofti* and *B. malayi*, 2 mg/kg tid of diethylcarbamazine is taken orally after meals for 5–7 days. Longer treatment (10–30 days) is required for eradication of adults and possible cure. Retreatment to kill the adult worms is sometimes necessary. Some authors advocate low doses for a prolonged period of time; 6 mg/kg weekly for prolonged periods has been shown to be effective. Treatment of chronic lymphatic obstruction is difficult; prolonged treatment with weekly doses is sometimes successful. *M. perstans* and *M. streptocerca* can be treated with the same dose used for other microfilaria. (Mebendazole, discussed above, is an effective alternative for *M. perstans* at a dose of 100 mg twice a day for 30 days.)

Severe initial reactions are more likely when treating loasis with diethylcarbamazine, and a test dose of 25 to 50 mg on the first day should be given, followed by 2 mg/kg tid for 3 to 4 weeks. Repeat courses are sometimes necessary, and should be separated by several weeks.

Ivermectin (see below) has largely replaced diethylcarbamazine for treatment of onchocerciasis. Diethylcarbamizine is not effective in killing adult worms, and initial toxic reactions can by severe. When lesions of the eye are present, or in heavily infected patients, the initial dose should not exceed 0.5 mg/kg. The dose is then increased to 0.5 mg/kg twice a day on the second day, 1 mg/kg twice a day on the third day, and then 2.5 mg/kg twice a day for 10 days.

*Ivermectin* is a semisynthetic mixture of two compounds derived from the fermentation broth of a soil actinomycete. The drug is active against at least some developmental stage of many nematodes, and is now the drug of choice for treating onchocerciasis. The drug produces a tonic paralysis of the peripheral musculature of susceptible parasites, possibly through the potentiation of the release and binding of $\gamma$-aminobutyric acid (GABA). Some recent studies support a mechanism involving chloride ion influx independent of GABA. The drug is rapidly absorbed after oral administration and is excreted in the feces. Ivermectin penetrates the CNS poorly, probably accounting for its lack of toxicity, as the CNS is the site of GABA producing neurons in humans. The drug is well tolerated with side effects limited to itching, tender lymphadenopathy, and rarely dizziness and hypotension. The drug does not provoke a Mazzotti like reaction, or exacerbate ocular lesions. The drug is contraindicated in pregnancy, in children less than 5 years old and in the first 3 months of lactation. Ivermectin does not kill adult worms, and administration must be repeated in order to control symptoms and tissue inflammation. A dose of 150 $\mu$g/kg taken orally once every 6 to 12 months is effective in controlling microfilaria.

Ivermectin is currently being evaluated for use in other microfilarial diseases and several studies support its usefulness as an alternative to diethylcarbamazine. The ability to give the drug in a single dose is an advantage, but the possible lack of activity against adult worms may prevent ivermectin from replacing diethylcarbamazine as the primary therapy for microfilarial diseases other than onchocerciasis. Recently ivermectin has been shown to be effective against strongyloides in a dose of 150–200 $\mu$g/kg given once orally. Its use as an agent against other gastrointestinal nematodes is being evaluated, and several studies show ivermectin to be efficacious against *Ascaris lumbricoides*, *Trichura trichiura*, and *Enterobius vermicularis*.

*Metronidazole*, discussed above, is often used as an adjunct to surgical removal in infection due to *Dracunculus medinensis* (guinea worm). It is not known whether the activity of metronidazole against guinea worm is due to a specific activity against the worm, or due to a nonspecific anti inflammatory response. Thiabendazole and mebendazole are also used in guinea worm infections.

## Agents active against trematodes and cestodes

*Praziquantel* is a broad spectrum anti-helminthic active against a wide spectrum of trematodes and cestodes. The drug acts by inducing a spastic paralysis, and by causing vacuolization and vesiculation of the tegement of susceptible worms, leading to the exposure of antigens and activation of host defenses. The molecular basis of this action is unknown, but is probably due to changes in membrane permeability to certain cations. Praziquantel is rapidly absorbed and has a plasma half life of 1.5 h. It undergoes extensive first pass metabolism; metabolites are excreted in the urine, most in the first 24 h after ingestion. Transient side effects that may occur shortly after ingestion include nausea and abdominal pain, malaise, headache, and dizziness. Fever, eosinophilia, and rash have also been noted. The drug is considered safe in pregnancy.

Praziquantel is active against all species of schistosomes that infect humans, as well as infection due to *Clonorchis sinensis*, *Opisthorchis viverrini*, *Paragonimus westermani*, *Diphylobothrium latum*, *Hymenolepis nana*, *Fasciolopsis buski*, *Nanophyetus salmincola*, and *Taenia saginata*. A single oral dose of 40 mg/kg or three oral doses of 20 mg/kg taken 4–6 h apart are effective for infection with *Schistosoma mansoni* and *S. haematobium*. Two oral doses 7 h apart are recommended for *S. japonicum*. The lung and liver flukes, *Paragonimus*, *Clonorchis* and *Opisthorchis*, respond well to three oral doses of 25 mg/per day for 2 days. The intestinal flukes *Fasciolopsis buski*, *Heterophyes heterophyes* and *Metagonimus yokogawai* are treated with three doses of 25 mg/kg given in 1 day. The adult cestodes respond to a lower dose: *Hymenolesis nana* (25 mg/kg once); *Diphyllobothrium latum*, and *Taenia* sp. (10–20 mg/kg once). Praziquantel is active against the larval form of *T. solium* (cysticercosis), but requires longer treatment, usually 20 mg/kg tid for 20 days. Therapy with praziquantel kill the cysticercaria, and the resulting inflammatory response may exacerbate symptoms. The drug is not reliable against infection with *Fasciola hepatica*. In the United States, praziquantel is approved only for the treatment of schistosomiasis.

*Niclosamide* is a halogenated salicylanilide derivative that is active against a variety of cestodes, and an alternative to praziquantel for treatment of *D. latum*, *H. nana*, *T. saginata*, and *T. solium*. The drug acts by inhibiting enzymatic steps involved in energy production. There is little systemic absorption, and with the exception of mild nausea, side effects are rare. Niclosamide is supplied as 500 mg chewable tablets and is given as one dose after a light meal. The adult dose is 2 g; for children under 2 years of age the dose is 500 mg and for children who weigh between 11 and 34 kg the dose is 1 g. Treatment of *H. nana* is an exception; the recommended daily dose should be taken once a day for 7 days to prevent autoinfection from larval cysticercoids. Because of the risk of cyctercicosis from release of viable ova from dying adult worms when niclosamide is used in therapy of *T. solium*, praziquantel is preferred. When used for *T. solium*, niclosamide should be followed by a purge 3–4 h after the drug is given.

*Oxamniquine* is an alternative agent for therapy of *S. mansoni*. The exact mechanism of action is unknown; oxamniquine does produce alterations in the tegement of adult worms which may account for its activity. It is absorbed after oral ingestion and excreted in the urine. Toxicities include headache, dizziness, nausea, and diarrhea. Rarely neuropsychiatric disturbance or seizures may occur. The drug may cause orange/red discoloration of the urine. For therapy of *S. mansoni* oxamniquine is active against all stages of infection and in patients with hepatosplenic involvement. The recommended dose varies by region due to intrinsic differences is susceptibility of various strains. In Brazil, 15 mg/kg is given as a single doses. Children less than 30 kg are given 20 mg/kg in two divided doses given several hours apart. In Africa, the dose is 15–60 mg/kg given over 1 to 3 days.

*Metrifonate* is an organophosphate inhibitor effective in treatment of *S. hematobium*. The drug is take orally and toxicities include mild vertigo and nausea. Patients treated with metrifonate should not receive neuromuscular blocking agents or be exposed to organophosphate inhibitors for several days following therapy. The dose is 7.5–10 mg/kg every 2 weeks for a total of 3 doses. The drug is not available in the United States.

*Bithionol* is the preferred drug for treatment of *F. hepatica* and is an alternative to praziquantel for paragonimiasis. The drug is administered orally in three doses of one gram on alternate days for 10–15 days. Adverse reactions include gastrointestinal upset, urticaria, photosensitivity reactions, and rarely, leukopenia and hepatitis. In the United States, the drug has not been approved by the FDA but is available from the CDC for use as in investigational agent.

As mentioned above, *albendazole* is the currently recommended agent for medical therapy of hydatid cyst disease (*Echinococcus* sp.). In this setting albendazole works by disrupting the germinal membranes of protoscolices. The recommended dose is 5 mg/kg bid for 28 days, with three-four course repeated at 14-day intervals. Approximately one-third of patients are cured with medical therapy alone.

## ANNOTATED BIBLIOGRAPHY

Bucher HC, Griffith L, Guyatt GH, Opravil M. Meta-analysis of prophylactic treatments against *Pneumocystis carinii* pneumonia and toxoplasma encephalitis in HIV-infected patients. J Acquir Immune Defic Syndr Hum Retrovirol 1997, 15(2):104–14.
*A good look at antiparasitic therapy in AIDS.*

De Vries PJ, Dien TK. Clinical pharmacology and therapeutic potential of artemisinin and its derivatives in the treatment of malaria. Drugs 1996, 52(6):818–836.
*An excellent review and an emerging class of antimaterials.*

Jernigan JA, Pearson RD. Antiparasitic agents. In: Principles and Practice of Infectious Diseases, 4th ed. Mandell GL, Bennett JE, Dolin R, eds. Churchill Livingstone, New York, pp 458–492, 1995.
*Excellent overview of antiparasitic therapy.*

Liu LX, Weller PF. Drug therapy: antiparasitic drugs. N Engl J Med 1996; 334:1178–1184.
*A succinct review of antihelminthic and intestinal antiprotozoan agents.*

Oldfield EC. Albendazole: new hope for treatment of microsporidiosis in AIDS. Am J Gastroenterol 1995; 90:159–161.
*A report of a possible therapy for microsporidiosis, a newly recognized cause of diarrhea in AIDS and other settings.*

Ottsesn EA, Campbell WC. Ivermectin in human medicine. J Antimicrob Chemother 1994; 34:193–203.
*An excellent and thorough review of an emerging anti-helminthic agent.*

Roos MH, Kwa MSG, Veenstra JG, Kooyman FNJ, Boersema JH. Molecular aspects of drug resistance in parasitic helminths. Pharmacol Ther 1993; 60:331–336.
*A review of the molecular biology of helminthic resistance; most of the data is from veterinary medicine, but much potentially applies to humans.*

Rosenblatt J. Antiparasitic agents. Mayo Clin Proc 1992; 67:276–287.
*A good general review.*

Warren KS, Mahmoud AAF. Tropical and Geographical Medicine, 2nd ed. McGraw-Hill, New York, 1990.
*Several excellent chapters dealing in depth with parasitic diseases and antiparasitic therapy.*

Webster LT. Chemotherapy of parasitic infections. In: The Pharmacologic Basis of Therapeutics, 8th ed. Goodman AG, Rall TW, Nies AS, Taylor P, eds. Pergamon Press, Elmsford, NY, pp 954–1017, 1990.

# 41

# Antifungal Drugs

PETER G. PAPPAS AND JOHN E. EDWARDS, JR.

Amphotericin B has been the mainstay of systemic antifungal therapy for decades, but the toxicity associated with parenteral administration of the drug has led to a search for effective, less toxic, and more easily administered alternative drugs. Flucytosine was among the first of the orally available antifungal compounds to be developed in the amphotericin B era, and it remains an important antifungal agent when used in conjunction with amphotericin B. The development of the azoles has resulted in several effective agents that are used commonly for the treatment of mucosal and systemic fungal infections. Among the azoles, intravenous miconazole has largely fallen into disuse, whereas ketoconazole, fluconazole, and the newest azole, itraconazole, have assumed a prominent role in systemic antifungal therapy, replacing amphotericin B in certain clinical situations. Lipid formulations of amphotericin B show promise of improved efficacy and lower toxicity than the standard compound. This chapter will focus primarily on the currently available systemic antifungal agents and their pharmacokinetics, mechanism of action, toxicities, spectrum of activity, and clinical use.

## Amphotericin B

Produced by *Streptomyces nodosus,* amphotericin B is a lipophilic compound which was released in 1960 as Fungizone, a colloidal suspension of amphotericin B and desoxycholate added as a solubilizing agent. Amphotericin B binds ergosterol in the cell walls of susceptible fungi altering membrane permeability allowing leakage of cellular contents eventually leading to cell death.

### Pharmacology

Amphotericin B is usually given intravenously since oral absorption is poor. Peak serum concentrations are 0.5 to 2.0 $\mu$g/ml after a 50 mg dose (Table 41.1). Amphotericin B is highly bound to serum proteins, principally to $\beta$-lipoproteins. The drug clears the circulation rapidly and is distributed in the liver, lungs, kidneys, and other tissues from which the drug appears to re-enter the circulation slowly. Only a small amount of the drug is excreted in bile and urine, and blood levels are not influenced by renal or hepatic failure. Hemodialysis does not influence blood levels. Penetration into inflamed areas such as pleura, joint, and peritoneum is excellent, though entry into the central nervous system and vitreous humor is minimal. Because of slow release from tissue stores, the drug may be detected in the serum for up to 8 weeks after cessation of treatment.

### Toxicity

The toxicity of chronic amphotericin B administration is well described and includes azotemia, hypokalemia, hypomagnesemia, renal tubular acidosis, and normochromic, normocytic anemia (Table 41.2). Much of the azotemia associated with amphotericin B can be reduced by avoidance of other nephrotoxic agents such as cyclosporine A and aminoglycosides, and avoiding hypovolemia and exposure to diuretic agents. Intravascular volume expansion with 0.5–1.0 L of normal saline daily may also be useful in reducing azotemia associated with amphotericin B. In spite of these measures, nephrotoxicity with amphotericin B is common, and moderate increases of serum creatinine should not necessarily lead to prompt discontinuation of drug. Renal damage is in part dose-related and usually reversible up to a cumulative dose of 2.0 to 5.0 g. In a patient with normal or near-normal renal function prior to therapy, the daily dose of amphotericin B should be decreased or drug temporarily discontinued when serum creatinine reaches 3.0 mg/dl. Alternate day dosing regimens reduce nephrotoxicity only if a reduced total dose is given. Normochromic, normocytic anemia is often encountered 2 to 3 weeks after initiation of amphotericin B therapy. The anemia is usually a consequence of a drug-induced decrease in erythropoietin production, and is reversible after discontinuation of the drug.

Infusion-related toxicities are common. Fever, chills, headache, nausea, myalgias, hypotension, and cardiac arrhythmias have all been associated with amphotericin B infusion. Many of these adverse events, especially fever and chills, can be ameliorated by premedicating with acetaminophen, aspirin or ibuprofen. If unsuccessful, meperidine or hydrocortisone may be useful. A test dose of 1 mg given over 15–30 min usually identifies individuals who will require premedication with the above regimen (s). Amphotericin B can be infused over a 1–4 h period safely. Rarely does the length of infusion require longer than 4 h. A full therapeutic dose should be given within the first 24 h to avoid underdosing. For most systemic infections, a daily dose of at least 0.5 mg/kg is administered, with doses up to 1.0–1.5 mg/kg for selected infections such as invasive aspergillosis and mucormycosis.

### Treatment indications

Most fungal pathogens are susceptible to amphotericin B (Table 41.3), and it remains the drug of choice for most patients with severe, life-threatening disease due to susceptible organisms. Notable exceptions include *Fusarium* sp., an opportunistic fungal pathogen resistant to most antifungal compounds, *Pseudallescheria boydii*, and many dermatiaceous fungi. Resistance to amphotericin B among normally susceptible fungi

**Table 41.1** Pharmacokinetics of amphotericin B and flucytosine

| | Amphotericin B | Flucytosine |
|---|---|---|
| Mechanism of action | Binds ergosterol, damages fungal cell membrane | Inhibits DNA and protein synthesis |
| Administration | Intravenous | oral |
| Daily dosage | .3–1.5 mg/kg | 100–150 mg/kg (normal renal function) |
| Dose adjustment for hepatic and/or renal dysfunction | No | Yes (renal) |
| Protein binding | 95% | Minimal |
| Serum half-life | 15 days | 3–5 h |
| Peak serum concentration | 2.0 $\mu$g/ml | 60–80 $\mu$g/ml |
| Excretion | Small amounts in bile and urine; largely unknown | Renal |

is usually due to altered membrane sterols and may be influenced by prior exposure to azole antifungal compounds.

Amphotericin B is the drug of choice for most serious and life-threatening systemic fungal infections such as invasive aspergillosis and mucormycosis. While amphotericin B, alone or in combination with 5-flucytosine, is effective therapy for invasive candidiasis, fluconazole is a reasonable alternative in some clinical situations. However, there have been no comparative studies between these regimens in overwhelming candida infection. Amphotericin B is still the initial agent of choice for patients with life-threatening invasive candidiasis including those with meningitis, endocarditis, or hepatosplenic disease. Amphotericin B combined with 5-flucytosine is the standard of therapy for non-HIV-infected patients with central nervous system cryptococcosis, but fluconazole is a reasonable alternative initial therapy in HIV-infected patients presenting with less severe manifestations of cryptococcal meningitis. Amphotericin B remains the drug of choice for all patients with serious or life-threatening forms of blastomycosis, histoplasmosis, and coccidioidomycosis while azole therapy is appropriate for mild to moderate forms of these endemic mycoses. Finally, amphotericin B is the antifungal agent of choice for the empiric treatment of the persistently febrile granulocytopenic host.

## Other Formulations of Amphotericin B

There are three amphotericin B formulations available and licensed in the United States: amphotericin B lipid complex (Abelcet), liposomal amphotericin B (AmBisome), and amphotericin B colloidal dispension (Amphotec). ABLC is an equimolar complex of amphotericin B and phospholipids; liposomal amphotericin B is a unilamellar liposome with a 9:1 ratio of cholesterol and phospholipid to drug; and ABCD contains equimolar amounts of cholesterol sulfate and drug. These formulations have been developed to increase the therapeutic index for amphotericin B therapy and improve delivery of drug to patients with deep-seated fungal infections such as hepatosplenic candidiasis and invasive aspergillosis. All of these compounds appear to be less nephrotoxic than deoxycholate amphotericin B. The spectrum of antifungal activity of the lipid formulations of amphotericin B is the same as the parent compound, but there are no clinical trials comparing efficacy. To date, only one randomized, prospective, double-blind study comparing a lipid formulation of amphotericin B (AmBisome) to conventional amphotericin B has been conducted. In this study, almost 700 neutropenic patients received either conventional or liposomal amphotericin B for persistent fever unresponsive to empiric antibacterial therapy. Overall efficacy was equivalent in both treatment arms, but there was far less infusion-related toxicity and nephrotoxicity in the liposomal amphotericin B recipients. Moreover, there was a significant reduction in emerging fungal infections among patients receiving liposomal amphotericin B. In addition to these data, clinical experience with the lipid formulations of amphotericin B suggests that these compounds may be useful for the treatment of invasive fungal infections refractory to therapy with conventional amphotericin B. The optimal dose for therapeutic efficacy while minimizing toxicity is unknown for these agents and probably varies between the different formulations. There is scant data to document serum and tissue levels but there appears to be considerable variation at similar doses of the lipid formulations of amphotericin B.

**Table 41.2** Toxicities of amphotericin B and flucytosine

| Drug | Toxicities |
|---|---|
| Amphotericin B | |
| Infusion-related | Chills, fever, hypotension, cardiac arrhythmias, thrombophlebitis |
| Other | Azotemia, renal tubular acidosis, azotemia, hypokalemia, hypomagnesemia, anemia, thrombocytopenia |
| Flucytosine | anemia, thrombocytopenia, leukopenia, hepatitis, abdominal pain, nausea, vomiting, diarrhea, gastrointestinal ulceration |

**Table 41.3** In vitro susceptibility of selected fungi to amphotericin B and flucytosine

| Organism | Amphotericin B | Flucytosine |
|---|---|---|
| *Aspergillus* sp. | S | R |
| *Blastomyces dermatitidis* | S | R |
| *Candida* sp. | S | S |
| *Coccidioides immitis* | S | R |
| *Cryptococcus neoformans* | S | S |
| *Fusarium* sp. | V | R |
| *Histoplasma capsulatum* | S | R |
| *Paracoccidiodes brasiliensis* | S | R |
| *Pseudallescheria boydii* | V | R |
| *Sporothrix schenckii* | V | R |
| *Trichosporon beiglii* | S | R |
| *Zygomycetes* | V | V |

S, susceptible; R, resistant; V, variable.

## Flucytosine

Flucytosine (5-fluorocytosine, 5-FC) is an orally administered antifungal agent which is the fluorine analogy of cytosine. Originally developed as an antitumor agent, the drug was found to have limited antifungal activity and was licensed in 1972 for the treatment of certain fungal infections. The mechanism of action of flucytosine is by intracellular deamination to 5-fluorouracil (5-FU) which is incorporated into cellular RNA and inhibits protein synthesis. Through several additional steps, flucytosine is also converted to fluorodeoxyuridine monophosphate, which interferes with DNA synthesis through the inhibition of thymidylate synthetase.

### Pharmacology

Flucytosine is a moderately water soluble white powder that is available in 250 and 500 mg capsules. Oral absorption is rapid and nearly complete. Protein and tissue binding is minimal resulting in a relatively short half-life of 3 to 5 h (Table 41.1). Abnormal renal function can increase the half-life to greater than 24 h, but hepatic dysfunction has no influence on serum half-life. Flucytosine concentration in the cerebrospinal fluid is about 75% of simultaneous serum concentrations. Approximately 90% of the drug is excreted unchanged in the urine, and the drug is removed by hemodialysis and peritoneal dialysis.

In patients with normal renal function, flucytosine is usually given as 100–150 mg/kg/day in four divided doses. The daily dose must be adjusted for patients with renal dysfunction (Table 41.4), and patients receiving hemodialysis are given a 37.5 mg/kg dose postdialysis. Serum levels of flucytosine should be measured routinely and maintained between 50 and 100 $\mu$g/ml, as toxicities are far more frequent in patients whose serum levels exceed 100 $\mu$g/ml.

### Toxicity

The toxicity of flucytosine is directed principally against the bone marrow, liver, and gastrointestinal tract (Table 41.2). Liver function abnormalities are seen in approximately 5% of patients. Diarrhea is not uncommon. Leukopenia, and thrombocytopenia may develop and can be severe. Flucytosine-induced hematologic alterations are usually reversible, but fatal bone marrow suppression has been reported. The combination of flucytosine and amphotericin B may be particularly suppressive to the bone marrow. Close monitoring of hepatic, renal and hematologic function is essential. The development of significant diarrhea or abdominal pain should prompt to withdrawal or reduction of flucytosine until symptoms improve or resolve.

### Treatment indications

The spectrum of activity of flucytosine is limited to *Candida* sp., *Cryptococcus neoformans*, and the agents of chromomycosis (Table 41.3). It is not the drug of choice for any fungal infection

**Table 41.4** Dosages of flucytosine in patients with renal insufficiency

| Creatinine clearance (ml/min) | Dose (mg.kg) | Interval (h) | Total daily dose (mg/kg) |
|---|---|---|---|
| >50 | 25–37.5 | 6 | 100–150 |
| 50–10 | 25–37.5 | 12–24 | 50–75 |
| <10 | 25–37.5 | 24 | 25–37.5 |
| Hemodialysis | 25–37.5 | After hemodialysis | |

[From Amsden GW, Schentag JJ. Tables of antimicrobial agent pharmacology. In: *Principles and Practice of Infectious Diseases*, 4th ed. Mandell GL, Bennett JE, Dolin R, eds. Churchill Livingstone, New York, pp 518–519, 1994.]

except chromomycosis. The development of resistance is common among patients treated with flucytosine alone, thus the drug is usually given in combination with amphotericin B, where an additive or synergistic effect is seen in the treatment of candidiasis and cryptococcosis. Data in the treatment of aspergillosis are conflicting, though some investigators have suggested a beneficial effect of combination therapy. Combination therapy with amphotericin B is generally accepted for patients with cryptococcal meningitis (including HIV-positive patients) and patients with severe forms of invasive candidiasis including meningitis, endocarditis, arthritis, endophthalmitis, and hepatosplenic disease.

## Imidazoles and Triazoles

Since their introduction in the late 1970s, the azole antifungal compounds have been increasingly used as less toxic alternatives to amphotericin B and flucytosine for the treatment of systemic and superficial fungal infections. These compounds are fungistatic and exert this activity by inhibiting P-450 cytochrome-dependent 14-$\alpha$-demethylization of lanosterol, leading to the accumulation of 14-$\alpha$-methylsterols and reduced ergosterol concentration in the cell membrane. This results in a more permeable cytoplasmic membrane and the leakage of intracellular contents. The imidazoles (ketoconazole and miconazole) contain two nitrogen atoms in the 5-member azole ring, while the triazoles (itraconazole and fluconazole) contain three. Inhibition of cytochrome P-450 in mammalian cells can lead to decreased synthesis of testosterone and cortisol, but the triazoles have more selective affinity for fungal than mammalian cytochrome P-450 enzymes; thus the triazoles are associated with fewer adverse events than the imidazoles.

## Ketoconazole

Ketoconazole was the first of the orally available systemic antifungal azoles. Released in 1981, the drug has broad antifungal activity and a low incidence of serious adverse effects; however, the newer azole compounds have largely replaced ketoconazole because of superior pharmacokinetics, fewer adverse events, and a broader spectrum of antifungal activity.

### Pharmacokinetics

The pharmacokinetics of ketoconazole and the other azoles are described in Table 41.5. Ketoconazole is available orally or topically. Oral ketoconazole is supplied as a 200 mg tablet, and absorption varies among individuals according to underlying gastrointestinal disease and the presence of gastric acidity. Thus, patients receiving antacids, H-2 receptor antagonists, or anticholinergics have poor absorption and lower serum levels. Important interactions between ketoconazole and other agents are well documented. For example, ketoconazole enhances the effects of anticoagulants and sulfonylureas, and decreases the clearance of cyclosporine, theophylline, chlordiazepoxide, and dilantin. Co-administration of rifampin and/or isoniazid may lead to lower ketoconazole levels through enhanced metabolism of the drug. Ketoconazole should not be co-administered with terfenadine and aztemizole because life-threatening arrhythmias due to QT interval prolongation may occur. Ketoconazole is metabolized in the liver and excreted in the bile as inactive drug. Serum protein binding is greater than 90%; and the drug is not removed by hemodialysis or peritoneal dialysis. Renal or hepatic dysfunction do not alter serum levels, and dosage adjustment is not necessary for these conditions. The half-life of ketoconazole is about 8 h.

### Toxicity

The most common adverse effects associated with ketoconazole are anorexia, nausea, vomiting, abdominal pain, and asymptomatic elevation of serum transaminase levels which is seen in up 10% of patients (Table 41.6). Symptomatic hepatotoxicity is rarely seen (about 1 in 10,000 to 15,000 patients). Rash, pruritus, and headache are occasional adverse events. At dosages of 400 mg daily or greater, ketoconazole may interfere with steroidogenesis resulting in suppression of testosterone synthesis causing decreased libido, gynecomastia, impotence, oligospermia, and menstrual irregularities.

### Treatment indications

Ketoconazole is effective therapy for superficial mycoses caused by *Candida* sp., *Epidermophyton*, *Trichosporon*, and *Microsporon* (Table 41.7). It is also effective therapy for less severe

**Table 41.5** Pharmacokinetics of ketoconazole, fluconazole, and itraconazole

| | Ketoconazole | Fluconazole | Itraconazole |
|---|---|---|---|
| Route of administration | Oral | Oral/intravenous | Oral |
| Solubility | Lipid | Water | Lipid |
| Protein binding | 90% | 11% | 99% |
| Serum half-life | 8 h | 30 h | 20–22 h |
| CSF concentration | Negligible | $\geq$70% | Negligible |
| Urinary excretion of active drug | Negligible | >90% | Negligible |
| Clearance | Hepatic | Renal | Hepatic |
| Dose adjustment for hepatic and/or renal dysfunction | None | Yes (renal) | None |

**Table 41.6** Toxicities of the azoles

| | Ketoconazole | Fluconazole | Itraconazole |
|---|---|---|---|
| Gastrointestinal distress (nausea, anorexia, vomiting) | ++ | + | + |
| Rash, Pruritus | + | + | + |
| Alopecia (reversible) | + | ++ | − |
| Transient elevation of liver enzymes | + | + | + |
| Severe hepatotoxicity | + | rare | − |
| Headache | + | − | + |
| Decreased steroidogenesis, libido, impotence | + | − | +/− |
| Mineralocorticoid excess | +/− | − | +/− |

forms of histoplasmosis, blastomycosis, coccidioidomycosis, paracoccidioidomycosis, chromomycosis, penicilliosis, and pseudallescheriasis. It has been replaced by the newer azoles for deep candidal infections. Ketoconazole is of no value in cryptococcosis or aspergillosis. The drug does not penetrate the cerebrospinal fluid well, and is not useful in treating mycoses of the central nervous system. Generally, ketoconazole is given as a 200 to 400 mg daily dose. For patients who demonstrate no response to therapy after 4 to 6 weeks, the dosage may be increased by 200 mg at weekly intervals to a total dose of 800 mg daily. Adverse events are significantly more common at daily doses exceeding 400 mg daily.

## Miconazole

Originally released in 1978 as a systemic antifungal agent, miconazole is now primarily used for the topical treatment of superficial mycoses. The drug is water soluble, and an intravenous form is available as a 20 ml ampule (10 mg/ml). The usual adult dose is 200 to 1200 mg every 8 h, which results in serum levels of 2 to 6 $\mu$g/ml. There is no oral formulation. Ninety percent of the drug is protein bound, and penetration into the cerebrospinal fluid is poor. Adverse effects are frequent during treatment with intravenous miconazole and include phlebitis, pruritus, nausea, vomiting, fever, chills, tremors, confusion, seizures, anemia, thrombocytosis, and rash. Rapid infusion has been associated with life-threatening cardiac arrhythmias. Intravenous miconazole is the drug of choice for invasive infections due to *Pseudallescheria boydii*, but it is rarely used for other systemic mycoses due the availability of more efficacious and less toxic alternatives.

## Fluconazole

Approved for use in Europe in 1988 and in the United States in 1990, fluconazole differs from the other azoles in that it is highly water soluble, has a longer half-life (approximately 30 h), has excellent penetration into the cerebrospinal fluid (at least 70%

**Table 41.7** In vitro susceptibility of fungal pathogens to the azoles

| | Ketoconazole | Fluconazole | Itraconazole | Miconazole |
|---|---|---|---|---|
| *Aspergillus* sp. | R | R | S | R |
| *B. dermatitidis* | S | S | S | S |
| *Candida* sp. | S | S | S | S |
| *C. immitis* | S | S | S | V |
| *C. neoformans* | R | S | S | V |
| *Fusarium* sp. | R | R | R | R |
| *H. capsulatum* | S | S | S | S |
| *P. brasiliensis* | S | S | S | S |
| *P. boydii* | V | V | S | S |
| *S. schenckii* | V | V | S | V |
| *Zygomycetes* | R | R | R | R |

S, susceptible; R, resistant; V, variable.

of serum levels), is weakly protein bound (approximately 11%), and is primarily excreted in the urine as active drug (Table 41.5). It is the only azole that is currently available in an intravenous and oral formulation. Oral absorption of fluconazole is rapid and complete and is independent of gastric acidity. Because of its renal excretion, the dose must be adjusted in patients with renal insufficiency. Hemodialysis removes 50% of the drug, thus fluconazole should be administered after dialysis. Fluconazole is available as intravenous solution (2 mg/ml) and as oral 50, 100, 150, and 200 mg tablets.

### Toxicity

Significant toxicity with fluconazole is relatively infrequent (Table 41.6). The most common adverse effect is gastrointestinal distress, especially nausea. Vomiting, abdominal pain, and diarrhea may occur. Headache and rash are seen occasionally. Alopecia has been described in patients receiving higher doses (≥400 mg/day) for at least 3 months. Mild asymptomatic elevation of transaminase levels is seen in approximately 1% of patients, however, fatal hepatic necrosis has been reported rarely with fluconazole. Fluconazole inhibits the metabolism and thus increases the plasma concentration of phenytoin, warfarin, and sulfonylureas. Cyclosporine levels may increase in patients receiving fluconazole. Co-administration with rifampin decreases fluconazole serum levels.

### Treatment indications

Fluconazole has broad-spectrum antifungal activity, especially against certain *Candida* sp. and *Cryptococcus neoformans* (Table 41.7). The drug is also active versus many of the dimorphic fungi including *Histoplasma capsulatum*, *Blastomyces dermatitidis*, *Sporothrix schenckii*, *Coccidioides immitis*, and *Paracoccidioides brasiliensis*. Fluconazole is one of the drugs of choice for mucosal candidiasis in normal and immunocompromised patients because of its efficacy and excellent pharmacokinetics. Based on clinical trials in non-neutropenic patients with candidemia, fluconazole is an acceptable alternative to amphotericin B in most circumstances; in contrast there is little comparative data exists to support its use in other forms of invasive candidiasis. For mucosal and cutaneous candidiasis, oral therapy with 100 to 200 mg daily is generally adequate. For patients with invasive candidiasis, 400 mg daily is an appropriate daily dose. Fluconazole is quite effective in cryptococcosis, and is the agent of choice for chronic suppression in patients with AIDS and cryptococcal meningitis. Its role among non-HIV-infected patients with cryptococcosis is unclear. The drug is effective in the treatment of non-life-threatening histoplasmosis, blastomycosis, and lymphocutaneous sporotrichosis, but it is a second-line drug for these conditions. It is highly effective in the treatment of coccidioidomycosis and is probably the drug of choice for coccidioidal meningitis. Patients with these conditions are usually initially treated with 400 mg daily, but doses of up to 2000 mg daily have been used and are reasonably well tolerated.

## Itraconazole

The newest of the orally available azoles, itraconazole was released in Europe in 1989 and in the United States in 1992 for the treatment of superficial and systemic mycoses. The drug is available as a 100 mg capsule and as an oral solution (10 mg/ml). There is currently no approved intravenous formulation of itraconazole, though investigational use of this formulation has recently begun. When taken with food and given as capsules, itraconazole is very well absorbed. The oral solution of itraconazole is maximally absorbed in the fasting state, and achieves a serum concentration 20% higher than the same dose of itraconazole capsule given to a fed individual. Maximal absorption appears to be dependent on gastric acidity. At steady state, the serum half-life is 20 to 22 h (Table 41.5). Ninety-nine percent of itraconazole is protein bound, and concentrations in the epidermis, kidneys, and lungs is about five times that of serum; however, penetration into the cerebrospinal fluid is minimal. Itraconazole is metabolized in the liver and excreted in the bile; little active drug appears in the urine. No dose adjustment is necessary for hepatic or renal dysfunction, and serum levels are uneffected by hemodialysis. As with the other azoles, itraconazole may elevate cyclosporine levels. Unlike the other azoles, the drug does not interact with phenytoin or oral anticoagulants. Rifampin enhances the metabolism of itraconazole and decreases serum levels.

### Toxicity

Significant adverse effects associated with itraconazole are rare (Table 41.6). Abdominal pain and nausea are the commonest toxicities, but rarely necessitate discontinuation of the drug. The drug does not appear to be significantly hepatotoxic nor does it suppress steroidogenesis at recommended doses. Hypokalemia with or without pedal edema has been reported.

### Treatment indications

Itraconazole is the drug of choice for nonlife-threatening histoplasmosis and blastomycosis, and has been effective in preventing relapse among patients with AIDS and histoplasmosis (Table 41.7). The drug is effective in the treatment of nonmeningeal coccidioidomycosis, and it is also an excellent agent for the treatment of lymphocutaneous sporotrichosis. The usual dose of itraconazole for these conditions is 200 to 400 mg daily. Itraconazole is the only azole with significant activity versus *Aspergillus* sp. and has been somewhat effective in indolent cases, but no comparative data with amphotericin B are available. Several noncomparative human trials suggest that itraconazole is effective in the treatment of onychomycoses, chromomycosis and paracoccidioidomycosis.

*Acknowledgments*—This work was supported in part by the NIAID Mycoses Study Group Contract NO1 AI 15082.

## ANNOTATED BIBLIOGRAPHY

Branch RA. Prevention of amphotericin B-induced renal impairment: review on the use of sodium supplementation. Arch Intern Med 1988; 148:2389–2394.
*This article focuses on the beneficial effects of volume expansion with intravenous saline or sodium loading by other means. The author suggests sodium loading in most patients receiving amphotericin B and avoidance of other nephrotoxins and diuretics together with close monitoring of serum electrolytes and renal function.*

Cauwenbergh G, De Doncker P, Stoops K, et al. Itraconazole in the treatment of human mycoses: review of three years of clinical experience. Rev Infect Dis 1987; 9 (Suppl 1):S146–S152.
*This is an early retrospective review of a large experience with itraconazole involving over 1000 patients. The study emphasizes its safety, tolerability and efficacy in selected superficial and deep mycoses.*

Como JA, Dismukes WE. Oral azole drugs as systemic antifungal therapy. N Engl J Med 1994; 330:263–272.

*An excellent review of the oral azole antifungal compounds, this well-written article covers pharmacokinetics, toxicities, spectrum of activity, and clinical indications for ketoconazole, fluconazole, and itraconazole. The authors also provide detailed comparisons with other available antifungal compounds including amphotericin B, miconazole, and flucytosine.*

Daneshmend TK, Warnock DW. Clinical pharmacokinetics of systemic antifungal drugs. Clin Pharmacokinet 1983; 8:17–42.

*This is an excellent review of the clinical pharmacology of ketoconazole, miconazole, and flucytosine.*

Fisher MA, Talbot GH, Maislin G, et al. Risk factors for amphotericin B-associated nephrotoxicity. Am J Med 1989; 87:547–552.

*This is a comparative study between 35 patients with amphotericin B-induced nephrotoxicity and 60 controls receiving amphotericin B to determine risk factors for nephrotoxicity. The authors identified higher daily doses, abnormal baseline serum creatinine, and diuretic use as important risk factors. The authors underscore the importance of maintaining adequate intravascular volume.*

Gallis HA, Drew RH, Pickard WW. Amphotericin B: 30 years of clinical experience. Rev Infect Dis 1990; 12:308–329.

*This is the best recent review of amphotericin B including its pharmacology, chemistry, clinical uses, and adverse reactions. In addition, the authors provide guidelines in the dosage and administration of the drug which should be helpful to most clinicians.*

Grant SM, Clissold SP. Fluconazole: a review of its pharmacodynamic and pharmacokinetic properties, and therapeutic potential in superficial and systemic mycoses. Drugs 1990; 39:877–916.

*This monograph is entirely dedicated to the description of fluconazole and its pharmacokinetics and clinical use. The chief importance of this article is its completeness in describing early pharmacokinetic studies with fluconazole.*

Grant SM, Clissold SP. Itraconazole: a review of its pharmacodynamic and pharmacokinetic properties, and therapeutic use in superficial and systemic mycoses. Drugs 1989; 37:310–344.

*Like the preceding article, this monograph describes itraconazole with an emphasis on clinical pharmacology.*

Sugar AM, Alsip SG, Galgiani JN, Graybill JR, Dismukes WE, Cloud GA, Carven PC, Stevens DA. Pharmacology and toxicity of high-dose ketoconazole. Antimicrob Agents Chemother 1987; 31:1874–1878.

*This is the best review of the pharmacology and toxicity of ketoconazole in therapeutic doses (400–2000 mg daily) in a large number of patients (160). The study demonstrates the poor penetration of ketoconazole into the CSF at any dose. Toxicities were reversible and included nausea and vomiting, gynecomastia, alteration in libido, alopecia, elevated liver function tests, and pruritus. Toxicity was much more common at doses exceeding 400 mg daily.*

Walsh T, Bodensteiner D, Hiemenz J, et al. A randomized, double-blind trial of AmBisome (liposomal amphotericin B) versus amphotericin B in the empirical treatment of persistently febrile neutropenic patients. Abstracts of the 37th Interscience Conference on Antimicrobial Agents and Chemotherapy, September 28–October 1, 1997; Toronto, Ontario, Canada. Abstract LM 90, pg 381.

*The largest comparative trial of AmBisome versus amphotericin B in 687 febrile neutropenic patients. AmBisome proved to be significantly less nephrotoxic, had fewer infusion-related toxicities, and was associated with significantly fewer emergent fungal infections on therapy. This study has been submitted for publication.*

# 42

## Selection of Antifungal Drugs for Deep Mycoses

PETER G. PAPPAS AND JOHN E. EDWARDS, JR.

Invasive fungal infections are among the most difficult infections to treat successfully. Furthermore, the incidence of invasive fungal infections has markedly increased over the last several years due to the increased use of broad-spectrum antibacterial agents and prosthetic devices, the large number of patients receiving cytotoxic chemotherapy, the growing number of solid organ and bone marrow transplant recipients, the acquired immunodeficiency syndrome (AIDS) pandemic, and other factors. Amphotericin B has been the cornerstone of systemic antifungal therapy since its release in 1960, but significant toxicities associated with its use plus the need for parenteral administration have created the need for safer, more easily administered agents. Flucytosine and the three licensed azoles for systemic use, ketoconazole, fluconazole, and itraconazole, have been studied extensively and represent important advances in the treatment of superficial and invasive fungal infections. In this chapter we review the current approach to antifungal therapy for the most common invasive fungal infections, emphasizing effective alternatives to amphotericin B.

### Candidiasis

*Candida* species are a significant cause of morbidity and mortality among both normal and immunocompromised hosts, causing mucosal and systemic disease. The treatment of candidiasis varies from topical therapy for mucosal disease such as oral thrush or vaginitis, to systemic therapy for invasive disease such as candidemia, endophthalmitis, and hepatosplenic candidiasis. A description of a therapeutic approach to the various forms of candidiasis follows and is outlined in Tables 42.1 and 42.2.

### Mucosal candidiasis

The primary treatment for thrush has been oral nystatin, a nonabsorbable polyene antifungal closely related to amphotericin B. Oral clotrimazole and miconazole are effective alternatives to nystatin. For thrush, all are given 3 to 5 times daily for about 7 days in acute cases, but they may be given chronically in patients with AIDS or other significant underlying conditions (Table 42.1). Ketoconazole, fluconazole, and itraconazole have also been used successfully for the treatment of thrush, and these compounds are probably preferable to topical therapy for the treatment of esophagitis. Among patients with AIDS, fluconazole is superior to ketoconazole for candida esophagitis; however, no comparative data with itraconazole are yet available.

Candida vaginitis in nonimmunocompromised women may be treated with a number of topical agents, most notably clotrimazole, miconazole, butoconazole, and terconazole (Chapter 72). For oral therapy, a single 150 mg oral dose of fluconazole has been shown to be as effective as topical azole therapy. Ketoconazole 400 mg daily for 5 days and a single 400 mg dose of itraconazole are also effective.

### Chronic mucocutaneous candidiasis

Although disease is limited to skin and mucous membranes, chronic mucocutaneous candidiasis (CMCC) is difficult to treat with topical therapy alone. Systemic therapy with amphotericin B is effective, but relapse rates are high. The use of immunotherapy, specifically transfer factor, in combination with antifungal therapy has been advocated by some. Other immunotherapies have undergone limited clinical evaluation, but their role in CMCC is unclear. Without question, the use of azoles, particularly ketoconazole and fluconazole, has been the most important therapeutic advance in the management of CMCC. Chronic therapy for months or years with ketoconazole or fluconazole at doses of 200 to 400 mg daily is often necessary.

### Candidemia

Candidemia, particularly intravenous catheter-related candidemia, is the most common form of invasive or systemic candidiasis. Until recently, there were no controlled trials comparing traditional therapy with amphotericin B to newer regimens. A recent study of 206 nonneutropenic patients with candidemia who were randomized to receive either fluconazole 400 mg/d or amphotericin B 0.5 mg/kg/d revealed no statistically significant difference in outcome, though toxicity was more common in the amphotericin B group. The majority of these patients had intravenous catheter-related candidemia. Based on these data, among stable nonneutropenic patients with candidemia, fluconazole appears to be roughly equivalent to amphotericin B in efficacy and is associated with less toxicity. Either regimen is given for about 2 weeks beyond clinical and microbiologic resolution of the infection (Table 42.2). When possible, intravenous catheters should be removed or replaced to decrease the duration of candidemia. For patients with more severe disease and in neutropenic patients, amphotericin B remains the drug of choice. Flucytosine may be added in more refractory cases, but serum levels should be monitored closely.

### Intra-abdominal candidiasis

Candida peritonitis due to peritoneal dialysis may be treated with intraperitoneal amphotericin B 2–4 $\mu$g/mL in dialysate fluid. Treatment is continued for 10 to 14 days. Fluconazole has also been successful in the treatment of candida peritonitis, although treatment is usually extended to at least 4 weeks. Catheter removal is usually necessary for cure. Postoperative intra-abdom-

**Table 42.1** Drugs of choice for noninvasive candidiasis

| Mucosal site | Topical | | | Systemic |
|---|---|---|---|---|
| Oral | Nystatin 100,000 U/mL | | | Fluconazole 200–400 mg/d |
| | (5 cc 3–5 × d) | | | Ketoconazole 400 mg/d |
| | Clotrimazole 10 mg troches | | | Itraconazole 200–400 mg/d |
| | (one 3–5 × d) | | | |
| Esophageal | Not recommended | | | Fluconazole 200–400 mg/d for 7–14 d |
| | | | | Ketoconazole 400 mg/d for 7–14 d |
| | | | | Itraconazole 200–400 mg/d for 7–14 d |
| | | | | Amphotericin B 0.3 mg/kg/d for 7–14 d |
| Vaginal | Clotrimazole | | | Fluconazole 150 mg, 1 dose |
| | 1% cream | 5 g | 7–14 d | Ketoconazole 200–400 mg/d for 5 d |
| | Suppository | 100 mg | 7 d | Itraconazole 400 mg, 1 dose |
| | | 500 mg | 1 d | |
| | Miconazole | | | |
| | 2% cream | 5 g | 7 d | |
| | Suppository | 100 mg | 7 d | |
| | | 200 mg | 3 d | |
| | Terconazole | | | |
| | 0.4% cream | 5 g | 7 d | |
| | Suppository | 80 mg | 3 d | |
| | Butoconazole | | | |
| | 2% cream | 5 g | 3–6 d | |

inal candidiasis is often suspected when *Candida* sp. is isolated from an abdominal drain, but this should not necessarily prompt antifungal therapy. However, *Candida* sp. isolated from ascites fluid or from tissue should prompt therapy with amphotericin B or fluconazole.

Hepatosplenic candidiasis has been traditionally treated with amphotericin B with or without flucytosine. Therapy for several weeks or months is often required and failure rates are high. Recent experience supports the use of long-term fluconazole in hepatosplenic candidiasis following initial therapy with amphotericin B, but no comparative data are available.

## Endocarditis

Candida endocarditis is best treated with combined antifungal therapy and surgical removal of the infected valve. Amphotericin B, usually combined with flucytosine, is given as antifungal therapy and may be necessary for up to 12 weeks after valve removal. Control of the disease without surgery is possible, but the relapse rate is very high, and valve replacement is usually necessary to effect a cure. Recent reports of treatment success with fluconazole are encouraging, but the experience has been limited to anecdotal reports in patients receiving chronic therapy.

## Central nervous system candidiasis

Amphotericin B plus flucytosine is the treatment of choice for meningitis, ventriculitis, and parenchymal disease due to *Candida* sp. The role for intraventricular or intrathecal amphotericin B is probably limited to the most severe cases which are refractory to parenteral therapy. Ventricular shunts, if present, should be removed when possible.

## Urinary tract infection

The ideal approach to urinary tract infection due to *Candida* sp. remains unclear. Persistent asymptomatic candiduria should be treated in immunocompromised patients and in patients in whom an upper tract infection is suspected. Asymptomatic patients with candiduria, particularly those with indwelling urinary catheters, should be observed without therapy. There are three therapeutic choices: amphotericin B local irrigation, flucytosine, and fluconazole. The latter two agents are excreted unchanged in the urine and achieve extremely high urine levels. Amphotericin B local irrigation in a concentration of 50 mg per liter of sterile water may be instilled continuously every 24 hours through a urinary catheter directly into the bladder or through nephrostomy tubes into the collecting system. Flucytosine given alone may be associated with the development of resistance while on therapy and is infrequently used for this purpose. The role of fluconazole in this infection is unclear, although the drug is frequently used in candidal urinary tract infections because of its antifungal activity and favorable pharmacokinetics.

## Endophthalmitis

Candida endophthalmitis is a serious and sight-threatening infection requiring aggressive intervention, often combining vitrectomy with antifungal therapy. Amphotericin B is the drug of

**Table 42.2** Drugs of choice for invasive candidiasis*

| Disorder | First choice | Alternative | Duration of therapy |
|---|---|---|---|
| Candidemia (uncomplicated) | Amphotericin B 0.5–0.6 mg/kg/d<br>or<br>Fluconazole 400 mg/d | Intraconazole<br>400 mg/d | 14 d |
| Intra-abdominal | Amphotericin B 0.5–1.0 mg/kg/d +/− flucytosine[a] 100–150 mg/kg/d | Fluconazole 400–800/d | 14 d after clinical, mycologic, radiographic improvement |
| Endocarditis | Amphotericin B 1.0 mg/kg/d +/− flucytosine 100–150 mg/kg/d | Fluconazole 400–800 mg/d | 6–8 w following removal of infected tissue; chronic therapy may be necessary |
| CNS | Amphotericin B 1.0 mg/kg/d +/− flucytosine 100–150 mg/kg/d | Fluconazole 400–800 mg/d | 4–6 w |
| Urinary | Fluconazole 100–400 mg/d<br>or<br>Amphotericin B bladder washout 50 mg/L sterile $H_2O$ | Flucytosine<br>150 mg/kg/d | 5–7 d |
| Endophthalmitis | Amphotericin B 0.5–1.0 mg/kg/d plus flucytosine if lesions are enlarging or near the macula | Fluconazole 400 mg/d | 4–6 w |
| Osteoarticular | Amphotericin B 0.5–1.0 mg/kg/d | Fluconazole 400 mg/d | 6–8 w |
| Hepatosplenic | Amphotericin B 0.7–1.0 mg/kg/d plus flucytosine 100–150 mg/kg/d | Fluconazole 400–800 mg/d | 2–6 mo (until clinical and radiographic resolution) |

*Except for nonneutropenic candidemic patients, no controlled trials are available to guide therapy. These recommendations are the authors' suggestions based on clinical experience and published reports.

[a]Flucytosine is given at doses of 100–150 mg/kg daily in four divided doses for patients with normal renal function.

choice for these infections; flucytosine is added for more refractory cases and in patients with involvement of the macula. Several recent reports suggest that fluconazole is effective in many cases of endophthalmitis due to *C. albicans*.

## Osteoarticular candidiasis

Vertebral osteomyelitis and septic arthritis are two of the more common manifestations of hematogenously disseminated candidiasis. Amphotericin B is the treatment of choice for these infections. Azole therapy has been successful in these situations, but comparative studies with amphotericin B are not available.

## Cryptococcosis

Cryptococcosis is an important infection among immunocompromised patients, but significant disease is also seen in immunologically normal patients. Clinical trials which address the therapy of cryptococcal infections are limited to the treatment of central nervous system cryptococcosis, and large studies have been performed in both patient populations infected with human immunodeficiency virus (HIV) and non–HIV-infected patient populations. Treatment recommendations are largely based on data from these trials, including recommendations for treatment of extraneural cryptococcosis, where only limited data are available (Table 42.3).

## Central nervous system cryptococcosis

The first studies to evaluate the efficacy of amphotericin B with or without flucytosine in the treatment of central nervous system (CNS) cryptococcosis were published in 1979. Based on data from these studies, the standard treatment for uncomplicated disease in non-AIDS patients became amphotericin B 0.3–0.4 mg/kg daily plus flucytosine 150 mg/kg daily for 4–6 weeks, and this remains the standard regimen in this group of patients. However, due to the relatively high rate of relapse on this regimen, particularly among transplant recipients and other immunocompromised patients, many investigators advocate the use of higher daily doses of amphotericin B (0.7 mg/kg/d) combined with flucytosine given for 6 weeks. Flucytosine levels must be followed carefully, particularly among patients with underlying renal dysfunction and those receiving higher daily doses of amphotericin B. The role of fluconazole in the treatment of non–HIV-infected patients with CNS cryptococcosis is under investigation.

Treatment of HIV-infected patients with CNS cryptococcosis has been extensively studied and continues to evolve. In an early study, treatment results with fluconazole 200 mg daily were found to be not statistically different from treatment with amphotericin B with or without flucytosine as initial therapy for cryptococcal meningitis in patients with AIDS. More recent data suggest that an initial course of amphotericin B 0.7 mg/kg and flucytosine 100 mg/kg/d for 10–14 days followed by long-term fluconazole may be the most effective therapy for the majority

**Table 42.3** Drugs of choice for the endemic mycoses

| Disorder | First choice | Alternative(s) | Duration |
|---|---|---|---|
| CRYPTOCOCCOSIS | | | |
| *HIV-INFECTED* | Amphotericin B 0.7 mg/kg/d and flucytosine 100 mg/kg/d for 14 d, followed by fluconazole 200–400 mg/d | Fluconazole 400 mg/d | Lifelong suppression with an azole |
| *NON-HIV-INFECTED* | | | |
| Central nervous system | Amphotericin B 0.7 mg/kg/d plus flucytosine 100–150 mg/kg/d | Fluconazole 400–800 mg/d | Combination therapy for 4–6 wk; for fluconazole at least 12 wk |
| Pulmonary and other | Amphotericin B 0.7 mg/kg/d plus flucytosine 100–150 mg/kg/d | Fluconazole 400–800 mg/d | Treat until clinical and radiographic resolution or stabilization |
| HISTOPLASMOSIS | Itraconazole 200–400 mg/d or Amphotericin B 0.5–1.0 mg/kg/d for life-threatening disease | Ketoconazole 400–800 mg/d Fluconazole 800 mg/d | 6–9 mo for most patients; chronic suppressive therapy in patients with AIDS and other immunodeficiency states |
| BLASTOMYCOSIS | Itraconazole 200–400 mg/d or Amphotericin B 0.5–1.0 mg/kg/d for life-threatening disease | Ketoconazole 400–800 mg/d Fluconazole 400–800 mg/d | 6 mo for most patients; longer treatment for patients with complicated disease |
| SPOROTRICHOSIS | | | |
| Lymphocutaneous | SSKI 5–40 qtts (drops) tid or Itraconazole 200–400 mg/d | Fluconazole 200–400 mg/d Ketoconazole 400 mg/d | At least 1 mo after clinical and mycologic resolution |
| Extracutaneous | Amphotericin B 0.5–1.0 mg/kg/d or Itraconazole 200–400 mg/d | Fluconazole 400–800 mg/d | 6–12 mo for extracutaneous disease |
| COCCIDIOIDOMYCOSIS | Fluconazole 400–800 mg/d or Amphotericin B 0.5–1.0 mg/kg/d (for severe cases) | Itraconazole 400 mg/d Ketoconazole 400–800 mg/d (non-meningeal) | 6 mos for nonmeningeal cases; lifelong therapy may be necessary for patients with meningeal involvement and immunocompromised hosts |
| PARACOCCIDIOIDOMYCOSIS | Itraconazole 100–200 mg/d | Sulfadiazine 4–6 g/d Amphotericin B 0.5–1.0 mg/kg/d Ketoconazole 400 mg/d Fluconazole 400 mg/d (?) | 6–12 mo for itraconazole; 3–5 yr of therapy with sulfadiazine may be necessary |

of these patients. Persistently positive cerebrospinal fluid cultures and frank relapses are not uncommon among patients with AIDS receiving fluconazole chronically; however, the chronic use of fluconazole 200–400 mg daily is associated with far less toxicity and fewer clinical relapses than chronic maintenance amphotericin B. Lifelong antifungal therapy is required in these patients.

There are fewer data regarding the use of itraconazole for cryptococcal meningitis in patients with AIDS, although preliminary studies have shown promising results. Following induction with amphotericin B and flucytosine, itraconazole 400 mg daily appears to be effective early therapy, but its role as an agent for chronic maintenance therapy is unclear. Finally, combination therapy with flucytosine and fluconazole in patients with AIDS and cryptococcosis has produced some promising results and probably warrants further investigation.

## Extraneural cryptococcosis

There are no controlled trials of antifungal therapy for extraneural cryptococcosis; thus treatment strategies are derived from data generated in the cryptococcal meningitis trials and from collective clinical experience. Patients with disease involving the skin, bone, prostate, and other organs (except the lungs) should probably be treated with combination therapy (amphotericin B and flucytosine) for at least 4 to 6 weeks or with fluconazole 400 mg daily until clinical, radiographic, and microbiologic resolution. Surgical therapy is probably unwarranted in nonpulmonary extraneural cryptococcosis.

The treatment of pulmonary cryptococcosis is in part dependent on the host underlying condition(s) and the risk of dissemination to the CNS. Among normal hosts with pulmonary cryptococcosis, observation alone is reasonable provided that there is no evidence of CNS involvement by examination of the cerebrospinal fluid (CSF) and the pulmonary lesion is stable or improving. Many such lesions resolve spontaneously following several months of observation. In contrast, virtually all immunocompromised patients require antifungal therapy because the risk of extrapulmonary dissemination is high. Combination therapy should probably be used for both the symptomatic normal host and the immunocompromised host. Surgical resection is advised for immunocompromised patients with persistent parenchymal disease unresponsive to antifungal therapy and for a small group of normal hosts with progressive pulmonary lesions. The role of fluconazole in this disorder remains unclear, but clinical experience suggests that it may be an effective agent.

## Histoplasmosis

The majority of cases of primary pulmonary histoplasmosis usually resolve spontaneously, with no therapy necessary. In patients with severe or progressive primary infection, a short course of amphotericin B (500–1000 mg), ketoconazole 400 mg daily for 3–6 months, or itraconazole 200–400 mg daily for 3–6 months is suggested. Among immunocompromised patients with acute pulmonary histoplasmosis, therapy with an azole for 6 to 12 months may be necessary following an induction course of amphotericin B.

The treatment of chronic pulmonary histoplasmosis is poorly standardized, partly because of the difficulty in clinically and radiographically distinguishing between chronic cavitary and pneumonitic disease. The early pneumonitis form of chronic pulmonary histoplasmosis often heals with rest and inactivity, and the use of antifungals in this setting is debatable. Antifungal therapy has traditionally been reserved for patients with progressive chronic cavitary disease with persistent or enlarging thick-walled cavities (Table 42.3). Amphotericin B (2.0–2.5 g) as well as ketoconazole and itraconazole (both given at 400 mg daily for 6–9 months) are effective. Relapse off therapy is common and requires retreatment, usually with an azole. Fluconazole has not been particularly useful in the treatment of chronic pulmonary disease.

In contrast to pulmonary histoplasmosis, all patients with disseminated (extrapulmonary) disease require antifungal therapy. For patients with severe, life-threatening disease, and for those with endocarditis or central nervous system involvement, amphotericin B (2.0–2.5 g) is the drug of choice. Among non-AIDS patients with milder disease, ketoconazole 400 mg daily or itraconazole 200 mg twice daily, given for at least 12 months, is effective. Fluconazole, when given at doses of 400–800 mg daily, is a reasonable alternative. Regardless of the initial therapy, relapses off therapy are common, particularly among patients with chronic immunodeficiency states, thus prolonged or even lifelong therapy may be required. Among patients with AIDS and severe histoplasmosis, induction therapy with amphotericin B (500–1000 mg) usually leads to a marked decrease in organism load and resolution of clinical illness, and this is followed by itraconazole 200 mg twice daily. In less severely ill patients, itraconazole may be given as initial therapy. Fluconazole given at 800 mg daily for patients with mild to moderate disease may be an alternative for primary therapy, but relapses on therapy are more common than with itraconazole. Ketoconazole is not recommended in patients with AIDS and histoplasmosis due to the possibility of inadequate absorption associated with HIV gastropathy.

All patients with HIV and disseminated histoplasmosis, regardless of the initial regimen, require lifelong antifungal suppression to prevent relapsing disease. Itraconazole 200–400 mg daily is the most widely used regimen for this purpose. This drug is well tolerated, and relapses on therapy are uncommon. Fluconazole at a dose of 400 mg may be an alternative for patients who cannot tolerate itraconazole, but it is less effective than itraconazole at this dose.

## Blastomycosis

Intravenous amphotericin B has traditionally been the standard of therapy for blastomycosis, but the development of effective oral azoles, specifically ketoconazole and itraconazole, has provided therapeutic alternatives for patients with non–life-threatening, non-CNS disease (Table 42.3). Ketoconazole is given at 400 mg daily, but it may be increased by 200 mg increments to as much as 800 mg daily in patients not responding to lower doses. Therapy is continued for at least 6 months. Itraconazole, given at doses of 200–400 mg daily, is even more effective than ketoconazole when given for at least 6 months. Success rates of 90%–95% can be expected in patients with chronic, indolent disease who are treated appropriately with itraconazole. Experience with fluconazole at the usual therapeutic doses of 200–400 mg daily suggests that it is not as effective as itraconazole. However, at higher doses (up to 800 mg daily) fluconazole appears to be roughly equivalent to itraconazole 200–400 mg daily.

Amphotericin B at a cumulative dose of 1.5–2.0 g should be given to patients with life-threatening or refractory disease and those with CNS blastomycosis. Some experts advocate a short course of "induction therapy" with amphotericin B (about 500 mg) to gain control of the disease followed by several months of ketoconazole or itraconazole. Fluconazole should be reserved for patients who cannot tolerate or who have failed other azole therapy. Patients should be given 400 mg daily, increasing to 800 mg daily in patients who fail to respond to the lower dose. Fluconazole may also have a role in the treatment of CNS blastomycosis in patients who have received an initial course of amphotericin B.

Controversy exists whether to treat all patients with acute pulmonary blastomycosis. For the majority of patients, this is a self-limited disease that requires no treatment. Thus many clinicians elect close observation without therapy provided that long-term follow-up is available to monitor for disease activity.

## Coccidioidomycosis

Primary infection with *Coccidioides immitis* is usually self-limited and requires no treatment. Therapy is usually reserved for patients with progressive disease and for immunocompromised patients with primary infection, although there are few published data to support treatment in the latter group. Amphotericin B has traditionally been the treatment of all forms of chronic progressive coccidioidomycosis at cumulative doses of 1–3 g. Intrathecal amphotericin B has been used successfully as chronic therapy for coccidioidal meningitis, although treatment-associated toxicity has limited its use. Azole antifungals have greatly expanded the treatment options for coccidioidomycosis (Table 42.3). Ketoconazole at doses of 400–800 mg daily is effective therapy for nonmeningeal disease, but relapses off therapy are common. Itraconazole at doses of 400 g daily, also effective for treatment of nonmeningeal disease, is better tolerated and less toxic than ketoconazole. Perhaps the most important new therapy, however, has been the use of fluconazole in doses of 400–800 mg daily for the treatment of chronic progressive coccidioidomycosis including coccidioidal meningitis. The length of therapy for all of the azoles is at least 6 months, and in some patients, particularly immunocompromised patients and those with meningeal involvement, lifelong therapy may be required. Among patients with AIDS and others with disorders of T-cell function, an induction course of amphotericin B (approximately 1 g) may be necessary to reduce organism load and gain control of the disease since it can be particularly aggressive and progress rapidly in this population.

## Paracoccidioidomycosis

Paracoccidioidomycosis is the only systemic mycosis for which sulfonamides are effective therapy. Sulfadiazine 4–6 g daily or one of the long-acting sulfonamides (1–2 g/d) can be used. After a clinical and mycologic response, the dose can be reduced but must be continued for prolonged periods, often for several years, to avoid relapse. Toxicities, especially fever and rash, are common. Amphotericin B is generally reserved for more severe and life-threatening forms of the disease and is given in cumulative doses of 1–3 g. Adjunctive therapy with a sulfonamide or an azole for months or years following completion of amphotericin B is necessary to prevent relapse.

Oral azole therapy represents a major advance in therapy of this disease (Table 42.3). Ketoconazole at doses of 200–400 mg daily given for 6–18 months compares favorably with amphotericin B plus sulfonamide therapy. Itraconazole at a dose of 100 mg daily for 6–12 months is associated with a lower relapse rate and less toxicity than ketoconazole. These considerations together with a shorter duration of therapy have led most clinicians to agree that itraconazole is the drug of choice for most forms of paracoccidioidomycosis. Experience with fluconazole is limited and appears to be favorable, but more data are necessary to determine the role of fluconazole in the treatment of this disease.

## Sporotrichosis

The traditional therapy of lymphocutaneous sporotrichosis has been a saturated solution of potassium iodide (SSKI), usually starting at 5 drops three times daily, increasing to as much as 120 drops daily in 3 to 5 drop increments daily. Although effective for most cases of lymphocutaneous sporotrichosis, this therapy is cumbersome and frequently toxic, causing rash, parotid enlargement, lacrimation, and gastrointestinal distress. Iodide therapy is given for at least 1 month following resolution of clinical findings.

Itraconazole in doses of 200–400 mg daily is an effective alternative to SSKI for cutaneous disease and is considerably less toxic, though more expensive. Itraconazole in doses of 200–400 mg daily is also moderately effective in the treatment of extracutaneous sporotrichosis, and it is more effective than either ketoconazole or fluconazole for both cutaneous and extracutaneous disease (Table 42.3).

Amphotericin B should be given to patients with cutaneous or extracutaneous disease who have failed conventional therapy with iodide or azoles and to immunocompromised patients with widely disseminated or life-threatening disease. Doses of 2.0–2.5 g may be required for patients with more refractory disease, including those with pulmonary or meningeal involvement. Surgical resection of involved synovium, lung, bone, or other tissue combined with antifungal therapy may be necessary in selected patients with extracutaneous disease. In some patients with extracutaneous sporotrichosis, an induction course of amphotericin B followed by long-term itraconazole therapy may be appropriate.

## Aspergillosis

Intravenous amphotericin B remains the drug of choice for invasive aspergillosis, but response to therapy remains poor in immunocompromised patients, particularly those with prolonged neutropenia. Daily doses of 1.0–1.5 mg/kg are generally advised for patients with proven or suspected invasive disease (Table 42.4). The addition of rifampin and/or flucytosine is commonly practiced based on in vitro data suggesting synergy with one or both of these compounds. However, clinical studies have never demonstrated a beneficial effect of combination therapy. Liposomal formulations of amphotericin B may play a significant role in the treatment of invasive aspergillosis in the future because they are less nephrotoxic and higher daily doses may be administered.

Itraconazole has demonstrated some benefit in patients with more indolent forms of the disease; however, no comparative studies with amphotericin B are available. When used, itraconazole should be given in a loading dose of 300–400 mg twice daily for 3 days, followed by 200 mg twice daily. The drug is probably not very effective in neutropenic patients and in patients with AIDS who have invasive aspergillosis.

Surgical resection of involved tissue is important in the management of invasive aspergillosis and has been successful in some cases involving brain, paranasal sinuses, and lung. Excision of infected heart valves, whether native or prosthetic, seems to be essential for providing a chance of cure. Among patients with pulmonary aspergillomata, surgical resection is generally reserved for those patients with recurrent, significant hemoptysis, but it should be undertaken with great caution since postoperative complications are common. Intracavitary amphotericin B has been used successfully in certain centers for inoperable aspergilloma, but it is not advised in usual cases.

## Zygomycosis

There are no controlled studies to evaluate the treatment strategies for zygomycosis (also known as mucormycosis). Because of the aggressive and necrotizing nature of the infection, surgical debridement, when possible, is advisable. Amphotericin B, given at doses of 1.0–1.5 mg/kg daily, is the antifungal drug of choice, although response to antifungal therapy alone is usually poor (Table 42.4). Once control of the disease is attained, alternate day amphotericin B given to a cumulative dose of 2.0–3.0 g is appropriate. The liposomal formulations of amphotericin B probably have a significant role in the management of zygomycosis, but this is as yet unproven. There is no role for the azole antifungals in the management of this disease.

**Table 42.4** Drugs of choice for invasive mold disease

| Disorder | First choice | Alternative | Duration |
|---|---|---|---|
| Aspergillosis | Amphotericin B 1.0–1.5 mg/kg/d or lipid Amphotericin B 5–7.5 mg/kg/d | Itraconazole 400–600 mg/d | No clear guidelines are established, but 6–8 wk after clinical radiographic and mycologic resolution of disease is reasonable. Debriding surgery is usually necessary for optional outcome in most cases of invasive aspergillosis, pseudallescheriasis, and zygomycosis |
| Pseudallescheriasis | Miconazole 200–800 mg 3 times/d | Itraconazole 400 mg/d<br>Ketoconazole 400–800 mg/d | |
| Zygomycosis (mucormycosis) | Amphotericin B 1.0–1.5 mg/kg/d or lipid Amphotericin B 5–7.5 mg/kg/d] | None | |

## Pseudallescheriasis

Pseudallescheriasis is an uncommon invasive fungal infection, and it is the only deep mycosis for which miconazole is the drug of first choice. The usual adult dose is 800 mg every 8 hours intravenously (Table 42.4). Ketoconazole and itraconazole have had limited success in a few cases. Amphotericin B is generally ineffective against *Pseudallescheria boydii*. Similar to aspergillosis and zygomycosis, surgical drainage and/or debridement, when possible, is important in the management of pseudallescheriasis.

## Other Emerging Fungi

The list of emerging, largely opportunistic fungi is rapidly increasing, and an extensive review is beyond the scope of this text. Chief among emerging organisms are *Fusarium* species and *Trichosporon beigelii*, but other fungi including the dermatiaceous fungi are also among the more commonly recognized pathogens. A brief description of selected emerging fungal pathogens is included in Table 42.5.

**Table 42.5** Emerging fungal pathogens

| Organism | Clinical manifestations | Therapy |
|---|---|---|
| *Fusarium* sp. | Localized or disseminated disease associated with skin lesions and positive blood cultures (60%) in patients with hematologic malignancy and neutropenia. | Conventional antifungal agents are generally inactive. Reconstitution of the immune system is essential to recovery. |
| *Paecilomyces lilacinus* | Localized cutaneous, ocular, or disseminated disease in immunocompromised hosts. | Surgical debridement is usually curative. Fluconazole or itraconazole may be useful adjuncts to surgery. |
| *Scedosporium prolificans* | Disseminated disease with positive blood cultures in neutropenic and other immunocompromised hosts. | Surgical resection of localized tissue involvement is essential. Resistant to all available antifungals. |
| *Trichosporon beigelii* | Pneumonia, cutaneous, and disseminated disease including chronic hepatosplenic involvement. | Immune reconstitution essential to recovery. Fluconazole probably more active than amphotericin B, long-term therapy often necessary. |
| *Malassezia furfur* | Fungemia in normal and immunocompromised patients receiving intravenous lipids at highest risk. | Removal of intravenous catheter essential and usually curative. Short-course therapy with amphotericin B or fluconazole in selected patients. |
| *Penicillium marneffei* | Disseminated hematogenous and cutaneous disease in patients with advanced HIV disease living in Southeast Asia. | Amphotericin B or itraconazole have been successful, but chronic antifungal suppressive therapy is essential. |

*Acknowledgment*—This work is supported in part by the NIAID Mycoses Study Group under Contract NO1 AI 15082.

## ANNOTATED BIBLIOGRAPHY

Denning DW, Lee JY, Hostetler JS, et al: NIAID Mycoses Study Group trial of oral itraconazole therapy for invasive aspergillosis. Am J Med 1994; 97:135–144.

*This is the largest published experience with itraconazole for the treatment of aspergillosis. Seventy-six patients were studied with a variety of underlying conditions including granulocytopenia, solid organ and bone marrow transplantation, glucocorticosteroids, and AIDS. The overall response rate of about 40% was similar to previous experience with amphotericin B.*

Dismukes WE, Bradsher RW, Cloud GC, et al. Itraconazole therapy for blastomycosis and histoplasmosis. Am J Med 1992; 96:489–497.

*This randomized, open-label study compared two doses of itraconazole (200 mg and 400 mg) in 48 patients with blastomycosis and 37 patients with histoplasmosis who had non–life-threatening, non–central nervous system disease. These results demonstrate a very favorable response to itraconazole in both disorders; successful outcome were seen in 95% of patients with blastomycosis and 81% with histoplasmosis, comparable to results seen with amphotericin B and superior to results seen with ketoconazole.*

Dismukes WE, Cloud G, Gallis HA, et al. Treatment of cryptococcal meningitis with combination amphotericin B and flucytosine for four as compared with six weeks. N Engl J Med 1987; 317:334–341.

*A classic antifungal clinical trial involving 194 patients with cryptococcal meningitis which compared 4 weeks to 6 weeks therapy with amphotericin B plus 5-flucytosine. The study defined the population for whom 4 weeks of therapy was appropriate, and remains the "gold standard" by which other trials in non–AIDS patients are measured.*

Galgiani JN, Cantanzaro A, Cloud GA, et al. Fluconazole therapy for coccidioidal meningitis. Ann Intern Med 1993; 119:28–35.

*Forty-seven patients with coccidioidal meningitis including 9 with HIV infection were treated with fluconazole 400 mg daily for up to 4 years. Almost 80% of patients responded to treatment and no one stopped drug due to toxicity. This represents major improvement over lifelong intravenous and/or intrathecal amphotericin B for treatment of this disorder.*

Graybill JR, Stevens DA, Galgiani JN, et al. Itraconazole treatment of coccidioidomycosis. Am J Med 1990; 89:282–290.

*Forty-seven patients with chronic nonmeningeal coccidioidomycosis were treated with itraconazole 100–400 mg daily for up to 3 years. Almost 60% of patients achieved remission and fewer than 10% relapsed off therapy. Itraconazole appears to be effective in nonmeningial coccidioidomycosis.*

National Institute of Allergy and Infectious Diseases Mycoses Study Group. Treatment of blastomycosis and histoplasmosis with ketoconazole. Ann Intern Med 1985; 103:861–872.

*The first large study to examine the efficacy and toxicity of ketoconazole in 80 patients with blastomycosis and 54 with histoplasmosis, this study demonstrated the efficacy of ketoconazole at doses of 400 mg and 800 mg daily in both disorders. Based on the results of this study, the recommendation for treatment of these two disorders included administering ketoconazole 400 mg daily for at least 6 months for nonmeningeal disease.*

Rex JH, Bennett JE, Sugar AM, et al. A randomized trial comparing fluconazole with amphotericin B for the treatment of candidemia in patients without neutropenia. N Engl J Med 1994; 331:1325–1330.

*This is the first and largest randomized study in the treatment of candidemia. It compared fluconazole to amphotericin B, and there were no statistically significant differences in outcome in 206 patients, most of whom had intravenous catheter-related candidemia. At least 2 weeks of therapy with fluconazole 400 mg daily or amphotericin B 0.6 mg/kg/d appears to be equivalent among nonneutropenic patients with intravenous catheter-related candidemia.*

Saag MS, Powderly WG, Cloud GA, et al. Comparison of amphotericin B with fluconazole in the treatment of acute AIDS-associated cryptococcal meningitis. N Engl J Med 1992; 326:83–89.

*In this open-label randomized trial, 194 patients with AIDS-associated cryptococcal meningitis received either fluconazole 200 mg daily (131 patients) or amphotericin B at least 0.3 mg/kg/d (63 patients) for 10 weeks. Although there was no significant difference in overall outcome, mortality in the first 2 weeks was higher in the fluconazole-treated group.*

Van der Horst CM, Saag MS, Cloud GA, Hamill RJ, et al. Treatment of cryptococcal meningitis associated with the acquired immunodeficiency syndrome. N Engl J Med 1997; 337:15–21.

*This is the largest study to date involving patients with AIDS and cryptococcal meningitis. The study suggests that amphotericin B plus flucytosine is equivalent to amphotericin B alone for induction therapy, and that fluconazole and itraconazole were equivalent for "consolidation therapy" in these patients. However, follow-up studies suggest that relapse rates are higher among patients not receiving flucytosine during the induction phase.*

Wheat J. Histoplasmosis: recognition and treatment. Clin Infect Dis 1994; 19(suppl 1):S19–27.

*An excellent review by one of the authorities on histoplasmosis, this article discusses current therapeutic and diagnostic approaches to this disorder in a succinct fashion.*

Wheat J, Hafner R, Wulfsohn M, et al. Prevention of relapse of histoplasmosis with itraconazole in patients with the acquired immunodeficiency syndrome. Ann Intern Med 1993; 118:610–616.

*Following successful induction therapy with amphotericin B (≥15 mg/kg) 42 patients with AIDS-associated histoplasmosis were given itraconazole 200 mg twice daily for at least 1 year. More than 90% of patients were successfully treated. Based on this and other studies, itraconazole has become the azole of choice for chronic suppression in patients with AIDS and histoplasmosis.*

# IV

## VACCINES AND IMMUNOMODULATORY AGENTS

# 43

# Principles of Vaccine Development and Immunoprophylaxis

GORDON L. ADA

The two principal attributes of a vaccine are safety and efficacy. Safety has become increasingly important and is now the decisive property; at the same time a substantial degree of efficacy must be demonstrated before a vaccine is used in humans. These properties are assessed in a series of steps. Following immunization studies in a susceptible nonhuman host to determine safety and conditions for inducing a protective response, a series of clinical trials is initiated in the following sequence:

- Phase I. Safety and limited immunogenicity studies.
- Phase II. More extensive studies measuring both properties, frequently in a more diverse group of recipients.
- Phase III. Efficacy studies in an endemic region.

If the candidate vaccine passes these tests, it is registered for general use. In the United States postregistration surveillance is carried out to detect unfavorable responses to the vaccination which may occur at a very low frequency.

For many years the sole measure of efficacy was the ability of a vaccine to prevent disease when the vaccinated host was later exposed to the wild-type infectious agent. This remains the major goal, but researchers increasingly look for evidence for correlates of protection, such as the level in the serum of vaccinees of antibodies capable of neutralizing the infectivity of the agent. With intracellular infections, it was found that there was not always a correlation between efficacy and antibody levels, so attention was directed first to determining the proliferative response of T lymphocytes to specific antigen, and, more recently, to measuring the level of T cell–mediated cytotoxicity. If such correlates could be demonstrated, vaccines could be designed to use the most effective way of inducing such responses. This has become the favored approach to the daunting task of developing vaccines to agents which cause chronic persisting infections, such as *Plasmodia* (malaria) and human immunodeficiency virus/acquired immunodeficiency syndrome (HIV/AIDS) (see Chapter 99).

## Vaccine Efficacy

The efficacy of a vaccine depends on the immune response it generates. Because vaccines for prophylaxis may be administered weeks, months, or even years before exposure to the wild-type agent occurs, efficacy depends on the response of mainly one cell type, the lymphocyte. Following activation, the lymphocyte displays two critical characteristics, specificity and memory—hence the term the *specific adaptive immune response*. Bone-marrow-derived lymphocytes (B cells) have specific immunoglobulin (Ig) receptors for antigen of two isotypes, IgM and IgD. Following stimulation, which leads to replication and differentiation, these cells, as plasma cells, may secrete other Ig isotypes, IgG, IgA, and IgE. Immunoglobulin G may be further subdivided into several more subgroups (see Chapter 11).

Recent studies have greatly expanded our understanding of the other class of lymphocytes, the T cells (thymus-derived cells), which are responsible for cell-mediated responses. The major cytokines produced by the three T-cell subsets and their actions are listed in Table 43.1. Chapter 11 also describes the properties of antigen-presenting cells (APCs) such as dendritic cells and macrophages and the recognition mechanisms of T and B cells.

## The Role of Immune Responses in the Prevention, Control, and Clearing of Intracellular Infection

During the course of an acute infection (one in which the immune response results in clearance of the infectious agent), immune responses generally are detected in the following sequence: regulatory T cells, effector T cells, and finally antibody.

Table 43.2 summarizes the roles of the different effector mechanisms before and during an acute infection. Specific antibody is the only mechanism that has the potential completely or largely to prevent an infection; thus an elaborate mechanism has evolved to ensure the continual presence of such antibody following infection or an effective vaccination.

Antibody also has the potential to control an intracellular infection by the lysis of infected cells (antibody-dependent cellular cytotoxicity, ADCC, or complement-dependent lysis) following the expression of foreign antigens at the surface of the infected cells (see Chapter 11). Except in rather special circumstances, however, there is little evidence that antibody in the absence of effector T cells can clear an intracellular infection. Furthermore, it is difficult to devise an immunization schedule that would generate antibody of sufficiently high affinity and specificity to clear a subsequent infection once it had become established.

Effector T cells are the *major* mechanism for controlling and clearing an *intracellular* infection. Evidence derived mainly from model systems, especially murine, indicates that peptides from newly synthesized foreign proteins in the cytosol of an infected cell combine with class I MHC (major histocompatibility complex) molecules. Once this complex is expressed on the cell surface, the infected cells are very likely to be destroyed by the induced cytotoxic T lymphocytes (CTLs). In some situations, such as murine leishmaniasis infections, the data suggest that a predominantly TH1 response confers protection by promoting macrophage activation. It is difficult to obtain conclusive evidence for a decisive role for TH1 cells in clearing an infection,

**Table 43.1** Cytokine profile and specific actions of T-cell subgroups

| Subgroup | Cytokine profile | Immune response |
|---|---|---|
| TH2 (CD4+) | IL-3, 4, 5, 6, 10, 13; TNF-$\alpha$ | Promotes antibody production by B cells |
| TH1 ($CD4^+$) | IL-2, 3; IFN-$\gamma$, TNF-$\alpha$, $\beta$ | Has direct antiviral effects; activates APCs; may promote CTL responses. |
| CTLs ($CD8^+$) | IL-2; IFN-$\gamma$, TNF-$\beta$ | May lyse infected cells and malignant cells. |

Abbreviations: IL, interleukin; IFN-$\gamma$, gamma interferon; TNF, tumor necrosis factor; CTLs, cytotoxic lymphocytes; APCs, antigen-presenting cells.

since there is currently no method for physically separating primary TH1 and TH2 cells.

Thus the outcome following infection of a naive host is determined by the timing and extent of the effector T-cell response. Persisting infections frequently occur because the effector T-cell response is inhibited or is bypassed in one or more of a number of possible ways.

## Four General Requirements for Successful Vaccination

Based on the preceding considerations, four general requirements for a vaccine to be successful can be proposed:

1. The foreign antigens should be "processed" correctly in the APC, resulting in the binding of several peptides to the host's MHC antigens, the expression of costimulator molecules at the surface of the APC, and probably the secretion of certain cytokines.

2. The vaccine should include peptide sequences containing several T- and B-cell epitopes, the latter especially of a specificity recognized by antibody capable of neutralizing the infectivity of the agent. If possible, these epitopes should come from conserved regions of the antigens. In this way, not only may the effects of antigenic variation be minimized, but the T-cell receptors in a majority of hosts in an outbred population recognize one or more of the MHC–peptide complexes and mount an effective immune response.

3. Both effector T and B cells have a short (days to weeks) half-life. Therefore, an effective vaccine should induce large pools of memory T and B cells. The memory T cells would ensure a more rapid T-cell response when a later challenge with the wild-type agent occurred; the memory B cells are necessary to provide a continuing production of antibody.

4. The localization of antigen (as antigen–antibody complexes) on the surface of follicular dendritic cells in the follicles in lymphoid tissues facilitates the formation of memory B cells. As these follicles turn into germinal centers, somatic hypermutation of B-cell receptors occurs, allowing those cells with receptors of higher affinity to be preferentially selected for activation and differentiation to antibody-secreting cells (ASCs) as the amount of antigen in the follicles decreases over time. This continual "recruitment" of B memory cells to form ASCs also depends on the longtime persistence of antigen. This persistence depends on the antigen being resistant to proteases, and this is favored if the antigen is present in its native conformation.

## Immunotherapy

Vaccines were designed for prophylaxis. Only two are currently used as a form of immunotherapy. Pasteur successfully used his rabies vaccine to treat a child bitten by a rabid dog, setting a precedent for the use of this vaccine, because some time may elapse between the bite and infection of nervous tissue. The hepatitis B vaccine is regularly given to newborn infants of an infected mother. Vaccine efficacy is enhanced if administered with convalescent serum which limits viral replication in the baby until the vaccination becomes effective.

The advent of HIV/AIDS, when a majority of infected people live a normal life for 8–10 years—the so-called (incorrectly) latent phase before immunodeficiency (induced by loss of $CD4^+$ T cells) becomes serious and opportunistic infections occur—presented the opportunity to introduce an immunization program to benefit infected people (see Chapter 103). The initial aim was to see if the level of $CD4^+$ T cells could be stabilized using an immunization schedule that should improve the overall immune

**Table 43.2** A summary of the role of different immune responses in preventing or controlling an intracellular infection

| Stage | Mechanism | | | |
|---|---|---|---|---|
| | Antibody | TH1 | TH2 | CTLs |
| 1. Prevention of infection | +++ | – | – | – |
| 2 .Control of replication | ++ | ++ | – | ++ |
| 3. Clearance of the infection | – | ++? | – | +++ |

response of infected people, thereby increasing T-cell activity. More recently, it has been noted that infected people with a predominantly TH1 response fare better (not unexpectedly; see Table 43.2) than those with predominantly a TH2 response, giving rise to the hope that an immunization program to preferentially induce a TH1-type response would delay the onset of immunodeficiency.

Similar approaches to immunotherapy of other persistent infections (eg., herpes) are in progress, perhaps as a result of the experiences with HIV-infected people.

## Current Vaccine Formulations

Currently, vaccines are available in mainly three formulations:

1. Live attenuated preparations, which are mainly viral but include a few bacterial preparations.
2. Whole inactivated virus or bacteria.
3. Subunit preparations, either in the form of isolated surface antigens of the microorganism or as "haptenic groups" (e.g., oligosaccharides) conjugated to different protein "carriers." A special situation is immunization with a "detoxified" toxin, such as diphtheria or tetanus toxoid.

Of these three, some live attenuated viral vaccines have been highly successful, giving long-lasting protection after one or two administrations (e.g., measles, yellow fever, and oral polio vaccines).

Most of these vaccines protect against agents that show no or only minor antigenic variation, they cause an acute infection in most instances (i.e., the natural immune response is protective), and the agent is not difficult to grow in bulk. With many, a suitable animal model was available to aid development. In contrast, the first hepatitis B virus vaccine, composed of the surface antigen isolated from the blood of infected people, was against a virus which could not be grown in bulk and could cause a persistent infection. It was a great advance when the surface antigen was made in DNA-transfected yeast cells as it heralded a new approach to making vaccines to many infectious agents which previously seemed beyond reach.

## New Approaches to Vaccine Development

Advances in four areas present great potential for making vaccines to otherwise difficult infectious agents and to enhance the induced immune responses (Table 43.3).

Two technologies dominate the newer approaches to antigen production. One is the synthesis of oligopeptides encoding T and B cell epitopes of important antigens of the agent. They may be formulated as linear conjugates, conjugated to carrier proteins (which usually provide the T-cell epitopes), or as repeated sequences (tandem arrays or as multiple antigenic peptides, MAPs). Furthermore, if the sequence contains a CTL epitope, it is now possible to add a lipid "tail," to induce a CTL response. Although no peptide preparation is currently licensed, several are in clinical trials, including malaria and HIV candidate vaccines.

The second technology, manipulation of DNA, has become increasingly popular. One approach is transfection of cells with DNA coding for the foreign antigen(s) as exemplified by the hepatitis B vaccine. However, the cell chosen for expression of the foreign DNA should be selected with care. For example, if the DNA product undergoes critical posttranslational modifications (e.g., viral glycoproteins), the cell in which the donor of the foreign DNA normally grows should be chosen for transfection so that an identical product may be made. Similarly, it may be desirable to use a bacterial vector to produce other bacterial proteins.

**Table 43.3** Different areas of research which have the potential to greatly enhance both vaccine development and usage

| |
|---|
| ANTIGEN PRODUCTION AND PRESENTATION |
| 1. *THE SYNTHESIS OF OLIGOPEPTIDES* |
| A synthetic approach in which only important peptide sequences coding for T- and B-cell epitopes form the basis of the vaccine |
| 2. *THE MANIPULATION OF DNA CODING FOR FOREIGN ANTIGENS* |
| Transfection of bacterial, yeast, or mammalian cells with DNA/RDNA coding for foreign proteins |
| The use of infectious agents as vectors of DNA from other agents |
| Viruses: Pox, adeno, polio, baculo (insect) |
| *Bacteria*: BCG, *Salmonella* |
| 'Naked' DNA (genetic vaccine) |
| The deletion of specific DNA sequences from some bacteria and complex viruses |
| IMMUNOPOTENTIATION |
| 1. *NEW ADJUVANTS* |
| The development of a range of adjuvants which, by the induction of different cytokine profiles, may selectively induce different responses (eg., TH2 vs. TH1 vs. CTLs) or different Ig isotypes (IgG vs. IgE vs. IgA) |
| 2. *ENHANCED ANTIGEN PERSISTENCE* |
| Controlled release formulations, immunostimulating complexes (ISCOMS), liposomes |

For many purposes, an even more attractive approach is use of a live attenuated virus or bacterium as a vector of the foreign DNA. In this way, a full spectrum of the desirable immune responses may be obtained. Poxviruses, especially vaccinia, have been studied in this way for many years. Because of the side reactions to this vaccine seen during the smallpox eradication campaign, there is much interest in the use of fowlpox viruses, especially canarypox, as a vector. These viruses undergo only abortive infections in humans (i.e., no infectious progeny is produced), but this may be sufficient to induce a strong immune response to the foreign antigen.

It is of interest that all of the foregoing approaches are being used to develop vaccines against HIV, perhaps the greatest challenge in the world today (see Chapter 103).

A recent, exciting development is the use of a DNA plasmid as a vector for foreign DNA by injecting the chimeric plasmid directly into muscle; by incorporation into a liposome; or, after adsorption onto tiny gold beads, by injection into skin cells using a "gene gun." Prolonged antibody and CTL responses have been obtained after a single administration to mice.

Finally, attenuation of viruses or bacteria may in certain cases become a much more precise procedure because of the ability to selectively delete specific DNA sequences which renders the product less virulent or avirulent without loss of immunogenicity.

## Immunopotentiation

Alum, first used as an adjuvant more than 50 years ago, remains the only product registered for general use. But as we have come to better understand what is expected of a vaccine, some of the newer products under trial seem promising.

Adjuvants are now thought to have three roles:

1. To act as a depot or reservoir of antigen. The new biodegradable formulations, composed of polyglycolides and lactides, allow controlled release of the antigen.
2. To direct the antigen to cell surfaces, for example, liposomes, or the $\beta$ subunit of cholera toxin (CT-$\beta$) binding to a cell receptor.
3. To act as an immunostimulant. This is increasingly being regarded as the ability to induce the synthesis and secretion of patterns of cytokines which favor different immune responses. For example, Freund's complete adjuvant, monophosphoryl lipid A, and lipopolysaccharide favor TH1 cell induction; alum, CT-$\beta$, and muramyl dipeptide (MDP) derivatives favor TH2 cell formation; inulin with alum and Quil A in immunostimulating complexes (ISCOMS) induce CTL formation; and interleukin-6 (IL-6) favors secretory IgA formation.

## Conclusion

Although with one exception these newer approaches have not yet resulted in licensed vaccines for human use, their application is certain to result in new vaccines over time, and particularly to those agents to which vaccines could not be developed using classical procedures.

There may also be spinoffs in other ways. The cost of vaccination with current vaccines is largely attributable to visits to or by the health care worker. Fewer administrations of individual vaccines and increased use of vaccines combined into a single "cocktail" (e.g., as with diphtheria–pertussis–tetanus and measles–mumps–rubella vaccines) could substantially reduce the expense. The newer approaches offer the potential of both minimizing antigenic competition (interference in the immune response to one vaccine by another) and avoiding the effects on replication patterns when different live agents, such as viruses, are mixed in a combined regimen.

However, a note of caution should be sounded. Although these new approaches potentially eliminate a previously major obstacle to the development of new vaccines, other factors that occur during natural infection can delay vaccine development. These include substantial antigenic variation of the agent; protective immunity not occurring naturally; escape mutants occurring during an infection; integration of DNA/cDNA into the infected host cell genome; and immune enhancement of infection by antibody. In addition, there may not be a suitable inexpensive and readily available animal model for vaccine development and testing. Combinations of these factors may prolong or obstruct vaccine development, as is clearly seen with vaccines to prevent malaria and AIDS.

## ANNOTATED BIBLIOGRAPHY

### General

Ada G, Ramsay A. Vaccines, Vaccination and the Immune Response. Lippincott-Raven, Philadelphia, pp 1–247, 1997.

Ada GL. Vaccines. In: *Viral Pathogenesis.* Nathanson N, ed. Raven Press, New York, pp 371–399, 1997.

Various authors. In: Strategies in Vaccine Design. Ada GL, ed. RG Landes Company, Austin, pp 1–217, 1994.

*The three preceding publications cover main aspects of the above topic in much greater detail, as seen by the author (first two references) and by 11 other (groups of) authors, respectively.*

### Specific

Birx DL, Redfield RR. Therapeutic HIV vaccines: concept, current status and future directions. In: Textbook of AIDS Medicine. Broder S, Merigan TC, Bolognesi D, eds. Williams and Wilkins, Baltimore, pp 693–712, 1994.

*This describes the approach taken by some leading workers to develop a therapeutic HIV vaccine, the results of clinical trials, and prospects for the future of this approach.*

Buller ML. 1994. Rational designs for attenuated live virus vaccines. In: Strategies in Vaccine Design. Ada GL, ed. RG Landes Company, Austin, pp 159–178, 1994.

*Most live attenuated vaccines have been developed empirically by multiple passages in different cell cultures or different hosts, the aim being to retain mmunogenicity while reducing virulence for humans. The new approach is to selectively delete certain DNA/RNA sequences, from the genome, thus providing a more reproducible product.*

Cadoz M, Strady A, Meigner B, et al. Immunization with canarypox virus expressing rabies glycoprotein. Lancet 1992; 339:1429–1432.

*Though canarypox undergoes only abortive infections in human cells, and thus is potentially safe to use as a vaccine, it still may generate a strong immune response in humans when used as a vector of foreign DNA.*

McDonnell WM, Askari FK. Molecular medicine. DNA vaccines. N Eng J Med. 1995; 334: 42–45.

*Immunization with DNA coding for foreign antigens rather than the antigens per se seems set to become a major new technique for vaccine development.*

Shearer GM, Clerici M. $CD4^+$ functional T cell subsets: their roles in infection and vaccine development. In: Strategies in Vaccine Design. Ada, GL, ed. RG Landes Company, Austin, pp 113–124, 1994.

*The development of a TH1-type response rather than a TH2-type response favors delayed progression to severe immunodeficiency and the resulting opportunistic infections*

Strauss SE, Corey L, Burke RL, et al. Placebo-controlled trial of vaccination with recombinant glycoprotein D of herpes simplex virus type 2 for immunotherapy of genital herpes. Lancet 1944; 343:1460–1463.

*The experience with immunotherapy of HIV infections (see above) has encouraged a similar approach to treating genital herpes infections by vaccination, with moderately encouraging results.*

# 44

## Passive Immunoprophylaxis and Treatment

JAMES E. PENNINGTON

The clinical use of antibodies from animal or human sources for treatment or prophylaxis of infection is not a new concept. The development in recent years, however, of methods to render human plasma–derived immunoglobulin G safe for rapid intravenous use has opened new opportunities for use of passive immunization for infectious diseases. Given the concerns over cost and safety of modern intravenous immunoglobulin G (IGIV) preparations, a carefully documented clinical trial literature is becoming available to determine the proper role of IGIV in treating or preventing infection. It is noteworthy that some rational uses of IGIV for acquired immunodeficiencies have been evaluated in controlled clinical trials with negative, or conflicting results, whereas other studies have proven these preparations to be quite effective. Although not entirely responsible for the clinical failures, the inability to deliver enough of the appropriate antibody using commercially available IGIV preparations is an important factor contributing to some failed studies. With this in mind, a number of IGIV preparations have been made in which antibody titers are enriched against a specific infectious pathogen. These so-called hyperimmune IGIV preparations usually contain four- to fivefold higher antibody titers against the target infectious agent, as compared to titers in usual IGIV preparations.

Even more recently, molecular biologic techniques have been employed to produce monoclonal antibodies (MAbs) directed against specific antigenic targets on infectious pathogens. The advantage of MAbs is the ability to deliver high titers of a specific antibody with a relatively low total dose of exogenous protein. In other words, one can avoid delivering the myriad unneeded antibodies present in pooled IGIV preparations made from human plasma donations. If broad-spectrum antibody prophylaxis is desired, such a collection of antibodies would be welcome. However, if a specific pathogen is being targeted, MAbs are an efficient method for antibody delivery. One potential problem with a monoclonal antibody is that the organism to which it is directed may via antigenic variation "escape." As such, a repertoire of different antibodies varying in epitope specificity, isotype, and complement binding capacity may be necessary for optimal therapy. Such monoclonal antibody "cocktails" (i.e., mixtures of MAbs) are being considered to address such situations.

An additional limitation in the utilization of MAb therapy directed at bacterial pathogens with a variety of serotype epitopes is that rapid serotyping would be needed in order to select the relevant MAb for that isolate. Unfortunately, most clinical diagnostic laboratories do not serotype bacterial isolates routinely. If the number of expected serotypes is limited (e.g., two to six), a cocktail approach again might be feasible with a MAb to each serotype included in the final preparation. Empiric treatment with a mixture of MAbs directed at all common serotypes could then be done with a reasonable assurance of correct therapy. For many pathogens, such as *Escherichia coli* and *Klebsiella* sp., too many serotypes occur in the clinical setting to make this a feasible strategy, however. As of 1994, no anti-infective MAbs were approved in the United States for general use. However, a number of MAbs were in clinical trials (Table 44.1).

Finally, the safety of antibody-based therapeutics must be considered. Use of human IGIV preparations has been remarkably well-tolerated; however, both acute and chronic side effects may occur. Most acute reactions, such as local pain at infusion site and fevers, can be diminished by slowing the rate of infusion. Rarely, serious allergic reactions can occur in individuals sensitized to trace contaminant proteins (e.g., IgA) in the IGIV preparations. Transmission of plasma-derived viral agents, such as hepatitis B and C, rarely occurs, and transmission of human immunodeficiency virus (HIV) has not been reported with IGIV preparations. Ironically, while the switch from old-fashioned horse serum– to modern human plasma–derived globulins eliminated serum sickness reactions associated with immunotherapy, the recent use of "high-technology" murine MAbs has reintroduced this risk. Fortunately, serum sickness has been rare and generally mild when associated with murine MAb therapy.

### Intravenous Immunoglobulin G Preparations

Commercially produced IGIV preparations are produced from pooled human plasma donations, and thus contain a repertoire of IgG antibodies which represents the normal antibody distribution in healthy adult humans. It is safe to say that many or even most of the antibodies existing in such preparations have not been identified or assayed for potency. However, for patients with primary humoral immunodeficiency, recurrent sinopulmonary infections of a wide variety of bacterial and viral etiologies are reduced by monthly replacement therapy with IGIV. For patients with acquired or relative antibody deficiencies, however, the picture is not so clear (Tables 44.2 and 44.3).

### Primary immunodeficiency

The original motivation for development of IGIV was to allow efficient and well-tolerated replacement therapy of patients with congenital hypogammaglobulinemia. Certainly the intravenous route of administration has been a welcome therapeutic advance over the use of immune serum globulins given by intramuscular injections. The respiratory tract is the most frequent organ system infected in such individuals and the causative organisms often include encapsulated bacteria such as pneumococcus and *Haemophilus influenzae*. Mycoplasma and viral infections also occur at increased frequency. Several studies have now docu-

**Table 44.1** Monoclonal antibodies in clinical development for treatment of infectious diseases

| |
|---|
| *Pseudomonas aeruginosa* (H) |
| Cytomegalovirus (H) |
| Antiendotoxin (M, H) |
| Anti–tumor necrosis factor (M, C, HI) |
| Respiratory syncytial virus (HI) |

Abbreviations: H, human; M, murine; C, chimeric; HI, humanized.

**Table 44.3** Conditions in which data are conflicting or negative for use of IGIV in infectious diseases

| Condition | Use of IGIV |
|---|---|
| Neonatal sepsis | Prophylaxis |
| Sepsis | Prophylaxis and treatment |
| Burns | Prophylaxis |
| Cancer chemotherapy | Prophylaxis |

mented that maintenance of serum IgG greater than 500 mg/dL will reduce the frequency and severity of respiratory tract infections in patients with primary immunodeficiency. It is not possible to achieve such concentrations unless an intravenous, rather than intramuscular, route of administration is employed.

A less well recognized form of congenital immunodeficiency is IgG subclass deficiency. Both $IgG_2$ and $IgG_4$ deficiencies are associated with recurrent bacterial respiratory tract infections, and the diagnosis is often missed if only total IgG is assayed. Replacement therapy with IGIV reduces infection rates.

## Chronic lymphocytic leukemia and multiple myeloma

Many patients with chronic lymphocytic leukemia (CLL) are known to have hypogammaglobulinemia and frequent respiratory tract infections. It was recently demonstrated that high-dose IGIV prophylaxis in patients with CLL is useful to reduce infectious complications. In that study, patients had profoundly low serum immune globulin and/or recurrent infections. Patients were randomized to receive either IGIV or placebo, with a dose of IGIV of 400 mg/kg every 3 weeks over a 17 dose trial period. The result was a significant reduction in bacterial infections for the IGIV prophylaxis group but no differences in viral or fungal infections. The beneficial effect in this study was limited almost exclusively to infections of the respiratory tract.

Patients with multiple myeloma are also known to be at increased risk of bacterial infections. Respiratory and urinary tracts are most frequently involved. The risk factors for infection are diverse, but one mechanism appears to be a dysfunctional humoral immune response. Early attempts to prevent infection in patients with multiple myeloma using low doses of intramuscular immunoglobulin failed. However, in a recent study, 83 stable patients were randomized to receive either 500 mg IGIV per kilogram per month or placebo, for at least 6 months. The mean number of infectious episodes occurring in controls was 2 versus 0.5 in the IGIV-treated group ($p = 0.021$). Septicemia and pneumonia were most notably decreased in the study. Thus it appears that higher doses of IGIV may be successful in prophylaxis of infection for this patient group.

In both CLL and multiple myeloma, the high cost of maintenance therapy with IGIV must be weighed against the demonstrated risk of serious infection in the individual patient.

**Table 44.2** Proven efficacy of IGIV in prophylaxis of infectious diseases

| Condition | Dose |
|---|---|
| Primary immunodeficiency | 400 mg/kg/mo |
| Bone marrow transplantation | 500 mg/kg/wk[a] |
| Pediatric AIDS | 400 mg/kg/mo |
| Chronic lymphocytic leukemia | 400 mg/kg/mo |
| Multiple myeloma | 500 mg/kg/mo |

[a]For initial 3 months posttransplantation.

## Bone marrow transplantation

Studies have been conducted with bone marrow transplant patients to explore the hypothesis that IGIV preparations may be used for prophylaxis against opportunistic infections, particularly cytomegalovirus (CMV) pneumonia. Most, but not all reports have described favorable results. Two recent reports, using randomized study designs, have shown clearly that weekly administration of 500–1000 mg/kg IGIV during the 3 months following bone marrow transplantation results in a significant reduction in CMV and bacterial infections, as well as in idiopathic interstitial pneumonia (see Chapter 88).

## Pediatric acquired immunodeficiency syndrome

A number of reports indicate that recurrent bacterial infections of the respiratory tract are particularly common in pediatric acquired immunodeficiency syndrome (AIDS) patients. It is also known that primary, as well as recall, B-cell functions against specific encapsulated bacteria are impaired more severely in HIV-infected children as compared to adults. To confirm several uncontrolled studies suggesting beneficial effects of IGIV prophylaxis in children with AIDS, 372 HIV-infected children were randomized to receive monthly IGIV (400 mg/kg) versus placebo. The mean length of follow-up was 17 months. Significant reductions in bacterial infections and days in the hospital were demonstrated for those receiving IGIV. Among the sites most protected were the lungs and sinuses. Reduction in pneumococcal infections was particularly noteworthy.

## Intensive care unit

The high mortality associated with nosocomial pneumonia has motivated a trial of IGIV prophylaxis among patients in the intensive care unit setting. Patients were randomized to receive IGIV 400 mg/kg/week, IGIV selected for high antiendotoxin antibodies (same dose), or placebo. The test groups numbered 109, 108, and 112 respectively. A significant reduction in nosocomial pneumonia was seen among IGIV recipients, 15 cases, as compared to placebo, 30 cases ($p = 0.02$). Surprisingly, this protective effect was not observed for the group receiving the selected antiendotoxin preparation.

## Neonates

Serum immunoglobulin concentrations in preterm infants are significantly below those in full-term infants. This relative hypogammaglobulinemic state may contribute to septic complications. Therefore, it has been proposed that prophylaxis with immunoglobulins might prevent septic complications in the premature infant. Several small clinical trials suggested that IGIV prophylaxis could reduce the incidence of sepsis in neonates, particularly in those less than 1500 g at birth. However, only recently have studies of adequate size been conducted to address the issue. Unfortunately, the studies reached opposite conclusions. In one report, 588 neonates, stratified by birth weight, were randomized to receive five infusions of IGIV 500 mg/kg, or placebo, over the first 5 weeks of life. For infants weighing between 500 and 1750 g, IGIV reduced significantly the incidence of nosocomial sepsis. In a separate study, 2416 low birth weight neonates were randomized to receive IGIV or placebo (or no infusion). Although dosages of IGIV were similar to the prior report, no benefit from IGIV prophylaxis could be demonstrated. Thus the use of IGIV in neonates remains controversial.

## Intravenous Hyperimmune Immunoglobulin G Preparations

Currently the only commercial hyperimmune IGIV preparation approved for clinical use in the United States is cytomegalovirus IGIV for prophylaxis of CMV infection in renal transplantation patients (see Chapter 87). However, several other preparations have been studied in clinical trials, with variable results.

### Cytomegalovirus IGIV

Cytomegalovirus pneumonia causes significant morbidity in solid organ transplant recipients and life-threatening infection after bone marrow transplantation. A randomized, placebo-controlled trial demonstrated that prophylaxis with CMV IGIV reduced significantly the incidence of CMV pneumonia in CMV seronegative recipients of renal transplants from seropositive donors. These results could not be repeated in liver transplant patients. Treatment of CMV pneumonia in bone marrow transplant patients with the combination of ganciclovir plus CMV IGIV resulted in survival rates superior to those previously reported for either agent when used alone.

### *Pseudomonas aeruginosa* IGIV

While the combination of antibiotics plus *Pseudomonas* IGIV in animal models of infection results in survivals superior to either agent alone, there are no clinical trials as of 1994 to verify the usefulness of *Pseudomonas* IGIV. One small uncontrolled trial in cystic fibrosis patients suggested beneficial effects of adding *Pseudomonas* IGIV to conventional treatment. However, until more clinical data are available, the clinical usefulness of *Pseudomonas* IGIV is open to question.

### Respiratory syncytial virus IGIV

A respiratory syncytial virus (RSV) IGIV has recently been prepared from human donors, screened for high plasma titers. In a randomized, but not placebo-controlled trial, infants at high risk of life-threatening RSV pneumonia (congenital heart disease, premature, bronchopulmonary dysplasia) received monthly prophylactic infusions during the peak season for RSV infections. Recipients of RSV IGIV experienced significantly fewer episodes of RSV pneumonia. No effect on mortality was seen, however.

### Antiendotoxin antibody preparations

The clinical syndrome of gram-negative sepsis and septic shock is reviewed in Chapter 50. Among a variety of innovative adjunctive therapies proposed to reduce mortality from gram-negative sepsis are antibody preparations in which the antigen target is the core glycolipid (endotoxin) portion of the gram-negative bacillus wall (see Chapter 53). A variety of antibody preparations have now been utilized in an attempt to neutralize endotoxin in such patients. Early studies using sera obtained from volunteers immunized with the J5 mutant of *E. coli* 0111:B4 resulted in lowering of mortality in patients with gram-negative bacteremia and shock. However, the subgroup in this study in which culture results proved a gram-negative bacterial etiology of sepsis could be analyzed only retrospectively. The effects of this therapy on patients enrolled on study but not found to have gram-negative infection are uncertain.

More recently, two hyperimmune IGIV preparations have been prepared containing high antibody titers against endotoxin. One preparation was prepared from human plasma donors hyperimmunized with J5 vaccine. In a randomized controlled trial, 100 patients with septic shock were randomized to standard care plus anti–J5 IGIV versus conventional IGIV. Seventy-one patients were eventually proven to have gram-negative sepsis. Overall mortality was 57% in the J5 group and 54% in the control group. In a separate study, an IGIV preparation was enriched for antiendotoxin antibodies by screening donors for antibody against the R595 mutant of *Salmonella minnesota*. That preparation was also studied in double-blind fashion, compared to conventional IGIV or placebo, to determine whether prophylactic administration to critical care unit patients could reduce infections. No reduction of infections was achieved using the antiendotoxin IGIV. As noted above, conventional IGIV did lead to reduced numbers of pneumonia.

Finally, two separate antiendotoxin monoclonal antibodies have been studied for the treatment of sepsis. Both reports suggested some protective effects when specific subgroups of the study population were analyzed retrospectively. However, no overall protective effect could be seen when an analysis of all enrollees with sepsis was performed.

## Conclusion

The ability to deliver immunoglobulin preparations containing high concentrations of a broad spectrum of IgG antibodies intravenously represents a major advance in passive immunotherapy. Monoclonal antibodies offer the potential advantage of precise targeting against virulence epitopes of infecting organisms. At present, the use of these agents has been proven beneficial only for a limited number of infections, however, and the high cost of the manufacture will make it imperative to assess cost-effectiveness of their use as part of future clinical trials.

## ANNOTATED BIBLIOGRAPHY


Baker CJ, Melish ME, Hall RT, et al. Intravenous immune globulin for the prevention of nosocomial infection in low-birth-weight neonates. N Engl J Med 1992; 327:213–219.

*A large, randomized trial, demonstrating a reduction in nosocomial sepsis for infants 500–1750 g in weight receiving IGIV prophylaxis.*

Calandra T, Glauser MP, Schellekens J, et al. Treatment of gram-negative septic shock with human IgG antibody to *Escherichia coli* J5: a prospective, double-blind, randomized trial. J Infect Dis 1988; 158:312–319.

*A randomized study of 100 patients with suspected or proven gram-negative septic shock. No significant difference in mortality was seen in recipients of hyperimmune anti-J5 IGIV vs. conventional IGIV.*

Casadevall A, Scharff MD. Serum therapy revisited: animal models of infection and development of passive antibody therapy. Antimicrob Agents Chemother 1994; 38:1695–1702.

*A historical overview of serum therapy of infectious diseases, with lessons that can be applied to contemporary research with monoclonal antibodies.*

Chapel HM, Lee M. The use of intravenous immune globulin in multiple myeloma. Clin Exp Immunol 1994; 97(suppl 1):21–24.

*A randomized study conducted in 83 patients with multiple myeloma demonstrated that IGIV prophylaxis given over 6 months led to a significant reduction in serious bacterial infections.*

Cometta A, Baumgartner J-D, Lee ML, et al. Prophylactic intravenous administration of standard immune globulin as compared with core lipopolysaccharide immune globulin in patients at high risk of postsurgical infection. N Engl J Med 1992; 327:234–240.

*Patients in the ICU were randomized to prophylaxis with conventional IGIV, hyperimmune antiendotoxin IGIV, or placebo. A significant reduction in nosocomial pneumonia was seen among those receiving conventional, but not hyperimmune, IGIV.*

Cooperative Group for the Study of Immunoglobulin in Chronic Lymphocytic Leukemia. Intravenous immunoglobulin for the prevention of infection in chronic lymphocytic leukemia. N Eng J Med 1988; 319:902–907.

*Patients with CLL demonstrated a significant reduction in bacterial infections when given prophylactic IGIV, as compared to a placebo.*

Fanaroff AA, Korones SB, Wright LL, et al. A controlled trial of intravenous immune-globulin to reduce nosocomial infections in very-low-birth-weight infants. N Engl J Med 1994; 330:1107–1113.

*More than 2400 low birth weight infants were randomized to prophylactic IGIV vs. placebo or no therapy. No reduction in nosocomial infections was seen among IGIV recipients.*

Greenman RL, Schein RMH, Martin MA, et al. A controlled clinical trial of E5 murine monoclonal IgM antibody to endotoxin in the treatment of gram-negative sepsis. JAMA 1991; 266:1097–1102.

*A randomized controlled trial of antiendotoxin monoclonal antibody vs. placebo showed no overall reduction in mortality in the treated group. Individuals retrospectively identified to have gram-negative sepsis without shock appeared to benefit.*

Groothius JR, Simoes AF, Levin MJ, et al. Prophylactic administration of respiratory syncytial virus immune globulin to high-risk infants and young children. N Engl J Med 1993; 329:1524–1530.

*Children at high risk of RSV experienced fewer episodes of RSV respiratory infection when prophylaxed over several months with RSV IGIV vs. placebo.*

Pennington JE. Newer uses of intravenous immunoglobulins as anti-infective agents. Antimicrob Agents Chemother 1990; 3:1463–1466.

*A review of clinical applications of IGIV for the treatment of infections.*

Reed EC, Bowden RA, Dandiker PS, et al. Treatment of cytomegalovirus pneumonia with ganciclovir and intravenous cytomegalovirus immunoglobulin in patients with bone marrow transplants. Ann Intern Med 1988; 109:783–788.

*Treatment of CMV pneumonia in bone marrow transplant patients with hyperimmune CMV IGIV plus ganciclovir resulted in survivals superior to those noted historically with either agent used alone.*

Snydman DR, Werner BG, Dougherty NN, et al. Cytomegalovirus immune globulin prophylaxis in liver transplantation. Ann Intern Med 1993; 119:984–991.

*Results of a randomized trial of prophylactic CMV IGIV vs. placebo in liver transplant patients were less impressive than previous results in renal transplant patients.*

Sullivan KM, Kopecky KB, Jocom J, et al. Immunomodulatory and antimicrobial efficacy of intravenous immunoglobulin in bone marrow transplantation. N Engl J Med 1990; 323:705–712.

*A randomized trial of weekly prophylactic IGIV vs. no prophylaxis in bone marrow transplant patients showed significant reductions in bacterial sepsis, viral infections, interstitial pneumonia and graft vs. host disease in IGIV recipients.*

National Institute of Child Health and Human Development Intravenous Immunoglobulin Study Group. Intravenous immune globulin for the prevention of bacterial infections in children with symptomatic human immunodeficiency virus infection. N Engl J Med 1991; 325:73–80.

*A randomized trial of monthly prophylactic IGIV vs. placebo in HIV-infected children showed that IGIV results in a significant reduction in serious bacterial infections.*

Van Wye JE, Collins MS, Baylor M, et al. Pseudomonas hyperimmune globulin passive immunotherapy for pulmonary exacerbations in cystic fibrosis. Pediatr Pulmonol 1990; 9:7–18.

*A small, uncontrolled study suggested that* Pseudomonas *IGIV may be of some benefit to cystic fibrosis patients.*

Winston DJ, Ho WG, Lin C-H, et al. Intravenous immune globulin for prevention of cytomegalovirus infection and interstitial pneumonia after bone marrow transplantation. Ann Intern Med 1987; 106:12–18.

*A randomized trial in bone marrow transplant patients demonstrated reduced CMV infections in those receiving prophylactic IGIV.*

Yap PL, Williams PE. The safety of IVIG preparations. In: Clinical Applications of Intravenous Immunoglobulin Therapy. Yap PL, ed. Churchill Livingstone, New York, pp 43–62, 1992.

*An excellent reveiw of the safety issues associated with the use of IGIV.*

Ziegler EJ, Fisher CJ, Sprung CL, et al. Treatment of gram-negative bacteremia and septic shock with HA-1A human monoclonal antibody against endotoxin. N Engl J Med 1991; 324:429–436.

*A randomized trial of antiendotoxin monoclonal antibody vs. placebo showed no overall reduced mortality in antibody recipients. A retrospective analysis showed some benefit in the subgroup found to have gram-negative bacteremia.*

Ziegler EJ, McCutchan JA, Fierer J, et al. Treatment of gram-negative bacteremia and shock with human antiserum to a mutant *Escherichia coli*. N Engl J Med 1982; 307:225–1230.

*A randomized trial demonstrated reduced mortality in patients with gram-negative bacteremia who received human antisera to endotoxin.*

# 45

## Specific Vaccines

PAUL T. HEATH AND E. RICHARD MOXON

Although improved socioeconomic circumstances, especially clean water and sanitation, must be credited as a major reason for drastic reductions in mortality from many infectious diseases, vaccination has been decisive in the control of at least 10 microbial diseases—smallpox, diphtheria, tetanus, yellow fever, pertussis, polio, measles, mumps, rubella, and most recently *Haemophilus influenzae* B. Thus vaccines provide one of the most compelling examples of the impact of public health measures in controlling mortality and morbidity from infectious diseases. These successes must be tempered by an appreciation of the enormous unfulfilled potential for preventing microbial diseases. The World Health Organization (WHO) recently recognized the escalating impact of tuberculosis as a global health emergency; the pandemic of disease caused by human immunodeficiency viruses (HIVs) poses huge threats to the infrastructures of several of the world's most important countries; millions of children die each year as a result of diarrheal disease or lower respiratory tract infection; and there is no successful immunoprophylactic strategy against any human parasite despite the infestation of about two-thirds of the world's population with various macroparasites that are collectively responsible for enormous morbidity. Finally, previously recognized or newly discovered infectious agents continue to pose novel threats (the so-called emerging infections), and increasing antimicrobial resistance has limited our ability to treat some infections.

To meet these challenges, there is a need to develop safe, effective, and inexpensive vaccines. But the availability of a vaccine is clearly only a first step in a complex set of activities which must be undertaken to ensure successful immunization of populations. In this chapter we summarize information on available vaccines and offer some guidelines for their use both in routine immunization programs and in subpopulations who, through unusual susceptibility, require special consideration concerning immunization.

### Special Risk Groups

### Immunocompromised patients

Existing vaccines may provide benefit for many immunocompromised patients, but the clinician must always be alert to the fact that vaccine response cannot be assumed and adjunctive measures such as antimicrobial prophylaxis, intravenous immunoglobulin, and immunization of family contacts and health care workers should be considered in some patients. If feasible, specific serum antibody titers or other immunological responses should be determined after immunization to assess immunity and to serve as a guide for future immunizations and the management of future exposures. However, one cannot conclude that immune responses associated with protection in normal hosts will necessarily be protective in individuals with impaired immunity.

For information on doses and schedules, see specific vaccines in Table 45.1.

#### Asplenia (Table 45.2)

The patients at highest risk from these infections appear to be those with thalassemia or sickle cell disease and those who have had splenectomy in association with hematologic malignancies (especially Hodgkin's disease).

#### Corticosteroid therapy

Experience with LV administration in patients on CS therapy is limited. In most situations theoretical considerations are the only guide. In principle, LV should be avoided if the dose of CS is sufficient to suppress the immune response and/or the underlying disease is associated with immunosuppression. The exact amount and duration of systemic CS needed to suppress the immune response in an otherwise healthy person is not known.

Moderate- to high-dose CS therapy is an absolute contraindication to LV administration, e.g., >2 mg/kg/day or (>20 mg/day) prednisone (or equivalent) for >2 weeks or >1 mg/kg/day for >1 month. Furthermore, LV should be avoided for >3 months after cessation of such therapy.

Aerosols, topical applications or intra-articular/bursal/tendon CS injections are not a contraindication.

Low-dose CS therapy, e.g., <2 mg/kg/day (or <20 mg/day if weigh >10 kg) or <1 mg/kg/day for <1 month is not a contraindication.

The decision to administer LV while on any dose or any duration of CS treatment should take into account the risk of exposure to the disease for that particular individual and the availability of safe alternatives, such as immunization of family members or use of specific immunoglobulin.

#### Human immunodeficiency virus infection (Table 45.3)

In general, live vaccines are contraindicated. Note the following cases:

- *BCG*—Contraindicated in symptomatic HIV patients. Recommended in asymptomatic HIV-infected infants who live in areas of high TB risk. Neonatal BCG immunization in children subsequently shown to be HIV positive is safe, but persistence of protection cannot be guaranteed.
- *Polio*—In general, OPV should be avoided. IPV should be given to patients and to household contacts that require immunization.

**Table 45.1** Guidelines for use of available vaccines

| Vaccine | Pathogen/ disease | Dose and schedule | | Comments |
|---|---|---|---|---|
| | | Infants and children | Adults | |
| TOXOIDS | | | | |
| Tetanus/ diphtheria adsorbed toxoids | Tetanus Diphtheria | 0.5 mL IM/ deep SC<br>Primary schedule: 3–4 doses<br>UK: 2, 3, 4, mo<br>USA: 2, 4, 6, 15–18 mo<br>WHO: 6, 10, 14 wk<br>Boosters: 2 doses (U.K.) 4–5 yr, 13–18 yr<br>USA: 4–6 yr, 11–16 yr every 10 years | 0.5 mL IM/ deep SC<br>Primary schedule: 3 doses<br>UK: 0, 1, 2 mo<br>USA: 0, 1–2, 6–12 mo<br>Boosters: 2 doses (U.K.): 10 yr after primary, 10 yr later<br>USA: every 10 yrs<br>WHO: pregnant women: 2 doses tetanus toxoid | Booster doses may be required at times of injury<br>Combined with pertussis vaccine (WCV, or USA: ACV) for primary series in children.<br>Use low-dose diphtheria toxoid: >7 yrs age (USA) >10 yrs (UK) |
| KILLED/SUBUNIT BACTERIAL VACCINES | | | | |
| Anthrax (cell-free filtrate of *B. anthracis* culture containing protective antigen) | Anthrax | No information | 0.5 mL IM<br>Primary schedule: 4 doses, 1–3 at 3 wk intervals with 6 mo between 3rd and 4th<br>Boosters: 1 yr intervals | Consider for workers at risk of exposure to the disease: those in contact with animal hides, wool, hair, bristle, bone, bonemeal, feeding stuffs, carcasses. |
| Cholera (heat-killed, phenol-preserved) | Cholera | Not recommended <1 yr of age<br>IM/SC/ID<br>Primary schedule: 2 doses<br>1st dose IM/SC<br>1–5 yr, 0.1 mL<br>5–10 yr, 0.3 mL<br>>10 yr, 0.5 mL<br>2nd dose (>1 wk later) IM/SC/ID<br>1–5 yr, 0.3 mL IM/SC<br>0.1 mL ID<br>5–10 yr, 0.5 mL IM/SC<br>0.1 mL ID<br>>10 yr, 1 ml IM/SC<br>0.2 mL ID<br>Booster (every 6 mo):<br>Same as 2nd dose above | Primary schedule: 2 doses<br>1st dose IM/SC<br>0.5 mL<br>2nd dose (>1 wk later) IM/SC/ID<br>1 mL IM/SC<br>0.2 mL ID<br>Booster (every 6 mo): IM/SC/ID<br>Same as 2nd dose above | No longer required under international health regulations; not routinely recommended for travelers.<br>Of limited efficacy (approx. 50%).<br>An attenuated *V. cholerae* O1 vaccine strain (CVD 103-HgR) with greater efficacy is licensed in some countries. |
| *Haemophilus influenzae* type b (polysaccharide conjugated to protein: tetanus toxoid = PRP-T; diphtheria toxoid = PRP-D; outer membrane protein of *Neisseria meningitidis* = PRP-OMP; mutant diphtheria toxin = HbOC); also available as plain unconjugated polysaccharide (PRP) | *Haemophilus influenzae* type b | 0.5 mL IM/ deep SC<br>Primary schedule<br>UK infants: 3 doses, 2, 3, 4 mo<br>USA infants: 2/3 doses, 2, 4, 6 mo<br>Booster<br>UK infants: not recommended<br>USA: 12–15 mo, 1 dose<br>UK >12 mo–4 yr, 1 dose only<br>USA ≥15 mo–5 yr 1 dose only | 0.5 mL IM/ deep SC<br>Unimmunized children and adults of any age with an increased risk of morbidity or mortality from Hib disease should be considered for Hib immunization<br>See Special Risk Groups | In the USA HbOC, PRP-T, and PRP-OMP are licensed for use <12 mo of age and all conjugate vaccines ≥12 mo of age.<br>Schedules for different conjugate vaccines vary.<br>When possible the Hib vaccine used at first immunization should be used subsequently.<br>However, any combination of conjugate vaccines should provide adequate protection. |

*(continued)*

**Table 45.1** Guidelines for use of available vaccines—*Continued*

| Vaccine | Pathogen/ disease | Dose and schedule: Infants and children | Dose and schedule: Adults | Comments |
|---|---|---|---|---|
| Meningococcal polysaccharide (1-valent/ 2-valent/ 4-valent) | *Neisseria meningitidis* Groups A+C/Y, W135 | 0.5 mL IM/ deep SC<br>Schedule: 1 dose.<br><br>2 doses of vaccine (3 mo apart) probably required to achieve adequate concentrations to group A in children ≤18 mo.<br>Booster: insufficient information.<br>Consider ≥5 yrs after initial immunization | 0.5 mL IM/ deep SC<br>Schedule: 1 dose<br>Booster: insufficient information.<br>Consider ≥5 yrs after initial immunization | Consider for travelers to endemic areas where the prevalent strain is included in the vaccine: (usually group A). May be useful for close contacts of cases of group A or C disease and in outbreaks due to groups A and C in closed or semiclosed communities. Consider in special risk groups with an increased risk of meningococcal sepsis (see Special Risk Groups). Efficacy has been demonstrated for the group A component from 3 mo of age and the group C component from 2 yr of age. In general consider immunization at ≥2 yr. A meningococcal C-protein conjugate vaccine is likely to be available in the near future. |
| Pertussis Whole cell vaccine Acellular component vaccine | Pertussis | 0.5 mL IM/ deep SC<br>Primary schedule: 3–4 doses<br>UK: 2, 3, 4 mo<br>USA: 2, 4, 6, 15–18 mo<br>WHO: 6, 10, 14 wk<br>Booster: 1 dose (USA) at 4–6 yr | Not currently recommended in adults | Combined with DT (DTP, DTaP).<br>DTaP preferred for use in USA but not UK.<br>DTP/DTaP can be initiated as early as 6 wk in areas of high endemicity or in outbreaks. |
| Plague (whole cell, formaldehyde-inactivated) | Plague | IM<br>Primary schedule: 3 doses, 0, 1, 6 mo<br>1st dose:<br><1 yr, 0.2 mL<br>1–4 yr, 0.4 mL<br>5–10 yr, 0.6 mL<br>>11 yr, 1.0 mL<br>2nd & 3rd dose:<br><1 yr, 0.04 mL<br>1–4 yr, 0.08 mL<br>5–10 yr, 0.12 mL<br>>11 yr, 0.2 mL<br>Boosters: 3 doses at 6 monthly intervals then 1 dose at 1–2 yearly intervals. Dose same as 2nd & 3rd doses[a]<br>There are no safety and efficacy data for this vaccine in children | IM<br>Primary schedule: 3 doses, 0, 1, 6 mo<br>1st dose: 1 mL<br>2nd & 3rd dose: 0.2 mL<br>Boosters:<br>3 doses at 6 monthly intervals, then 1 dose at 1–2 yearly intervals.<br>Dose same as 2nd & 3rd doses[a]<br>Accelerated schedule: ×3, 0.5 mL at weekly intervals[b] | Consider for those at high risk of exposure: laboratory workers handling *Y. pestis* and field personnel and workers engaged in operations in areas in which preventing exposure to rodents and fleas is impossible. It is not indicated for most travelers to countries reporting cases. |

(*continued*)

**Table 45.1** Guidelines for use of available vaccines—*Continued*

| Vaccine | Pathogen/ disease | Dose and schedule: Infants and children | Dose and schedule: Adults | Comments |
|---|---|---|---|---|
| Pneumococcal polysaccharide (23-valent) | *Streptococcus pneumoniae* | 0.5 mL SC/IM<br>Booster: see Special Risk Groups | 0.5 mL SC/IM<br>Booster: see Special Risk Groups | Consider in persons in whom there is an increased risk or morbidity and mortality from pneumococcal disease. See Special Risk Groups. Will immunize only against pneumococcal types present in the vaccine. Response is age-dependent and age at response varies between serotypes. Consider in persons ≥2 yr of age. A pneumococcal-protein conjugate vaccine is likely to be available in the near future. |
| Q Fever (*Coxiella burnetti*) (Whole cell, formalin inactivated) | Q Fever (*Coxiella burnetti*) | | 0.5 ml (30 $\mu$g)<br>SC<br>1 dose*<br>Protection lasts >5 yr | Consider for those at high risk of exposure: abattoir workers, shearers, livestock, dairy and laboratory workers, veterinarians and farmers. |
| Typhoid Vi polysaccharide | Typhoid fever | Not generally recommended <18 mo (see Comments)<br>0.5 mL IM/deep SC<br>Primary schedule: 1 dose<br>Booster: every 2–3 yr | 0.5 mL IM/deep SC<br>Primary schedule: 1 dose<br>Booster: every 2–3 yr | Consider in travelers to endemic areas. Children <18 mo may show suboptimal antibody responses to polysaccharide antigens. |
| Typhoid whole cell (heat-killed phenol-preserved) | Typhoid fever | Not recommended <1 yr<br>IM, deep SC, ID (see Comments)<br>Primary schedule: 1–10 yr, 0.25 mL IM/deep SC then 0.25 mL IM/deep SC or 0.1 mL ID 4–6 wk later<br>Booster: 0.25 mL IM/deep SC or 0.1 mL ID every 3 yr | IM, deep SC, ID (see Comments)<br>Primary schedule: 0.5 mL IM/deep SC then 0.5 mL IM/deep SC or 0.1 mL ID 4–6 wk later<br>Booster: 0.5 mL IM/deep SC or 0.1 mL ID every 3 yr | Consider in travelers to endemic areas.<br>The 1st dose of the primary course must be given by IM/deep SC injection. Subsequent doses may be given by ID injection, which may reduce severity of adverse reactions. |
| ATTENUATED, LIVE BACTERIA[C]<br>BCG (Bacille Calmette-Guérin) | Tuberculosis | ≤3 mo: 0.05 mL ID<br>≥3 mo: 0.1 mL ID<br>Primary schedule: 1 dose<br>Booster: insufficient information available<br>WHO: at birth<br>USA: not routine unless at-risk group (see Comments)<br>UK: not routine in neonatal period unless at-risk group; routine in all individuals at normal risk between 10 and 13 yr (see Comments) | 0.1 mL ID<br>Primary schedule: 1 dose<br>Booster: insufficient information available.<br>USA, UK: not indicated unless in at-risk group | Information is not available on the age at which it is safe to give BCG without a prior tuberculin test. It would be reasonable to vaccinate infants ≤3 mo without such testing.<br>All other individuals should only be immunized if (*1*) there are no contraindications to live vaccine administration and (*2*) tuberculin skin test is negative. Indications for neonatal, childhood and adult immunization vary widely between countries. |

**Table 45.1** Guidelines for use of available vaccines—*Continued*

| Vaccine | Pathogen/ disease | Dose and schedule: Infants and children | Dose and schedule: Adults | Comments |
|---|---|---|---|---|
| *Francisella tularensis* | *Francisella tularensis* (tularemia) | | 1 dose<br>Protection lasts >5 yrs | Consider for those at high risk of exposure: those with occupational or recreational exposure to infected animals or their habitat, such as rabbit hunters and trappers, those with tick or insect bites and laboratory technicians working with *f. tularensis*. |
| Oral typhoid (Ty 21a) | Typhoid fever | Not recommended <6 yr<br>Primary schedule: 4 doses (USA), 3 doses (UK) given on alternate days<br>Booster: 3 dose course annually (UK) (*for residents of nonendemic areas*); 4 dose course every 5 yr (USA) | Primary schedule: 4 doses (USA), 3 doses (UK) given on alternate days<br>Booster: (see Comments) 3 dose course annually (UK) (*for residents of nonendemic areas*); 4 dose course every 5 yr (USA) | Enteric coated capsules. Consider in travelers to endemic areas. In conditions of continued exposure to *S. typhi* protection may persist for ≥3 yr. New liquid formulation with greater efficacy will shortly be available. |
| INACTIVATED/SUBUNIT VIRUS VACCINES<br>Hepatitis A (whole-virion formaldehyde-inactivated) | Hepatitis A | 360 ELISA U (0.5 mL)[d] IM<br>Primary schedule 2 doses, 0, 2–4 wk<br>Dose 720 ELISA u (0.5 mL)*<br>Primary schedule: 1 dose<br>Booster: 1 dose, 6–12 mo after primary course[e] | 1440 ELISA U (1 mL)[d] IM<br>Primary schedule: 1 dose,<br>Booster: 1 dose 6–12 mo after primary course[e] | Consider for travel to areas of moderate or high HAV endemicity. Insufficient information available on possible use in other situations, e.g., sewerage workers and outbreak situations. When practicable, testing for anti-HAV may be worth while in those ≥50 y, those born in endemic areas, and those with a history of jaundice. |
| Hepatitis B (recombinant surface antigen) | Hepatitis B | Age <12 yr: 10 μg[f] IM<br>Schedule: 3 doses<br>WHO: 0, 6, 14 wk or 6, 10, 14 wk<br>UK/USA: Infant (mother HBsAg negative), 0, 1–2, 6–18 mo or 2, 3–4, 6–18 mo Infant (mother HBsAg positive), 0, 1, 6 mo [& HBV immunoglobulin at 0 unless mother shown to be anti-HBe positive (UK)]<br>Booster: see Comments | 20 μg[f] IM<br>Schedule: 3 doses, 0, 1, 6 mo<br>Accelerated: 4 doses, 0, 1, 2, 12 mo<br>Booster: see Comments | Recommendations for use in normal individuals vary between countries. Routine infant immunisation in USA. See Special Risk Groups. Accelerated schedule may be used to provide earlier protection. For high-dose exposure consider HBV immunoglobulin. Need for routine testing/booster doses following primary immunization is not clear, although infants of HBsAg-positive mothers should have antibodies determined ≥1 mo after 3rd dose. Antibody levels >10 U/L are considered protective. Individuals who continue to be at risk should receive a booster dose 3–5 yr after the primary course. |

(*continued*)

**Table 45.1** Guidelines for use of available vaccines—*Continued*

| Vaccine | Pathogen/ disease | Dose and schedule: Infants and children | Dose and schedule: Adults | Comments |
|---|---|---|---|---|
| Inactivated polio virus vaccine (trivalent) | Polioviruses types 1, 2, 3 | 0.5 mL IM/ deep SC Primary schedule and boosters: sequential IPV/OPV may be given See OPV schedules. | 0.5 mL IM/ deep SC Primary schedule and boosters: sequential IPV/OPV may be given (see Comments) See OPV schedules | IPV preferred in USA for primary immunization of adults ≥18 yr. |
| Influenza A & B (whole virus, split virus and surface antigen vaccines) | Influenza A & B | Use split virus vaccine 6 mo–3 yr, 0.25 mL 4–12 yr, 0.5 mL IM/deep SC Booster: Repeat 4–6 wk later if receiving vaccine for first time Annual vaccination with current vaccine | 0.5 mL IM/ deep SC Annual vaccination with current vaccine | Consider immunization of family members of child/adult in special risk group. |
| Japanese B encephalitis. (formalin-inactivated mouse brain–derived) | Japanese B encephalitis | <3 yr, 0.5 mL SC >3 yr, 1 mL deep SC Primary schedule: 3 doses, 0, 7–14 + 28 d (see Comments) Booster: 1 dose at 1 yr | 1 mL, deep SC Primary schedule: 0, 7–14 + 28 days (see Comments) Booster: 1 dose at 1 yr Consider every 1–3 yr | Not licensed in the UK. Consider for travelers to infected areas. Two-dose schedule at 0 and 7–14 d gives protection for up to 3 mo. |
| Rabies (human diploid cell) | Rabies | No information <1 yr of age >1 yr, 1 mL IM, deep SC, ID. Preexposure schedule: 3 doses, 0, 7 + 28 d Booster: every 2–3 y (rabies serum antibody titers can be monitored) | 1 mL IM, deep SC, ID Preexposure schedule: 3 doses, 0, 7 + 28 d Booster: every 2–3 y (rabies serum antibody titers can be monitored). | Consider in those at risk from disease (see Special Risk Groups) and those living in or traveling to enzootic areas. Intragluteal administration may be associated with reduced efficacy. |
| Tick-borne encephalitis (formaldehyde-inactivated; propagated in chick embryo cells) | Tick-borne encephalitis | 0.5 mL IM Primary schedule: 3 doses, 0, 4–12 wk, 9–12 mo Booster: 1 dose after 3 yr | 0.5 mL IM Primary schedule: 3 doses, 0, 4–12 wk, 9–12 mo Booster: 1 dose after 3 yr | Not licensed in the UK and USA. Consider for individuals with prolonged exposure in at-risk areas. |
| ATTENUATED LIVE-VIRUS VACCINES[c] | | | | |
| Adenovirus (enteric-coated tablets) | Adenovirus (types 4, 7, 21) | | | Currently used only in military personnel. |
| Measles (various strains) | Measles | 0.5 mL IM/ deep SC Primary schedule UK/USA: 1 dose, 12–15 mo WHO: 1 dose, 9 mo Booster: UK/USA ×1 dose 4–6 yrs | 0.5 mL IM/ deep SC Primary schedule UK: 1 dose USA: 1 dose Any age if not immunized or not developed immunity Booster: (USA) ×1 dose (>1 mo later) | Usually combined as MMR.[g] Measles vaccine can be used to protect susceptible contacts during a measles outbreak. A further dose of measles vaccine should be provided (usually at 15 mo) if the 1st dose is given at <12 mo. |
| Mumps (various strains) | Mumps | 0.5 mL IM/ deep SC Primary schedule UK/USA: ×1 dose, 12–15 mo Booster: UK/USA ×1 dose 4–6 yr | 0.5 mL IM/ deep SC Primary schedule: 1 dose any age if not immunized or not developed immunity Booster: none | Usually combined as MMR.[g] |

**Table 45.1** Guidelines for use of available vaccines—*Continued*

| Vaccine | Pathogen/ disease | Dose and schedule: Infants and children | Dose and schedule: Adults | Comments |
|---|---|---|---|---|
| Polio virus (oral, trivalent) | Polioviruses types 1, 2, 3 | Dose: contents 1 container<br>Primary schedule: 3 or 4 doses UK: 2, 3, 4 mo<br>USA: 2, 4, 6–18 mo<br>WHO: 0, 6, 10, 14 wk<br>Boosters: 1 or 2 doses<br>UK: 4–5 yr, 15–19 yr<br>USA: 4–6 yr | Dose: contents 1 container<br>Primary schedule: 3 doses<br>UK: 0, 1, 2 mo<br>USA: 0, 1–2, 6–12 mo (see Comments)<br>Boosters: if continuing risk of infection, a single booster every 10 y | See IPV comments. Sequential IPV/OPV may be given (USA) OPV contraindicated in contacts of immunosuppressed patients. USA: routine primary immunization of previously unimmunized adults residing in the USA not indicated. IPV preferred |
| Rotavirus (oral, rhesus reassortant, tetravalent) | Rotavirus | Primary schedule: 3 doses used in published trials<br>Booster: no data available | Not indicated at present | Other candidate vaccines likely to be licensed in near future. |
| Rubella (various strains) | Rubella | 0.5 mL IM/ deep SC<br>Primary schedule: UK/USA: 1 dose, 12–15 mo<br>Booster: ×1 dose 4–6 yr | 0.5 mL IM/ deep SC<br>Primary schedule: 1 dose, any age if not immunized or not developed immunity (females) | Usually combined as MMR.[g] Before the onset of puberty susceptible girls should have been immunized. |
| Varicella (OKA strain) | Varicella Zoster | 0.5 mL SC<br>Primary schedule (USA): 12 mo–13 y: 1 dose<br>>13 y: 2 doses (4–8 wk apart)<br>Primary schedule for children with malignancies: 2 doses with an interval of 3 mo<br>Booster: insufficient information | Inadequate information available | See Special Risk Groups. Consider also family members of any child in special risk group. |
| Yellow fever (17D strain) | Yellow fever | 0.5 mL deep SC<br>Primary schedule: 1 dose<br>WHO: at 9 mo.<br>Booster: every 10 yr for those at risk.<br>Generally recommended for infants ≥9 mo; immunization ≤9 mo may be performed if exposure cannot be avoided but should not be given <4 mo | 0.5 mL deep SC<br>Primary schedule: 1 dose<br>Booster: every 10 yr for those at risk | Consider for those at risk: laboratory workers handling infected material, travelers to infected areas. |

The age of which vaccines are given and the exact schedules vary between counties.

*Administer if shown to be unsensitized (antibody test/skin test).

[a]Half the usual dose may be used if severe side effects are expected.

[b]The efficacy of this schedule has not been determined.

[c]Contraindications to live vaccine administration include malignancy, immunodeficiency, immunosuppression from disease or therapy (see also Special Risk Groups).

[d]Refers to Havrix (SKB). Other preparations available. Refer to relevant literature.

[e]Provides persistent immunity for up to 10 years.

[f]Refers to Engerix B (SKB). Other preparations available. Refer to relevant literature.

[g]There is no evidence to suggest adverse consequences from giving MMR to a person who is already immune to one or more of its components as a result of earlier immunization or natural disease.

**Table 45.2** Guidelines for vaccine use for asplenia patients

| Recommended vaccines | Pathogen/disease | Vaccine | Comments |
|---|---|---|---|
| All routine vaccinations should be given unless otherwise stated | *Streptococcus pneumoniae* | Pneumococcal polysaccharide (23-valent) | Immunization should be performed at least 2 wk before splenectomy. Indicated in children >2 yr. Consider antimicrobial prophylaxis. Booster doses recommended after 6 yr in adults and 3–5 yr in children who will be <10 yr at revaccination. |
| | *Neisseria meningitidis* (A/C/Y/W135) | Meningococcal polysaccharide (4-valent) | Immunogenicity has been demonstrated with the meningococcal vaccine. Insufficient information available on the need for boosters. |
| | *Haemophilus influenzae* type b | Hib polysaccharide conjugated to protein | Immunogenicity has been demonstrated with Hib conjugate vaccines. Although the timing of boosters may be guided by anti-PRP levels (e.g., <0.15–0.5 μg/mL), there are no data to support any particular serum antibody level as protective following immunization with conjugate vaccines. |

### Malignancies (Table 45.4)

Note the following:

• *Polio*—OPV should be avoided in patients and their immediate contacts. IPV can be safely used in both patients and contacts whenever polio immunization is indicated.
• *Hepatitis B*—Active immunization offers only moderate benefit for patients receiving chemotherapy for leukaemia or lymphoma. Passive protection should be considered in any setting with high risk of infection by HBV.

• *Influenza A and B*—Immunogenicity is poor in those receiving chemotherapy regardless of the number of doses provided. Children in whom chemotherapy has been stopped (≥1 month) achieve equivalent titers to normal children. Response is better in those with solid tumors. In general, immunization is probably not indicated. It may be considered in situations in which there is another reason for vaccination. Immunization of normal contacts should be strongly considered.

• *Measles*—Not recommended. Since previously immunized children may become antibody-negative during therapy, clinicians may consider

**Table 45.3** Guidelines for vaccine use for HIV-infected patients

| Recommended vaccines | Pathogen/disease | Vaccine | Comments |
|---|---|---|---|
| All routine vaccinations should be given unless otherwise stated; vaccination early in the disease is recommended (See note on BCG.) | Measles, mumps, rubella | MMR live, attenuated | Measles vaccination (as measles vaccine ≤12 mo, MMR ≥12 mo) should be considered for all HIV-infected children, at the age recommended for non-HIV infected children or younger if there is an increased risk of exposure. It should probably be avoided if severely immunocompromised. Response may be suboptimal, however, and cannot be relied on to provide protection. If facilities exist for antibody determination, this should be performed. If there is no antibody response after 2 doses of vaccine, then monthly immunoglobulin should be considered. |
| | *Streptococcus pneumoniae* | Pneumococcal polysaccharide (23-valent) | As pneumococcal disease is important in children and adults with HIV, immunization should be considered but not relied on. Antibody responses may be suboptimal both immediately and in the longer term. |
| | *Haemophilus influenzae* type b | Hib polysaccharide conjugated to protein | Antibody response to vaccination should be measured. (see Hib comments in Table 45.2) |
| | Influenza A&B | Inactivated whole and split virus | Antibody response may be suboptimal. Consider immunization of household contacts. |
| | Hepatitis B | Hepatitis B recombinant | Advisable in patients with other risk factors for HBV, especially male homosexuals and their partners and intravenous drug users and their partners. Suboptimal responses to the vaccine are seen. Antibody response to vaccination should be measured. The use of larger doses of vaccine or more frequent booster doses has not been explored. |

**Table 45.4** Guidelines for vaccine use in patients with malignancies

| Recommended vaccines | Pathogen/disease | Vaccine | Comments |
|---|---|---|---|
| All routine vaccinations should be given unless otherwise stated | Varicella zoster | Live attenuated OKA strain | Most experience has been for children with hematological malignancies or malignant solid tumors (especially leukemia). Immunosuppressive therapy must be stopped from 1 wk before until 1 wk after the first vaccination, although equivalent immunogenicity is seen when 6-mercaptopurine is continued. Administration of CS must be postponed for at least 2 wk after vaccination. Lymphocyte count and neutrophil count should be $>500/mm^3$ respectively at the time of vaccination. |
| | *Haemophilus influenzae* type b | Hib polysaccharide conjugated | Consider booster doses according to anti-PRP level (see Hib comments in Table 45.2) |

booster measles immunization after the completion of therapy (≥3 months). Given the relative safety of live VZ vaccine in children with malignancies and of the measles vaccine in symptomatic patients with HIV, the vaccine may be relatively safe. There are no clinical data to support this, however.

• *Pneumococcus*—The degree and duration of protection provided by the currently available pneumococcal vaccine does not warrant its use for most patients. Patients at risk because of splenectomy should be immunized prior to splenectomy and prior to the initiation of chemotherapy or radiotherapy.

Other LV should be avoided until at least 3 months after chemotherapy has been stopped.

## Renal disease (Table 45.5)

In general, LV should be avoided in renal patients who are on immunosuppressive medication. The inactivated form of the vaccine, e.g., IPV, can be given if available. In addition, risk can be reduced by vaccinating close susceptible contacts (the exception is OPV). If the only immunosuppressive factor is CS, patients may be immunized if they are receiving less than 1 mg/kg/d of prednisone or its equivalent or if the steroids are stopped for 1 week before and 2 weeks after the vaccine has been administered. This strategy is predicated on clinical judgment that the child is not otherwise immunosuppressed. Otherwise live attenuated vaccines may be given ≥3 months after stopping immunosuppressive medication. Immunogenicity and safety have been demonstrated with the VZ vaccine in chronic renal failure prior to transplantation.

## Transplants (Table 45.6)

It is preferable to give vaccines prior to transplantations (≥2 weeks before). In general, LV should not be given until ≥3 months after immunosuppressive therapy has been stopped. Limited data are available on the VZ vaccine.

**Table 45.5** Guidelines for vaccine use in patients with renal disease

| Recommended vaccines | Pathogen/disease | Vaccine | Comments |
|---|---|---|---|
| All routine vaccinations should be given unless otherwise stated; vaccination early in the course of the disease is recommended | Hepatitis B | Hepatitis B recombinant | Strongly recommended in all patients at risk of developing end-stage renal failure, and for those on renal replacement therapy. For patients on hemodialysis a dose double the normal dose given at 0, 1, 2, 6 mo is recommended. Antibody level should be checked 2–4 mo after completion of the vaccine course and at regular intervals to guide timing of booster doses (when anti-HBsAg < 10 mU/L). |
| | Influenza A&B | Inactivated whole and split virus | Recommended annually for all patients in chronic renal failure. Antibody response may be less in patients on hemodialysis. |
| | *Streptococcus pneumoniae* | Pneumococcal polysaccharide (23-valent) | Strongly recommended in all patients with nephrotic syndrome and consider in patients with chronic renal failure. Consider revaccination after 3–5 yr in children and 6 yr in adults. Regular booster doses required in hemodialysis patients. |

**Table 45.6** Guidelines for vaccine use in transplant patients

| Recommended vaccines | Pathogen/disease | Vaccine | Comments |
|---|---|---|---|
| All routine vaccinations should be given unless otherwise stated | Influenza A&B | Inactivated whole and split virus | Satisfactory antibody levels achieved. Antibody response impaired by cyclosporin but not azothioprine. |
| | *Streptococcus pneumoniae* | Pneumococcal polysaccharide (23-valent) | Suboptimal antibody response seen when given after transplantation. |
| | *Haemophilus influenzae* type b | Hib polysaccharide conjugated to protein | Good antibody responses seen after primary and booster doses. Consider booster dose (≥1 mo later). |

### Other immunodeficiencies

#### *Congenital disorders of immune function*

Live viruses are contraindicated. Inactivated vaccines should be administered but their efficacy may be substantially reduced and they cannot be relied on to provide protection. Consider immunization of family members (OPV contraindicated) and specific immunoglobulin following exposure.

#### *Hypogammaglobulinemia/Agammaglobulinemia*

Active immunization is of no value. Immunoglobulin infusions are appropriate with consideration of specific immunoglobulin following exposure. OPV is specifically contraindicated.

#### *Complement deficiencies*

Immunizations against the pneumococcus, meningococcus, and Hib should be offered and antibiotic prophylaxis should be considered.

## Patients defined by condition

### Chronic heart disease

Pneumococcal and influenza vaccines should be considered. In children, consideration should be given to those with congenital heart disease, although the data on the need for and efficacy of these vaccines are insufficient.

### Chronic liver disease

Pneumococcal vaccine should be offered.

### Chronic lung disease

Pneumococcal and influenza vaccines should be considered in adults and children, although there are insufficient data on the need for and efficacy of these vaccines in children, especially in asthma. It would be reasonable to offer the influenza vaccine to children with CS-dependent asthma, bronchopulmonary dysplasia, and cystic fibrosis.

### Diabetes mellitus (Table 45.7)

### People 65 years and older and nursing home residents (Table 45.8)

### Pregnant women

Live vaccines should generally be avoided in pregnancy (there are theoretical risks). Oral polio vaccine and yellow fever vaccine may be given for travel in high-risk areas.

Among other vaccines, DT is safe. Although there are insufficient data on other vaccines, rabies vaccine, hepatitis B vaccine, and influenza vaccine may be given if the risk of these conditions is high. When any vaccine or toxoid is to be given, delaying until the second or third trimester when possible is a reasonable precaution to minimize concern about possible teratogenicity. The rubella vaccine should be administered in the postpartum period to women who are not rubella-immune.

**Table 45.7** Guidelines for vaccine use in diabetes patients

| Pathogen/disease | Vaccine | Comments |
|---|---|---|
| Influenza A&B | Inactivated whole and split virus | Influenza and pneumococcal immunizations should be considered in adult diabetic patients, particularly if they have other risk factors for |
| *Streptococcus pneumoniae* | Pneumococcal polysaccharide (23-valent) | morbidity from these infections. |

**Table 45.8** Guidelines for vaccine use in the elderly

| Pathogen/disease | Vaccine | Comments |
|---|---|---|
| Influenza A&B | Inactivated whole and split virus | Shown to be effective in the reduction of hospitalizations and death from influenza and its complications. |
| *Streptococcus pneumoniae* | Pneumococcal polysaccharide (23-valent) | Consider revaccination after 6 yr. Both vaccinations are particularly indicated if there is associated medical illness that predisposes to complications from these infections. |

### Preterm infants

All routine vaccinations should be given at full dose and according to chronological age, regardless of weight. Administer when the infant is clinically stable.

Oral polio vaccine should be witheld until discharge from the nursery to avoid cross-infection of other premature infants. As an alternative, IPV may be given while an inpatient and the routine course can be completed with OPV or IPV.

Tuberculin (BCG) conversion rates may be lower in preterm and/or growth-retarded infants immunized at birth.

With *Haemophilus influenzae* type b conjugate vaccines, suboptimal antibody responses may occur in sick preterm infants.

With hepatitis B vaccine, seroconversion rate may be reduced in preterm infants. Antibody levels should be assessed.

Influenza A and B vaccine has been recommended for preterm infants with risk factors for severe influenza infection (e.g., bronchopulmonary dysplasia, congenital heart disease). Suboptimal antibody response may be seen in young infants (≤6 months of age) and in infants who are chronically sick, so that immunization cannot be relied on. Immunization of family members should be considered.

## Patients defined by occupation

### Health care workers (Table 45.9)

### Veterinarians and animal workers

Consider rabies, BCG, anthrax, plague, tularemia and Q fever vaccines in veterinarians and other animal workers who may come in contact with these infections.

## Abbreviations

| | |
|---|---|
| ACV | Pertussis acellular component vaccine |
| Anti-HAV | Antibody to HAV |
| Anti-HBsAg | Antibody to HBsAg |
| Anti-PRP | Antibody to polyribosyl-ribitol-phosphate |
| BCG | Bacille Calmette-Guérin |
| CS | Corticosteroid |
| DT | Diphtheria/tetanus toxoid |
| DTP | Diphtheria/tetanus/pertussis (whole-cell) |
| DTaP | Diphtheria/tetanus/pertussis (acellular, component) |
| ELISA | Enzyme-linked immunosorbent assay |
| HAV | Hepatitis A virus |
| HBV | Hepatitis B virus |
| HBsAg | Hepatitis B surface antigen |
| HCW | Health care worker |
| Hib | *Haemophilus influenzae* type b |
| HIV | Human immunodeficiency virus |
| ID | Intradermal |
| IM | Intramuscular |
| IPV | Inactivated polio vaccine |

**Table 45.9** Guidelines for vaccine use in health care workers

| Vaccine | Occupation | Comments |
|---|---|---|
| Hepatitis B | Strongly recommended in all HCWs who have contact with blood or bloodstained body fluid or patients tissues. | See Table 45.1, Inactivated Virus Vaccines, adult column. Accelerated schedule may be appropriate. Booster doses may be provided every 5 yr for those who continue to be at risk. |
| Influenza A&B | Consider in HCWs in contact with special groups at risk from influenza | Particularly important if patients at risk also have suboptimal response to influenza vaccines. |
| Measles, rubella, (varicella) | Consider in HCWs in contact with paediatric, obstetric, and immunosuppressed patients. | Proof of immunity should be sought. Live measles and rubella vaccines can be offered. VZ vaccine not currently indicated for HCWs. |
| BCG | Consider in HCWs who may come in contact with patients with tuberculosis or with their secretions. | |
| Diphtheria | All HCWs should have received primary and reinforcing doses. | |

| | |
|---|---|
| LV | Live vaccine |
| MMR | Measles/mumps/rubella vaccine |
| OPV | Oral polio vaccine |
| SC | Subcutaneous |
| SKB | SmithKline Beecham Pharmaceuticals |
| TB | Tuberculosis |
| u | Unit |
| UK | United Kingdom |
| USA | United States of America |
| WCV | Pertussis whole-cell vaccine |
| WHO | World Health Organization |
| VZ | Varicella zoster |

## ANNOTATED BIBLIOGRAPHY

Cherry J. Comparative efficacy of acellular pertusis vaccines: an analysis of recent trials. Pediatr Infect Dis J 1997; 16:S 90–96

*A review of the paediatric trials of this new vaccine.*

Gershon AA, Steinberg SP, and the Varicella Vaccine Collaborative Study Group. Persistence of immunity to varicella in children with leukemia immunized with live attenuated varicella vaccine. N Engl J Med 1989; 320:892–897.

*Provides evidence of the safety, efficacy, and persistence of immunity following administration of the varicella vaccine.*

Johnson DW, Fleming SJ. The use of vaccines in renal failure. Clin Pharmcokinet 1992; 22:434–446.

*Good review of the basis for impaired immunity in renal failure and consideration of the efficacy of common specific vaccines.*

Monto AS. Editorial. Influenza vaccines for the elderly. N Engl J Med 1994; 331:807–808.

*A clear summary of the available data prompted by a serial cohort study assessing efficacy and cost-effectiveness of the vaccine in a large number of elderly subjects and published in the same edition (pp 778–784).*

Pirofski L, Casadevall A. Use of licensed vaccines for active immunization of the immunocompromised host. Clin Micro Rev 1998; 11(1):1–26

*A thorough review of the literature.*

Wolfe MS. Protection of travelers. CID. 1997; 25:177–186.

*Guidelines for immunisation of travelers.*

*See also:*

Salisbury DM, Begg NT, eds. Immunisation against infectious disease. HMSO, UK, 1996.

Peter G, ed. Red Book: Report of the Committee on Infectious Diseases. 24th edition. Elk Grove Village, IL: American Academy of Pediatrics, 1997.

# 46

# Growth Factors, Immunomodulators, and Cytokines

BRIGITTA U. MUELLER AND PHILLIP A. PIZZO

Knowledge about the actions and interactions of cytokines and their therapeutic indications as recombinant growth factors has expanded rapidly. The word cytokine (from Greek *cyto* "cell" and *kinesis* "movement") can be used to describe all the biologic response modifiers, including the hematopoietic growth factors, the interferons, interleukins, and tumor necrosis factor. Initially the cytokines were named according to their perceived functions (granulocyte colony-stimulating factor, tumor necrosis factor, etc.), but newer cytokines have been numbered sequentially as interleukins. This appears to be a more rational nomenclature, since most cytokines have more than one function and are part of a cascade of host defense mechanisms against endogenous abnormalities (e.g., neoplastic cells), exogenous invaders (e.g., microorganisms, alloimmune response) or other stimuli (allergic reaction).

More than 20 interleukins or colony-stimulating factors (CSFs) have been described to date. Table 46.1 lists the cytokines that play a role in infectious diseases. Some of them have pathophysiologic or therapeutic functions in other diseases as well (e.g., cancer, graft-versus-host disease, or autoimmune reactions). The myelopoietic growth factors, especially granulocyte-macrophage colony-stimulating factor (GMCSF), granulocyte colony-stimulating factor (GCSF), monocyte colony-stimulating factor (MCSF), and interleukin 3 (IL-3) increase the number of activated neutrophils in the circulation, simulating and enhancing the physiologic events triggered by acute infections. When an invading microorganism or the presence of an endotoxin is detected, the body responds with the production of interleukin 1 (IL1), tumor necrosis factor (TNF), and other cytokines, which in turn stimulate regulatory T cells and bone marrow stroma cells to release the hematopoietic growth factors, including GMCSF, IL-3, and IL-6. Certain cytokines, such as GMCSF, GCSF, IL-1, and interferon gamma (IFN-$\gamma$) can also enhance the bactericidal and fungicidal activity of mature granulocytes or macrophages.

Immunomodulatory agents can be defined as drugs that can normalize an impaired, hyperactive, or deficient immune response, improving the host's defenses against an infection. Several cytokines (e.g., IL-1, IL-2, IL-4, IL-6, IL-12, TNF) have an immunomodulatory effect on T and B lymphocytes. The functions of many cytokines are overlapping and often synergistic, although the cellular receptors are specific for each CSF. Other agents that have an effect on the immune system include corticosteroids, nonsteroidal anti-inflammatory agents, thymic hormones, chemical immunomodulators (glutathione, levamisole, *N*-acetyl-cysteine), specific T-cell immunosuppressants (cyclosporin A), and certain cytotoxic chemotherapeutics (cyclophosphamide).

Because of advances in recombinant DNA technology, an increasing number of cytokines have been synthesized for clinical use. Table 46.2 lists the cytokines and immunomodulators that are of potential importance for the treatment of infectious diseases, along with their current licensed indications, side effects, and suggested dosages. To date, most of the clinical experience with these cytokines is based on the treatment of patients with congenital or acquired immunodeficiency syndromes, especially patients with cancer, bone marrow failure syndromes, or infection with the human immunodeficiency virus (HIV). It is probable that some of these agents will also prove useful for the treatment of various infectious diseases in immunocompetent patients.

## Cytokines and Immunomodulators in Bacterial and Fungal Infections

The therapy of severe bacterial or fungal infections, especially in the immune-compromised host, remains a significant problem despite advances in the development of new antimicrobial or antifungal agents. The clear role of cytokines in the treatment of bacterial and fungal infections stems from their stimulatory effect on myelopoiesis and their ability to enhance the function of mature granulocytes and monocytes/macrophages. In patients receiving cytotoxic therapy as well as in those with primary bone marrow failure, prolonged neutropenia (especially with neutrophil counts below 100 cells/mm$^3$) is associated with an increased risk for recurrent bacterial as well as invasive fungal infections. Resolution of the infection is often dependent on the recovery of the neutrophil count and immunoreconstitution. Hematopoietic cytokines have been successfully utilized to increase the number of circulating neutrophils (GMCSF, GCSF, IL-3) and macrophages/monocytes (GMCSF, IL-3), decreasing the duration of neutropenia. In addition, GMCSF, GCSF, MCSF, and IFN-$\gamma$ can enhance the bactericidal and fungicidal activity of mature granulocytes or macrophages, and potentially might reduce the number and severity of bacterial and fungal infections.

It has been known since the beginning of the twentieth century that a nonspecific resistance to infection can be achieved by the administration of killed micro-organisms such as *Mycobacterium bovis* (bacille Calmette-Guérin, BCG), *Propionibacterium acnes*, *Listeria monocytogenes*, or *Candida albicans*. It is now recognized that the probable mediation of this effect is through the release of IL-1, IL-6, and TNF. These interleukins are under investigation as adjunctive therapy for the treatment of a wide variety of infections, especially those caused by intracellular organisms. Other CSFs that have shown promising activity in preclinical studies are IL-2, IL-8, and IL-12.

The use of cytokines in nonneutropenic patients remains investigational, although there are preliminary data indicating that GCSF may be of benefit in patients with diabetes mellitus, alcoholism, or renal disease who develop septicemia, presumably because these patients are less able to mount a quantitatively and

**Table 46.1** Cytokines with a potential role in infectious diseases

| Cytokine (abbreviation) | Cellular source | Target cells | Function |
|---|---|---|---|
| Granulocyte–macrophage colony-stimulating factor (GMCSF) | T lymphocytes, macrophages, endothelial and epithelial cells, fibroblasts | Myeloid progenitor cells, neutrophils, eosinophils, macrophages | Stimulates proliferation of hematopoietic progenitor cells<br>Enhances differentiation and terminal maturation of granulocytes and macrophages |
| Granulocyte colony-stimulating factor (GCSF) | Monocytes, endothelial and epithelial cells, bone marrow stroma, fibroblasts, neutrophils | Neutrophils, promyelocytes | Stimulates proliferation of myeloid progenitor cells<br>Enhances neutrophil survival and chemotactic function |
| Macrophage colony-stimulating factor (MCSF) | Fibroblasts, endothelial cells, monocytes/ macrophages | Monocyte progenitor cells, macrophages | Stimulates proliferation, differentiation, survival and function of monocytes/macrophages<br>Enhances production of IL-1, IFN-$\gamma$, and TNF-$\alpha$ |
| Interleukin-1 (IL-1, $\alpha$, and $\beta$) | Macrophages, fibroblasts, T lymphocytes, vascular endothelial cells, hepatocytes, osteoclasts | Fibroblasts, T lymphocytes, monocytes, granulocytes | Induces cytokines (IL-2, IFNs, IL-3, IL-6, TNF)<br>Induces B- and T-cell activation, growth, and differentiation<br>Induces bone marrow cell proliferation<br>Synthesis of acute phase reactants, induces fever, catabolism |
| Interleukin-2 (IL-2) | Activated T cells | Activated lymphoid cells | Enhances B- and T-cell immune responses<br>Promotes generation of cytotoxic T cells<br>Induces IFN-$\gamma$, TNF |
| Interleukin-3 (IL-3, multi-CSF) | Activated T cells | Myeloid progenitors, macrophages | Promotes growth of stem cells, erythroid and myeloid progenitors |
| Interleukin-4 (IL-4, B-cell stimulatory factor) | TH2 lymphocytes | B and T lymphocytes, macrophages, mast cells | Induces B-cell activation, proliferation, and differentiation and IgE and IgG1 production<br>Enhances MCH class II and IgE receptors |
| Interleukin-5 (IL-5, eosinophil differentiation factor) | TH2 lymphocytes | Eosinophils | Stimulates proliferation, differentiation, and function of eosinophils<br>Induces production of IgA and IgM |
| Interleukin-6 (IL-6) | Macrophages, fibroblasts, TH2 lymphocytes | Lymphocytes, monocytes | Stimulates B-cell growth, differentiation, activation<br>Induces synthesis of acute-phase reactants |
| Interleukin-8 (IL-8) | Monocytes, fibroblasts, endothelial cells | Neutrophils, monocytes | Enhances neutrophil activity (chemotaxis, lysosomal enzyme release) and basophil chemotaxis and histamine release |
| Interleukin-11 (IL-11) | Bone marrow stromal cells | | Augments IL-3–dependent proliferation of primitive hematopoietic cells<br>Stimulates synthesis of acute-phase reactants<br>Improves mucosal integrity |
| Interleukin-12 (IL-12, natural killer cell stimulating factor) | Macrophages, B cells | T cells | Induces differentiation of TH1 cells<br>Initiates production of IFN-$\gamma$ by TH1 cells and natural killer cells |

(*continued*)

**Table 46.1** Cytokines with a potential role in infectious diseases—*Continued*

| Cytokine (abbreviation) | Cellular source | Target cells | Function |
|---|---|---|---|
| Interferon alpha (IFN-$\alpha$, leukocyte interferon) | Leukocytes, lymphocytes, fibroblasts, macrophages | Neutrophils, macrophages | Antiviral function<br>Neutrophil and monocyte/macrophage function<br>Increases MHC class II expression<br>Enhances production of IgG subclasses |
| Interferon beta (IFN-$\beta$, fibroblast interferon) | Fibroblasts, epithelial cells, lymphocytes | Same as IFN-$\alpha$ | Same as IFN-$\alpha$<br>Increases natural killer cell function |
| Interferon gamma (IFN-$\gamma$, immune interferon) | T cells | Macrophages, monocytes<br>T cells, B cells | Similar to IFN-$\alpha$, but more pronounced monocyte/macrophage activation<br>Increases MHC class II expression |
| Tumor necrosis factor (TNF, cachectin [= TNF-$\alpha$], lymphotoxin [= TNF-$\beta$]) | Monocytes, macrophages, leukocytes, lymphocytes, mast cells | Monocyte/macrophages, lymphocytes, neutrophils, fibroblasts | Macrophage and neutrophil activation<br>Immunomodulatory effects<br>Induces cascade of inflammatory reactions (fever, catabolism, acute-phase proteins)<br>Mediates endotoxic shock<br>Induces multiple cytokines (e.g., IL-1, GMCSF)<br>Increases MHC class I expression<br>Enhances B-cell proliferation and Ig production |

qualitatively successful response to an infectious challenge. It has been shown clearly that IFN-$\gamma$ provides a benefit to patients with chronic granulomatous disease (CGD). Moreover, the role of IFN-$\gamma$ has been extended to patients with disseminated *M. avium* complex infection. Corticosteroids, with their nonspecific anti-inflammatory effect, are now used as adjunctive therapy in the treatment of severe *Pneumocystis carinii* pneumonia and bacterial meningitis.

## Cytokines and Immunomodulators in Viral Infections

The only cytokine that has been licensed to date for the use in viral infections is IFN-$\alpha$ for the treatment of chronic hepatitis B and C infections and genital papillomavirus infection. Whether the effect of interferon in these infections is due to its immunomodulatory or antiviral effect is unclear. Hepatitis B and C infections require prolonged therapy and are often associated with side effects such as fatigue, malaise and headaches (Table 46.2). Relapse, once therapy is withdrawn, can occur. Interleukins under clinical investigation include IL-2 for the treatment of human immunodeficiency virus disease, IL-1 as a protection against influenza virus infection, and IFN-$\alpha$ or IFN-$\beta$ against herpes infections (*H. simplex*, *H. zoster*, cytomegalovirus).

The importance of host response in containing HIV-1 has created an interest in evaluating interleukins as adjunctive therapy for HIV infection. Whereas several cytokines inhibit HIV replication directly (IFN-$\alpha$ and IFN-$\beta$), others, including IL-1, IL-3, and IL-6, as well as GMCSF and MCSF, can stimulate HIV replication. Tumor necrosis factor appears to have antiviral activity as well as toxic effect. Furthermore, it seems likely that cytokines (TNF-$\alpha$ and IL-1) may contribute to disease progression, including the wasting syndrome and the encephalopathy associated with HIV infection in children and adults, or the acute neurologic symptoms that accompany bacterial meningitis. Accordingly, attempts to suppress or modify cytokine production are also being pursued as an adjunctive therapy. This can be achieved in several ways, including the use of a soluble receptor antagonist to IL-1 or TNF receptors or direct inhibition of TNF-$\alpha$ release with thalidomide or pentoxifylline.

Other immunomodulatory agents with a still unclear role in viral diseases are the corticosteroids, antioxidants such as *N*-acetyl-L-cysteine, and retinoic acid, which are all currently investigated for the treatment of HIV infection. Corticosteroids may have a role in the treatment of HIV-associated encephalopathy in selected patients or the treatment of oxygen-dependent lymphocytic interstitial pneumonitis.

## Myelopoietic Growth Factors

The clinical indication for the use of hematopoietic cytokines is based on the observation that prolonged neutropenia, especially with neutrophil counts below 100 cells/mm$^3$, is associated with an increased risk for infections. Current antineoplastic regimens often result in neutrophil nadirs below this level, and GMCSF and GCSF have been shown to shorten the duration of this neutropenia. In addition, the use of hematopoietic cytokines has been associated with reductions in the number of hospitalization days and antibiotic use, potentially reducing the incidence of documented infections. However, no study to date has demonstrated an impact on survival. Furthermore, the implications of costs

**Table 46.2** Therapeutic indications of cytokines and immunomodulators for infectious diseases

| Cytokine | Licensed indication (infectious diseases) | Dose | Investigational indication | Side Effects |
|---|---|---|---|---|
| GMCSF | Myeloid reconstitution after autologous bone marrow transplant | 250 $\mu$g/m$^2$/d for 21 d as a 2 h IV infusion | Neutropenia associated with HIV infection or its treatment<br>Clinical trials with the combination of GMCSF and IL-3 (PIXY) | Fever, flulike symptoms, capillary-leak syndrome, fluid retention, large-vessel thrombosis |
| GCSF | Decrease the incidence of infections (febrile neutropenia) in patients with nonmyeloid malignancies receiving myelosuppressive anticancer therapy | 5 $\mu$g/kg (or higher if tolerated and needed) | Widely used as supportive treatment in other neoplastic diseases or bone marrow failure syndromes<br>Mobilization of myeloid precursors for peripheral stem cell harvest | Mild bone pain, occasionally increased alkaline phosphatase and lactate dehydrogenase levels<br>Thrombocytopenia with prolonged use; rarely disseminated intravascular coagulation |
| MCSF | None | Unknown | Possible role in combination with other growth factors or for invasive mycosis | Transient thrombocytopenia and lymphopenia at high doses |
| IL-1 | None | Unknown | In combination with other factors to ameliorate chemotherapy-induced neutropenia<br>As an adjunct to antimicrobial therapy | Fever, anorexia, hypotension, capillary-leak syndrome, fluid retention, hemodynamic shock |
| IL-2 | No current infectious disease indications | Unknown | As potential immunoenhancing factor in the treatment of HIV disease | Fluid retention, hypotension, capillary-leak syndrome, chemotactic and Fc receptor defects of neutrophils |
| IL-3 | None | Unknown | In combination with GMCSF (PIXY) to shorten duration of neutropenia in patients with aplastic anemia or chemotherapy-induced aplasia | Low-grade fever, headache, bone pain, transient thrombocytopenia at high doses |
| TNF | None | Unknown | Role as immunoenhancing agent | Fever, hypotension, capillary-leak syndrome |
| IFN-$\alpha$ | Condylomata acuminata (intralesional treatment) | 1 million IU/lesion 3 times/wk for 3 wk; repeat every 12–16 wk if needed | HIV infection in combination with zidovudine | Fever, flulike symptoms |
| | Hepatitis B | 6 million IU/d IV or SC | | |
| | Chronic hepatitis C | 3 million IU/m$^2$ 3 times/wk IV or SC | | |

| Cytokine | Licensed indication (infectious diseases) | Dose | Investigational indication | Side Effects |
| --- | --- | --- | --- | --- |
| IFN-$\gamma$ | Reducing frequency and severity of infections associated with chronic granulomatous disease | 50 $\mu g/m^2$ for BSA $>0.5\ m^2$; 1.5 $\mu g/kg$ for BSA $< 0.5\ m^2$, 3 times/wk SC | *Leishmania donovani*<br>*Listeria monocytogenes*<br>Disseminated MAC infection in patients with AIDS<br>*Mycobacterium leprae* | Fever, headaches, chills, erythema and tenderness at injection site |
| Corticosteroids | Concomitant with specific antimicrobial therapy<br>Meningitis (especially for *M. tuberculosis*)<br>*Pneumocystis carinii* pneumonia<br>Acute eye infection with *H. zoster* | Depends on indication (generally 0.5–2 mg/kg 2 times/d | HIV-related encephalopathy | Hyperglycemia, glucosuria, hypertension, electrolyte disturbances |
| Levamisole | No infectious disease indications to date | | Chronic active hepatitis B<br>T-cell immunodeficiency (against opportunistic infections)<br>Parasitic intestinal disease | Neutropenia, flulike symptoms |

Abbreviations: BSA, body surface area; MAC, *Mycobacterium avium* complex.

versus benefits have not yet been fully assessed. Another potential problem is the lack of clear efficacy studies in children; moreover, the side effects of long-term use of these agents (e.g. in HIV-infected patients) are unknown.

## Granulocyte-macrophage colony-stimulating factor

Naturally occurring GMCSF is a glycoprotein, produced by a number of cells, and its gene is encoded on the long arm of chromosome 5 (5q21-5q32). It acts locally in a paracrine fashion. Because its actions are local, GMCSF is usually not detected in measurable amounts in the blood of healthy adults, although it is detectable in umbilical cord blood and in the blood of some adults with hematologic disorders. The synthesis of GMCSF is induced by other cytokines, such as IL-1 and TNF-$\alpha$, in response to severe infections or an inflammatory event.

As a multilineage colony-stimulating factor, GMCSF has a proliferative effect, predominantly on intermediately mature hematopoietic precursor cells. It is even more active when combined with other cytokines (e.g., IL-3 or GCSF), resulting in increased numbers of granulocytes, monocytes, eosinophils, and megakaryocytes in the circulating blood. GMCSF enhances the phagocytic activity of polymorphonuclear cells (PMNs) against bacteria and yeast cells, and it increases antibody-dependent cell cytotoxicity (ADCC) of PMNs and the release of lysozymes. In addition, GMCSF is a potent inhibitor of neutrophil migration and may concentrate the granulocytes at the site of infection. In animal models, GMCSF enhances resistance to a lethal challenge with *Pseudomonas aeruginosa*, *Staphylococcus aureus*, or *Candida albicans*.

Recombinant GMCSF has been produced in bacteria, yeast cells, and mammalian cell systems. It can be administered either subcutaneously or intravenously on a daily basis. For both routes of administration there is a marked dose-dependency in peak levels as well as half-life.

Granulocyte-macrophage-CSF is licensed for myeloid reconstitution after autologous bone marrow transplant, but it is also commonly used to ameliorate the duration and depth of neutropenia during chemotherapy as well as to support patients with myelodysplastic syndromes, aplastic anemia, idiopathic neutropenia, or HIV-associated neutropenia. In a randomized double-blind study of patients with neutropenia after chemotherapy and autologous bone marrow transplant for lymphoid cancer, it was found that the patients given GMCSF had a recovery of their neutrophil count to >500 cells/mm$^3$ a mean of 7 days earlier than the patients who received placebo, had fewer infections, required less antibiotics (3 days less) and days of hospitalization (6 days less). In patients with HIV infection and zidovudine-associated neutropenia, an increase in white blood cell count can be achieved with GMCSF, but it is important to recognize that this cytokine can upregulate HIV replication (reflected by increased serum p24 antigen levels in patients receiving GMCSF alone), underscoring the importance of administering it together with an antiretroviral agent.

The major toxicities associated with GMCSF include fever (which can pose diagnostic problems in patients who are neutropenic), rash, and, at higher doses, a transient respiratory distress syndrome (probably secondary to a pulmonary sequestration of neutrophils), which can be difficult to differentiate from an infectious etiology. Because some malignant cell lines express receptors for both GMCSF and GCSF, there is also the theoretical concern that these cytokines might stimulate a neoplastic clone if the receptors are present on the tumor cells.

## Granulocyte colony-stimulating factor

Serum levels of GCSF may be elevated and measurable in human plasma during infection and in patients with aplastic anemia or cyclic neutropenia. Granulocyte colony-stimulating factor, also a glycoprotein, whose gene is located on chromosome 17, is relatively specific, stimulating the proliferation and maturation of progenitors already committed to the neutrophil lineage. A dose of 5 $\mu$g/kg, administered either subcutaneously or in an albumin solution which is infused intravenously over several hours, has become commonly used during the therapy of chemotherapy-associated neutropenia, but doses up to 20 $\mu$g/kg have been given safely to adults and children.

Granulocyte colony-stimulating factor can be given either as prophylaxis or therapeutically to patients receiving myeloablative treatment for cancer. Administration of this cytokine has been shown to decrease the duration and severity of neutropenia, as well as the length of antibiotic therapy and hospitalization. Beneficial effects have also been demonstrated in some patients with aplastic anemia and commonly in patients with chronic neutropenia or HIV-associated neutropenia. Side effects appear to be less frequent with GCSF than with GMCSF, the major toxicity being mild bone pain. However, rare cases of leukoclastic vasculitis, large vessel thrombosis, and disseminated intravascular coagulation have also been reported. Although patients with myelodysplastic syndrome respond to GCSF therapy with an increase in neutrophil counts, there is a concern that the risk of developing acute leukemia may be increased.

Several animal models of acute bacterial infection without neutropenia have been employed to demonstrate improved survival when GCSF is added to antimicrobial management. Furthermore, GCSF is being investigated as an adjunct to therapy in patients with bacterial pneumonia. The drug appears to be well tolerated in these patients and has not induced adult respiratory distress syndrome. Since GCSF was licensed in the United States, it has become widely used for a variety of indications despite its high costs. Although it has a role in patients anticipated to have periods of neutropenia exceeding 7–10 days, its indiscriminate use is costly and unwarranted, especially in patients whose duration of neutropenia is short. In recently published guidelines the American Society for Clinical Oncology recommends the use of cytokines in the following situations: if the likelihood of neutropenia is expected to be more than 40%; after an episode of fever and neutropenia in a prior cycle when dose reduction is not an option; after high-dose therapy with autologous bone marrow transplant.

## Interferons

The IFNs are proteins consisting of 165–187 amino acids, with their genes clustered on chromosomes 9 (IFN-$\alpha$ and IFN-$\beta$) and 12 (IFN-$\gamma$). Interferon production is induced by such common stimuli as viruses, bacteria, and double stranded RNA, as well as other cytokines (TNF, IL-1, IL-2, and CSFs). After binding to their cellular receptors the IFNs induce at least two enzymes that inhibit protein translation, a synthetase and a protein kinase. In addition, they induce or enhance expression of cell surface antigens for the major histocompatibility complexes (MHCs). The regulatory actions of IFNs include the establishment of a resistance to viral infection by interacting at different stages of the viruses' life cycles, enhancement of the cytotoxic activity of natural killer (NK) cells, and induction of other growth hormones.

In addition, the IFNs have potent inhibitory activity of normal and malignant cell growth.

## Interferon alpha

There are more than 15 subtypes of naturally occurring IFN-$\alpha$, and the recombinant forms (IFN-$\alpha$-2a and IFN-$\alpha$-2b) are produced in *Escherichia coli*. Interferon alpha increases MHC class I expression and has direct antiviral activity against hepatitis C and papovavirus-induced condylomata. The elimination half-life of IFN-$\alpha$ is only 4–5 hours, but the biological activity lasts for 2–3 days, which justifies a thrice weekly administration. Interferon alpha is well absorbed after subcutaneous or intramuscular injection, and is eliminated through renal secretion and catabolism.

Interferon alpha has been shown to be active for the treatment of hepatitis C (HCV). For example, 80% of patients with HCV who received 2 million units of IFN-$\alpha$ subcutaneously three times a week for 6 months had a marked reduction in serum HCV RNA, whereas the viral genome remained detectable in all patients who did not respond or who received a placebo. These findings suggest a direct effect of IFN-$\alpha$ on the rate of viral replication. However, the overall response rate (about 40%–50% of the patients) is dose-dependent and long-term remissions are rare.

In patients with hepatitis B (HB) the overall response rate, as measured by loss of HB surface antigen, HB viral DNA, and HBe antigen, as well as normalization of liver enzymes, was 46% in a group receiving 5 million units of INF-$\alpha$ per day for 4 months and 25% in the group receiving 1 million units per day. Histologically the response was manifested by regression of periportal necrosis and reduced portal inflammation. In both hepatitis B and C infection response to INF-$\alpha$ appears to be inversely related to "viral load."

The intralesional application of IFN-$\alpha$ is approved by the Food and Drug Administration for the treatment of condylomata acuminata, genital or venereal warts caused by infection with human papilloma virus. One million units of interferon per wart, injected intralesionally three to four times per week, resulted in the disappearance of 35%–60% of the warts compared to 20% when treated with placebo.

In cells infected with HIV, IFN-$\alpha$ appears to block the late (i.e., posttranslational) stages of virus production. It has been used, sometimes in combination with zidovudine, for the treatment of HIV disease, especially in patients with Kaposi's sarcoma, taking advantage of the antiviral and antiproliferative activity of the compound. The combination of zidovudine and IFN-$\alpha$ was well tolerated with hematologic toxicity (mainly neutropenia) being the dose-limiting side effect. This therapy resulted in improved immune function as measured by CD4 counts and had an antitumor effect in about 40% of the patients.

The major side effects of IFN-$\alpha$ are dose-related flu-like symptoms including fever, headaches, and malaise. When combined with zidovudine, IFN-$\alpha$ enhances the bone marrow toxicity of this agent and neutropenia becomes dose-limiting. Neutralizing antibodies to IFN-$\alpha$ have been described and may interfere with the biologic activity of the compound.

## Interferon beta

Interferon beta has a spectrum of in vitro activities similar to IFN-$\alpha$, including antiviral, antiproliferative, and immunomodulatory effects, but limited clinical trials showed only minimal benefits in the treatment of infectious diseases. However, IFN-$\beta$ appears to have a role in the treatment of multiple sclerosis. In a study of subcutaneous IFN-$\beta$ every other day it reduced the rate and severity of disease exacerbations in patients with relapsing multiple sclerosis.

## Interferon gamma

Interferon gamma has synergistic activity with TNF in vitro in inhibiting the replication of several viruses, including HIV. It also has an effect on a number of intracellular organisms, including *Toxoplasma gondii*, *Leishmania donovani*, *Chlamydia*, and *Plasmodia*. It triggers the $O_2^-$ and $H_2O_2$ release (respiratory burst) of PMNs, which is critical for the intracellular digestion of microorganisms.

Patients with chronic granulomatous disease have a NADPH oxidase deficiency, preventing the production of superoxide via the respiratory burst mechanism in their phagocytes. This leads to an impaired ability to kill intracellular microorganisms, and consequently these patients suffer of recurrent pyogenic infections. Treatment with IFN-$\gamma$ leads to a normalization of the microbicidal activity, albeit without directly affecting the NADPH oxidase or improving its function, decreasing the risk for serious infection by 67%. Further studies are needed to elucidate the mechanism of action of IFN-$\gamma$ in these patients.

Interferon gamma may also have a role in the prophylaxis or treatment of fungal infections, because the in vitro fungicidal activity of PMNs against *C. albicans* and *Aspergillus fumigatus* hyphae has been demonstrated to be increased. In clinical trials IFN-$\gamma$ has been shown to have activity against *M. leprae* infection. Clinical trials are currently planned to evaluate the use of IFN-$\gamma$ as an adjunct to the treatment of *M. avium* complex infection in patients with AIDS. This is based on the recognition that T lymphocytes from patients with HIV infection produce subnormal levels of IFN-$\gamma$ and that the in vitro microbicidal activity of the patients' PMNs was restored to normal when IFN-$\gamma$ was added.

## Interleukins

More than a dozen different interleukins have been described, and their functions are often overlapping, additive, or synergistic. In this chapter, only the interleukins with a defined role in the pathogenesis or treatment of infectious diseases are considered. Interleukins 1, 6, and 8 are produced by the body in response to an inflammation or infection, and in turn they induce the synthesis of acute phase proteins and prostaglandins and can act as pyrogens. Interleukin 2 is a growth and maturation factor for mature T cells, inducing cytotoxicity and natural killer cell activity. Interleukins 4 and 5 are B-cell stimulators.

A single intravenous dose of IL-1 rapidly results in arterial hypotension, similar to septic shock, in which hypotension is induced by the combined action of IL-1 and TNF. Blocking this effect with soluble IL-1 receptors or IL-1 receptor antagonists has shown promising results in vitro and resulted in improved survival of mice and rabbits injected with endotoxin or bacteria. Both molecules act like antibodies and prevent the binding of IL-1 with its cellular receptors, thereby reducing the severity or manifestations of disease. However, preliminary evaluations of clinical trials in humans have shown only limited efficacy, probably related to the complex interactions of other interleukins in sepsis syndrome.

Interleukin 2 and the interaction with its receptor induce a cascade of cytokines, including various interleukins, interferons, and tumor necrosis factor. Interleukin-2 is produced by $CD4^+$ and $CD8^+$ T lymphocytes in response to antigenic and mitogenic stimuli. In animals, IL-2 increases the primary immune response after immunization, restores T-cell activity, and induces NK cell activity. Production of IL-2 is deficient in HIV-infected individuals, and clinical trials are currently evaluating the role of IL-2 therapy as an immune stimulating agent. However, high doses of IL-2 are complicated by fever, hypotension, and pulmonary edema, limiting its clinical applications. Current studies in patients with HIV infection use a combination of antiretroviral agents and IL-2, and preliminary results indicate a transient increase in T-helper cells and a decrease in viral burden.

In vitro, IL-4 has a potent stimulatory effect on the production of HIV-1 by peripheral blood mononuclear cells. It may have a role in other infectious disease, by virtue of its suppressive effect on the release of IL-1 and TNF and the oxidative burst of monocytes. Conversely, inhibition of IL-4 activity in animal models of intracellular infection (e.g., leishmaniasis) has led to their limitation and resolution by enhancing the production of IL-1, TNF, and IFN-$\gamma$.

The role of IL-6 in infectious diseases is not yet well understood, but it appears to represent an acute inflammatory response mediator in the host defense against infectious agents, and it acts synergistically with TNF and IL-1 in this regard. Expression of HIV in chronically infected cells is stimulated by IL-6, and HIV infection itself increases IL-6 production in the presence of IL-4.

A recently characterized cytokine—IL-12, or natural killer cell stimulatory factor (NKSF)—appears to play a key role in the immune response against infections and some neoplastic processes. It enhances the cytolytic activity of T cells, natural killer cells, and macrophages; induces the secretion of IFN-$\gamma$; and presumably induces a switch from a TH2 to a TH1 state. Interleukin-12 has shown efficacy in the treatment of murine leishmaniasis and toxoplasmosis.

## Tumor Necrosis Factor (TNF)

Tumor necrosis factor alpha (cachectin) is produced by macrophages, T cells and B cells, and TNF-$\beta$, a functionally related cytokine, is produced by T cells. Both cytokines have similar biological activities and bind to the same receptors on target cells, although they show only 28% sequence homology. Further, TNF-$\alpha$ and TNF-$\beta$ have a stimulatory effect on the production of GM-CSF, IL-1, and IL-6, the phagocytic activity of PMNs, their degranulation, and release of $O_2^-$ and $H_2O_2$. The fungicidal activity of PMNs against *C. albicans* blastoconidiae, but not against *C. albicans* hyphae, is increased by TNF-$\alpha$. Both TNF-$\alpha$ and TNF-$\beta$ enhance HIV replication but also selectively kill HIV-infected cells, presumably through direct lysis or an immune mediated action. Wasting, B-cell activation with subsequent hypergammaglobulinemia, T-cell death, and oligodendrocyte killing and inflammation are HIV-associated symptoms that have been attributed to TNF-$\alpha$. As mentioned earlier a novel therapeutic approach in advanced HIV infection is therefore the suppression of TNF production with agents such as pentoxifylline.

## Other Immunomodulatory Agents

Chemical immunomodulators include imidazoles such as levamisole, which was found to augment delayed hypersensitivity to recall antigens. It may have a role in the treatment of opportunistic infections caused by T-cell deficiency states.

The thiols diethyldithiocarbamate (DTC) and *N*-acetylcysteine exert their immunorestorative effect via their sulfur group. They restore both T- and B-cell function and induce T-cell differentiation, and DTC has been shown to reduce bacterial infections in surgical patients and appears to improve the efficacy of antituberculous therapy. Both drugs are currently being investigated for their role in HIV disease, because some data indicate that they inhibit in vitro the cytokine-stimulated replication of HIV-1. Limited clinical studies indicated a beneficial effect in reducing the incidence of opportunistic infections.

Isoprinosine, a nucleic acid analogue, has been shown to enhance the function of various cells of the immune system. The drug is licensed in some countries for the treatment of viral diseases such as Herpes simplex infection, although there is no conclusive evidence supporting its use in this setting. While one study has suggested a therapeutic effect in HIV infection, the results are not convincing enough to justify its use for the therapy of HIV infection.

The role of vascular endothelial growth factor (VEGF) and vascular endothelial permeability factor (VEPF) in infection and sepsis is currently being defined.

## Adjuvants

Immunoadjuvants are an important component of vaccine development because of their ability to stimulate $CD4^+$ subpopulations (TH1 and TH2) as well as cytotoxic $CD8^+$ lymphocytes, thus enhancing the immunogenicity of the vaccine. The only approved agents for clinical use are the aluminum-containing compounds, the alums (hydroxides and phosphates). Another group are the immunostimulating complexes (ISCOMS) and saponins, structures that can increase the humoral response and induce a delayed hypersensitivity response. Nonionic block polymer surfactants and monophosphoryl lipid A, a less toxic derivative of lipopolysaccharides, as well as muramyl dipeptides, have undergone preliminary clinical trials with promising results. Freund's complete adjuvant, a strong activator of TH1 cells, was previously used for vaccine trials for influenza, poliomyelitis, and cholera, but it is now considered to be too toxic for clinical indications. Cytokines, especially IL-2 in a polyethylene glycol or liposome form, are currently being assessed for their function as immunoadjuvants.

## Conclusions

The cascade of effects and multitude of interactions makes the understanding and rational use of cytokines a challenge. However, used judiciously, they can be powerful tools in the treatment of infections and their complications. Clearly, further studies are needed to define the role of the different cytokines in physiologic and pathophysiologic events as well as their indications in the treatment of infections.

## ANNOTATED BIBLIOGRAPHY


Audibert FM, Lise LD. Adjuvants: Current status, clinical perspectives and future prospects. Immunol Today 1993; 14:281–284.
*Summary of current knowledge and discussing problems of adjuvants.*

Balkwill FR. Interferons. Lancet 1989; i1060–1063.
*Review of molecular biology of interferons and their role in disease.*

Curnutte JT. Conventional versus interferon-γ therapy in chronic granulomatous disease. J Infect Dis 1993; 167(suppl 1):S8–S12.
*Summary of clinical experience with interferon gamma in the treatment of CGD. Important publication for the clinician.*

Hersh EM. Immunomodulatory drugs of relevance to the management of microbial infections. Adv Exp Med Biol 1992; 319:1–11.
*One of the few reviews summarizing current knowledge on immunomodulatory drugs different from cytokines.*

Lieschke GJ, Burgess AW. Granulocyte colony-stimulating factor and granulocyte-macrophage colony-stimulating factor. First part: N Engl J Med 1992; 327:28–35; Second part: N Engl J Med 1992; 327:99–106.
*Review articles summarizing the current knowledge on GM-CSF and G-CSF. The first part discusses physiology and pathophysiology, the second part the clinical indications.*

Miles S. The use of hematopoietic growth factors in treating HIV infection. Curr Opin Hematol. 1995 May; 2(3):227–233.
*Concise review of the indications for growth factors in HIV disease.*

Nemunaitis J. A comparative review of colony-stimulating factors. Drugs. 1997 Nov; 54(5):709–729.
*Comprehensive discussion of CSFs.*

Paul WE, Seder RA. Lymphocyte response and cytokines. Cell 1994; 76:241–251.
*Review of physiology of cytokine response and their interactions.*

Pizzo PA. Management of fever in patients with cancer and treatment induced neutropenia. N Engl J Med 1993; 328:1323–1332.
*Review of the problems in the management of immunocompromised cancer patient, including the use of cytokines. Especially helpful for the clinician.*

Poli G, Fauci AS. Cytokine modulation of HIV expression. Semin Immunol 1993; 5:165–173.
*Detailed discussion of the involvement of cytokines in HIV infection, including their role in pathogenesis.*

Roilides E, Pizzo PA. Modulation of host defense by cytokines: evolving adjuncts in prevention and treatment of serious infections in immunocompromised hosts. Clin Infect Dis 1992; 15:508–524.
*Clinically oriented review of the current knowledge of pathophysiology and therapeutic indications of cytokines, focused on the immunocompromised host.*

Warren RP, Sidwell RW. The potential role of cytokines in the treatment of viral infections. Clin Immunother 1994; 1:15–30.
*Detailed review of the role of cytokines in viral infections with extensive references.*

# V

# INFECTIOUS DISEASE SYNDROMES

# 47

# Approach to the Patient with Fever: Acute Febrile Illness

ETHAN RUBINSTEIN AND DAVID HASSIN

Acute febrile illnesses usually develop within a 24 h period, and either subside in a few days (e.g., viral upper respiratory tract infection [URI]) or, because of their severity or associated symptoms, lead to early medical evaluation and diagnosis. While any process that can cause fever may have an acute onset and could involve a wide variety of infectious, inflammatory, or other disorders (Chapter 10), the vast majority of acute febrile illnesses are due to infection (Table 47.1). Chronic febrile illnesses, i.e., those lasting several weeks, often have a subtle onset; they may be more difficult to diagnose, and when infectious that are most often caused by pathogens that are sheltered from host defenses (e.g., intracellular or in abscesses, bone, or endocardium). In addition, more often than not, chronic febrile illnesses are noninfectious in etiology (Table 47.2).

Regardless of whether the febrile illness is acute or chronic, understanding and managing a patient with fever cannot be successful unless a thorough, systematic approach is adopted which first considers the possibility of infection. Shortcuts, associations, and ungrounded diagnoses can lead to an erroneous working hypothesis. As a result, therapy that is incorrect, or dangerous, or which obscures the case, may be instituted. This chapter focuses primarily on the approach to patients with acute fevers due to infectious agents acquired in the community, and it outlines a process that can be followed in the evaluation of any febrile patient. Chapter 48 does the same for the patient in the hospital and Chapter 49 for the patient with a chronic febrile illness often labeled as "fever of unknown origin."

## Medical History

The principal objectives in obtaining the history in patients with possible infectious diseases (with or without fever) are summarized schematically in Figure 47.1. First, the major clinical manifestations that are associated with the illness must be ascertained and defined. Second, the presence and potential interplay of any unique epidemiological and host factors must be elucidated. For example, fever, cough, and a pulmonary infiltrate in an elderly patient whose mother died of tuberculosis during his childhood will generate a much different diagnostic approach than the same manifestations in a young military recruit in the middle of an outbreak of respiratory illness. In turn, both of these patients will be considered differently from a middle aged man with fever and cough who is receiving cytotoxic chemotherapy for malignancy.

### Age

Certain infections are most common in childhood and may only appear later in life or in patients with immunosuppressing conditions. The immune response following immunization or natural exposure limits the following etiologic agents mostly to children and adolescents: measles, mumps, varicella, Epstein-Barr virus (EBV), parvovirus $B_{19}$, enteroviruses, and *Hemophilus influenzae*. Older family members may be reexposed to these pathogens when they are acquired by children in day care centers or schools, making this important information to gather when evaluating an acute febrile illness.

Elderly patients experience a variety of physiological modifications due to aging, including a decline in certain host defenses—in particular, cellular immunity. They may also be more likely to suffer from nutritional deficiencies if they are unable to care for themselves. Protein-calorie malnutrition leads to a further suppression of cellular immunity. Thus, elderly are more likely to activate quiescent tuberculosis or to develop malignancies than younger individuals. Impairment of bladder emptying by prostatism, prolapse, or neurogenic disease is also more common in the elderly, leading to a higher incidence of urinary tract infection. Finally, elderly patients may have dampened febrile and inflammatory responses to infection, making their presentation with potentially serious illness more subtle or less specific.

### Occupation

The potential for occupational infectious diseases should always be considered. Farmers, livestock handlers, veterinarians, and market and abattoir workers may be exposed to *Brucella*, *Coxiella burnetti*, *Leptospira*, *Campylobacter fetus*, and *Pasteurella multocida* as causes of infection and fever. Bird and poultry breeders can be exposed to *Chlamydia psittaci* and *Cryptococcus neoformans*. *Erysipelothrix rhusiopathiae* and aeromonas infections are encountered in fishermen, fish handlers, and individuals exposed to contaminated water. Hunters and individuals exposed to wildlife can be infected with *Francisea tularensis* or other agents carried by ticks and mosquitoes. Medical staff are exposed to blood-borne infections such as viral hepatitis types B and C, cytomegalovirus (CMV), and human immunodeficiency virus (HIV). Tuberculosis, particularly with resistant organisms, has also become a recent significant occupational hazard for health care personnel and prison guards.

### Present residence, place of origin, and travel history

These points, as well as vaccination before travel and prophylactic treatment during travel, should be elicited. The incubation period of the various infectious diseases should be considered: For example, *Vivax malaria*, amoebic liver abscess, and kala azar can manifest themselves even months after leaving the endemic area. Typhoid fever and Lyme disease usually present 1 wk to several weeks, Katayama fever 4–8 wk, and dengue and yellow

**Table 47.1** Common infectious acute febrile illnesses

| |
|---|
| Upper respiratory infections |
| Lower respiratory infections |
| Gastroenteritis |
| Cellulitis and soft tissue infections |
| Genitourinary tract infections |
| Viral exanthems (children) |
| Bacteremias |
| Meningitis |

fever 2 wk after exposure. Tuberculosis may not be manifested clinically until months to many years after the primary infection.

Some infectious diseases are directly related to certain geographical regions (Table 47.3): For example, malaria should be considered after travel in Africa, Southeast Asia, and Latin America but not after trips to Jamaica, Antilles, Chile, Israel, Lebanon, Japan, Taiwan, North Korea, and Australia, where the disease has presently been eliminated. Table 47.3 provides a summary of some important infectious diseases causing fever by country of origin. Chapter 92 focuses on febrile disorders in travelers returning from tropical countries. Chapters 92 to 94 deal specifically with infections seen in tropical countries that may infect the tourist or returning traveler.

## Present illness

The patient's complaints or direct questioning regarding specific symptoms will help to localize the infectious site and give clues to the diagnosis. The pattern of fever and its duration should be investigated and plotted; they are occasionally useful in suggesting certain diagnoses. Intermittent or septic fever is characterized by wide swings in temperature from very high to normal or almost normal over a 24 h period. Such a fever pattern may be exhibited in pyogenic abscesses, empyema, bacteremia, pyelonephritis, and military tuberculosis. Sustained (continuous) fever frequently accompanies brucellosis, Q fever, typhoid fever, tularemia, endocarditis, infectious mononucleosis, CMV, psittacosis, pneumococcal pneumonia in the later stages, rickettsial infections, acquired immunodeficiency syndrome (AIDS), and cryptococcal meningitis. Remittent fever which is similar to intermittent fever but with less prominent fluctuations of temperature is common in many infections, particularly if the patient has used antipyretics. Relapsing fever (i.e., periods of fever and normal temperature alternating cyclically) is seen in malaria. A fever spike every third day (tertian fever) may occur in *Plasmodium vivax* and *falciparum* infections. A relapsing or recurrent fever pattern is a feature of rat-bite fever, borreliosis, and dengue fever. Shaking chills can be an important clue that the patient with an acute febrile illness has bacteremia or parasitemia. It should be observed, however, that previous antibiotic or antiparasitic

**Table 47.2** Common etiologies of chronic febrile states*

| Patient % | | | | |
|---|---|---|---|---|
| 36% | 23% | 13% | 20% | 9% |
| Infection | Neoplasm | Collagen vascular disease | Miscellaneous | Undiagnosed |
| CI (31%–40%) | CI (19%–31%) | CI (9%–15%) | CI (9%–23%) | CI (5%–12%) |
| Tuberculosis | Lymphoma | Rheumatoid Arthritis | Granulomatous hepatitis | |
| Liver and biliary tract infection | Leukemia | Systemic Lupus erythematosis | Drug fever | |
| Infective endocarditis | Localized Tumor | Rheumatic fever | Inflammatory bowel disease | |
| Abdominal abscess | Disseminated carcinomatosis | Temporal arteritis | Pulmonary embolism | |
| Pyelonephritis | | Polyarteritis nodosa | Familial Mediterranean fever | |
| Prostatic abscess | | Wegener granulamatosis | Hematoma | |
| Sinusitis | | | Myxoma | |
| Osteomyelitis | | | Sarcoidosis | |
| Catheter infection | | | Pericarditis | |
| Amebic hepatitis | | | Factitious fever | |
| Psittacosis | | | Laennec's cirrhosis | |
| Brucellosis | | | Whipple's disease | |
| Gonococcemia | | | Periodic fever | |
| Chronic meningococcemia | | | Thyroiditis | |
| Toxoplasmosis | | | Erythema multiforme | |
| Cytomegalovirus | | | Weber-Christian disease | |
| Disseminated mycosis | | | Myelofibrosis | |
| Cirrhosis with bacteremia | | | Pancreatitis | |
| Wound infection | | | | |

*See Chapter 49 for details and references.

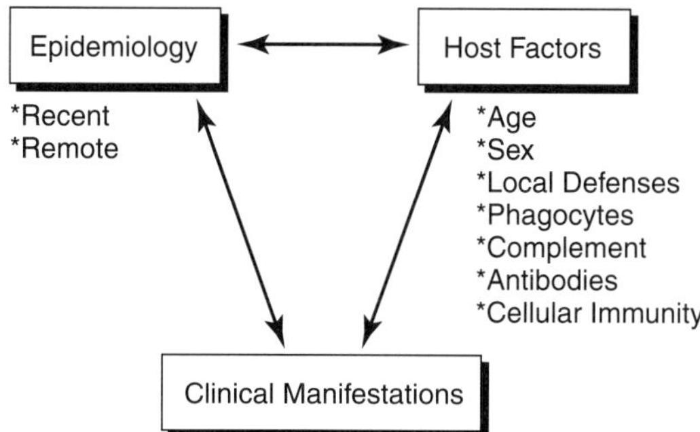


**Fig. 47.1** Approach to the patient with infectious disease: "The Historical Triangle."

therapy may mask the typical fever pattern, as will the use of antipyretics or glucocorticosteroids. Febrile responses to infection may be blunted in the elderly patient, in those with burns or spinal cord injury, and in those with severe renal or hepatic failure (Chapter 9).

## Headache

**Headache** can be a prominent symptom in some self-limited viral illnesses such as influenza and is a consistent feature of sinusitis. It can also signify more serious intracranial or systemic disease. For example, headache can be the leading complaint in patients with meningitis or encephalitis (see Chapters 73 and 74). Osteomyelitis of the skull and lateral and sigmoid venous thrombosis may also present with headache as a major symptom. Subdural empyema and cervical epidural abscess may present with fever and headache followed later by the appearance of neurological deficits. In contrast, brain abscesses often present with focal neurologic signs whereas fever and headache may be initially absent (see Chapter 76). In AIDS patients, sinusitis with headache is common and may present as a chronic or acute febrile condition; it must be distinguished from more serious intracranial disorders such as toxoplasmosis and cryptococcus (see Chapter 97). Among other systemic infections, headache is a common complaint in rickettsial diseases and infections with *Chlamydia psittaci*, *Borrelia recurrentis*, leptospira, and *Salmonella typhi*.

**Table 47.3** Selected important infections according to country of origin

| Disease | Distribution | Clinical presentation | Diagnosis |
|---|---|---|---|
| Babesiosis | Egypt, France, Ireland, Yugoslavia, Mexico, Russia, Spain, U.K., U.S. | Fever, myalgia, hemolysis, jaundice, renal failure, relapsing course | Blood smear |
| Bartonellosis (Oroya fever) | South America | Myalgia, hepatosplenomegaly, anemia, fungating skin lesions (verruga pervana) | Culture, blood smear |
| Brucellosis | Mediterranean countries, Peru | Fever, hepatosplenomegaly, osteomyelitis | Serology, blood culture |
| Cholera | Disease in epidemics which change locations worldwide | Watery diarrhea, stupor, shock, acidosis | Stool culture |
| Dengue | Southeast Asia, Central America, Caribbean, Southwest Pacific | Headache, myalgia, arthralgia, bradycardia, shock, DIC | Serology |
| Eastern equine encephalitis | United States, Central America | Headache, fever, seizures, neurological sequela | Viral cultures |
| Ebola fever | East and West Africa | Myalgia, sore throat, bloody diarrhea, conjunctivitis, hemorrhagic rash, hepatic dysfunction, DIC | Viral culture |
| Ehrlichiosis | United States | Headache, myalgia, arthralgia following tick bite, hepatic dysfunction | Blood smear |
| Hantaan virus | United States, Central Europe, Asia | Fever, myalgia, renal failure, respiratory failure (U.S.) | PCR + serology |
| Lassa fever | Africa | Pharyngitis, conjunctivitis, chest pain, protein urea, G. I. symptoms | Viral culture |
| Lyme disease | Northern Europe, U.S. (New England, Middle Atlantic States, Wisconsin, Minnesota, Northern California, Oregon Washington), Zaire | Fever, circular erythematous skin lesions, arthralgia, arthritis, Bell's palsy, meningitis myocarditis | Serology |
| Meliodosis | Southeast Asia, India, West Pacific, Australia | Multisystem disease | Blood culture |
| Rift valley fever | Mediterranean countries, Africa | Headache, photophobia, rash, arthralgia | Viral Culture |
| Tularemia fluorescence | Europe, U.S., Mexico, Japan | Fever, lyphadenopathy, skin escar, sepsis, pneumonia | Culture, direct |
| Western equine encephalitis | U.S., South America | Late summer meningoencephalitis | Serology |
| West Nile fever | Mediterranean countries, Africa, Russia | Fever, conjunctivitis, rash myalgia, arthralgia, lymphadenopathy | Serology |
| Yellow fever | Africa, Central and South America | Headache, vomiting, jaundice, DIC, bradycardia, leukopenia | Viral culture |

### Ear pain, ear drainage, an hearing loss

**Ear pain, ear drainage, and hearing loss** should direct the physician's attention to otitis media, mastoiditis, or to the Ramsay Hunt syndrome that accompanies herpes zoster involving the seventh and eight cranial nerves. *Mycoplasma pneumoniae* infection can be associated with ear pain because of bullous myringitis, a condition that is only rarely seen in adults.

### Visual and eye symptoms

A number of infectious agents may cause conjunctivitis including *H. influenzae*, *Neisseria gonorrhea*, *Staphylococcus aureus*, *Chlamydia trachomatis* and adenovirus. Fever in these patients is usually indicative of a larger systemic process. Scleral hemorrhage is a feature of leptospirosis and of the hemorrhagic fevers and is usually painless. Bacterial endophthalmitis presents with decreased visual acuity, photophobia, and pain. Hematogenous bacterial endophthalmitis usually originates from an obvious septic focus, but fungal endophthalmitis may be the only presenting symptom of systemic fungal infection other than fever. Sudden visual loss can indicate an embolus to the ophthalmic artery or to the visual cortex originating from infective endocarditis. Chapter 77 presents the approach to differential diagnosis and management of ocular and orbital infections. Fever and eye manifestations including vision loss are prominent features of noninfectious illness such as giant-cell arteritis.

### Sore throat

**Sore throat** is usually indicative of pharyngitis either of viral or bacterial origin. Stridor, aphonia, and dry cough with signs of upper respiratory infection are suggestive of epiglottitis. Acute laryngotracheobronchitis (croup), a viral disease in children aged 3 mo to 3 yr is associated with hoarseness, typical barking cough, and stridor. Chapter 54 discusses the etiology, diagnosis, and management of upper respiratory infections.

### Chest and pulmonary symptoms

Chest pain made worse on inspiration is common in pleuritis, pneumonia, and infective endocarditis with septic embolization. Pleuritic chest pain and fever can also signify pulmonary embolization with or without infarction, or a variety of noninfectious causes of pleuritis (e.g., systemic lupus erythematosis). Central chest pain relieved by sitting up is typical of pericarditis, which may be infectious or noninfectious with associated fever. As with any other process that interferes with ventilatory function, dyspnea and tachypnea are common manifestations of pneumonia. Wheezing with fever may be a prominent manifestation of bronchitis.

### Abdominal symptoms

Abdominal pain in the patient with febrile illness may be associated with a large number of infectious disorders, including acute appendicitis, cholecystitis, intraabdominal abscesses, acute diverticulitis, peritonitis, pyelonephritis, pelvic inflammatory disease, and infectious enteritis. Noninfectious diseases causing fever and abdominal pain include pancreatitis, perforated viscus, and inflammatory bowel disease. Psoas abscess can manifest itself as pain in the anterior aspect of the thigh (femoral nerve irritation) or lower back pain. The local symptomatology of hepatic, splenic, perinephric and intraperitoneal abscesses, gastrointestinal tuberculosis, and infected aortic aneurysms may be absent or minimal, particularly in the aged, in quadriplegic patients, and in those on glucocorticosteroids. These diagnoses may therefore represent a difficult challenge (see Chapter 65).

Pyelonephritis usually presents with flank pain, dysuria, frequency, and urgency and is not difficult to diagnose (Chapter 69). In some patients with pyelonephritis central abdominal pain with nausea and vomiting and diarrhea suggest an intraabdominal process. In the hospitalized and handicapped elderly, however, symptoms of a urinary tract infection [UTI], apart from fever may be lacking.

Pelvic inflammatory disease typically presents with lower abdominal pain accompanied by vaginal discharge and is a disorder of sexually active women. Occasionally women with intrauterine devices or postabortion may develop pelvic inflammatory disease (see Chapter 72).

Infectious enteritis is usually characterized by nausea, diarrhea, and fever is most often caused by enteroinvasive *E. coli*, *Shigella*, *Salmonella*, *Campylobacter* species or *Clostridium difficile* or viruses such as the Norwalk agent (see Chapter 61). The type and place of food intake over the preceding 48 h should be questioned in the evaluation of a patient with gastroenteritis; for example, *Vibrio parahemolyticus* gastroenteritis is usually associated with saltwater or seafood exposure. A prior history of antibiotic therapy suggests *C. difficile* infection. Nausea, vomiting, and fever are manifestations of infection with Norwalk agent or rotavirus. When abdominal pain is prominent clostridial food poisoning may be the cause.

### Back pain

**Back pain** with fever, particularly if severe and localized, should direct diagnostic efforts to exclude discitis, vertebral osteomyelitis and, most importantly, spinal epidural abscess (see Chapter 78). Occasionally, endocarditis presents with back pain as a major symptom (see Chapter 66). Persistent lower back pain is a characteristic of brucellosis.

### Joint or skeletal pain

**Joint or skeletal pain** with fever may result from septic arthritis and osteomyelitis. Dengue fever, trichinosis, and leptospirosis should be considered in a patient with generalized muscle pain and tenderness and the appropriate epidemiologic exposure. Myalgia is a prominent feature of a variety of infectious diseases such as influenza, dengue, typhus, trichinosis, and, rarely, toxoplasmosis.

## Past illnesses

Past medical history may provide important clues to the diagnosis of the patient with acute febrile illness: Splenectomy predisposes the patient to life-threatening infections caused by *Streptococcus pneumoniae*, *H. influenzae*, and occasionally *Babesia*. These may present with symptoms very similar to influenza in a normal individual. A blood transfusion received before 1985, the year in which routine testing of HIV was started in many countries, can point to the diagnosis of an AIDS-related febrile illness. Surgical implantation of prostheses—for example, an artificial ileofemoral or abdominal aortic graft—can be complicated by infection years later (see Chapter 85). Hip or knee prosthetic joints can become infected as a result of a distant focus of infection. Infected ventriculoatrial or ventriculoperitoneal cerebrospinal fluid (CSF) shunts may give rise to meningitis, endocarditis, pleuritis, or peritonitis. Placement of a stent in an obstructed biliary duct or papillotomy may lead to ascending cholangitis (see Chapter 63). Artificial heart valves, patches, and pacemaker insertion can predispose to early or late infective endocarditis (Chapter 66). Trivial skin and skin appendage infections—for example, hydradenitis and furunculosis—may lead to metastatic, deep-seated infections. Mild intestinal infections caused by *Salmonella* can, in rare cases, cause secondary infection of arterial aneurysms of the large blood vessels or osteomyelitis. Amebic colitis can give rise to an amebic liver abscess. Genital infections with the gonococcus can evolve into disseminated gonococcal infection and cause septic arthritis and tendonitis.

A number of chronic diseases can be complicated by acute infections. For example, chronic venous or lymphatic insufficiency of the legs predisposes to recurrent erysipelas. Conditions causing ascites, especially cirrhosis of the liver, predispose to primary bacterial peritonitis. Wegener's granulomatosis is often associated with recurrent sinusitis. Bronchiectasis may lead to brain abscess. Previous head trauma with occult fracture of the cribriform plate can be a predisposing condition to recurrent pneumococcal meningitis. Rare congenital conditions, such as complement deficiencies, have also been associated with recurrent meningeal infections, particularly by *Neisseria meningitidis* and *H. influenzae*. Patients with hypogammaglobulinemia will have repeated sinopulmonary infections, as will those with congenital defects of the respiratory cilia. In these and other patients with congenital deficiencies of host defense there is usually a history of repeated infectious episodes since early childhood (see Chapter 86).

Finally, medications taken acutely or chronically can dramatically affect the clinical presentation of infections (antipyretics) or host defense systems against infection (glucocorticoids and other immunosuppressants) or alter the infecting flora (antibiotics). Chapters 86–88 deal with immunosuppressive therapy and resulting infections. Superinfections with resistant species can be a major complication of prolonged antimicrobial therapy in an individual patient or alter the infecting flora in a community or hospital in which the patient develops a febrile, bacterial illness.

### Family history

A pattern of specific infectious diseases in the family can suggest an inherited disorder of the host defense systems. Inquiries about tuberculosis in the patient's family even years previously may provide an epidemiological link to tuberculosis. The occurrence of recent infectious diseases in the family can at times be helpful in the diagnosis of the patient with an acute febrile illness.

### Habits

Sexual practices should be ascertained since promiscuity and male homosexuality are associated not only with sexually transmitted diseases but also with viral hepatitis (B and C), some intestinal diseases, and HIV infection. Injection drug abuse predisposes to HIV infection, hepatitis type C, soft-tissue abscesses, bacteremia, endocarditis, peripheral vascular infections, bone and joint infection, and rarely, tetanus (see Chapter 90). Excessive alcohol use can lead to a high incidence of tuberculosis, aspiration pneumonia, and primary bacterial peritonitis in the patient with alcoholic cirrhosis (see Chapter 91).

## Physical Examination

Just as a detailed medical history is of paramount importance, so is a meticulous physical examination, depending upon the nature of the disease considered.

### Pulse

Tachycardia usually accompanies fever (Chapter 9), but in brucellosis, typhoid fever, psittacosis, and Legionnaire's disease there may be a high temperature accompanied by a relatively slow pulse. In patients taking beta blockers there may also be a failure to increase the heart rate with fever.

### Blood pressure

In most infections a low blood pressure is indicative of volume loss, particularly if there has been high fever with poor fluid intake, diarrhea, or vomiting. In some patients this will signify sepsis and septic shock (see Chapter 50), and should be dealt with rapidly.

### Respiration

Tachypnea, cyanosis, and cough in the febrile patient are key manifestations of pneumonia. However, pneumonias of various etiologies may occur without fever (see Chapter 56), and tachypnea and cyanosis may indicate massive pulmonary embolism or the development of ARDS (adult respiratory distress syndrome) (see Chapter 58). Left cardiac failure can develop as a complication of infection, involving either the endocardium or myocardium or because of infection-induced decompensation of previous heart disease or acute myocardial infarction.

### Jaundice

Three major diagnostic categories should be considered in investigating a patient with possible infectious causes of fever with jaundice: (*1*) infection of the biliary tract, (*2*) hepatitis, and (*3*) hemolysis. Ascending cholangitis usually presents with fever, shaking chills and jaundice, with or without upper quadrant abdominal pain or tenderness (Chapter 63). Viral hepatitis type A can present as an acute febrile illness, often without marked jaundice, whereas hepatitis type B and hepatitis type C are more often insidious initially (Chapter 62). Yellow fever should be considered when the patient returns from endemic areas and has not been previously vaccinated. Rarely, EBV and CMV infection should be considered in the patient with fever and jaundice, although jaundice is usually mild. Infectious diseases that cause granulomatous hepatitis such as tuberculosis, Q fever, brucellosis, histoplasmosis, and syphilis usually do not cause frank jaundice. Intraabdominal sepsis or pylephlebitis of the portal vein in elderly or debilitated patients may at times present as jaundice with fever. Ischemic liver injury can cause jaundice in a patient with, or after, septic shock.

Hemolysis should be considered in a patient with fever and jaundice. Viral URI or a self-limited infectious disease such as tonsillitis can be the cause of a hemolytic crisis in patients with glucose-6-phosphate-dehydrogenase (G-6PD) deficiency, sickle cell disease, or other hemoglobinopathies. Infectious diseases which characteristically cause hemolysis include leptospirosis, *Clostridium welchii* septicemia, bartonellosis, babesiosis, malaria, and occasionally *Mycoplasma pneumoniae* infection. In the differential diagnosis of the causes for hemolysis, antibiotics, antimalarials, antipyretics, and other medications used to treat infections should also be considered. Finally, in patients with bloody diarrhea, the possibility of an infectious hemolytic uremic syndrome should be considered (see Chapter 61).

## Skin examination

It has been stated that a rash, if "characteristic," is the "identity card" of an infection. A skin rash is an extremely important diagnostic clue in the patient with an infection. A rash is of value not only through its morphology; it also may serve as a source for diagnostic biopsy or culture. The appearance, differential diagnosis, and approach to patients with fever and skin lesions are discussed in detail in Chapter 51.

## Lymphadenopathy

Lymph node examination in febrile patients should determine if enlargement or tenderness is present and if it is localized or generalized. Localized and diffuse lymphadenopathy and their relationship to infection are discussed in detail in Chapter 53.

## Eyes

The eyes may be involved in systemic infectious diseases causing fever. Detailed ophthalmic examination including eye ground examination is therefore important in the evaluation of many patients with an acute febrile illness. Chapter 77 presents local and systemic infections which involve the eyes, including their presentation, differential diagnosis, and management.

## Ear, nose, and throat

The ears, nose, and throat as well as the paranasal sinuses are the sites most commonly involved by the respiratory viruses and certain bacteria, in particular group A streptococci, pneumococci, and *H. influenza*; thus they are very frequently involved in an acute febrile illness. The clinical manifestations of infections in these sites are discussed in Chapter 54. Sinusitis, a very common infection, is not always accompanied by fever. Awareness of the possibility of sinusitis in the febrile patient can prevent serious complications such as orbital cellulitis, septic sinus thrombosis, meningitis, epidural abscess, subdural empyema, and brain abscess. Upper respiratory infection can also result in sinusitis with purulent nasal discharge and postnasal drip and cause a prolonged productive cough leading to a misdiagnosis of "bronchitis." Blocked nostrils and tenderness over the maxillary and frontal sinuses are important diagnostic clues for sinusitis. There may also be pain on percussion of the upper dental plate with maxillary sinusitis.

Laryngitis, a disease usually of viral etiology, is diagnosed by typical hoarseness, dry cough, and, sometimes, stridor. Epiglottitis, a disease of children 2–4 yr old, is an emergency situation that can evolve into respiratory obstruction with high mortality. It is diagnosed by the typical edematous cherry red epiglottis along with dysphagia, sore throat, stridor, and fever. It can occasionally occur in adults as well (see Chapter 54).

The presence of bullous myringitis, characterized by reddened vesicles in the external auditory canal and on the tympanic membrane, can assist in the diagnosis of *Mycoplasma pneumoniae* infection. Otitis media, a common febrile illness mainly of childhood, accompanied by fever, otalgia, and hearing loss, is diagnosed by demonstrating the loss of shine and redness of the tympanic membrane along with a presence of fluid in the middle ear. Swelling, redness, and tenderness over the mastoid bone can indicate mastoiditis, complicating otitis media.

Infections in the oral cavity, neck, and head can result in pain and swelling of the mandibular area, cheek, upper lip, periorbital, submandibular, sublingual, temporal, and parotis areas with or without dysphagia and trismus. Fever is usually present and immediate therapy is mandatory. At times, dental root infections can present as a febrile disease of prolonged duration, sometimes without local signs. Swelling of the parotid gland is bilateral as in mumps or unilateral as in septic parotitis and should call for a careful oral examination. A reddened Stensen's duct opening with purulent discharge can establish the diagnosis of septic parotitis. This may be a complication of the postoperative state following general anesthesia or be indicative of parotid duct stones.

## Neck

Nuchal rigidity as a sign of meningeal irritation should be sought in suspected meningitis (see Chapter 73). It is important to both rotate and flex the neck and head, particularly in elderly patients who may have cervical arthritis or spondylolisthesis. Nuchal rigidity as a manifestation of meningeal irritation cannot be properly assessed and interpreted in patients whose heads do not rotate fully. Rare infectious diseases of the neck structures such as purulent thyroiditis, suppurative jugular thrombophlebitis, and retropharyngeal space infection will result in tenderness and pain in the related area. At times, esophageal diverticula and pharyngeal pouches may become infected and cause similar symptoms.

## Chest and lungs

Cough is often the only sign of bronchitis. It can be associated with fever and other signs of upper respiratory infection in influenza, adenovirus, *Mycoplasma pneumoniae*, *Chlamydia pneumoniae* and *Bordetella pertussis* infections. Besides a productive cough, bronchitis causes rhonchi, and if there is associated bronchospasm, inspiratory and expiratory wheezes may be found.

Pneumonia is a very common infectious disease and as such should be a major diagnostic consideration in any patient with a febrile illness. The clinical patterns and manifestations of different agents causing bronchitis or pneumonia are discussed in Chapters 55 and 56. The physical findings in pneumonia vary with the extent of the disease and the pattern of involvement. Lobar pneumonias create the classic findings of dullness to percussion, tubular breath sounds with egophony, increased vocal fremitus, and "sticky" inspiration rales. If there is an accompanying effusion, the breath sounds and vocal fremitus may be diminished. If there is pleuritis there may be splinting with decreased respiratory excursions on the involved side. Bronchopneumonias are often accompanied by the physical findings of bronchitis plus scattered inspiratory rales. Diffuse pneumonias with interstitial involvement usually have few abnormal airway sounds; diffuse inspiratory rales may be present. In some interstitial pneumonias or with granulomatous pulmonary involvement there may be no abnormal physical findings on chest examination. This is also true in neutropenic patients.

Mediastinitis may result from descending oropharyngeal infection or perforation of the esophagus or occur after sternotomy for cardiac surgery. It can present as a severe febrile illness. Physical findings that suggest mediastinitis can include excruciating pain on neck hyperextension, subcutaneous crepitus, edema of the neck, a pericardial "crunch" or rub, and other manifestations of pericardial effusion (see below).

A patient with a central catheter or permanent indwelling right atrial catheter such as of the Broviac and Hickman types can develop line sepsis or septic thrombophlebitis of the large veins as a cause of febrile illness. These catheter sites should be examined carefully for signs of inflammation. If inflammation is present, management involves line removal and culture in addition to antibiotic treatment (see Chapter 67).

## Heart

In any febrile patient with valvular heart disease, prosthetic heart valve, drug addiction, or a permanent pacemaker, the possibility of infective endocarditis should be thoroughly evaluated. The clinical presentation and peripheral signs of infective endocarditis are discussed in Chapter 66. Changes in heart murmurs, the appearance of a new diastolic murmur, or symptoms of congestive heart failure may indicate a destructive process of the valve and the need for surgical intervention. Myocarditis is suggested by diffuse anterior chest pain, tachycardia, S3 gallop, arrhythmias, and congestive heart failure (see Chapter 68). Pericarditis often causes a pericardial friction rub, a rubbing "leathery" sound heard in both systole and diastole; it may rarely present as pericardial tamponade with quiet heart sounds, elevated neck veins, tachycardia, and marked pulsus paradoxus or hypotension.

## Abdomen

Abdominal, retroperitoneal, and pelvic infections can present with various signs of intraabdominal inflammation including localized or diffuse, tenderness, rebound tenderness (sign of peritoneal irritation), ileus with distention, or ascites. Intraabdominal abscesses may present as tender masses or organomegaly with overlying peritonitis (Chapter 65). Hepatitis is often characterized by tender hepatomegaly (Chapter 62). Cholecystitis may present with an enlarged tender gallbladder in the right upper quadrant or a positive Murphy's sign on inspiration (Chapter 63). On the other hand, typhoid fever, psoas abscess, infection of an abdominal aortic graft, a mycotic aneurysm of the large blood vessels, and various organ abscesses may be associated with fever only, without additional localizing signs. A variety of noninfectious inflammatory diseases such as pancreatitis, familial Mediterranean fever (FMF), porphyria, lead intoxication, hemolytic crisis, and tabes dorsalis may also cause abdominal pain with tenderness or ileus and fever.

Splenomegaly accompanied by fever is frequent in infectious mononucleosis, CMV infection, infective endocarditis, typhoid fever, splenic abscess, typhus, malaria, and visceral leishmaniasis. In most cases the spleen is not tender unless the enlargement has been rapid or there is a splenic abscess or infarction; with abscess or infarction a splenic friction rub with respiration may be present. Nontender splenomegaly and fever may be characteristic findings in acute leukemias, lymphoma, or, rarely, systemic lupus erythematous.

## Genitalia, pelvic, and rectal examinations

Characteristic skin and mucosal lesions of primary infectious sexually transmitted diseases are described in Chapters 70 to 71. Many of these do not have fever as a major manifestation. Pelvic inflammatory disease or salpingitis can result in localized peritonitis of the pelvis and inguinal regions with vaginal discharge and tenderness on movement of the uterine cervix, or with a palpable swollen adnexa on bimanual pelvic examination (see Chapter 72). Acute prostatitis or prostatic abscess can be palpated by rectal examination as a swollen and extremely tender prostate. With epididymitis there is a tender swelling above the testis. With orchitis the testis itself is swollen.

## Musculoskeletal system

Septic arthritis and osteomyelitis often present with fever and localized swelling with tenderness and erythema over the involved joint(s) or bone. A careful search for tenderness, local warmth, and swelling of all joints and bones should be performed routinely. Acute or subacute polyarthritis may be a feature of several viral diseases in the adult (parvovirus $B_{19}$, rubella, hepatitis B), disseminated gonococcal disease, Lyme disease or endocarditis. Polyarthritis and fever are also typical manifestations of immunologic disorders—in particular, systemic lupus erythematous, acute rheumatoid arthritis, and postinfectious arthritides, including Reiter's syndrome. Tenosynovitis, if found, is a prominent feature of disseminated gonococcal infection. Percussion with a fist can assess possible tenderness along the spine, sacroiliac joints, and symphysis pubis. Septic joints are not always red, warm, and tender, and only awareness of the condition and careful examination will lead to the correct diagnosis. The clinical presentation and differential diagnosis of infectious and postinfectious arthritis are discussed in Chapter 79.

Hematogenous osteomyelitis frequently involves the long bones in children, whereas in adults the vertebrae are more often the site of infection (see Chapter 78). The source of infection is often obscure; infective endocarditis should be sought as a possible origin. The clinical presentation of vertebral osteomyelitis can be subtle with only back pain and local tenderness. Complications such as spinal epidural abscess can result in paraparesis or paraplegia, sensory loss, or loss of bladder and rectal function. Epidural abscess often causes a peripheral and usually symmetrical neuropathy at the local site. In osteomyelitis secondary to a contiguous focus of infection such as soft-tissue infection, sinusitis, or infected teeth, the source of infection is obvious but awareness of the possible involvement of the adjacent bones is important for a correct therapeutic approach.

Pyomyositis presents with fever, local muscle pain, swelling and tenderness, frequently of deep muscle compartments in the leg and buttock. Clinically, it may be difficult to distinguish from fasciitis (see Chapter 80).

Gas gangrene or *Clostridial myonecrosis* and other nonclostridial myositis such as caused by streptococci, mixed anaerobes, or *Aeromonas hydrophilia* are devastating febrile illnesses in which the involved area is painful and tender with tense edema. There may be a foul discharge containing gas bubbles leaking from the portal of entry in the skin in patients with polymicrobial anerobic infection (see Chapter 80).

Signs of diffuse muscle tenderness and swelling can accompany several infections such as leptospirosis, toxoplasmosis, and trichinosis. Acute rhabdomyolysis has been reported with influenza A virus, Legionnaire's disease, Echo virus, coxsackievirus, Epstein-Barr, and adenovirus infections as well as primary HIV infection. Influenza A may also cause the clinical picture of polymyositis, with generalized weakness. This usually develops after the acute respiratory illness and fever have subsided.

### Neurological system

Diseases which involve the central nervous system can produce a variety of findings ranging from altered mental status with encephalopathy to meningitis to localized motor or sensory defects and cranial or peripheral neuropathies (see Chapters 73–76). In addition, the patient with severe sepsis or septic shock may have altered mental status and obtundation (Chapter 50), as can the severely hypoxic patient with pneumonia and respiratory failure (Chapters 56, 58). One purpose of the neurologic examination is to detect findings that may be unique to intracranial or CNS disorders and to differentiate them from diseases which may affect the nervous system from peripheral locations or through toxemia or toxins.

The approaches to the patient with altered mental status and fever are discussed in detail in Chapters 74, 75, and 77. Infectious disorders which affect the spinal cord or peripheral nervous system are discussed in Chapter 76.

## Laboratory Studies

Laboratory studies obtained in patients with suspected infectious diseases fall into three categories: (*1*) those that assess the extent and severity of the inflammatory response to infection; (*2*) those that help determine the site(s) and complications of organ involvement by the process; and (*3*) those that are designed to determine the etiology of the infectious agents either by direct culture or histology or by a specific immune response. Almost all patients with suspected acute infectious processes (unless clearly limited to acute, benign illnesses such as viral URI or uncomplicated UTI) should have a complete blood count (CBC). In selected patients measurement of the erythrocyte sedimentation rate (ESR) or determination of the C-reactive protein (CRP) concentration may allow quantitation of the acute phase response to infection or even distinguish between bacterial and other etiologies. These tests are discussed in detail in Chapter 13. The use of specific radiologic studies will be guided by the physical examination and clinical presentation. Chest radiograms are a useful screening tool for pulmonary disease even in the absence of physical findings and certainly should be done in any patients with suspected pneumonia. The indications for using more sophisticated imaging approaches to localize and define disease are covered in Chapter 12 as well as in the individual organ-centered chapters. Besides selecting tests that will aid in defining the site of infection and extent of alterations in organ function (e.g., hepatic enzymes, bilirubin, and prothrombin time in patients with suspected hepatitis) it is important to characterize the degree of alteration in normal physiology to assist in appropriate supportive care. For example, all patients with pneumonia severe enough to require hospitalization should have oxygenation evaluated (see Chapter 56).

The selection of laboratory studies to isolate infectious agents and to specifically diagnose the type of infection will be determined both by the infectious sites and the availability of secretions or tissues for analysis. In general, all patients with suspected severe systemic bacterial infections should have blood cultures performed. Ideally, in the case of suspected bacteremia, two blood samples should be obtained with a 20 to 30 min interval between the collections (see Chapter 50). Urinary tract infections may not give localized symptoms, particularly in elderly patients; thus a routine urinalysis with microscopic examination of a spun sediment and gram stain of an unspun sample are routinely indicated in most febrile patients without an obvious other source for their infections (see Chapter 69).

Instructions on how to obtain specimens and the microbiologic and serologic procedures used to make a specific diagnosis are covered in Chapters 15–20. In general, exudates and sputum, if available, should be examined with appropriate stains and cultures *before* initiating antimicrobial therapy to both guide antibiotic choice and improve the likelihood of recovery of the infecting agents. Skin lesions should be unroofed or biopsied. If it is not possible to obtain sputum from patients with pneumonia, cases with diffuse disease should undergo bronchoscopy and lavage since many different organisms can cause a similar clinical picture (see Chapter 58).

## Management

The management of patients with acute febrile illnesses centers on providing answers to these questions:

1. Is the illness of infectious or of some other etiology?
2. Is the severity of illness likely to cause significant organ dysfunction or death?
3. Is there a specific treatment available to inhibit or eradicate the likely infecting agents?
4. Has there been an adequate attempt made to document and isolate the potential pathogen?
5. Are the supportive care procedures adequate?

Blind or empiric antipyretic or antibiotic therapy should be discouraged as a general response to acute febrile illnesses until the possible answers to these questions have been addressed in the individual patient. Excessive antibiotic usage in patients for which no indication exists (e.g., for treatment of viral URIs) has contributed to the worldwide increase of antimicrobial resistance (see Chapter 26) and may cause unwanted reactions. Conversely, if it is likely that the patient has a severe or life-threatening illness for which antibiotic therapy would be indicated as part of treatment, it is quite appropriate to initiate treatment before culture results are known. The approach to antimicrobial therapy of infections involving different organ systems is discussed generally in Chapter 24 and in each of the individual sections. The management of fever per se is covered in Chapter 10.

An algorithm which summarizes the steps to be taken in the evaluation and management of patients with febrile illnesses is presented in Figure 47.2. An early decision involves defining whether it is an acute (i.e., several hours to several days) or chronic (several weeks) illness. Subacute illnesses are those which last longer than 7 to 10 d; they show a diagnostic profile which usually does not include acute infections of the respiratory or urinary tract (cystitis), or acute, fulminating systemic infections likely to cause mortality if not treated promptly within the first 24 to 36 h. As such, they resemble more the illnesses causing chronic fever. The second decision which must be undertaken is determining whether or not the patient qualifies for prompt therapy before the results of specific diagnostic tests are available. The two types of patients who fall into this category are (*1*) those who manifest signs of a major infectious illness, an indication of which can be assessed by the nature of the systemic response—that is, the presence of sepsis or septic shock, as well as the extent of organ involvement; and (*2*) those who

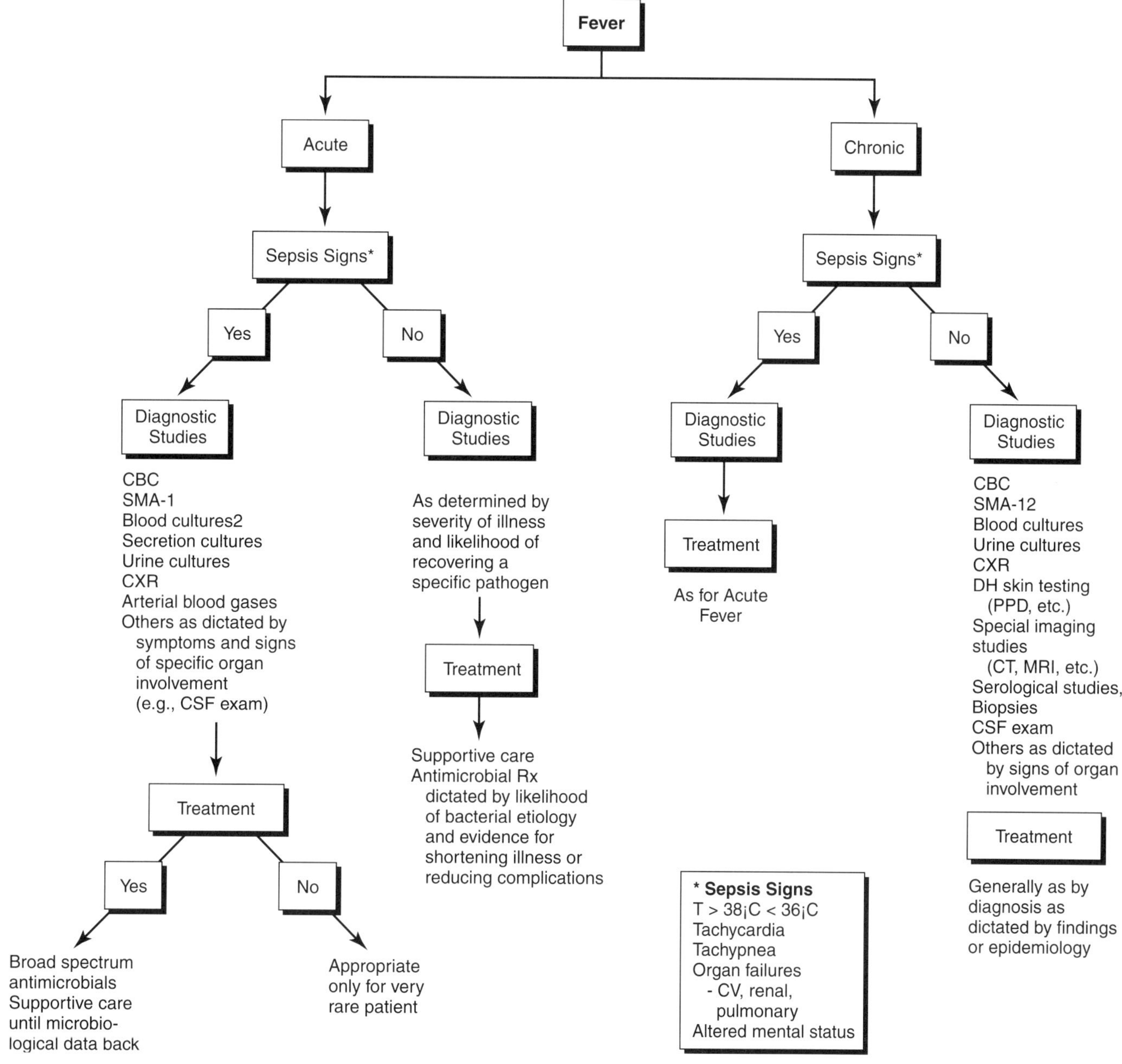


**Fig. 47.2** Fever workup algorithm.

have major impairments in host defense, such as severe neutropenia, in whom a delay in specific antimicrobial therapy could prove fatal.

Similar decision-making must be undertaken in patients with subacute or chronic febrile illnesses. Each chapter in this book that focuses on organ system involvement with infection or unique situations of host alteration provides necessary guidelines for the extent of specific diagnostic studies as well as appropriate empiric or definitive therapy.

## ANNOTATED BIBLIOGRAPHY

Isselbacher KJ, Braunwald E, Wilson JD, Martin JB, Fauci AS, Kasper DL. Harrison's Principles of Internal Medicine, 13th ed. McGraw-Hill, New York, 1994.

*See the chapters on fever, basic considerations in infectious diseases, and acute infectious disease syndromes.*

Mackowiak P, ed. Fever: Basic Mechanisms and Management. Lippincott-Raven, Philadelphia PA, 1997.

*A comprehensive monograph which covers causes of both acute and chronic fevers including evaluation and management as well as underlying mechnisms in fever production.*

Mandel GL, Bennett JE, Dolin R. Principles and Practice of Infectious Diseases. 4th ed. Churchill-Livingstone, New York, 1995.

*Excellent, well-referenced, encyclopedic review of all aspects of infecitous diseases including the mechanisms, evaluation, and management of acute and chronic conditions causing fever.*

Wilson ME. A World Guide to Infections: Diseases, Distribution, Diagnosis. Oxford University Press, New York, 1991.

*An excellent and succinct text that covers the approach to the patient with fever and other manifestations of infectious diseases and relates them to the country of origin or travel. Includes a nice summary of the major infectious diseases in different regions of the world and their manifestations, diagnosis, and management.*

# 48

## Fever in Hospitalized Patients

DAVID N. SCHWARTZ AND ROBERT A. WEINSTEIN

Few clinical parameters in hospitalized patients are followed as routinely or have as much clinical import invested in them as the presence of an elevated body temperature. As a cardinal manifestation of localized or systemic inflammation (see Chapter 10), fever is an important correlate of the severity, and response to therapy, of many of the diseases that prompt hospital admission. In addition, because hospitalized patients are often acutely ill and are exposed to a variety of invasive procedures and immunocompromising therapies, they are highly susceptible to a broad array of infectious and noninfectious complications for which fever is often an important marker. However, there is wide variation in the frequency with which fever is associated with these hospital-acquired diseases. Moreover, an individual patient's risk of developing one of these nosocomial diseases and the resultant fever depends upon a complex set of variables including host factors, such as age and underlying diseases, hospital service, interventions or treatments received, and the local hospital-specific epidemiology of nosocomial infections and iatrogenic illnesses. In this chapter we will describe the causes of fever in hospitalized patients, the epidemiology of fever among specific patient populations, and an approach to diagnosis and therapy. Our discussion will be restricted to adult patients.

The complexity of this topic is compounded by the lack of consensus regarding the definition of fever (see Chapter 9). Unfortunately, in published reports describing the association between fever and various diseases and procedures, investigators have variously defined fever as ranging from 37.0° C to 39.0° C, have rarely specified the time of day or body site at which the temperature was measured, and have included minimal durations of temperature elevation ranging from 0 to 48 h in their fever definitions. Consequently, the data in these reports are not strictly comparable.

Additionally, all of the disorders associated with fever, including infections, can also occur in the absence of body temperature elevation. In one prospective survey of fever and nosocomial infection in general surgical patients, for example, 26 of the 51 documented postoperative infections occurred without fever (restrictively defined as a rectal temperature greater than or equal to 38° C lasting at least 48 h). Approximately 10% of nosocomial bacteremias occur without fever, although the true prevalence may be higher given the clinical bias against drawing blood cultures in afebrile patients. Furthermore, elderly patients and those with underlying diseases such as cirrhosis or renal failure may exhibit blunted or absent febrile responses to infection (Chapter 9). These and other data suggest that nosocomial infections occur without fever in a substantial proportion of patients.

Thus, from an operational standpoint, there is no discrete body temperature threshold below which the absence of any of the recognized causes of fever can be assured. The recognition of infection in afebrile patients may be particularly important, however, particularly in patient groups who are at the greatest risk and suffer the greatest morbidity from nosocomial infections. In clinical practice, therefore, we believe it is prudent to employ a lower temperature threshold to define fever in elderly patients and in those with major underlying diseases, and to be vigilant for disturbances in other clinical parameters, such as blood pressure, pulse, respiratory rate, and mental status, in screening patients for the presence of nosocomial infections and other diseases associated with hospital-acquired fever.

### Etiologies

Among the categories of diseases causing hospital-acquired fever (Table 48.1), nosocomial infection is encountered most often. Since nosocomial infections are described both generally and individually elsewhere in this book, they will be discussed only briefly here, to be followed by a discussion of selected noninfectious causes of fever.

### Infectious causes

Nosocomial infections most often involve the urinary or lower respiratory tracts, or surgical wounds (see Chapter 8). However, since infections at these sites are usually detected readily by routine clinical evaluations such as physical examination, urinalysis, and chest radiography, it is worth considering the infectious causes of hospital-acquired fever that are most often missed by the initial workup. Although few data directly address this issue, several generalizations can be offered. First, colitis due to *Clostridium difficile* is associated with fever in 25%–45% of cases. It therefore may become a preeminent cause of hospital-acquired fever in the many institutions in which it has reached epidemic proportions (Chapter 8). It may cause little diarrhea or occur in patients who are too ill to report this symptom, and it may sometimes be associated with severe systemic manifestations. Second, other intraabdominal processes—hepatobiliary disorders, abscesses, septic thrombophlebitis, or infarction or perforation of a viscus—are important to consider in elderly, immunocompromised, steroid-treated, or critically ill patients who may have few signs or symptoms referable to the abdomen. Third, bacteremias that arise in the absence of a clinically apparent source have become common. They may be primary, a phenomenon observed most often in neutropenic or other immunocompromised patients, or secondary to clinically occult infections of central venous catheters (CVCs) or other prosthetic devices. Septic thrombophlebitis of central veins and infectious endocarditis are complications of CVC infections that are sometimes overlooked as well. Finally, sinusitis and otitis media are important causes of hospital-acquired fever in patients receiving

**Table 48.1** Etiologies of nosocomial fever

| Common etiologies | Less common etiologies |
|---|---|
| INFECTIOUS | |
| Urinary tract | Endocarditis |
| Surgical wound | Mediastinitis |
| Lower respiratory | Intraabdominal abscess |
| Vascular catheter-associated or primary bacteremia | Pelvic vein thrombophlebitis |
| Diarrhea due to *Clostridium difficile* | CNS infection |
| Postpartum endometritis | Biliary tract infection |
| Sinusitis (intubation associated) | Viral hepatitis |
| Decubitus ulcers and other skin infections | CMV infection |
| TISSUE ISCHEMIA/INFARCTION | |
| Venous thromboembolism | Intestinal infarction |
| Myocardial infarction | Renal infarction |
| Hematoma | Splenic infarction |
| Stroke | Pancreatitis |
| Subarachnoid hemorrhage | Atheroembolic syndrome |
| Infusion-related phlebitis or chemical injury | Heterotopic ossification |
| Cholecystitis | |
| Intramuscular injections | |
| POSTOPERATIVE OR POSTPROCEDURE | |
| Trauma | |
| Major surgery | |
| Endoscopy | |
| Transfusion reaction | |
| IDIOPATHIC INFLAMMATORY | |
| Drug fever | Dressler's syndrome |
| | Postpericardiotomy syndrome |
| | Pulmonary fibroproliferation |
| | Malignancy |
| AUTONOMIC AND ENDOCRINE DYSFUNCTION | |
| Delerium tremens | Central/spinal cord fever |
| | Thyrotoxicosis |
| | Addison's disease |

long-term mechanical ventilation, occurring in 3%–18% of such patients according to prospective surveys.

Pelvic vein thrombophlebitis is a rare but important cause of fever in obstetric and gynecologic patients. Septic thrombophlebitis, usually of the right ovarian vein, is seen in the setting of pelvic infection related to childbirth, gynecologic surgery, or pelvic inflammatory disease. The most common clinical presentation involves steadily worsening lower abdominal pain and persistent fever in a patient receiving appropriate antibiotic therapy for endomyometritis or pelvic cellulitis; the thrombosed right ovarian vein forms a mass that is often palpable on examination. Less commonly seen is "enigmatic fever" in which fever persists in patients with pelvic infection who respond appropriately to therapy in other respects; physical examination is usually negative. Both forms of the disease can be complicated by bland or septic pulmonary emboli.

## Noninfectious causes

### Tissue ischemia, infarction, and inflammation

The death or devitalization of tissues provokes an inflammatory response similar to the response to pyogenic infection. Hence, fever should be anticipated in diseases that cause tissue infarction or inflammation. This is well illustrated by embolization of the hepatic artery for the treatment of hepatic malignancy, after which fever and abdominal pain in the absence of infection are common, or by acute pancreatitis in which fever and other findings associated with the systemic inflammatory response syndrome (SIRS) often occur. However, the association of fever with other common and important complications of hospitalization such as myocardial infarction and pulmonary embolism is less well appreciated. Indeed, because of the tendency to assume that fever reflects the presence of infection, an elevated temperature can sometimes delay the diagnosis of these diseases.

#### *Myocardial infarction*

Fever occurs in the majority of patients with myocardial infarction. Approximately 50% will develop a temperature of 38° C or more at some point during the hospital stay, although few exceed 38.5° C. In general, the degree of temperature elevation parallels the severity of the infarction. Because the maximal temperature is nearly always achieved after the first hospital day, fever in these patients could appear to be "hospital-acquired" even when the infarction occurred before hospital admission.

### *Venous thromboembolism*

Deep venous thrombosis (DVT) and pulmonary embolism (PE) are considered together here because of the association between the two diseases and because recent data suggest that up to 40% of patients with DVT who lack pulmonary symptoms have evidence of PE on ventilation-perfusion scanning and chest roentgenography. It seems reasonable, therefore, to consider venous thromboembolism as a single disease entity, and, in the context of investigating the cause of fever in a hospitalized patient, to consider the diagnosis of PE if DVT is discovered.

PE is strongly associated with fever. In a series of 35 patients with angiographically proven PE and no evidence of infection on careful evaluation, 20 (57%) had a rectal temperature ≥38.0° C, with a mean peak temperature of 38.4° C (range, 38.0° to 40.2° C). Fever was most common in the first 3 d following diagnosis, rarely lasted longer than 7 d, and was significantly associated with pleuritic chest pain, an elevated serum lactate dehydrogenase (LDH), and pulmonary infiltrates and pleural effusions on chest roentgenography, all findings suggestive of pulmonary infarction. Patients with PE and fever were also more likely to have had a white blood cell (WBC) count exceeding 10,000/mm$^3$, and more severe hypoxemia.

The clinical features of febrile PE make it difficult to distinguish from pneumonia. Moreover, many patient populations are at high risk for both processes, and because the usual time-course of PE-associated fever—gradual resolution over several days—mirrors the response of pneumonia to antibiotic therapy, occasional confusion between the two diseases is likely to occur, with potentially disastrous consequences. Indeed, autopsy studies of hospitalized patients consistently have identified clinically occult PE in about 5% of cases; in about half of these cases, PE was thought to have been an important contributor to death.

### *Pulmonary fibroproliferation complicating the acute respiratory distress syndrome (ARDS)*

Survivors of the acute phase of ARDS (d 3–7 after onset) suffer high mortality, often because of subsequent infection, usually pneumonia or intraabdominal sepsis. However, patients have been described whose ARDS was complicated by the new onset of fever, leukocytosis, and worsening pulmonary function, often accompanied by purulent lower respiratory secretions and diffuse or localized worsening of the chest roentgenogram, but in whom pneumonia was excluded by negative quantitative bronchoscopic cultures and/or open lung biopsy. In this syndrome, biopsy specimens reveal exuberant interstitial and intraalveolar fibrosis similar to that seen in idiopathic pulmonary fibrosis. Significant improvements in pulmonary function and survival after the administration of high doses of corticosteroids have been shown in these patients in uncontrolled, open-label trials.

### *Stroke*

About 40% of strokes are accompanied by fever which is independently associated with an increased risk of poor neurologic outcome or death. Although stroke has been cited as a common noninfectious cause of hospital-acquired fever on medical wards, the extent to which stroke-associated fever is caused by cerebral infarction per se or is due to complications such as venous thromboembolism or infection of the urinary or lower respiratory tract is unclear. Fever is also a common consequence of subarachnoid hemorrhage and subdural hematoma.

### *Hematoma*

The association between fever and hematoma has long been recognized by experienced clinicians. Although the incidence of fever as a complication of hematoma is unknown, the importance of hematoma in causing fever is illustrated by the recent finding that pelvic hematomas may account for up to 20% of episodes of puerperal fever that is unresponsive to empiric antibiotic therapy.

### *Heterotopic ossification*

Heterotopic ossification (HO) is the abnormal formation of new bone in tissues that do not normally ossify, most often in the periarticular soft tissues of joints immobilized by neurologic disease or trauma. It complicates spinal cord injury in up to 50% of patients, usually within 4 months of injury, and may contribute to joint ankylosis and immobility. A local inflammatory response, manifested by erythema, warmth, swelling, and fever is variably encountered. Fever has been attributed to HO in up to 10% of febrile spinal cord injury patients undergoing rehabilitation, making HO an important diagnostic consideration in febrile, at-risk patients. Diagnosis is made by a variety of imaging studies, of which radionuclide bone scan is most sensitive. Treatment with indomethacin or other antiinflammatory agents usually results in resolution of fever and the other inflammatory manifestations of HO but without affecting the associated joint immobility.

### *Intramuscular injections and intravenous catheters*

Although bacterial abscesses are rare complications of intramuscular injections, sterile inflammation appears to be far more common, and associated fever has been well documented. Up to one-third of patients who receive multiple intramuscular analgesic injections during hospitalization for back pain may have fever without the identification of alternative causes. Clinical evaluation may disclose areas of subcutaneous induration at injection sites and leukocytosis, and positive uptake in the gluteal and quadriceps regions on gallium scanning has been recorded. Of note, computed tomography studies have shown that standard 3.5 cm needles are not long enough to reach muscle when intragluteal drug administration is attempted in the vast majority of adults, and that calcification and fibrosis in the overlying fat is a common consequence.

Thrombosis of peripheral intravenous catheters—so-called *infusion-related phlebitis*—is a common problem whose incidence is increased by certain types of infusates (e.g., peripheral alimentation, antibiotics), prolonged duration of use, and anatomic site, among other factors. Although it is rarely associated with localized or systemic catheter-related infection, it is recognized as a cause of fever by many clinicians. However, the importance of infusion-related phlebitis as a cause of hospital-acquired fever is difficult to gauge because there are few data detailing the frequency with which it is accompanied by fever.

## Procedure-related fever

Fever in the first 2 or 3 postoperative d occurs in 2%–80% of surgical patients and has long been recognized as being self-limited and noninfectious in the majority of patients. The likelihood of fever is proportionate to the invasiveness of the procedure. It has often been attributed to pulmonary atelectasis, although this association has recently been refuted convincingly. More compelling is the observation that surgical and nonsurgical trauma provoke rapid increases in the serum levels of acute phase reactants and cytokines, such as C-reactive protein (CRP) and interleukin-6 (IL-6); such increases have been correlated with the development of fever, and sustained increases have been shown to be important correlates of severe trauma or of postoperative infections that may not become clinically manifest for days. Thus, surgical procedures appear to induce a systemic inflammatory state of which fever may be an expected result. Unless complications ensue, recovery from this inflammatory state and defervescence are rapid.

A variety of surgical and endoscopic procedures involving tissues that are colonized or infected with bacteria have been associated with substantial rates of transient bacteremia in conjunction with procedure-related fever. Examples include oral surgical procedures, rigid bronchoscopy, esophageal dilatation, sclerotherapy for esophageal varices, endoscopic retrograde cholangiography in the presence of biliary obstruction, and instrumentation of the genitourinary tract, including lithotripsy, in the presence of urinary tract infection. Heightened awareness of the possibility of bacterial infection causing or contributing to postprocedure fever is therefore justified in these settings.

## Fever related to medications

A broad range of medications have been reported to cause a variety of febrile syndromes (Tables 48.2, 48.3). Although organ-specific drug toxicities are often considered separately, fever is a prominent feature of nearly all such syndromes and often precedes the development of any localizing manifestations. It is therefore important to be aware of the association of medications with each of these syndromes and not simply those drugs that can cause undifferentiated fever.

Drug fever is described stereotypically as a relatively benign disorder in which the patient is nontoxic in appearance and has a relative bradycardia and an accompanying drug rash and/or eosinophilia. Although helpful when present, these classic characteristics of drug fever are uncommon. Rash and eosinophilia each occur in only about 20% of cases, and relative bradycardia in about 10%, whereas rigors occur about half the time, and syndromes of organ-specific inflammation and even shock (Table 48.3) may also be seen. Thus, apart from the temporal association between the administration and/or withdrawal of medications and the occurrence of fever, there are no clinical features which readily distinguish most drug fevers from other kinds of febrile illness.

## Fever associated with blood transfusions

Although hemolytic transfusion reactions are now rare, fever is still a common and important complication of these procedures. Febrile, nonhemolytic transfusion reactions, characterized by fever, rigors, chills, and nausea during or shortly after transfusion, occur in 5%–30% of platelet transfusions but are much less frequently seen with transfusions of other blood products. Recent studies have shown that the risk of febrile, nonhemolytic transfusion reactions is directly correlated with the age of the transfusate and the number of leukocytes and the concentrations of TNF-$\alpha$, IL-1$\beta$, and IL-6 contained in the transfusate. Because these reactions are largely avoided by removing the plasma supernatant from the cellular fraction before transfusion, the reactions appear to be caused by cytokines released by the white cells during storage rather than by the white cells themselves. Bacterial contamination, most often with gram-positive skin flora, has been reported in up to 10% of platelet concentrates tested, although sepsis as a consequence is very rare. This high rate of contamination presumably is due to contamination of blood at the time of collection, with subsequent multiplication of bacteria during the storage of platelets at room temperature for up to 5 d prior to infusion. Contamination of red blood cell products, which are stored at 4° C, is considerably rarer, is usually due to *Yersinia enterocolitica* or psychrophilic pseudomonads, and is frequently associated with clinical sepsis.

**Table 48.2** Agents associated with drug fever (The agents listed have been reported to cause fever with or without rash)

| Common agents | Uncommon agents |
|---|---|
| CARDIOVASCULAR AGENTS | |
| $\alpha$-methyldopa | Diltiazem |
| Procainamide | Hydralazine |
| Quinidine | Hydrochlorothiazide |
| | Nifedipine |
| | Labetolol |
| | Triamterene |
| ANTIINFECTIVES | |
| Amphotericin B | Aminoglycosides |
| Cephalosporins | Clindamycin |
| Isoniazid | Ciprofloxacin |
| Penicillins | Dapsone |
| Sulfonamides | Griseofulvin |
| Trimethoprim-sulfamethoxazole | Metronidazole |
| | Nitrofurantoin |
| | Rifampin |
| | Teicoplanin |
| | Tetracyclines |
| | Vancomycin |
| | Zidovidine |
| ANTINEOPLASTICS, IMMUNOSUPPRESSIVES | |
| Bleomycin | all-*trans* retinoic acid |
| $\alpha$-Interferon | L-asparaginase |
| | Azathioprine |
| | Chlorambucil |
| | Cisplatin |
| | Cyclophosphamide |
| | Cytarabine |
| | Daunorubicin |
| | Hydroxyurea |
| | Mercaptopurine |
| | Methotrexate |
| | Procarbazine |
| | Streptozocin |
| MISCELLANEOUS | |
| Carbamazepine | Acetaminophen |
| Phenytoin | Acetylcysteine, inhaled |
| | Allopurinol |
| | Aminophylline |
| | Cimetidine |
| | Clofibrate |
| | Codeine |
| | Fluoxetine |
| | Methimazole |
| | NSAIDs |
| | Penicillamine |
| | Propylthiouricil |
| | Thyroxine |

**Table 48.3** Syndromes of drug-induced organ disease and associated fever

HEPATITIS

Allopurinol
α-Methyldopa
Amiodarone
Carbamazepine
Cimetidine
Fluconazole
Hydralazine
Isoniazid
Itraconazole
Ketoconazole
Methimazole
Methotrexate
Penicillins
Phenytoin
Propylthiouracil
Pyrazinamide
Quinidine
Rifampin
Sulfonamides
Trimethoprim-sulfamethoxazole
Trimethoprim-sulfamethoxazole

PNEUMONITIS

All-*trans* retinoic acid
Amiodarone
Bleomycin
Carbamazepine
Cyclophosphamide
Hydrochlorothiazide
Isoniazid
Methotrexate
NSAIDs
Nitrofurantoin
Penicillins
Phenytoin
Procarbazine
Propylthiouracil
Sulfonamides
Rifampin
Salicylates
Sulindac
Tetracycline

SHOCK

Azathioprine
Ciprofloxacin
Cytarabine
Nitrofurantoin
Penicillins
Rifampin
Streptomycin
Trimethoprim-sulfamethoxazole

OTHER MECHANISMS OF SELECTED DRUGS:

Enteric ulceration: corticosteroids, NSAIDs, zalcitabine
Destruction of tissues (antineoplastics) or microorganisms (Jarisch-Herxheimer reaction due to penicillin)
Cytokine activation: interleukin 2
Hyperthermia due to muscle hypermetabolism: Neuroleptic malignant syndrome (antipsychotics), malignant hyperthermia (general anesthetics)
Hyperthermia due to failure to dissipate heat: Drugs with anticholinergic activity (antihistamines, antidepressants, anticholinergics, antipsychotics)

NEPHRITIS

Allopurinol
Aminoglycosides
Amphotericin B
α-Methyldopa
Azathioprine
Carbamazepine
Cephalosporins
Cimetidine
Cisplatin
Clofibrate
Hydrochlorothiazide
NSAIDs
Penicillamine
Penicillins
Phenytoin
Propylthiouracil
Rifampin
Sulfonamides
Tetracyclines
Triamterene
Trimethoprim-sulfamethoxazole

PANCREATITIS

α-Methyldopa
Azathioprine
Cimetidine
Didanosine
Erythromycin
Estrogens
Furosemide
Isoniazid
Mercaptopurine
Metronidazole
Nitrofurantoin
Pentamidine
Pentavalent antimonials
Ranitidine

ASEPTIC MENINGITISM

Azathioprine
Ibuprofen
Intravenous immunoglobulin
Isoniazid
Metronidazole
OKT3 monoclonal antibody
Penicillin
Trimethoprim-sulfamethoxazole

A host of other blood-borne infections may be transmitted via transfusion of blood products, including viruses (e.g., hepatitis B and C, cytomegalovirus [CMV], HIV), spirochetes (syphilis, borellia species), and protozoa (malaria, toxoplasmosis, African and American trypanosomiasis). However, the interval between transfusion and onset of symptoms varies from days to months in these infections, with fever rarely occurring during or immediately following transfusion.

Finally, transfusion of nonirradiated, allogeneic blood to immunocompromised patients or from human leukocyte antigen (HLA)-homozygous donors to recipients heterozygous for that HLA haplotype can cause transfusion-associated graft-versus-host disease in which donor-derived cytotoxic T cells infiltrate recipient organs, dermis, and bone marrow. The ensuing clinical syndrome, consisting of high fever, generalized erythematous rash, and liver function abnormalities, typically begins 1–2 wk following transfusion and is associated with a high mortality rate.

#### Fever associated with central nervous system dysfunction

Noninfectious fever is a common consequence of both accidental and operative trauma to the brain, although data pertaining to the actual incidence of fever in these settings are not available. There appear to be two basic mechanisms by which fever occurs. First, aseptic meningitis predictably ensues after bleeding into the subarachnoid space. It is therefore frequent in patients with spontaneous subarachnoid hemorrhage, although it can also complicate the postoperative course of a wide range of neurosurgical procedures, especially those involving the posterior fossa. Distinguishing postoperative bacterial or fungal meningitis from this aseptic meningitis syndrome is very difficult: Only the presence of new neurological deficits, a cerebrospinal fluid (CSF) leak, or a positive CSF gram stain reliably predicts the presence of bacterial infection; other CSF parameters are not sufficiently sensitive or specific to distinguish the two entities. Second, damage to hypothalamic or thalamic nuclei can disturb central thermoregulation and cause an elevated temperature, either by increasing the temperature setpoint or by interfering with mechanisms of heat dissipation (Chapter 9). This "central fever" is more common in severe and widespread cerebral damage, is usually short-lived but can be persistent, and can occur with or without other manifestations of autonomic dysfunction such as sudden changes in blood pressure, respiratory rate, or diaphoresis (so-called *diencephalic seizures*). Again, exclusion of an infectious cause of fever can be difficult, although a sustained or unremittent fever pattern is more characteristic of central fever than of most other infectious or noninfectious etiologies.

Severe injury or disease of the spinal cord may also cause thermoregulatory dysfunction to which temperature elevation has occasionally been attributed after exclusion of the more common infectious and noninfectious causes of fever. That normal vaginal deliveries achieved with the use of epidural anesthesia are often complicated by noninfectious maternal fever may be attributable in part to transient, pharmacologically induced spinal cord dysfunction.

## Epidemiology of Hospital-Acquired Fever

The incidence and clinical significance of fever in hospitalized patients are largely dependent upon their severity of illness and the number and type of interventions they endure. Increased number and severity of comorbid diseases clearly predisposes patients to nosocomial infection, although few data pertain to the relationship between comorbidities and hospital-acquired fever. Because the risk of each of the causes of hospital-acquired fever varies according to hospital service, and because most studies have segregated patients along these lines, we will consider separately the incidence and distribution of etiologies of nosocomial fever among general medical, surgical, obstetric and gynecologic, immunocompromised, and intensive care unit (ICU) patients.

### General medical patients

Hospital-acquired fever occurs in about 10% to 20% of patients hospitalized on general medical wards. Between 30% and 60% of episodes are caused by infections, about 5% are caused by noninfectious diseases which generally require specific therapy (e.g., pulmonary embolism, myocardial infarction, cancer), drug fever is implicated in up to 5%, and the cause of fever eludes identification in up to one-fifth of patients. The most common infectious causes of fever, in descending order of frequency, are infections of the lower respiratory tract, and urinary tract, and catheter-associated and primary bacteremias. Although patients who develop fever have longer hospital stays than do afebrile controls, nosocomial fever does not confer a higher risk of in-hospital mortality when the control population is matched according to the level of comorbidity.

Early identification of patients at high risk of bacterial infection is desirable in order to guide the use of empiric antimicrobial therapy. In general, the majority of febrile medical patients have localizing signs and/or symptoms which provide direction to both the diagnostic workup and the use of antimicrobial therapy. However, up to 20% of patients with bacterial infection lack these findings, a circumstance observed most often in the elderly and in patients with important comorbidities. In addition, the presence of diabetes mellitus, a length of stay to fever onset of >10 d, a maximal temperature of >38.7°C, and a leukocyte count of >10,000/mm have been found to be independent predictors of bacterial infection on multivariate analysis.

### General surgical patients

Fever can be anticipated to occur more often in patients subjected to invasive procedures, both because of the inflammatory state incited by the procedure itself and because of heightened susceptibility to infection due to wounds and anesthesia. The reported incidence of fever in postoperative patients ranges from 15% to 90% depending upon the definition of fever used and the type of population studied. An infectious cause of temperature elevation is found in 10% to 50% of febrile patients; the most common sites of infection are surgical wounds, urinary tract, and lower respiratory tract.

The likelihood that postoperative fever is infectious is critically dependent on the timing of the fever with respect to the operation (Fig. 48.1). Early postoperative fever is most often noninfectious and self-limited, whereas fevers beginning on or after the fifth postoperative day are usually due to infection. However, although uncommon, some exceptions to the benignity of early postoperative fever are worth emphasizing. For example, necrotizing wound infections due to *Clostridia* or streptococcal species often present in the first 48 h (Chapter 82), and anastomotic leaks or dehiscences can occur at any time in patients recovering from major abdominal or thoracic operations. Patients with early postoperative fever must therefore undergo careful clinical evaluation to exclude such potentially catastrophic complications.

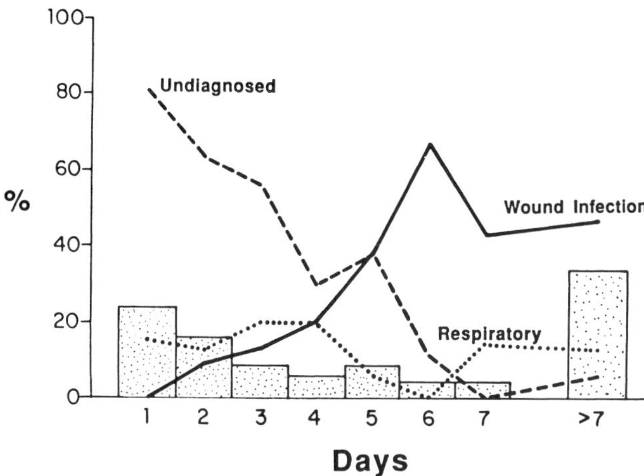


**Fig. 48.1** The percentage of new fevers that appear each postoperative day is indicated by vertical bars. The percentages of new fevers on each day that are due to wound infection or respiratory infection or are unexplained are indicated by the solid, dotted, and hatched lines, respectively. [Reprinted with permission from Garibaldi, Infection Control 6:273, Slack Publishing, Thorofare, NJ, 1985.]

## Obstetric and gynecologic patients

Maternal fever complicates up to 15% of vaginal deliveries in which epidural anesthesia is employed, almost all of which is noninfectious, while fever occurs in only 1%–2% of vaginal deliveries without epidural anesthesia. Cesarean section is associated with postoperative fever in 12% to 20% of deliveries; postoperative fever occurs in about 15% of patients undergoing abdominal hysterectomy. Puerperal fever not associated with epidural anesthesia is caused by bacterial infection in 40% to 100% of episodes; endomyometritis, wound infection, urinary tract infection, and pelvic abscesses are most commonly observed; pelvic vein thrombophlebitis is an important but rare cause. An increased risk of puerperal infection has been associated with amnionitis, prolonged labor and rupture of membranes, the use of transvaginal monitoring devices, repetitive pelvic and rectal examinations during labor, and maternal obesity.

## ICU patients

Although nosocomial infections in ICUs have been studied intensively, there is remarkably little data available on the incidence and distribution of etiologies of fever in the ICU setting. Extrapolation from studies of nosocomial infection would suggest that fever, like infection, is likely to be more frequent in the ICU than elsewhere and that it is more likely to occur in patients with multiple comorbidities and in patients whose acute illnesses are most severe and require the most frequent and prolonged use of invasive devices. Indeed, the same features that correlate with the risk of nosocomial infection in ICU patients are also likely to predispose to noninfectious causes of fever such as tissue ischemia, venous thromboembolism, hematoma, and postprocedural fever. Furthermore, the intensive use of antimicrobials, antiarrhythmics, and anticonvulsants in the ICU suggests that drug fever should be relatively more common as well. Clearly, heightened vigilance for both infectious and noninfectious complications of ICU care is warranted and should be based upon the totality of clinical and physiological data that are available, of which patient temperature is a component.

Determining the causes of fever and pulmonary infiltrates in mechanically ventilated patients is particularly difficult. As noted above, both pulmonary emboli and pulmonary fibroproliferation, among other disorders, can present in a manner that is clinically indistinguishable from pneumonia; in addition, the development of purulent endotracheal secretions harboring potentially pathogenic bacteria commonly occurs in mechanically ventilated patients with no evidence of pneumonia. Indeed, in patients from whom specimens for quantitative culture were obtained during bronchoscopy, conventional clinical criteria for ventilator-associated pneumonia such as fever, leukocytosis, purulent sputum, and new radiographic infiltrates have been shown by many investigators to be inaccurate (Chapter 58). A recent prospective study employing a comprehensive diagnostic protocol found that one or more infections—primarily pneumonia, sinusitis, catheter-related infection, or urinary tract infection—were present in over 80% of febrile ICU patients, that multiple infections were common, and that noninfectious causes of fever were more common in patients with ARDS, with pulmonary fibroproliferation identified as the sole etiology in five of 35 ARDS patients.

## Immunocompromised patients

Fever occurs in 30%–90% of patients with chemotherapy-induced neutropenia and is attributable to documented infection in about half the cases. The incidence of neutropenic fever and associated infection is related to the type of malignancy (solid tumors less often than acute leukemias), the intensity of chemotherapy, and the duration of neutropenia. By contrast, fever in organ transplant recipients, and in patients with congenital and acquired immunodeficiency syndromes, as an accompaniment of either infectious or noninfectious diseases—for example, the incidence and causes of hospital-acquired fever in HIV-infected patients—has received relatively little attention. In addition to infections, acute rejection and graft-versus-host disease must be considered in solid organ and allogeneic bone marrow transplant recipients, respectively. Among AIDS patients, drug-induced fever (Tables 48.2, 48.3) is probably more common given the high incidence of adverse drug reactions in this patient population.

# Management of the Patient With Hospital-Acquired Fever

Detailed approaches to the evaluation and treatment of hospital-acquired fever due to specific infections syndromes are presented elsewhere in this textbook. Here, we provide a more general framework for the approach to hospital acquired fever (Tables 48.4, 48.5).

A carefully performed history and physical examination suggests the source of fever in up to 80% of patients. In addition to eliciting the patient's symptoms, a thorough history should include an assessment of the patient's immune status, comorbidities, risk factors for sources of fever (Tables 48.1–48.3), a review of recent invasive procedures and medications, and an inventory of indwelling catheters in use.

The physical examination should begin with assessment of the patient's blood pressure, pulse, respiratory rate, mental status, and, if possible, urine output, as perturbations in any of these parameters increase the likelihood of a serious infection or inflammatory disorder. The examination should then focus on any

**Table 48.4** Diagnostic options for hospital-acquired fever*

ALL PATIENTS: Careful history and physical examination (see text for details)
Close observation[a]

SELECTED PATIENTS:[b] WBC count and differential
Two sets of blood cultures

| In the setting of | Obtain or consider |
|---|---|
| Urinary catheterization<br>Genitourinary instrumentation<br>Genitourinary complaints | Urinalysis<br>Urine culture |
| Nosocomial diarrhea | *Clostridium difficile* toxin assay<br>Stool culture (in outbreak only)<br>Stool for ova & parasites<br>(AIDS and other susceptible patients)<br>Sigmoidoscopy<br>Abdominopelvic CT |
| Abdominal pain or tenderness<br>Nausea, vomiting | LFTs, amylase, pregnancy test<br>CXR, KUB, EKG<br>*Clostridium difficile* toxin assay<br>Ultrasound and/or CT<br>Nuclear medicine study<br>Surgical consultation |
| Postpartum<br>Thoracic signs/symptoms<br>Mechanical ventilation<br>Immunocompromised | Pelvic ultrasound<br>CXR, EKG<br>Arterial blood gas<br>Sputum gram stain and culture<br>Sinus CT<br>Noninvasive test for DVT<br>V/Q scan, pulmonary angiogram<br>Bronchoscopy<br>Chest CT |
| Central venous catheter<br>High risk for drug fever | Removal and quantitative culture<br>Withdrawal of drug in question |

[a]For patients <48 h ostoperative with negative histories and examinations, observation without further testing may be appropriate.

[b]For patients whose acute illness and/or comorbid diseases are severe, or who are otherwise at high risk of blood-borne infection as described in the text.

*Abbreviations: CT = computed tomography scan; CXR = chest roentgenogram; DVT = deep venous thrombosis; EKG = electrocardiogram; KUB = plain roentgenogram of the abdomen; LFTs = liver function tests; V/Q = nuclear medicine ventilation/perfusion.

localizing symptoms offered by the patient and should include careful inspection of integument, including surgical wounds, possible sites of decubiti, and catheter sites for the presence of inflammation or infection. Inspection of the lochia for purulence or malodorousness in postpartum women contributes to the diagnosis of endometritis. In mechanically ventilated patients, changes in ventilatory parameters can provide clues to the presence of local pulmonary or systemic disorders; in addition, changes in the quantity and quality of endotracheal and nasal secretions should be assessed, and otoscopy should be performed, as otitis media is well described in this setting, and the presence of a middle ear effusion is predictive of sinusitis. In patients who have undergone elective and/or uncomplicated surgery in the previous 48 h, a negative evaluation as described above is probably sufficient to exclude infection or other important treatable causes of fever, and observation is appropriate, with further diagnostic testing and/or empiric therapy reserved for patients in whom fever persists beyond the third postoperative day.

Clinicians have long employed an intuitive judgment of the level of sickness or toxicity manifested by febrile patients in assessing the likelihood of serious underlying diseases, especially bacterial infections. However, when studied formally, assessments of "toxicity" have been neither sensitive nor specific in predicting the presence of occult bacterial infection or bacteremia. The only component of a general evaluation of the patient's appearance that has been found to be predictive of bacteremia is the presence of chills. However, noninfectious causes of fever can also present with chills: drug fever, for example, is accompanied by rigors in about 50% of patients and is sometimes accompanied by hemodynamic compromise as well.

Similarly, the pattern of fever is generally unreliable in distinguishing among its possible causes. In the only recent systematic study of fever patterns in hospitalized patients, 240 of 306 (78%) patients had fever patterns in which the temperature fell between 0.3° C and 1.4° C each day, either to normal or below ("intermittent") or with the nadir staying above normal ("remittent"); in over 90% of these, there was normal diurnal variation in which the peak temperature occurred in the afternoon or evening, and the nadir temperatures occurred in the morning hours. The only diseases that were strongly associated with unusual fever patterns were gram-negative pneumonia and central fever in which, taken together, a "sustained" pattern (i.e.

**Table 48.5** Therapeutic options for hospital-acquired fever*

| Option | Indication |
|---|---|
| Empiric antimicrobials | Suggestive syndrome<br>High risk host, e.g., neutropenia<br>High risk setting, e.g., outbreak of *Clostridium difficile* |
| Therapeutic antimicrobials | Diagnosis is certain<br>Significance of diagnosis is uncertain, e.g., urinary tract infection |
| Empiric antiinflammatory drugs | Suspected inflammatory and/or malignant disease |
| Empiric anticoagulants | Suspected thromboembolic disease<br>Suspected pelvic vein thrombophlebitis |
| Surgical exploration, drainage, debridement | Suspected or proven surgical problem |
| Removal of intravascular catheter or other device | Signs of inflammation and/or thrombosis<br>High risk of infection (Chapters 67, 85) |
| Withdrawal of suspected cause of drug fever | Absence of alternative cause of fever<br>Exposure to high-risk drug (Tables 48.2, 48.3) |

*Specific antimicrobial regimens should be tailored according to the syndrome and/or suspected pathogens as outlined in the relevant chapters in this textbook.

daily temperature fluctuation of 0.3° C or less) was 99% specific, though only 66% sensitive (19 of 29) for the presence of one of these disorders.

Beyond the history and physical examination, the tests most often used to investigate the cause of fever in hospitalized patients include the WBC count, urinalysis, chest roentgenogram, and cultures of blood and/or other specimens as indicated. Determination of the WBC count and differential to exclude neutropenia is clearly important, and the presence of eosinophilia is a specific though insensitive indicator of a drug reaction. The presence of leukocytosis and/or a "left shift" of the myeloid series on peripheral smear has been found to predict bacterial infection in some studies, although they are neither sensitive nor specific in this regard. Monitoring trends in the WBC count can sometimes help in evaluating the patient's response to therapy, although the extent to which it adds meaningfully to the assessment of more basic clinical parameters is unknown but is probably small. Conversely, the correlation between the risk of infection and the presence of neutropenia is well known (Chapter 86).

Blood cultures are an important component of the evaluation of many hospitalized patients with fever. They are particularly valuable in patients who are seriously ill, are immunocompromised, have indwelling catheters, or have multiple comorbidities. And although a number of studies have shown that the likelihood of a blood culture being positive is correlated with high fever and leukocytosis, the absence of these findings in no way provides assurance against the presence of bacteremia when other risk factors are present. For example, nearly one-fourth of AIDS patients with community-acquired bacteremia presented with normal vital signs in one study.

The chest roentgenogram is clearly important in evaluating febrile patients with cardiopulmonary symptoms or signs. It is also important in the assessment of febrile patients who lack localizing findings but who are debilitated or immunocompromised. Its main limitation is the lack of specificity of abnormal findings. The interpretation of abnormal chest roentgenograms is particularly difficult in mechanically ventilated patients with fever in whom the accuracy of standard clinical criteria for the diagnosis of nosocomial pneumonia has come under question.

Since nearly 100% of nosocomial urinary tract infections occur in patients with indwelling urinary catheters or who have undergone recent urological instrumentation, a urinalysis and/or urine culture should be obtained routinely only in febrile patients with these risk factors. These tests should be interpreted with caution, however, because the high prevalence of bacteriuria in catheterized patients (about 50% after 7 to 10 d) coupled with the low incidence of fever attributable to this bacteriuria (about 1%) suggests that alternative sources of fever should be considered in febrile, bacteriuric patients.

In evaluating patients with hospital-acquired diarrhea and fever, the only stool test that has been shown to be consistently worthwhile is an assay for the toxin produced by *Clostridium difficile*. It has been shown, for example, that in U.S. hospitals routine stool cultures and examinations for ova and parasites are rarely, if ever, positive when employed for the evaluation of diarrhea that begins during hospitalization. In evaluating febrile nosocomial diarrhea, therefore, tests for ova and parasites are appropriate only in patients who have AIDS or are otherwise at risk because of their community exposures or other epidemiologic factors, such as known or suspected outbreaks of diarrhea due to bacterial pathogens or exposure to pathogens (e.g., *Strongyloides stercoralis*) known to cause disease in the setting of stress or compromised immunity. One must also be mindful of the fact that diarrhea is sometimes a response to adjacent pelvic inflammation or infection or a nonspecific manifestation of systemic illnesses, and that important noninfectious diseases, such as intestinal ischemia or infarction, can also present with fever and diarrhea.

The proper pace and scope of the evaluation of the patient with other abdominal findings such as pain, bleeding, or emesis, depends on the severity of the patient's illness—for example, is an acute abdomen present?—and whether comorbid risk factors such as recent abdominal surgery or known intraabdominal malignancy are present. An appropriate screening evaluation includes measurement of liver function tests and serum amylase and/or lipase levels and roentgenograms of the chest and abdomen. Pregnancy testing is essential in women of child-bearing potential, and surgical consultation should be sought in any patient for whom surgical therapy may be necessary. Further imaging studies that may be helpful in patients for whom this preliminary workup is nondiagnostic include ultrasonography, computed tomography (CT), and nuclear medicine scanning using gallium- or indium-labeled white blood cells. The most efficient deployment of these tests has yet to be defined; a popular algorithm recommends ultrasound as the initial test in patients with findings localized to the right upper quadrant or pelvis, CT for patients with findings localized elsewhere in the abdomen or with suspected retroperitoneal disease, and nuclear medicine scanning if the findings are not localized.

Treatment for most causes of hospital-acquired infection is straightforward once the diagnosis is made and is detailed elsewhere in this text (Chapter 8). The treatment of fever itself as a management problem in hospitalized patients is covered in Chapter 9. Of greater challenge to the clinician are whether and when to administer therapies before the cause of fever has been determined (Table 48.5). Empiric therapy is sometimes valuable diagnostically, as with the use of heparin in women with suspected pelvic vein thrombophlebitis or naproxen in patients with fever suspected to be caused by an underlying malignancy. More often, though, empiric therapy is given because the consequences of delaying treatment until a diagnosis is made are felt to be prohibitive. Examples include exploratory surgery for the patient with an acute abdomen and broad-spectrum antibiotics in febrile patients with neutropenia. Beyond these narrowly defined circumstances, the proper use of empiric treatments, especially antibiotics, is ambiguous and must be evaluated on a case-by-case basis. Important considerations include the degree of immune impairment present and the extent to which the patient's syndrome resembles a treatment-responsive disease.

## ANNOTATED BIBLIOGRAPHY


Arbo MJ, Fine MJ, Hanusa BH, Sefcik T, Kapoor WN. Fever of nosocomial origin: etiology, risk factors, and outcomes. Am J Med 1993; 96:505–512.
*Prospective analysis of 100 general medical patients with hospital-acquired fever. Risk factors for bacterial infection are elucidated, and cohort mortality is compared with a control group carefully matched for age, sex, and level of comorbidity.*

Clarke DE, Kimelman J, Raffin TA. The evaluation of fever in the intensive care unit. Chest 1991; 100:213–220.
*Comprehensive and careful review of the literature.*

Dellinger EP. Approach to the patient with postoperative fever. In: Infectious Diseases. Gorbach SL, Bartlett JG, Blacklow NR, eds. WB Saunders, Philadelphia, PA, pp 753–758, 1992.
*Comprehensive review of the approach to the postoperative patient with fever. The discussion on the implications of the timing of fever with respect to surgery is particularly helpful.*

Klimek JJ, Ajemian ER, Gracewski J, Klemas B, Quintilliani R. A prospective analysis of hospital-acquired fever in obstetric and gynecologic patients. JAMA 1982; 247:3340–3343.
*Prospective study of 427 febrile patients seen over 12 months.*

Lieberman E, Lang JM, Frigoletto F, Richardson DK, Ringer SA, Cohen A. Epidural analgesia, intrapartum fever, and neonatal sepsis evaluation. Pediatrics 1997; 99:415–419.
*Prospective analysis of the incidence of fever complicating routine childbirth in 1,657 women and the outcomes of their children.*

Lofmark R, Nordlander R, Orinius E. The temperature course in acute myocardial infarction. Am Heart J 1978; 96:153–156.
*Careful longitudinal analysis of body temperature in 160 patients with acute myocardial infarction demonstrating the strong association between myocardial infarction and fever.*

Mackowiak PA, LeMaistre CF. Drug fever: a critical appraisal of conventional concepts. Ann Intern Med 1987; 106:728–733.
*Retrospective analysis of the causes and clinical manifestations of drug fever in 148 patients.*

Mackowiak PA, Wasserman SS, Levine MM. A critical appraisal of 98.6°F, the upper limit of the normal body temperature, and other legacies of Carl Reinhold August Wunderlich. JAMA 1992; 268:1578–1580.
*Descriptive analysis of baseline oral temperature data from volunteers that calls into question long-held assumptions about the range of normal human body temperatures.*

Meduri GU, Mauldin GL, Wunderink RG, Leeper KV, Jones CB, Tolley E, Mayhall G. Causes of fever and pulmonary densities in patients with clinical manifestations of ventilator-associated pneumonia. Chest 1994; 106:221–235.
*Presents the results of a comprehensive diagnostic protocol, including quantitative culture of bronchoalveolar lavage, applied prospectively to 50 consecutive mechanically ventilated patients with fever and pulmonary infiltrates. Demonstrates that such patients commonly have multiple sources of fever, and that pulmonary fibroproliferation may be an important consideration in patients with ARDS.*

Musher DM, Fainstein V, Young EJ, Pruett TL. Fever patterns: their lack of clinical significance. Arch Intern Med 1979; 139:1225–1228.
*Descriptive study of the correlation between fever patterns and causes of fever; demonstrates that fever patterns are rarely helpful in suggesting a specific cause.*

Murray HW, Ellis GC, Blumenthal DS, Sos TA. Fever and pulmonary thromboembolism. Am J Med 1979; 67:232–236.
*Describes the body temperature course of 35 consecutive patients with angiographically proven pulmonary embolism.*

# 49

## Fever of Unknown Origin

RICHARD K. ROOT AND ROBERT G. PETERSDORF

As a cardinal manifestation of the inflammatory process that accompanies infection, fever is often the major symptom that causes patients to seek medical attention. The majority of febrile disorders are short-lived and produced by intercurrent viral respiratory infections. Less commonly fever may be prolonged and last for weeks or months as part of a chronic infectious disease, a diffuse inflammatory disorder or an occult neoplasm. If initial evaluation fails to disclose a cause the disorder is stated to be a "fever of unknown origin (FUO)". In 1960 Petersdorf and Beeson provided a working definition of FUO that described a series of hospitalized patients who had "fever higher than 101 degrees Fahrenheit (38.3 degrees Centigrade) on several occasions, persisting without diagnosis for at least 3 weeks, including at least one week's investigation in the hospital." With changes in medical practice that increasingly call for extensive outpatient evaluations and the advent of immunosuppressive or cytotoxic therapy as well as AIDS it has been suggested that we delete the requirement for in-hospital investigation and further define patients with FUO based upon the setting and whether or not they are immunocompromised (Table 49.1). This approach permits a more targeted series of investigations based upon disorders that are more likely to be prevalent in the host populations. Because the problems of undiagnosed fever in patients who are hospitalized or who have neutropenia or HIV infection are discussed in detail elsewhere in the book (see Chapters 48, 86–88 and 100), this chapter will focus on *classical FUO*.

### Pathogenesis

The basic mechanisms in the pathogenesis of fever are presented and discussed in Chapter 9. In brief, while elevation of body temperature is the measurable characteristic of fever, it is important to distinguish true *fever* from *hyperthermia*. Fever reflects a change in the hypothalamic set point for body temperature under the influence of the inflammatory cytokines which serve as endogenous pyrogens ( interleukin-1, tumor necrosis factor $\alpha$, interferon $\gamma$, interleukin-6). Their release has usually been triggered by exposure to exogenous pyrogens, such as bacterial endotoxin or other microbial products. Hyperthermia refers to the elevation of body temperature seen when heat production mechanisms exceed those of heat dissipation. As such, since most hyperthermic conditions are short lived, it is unusual to have hyperthermia sustained for weeks or months. Exceptions to this rule may be seen in patients with hyperthyroidism in whom cellular thermogenesis remains increased until euthyroidism is attained by successful therapy. Sustained hyperthermia can also be seen in patients who have a central disorder of thermoregulation, caused, for example, by an encephalitis, or other hypothalamic injury, but these conditions are rare.

When prolonged fever is due to infection, almost always the infecting agent is in a sanctuary where it is not easily eradicated by host defenses, thereby leading to the continuous production of inflammatory cytokines. Similarly, involvement of macrophages and lymphocytes in autoimmune or other causes of chronic inflammation leads to persistent pyrogen production and sustained or episodic fevers. Certain neoplasms, particularly those derived from macrophages or lymphocytes, may also have uncontrolled release of inflammatory cytokines and give rise to prolonged fevers. Given the central involvement of these common mechanisms it is not surprising that the majority of cases of "classical" FUO are caused by infection, autoimmune disorders, or neoplasms. In addition, other manifestations of disorders characterized by prolonged fever can include weight loss progressing to cachexia, elevated acute phase reactant proteins and erythrocyte sedimentation rate, depressed serum iron and albumin, inflammatory block anemia, and hyperlipidemia, all due to the actions of the cytokines involved in a sustained inflammatory process (see Chapters 13 and 14.)

### Etiologies

Over 200 separate diseases have been reported to produce prolonged fever or recurrent febrile episodes which have defied easy diagnosis (Table 49.2). Despite the large number, almost all can be classified into the original five categories proposed by Petersdorf and Beeson: *infections*, *neoplasms*, *collagen vascular disorders*, a *miscellaneous* group, and a final category in which the cause of the fever remains *undiagnosed*. The proportion of patients reported (and expected) in each category has varied with the geographic locale (Table 49.3), with the age group under consideration, the duration of the febrile disorder, and whether or not the patient has a known underlying disease, such as HIV infection. Infections account for FUO in 25%–50% of reported cases; the highest percentages are found in developing countries in tropical and subtropical areas of the world. Neoplasms have accounted for 20%–30% of cases in most series. In about a third of the patients with neoplasms the fever is due to the tumor itself, whereas complicating infections are responsible for fever in more than half of the cases. The category of collagen-vascular diseases accounts for 15%–30% of reported cases in developed countries and ranges from younger patients with Still's disease or systemic lupus erythematosus to elderly patients who have giant cell arteritis or polymyalgia rheumatica. With the development of more effective methods to diagnose certain viral or bacterial infections, improved serologic assessment of collagen vascular disorders, and better imaging techniques to detect occult neoplasms, the proportion of cases with FUO in the miscellaneous and undiagnosed cat-

**Table 49.1** Definitions for fever of unknown origin (FUO)*

| |
|---|
| CLASSICAL FUO |
| Fever 38.3° C (101° F) or higher on multiple days |
| Duration more than 3 wk |
| Diagnosis uncertain after appropriate initial investigations 3 d into hospitalization or 3 outpatient visits |
| NOSOCOMIAL FUO |
| Fever 38.3° C (101° F) or higher on several occasions in a hospitalized acute care patient |
| Infection not present or incubating on admission |
| Diagnosis uncertain after 3 d evaluation, including 2 d of microbiologic culture incubation |
| NEUTROPENIC FUO |
| Fever 38.3° C (101° F) or higher on several occasions |
| Neutrophil counts <500/μl |
| Diagnosis uncertain after 3 d evaluation including 2 d of microbiologic incubation |
| HIV-ASSOCIATED FUO |
| Fever 38.3° C (101° F) or higher on several occasions |
| Confirmed positive serology for HIV infection |
| Fever more than 4 wk (outpatients) or more than 3 d (inpatients) |
| Diagnosis uncertain after 3 d evaluation including 2 d of microbiologic culture incubation |

*Modified with permission from Durack and Street (1994).

egories has increased to up to a third of the total reported in developed countries.

The longer febrile episodes persist without specific diagnosis or appropriate therapy the less likely they are to be caused by an infectious process. In a study of 347 patients referred to the U.S. National Institutes of Health who had FUO lasting more than 6 months only 6% were found to have infection as a cause. The largest category of patients (27%) had no documented true fever and included a number of children who had exaggerated circadian temperature swings or exercise-induced hyperthermia. Nine percent of the patients were found to have *factitious fever* (see below). Granulomatous hepatitis, in some cases without abnormalities of liver function tests, accounted for 8% of the cases; neoplasms for 7%; 6% were due to Still's disease in adults and 4% to other collagen vascular diseases; 3% were due to familial Mediterranean fever and the remaining 13% to a variety of miscellaneous causes.

Elderly patients with FUO are more likely to have neoplasms or connective tissue diseases, such as giant cell arteritis, as a cause for fever than infections. Recurrent respiratory tract infections are the most likely cause of FUO in infants under 12 months. Noninfectious disorders such as Kawasaki's syndrome, Still's disease, systemic lupus erythematosus (SLE), and hematologic or lymphatic malignancies become progressively more important in older children and young adults.

## Clinical Features

The clinical features of a FUO will be dictated by a number of factors including the specific etiology, the age and condition of the patient, accompanying diseases, and the influences of antibiotic or antiinflammatory therapy. Conversely, because fever and other expressions of the inflammatory response may be shared manifestations of almost all of the diseases causing FUO, in the absence of focal symptoms and signs it may be very difficult to differentiate between different disorders on the basis of history and physical examination alone. This may lead to an overly comprehensive and needlessly expensive evaluation or to various attempts at ill-conceived "shotgun" antimicrobial or antiinflammatory therapeutic trials. Some general principles can be applied to the major diseases in each diagnostic category. For those disorders presenting as FUO with prominent localizing symptoms and signs the reader is referred to the specific organ-system chapters in this book.

## Infections

Whether infections are localized or generalized, they may cause prolonged fever if they are not readily controlled by an effective inflammatory and immune response. Furthermore they frequently lack characteristic localizing features that may help focus the evaluation. Table 49.4 lists the most common infectious causes for classical FUO from studies conducted in different parts of the world.

*Bacterial species* are the most common infectious cause for prolonged FUO in most areas of the world. These infections are either generalized or localized. In the case of generalized infections the organism has usually adapted to the host immune and inflammatory defenses as a virulence factor and is not readily eradicated without specific antimicrobial treatment. Localized bacterial infections that cause FUO often involve sites of the body where the inflammatory response is blunted or nonexistent (e.g., heart valves).

*Mycobacterial infections* make up the largest category of generalized bacterial infections that cause prolonged FUO. The vast majority of these are caused by *Mycobacterium tuberculosis*, rather than atypical organisms (see Chapter 57), and it remains the most common infectious cause for FUO worldwide. *M. tuberculosis* is the classic intracellular bacterial pathogen, protected from the action of antibodies by its intracellular location and resistant to the microbicidal mechanisms of phagocytes by inhibition of phagolysosomal fusion. It requires activation of macrophage function by cellular immune processes to contain the number of viable bacilli. These processes typically takes weeks to months to develop and in about 10% of active tuberculosis cases fail, leading to disseminated and ultimately fatal disease unless successful treatment is instituted. Any suppression of cellular immunity by coexistent disease or therapy increases the likelihood of dissemination and a fatal outcome and makes the diagnosis of tuberculosis more difficult. When tuberculosis presents as FUO it is frequently disseminated, and over half of the patients may lack characteristic chest radiographic abnormalities and have negative tuberculin skin tests, usually due to anergy (see Chapter 57). The lack of typical identifying features for tuberculosis is a particularly prominent feature of patients who are immunosuppressed by disease (e.g., AIDS, end-stage renal disease) or who are receiving immunosuppressive therapy (in particular, high-dose glucocorticosteroids).

Other bacterial infections caused by organisms that have adapted to survive in the intracellular location and cause chronic or relapsing fevers include salmonella enteric fever (caused by *Salmonella typhi* and *paratyphi* ), brucellosis, Q fever (caused by *Coxiella burnettii*), and psittacosis. Still other bacteria undergo frequent changes in surface antigens so that they are not

**Table 49.2** Diseases causing classical FUO in adults in the United States*

INFECTIONS

*LOCALIZED PYOGENIC INFECTIONS*

Appendicitis
Cat scratch disease
Cholangitis
Cholecystitis
Dental abscess
Diverticulitis/abscess
Lesser sac abscess
Liver abscess
Mesenteric lymphadenitis
Osteomyelitis
Pancreatic abscess
Pelvic inflammatory disease
Perinephric/intrarenal disease
Prostatic abscess
Sinusitis
Subphrenic abscess
Suppurative thrombophlebitis
Tuboovarian abscess

*INTRAVASCULAR INFECTIONS*

Bacterial aoritis
Bacterial endocarditis
Vascular catheter infections

*SYSTEMIC BACTERIAL INFECTIONS*

Brucellosis
*Campylobacter*
Gonococcemia
*Legionella*
Leptospirosis
Listeriosis
Lyme disease
Melioidosis
Meningococcemia
Rat bite fever
Relapsing fever
Salmonellosis
Syphilis
Tularemia
Typhoid
Vibriosis
*Yersinia*

*MYCOBACTERIAL INFECTIONS*

Mycobacterium-avium-intracellulare (MAI)
Other atypical mycobacteria
Tuberculosis

*FUNGAL INFECTIONS*

Aspergillosis
Blastomycosis
Candidiasis
Coccidioidomycosis
Cryptococcosis
Histoplasmosis
Mucormycosis
Paracoccidioidomycosis
Sporotrichosis

*OTHER BACTERIA*

Actinomycosis
Cat-scratch disease (*Bartonella henselae*)
Nocardiosis
Whipple's bacillus

*RICKETTSIAL INFECTIONS*

Ehrlichiosis
Murine typhus
Q fever
Rickettsialpox
Rocky Mountain spotted fever

*MYCOPLASMA*

*CHLAMYDIAL INFECTIONS*

Lymphogranuloma venereum (LGV)
Psittacosis

*VIRAL INFECTIONS*

Colorado tick fever
Coxsackie group B
CMV
Dengue
EBV
Hepatitis A, B, C, D and E
HIV
Lymphocytic choriomeningitis (LCM)
Parvovirus $B_{19}$

*PARASITIC*

Amebiasis
Babesia
Chagas's disease
Leishmaniasis
Malaria
*Pneumocystis carinii*
*Strongyloides*
Toxoplasmosis
Toxocariasis
Trichinosis

*PRESUMED INFECTIONS, AGENT UNDETERMINED*

Kawasaki's disease (mucocutaneous lymph node syndrome)
Kikuchi's disease (necrotizing lymphadenitis)

NEOPLASMS

*MALIGNANT*

Colon
Hodgkin's lymphoma
Immunoblastic lymphadenopathy
Kidney
Leukemia
Liver
Lymphomatoid granulomatosis
Malignant histiocystosis
Non-Hodgkin's lymphoma
Pancreas
Sarcoma

*BENIGN*

Atrial myxoma
Renal angiomyolipoma

COLLAGEN VASCULAR DISEASES/HYPERSENSITIVITY DISEASES

Adult Still's disease
Behçet's disease
Erythema multiforme
Erythema nodosum
Giant cell arteritis/polymyalgia rheumatica
Hypersensitivity pneumonitis (e.g., "metal fume fever," "farmer's lung," "air-conditioner lung")
Hypersensitivity vasculitis
Mixed connective tissue disease
Polyarteritis nodosa
Relapsing polychondritis
Rheumatic fever
Rheumatoid arthritis



(*continued*)

**Table 49.2** Diseases causing classical FUO in adults in the United States*—*Continued*

Systemic lupus erythematosus
Takayasu's aortitis
Weber-Christian disease
Wegener's granulomatosis

GRANULOMATOUS DISEASES

Crohn's disease
Idiopathic granulomatous hepatitis
Midline granuloma
Sarcoidosis

MISCELLANEOUS DISEASES

Aortic dissection
Drug fever
Gout
Hematomas
Hemolytic diseases/hemoglobinopathies
Laennec's cirrhosis
Postmyocardial infarction syndrome
Recurrent pulmonary emboli
Subacute thyroiditis (deQuervain's)
Tissue infarction/necrosis

INHERITED AND METABOLIC DISEASES

Adrenal insufficiency
Cyclic neutropenia
Deafness, urticaria and amyloid
Fabry's disease
Familial Mediterranean fever
Hyperimmunoglobulinemia D and periodic fever
Type V hypertriglyceridemia

THERMOREGULATORY DISORDERS

*CENTRAL*

Brain tumor
Cerebrovascular accident
Encephalitis
Hypothalmic dysfunction

*PERIPHERAL*

Hyperthyroidism
Pheochromocytoma

FACTITIOUS FEVERS

"Afebrile" FUO (<38.3° C)
Habitual hyperthermia (exaggerated circadian rhythm)

*Reprinted with permission from Isselbacher et al, Harrison's Principles and Practice of Internal Medicine. 13th edition, McGraw-Hill, New York, 1994.

readily eradicated by immune mechanisms: These include *Bartonella* species (the causes of bartonellosis, cat scratch fever, bacillary angiomatosis, and Lyme disease); *Borellia* sp. (the cause of relapsing fevers); and perhaps spirochetes such as *Treponema pallidum*, the cause of syphilis, which may present as FUO during the secondary phase (see Chapter 70).

The most frequent localized infections causing FUO are *cryptic abscesses*, particularly in an intraabdominal location (see Chapters 63 and 65). Worldwide, abscesses are second only to tuberculosis as a cause of FUO. A well-encapsulated abscess may prevent the systemic spread of infecting organisms, giving rise to negative blood cultures but creating conditions where responses to antibiotic therapy are impaired. Furthermore, the physical conditions within abscess cavities (low pH, high osmolarity and low $pO_2$) inhibit effective antimicrobial activity by neutrophils, resulting in a standoff between the pathogen and the host. While localizing pain and tenderness are usually prominent in early abscess formation, they are often blunted in the chronic encapsulated state. Complete eradication of the infecting organisms and the febrile response is usually not achieved until the abscess is identified and drained surgically. Besides intraabdominal cryptic abscesses causing FUO, dental, sinus, and middle ear or mastoid infections occasionally produce prolonged fevers that may not be accompanied by prominent localizing symptoms.

*Endocarditis* accounts for 3% to 5% of cases of FUO in most series. The presentation of this disease, the etiologic agents, the diagnosis, and the management are thoroughly discussed in Chapter 66. Continuous bacteremia is a hallmark of bacterial endocarditis. This occurs because the vegetation on heart valves consisting of clumps of bacteria, platelets, and fibrin is constantly bathed by blood and is devoid of a phagocytic inflammatory response. Bacteremia may be obscured by intermittent antimicrobial therapy or fail to be detected unless special media are employed (e.g., *Legionella* species, *Chlamydia* species, *Coxiella burnetti*, fungi). In addition, certain pathogens (e.g., members of the HACEK group of bacteria (*Hemophilus*, *Actinobacillus*, *Cardiobacterium*, *Eikenella*, *Kingella* sp.)—nutritionally fastidious streptococci) may grow slowly under standard culture con-

**Table 49.3** Diagnostic categories for FUO in different countries*

| Country | No. patients (studies) | % Infection | % Neoplasm | % CVD† | % Other | % No DX |
|---|---|---|---|---|---|---|
| USA | 191 (2) | 30–33 | 24–31 | 9–16 | 17–18 | 9–12 |
| Europe[a] | 332 (2) | 23–31 | 7–18 | 13–22 | 17–24 | 21–26 |
| Japan | 381 (5) | 25–52 | 14–27 | 16–29 | 6–20 | 10–22 |
| India | 150 (1) | 50 | 21 | 9 | 16 | 4 |

*Data for studies reported between 1980 and 1994 and reviewed by Iikuni et al. Int Med 1994; 33:67–73, and Durack In Fever: Mechanisms and Management, 2nd ed. P.A. Mackowiak ed. Lippincott-Raven, Philadelphia, PA, 1997, p 237.

†Collagen vascular diseases

[a]Belgium (199 cases) and Spain (133 cases).

**Table 49.4** Proportion of infectious etiologies causing FUO*

| Cause | Rate (%) |
|---|---|
| Abscess | 28 |
| Mycobacterial | 40 |
| Endocarditis | 12 |
| Urinary tract | 4 |
| Viral | 8 |
| Amebic | 4 |
| Others | <4 |

*Data derived from 193 cases reviewed by Durack (1997).

ditions and delay the diagnosis. While the development of echocardiographic approaches (particularly transesophageal echocardiography) has greatly facilitated the detection of vegetations, both false positives and false negatives may occur. Successfully treated endocarditis is not necessarily accompanied by eradication of vegetations and not all vegetations are infectious in etiology (e.g., the fibrin-platelet thrombi that occur in SLE or other chronic diseases, such as malignancy). Many of the diseases that cause marantic (noninfectious) endocarditis may present as FUOs and mimic an infectious disease.

*Urinary tract infections* (*UTI*), while usually easy to diagnose and treat during their acute presentation (see Chapter 69), may not be appreciated as causes for recurrent or persistent fever when they are chronic, complicate urinary stones, or produce intrarenal or perinephric abscesses. The renal medulla is hyperosmolar and the tissue $pO_2$ levels may be low, both conditions that inhibit effective neutrophil function. When stones are present they constitute a foreign body that provides protection against phagocyte antimicrobial activity. Under each of these conditions localizing symptoms may be minimal and not direct attention to the urinary tract. Surprisingly, in the series of cases of chronic FUO seen at the National Institutes of Health (NIH, see above), chronic UTIs constituted the most frequent infectious cause.

While osteomyelitis is an example of a localized infection that is sheltered from the normal host defenses (see Chapter 78) it is a relatively rare cause of FUO, probably because localizing findings are usually prominent. In adults, vertebral osteomyelitis is the most likely form to present as FUO; localized back pain and tenderness provide clues to its presence, although if there is nerve root involvement with early epidural abscess formation, the pain may radiate in a girdling fashion to the abdomen.

*Chronic viral infections* constitute a small but readily identifiable subset of patients who present with FUO. The classic viruses to do this in developed countries are members of the herpes group (Epstein-Barr virus [EBV], cytomegalovirus [CMV]), HIV, and hepatitis viruses. While the presence of antibodies may prevent new infection with any of these viruses, once infection is established the cellular immune response may result in latent infection after a prolonged time period (EBV and CMV) or may actually contribute to the pathology (e.g., hepatitis B, C?) (see Chapter 62). In the case of HIV the immunosuppressive actions of the virus cripple the immune defenses (see Chapter 99). Acutely, EBV, CMV, and HIV primary infections in normal hosts present as variants of the mononucleosis syndrome (see Chapter 53) with fever, lymphadenopathy, and a mild hepatitis being common features. Modern techniques now readily detect active infection by all of these viruses. It is likely that they will decrease in frequency in the future as a cause of chronic fevers in which the diagnosis is obscure.

*Fungi* are an infrequent cause of FUO in normal hosts because they are usually readily contained by the phagocytic defenses and cellular immunity (see Chapter 6). However, some, notably, *Histoplasma capsulatum* and *Coccidiodes immitis*, may become reactivated at a later time or disseminate. Both may remain latent for years and only reactivate when cellular immunity is suppressed by immunosuppressive therapy or disease. Both of these disorders are sharply localized geographically in the United States but may reactivate under the right conditions when the patient has left the endemic areas. Reactivation or dissemination is also more frequent in persons of Asian or African descent. Lymphocytic meningitis is a characteristic feature of CNS disease. Disseminated histoplasmosis often has profound effects on the bone marrow and may be a cause of pancytopenia. Both of these agents, but particularly histoplasmosis, may mimic disseminated tuberculosis. While disseminated histoplasmosis or coccidiomycosis may occur in immunologically intact hosts, other fungal infections that might cause FUO, such as candidiasis, aspergillosis, and cryptococcosis, are almost always restricted to patients with seriously impaired host defenses.

*Parasitic infections* as a cause for FUO will vary in frequency according to their geographic prevalence. In Africa, Asia, and portions of Central and South America malaria is the most common cause for sustained or recurrent fevers. Other disorders to consider are trypanosomiasis, visceral forms of leishmaniasis, hepatic amebiasis, and fascioliasis. Diagnosis of these diseases should be considered in residents who live in the specific regions or those who give a travel history to the endemic areas (see Chapter 92). In North America and Europe, toxoplasmosis and *Pneumocystis carinii* infection can both present as FUO. Toxoplasmosis can present as a mononucleosis syndrome in seronegative normal individuals who have been exposed to cat feces or who fancy raw meat ingestion. The vast majority of patients with *P. carinii* infection are immunosuppressed by treatment with glucortocicosteroids or have HIV infection, and this diagnosis should be considered in these patient populations, sometimes even when the chest radiograph is normal (see Chapters 87, 100).

## Neoplasms

Neoplasms can cause prolonged fever by two mechanisms. Either they directly produce inflammatory cytokines or they undergo necrosis and secondary inflammation. They can also cause fever because of complicating infections. The most common neoplastic disease to cause fever is *lymphoma*, either Hodgkin's-type or non-Hodgkin's (Table 49.5). These are examples of neoplasms that spontaneously release inflammatory cytokines. The fevers usually occur daily and are unremitting, although a small group of subjects may exhibit a relapsing pattern of several days of increasing fever, followed by a number of afebrile days (Pel-Ebstein fever). *Leukemias* that present as FUO are usually of the nonlymphocytic type and may not have definitive findings on smear, necessitating diagnosis by bone marrow examination. In older adults preleukemic conditions such as the *myelodysplastic syndromes* may rarely have fever as a prominent feature. Most of these patients will have evidence of abnormalities of more than one hematopoietic cell lineage with severe anemia, variable thrombocytopenia, and, usually, neutropenia (rarely neutrophilia) and a variety of morphologic abnormalities involving the different cell lines.

**Table 49.5** Proportion of neoplasms causing FUO*

| Neoplasm | % |
|---|---|
| LYMPHOMA | 41 |
| Non-Hodgkin's | 19 |
| Hodgkin's | 21 |
| LEUKEMIA | 11 |
| OTHER HEMATOLOGIC | 7 |
| SOLID TUMORS | 34 |
| OTHERS | <5 |

*Data derived from 231 cases reviewed by Durack (1997).

**Table 49.6** Collagen-vascular diseases causing FUO*

| Disease | % |
|---|---|
| Still's Disease | 19 |
| Polyarteritis nodosa | 15 |
| SLE | 24 |
| Temporal arteritis/PMR | 16 |
| Rheumatic fever | 10 |
| Others | 15 |

*Data derived from 70 cases reviewed by Durack (1997). SLE = systemic lupus erythematosis, PMR = polymyalgia rheumatica.

Fever may be a presenting feature of certain *solid tumors*, the most heralded being hypernephroma. Even though it is an infrequently reported tumor, in FUO series the frequency of fever as a presenting symptom may be as high as 15% in patients with this neoplasm. Many other solid tumors have been reported as causes of FUO, particularly those of the GI tract, the liver, and, rarely, sarcomas at other sites. There is some debate about the significance of fever associated with cancer. While in most cases fever is associated with metastatic disease, it is clear that fever may occur in the absence of metastases. In one series of patients reported from a European cancer center, the cause for fever as a presenting complaint was due to secondary infection in over half of the patients with malignancy, including some who had leukemias or lymphomas. Last, but not least, *atrial myxoma* is a rare but distinctive tumor that can present with fever along with a number of systemic complaints, including malaise, myalgias, arthralgias, and weight loss. When peripheral embolization and changing murmurs are present together with these other manifestations, these tumors can masquerade as culture negative endocarditis. Echocardiography has been extremely helpful in identifying these tumors.

## Collagen vascular disorders

These immunologically mediated inflammatory disorders are often characterized by primary cytokine dysregulation and secondary vascular inflammation, leading in some cases to tissue infarction or inflammation of serosal and joint surfaces. Any of these phenomena can produce fever which may be a very prominent feature of the illness.

In recent FUO series *adult Still's disease* has been the leading rheumatologic disorder responsible for presenting as FUO (Table 49.6). This is the adult variant of the childhood disease, which is diagnosed clinically by the constellation of recurring febrile episodes (in some cases the fever may be as high as 42°C [107.6°F]), myalgias, arthralgias, arthritis, and leukocytosis. Some patients may have lymphadenopathy, splenomegaly, or pharyngitis. There may be a fleeting salmon-colored rash. Most patients are young and between age 16 and 35. There is no serologic marker for the disease as in other collagen-vascular disorders, and the diagnosis frequently becomes one of exclusion.

Although the diagnosis has been made easier with the profusion of serologic tests for circulating autoantibodies, *SLE* is still an occasional cause of FUO, particularly if it presents atypically. It should be considered in any young woman who has fever, arthralgias, or nondeforming arthritis involving small joints, episodic pleurisy or pericarditis, nephrotic syndrome, coagulation abnormalities, or signs of a cerebral vasculitis and a lymphocytic meningitis.

*Temporal arteritis* and the related disorder, *polymyalgia rheumatica*, two diseases which are almost exclusively seen in patients over the age of 50, have been increasingly identified as a cause for FUO in the elderly. In a recently reported series from Belgium they accounted for 9% of all the cases of FUO. Systemic complaints of persisting fever, myalgias, and weakness, particularly of the shoulder girdle musculature, are prominent features of both disorders. In addition, patients with temporal arteritis will have complaints related to ischemia of the cranial musculature or the scalp. These can include bitemporal headache, scalp tenderness, jaw claudication, and opthalmoplegias. The sedimentation rate is very high, and an inflammatory block anemia is common. The diagnosis is made by temporal artery biopsy, even if the vessels are not palpably abnormal to exam. Most patients respond dramatically to glucocorticosteroid therapy.

Other rarer causes of FUO include polyarteritis nodosa, the mixed cryoglubulinemia syndromes (both complications of either type B or C hepatitis), and polymyositis.

## Miscellaneous

Several broad categories of disease fall into this realm. The mechanisms for fever production can include granulomatous inflammation, vascular inflammation with infarction, drug allergies, and genetic inflammatory disorders. In addition, certain endocrine disorders may cause persistent or recurrent hyperthermic states that are perceived as fevers.

### Granulomatous diseases

These can include *sarcoidosis*, *Wegener's granulomatosis*, *Crohn's disease*, and *granulomatous hepatitis*. Presumably the formation of granulomas to unknown inciting agents represents a variant of the cellular immune response in which type 1 cytokines (interferon $\gamma$, tumor necrosis factor [TNF], interleukin [IL]-1, IL-6), play an important role in the pathogenesis of both the tissue response and fever. When the characteristic pulmonary infiltrates and bilateral hilar adenopathy are present the diagnosis of sarcoidosis is not difficult. Similarly , Crohn's disease typically presents with diarrhea, which may be bloody, and abdominal pain. Occasionally, when the disease is limited to the ileum, diarrhea may not be a prominent feature, abdominal pain and tenderness may be minimal, and fever may appear to be out of proportion to the localizing findings. Wegener's granulomatosis is a granulomatous arteritis which most often is localized to the sinopulmonary tract and presents with recurrent sinusitis, otitis media, and nodular pulmonary infiltrates. Rarely, destruction of the nasal cartilage can give rise to a saddle nose deformity. With more generalized disease a glomerulitis develops that can progress to advanced renal failure. Arthritis may also be a feature. The fever that accompanies Wegener's granulomatosis is often due to superimposed infection in the sinuses or lung, resulting in cavitation and air fluid levels on radiographs. Patients with granulomatous involvement of the liver that is not due to tuberculosis, fungal disease, or lymphoma have made up a surprisingly high percentage of FUO cases in some series (e.g., 6% of the NIH cases of fever prolonged for over 6 mo). Hepatomegaly is variable and the liver is not usually tender. The liver function tests are not strikingly abnormal; moderate to marked elevations of alkaline phosphatase are the most common finding. The diagnosis depends upon finding granulomas on liver biopsy and excluding other causes for hepatic granulomatosis. This disease responds to glucocorticosteroid and immunosuppressant therapy and eventually the patients recover completely.

### Alcohol-related diseases

Two diseases that complicate alcoholism and can give rise to chronic or recurring fevers are *alcoholic hepatitis* and *chronic pancreatitis*. Patients may not readily admit to excessive alcohol intake. With alcoholic hepatitis there is usually tender hepatomegaly and there may be other stigmata of chronic liver disease, such as spider angiomas, palmar erythema, parotid enlargement, and testicular atrophy. Typically, elevations of the aspartase transaminase (AST) are greater than the alanine transaminase (ALT) often by a ratio of more than 2:1. In chronic pancreatitis abdominal findings may not be striking, unless a pseudocyst is present, creating a midepigastric mass, and the amylase levels may be normal. Lipase levels are usually elevated and findings on abdominal CT exam are usually definitive.

### Vascular diseases

The most common vascular disease to cause fever is pulmonary embolization. Short-lived fever is usually, but not always, due to pulmonary infarction, and is seen in about 50% of patients with embolization. True prolonged fevers, falling into the category of FUO, are ususally associated only with multiple pulmonary emboli. Occasionally embolization may be cryptic and recurrent, giving rise to recurrent febrile episodes and ultimately pulmonary hypertension. Episodic dyspnea, pleuritic chest pain, and hemoptysis provide historical clues, and the chest X-ray may disclose areas of atelectasis or enlarged pulmonary arteries. The diagnosis is established by ventilation/perfusion scanning, "spiral" CT scanning, or pulmonary angiography. Fever associated with pulmonary emboli usually remits on heparin therapy. Other vascular causes of cryptic fever include intrabominal or retroperitoneal hematomas, which sometime arise from a contained rupture of an abdominal aneurysm or from aortic dissection.

### Drug fever

A key question to ask any patient with FUO is if they are taking any medication, whether prescribed by a physician, purchased over the counter, or obtained from a friend, relative, or some other source. This query should include health food additives, vitamins, etc. In a susceptible patient, almost any medication may produce an allergic reaction, in which fever may be the only manifestation. Table 49.7 lists the drugs most commonly associated with drug fever. In about 20% of cases there may be other manifestations of allergy, such as rash or eosinophilia. Drug fevers may develop at any time during therapy and can include medications that patients have been taking for years. Furthermore, they may be variable in their presentation and range from persistent low-grade fevers to more dramatic "hectic"-type patterns, or even mimic sepsis with high fever, chills, rigors, and hypotension. The fever usually resolves when the offending drug is discontinued, although it may take 48 to 72 h.

### Hereditary conditions

Recurrent fevers can be a prominent part of certain familial disorders. The most prominent of these is the complex of recurring symptoms seen predominantly in patients of Mediterranean ancestry, known as *familial Mediterranean fever* (*FMF*). Typically this disease has its onset during late childhood or adolescence. Besides fever and leukocytosis the patients have bouts of self-limited serosal inflammation, including peritonitis, or less commonly pleuritis and synovitis. They may undergo abdominal exploratory surgery, where the only finding is a small amount of sterile peritoneal exudate. Severe cases may be complicated by

**Table 49.7** Agents responsible for episodes of drug fever*

| | |
|---|---|
| ANTIMICROBIAL | Naproxyn |
| Penicillins | Tolmetin |
| Cephalosporins | Sulfosalazine |
| Sulfonamides | Corticosteroids |
| Trimethoprim | |
| Tetracyclines | ANTINEOPLASTIC |
| Clindamycin | Asparaginase |
| Chloramphenicol | Azathioprine |
| Macrolides | Bleomycin |
| Aminoglycosides | Cytarabine |
| Nitrofurantoin | Chlorambucil |
| Isoniazid | Daunorubicin |
| Rifampin | Hydroxyurea |
| Para-aminosalicylic acid | 6-Mercaptopurine |
| Pyrazinamide | Streptozocin |
| Amphotericin B | Procarbazine |
| Pentamidine | |
| Pyramethamine | CARDIOVASCULAR |
| Dapsone | $\alpha$-Methyldopa |
| Primaquine | Quinidine |
| Zidovudine | Procainamide |
| Mebendazole | Hydralizine |
| | Nifedipine |
| CENTRAL NERVOUS SYSTEM | Oxprenolol |
| Phenytoin | Atropine |
| Carbemazepine | |
| Phenothiazines | OTHER |
| Haloperidol | Allopurinol |
| Triamterene | Cimetidine |
| Amphetamine | Propylthiouracil |
| Ritalin | Metaclopramide |
| Cocaine | Clofibrate |
| Barbiturates | Iodide |
| | Phenolphthalein |
| ANTIINFLAMMATORY | Interferon |
| Aspirin | Interleukin-2 |
| Ibuprofen | |

*Updated and revised from Mackowiak and LeMaistre. Ann Intern Med 1987;106:728–33.

one of the sequelae of chronic inflammation, amyloidosis, which in turn leads to renal failure. The symptoms can often be aborted or controlled with colchicine therapy. Similar disorders have been seen in patients from northern European countries (e.g., "familial Hibernian fever").

### Endocrine disorders

While not always indicative of true fever, two thyroid disorders may give rise to prolonged fever: *subacute thyroiditis* and *hyperthyroidism.* In both conditions excess production of thyroid hormone can increase the activity of the sodium–potassium ATPase that is universal to all cells and responsible for maintaining intracellular to extracellular gradients of these cations. The heat generated by this activity is responsible for basic thermogenesis (see Chapter 9). In thyroid storm the temperatures reached may be extremely high and threaten survival. The majority of patients with subacute thyroiditis are not hyperthyroid; fever is due to the inflammatory process. While the thyroid may not be tender, it is almost always diffusely enlarged.

Another endocrine disorder that can cause recurrent febrile episodes with diaphoresis is *pheochromocytoma.* During acute discharges of adrenal catechols there is often an accompanying leukocytosis, and in the majority of cases hypertension. The temperature elevation is most likely due to an abrupt increase in metabolic rate and a decrease in heat dissipation due to vasoconstriction. Occasionally *adrenal insufficiency* is associated with fever. This may be due to tuberculous involvement of the adrenals, part of disseminated tuberculosis, or, rarely, be due to the autoimmune process underlying Addison's disease.

### Factitious fever

In this psychiatric disorder, often for unclear reasons, patients manufacture temperature elevations: They manipulate or switch thermometers or they induce infections or inflammation by self-injection of bacteria or other pyrogens. The majority of reported patients have been female, and many are in medical or paramedical professions. When the temperature is artificially elevated (made much more difficult in medical settings by the advent of electronic thermometry) there is a disparity between the physical examination and the recorded temperatures. The patients appear normal, the skin is cool, and there is not the usual tachycardia seen in most patients with fever. An important subgroup in this category are children and adolescents who have school phobias. Patients who self-inject or self-mutilate will often give a long history of repetitive medical care for similar conditions and may have abscesses in easily accessible locations, disturbed wound dressings, or other signs of self manipulation. Many of these patients have major psychopathology which may be unmasked when confronted with their behavior and role in their disease. This syndrome is very refractory to psychotherapy. Usually when confronted with their decption, patients sign out of the hospital, leave their physician's care, and often end up in another location with similar symptoms and signs.

### Habitual hyperthermia

This is not a febrile illness or a disease. It is a condition that is usually seen in children or young adults and represents an extreme of normal swings in the circadian temperature rhythm (see Chapter 9), or in some cases exercise-induced or postovulation hyperthermia. The patients grow and develop normally and have no abnormal physical or laboratory findings. Patients who fit this general description constituted a sizable subgroup of those admitted to the NIH with FUO for over 6 mo. Perhaps because of the occasional relationship to ovulation, women are more frequently identified with this condition than men.

## Evaluation and Diagnosis of FUO

While the original working definition of classical FUO included a period of observation and evaluation while in the hospital, many diagnostic studies can now be carried out in the ambulatory setting. The need for hospitalization should depend mainly upon the pace of the disease and the severity of illness. A period of hospitalization can be useful to document the presence of fever and its pattern and may facilitate organizing the evaluation, particularly where multiple procedures and consultants are involved. There are certain logical steps that can be taken in the workup of any patient with FUO. However, it is difficult to come up with a precise algorithm that will account for a myriad of possibilities and branch points given the array of diseases that may be responsible.

Before embarking on what may be a time-consuming and expensive series of diagnostic tests and procedures it is extremely important to review the list of medications that a patient might be receiving for other medical conditions and to discontinue all nonessential ones, in particular if they have a track record of causing drug fever as part of a hypersensitivity response (see Table 49.7). If continued treatment of a medical condition is necessary, then switching to a structurally unrelated drug with similar actions is warranted. Most drug fevers will disappear within 48–72 h, which in many cases can serve as an appropriate waiting period before going on to more tests.

## History and physical examination

Perhaps more than in most other medical conditions, the carefully performed history and physical examination plays a major role in documenting the nature of the problem and in providing important diagnostic clues that can direct the remainder of the investigations. The initial objective is to characterize the nature of the presenting illness and the important host and epidemiologic factors that must be considered. It also usually takes repeated exposure to the patient to tease out further historical information or to document important features or changes in the physical examination.

### History

Not only should the characteristics of the febrile pattern be clarified, but the extent of involvement of the various organ systems should be rigorously assessed by a careful review of systems. Ascertaining any important previous medical conditions or those being managed currently as well as major trauma and surgeries will help to determine if there is any predisposition to specific infections, malignancies, or inflammatory disorders. With young people in particular the immunization history should be reviewed and the results of previous tuberculin testing should be determined. A careful recording of medications, health additives, and dietary habits is essential, particularly regarding potential allergens or dietary sources for infection. Other epidemiologic points include recent or remote travel, residence in endemic areas for certain infectious diseases, and exposure to animals or ill people, such as previous contact with tuberculosis in family members or housemates. A detailed occupational and recreational history can detect the presence of any unique exposures. These should include sexual contacts and habits as well as the use of alcohol or illicit drugs.

### Physical examination

Particular attention should be paid to documenting that fever is actually present. When determining fever, the temperature should be taken at least four to six times in a 24 h period. Twice-daily temperatures are insufficient in assessing FUO. While there is not a good general correlation between febrile characteristics and specific diseases due to considerable variation and the common use of antipyretics, at times the febrile pattern may be useful in suggesting a particular diagnosis (e.g., the tertian fever pattern of vivax malaria).

The examiner should ask him or herself a series of questions that often reveal the source of the problem. They include: What other changes in vital signs accompany the fever? Is there a tachycardia? Blood pressure or respiratory pattern changes? Does the patient have evidence of weight loss? Muscle wasting? Are there any skin lesions? Lymphadenopathy? Is there evidence of hearing loss or otitis media? Sinusitis? Dental caries? Mouth ulcers or other lesions? Is the thyroid gland enlarged or tender? Are there abnormalities on chest or rib examination? Cardiac murmurs? Is there enlargement of the liver or spleen? Abdominal tenderness? Masses? Is the prostate enlarged or tender? Is there uterine enlargement? Adnexal tenderness or masses? Are the joints tender or swollen? Is there any muscle tenderness or weakness? Are there changes in mental status or focal neurologic abnormalities? The answers to these questions during physical examination can help target the subsequent evaluation.

## Laboratory and imaging studies

The purpose of the initial studies is to determine if an inflammatory process is present, to localize any organ system abnormalities, and to screen for systemic infection. The initial blood studies should include a complete blood count, evaluation of total protein and albumin, liver function tests, thyroid functions, measurement of the erythrocyte sedimentation rate (ESR), performance of blood cultures, urinalysis and urine culture, and chest radiograph. An intermediate-strength purified protein derivative (PPD) should be placed along with appropriate controls to detect anergy in the case of a negative reaction (see Chapter 11). Usually individuals who give a history of strongly positive PPD reactions should not be tested unless they are being evaluated for possible anergy.

More than 90% of patients with endocarditis will have positive blood cultures if two sets are obtained, and >95% with three sets (see Chapter 66). The only reason to extend the number beyond three is if the patient has received antibiotic therapy in the preceding 48 h. Then, obtaining the third and perhaps a fourth culture at least 24 to 48 h after discontinuing therapy is reasonable. In patients who have prosthetic valves, endocarditis caused by coagulase-negative staphylococci may give rise to an intermittent bacteremia and justify obtaining more cultures if the original ones are negative. If the cultures are negative at 24 to 48 h and the index of suspicion for endocarditis is high, the laboratory should be notified to look for fastidious organisms by staining a sample of the cultures and holding them for up to several weeks. Analysis using lysis centrifugation may also help to reveal fastidious pathogens (see Chapter 16).

An ESR in excess of 100 mm/h suggests a major systemic disease, which could be in any of the major FUO categories. ESR values in the moderately elevated range (20–40) are found commonly in FUO series, particularly in the elderly, and have little diagnostic utility. Normal ESR values usually are incompatible with most collagen vascular diseases, and in the case of prolonged fever should suggest a thermoregulatory cause or even factitious fever.

Beyond the screening chest radiograph the only other radiological test that should be considered for routine use in the evaluation of FUO is the abdominal CT scan (see Chapter 12). This is particularly true in any patient where there is a suggestion of intraabdominal pathology or in elderly patients in whom intraabdominal problems (abscesses, tumors, aneurysms) make up a high percentage of FUOs. Besides identifying the cause for fever the CT scan findings can help identify the site for invasive procedures such as percutaneous needle biopsy, aspiration or catheter placement, laparoscopy, or, in rare instances, laparatomy to firmly establish the diagnosis and in some cases initiate therapy.

Unless the patient is acutely or severely ill or debilitated and requires hospitalization most of these studies can be conducted in the outpatient setting. At their conclusion the clinician is frequently able to decide on a further course of action involving more diagnostic procedures or in some cases specific therapy.

## Special tests

While the precise selection of further diagnostic tests or procedures should be guided by the results of the initial evaluation, certain approaches have frequently been used in the evaluation of patients with FUO.

### Radionuclide scanning

Various scanning techniques have been employed to detect sites of inflammation or possible neoplasms, but in general, they have not served a useful purpose in revealing information beyond that disclosed by CT scanning (see Chapter 12). Magnetic resonance imaging (MRI) may occasionally reveal brain lesions that are not well defined by CT scanning (particularly useful in AIDS patients with CNS toxoplasmosis or white matter disease). Usually some aspect of the initial evaluation will suggest intracranial disease, justifying brain CT and perhaps MRI scanning. MRI may also be helpful in defining lesions affecting vertebral bodies, the spinal cord, and adjacent soft tissues (e.g., epidural abscess or neoplasms). Gallium-67 scintigraphy can reveal inflammation or certain neoplasms; however, there are abundant examples of false-negative and -positive studies, and the nonspecific retention of the isotope in the bowel has made its utility for intraabdominal evaluation difficult. Indium-111 leukocyte scanning is restricted to detecting sites of pus; its major utility is in the evaluation of postoperative sites, and occasionally areas of osteomyelitis with surrounding soft-tissue inflammation. Both false negatives and positives have been reported when it has been used randomly in evaluations of FUO. Bone scanning with technetium-99 can detect cryptic sites of osteomyelitis or bone metastases. However, these may be difficult to differentiate from old fractures. In any case, with any of these scanning techniques, areas of abnormal or increased activity should focus further exploratory studies to define their nature.

### Tissue biopsies

Usually these will be guided by preliminary data that suggest abnormalities in the sites in question. In up to 15% of FUO cases, however, biopsies of the bone marrow or liver have been useful in providing specific diagnostic information, even in the absence of hematologic or liver function abnormalities or hepatic enlargement. This seems to be a feature of diseases that cause granuloma formation in either of these organs. In the elderly patient with FUO, particularly if anemia and marked elevation of the ESR are present, biopsies of the temporal arteries may disclose evidence of giant cell arteritis, even in the absence of palpable enlargement or tenderness of the vessels. Biopsies of enlarged or abnormal lymph nodes (CT guided in the abdomen or via mediastinoscopy in the thorax) should be vigorously pursued as a way to establish a diagnosis of infection or neoplasm at these sites.

### Exploratory laparotomy

In older reports it was possible to make a specific diagnosis of FUO in up to 60% of cases by exploratory laparotomy, even without striking findings that pointed to intraabdominal pathology. The need for this approach and the definition of which patients might benefit diagnostically have been greatly modified by the advent of CT scanning. Furthermore, laparoscopy can now often provide the same information about the status of the peritoneum, lymph nodes, and organs from which biopsies can be obtained with less morbidity than laparotomy. In the vast majority of patients who have absolutely no evidence of intraabdominal pathology by organ function tests or CT scanning, laparotomy is not indicated because of the low diagnostic yield and morbidity and expense of the procedure. If laparotomy for FUO is carried out, the attending or consulting physician should be present to be sure that the proper specimens and cultures are taken.

## Therapeutic trials

In about 5 to 15% of cases a precise diagnosis for FUO is not made with the initial studies, even when they are extensive. The clinician then faces a decision about whether to continue to observe the patient without therapeutic intervention or to conduct a careful therapeutic trial with either an antibiotic or antiinflammatory agent. If the patient is stable clinically, has no evidence of a major life-threatening disease process (e.g., weight loss), and has not shown any deterioration over several weeks of observation, it is probably best to do nothing except to offer supportive care and to reevaluate the patient periodically for changes in physical signs or laboratory findings. The longer that a patient shows a stable clinical pattern, the less likely he is to have a cryptic infection or a neoplasm and the more likely there is spontaneous resolution of the fever. If the fever resolves spontaneously during an ill-conceived therapeutic trial it is likely that this will be misinterpreted as a response to treatment, resulting in unnecessary and sometimes dangerous prolongation of treatment. Most antiinflammatory drugs, in particular glucocorticosteroids, are potent antipyretics, and may suppress fever without changing the course of a disease. Their use may have the undesirable effect of lulling the physician and the patient into a sense of false security, reducing the level of surveillance needed to establish the proper diagnosis and exposing the patient to unwanted drug toxicities.

In patients who appear to be actively deteriorating during the evaluation process, a well-targeted therapeutic trial can be justified. A good example is a patient who has disseminated, cryptic tuberculosis and who often has cutaneous anergy. With this disease it may take weeks for diagnostic specimens to be culture positive. Given this delay and the high mortality rate, without prompt effective therapy a trial of optimum multidrug treatment can be justified once the appropriate diagnostic specimens are obtained (see Chapters 37, 57). In this setting almost half of patients will remain febrile for over 2 wk, and it may take a month for defervescence to occur. In contrast to the situation with tuberculosis, blind broad spectrum antibiotic trials for febrile patients should not be undertaken unless there is good diagnostic evidence for culture-negative endocarditis or systemic infection with some other fastidious organism. In each of these situations an appropriate antibiotic regimen can be designed (see, e.g., chapter 66), and treatment should be given for a sufficient period of time (at least 2 wk) to allow a therapeutic response to occur.

Two conditions that may produce little in the way of specific diagnostic pathology are Still's disease in young adults and polymyalgia rheumatica (PMR) in elderly individuals. In both conditions the diagnosis is often made clinically (see above) and is usually accompanied by nonspecific evidence of inflammation ( inflammatory block anemia and elevated ESR). In the case of Still's disease there may be a dramatic response to treatment with nonsteroidal antiinflammatory agents and in PMR patients to low dose glucocorticosteroids. In both conditions there should be solid evidence of a response to treatment as early as 1 week after the drugs are given. Evidence for such a response is defervescence, improvement in systemic symptoms, a fall in the ESR, and a resolution of the anemia. Without these expected changes it becomes fruitless to continue treatment or increase the dosage level of treatment without running the risk of substantial toxicity or obfuscation of the true nature of the cause for the FUO.

While cautious observation with frequent reevaluation is an acceptable approach in the clinically stable patient, in those who progress rapidly to a critical illness, both the tempo of the evaluation and the need to intervene with potentially curative therapy become much more urgent. Under these conditions obtaining all the necessary diagnostic specimens before initiating potentially obscuring broad-spectrum antibiotic or antiinflammatory therapy is important. Often the nature of an offending pathogen or a specific vasculitic process can be discovered even after treatment has been instituted, allowing the therapeutic approach it to made more specific.

## FUO in Special Groups

Besides patients with "classical" FUO, several other categories of patients with fever in whom the diagnosis is not immediately apparent have been proposed as deserving special attention. The importance of these categories is highlighted by the fact that they are much more frequently encountered in clinical practice than classical FUO patients. These include patients who have what has been labeled as *nosocomial FUO*, *neutropenic FUO*, or *HIV-associated FUO*. Definitions for these groups in comparison to classical FUO are given in Table 49.1.

## Nosocomial FUO

Patients in this group are hospitalized; most have significant underlying disorders which led to hospitalization and, often complex, treatment. The combination of the hospital environment (e.g., ICU), the selective pressure of previous or ongoing antibiotic therapy, the alteration of the host defenses by various intravenous lines and invasive procedures, and the immunosuppressive effects of underlying diseases or therapy set the stage for potentially unique infectious complications. These can entail significant morbidity, prolonging the hospitalization and its attendant costs. When sepsis results (see Chapter 50) the mortality may be considerable. Besides bacterial and opportunistic fungal infections, prominent causes for fever include tissue injury or infarction and febrile drug reactions. If no infectious agent is isolated or another cause for fever is not defined within 3 d, then the patient is defined as having a *nosocomial FUO*. A detailed consideration of the pathogenesis and etiologies for infection and fever in hospitalized patients, including those with nosocomial FUO, is presented in Chapter 48.

## Neutropenic FUO

This entity refers to the problem of undiagnosed fever in patients who have severe neutropenia. In clinical practice the majority of patients with this entity will have received recent cytotoxic and immunosuppressive therapy for their underlying diseases. The diseases or treatment may also produce a broad alteration in the host defenses in addition to neutropenia. Less frequent causes for neutropenia include drug reactions, coexistent disease (e.g., HIV infection), and various congenital disorders. Regardless of the cause, complicating infections are not commonly seen until the circulating neutrophil counts fall below 1000/$\mu$l. Bacteria are the most frequent species causing acute infection with fever in these patients, and deterioration may be rapid. For these reasons, broad spectrum antibiotic treatment is routinely given empirically to febrile neutropenic patients after obtaining the appropriate initial cultures. If no pathogens have been isolated and the patient is still febrile after 3 d of treatment then the patient is determined to have a *neutropenic FUO*. Chapter 86 outlines the approach to be taken in these patients and includes the various diagnostic and therapeutic options. The problems imposed by infection that may complicate neutropenia in patients with solid organ or bone marrow transplantation are also discussed in Chapters 87 and 88, respectively.

## HIV-associated FUO

Fever is one of the most common symptoms experienced by HIV-infected patients and can occur at any stage of the disease. Fever may be due to the disease itself, or, more commonly, to a broad variety of complicating infections, neoplasms, or drug reactions. When fever has persisted for more than 4 wk as an outpatient or 3 d in the hospital without a defining diagnosis, this is termed *HIV-associated FUO*. The most likely causes vary according to the stage of disease and the nature of the treatment that the patient is receiving. The problem of HIV-associated FUO is discussed in detail in Chapter 100.

## ANNOTATED BIBLIOGRAPHY


Arnow PM, Flaherty JP. Fever of unknown origin. Lancet 1997; 350:575–580.
*An up-to-date review of the subject.*

Bayard PJ, Berger TG, Jacobson MA. Drug hypersensitivity reactions and human immunodeficiency virus disease. J Acquir Immunodefic Syndr 1992; 5:1237–1257.
*This article points out the high frequency of drug reactions in patients with HIV infection including fever.*

Bissuel P, Leport C, Perronne C et al. Fever of unknown origin in HIV-infected patients: a critical analysis of a retrospective series of 57 patients. J Int Med 1994; 236:529–535.
*Twenty-one percent of 270 patients with HIV infection hospitalized in a Paris hospital had FUO. An etiology was found in 86% of cases, with mycobacterial infections accounting for the majority. Liver biopsy helpful in making a specific diagnosis.*

Durack DT. Fever of unknown origin. In: Fever: Basic Mechanisms and Management, 2nd ed. Mackowiak P, ed. Lippincott-Raven, Philadelphia, PA, p. 237, 1997.
*A thorough and well-referenced review of concepts, etiologies, and evaluation of patients with FUO.*

Durack DT, Street AC. Fever of unknown origin—reexamined and redefined. Curr Clin Topics Infect Dis 1991; 11:35–51.
*The authors expand the concept of FUO beyond the original "classical" definition proposed by Beeson and Petersdorf in 1960 to include patients who are in the hospital (noscomial FUO), those who are neutropenic (neutropenic FUO), and those who have HIV infection (HIV-associated FUO). This is a useful way of categorizing patients in different settings on the basis of likely etiologies and a directed workup.*

Engels E, Marks PW, Kazanjian P. Usefulness of bone marrow examination in the evaluation of unexplained fevers in patients infected with the human immunodeficiciency virus. Clin Inf Dis 1995; 21:427–428.
*Thirty-two percent of 65 HIV-infected patients with prolonged fevers had a diagnosis made by bone marrow biopsy. Mycobacteria were the most frequent cause for fever.*

Hirschmann JW. Fever of unknown origin. Clin Infect Dis 1997; 24:291–302.
*A "state-of-the-art" article which reviews recent literature on etiologies, diagnostic approaches, and management of patients with classical FUO.*

Iikuni Y, Okada J, Kondo H, Kashiwazaki S. Current fever of unknown origin 1982–1992. Intern Med 1994; 33:67–73.
*A thorough review of the Japanese experience, contrasting it with other geographic areas in the world.*

Knockaert DC, Vanneste LJ, Bobbaers HJ. Fever of unknown origin in elderly patients. J Am Geriatr Soc 1993; 41:1187–1192.
*A subgroup of 47 elderly patients is described from a larger 199-patient study in Belgium. The elderly patients were more likely to have malignancies or multisystem diseases responsible for FUO.*

Mackowiak PA, LeMaistre CF. Drug fever: a critical appraisal of conventional concepts. An analysis of 51 episodes in two Dallas hospitals and 97 episodes reported in the English literature. Ann Int Med 1987; 106:728–733.
*A nice study which classifies drugs most likely to be associated with causing fever as an idiosyncratic or clearly allergic response during therapy. Most drug fevers were noted to resolve within 72 h of stopping the offending agent.*

Miller WC, Durack DT. FUO: a rational diagnostic approach. Hosp Med 1994; 30:49–56.
*Using the Durack classification system, the most likely etiologies for FUOs are reviewed and a logical cost-effective diagnostic approach is outlined.*

# 50

## Bacteremia, Sepsis, and Septic Shock

GIORGIO ZANETTI, JEAN-DANIEL BAUMGARTNER,
AND MICHEL-PIERRE GLAUSER

For almost every type of infection, there is a continuous spectrum ranging from purely local manifestations to severe systemic involvement with multiple organ dysfunction and shock. Most systemic symptoms of infections are not due to the proliferation of bacteria themselves but to inflammatory reactions triggered by the infectious process. A paradox of the defense against infection is that the same inflammatory systems responsible for defending against microbial invasion may produce severe local and/or systemic symptoms when they are activated excessively. The administration of antibiotics, together with surgical procedures when needed, remains the cornerstone of the treatment of sepsis. Antibiotics can kill bacteria, but they do not inhibit bacterial and host mediators. Modern antibiotics are characterized by broad spectra of antibacterial activities and by powerful bactericidal effects. Patients may thus survive infections that are more severe and last longer than seen before, so some of these patients may develop septic shock and multiple organ dysfunction. The need to develop effective new adjunctive therapies against sepsis is thus a major challenge to modern medicine.

Clinicians have been confused by the imprecise nature of the definitions generally used to describe the systemic manifestations observed during infections. In an effort to clearly define the roles of various new strategies for septic shock, a standardization of these definitions has been recently attempted by a consensus conference of the American College of Chest Physicians and the Society of Critical Care Medicine (Table 50.1). To describe systemic responses to inflammatory processes, regardless of their etiology, a *systemic inflammatory response syndrome* (*SIRS*) was defined. SIRS may be provoked as well by noninfectious diseases such as pancreatitis or postoperative inflammatory processes. The other definitions proposed by the consensus conference allow a classification of the systemic responses to infection according to their severity (*sepsis*, *severe sepsis*, *septic shock*). However, they also designate nonspecific symptoms which may be due to broadly different infections, which extend from meningococcal purpura fulminans to necrotizing fasciitis, peritonitis, nosocomial pneumonia, and pyelonephritis. In addition, these definitions do not take into account the fact that the consequences of septic shock in a patient with pyelonephritis are certainly not as severe as those in a patient with nosocomial pneumonia, for instance, demonstrating the importance of the primary focus of infection. Thus, these criteria of sepsis or septic shock have not been accepted by some experts. They should be used as an adjunct to the microbiological and clinical diagnosis of infection but should not be the sole criteria for describing patients' illnesses.

*Bacteremia* is defined as the presence of viable bacteria in the blood as demonstrated by positive blood cultures. This is not a clinical definition. Indeed, bacteria may circulate without inducing a detectable response. On the other hand, the most severe septic shock may be present without detectable circulating bacteria. Thus, bacteremia and sepsis are different entities which overlap only partially. The term *septicemia* was sometimes used to describe the presence of severe clinical manifestations in a bacteremic patient. However, this term was considered to be largely dependent on subjective interpretation, and its use was not recommended by the consensus conference of the American College of Chest Physicians and the Society of Critical Care Medicine.

### Epidemiology

Symptomatic bacteremia was recently estimated to occur in one in 100 patients in tertiary care hospitals, leading in the United States to a total of between 70,000 and 400,000 patients with documented bacteremia per year. Moreover, the true incidence of bacteremia is probably underestimated because blood cultures are not always performed in clinical circumstances where bacteria could be found in blood, particularly in outpatients.

The true epidemiology of sepsis and septic shock is unknown because these entities are defined by clinical features and not by laboratory values. Thus, establishing precise epidemiologic data would require large-scale prospective studies. One indirect way to estimate their frequency is to look at patients with documented bacteremia. On the one hand, it is known that 27% to 62% of bacteremic patients develop severe sepsis or septic shock. On the other hand, about half of the patients with severe sepsis or septic shock are bacteremic. Based on these figures and on the analysis of frequency of sepsis or septic shock in particular settings, such as intensive care units and teaching hospitals, the incidence of sepsis has been estimated to increase gradually over the last several decades from 0.75 cases per 1000 admissions in 1951 to about 14 in 1993; the Center for Disease Control in Atlanta reported an incidence of 73.6 cases for 100,000 patients per year in 1979 and of 176 cases in 1987. Sepsis now represents the 13th cause of mortality in the United States. It is the most common cause of death in intensive care units.

The increase in the frequency of bacteremia, sepsis and septic shock is due to multiple factors. A rise of gram-negative sepsis followed the introduction of antibiotics of the first generation, which were more active on gram-positive than on gram-negative bacteria. In more recent years concommitant with improved antibiotic activity against gram-negative bacteria, gram-positive organisms are increasing in frequency as a cause of severe sepsis and septic shock. Other factors undoubtedly play a major role in the increased rate of sepsis; they include more aggressive surgical interventions, widespread use of invasive procedures and de-

**Table 50.1** Definitions of severity of response to infections (Consensus Conference of the American College of Chest Physicians and the Society of Critical Care Medicine, 1992)*

| Term | Definition | Comments |
|---|---|---|
| Bacteremia | Presence of viable bacteria in the blood | May be accompanied or not by symptoms |
| Systemic inflammatory response syndrome (SIRS) | Two or more of the following conditions:<br>• temperature >38°C or <36°C<br>• heart rate >90 per minute<br>• respiratory rate >20 per minute or $PaCO_2$ <32 mm Hg<br>• white blood cell count >12 G/L or <4 G/L or >10% immature forms | The SIRS was included in the original consensus, but has remained controversial in the U.S. and is not accepted by a panel of experts in Europe, because of its lack of specificity |
| Sepsis | Same as SIRS, with evidence of infection | Also called sepsis syndrome |
| Severe sepsis | Sepsis associated with at least one organ dysfunction (hypoxemia, oliguria, acute alteration in mental status . . .), lactic acidosis, coagulation abnormalities, or hypotension not due to another cause | |
| Septic shock | Severe sepsis with hypotension despite adequate fluid resuscitation (systolic blood pressure <90 mmHg or reduction of >40 mmHg from baseline) | |

*Source: The ACCP/SCCM Consensus Conference Committee. Definitions for sepsis and organ failure and guidelines for the use of innovative therapies in sepsis. Chest 1992; 101: 1644–1655. Used with permission.

vices, a growing population of patients with serious underlying diseases, especially in intensive care units, greater use of immunosuppressive therapy for organ transplant recipients, and radiation and chemotherapy for patients with malignancies.

## Etiology

Data on the microbiological etiologies of sepsis and septic shock are often biased because numerous studies addressed patient populations selected for their likelihood of being infected by organisms to which a treatment was targeted, such as gram-negative bacteria. Table 50.2 shows data from three studies aimed at treating sepsis and septic shock whatever the causative organism. In blood cultures, gram-negative organisms were recovered from 57% to 64% of the cases and gram-positive organisms from 35% to 40%, with a few cases of mixed infections or fungemias. For cultures taken from the local sites of infections, the proportion of gram-negative to gram-positive bacteria remained similar (3:2), but the number of mixed infections was much higher. In the most recent studies, the number of cases of sepsis due to fungal infections increased, reaching a proportion of 5% to 10% of the cases. Parasitic or viral infections may also occasionally be responsible for clinical pictures of sepsis or septic shock.

## Host Factors

Sepsis or septic shock may occur in patients without underlying disease. In this case, highly virulent organisms, such as meningococci, are most often responsible, or alternatively, sepsis occurs during infections which are inadequately treated, such as urinary tract infections or pneumonias. However, most cases of sepsis or septic shock occur in patients with underlying conditions which make them more susceptible to infections, such as lesions of an anatomical barrier, multiple trauma or burns, malignancies, renal or hepatic failure, diabetes, splenectomy, drug abuse, AIDS, and chemotherapies. Table 50.3 shows the most prevalent underlying conditions reported in two large studies of sepsis and septic shock. Of note, neutropenia is a predisposing condition to sepsis but not not to septic shock, since less than 2% of febrile episodes in neutropenic patients are complicated by shock if they are promptly treated with antibiotics.

## Pathogenesis of Sepsis and Septic Shock

Sepsis results from the activation of inflammatory systems by bacterial components. Initial studies concentrated on the interactions of lipopolysaccharide (LPS, also called endotoxin), a component of the gram-negative cell wall, with various humoral pathways. It is now recognized that exotoxins and other cell wall components are also potent activators of inflammatory mediators and that macrophages and other cells involved in inflammatory processes may play an even more important role than humoral pathways.

### Bacterial components and sepsis

The prime initiator of *gram-negative bacterial sepsis* is endotoxin, an LPS component of the bacterial outer membrane. The outermost part of the endotoxin molecule consists of a series of structurally and antigenically diverse oligosaccharides that are responsible for the O serotypes of gram-negative bacteria (Figure 50.1). Internal to the O-side chains are the core oligosaccharides, which have similarities among groups of bacteria. Lipid A, which

**Table 50.2** Microbiological documentation in three large studies of sepsis and septic shock

| Characteristic | Veterans administration[a] | Bone et al.[b] | Fisher et al.[c] |
|---|---|---|---|
| TOTAL NUMBER OF PATIENTS | 223 | 382 | 893 |
| NO. OF PATIENTS (%) WITH SHOCK | 100 (*45*) | 148 (*39*) | 714 (*80*) |
| NO. OF PATIENTS (%) WITH: | | | |
| • Positive blood culture | 107 (*48*) | 179 (*49*) | *N.R.*[d] |
| • Microbiologically documented focal infection | *N.R.* | *N.R.* | 718 (*80*) |
| NO. OF SPECIES (%) GROWN: | | | |
| • Gram-positive bacteria | 36[e] (*40*) | 59[e] (*35*) | 413[f] (*46*) |
| • Gram-negative bacteria | 51[e] (*57*) | 115[e] (*64*) | 491[f] (*55*) |
| • Fungi | 3[e] (*3*) | 5[e] (*3*) | 68 (*9*) |

[a]Veterans Administration Systemic Sepsis Cooperative Study Group. Effects of high-dose glucocorticoid therapy on mortality in patients with clinical signs of systemic sepsis. N Engl J Med 1987; 317:659–665.

[b]Bone RC, Fisher CJ, Clemmer TP et al. A controlled clinical trial of high-dose methylprednisolone in the treatment of severe sepsis and septic shock. N Engl J Med 1987; 317:653–658.

[c]Fisher CJ, Dhainaut JF, Opal SM et al. Recombinant human Interleukin 1 receptor antagonist in the treatment of patients with sepsis syndrome. JAMA 1994; 271:1836–1843.

[d]N.R.: not reported.

[e]Only the organisms cultured in blood at study entry were reported.

[f]Among whom 254 cultures grew both gram-positive and gram-negative bacteria.

is bound to the core oligosaccharide, has a highly conserved structure and is responsible for most of the toxicity of endotoxin. Endotoxin circulating in the blood appears to be a predictor of poor outcome in some clinical settings such as meningococcemia, but the levels of endotoxin required to trigger the cascade of events in sepsis may vary greatly. Indeed it has been observed that bacterial products other than LPS may profondly increase the host's sensitivity to endotoxin, thereby rendering toxic otherwise harmless levels. Hence, the measurement of endotoxin has not become standard clinical practice.

In *sepsis due to organisms other than gram-negative bacteria*, the triggering agents have not been studied to the same extent. The exotoxins produced by some bacteria can initiate sepsis and septic shock. Some of these exotoxins produce a peculiar form of septic shock, called toxic shock syndrome (TSS). TSS is characterized by fever, desquamative skin rash, hypotension, vomiting and diarrhea, and multisystem involvement. It is triggered by several exotoxins of *Staphylococcus aureus* (including TSS toxin-1 and enterotoxins, mainly of the B and C serotypes) and of *Streptococcus pyogenes*. These 20–30 kDa polypeptides belong to the family of superantigen molecules, which are able to bind class ll major histocompatibility complex on antigen-presenting cells and the $V_\beta$ region of the T cell receptor, resulting in non-antigen-restricted stimulation of T cells with production of cytokines (see Chapter 10). In addition to the effects of exotoxins, bacteria themselves—and in particular some of their cell wall components—are potent activators of numerous humoral or cellular pathways. Mannan, a major cell wall component of some fungi, can also trigger sepsis responses.

**Table 50.3** Underlying conditions in two studies of sepsis and septic shock

| Reference | Bone et al.[a] | Fischer et al.[b] |
|---|---|---|
| NUMBER OF PATIENTS | 382 | 893 |
| MEAN AGE (YR) | 536 | 578 |
| NO. OF UNDERLYING CONDITIONS (%) | | |
| None | 7 (*2*) | Not given |
| Cancer | 71 (*19*) | 159 (*18*) |
| Diabetes | 10 (*3*) | 155 (*17*) |
| Pulmonary Disease | 17 (*4*) | 138 (*15*) |
| Renal Disease | 12 (*3*) | 70 (*8*) |
| Other Medical Condition[c] | 99 (*26*) | 291 (*33*) |
| Trauma | 44 (*12*) | 137 (*15*) |
| Recent Surgery | N.R. | 497 (*56*) |

[a]Bone RC, Fisher CJ, Clemmer TP et al. A controlled clinical trial of high-dose methylprednisolone in the treatment of severe sepsis and septic shock. N Engl J Med 1987; 317:653–658.

[b]Fisher CJ, Dhainaut JF, Opal SM et al. Recombinant human Interleukin 1 receptor antagonist in the treatment of patients with sepsis syndrome. JAMA 1994; 271:1836–1843.

[c]Included cardiovascular diseases, hepatic failure, pancreatitis, neurologic diseases, alcohol abuse, intravenous drug abuse.

## Interactions of bacterial cell wall components with humoral pathways

Bacterial cell wall components can directly activate the complement system, the coagulation/ fibrinolysis system, and the kallikrein/bradykinin system (Fig. 50.2). These humoral systems can also be indirectly activated following the activation of cellular targets (see next paragraph).

Both the *alternative* and the *classic complement pathways* can be activated by LPS and gram-positive bacterial cell wall components. The classic pathway is activated mainly by complexes of cell wall components and antibodies, whereas the alternative

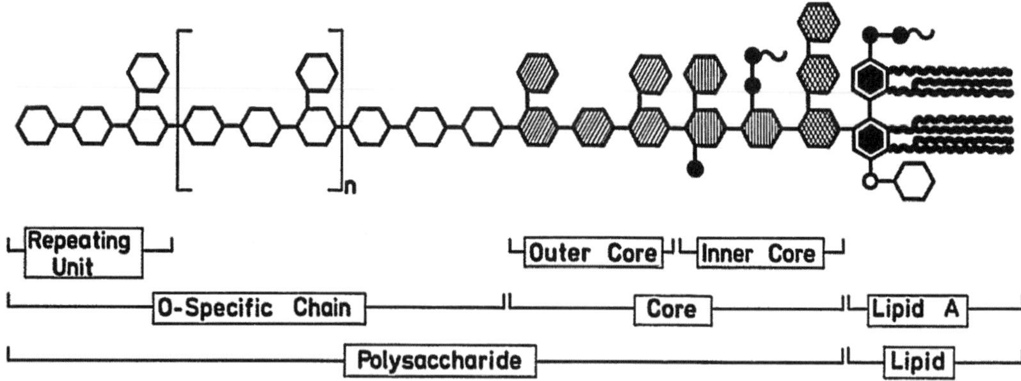


**Fig. 50.1** Diagrammatic representation of the structure of endotoxin.

pathway is activated through direct interactions with cell wall components. The anaphylatoxins $C_{3a}$ and $C_{5a}$, produced as a result of activation of these pathways, induce vasodilatation and increased vascular permeability, resulting in hemodynamic changes and aggregation of platelets; in addition, $C_{5a}$ is a potent chemotactic agent which provokes an aggregation and activation of neutrophils. All these processes have been implicated in the pathogenesis of the adult respiratory distress syndrome. Levels of free $C_{5a}$ have been directly associated with TNF and LPS levels in hemorrhagic necrosis of the gut observed in some experimental models of sepis. An increased concentration of activated complement has been associated with a fatal outcome in septic shock of both gram-positive and gram-negative origin.

The *coagulation cascade* has long been known to play a central role in the pathogenesis of septic shock. The contact system is activated directly when factor XII (Hageman factor) comes in contact with negatively charged surfaces, such as peptidoglycan residues and teichoic acid from the cell wall of gram-positive organisms, or LPS from gram-negative bacilli. Activated factor XII activates factor XI which in turn triggers the production of tissue factor by the intrinsic coagulation pathway and by endothelial cells and macrophages. Activation of tissue factor in turn activates the extrinsic coagulation pathway. Tissue factor is also produced by the stimulation of macrophages and endothelial cells by LPS or other cell wall components. The activation of these pathways leads to activation of *fibrinolysis*, thus resulting in consumption of coagulation factors and disseminated intravascular coagulation (DIC). The fact that tissue factor plays a major role in inducing DIC is indicated by the prevention of LPS-induced DIC by antibody to tissue factor in animals. Evidence also ex-

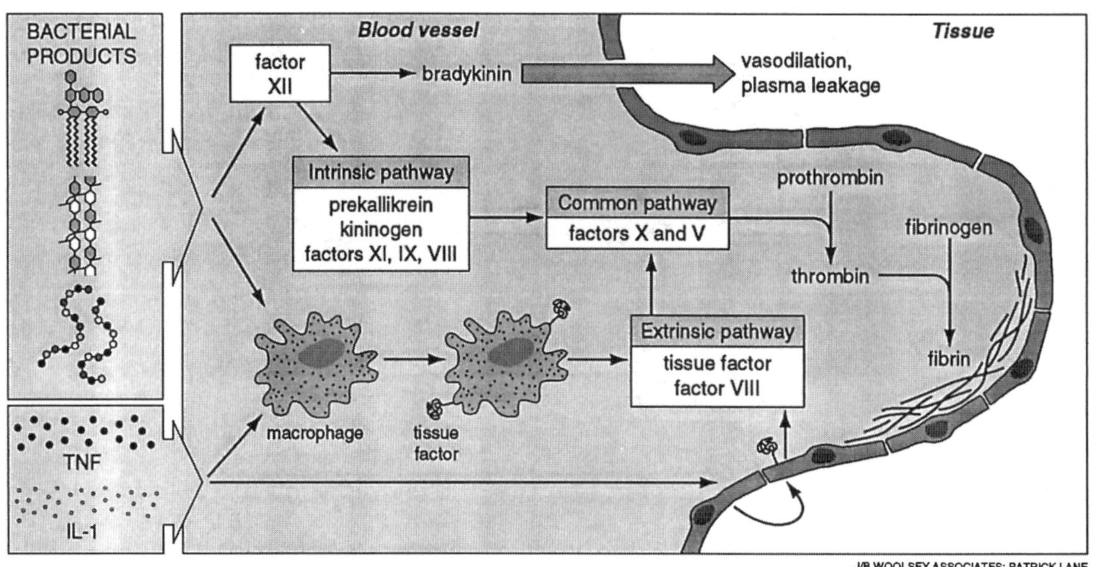


**Fig. 50.2** Induction of kinins and clotting in sepsis. Bacterial products and cytokines produce hypotension and plasma leakage by allowing release of the vasodilator bradykinen. They also induce intravascular coagulation.

ists that protein C can be activated during gram-negative bacteremia and that activated protein C can prevent the coagulation disorders and lethal effects of *E. coli* infusion in baboons.

Finally, the activation of the contact system results in the *conversion of prekallikrein* to *kallikrein*. In turn, kallikrein cleaves high molecular weight kininogen to release bradykinin, a potent hypotensive agent which, like $C_{3a}$ and $C_{5a}$, causes vasodilation and increases capillary permeability. The resulting leakage of fluid into interstitial space can be a prominent feature of sepsis and septic shock.

## Role of cellular pathways

Monocytic cells, endothelial cells, and neutrophils play a major role in the pathogenesis of sepsis and septic shock (Fig. 50.3).

### Monocytic cells

Monocytic cells have at least two roles in sepsis. They were first recognized as *phagocytic cells*. As such, they can remove and destroy bacteria and bacterial products, minimizing the response to infection. More recently, they were found to *produce potent mediators of inflammation* such as various cytokines. Several cytokines are produced not only by these cells but also by lymphocytes, endothelial cells, and other cells stimulated by microbial products. The pro-inflammatory cytokines are crucial in the regulation of the host defenses against infections, but their overproduction can lead to an excessive stimulation of the inflammatory cascade, which is responsible for the clinical picture of septic shock.

Monocytic cells can be triggered by various bacterial components, both from gram-positive and gram-negative bacteria. The mechanism of stimulation by LPS has been extensively studied. LPS can interact with monocytes after binding to an acute-phase protein called LPS-binding protein (LBP). The LPS–LBP complex is a ligand for the CD14 receptors on monocytic cells and on primed neutrophils, resulting in increased expression of LPS-inducible genes. When complexed with LBP, LPS can activate CD-14–bearing cells at concentrations far below those required for stimulation by LPS alone. Therefore, a principal function of LBP may be to enhance the ability of the host to detect LPS early in infection. Furthermore, a soluble form of the CD14 receptor in serum has been shown to promote the binding of LPS to endothelial cells and to stimulate these cells to produce cytokines and adhesion molecules. The precise roles played by CD14, soluble CD14, and LBP in vivo during sepsis are under investigation.

Among the *pro-inflammatory cytokines* produced by monocytic cells, *tumor necrosis factor-α* (TNF) is regarded as a central mediator of the pathophysiological changes associated with sepsis. Injection of TNF into animals can mimic most of the effects of LPS challenges. Moreover, antibodies to TNF have effectively decreased mortality in some, but not all, animal models of sepsis. Cytokines other than TNF are also involved in the induction of a shock-like state in animals. Considerable interest has focused on *interleukin-1* (IL-1), previously called *endogenous pyrogen* (see Chapter 10). TNF and IL-1 exert pleiotropic biological effects, many of which are common to both cytokines. Both can activate various cells (monocytic cells, neutrophils, B and T lymphocytes, hepatocytes); increase adherence of endothelial cells; induce colony-stimulating factors, IL-6, IL-8, and cyclooxygenase; and produce an endogenous pyrogenic effect, lypolysis, and cachexia—a nonexhaustive list. Circulating levels of IL-1, like levels of TNF, are elevated in shock.

Evidence for the role of IL-1 in septic shock comes from experiments with animals in which blocking of the binding of IL-1 to its cell receptor by a specific receptor antagonist (IL-1ra) prevented the detrimental effects of inoculation of LPS or live *E. coli*, as well as heat-killed gram-positive cocci. The overlap of the proinflammatory effects of various cytokines and the synergy between different mediators are important clues to the pathogenesis of septic shock. For instance, when IL-1 is combined with TNF, the former increases the toxicity of the latter. LPS itself potentiates the lethal effects of TNF.

*γ-Interferon* has also been implicated in the synergy of TNF and IL-1; one of its actions is to increase expression of cellular receptors for TNF. Interleukin-6 is a cytokine produced by a number of lymphoid and nonlymphoid cells in response to various

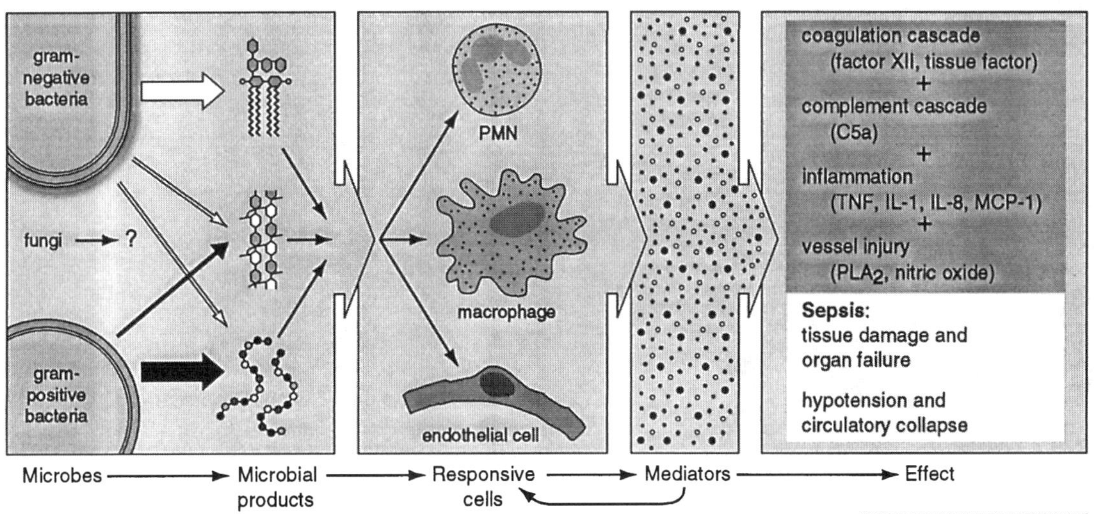


**Fig. 50.3** Microbial products activate host cells to produce a number of mediators with specific and interdependent tissue effects. PMN: polymorphonuclear cells; TNF: Tumor Necrosis Factor; IL-1: Interleukin 1; IL-8: Interleukin 8; $PLA_2$: phospholipase-A2; MCP-1: monocyte chemotactic protein 1.

stimuli, including LPS, TNF, and IL-1. Interleukin-6 plays a major role in the mediation of inflammatory and immune response to infection. Among its pleiotropic biological effects, IL-6 enhances the production of hepatic acute phase proteins, expands the production of hematopoietic cells, stimulates differentiation of B lymphocytes and antibody secretion, and induces an elevation in body temperature. High levels of IL-6 have been correlated with death in patients with septic shock. Currently, other cytokines are being evaluated as possibly important mediators in shock.

Naturally occuring antiinflammatory mechanisms are elicited in sepsis to control the intensity of the inflammatory response. For instance, IL-1ra competes with IL-1 for binding to IL-1 receptors; IL-10 inhibits the proliferation of helper T cells and their production of cytokines and downregulates the expression of major histocompatibility class (MHC) II molecules on monocytes. The soluble TNF receptors (p55 and p75) neutralize circulating TNF.

### Neutrophils

Activated neutrophils, a key element in the inflammatory response, probably play an important part in the pathogenesis of septic shock by contributing to vascular and tissue injuries. Strong evidence indicates that neutrophils are activated either directly by LPS or indirectly through the action of cytokines. As a result, activated neutrophils may damage tissues by releasing oxygen metabolites and lysosomal enzymes, or they may cause microemboli after aggregation. Activated leukocytes adhere to one another, to endothelial cells, and to tissues through interactions of receptors (on endothelial cells) and ligands (on inflammatory cells) that are mediated by specific adhesion molecules (see Chapter 10).

### Endothelial cells

It is now widely recognized that the vascular endothelium is both a key target for various inflammatory mediators and an important producer of active mediators. The systemic effects of high doses of intravenously administered TNF or IL-1 into animals include hypotension, decreased systemic vascular resistance, vascular leak, and infiltration of polymorphonuclear cells (PMN) into tissues. TNF and IL-1 enhance the expression of adhesion molecules on endothelial cells, facilitating PMN margination. TNF and IL-1 increase the procoagulant activiy of endothelium and depress the expresssion of fibrinolytic activity, resulting in a trend toward intravascular coagulation.

### Other mediators produced by activated cells

Various humoral factors are currently being evaluated for their role as mediators of septic shock, among which are *platelet activating factor* (PAF) and *nitric oxide* (NO).

PAF is produced by macrophages, neutrophils, platelets, and endothelial cells in response to injury. It is a potent phospholipid mediator of inflammation that amplifies cytokine release. Elevated levels of PAF have been found in models of endotoxin-induced hypotension and endotoxin-induced lung injury in rats.

NO is a potent physiologic vasodilatator that is essential for the regulation of blood flow and pressure. It is synthetized by a calcium- and calmodulin-dependent enzyme in endothelial cells, the NO synthase. Beside this constitutive enzyme, there is an calcium-independent isoform called inducible NO synthase (INOS) that has been found in endothelial and smooth-muscle cells and in many other cells including myocardium, neutrophils and murine macrophages. INOS can be induced by LPS and various cytokines such as TNF and IL-1, a phenomenon that might contribute to the rapid decrease in blood pressure associated with endotoxic shock. NO may also be involved in the pathophysiology of sepsis by its inhibitory effect on platelet adhesion and leukocyte activation. An increasing number of reports deal with the inhibition of this pathway in animal models, but the benefit of this inhibition remains questionable.

Finally, it is well known that *arachidonic acid metabolites* cause vasodilatation, platelet aggregation, and neutrophil activation, which may contribute to the pathogenesis of septic shock. These substances are found in increased concentrations after experimental endotoxin challenge and during septic shock in patients.

## Clinical Manifestations

The clinical picture of sepsis and septic shock is composed of nonspecific signs, as described in Table 50.1. Typically, fever may be preceded by chills. Skin is warm in the early stage, with a short capillary recoloration time, reflecting vasodilation. In advanced stages of shock, skin becomes cold, pale, and marbled. These clinical signs are most often associated with the signs due to the primary focus of infection, which are described elsewhere in this book. In addition, some clinical clues may suggest specific microorganisms (Table 50.4). It should be emphasized that immunocompromised hosts, such as neutropenic patients and transplant recipients, may have serious focal infections without obvious clinical signs. In the elderly, the typical clinical signs of sepsis may be attenuated or absent.

Septic shock may result in the failure of virtually any organ or system. It is beyond the scope of this chapter to discribe each organ dysfunction. However, alterations of the cardiovascular system represent key points in the clinical manifestations of septic shock. Hemodynamic study, by clinical examination and sometimes by use of a Swan-Ganz catheter, is of crucial importance in differentiating septic shock from other causes of shock. The main cardiovascular alterations in septic shock are rather similar whatever the causative organism. They consist of (*1*) absolute or relative hypovolemia due to both venous and arterial dilation and leakage of plasma in the extravascular space, leading to low systemic vascular resistance, tachycardia, and normal or increased cardiac output; (*2*) a decreased oxygen extraction mainly due to arteriovenous shunting and microvascular alterations; this is peculiarly harmful for tissues, given the increased oxygen demand due to increased cellular metabolism induced by inflammation; and (*3*) a decreased oxygen transport resulting from relative myocardial depression, in addition to hypovolemia; these problems are often worsened by a decrease in oxygen saturation of hemoglobin due to respiratory failure. Despite the fact that cardiac output is normal or increased in the early phase of septic shock, ventricular function is abnormal. It is characterized by reduction of left and right ventricular ejection fraction, biventricular dilation, and normal stroke volume.

## Laboratory Studies

*Microbiological investigations* should be performed whenever possible before the beginning of the antibiotic therapy, with exceptions when immediate treatment is mandatory, such as in the

**Table 50.4** Clinical findings in the setting of sepsis may suggest possible sources of infection

| Clinical finding | Possible source of sepsis |
|---|---|
| SKIN | |
| Purpuric or petechial rash | Meningococcemia |
| Petechial rash and history of tick bite | *Rickettsia rickettsii* |
| Generalized papular rash, history of tick bite or presence of an inoculation eschar | *Rickettsia conorii* |
| Scarlatiniform rash and diarrhea | Toxic shock syndrome |
| Maculopapular rash | Candidemia |
| Necrotic ulcer with erythematous halo (*Echtyma gangrenosum*) | *Pseudomonas* bacteremia (occasionally other gram-negative bacteria) |
| I.V. line | Catheter-related sepsis |
| I.V. drug abuse marks | *Staphyloccocus aureus*, *Pseudomonas aeruginosa*, *C. albicans* |
| Furuncles | *S. aureus* |
| Embolic lesions (Janeway lesions, Osler nodes) | Endocarditis |
| Postsplenectomy scar and diffuse hemorragic suffusions | Fulminant pneumococcal sepsis |
| Soft-tissue gas | Clostridial infection (occasionally other anaerobes, *Klebsiella*, *E. coli*) |
| Decubitus ulcer | Mixed anaerobic–aerobic infection |
| Diabetic foot | Mixed anaerobic–aerobic infection |
| Erysipelas | Group A *streptococcus*, *S. aureus* |
| CENTRAL NERVOUS SYSTEM | |
| Sudden focal neurologic event | Endocarditis, cerebral abscess |
| Signs of meningeal irritation | Meningitis (organism depending on age and underlying conditions) |
| RETINA | |
| Roth's spot | Endocarditis |
| Retinal abscess | *C. albicans* |
| HEART | |
| New murmur | Endocarditis |
| LUNGS | |
| Rales | Pneumonia |
| DIGESTIVE SYSTEM | |
| Rectal abscess | Enterobacteriaceae, anaerobes |
| Murphy's sign or icterus | Cholecystitis or cholangitis |
| URINARY TRACT | |
| Flank tenderness | Pyelonephritis |
| GENITAL TRACT | |
| Metrorrhagia | Septic abortion |

case of meningococcemia, severe bacterial meningitis, or suspicion of fulminant pneumococcal sepsis in a splenectomized patient. In these settings, parenteral antibiotics should be administered within minutes after the first clinical examination, sometimes before arrival at the hospital. *Blood cultures* are essential in the workup of sepsis. The processing and interpretation of blood cultures have been discussed previously in this book (see Chapter 16). At least two samples, drawn a few minutes apart, should be obtained before the administration of antibiotics. *Specimens for direct examination and cultures* must be obtained from any primary or metastatic sites of infection. These include urine, respiratory tract secretions (sputa, tracheal aspiration, bronchoalveolar lavage, brush), peritoneal or pleural effusions, cerebrospinal fluid, cutaneous lesions, joint fluid, intravascular device, or swab from puncture site.

*Other laboratory determinations*, useful to diagnose the systemic inflammatory process and to evaluate its severity, are listed in Table 50.1. They include differential blood cell count; coagulation tests (such as prothrombin time, partial thromboplastin time, levels of fibrinogen, and fibrin degradation products); tests reflecting organ dysfunction such as blood gas measurements and serum levels of lactic acid, creatinine, aminotransferase, and amylase; and tests of cholestasis. Blood gas measurement will often show hypoxemia, lactic acidosis with respiratory compensation. An electrocardiogram is important both to exclude cardiogenic causes for hypotension and to evaluate cardiac involvement in organ failures. Some of these laboratory values are needed to calculate scores of severity, such as the Acute Physiology and Chronic Health Evaluation (APACHE) score and the Simplified Acute Physiology Score (SAPS). These scores are useful to statistically compare the severity of disease among groups of patients, but, although they have been shown to correlate with mortality to some extent, they are not reliable to predict the probability of death for individual patients.

Among other laboratory studies which are currently under investigation, levels of various mediators of inflammation as well as levels of LPS are extensively evaluated for clinical use. To date, however, none has definitely been found to be of interest for diagnosis or follow-up of sepsis and septic shock.

## Treatment of Sepsis and Septic Shock

The treatment of sepsis and septic shock consists of measures aimed at the infectious process itself (antibiotics and surgical management if needed), together with supportive care. In addition, interventions at the level of microbial or host mediators are under investigation.

### Antibiotic therapy

Although early retrospective studies failed to demonstrate it, more recent studies have clearly shown that the outcome of bacteremic patients is significantly improved and the occurrence of septic shock is reduced by half when appropriate antibiotic therapy is administered early. The choice of antibiotics relies on therapeutic guidelines discussed in the sections of this book dealing with the primary foci of infection. When a primary focus of infection is complicated by sepsis or septic shock, emphasis should be given to the administration of high doses of antibiotics by the parenteral route. We will focus here only on the empirical treatment of sepsis of unknown origin. The following considerations are important for an adequate choice.

#### Origin of the patient

Hospital-acquired infections may be due to a wider spectrum of bacteria than community-acquired infections. Empirical treatment of sepsis occurring after more than 2 d in the hospital must cover nosocomial agents such as *S. aureus* and resistant enterobacteriaceae, and sometimes *Pseudomonas aeruginosa*. The pattern of resistance to antibiotics varies greatly among different institutions. For instance, in a survey of *S. aureus* in Europe in 1993, methicillin resistance was observed in only 2% of the strains in some hospitals, whereas it was observed in more than 50% in others.

#### Previous antibiotic therapy

When sepsis occurs in a patient recently treated with antibiotics, the likelihood of a bacterial resistance to this antibiotic or of a fungal infection is high.

#### Colonization

In hospitalized patients, infections are often heralded by previous colonization of mucosal surfaces with the same organisms. Thus, the results of previous cultures from sites such as upper respiratory tract, skin, or urine must be taken into account when choosing an antibiotic for empiric treatment.

#### Dosage

In the treatment of sepsis and septic shock, a rapid killing of bacteria is desirable. Concerns have been raised that a rapid bactericidal effect may result in increased release of cell wall components, such as endotoxin. However, there is so far no evidence that this concern is of clinical importance. Appropriate antibiotic therapy in adequate doses remains the most effective intervention in sepsis and, with a few exceptions such as typhoid fever or borelliosis, should not be compromised by concerns regarding the release of endotoxin induced by antibiotics. Bactericidal antibiotics with high serum levels are preferred. Relapses of infection or so-called "breakthrough bacteremias" can occur in patients with subinhibitory serum levels. When the pharmacokinetics is dependent on renal function and the therapeutic margin is narrow, such as with aminoglycosides and vancomycin, monitoring of serum levels is necessary (see Chapters 30 and 31).

#### Combination versus single-agent therapy

Most antibiotics available in the past had a narrow or intermediate antibacterial spectrum. Their bactericidal activity on many bacteria was weak, and resistance rapidly became a problem. The rationale for administering a combination of antibiotics was to extend the antibacterial spectrum, to obtain a synergistic effect, and to diminish the emergence of resistant bacteria. The standard treatment of patients with sepsis of unknown origin was thus a combination of $\beta$-lactams plus an aminoglycoside. This approach has been challenged by the advent of more potent antibiotics with an extended antibacterial spectrum, such as the third-generation cephalosporins and the carbapenems. Recent studies with ceftazidime and imipenem/cilastatin have suggested that both drugs were as effective and less nephrotoxic than combination therapies for the empirical treatment of sepsis. However, the addition of an aminoglycoside probably remains necessary in infections where *P. aeruginosa* or multiresistant organisms are suspected, and in neutropenic patients with gram-negative bacteremia, especially that caused by *P. aeruginosa*. A choice for empirical treatment of sepsis of unknown origin is listed in Table 50.5. Treatment should be adjusted as soon as microbiological data are available.

## Supportive care

Septic shock is one of the most common causes of multiple organ failure in intensive care units. It is beyond the scope of this chapter to review the management of each organ dysfunction. Only the cardiovascular, the respiratory, and the coagulation systems will be briefly discussed.

### Cardiovascular management

The goals of the cardiovascular management of septic shock are aimed at reversing tissue hypoxia and include restoration of intravascular volume, tissue perfusion, and oxygen delivery. Restoration of intravascular volume can be achieved by administration of colloid or crystalloid solutions. The advantage of one type of solution over the other is still a matter of controversy. Fluid should be administered until the pulmonary artery wedge pressure reaches the lowest value allowing adequate cardiac output and oxygen delivery associated with reversal of shock. This value is often close to 12 mmHg. In the presence of acute renal failure, a consequence of an aggressive fluid replacement is the frequent need to decrease fluid overload by hemodialysis or hemofiltration.

In 30% to 40% of the cases, fluid therapy alone is sufficient to restore a normal pressure. If this is not the case, adrenergic agents are required, aiming at achieving a mean arterial pressure of 70 to 75 mmHg. Dopamine is usually given first because, due to its weak $\alpha$-adrenergic effect, organ perfusion is better preserved. If hypotension persists despite doses of 25 $\mu$g/kg/min, noradrenaline should be added or used instead of dopamine. A small dose 2 $\mu$g/kg/min of dopamine is often maintained in an attempt to preserve renal perfusion. In addition, dobutamine may be given because myocardial depression can limit the oxygen supply to the tissues. The optimal cardiac output is difficult to determine, however, because high doses of dobutamine can increase oxygen demand. To increase oxygen delivery, it is also mandatory to maintain the hemoglobin oxygen saturation above 90% and the oxygen partial pressure above 60 mmHg in arterial blood, and to achieve an hematocrit of 30% to 35%. Determination of blood lactate may be an useful parameter to determine appropriate oxygen delivery.

### Ventilatory support

Respiratory failure attributable to the adult respiratory distress syndrome (ARDS) generally requires the use of mechanical ventilatory support, high inspired oxygen concentration, and positive end expiratory pressure (PEEP) (see Chapter 58). The "optimal" PEEP must be chosen with consideration for its harmful effects on cardiac output and the increased risk of barotrauma. Recent developments in ventilatory support include high-frequency ventilation, aerosolized nitric oxide, and various techniques for extrapulmonary oxygenation or $CO_2$ removal.

### Management of coagulopathy

Disseminated intravascular coagulation (DIC) occurs in about 10% to 20% of patients with septic shock, ranging from a mild laboratory disorder to the full clinical syndrome characterized by thrombosis, hemorrhage, or both. The most important component of treatment is directed toward reversal of shock and removal of the septic source. Supportive measures include administration of fresh frozen plasma. In addition, low doses of heparin (5000 to 10,000 units per day) are often administered to "switch off" the coagulation cascade by neutralizing serine proteases, but its use remains controversial. Heparin has been shown to be effective mostly in the less acute forms of DIC and should be considered on an individual basis when the condition is not rapidly reversible and in the absence of bleeding.

**Table 50.5** Empirical treatment of sepsis of unknown origin*

| Place of acquisition | Pathogens to consider | 1st treatment choice | 2nd treatment choice[a] |
|---|---|---|---|
| Community-acquired | Pneumococci, streptococci, *S. aureus*, meningococci, *H. influenzae*, enterobacteriaceae | • 2nd- or 3rd-generation cephalosporin<br>• Or a penicillin + a $\beta$-lactamase inhibitor | • Vancomycin + an aminoglycoside,<br>• Or vancomycin + a quinolone |
| Hospital-acquired | Same as above + *S. epidermidis*, multi-resistant enterobacteriaceae, *P. aeruginosa* | • Imipenem<br>• Or an antipseudomonas penicillin + a $\beta$-lactamase inhibitor<br>• Or ceftazidime + an antistaphyloccocal drug[b] | • Vancomycin + an aminoglycoside<br>• Or vancomycin + a quinolone<br>• Or vancomycin + aztreonam |

*Note: These guidelines apply to empirical treatment when the primary focus of infection is unknown. (See related chapters for empirical treatments of the various foci of infections.) When multiresistant organisms are suspected in a severely ill patient, the addition of an aminoglycoside should be considered.

[a]Allergy to $\beta$-lactams or special epidemiological settings.

[b]A beta-lactamase resistant penicillin, a penicillin + a $\beta$-lactamase inhibitor, or vancomycin.

## Antimediator approaches

Antibiotics can suppress bacterial proliferation or kill bacteria, but they cannot neutralize bacterial toxins, nor can they downregulate the inflammatory cascade. Thanks to progress in biotechnology, monoclonal antibodies, soluble receptors, receptor antagonists, and constructs of receptors attached to immunoglobulin molecules can now be synthesized on a large scale, suitable for study in patients. The neutralization of mediators of bacterial origin or of mediators of inflammation could be a very useful adjunctive therapy of sepsis. Numerous investigations have recently been performed in this field; some of them are cited below. However, at the time this chapter was written, none of these approaches had led to therapeutic modalities that can be applied routinely to patients.

### Inhibition of endotoxin

The O-specific oligosaccharide side chains of endotoxin are very immunogenic. Anti-O antibodies are effective in inhibiting the effects of endotoxin and, by virtue of their opsonophagocytic properties, in eradicating the corresponding organism. However, because the antibodies are specific for a particular O serotype and because there are hundreds of different O serotypes, their clinical application is limited.

An alternative approach has been to develop antibodies against the structurally conserved core glycolipid of endotoxin or against lipid A itself, with the purpose of cross-protecting against all gram-negative bacteria. The initial clinical trials were performed with antisera or hyperimune polyclonal intravenous immunoglobulins raised against core glycolipid. Some of these studies suggested a benefit, although the precise epitope responsible for cross-protection was not demonstrated.

These promising results stimulated subsequent trials with anti–lipid A monoclonal antibodies (although it was not formally demonstrated that antibodies to lipid A were indeed responsible for the protection observed in the clinical trials with the polyclonal anti-core glycolipid antibodies). Two monoclonal IgM anti–lipid A antibodies, called E5 and HA-1A, have been investigated in patients. In both cases, the first clinical trials suggested that these antibodies could protect some subsets of septic patients. In the case of HA-1A, the initial report of a reduced mortality in a subgroup of patients given the antibody led to its licensure under the name of Centoxin in some European countries. However, the licensure applications were not approved by the Federal Drug Administration in the United States for several reasons. Second trials of both antibodies were therefore done, which did not confirm their efficacy, leading to the removal of Centoxin from the market in Europe. These disappointing results were perhaps not totally unexpected when critically reviewing the data that led to their development. It now appears that clinical trials with anti–lipid A antibodies were initiated before the immunological reactivity of these monoclonal antibodies for LPS substructures were known and despite many controversies concerning their in vitro and in vivo experimental evidences of efficacy.

Despite these disappointing results, LPS remains an important target for therapies of septic shock. Research has moved now toward new monoclonal antibodies with a cross-reactivity pattern intermediate between the narrow range of type-specific antibodies and the broad range of anti–lipid A antibodies. The administration of a mixture of a few antibodies with a complementary spectrum might be worth studying. In addition, some synthetic analogues of lipid A with a low toxicity can induce a state of tolerance to LPS or can compete with LPS-binding sites. The role of these analogues in the adjunctive treatment of septic shock is under study.

Substantial progress has been made recently in understanding how LPS can trigger the immune system. Two members of a family of proteins possessing LPS-binding sites—LPS-binding protein (LBP) and bactericidal permeability-increasing protein (BPI)—have been recognized. These proteins have a striking homology in DNA sequence, but they have different functions. Both form high-affinity complexes with LPS in blood. However, whereas LPS–LBP complexes bind to CD14 on monocytic cells and on primed neutrophils, resulting in increased expression of LPS-inducible genes, the formation of LPS–BPI complexes inhibits the LPS-induced triggering of CD14-possessing cells. BPI is found in neutrophil azurophilic (primary) granules. It may be released in small amounts during degranulation of activated neutrophils, which might represent a possible negative feedback mechanism of LPS-mediated events. The biological roles of LBP, BPI, and CD14 are now being actively investigated, as is their modulation by soluble receptors and antibodies.

### Inhibition of host inflammatory mediators

The role of *proinflammatory cytokines* in the pathophysiology of septic shock *in experimental animals* has been most convincingly demonstrated. This has led to the hypothesis that the blockade of some of these cytokines could be useful in patients. A potentially important advantage of this approach over the antiendotoxin approach arises from the fact that the same cytokines also play a part in the pathogenesis of shock due to gram-positive bacteria. Many studies have reported benefit from the blockade of TNF or IL-1 in animals, including mice, rats, pigs, rabbits, and baboons. Several large trials have been performed recently in patients. Several anti-TNF monoclonal antibodies and two constructs of a TNF receptor linked to a human IgG have been studied in patients presenting with sepsis or septic shock. Up to now, and although some studies are still ongoing the results were considered as disappointing because no statistically significant improvement in survival was observed. Similarly, the blockade of IL-1 with IL-1 receptor antagonist (IL-1ra) did not result in a significant improvement in survival. Most recently, the antiinflammatory IL-10 has also been suggested as a candidate for treatment of sepsis. Indeed, IL-10 decreased the production of IL-1, IL-6, and TNF in vitro and protected mice challenged with lethal doses of endotoxin. However, as mentioned above, the synergy and overlapping biological effects between cytokines, especially TNF and IL-1, as well as between cytokines and cell wall fragments, suggests that a combined approach aimed at blocking various triggers and mediators may offer the best potential for improving the outcome of septic shock. In addition, the population of patients that might benefit from these approaches still has to be defined.

In addition to anticytokine approaches, a number of molecules and monoclonal antibodies are currently under investigation, involving almost all pathways shown to be involved in septic shock so far. These include inhibitors of arachidonic acid metabolites, monoclonal antibodies blocking the adhesion process of neutrophils, PAF antagonists, inhibitors of NO synthase, monoclonal anti–factor XII, monoclonal antibody to tissue factor, and activated protein C. More studies will be needed both experimentally and clinically to explore the role of these approaches in septic shock.

## ANNOTATED BIBLIOGRAPHY

Baumgartner JD. Anti-endotoxin antibodies as treatment for sepsis—lessons to be learned. Rev Med Microbiol 1994; 5:183.

*A story of antiendotoxin antibodies as treatment for sepsis, with emphasis on anti–lipid A antibodies.*

Bryan CS, Reynold KL, Brenner ER. Analysis of 1186 episodes of gram-negative bacteremia in non-university hospitals: the effects of antimicrobial therapy. Rev Infect Dis 1983; 5:629.

*With reference by McCabe et al, classical studies of gram-negative bacteremia, showing the importance of appropriate antibiotic therapy for the outcome of patients.*

Cohen J, Glauser MP. Septic shock: treatment. Lancet 1991; 338:736.

*An update on steroids, anti-endotoxin antibodies, and anti-TNF approaches in the treatment of septic shock.*

Glauser MP, Zanetti G, Baumgartner JD, Cohen J. Septic shock: pathogenesis. Lancet 1991; 338:732.

*Review on mediators of septic shock.*

Heumann D, Glauser MP. Pathogenesis of sepsis. Sci Am Sci Med 1994; 1(5):28.

*Review mainly devoted to interactions between microbial products and immune system.*

Marrack P, Kappler J. The staphylococcal enterotoxins and their relatives. Science 1990; 248:705.

*A review on microbial superantigens, their association with T cells, and their significance.*

McCabe WR, Jackson GG. Gram-negative bacteremia. Arch Intern Med 1962; 10:92.

Mocada S, Higgs A. The L-arginine-nitric oxide pathway. N Engl J Med 1993; 329(27):2002.

*An update on our knowledge of the pathophysiologic implications of nitric oxide.*

Parillo JE. Pathogenetic mechanisms of septic shock. N Engl J Med 1993; 328 (20):1471.

# 51

# Infections with Rash

MORTON N. SWARTZ

The patient with fever and a rash represents an important diagnostic challenge, since causes of this syndrome include acute systemic infections requiring early diagnosis and prompt therapy. For purposes of this discussion we will consider only systemic infections in which rash is a significant element. Infections originating in the skin or its appendages (e.g., pyodermas such as impetigo, erysipelas, cellulitis) are often accompanied by fever, but they have a different pathogenesis and will be considered elsewhere (Chapters 52 and 53). While the febrile rash syndrome (FRS) should initially raise the concern of an infectious etiology, the differential diagnosis can be broad, including drug eruptions, vasculitides of various types, and infiltrative processes including leukemias and Sweet's syndrome.

Systemic infections associated with a rash include those of bacterial, spirochetal, mycobacterial, fungal, chlamydial, mycoplasmal, rickettsial, ehrlichial, and viral etiologies. However, since the skin often serves as a ready mirror of systemic infection, the practical "first pass" at differential diagnosis is reasonably based on the morphology of the skin lesions. Subsequent classification would then involve consideration of the various microorganisms previously noted. Although the appearance of a rash may suggest several diagnostic possibilities, it is usually not definitive per se. Epidemiologic considerations may sharpen the differential diagnosis. These include (*1*) season of the year (e.g., enteroviral infections in the summer), (*2*) recent travel (e.g., dengue acquired in the Caribbean or Southwest Pacific areas), (*3*) recent exposure to infectious diseases (e.g., measles, varicella), (*4*) animal contacts (e.g., leptospirosis), (*5*) insect or tick bites (e.g., tularemia, Rocky Mountain spotted fever, Lyme borreliosis), and (*6*) specific exposures of particularly predisposed individuals (e.g., ingestion of raw oysters by a person with chronic liver disease, and ensuing bacteremic *Vibrio vulnificus* infection). Of particular help in sharpening the focus on initial diagnosis for the patient with FRS is a full history (including HIV risk factors, medications taken, acute or subacute nature of the illness), observation of physical findings (e.g., arthritis, stiff neck, heart murmurs, jaundice), and the results of the initial blood count (leukocytosis, suggesting bacterial infection; leukopenia, suggesting viral infection; eosinophilia, suggesting parasitic infection or hypersensitivity response). In some instances, the diagnosis may be established only with skin biopsy and histologic examination.

In approaching the patient with FRS several caveats are in order. The first is that common entities are more frequently seen and should take a higher priority in one's thinking unless ancillary (e.g., epidemiologic) considerations have come to the fore. The second is that while the cutaneous lesions of certain systemic infections generally assume a characteristic morphology, they may appear differently in specific circumstances or at other stages of an illness. Thus, a generalized maculopapular eruption may become vesiculobullous on the lower extremities due to the effects of dependency and edema; or an area of purpura may undergo necrosis and ulceration, as in meningococcemia with disseminated intravascular coagulation. The third is that the host's immune state may alter the classic appearance of certain infections involving the skin. For example, in the immunocompromised host, skin lesions of gram-negative bacteremia or cryptococcal fungemia may resemble cellulitis or erysipelas-like processes, commonly due to gram-positive cocci. Finally, it is always important to remember that the same ultimate histologic picture may be presented by quite different entities pathogenetically. Thus, the pathologic appearance described as "leukocytoclastic angiitis" may be due, on the one hand, to small vessel hypersensitivity vasculitis, and, on the other hand, to bacteremic infection as in chronic meningococcemia or subacute infective endocarditis.

## Etiologies

The patterns of the skin lesions accompanying systemic infections can conveniently be placed in several categories convenient for organizing these clues to etiologic diagnosis: diffuse maculopapular lesions, maculopapular rash with primary herald plaque or initial solitary eschar, generalized confluent erythema, vesicular or bullous lesions, petechial-purpuric rash, urticarial syndromes, multiple nodules, or nodular lymphangitis syndrome. Additional characteristics can serve to further refine these categories. These include the distribution of lesions (e.g., the more truncal distribution of the maculopapular rash of epidemic or murine typhus, the more peripheral rash of Rocky Mountain spotted fever on the extremities); the distinctive targetoid or iris lesions of erythema multiforme; the grouping of vesicular lesions of herpes simplex or zoster; the emergence of new lesions in crops, as in chicken pox, resulting in the presence of all stages (macules, papules, clear and clouded vesicles, and crusts) in a given area; presence of an enanthem as well as an exanthem as in scarlet fever or the toxic shock syndrome; the evolution of lesions (e.g., infarct necrosis or purulent purpura in acute *Staphylococcus aureus* endocarditis). While the organization of one's initial approach to a patient with a fever and a rash can benefit from a categorization of the gross features of the cutaneous lesions, it is important to remain aware that many different infectious or noninfectious processes may be associated with similar-appearing lesions. Only evaluation of the full clinical picture along with microbiologic study of the blood and/or skin biopsy can provide the specific diagnosis. Tables 51.1 through 51.7 can provide a framework for differential diagnosis.

**Table 51.1** Systemic infections with maculopapular lesions

| Diffuse maculopapular lesions | Maculopapular rash with herald plaque/eschar |
|---|---|
| VIRAL INFECTIONS | |
| Rubella (German measles) | Pityriasis rosea |
| Rubeola (Measles) | |
| Atypical measles | |
| Enteroviruses (echovirus; coxsackie); rashes include maculopapules in "hand-foot and mouth disease" as well as more typical vesicles | |
| Erythema infectiosum (fifth disease, parvovirus $B_{19}$, slapcheek disease) | |
| Roseola infantum (exanthem subitum; HHV-6 infection) | |
| HIV infection (acute mononucleosis-like syndrome) | |
| Dengue | |
| Epstein-Barr virus infection (infectious mononucleosis, commonly if ampicillin administered) | |
| Varicella (chickenpox, early stage) | |
| Lymphocytic choriomeningitis | |
| Colorado tick fever (*Orbivirus* infection; rash in 5%–10%) | |
| Hepatitis B (uncommonly in adults; in children, Gianotti-Crosti syndrome occasionally, with erythematous papules) | |
| CMV-associated mononucleosis | |
| RICKETTSIA/EHRLICHIA INFECTIONS | |
| Rocky Mountain spotted fever (*Rickettsia rickettsii*) | Rickettsialpox (*R. akari*) |
| Epidemic typhus (*R. prowazekii*) | Boutonneuse fever (*R. conori*; designated by many geographic names; e.g., *S. African* tick fever, Mediterranean tick fever, etc.) |
| Endemic (murine) typhus (*R. typhi*) | |
| Q fever (5%–18% with rash) | Scrub typhus (*R. tsutsugamushi*) |
| Ehrlichiosis (*Ehrlichia chaffeensis*) (nonspecific rash in 20%) | |
| MYCOPLASMA/CHLAMYDIA INFECTIONS | |
| *Mycoplasma pneumoniae* pneumonia | |
| *Chlamydia psittaci* pneumonia (pale, macular rash; Horder spots) | |
| BACTERIAL INFECTIONS | |
| Secondary syphilis | *Spirillum minus* infection (rat bite fever) |
| Leptospirosis (*Leptospira interrogans*) | Tularemia (*Franciscella tularensis*) |
| Meningococcemia (early in acute infection; in chronic meningococcemia) | |
| Typhoid fever (*Salmonella typhi*; rose spots) | |
| Pseudomonas aeruginosa bacteremia | |
| Brucellosis (1%–9%; may be erythematous or papular; transient) | |
| *Streptobacillus moniliformis* infection (Rat bite fever) | |
| Relapsing fever (*Borrelia recurrentis*; *Borrelia hermsii*) | |
| Scarlet fever (*Streptococcus pyogenes*) | |
| Lyme disease (giant figurate erythema of erythema chronicum migrans; *B. burgdorferi* infection) | |
| Tuberculosis (miliary tuberculosis of the skin, most often in infants; papulonecrotic tuberculid, a hypersensitivity phenomenon) | |
| PARASITIC DISEASE | |
| Acute acquired toxoplasmosis | |
| Trichinosis | |
| African trypanosomiasis (during acute phases of W. African [*Trypanosoma brucei gambiense*] and E. African [*T.b. rhodesiense*] trypanosomiasis | |
| NONINFECTIOUS MIMICS OF INFECTIOUS RASH | |
| Erythema multiforme | |
| Juvenile rheumatoid arthritis | |
| Kawasaki disease (mucocutaneous lymph node syndrome) | |
| Connective tissue disease (SLE; dermatomyositis) | |
| Vasculitis | |
| Drug eruption with fever | |
| Sweet's syndrome (acute febrile neutrophilic dermatosis) | |
| Eosinophilic folliculitis | |

**Table 51.2** Systemic infections with vesicular-bullous eruptions

| INFECTIONS |
|---|
| Varicella (chickenpox) |
| Disseminated herpes zoster |
| Generalized vaccinia |
| Disseminated herpes simplex |
| [Smallpox] |
| Monkeypox virus infection |
| *Mycoplasma pneumoniae* infections (bullous erythema multiforme) |
| Rickettsialpox |
| *Pseudomonas aeruginosa* bacteremia; evolution into ecthyma gangrenosa |
| *Vibrio vulnificus* bacteremia |
| Hand-foot and mouth disease (coxsackie A16, other serotypes less commonly) |
| Echovirus 11 (generalized vesicular eruption) |
| NONINFECTIOUS MIMICS |
| Toxic epidermal necrolysis |
| Pyoderma gangrenosa |
| Pustular psoriasis |

## Pathogenesis of Skin Rash

The cutaneous changes that occur with systemic infections may be produced in a number of ways: (*1*) the vesicular eruption characteristic of varicella or disseminated herpes zoster is due to multiplication in the skin of varicella-zoster virus; (*2*) the diffuse erythema of scarlet fever or the toxic shock syndrome results from the impact on the skin of toxins produced elsewhere (pharynx in streptococcal scarlet fever; any site of *S. aureus* infection for toxic shock syndrome); (*3*) the role of hypersensivity (cellular immunity) is important in the production of the rash of measles which appears contemporaneously with the appearance of circulating antibody and the cessation of the period of communicability; (*4*) vasculitis or vaso-occlusive processes are responsible for the petechial or purpuric lesions occurring during systemic infections such as meningococcemia, *Pseudomonas aeruginosa* bacteremia, Rocky Mountain spotted fever, and disseminated intravascular coagulation (DIC) associated with many types of infections. The cutaneous stigmata of bacterial endocarditis (petechiae, purpura, Osler nodes, Janeway lesions) may result from either vasculitis or infective embolization. Thus, the Osler nodes and petechiae of subacute bacterial endocarditis (SBE) are a consequence of noninfected lesions of vasculitis, whereas the Osler nodes and purulent purpura (central purulent area with surrounding hemorrhage) of acute *S. aureus* endocarditis represent the consequences of infective embolization.

**Table 51.3** Systemic infections with diffuse erythroderma

| Infection-related | Noninfectious mimics |
|---|---|
| Scarlet fever syndrome | Toxic epidermal necrolysis (Lyell's disease) |
| Streptococcal toxic shock | Kawasaki syndrome |
| Staphylococcal scalded skin syndrome | Diffuse erythroderma due to drug hypersensitivity |
| Staphylococcal toxic shock syndrome | |

**Table 51.4** Systemic infection with petechial-purpuric or polymorphic rashes

| PETECHIAL-PURPURIC LESIONS |
|---|
| Acute meningococcemia |
| Rat-bite fever (*Streptobacillus moniliformis*) |
| Viral hemorrhagic fevers such as dengue, Argentine (Junin), Bolivian (Machupo), Sabia and |
| Venezuelan (Guanarito) hemorrhagic fevers |
| Yellow fever |
| Echo virus (particularly echo virus 9) |
| Epidemic (louse-borne)typhus |
| Rocky Mountain spotted fever |
| African tick fever |
| Atypical measles |
| Infectious mononucleosis (EBV) |
| Congenital rubella |
| Congenital cytomegalic inclusion disease |
| Relapsing fever (*B. recurrentis*, *B. hermsii*) |
| *S. aureus* endocarditis or bacteremia |
| Purpura fulminans or symmetrical gangrene complicating infections due to varicella, group A |
| streptococci, meningococci, pneumococci, etc. |
| Henoch-Schönlein purpura |
| Trichinosis (subungual splinter hemorrhages) |
| POLYMORPHIC LESIONS |
| *N. meningitidis* bacteremia (scattered macules, papules, vesicles, petechiae in chronic |
| meningococcemia) |
| *N. gonorrhoeae* bacteremia (scattered macules, papules, vesicles, petechiae) |
| Subacute bacterial endocarditis (Janeway lesions, petechiae and subungual splinter hemorrhages, |
| Osler nodes |

## Clinical Manifestations

### Diffuse maculopapular lesions (Table 51.1)

In evaluating a patient with diffuse maculopapular lesions it is important to recognize that while in the majority of instances a viral infection (often not requiring specific treatment) is the etiology, rickettsial and bacterial etiologies, often requiring prompt diagnosis and treatment, also can be responsible. Viral infections also require prompt diagnosis in order to avoid exposure of susceptible individuals to the highly contagious childhood exanthems.

#### Viral infections

*Rubella* produces an exanthem of discrete, irregular pink macules, appearing first on the face and then spreading peripherally to the trunk and extremities (Plate 8). The rash may rapidly become diffuse and suggest scarlet fever. Fever is only low grade (or absent); malaise and coryza may have been present prior to the exanthem; and lymphadenopathy is common, particularly enlargement of postauricular and suboccipital lymph nodes. The character of the rash, the low-grade fever, the lymphadenopathy, the lack of immunization, and the possible exposure to someone with the disease strongly suggest the diagnosis. The rash usually disappears in 2–4 d. There may be limited, fine desquamation, easily distinguishable from the more prominent desquamation on the hands and feet following scarlet fever or the toxic shock syndrome.

**Table 51.5** Systemic infections with nodular lesions or annular erythema/urticaria

NODULAR LESIONS (CUTANEOUS OR SUBCUTANEOUS)

*S. aureus* bacteremia
Candidemia (disseminated candidiasis)
Sporotrichosis (nodular lymphangitis)
Bacillary angiomatosis (*Bartonella henselii*, *B. quintana*)
Mycobacteria (*M. tuberculosis*, *M. marinum*, *M. hamophilum*, *M. chelonae*)
*Nocardia* (*N. brasiliensis*, *N. asteroides*) nodular lymphangitis
Melioidosis
American cutaneous leishmaniasis (nodular lymphangitis)
Cryptococcus fungemia
Histoplasmosis
Coccidioidomycosis
*Fusarium* species infection
Erythema nodosum leprosum
Erythema nodosum secondary to infections with group A streptococci, *Yersinia enterocolitica*, *Coccidioides immitis*, *L. autumnalis*, *M. tuberculosis*, *Blastomyces dermatitidis* etc. as well as secondary to drug hypersensitivity and sarcoidosis
Noninfectious processes: Weber-Christian disease, factitial panniculitis, Sweet's syndrome

ANNULAR ERYTHEMA/URTICARIA

Erythema chronicum migrans of Lyme disease
Erythema marginatum (rheumatic fever)
Erythema multiforme (associated with *M. pneumoniae*, *Herpes simplex*, and other infections
Acute hepatitis B infection (urticaria)
Trichinosis (urticaria)
Coxsackie A-9 (urticaria)
Strongyloidiasis (larva currens; urticaria)
Onchocerciasis (urticaria)
Loiasis (filariasis, urticaria)
Katayama fever of acute schistosomiasis (*Schistosoma japonicum*, *S. mansoni*, (urticaria)
Echinococcal cyst leakage or rupture (urticaria)
Noninfectious causes of febrile urticaria: drug hypersensitivity, serum sickness,
hypocomplementemic urticarial vasculitis

*Measles* (*rubeola*) has an incubation period of 8–12 d, followed by a 2–6 d prodrome of nonproductive cough, coryza, fever, and conjunctivitis. Then a rash, consisting of pink macules and papules, appears first on the face and spreads to the trunk and extremities (Plate 9). It reaches its maximum (with coalescence about face and trunk) in extent and severity in 3–4 d. Koplik spots, irregular small bright red lesions with tiny bluish-white centers, appear on the buccal mucosa opposite the second molar teeth during the prodromal phase and last for several days after the skin eruption develops. This enanthem, in combination with the exanthem, is highly suggestive of the diagnosis, but similar lesions can be seen in echovirus infections. With progression of the rash, fever may reach 105° F. In rare instances thrombocytopenia accompanying measles may be marked and produce widespread cutaneous hemorrhages about the rash. "Atypical measles" has occurred in patients who received killed measles vaccine and later were exposed to natural measles virus and were infected with it. Such atypical measles is characterized by a 1–2 d prodrome of fever, followed by a rash which, in contrast to ordinary measles, begins on the extremities. The rash may be urticarial, petechial, maculopapular, and/or vesicular and accompanied by edema of the hands and feet. The disease tends to be quite severe, with high fever. The nature and severity of manifestations may suggest the diagnoses of Rocky Mountain spotted fever, Henoch-Schönlein purpura, toxic shock syndrome, or an intense drug eruption. The pathogenesis of the process is thought to be hypersensitivity to measles virus in an incompletely immune host.

*Enteroviruses* are commonly the cause of FRS, particularly in children. They often produce rubella-like eruptions. Enterovirus infections, particularly echovirus 9, can occur as sporadic cases or as epidemic outbreaks of a syndrome of fever, rash, and aseptic meningitis. The macular rash progresses to petechiae. The clinical picture may mimic that of acute meningococcemia and meningitis, especially since the initial CSF formula may show up to 500–800 WBC per mm$^3$ with 40%–70% polymorphonuclear leukocytes (PMNs). Clinical clues that may help to distinguish this process from meningococcemia are the early appearance of the echovirus 9 rash about the face and neck rather than on the extremities, the occasional presence of an enanthem consisting of Koplik spot-like lesions, and a peripheral WBC that is more typical of a viral than a bacterial infection. However,

**Table 51.6** Additional systemic infections with rash to consider in travelers recently abroad

LATIN AMERICA OR CARIBBEAN AREA

Dengue
Yellow fever
Argentine, Bolivian, Venezuelan hemorrhagic fevers
Mayaro virus infection (fever, maculopapular rash at defervescence)
Acute HIV infection syndrome
Typhoid fever
Leptospirosis
Relapsing fever (louse-borne, tick-borne)
Bartonellosis
Brucellosis
Brazilian purpuric fever
Melioidosis
Trench fever (*Bartonella* [formerly *Rachalimaea*] *quintana*)
Epidemic typhus
Murine typhus
Tick-borne spotted fever (Sao Paulo fever, Brazil; fiebre manchada, Mexico; fiebre petequial, Columbia)
Paracoccidioidomycosis (macules, papules in acute disease in children; nodules,ulcers in chronic disease)
Histoplasmosis and coccidioidomycosis
Visceral leishmaniasis
Chagas disease (chagoma; erythema multiforme-like)
Schistosomiasis
Filariasis (*Wuchereria bancrofti*; retrograde lymphangitis)
Echinococcal disease

MIDDLE EAST

Sandfly fever (*Phlebotomus* fever, pappataci fever; phlebovirus; erythema at bite site, facial flush)
Congo-Crimean hemorrhagic fever (nairovirus; petechiae/purpura)
West Nile fever (flavivirus; macular rash)
Rift Valley fever (phlebovirus)
Typhoid fever
Brucellosis
Epidemic typhus (louse-borne)
Endemic typhus (flea-borne)
Schistosomiasis (Katayama fever; *S. mansoni*, *S. hematobium*)
Echinococcal disease

**Table 51.7** Additional systemic infections with rash to consider in travelers recently abroad

| |
|---|
| SOUTHEAST ASIA AND OCEANIA |
| Dengue fever |
| Dengue hemorrhagic fever and shock syndrome |
| Korean hemorrhagic fever (Hantaan virus; erythematous flush, petechiae) |
| Chikungunya fever (alphavirus; maculopapular rash) |
| Ross River fever (alphavirus; maculopapular rash) |
| HIV (acute infection syndrome) |
| Leptospirosis |
| Meliodosis |
| Brucellosis |
| Endemic (murine) typhus |
| Scrub typhus |
| Q fever |
| Rat-bite fever (sọdoku; *Spirillum minor*) |
| Relapsing fever (*B. recurrentis*) |
| Schistosomiasis (Katayama fever; *S. japonicum*; urticaria) |
| Strongyloidiasis (urticaria; larva currens) |
| Filariasis (*Wuchereria bancrofti*; *Brugia malayi*; *B. timori*; filarial fevers with retrograde lymphangitis) |
| Visceral leishmaniasis (kala-azar); in India, Pakistan, and China |
| AFRICA |
| Dengue fever |
| Yellow fever |
| Chikungunya fever |
| O'nyong-nyong fever (alphavirus) |
| Congo-Crimean hemorrhagic fever |
| Marburg hemorrhagic fever (filovirus; macular rash; skin hemorrhages) |
| Ebola hemorrhagic fever (filovirus; macular rash; skin hemorrhages) |
| Lassa fever (arenavirus; facial edema; skin hemorrhages) |
| HIV infection (acute syndrome) |
| Leptospirosis |
| Louse-borne relapsing fever (borreliosis) |
| Typhoid fever |
| Brucellosis |
| Typhus (endemic or murine) |
| Typhus (epidemic or louse-borne) |
| Tick typhus (*R. conorii*): S. African tick bite fever; Kenya tick typhus; |
| Mediterranean or boutonneuse spotted fever in Mediterranean littoral |
| Visceral leishmaniasis (kala-azar): *L. donovani; L. infantum* |
| Schistosomiasis (Katayama fever): *S. mansoni*; *S. haematobium* |
| East African trypanosomiasis (*T. brucei rhodesiense;* erythema multiforme-like) |
| West African trypanosomiasis (*T. brucei gambiense*; erythema multiforme-like) |

with petechial skin lesions and with a PMN predominant pleocytosis, the clinical picture suggesting meningococcemia should prompt immediate antimicrobial therapy.

*Erythema infectiosum*, or fifth disease, due to parvovirus $B_{19}$, is a mild exanthematous disease, primarily of children. It begins with a prodrome of low-grade fever followed upon defervescence by appearance of an erythematous rash, initially on the face, producing the appearance of "slapped cheeks" (hence, *slapped cheek disease*) (Plate 10A). A morbilliform rash (Plate 10B) appears on the extremities 1–4 d later. Sore throat, mild fever, and headache occur in about 25% of patients. Arthritis, primarily of the knees and wrists, is more common in adults. The timing of the rash and the arthritis is consistent with immune-complex-mediated phenonoma.

*Roseola infantum*, (*exanthem subitum*) is an infection of infants or young children caused by human herpes virus type 6 (HHV-6). It begins with fever, often to 104–106°F, which lasts for about 3 d, during which the infant may be irritable but does not appear acutely ill. Upon defervescence the typical rash appears, consisting of maculopapular pink lesions first noted on the anterior abdomen, behind the ears, or on the neck (sparing the face). The rash fades within 1–3 d.

The *acute retroviral syndrome*, a mononucleosis-like illness with rash, occurs 1–6 wk after exposure to the virus in 30%–60% of persons who acquire HIV infection. The rash is truncal in distribution and consists of maculopapules or urticaria accompanied by fever, sweats, lymphadenopathy, malaise, and headache. A minority of patients have aseptic meningitis.

The rash of *varicella* is polymorphous, beginning as macules, quickly becoming papules, and rapidly progressing to vesicles. Chickenpox is mentioned here under macular rashes since the macular lesions appear abruptly early in the illness before the more distinctive components of the rash become evident. Chickenpox will be considered more fully with vesicular bullous eruptions.

*Infectious mononucleosis* is associated with rash in 5%–10% of cases. It is usually located on the trunk and arms, and it appears during the first few days of febrile illness. It is usually macular or maculopapular (morbilliform). Periorbital edema is present in about 30% of patients, and a nonspecific enanthem (palatal petechiae) is present in 10%–25%. A second type of rash, an extensive pruritic, maculopapular, brightly erythematous one, can develop in patients with mononucleosis given ampicillin. This drug reaction may become confluent, last for up to a week, and be followed by some desquamation.

*CMV mononucleosis* may occasionally be associated with maculopapular rashes. *Hepatitis B infection* may be accompanied by several types of rashes: urticaria (in about 20% of patients, with arthralgias or polyarthritis resembling transient serum sickness–like syndrome), vasculitic lesions (polyarteritis nodosa or leukocytoclastic angiitis), purpura (with arthralgias and renal involvement of essential mixed cryoglobulinemia), and papular acrodermatitis (Gianotti-Crosti syndrome). The latter occurs uncommonly and is an erythematous papular rash of about 3 wk duration on the extremities and face of children with acute hepatitis B infection. Rarely, *lymphocytic choriomeningitis*, an arenavirus infection, is accompanied by a maculopapular eruption. The illness is usually acquired in the summer and is commonly related to exposure to rodents or aerosols of their excreta. The illness may be a nonspecific febrile one or take the form of aseptic meningitis.

*Dengue fever* can take either of two forms: classic dengue fever or dengue hemorrhagic fever (DHF). The former is a self-limited, nonfatal disease that is endemic in tropical South and Central America, Africa, and Southeast Asia. This form of mosquito-borne (*Aedes aegypti*) disease results from initial infection with one of the four serotypes of this virus. DHF occurs in the setting of circulating immunity to another dengue serotype, with the development of immune enhancement. Classic dengue fever is a febrile illness that follows an incubation period of 5–8 d. Backache, prostration, retroorbital headache, and arthralgias are prominent features. The initial febrile period lasts about a week and may be accompanied by facial flushing and a transitory generalized macular rash. Shortly after defervescence the fever often recurs, a biphasic febrile course that is characteristic. Lymphadenopathy may be present. During the second febrile period a generalized maculopapular rash (sparing palms and soles) appears and lasts for 2–5 d. DHF is a much more serious illness characterized by fever, petechiae and purpura, thrombocytopenia, and other hemorrhagic manifestations such as gastrointestinal bleeding and epistaxis. DIC may be present and severe hypotension may supervene (dengue shock syndrome).

*Colorado tick fever* (*orbivirus*) occurs during the spring and summer in the western states following a tick (*Dermacentor andersoni*) bite. The illness resembles classic dengue fever with a biphasic fever pattern. A macular, maculopapular, or petechial (rarely) rash occurs with remission of the initial febrile period or during the second febrile phase.

### Rickettsial and ehrlichial infections

The highest prevalence of Rocky Mountain spotted fever (RMSF) in the United States is in the south Atlantic states (North and South Carolina, Virginia), in the Midwest (Oklahoma, Missouri), and on Cape Cod and Martha's Vineyard in Massachusetts. Less than 1%–2% of cases now occur in the Rocky Mountain states. The principal vector is the tick (dog tick, *Dermacentor variabilis*, in the eastern states). After an incubation period (median, 7 d) the illness begins with fever, severe headache and myalgias, nausea, vomiting, and abdominal pain. Rash is the sign that first suggests the diagnosis and becomes evident 3–5 d after the onset of the fever. The pink macular rash begins on the wrists, ankles and forearms and proceeds to involve the palms and soles, thighs, trunk, and face (Plate 11). Within 2–3 d of its onset the rash becomes petechial, but in some patients the rash is petechial from its onset. Petechiae can progress to ecchymoses. Other organs that may be involved in RMSF include the lungs (noncardiogenic pulmonary edema, interstitial pneumonia), kidney (renal failure), and central nervous system (aseptic meningitis, meningoencephalitis) and liver (hepatomegaly, jaundice) and heart (myocarditis). In fulminant RMSF the clinical presentation may involve encephalopathy, shock, and prominent hemorrhagic rash. Skin necrosis requiring multiple skin grafts may develop as a result of rickettsial damage to microvascular endothelium. Untreated RMSF can be fatal in 5–15 d if appropriate therapy has not been administered promptly. A tetracycline or chloramphenicol is the drug of choice.

Other rickettsial infections characterized by macular or maculopapular eruptions are *epidemic* and *endemic* typhus. Epidemic typhus is spread from person to person by the body louse. It is a rare disease in the United States but still occurs in parts of Asia, South America, and North Africa. A few indigenous cases, usually milder than classical epidemic typhus, have occurred in the eastern United States as a result of transmission by fleas or squirrel lice from a nonhuman reservoir of *Rickettsia prowazekii* in flying squirrels. Crowding, inadequate housing, infrequent bathing and changing of clothes, particularly during winter in times of war or natural disasters, predispose to proliferation of lice and spread of epidemic typhus. During World War I major outbreaks occurred in Eastern Europe; during World War II, concentration camps were hard hit. Typhus begins acutely with fever, chills, myalgias, and severe headache. After 4 or 5 d pink macules appear on the upper trunk. There is no eschar. The rash spreads centrifugally (sparing palms, soles, and face), becoming maculopapular, more confluent, deeper in color, with interspersed petechiae. Infection by *R. prowazekii* of endothelial cells produces vascular damage, sometimes with interstitial pulmonary infiltrates and prominent central nervous system manifestations (confusion, delirium, lymphocytic pleocytosis). Untreated, the fever subsides over 2 wk in uncomplicated cases; but the overall mortality rate is 10%–40%. Treatment with a tetracycline or chloramphenicol is highly effective.

A mild form of epidemic typhus, Brill-Zinsser disease, is a recrudescence of a previous episode of *R. prowazekii* infection occurring two to five decades after the initial infection. It has been seen in immigrants to this country from Eastern Europe who acquired their infection during World War II.

Endemic (murine) typhus is worldwide in distribution. Rats are the principal reservoir and infection with *R. typhi* is spread by rat fleas. In the United States most cases occur in urban areas in the Gulf Coast and in the Rio Grande area of southern Texas. The illness begins following an incubation period of 1–2 wk with fever, prominent headache, and myalgias. A macular rash is present in most patients and appears on the trunk 3–5 d later. It becomes maculopapular, mainly central in location, and persists for a total of 4–8 d, sparing palms and soles. No eschar is present. If untreated, the disease lasts for about 2 wk. It is generally milder than epidemic typhus with fewer pulmonary or CNS complications. Therapy with a tetracycline or chloramphenicol produces a prompt response in fever.

*Q fever*, caused by the rickettsia *Coxiella burnetii*, is worldwide in occurrence. The principal syndromes consist of a self-limited febrile illness, atypical pneumonia or hepatitis. Other forms of *C. burnetii* infection include infective endocarditis and meningoencephalitis. Q fever is acquired via inhalation of aerosols generated from tissues or excreta of cattle, sheep, and goats. This most often occurs among slaughterhouse workers, ranchers, and veterinarians. Occasionally, Q fever has been contracted by ingestion of contaminated unpasteurized milk, exposure to parturient cats, or from skinning infected wild rabbits. Generally, Q fever is considered the one rickettsial illness that does not have a characteristic rash. However, a centrally located maculopapular rash has been described in about 5%–20% of patients with acute Q fever. A tetracycline or chloramphenicol are the drugs of choice.

*Human ehrlichiosis* is due to *Ehrlichia chaffeensis*, a rickettsia-like intracellular organism. Ehrlichiosis occurs most commonly in the central and southwestern United States and is tick-borne. The clinical manifestations are generally like those of rickettsial infections, but without a rash. However, occasionally a central maculopapular rash is present. Leukopenia and thrombocytopenia are common, and the organism may occasionally be seen in the cytoplasm of polymorphonuclear leukocytes in Wright-Giemsa–stained smears of peripheral blood. Tetracyclines are effective therapy.

### *Mycoplasma* and chlamydial infections

*Mycoplasma pneumoniae* infections take the form of pharyngitis, tracheobronchitis, or atypical pneumonia. The incubation period is 21 d. The pneumonia is usually gradual in onset with fever, malaise, and prominent headache; a nonproductive cough follows a few days later. Rashes may develop in *M. pneumoniae* infections: maculopapular, vesicular, urticarial, petechial, erythema multiforme-like, Stevens-Johnson syndrome. The eruptions can occur during the atypical pneumonia syndrome or in the absence of clinically evident pneumonia. While antimicrobial treatment with a tetracycline or erythromycin may ameliorate clinical and radiologic manifestations, it does not appear to significantly alter the course of erythema multiforme.

*Psittacosis*, infection with *Chlamydia psittaci*, is transmitted to humans from birds. Human cases have been associated with exposure not only to psittacine birds (canaries, parrots, parakeets) but also to other avian species such as pigeons and sparrows. Illness begins either acutely with chills and high fever or more

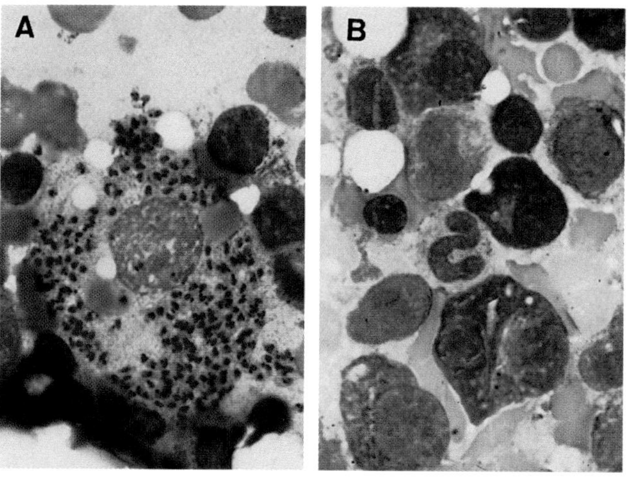


**Plate 1.** *Leishmania donovani.* Polyclonal reactional plasmacytosis is seen in *part B.* Bone marrow. Wright staining, x1000.

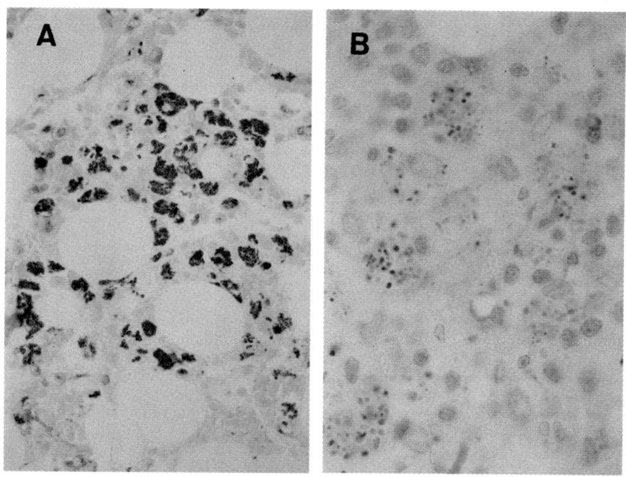


**Plate 2.** *Penicillium marnsei* in bone marrow of a patient with AIDS (*A*: Grocott staining; *B*: Prussian blue staining, x200).

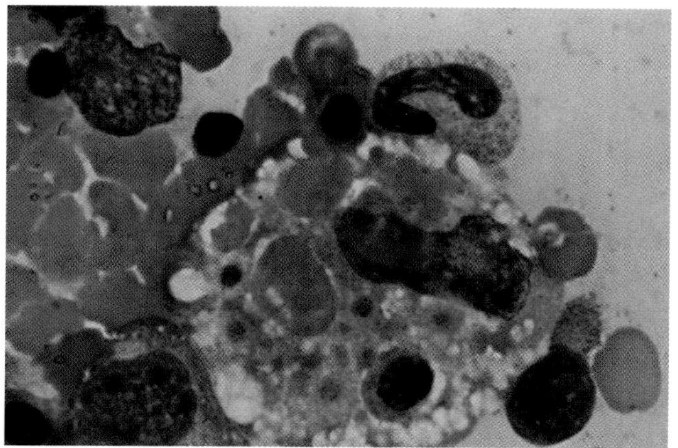

**Plate 3.** Hemophagocytosis in a case of EBV infection. Wright staining, x1000.

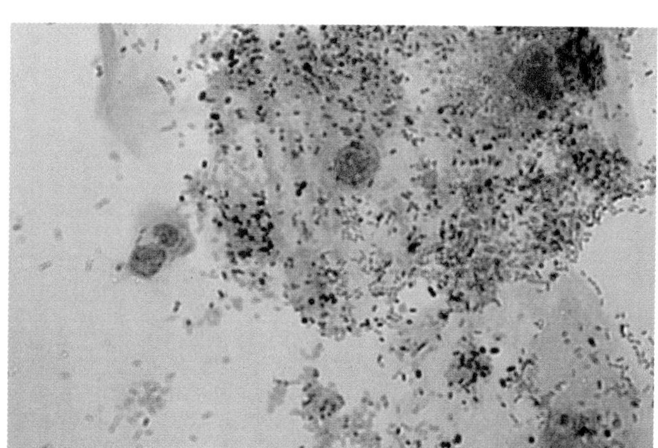

**Plate 4.** Polymicrobial flora—abscess.

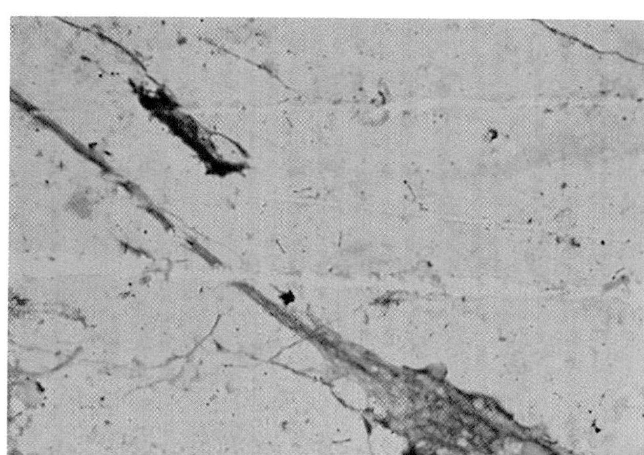

**Plate 5.** AFB—Kinyoun stain.

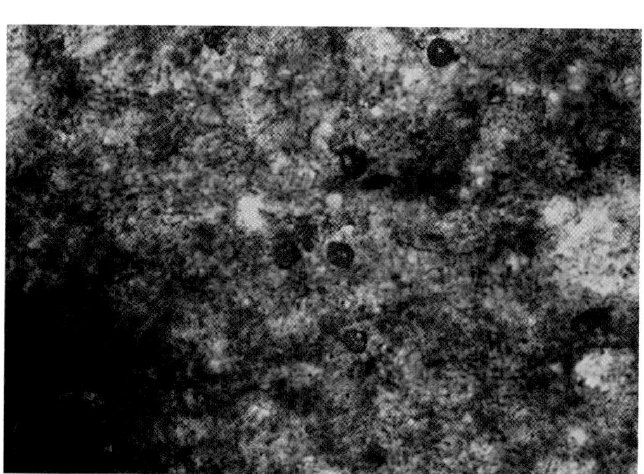

**Plate 6.** *Cryptosporidium*—Ziehl-Neelsen.

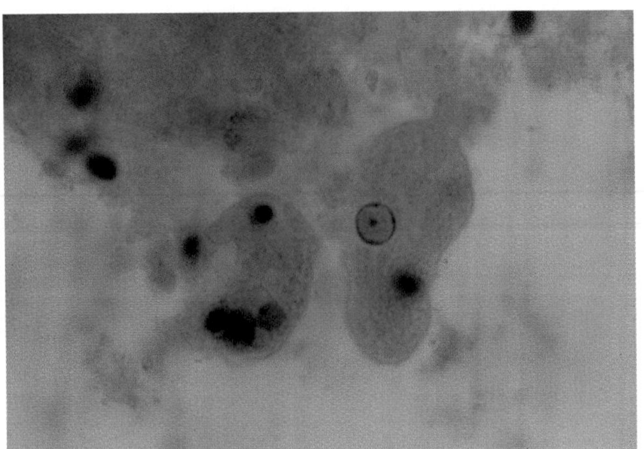

**Plate 7.** *E. histolytica* trophozoites—trichrome stain.

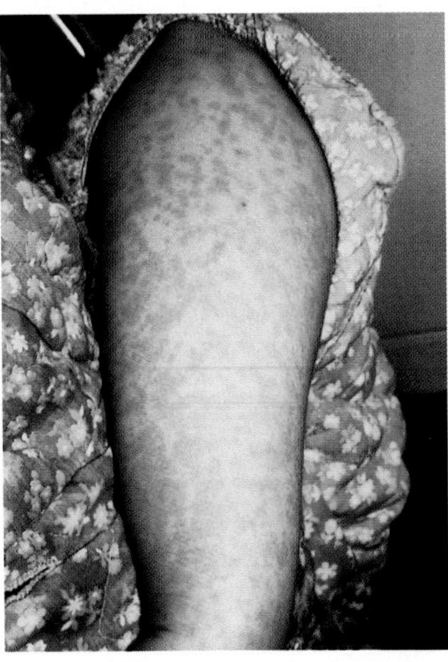

**Plate 8.** *Rubella* with diffuse irregular pink macules.

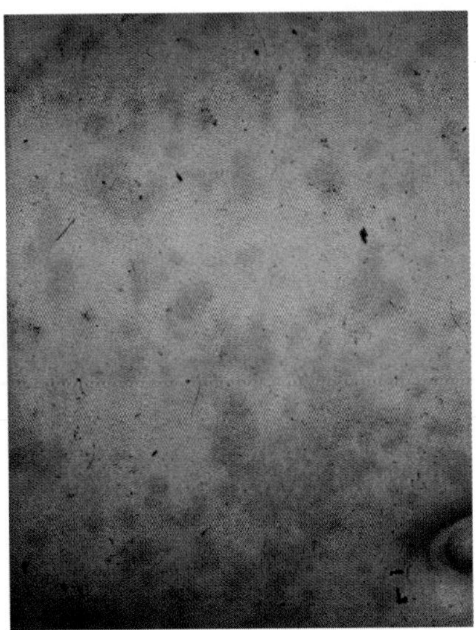

**Plate 9.** Measles showing pink macules on the abdomen of a child whose illness began with coryza, cough, fever, and conjunctivitis 4 d earlier.

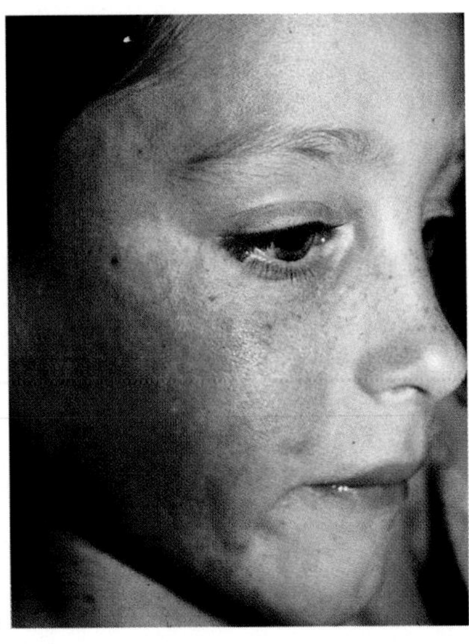

A

B

**Plate 10.** *A* Child with fifth disease showing "slapped cheek" appearance. *B* Child with fifth disease and lacy reticulate erythematous macules on forearm. [Reproduced with permission from "Dermatology in General Medicine," Fitzpatrick et al, eds. Chap. 202, 4th edition.]

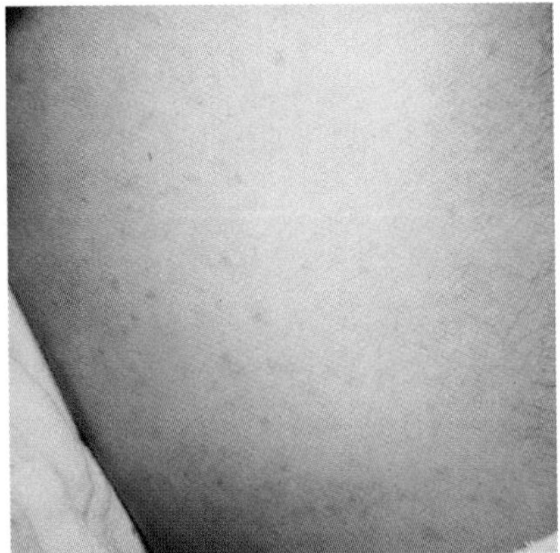

**Plate 11.** Pink macular rash on the trunk of a patient with Rocky Mountain spotted fever from Martha's Vineyard, an endemic area. Rash became petechial over next 24 h.

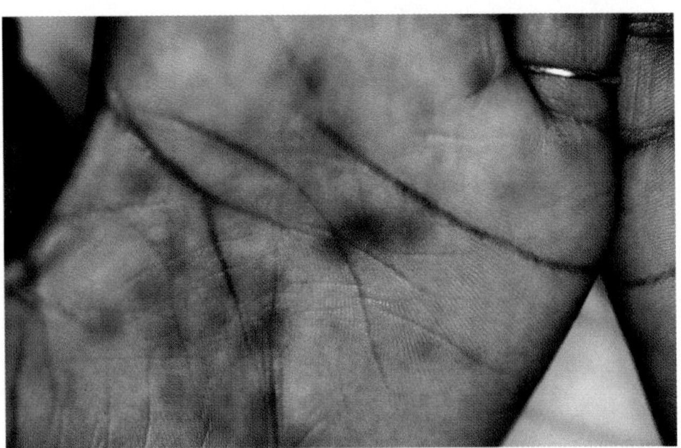

**Plate 12.** Pink palmar macules, some crossing palmar creases, in a patient with secondary syphilis. [Courtesy of Dr. Bonnie Mackool.]

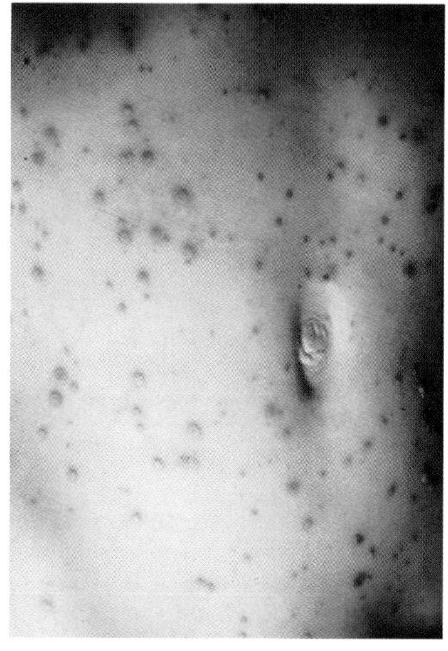

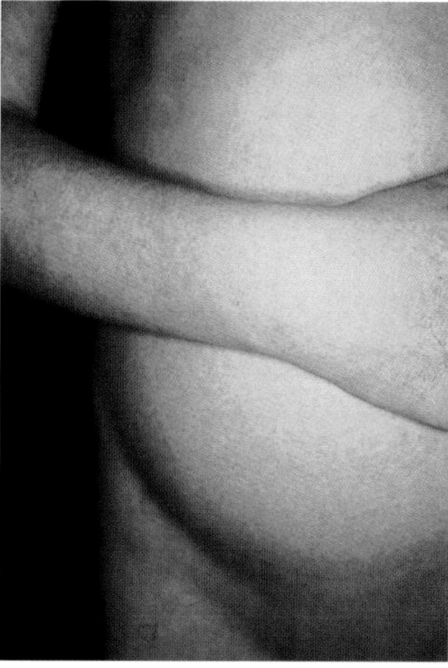

**Plate 13.** *Far left* Child with chickenpox showing all stages (macules, papules, vesicles, and crusts) of the rash in the same area of the trunk. [Courtesy of Dr. Louis Weinstein.]

**Plate 14.** *Left* Child with scarlet fever showing diffuse erythema on trunk and arm. Punctate papular elevations (1–2 mm), representing engorged dermal papillae, are present. [Courtesy of Dr. Louis Weinstein.]

A 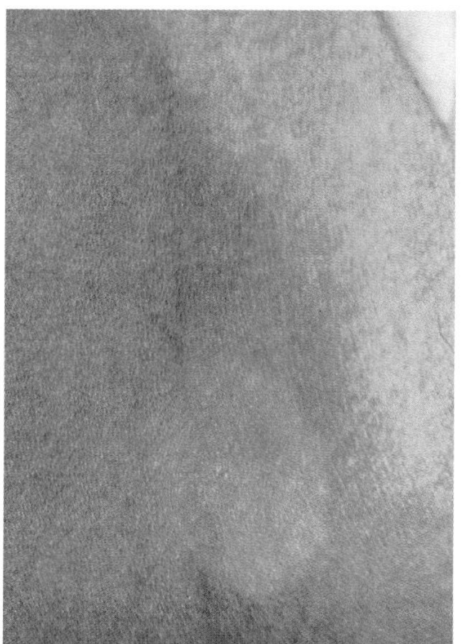

B 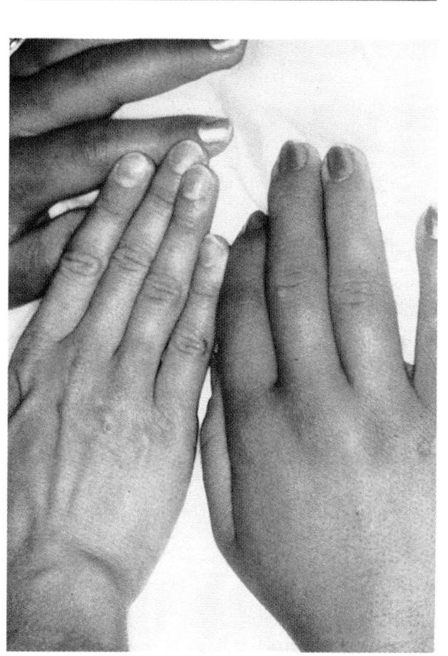

C 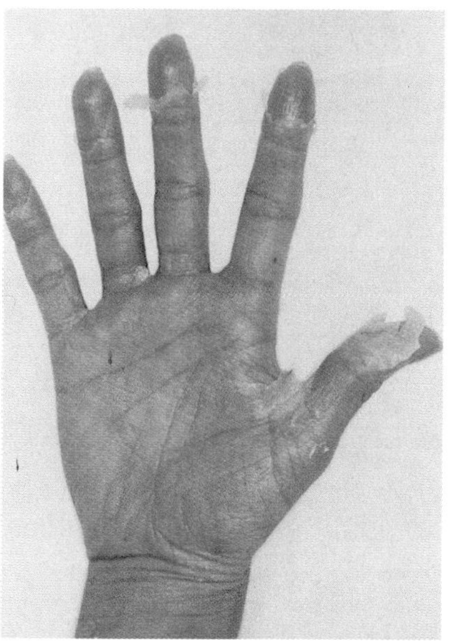

**Plate 15.** *A* Diffuse erythema of toxic shock syndrome, showing area of blanching where thumb pressure had been applied. [Courtesy Dr. Michael Bach.] *B* Hands of patient with toxic shock syndrome compared to hand of a normal individual in the center [Courtesy of Dr. Michael Bach.] *C* Desquamation of the fingers during convalescence from toxic shock sydrome [Courtesy of Dr. Michael Bach.]

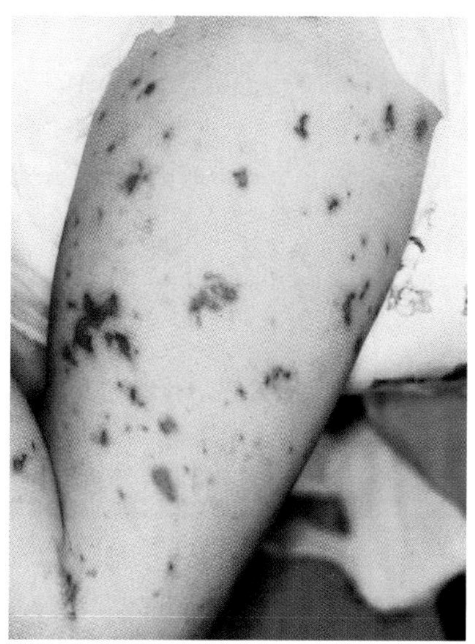

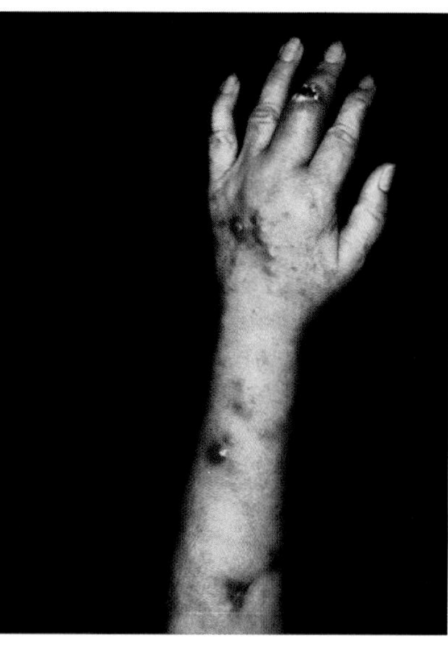

**Plate 16.** *Far left* Petechial-purpuric rash (36 h after onset) in a young child with meningococcemia and meningitis. Area of suggillation (gunmetal gray area of necrosis) visible in largest lesion. [Courtesy of Dr. Edward Lewin.]

**Plate 17.** *Left* Chancriform initial lesion and linear nodular lymphangitis extending over dorsum of hand and involving forearm in a gardener with sporotrichosis. [Courtesy of Dr. Newton Hyslop.]

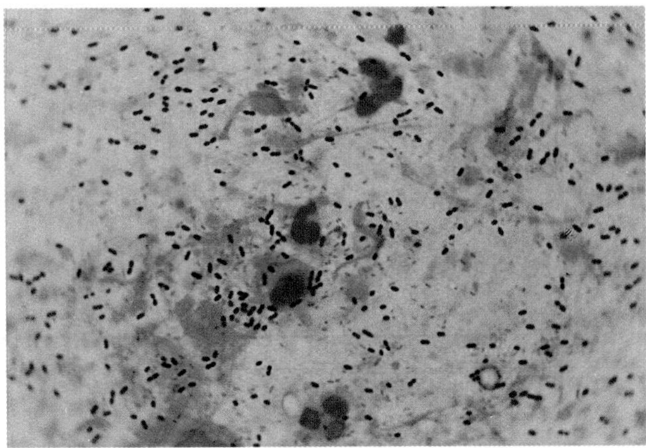

**Plate 18.** Gram stain showing both gram-positive cocci *(S. pneumoniae)* and small, faintly staining gram-negative coccobacillary forms *(H. influenzae).* Housestaff physicians identified the gram-positive cocci but overlooked the gram-negative organisms. [Reprinted with permission from Fine MJ, Orloff JJ, Rihs JD et al. Evaluation of sputum gram stains for community-acquired pneumonia: J Gen Int Med 1991; 6:189–198.]

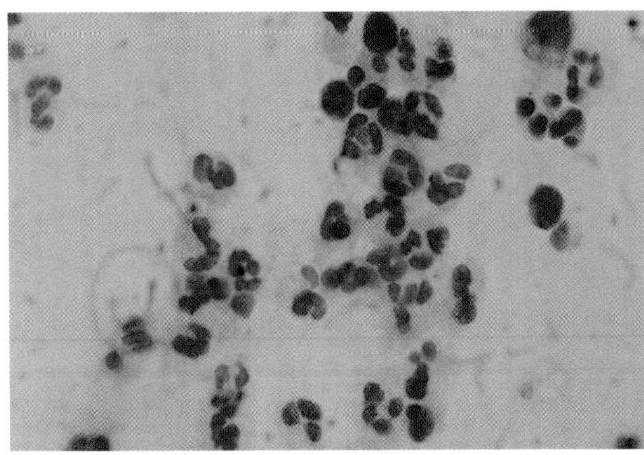

**Plate 19.** Gram stain showing numerous leukocytes but no organisms. This gram stain can be seen in patients with *Legionella, Chlamydia,* or viral pneumonia. Fourfold seroconversion to *Chlamydia pneumoniae* was demonstrated in this patient. [Reprinted with permission from Fine MJ, Orloff JJ, Rihs JD et al. Evaluation of sputum gram stains for community-acquired pneumonia: J Gen Int Med 1991; 6:189–198.]

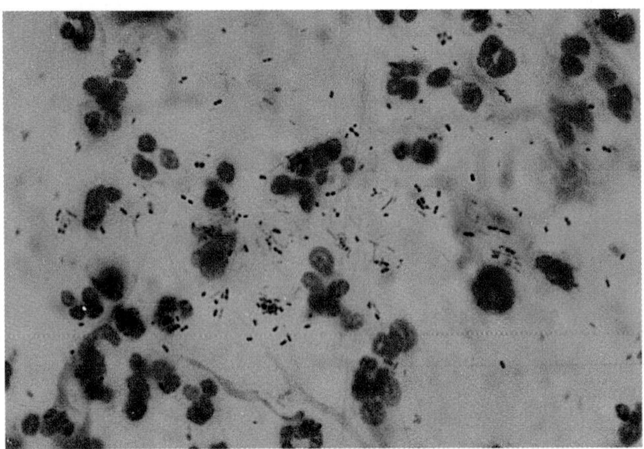

**Plate 20.** Gram stain showing gram-positive cocci, gram-negative bacilli, and gram-negative cocci that are characteristic of oropharyngeal bacteria. The presence of leukocytes confirmed that the sputum specimen was adequate for interpretation. Evaluation of the patient was consistent with aspiration pneumonia. [Reprinted with permission from Fine MJ, Orloff JJ, Rihs JD et al. Evaluation of sputum gram stains for community-acquired pneumonia: J Gen Int Med 1991; 6:189–198.]

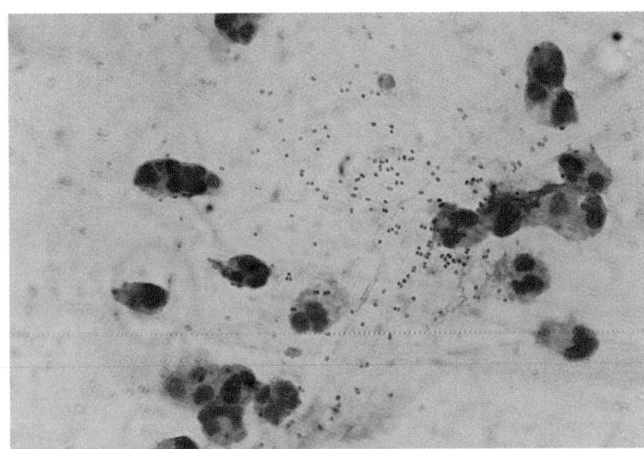

**Plate 21.** Gram stain shows large numbers of gram-negative cocci. Sputum culture revealed pure culture of *Moraxella catarrhalis.* [Reprinted with permission from Fine MJ, Orloff JJ, Rihs JD et al. Evaluation of sputum gram stains for community-acquired pneumonia: J Gen Int Med 1991; 6:189–198.]

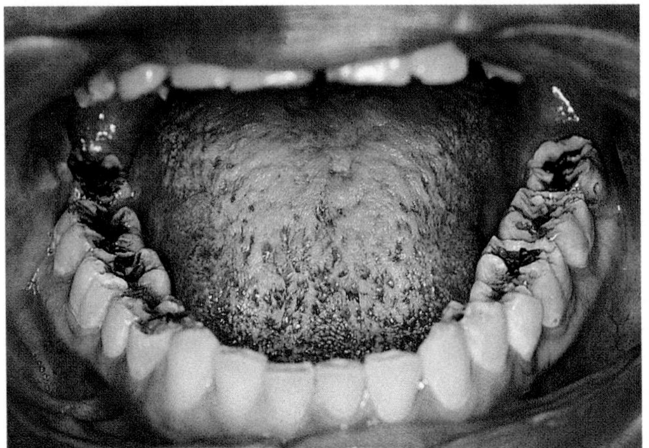

**Plate 22.** Widespread dental caries associated with irradiation for pharyngeal carcinoma.

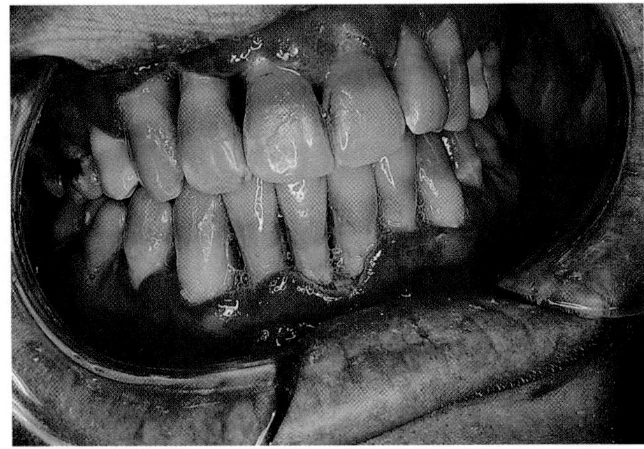

**Plate 23.** Necrotizing ulcerative periodontitis associated with HIV infection.

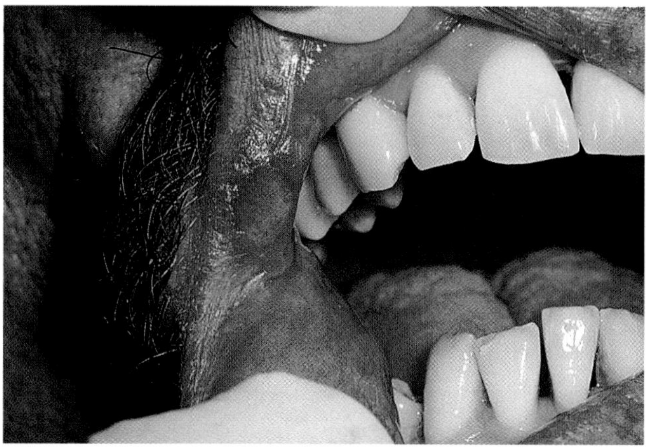

**Plate 24.** Syphilis, mucous patch of vermilion border and labial mucosa.

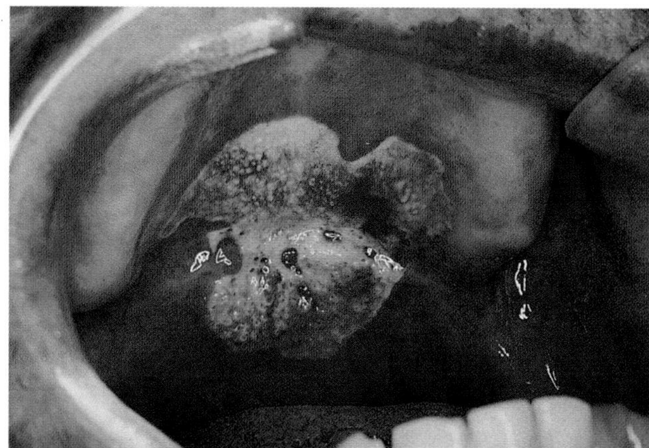

**Plate 25.** Pseudomembranous candidiasis, palate, 80-y-old female.

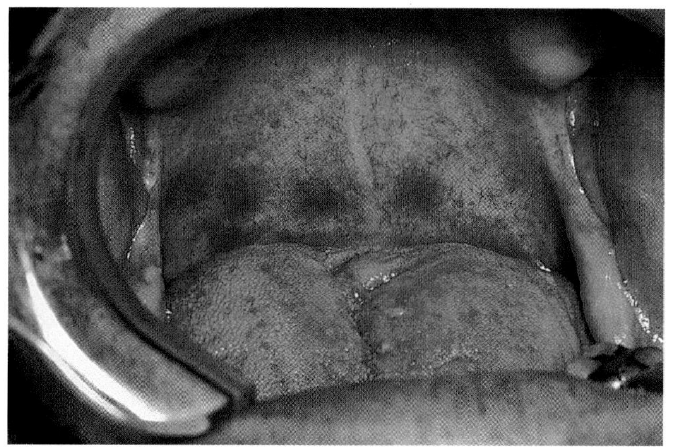

**Plate 26.** Erythematous candidiasis, palate; HIV infection.

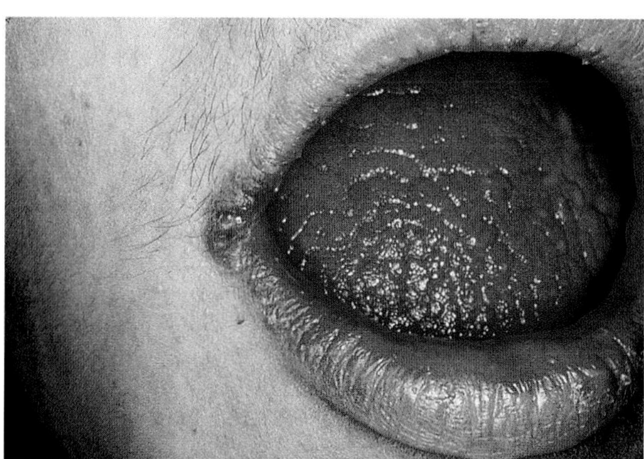

**Plate 27.** Angular cheilitis and mucosal dryness in Sjogren's syndrome. [Courtesy of Dr. T.E. Daniels.]

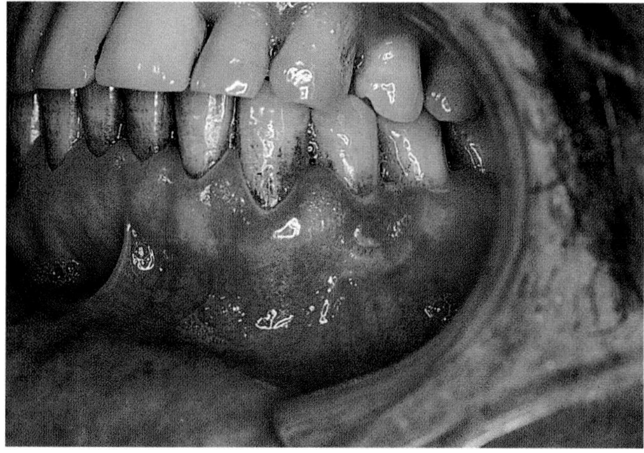

**Plate 28.** Histoplasmosis, gingiva; HIV infection.

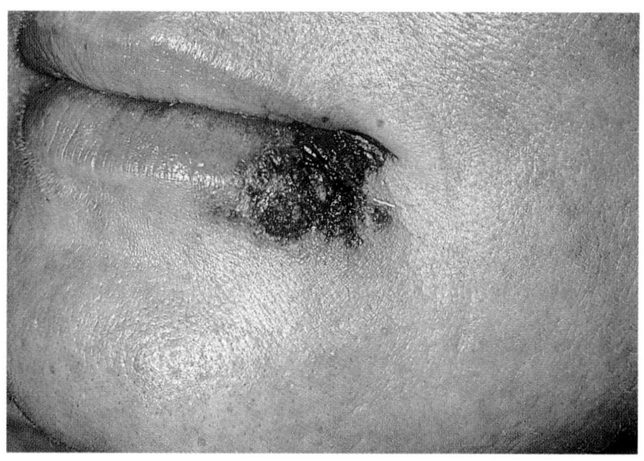

**Plate 29.** Herpes labialis due to HSV-2; HIV infection.

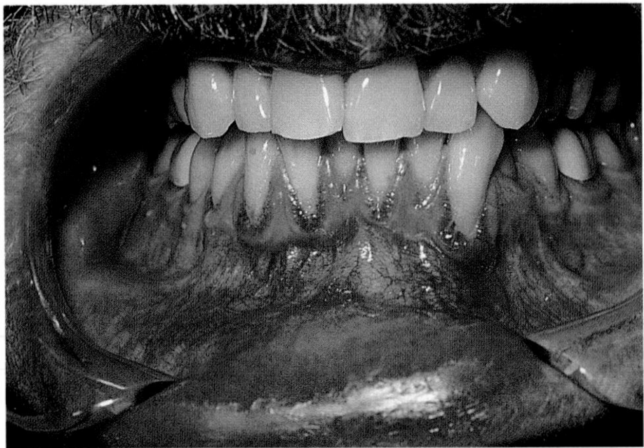

**Plate 30.** Recurrent intraoral herpes simplex, mandibular gingiva; HIV infection.

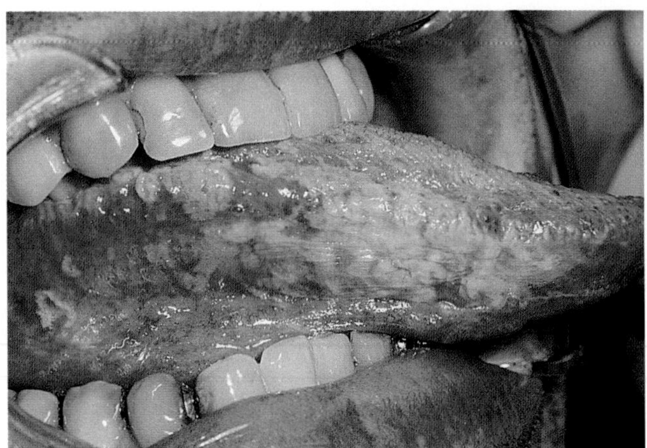

**Plate 31.** Hairy leukoplakia; HIV infection.

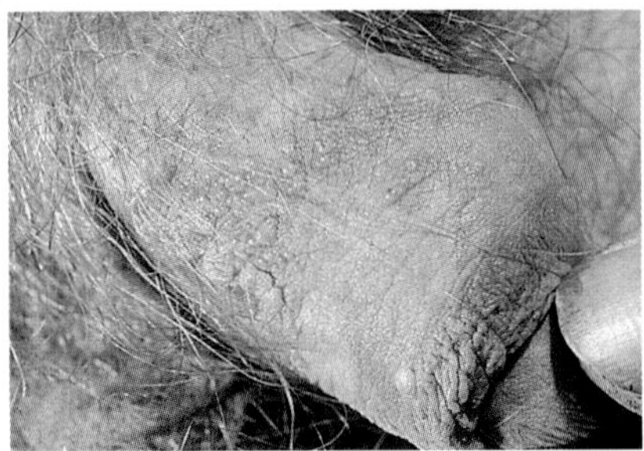

**Plate 32.** Classical genital herpes, with multiple penile vesicles on erythematous bases. [Reproduced with permission from Handsfield HH. Color Atlas and Synopsis of Sexually Transmitted Diseases. New York, McGraw-Hill, 1992.]

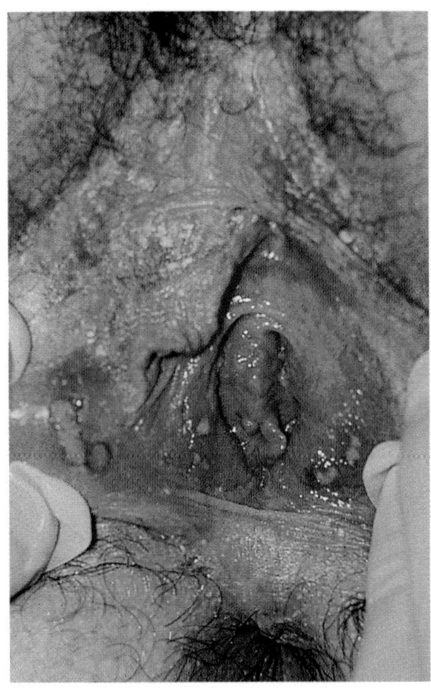

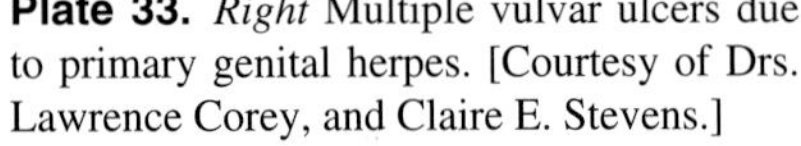

**Plate 33.** *Right* Multiple vulvar ulcers due to primary genital herpes. [Courtesy of Drs. Lawrence Corey, and Claire E. Stevens.]

**Plate 34.** Genital herpes mimicking chancroid; type 1 herpes simplex virus was isolated from the lesion and culture for *Hemophilus ducreyi* and darkfield microscopy were negative. [Reproduced with permission from Handsfield HH. Color Atlas and Synopsis of Sexually Transmitted Diseases. New York, McGraw-Hill, 1992.]

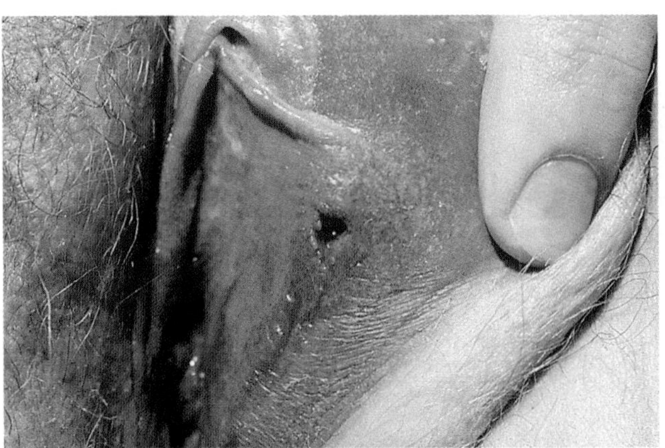

**Plate 35.** Asymptomatic vulvar lesion due to recurrent genital herpes; type 2 herpes simplex virus was isolated, following which the patient recognized subsequent recurrences. [Reproduced with permission from Handsfield HH. Color Atlas and Synopsis of Sexually Transmitted Diseases. New York, McGraw-Hill, 1992.]

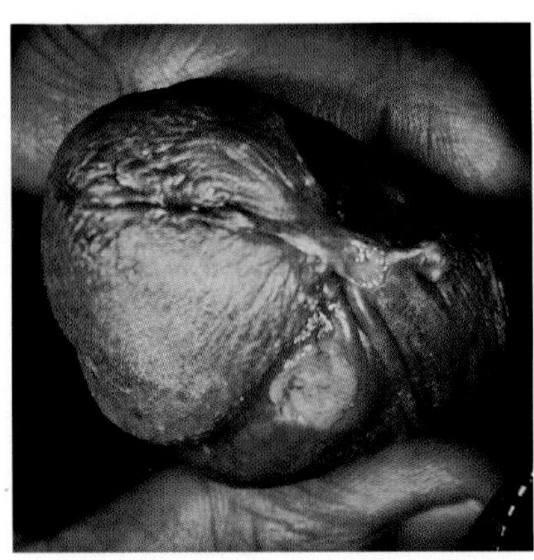

**Plate 36.** Two chancres of the penis in primary syphilis.

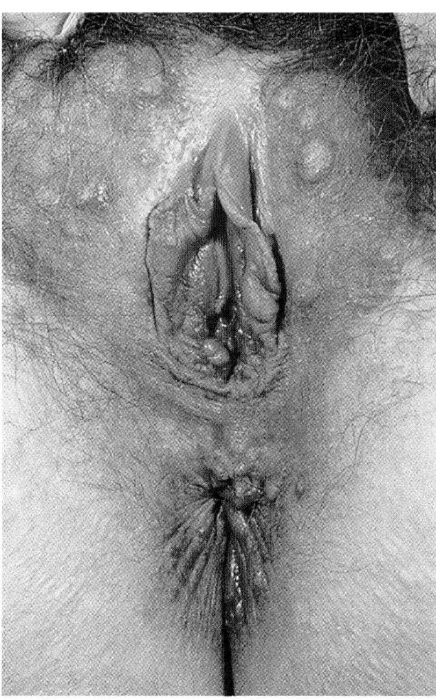

**Plate 37.** *Left* Secondary syphilis with condylomata lata with superficial ulcerations suggestive of genital herpes; the lesions were dark-field-positive and culture-negative for herpes simplex virus. [Reproduced with permission from Handsfield HH. Color Atlas and Synopsis of Sexually Transmitted Diseases. New York, McGraw-Hill, 1992.]

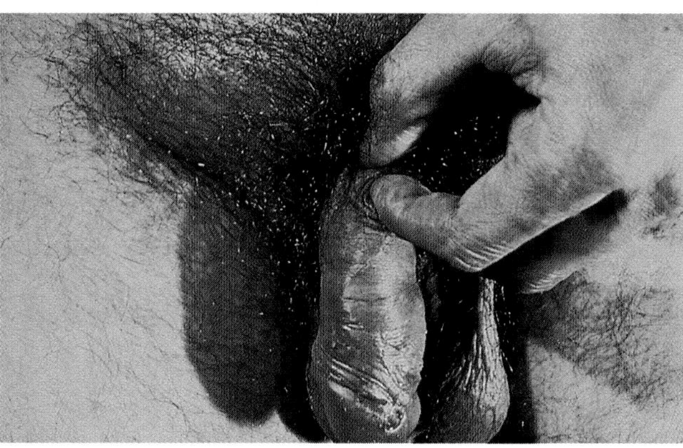

**Plate 38.** Chancroid, with penile ulcers and prominent inguinal lymphadenopathy; the small eschars adjacent to the bubo mark the sites of needle aspiration of the fluctuant lymph node.

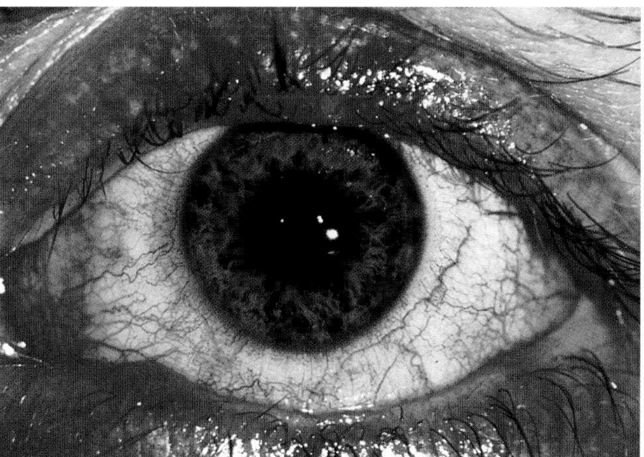

**Plate 39.** Blepharitis. Swollen, inflammed eyelids.

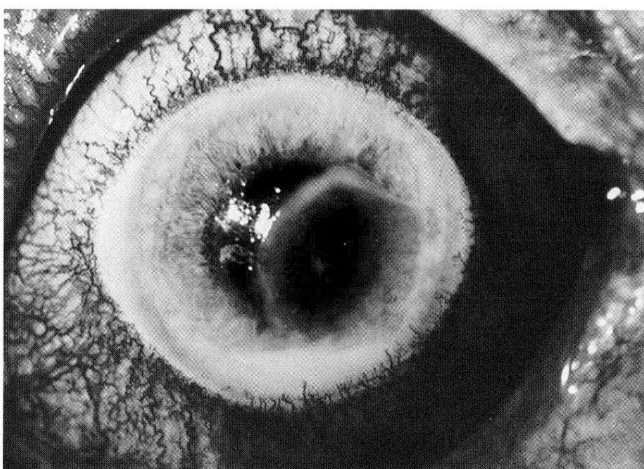

**Plate 40.** Corneal ulcer with hypopyon. Opacification of the cornea and white blood cells layered in the anterior chamber in a patient with pneumococcal keratitis.

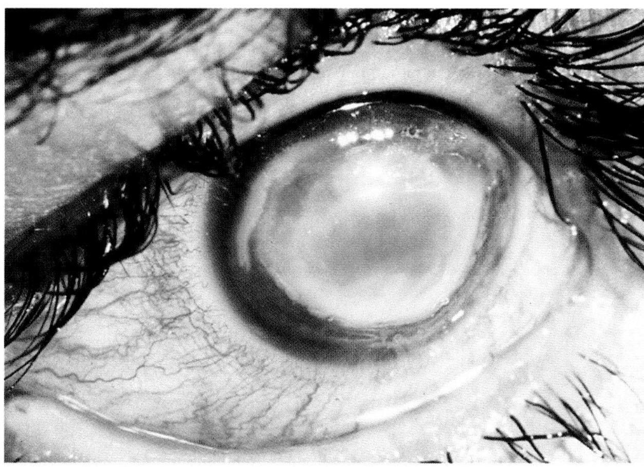

**Plate 41.** Acanthomoeba corneal ulcer. Opacification of the cornea with parasitic infection.

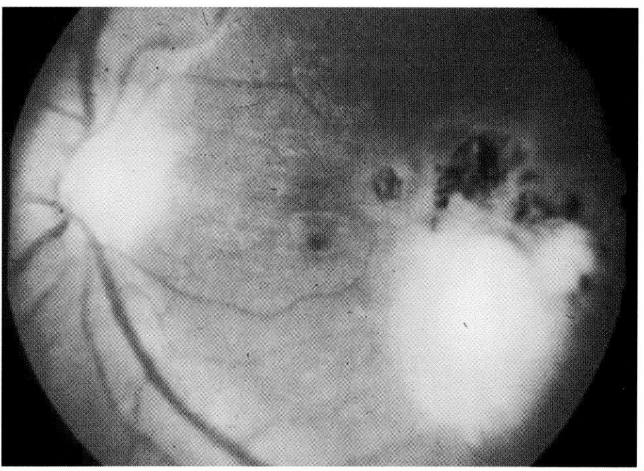

**Plate 42.** Toxoplasma chorioretinitis. A new fluffy lesion next to an old pigmented scar in the fundus.

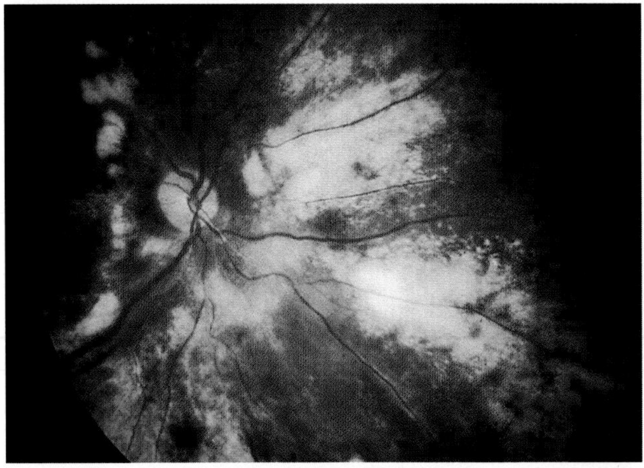

**Plate 43.** Cytomegalovirus retinitis. Typical brush-fire borders of the hemorrhagic form of the disease.

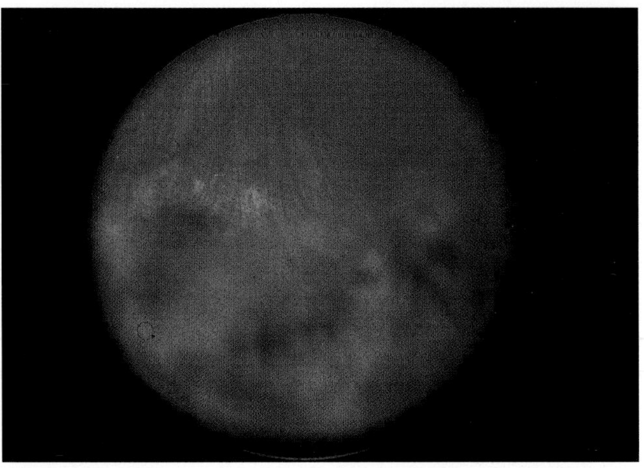

**Plate 44.** Acute retinal necrosis. Hemorrhage, edema of retina.

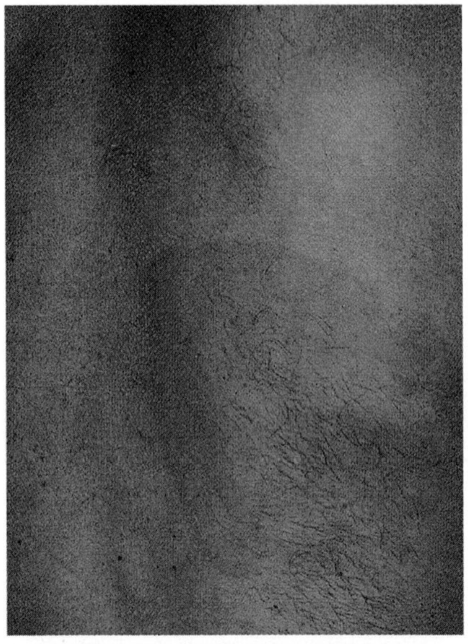

**Plate 45.** Erythma migrans rash in patient with Lyme disease. [Reproduced with permission from Spach DH, et al.]

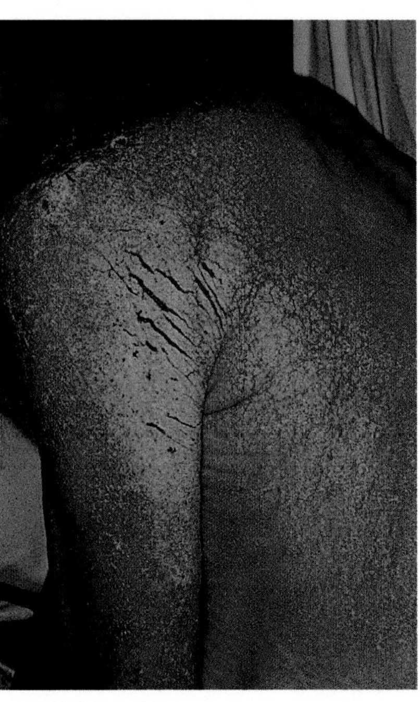

**Plate 46.** *Left* Crusted (Norwegian) scabies. AIDS patient with crusted hyperkeratotic, fissured lesions typical of crusted scabies. [Reproduced with permission from Spach DH, Fritsche TR. Norwegian scabies in a patient with AIDS. N Engl J Med 1994;331:777.]

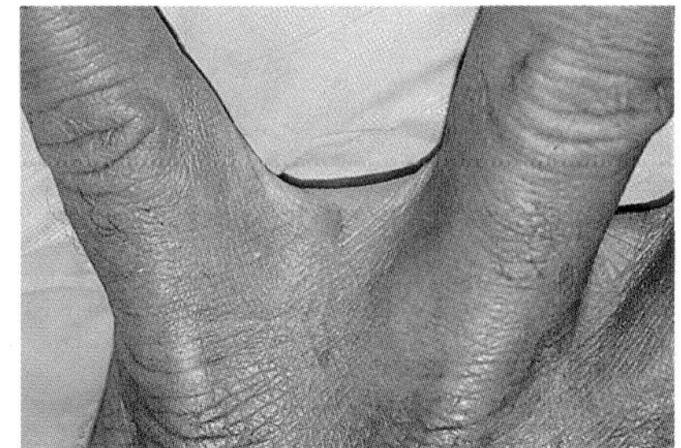

**Plate 47.** Typical scabies burrow in the space between fingers.

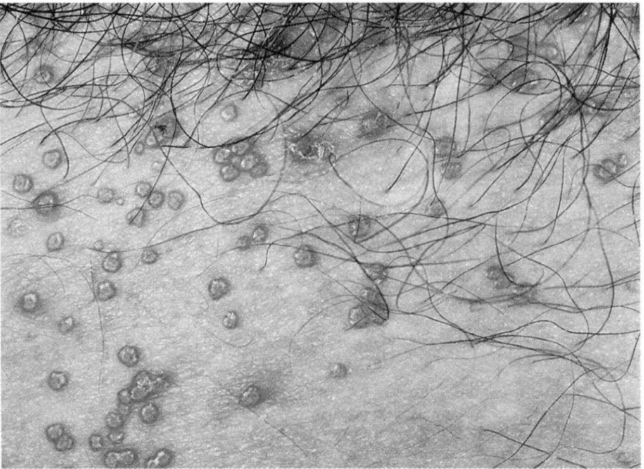

**Plate 48.** Skin lesions of molluscum contagiosum, showing multiple umbilicated papules. [Courtesy of Dr. Hunter Handsfield.]

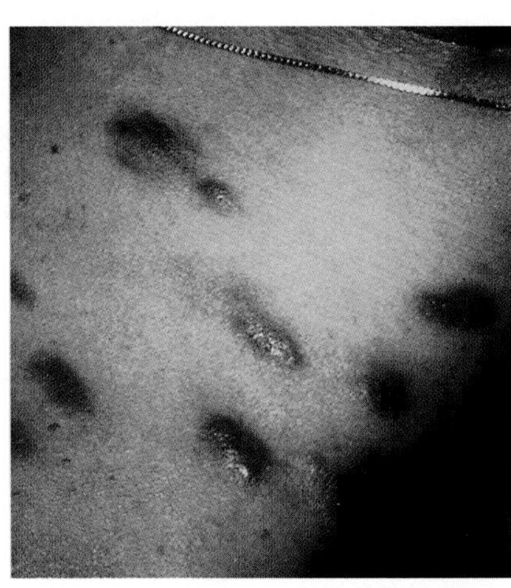

**Plate 49.** Skin lesions of Kaposi's sarcoma, showing multiple nontender, erythematous macules.[Credit: Phil Kirby, M.D.]

gradually with increasing malaise, myalgias, and fever. Headache is commonly present. Persistent dry cough may be present from the beginning or develop several days after the onset of fever. Splenomegaly is sometimes present. The clinical and radiologic features of atypical pneumonia are usually evident. Clustered, pink macular lesions (Horder spots) on the trunk are observed rarely and closely resemble the rose spots of typhoid fever.

### Bacterial infections

Along with rickettsial/ehrlichial infections, bacterial infections causing fever and a rash are the most important to promptly identify because of the need for specific antimicrobial treatment. *Secondary syphilis* begins 2–8 wk after the appearance of the chancre. Most common manifestations consist of macular, maculopapular, papular, or pustular lesions. The initial lesions are usually 3–10 mm pink macules on the torso and proximal extremities. These lesions can evolve to red papules and even progress to pustules. Involvement of palms and soles, particularly with papules crossing palmor creases, suggests secondary syphilis (Plate 12). Occasionally, maculopapular lesions develop superficial scaling, a papulosquamous syphilid. Vesicular or bullous lesions do not occur. Often, several types of lesions are present simultaneously. Although typically the lesions of secondary syphilis are nonpruritic, pruritis has been reported recently in 10% of patients. In warm, moist, intertriginous areas (e.g., axilla, perianal area, vulva) painless papular lesions enlarge, producing flat, moist, gray-white to erythematous lesions covered with a thick mucoid exudate (*condyloma latum*). Such highly infectious lesions teem with spirochetes. On mucous membranes similar highly infectious lesions (*mucous patches*) may be present and consist of rounded, flat, gray-white, superficial erosions with a red periphery.

Constitutional manifestations are common in secondary syphilis and include low-grade fever, malaise, and generalized lymphadenopathy. Occasionally, the fever may be so high and constitutional manifestations so prominent as to suggest sepsis. Hepatitis or lymphocytic meningitis may be prominent features in the secondary stage. Therapy utilizes penicillin G parenterally. Treatment is often accompanied within 12 h by the Jarisch-Herxheimer reaction (fever, flare of mucocutaneous lesions).

*Leptospirosis* is acquired from oral or cutaneous exposure to water contaminated with infected animal (rodents, dogs) urine or from direct animal contact (farmers, abattoir workers). The forms this illness may take are anicteric (undifferentiated fever, aseptic meningitis) or icteric (Weil's disease) leptospirosis. Features include high fever (sometimes biphasic), chills, headache, myalgias, nausea, and vomiting. Findings in the anicteric form may include lymphadenopathy, splenomegaly, scleral conjunctival suffusion, pulmonary involvement (cough, radiologic infiltrates), and rash. The latter occurs in less than half the cases, is truncal in distribution, and consists of erythematous macules, papules, and scattered petechiae. An uncommon form of anicteric leptospirosis ("Fort Bragg fever") due to *L. interrogans* serovar *autumnalis* has been associated with slightly raised, erythematous, 1–5 cm tender lesions on the pretibial areas. Icteric leptospirosis, a more severe form of the disease, is characterized by prominent hepatic and renal (hematuria, azotemia) dysfunction with hepatomegaly, obtundation, hypotension, and hemorrhagic manifestations in many organs including the skin (petechiae, ecchymoses). Treatment of mild (nonicteric) leptospirosis involves use of doxycycline. Treatment of more severe leptospirosis (Weil's disease) employs intravenous penicillin or ampicillin.

Patients with *acute meningococcemia* or the *meningococcemia/meningitis syndrome* may occasionally have an initial pink macular eruption with a few scattered petechiae, predominantly on the extremities. The macular lesions are followed by the prominent petechial-purpuric eruption of meningococcemia (see below). Chronic meningococcemia is characterized by recurrent fevers and migratory arthralgias or arthritis and polymorphous skin lesions (see below), the scattered skin lesions may initially be only maculopapular.

*Typhoid fever* is a systemic infection with *S. typhi* that is characterized by rising fever (104–106°F), headache, myalgias, constipation, bronchitis, and a relative bradycardia. Skin lesions (rose spots) occur after about 7–10 d of high fever and are not a prominent feature, but their presence may be helpful in diagnosis. Rose spots consist of nontender, 2–3 mm, slightly raised pink papules which blanch on pressure. They appear in crops of 10–20 lesions on the lower anterior chest and upper abdomen. Antimicrobial choices include ciprofloxacin and chloramphenicol.

Although the typical skin eruption of *Pseudomonas aeruginosa* bacteremia consists of either vesicles/bullae or ecthyma gangrenosa or gangrenous cellulitis, occasionally small maculopapular lesions resembling the rose spots of typhoid fever occur on the trunk.

The reservoir of *Brucella* is in cattle, sheep, and swine; human infection stems from ingestion of unpasteurized milk or cheese or from direct animal contact. Acute brucellosis is a bacteremic illness with high fever, headache, and skeletal symptoms. Hepatosplenomegaly may be a feature. In some patients brucellosis is a more indolent infection. Nonspecific erythematous maculopapular lesions have been reported, but in less than 10% of patients. Treatment consists of the combination of doxycycline with streptomycin or the combination of doxycycline with rifampin.

*Streptobacillus moniliformis infection* (*rat-bite fever*) is characterized by fever, polyarthralgias or arthritis, and a rash 1–5 d following a rat bite. Rarely, it has occurred following ingestion of contaminated milk. The rash consists of erythematous macules, papules, and scattered petechiae. It is most concentrated on the distal extremities, particularly about joints, and on the palms and soles. Treatment with penicillin or ampicillin is curative.

*Relapsing fever* is louse-borne or tick-borne. The former, due to *Borrelia recurrentis*, is worldwide in distribution, often occurring in epidemics in wartime or during natural disasters. The latter, due to *B. hermsii* and other species, is endemic in the western United States. Recurrent cycles of high fever, chills, severe headache, myalgias, and cough occur at intervals of 7–10 d and last for 3–6 d if untreated. Findings include conjunctival injection, tachycardia, abdominal tenderness, and hepatosplenomegaly. Borrelia spirochetes can be seen on Wright-stained smears of peripheral blood. A maculopapular rash with petechiae is often seen on the trunk for 1–2 d during the initial period of fever. Tetracycline and erythromycin are the drugs of choice but penicillin also has been used.

*Scarlet fever*, due to infection with a group A streptococcal strain producing a pyrogenic (erythrogenic) exotoxin, is characterized by a diffuse erythematous blush-like eruption (see *diffuse erythroderma*). Mention is made here because of the superimposed presence of numerous deeper red, punctate elevations (engorged dermal papillae) suggesting a maculopapular eruption.

Infection with *B. burgdorferi* (*Lyme disease*) is tick-borne and particularly endemic in southeastern New England, New York, New Jersey, and Wisconsin. It is included among febrile infections with maculopapular lesions since an initial red macule or papule develops at the site of the tick bite. Between 3 and 32 d later the characteristic large (10–15 cm), flat, ring-like erythematous lesion of erythema chronicum migrans (ECM) develops. ECM is often accompanied by fever, fatigue, headache, and generalized lymphadenopathy. Dissemination of infection may be evidenced by the appearance of multiple ECM lesions, carditis, Bell's palsy, and lymphocytic meningitis.

*Miliary tuberculosis*, rarely, may be associated with an erythematous, maculopapular eruption on the trunk.

### Parasitic infections

A few parasitic diseases may be associated with fever and an accompanying maculopapular rash. Rarely, acute acquired *toxoplasmosis* in the immunocompetent individual may produce the picture of mononucleosis with a maculopapular rash.

Symptoms associated with systemic invasion by larvae of *Trichinella* (*trichinosis*) follow ingestion of inadequately cooked meat, principally pork. They include fever, myalgias, periorbital edema, and weakness. Subconjunctival and subungual splinter hemorrhages may be seen. Maculopapular, urticarial, or petechial rashes occur. Eosinophilia is common.

*West and East African trypanosomiasis* (due to *Trypanosoma brucei gambiense* and *T. b. rhodesiense*, respectively) are transmitted by tsetse flies. The latter illness tends to be more acute. At the site of the fly bite a painful trypanosomal chancre sometimes develops but resolves spontaneously. Systemic invasion weeks or months later is characterized by intermittent fever and posterior cervical lymphadenopathy (Winterbottom's sign). During this acute phase, hepatosplenomegaly may be evident. Cutaneous involvement consists of transient facial edema and swelling of hands and feet, pruritus, and large erythematous (often circinate) areas on the trunk and proximal extremities. Untreated, the illness progresses to a meningoencephalitic phase (*sleeping sickness*) weeks to months later.

### Noninfectious causes of diffuse maculopapular rashes

*Erythema multiforme* may present with high fever and suggest a serious infectious disease. It may be associated with specific infections such as those due to *M. pneumoniae*. It also may be associated with hypersensitivity reactions to a number of drugs (e.g., barbiturates, sulfonamides, penicillin, phenytoin). Lesions are usually monomorphous initially: (*1*) target or iris macular erythematous lesions, particularly on the extensor surfaces and often on the palms and soles, (*2*) urticarial, nonchanging plaques, and (*3*) bullous-erosive lesions with prominent involvement of oral and conjunctival mucosa.

*Juvenile or adult Still's disease* (systemic juvenile rheumatoid arthritis) may present initially with an acute onset with fever and a rash, but the true nature of the process may not be apparent until later with the development of articular abnormalities. The rash, consisting of small erythematous macules on the trunk and extremities, is more prominent at the height of fever.

*Kawasaki disease* (*mucocutaneous lymph node syndrome*) (see below) is an acute febrile illness occurring in children, characterized by cervical lymphadenopathy, scarlatiniform or maculopapular eruption, conjunctival injection, erythema of lips, and strawberry tongue.

*Connective tissue diseases* may present initially as an FRS, or an exacerbation of an established connective tissue disease may involve fever and a rash, suggesting a superimposed infection. Diffuse macular erythema on the trunk and extremities may occur in systemic lupus erythematous (SLE), or a maculopapular erythematous rash may be induced by sunlight or a drug. Fever is more common in childhood dermatomyositis than in the adult form. An erythematous rash on the trunk and arms often occurs along with a lilac (heliotrope)-colored rash on the upper eyelids and erythematous scaly plaques on the extensor surfaces of the interphalangeal joints of the hands (Gottron's sign).

In *hypersensitivity vasculitis* the typical skin lesion is that of palpable purpura, but maculopapular lesions, vesicles, ulcers, and recurrent urticaria may occur. The most common forms of cutaneous lesions in drug reactions are macular, morbilliform, and papular. Others include urticaria, erythema multiforme, erythema nodosum and vasculitic lesions, and toxic epidermal necrolysis. Fever often accompanies such drug reactions.

*Sweet's syndrome* (acute febrile neutrophilic dermatosis) is a recurrent febrile illness with arthralgias, red papules or nodules which tend to coalesce into irregular sharply outlined plaques, conjunctivitis, and leukocytosis. The cause is unknown but it is sometimes associated with chronic myelogenous leukemia, or inflammatory bowel disease. *Eosinophilic pustular folliculitis* consists of pruritic nodules with a pustular head on an erythematous base about hair follicles, occurring more often, but not exclusively, in HIV-infected patients. Fever is not intrinsic to the skin eruption but may be present due to opportunistic infections.

## Maculopapular rash with herald plaque or initial eschar (Table 51.1)

### Viral infections

*Pityriasis rosea* often follows prodromal symptoms of mild fever, malaise, and arthralgia during the spring–summer–fall period. While an infectious etiology is suggested, proof has not been obtained. The primary plaque (herald patch) develops on the trunk in most cases. It is oval with a central salmon-colored area, surrounded by a darker peripheral area, and separated from it by a collarette of fine scale. A secondary eruption appears 2–21 d later and consists of crops of new maculopapular lesions or miniature versions of primary plaques. Lesions are mainly on the trunk, oriented along the lines of cleavage of the skin in a "Christmas tree" pattern.

### Rickettsia/ehrlichia infections

*Rickettsialpox*, due to *R. akari*, is transmitted by mouse mites. An asymptomatic papule develops at the site of a mite bite, ulcerates, and evolves into a black eschar with mild regional lymphadenopathy. Systemic symptoms, consisting of chills, fever, headache, and myalgias, develop acutely 9–14 d after the insect bite. Several days after the onset of fever a generalized erythematous papular rash occurs and becomes papulovesicular, resembling varicella. The illness is mild, resolving in 2–3 wk.

A variety of tick-borne rickettsial diseases with eschar and spotted fever pattern occur in different geographic areas: *Fievre boutonneuse* or Mediterranean spotted fever due to *R. conorii* along the Meditterranean littoral; *Kenya and South African tick fever*, both due to *R. conorii*; *Queensland tick fever* (*R. australis*); *North Asian spotted fever* (*R. ubirica*) in China, Pakistan, and Russia; and *Oriental spotted fever* (*R. japonica*) in Japan. All produce a similar clinical syndrome. Five days after the tick bite a black eschar (tache noire) with a red halo may become evident at the bite site, or it may not be noted for another 2–5 d until the onset of systemic symptoms: fever, myalgias, headache, rash and regional lymphadenopathy. The rash is generalized, maculopapular, erythematous, and often spreads from the trunk to involve palms and soles.

*Scrub typhus* (*tsutsugamushi fever*) is due to infection with *R. tsutsugamushi* transmitted by larval mites (chiggers) of small rodents. It is endemic in a region extending from Japan to Australia, including the South Pacific islands and Indonesia. Humans are exposed when they enter partially cleared areas that maintain the rodent hosts to build roads, clear forests, or for military maneuvers. A primary papular lesion develops at the bite site after 6–18 d. Systemic illness then develops with an acute onset of headache, chills, fever, and malaise. Fever increases over the next few days, and signs of meningoencephalitis may develop if treatment is not initiated. After 5–7 d of illness a faint pink maculopapular rash appears on the trunk and spreads to the extremities. Interstitial pneumonia and myocarditis may be complications. Treatment with a tetracycline or chloramphenicol is rapidly curative.

### Bacterial infections

*Spirillum minus rat-bite fever* (*sodoku*) is similar to streptobacillary rat bite fever in its initiation through a bite wound. The wound heals promptly but 1–4 wk later this site becomes swollen, purple, and painful, associated with lymphangitis and regional lymphadenitis. This is accompanied by fever, chills, headache, and malaise. A leukocytosis is often present. A chancre-like ulceration with a dark crust develops at the original bite site. A blotchy central, then generalized, deeply erythematous rash appears during the first 3–4 d of fever. The fever thereafter becomes cyclic, with febrile periods alternating with afebrile ones of 3–9 d. With recurrences of fever recrudescent rash may develop. If untreated, three to six such cycles may occur before spontaneous cure. Clinically, *Spirillum minus* rat-bite fever differs from that due to *S. moniliformis* in that the latter has a rash on the distal extremities (central with the former), accompanying arthritis, and no eschar. Penicillin is the treatment of choice for both.

*Tularemia* is an infection with *Franciscella tularensis* acquired through direct animal (wild rabbits, beavers, voles) contact or through bites of tick or fly vectors, particularly in endemic areas of Missouri, Arkansas, Oklahoma, and Tennessee. Tularemia may present in any of six clinical forms: ulceroglandular, glandular, oculoglandular, pharyngeal, typhoidal, or pneumonic. After an incubation period of 3–5 d the illness begins acutely with chills, fever, headache, and malaise. Cough, pharyngitis, abdominal pain, and an inappropriately slow pulse rate for the level of fever may be present. Other clinical manifestations relate to the site of entry of *F. tularensis*, roughly concordant with the six clinical forms. With systemic infection during the first 1–2 wk of symptoms, various skin eruptions have been noted in up to one-third of cases: diffuse maculopapular, vesiculopapular, erythema multiforme, erythema nodosum. The preferred treatment for tularemia is streptomycin, but gentamicin is an effective alternative.

## Vesicular-bullous eruptions (Table 51.2)

### Viral infections

*Varicella* is a common childhood viral infection spread by the respiratory route. After an average incubation period of 12–14 d, 1–2 d of malaise and low-grade fever follow. The rash appears abruptly, initially on the trunk. The first lesions are macular, rapidly becoming papular, then quickly vesiculating (Plate 13). The vesicles are surrounded by a halo of erythema and are clear initially, becoming cloudy 2–3 d later. The eruption is most prominent on the trunk, but lesions do appear on the face and extremities, and frequently on the scalp, palms, and soles. Lesions are pruritic. Over the next 4–5 d new crops of lesions develop, resulting in the appearance in any given area of all stages of lesions (macules, papules, clear and clouded vesicles, and crusts). In most cases constitutional symptoms are mild, but in some adults fever is high and the general reaction is profound. Varicella can be a life-threatening infection in immunocompromised patients. Complications of chickenpox include secondary bacterial (*S. aureus*, Gp A streptococcus) infection of the skin, uncommonly encephalitis, Reye's syndrome in children, DIC, and pneumonia. In children the pneumonia is usually due to secondary bacterial infection, whereas in adults it results from primary varicella infection. Acyclovir is recommended therapy for varicella in adolescents, adults or children at high risk for severe infection.

*Herpes zoster* (*shingles*) represents a recurrence of active infection with varicella virus in a unilateral, dermatomal distribution. Pain in the distribution of the involved dermatome is the initial manifestation, followed within 2–3 d by erythematous maculopapular lesions evolving locally over 3–5 d into vesicles and then crusting. Unlike chickenpox, vesicles often coalesce into bullae. In the immunocompromised individual new lesions may continue to develop for several weeks, and crusting may not take place for a further 1–2 wk. Zoster occurs particularly in the elderly and in the immunocompromised (particularly with HIV infection). Widespread dissemination may occur in patients with lymphoproliferative disease. Treatment is with intravenous acyclovir.

Severe *disseminated herpes simplex* infections can occur in patients with underlying immunocompromise of T cell function (e.g., HIV infection, iatrogenic immunosuppression for organ transplantation) or various skin disorders (e.g., burns, eczema). Visceral involvement can occur. Dissemination occurs from genital herpes or herpes labialis or from external contact of lesions of preexisting skin disorders with herpes simplex virus (HSV). Eczema herpeticum begins as clusters of umbilicated vesicles in eczematized skin. These coalesce and become eroded. Fever is a feature with disseminated HSV infection. Necrotic, gangrenous lesions may be a feature of HSV infection in patients with AIDS. Acyclovir is the treatment of choice.

Hand-foot and mouth disease (HFM) is a vesicular eruption, predominantly in children, caused by coxsackievirus A 16 (less commonly other A and B serotypes) and by enterovirus 71, sometimes accompanied by aseptic meningitis or meningoencephalitis. Fever and sore throat for several days are early features. Vesicles appear on the oral mucosa and tongue, sometimes coalesce to form bullae, and then collapse, causing mucosal erosion. The cutaneous lesions of HFM are peripherally distributed mixed papules, clear vesicles, and occasionally bullae. The extensor surfaces of the hands, feet, palms, and soles are most commonly involved.

Vesicular-bullous forms of *erythema multiforme* with erosive lesions of the mucous membranes of the lips and conjunctivae (Stevens-Johnson syndrome) have been associated with *M. pneumoniae* and *HSV infections*. Rickettsialpox has a papulovesicular appearance of chickenpox but is distinguished from the latter by the distinctive eschar.

### Bacterial infections

Four types of skin lesions may be associated with the acute febrile course of *Pseudomonas aeruginosa* bacteremia: (*1*) maculopapular lesions resembling rose spots, (*2*) gangrenous cellulitis, (*3*) bullae, and (*4*) ecthyma gangrenosum. Isolated bullae occur anywhere on the skin surface. A narrow halo of dusky erythema surrounds the bulla, the contents of which rapidly become hemorrhagic. The lesion goes on to necrosis and ulceration; it is covered with a gray-black eschar and surrounded by a narrow zone of erythema. This necrotic ulcer is called *ecthyma gangrenosa*.

*Vibrio vulnificus* is a halophilic vibrio found in saltwater or brackish inland waters. It is responsible for the rapid development of cellulitis (often eventuating in bacteremia) following contamination of a superficial laceration by warm seawater. Hemorrhagic bullae may develop in the skin as a manifestation of subsequent bacteremia. In compromised patients, particularly those with hepatic cirrhosis, life-threatening *V. vulnificus* bacteremia can follow ingestion of raw oysters. Fever and cellulitis with large hemorrhagic bullae may develop rapidly after onset of bacteremia. A tetracycline is the usual treatment, with cefotaxime an alternative.

## Noninfectious causes of vesicular-bullous eruptions

Toxic epidermal necrolysis (TEN) is an initially diffuse erythema with vesicles that become confluent as large flaccid bullae that easily rupture leaving denuded areas resembling scalded skin (Table 51.2).

*Pyoderma gangrenosum* is an irregular ulcer with a bright erythematous border and a necrotic base. It commonly begins with a subcutaneous painful nodule, a hemorrhagic pustule, or a bulla containing cloudy fluid. At the pustular or bullous stage cultures are negative, but secondary colonization with a variety of bacteria occurs following necrosis and ulceration. The process may be idiopathic or associated with inflammatory bowel disease, rheumatoid arthritis, or lymphoproliferative disease.

*Pustular psoriasis* is an acute eruptive form of psoriasis. It begins with fever and a sudden outpouring over the extremities and trunk of small (2–3 mm) erythematous pustules which subsequently become confluent in patches. Characteristically, recurrent brief cycles of fever to 103°F are followed by a new crop of sterile pustules The high fever, cutaneous pustules, and associated leukocytosis mimic acute infection.

## Infections with diffuse erythroderma (Table 51.3)

### Specific infections

*Scarlet fever* is a group A streptococcal infection with a diffuse erythematous eruption due to erythrogenic (pyrogenic) exotoxin. The clinical onset is usually abrupt with sore throat and fever. Rash appears 24–48 h after pharyngeal symptoms. Other clinical manifestations include nausea, vomiting, headache, and generalized lymphadenopathy. The rash consists of diffuse erythema beginning about the face and neck and rapidly involving the trunk and extremities (Plate 14). Distinctive features of the exanthem include blanching on pressure, punctate 1–2 mm papular elevations producing a sandpaper quality, circumoral pallor, prominent linear and petechial character of rash (Pastia's lines) in antecubital and other skin folds, and desquamation during the second week of illness. An enanthem, consisting initially of reddened engorged papillae projecting through the white furred surface of the tongue, is followed by a diffusely reddened ("strawberry") appearance of the tongue.

Pharyngitis due to *Arcanobacterium haemolyticum* is a rare cause of a febrile illness with scarlatiniform rash that closely mimics scarlet fever.

*Streptococcal toxic shock syndrome* is associated with invasive GpA streptococcal infection (e.g., cryptogenic bacteremia or necrotizing fasciitis), rapid progression, and marked severity of manifestations. The latter include a scarlatiniform rash, conjunctivitis, hypotension, and multiorgan involvement as in staphylococcal toxic shock syndrome.

*Staphylococcal toxic shock syndrome* (*TSS*) is an acute febrile illness caused by strains of *S. aureus* producing a toxin that acts as a superantigen. The defining elements of the syndrome are a generalized erythroderma followed by some desquamation (Plate 15) after about 1 wk, hypotension, and functional abnormalities in at least three organ systems. The latter may include the nervous system (toxic encephalopathy), kidney (renal failure, hematuria), liver (bilirubin and ALT elevation), blood (thrombocytopenia), heart (pulmonary edema), and skeletal muscle (myalgias, rhabdomyolysis). Other early clinical features include subjective sore throat, pharyngeal and oral erythema, conjunctival injection, diarrhea, and vomiting. The site of staphylococcal colonization or infection may be in the vagina (particularly associated with use of highly absorbent tampons), surgical wounds, or nasopharynx. Bacteremia is uncommon. Antibiotic therapy involves use of nafcillin intravenously; alternatives include a first-generation cephalosporin or vancomycin.

*Staphylococcal scalded skin syndrome* (*SSSS*) is a diffuse erythroderm rapidly progressing to bulla formation and exfoliation caused by an exfoliative exotoxin produced by *S. aureus*. It is more common in children and begins abruptly with a diffuse erythema resembling sunburn or scalding, skin tenderness, and fever. Nikolsky sign (sheet-like separation of epidermis on gentle traction) can be elicited. Large flaccid bullae develop and immediately collapse, exposing a bright red, moist surface. The initiating *S. aureus* infection is usually not on the skin but involves a distant abscess, purulent conjunctivitis, sinusitis, or bacteremia. The development of extensive areas of superficial skin sloughing and exfoliation can present problems in thermal regulation and fluid balance.

A forme fruste of SSSS is the rare so-called *staphylococcal scarlet fever*. The fever, diffuse erythema with a sandpaper feel, Pastia's lines, and subsequent mild desquamation (without bulla formation) resemble scarlet fever.

### Noninfectious causes of diffuse erythroderma

Toxic epidermal necrolysis (TEN, Lyell's syndrome) is a severe widespread erythema and detachment of the skin, most often due to drug allergy. The skin changes are difficult to distinguish from SSSS, but on histologic examination the cleavage plane in TEN is at the basal cell layer, whereas in SSSS it is located just under the granular cell layer.

*Kawasaki disease* is an illness of children of unknown etiology, usually in the first several years of life and rarely after the age of 10. Acute clinical manifestations include fever, conjunctival injection, diffuse scarlatiniform or polymorphous rash (maculopapular, erythema multiforme-like), cervical lymphadenopathy, erythema and fissuring of the lips and oral cavity, strawberry tongue, and erythema of palms and soles with swelling of the fingers and toes. When the fever begins to subside, after 1 or 2 wk, peeling of the fingers or toes occurs. Kawasaki disease has features of a vasculitis, with a striking involvement of the coronary arteries with aneurysm formation or occlusions. Treatment involves use of IV immunoglobulin and salicylates.

## Systemic infections with petechial-purpuric lesions or polymorphic rashes (Table 51.4)

*Acute meningococcemia* is often preceded by mild upper respiratory symptoms or malaise and myalgias. The rash of acute meningococcemia may begin in a minority of patients with macular or papular lesions, but these are followed rapidly by numerous small petechiae on the trunk and extremities. Petechiae may also occur on palms and soles, face, and on conjunctivae and buccal mucous membranes. Petechiae may enlarge and become confluent, forming purpuric lesions (Plate 16). Purpura may become extensive over a few hours. Such lesions tend to have gunmetal gray centers (sugillations) and may become bullous and undergo necrosis. With fulminant meningococcemia, DIC and shock occur. The cutaneous lesions of DIC (purpura fulminans) consist of large ecchymoses with sharp, irregular ("geographic") borders outlined by a narrow zone of erythema. Similar lesions on the digits, ears, and nose may blacken and go on to gangrene and spontaneous amputation. Patients are acutely ill with high fever and tachycardia. Meningitis may be simultaneously present, but often with fulminant meningococcemia, meningitis has not yet developed. Antibiotic treatment involves use of ampicillin or a third-generation cephalosporin.

*Henoch-Schönlein* (*anaphylactoid*) *purpura* is a systemic necrotizing small-vessel vasculitis of immunologic origin (IgA deposition) occurring more frequently in children. Onset is acute with skin lesions and arthralgias, but patients also may have gastrointestinal symptoms (abdominal pain, bleeding, diarrhea) and acute glomerulonephritis. Typical cutaneous lesions are those of palpable purpura, which may have begun as urticaria and a maculopapular rash, occurring predominantly over the extensor aspects of lower extremities and buttocks.

The *congenital rubella syndrome* (cardiac malformations, microcephaly, cataracts, deafness, splenomegaly, hepatitis) may also be associated at birth with thrombocytopenia and prominent cutaneous petechiae and purpura ("blueberry muffin baby"). Similar petechial rashes may be observed in fulminant congenital cytomegalovirus (CMV) disease characterized by jaundice, hepatosplenomegaly, microcephaly, cerebral calcifications, respiratory distress, and seizures.

*Subacute bacterial endocarditis* is sometimes accompanied by subungual splinter hemorrhages, conjunctival hemorrhages, and scattered petechiae. In occasional patients the petechiae may be quite numerous, particularly on the lower extremities, and suggest a primary hematologic or vasculitic process. In acute endocarditis, particularly when due to *S. aureus*, distinctive skin lesions may occur in addition to petechiae. One is a Janeway lesion, a painless hemorrhagic, plaque-like macular lesion, occurring most commonly on palms or soles. The second is purulent purpura, consisting of a white-yellow purulent center with a surrounding hemorrhagic halo. Gram-stained smears of an aspirate of the latter will usually show gram-positive cocci in clusters.

### Polymorphic lesions

The syndromes of meningococcemia-meningitis and fulminant meningococcemia have already been described. Two other syndromes of *meningococcal bacteremia* with polymorphic skin lesions also occur but uncommonly. The first is a more subacute illness with malaise, fever, arthralgias, or joint effusions accompanied by a few macular and petechial skin lesions. These symptoms may persist for about a week, but promptly subside on treatment with penicillin. The second is *chronic meningococcemia*, consisting of intermittent, recurrent febrile episodes (usually lasting less than a week), migratory arthralgias, headache, and a transient polymorphic rash. Toxity is minimal. The rash consists of scattered nonpruritic erythematous macules, papules, rare petechiae (some with vesicular or pustular centers), purpuric nodules, reappearing with subsequent febrile episodes. Splenomegaly may be present. Gram stain of skin lesions only rarely discloses the etiologic agent; blood cultures are likely to be positive during the febrile, but not the apyrexial, periods. Biopsy of the skin lesions shows leucytoclastic angiitis which mistakenly may be considered to represent a primary hypersensitivity vasculitis. Penicillin therapy is curative.

Spread of *N. gonorrhoeae* to the bloodstream occurs in 1%–3% of patients, (usually female) with gonorrhea, and this commonly produces a clinical picture known as a *disseminated gonococcal infection* (*DGI*) *or the dermatitis-arthritis syndrome*. The onset of bacteremia often coincides with menstruation. Chills, fever, arthralgias, arthritis and tenosynovitis, and skin lesions make up the syndrome. The latter are typically few in number (ten or less), located on extremities about joints, and consist of a combination of papules, petechiae, vesicles or pustules, and rare hemorrhagic bullae. Ceftriaxone is recommended initial therapy.

The petechial-purpuric skin lesions of *acute and subacute bacterial endocarditis* can be considered polymorphic when accompanied by Osler nodes—2–10 mm, painful, often erythematous, nodular lesions commonly located on the pads of the fingers and toes. They are transient, lasting up to several days, sometimes multiple, and are rare in acute endocarditis but occur in 10%–20% of patients with SBE.

## Systemic infections with nodular lesions or annular erythema/urticaria (Table 51.5)

Nodular cutaneous or subcutaneous lesions in a patient with fever can provide clues to the underlying infection. Sharpening of the differential diagnosis can be provided by the location of the nodules (disseminated, arrayed in a linear lymphangitic distribution, primarily pretibial distribution), the nature of the host (immunocompetent or immunosuppressed), and epidemiologic factors (residence in or travel to areas in the United States endemic for primary invasive mycoses; foreign travel; exposure to tuberculosis; occupational exposure to particular pathogens).

Although cutaneous manifestations of *S. aureus endocarditis* and bacteremia have been described (Table 51.4), subcutaneous nodules with normal or erythematous overlying skin may occasionally be noted early in the course of such bloodstream infections. These inflammatory nodules contain staphylococci, and, if the febrile illness is not treated appropriately, go on to suppuration.

Settings predisposing for *disseminated candidiasis* include underlying malignancies (particularly with granulocytopenia), immunosuppression, corticosteroid therapy, intravenous drug abuse, and nosocomial features (broad-spectrum antibiotics, indwelling catheters). Skin lesions occur in 10%–13% of patients with disseminated candidiasis and prolonged candidemia. Such skin lesions consist of 0.3–1.0 cm erythematous papules and papulonodules. They sometimes appear in large numbers over a few hours on the trunk and extremities in a patient with fever and myalgias. The lesions may become hemorrhagic, particularly in thrombocytopenic patients. Occasionally, nodular hemorrhagic lesions become necrotic, resembling lesions of ecthyma gangrenosa. Skin biopsy with gram-stained smears, histologic sections with fungal stains, and culture provide the diagnosis. White, cotton-ball-like chorioretinal lesions may be found in up to 25% of patients with candidemia. Candidemia and disseminated candidiasis, particularly in neutropenic patients, require initial antifungal therapy with intravenous amphotericin B.

*Disseminated cryptococcosis*, particularly in immunosuppressed transplant recipients or patients with AIDS, may be accompanied by skin lesions in about 10% of patients. These may take the form of small papules (umbilicated and resembling molluscum contagiosum), pustules, areas of cellulitis, subcutaneous abscesses, or ulcers with undermined edges. With thrombocytopenia some lesions may mimic palpable purpura. Major organ involvement includes pulmonary cryptococcosis and meningitis. Initial antimicrobial treatment consists of amphotericin B with or without flucytosine.

*Acute progressive disseminated histoplasmosis* (PDH) occurs particularly in patients with AIDS, very young children, and patients with hematologic malignancies. Skin lesions are present in about 10% of patients with AIDS and acute PDH. Most commonly these lesions are erythematous maculopapules or small nodules. Purpuric lesions, skin ulcers, and proliferative lesions sometimes occur. Residence in an endemic area (e.g., Midwestern states) at some time is an important epidemiologic factor.

Skin involvement in *coccidioidomycosis* occurs in two stages of infection. Erythema nodosum or, occasionally, erythema multiforme associated with fever, malaise, night sweats, and arthralgias occurs with initial pulmonary infection. In later disseminated coccidioidomycosis various skin lesions (papules, pustules, nodules, subcutaneous abscesses, and ulcers as well as large proliferative verrucous lesions) may be a feature.

Disseminated skin lesions may occur in *disseminated mycobacterial infections*. In miliary tuberculosis a maculopapular rash (Table 51.1) occurs rarely. Occasionally, firm subcutaneous nodules (0.5–5 cm) develop subcutaneously. Initially there is no overlying erythema, but with time the lesions become softer with overlying erythema. Fluctuation may develop, and spontaneous drainage of such tuberculous abscesses occurs, occasionally despite antituberculous therapy. With disseminated infection in patients with AIDS due to *Mycobacterium avium complex* (MAC), a variety of skin lesions have been observed: These include deep-seated inflammatory nodules, subcutaneous abscesses, infiltrated erythematous plaques, and pustular lesions. Disseminated infection with *M. chelonae* (a rapidly growing mycobacterium), an uncommon infection but one which may occur in the setting of granulocytopenia, may produce erythematous macronodular skin lesions involving extensor surfaces. The lesions frequently suppurate and drain. Another uncommon mycobacterial species, *M. hemophilum*, one with a growth requirement for added iron, has been responsible for multiple raised, violaceous, nodular, or fluctuant skin lesions that spontaneously drain and ulcerate. The lesions occur predominantly on the extremities and in patients with AIDS.

*Nodular lymphangitis*, usually associated with a chancriform initiating site of inoculation, may present as a subacute or chronic process with multiple cutaneous nodules in linear arrangement along the course of thickened lymphatics, usually on an upper extremity (Plate 17). The nodules are from 2 to 15 mm in size and appear to be in the dermis. The overlying skin may be erythematous or violaceous or may appear normal. The lesions are minimally painful. There is usually little systemic evidence of infection. Among the causes of the nodular lymphangitis syndrome are a variety of infectious agents. *Sporothrix schenckii* (a fungus present in plants, sphagnum moss, and bushes) is introduced into the skin of a gardener by a splinter or thorn. This (sporotrichosis) form of nodular lymphangitis is the most common one. A similar sporotrichoid picture is produced by cutaneous infection ("*swimming pool granuloma*") with *M. marinum*, an atypical mycobacterium that grows best at 25–32° C and has its ecologic niche in fresh- and saltwater. Human infection results commonly from minor trauma sustained in a swimming pool or from cleaning a fish tank. Similar findings of a verrucous or ulcerative lesion at the site of inoculation and nodular lymphangitis can be produced, but much less commonly, by other etiologic agents: *M. kansasii* or *chelonae*, *Nocardia brasiliensis* or *asteroides*, *S. aureus* (in the form of botryomycosis), and several filarial and American leishmanial species in endemic areas.

Disseminated bloodstream infection with the *fungus Alternaria* occurs rarely, usually in the setting of extensive burns, hematologic malignancy, or bone marrow transplantation. Tender, erythematous nodules develop on the extremities, vesiculate, and then undergo necrosis, producing black eschars. Scattered similar lesions occasionally occur with cutaneous dissemination by the hematogenous route of *Aspergillus* or *Mucor.*

Cutaneous lesions of *bacillary angiomatosis*, seen principally in patients with AIDS but also in other immunosuppressed patients, are manifestations of infection with *Bartonella henselae* or *B. quintana*. The dermal or subcutaneous nodules of neovascular proliferation begin as either solitary dome-shaped red or purple papules, or appear in crops. The cutaneous lesions vary considerably in form from fixed to mobile, in number from several to hundreds, in size from a few millimeters to several centimeters, and in location from wide distribution on skin and mucosa to visceral involvement (peliosis hepatis). They resemble those of Kaposi's sarcoma and pyogenic granuloma. *B. henselae* is responsible for the majority of cases of *cat-scratch disease* as well. The epidemiologic role of contact with cats in both bacillary angiomatosis and cat-scratch disease is emphasized by the demonstration of bacteremia with *B. henselae* in about 40% of apparently healthy cats. Initial antibiotic therapy for cutaneous bacillary angiomatosis involves use of oral doxycycline or erythromycin for 8–12 wk.

*Erythema nodosum* is characterized by erythematous tender nodules or raised plaques primarily on pretibial areas but also occasionally on the thighs, arms, and other areas with subcutaneous fat. It is more common in women. The initial appearance of the lesions is frequently accompanied by fever and malaise. Symmetrical pain and swelling (of the ankles and knees ) is common. The nodules become violaceous over several weeks but do not ulcerate, and healing without scarring occurs in 3–6 wk. Erythema nodosum is believed to be a consequence of an immunologic reaction to a large variety of possible antigenic stimuli: infections, drugs, systemic diseases. Among infectious agents associated with erythema nodosum are group A streptococci, *Mycobacterium tuberculosis*, *Coccidioides immitis* (in the southwest), *Histoplasma capsulatum* (in the Midwest), *Blastomyces dermatitidis*, *Leptospira interrogans* serotypes (particularly *L. autumnalis*), *Chlamydia trachomatis* (LGV serovars), *Yersinia enterocolitica* and *pseudotuberculosis*. A form of erythema nodosum (*erythema nodosum leprosum*) occurs in almost 50% of patients with lepromatous leprosy, and the painful lesions are not confined to the extensor surfaces of the legs but appear on arms, thighs, trunk, and face. Fever, often high, is accompanied by polyneuritis, polyarthritis, lymphadenitis, and sometimes iridocyclitis. Drugs associated with erythema nodosa commonly include sulfonamides, penicillin, and oral contraceptives. Systemic diseases in which erythema nodosum may be a manifestation include sarcoidosis, inflammatory bowel disease, and Behcet's syndrome.

Other noninfectious processes that produce fever, malaise, and nodular skin lesions mimicking systemic infections include *Weber-Christian disease* (acute, febrile, nonsuppurative relapsing idiopathic panniculitis), *pancreatic fat necrosis*, *factitial panniculitis*, and *Sweet's syndrome*. *Weber-Christian disease* is characterized by recurrent crops of erythematous, often tender, subcutaneous nodules, most often on the thighs and lower legs. Fat necrosis is often followed by necrosis of the overlying epidermis and discharge of an oily brown liquid. Crops of painful erythematous nodular lesions with subsequent oily discharge may be a feature of pancreatitis-associated distant subcutaneous fat necrosis. Sweet's syndrome has been described earlier (Table 51.1) in association with maculopapular lesions but larger erythematous cutaneous nodules are commonly present. Multiple, 2–5 mm nonerythematous subcutaneous nodules located over bony prominences, particularly about the elbow, occur in about one-third of patients with *acute rheumatic fever*. Since they occur later in the course of the active illness, often when manifestations of carditis are already present, it is not commonly considered in the differential diagnosis of acute systemic infection with nodular skin lesions. *Factitial panniculitis* may be associated with fever. Self-injection of bacteria-laden or foreign materials (e.g., milk, cotton fibers) has resulted in subcutaneous inflammatory nodules.

### Annular erythemas/urticaria

Several of the annular erythemas (erythema chronicum migrans, erythema multiforme) have been considered earlier with maculopapular lesions (Table 51.1). *Erythema marginatum* is a distinctive rash in acute rheumatic fever. It consists of rapidly spreading (over the course of 6–12 h), often evanescent, erythematous ringed lesions with slightly raised margins. As the rash enlarges it may develop an irregular geographic outline. The rash follows the onset of migratory polyarthritis by a few days and is commonly associated with carditis. A rash resembling erythema marginatum may occur infrequently with enteroviral infections.

Urticarial lesions occur with a variety of infectious fevers. These include viral infections such as *acute hepatitis* B (Table 51.1) and *coxsackie A9 infection*. Rashes caused by the latter are vesicular and often resemble those of hand-foot and mouth disease. However, occasionally outbreaks of coxsackie A9 infection have been associated with fever and a diffuse urticarial rash.

Urticaria may accompany a variety of parasitic infections. In trichinosis the accompanying rash sometimes seen may be maculopapular or urticarial (see Table 51.1). Gastrointestinal infection *with Strongyloides stercoralis*, a soil-transmitted nematode, is characterized by abdominal pain, diarrhea, eosinophilia, and cutaneous lesions. Infection is endemic in the tropics, subtropics, and in the southern United States. Two types of rash occur: generalized urticaria and larva currens. The latter is a distinctive overlying rash due to the rather rapid subcutaneous migration of larvae. It consists of pruritic urticarial wheals beginning perianally and moving to buttocks, abdomen and thighs. Treatment is with oral thiabendazole.

*Onchocerciasis* (river blindness) is caused by the filaria *Oncocercus volvulus*, transmitted to humans by the bite of blackflies. It is endemic in West, Central, and East Africa, where the fly vector breeds in fast-flowing streams, and in scattered areas of Central and South America. Clinical findings consist of scattered, firm, nontender subcutaneous nodules (containing adult worms), impaired vision due to punctate keratitis (with microfilaria in the cornea) and iridocyclitis, musculoskeletal pain, and pruritic skin lesions consisting of papules or urticaria. Fever is uncommon. Oral ivermectin or diethylcarbamazine is the treatment of choice.

*Loiasis* is another filarial infection, endemic in West and Central Africa, transmitted to humans by the bite of tabamid flies. Clinical features consist of distinctive transient pruritic and painful nonerythematous subcutaneous swellings of up to 5 cm in diameter (Calabar swellings) at the site of migration of the adult worm. Urticaria may be seen with newly acquired but not chronic infection. The worm may occasionally be seen passing through inflamed subconjunctivae. Peripheral blood eosinophilia may be marked, and daytime blood samples reveal the presence of microfilaria. Diethylcarbamazine or ivermectin is effective in eliminating the microfilaremia but does not kill the adult worm.

*Schistosomiasis* is due to infection with parasitic trematodes. Endemic areas for *Schistosoma mansoni* are in Africa, Arabia, South America, and the Caribbean; for *S. hematobium*, in Africa and the Middle East; for *S. japonicum*, in Japan, China, and the Phillipines; for *S. mekongi*, in Southeast Asia; and for *S. intercalatum* in West and Central Africa. Infection is initiated when cercariae enter the skin of humans bathing in fresh water. A pruritic papular rash is associated with this initial cercarial penetration of the skin. Katayama fever is an acute serum sickness-like syndrome that occurs with heavy primary infection with *S. japonicum* primarily, but also sometimes with *S. mansoni*. Clinical features include fever, chills, headache, cough, myalgias, lymphadenopathy, hepatosplenomegaly, and occasionally angioedema and urticaria.

*Echinococcosis* (hydatid disease) in humans results from ingestion of food contaminated with eggs of the dog tapeworm, *Echinococcus granulosus*. In the human intestinal tract the eggs hatch to oncospheres which enter the circulation and encyst in host organs, particularly liver and lung. Urticaria may be a complication of sensitization to cyst fluid components absorbed systemically; cyst leakage or rupture may be associated with a severe allergic reaction with fever and hypotension.

## Systemic infections with rash to consider in travelers recently abroad (Tables 51.6, 51.7)

Because of the millions of U.S. citizens travelling abroad and foreigners entering this country, and in view of the rapidity of air travel, febrile illnesses with associated skin lesions acquired abroad are not unusual occurrences in this country. In making a diagnosis in such individuals it is helpful to have insights into endemic infections in specific areas. Also, it is important to recognize that infections that are common in this country, such as meningococcemia, hepatitis B virus (HBV) infection, and secondary syphilis, also occur abroad. Such causes of FRS are not shown on Tables 51.6 and 51.7. Other causes of FRS typically found abroad that have been considered earlier such as dengue, typhoid fever, and leptospirosis will not be considered here; uncommon specific endemic FRSs not described earlier will be mentioned.

### Latin America or Caribbean areas (Table 51.6)

*Yellow fever* is a mosquito-borne flavivirus infection endemic in tropical Africa and in the Amazon region of South America. Unimmunized individuals clearing forests in the Amazon area are infected (jungle yellow fever) following bites from tree-hole breeding *Hemagogus* mosquitoes which acquired the virus from monkeys. Urban yellow fever has developed in South America in the past two decades as a result of the reemergence of domestic *Aedes aegypti* mosquitoes serving as vectors for spread of the virus from viremic humans. The clinical features of yellow fever consist of fever, headache, severe myalgias, and prostration. Relative bradycardia and conjunctivitis are common. The course is biphasic, with remission of symptoms after a few days and then recurrence of fever with development of jaundice, upper GI bleeding, petechiae, epistaxis, oliguria, and coma.

*Argentine, Bolivian, and Venezuelan hemorrhagic fevers*, due to the arenaviruses Junin, Machupo, and Guanarito, are endemic in the respective countries. Rodents are vectors. Fever, myalgia, conjunctival injection, and lymphadenopathy are initial findings. A petechial rash, most prominent in the axilla, develops, and in the more severely ill, a capillary leak syndrome ensues. Mayaro (an alphavirus) infection is characterized by fever, macular rash, and occasionally arthropathy, and occurs in the Caribbean area, Brazil, and Columbia.

*Bartonellosis* (*Carrion's disease*) occurs in the valleys of the Andes Mountains, particularly in Columbia, Ecuador, and Peru. It is due to a gram-negative coccobacillus, *Bartonella bacilliformis*, spread by the bite of an infected sandfly. The disease occurs in two phases: (*1*) an acute febrile illness with hemolytic anemia (Aroya fever) and (*2*) a benign nodular cutaneous eruption known as verruga peruana. In the first phase the infecting bacteria can be readily visualized attached to red blood cells. In the second phase 30–60 d later erythematous macules, papules, and vascular nodules appear on the face and extensor surfaces of the extremities.

An acute life-threatening bacteremic infection due to *H. influenzae* biogroup *aegyptius* occurs in Brazil and is known as *Brazilian purpuric fever*. It occurs in young children and is characterized by high fever, purulent conjunctivitis, vomiting, shock, and purpura.

*Melioidosis*, due to *Pseudomonas pseudomallei*, is endemic in Southeast Asia but also occurs in South America and Africa between 20° north and south of the equator. The disease is transmitted by contamination of abraded skin with infected soil. Septicemia may complicate initial cellulitis or ulceration. Acute pneumonia may result from initial infection by the respiratory route or subsequent bacteremic spread of infection. Subcutaneous abscesses may occur initially secondary to bacteremia or later as a result of spread from suppurating lymphadenitis or osteomyelitis. Antimicrobrial treatment of the septicemic form of the disease involves combined intravenous therapy with ceftazidime (or imipenem or piperacillin-tazobactam) plus trimethoprim-sulfamethoxazole.

*Trench fever* is a louse-borne infection with *Bartonella* (formerly *Rochalimaea) quintana*. It is characterized by recurrent 4–5 d cycles of fever associated with headache, conjunctival injection, myalgias, arthralgias, hepatosplenomegaly and an erythematous macular rash on the trunk.

*Paracoccidioidomycosis* (due to *Paracoccidioides brasiliensis*) is a systemic fungal disease endemic to South America (primarily Brazil) and Central America. The initiating lesion is pulmonary. The acute form of the disease is uncommon and affects mainly children, who develop generalized lymphadenopathy, hepatosplenomegaly, bone marrow dysfunction, and gastrointestinal symptoms. Associated skin lesions may be present in up to 20% of juvenile cases and consist of subcutaneous nodules, abscesses and ulcerations, or, occasionally, disseminated maculopapules. The chronic (adult) form of paracoccidioidmycosis is more common and involves primarily the lung. Occasionally a chronic multifocal form of disease develops with secondary metastatic infection in lungs, lymph nodes, liver, spleen, mucosal surfaces, and skin. The latter consist of warty or ulcerated lesions and subcutaneous nodules or abscesses.

*Visceral leishmaniasis* (*kala-azar*), caused by *Leishmania donovani chagasi*, is endemic in the dry tropical regions of Mexico, Central America, northern South America, Africa, the Middle East, and Asia. It occurs principally in undernourished children exposed to the sandfly vector. Hepatosplenomegaly and pancytopenia accompany fever. Papular, nonulcerative skin lesions may be present.

*Acute Chagas' disease* (*American trypanosomiasis*) is due to *Trypanosoma cruzi* usually acquired through the bite of a reduviid ("kissing") bug or through blood transfusions from asymptomatic infected donors. The endemic area is South and Central America and Mexico. When transmitted by the reduviid through a break in the skin, a chagoma develops consisting of localized erythema, induration, and swelling. When entry has been through the conjunctiva, painless edema of the eyelids and periocular tissues are features (Romaña sign). Fever, generalized lymphadenopathy, and hepatosplenomegaly follow. Occasional patients develop myocarditis or meningoencephalitis. In children various eruptions, some resembling erythema multiforme, may occur.

*Lymphatic filariasis* is a mosquito-borne infection with *Wuchereria bancrofti*, *Brugia malayi*, or *B. timori*. The latter two are restricted to South and Southeast Asia. *W. bancrofti* is widely distributed in the tropics and subtropics; in the Western Hemisphere endemic foci exist in Brazil, Central America, Trinidad, and Haiti. The disease occurs only after prolonged residence in endemic areas. Clinical features are associated with either acute inflammation (lymphangitis, fever) or chronic lymphatic obstruction (lymphedema, chronic lymphadenitis).

### Middle East (Table 51.6)

*Sandfly* (*Phlebotomus*) *fever* is an acute sandfly-borne illness due to phleboviruses of the family Bunyaviridae. Skin manifestations consist of a punctate hemorrhage at the sandfly bite site and surrounding erythema. Fever begins abruptly 3–6 d later, accompanied by frontal headaches, severe myalgias, abdominal pain, nausea, conjunctival suffusion, photophobia, pain on eye movement, and prominent facial flushing. The acute illness is over in 2–4 d but postviral asthenia may persist for weeks.

*Congo-Crimean hemorrhagic fever* is a tick-borne *Nairovirus* infection endemic in the Middle East, former Soviet Republics, Balkans, and Africa. Infections occur in the spring–summer among those in contact with domestic animals which the ticks infest. After an incubation period of 6–14 d, the illness begins with fever, headaches, nausea, vomiting, severe myalgias, abdominal pain. Hepatitis and disseminated intravascular coagulation occur in severe cases. Petechiae and ecchymoses are cutaneous manifestations.

*West Nile fever* resembles sandfly fever in its clinical onset and features but the cutaneous involvement consists of a macular rash on the trunk and extremities. The disease is mosquito-borne, due to a flavivirus, and is self-limited.

*Rift Valley fever* is a mosquito-borne (*Aedes*) phlebovirus disease, endemic along the Nile River, but often occurs in epidemics. The illness is usually an undifferentiated fever, but severe cases involve hepatitis, DIC, retinitis (with blindness), and encephalitis.

### Southeast Asia and Oceania (Table 51.7)

Most of the febrile infections with rash listed in Table 51.7 have been considered previously. Among others is *Korean hemorrhagic fever* (*hemorrhagic fever with renal syndrome*) due to *Hantaan* virus, one of the Hanta viruses. Infection is acquired through inhalation of aerosols of excreta of chronically infected rodents. After an incubation period of about 2 wk patients develop fever, headache, and abdominal and back pain. Cutaneous lesions consist of petechiae and an erythematous flush on the trunk and face. More severe cases go on to develop shock, oliguria, and renal failure.

*Chikungunya fever*, a mosquito-borne alphavirus infection occurring in Southeast Asia and Africa, is characterized by chills, fever, headache, myalgias and arthralgias, and lymphadenopathy. Joint pains are intense and are the most striking feature. Skin involvement consists of a diffuse maculopapular eruption on the trunk, extending to the limbs, palms, and soles. The febrile course may have a "saddle back" character. Mild leukopenia with relative lymphocytosis may be present.

*Ross River fever* also is due to a mosquito-borne alphavirus and occurs in epidemics in Australia, Papua New Guinea, and the Pacific islands. Clinical features include fever, headache, symmetric arthralgias, and a diffuse maculopapular rash. Joint pains are prominent, commonly involve small joints of hands and feet, and frequently progress to polyarthritis.

### Africa (Table 51.7)

Most of the febrile illnesses with cutaneous eruptions have been described earlier and included in previous tables. Several other FRSs unique to Africa will be mentioned here. *Ebola virus* is a filovirus that has produced hemorrhagic fever in southern Sudan and Zaire. Illness is characterized by abrupt onset of fever, myalgia, headache, photophobia, conjunctival injection, and lymphadenopathy. A few days later a trunkal maculopapular rash appears. As the disease progresses, petechiae and ecchymoses and bleeding from mucous membranes develop. Epidemics in Zaire have occurred through use of improperly sterilized needles, and spread has occurred among medical staff caring for patients with the disease. Mortality is over 50%. *Marburg virus*, another filavirus causing hemorrhagic fever, produces a similar illness. Primary cases have occurred following close contact with monkey blood or monkey cell lines in culture, and secondary cases have occurred in hospital personnel associated with exposure to blood from the primary cases.

*O'nyong-nyong fever* is due to a mosquito-borne alphavirus antigenically related to Chikungunya virus. The clinical picture of O'nyong-nyong fever closely resembles that of Chikungunya fever.

*Lassa fever* is caused by an arenavirus endemic in Central and West Africa. It is transmitted by multimammate rats, and human-to-human spread can subsequently occur within hospitals. The clinical picture includes fever, pharyngitis, retrosternal pain, and proteinuria. Skin lesions are uncommon, but facial edema, hemorrhages, petechiae, and mucosal bleeding may occur as the disease develops. Capillary leak syndrome, hypotension, and liver dysfunction are prominent features in the more seriously ill patients. The case fatality rate is 14%–52%.

## Approach to Diagnosis

Initial evaluation of the patient with fever and a rash involves several important considerations. First, are isolation precautions indicated on the basis of the epidemiologic history, the appearance of the rash, immune status of the host, and the initial physical examination? Second, are systemic features (e.g., hypotension or shock, organ dysfunction, dehydration) those that require immediate resuscitative or therapeutic interventions? Third, does the combination of the general examination findings, the height of the fever, the immune status of the patient, epidemiologic factors, and the morphology, distribution, and progression of skin lesions indicate the need for immediate parenteral antimicrobial therapy after prompt performance of blood and other (e.g., CSF) cultures? This applies particularly to patients with hemorrhagic lesions (petechiae, purpura, or DIC) in whom life-threatening bacterial or rickettsial infections may be present. In a splenectomized patient, high-grade bacteremia due to *S. pneumoniae* (or other encapsulated bacteria) or bacteremia due to *Capnocytophaga canimorsus* (following a dog bite) may produce a similar picture. Purulent purpura is another important cutaneous clue that suggests the presence of bacteremia due to pyogenic bacteria (e.g., *S. aureus* or *P. aeruginosa*) requiring prompt institution of antimicrobial therapy (possibly modified by results of gram-stained smears of such lesions).

### Important aspects of patient history

The history can often provide clues for determining the etiology of the FRS syndrome (Table 51.8). For example, a diffuse maculopapular rash in a senior citizen with fever returning from travel in the Caribbean might suggest a different disease (dengue) than a similar rash in a young adult male who has not travelled abroad but has indulged in high risk behavior (acute HIV syndrome, secondary syphilis). Hemorrhagic bullae in a febrile patient with cirrhosis who has eaten raw oysters within the past few days will suggest a different etiology (*V. vulnificus*) than similar skin lesions in a hospitalized burn patient (*P. aeruginosa*).

The timing of the onset of the rash after the onset of febrile illness may be informative regarding the cause of a FRS. For example, the petechial and purpuric lesions of bacteremia due to *N. meningitidis* develop 8–24 h after the onset of illness, whereas similar lesions in Rocky Mountain spotted fever usually appear 1–5 d after the clinical onset of febrile illness. Whereas the diffuse erythroderma of streptococcal or staphylococcal toxic shock syndromes usually are present at the time of clinical presentation, in contrast, the rose spots of typhoid fever appear after 7–10 d of high fever.

### Important aspects of the physical examination apart from the skin

Evaluation of vital signs is important since hypotension or shock early in FRS might suggest acute meningococcemia (or other bacteremias), toxic shock syndrome, dengue shock syndrome, or Rocky Mountain spotted fever, among others. Relative bradycardia would raise the possibility of typhoid fever, psittacosis, and viral infections. General appearance of the patient is helpful

**Table 51.8** Important aspects of history in febrile-rash syndrome

|  |
|---|
| Exposure to febrile or ill patients, particularly with exanthems |
| Immunizations: particularly to rubella, measles, chickenpox, *N. meningitidis*, *S. pneumoniae*, *H. influenzae* |
| Prior illnesses: particularly childhood diseases, rheumatic fever, valvular heart disease |
| Recent travel: elsewhere in U.S. or abroad |
| Season of the year: timing of respiratory viral and enteroviral infections |
| Recent medications |
| Drug allergies: particularly to antimicrobial agents |
| Immune status: hematologic malignancy, asplenia, corticosteroid use, chemotherapy, immunoglobulin deficiency, solid organ or bone-marrow transplantation |
| Risk factors for sexually transmitted diseases, including HIV infection |
| Occupational exposures: chemical plant workers, health care providers, veterinarians |
| Exposure to wild animals and the outdoors (ticks, mosquitoes) |
| Pets: animal bites, licks, scratches |
| Recent invasive procedures: dental manipulations, surgery of any kind |
| Parenteral drug abuse |
| Time of onset of rash in relation to onset of febrile illness |
| Sun exposure |

in ascertaining degree of toxicity and can provide information about the severity of myalgias (as in dengue). Impaired mentation might suggest early shock (as in meningococcemia), diffuse capillary endothelial disease (as in various spotted fevers and typhus), or meningoencephalitis (as in Lyme borreliosis or enteroviral diseases). Frank meningeal signs (nuchal rigidity), cranial nerve signs, and localizing cerebral signs might suggest meningococcemia-meningitis syndrome, secondary syphilis, and infective endocarditis, respectively.

The presence of *lymphadenopathy* may be helpful. Generalized lymphadenopathy would be consistent with secondary syphilis, scarlet fever, infectious mononucleosis, acute HIV syndrome, or dengue, among others. Specific localized lymphadenopathy in the posterior cervical chain (Winterbottom sign) in a patient who has been bitten by a tsetze fly while in West Africa would suggest West African trypanosomiasis. Regional lymphadenopathy associated with a chancriform lesion on the hand and a maculopapular rash in a hunter in Tennessee would suggest the diagnosis of tularemia.

*Hepatosplenomegaly* in a patient with FRS would be an important finding. It might suggest typhoid fever, brucellosis, miliary tuberculosis, hepatosplenic candidiasis, or visceral leishmaniasis in a patient from Latin America, Africa or the Indian subcontinent.

*Arthritis* (synovial thickening or effusion) with FRS might suggest acute (or chronic) meningococcemia, Still's disease, *Streptobacillus moniliformis* rat-bite fever, parvovirus $B_{19}$ infection, or Ross River fever (in a person recently in Australia), among others. Arthritis may also be manifest in patients with the gonococcal dermatitis-arthritis syndrome. Arthralgias or arthritis may be features of bacterial endocarditis.

*Mucosal lesions* in a patient with the FRS may suggest a variety of etiologies. If present in the oral mucosa as "mucous patches" or about the vulva or perineum secondary syphilis would be suggested. A "strawberry tongue" associated with an erythematous rash might be suggestive of scarlet fever or Kawasaki disease, or bullous lesions of the lips and oral mucosa associated with erythema multiforme might be suggestive of *Mycoplasma pneumoniae* or *Herpes simplex* infection.

*Conjunctivitis* as part of the FRS might suggest leptospirosis, bullous erythema multiforme, early measles, varicella, toxic shock syndrome, or Brazilian purpuric fever, among other causes.

## Laboratory studies to aid in diagnosis

### Early diagnosis

In acutely ill patients where high-grade bacteremia is likely (asplenic patients, patients with DIC), examination of Wright-Giemsa- and gram-stained smears of buffy coat may rapidly demonstrate *S. pneumoniae* and *N. meningitidis*, or, occasionally, *C. albicans*. Blood cultures can reveal the etiologic agent in acute bacteremias due to common pathogens or uncommon bacteria such as *S. typhi* and *Streptobacillus moniliformis*. In the acutely ill patient with petechial or purpuric skin lesions and a stiff neck or confusion, CSF examination (including gram-stained smear and testing for capsular antigens of *H. influenzae*, *S. pneumoniae*, *N. meningitidis*) may provide prompt etiologic diagnosis.

Peripheral WBC and differential may provide important clues in FRS. A polymorphonuclear leukocytosis might suggest a pyogenic infection, whereas a leukopenia might be suggestive of a viral or rickettsial infection or of typhoid fever. A lymphopenia, without a leukocytosis or shift to the left in neutrophils, might suggest the acute HIV infection syndrome, whereas a prominent atypical lymphocytosis might be suggestive of EBV or CMV mononucleosis. Wright-Geimsa-stained smears of peripheral blood may provide the diagnosis in human granulocytic ehrlichiosis (intracytoplasmic inclusions within neutrophils), in tick or louse-borne relapsing fever (*Borrelia* visible extracellularly), and in African trypanosomiasis. Eosinophilia might provide a clue to consider a drug hypersensitivity reaction, an allergic vasculitis, or a number of parasitic diseases (e.g., strongyloidiasis, filariasis, trichinosis).

In the acutely ill patient with FRS and certain types of skin lesion, prompt aspiration, with gram-stained smear and culture, of the lesion may provide the necessary information to direct appropriate initial antimicrobial therapy. Such lesions include those of purulent purpura (e.g., *S. aureus*, *P. aeruginosa*), soft subcutaneous nodules or abscesses, and suspicious bullae (gray, dark, or cloudy contents). FRS with multiple small vesicular lesions might be due to systemic infection with Herpes simplex virus (HSV) or varicella-zoster virus (VZV). Rapid diagnosis of suspicious skin lesions can be provided by smears from the base of the lesion, fixed with ethanol or methanol, and stained with Wright-Giemsa stains. Multinucleated giant cells indicate infection with HSV or VZV. Viral culture or direct fluorescent antibody staining will provide confirmation and specific diagnosis.

In the patient with FRS and a diffuse erythema suggestive of scarlet fever, a throat culture might be informative, but not diagnostic, if it revealed the presence of group A streptococci. In a patient with FRS and erythema multiforme the demonstration of cold agglutinins may provide early evidence suggestive of *M. pneumoniae* infection.

In the patient with purpuric and ecchymotic lesions, disseminated intravascular coagulation is an important consideration, and determination of the coagulation parameters (prothrombin time

(PT), partial thromboplastin time (PTT), platelet count, fibrinogen, fibrin split products or D-dimer) can confirm the diagnosis.

A *skin punch or surgical biopsy* can provide early information as to specific diagnosis of the etiology of FRS in several ways. It can provide material for culture. It can also help define the nature of atypical skin lesions on the basis of histology. In addition, fluorescent antibody stains of the histologic sections may provide the diagnosis: demonstration of IgA in the skin lesions of Henoch-Schönlein purpura; demonstration of *R. rickettsii* in capillary endothelial cells in Rocky Mountain spotted fever.

Although serologic testing provides later diagnosis, a few serologic studies may be positive at the time of clinical presentation of FRS. The serologic tests for syphilis (VDRL and MHA-TP) are positive in patients with the rash of secondary syphilis; antistreptolysin O or anti-DNAase B antibodies usually are present by the time of appearance of erythema marginatum in acute rheumatic fever.

### Later diagnosis

Specific diagnosis for many causes of FRS can be established only in retrospect by showing a ≥4-fold rise in antibody titer to antigen(s) of the infecting agent. Antibody titer rises can be used to make a diagnosis in certain acute viral diseases (e.g., dengue, parvovirus $B_{19}$), rickettsial and ehrlichial infections, mycoplasmal and chlamydial infections, specific bacterial infections (e.g., leptospirosis, brucellosis, Lyme disease), and parasitic diseases (e.g., trichinosis, toxoplasmosis, African trypanosomiasis, filariasis).

Culture of slow-growing organisms may require weeks of incubation before definitive results (e.g, *M. tuberculosis*, *Bartonella henselii* or *B. quintana*, *Histoplasma capsulatum*) establish the diagnosis.

## Treatment

The treatment of individual conditions has been mentioned with the clinical manifestations.

## ANNOTATED BIBLIOGRAPHY


Cherry JD. Cutaneous manifestations of systemic infections. In: Textbook of Pediatric Infectious Diseases, 3rd ed. Feigin R, Cherry J, eds. WB Saunders, Philadelphia, PA, chap 81, pp 755–782, 1992.
*Extremely detailed coverage of skin manifestations in systemic infections. Particularly good regarding viral infections in children, with ample color photographs.*

Lambert HP, Farrar WE. Cutaneous manifestations of infection. In: Infectious Diseases Illustrated. An Integrated Text and Colour Atlas. Gower Medical, London, chaps 4–6, 1982.
*An outstanding collection of color photographs of cutaneous manifestations of many of the common as well as exotic systemic infections (viral, bacterial, fungal, parasitic).*

Levin S, Goodman LJ. An approach to acute fever and rash (AFR) in the adult. In: Current Clinical Topics in Infectious Diseases, vol 15. Remington JS, Swartz MN, eds. Blackwell Science, Cambridge, MA, pp 19–75, 1995.
*This is an excellent, comprehensive overview of infectious causes of fever and a rash. Despite the title the discussion includes consideration of many exanthematous diseases of childhood as well.*

Liu LX, Weller PF. Approach to the febrile traveler returning from Southeast Asia and Oceania. In: Current Clinical Topics in Infectious Diseases, vol 12. Remington JS, Swartz MN, eds. Blackwell Scientific, Cambridge, MA, pp 138–164, 1992.
*This article provides a broad view of infections endemic to Oceania and Southeast Asia, including those with cutaneous manifestations.*

Maguire JH. Epidemiologic considerations in the evaluation of undifferentiated fever in a traveler returning from Latin America or the Caribbean. In: Current Clinical Topics in Infectious Diseases, vol 13. Remington JS, Swartz MN, eds. Blackwell Science, Cambridge, MA, pp 26–56, 1993.
*Good coverage of dengue, yellow fever, and undifferentiated arboviral fevers as well as FRSs unique to the Southern Hemisphere, such as bartonellosis and Brazilian purpuric fever. Extensively referenced.*

Oster CN, Tramont EC. Fever in a recent visitor to the Middle East. In: Current Clinical Topics in Infectious Diseases, vol 13. Remington JS, Swartz MN, eds. Blackwell Scientific, Cambridge, MA, pp 57–73, 1993.
*Authoritative discussion of endemic infectious fevers in the Middle East, based to a large extent on experiences gained from Desert Shield/Desert Storm military operations.*

Swartz MN, Weinberg AN. Miscellanous bacterial infections with cutaneous manifestation. In: Dermatology in General Medicine, 4th ed. Fitzpatrick TB, Eisen AZ, Wolff K, Freudberg IM, Austen KF, eds. McGraw-Hill, New York, chap 190, pp 2354–2369, 1993.
*The emphasis here is on those bacterial infections, both localized in the skin and systemic in nature (but with cutaneous manifestations), in which epidemiologic clues are of particular importance in diagnosis.*

Weinberg AN, Swartz MN. Gram-negative coccal and bacillary infections. In: Dermatology in General Medicine, 4th ed. Fitzpatrick TB, Eisen AZ, Wolff K, Freedberg IM, Austen KF, eds. McGraw-Hill, New York, chap 188, pp 2334–2350, 1993.
*This is a detailed description of gram-negative bacillary infections involving the skin. The discussion includes both local infections of the skin and various systemic infections with cutaneous manifestations.*

Wilson ME. Fever. In: A World Guide to Infections: Diseases, Distribution, Diagnosis. Oxford University Press, Oxford, chap 5, pp 80–115, 1991.
*Covers infectious fevers from around the world in an organized fashion with many helpful tables. Considerable emphasis on epidemiology.*

Wyler DJ. Evaluation of cryptic fever in a traveler to Africa. In: Current Clinical Topics in Infectious Diseases, vol 12. Remington JS, Swartz MN, eds. Blackwell Scientific, Cambridge, MA, pp 329–347, 1992.
*This article takes up the problem of fever in a returning traveler from Africa. The approach to the broad problem is well covered, and the specific issue of fever and an exanthem is included. Exotic viral infections endemic in Africa are discussed.*

# 52

## Cellulitis and Abscesses

DENNIS L. STEVENS

Infections in the skin and subcutaneous tissue may be caused by viruses, fungi, bacteria, rickettsia, and parasites. Literally hundreds of different etiologies have been described in normal individuals, and more recently in compromised patients such as bone marrow transplant recipients and patients with AIDS. Thus, the clinician is faced with the formidable task of establishing a specific diagnosis and prescribing a definitive treatment. The most important points in establishing the diagnosis are the general appearance of the infected site, the patient's symptoms, a history of contact with arthropods or animals (including bites), hot tub exposure, specific geographical areas in which the patient has traveled, occupation, the immune status of the host, and the chronicity and anatomical distribution of the infection. Soft-tissue infections may range in severity from life-threatening to minor annoyances and may be recurrent or single episodes. If the diagnosis cannot be established based upon the history, signs, and symptoms, then needle aspiration, appropriate staining of aspirated fluid, skin biopsy, or surgical exploration may be necessary. Infections in the soft tissues produce local pathologic changes early in the course of infection and invariably as the process continues there may be regional effects—invasion of deeper structures such as lymph channels and capillary beds that ultimately results in systemic manifestations such as bacteremia or shock. The skin manifestations of viral, parasitic, and fungal infections will be discussed in other chapters.

### Folliculitis, Carbuncles, and Abscesses

Abscesses can develop from skin organisms introduced into the deeper tissue, from seeding of the skin from hematogenous sources such as bacteremia associated with endocarditis, or contiguously from infectious foci in the lung or gastrointestinal tract. In the former case, hair follicles serve as a portal of entry for a number of bacterial species, though *Staphylococcus aureus* is the most common cause of localized folliculitis. Recurrent folliculitis is most common in black males in association with shaving (folliculitis barbae). Folliculitis can progress to small subcutaneous abscesses (furuncles) which either resolve with antibiotic treatment alone or progress to form very large, exquisitely painful carbuncles which require surgical drainage as well as antibiotics. Certain individuals seem predisposed to develop recurrent *Staphylococcus aureus* infections (recurrent furunculosis) and most have underlying factors such as poor hygiene, nasal carriage of staphylococcus, or neurodermatitis. Though it is suggested that diabetic patients are prone to such infections, there is little data to support this concept. In contrast, patients with Job's syndrome classically have recurrent *Staphylococcus aureus* infections. In addition, these patients have eosinophilia and high levels of IgE antibody in serum.

Treatment of recurrent furunculosis may require surgical incision and drainage as well as antistaphylococcal antibiotics such as nafcillin parenterally or dicloxacillin orally. Prevention is difficult but some success has been realized with intranasal bacitracin or mupirocin ointment and pHisohex baths (in adults). Prophylactic antibiotics should be used only in severe cases.

Sebaceous glands empty into hair follicles, and the ducts, if blocked (sebaceous cyst), may resemble staphylococcal abscess or may become secondarily infected. Chronic folliculitis is uncommon except in acne vulgaris, where normal flora, e.g., *Propionibacterium acnes*, may play a role. Hidradenitis suppurativa occurs in either acute or chronic forms and can lead to recurrent axillary or pudendal abscesses.

Diffuse folliculitis occurs in two distinct settings. The first, "hot tub folliculitis," is caused by *Pseudomonas aeruginosa* in waters that are insufficiently chlorinated and maintained at temperatures between 37° and 40° C. Infection is self-limited though patients with bacteremia and shock have occasionally been reported. The second type of diffuse folliculitis, swimmer's itch, occurs when the skin is exposed to water infected with avian freshwater schistosomes. Free-swimming cercariae readily penetrate human hair follicles or pores but quickly die. This triggers a brisk allergic reaction causing intense itching and erythema. Warm water temperatures and alkaline pH are suitable for mollusks that are the intermediate host between bird and human. The infestation is self-limited, secondary infection is uncommon, and antipruritics and topical steroid cream relieve symptoms promptly.

### Cellulitis

*Cellulitis* is a term commonly used by physicians but poorly defined in the literature. It is characterized by leukocytic infiltration of the dermis, capillary dilation, and proliferation of bacteria in the dermis. Patients typically present with areas of skin which are red to pink in color, hot, tender, swollen, and painful. Cellulitis is most commonly due to normal skin flora such as *Staphylococcus aureus* or group A streptococci. Recently, recurrent cellulitis has been described in patients with coronary artery bypass surgery at the saphenous vein donor site. Such infections have largely been caused by group C and group G streptococci.

Cellulitis is also more common in conditions associated with chronic venous insufficiency and lymphedema. Though the causative organisms are likely streptococci, in most cases an organism cannot be isolated. In fact, aspiration of cellulitic skin or even punch biopsy fails to identify a bacterium 80% to 85% of the time. Thus, our knowledge of causes of cellulitis is far from complete.

A number of conditions predispose to infection by specific

pathogens (Table 52.1). In addition, bites of various types may introduce specific organisms into the deeper tissues, resulting in soft-tissue infections (see next section).

## Soft-Tissue Infections Associated with Bites

### Insect bites

Soft-tissue infections may result from the bites of mosquitos, horse flies, and spiders; usually they cause only local allergic reactions with itching, swelling, and erythema. The brown recluse spider bite may resemble acute infection early, but later there is primary tissue destruction and central necrosis due to dermonecrotic toxins produced by the spider. These infections may resemble pyoderma gangrenosa or they may be secondarily infected with skin organisms. Mosquito bites may serve as portals of entry for skin organisms such as *Staphylococcus aureus* or *Streptococcus pyogenes*. Such infections are not uncommon in clinical practice, yet given the number of individuals bitten by mosquitos, infection is a rare complication of insect bites.

### Animal bites and human bites

A vast array of bacteria may be isolated from bites from dogs, cats, and other animals. This subject is discussed in detail in Chapter 95.

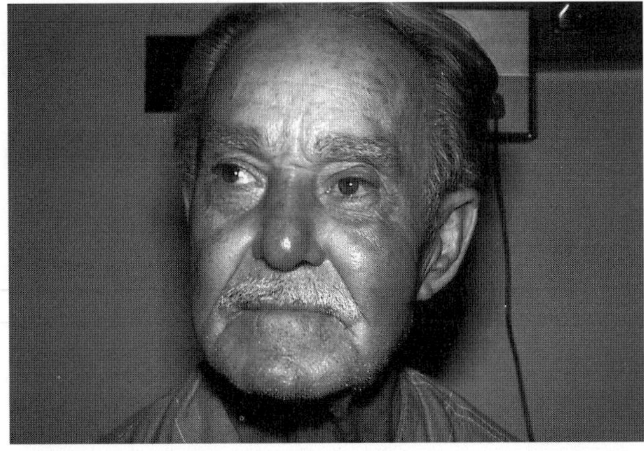

**Fig. 52.1** Erysipelas. In the characteristic appearance of erysipelas, a brilliant red or salmon red, painful confluent erythema in a "butterfly" distribution involves the nasal eminence, cheeks, and nose with abrupt borders along the nasolabial fold. The erythema increases over a course of 3–6 days and usually resolves in 7–10 days. Erysipelas has been associated with high fevers, bacteremia, and possible death, even in modern times. The fluctuation in severity may reflect cyclical changes in the virulence of group A $\beta$ hemolytic streptococci. [Reproduced with permission from Atlas of Infectious Diseases. Vol. 2: Skin, Soft-Tissue, Bone, and Joint Infections. DL Stevens, ed. Current Medicine, Philadelphia, PA, 1995.]

## Erysipelas

Erysipelas is caused exclusively by *Streptococcus pyogenes* and is characterized by an abrupt onset of fiery, red swelling of the face or extremities. Distinctive features are its well-defined margins, particularly along the nasolabial fold, its rapid progression, and its intense pain (see Fig. 52.1). Flaccid bullae may develop during the second to third day of illness, but extension to deeper soft tissues is rare. Surgical debridement is rarely necessary, and treatment with penicillin is effective. Swelling may progress despite appropriate treatment, though fever, pain, and the intense red color diminish. Desquamation of the involved skin occurs 5 to 10 d into the illness. Infants and elderly adults are most commonly afflicted, and the severity of systemic toxicity may vary. Erysipelas may be less severe today than it was at the turn of the century.

**Table 52.1** Etiology of soft tissue infections associated with specific risk factors

| Risk factor | Etiologic agent |
|---|---|
| Cat bite | *Pasteurella multocida* |
| Dog bite | *Pasteurella multocida*, DF-2 |
| Hot tub folliculitis | *Pseudomonas aeruginosa* |
| Diabetes mellitus | Group B Streptococcus |
| Periorbial cellulitis | *Hemophilus influenza* |
| Saphenous vein donor site | Group C, G streptococcus |
| Freshwater laceration | *Aeromonas hydrophila* |
| Sea water/cirrhosis | *Vibrioc vulnifica* |
| Stasis Dermatitis | Group A, C, G streptococcus |
| Lymphedema | Group A, C, G streptococcus |
| Cat scratch | *Rochalimea quintana* |
| | *Rochalimea hensela* |
| | *Bartonella* |
| Fish cleaning, bone rendering | *Erysipelothrix rhusiopathia* |
| Fish tank exposure | *Mycobacterium marinum* |
| Peripheral vascular disease | Group B streptococcus |
| Compromised hosts | Gram-negative rods |

## Impetigo

Impetigo contagiosa is caused by *Streptococcus pyogenes*, and bullous impetigo is due to *Staphylococcus aureus*. Both skin lesions may have an early bullous stage, but they then appear as thick crusts with a golden brown color. Streptococcal lesions are most common in children 2–5 yr of age, and epidemics may occur in settings of poor hygiene and particularly in children from lower socioeconomic conditions in tropical climates. It is important to recognize impetigo because of its potential relationship to post-streptococcal glomerulonephritis.

## Treatment

Because of the diverse etiologies responsible for cellulitis, empiric choices of antibiotic therapies depend greatly on the clinical factors described previously. Once cultures and sensitivities are available, choices are much easier and more specific. The physician must first decide if the patient's illness is severe enough to require parental treatment either in the hospital or on an outpatient basis. For presumed streptococcal or staphylococcal cellulitis, nafcillin, cephalothin, cefuroxime, vancomycin, and erythromycin are good choices. Cefazolin and ceftriaxone have less activity against *Staphylococcus aureus* than cephalothin, though clinical trials have shown a high degree of efficacy. Ceftriaxone may be a useful choice for outpatient treatment because of once per day dosing. Similarly, teicoplanin, like vancomycin, has excellent activity against *S. pyogenes* and both *S. aureus* and *S. epidermidis* and may be given once per day by intravenous or intramuscular injection. For patients being treated with oral drugs, dicloxacillin, cefuroxime axetil, cefpodoxime, and erythromycin (or clarithromycin or azrithromycin) are all effective treatments. For known group A, B, C, or G streptococcal infections, penicillin or erythromycin should be used orally or parenterally. In serious group A streptococcal infections, clindamycin is superior to penicillin. This is probably because in this type of infection where large numbers of bacteria are present, streptococci are in a stationary phase of growth and do not express a full complement of penicillin binding proteins. In contrast, clindamycin is not affected by inoculum size or stage of growth. In addition, clindamycin suppresses synthesis of many streptococcal exotoxins.

For cellulitis associated with *Eikenella corrodens*, penicillin, ceftriaxone, sulfamethoxazole-trimethoprim, tetracyclines, and fluoroquinolones are all useful. Interestingly, this organism is resistant to oxacillin, cefazolin, clindamycin, and erythromycin. Cellulitis associated with cat bites may fail with treatment with oral cephalosporins, erythromycins, and dicloxacillin. Reasons for failure include *Pasteurella multocida*'s resistance to oxacillin/dicloxacillin and failure of oral cephalosporins and erythromycins to attain adequate serum and tissue levels.

## ANNOTATED BIBLIOGRAPHY

Duvanel T, Auckenthaler R, Rohner P, Hurms M, Saurat JH. Quantitative cultures of biopsy specimens from cutaneous cellulitis. Arch Intern Med 1989; 149:293.
*Describes the technique of using punch biopsy to establish a diagnosis of cellulitis.*

Goldstein EJC. Bite wounds and infection. Clin Infect Dis 1992; 14:633.
*Excellent review of soft-tissue infection associated with many different types of animal bites.*

Hook EW et al. Microbiologic evaluation of cutaneous cellulitis in adults. Arch Intern Med 1986; 146:295.
*This paper also describes the punch biopsy technique as a way to evaluate the etiology of cellulitis.*

Stevens DL. Streptococcal infections of the skin. *In*: Atlas of Infectious Diseases: Skin, Soft-Tissue, Bone and Joint Infections. Stevens DL, ed. Current Medicine, Philadelphia, PA, 1994.
*This atlas has color plates and extensive descriptions of all types of group A soft-tissue infection including necrotizing fasciitis, myonecroses, and streptococcal toxic shock syndrome.*

Stevens DL. Infections of the skin, muscle & soft tissues. *In*: Harrison's Principles of Internal Medicine, 13th ed. KJ Isselbacher, E Braunwald, JD Wilson, JB Martin, AS Fauci, DL Kaspar, eds. McGraw-Hill, New York, 1994, pp 561–563.
*This chapter is an anatomical approach to soft-tissue infections. It provides an overview of skin, fascial, and muscle infection.*

Stevens DL. Group A streptococcal infections. *In*: Stein's Textbook of Internal Medicine, JH Stein ed. Mosby, St Louis, 1993.
*This chapter discusses the epidemiology, pathogenesis, clinical manifestation, and treatment of all types of group A streptococcal infections.*

# 53

# Infectious Diseases with Lymphadenopathy

IVOR BYREN

Lymph nodes, together with the spleen, are a major site of interaction between antigen and the immune system and are involved in a broad spectrum of disease processes including infection, neoplasia, immune diseases, infiltrative conditions, endocrine diseases and a number of idiopathic conditions (Table 53.1). Afferent lymph from the circulation containing antigens, microorganisms, macrophages, and lymphocytes is processed in lymph nodes, and efferent lymph containing sensitized T cells, B cells, and antibody-secreting plasma cells is returned to the circulation via the thoracic duct. Lymph node structure includes the cortex, paracortex, and medulla. The cortex contains primary lymphoid follicles which, on exposure to afferent lymph, develop into secondary lymphoid follicles containing germinal centers, which are the major site of B cell proliferation. The cortical area also contains macrophages, including Langerhans cells and histiocytes, which are responsible for antigen presentation to B and T cells. The paracortex is the major site of T cell localization of which 80% are $CD4^+$ T helper cells and 20% are $CD8^+$ suppressor/cytotoxic T cells. The medulla consists of macrophage rich sinuses which remove microorganisms and unite to form the efferent lymphatics. Lymphatic channels are distributed regionally, and this anatomical consistency results in predictable patterns of lymph node enlargement. This system engages the humoral and cellular components of the immune system in a process designed to eliminate foreign antigens (Fig. 53.1).

The infectious causes of lymphadenopathy are characterized by benign proliferation of lymphocytes and macrophages, or infiltration with inflammatory and phagocytic cells. The latter infiltrate is a feature of lymphadenitis and is invariably associated with infection. In this chapter the term lymphadenopathy will be used to include both lymph node enlargement and the specific condition of lymphadenitis.

## Etiology

Lymph node enlargement, the most common manifestation of lymphadenopathy, is not a disease but a clinical sign and as such has a number of causes. Infection is the most common cause of lymph node enlargement, and this sign may occur as a pathognomonic feature of a common disease, a pathognomonic feature of a rare disease, or a nonspecific feature of either (Table 53.2). The prevalence of infectious diseases associated with lymphadenopathy is not constant and reflects historical trends, changing social structures, and geographical location. The pandemic of tuberculosis that involved Europe in the 18th and 19th centuries has disappeared with improved social circumstances, while in developing countries there is an epidemic of tuberculosis linked to the human immunodeficiency virus pandemic.

Noninfectious causes of lymphadenopathy, although less common, need to be considered in the differential diagnosis (Table 53.1). These include a number of idiopathic conditions, some of which may ultimately be shown to be infectious in origin, in particular Kawasaki syndrome (mucocutaneous lymph node syndrome) and Kikuchi's histiocytic necrotizing lymphadenitis. Both present with cervical lymphadenopathy, the former a disease of children and the latter a disease of young adults. The infectious etiology of roseola infantum, human herpesvirus 6, was identified in 1988. More recently human herpesvirus 8 has been identified as the cause of Kaposi's sarcoma and possibly also giant follicular lymph node hyperplasia (Castleman's disease). A number of reactive conditions, not in themselves infections, may be triggered by infection or associated with infection. Secondary amyloidosis (AA type) has been associated with underlying infections—in particular, bronchiectasis, leprosy, osteomyelitis, and tuberculosis. Infection associated erythrophagocytic lymphohistiocytosis, which may present with fever and lymphadenopathy, has been linked to viruses (adenovirus, EpsteinBarr virus, cytomegalovirus, herpes simplex virus, human parvovirus $B_{19}$, parainfluenzavirus, and varicella-zoster virus), viral immunization, bacterial sepsis (*Escherichia coli* and other gram-negative organisms), leishmaniasis, tuberculosis, and fungi (candidiasis and histoplasmosis).

## Epidemiology

There is no descriptive epidemiology for lymphadenopathy and the relevant epidemiology is that of the underlying etiology (Table 53.2). Within this context there are, however, a number of important factors to consider which will provide clues as to the likely etiology. The age of the patient will determine the relative likelihood of infection as a cause for the lymphadenopathy. Neoplasia accounts for lymphadenopathy in only 20% of patients under age 30 years, but 60% of those over age 50 years, and in this group neoplastic lesions must always be considered. Neoplasia is almost never the cause of lymphadenopathy in the neonate.

A thorough enquiry regarding animal contact, receipt of blood products, diet, human immunodeficiency virus status, immunosuppression, injecting drug use, family history, institutionalization, occupation, recreation, hobbies, pregnancy, sexual history, travel history, country of origin, immunization history, antecedent trauma, and coincident medical conditions can narrow the dif-

**Table 53.1** Noninfectious causes of lymphadenopathy

| | |
|---|---|
| NEOPLASIA | ENDOCRINE DISEASE |
| Metastatic<br>Reticuloendothelial | Hyperthyroidism |
| IMMUNE DISORDERS | IDIOPATHIC AND MISCELLANEOUS CAUSES |
| Angioimmunoblastic lymphadenopathy<br>Common variable immunodeficiency<br>Dermatomyositis<br>Drug reactions (allopurinol, hydralizine, phenytoin)<br>Primary biliary cirrhosis<br>Rheumatoid arthritis<br>Serum sickness/immune complex disease<br>Sjogren's syndrome<br>Systemic lupus erythematosus | Familial Mediterranean fever<br>Giant follicular lymph node hyperplasia (Castleman's disease)<br>Histiocytic diseases (Sinus histiocytosis, Letterer-Siwe disease, erythrophagocytic lymphohistiocytosis, histiocytic medullary reticulosis, malignant histiocytosis)<br>Kawasaki disease (Mucocutaneous lymph node syndrome)<br>Kikuchi's histiocytic necrotizing lymphadenitis<br>Lymphatoid granulomatosis<br>Multifocal Langerhans cell granulomatosis<br>Sarcoidosis<br>Vaccination (smallpox) |
| INFILTRATIVE DISEASES | |
| Amyloidosis<br>Gaucher's disease<br>Niemann-Pick disease | |

ferential diagnosis. In particular, the spectrum of infectious diseases associated with lymphadenopathy should be expanded in light of the travel history and country of origin. The frequency of international travel may increase the incidence of certain infections, and this is particularly well illustrated by increasing reports of dengue in travelers. Infections of travelers to tropical countries is discussed further in Chapters 92–94. The family and immunization history are particularly important considerations in the childhood viral exanthems and conditions associated with overcrowding such as tuberculosis. Pregnancy, immunosuppression, and the consumption of contaminated foods are strongly associated with the acquisition of listeriosis. Occupation, animal contact, sports, and hobbies highlight certain infections as potential causes of lymphadenopathy. Infections complicating contacts with animals and insects are discussed in Chapters 95 and 96. The sexual history, including the country of origin of partners, is of particular importance in inguinal lymphadenopathy and in generalized lymphadenopathy, which is a feature of infectious mononucleosis and secondary syphilis. High-risk sexual behavior and injecting drug use may require exclusion of human immunodeficiency virus and hepatitis B and C.

## Host Factors

Host factors are rarely relevant to lymphadenopathy per se, except in chronic granulomatous disease, which is characterized by neutrophil and monocyte dysfunction and recurrent infection of

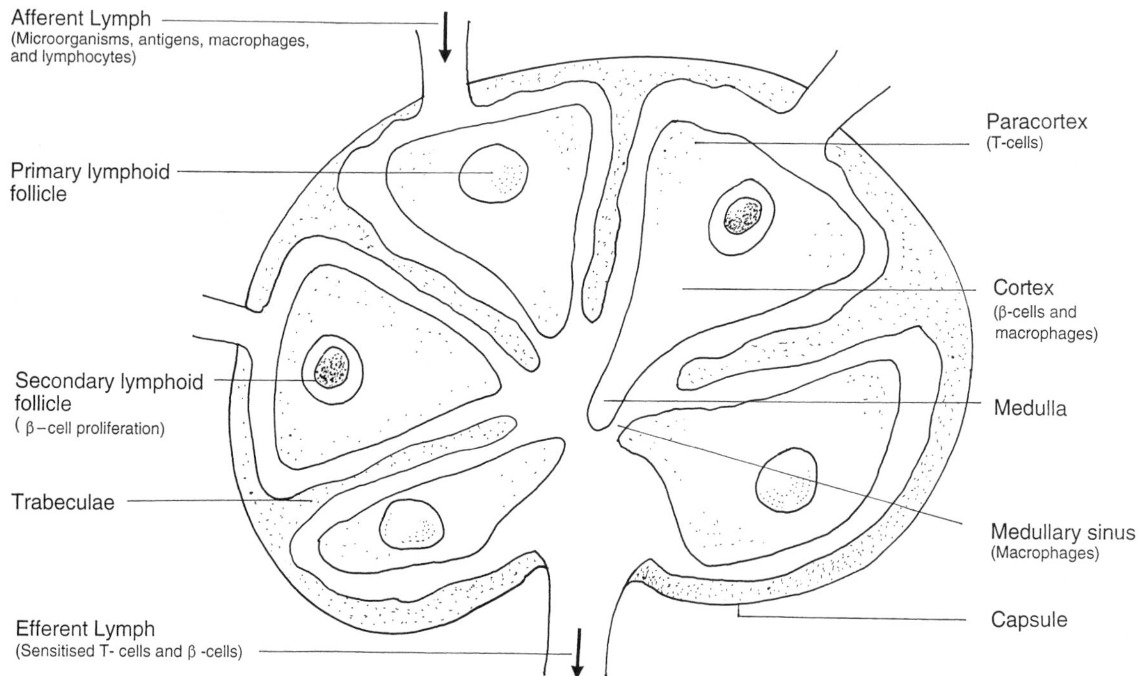


**Fig. 53.1** Lymph node structure and function.

**Table 53.2** Infectious causes of lymphadenopathy and their epidemiological factors

| Disease | Organism | Epidemiology[a] |
|---|---|---|
| BACTERIAL | | |
| Anthrax | *Bacillus anthracis* | A, O |
| Brucellosis | *Brucella* species | A, O, D |
| Cat scratch | *Bartonella (Rochalimaea) henselae* | A, O |
| Chancroid | *Hemophilus ducreyi* | S, T |
| Diphtheria | *Corynebacterium diptheriae* | In, V |
| Glanders | *Pseudomonas mallei* | A, O |
| Gonorrhoea | *Neisseria gonorrhoea* | S |
| Granuloma inguinale | *Calymmatobacterium granulomatis* | S, T |
| Granulomatous lymphadenitis | *Corynebacterium pseudotuberculosis* | A, O |
| Leptospirosis | *Leptospira* species | A, O |
| Listeriosis | *Listeria monocytogenes* | D, I, P |
| Lymphogranuloma venereum | *Chlamydia trachomatis* | S, T |
| Melioidosis | *Pseudomonas pseudomallei* | T |
| Mesenteric lymphadenitis | *Yersinia* species | Undefined |
| Necrotizing pharyngitis | Mixed anaerobes<br>Spirochetes<br>*Fusobacterium necrophorum* | In |
| Nocardiosis | *Nocardia* species | I |
| Non-venereal treponematoses | *Treponema pallidum* | T |
| Plague | *Yersinia pestis* | A, O, T |
| Pyogenic lymphadenitis | Group A streptococci<br>*Staphylococcus aureus* | O |
| Rat-bite fever | *Spirillum minor*<br>*Streptobacillus moniliformis* | A, O |
| Scarlet fever | Group A streptococci | In |
| Scrofula | *Mycobacterium tuberculosis*<br>Atypical mycobacteria<br>Calmette-Guerin bacillus (BCG) | I, T, V |
| Syphilis | *Treponema pallidum* | S |
| Tuberculosis | *Mycobacterium tuberculosis*<br>Atypical mycobacteria | I, T |
| Tularemia | *Francisella tularensis* | A, O, T |
| VIRAL | | |
| Acquired immune deficiency Syndrome | Human immunodeficiency virus | B, IDU, In, S, T |
| Adult T-cell leukemia-lymphoma | Human T-cell lymphotropic virus | B, S, T |
| Cytomegalovirus | Cytomegalovirus | B, I |
| Dengue | Dengue virus | T |
| Epidemic keratoconjunctivitis | Adenovirus | In |
| Hemorrhagic fevers | Arenaviruses | A, T |
| Hepatitis | Hepatitis B, C | B, IDU, In, S, T, V, |
| Herpes genitalis | Herpes simplex virus 1, 2 | I, S |
| Herpes zoster | Varicella zoster virus | Latency |
| Infectious mononucleosis | Epstein-Barr virus | S |
| Kaposi's sarcoma | Human herpesvirus 8 | S |
| Measles | Measles virus | In, V |
| Pharyngoconjunctival fever | Adenovirus | In |
| Postvaccinial lymphadenitis | Vaccinia virus | V |
| Roseola infantum | Human herpes virus 6 | Sporadic |
| Rubella | Rubella virus | In, V |
| West Nile fever | West Nile virus | T |
| FUNGAL | | |
| Aspergillosis | *Aspergillus* species | I |
| Blastomycosis | *Blastomyces* dermatitidis | O |
| Candidiasis | *Candida* species | I |
| Coccidioidomycosis | *Coccidioides immitis* | I, T |
| Cryptococcosis | *Cryptococcus neoformans* | I, T |
| Histoplasmosis | *Histoplasma capsulatum* | O, T |
| Pneumocystis carinii pneumonia | *Pneumocystis carinii* | I |
| Paracoccidioidomycosis | *Paracoccidioides brasiliensis* | T |
| Sporotrichosis | *Sporothrix schenkii* | O |

*(continued)*

**Table 53.2** Infectious causes of lymphadenopathy and their epidemiological factors—*Continued*

| Disease | Organism | Epidemiology[a] |
|---|---|---|
| PARASITIC | | |
| Filariasis | *Wuchereria bancrofti* | T |
| | *Brugia* species | T |
| Leishmaniasis | *Leishmania* species | O, T |
| Loiasis | Loa loa | T |
| Onchocerciasis | *Onchocerca volvulus* | T |
| Toxoplasmosis | *Toxoplasma gondii* | D, O |
| Trypanosomiasis | *Trypanosoma brucei* | T |
| | *Trypanosoma cruzi* | |

[a]Key: A = animal contact, B = blood products, D = diet, I = immunosuppression, IDU = injecting drug use, In = institutionalization, O = occupation and recreation, P = pregnancy, S = sexual history, T = travel, V = vaccination history.

lymph nodes (as well as bones, lungs, liver, and skin), particularly with *Staphylococcus aureus* and gram-negative bacilli. Other immune dysfunction may predispose patients to acquiring infections which may be predictably associated with lymphadenopathy. Iatrogenic immunosuppression and human immunodeficiency virus infection are the most common circumstances where this occurs, but congenital and other acquired immunodeficiencies also need to be considered. Generalized lymphadenopathy may be a prominent feature of common variable immunodeficiency, and treatment with $\gamma$-globulin will reverse the lymphadenopathy. Infections complicating immunodeficiency and immunosuppression, including human

**Table 53.3** Distribution of lymphadenopathy and characteristic infectious causes

CERVICAL

Cat scratch disease
Cytomegalovirus
Herpes simplex virus
Infectious mononucleosis
Listeriosis
Roseola infantum
Rubella
Scrofula
Sporotrichosis
Toxoplasmosis
Tularemia

AXILLARY AND EPITROCHLEAR

Brucellosis
Cat scratch disease
Filariasis
Infectious mononucleosis
Rat bite fever
Sporotrichosis
Tuberculosis
Tularemia

INGUINAL

Brucellosis
Cat scratch disease
Chancroid
Filariasis
Gonorrhoea
Granuloma inguinale
Herpes simplex virus
Lymphogranuloma venereum
Nonvenereal treponematoses
Onchocerciasis
Plague
Syphilis
Toxoplasmosis
Tuberculosis
Tularemia

HILAR, MEDIASTINAL, AND PARATRACHEAL

Coccidioidomycosis
Cryptococcosis
Cytomegalovirus
Histoplasmosis
Infectious mononucleosis
Pneumocystis carinii pneumonia
Toxoplasmosis
Tuberculosis

GENERALIZED

Adult T-cell leukemia-lymphoma
Brucellosis
Cytomegalovirus
Dengue
Infectious mononucleosis
Filariasis
Glanders
Hemorrhagic fevers
Hepatitis B,C
Histoplasmosis
Human herpesvirus 6
Human immunodeficiency virus
Leishmaniasis
Leptospirosis
Lymphogranuloma venereum
Measles
Melioidosis
Rubella
Scarlet fever
Syphilis
Toxoplasmosis
Trypanosomiasis
Tuberculosis (including atypical mycobacteria)
Tularemia
Typhus
West Nile fever

immunodeficiency virus infection, are discussed further in Chapters 86 to 89.

## Clinical Manifestations

The distribution of lymphadenopathy must be evaluated in the context of the overall clinical picture, which will often allow a diagnosis to be reached rapidly and accurately. These clinical patterns are discussed further in Chapters 47 to 49 dealing with the approach to the patient with fever and in Chapter 51 dealing with infections associated with rash. Tables 53.2 and 53.3 must therefore not be interpreted as suggesting that lymphadenopathy is necessarily a common or a prominent feature of the clinical presentation. The relevant chapters should be consulted for a detailed description of each disease.

The presence of some degree of lymphadenopathy may be normal; benign inguinal lymphadenopathy of up to 2 cm is a frequent finding in adults. Submandibular lymphadenopathy of up to 1 cm is a frequent finding in children and young adults. Both of these findings reflect previous infection within the draining anatomy. The differential diagnosis of mass lesions occurring at specific lymph node sites must also be considered, and in particular childhood neck masses may represent congenital lesions. After assessing the epidemiological and host factors, lymphadenopathy associated with infectious diseases is best considered as either an acute or chronic process, with specific physical characteristics, presenting with an anatomical distribution that may involve a single node, regional lymphadenopathy, or generalized lymphadenopathy. Lymphadenopathy in the presence of fever and local or other systemic signs of infection is highly suggestive of an infectious cause for the lymphadenopathy, although the constellation of night sweats, low grade fever, weight loss, and pruritus must also prompt consideration of lymphoma. Neoplastic conditions typically produce nodes that are hard or firm, occasionally rubbery, nontender, and may be matted or fixed to adjacent structures. Symmetry is a classical feature of the lymphomas but may also be seen with the infectious causes of generalized lymphadenopathy, intrathoracic lymphadenopathy, and inguinal lymphadenopathy. Transient lymphadenopathy is a particular feature of the childhood viral exanthems, minor trauma, and subclinical infection, and these circumstances are usually readily identified.

Lymphangitis is characterized by red streaking of the skin due to infection tracking along subcutaneous lymphatic channels and is usually associated with lymph node enlargement. If presenting as an acute process, it is most commonly associated with group A streptococci but may also occur with *Staphylococcus aureus*, *Pasteurella multocida*, *Spirillium minor*, *Wuchereria bancrofti*, and *Brugia malayi*. If presenting as a chronic process it is most commonly associated with *Sporothrix schenckii*, *Mycobacterium kansasii*, *Mycobacterium marinum*, *Nocardia brasiliensis*, *Nocardia asteroides*, *Wuchereria bancrofti*, and *Brugia malayi*.

The physical characteristics of lymphadenopathy provide clues to the etiology. Infection typically produces suppurative, nonsuppurative, or caseous changes in lymph nodes; on examination they are are tender, asymmetrically enlarged, and occasionally matted, and the overlying skin may show erythema and swelling. Lymph node enlargement of acute onset suggests an infectious cause, and the rapid stretching of the lymph node capsule is usually accompanied by tenderness to palpation. This may also be a feature of the acute leukemias, which may themselves be associated with infections typical of the immunocompromised host. Abscess, bubo, and sinus formation suggest an infectious cause and are most commonly associated with regional lymphadenopathy. Sinus formation is a particular feature of infection with *Mycobacterium tuberculosis* and atypical mycobacteria. Acute suppurative lymphadenitis, involving cervical, inguinal, or axillary lymphadenopathy, is more common in children, and *Staphylococcus aureus* or group A streptococci are usually involved. A single tender large node with fluctuation and accompanying systemic signs is typical. A chronic presentation, possibly accompanied by suppuration and the development of abscesses or sinuses, may be seen with cat scratch disease, chancroid, granuloma inguinale, lymphogranuloma venereum, and tuberculosis. A similar appearance may be seen in neutropenic patients (aspergillus species and *Candida albicans*) and chronic granulomatous disease (Calmette-Guerin bacillus, *Chromobacterium violaceum*, enterbacteriaceae, *Nocardia* species, *Pseudomonas*, and *Staphylococcus aureus*). Lymphedema may occur with recurrent attacks of suppurative lymphadenopathy involving inguinal and axillary nodes. It is also a particular feature of filariasis and lymphogranuloma venereum.

It is important to define the distribution of lymphadenopathy as this may narrow the differential diagnosis. The presence of a single node or regional lymphadenopathy invites consideration of the drainage pattern and a search for a focus of infection. Specific infections may present with a predictable anatomical distribution of lymphadenopathy, and this approach, although limited, is used below (Table 53.3).

### Cervical lymphadenopathy

The cervical group of nodes, draining head and neck structures (including supraclavicular draining intrathoracic and intraabdominal structures), are located as follows: submental nodes under the chin and close to the midline, submandibular nodes underneath and close to the angle of the jaw, jugular nodes along the anterior border of the sternocleidomastoid muscle, supraclavicular nodes behind the clavicle, suboccipital nodes at the apex of the posterior cervical triangle, and pre- and postauricular nodes, respectively, anterior and posterior to the ears (Fig. 53.2). In the elderly, cervical lymphadenopathy may be neoplastic in origin, particularly if unilateral and involving submandibular, jugular, supraclavicular, or scalene nodes, but in children and young adults it is almost always secondary to infection. The most common infections responsible for nonsuppurative cervical lymphadenopathy are pharyngitis (group A streptococci, adenovirus, *Corynebacterium diptheriae*, enterovirus, herpes simplex virus, and parainfluenza virus), tonsillitis, otitis media, dental infection, and scalp infections. Mononucleosis syndromes (cytomegalovirus, Epstein-Barr virus, and toxoplasmosis) and rubella, often accompanied by generalized lymphadenopathy and rash, also need to be considered. Postauricular lymphadenopathy is often a particular feature of rubella. Postvaccinial lymphadenopathy following smallpox immunization and involving, typically, left sided cervical and axillary nodes is now extremely rare but should be suspected in recently vaccinated military or laboratory personnel. Necrotizing infections involving the pharynx, gingiva, and related structures caused by anaerobes, spirochetes, and, rarely, *Fusobacterium necrophorum* may present with marked neck swelling and a sepsis syndrome. Various eponyms are attached to the different presentations including Lemiere syndrome, Ludwig's angina, and Vincent's angina (see Chapter 84). The oculoglandular syndrome

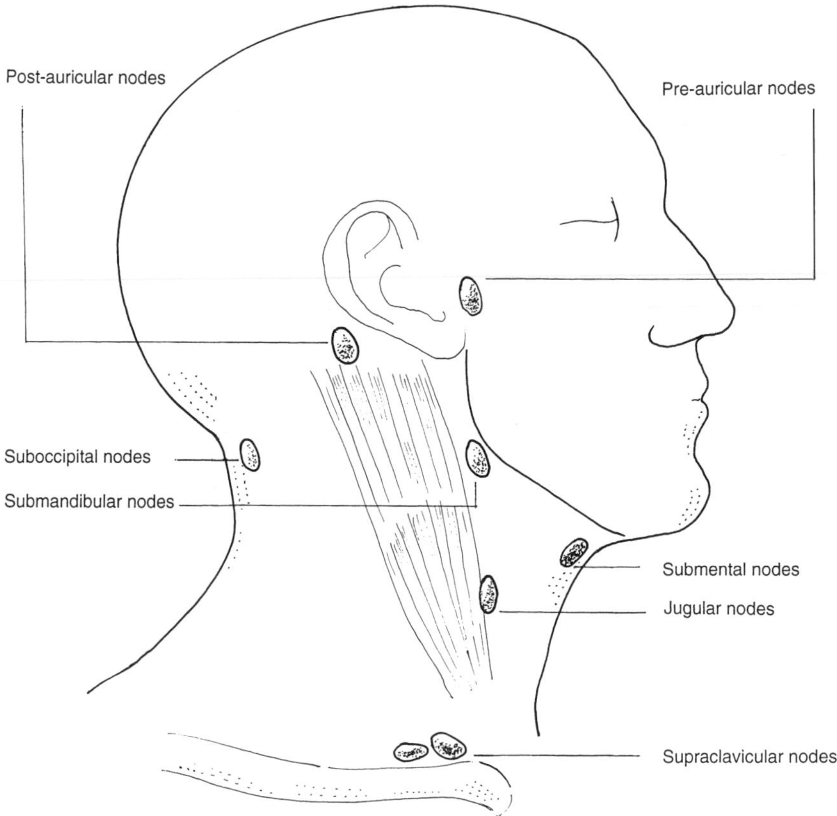


**Fig. 53.2** Location of cervical lymph nodes.

presents with preauricular lymphadenopathy secondary to the conjunctival infection occasionally associated with adenoviruses, cat scratch disease, listeriosis, lymphogranuloma venereum, sporotrichosis, and tularemia. Bubo formation involving cervical nodes is uncommon but is seen occasionally with plague or tularemia. Tuberculous cervical lymphadenopathy (scrofula) was uncommon in developed countries, but since 1984 there has been a resurgence of extrapulmonary tuberculosis associated with the human immunodeficiency virus. Presentation is typically accompanied by a slowly enlarging, nontender mass of cervical nodes which become fluctuant and finally chronically discharge caseous material. There may be a paucity of systemic symptoms. A number of mycobacterial species have been implicated, including *Mycobacterium tuberculosis*, mycobacterium avium complex, *Mycobacterium bovis*, *Mycobacterium kansasii*, and *Mycobacterium scrofulaceum*. The condition may also present after immunisation with *Calmette-Guerin bacillus*, in which case it is usually self limiting.

Cat scratch disease is probably the most common cause of chronic benign cervical lymphadenopathy in children and young adults (see Chapter 95). Any age group may be affected, but 80% of patients are under the age of 20 years and in 80% of cases present with lymphadenopathy in the cervical or axillary region and less frequently in the inguinal region, reflecting the site of inoculation. Other patterns of lymphadenopathy include the oculoglandular syndrome, hilar lymphadenopathy, mesenteric lymphadenitis, and abdominal lymphadenopathy. The etiological agent in most cases appears to be *Bartonella* (*Rochalimaea*) *henselae*, which is also responsible for bacillary angiomatosis, bacillary peliosis hepatis, and a chronic bacteremia syndrome. Together with *Bartonella* (*Rochalimaea*) *quintana* (trench fever) and *Bartonella* (*Rochalimaea*) *elizabethae* these gram-negative rods have been recently assigned to the genus *Bartonellaceae*. The salient epidemiological feature of cat scratch disease is an almost invariable history of cat—typically a kitten—scratch, bite, or ownership. Some two-thirds of patients develop a papule or pustule at the site of inoculation, which is followed some 7 d to 7 weeks later by regional lymphadenopathy. The lymphadenopathy lasts from 1 to 4 wk, and in only the minority of cases is it accompanied by a low-grade fever. The features of bartonella (rochalimaea) bacteremia are discussed in Chapters 50, 95 and 100.

## Axillary and epitrochlear lymphadenopathy

The axillary group of nodes, draining chest wall, breast, upper extremity, and intrathoracic structures, are located as follows: central axillary nodes on the thoracic wall of the axilla and the lateral group along the axillary vein close to the proximal humerus, subscapular nodes along the anterior edge of the latissimus dorsi muscle, pectoral nodes along the lateral border of the pectoralis muscle, and infraclavicular nodes underneath the distal aspect of the clavicle. Lymphadenopathy at these sites is typically secondary to upper limb infections, often following minor trauma, but it is also a feature of cat scratch disease, brucellosis, sporotrichosis, miliary tuberculosis, and tularemia. Rarely, suppurative subpectoral lymphadenopathy, with cellulitis involving the trunk, is seen with staphylococcal or streptococcal thumb infections as a result of the unique lymphatic drainage from this site. Epitrochlear nodes, draining forearm and hand, are found proximal to the medial epicondyle of the humerus and are typically associated with upper limb inoculations or infections, including cat scratch disease and rat bite fever, but they may also be a feature of brucellosis, infectious mononucleosis, sporotrichosis, secondary syphilis, miliary tuberculosis, or tularemia.

## Inguinal lymphadenopathy

Inguinal nodes, draining genitalia and lower extremities, are palpable along the inguinal ligament and femoral nodes within the femoral triangle. Their presence requires assessment of the genital area to identify a sexually transmitted infection. In a sexually active patient, genital herpes simplex virus and primary syphilis are common causes of lymphadenopathy at this site. Bubo formation suggests chancroid, granuloma inguinale, or lymphogranuloma venereum and only rarely gonorrhoea or syphilis. Herpes simplex virus rarely causes a suppurative inguinal lymphadenitis. Sexually transmitted diseases are discussed in detail in chapters 70 to 72. Lymphadenopathy at this site may also be a feature of nonsexually transmitted diseases including brucellosis, cat scratch disease, mycobacteria, onchocerciasis, plague, toxoplasmosis, tularemia, and, if suppuration is present, *Staphylococcus aureus*, streptococci, and yersinia. Nonvenereal treponematoses—in particular, endemic syphilis and yaws—are also characterized by lymphadenopathy although not limited to the inguinal region. Suppurative lymphadenopathy at this site is also a particular feature of injecting drug use and the infective complications of intravenous drug abuse are discussed in Chapter 90.

## Intrathoracic and intraabdominal lymphadenopathy

Hilar, mediastinal, and paratracheal nodes, draining intrathoracic structures and superficial node groups, are never palpable and abdominal and pelvic, draining intraabdominal structures, pelvic structures, and lower extremities, only rarely. Lymphadenopathy at these sites is usually detected by imaging techniques and, particularly with abdominal and retroperitoneal nodes, should raise the possibility of neoplasia (see Chapter 12). The intrathoracic infections associated with lymphadenopathy include tuberculosis, bronchiectasis, coccidioidomycosis, cryptococcosis, histoplasmosis, mononucleosis syndromes, and *Pneumocystis carinii*. Coccidioidomycosis or histoplasmosis can be associated with epidemics linked to environmental disturbance such as that affecting the western United States in 1991–1992. Rarely a gumma of late benign syphilis is responsible for intrathoracic lymph node enlargement.

Mesenteric lymphadenitis typically presents in childhood with features suggesting acute appendicitis, and the most commonly identified organisms include *Yersinia enterocolitica*, *Yersinia pseudotuberculosis*, *Staphylococcus aureus*, and streptococci, but it is also described with cat scratch disease, *Giardia lamblia*, and tuberculosis. Suppurative iliac lymphadenopathy may occur at any age, and the organisms most commonly implicated are *Staphylococcus aureus* and streptococci. Typically an abscess develops over weeks between the psoas and iliacus muscles, producing a limp, back or hip pain, and eventually hip flexion.

Compression syndromes are an uncommon feature of expanding infectious lymphadenopathy in the rigid thoracic cavity and only rarely a feature of intraabdominal lymphadenopathy. Symptoms may include cough and wheeze from airway compression, dysphagia from esophageal compression, hoarseness from recurrent laryngeal compression, diaphragmatic paralysis, swelling of face, neck, and arms from superior vena caval or subclavian compression, and swelling of the lower limbs and genitals from venous or lymphatic obstruction.

## Generalized lymphadenopathy

Generalized lymphadenopathy, involving two or more noncontiguous sites, is typical of certain infections, usually accompanied by bloodstream dissemination and nodal invasion, but rarely produces suppuration or sinus formation (Table 53.3). Generalized lymphadenopathy can be a feature of infections with cytomegalovirus, Epstein-Barr virus, human immunodeficiency virus, tuberculosis, atypical mycobacteria, syphilis, histoplasmosis, and toxoplasmosis. It may also be a feature of endocarditis independent of whether the causative organism is one usually associated with generalized lymphadenopathy. Dermatopathic lymphadenitis is common with chronic exfoliative dermatides and may present with generalized or regional lymphadenopathy and usually resolves with treatment of the skin condition. Lymphadenopathy may be a prominent feature of infection with retroviruses including the human immunodeficiency virus and may be seen with seroconversion, persistent generalized lymphadenopathy, opportunistic infections, and neoplasia. The epidemiology and clinical features of human immunodeficiency virus infection are now well described; the condition is usually recognized early and is discussed in detail in Chapters 97 to 103. Lymphadenopathy, developing after a prolonged asymptomatic phase, is a feature of adult T-cell leukemia-lymphoma which is now known to be associated with an oncogenic retrovirus, human T-cell lymphotropic virus type 1.

## Laboratory studies and diagnosis

The investigation of lymphadenopathy potentially involves the exclusion of a large number of causes and must be guided by the salient epidemiology, host factors, and clinical features (Tables 53.2, 53.3). On the basis of this information a single appropriate investigation may clinch the diagnosis without recourse to more extensive investigation. Lymphadenopathy of recent onset, producing minimal enlargement, unaccompanied by other diagnostic clinical features and not producing significant systemic upset can reasonably be observed and reassessed 2 wk later. The specific investigations are not unique to lymphadenopathy associated with infection, except that the condition often requires access to tissue for specific diagnosis. The various approaches are discussed in detail in Chapters 12 to 20. Investigations should assess the host response to infection, establish the site of infection if appropriate, using imaging techniques, and identify the organism by direct microscopy, culture, or serology. Serology plays a particularly useful role in the assessment of generalized lymphadenopathy in young adults where Epstein-Barr virus, cytomegalovirus, human immunodeficiency virus, syphilis, and toxoplasmosis are common causes.

The host response to infection should be assessed with a routine blood count, peripheral blood film, routine biochemistry, and measurement of acute phase reactants such as C reactive protein or the erythrocyte sedimentation rate. These investigations may point to chronicity or underlying disease or establish the diagnosis, for example, with the mononucleosis syndromes and trypanosomiasis. The acute phase reactants may play a useful role in discriminating between transient or normally palpable lymph nodes and significant disease. Blood cultures are an important investigation in the presence of fever and disseminated lymphadenopathy and should be done using the appropriate culture medium. Prolonged incubation and repeated culture may be necessary to isolate fastidious organisms such as bartonella (rochalimaea). Skin testing plays a limited role in the diagnosis except in the case of the purified protein derivative test for tuberculosis. Regional lymphadenopathy may limit both the range of likely organisms and the necessary investigations to a search for a definable focus of infection or inoculation. This is particularly true of inguinal lymphadenopathy, which will often require investigations for a limited range of sexually transmitted infections (see Chapters 70 to 72).

Imaging is required where a focus of infection is suspected, or needs further definition, within the drainage area of regional lymphadenopathy. In generalized lymphadenopathy it may be necessary to establish the presence of lymphadenopathy in the chest or abdominal cavity. Various techniques may be used including X-ray, ultrasound, computed tomography, or magnetic resonance imaging. Radionuclide scans, using gallium- or indium-labeled leukocytes, are occasionally useful in locating an occult focus of infection and are discussed in Chapter 12. Lymph node enlargement can be evaluated by excision biopsy, fine needle biopsy, or image-guided fine needle biopsy, and a biopsy should be performed when noninvasive investigations have failed to establish the diagnosis. The complication rate for these techniques is low and biopsy should not be delayed if the patient's clinical condition is deteriorating or a diagnosis cannot be arrived at by noninvasive means. Tissue should be sent for microscopy, culture, cytology, and histology, specifying the differential diagnosis. Fungal, mycobacterial, and viral isolation should be requested if appropriate. The histopathology of infection-associated lymphadenopathy is characterized by preservation of the nodal architecture, with the diagnosis established by direct visualization of organisms, culture, or pathognomonic histological appearance. This assessment also helps to exclude neoplasia as a potential cause of lymphadenopathy.

## Treatment

The treatment of lymphadenopathy is dictated by the underlying condition identified and may include a drainage or excision procedure in the presence of an abscess or lymphadenitis. Antimicrobial choice is discussed by organism and disease in Chapters 38 to 41. The difficult management decisions relate to failure to identify an organism. This may suggest that the etiology is not infectious or that the lymphadenopathy is caused by a fastidious agent or virus. Transient benign lymphadenopathy is a feature of the childhood viral exanthems and minor trauma or subclinical infection involving the extremities, and seldom requires extensive investigation or treatment. Significant lymphadenopathy, with no identified organism, requires repeated investigation and observation, or consideration of the noninfectious causes of lymphadenopathy. Empirical therapy may be required and is usually dictated by clinical features other than lymphadenopathy and may be appropriate in the setting of suspected tuberculosis, the sepsis syndrome, immunosuppression, or progressive signs of infection. Once again consideration of the epidemiology, host factors, and clinical features must dictate the choice of antimicrobial used, and the principles underlying empirical therapy are discussed further in Chapter 24. The duration of empirical therapy should be based on serial evaluation of the clinical features—in particular, fever, lymph node size, and the response of acute phase reactants. Where appropriate intrathoracic or intraabdominal lymphadenopathy should also be monitored with imaging techniques.

## ANNOTATED BIBLIOGRAPHY

Adal KA, Cockerell CJ, Petri WJ. Cat scratch disease, bacillary angiomatosis, and other infections due to rochalimaea. N Engl J Med 1994; 330:1509–1515.

*An excellent review of the clinical spectrum of bartonella (rochalimaea) infections.*

Baroni CD, Uccini S. The lymphadenopathy of HIV infection. Am J Clin Pathol 1993; 99:397–401.

*A histopathological review.*

Burton MD, Pransky SM. Practical aspects of managing non-malignant lumps of the neck. J Otolaryngol 1992; 21:398–403.

*Provides a practical approach to neck masses occurring in childhood.*

Carithers HA. Cat scratch disease; an overview based on a study of 1200 patients. Am J Dis Child 1985; 139:1124–1133.

*A detailed description of the clinical features of cat scratch disease.*

Grossman M, Shiramizu B. Evaluation of lymphadenopathy in children. Curr Opin Pediatr 1994; 6:68–76.

*Provides a broad approach for the assessment of children.*

Irizarry L. Fever and lymphadenopathy. In: Infectious Diseases in Emergency Medicine. Brillman JC, Quenzer RW, eds. Little, Brown, Philadelphia, pp 197–215, 1992.

*Provides algorithms for the investigation of fever and lymphadenopathy in the emergency room.*

Loutit JS. Bartonella infections. In: Current Clinical Topics in Infectious Diseases. Boston, Blackwell Science, 1997, pp. 269–290.

*An excellent review of the clinical spectrum of bartonella infections.*

Pastores SM, Naidich DP, Aranda CP, McGuinnes G, Rom WM. Intrathoracic adenopathy associated with pulmonary tuberculosis in patients with human immunodeficiency virus infection. Chest 1993; 103:1433–1437.

*Presents the computed tomography features of a series of patients with pulmonary tuberculosis.*

Rieder HL, Snider DE, Cauthen GM. Extrapulmonary tuberculosis in the United States. Am Rev Respir Dis 1990; 141:347–351.

*Reviews the epidemiology of extrapulmonary tuberculosis.*

Wolinskey E. Mycobacterial diseases other than tuberculosis. Clin Infect Dis 1992; 15:1–12.

*Reviews the clinical features of atypical mycobacteria.*

# 54

# Upper Respiratory Tract Infections

CHARLES B. SMITH

The most common infectious diseases of man are those that involve the upper respiratory tract and adjacent sinuses, middle ear, pharynx, epiglottis, and larynx. Although the severity of most upper respiratory tract infections (URIs) is limited to the "temporarily annoying" category, these illnesses are the leading causes of time lost from work in most developed societies, and the resources spent on finding relief represent a significant health care expenditure. Occasionally these minor infections can become severe and lead to organ damage or death.

Upper respiratory infections are usually caused by a large variety of viruses; bacteria more frequently cause complicating infections, but occasionally they are primary pathogens. There is little role for specific antimicrobial therapy unless bacterial infection is suspected or documented. This chapter will focus on the relevant etiologies, epidemiology, pathogenesis, clinical presentations, and management of acute rhinitis, sinusitis, otitis, pharyngitis, and laryngitis, all of which are examples of acute upper respiratory tract infections.

## Acute Rhinitis

The common cold is usually due to viral infection causing acute rhinitis or inflammation of the nasopharyngeal passages.

### Etiology (Table 54.1)

Rhinoviruses are the most common causes of colds, particularly in adults, and the more than 100 serotypes that have been identified present a challenge to investigators exploring preventive vaccines. Rhinoviruses propagate best at temperatures several degrees lower than core body temperature, which explains why rhinovirus infections and illnesses are almost always confined to the cooler surfaces of the upper respiratory tract. On the other hand, other respiratory viruses, such as influenza virus, parainfluenza viruses, and respiratory syncytial virus, which grow well at core body temperature, typically cause both upper and lower respiratory tract infection and illnesses in immunologically naive individuals. Reinfections of older persons with these agents are often limited to the upper respiratory tract because of partial retained immunity. A small number of colds are caused by *Mycoplasma pneumoniae* or *Chlamydia pneumoniae* infections. Although potential respiratory pathogens such as *Streptococcus pneumoniae* and *Haemophylus influenzae* are commonly cultured from respiratory tract secretions in patients with colds, they are not believed to be significant causes of acute rhinitis, and there is no evidence that antimicrobial agents are effective in treating the common cold.

### Epidemiology

Acute respiratory viral infections occur worldwide and throughout the year. Because these infections are acquired from other infected persons, they are more common during the fall, winter, and spring months when schools are in session and the weather causes people to congregate indoors. Although folklore has related colds to cold weather and chilling, volunteer experiments indicate that lowering air and body temperature has no effect on susceptibility to respiratory viral infection.

Cold viruses are shed in the nasal secretions of infected patients for several days after the onset of symptoms, and spread to others occurs by the droplet route, particularly during coughing or sneezing, and by direct or indirect contact with infected secretions. Hands of patients with colds are often contaminated with the offending virus, and the infection can be spread by hand to hand or by contact with contaminated surfaces. The susceptible person is typically self-inoculated by contact between their infected fingers and the susceptible tissues of their nose or conjunctiva.

### Host factors

Immune status is the most important host factor in determining susceptibility to infection with respiratory viruses. Breast-fed infants enjoy relative protection against infection with respiratory viruses because of transmission of maternal antibodies, and susceptibility becomes greatest after breast feeding stops and infants begin the gradual process of developing their own immunity. Inborn defects of immunoglobulin synthesis, particularly of IgG, are often first manifest by the appearance of repeated and prolonged upper respiratory tract infections. In most instances, the prolongation of symptoms is related to secondary bacterial infections in the immune-deficient child. Patients with atopic allergies and hay fever are more likely to complain of rhinitis, but there is no evidence that they are more frequently infected with respiratory viruses. On the other hand, acute respiratory viral infections do stimulate exaggerated and prolonged allergic responses in atopic patients.

The most important susceptibility factor that the host can control is exposure to cigarette smoke; both active and passive exposure is associated with more frequent and more severe URIs. Dietary supplements beyond a generally nutritious diet are not associated with reduced susceptibility to colds. In particular, avoiding milk or milk products does not reduce mucus production. There is a single report that patients who are regular users of saunas have fewer colds, but other variables that might also influence susceptibility were not studied. In nonsmokers, moderate alcohol consumption (up to three drinks per day) has been

**Table 54.1** Common upper respiratory tract pathogens

| | % ARD[a] | Rhinitis | Sinusitis | Otitis media | Pharyngitis | Epiglottitis | Croup |
|---|---|---|---|---|---|---|---|
| Rhinovirus | 30–40 | + | + | + | + | | + |
| Parainfluenza virus | 15–20 | + | + | + | + | | + |
| Respiratory syncytial | 5–10 | + | + | + | + | | + |
| Adenovirus | 3–5 | + | | + | + | | + |
| Corona virus | 10+ | + | | | + | | |
| Influenza A | 5–15 | + | | + | + | | + |
| Other | 10 | + | | | + | | |
| Herpes simplex virus | <5 | | | | + | | |
| Epstein-Barr virus | <5 | | | | + | | |
| *Mycoplasma pneumoniae* | – | + | + | + | + | | + |
| *Mycoplasma hominis* | – | | | | + | | |
| *Chlamydia pneumoniae* | – | + | + | + | + | | |
| *Streptococcus pneumoniae* | – | | + | + | | + | |
| *Streptococcus pyogenes* | – | | + | + | + | | |
| *Haemophylus influenzae* | – | | + | + | | + | |
| *Moraxella catarrhalis* | – | | + | + | | | |

[a]Acute respiratory disease

associated with reduced clinical colds, although susceptibility to viral infection was not altered.

The emotional state of the host is also an important factor in determining the host's response to acute upper respiratory viral infection. Psychological stress has been associated with an increased risk of acute respiratory illness following experimental viral infections. It is not clear whether or not the increased symptomology is due to increased susceptibility to viral infection. The fact that blood flow through nasal tissues is influenced by stress and emotional state via the cholinergic nervous system provides a pathway linking emotional state to clinical symptomatology in response to respiratory viral infections.

## Pathophysiology

Respiratory viruses infect and multiply in cells lining the surface of the nasal mucosa. The degree of damage to these cells varies with the viral pathogen. Rhinoviruses produce surprisingly little change in the histological appearance of the nasal mucosa, and the only common detectable abnormality is the appearance of sloughed ciliated epithelial cells in nasal secretions of infected individuals. Corona virus infections cause alterations in ciliary function of organ cultures of nasal mucosa, while influenza viruses are much more damaging to respiratory tract mucosal cells. Clinical colds following respiratory viral infection are associated with increased levels of inflammatory mediators such as interleukins, kinins, and prostaglandins and a secondary outpouring of serum proteins and neutrophils in nasal secretions. These inflammatory mediators also have a systemic effect, causing a slight neutrophilia in about half of patients with viral colds and the common systemic symptoms of headache, myalgias, and occasional fever. Except in atopic patients, histamine levels are not increased in the secretions of patients with viral colds.

## Clinical manifestations

In studies of human volunteers experimentally infected with rhinoviruses the incubation period before the first symptoms of the common cold is 2 to 3 d. Acute rhinitis is the hallmark of the uncomplicated common cold. It first appears as an itching or scratchiness of the nose accompanied by sneezing and is soon followed by an outpouring of clear nasal secretions that can flow at the rate of 10–15 g per day. Nasal obstruction or stuffiness is an early complaint. On examination, the nasal mucosa is erythematous at first and as swelling increases it becomes pale and boggy. Approximately 50% of patients will also complain of sore throat and on examination a mild erythema may be seen. Thirty percent of patients will also experience hoarseness or cough and examination of the chest is usually normal except for patients with chronic bronchitis who often exhibit increased wheezes and ronchi. Generalized headache is the most common systemic complaint while fewer than one in five patients will complain of feverishness and myalgias. When abnormal, the temperature elevation rarely exceeds one degree Fahrenheit. The symptoms and signs of the uncomplicated common cold usually resolve within 5 to 7 d, although some patients will complain of persistent cough for longer periods of time.

Complications of the common cold occur in 1–5% of normal patients and are more common in patients with reduced defenses against bacterial infections. These are generally due to bacterial infection of the paranasal sinuses, the middle ear, or the lungs. If the symptoms of the cold persist after 7 days, the normally clear nasal secretions become purulent, and the patient develops pain over the sinuses or in the ear or cough productive of purulent sputum, it is appropriate to explore the diagnosis of a complicating bacterial sinusitis, otitis media, or bronchitis.

## Laboratory studies and diagnosis

The common cold can be readily diagnosed clinically and there is little value in pursuing routine laboratory or radiological tests. Apart from a transient slight increase in the neutrophil count and the sedimentation rate, there are no abnormalities in nonspecific laboratory tests. A recent evaluation of adults with rhinovirus colds found that more than 75% had transient abnormalities of the paranasal sinuses by computed tomographic scanning, suggesting that sinus inflammation is a usual part of the common cold. In the absence of symptoms and signs suggesting acute bacterial sinusitis, radiographic examination of the paranasal sinuses is not recommended in evaluating the common cold.

Specific diagnosis of the viral etiology of common colds is possible using cell cultures, using methods for detecting viral antigens or genomes in nasal cells, and by demonstrating specific serum antibody responses. These methods are all expensive and laborious and their use is currently justified only in experimental situations or when there is a need to document a hospital or community outbreak of infection with influenza A or respiratory syncytial viruses.

## Treatment

Although studies in volunteers indicate some effect against respiratory viruses of interferon and other antiviral agents, the generally benign and time limited course of the common cold does not yet warrant specific antiviral therapy. However, some of the symptoms of the common cold can be ameliorated by nonspecific therapies. Nonsteroidal antiinflammatory agents such as aspirin (600 mg four times a day for adults, avoid in children), acetaminophen (650 mg four times a day for adults) or propprionic acids such a naproxen (250 mg three times a day) can reduce the systemic symptoms of headache, myalgias, and malaise. Nasal obstruction and rhinorrhea can be temporarily relieved by the use of vasoconstrictors applied topically as drops or spray (phenylephrine 0.125% for children, 0.25 to 1% for adults every 4 h). Use of vasoconstrictors for more than 5 d can lead to habituation, and their use is contraindicated in patients with hypertension, cardiovascular diseases, and those taking antidepressants. Cough suppressants are useful in patients whose sleep is interrupted by cough (dextromethorphan 15 mg, adults or 1 mg/kg, children, four times a day). Antihistamines may be effective in relieving sneezing and rhinorrhea symptoms of the common cold, but they have the unpleasant side effects of drying and thickening secretions and can cause drowsiness. Because bacteria are rarely etiologic agents for the common cold, there is no reason to treat patients with antibiotics.

A multitude of lay therapies are promulgated for the common cold. Vitamin C in large doses is perhaps the most popular of these therapies. The few reports suggesting a clinical effect were flawed by loss of true blindness in controls and the positive responses are believed to be due to placebo effect. In environments where the humidity is unusually low, humidification of the air can relieve an annoying drying and crusting of nasal secretions. Inhalation of hot humidified air has not been effective against respiratory viruses or in relieving the symptoms of the common cold. Home-made chicken soup tastes good and provides valuable comfort to patients suffering from the common cold.

## Prevention

Reduced spread of the common cold can be achieved by use of disposable paper tissues rather than secretion-sodden cloth handkerchiefs to control nasal secretions. In addition, patients suffering colds should frequently wash their hands as should those wishing to reduce their chances of becoming infected. Common disinfectants such as Lysol can destroy respiratory viruses on contaminated surfaces; however, their usefulness in reducing colds in the family has not been proven. Droplet spread may be reduced by covering the mouth and nose with disposable tissues during sneezes and coughing.

Upper respiratory infections due to influenza virus types A and B can be reduced by the regular use of influenza vaccine. Because of the multiple serotypes of the common rhinoviruses, vaccines are not a likely future prospect. Most immunoglobulin deficiency syndromes are characterized by increased susceptibility to respiratory bacterial infections but not to respiratory viral infections. Prescription of immunoglobulin injections for nonimmunoglobulin-deficient children with frequent colds is costly and does not reduce their frequency, and infection with hepatitis C virus can be a complication of this therapy.

## Sinusitis

The broad spectrum of clinical illnesses associated with inflammation of the paranasal sinuses extends from transient and clinically benign inflammation associated with common colds to acute bacterial sinusitis that may spread to adjacent vital structures or to chronic inflammation associated with anatomic abnormalities, immune deficiencies, and allergies.

## Etiologies

Acute sinusitis is most often a complication of primary respiratory viral infection and a secondary infection with one of the common respiratory bacterial pathogens listed in Table 54.1. Direct needle aspiration of the maxillary sinuses in over 300 adults with acute sinusitis detected bacteria in 60% and *S. pneumoniae* and *H. influenzae* together accounted for 75% of the positive bacterial cultures. *M. catarrhalis*, anaerobes, other streptococcal species, and *S. aureus* were each found in fewer than 10% of patients. Acute nosocomial sinusitis occurs in patients who are intubated in critical care units, and needle aspiration of infected maxillary sinuses in these patients has revealed highly antibiotic-resistant hospital strains of gram-negative bacteria in 47%, *S. aureus* in 18% and *Candida* species of yeast in 18%. Immunocompromised patients are subject to acute sinusitis due to the bacterial pathogens listed above and also to sinusitis due to *Aspergillus*, *Phycomycetes*, and other invasive fungal pathogens. Chronic sinusitis is more likely to be associated with gram-negative bacteria and anaerobes than is acute sinusitis, and it is occasionally caused by fungal infection with *Aspergillus* or *Curvularia* sp. that can be noninvasive, slowly invasive, or associated with allergic reactions to the fungal antigens.

## Epidemiology and pathogenesis

Although the majority of adults with the common cold have transient abnormalities of the paranasal sinuses on computed tomographic scanning, fewer than 1% of patients with viral colds develop acute bacterial sinusitis. Conversely, a recent history of a cold commonly precedes the development of acute sinusitis, particularly in children. While the nasal airways are normally bacterialogically not sterile, the paranasal sinuses are, and the occurrence of acute bacterial sinusitis implies that the normal clearance and antibacterial properties of sinus secretions have been impaired. The importance of physical obstruction to normal sinus drainage in the pathogenesis of acute sinusitis is illustrated by the greater than 90% incidence of acute sinusitis in critical care patients who had nasotracheal intubation. Similar acute obstruction to the normal clearance mechanisms of the sinuses explains the association between recent viral infections or allergic rhinitis and acute bacterial sinusitis. Chronic sinusitis can result from persistent anatomic obstruction of sinus drainage, as might occur after nasal trauma or with chronic allergy, with ciliary dyskinesia syndromes that impair normal clearance mechanisms or from inborn or acquired deficiencies in host cellular or humoral immunity. Acute maxillary sinusitis may be a complication of a spreading dental infection.

## Clinical manifestations

The patient with acute sinusitis typically complains of a cold that has persisted longer than the usual 5 to 7 d and of purulent nasal and postnasal discharge, nasal obstruction, fever, persistent cough, and headache or facial discomfort. Patients with acute frontal and maxillary sinusitis may have pain over these sinuses, and the pain of maxillary sinusitis can be referred to an upper tooth. The pain of ethmoid sinusitis is often behind the eyes or over the mastoids while sphenoid sinusitis gives a generalized or suboccipital headache. In some patients acute sinusitis is clinically unimpressive, and only two or three of the above symptoms may be noticed. The examiner often finds purulent discharge from the sinus ostia and in the upper nasopharynx, halitosis, and occasionally tenderness over the maxillary or frontal sinuses. Transillumination of the maxillary and frontal sinuses is helpful if unilateral failure to illuminate is observed. Observation of swelling of the face over the maxillary or frontal sinuses supports the diagnosis, while unilateral puffiness around the eye and impaired ocular movements are ominous signs indicating the infection has extended into the orbit. Worsening headache or the appearance of obtundation or focal neurologic signs indicate possible spread of the infection to the subdural space or brain (Table 54.3).

Chronic sinusitis is defined as persistence of the above symptoms and signs beyond 3 months, despite treatment with antimicrobials. Systemic symptoms of fever and malaise and pain are less common while persistent purulent drainage and cough are characteristic of chronic sinusitis.

## Laboratory and radiologic diagnosis

Radiographic examination of the sinuses is helpful in confirming the diagnosis of acute sinusitis when the clinical presentation is confusing. The sinuses are still developing in children less than 1 yr of age and radiographic examination is of less value in this age group. CT or MRI techniques add clarity to the examination, particularly when visualizing the ethmoid and sphenoid sinuses and looking for evidence of extension to the orbit. In most patients, however, sinusitis can be diagnosed and managed without radiological imaging.

Microbiological cultures are not usually needed for management of patients with uncomplicated sinusitis. Identification of specific etiologic agents becomes helpful when the infection is rapidly progressing and threatening vital structures, when patients fail to respond to usual therapy, in patients likely to be infected with resistant hospital-acquired pathogens, and in immunocompromised patients with suspected fungal sinusitis. Culture of sinus secretions or fluids obtained by irrigation of sinuses is of little value because of contamination with bacteria present in normal nasal secretions. Cultures should be obtained by direct needle puncture of the sinuses, and they should be immediately taken to the laboratory to enhance the likelihood of culturing anaerobic bacteria.

## Treatment

Placebo-controlled trials indicate a positive effect of antimicrobial treatment for acute bacterial sinusitis in children and adults. Treatment should be directed against the common respiratory bacterial pathogens identified in Table 54.1, and selection of antimicrobials and dosage are as outlined in Table 54.2. Acute uncomplicated sinusitis usually responds rapidly to antimicrobial treatment, and the duration of therapy does not need to exceed 3 to 5 d. Choice of antimicrobials for treatment of nosocomial sinusitis should be initially based on knowledge of the susceptibility of local hospital-acquired gram-positive and gram-negative bacteria and the antimicrobial choice should be adjusted later based on culture and sensitivity results. Because the pathogens associated with hospital-acquired sinusitis are often less susceptible to antimicrobials, treatment should be continued for at least 14 d and until there is clear clinical improvement. Antimicrobial selection for treatment of chronic sinusitis, can await the culture results because of the chronicity of the infection. Infection with

**Table 54.2** Oral antimicrobial agents for treating common bacterial pathogens (Table 54.1) causing acute sinusitis and acute otitis media

| | | Dose | |
|---|---|---|---|
| Therapy | Antimicrobial | Children | Adults |
| Primary | Amoxicillin | 40 mg/kg/d in TID doses | 0.5 g TID |
| Alternative[a] | Amoxicillin/clavulanic acid | 5–7.5 ml, TID | 0.5 g TID |
| | Cefaclor[a] | 20 mg/kg/d in TID doses | 0.5 g TID |
| | Cefixime[a] | 8 mg/kg/d single dose | 400 mg/qd |
| | Trimethoprim (TMR)/ sulfamethoxazole (SMO)[a,b] | 8 mg/kg/d TMP 40 mg/kg/d SMO in BID doses | 160 mg TMP 800 mg SMO BID |
| | Erythromycin (ERY)/ sulfisoxazole (SSX)[a,b] | 40 mg/kg/d ERY 150 mg/kg/d SSX in QID doses | — |

[a]Suspected $\beta$-lactamase-producing strains of *H. influenzae* or *M. catarrhalis*.

[b]History of allergy to penicillin.

multiple species of bacteria is common in chronic sinusitis, and a broad-spectrum antimicrobial which includes coverage for respiratory anaerobes, such as amoxicillin/clavulanate, is commonly used. Duration of treatment for chronic sinusitis should extend to at least 4 wk to give maximal opportunity for the sinuses to heal before surgical intervention is considered.

Although use of antimicrobials is recommended for treatment of acute sinusitis, it is important to note that as many as 40% of patients who received placebo in antimicrobial trials had resolution of their sinusitis. This observation supports the importance of therapy directed at reducing obstruction and improving drainage of the sinuses. Topical application of decongestants such as phenylephrine drops or nasal spray, as noted for the common cold, is helpful in reducing swelling and promoting drainage. Because of tolerance and rebound vasodilation, topical decongestant therapy should be limited to 5 d. Oral decongestants are of limited effect and are more likely to cause undesirable side effects. Secretions in patients with sinusitis are often thick, and the patient may benefit from regular irrigation of the nose with sterile physiologic saline solutions. Although antihistamines may reduce secretions in allergic patients, they should not be used in therapy of sinusitis because of their drying effect on the nasal mucosa and tendency to thicken secretions. Chronic sinusitis may be the result of nasal allergy, and thorough evaluation and treatment for allergic rhinitis is an important aspect of therapy in these patients.

Surgical drainage, either by direct intervention or by endoscopy, may be required in patients with rapidly progressive sinusitis that has invaded adjacent vital structures. Chronic sinusitis in immunologically normal patients is usually the result of anatomic abnormalities and surgical approaches to drainage are often indicated.

## Pharyngitis

Sore throat or pharyngitis is one of the most common complaints bringing patients to the physicians office. While most sore throats are due to respiratory viral infection and are transient and benign, the importance of group A streptococci as a cause of rheumatic fever requires specific diagnostic tests and therapy.

### Etiology

Respiratory viruses that cause the common cold (Table 54.1) are also the most common causes of sore throat. Pharyngitis is also a common finding in patients infected with *M. pneumoniae* or *C. pneumoniae.* Less commonly, primary infection with herpes simplex virus is associated with acute vesicular stomatitis and pharyngitis, and Epstein-Barr virus infection may cause severe sore throat as a common manifestation of the mononucleosis syndrome. Group A streptococci are the most common bacterial causes of sore throat, accounting for 15%–40% of cases. Groups C and G streptococci are less common causes of sore throat. Gonococci are occasional causes of sore throat in sexually active young people, and infection with *Corynebacterium diptheriae* needs to be considered in elderly patients or unimmunized populations.

### Epidemiology

For most patients complaining of sore throat due to infection with common cold viruses, epidemiological factors that predispose to infection are the same as those discussed for the common cold. Similarly, group A streptococcal infections are acquired by intimate person-to-person contact, and the environmental factors that predispose to this bacterial infection include crowding, day care, and school exposures. The organism is a common resident of the human pharynx and can be cultured from the throats or tonsils of 10% to 15% of normal persons. Colonization is particularly common in school-age children, who often serve as the initial source of family outbreaks. Chronically swollen and inflamed tonsils are the major host factor influencing susceptibility to recurrent group A streptococcal infections, presumably due to difficulty in eradicating the pathogen from damaged or necrotic tissues. Although spread is usually by the respiratory route, food borne epidemics are regularly described.

### Pathophysiology

Group A streptococci are remarkably well adapted to infect and invade the tissues of the human pharynx. Surface proteins such as the M protein are involved in initial infection and are a virulence factor because they inhibit the host phagocytic defense. Antibodies to M protein are associated with decreased infection. Other extracellular enzymes such as hyaluronidases assist the organism in its spread through tissues, and a variety of hemolysins and other exotoxins are involved in damaging host tissues and in the pathogenesis of scarlet fever and the toxic shock syndrome which may be associated with group A streptococcal infection. Delayed responses to group A streptococcal infection, such as acute rheumatic fever, are immunologically mediated, and a sharing of antigenic determinants between bacterial proteins and polysaccharides and those of host tissues is undoubtedly involved in the pathogenesis of this autoimmune disease.

### Clinical manifestations

Pharyngitis is often a manifestation of upper respiratory tract viral infections. The pharynx is mildly erythematous and exudate that may be seen is usually related to postnasal discharge rather than direct inflammation of the pharynx or tonsils. Rhinorrhea is often present and cervical lymphadenopathy is uncommon. Among the common respiratory viruses, adenoviruses are associated with the most severe clinical findings, and some patients will exhibit exudate, cervical lymphadenopathy, and a prolonged course that clinically resembles group A streptococcal pharyngitis. Respiratory adenoviral infections are often associated with prominent bronchitis, atypical pneumonia, and conjunctivitis, assisting in the diagnosis. Herpes simplex virus pharyngitis can be quite disabling, with severe pain associated with exudate and cervical adenopathy. A pathognomic finding is the associated stomatitis and the finding of shallow ulcers over the soft palate and/or the lip. Coxsackie virus infection in young children can sometimes mimic herpes virus pharyngitis with associated vesicles and shallow ulcers on the soft palate and pharynx. The pharyngitis associated with mononucleosis due to Epstein-Barr virus infection can also be severe with marked cervical lymphadenopathy and pharyngeal swelling threatening respiratory obstruction.

Group A streptococcal pharyngitis is the most important to diagnose because of the potential for rheumatic fever or spread to the sinuses, middle ear, or parapharyngeal tissues (Table 54.3). The classical findings of fever with severe exudative pharyngitis and cervical lymphadenopathy are unfortunately found in fewer than one-third of patients with microbiologically confirmed group A streptococcal pharyngitis, and many patients will only manifest a mild sore throat with unimpressive findings on

**Table 54.3** Complications of upper respiratory tract infections

| |
|---|
| SINUSITIS AND OTITIS |
| Osteomeyelitis |
| Orbital cellulitis |
| Rhinocerebral mycoses |
| Epidural abscess |
| Subdural abscess |
| Brain abscess |
| Intracranial venous thrombosis |
| Meningitis |
| OTITIS |
| Mastoiditis |
| Hearing loss |
| Labrynthitis |
| Malignant (necrotizing) otitis externa |
| PHARYNGITIS AND EPIGLOTTITIS |
| Peritonsillar abscess |
| Retro- or parapharyngeal abscess |
| Vincent angina (acute ulcerative necrotizing mucositis) |
| Lemierre's disease (retropharyngeal involvement with jugular thrombophlebitis and/or mediastinitis) |

clinical examination. Because the clinical picture is so unreliable in diagnosing this infection, the threshold for laboratory testing should be low.

There are several other bacterial causes of pharyngitis that are uncommon but important to diagnose because of the potential for serious complications. Diphtheria still occurs in unimmunized populations, and this diagnosis should be considered in susceptible patients who have pharyngitis with a gray exudate over the tonsils that is adherent and who may have associated myocarditis. Several outbreaks of diphtheria have recently been described in the United States in inner-city alcoholic populations and in Russia and the other countries of the former USSR where immunization rates have fallen. Gonococci can cause acute pharyngitis, and this diagnosis needs to be considered in patients who are at risk because of multiple sexual contacts or practice of oral-genital sex, or who have other manifestations of gonorrhea. Peritonsillar abscess can complicate group A streptococcal pharyngitis or may occur secondary to mixed infection with oral anaerobes, fusobacteria, and spirochetes (Vincent's angina). Asymmetric swelling of the peritonsillar tissues and palpable fluctuance in the peritonsillar area are characteristic of this diagnosis. If untreated this infection may spread to the adjacent tissues of the neck and the mediastinum.

*Mycoplasma pneumoniae* and *Chlamydia pneumoniae* infections are often associated with pharyngitis both during the acute and chronic phases. Clinical diagnosis is suggested by associated cough or atypical pneumonia and the greater incidence of these infections in adolescents and the elderly.

## Diagnosis

Group A $\beta$-hemolytic streptococci are most reliably diagnosed by direct culture of the organism on blood agar plates. This test can be successfully applied by physicians in their office practices, and it is important to have access to it as a backup when other more rapid office tests fail to detect the organism. There are now many commercially available rapid tests for detecting group A streptococcal antigens that are appropriate for use in the practitioner's office. These direct antigen detection tests generally have more than 90% specificity but are less than 90% as sensitive as cultures in detecting the organism. Thus a positive test does not need to be confirmed by culture, but a culture should be done when the rapid test is negative and the clinical picture suggests group A streptococcal infection. Repeat rapid tests or cultures are not recommended after the usual course of therapy, except perhaps in patients with a history of rheumatic fever.

Tests for antibodies to group A streptococci, such as the anti-streptolysin O test and the anti-DNAase tests, are not diagnostically useful in the acute situation but are helpful in confirming a recent infection in patients who are suspected of having rheumatic fever or acute poststreptococcal glomerulonephritis.

## Therapy

Group A streptococci are still highly susceptable to penicillin, and this antimicrobial remains the therapy of choice for initial treatment of these infections in patients who are not allergic to penicillin. Both children and adults can be treated orally with penicillin V, 250 mg three times a day for 10 d. The 10 d course is important for success, and patients who are suspected of poor compliance, or patients with past history of acute rheumatic fever, should be given an IM injection of benzathine penicillin G. The dose for children who weigh less then 60 lb is 600,000 units and the dose is 1.2 million units for larger children and adults. Prophylaxis against recurrent infections with the above oral or IM therapies is recommended for children and some adults who have recurrent attacks of rheumatic fever. Patients who are allergic to penicillin can be treated with erythromycin. It important to remember that several commonly used antimicrobials, such as sulfonamides, trimethoprim, and tetracyclines, are not effective against group A streptococci.

Approximately 10% of patients treated for group A streptococcal infections with oral penicillin will have recurrent pharyngitis and positive cultures or will become asymptomatic carriers. Poor compliance with oral therapy is the most common cause of these failures, and prompt reinfection from schoolmates or other infected family members is also important. It has been suggested that these failures are due to protection of penicillin-sensitive group A streptococci by other bacteria in the pharynx that produce penicillin-destroying $\beta$-lactamases such as staphylococci or *H. influenzae*. When this explanation for failure is suspected, patients can be treated with a $\beta$-lactamase-resistant oral cephalosporin such as cephalexin, cephaclor, or cephadroxil. At one time tonsillectomy was widely practiced as therapy for children with recurrent group A streptococcal infections or tonsillitis. Because of the recognition that the tonsils play a significant role in development of local immune defenses, this practice has become much less common, and it now is reserved for children with severe recurrent tonsillitis and with tonsils that are of such size as to compromise respiration.

Pharyngitis due to *Chlamydia pneumoniae* should be treated with tetracycline hydrochloride 500 mg four times a day (or doxycycline 100 mg BID) for 10 d. Tetracycline or erythromycin should both be effective in treating the pharyngitis associated with *Mycoplasma pneumoniae* infection, and the duration of therapy should be extended to 14 d. Treatment for gonococcal pharyngitis is the same as that recommended for genital infections (Chapter 70). Diphtheria does not respond clinically to antimicrobial therapy, and these patients should receive 50,000–100,000 units of equine antiserum. Erythromycin, 500 mg orally four times a day for 7 d is effective in eliminating the carrier state.

## Epiglottitis, Laryngitis, and Laryngotracheitis (Croup)

Acute respiratory viral infections can descend down the upper airways and cause acute inflammation of the larynx, or acute laryngotracheitis (croup). The epiglottis is particularly susceptible to acute bacterial infection with *H. influenzae*. Acute croup in young children, and acute epiglottitis at all ages can be associated with life-threatening respiratory obstruction.

### Etiologies

In children, croup is a common complication of acute infection of the upper respiratory tract with parainfluenza viruses, respiratory syncytial virus, or influenza viruses. Secondary infection with one of the common respiratory bacterial pathogens occurs in less than 5% of children, and when bacterial infection occurs it is usually associated with acute bacterial bronchitis or pneumonia. There have been a few reports of atypical or prolonged croup due to infection with herpes simplex virus or to *Candida* sp. in children who were receiving corticosteroids for croup. In adults, laryngitis is also usually a complication of acute respiratory viral infection. When symptoms extend beyond 7 d, other etiologies such as *M. tuberculosis* infection or laryngeal cancer need to be considered.

Epiglottitis in most cases is due to acute infection with *H. influenzae* or less commonly with one of the other common respiratory bacterial pathogens (Table 54.1). There are a few reports of epiglottitis due to respiratory viral infection. In immunologically deficient patients, epiglottitis can be due to herpes simplex virus or to opportunistic fungi such as aspergillus or *Candida* sp.

### Epidemiology

Croup is a common condition in children, occurring at an annual rate of 3% in children less than 3 yr of age. As with the other respiratory syndromes, the incidence of croup increases with exposure to air pollutants. Until the past decade, epiglottitis was more common in children than adults, but the ratio has recently reversed because of a reduction in the incidence of encapsulated *H. influenzae* infection in children. This is presumably due to the effectiveness of *H. influenzae* type b vaccine. Epiglottitis occurs more often in males than females.

### Pathophysiology

Young children are more susceptible to croup because of the greater incidence of acute respiratory viral infections at this age and also because of the small diameter and collapsibility of the subglottic airways at this age. Croup is due to acute swelling and inflammation of the subglottic tissues, and because of the narrowness of this part of the airway, this swelling leads to obstruction of airflow and the typical symptoms and signs of croup. The epiglottis also occupies a narrow space in the upper airway, and acute inflammation and swelling of this tissue can rapidly lead to acute airway obstruction.

### Clinical manifestations

The illness in a young child with croup typically begins with rhinorrhea with mild cough. After a few days the cough becomes more noisy and takes on a barking sound. The full attack of croup often occurs at night when the cough becomes associated with the typical crowing or barking sound of croup and inspiratory stridor. On examination the child often has low grade fever, signs of nasal congestion, a normal epiglottis, and acute respiratory distress with an increased respiratory rate and retraction of the supraclavicular and intracostal tissues during inspiration. Auscultation of the chest reveals sounds of inspiratory stridor and occasionally wheezes and ronchi or rales.

Epiglottitis, in contrast to croup, typically occurs in children over the age of 2 yr and most often in adult males. The onset is more sudden than that of croup and the course can progress to severe respiratory obstruction over a few hours. Severe sore throat and dysphagia are the most common initial complaints, and as the illness progresses the patient will complain of respiratory distress. On examination the patient is usually febrile and has tenderness to palpation over the larynx; the voice may be hoarse or absent. As the illness progresses, the inability to swallow may be associated with drooling, and the appearance of inspiratory stridor and obvious respiratory distress is an ominous sign indicating the need for interventions to preserve the airway. In some adults, the swollen epiglottis can be visualized by direct examination using a tongue depressor. Indirect laryngoscopy using a mirror or examination using a flexible laryngoscope or nasolaryngoscope is preferable and more likely to establish the diagnosis. In young children direct examination using a tongue depressor can reveal the typical cherry-red enlarged epiglottis; however, this procedure has initiated acute respiratory obstruction, and the indirect routes for examination are preferred. In both adults and children, examination of the epiglottis should only be attempted in situations where rapid intubation or tracheotomy can be performed.

### Laboratory diagnosis

In the child with croup, the leukocyte count is usually low, as is typical of viral infections, and an elevated count should initiate a search for complicating bacterial pneumonia. In hospitalized patients, measurement of $PaO_2$ and $PaCO_2$ can be helpful in assessing the effectiveness of therapy and in identifying the unusual child who needs airway intervention. Anteroposterior soft-tissue radiographic examination of the neck is reasonably sensitive in identifying the swollen subglottic tissues characteristic of croup (Fig. 54.1). This examination may be helpful in the unusual child where differentiation between croup and epiglottitis is not possible based on clinical findings.

The leukocyte count is usually elevated in the patient with acute epiglottitis, and cultures of the blood are positive for *H. influenzae* in about 15% of patients. As with croup, measurement of blood gases is helpful in assessing the severity and course of the illness. Lateral soft-tissue radiographic examination of the neck may be helpful in identifying the swollen epiglottis (Fig. 54.2); however, direct or indirect laryngoscopic examination has been found to be more sensitive and specific for the diagnosis. If radiographic examination is attempted the patient should remain in the hands of the physician so that immediate intubation or tracheotomy can be performed if necessary.

### Therapy

The natural course of croup is to wax and wane over a period of several hours, and many children will improve at home after a few hours of observation. Exposing the child to humidified air or steam by the shower or bathroom is often practiced, but is of little proven value. In fact, the common experience of the child

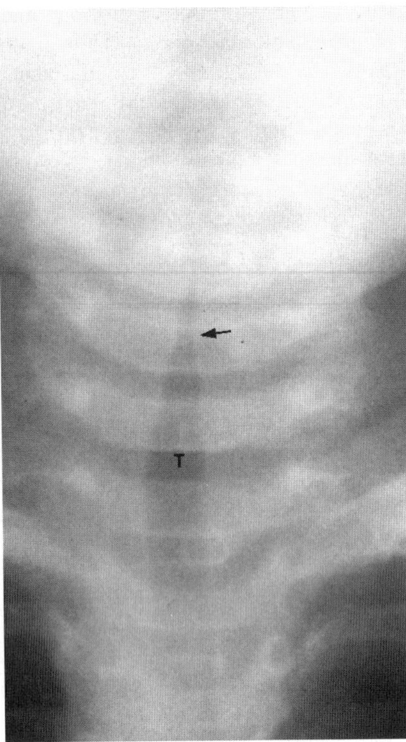


**Fig. 54.1** Anteroposterior radiograph of the neck showing narrowing (arrow) of the subglottic space characteristic of croup. (T = trachea). [Courtesy of Dr. L. Quan from Quan, L., "Diagnosis and treatment of croup." American Famil. Physic. 46(3):747–755, 1992.]

improving in the car on the way to the hospital suggests that exposure to colder air may be effective. When the attack lasts longer than an hour, or the child appears to be worsening and showing obvious signs of respiratory distress over this period of time, it is reasonable to take the child to an emergency room or physician's office for further examination and therapy. If hypoxemia is detected on initial evaluation, the child should receive humidified 40% oxygen. Aerosolized administration of racemic or L-epinephrine (dose equivalent to 5 mg of the LE isomer) has been shown to lead to more rapid improvement of signs and symptoms of croup, and most children can be discharged 3–4 h after initiating this therapy. It should be noted, however, that this therapy is only transiently effective; patients may worsen 2 h after this therapy; and it does not alter the natural course of croup, which tends to persist for 3 or 4 d. Some studies suggest that a single dose of corticosteroids (0.5 mg/kg dexamethasone, up to 10 mg) becomes effective after 6 h in relieving the symptoms of croup and the effect lasts for 12 to 24 h. This therapy remains controversial and is best reserved for the more serious cases that require hospitalization.

Approximately 15% of children with croup will progress to have worsening respiratory distress, develop respiratory fatigue and an elevated $PaCO_2$, and require hospitalization for intensive respiratory therapy. A small number of these will require intubation, and this is least traumatically done by the nasotracheal route. Some studies indicate that the duration of intubation and need for reintubation are improved if corticosteriods are administered along with intubation. This may be by the parenteral route (0.5 mg/kg dexamethasone; up to 10 mg) or by the aerosol route (nebulized budesonide, 2 mg in 4 ml). Tracheotomy is rarely needed to control children with croup.

In contrast to croup, epiglottitis is often a rapidly progressive infection that commonly requires intubation or tracheotomy. Even in optimal health care environments the mortality from this infection exceeds 5%, indicating that the diagnosis and appropriate therapy are not made as often as they should be. Once the diagnosis of epiglottitis is considered, the patient should be hospitalized and kept under intense observation. Blood and pharyngeal cultures should be obtained. When there is evidence of respiratory distress (respiratory rate >20/min, or obvious stridor) the patient should be prepared for urgent elective intubation under controlled conditions. When there is obvious evidence of respiratory difficulty with the respiratory rate >30/min, $pCO_2$ >45 mmHg, cyanosis, and obvious respiratory distress and stridor, the patient should be prepared for immediate intubation. If intubation is unsuccessful, the airway should be secured by emergency tracheostomy. The many case reports of patients suddenly expiring while under intense observation indicate that most errors are on the side of delay rather than too aggressive an approach to this infection.

In contrast to croup, there is no evidence that nebulized epinephrine or use of corticosteroids is effective in treating epiglottitis. Because this infection is usually due to type b *H. influenzae*, and a significant percent of these organisms are now resistant to ampicillin, patients should be treated intravenously with a $\beta$-lactamase-resistant antimicrobial such as cefuroxime, 1 g IV every 8 h or cephtriaxone 1 g IV every 12 h.

Regular use of the *H. influenzae* type b vaccine has been shown to be effective in reducing the incidence of epiglottis in children. It will take a few more years to tell us if this vaccine will be

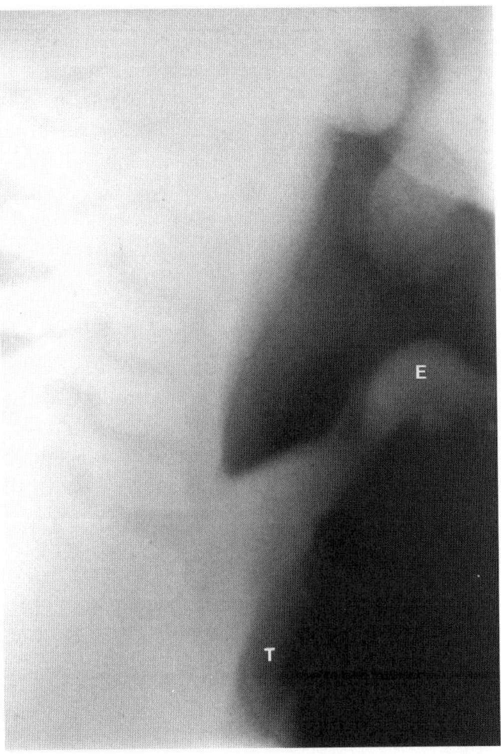


**Fig. 54.2** Lateral radiograph of the neck showing swollen epiglottis. (E = epiglottis). [Courtesy of Dr. L. Quan from Quan, L. "Diagnosis and treatment of croup." American Famil. Physic. 46(3):747–755, 1992.]

effective in reducing the incidence in adults. A significant percentage of adults with epiglottitis will have *S. pneumoniae* isolated from the pharynx or blood.

## Otitis

Inflammation of the middle ear (otitis media) is best understood by considering two common syndromes: *Acute otitis media* which is fluid in the middle ear, accompanied by signs or symptoms of acute infection, and *otitis media with effusion*, which is fluid in the middle ear without signs and symptoms of infection. Untreated acute otitis media may spread to adjacent structures and cause mastoiditis (Table 54.3). Inflammation of the external ear canal is labeled *otitis externa*.

### Etiology

Acute otitis media usually occurs in young children as a complication of infection with one of the common respiratory viruses (Table 54.1). While viruses such as influenza A and respiratory syncytial viruses have been isolated as the sole pathogens from middle ear fluids, cultures of middle ear fluid yield a common respiratory bacterial pathogen in the majority of cases; *S. pneumoniae* is the most common bacterial pathogen, followed in importance by nontypable strains of *H. influenzae* and by *M. catarrhalis*. Staphylococci and group A streptococci are implicated in less than 5% of cases. In contrast to the important role of bacteria in the pathogenesis of acute otitis, a minority of children with otitis with effusion will show bacteria on culture of middle ear fluids. Otitis externa is usually due to infection with *Pseudomonas aerugenosa*, which is associated with excessive moisture and poor drainage of the external ear. Other bacterial pathogens which commonly cause skin infections, such as group A streptococci or staphylococci, also cause otitis externa.

### Epidemiology

Acute otitis media is almost a universal infection of children during their first 3 yr, and it has been estimated that 30% of visits to pediatricians are for this condition. Risk factors are similar to those for acute respiratory viral infections, and they include bottle rather than breast feeding, exposure to tobacco smoke, and crowded environments such as day care centers. Children who have anatomic defects that are associated with dysfunction of the eustachian tube, such as cleft palate, are at increased risk of developing acute otitis media. Although some children with severe allergies appear to be more susceptible to acute otitis media, the importance of allergies in this infection is relatively small compared to the role of allergies in sinusitis. External otitis occurs most often in children during the swimming season (swimmer's ear) or occasionally in immunosuppressed patients or those with diabetes mellitus.

### Pathogenesis

Acute otitis media is almost always a manifestation of impairment of the normal functions of the eustachian tube which are designed to allow for equilibration of pressures in the middle ear, to permit drainage of normal middle ear secretions, and to protect the middle ear from normal respiratory tract pathogens. The high incidence of acute otitis media in young children is due to underdevelopment of the protective mechanisms of the eustachian tube at this age. In addition, the high incidence of acute respiratory infections at this age has the effect of directly infecting the middle ear and of causing obstruction of the eustachian tube, impairing normal drainage and clearance of pathogens. Children with cleft palate and other anatomic abnormalities have abnormally patent eustachian tubes and increased incidence of acute otitis media because of loss of their protective function. In a small percent of children, recurrent bouts of acute otitis appear to be related to physical obstruction of the eustachian tube by greatly enlarged adenoids.

### Clinical manifestations

The child or adult with acute otitis media has symptoms that usually refer to the ear such as ear pain, fullness, hearing loss, and sometimes discharge from the external otic canal. General signs and symptoms of infection are also usually present, and these include fever, fussiness, headache, and sometimes nausea and vomiting. The diagnosis of acute otitis media is confirmed by demonstrating fluid in the middle ear by use of pneumatic otoscopy. This examination should show that the tympanic membrane is red, retracted or bulging, and is relatively immobile in response to pneumatic manipulation. Otitis media with effusion differs from acute otitis media in the absence of signs or symptoms of infection and in the presence of a slightly red or normally gray-appearing membrane, with similar evidence of effusion with bulging or retracted membrane and reduced mobility. In occasional patients where pneumatic otoscopy findings are equivocal, tympanometry or acoustic reflectometry may be helpful in detecting and monitoring the effusion.

Generalized otitis externa is characterized by pain or itching of the external canal, and the canal is red and swollen with serous or purulent discharge. A milder form of otitis externa with chronic discharge but less swelling and inflammation may be associated with chronic drainage from a perforated tympanic membrane as the residual from a bout of acute otitis media. Focal infection of the external canal by staphylococci is characterized by localized swelling and pain in the outer canal.

### Laboratory diagnosis

The microbiology laboratory can help identify the etiologic agent and its antimicrobial sensitivities in patients with acute otitis media who fail to respond to usual antimicrobial therapy. Because bacteria present in the external canal or nasopharynx do not predict the findings on culture of middle ear fluids, it is important that cultures be taken either by needle aspiration of middle ear fluid or during tympanostomy. Direct culture of exudate in the external canal is helpful in identifying the cause of otitis externa. Radiographic examination may be required to evaluate the extent of mastoiditis in patients who develop pain and swelling over the mastoids as a complication of acute otitis media.

### Therapy

Although some experts have recently questioned the routine use of antimicrobials for acute otitis media because of uncertain benefits and their contribution to the growing problem of antibiotic resistance, most experts still believe that acute otitis media should be treated with an antimicrobial that is effective against the most common bacterial pathogens—*S. pneumoniae*, *H. influenzae*, *M. catarrhalis*, and group A streptococci (Table 54.2). Amoxicillin is effective in over 85% of patients and it should be the initial choice for therapy in most communities because of its low toxicity and cost. In communities where a high percent of strains of *H. influenzae* are known to be $\beta$-lactamase producers or where a high percent of pneumococci are known to be resistant to penicillins, and in patients who fail to respond promptly to therapy, an alternative antimicrobial which is more likely to be effective against resistant organisms should be selected (Table 54.2). Therapy should be continued for at least 10 d. Oral analgesics should be prescribed during the first few days if the patient is complaining of pain. There is no evidence that decongestants, antihistamines, or corticosteroids are beneficial in treating acute otitis media. Myringotomy may be required during the acute phase in patients who have unusually severe pain or whose illness is progressive despite therapy. This surgical procedure usually provides prompt relief from pain and provides valuable material for culture.

Therapy for otitis media with effusion in young children remains controversial because few therapies have been convincingly more effective than watchful waiting. A clinical practice guideline for this condition published by the U.S. Department of Health and Human Services in 1994 has been helpful in sorting out the conflicting medical literature and outlining a rational approach to treatment of these patients. This guideline recommends two options for treating the child who either has asymptotic effusion at the end of 2 wk of therapy for acute otitis media or who has a new diagnosis of otitis media with effusion without history of recent acute disease. One option is to simply examine the patient at 6 wk intervals for 3 mo since the condition will resolve in the majority of patients without intervention. The other option is to give a trial of 10 d of antimicrobial therapy every 6 wk for 3 mo. This approach is associated with a 14% improvement in the rate of clearing of the effusion, but it is costly, and most antimicrobials have some side effects. If the effusion is still present at 3 mo the child should be tested for hearing loss. If the loss is greater than 20 db, this author's opinion is to give a trial of antimicrobial therapy. If the effusion is still present at 4 mo, there is consensus that the child should have a myringotomy with insertion of tubes. This procedure usually results in immediate improvement in hearing. These guidelines do not support tonsillectomy or adenoidectomy as therapy in young children with otitis with effusion.

External otitis, or swimmer's ear, is best managed by no longer swimming, keeping the ears dry, and topical treatment for *P. aeruginosa*. This can done either by lowering the pH with 2% acetic acid drops or by topical application of a solution containing both polymyxin B sulfate 10,000 U/ml and neomycin sulfate 0.5% four times a day for a week. Malignant external otitis externa in the immune-deficient patient should be treated with parenteral antibiotics selected to cover *P. aeruginosa* or other pathogens identified by the laboratory.

## ANNOTATED BIBLIOGRAPHY


Berman S. Otitis media in children. N Engl J Med 1995; 332:1560–1565.
*An excellent algorithm for the diagnosis and management of otitis media in children.*

Cohen S, Tyrrell DAJ, Russell MA, Jarvis MJ, Smith AP. Smoking, alcohol consumption, and susceptibility to the common cold. Am J Public Health 1992; 83(19):1277–1283.
*While smoking increased risk of infection and illness following experimental infection with common cold viruses, moderate alcohol consumption decreased illness in nonsmokers.*

Culpepper L, Froom J. Routine antimicrobial treatment of acute otitis media. Is it necessary? J Am Med Assoc 1997; 278:1643–1645.
*A thoughtful critique of the benefits and costs of the routine use of antimicrobials for acute otitis media.*

Franz TD, Rasgon BM, Quesenberry CP. Acute epiglottitis in adults. JAMA 1994; 272(17):1358–1360.
*The authors' approach to diagnosis and treatment of epiglottitis resulted in no deaths in 129 patients.*

Gwaltney JM, Scheld WM, Sande MA, Sydnor A. The microbial etiology and antimicrobial therapy of adults with acute sinusitis: a fifteen-year experience at the University of Virginia and review of other selected studies. J Allergy Clin Immunol 1992; 90(3):457–462.
*These authors found that* S. pneumoniae *and* H. influenzae *were the most common bacterial isolates detected by needle aspiration of acute maxillary sinusitis.*

Gwaltney JM, Phillips CD, Miller RD, Riker DK. Computed tomographic study of the common cold. N Engl J Med 1994; 330(1):25–30.
*Documents asymptomatic sinus involvement by CT scan in more than 80% of patients with the common cold.*

Kairys SW, Olmstead EM, O'Connor GT. Steroid treatment of laryngotracheitis: a meta-analysis of the evidence from randomized trials. Pediatrics 1989; 83(5):683–693.
*This meta-analysis of ten randomized studies indicated that adrenocorticoids reduced the morbidity of children hospitalized with croup.*

Klassen TP, Feldman ME, Watters LD, Sutcliffe T, Rowe PC. Nebulized budesonide for children with mild-moderate croup. N Engl J Med 1994; 331(5):285–289.
*Establishes the beneficial effect of aerosolized steroids for children with croup who were managed as outpatients.*

Klein JO. Current issues in upper respiratory tract infections in infants and children: rationale for antibacterial therapy. Pediatr Infect Dis J 1994; 13(1):S5–8.
*A thorough review of the literature supporting the use of antimicrobials in treating upper respiratory tract infections.*

Klein JO. Otitis media. Clin Infect Dis 1994; 19:823–833.
*An extensive review of the diagnosis and therapy of otitis media.*

Kozyrskyj AL, Hildes-Ripstein GE, Longstaffe SE, et al. Treatment of acute otitis media with a shortened course of antibiotics. J Am Med Assoc 1998; 279:1736–1742.
*A meta-analysis of randomized trials of antibiotic treatment of acute otitis media in children suggested that 5 days of short-acting antibiotic use is effective treatment for uncomplicated acute otitis media in children 2 years of age or older.*

Monto AS, Ullman BM. Acute respiratory illness in an American community. The Tecumseh Study. JAMA 1974; 227(2):164–169.
*A classic study illustrating the prevalence of acute respiratory illnesses in a community of 5000 observed for 6 yr.*

Morrison VA, Pomeroy C. Upper respiratory tract infections in the immunocompromised host. Semin Respir Infect 1995; 10:37–50.
*An excellent review of the diagnostic and therapeutic considerations unique to patients with impaired immunity.*

Quan L. Diagnosis and treatment of croup. Am Fam Physician 1992; 46(3):747–755.
*An excellent review of the diagnosis and therapy of croup and epiglottitis.*

Rouby JJ, Laurent P, Gosnach M, et al. Risk factors and clinical relevance of nosocomial maxillary sinusitis in the critically ill. Am J Respir Crit Care Med 1994; 150:776–783.
*After 7 d of nasotracheal and nasogastric intubation 95% of patients developed radiologic evidence of sinusitis.*

Shulman ST, Gerber MA, Tanz RR, Markowitz M. Streptococcal pharyngitis: the case for penicillin therapy. Pediatr Infect Dis J 1994; 13(1):1–7.
*A convincing argument that penicillin is still the first-choice antimicrobial for treating streptococcal pharyngitis.*

U.S. Department of Health and Human Services, Public Health Service, Agency for Health Car Policy and Research Publication No. 94-0622. Clinical Practice Guidelines #12, Managing Otitis Media with Effusion in Young Children. 1994.
*A well-documented guideline for managing otitis media with effusion in young children.*

Williams JW Jr, Holleman DR Jr, Samsa GP, Simel DL. Randomized controlled trial of 3 vs 10 days of trimethoprim/sulfamethoxazole for acute maxillary sinusitis. JAMA 1995; 273:1015–1021.
*By d 14 of therapy 77% of 40 adults treated for 3 d were cured compared to a 76% cure rate in 40 patients treated for 10 d.*

# 55

# Bronchitis and Bronchiectasis

CHRISTOPH M. TANG AND CHRISTOPHER P. CONLON

## Bronchitis

The term *bronchitis* implies an inflammation of the bronchi without involvement of the lung parenchyma and is usually associated with cough. There is often an associated tracheitis. Acute bronchitis is a short-lived condition, usually infective in origin, that can occur in individuals with previously normal airways. Chronic bronchitis, on the other hand, is not primarily infective but infection may cause a worsening of symptoms in already damaged airways. Chronic bronchitis, which usually does not involve the trachea, is defined clinically as the occurrence of cough with sputum production for at least 3 consecutive mo for more than 2 yr in succession. The terms *chronic obstructive airway disease* (*COAD*) and *chronic obstructive pulmonary disease* (*COPD*) are often used to describe chronic bronchitis.

## Etiology

### Acute bronchitis

This condition is usually caused by respiratory viruses although occasionally bacterial causes, such as *Mycoplasma pneumoniae*, *Bordetella pertussis*, and *Chlamydia pneumoniae*, are implicated (Table 55.1). Bacteria that may colonize the upper airways, such as *Streptococcus pneumoniae* and *Hemophilus influenzae*, do not cause acute bronchitis.

### Chronic bronchitis

Cigarette smoking and to a lesser extent, air pollution and inhaled dust are the main factors responsible for chronic airway damage. These environmental irritants damage the respiratory mucosa causing inflammatory changes that may narrow the airways and make them more susceptible to bacterial colonization. In such circumstances, secondary infection may occur and lead to a worsening of symptoms in patients with chronic bronchitis. The most common organisms associated with such exacerbations are *S. pneumoniae*, nonencapsulated strains of *H. influenzae*, and *Moraxella catarrhalis*. In addition, respiratory viruses may be responsible for up to 50% of acute exacerbations. *Mycoplasma pneumoniae* may cause some flare-ups but other bacteria such as *Staphylococcus aureus* and enterobacteriacae only rarely cause acute exacerbations.

## Epidemiological and host factors

Acute bronchitis most commonly occurs in children, usually those under the age of 5 yr, with a smaller peak in the elderly. The disease has marked seasonal variation with peak prevalence occurring in the middle of winter and a trough in midsummer. In the United Kingdom, the annual attack rate is about 45 per 100,000 population but can rise to 170 per 100,000 in the winter. There are no particular host factors that predispose individuals to acute bronchitis other than extremes of age.

Chronic bronchitis is common and is estimated to affect up to 25% of the adult population. The disease is most common in men over the age of 40 and is highly associated with cigarette smoking. There is some evidence that lower respiratory tract infection in early childhood may predispose to the later development of chronic bronchitis in adult life.

Repeated chest infections and persistent chronic bronchitis are sometimes the presenting features of an underlying immunodeficiency, such as common variable hypogammaglobulinaemia or specific IgA deficiency. In addition, disorders of epithelial ciliary function and cystic fibrosis should be considered.

## Pathophysiology

### Acute bronchitis

The degree of inflammation in the bronchi varies according to pathogen involved. Some, such as rhinoviruses, may cause little damage to the epithelium whereas others, like influenza viruses, may result in extensive epithelial inflammation and cell destruction. The trachea and bronchi are often edematous, and there may be associated bronchospasm. Environmental factors, such as air pollution and smoking, may exacerbate symptoms.

### Chronic bronchitis

Patients with chronic bronchitis, probably as a consequence of smoking, have an increased number of mucus-producing goblet cells in the bronchial epithelium, in some cases almost entirely replacing the normal ciliated epithelial cells. In addition, chronic inflammation leads to mucosal gland hypertrophy in the bronchial wall, resulting in narrowing of the airway. In chronic bronchitis, the airways appear to be more irritable than normal, leading to excessive secretions and bronchospasm. Normally the bronchi are sterile but, as a result of the damage seen in chronic bronchitis, the bronchi become colonized with bacteria, usually pneumococci and nontypable *H. influenzae*. Colonization may be enhanced by bacterial adhesins, such as pili in *H. influenzae*, which have a prediliction for respiratory mucosa. It is likely that bacterial products and the neutrophil and cytokine response to these products may contribute to the epithelial damage.

**Table 55.1** Infective causes of acute bronchitis

| |
|---|
| Adenovirus |
| *Bordetella pertussis* |
| *Chlamydia pneumonia* |
| Coronavirus |
| Coxsackievirus |
| Influenza A and B |
| *Mycoplasma pneumoniae* |
| Parainfluenza virus |
| Respiratory syncitial virus |
| Rhinovirus |

## Clinical features

### Acute bronchitis

The cardinal feature of acute bronchitis is cough. The onset of symptoms is usually fairly abrupt. There may be preceding coryzal symptoms with some viral infections. Fever is not usually a feature unless the bronchitis results from influenza or *Mycoplasma pneumoniae* infection. Although acute bronchitis often starts with a dry cough, about half of those affected produce some, usually mucoid, sputum which may later become frankly purulent. Retrosternal burning pain occurs if tracheitis is marked.

Clinical signs are few. There may be a few coarse crackles heard in the chest with occasional wheeze. Peak flow rate may be reduced. Signs of pleurisy or consolidation are not found.

### Chronic bronchitis

Most patients with chronic bronchitis have a productive cough, often worse in the morning, and they may be breathless on exertion depending on the severity of their disease. Often symptoms are mild until there is an acute exacerbation. These occur more commonly in the winter months and are characterized by increased cough, increased dyspnea, and increased sputum production with sputum changing from mucoid to purulent.

Clinical signs depend on the severity of the obstructive lung disease. The peak expiratory flow rate is usually markedly reduced, and there may be crackles and wheezes on auscultation of the chest. Chronic hypoxia may lead to right heart failure, or cor pulmonale. Such patients are sometimes referred to as "blue bloaters" as they usually retain carbon dioxide and are centrally cyanosed, dependent upon hypoxia to maintain their respiratory drive. At the other end of the spectrum are the so-called "pink puffers" with severe emphysema who maintain near-normal arterial oxygen concentrations by increased respiratory effort. Sputum production usually only occurs in this group during acute infective exacerbations. In practice, most patients fall between these two extremes.

## Laboratory findings

Acute bronchitis is usually dealt with in community practice and does not need laboratory investigation. There are no predictable blood test abnormalities and the chest X-ray is normal. Although cultures of sputum may occasionally reveal the causative pathogen, these are not routinely performed. Investigation is only warranted in those whose cough persists beyond 3 to 4 wk.

In chronic bronchitis, blood gas analysis often shows hypoxia with or without hypercapnia. Routine bloods are normal although the white cell count may be raised in severe infective exacerbations. The chest X-ray is often normal but may show emphysema, streaky fibrosis, or an enlarged heart in advanced cor pulmonale. Pulmonary infiltrates indicate a complicating pneumonia.

Most interest and controversy surrounds the analysis of expectorated sputum. Because the airways of the majority of chronic bronchitics are colonized with potentially pathogenic bacteria, the finding of pneumococci, *M. catarrhalis*, or *H. influenzae* in sputum cultures is difficult to interpret. However, gram staining of sputum can be helpful and is often considered indicative of infection if there are numerous neutrophils together with predominance of one type of organism on the gram stain; *S. pneumoniae* appears as gram-positive diplococci, *M. catarrhalis* as gram-negative intracellular diplococci, and *H. influenzae* as small gram-negative coccobacilli. Viral and mycoplasma infections are usually diagnosed serologically.

## Diagnosis

The diagnosis of acute or chronic bronchitis is a clinical one and is not usually difficult. Symptoms and signs are limited to the respiratory system and the chest X-ray is normal. Sometimes, particularly in children, it may be difficult to distinguish between acute bronchitis and asthma. There are also real difficulties in determining whether exacerbations of chronic bronchitis are due to infection or not though most clinicians make the assumption that they are.

## Treatment

### Acute bronchitis

Treatment is largely supportive with encouragement to give up or limit smoking. Antitussives sometimes help and advice should be given about maintaining hydration to help loosen bronchial secretions. There is no role for antibiotics in most cases.

Influenza vaccination for the elderly and those with chronic cardiopulmonary disease or immunosuppression will prevent some episodes of acute bronchitis, as will pertussis vaccination for children. One of the most important prophylactic measures is the discouragement of cigarette smoking.

### Chronic bronchitis

Here again, cessation of smoking is important. The role of antibiotics in acute exacerbations is controversial. However, some studies have shown that in the most severely affected patients with increased dyspnea, increased sputum production, and purulent sputum, antibiotics have a better success rate than placebo with earlier improvement in cough, sputum purulence, and peak flow. Most clinicians give antibiotics to those patients ill enough to be hospitalized. Antibiotics that cover both *H. influenzae* and *M. catarrhalis* and the pneumococcus are usually selected. Most studies have shown no difference between cotrimoxazole, $\beta$-lactams, and tetracyclines. Between 10% and 15% of nontypable *H. influenzae* isolates and up to 75% of *Moraxella* isolates are $\beta$-lactamase producers. In addition, sputum may contain $\beta$-lactamases from other organisms so $\beta$-lactamase–stable antibiotics should be chosen. Typically antibiotics are given for 7 to 10 d.

Other therapeutic measures include judicious oxygen therapy and bronchodilators. Many patients show considerable reversibility with inhaled $\beta_2$-agonists such as salbutamol and with anticholinergics like ipatropium. Phosphodiesterase inhibitors, such as theophylline, are sometimes used for added bronchodilator effect. These drugs have a narrow therapeutic window, and blood levels may be dangerously increased by concomitant use of fluoroquinolone antibiotics or be inadequately low in smokers. It is also often worth giving a trial of systemic steroids to improve bronchospasm.

Prophylactic measures are similar to those used with acute bronchitis, including influenza immunizations and advice about smoking. There are no data to suggest that immunization against pneumococci prevents exacerbations. In a few highly selected patients who get frequent exacerbations (more than three per year), it may be worth considering prophylactic antibiotics. Some patients may take them continuously during the winter months, but a better strategy may be for patients to start antibiotics at the first sign of a cold or if the sputum becomes purulent.

## Bronchiectasis

Bronchiectasis is the permanent dilatation of airways including and distal to the subsegmental bronchi; this pathological endpoint can result from a wide variety of insults though in a significant number of cases the cause is never identified. Bronchiectasis has received little attention recently and remains an underresearched topic. This is probably because it is perceived as condition of declining prevalence which carries a relatively low mortality and is easily managed conservatively. Longitudinal hospital-based studies demonstrated that the prevalence of bronchiectasis fell dramatically in developed countries when broad-spectrum antibiotics became available and when vaccination against measles and pertussis was introduced. However, bronchiectasis is now emerging as a problem in patients with the acquired immunodeficiency syndrome (AIDS); the increased longevity of patients with AIDS is associated with chronic and recurrent bacterial pneumonias. Bronchiectasis is frequently debilitating, causing progressive respiratory failure, and more refined imaging of the chest, particularly with computerized tomographic (CT) scanning, has demonstrated that bronchiectasis is often underdiagnosed. Therefore, in a significant number of affected patients the diagnosis is not established and they do not receive appropriate therapy.

## Etiology

The major causes of bronchiectasis are listed in Table 55.2. A few points are worth emphasizing. The presence of localized disease suggests a focal etiology; for instance, occlusion of an airway by a foreign body or an extrabronchial neoplasm will result in bronchiectasis distal to the obstruction only. In this context, the right middle lobe bronchus is particularly vulnerable given its relatively long course in the lung and its close relationship to mediastinal lymph nodes. The underlying insult remains unidentified in 30% to 70% of patients though usually this has little bearing on the subsequent management of the patient. However, there are a number of potentially reversible conditions which should be excluded in all cases. These include obstruction of an airway, immunodeficiency syndromes, chronic upper respiratory tract sepsis, and active tuberculosis. Additionally, while the presence of a disease such as $\alpha$-1-antitrypsin deficiency or Kartagener's syndrome has no implications for the treatment of the affected individual, the identification of such inherited conditions is worthwhile so that genetic counselling can be offered. There is no evidence that smoking *per se* causes bronchiectasis, but, given its detrimental effect on both mucocilary clearance and the balance of proteases and antiproteases in the lung, smoking should be actively discouraged in all patients with bronchiectasis.

**Table 55.2** Causes of bronchiectasis

| |
|---|
| 1) POSTINFECTIOUS |
| Tuberculosis |
| Allergic bronchopulmonary aspergillosis |
| Whooping cough |
| Measles |
| Aspiration pneumonia |
| Chronic upper respiratory tract sepsis |
| 2) SECONDARY TO OBSTRUCTION OF A MAJOR AIRWAY |
| Foreign body |
| Endobronchial or extrabronchial compression |
| 3) ABNORMAL HOST DEFENSE |
| *CONGENITAL* |
| Agzaglobulinemia |
| Alpha-1-antitrypsin deficiency |
| Immotile cilia syndrome |
| IgG subclass deficiencies |
| Cystic fibrosis |
| *ACQUIRED* |
| Chronic lymphatic leukemia |
| Multiple myeloma |
| HIV infection |
| 4) IDIOPATHIC |

## Pathophysiology

Histological examination of lung tissue from patients with bronchiectasis often reveals partial obstruction of the airways by viscid secretions which have not been cleared by mucociliary transport. There are inflammatory cells present in the airways with accompanying edema of the respiratory mucosa; the bronchial epithelium may be swollen and ulcerated, and occasionally squamous metaplasia can be detected. In long-standing bronchiectasis, peribronchial regions may be replaced by fibrous tissue. One way of classifying bronchiectasis is by the pattern of airway dilatation. Three predominant patterns are recognized: saccular, cystic, and tubular. These distinctions can be made easily by bronchography but are not particularly helpful to the clinician as there appear to be no important clinical correlates with these histological patterns.

The precise sequence of events leading to bronchiectasis has not been determined, as this is difficult to determine experimentally or by longitudinal histopathological studies. There are two major theories which explain the progression to airway dilatation. The first is that proinflammatory cytokines are liberated in response to an inflammatory stimulus within the airway, causing neutrophil activation and degranulation with the release of proteolytic enzymes. The enzymes partially degrade the bronchial wall, resulting in an area of weakness which then dilates in response to negative intrathoracic pressure during inspiration. This hypothesis is supported by the high prevalence of bronchiectasis in patients with $\alpha$-1-antitrypsin deficiency in whom there is uncontrolled and excessive proteolytic activity in the lung parenchyma. Inhaled antiproteases have, however, failed to prevent disease progression. Second, it has been proposed that when parenchymal lung damage heals by fibrosis, traction is exerted on the wall of the airway with subsequent dilatation. Whatever the primary mechanism, sites of airway constriction proximal to the dilated bronchial segments can impede the effectiveness of cough and the mucociliary elevator in draining inflammatory debris and mucus.

## Clinical manifestations

The clinical picture of bronchiectasis is largely dependent upon the site and extent of disease. Patients with extensive bronchiectasis present with a chronic cough productive of copious amounts of purulent sputum and occasional hemoptyses. Physical examination of these patients reveals a number of abnormalities such as coarse crackles over the affected areas, finger clubbing, and widespread expiratory wheeze. Individuals with end-stage disease may have signs of associated emphysema, cor pulmonale, or other complications such as empyema, lung abscess, and amyloidosis. However, in the majority of individuals the findings are less florid; the most frequent complaint is of cough which may be purulent only intermittantly, and occasionally even nonproductive. ("Dry bronchiectasis" is a feature of disease in the upper lobes which drain effectively by gravity.) There may be few clinical pointers to the disease and the patient may present with a recurrent cough alone with no abnormal physical signs, making it impossible to diagnose bronchiectasis on clinical grounds.

The assessment of the patient should also be directed at determining the cause of bronchiectasis and include careful inquiry for the symptoms of chronic sinus infection, a history of severe childhood respiratory infection or inhalation of a foreign body, and a family history of recurrent lung infection. Examination of the nasopharynx should be performed in all patients with bronchiectasis to exclude an upper respiratory tract source. The development of diffuse bronchiectasis in a child or young adult without a clear precipitating factor should prompt investigation for cystic fibrosis and immunodeficiency syndromes.

## Laboratory studies

A differential white cell count may provide an indication of active infection or identify an underlying lymphoproliferative disease, and an anemia of chronic disease is found in chronically affected patients. Gram stain of the sputum usually shows a large number of polymorphonuclear leucocytes and a variety of bacteria. Culture of sputum is often of limited value as specimens are frequently contaminated with upper respiratory tract flora, and overgrowth of these species may obscure the isolation of the pathogen. Culture for anaerobic bacteria may be helpful in patients with foul-smelling breath and in those with an acute exacerbation which fails to respond a conventional course of antibiotics (see below). In this latter group, more invasive tests, including lung aspiration, should be considered. Isolation of *Aspergillus* spp. from sputum and the detection of IgG and IgE antibodies against this genus indicate that the patient may have allergic bronchopulmonary aspergillosis (ABPA), which is often associated with airways obstruction and has a characteristic central distribution.

Clearly, detailed immunologic investigation of all patients with bronchiectasis for total IgA or IgG subclass deficiencies is inappropriate. These tests should be reserved for those in whom the clinical suspicion for immunodeficiency is high; that is, early onset of diffuse disease or in association with recurrent infections outside the lung. In a significant proportion of patients with bronchiectasis, reversible airway obstruction is a feature of their illness, and this can be detected by lung spirometry before and after bronchodilators.

## Diagnosis

There is no great diagnostic difficulty in a patient with the typical symptoms and signs of severe bronchiectasis in whom the diagnosis is virtually certain without need for further investigation. Clearly, the situation is more difficult when there is less extensive disease. In the past, the diagnosis has relied upon bronchography, but in recent years, this has been superceded by less invasive techniques. There remain only a few indications for bronchography, and these include the identification of a congenital lung abnormality and the assessment of patients prior to surgery. Chest radiography may show the characteristic changes of increased lung markings (with evidence of tramlining of the markings and ring or cystic lesions), but can be entirely normal. Where the clinical suspicion of chronic sinusitis is high, X-ray of the sinus cavities may reveal opacification or fluid levels. CT scanning is a much more reliable method of detecting bronchiectasis than chest X-ray, and saccular disease is most easily recognized. The major reason for performing bronchoscopy is not to diagnose bronchiectasis but rather to exclude mechanical obstruction of an airway in a patient with localized bronchiectasis. Bronchoscopy may also be used to obtain reliable bacteriological specimens.

## Treatment

Before discussing the therapy of bronchiectasis, it is important for the clinician to consider the need to direct treatment at the underlying cause (e.g., the removal of an obstructive endobronchial tumor or regular immunoglobulin replacement in patients with specific deficiencies). Otherwise, the principal aims of therapy are to alleviate symptoms and to prevent disease progression. There is no doubting the need for antimicrobial therapy in an individual with an acute febrile exacerbation of bronchiectasis with increased production of purulent sputum, pleuritic chest pain, and/or hemoptysis. Under these circumstances, a course of antibiotics often results in a resolution of the acute symptoms. In certain patients, such exacerbations are heralded by a viral upper respiratory tract infection (URTI); there is a clinical experience which suggests that preemptive therapy, initiated at the earliest sign of an URTI, is effective. Some recent research has been conducted into the recommended dose of antibiotics, as it is recognized that conventional doses often appear to be ineffective in treating acute exacerbations. This treatment failure appears to have two causes; first, the penetration of antibiotics into lung secretions is reduced in patients with inflammation of the airways. Second, there is evidence that $\beta$-lactamase is secreted by organisms colonizing the airways of patients with bronchiectasis. Therefore, it is possible to isolate a respiratory pathogen which is fully sensitive *in vitro* but which is relatively unresponsive *in vivo*. These considerations have led to the use of high-dose antibiotic regimens (e.g., 3 g amoxycillin twice a day) in the therapy of bronchiectasis. The optimum duration of antibiotic courses has not been evaluated in any randomized controlled trials but a 7–14 d course is usually sufficient. The selection of antimicrobial agent is dependent upon the results of sputum culture if available, or the likeliest causative organisms if not. As *Streptococcus pneumoniae* and *Hemophilus influenzae* are the predominant pathogens in febrile exacerbations, treatment with amoxycillin or cotrimoxazole is usually appropriate.

Major controversies arise in the strategies used for patients with chronic, progressive disease whose sputum is continually purulent. A trial in the 1950s showed that oral tetracycline (500 mg twice a day, taken for 2 d per week for a year, Medical Research Council, 1957) can reduce the number of acute exacerbations, the volume of sputum production, and the amount of absenteeism from work. However, these benefits were only marginal, and this approach is no longer favored given the relatively high risk of acquiring infections with resistant organisms. One approach is that these patients should receive a 4 mo course of antibiotics in an attempt to eliminate respiratory tract sepsis. Subsequent relapses are then treated with further 2 wk courses.

Postural drainage and chest percussion are widely used adjunctive therapies for bronchiectasis, although their superiority over coughing in clearing respiratory secretions is far from proven. The usual practice is to advise postural drainage of pulmonary segments twice daily. The incidence of reversible airway obstruction in patients with bronchiectasis ranges from 5% to 10%; this group of patients should receive regular bronchodilators. Many other individuals have both a restrictive and an obstructive component to their lung function, and the role of bronchodilators in these individuals is not as clear. Inhaled corticosteroids may have a place in the management of bronchiectasis. A recent study demonstrated that treatment of stable disease with inhaled steroids led to a reduction both in the amount of sputum produced and coughing when compared with those given placebo. These observations need to be extended to include longer follow-up (only 3 wk in this study) and to see if therapy has any influence on the frequency of exacerbations.

Administration of the polyvalent pneumococcal and the conjugate *Hemophilus influenzae* type B vaccines should be considered in all patients with bronchiectasis. It would be of considerable interest to examine the effect of vaccination on the respiratory flora of patients, the frequency of exacerbations, and the natural history of disease. There are, however, no long-term studies of patients which evaluate measures to reduce the progression of bronchietasis.

Surgical excision of the affected lung offers the only curative therapy for bronchiectasis. The only generally accepted indications for surgical intervention in bronchiectasis are localized symptomatic disease and recurrent troublesome hemoptysis related to a single segement in extensive disease.

## Cystic fibrosis

Cystic fibrosis (CF) is the most common hereditary lethal disease in Caucasian populations: Mutations detected in the affected gene—the cystic fibrosis transmembrane conductance regulator (CFTR), which affects development of a critical chloride ion channel—occur in 2%–4% of the population. This condition should be considered in young patients with extensive bronchiectasis in whom there is no clear precipitating illness. The diagnosis can usually be established by detecting elevated chloride ion concentrations in the sweat (>70 mEq/l in adults), and more recently, by identifying the associated mutation in the CF gene. About 1% of patients with clinical CF have normal sweat tests and about half of these have a well-described single mutation in the gene. Measuring the nasal transepithelial potential difference and the response of sweat gland to $\beta$-adrenergic agonists may help to diagnose these cases.

Pulmonary pathology accounts for the majority of the morbidity and mortality associated with CF. The difference between bronchiectasis caused by CF as opposed to other conditions is the organisms which cause infective exacerbations. Initially the respiratory tract of individuals with CF is colonized with *Staphylococcus aureus* and very mucoid *Pseudomonas* species. Later in the course of the illness, *Berkholderia* (formerly *Pseudomonas*) *cepacia* may be isolated; this species, which may be resistant to multiple antibiotics, is associated with rapid deterioration of pulmonary function. The therapy for pulmonary exacerbations of cystic fibrosis is guided by the severity of the episode. For mild attacks, oral antibiotics may be sufficient; some fluoroquinolones are useful in this situation because of their antipseudomonal activity. These antibiotics should only be used in short courses (up to 14 d) because of the potential for rapid emergence of resistance. Inhaled antibiotics, such as colistin, can be given over longer periods and be used for maintainence therapy. Parental antibiotics are required both in severe attacks and when oral treatment has failed to alleviate the symptoms. If *Pseudomonas* spp. are isolated from respiratory specimens, patients should receive a combination of agents with good antipseudomonal activity (e.g., an aminoglycoside and a third-generation cephalosporin such as ceftazidime) to reduce the chances of selecting for resistant strains. CF patients have a larger volume of distribution and increased clearance of antibiotics than normal, so often larger doses of aminoglycosides need to be given, with appropriate monitoring of peak, as well as trough, serum levels.

## ANNOTATED BIBLIOGRAPHY

### Bronchiectasis

Barker AF, Bardana EJ. Bronchiectasis: update of an orphan disease. Am Rev Respir Dis 1988; 137:969–978.
*Good review of the pathogenesis of this condition highlighting the need for further research. Contains little on the treatment of bronchiectasis.*

Elborn JS, Johnston B, Allen F, Clarke J, McGarry J, Varghese G. Inhaled steroids in patients with bronchiectasis. Respir Med 1992; 86:121–124.
*A small randomized control trial examining the effect of inhaled steroids on symptoms; positive benefit was seen in terms of an increase in peak expiratory flow rates and a reduction in sputum production. Follow-up period limited.*

Hill SL, Burnett B, Lovering AL, Stickley RA. Use of an enzyme-linked immunosorbent assay to assess penetration of amoxycillin into lung secretions. Antimicrob Agents Chemother 1992; 36:1545–1552.
*Demonstration of low penetration of amoxycillin into the sputum of patients with bronchiectasis taking standard doses of the drug and inactivation by local* $\beta$*-lactamases.*

Medical Research Council. Prolonged antibiotic treatment of severe bronchiectasis. Br Med J 1957; 2:255–259.
*Large randomized control trial showing marginal benefit in symptoms and time lost to work with regular tetracycline. The influence of therapy on disease progression and respiratory tract flora was not studied.*

### Bronchitis


Anthonisen NR, Manfreda J, Warren CPW, Hershfield ES, Harding GK, Nelson NA. Antibiotic therapy in exacerbations of chronic obstructive pulmonary disease. Ann Intern Med 1987; 106:196–204.
*One hundred seventy-three patients with 362 exacerbations of chronic obstructive pulmonary disease were randomized in a double-blind, crossover trial to antibiotic therapy (either trimethoprim-sulfamethoxazole or amoxicillin or doxycyline) or placebo. Patients on antibiotics showed a modest improvement in terms of duration of symptoms, cough, sputum production, and peak flow compared to those on placebo. Benefits were most marked in those with the most severe exacerbations, and side effects were minimal in both groups.*

Ayre JG. Seasonal pattern of acute bronchitis in general practice in the United Kingdom 1976–83. Thorax 1986; 41:106–110.
*An analysis of weekly reports of respiratory illness from sentinel British family practices to look for trends in attack rates of acute bronchitis. There was a consistent peak in January and February and a trough in August. Most cases were diagnosed in children under 5 yr and adults over 50. Interpretation is limited by lack of a good definition of acute bronchitis and the difficulty in distinguishing bronchitis from asthma in young children.*

Lees AW, McNaught W. Bacteriology of lower-respiratory-tract secretions, sputum and upper-respiratory-tract secretions in "normals" and chronic bronchitics. Lancet 1959; ii:1112–1115.
*The "normal" patients were those recovering from tuberculosis who had never had symptoms of chronic bronchitis. The airways were sampled with a sterile protected specimen swab via a rigid bronchoscope. Swabs from upper airways and pharynx frequently grew* Hemophilus influenzae *and* Streptococcus pneumoniae *from both groups. However, the lower airways were sterile in the "normals" but often grew* H. influenzae *and/or* S. pneumoniae *in those diagnosed with chronic bronchitis.*

Murphy TF, Sethi S. Bacterial infection in chronic obstructive pulmonary disease. Am Rev Resp Dis 1992; 146:1067–1083.
*An excellent review of the role of bacterial infection in chronic obstructive pulmonary disease in causation and exacerbation of the disease. The roles of nontypable* Hemophilus influenzae, Streptococcus pneumoniae, *and* Moraxella catarrhalis *are examined in detail and an algorithm for use of antibiotics in exacerbations is provided.*

Orr PH, Scherer K, MacDonald A, Moffat ME. Randomized placebo-controlled trials of antibiotics for acute bronchitis: a critical review of the literature. J Fam Pract 1993; 36:507–512.
*This is an analysis of six published randomized clinical trials of a variety of antibiotics to treat acute bronchitis. Those trials with the best methodology do not support the use of antibiotics. While not being a proper meta-analysis of the data on the treatment of acute bronchitis, this is a well-reasoned assessment of the data currently available.*


### Cystic fibrosis


Harris CE, Wilmott RW. Inhalation-based therapies in the treatment of cystic fibrosis. Curr Opin Pediatr 1994; 6:234–238.
*Discussion of the administration of drugs by aerosol. This paper includes recent data on the use of agents altering ion flux, such as amiloride, recombinant DNase, and antiproteases.*

Zabner RL, Quinn JP. Antimicrobials in cystic fibrosis: emergence of resistance and implications for treatment. Semin Respir Infect 1992; 7:210–217.
*A review of the difficulties of antibiotic resistance in treating exacerbations of cystic fibrosis.*

# 56

# Acute Pneumonia

FENG YEE CHANG AND VICTOR L. YU

Pneumonia is not only a common infection; it is the leading cause of death from infectious diseases in the developed countries. Correct diagnosis is paramount if cost-effective antimicrobial agent therapy is to be prescribed. With an increase in the number of potential microbial etiologies and emerging resistance to antibiotics, controversies regarding empiric antibiotic therapy and use of invasive diagnostic procedures have arisen. On the other hand, the modern era which brought us effective antimicrobial agents now also promises to bring newer diagnostic methods based on molecular biology.

## Host Defenses

In order for pulmonary infection to be initiated, the microorganisms must first gain access to the lung. The host defense mechanisms that protect the lung from infection are impressively diverse. In the nasopharynx, the anterior nasal hairs provide a filter for coarse particles. The large surface area of the nasal septum and turbinates and the sharp directional change of the incoming air at the nasopharynx constitute a barrier for entry of foreign particles and microorganisms. The cough reflex expels particulate matter and foreign objects. The epiglottis protects the airway from aspiration. Reflex bronchoconstriction minimizes entry of particles into the alveoli. The respiratory tract is lined by a mucous blanket that entraps microorganisms and particles, and upward-beating cilia continuously provide clearance. Respiratory secretions contain nonspecific inhibitors of microorganisms including $\alpha$-1-antitrypsin, lysozyme, lactoferrin, and secretory IgA. Fibronectin is a glycoprotein within respiratory secretions that inhibits adherence of some bacteria to cell surfaces preventing colonization, an important initial step to subsequent infection. If the microorganism can finally reach the alveoli, alveolar macrophages are available to phagocytose these invaders. An inflammatory response is provoked with an influx of neutrophils from the lymphatics and the vascular system. As neutrophils and microorganisms accumulate, the local area becomes acidic and hypoxic, since ventilation is impaired by alveolar filling. These conditions impair killing by phagocytes such that viable organisms might persist and multiply.

Conditions that depress local host defenses will predispose the host to pneumonia. Viral infections, especially influenza, alter the physical and chemical characteristics of the mucous blanket. Viral upper respiratory tract infections increase colonization of the oropharynx by *Staphylococcus aureus*. Impaired consciousness caused by alcoholism and neurologic disorders can depress the gag reflex and permit aspiration of oropharyngeal bacteria into the alveoli. Foreign bodies and lung neoplasms may impair bronchial drainage predisposing to infection behind the obstruction.

## Pathogenesis

The three major modes of transmission of microorganisms into the lung are aerosolization, aspiration, and bloodborne delivery.

### Aerosolization

In general, infectious particles with a diameter of 10 $\mu$m or greater are trapped in the upper respiratory tract passages and do not reach the terminal airway system. The trachea and conducting airways are usually effective in entrapping particles from 2 to 10 $\mu$m. Particles in the range of 0.5 to 2 $\mu$m may reach the terminal airways and alveoli. "Droplet nuclei" refers to particles 1–3 $\mu$m in diameter containing a single bacterium, the likely infecting unit for organisms transmitted by aerosolization. Interestingly, relatively few bacteria are transmitted by the airborne route; exceptions include *Mycobacterium tuberculosis* and the plague bacillus *Yersinia pestis*. The infective dose may be as low as a single organism, most often resulting in only a positive skin test as evidence for infection (see Chapter 60). On the other hand, many viruses including influenza are transmitted by the airborne route. Fungi that produce spores which are spread via the airborne route include *Coccidioides immitis*, *Blastomyces dermatitidis*, and *Histoplasma capsulatum*. One universal characteristic of organisms capable of airborne transmission is their high degree of infectivity, so outbreaks of such pneumonias are common.

### Aspiration

Pneumonias developing from this mechanism require colonization of the oropharynx by potential pathogens. Most bacterial pneumonias occur via this mode of transmission, including pneumococcal and aerobic gram-negative bacillary pneumonia. Disorders that impair consciousness and depress the gag reflex permit aspiration of colonizing bacteria; these disorders include neurologic disorders and alcoholism. Patients with chronic obstructive pulmonary disease have frequent bouts of pneumonia because of ciliary dysfunction caused by cigarette smoking and inefficient cough reflex. Ciliary function may also be depressed by alcohol or antecedent viral infections, such as influenza. Finally, some patients who develop recurrent pneumonias will have genetic deficiencies in ciliary function (e.g., Kartagener's syndrome).

### Bloodborne

In bloodborne delivery, the lung is a secondary site of infection. Right-sided endocarditis and purulent phlebitis caused by *S. aureus* can produce pneumonia from metastatic seeding.

Bloodborne delivery has also been implicated in pneumonia caused by gram-negative bacilli.

## Epidemiology

In the pre-antibiotic era, pneumonia was easy to diagnose (*Streptococcus pneumoniae* was the most common etiology) but difficult to treat. Antibiotics have greatly modified the natural history of pneumonia and sharply reduced the morbidity and mortality of this common infection. The demographics have also changed. The populations at risk are increasing in number, both neonates and elderly. Pneumonia acquired in the nursing home is a major clinical problem. The increase in immunosuppression caused by disease or treatment (e.g., AIDS patients, patients with malignancies, organ transplants) has expanded the number of susceptible hosts in an era of new and emerging opportunistic pathogens. Furthermore, widespread antibacterial agent use is predisposing to pneumonias caused by antibiotic-resistant bacteria and nonbacterial pathogens.

Pneumonias can be classified by their distinctive epidemiology: community-acquired, nosocomial, nursing home, and occurrence in immunocompromised hosts.

## Community-acquired pneumonia

Community-acquired pneumonia refers to pneumonia originating in the community in contrast to occurring within the hospital (Fig. 56.1). This is the most common cause of infections that require hospitalization. The attack rates for community-acquired pneumonia are highest at the extremes of age (ages less than 4 and greater than 65 yr). The incidence is highest in the winter because of a seasonal increase in viral infections with confinement indoors and closer contact of people. *S. pneumoniae* accounts for most of the identified cases of community-acquired pneumonia in immunocompetent hosts. Other common etiologies are given in Table 56.1 for patients requiring hospitalization. *Mycoplasma pneumoniae*, *Chlamydia pneumoniae*, and viral etiologies are more common in patients treated as outpatients ("walking" pneumonias).

Interestingly, about 30% to 50% of patients with community-acquired pneumonia have no identifiable pathogen despite intensive microbiologic studies. This includes patients with bacterial pneumonias in whom prior antibiotic therapy rendered microbiologic studies unrevealing or patients with pathogens that are as of today unrecognized. It should be kept in mind that *Legionella* and *Clamydia pneumoniae* were not recognized as pathogens until the late 1970s and 1980s, respectively.

## Nosocomial pneumonia

Nosocomial pneumonia refers to pneumonia acquired during hospitalization, i.e., 3 d or more after admission. The prevalence is increasing in part due to the ability of high-technology management to prolong life in severely ill patients; in the developed countries, it is the second most common hospital-acquired infection.

The etiologies of nosocomial pneumonia differ from those of community-acquired pneumonia. Most cases are polymicrobial with aerobic gram-negative bacilli, oropharyngeal anaerobes, and occasionally *S. aureus* playing an important role. *Legionella* is a

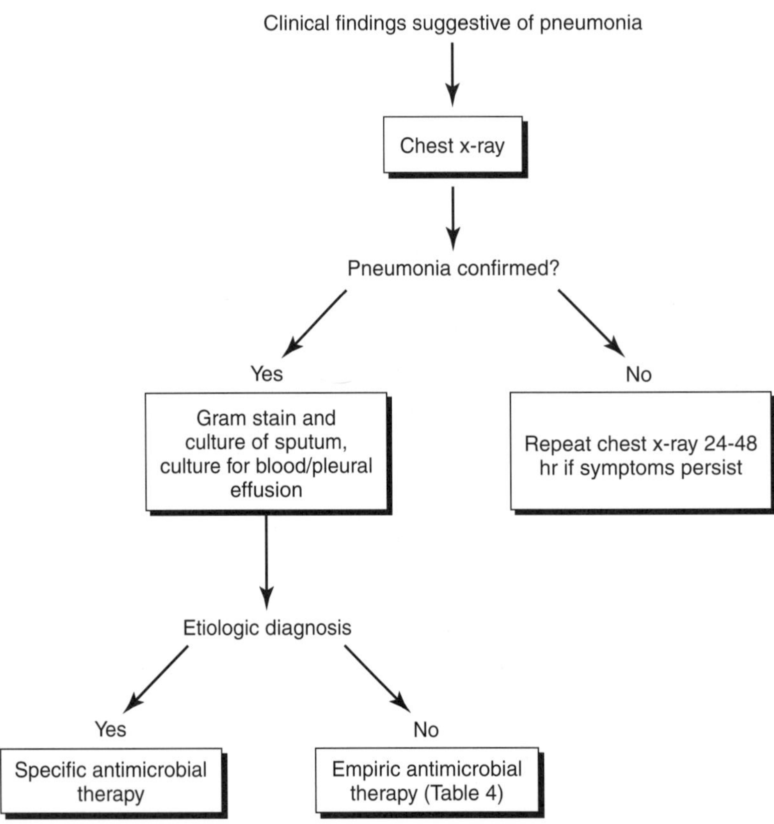


**Fig. 56.1** Approach to the patient with community-acquired pneumonia.

**Table 56.1** Causes of community-acquired pneumonia requiring hospitalization*

| Cause of pneumonia | Percent |
|---|---|
| *Streptococcus pneumoniae* | 10–20 |
| *Haemophilus influenzae* | 6–10 |
| *Chlamydia pneumoniae* | 6 |
| *Legionella pneumophila* | 2–7 |
| Aerobic gram-negative bacilli | 3–6 |
| *Staphylococcus aureus* | 3 |
| Influenza | 1–9 |
| *Mycoplasma pneumoniae* | 2–8 |
| *Moraxella catarrhalis* | 1 |
| *Coxiella burnetii* | 1–3 |
| *Pneumocystis carinii* | 2–5 |
| *Mycobacterium tuberculosis* | 1–3 |
| Unknown etiology | 30–50 |

*Data derived from numerous prospective studies including Fang GD, et al. Medicine 1990;69:307–316; Marrie TJ, et al. Rev Infect Dis 1989; 11:586–599; Blanquer J, et al. Thorax 1991;46:508–511; Karalus NC, et al. Thorax 1991;46:413–418; Bates JH, et al. Chest 1992;101:1005–1012.

major pathogen if the hospital water distribution system is contaminated with *Legionella*.

Aspiration is the most frequent mode of transmission in this setting. Host factors include advanced age, depressed consciousness, chronic lung disease, and previous use of antibiotics. Exogenous risk factors include respiratory tract manipulation, endotracheal intubation with mechanical ventilation, presence of nasogastric tubes, and surgery. In one study, pneumonia developed in 28% of patients after 30 d of mechanical ventilation. Antacids and histamine type 2 blockers increase the risk of bacterial colonization of the upper GI tract by decreasing gastric acidity. An increased incidence in gram-negative bacteria pneumonias in critically ill patients has been attributed to their use. At the molecular level, fibronectin—a glycoprotein present in respiratory secretions—has been shown to inhibit adherence of bacteria to respiratory tract cells. This substance is decreased in seriously ill patients, predisposing to colonization of bacteria in the tracheobronchial tree.

### Nursing home pneumonia

The etiology of nursing home pneumonias is similar to that of nosocomial pneumonias. Aerobic gram-negative bacilli account for an appreciable proportion of cases, in addition to usual pathogens such as *S. pneumoniae* and *H. influenzae*. Aerobic gram-negative bacilli are more common in debilitated patients in nursing homes because colonization readily occurs in patients with bowel incontinence or in patients with chronic bladder catheters. Outbreaks of influenza, respiratory syncytial virus, and tuberculosis are more common in a nursing home setting than in a home setting.

### Pneumonia in the immunocompromised host

Immunocompromised patients not only can be infected by the pathogens commonly involved in community-acquired and nosocomial pneumonia, but their compromised immune status makes them vulnerable to the "opportunistic" microorganisms that are nonpathogenic to the immunologically competent person. Pneumonias constitute 25%–50% of serious infections in patients with hematologic malignancies or recipients of solid organ or bone marrow transplants. Although aerobic gram-negative bacilli and *Legionella* are major pathogens, fungi and cytomegalovirus are particularly problematic (Table 56.2).

Specific defects in the immune system will predispose to infections by certain organisms. Neutropenia as a consequence of leukemia or a complication of cancer chemotherapy predisposes to infection by *Pseudomonas aeruginosa* and aspergillus. Defects in cell-mediated immunity seen in lymphomas, AIDS, or caused by corticosteroid or other immunosuppressive medications predispose to primary or reactivation infection by *Pneumocystis carinii*, *M. tuberculosis*, *Cryptococcus neoformans*, and cytomegalovirus. Defects in humoral immunity seen in lymphocytic leukemias and multiple myeloma predispose to infection by *S. pneumoniae*. Patients with mixed defects in humoral and cellular immunity (e.g., AIDS patients) are subject to infection by the entire range of microbial species (see Chapter 99).

## Clinical Manifestations

### Symptoms

Historically, the terms *typical* and *atypical* were used to differentiate the causes of pneumonia based on the clinical presentation of the patient. In *typical* pneumococcal pneumonia, patients

**Table 56.2** Pneumonia occurring in immunocompromised patients caused by opportunistic pathogens

BACTERIA

*GRAM-NEGATIVE BACILLI*
- *Klebsiella pneumoniae*
- *Escherichia coli*
- *Pseudomonas aeruginosa*
- *Haemophilus influenzae*

*Legionella* spp.
*Staphylococcus aureus*
*Nocardia asteroides*
*Mycobacterium tuberculosis*
*M. avium intracellulare*

FUNGI

*Aspergillus* spp.
Zygomycetes including mucor
*Candida* spp.
*Pneumocystis carinii*
*Cryptococcus neoformans*
*Histoplasma capsulatum*
*Coccidioides immitis*

PARASITES

*Toxoplasma gondii*
*Strongyloides stercoralis*

VIRUSES

Cytomegalovirus
Varicella zoster virus
Herpes simplex
Adenovirus
Respiratory syncytial virus

presented with a productive cough, high temperature, and a single rigor, whereas patients with *atypical* pneumonia were supposedly less toxic and classically presented with a dry, nonproductive cough and constitutional symptoms of malaise, headache, and myalgia. A diverse group of organisms have been classified as causing atypical pneumonia, including *M. pneumoniae*, *Legionella* spp., *C. pneumoniae*, *Coxiella burnetii* (rickettsia), and viruses. However, considerable overlap is, in fact, seen between the clinical presentation of "typical" pneumococcal pneumonia and that of "atypical" pneumonia, especially in the elderly. Recent rigorous studies have confirmed that neither clinical features nor radiographic characteristics can be reliably used to establish the etiologic diagnosis of pneumonia.

Cough is the predominant symptom in pneumonia; 90% of patients with pneumonia complain of cough. Mucopurulent sputum is most commonly found with bacterial pneumonia, although it occurs in 30% to 50% of patients with pneumonia caused by *M. pneumoniae* or adenovirus. Scanty or watery sputum is more often noted with atypical pneumonia. Rusty sputum suggests alveolar involvement and has been most commonly associated with pneumococcal pneumonia. Foul-smelling sputum is associated with mixed anaerobic infections most commonly seen with aspiration.

Fever may be sustained, remittent, or at times hectic. Fever patterns per se, however, are not useful for establishing a specific diagnosis and may even be absent in elderly patients. Chills occur in about 50% of patients. Pleuritic chest pain occurs in 40%. A variety of nonspecific symptoms including headache, anorexia, nausea, vomiting, sore throat, myalgias, arthralgias, rigors, abdominal pain, and diarrhea are common.

Advanced age and comorbid illness are important factors that affect the clinical presentation of pneumonia. Elderly patients with pneumonia may be less likely to develop cough, fever, or leukocytosis and may occasionally present with mental status changes rather than respiratory tract symptoms.

### Physical examination

The examination should focus on signs of consolidation and pleural disease and assessment of the adequacy of gas exchange. Cyanosis, rapid respiratory rate, the use of accessory muscles of respiration, sternal retraction, and nasal flaring suggest serious respiratory compromise. Early in the disease process, crackling rales may be the only abnormality. Examination of the chest may reveal crackles (78%), rhonchi (34%), and consolidation (29%). Evidence of consolidation (dullness on percussion, bronchial breath sounds, and egophony) is suggestive of bacterial infection. Patients with mycoplasmal or viral infection may exhibit few abnormalities on physical examination despite the presence of impressive infiltrates on the chest film.

Some physical findings may be associated with specific causes of pneumonia. Rashes or petechiae are seen in both viral or bacterial etiologies. Other cutaneous findings include furuncles in staphylococcal pneumonia, erythema multiforme in *M. pneumoniae*, erythema nodosum in pneumonia caused by *C. pneumoniae*, *H. capsulatum*, *C. immitis*, or *M. tuberculosis*, ecthyma gangrenosum in pneumonia caused by *P. aeruginosa* or *S. aureus*, and maculopapular rash in measles. Herpes labialis occurs commonly in the patients with pneumococcal pneumonia. The presence of periodontal disease and foul-smelling sputum are classical signs for an anaerobic pneumonia associated with aspiration. Bullous myringitis is an infrequent although significant finding in pneumonia caused by *M. pneumoniae*.

### Chest Radiography

The chest radiograph is the key study in the diagnosis of pneumonia. An infiltrate must be seen on the chest radiograph to substantiate its presence. Radiographic findings can assist in differentiating pneumonia from other noninfectious entities including pulmonary emboli, congestive heart failure, tumor, and collagen vascular disease. It is less reliable in pinpointing a specific microbial etiology. The chest radiograph can also assess severity of illness by identifying multilobar involvement, which is an objective indication of advanced pneumonia.

Several common radiographic patterns are seen in patients with pneumonia: lobar or segmental consolidation (Fig. 56.2), bronchopneumonia, interstitial infiltrates, and cavitary lesions. Radiologic associations suggestive of microbial etiology include bilateral diffuse interstitial infiltrates in *P. carinii* pneumonia (Fig. 56.3), cavitary lesions in anaerobic infections, lobar consolidation in pneumococcal pneumonia, multiple nodular abscesses in *S. aureus* pneumonia, and apical fibrosis with infiltrates in tuberculosis. Pneumocystosis, viral, and mycoplasmal pneumonias generally show interstitial infiltrates (Fig. 56.4). However, no radiographic picture is so distinct as to reliably establish an etiologic diagnosis. The differential diagnosis of cavitary lesions is discussed in Chapter 57 and that of diffuse infiltrates in Chapter 58.

## Laboratory Studies

### General

The white blood cell (WBC) count is often in the range of 15,000 to 20,000/mm$^3$. A left shift with immature forms is characteristic of bacterial pneumonia. Normal WBC counts are the rule in viral pneumonias, while infection with *M. pneumoniae* has been associated with WBC counts up to 15,000/mm$^3$ in about one-fourth of patients. Serum chemistries commonly show mild hepatic or renal dysfunction. Hyponatremia has been associated with Legionnaires' disease.

The specific laboratory diagnosis of etiologies depends upon either isolation of organism, antigen detection by antibody or DNA probe, or serology.

### Gram stain of respiratory secretions or pleural fluid

Most authorities believe that a properly performed gram stain provides invaluable information (Plate 18). However, it is imperative that patients be given adequate instruction to encourage them to produce a respiratory tract sample rather than saliva and that the results be confirmed by experienced microbiologists. Purulent sputa free of oropharyngeal contamination will yield more reliable information. The number of neutrophils and epithelial cells should be quantitated under low power (100×), with further examination reserved only for sputa containing ≥25 neutrophils and ≤10 epithelial cells.

### Isolation of organism

The utility of the sputum culture as a means of diagnosing pneumonia is controversial. Reliability has been questioned due to the ease of contamination of sputum with oropharyngeal flora. The sensitivity of sputum culture for the diagnosis of pneumococcal

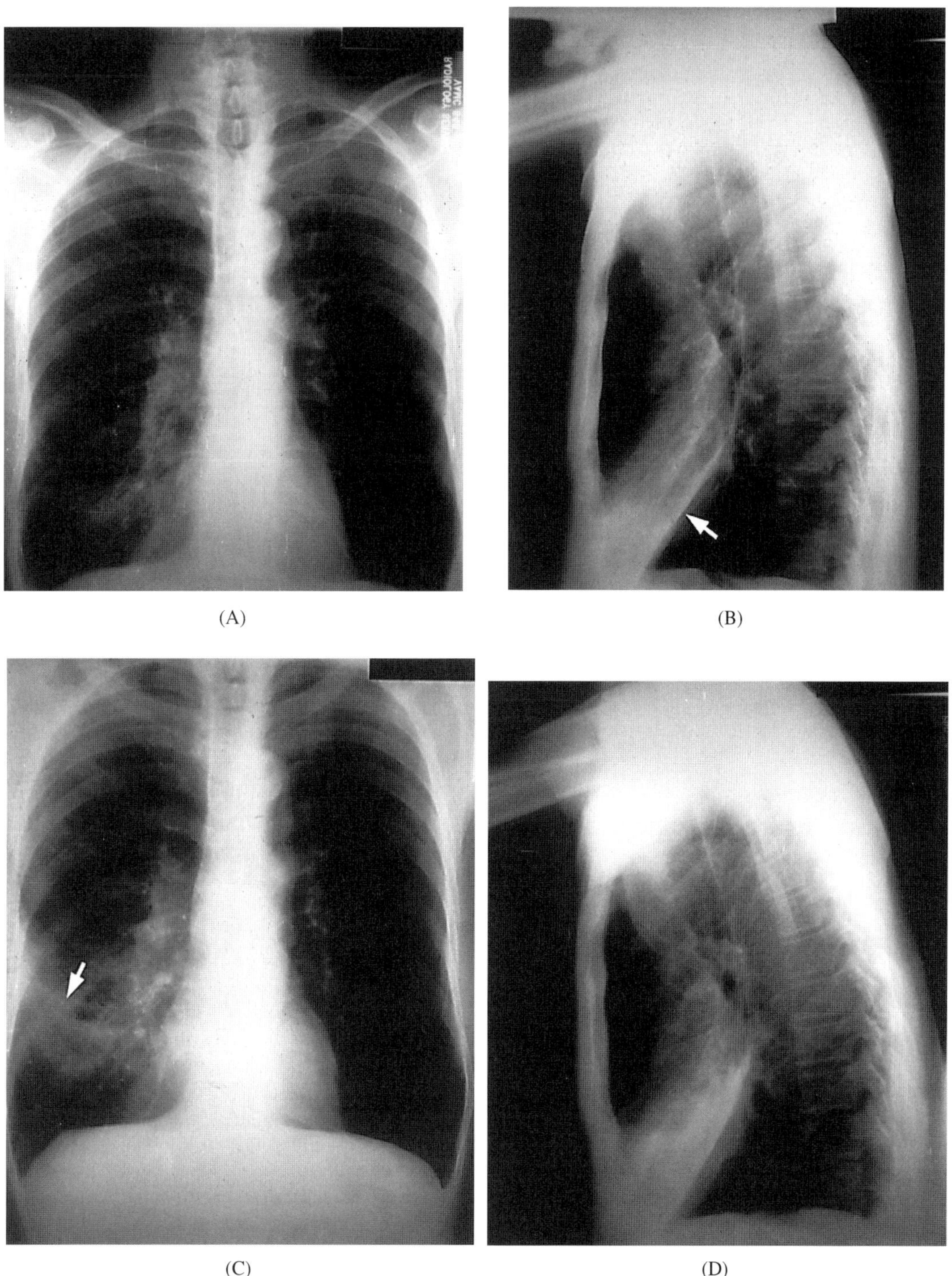


**Fig. 56.2** *A* An elderly male with a history of chronic obstructive pulmonary disease presented with a chief complaint of fever, night sweats, malaise, and a loss of appetite. He had a chronic nonproductive cough which was unchanged. The PA chest radiograph on admission shows a subtle patchy density which was overlooked by the admitting physician. Note that the right heart border is obscured showing that the infiltrate is in the right middle lobe (silhouette sign). *B* The lateral view of Figure 56.2A shows an infiltrate in the right middle lobe. The major fissure dividing the right upper lobe and right middle lobe is seen as a dense white streak (arrow). *C* The PA chest radiograph 2 d later shows marked progression of the infiltrate in the right middle lobe (lateral segment) (see arrow). Sputum and blood culture yielded *S. pneumoniae*. *D* The lateral view of C shows that the infiltrate is more dense when compared to B.

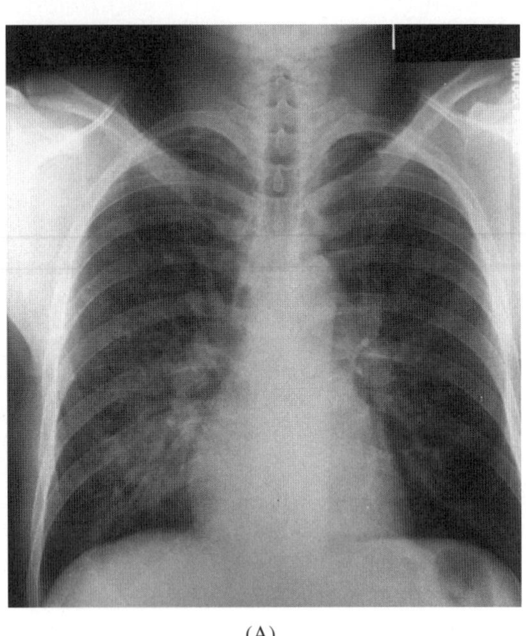

(A)

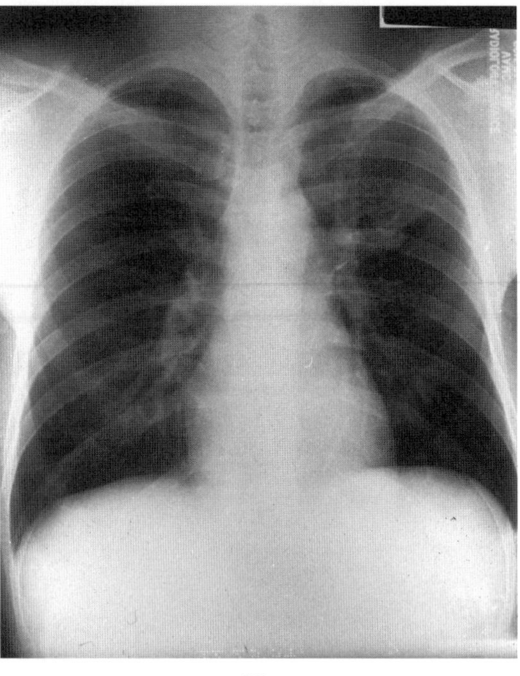

(B)

**Fig. 56.3** *A* A 37-yr-old intravenous drug user presented with a 3 wk history of fever and nonproductive cough. Chest X-ray revealed diffuse interstitial infiltrates especially marked on the right side. He was found to be HIV positive with a CD4 count of 20. Bronchoalveolar lavage yielded *Pneumocystis carinii.* He received 2 wk of trimethoprim-sulfamethoxazole. *B* Chest X-ray 19 days later after completion of trimethoprim-sulfamethoxazole therapy shows resolution of infiltrates.

pneumonia is only about 50%–70%. However, the diagnostic yield may greatly improve with careful collection of sputa (discussed later) and prompt culture of specimens. The diagnosis of *Hemophilus influenzae* infections relies on isolation of the organism. Culture of *M. pneumoniae* is a difficult procedure requiring specialized media; 1–2 wk is required for isolation and identification. Isolation of *C. pneumoniae* can be performed using cell lines, but both the sensitivity and specificity remain uncertain. The definitive test for diagnosis of Legionnaires' disease is isolation of the organism from respiratory secretions; special selective media with dyes is required.

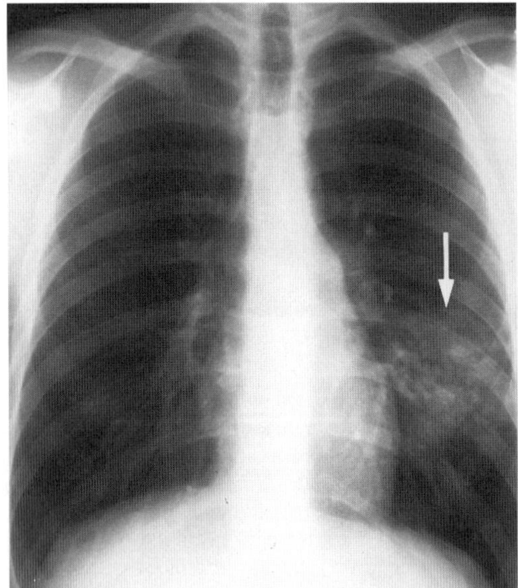

**Fig. 56.4** Chest X-ray of a 19-yr-old college student showing a fan-shaped infiltrate (arrow) in the right lower lobe. Serology revealed elevated titer to *C. pneumoniae.* The infiltrate resolved on antibiotic therapy. [Reprinted with permission from Grayston JT, et al, N Engl J Med 1986;315:164.]

Approximately 20% of patients with bacterial pneumonia are bacteremic. Positive blood cultures offer definitive proof of the etiology for an associated pneumonia. The frequency with which the pleural fluid becomes infected depends in part on the etiologic agent. Approximately 35% of patients with anaerobic pneumonia have culture-positive pleural effusion, but only 5% of patients with pneumococcal pneumonia have culture-positive effusion. Chapter 59 gives the necessary recommendations for diagnostic thoracocentesis.

## Antigen detection

Various immunoassays including counterimmunoelectrophoresis (CIE), agglutination, and enzyme-linked immunosorbent assay (ELISA) have been used for antigen identification of *S. pneumoniae.* Yields have been highest for pneumococcal antigen detection in sputum, with reported sensitivities of 70% and specificity of 80%. This test is used in Europe, but not in the United States. Detection of *M. pneumoniae* antigens in sputum by indirect enzyme immunoassay is reported to be highly specific. Sensitivity was also high (91%) when the assay was used on sputum and nasopharyngeal aspirates from patients who were shown either by culture or serologically to have *M. pneumoniae* infection. CIE and latex agglutination have been used for the detection of *H. influenzae* and *Pseudomonas* antigens in patients with pneumonia, but the results have been inconsistent. Soluble *L. pneumophila* antigen can be detected in urine by radioimmunoassay and ELISA; this test is sensitive (80%) and specific (100%) for detecting *L. pneumophila* serogroup 1. It is often easier to obtain urine than adequate sputum, and since serogroup 1 accounts for about 80% of *Legionella* infections, this rapid diagnostic test should be routinely available for cases of pneumonia.

Monoclonal antibodies in the immunofluorescence assay have been used to rapidly detect a variety of viruses, *Chlamydia* spp., and *Legionella* spp. in respiratory secretions. The sensitivity of the direct fluorescent antibody for *Legionella* spp. has ranged from 50% to 70%. The utility of monoclonal antibody tests for other pathogens remains under evaluation and their general applicability has yet to be determined.

## Serology

Antibody tests have been used to diagnose a variety of pulmonary pathogens, including *L. pneumophila*, *L. micdadei*, *M. pneumoniae*, *Chlamydia* spp., and *Coxiella burnetti*. The sensitivities and specificities of these serologies are variable, and many have not been completely standardized. Antibody titers are of more help in confirming a clinical diagnosis rather than making a decision for therapy, since a second specimen 2 to 4 wk later is mandatory for showing changes in antibody titers.

The specificity and sensitivity of serologic tests for *M. pneumoniae* are uncertain. Although the cold agglutination phenomenon is neither sensitive nor specific, this assay is the most widely used laboratory test for *M. pneumoniae*. Complement-fixing antibodies, although more specific, do not arise early enough in infection to be helpful in guiding therapeutic decisions. A titer of 1:32 or greater is highly suggestive of infection with *M. pneumoniae*.

Serologic diagnosis for *Legionella* with a fourfold rise in antibody titer to 1:128 is useful for epidemiologic purposes. In some outbreak settings of Legionnaires' disease in which specific antibiotic therapy was not given, sensitivity has been almost 90%. However, recent studies show a sensitivity of 60% for community-acquired cases and 40% for nosocomial cases.

The microimmunofluorescence test is the most sensitive method for the diagnosis of *C. pneumoniae*. The use of IgM- and IgG-specific conjugates helps distinguish current infection from past infection. Reinfection with *C. pneumoniae* is common, especially in adults. In reinfection, the frequent absence of IgM and complement fixation antibodies makes serologic diagnosis less clear-cut, although IgG often rises to >1:512 in 1 to 3 wk after reinfection. The complement-fixation serology is genus-specific and does not distinguish between *C. trachomatis*, *C. pneumoniae*, or *C. psittaci*. In persons with a clear history of exposure to a sick bird, complement-fixation antibody elevation may be diagnostic of infection with *C. psittaci*.

## Nucleic acid probe

DNA hybridization techniques have been used to detect herpes simplex virus, cytomegalovirus, mycoplasma, *Legionella* spp., *M. tuberculosis*, and nontuberculous mycobacteria. Polymerase chain reaction (PCR) techniques combined with DNA probes have been used to detect *C. pneumoniae* and *Legionella* spp. in throat swabs and sputum (see Chapter 15). Early results suggest that PCR may be more sensitive than culture.

## Management

### Approach to the immunocompetent patient with community-acquired pneumonia (Fig. 56.1)

#### History

History can furnish important clues including family history of respiratory infection, travel history, animal contact, clinical setting, and underlying disease (Table 56.3).

#### Chest radiography

A PA and lateral chest radiograph should be performed in patients whose symptoms and physical examination suggest the possibility of pneumonia. If the clinical findings support a diagnosis of pneumonia but the chest radiograph is negative, repeat radiographs should be obtained in 24 to 48 h if symptoms do not abate. The frequency with which follow-up radiographs should be obtained is dictated by the clinical status of the patient. Patients who are responding to antibiotic therapy may need only one follow-up film at conclusion of antimicrobial agent therapy for use as a baseline should clinical symptoms relapse. Elderly patients with chronic obstructive lung disease may require many months for radiographic resolution of the pneumonia. Patients who are not improving or whose condition is deteriorating may require multiple chest radiographs. The computed tomographic scan of the thorax is useful for detecting empyema and small abscesses (see Chapter 59).

#### Laboratory studies

Two sets of blood cultures should be performed on every hospitalized patient. Patients with a moderate or large pleural effusion should have a diagnostic thoracentesis. Pleural fluid examination should include white blood cell count and differential, measurement of protein, glucose, LDH, and pH, gram stain and acid-fast stain, and culture for bacteria, fungi, and mycobacteria (see Chapter 59). All patients with pneumonia complicated by cyanosis, severe dyspnea, hypotension, or mental status changes should undergo blood gas analysis. A $PaO_2$ of less than 60 mmHg while breathing room air is a poor prognostic sign.

If sputum is available, gram stain and culture of sputum should be routinely performed. Invasive diagnostic procedures are not indicated in most patients with community-acquired pneumonia. However, in patients who are immunocompromised or have multilobar infiltrates or progressive infiltrates on chest radiograph while receiving antibacterial agents, morbidity is substantial if incorrect antimicrobial agent therapy is administered or if unusual opportunistic pathogens are present. Thus, bronchoscopy with bronchoalveolar lavage, or protected specimen brush, and direct needle aspiration of the lung may be useful in these specific clinical situations.

#### Empiric antibiotic therapy

Guidelines for the initial empiric antimicrobial treatment of community-acquired pneumonia now emphasize the severity of the pneumonia and site of treatment (home or hospital) rather than clinical syndromes (Table 56.4). The empiric therapies recommended in Table 56.4 are for clinical situations in which the gram stain is unrevealing or if no sputum is available for examination.

**Table 56.3** History in suggesting etiologies

| | |
|---|---|
| Family history of respiratory illness | Respiratory syncytial virus<br>*Mycoplasma pneumoniae* |
| TRAVEL HISTORY | |
| Southeast Asia | *Burkholderia pseudomallei* |
| Asia, West Africa, South America | *Paragonimus westermani* |
| Ohio and Mississippi River Valleys, tropical areas | *Histoplasma capsulatum* |
| Southwestern U.S. | *Coccidioides immitis* |
| ANIMAL CONTACT | |
| Birds, parakeets, turkeys | *Chlamydiae psittaci* |
| Cats, cows, sheep, goats | *Coxiella burnetii* |
| CLINICAL SETTING | |
| Recent influenza infection | *Streptococcus pneumoniae*, *Staphylococcus aureus*, *Haemophilus influenzae* |
| Altered mental status | Oropharyngeal flora including anaerobes (aspiration pneumonia) |
| Intravenous drug abuse | *S. aureus*, *Pseudomonas aeruginosa* |
| UNDERLYING DISEASE | |
| Chronic alcoholism | Oropharyngeal flora (aspiration pneumonia)<br>Aerobic gram negative bacilli,<br>*S. pneumoniae* |
| Chronic obstructive pulmonary disease | *S. pneumoniae*, *H. influenzae*,<br>*Moraxella catarrhalis*, *Legionella pneumophila* |
| Cystic fibrosis | *P. aeruginosa*<br>*Burkholderia cepacia*, *S. aureus* |
| Sickle cell anemia | *S. pneumoniae* |

Note that empiric therapies for hospitalized patients cover both "typical" and "atypical" pathogens. Therapy should be altered when culture and sensitivity results become available.

### Hospitalization and intensive care unit admission

In-patient treatment of pneumonia is 15- to 20-fold more expensive per patient than for outpatients. Patients are also generally more comfortable at home. The advantages of care at home are offset by the fact that pneumonia is the most common cause of death due to infection in the United States. Severity of illness and underlying disease are the important factors in deciding on hospitalization. The following factors are indications for hospitalization: (*1*) immunosuppression, (*2*) altered mental status, (*3*) abnormal vital signs, especially tachypnea and hypotension, (*4*) advanced disease on chest radiograph (more than one lobe involvement, presence of a cavity, rapid radiographic spreading, and the presence of a pleural effusion), (*5*) severe metabolic and physiologic abnormalities (especially hypoxia). Relative indications for hospitalization include absence of a reliable adult in the home who can care for and monitor the patient. Comorbid disorders, such as ischemic cardiac disease, liver disease, chronic pulmonary disease, renal failure, or insulin-dependent diabetes mellitus may be exacerbated in patients with pneumonia and are also relative indications for hospitalization.

**Table 56.4** Initial empiric treatment of community-acquired pneumonia in immunocompetent patients*

A. Age $\leq$ 60 yr; no comorbid disease; outpatient therapy (oral): macrolide or tetracyclines

B. Age > 60 yr; comorbid disease; outpatient therapy (oral): a) second-generation cephalosporin, trimethoprim-sulfamethoxazole, or amoxicillin/clavulanate combined with b) a macrolide

C. Therapy in hospital (parenteral): a) cefuroxime or ampicillin/sulbactam combined with b) a macrolide, or c) azithromycin alone

D. Therapy in intensive care unit—severe pneumonia (parenteral): a) antipseudomonal antibiotic such as ceftazidime, ciprofloxacin, ticarcillin/clavulanate, piperacillin/tazobactam or imipenem/cilastatin combined with b) azithromycin

*Modified from Mandell LA, Niederman MS, The Canadian Community-Acquired Pneumonia Consensus Group: Antimicrobial treatment of community-acquired pneumonia in adults: A conference report. Reproduced with permission of Canadian Journal of Infectious Diseases 1993;4:25.

The presence of at least one of the following conditions justifies defining the pneumonia as severe and indicates that admission to the intensive care unit is appropriate: (*1*) severe tachypnea: respiratory frequency > 30 breaths/min at admission, (*2*) respiratory failure defined by a $PaO_2$ less than 50–60 mmHg while breathing room air, a $PaO_2/FiO_2$ ratio < 250 mmHg or requirement for mechanical ventilation, (*3*) chest radiograph showing bilateral involvement or marked increase in infiltrate while receiving outpatient antibiotic therapy, (*4*) hypotension (systolic blood pressure below 90 mmHg or diastolic blood pressure below 60 mmHg) or requirement for vasopressors, and (*5*) oliguria or acute renal failure.

## Approach to nosocomial pneumonia

Precise identification of bacterial pathogens in this setting has been difficult given the fact that colonization of the respiratory tract confounds the interpretation of sputum cultures. Nevertheless, common sense dictates that antimicrobial therapy should be directed at the potential pathogens isolated from cultures of sputum. Obtaining specimens by bronchoscopy including quantitative culture of protected brush specimens and bronchoalveolar lavage can be useful in selected situations but is not routinely indicated; standardization of the culture methods and clinical trials are needed to define their utility in diagnoses.

*Klebsiella* spp., *Enterobacter* spp., *Escherichia coli*, *Proteus* spp., *Serratia marcescens*, and *S. aureus* can cause nosocomial pneumonias and often require coverage. Options for empiric therapy include cefazolin plus gentamicin, second-generation cephalosporin agents, and third-generation cephalosporin agents. In patients with risks of aspiration or thoracoabdominal surgery, extension of the antibiotic spectrum to cover anaerobes is appropriate. Options include ticarcillin-clavulanic acid or imipenem. In patients with prolonged hospitalization and prior antibiotic usage, resistant aerobic gram-negative bacilli require coverage; options include a broad spectrum $\beta$-lactam agent or ciprofloxacin; either one should be combined with an aminoglycoside. The isolation of *P. aeruginosa* from sputum requires that combination therapy be given: a $\beta$-lactam agent (ceftazidime, imipenem, piperacillin-tazobactam, ticarcillin-clavulanate) or ciprofloxacin is appropriate; either one should be combined with an aminoglycoside (tobramycin, amikacin). Empiric coverage for *Legionella* is indicated if the hospital water supply is known to be colonized with the organism or infiltrates progress on $\beta$-lactam and aminoglycoside therapy. The newer macrolides (especially azithromycin) and quinolones (such as ciprofloxacin) are effective against *Legionella*. Erythromycin is less active and more toxic when compared to the newer macrolides (azithromycin, clarithromycin, and roxithromycin) and the quinolone agents.

The antibiotics used for patients in nursing homes with pneumonia are similar to those for nosocomial pneumonia. Elderly patients in nursing homes are infected by the pathogens commonly seen for community-acquired pneumonia, but aerobic gram-negative bacilli are more frequent, as mentioned previously. If the patient is clinically stable, an oral empiric regimen can be given, including ciprofloxacin (coverage for *H. influenzae*, gram-negative rods, and *Legionella*) plus penicillin (coverage for oropharyngeal anaerobes and *S. pneumoniae*), or a third-generation cephalosporin agent (cefixime or cefpodoxime) plus a macrolide. Patients on oral therapy must be monitored closely. Intramuscular ceftriaxone plus an oral macrolide (azithromycin) is a regimen that is both convenient and broad-spectrum in a nursing home setting.

## Approach to pneumonia in the immunocompromised host

Given the multiplicity of potential pathogens in an immunocompromised host (Table 56.2, Fig. 56.3), greater emphasis should be directed at obtaining specimens for definitive microbial diagnosis. While empiric antibacterial agent therapy may be initiated in selected patients, bronchoscopy with bronchoalveolar lavage and occasionally biopsy should be performed if infiltrates progress on such therapy. Needle biopsy under CT guidance or thoracoscopy can be implemented if bronchoscopy is unrevealing. The type of antibacterial agent therapy selected should cover the bacteria seen on the gram stain of sputum and associated with the specific immune defect in the individual patient.

Bronchoalveolar lavage has proven to be most useful in evaluation of AIDS patients with pulmonary infiltrates (see Chapter 99); *P. carinii* is the most common cause of pneumonia in such patients with diagnostic yields of greater than 90%. The sensitivity decreases to 60% if the patient is receiving inhaled pentamidine prophylaxis. Bronchoalveolar lavage also is useful in detecting cytomegalovirus pneumonia in patients with AIDS as well as in bone marrow and solid-organ transplant recipients. Results can be available immediately with monoclonal antibody stains. Invasive fungal infections in leukemic patients and transplant recipients have been diagnosed by bronchoscopy cultures and histopathology when sputum cultures were unrevealing. The approach to the diagnosis and treatment of pneumonia in transplant recipients and AIDS patients is presented in Chapters 91, 92, and 99.

## Prevention

Given the morbidity, mortality, and expense associated with pneumonias, preventive measures should be applied whenever possible. Cigarette smoking should be discouraged. Influenza A and pneumococcal vaccines should be administered to high-risk patients including the elderly, those with underlying lung disease, and those with immunocompromised condition (see Chapter 45). Infection control guidelines should be strictly enforced in hospitals and manipulation of the respiratory tract should be minimized.

### ANNOTATED BIBLIOGRAPHY


American Thoracic Society Consensus Statement. Guidelines for the initial management of adults with community-acquired pneumonia: diagnosis, assessment of severity, and initial antimicrobial therapy. Am Rev Respir Dis 1993; 148:1418–1426.

*Experts discuss management including empiric antibiotic therapy and decisions on hospitalization. Controversies are acknowledged, but a coherent approach is presented.*

Bartlett JG, Breiman RF, Mandell LA, File TM. Community-acquired pneumonia in adults: guidelines for management. Clin Infect Dis 1998; 26: 811–838.

*This article presents a reasoned approach to community acquired pneumonia that differs somewhat from the ATS Consensus Statement.*

Donowitz GR, Mandell GL. Acute pneumonia. In: Principles and Practice of Infectious Diseases, 4th ed. Mandell GL, Bennett JE, Dolin R, eds. Churchill Livingstone, New York, pp 619–637, 1995.

*This chapter gives a comprehensive review on general aspects of diagnosis and treatment in patients with acute pneumonia.*

Mandell LA, Niederman MS, and the Canadian Community-acquired Pneumonia Consensus Group. Antimicrobial treatment of community-acquired pneumonia in adults: a conference report. Can J Infect Dis 1993; 4:25–28.

*Experts provide the practicing physician with specific empiric antibiotic regimens for community-acquired pneumonia based on severity of illness and underlying diseases.*

Niederman MS, Sarosi GA, Glassroth J, eds. Respiratory Infections: A Scientific Basis for Management. WB Saunders, Philadelphia, PA, 1994.

*A multi-authored textbook with chapters on pathogenesis, clinical syndromes, etiologic agents, diagnostic methods, and therapy.*

Pomilla PV, Brown RB. Outpatient treatment of community-acquired pneumonia in adults. Arch Intern Med 1994; 154:1793–1803.

*A review of the diagnosis, etiology, and treatment of nonhospitalized adults with community-acquired pneumonia.*

Proceedings of the First International Consensus Conference on the Clinical Investigation of Ventilator-associated Pneumonia. Infect Control Hosp Epidemiol 1992; 13:633–677.

*A consensus review of invasive diagnostic methodologies used for nosocomial pneumonia with recommendations.*

Tablan OC, Anderson LJ, Arden NH et al. Centers for Disease Control guidelines for prevention of nosocomial pneumonia. Respir Care 1994; 39:1191–1236.

*The Centers for Disease Control advisory panel presents a comprehensive review of nosocomial pneumonia with focus on infection control measures; Legionnaires' disease, aspergillus, and viruses are discussed in detail.*

# 57

## Cavitary Pulmonary Disease

JOHN L. JOHNSON AND JERROLD J. ELLNER

A myriad of diseases involve the lower respiratory tract; however, only a limited number of these diseases, processes, and microbial pathogens typically result in lung tissue necrosis and cavity formation. Recognizing the presence of cavitation, therefore, can be very valuable in the differential diagnosis of pulmonary disease (Table 57.1). Specific physical examination findings of cavitary pulmonary disease are infrequent; cavitary lung disease is primarily a radiographic diagnosis.

A cavity is a gas-containing space within the lung parenchyma surrounded by a wall greater than 1 mm thick; the wall usually is irregular in contour. This wall thickness distinguishes cavities from air cysts and bullae that are thin-walled structures usually due to degenerative, inflammatory, or other noninfectious causes. The term *abscess* is generally used to refer to lesions of infectious origin filled with pus or inflammatory debris. A fluid-filled abscess has the radiographic appearance of a homogenous opacity indistinguishable from a solid mass or hematoma; only when the liquefied contents of a lesion drain into the bronchial tree or pleural space does the cavity become visible. Cavities may be partially filled with necrotic lung tissue, blood, pus, or fungal hyphae. Cavities may be large or small, thin or thick-walled, single or multiple. Each of these radiographic features may be valuable in differential diagnosis.

This definition of a cavity emphasizes the central features of the pathogenesis of most cavitary lesions. Cavity formation is most commonly the end result of severe inflammatory, infectious, or neoplastic lung diseases that cause tissue necrosis by ischemia, direct toxic effects of the offending microorganism or its products, or indirect effects due to the products of host–pathogen interactions such as cytokines. Drainage of the necrotic lesion results in an air-filled space or cavity.

The most common causes of cavitary pulmonary disease are infectious diseases. Mycobacteria, staphylococci, gram-negative bacilli, and fungi frequently result in lung necrosis and formation of cavities. Tuberculosis (TB) is probably the most common cause of cavitary lung disease globally. In the United States pyogenic lung abscesses, endemic deep mycoses, and necrotizing bacterial pneumonia are common etiologies. Viruses, rickettsiae, and mycoplasmas generally do not cause necrotizing pneumonia and cavity formation.

The initial evaluation of patients with cavitary lung disease should include a complete history and physical examination including travel, exposure, occupational, and recreational histories, review of chest X-rays, and appropriate sputum examinations and cultures. Identification of host factors such as HIV infection, prior TB, emphysema, and chronic treatment with glucocorticosteroids or other immunosuppressive medications is important in shifting the differential diagnosis toward certain diseases. Additional diagnostic procedures such as computerized chest tomography, skin tests, serologic testing, fiberoptic bronchoscopy, transthoracic needle aspiration, and transbronchial or open lung biopsy should be individualized based on initial diagnostic impressions.

### Radiographic Differential Diagnosis

Cavitary lesions can be described based upon their size, location, number, wall thickness, appearance of their inner wall, and contents. Although these features are not pathognomonic for any single entity, a number of useful etiologic associations can be made. Apical infiltrates are most common in mycobacterial or chronic fungal infections. Aspiration pneumonia and lung abscesses most commonly occur in gravity-dependent lung segments. Septic emboli appear as peripheral lesions.

Maximum wall thickness on chest X-ray is useful in discriminating benign from neoplastic etiologies of solitary pulmonary cavities. In one prospective series, 95% of solitary cavities without surrounding infiltrates and a maximum wall thickness of 4 mm or less were due to benign causes whereas 84% of lesions with a maximum wall thickness of 16 mm or greater were malignant neoplasms. Thick cavity walls are typical of acute lung abscess, primary lung cancer, pulmonary metastases, and Wegener's granulomatosis. Thin-walled lesions are frequent in coccidioidomycosis, infected bullae, and post-traumatic lung cysts. The inner wall of the cavity appears thick and nodular in primary lung cancer and "shaggy" in acute lung abscess and Wegener's granulomatosis and is smooth in most other diseases. An air-meniscus sign or irregularly shaped mass visible within a cavity may indicate the presence of a mycetoma, blood clot, or sloughed necrotic lung tissue in the cavity. Solitary lesions are suggestive of primary lung cancer, pyogenic lung abscess, and post-traumatic lung cyst. Multiple lesions often are present with necrotizing pyogenic pneumonia, septic pulmonary embolism, Wegener's granulomatosis, metastatic cancer, coccidioidomycosis, and other chronic fungal and mycobacterial diseases (Table 57.1).

The presence and characteristics of pulmonary infiltrates associated with cavitary lesions are extremely helpful in differential diagnosis (Table 57.2). Isolated cavitary lesions with little surrounding lung infiltrate or fibrosis are characteristic of primary or metastatic pulmonary neoplasms, vasculitis, and immunologically mediated lung diseases. Lung abscesses and cavitating pyogenic pneumonias originate as areas of acute necrosis within preexisting alveolar (air space) infiltrates and thus usually present as cavities within infiltrates. In chronic lung abscess, surrounding infiltrates may resolve leaving single or multiple cavities.

Air space consolidation surrounding a cavity is indicative of acute tissue edema, pneumonia, inflammation, or hemorrhage. This pattern must be distinguished from fibrocavitary disease. Fibrocavitary disease refers to a radiographic pattern of pul-

**Table 57.1** Causes of single and multiple pulmonary cavities

| | Infectious diseases | Developmental lesions | Neoplasms | Inflammatory diseases | Miscellaneous diseases |
|---|---|---|---|---|---|
| SINGLE LESIONS | Aspergillosis<br>Coccidioidomycosis<br>Histoplasmosis<br>Nocardiosis<br>Putrid lung abscess | Bronchogenic cyst<br>Pulmonary sequestration | Primary lung cancer<br>Pulmonary metastases (usually multiple) | Rheumatoid nodule<br>Wegener's granulomatosis (usually multiple) | Bland pulmonary infarct<br>Pneumatocele (postinfectious or traumatic) |
| MULTIPLE LESIONS | Aspergillosis<br>Atypical mycobacterial disease<br>Blastomycosis<br>Coccidioidomycosis<br>Cryptococcosis<br>Hisotplasmosis<br>Necrotizing bacterial pneumonia (staph, gram-negative bacilli, anaerobes)<br>Tuberculosis | Cystic adenomatoid malformation<br>Diaphragmatic herniae | Lymphoma<br>Pulmonary metastases | Rheumatoid nodule<br>Wegener's granulomatosis | Pneumatocele (postinfectious) or traumatic)<br>Sarcoidosis (rare)<br>Silicosis (must exclude TB) |

monary infiltrates characterized by nodular densities, linear fibrous scars, volume loss due to scarring and contraction of lung tissue, and cavitation. Fibrocavitary disease indicates chronic inflammation and lung necrosis of weeks to months in duration and is typical of chronic necrotizing infections such as TB and the endemic mycoses.

Pseudocavitation may occur when pneumonia and consolidation involve areas of lung surrounding bullae or ectatic airways. The air-filled bullous lesions become visible when outlined by surrounding areas of consolidation and simulate the radiographic appearance of cavitation. This pattern of "emphysema pneumonia" may be mistaken for necrotizing pneumonia or TB.

As with single cavities, the most common causes of multiple pulmonary cavities are infectious diseases. Multiple cavities due to infectious diseases usually manifest as cavitary lesions within pulmonary infiltrates. The rapid appearance of cavitation in alveolar infiltrates suggests necrotizing bacterial pneumonia; multiple cavities with associated fibronodular lesions, scarring, and volume shrinkage indicate chronic inflammation and are suggestive of mycobacterial and fungal infections.

**Table 57.2** Roentgenographic differential diagnosis of cavitary lung disease based on presence and characteristics of adjacent pulmonary infiltrate

| | No surrounding pulmonary infiltrate | Surrounding pulmonary infiltrate (air space consolidation) | Surrounding fibronodular lesions |
|---|---|---|---|
| INFECTIOUS ETIOLOGIES | Chronic lung abscess<br>Coccidioidomycosis<br>Echinococcal cyst | Aspergillosis and other saprophytic fungal infections (acute)<br>Actinomycosis<br>Aspiration pneumonia/acute lung abscess<br>Cystic fibrosis (pseudocavitation due to consolidation surrounding areas of bronchiectasis)<br>Endemic mycoses<br>Infected bullae (pseudocavitation)<br>Necrotizing pyogenic pneumonia<br>Nocardiosis<br>Septic pulmonary embolism | Aspergillosis and other saprophytic fungal infections (chronic)<br>Atypical mycobacterial infections<br>Endemic mycoses<br>Melioidosis<br>Tuberculosis |
| NONINFECTIOUS ETIOLOGIES | Bronchogenic cyst<br>Cystic adenomatoid<br>Diaphragmatic herniae<br>Eosinophilic granuloma<br>Metastatic cancer (frequently from squamous cell carcinomas)<br>Necrobiotic rheumatoid nodules<br>Primary lung cancer<br>Traumatic pneumatocele<br>Wegener's granulomatosis | Bland pulmonary embolism with infarction (rare)<br>Lymphoma<br>Pulmonary sequestration | Ankylosing spondylitis (apical lesions)<br>Sarcoidosis (rare)<br>Silicosis (rare; must exclude TB) |

Multiple discrete cavitating nodules with little surrounding pulmonary infiltration are highly suggestive of metastatic malignancy. The borders of these lesions usually are sharply circumscribed and there is a significant predilection for the lower lobes. Squamous cell carcinomas of the head and neck, esophagus and cervix, and adenocarcinomas of the gastrointestinal tract account for approximately two-thirds and one-third of these lesions, respectively. Metastatic melanoma, osteosarcoma, and lymphoma are rarer etiologies. The presence of multiple small cavitating and noncavitating peripheral pulmonary nodules with asymmetrical hilar or mediastinal lymphadenopathy is highly suggestive of lymphoma.

## Noninfectious Causes of Cavitary Lung Disease

Cavitation has been reported to occur in 2%–15% of primary lung cancers; greater than 90% of these are squamous cell carcinomas. Pathologically, cavitation in neoplastic masses represents central necrosis of tumors that have compromised their vascular supply. These lesions typically are thick-walled without surrounding pulmonary infiltrates. Primary lung cancer also may present with cavitary lung disease due to postobstructive pneumonia and lung abscess formation distal to a bronchus that is partially obstructed by tumor. Metastatic cancer may occasionally appear as multiple cavitating nodules or masses with little surrounding infiltrate.

Systemic vasculitides such as Wegener's granulomatosis, vascular processes such as bland pulmonary embolism with infarction, and developmental anomalies including bronchogenic cysts, diaphragmatic herniae, and pulmonary sequestrations also may present with cavitary lesions. Other noninfectious etiologies of cavitary lung disease that must be considered in the differential diagnosis of cavitary pulmonary disease are listed in Table 57.2. The absence of fever (in nonimmunosuppressed patients) and peripheral leukocytosis is suggestive of noninfectious etiologies of cavitary pulmonary disease.

## Specific Infectious Etiologies of Cavitary Lung Disease

### Cavitary lung disease in bacterial pneumonia

Most common respiratory viruses (in the nonimmunosuppressed host), chlamydiae, mycoplasmas, and common encapsulated bacteria such as the pneumococcus and *H. influenzae* can cause extensive, severe acute bronchopneumonia (or in the case of *S. pneumoniae* lobar pneumonia) but rarely result in cavity formation. The presence or evolution of cavitation on chest radiographs, therefore, can serve as an important clue in narrowing the differential diagnosis of the etiology of pneumonia in individual patients. Certain bacteria such as *Staphylococcus aureus*, gram-negative enteric bacilli including *Klebsiella pneumoniae*, *Pseudomonas aeruginosa*, and *Escherichia coli*, and anaerobes typically produce acute necrotizing pneumonia and pulmonary cavitation. Cavitation is unusual in normal hosts with *Legionella* species pneumonia but occurs in 13%–70% of cases in immunocompromised and renal transplant patients. The diagnosis and management of clinically important representative infectious diseases causing cavitary pulmonary disease will be discussed in the remaining sections of this chapter. Chapters 38–42 provide detailed information regarding treatment of specific infections.

### Pyogenic lung abscess secondary to aspiration pneumonia

#### Pathogenesis

Putrid lung abscesses begin as multiple areas of tissue necrosis and microabscesses in regions of consolidation secondary to anaerobic or mixed aerobic–anaerobic aspiration pneumonia. The microabscesses may coalesce to form a larger cavity and drain intrabronchially, creating a visible air-filled cavity within the infiltrate (Figure 57.1). With time or treatment, the surrounding

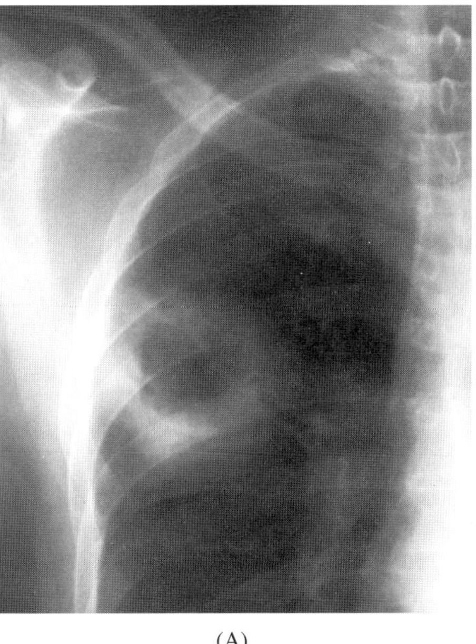

(A)

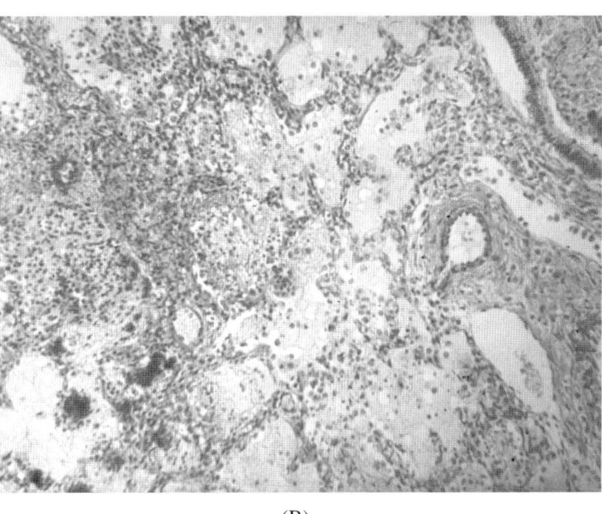

(B)

**Fig. 57.1** Pyogenic lung abscess. Representative (*A*) chest X-ray and (*B*) photomicrograph of early lung abscess showing destruction of normal alveolar architecture and multiple microabscesses (100×, hematoxylin and eosin).

pulmonary infiltrate may clear, leaving only the cavity with its thick fibrous wall visible. The role of aspiration of infected oropharyngeal secretions in the genesis of pyogenic lung abscess is widely accepted. This role is well supported by observations including the production of lung abscess following intratracheal inoculation of anaerobic microorganisms in animal models, the frequent association of severe periodontal disease with anaerobic pleuropulmonary disease, the frequent occurrence of these infections in gravity-dependent pulmonary segments, and the frequent association of conditions such as alcoholism or seizures leading to impairment of normal upper airway reflexes protective against aspiration. The nature and volume of the aspirated inoculum material also are important contributing factors. Minor episodes of silent aspiration are frequent events although they do not often lead to pneumonia. In one study using radiolabeled tracer instilled into the posterior nasopharynx during sleep, silent aspiration occurred in 70% of subjects with a depressed sensorium due to metabolic or cerebrovascular disease and in 45% of healthy volunteers. The volume of material aspirated into the lung during these silent aspiration episodes is small and efficiently cleared by cough, mucociliary transport and other local pulmonary defenses. The aspiration of larger volumes of material with increased bacterial burden due to concomitant pyorrhea or oropharyngeal colonization is presumed to overwhelm these defenses and establish a nidus for bacterial replication and progressive pneumonia.

### Clinical manifestations

The clinical presentation of aspiration pneumonia and lung abscess is variable. Many patients present with acute fever, productive cough, and chest pain similar to other pyogenic pneumonias. Rigors are uncommon. A chronic presentation with several weeks to months of chronic cough with low-grade fever, anemia and weight loss, and an indolent clinical course also is frequent.

Due to the central role of aspiration in its pathogenesis, pyogenic lung abscesses most commonly occur in gravity-dependent lung segments. As most episodes of aspiration occur with the individual in the supine position, pyogenic lung abscesses show a marked predilection for the posterior segments of the upper lobes and the superior segments of the lower lobes. Because pyogenic lung abscesses develop as areas of necrosis within acute pulmonary infiltrates, they lack the surrounding fibrosis, linear scarring, pleural thickening, and other signs of longstanding inflammation and volume loss typical of chronic necrotizing infections such as TB. One to 2 weeks usually is necessary for progression from an acute infiltrate to the appearance on chest X-ray of a distinct cavity with air-fluid levels. Patients with chronic symptoms are more likely to present with thick-walled cavities and foul-smelling sputum.

### Diagnosis

Pyogenic lung abscesses are usually anaerobic or mixed aerobic-anaerobic infections reflecting their origin in material aspirated from the oropharynx. Anaerobic organisms were the sole isolates recovered in one-half of a series of 193 cases of aspiration pneumonia and lung abscess; mixed anaerobic and aerobic species were recovered from the remainder. *Fusobacterium nucleatum*, *Bacteroides melaninogenicus*, and peptostreptococci were the most common anaerobes isolated. Since these organisms constitute normal flora of the upper respiratory tract, it is difficult to make a specific etiologic diagnosis using expectorated sputum or routine bronchoscopic specimens. Techniques such as transtracheal aspiration (TTA) formerly used to obtain uncontaminated lower respiratory secretions for culture are rarely performed today. Newer bronchoscopic methods combining the use of double lumen protected brushes with appropriate aerobic and anaerobic transport media and quantitative culture may be helpful; however, their diagnostic accuracy is not as well documented as TTA or transthoracic needle aspiration. Bronchoscopy is rarely essential for the management of lung abscess unless patients are failing antibiotic therapy.

### Treatment

Penicillin G was formerly the drug of choice for the treatment of pyogenic lung abscess. Prolonged treatment was necessary with penicillin, however, overall outcomes were good. Reports of increased in vitro resistance of common anaerobic pathogens to penicillin and improved cure rates in randomized studies comparing clindamycin and penicillin for the treatment of community-acquired putrid lung abscess have led to the current widespread practice of using clindamycin as the initial antimicrobial agent in severely ill patients with lung abscess. The combination of ampicillin and sulbactam is a reasonable alternative.

### Complications

Aspiration pneumonia and lung abscess frequently transgress the pleural space, resulting in complicated effusion or empyema. Rupture of a focus of necrotizing pneumonia into the pleural space may result in pyopneumothorax with a visible air-fluid level in the pleural space. Pyopneumothorax must be distinguished from air-fluid levels occurring within lung abscesses as the former requires chest tube drainage or decortication for successful treatment as well as antibiotic therapy. On plain chest X-ray, air-fluid levels in empyema tend to be longer than those in lung abscess, generally extend to the chest wall, and form an obtuse angle with the adjacent pleura. Empyemas have an oval appearance whereas abscesses are round. Chest CT scanning is frequently useful in distinguishing between empyema and lung abscess in some, but not all cases where the plain chest X-ray film findings are equivocal (see Chapter 59). The penetration and activity of antimicrobial agents into such empyema spaces is poor. Early thoracentesis to exclude empyema formation is indicated whenever pleural effusion complicates aspiration pneumonia or lung abscess. If gross pus, fluid with visible organisms on gram stain, or fluid with pH less than 7.20 is recovered, prompt drainage by tube thoracostomy should be attempted. Chest tube drainage may be unsuccessful if pleural loculations or a fibrous peel have already formed; thoracotomy with decortication may be required in these cases.

### Bronchoscopy

The role and timing of bronchoscopy and other drainage procedures in the management of lung abscess are controversial. There are three general indications for bronchoscopy—exclusion of concomitant pulmonary malignancy, bacteriological diagnosis, and internal drainage of an abscess cavity. The first indication is the most widely accepted. Between 8% and 17% of patients with cavitating pulmonary infiltrates or lung abscesses have been found to have an underlying primary lung cancer; the frequency of associated lung cancer increases with age. An anterior location of the cavity is more common in patients with underlying primary lung cancer than benign abscess; however, this finding is not absolutely specific. Diagnostic fiberoptic bronchoscopy is indicated in cases highly suspicious for malignancy or those cases failing to respond to antimicrobial therapy. Early bronchoscopy with topical airway anesthesia is not without risk; several case reports document severe morbidity due to intrabronchial spillage and spread of pus into noninvolved lung regions, and thus early bronchoscopy cannot be routinely recommended for all patients with apparent putrid lung abscess. When performed in patients who fail to respond to medical therapy, bronchoscopy has a high yield for the diagnosis of bronchogenic carcinoma and also allows identification and removal of aspirated nonradiopaque foreign bodies that may be interfering with bronchial drainage.

The role of therapeutic bronchoscopy, percutaneous drainage procedures, and surgical resection is much more controversial, with a sharp dichotomy of opinions between the medical and surgical literature regarding patient selection and tolerable waiting periods for clinical improvement before surgical treatment is necessary. The effectiveness of bronchoscopic manipulation in promoting bronchial drainage is questionable, associated with significant risks, and of unproven benefit. Occasionally therapeutic bronchoscopy may allow laser photoresection or brachytherapy catheter placement for treatment of nonresponsive lung abscesses occurring distal to obstructing neoplasms.

Prolonged appropriate antimicrobial therapy will result in healing and eventual closure of most pyogenic lung abscesses. The clinician must be patient—cavity closure may require 3 or more mo of oral antimicrobial treatment. A prolonged course of antibiotics is advisable before considering surgical treatment in nontoxic patients. Surgical treatment may be required for true medical failures. Medical failures with inadequate pulmonary function reserve for lung resection surgery or who are prohibitive operative risks for other reasons may be treated alternatively with percutaneous drainage using either a CT-guided or fluoroscopically guided tube or by the creation of a surgical fistula into the lung abscess cavity.

## Staphylococcal pneumonia

### Pathogenesis

Among the common bacteria causing community acquired pneumonia, only *Staphylococcus aureus* is frequently associated with tissue necrosis, cavitation, and abscess formation. This is due to the action of toxins (e.g., $\alpha$ toxin) with necrotizing activity that are produced by *S. aureus*; *S. aureus* is a more frequent cause of pneumonia in children than adults and can produce fulminant pneumonia with the development of multiple abscesses and pneumatoceles.

Secondary staphylococcal pneumonia is a major cause of mortality during influenza pandemics; pneumonia may develop in the setting of impaired pulmonary defenses resulting from severe inflammation and tracheobronchiolitis due to influenza. An extremely high mortality rate (up to 50%) has been reported in pregnant women developing staphylococcal pneumonia following influenza; the reasons underlying this association are unknown.

Staphylococcal pneumonia also may develop from hematogenous spread from another site of infection. When cavitation is peripheral or multiple, the possibility of septic embolization from the heart must be considered.

### Clinical manifestations

Staphylococcal pneumonia usually presents as an acute pneumonia with serious clinical toxicity and prostration, high fever, and productive cough. Rigors are said to be less common than in pneumococcal pneumonia. Subacute or chronic presentations may be seen in hematogenous staphylococcal pneumonia and in elderly patients.

The chest X-ray appearance of an acute, rapidly progressive, necrotizing pneumonia with multiple large abscesses or pneumatoceles is highly suggestive, although not pathognomonic, of staphylococcal pneumonia. Pneumatoceles are lucent areas appearing in areas of dense consolidation due to bacterial pneumonia. Pneumatoceles are classically seen as a complication of staphylococcal pneumonia in children, where they are an important clue to the underlying etiology of the pneumonia. The early radiographic appearance of a pneumatocele may be indistinguishable from an abscess; pneumatoceles are, however, often multiple, occur during the healing phase of pneumonia when the patient is clinically improving, and tend to progressively enlarge. Pneumatoceles represent dilated airspaces rather than areas of lung necrosis, rarely produce clinically significant symptoms by themselves, and tend to resolve spontaneously over weeks to months. Peripheral cavitation is suggestive of septic embolization from an infected endovascular source.

Parapneumonic pleural effusions complicate staphylococcal pneumonia in 40% of adult cases and one-half of these effusions progress to empyemas. Prompt diagnostic thoracocentesis is indicated to evaluate this possibility followed by immediate pleural drainage if pus is found.

### Diagnosis

The etiological role of staphylococci in pneumonia may be difficult to confirm as *S. aureus* frequently colonizes the upper airway, especially in hospitalized or immunocompromised individuals. Numerous polymorphonuclear leukocytes and predominant plump gram positive cocci in clusters on sputum gram stain and a sputum culture growing *S. aureus* as the sole or predominant organism are highly suggestive. Isolation of the organism from blood cultures or pleural fluid is diagnostic.

### Treatment

Most staphylococcal species produce $\beta$-lactamase. Beta-lactamase resistant penicillins such as oxacillin or nafcillin are the drugs of choice for susceptible organisms. First-generation cephalosporins such as cephalothin are useful alternative agents (see Chapters 27–29 and 38). In many areas, the prevalence of methicillin resistant *S. aureus* (MRSA) has increased significantly in recent years; treatment with intravenous vancomycin is necessary in this instance. In order to promote a cure and lessen the likelihood of relapse, treatment is usually prolonged for at least 4 wk, particularly if there is a complicating bacteremia or the pneumonia is secondary to hematogenous spread.

## Septic pulmonary embolism

Severe inflammation and infection of adjacent lung tissue due to trapping of infected emboli originating from right-sided endocarditis or suppurative thrombophlebitis may result in pulmonary infarction. Septic embolism most often occurs in intravenous drug users and individuals with indwelling vascular access devices such as central venous catheters (including Hickman and Broviac catheters) and hemodialysis shunts. Staphylococci are the most frequently isolated pathogens. Septic pulmonary emboli have a very characteristic radiographic appearance and temporal evolution. Septic pulmonary emboli present as solitary or multiple rounded or flame-shaped peripheral infiltrates which undergo rapid central cavitation (Fig. 57.2). Cavitating and noncavitating lesions usually are present simultaneously as the lesions are of different ages. Lesions are more common in the lower lobes due to higher pulmonary blood flow to the lung bases. In cases of massive or repeated embolization, the lesions may coalesce to form large dense pulmonary infiltrates.

Most patients with septic pulmonary embolization will have positive blood cultures and they must be evaluated for possible right-sided endocarditis (see Chapter 66). Treatment of septic embolism includes appropriate antimicrobial therapy with bactericidal antibiotics specific for isolated organisms for 2 to 4 wk, removal of infected endovascular devices, and surgical debridement of suppurative thrombophlebitis. Systemic heparin therapy is not recommended.

## Necrotizing gram-negative pneumonia

### Pathogenesis

Parenchymal lung necrosis is a common clinical feature of all gram-negative bacillary pneumonias. Any of the Enterobacteriaceae and especially *Pseudomonas aeruginosa* can produce necrotizing bronchopneumonia and pulmonary cavitation due to the formation and action of proteolytic toxins. These microorganisms generally produce serious life-threatening pneumonia in elderly or neutropenic patients and those with serious underlying illnesses such as alcoholism or diabetes mellitus. Elderly nursing home residents, diabetics, alcoholics, and patients with chronic obstructive pulmonary disease frequently have chronic oropharyngeal colonization with gram-negative enteric bacilli. Acutely ill and severely debilitated patients in tertiary hospitals and intensive care units also may become rapidly colonized with these pathogens due to alterations in oral epithelial cell surface adhesion receptors that prevent removal of these organisms by normal mechanisms. The most common mechanism for the development of gram-negative pneumonia is aspiration of infected oropharyngeal or refluxed gastric secretions. Hematogenous spread from the genitourinary or gastrointestinal tracts also may occur. Aerogenous spread from infected respiratory therapy equipment is now primarily of historical interest. Interestingly, mucoid *P. aeruginosa* and *P. cepacia* are frequently present in enormous numbers in the ectatic airways of patients with cystic fibrosis but uncommonly produce invasive necrotizing pneumonia in these patients.

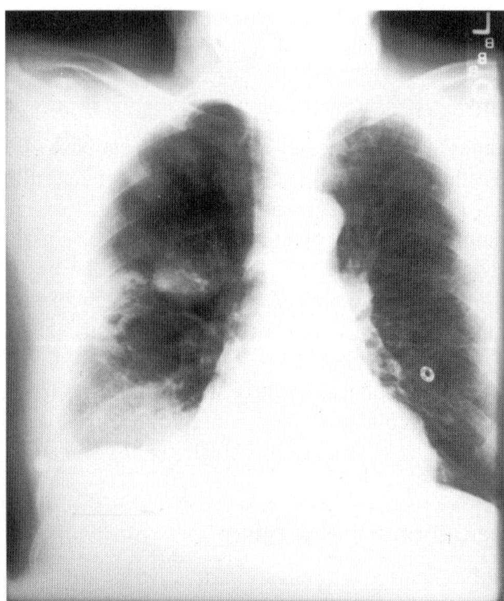

**Fig. 57.2** Septic emboli due to staphylococcal tricuspid endocarditis. Note differing appearance and presence of cavitation in lesions of different ages.

### Clinical manifestations

The clinical presentation of gram-negative bacillary pneumonias is indistinguishable from other severe acute bacterial pneumonias. Fever, rigors, dyspnea, productive cough, and pleuritic chest pain are variably present. Physical findings and sputum production may be minimal or absent in granulocytopenic patients, a high-risk group for overwhelming gram-negative pneumonia.

The most frequent radiographic presentation of gram-negative pneumonia is patchy focal or diffuse bronchopneumonia with subsequent cavitation. Parapneumonic pleural effusions have a high predilection for progression to empyema. Classically, *Klebsiella pneumoniae* pneumonia presents as an acute lobar pneumonia with dense upper lobe consolidation and bulging interlobar fissures due to increased lobar volume. Rapid cavitation often ensues and lung abscess formation occurs in 40%–50% of patients with *K. pneumoniae* pneumonia. *Pseudomonas aeruginosa* pneumonia (Fig. 57.3) characteristically presents as a diffuse lower lobe necrotizing pneumonia with multiple small abscesses.

### Diagnosis

Unfortunately, the radiographic and clinical manifestations of the gram-negative bacillary pneumonias are relatively nonspecific. The classic radiographic findings described above occur in a mi-

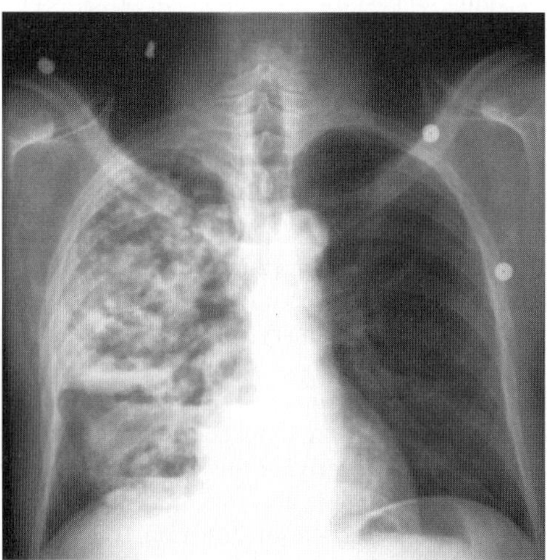

**Fig. 57.3** *Pseudomonas* pneumonia with extensive lung necrosis.

nority of cases. Sputum gram staining is also of limited diagnostic specificity due to the frequent colonization of hosts at risk and contamination of sputum specimens by endogenous microflora in the upper airway. Gram stains exhibiting <10 epithelial cells and >25 neutrophils per low-power field indicate a deep respiratory specimen likely to be representative of the lower respiratory tract. The likelihood that gram-negative organisms are etiologic agents in pneumonia is increased if gram-negative bacilli constitute a predominance of visible organisms or if intracellular bacilli are visible within phagocytes in adequate specimens of deep respiratory secretions. Sputum cultures must be correlated with sputum gram stain results for optimal diagnostic assessment; reliance on sputum culture alone may lead to overdiagnosis of gram-negative pneumonia. A definitive diagnosis of gram-negative bacillary pneumonia can be made only by the isolation of the pathogen from blood or pleural fluid cultures or (more controversially) by the recovery of greater than $10^3$ to $10^5$ colony-forming units per ml of the organism on protected bronchial brush or bronchoalveolar lavage (BAL) fluid specimens.

Sputum examination for elastin fibers after digestion with 40% KOH also may be helpful in confirming the significance of sputum gram stain and culture results for the diagnosis of pneumonia in immunosuppressed and intubated, mechanically ventilated patients. Detection of elastin fibers with their characteristic "split end" appearance is highly correlated with the presence of necrotizing pneumonia and is simple, quick, and inexpensive to perform.

#### Treatment

Gram-negative bacillary pneumonia is associated with a high mortality. The approach to antimicrobial therapy in suspected gram-negative pneumonia must be guided by knowledge of common local pathogens and antimicrobial susceptibility patterns. Broad-spectrum antimicrobial coverage with a third-generation cephalosporin or carbapenem active against *P. aeruginosa* in combination with an aminoglycoside is a reasonable initial approach pending culture and sensitivity results. Additional anaerobic or staphylococcal coverage should be added if warranted by the clinical situation. Empyemas require chest tube drainage as well as appropriate antimicrobial therapy.

### Pulmonary gangrene

Pulmonary gangrene refers to rapid necrosis and sloughing of extensive areas of infected lung tissue resulting in a large cavity containing a mobile necrotic mass. Pulmonary gangrene usually develops in areas of densely consolidated lung as a result of intense local inflammation with vascular thrombosis or compromise. Most reported cases have been due to *K. pneumoniae*, *S. pneumoniae*, *H. influenzae*, *M. tuberculosis*, and *Zygomycetes*. The presence of pulmonary gangrene limits the number of potential etiologic pathogens in the differential diagnosis and is associated with a poor prognosis and frequent need for surgical resection or pleural drainage.

### Pneumococcal pneumonia

Cavitary pulmonary disease is a rare complication of pneumococcal pneumonia occurring in only 1%–2% of cases in clinical series of hospitalized adults. In older series, capsular serotype III was most frequently associated with cavitation although higher serotypes infrequently may cause necrotizing pneumonia. Serotype III is associated with the production of large quantities of capsular polysaccharide and requires the presence of type-specific antibody prior to activation of the alternative complement pathway and efficient phagocytosis of the organism. The role of mixed infections with other organisms capable of producing cavitation, such as anaerobes, cannot be excluded in many earlier reports.

## Pulmonary Cavitation Due to Other Uncommon Bacterial Pathogens

### Actinomycosis

#### Pathogenesis

*Actinomyces* species are gram-positive obligate or facultative anaerobic filamentous microbes normally inhabiting the human oral cavity. Most human disease is caused by *A. israelii*; colonization of the oropharynx is common in individuals with poor dental hygiene. Invasive actinomycosis has only rarely been described in edentulous patients.

Intrathoracic involvement is seen in 15%–20% of all patients with actinomycosis and occurs by either contiguous spread from cervical or facial disease or more commonly by aspiration of infected oropharyngeal material similar to the pathogenesis of anaerobic or mixed aerobic/anaerobic lung abscesses. Presenting clinical symptoms include cough, fever, weight loss, and chest pain due to chest wall abscess or fistula. The clinical picture usually is one of an indolent lower lobe pneumonia which spreads across the visceral pleura into other lung regions or the pleural space; cavitation with surrounding fibrosis, volume loss, osteomyelitis of adjacent ribs, empyema, and, notably, invasion through the contiguous chest wall (empyema necessitans) with formation of open draining sinus tracts and fistulae are other important suggestive findings. "Wavy" periosteal inflammation involving multiple adjacent ribs without visible empyema is said to pathognomonic of actinomycosis. The most characteristic clinical finding is the drainage of gritty 1–2 mm yellow or brown "sulfur granules" representing tightly packed colonies of the organism in purulent material from an abscess or chest wall sinus. Due to its frequent presentation as a cavitating pulmonary mass, actinomycosis is often initially misdiagnosed as a cavitating pulmonary neoplasm.

#### Diagnosis

The diagnosis of actinomycosis is confirmed by visualization or culture of the organism; no reliable serologic or skin tests are available. *Actinomyces* species are gram-positive filamentous bacteria that also stain well with the Grocott methenamine silver method but not with modified acid-fast stains. As *Actinomyces* species are members of the endogenous oral microflora, it is important to remember that the mere isolation of the organism from a sputum or oral specimen does not establish the diagnosis of invasive actinomycosis; consistent clinical and radiographic findings also must be present.

#### Treatment

Treatment of pulmonary actinomycosis requires prolonged treatment with penicillin or tetracycline. Empyemas must be drained.

Surgical resection of severely compromised lung tissue or chest wall sinus tracts must be considered on an individual basis.

## Nocardiosis

### Pathogenesis

Nocardiosis is an opportunistic infection associated with lymphoreticular neoplasms, renal and other solid-organ transplantation, alveolar proteinosis, and chronic glucocorticosteroid use. Human infection occurs primarily via the respiratory tract. Nocardiosis produces suppurative tissue necrosis and abscess formation typical of pyogenic infections. *Nocardia asteroides* is the predominant human pathogen but disease is occasionally caused by *N. brasiliensis* or *N. caviae*.

### Clinical manifestations

Common radiographic lesions include solitary or multiple pulmonary masses or infiltrates, air-space pneumonia, pleural thickening, and chest wall involvement. Central nervous system involvement including brain abscess occurs in up to one-third of patients. Subcutaneous abscesses also may occur. Pulmonary nocardiosis often presents as an indolent or subacute chest syndrome with chronic nonproductive cough with or without pleurisy. Nocardiosis is often mistaken for bronchogenic carcinoma, pulmonary TB, or the endemic pulmonary mycoses given the chronic clinical course and overlapping radiographic features.

### Diagnosis

The diagnosis of pulmonary nocardiosis is made by visualization or culture of the organism in respiratory secretions or tissue biopsies. The organism is a weakly gram-positive aerobic rod with a beaded appearance that forms branching filaments 5–10 $\mu$m in length. Examination of expectorated sputum has limited diagnostic sensitivity; transthoracic needle aspirates, bronchoscopic washings, and transbronchial or open lung biopsy have higher yields. Modified acid-fast staining is the preferred method for demonstrating the organism in deep respiratory specimens. The organism is not stained by routine hematoxylin and eosin stains in tissue biopsies but is well demonstrated by modified gram stain or Grocott silver stain. The organism is typically very slow growing, and it is essential that the clinician communicate directly with the microbiology laboratory when nocardial infection is suspected so that cultures can be observed for up to 3 weeks. Sulfur granules have occasionally been reported in clinical materials of patients with nocardiosis as well as actinomycosis.

### Treatment

Sulfonamides are the drugs of choice for the treatment of nocardial infections; prolonged treatment is necessary. Oral sulfonamides are well absorbed and adequate in most instances. Minocycline, amikacin, and imipenem also have excellent activity against the organism. The optimal duration of treatment is unknown. Relapses rarely occur in patients treated for 3 or more mo with sulfonamides. Drainage of metastatic nocardial abscesses is important for the prevention and treatment of late relapses.

## Melioidosis

*Pseudomonas pseudomallei*, a small gram-negative water-borne saprophytic bacillus, causes melioidosis, a necrotizing pneumonia endemic in tropical regions between 20° north and south latitude especially Southeast Asia. The chronic form of the disease may resemble reactivation TB with upper-lobe fibrocavitary lesions, fever, cough, weight loss, and hemoptysis. The diagnosis is made by visualizing small bipolar gram-negative bacilli on smears of respiratory secretions, culture, and indirect hemagglutination serology. Prolonged treatment with ceftazidime or combinations including trimethoprim-sulfamethoxazole, imipenem, or doxycycline are effective.

## Mycobacterial Diseases

## Tuberculosis

TB is the prototypical pulmonary infection associated with chronic tissue destruction and pulmonary cavitation. TB produces disease in many organ systems; however, most serious morbidity is due to pulmonary disease. Approximately one-third of the world's population is infected with *Mycobacterium tuberculosis* and about 2.8 million deaths each year are due to this pathogen.

### Pathogenesis

TB is transmitted by the aerogenous spread of *M. tuberculosis*, a small beaded acid-fast bacillus, in droplet nuclei created by coughing or expectoration of infected pulmonary secretions. After reaching the alveolar space, in the nonimmune host, the organism is phagocytosed by alveolar macrophages, where it multiplies intracellularly. Spread to local lymph nodes and a transient diffuse mycobacteremia follow with wide dissemination of the organism. In the majority of patients an effective cell-mediated immune response by coordinated macrophage–T-lymphocyte interactions develops in response to mycobacterial antigens. This is marked by clonal proliferation of antigen-specific lymphocytes and the production of cytokines such as interferon-$\gamma$ and granulocyte-monocyte colony-stimulating factor. These promote activation of macrophages, formation of tissue granulomata, and control of the infection without evident disease in immunocompetent individuals. The appearance of specific cell-mediated immunity is temporally associated with the development of cutaneous delayed-type hypersensitivity responses (positive tuberculin skin test). In more than 90% of normal hosts, *M. tuberculosis* infection is adequately controlled, leaving only the positive tuberculin reaction and (less commonly) radiographically visible calcification of thoracic lymph nodes and the initial site of parenchymal infection (Ghon complex) as stigmata of primary infection. In a few persons the primary infection progresses to active TB typically with lower lung field infiltrates and intrathoracic adenopathy. Only 3%–4% of individuals develop progressive primary TB during the first year after *M. tuberculosis* infection. The risk of progressive primary disease varies with age at the time of infection with *M. tuberculosis*; infants, young adults, and the elderly are at highest risk.

Classically, the development of late TB in the adult has been ascribed to reactivation of residual latent tuberculous foci from earlier primary infection in the presence of waning cell-mediated immunity due to aging or other comorbid illnesses. The lifetime risk of developing active TB after TB infection is approximately 5%–10% in normal individuals. This risk is greatly increased in immunocompromised patients and is highest in HIV-infected subjects who have an estimated 3%–7% annual risk of developing active TB.

### Clinical manifestations

TB presents as a subacute or chronic illness with fever, weight loss, night sweats, pleuritic chest pain, productive cough, anorexia, and weight loss, and less commonly with hemoptysis, suppurative lymphadenitis, and CNS symptoms. Findings on chest examination are frequently limited to localized rales indicative of focal consolidation. Three-fourths of patients with extrapulmonary disease have chest radiographic findings consistent with pulmonary TB.

The radiographic manifestations of pulmonary TB are broad and the subject of many excellent reviews and monographs. There are two basic patterns of disease (Fig. 57.4). Primary TB presents with mid and lower lung field lobar or segmental infiltrates, often with associated hilar or mediastinal lymphadenopathy, pleural effusion, and miliary disease. Infiltrates generally involve one or two lobes and characteristically require months to resolve. Cavitation is infrequent. Lymphadenopathy may occur without visible parenchymal infiltrates. Enlarged hilar lymph nodes also may compress central bronchi, resulting in lobar or segmental atelectasis.

Primary disease patterns have been reported with increased frequency among patients in the later stages of HIV infection. Whether these findings represent an atypical pattern of reactivation in profoundly immunocompromised patients or true progressive primary disease due to exogenous reinfection is controversial and a matter of intense current research interest. Recent analyses of restriction-fragment-length polymorphisms (RFLP) of *M. tuberculosis* isolates from newly diagnosed TB cases in New York City and San Francisco demonstrated clustering of isolates in approximately 40% of cases, suggesting a greater role of recent infection in TB in adults than had been suspected previously, at least in urbanized, industrialized areas of the world.

Typical reactivation TB occurring in the immunocompetent, HIV-noninfected adult patient usually presents with bilateral fibrocavitary infiltrates involving the apical and posterior segments of the upper lobes or the superior segments of the lower lobes. Soft, fluffy opacities and nodular infiltrates with indistinct borders are associated with pulmonary fibrosis, linear scarring, and adjacent pleural thickening or localized empyemata.

Vigorous granulomatous inflammation may lead to caseous necrosis of lung tissue followed by cavitation. Cavitation is a critical event in the natural history of pulmonary TB as the walls of the cavity and its liquefied caseous contents provide an ideal environment for rapid mycobacterial replication. Cavities in pulmonary TB are usually multiple, irregular in size and internal contour, and associated with dense surrounding fibrosis or infiltration; calcified lymph nodes or parenchymal granulomata also may be present. Air-fluid levels are less commonly evident in cavities due to pulmonary TB than to pyogenic lung abscess; however, this rule is not absolute, as up to 20% of cavitary lesions due to pulmonary TB in older series had demonstrable air-fluid levels using plain tomography. Spillover of infected contents from open cavities with intrabronchial spread may result in widespread infiltrates.

### Diagnosis

These radiographic features are highly suggestive although not pathognomonic for TB. Fungal infections such as histoplasmosis, blastomycosis, cryptococcosis, and chronic necrotizing aspergillosis and chronic bacterial infections including melioidosis also must be considered. The diagnosis of TB is made by the demonstration of typical acid-fast bacilli on smears and cultures from infected body secretions or tissues. Up to 25%–50% of patients with active TB have negative tuberculin skin tests. A positive tuberculin skin test only indicates infection by the tubercle bacillus. Serodiagnostic tests for TB have been of little value.

Multiple expectorated or induced sputa should be concentrated

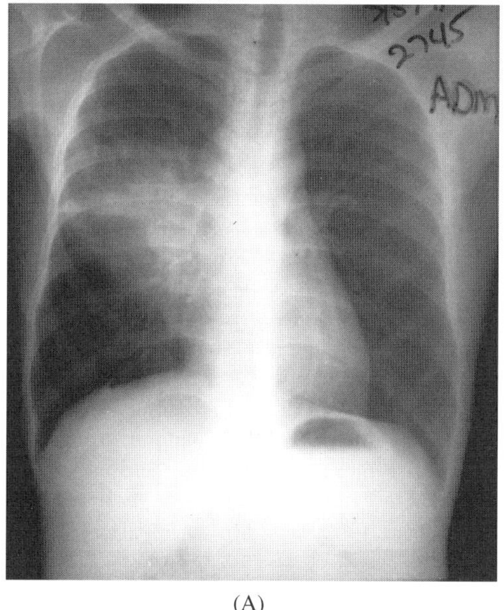

(A)

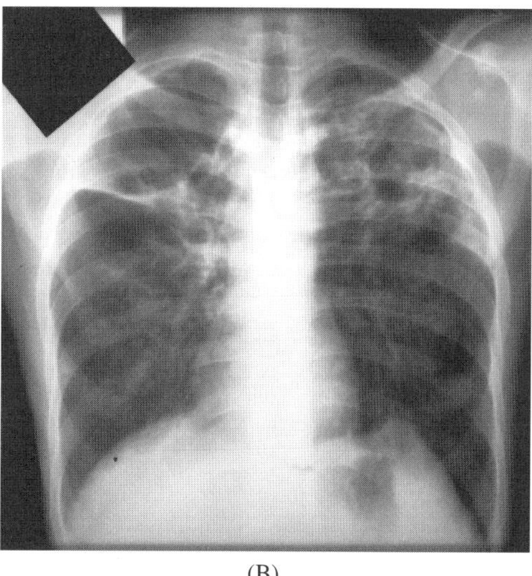

(B)

**Fig. 57.4** Radiographic appearance of (*A*) primary and (*B*) reactivation TB.

and examined via fluorochrome (auramine-rhodamine) or modified carbol fuchsin acid-fast staining methods. The diagnostic yield is slightly higher with overnight collections or early morning sputum specimens. Fluorochrome and carbol fuchsin staining methods have comparable sensitivity; fluorochrome-stained specimens can be reviewed faster and are most valuable in laboratories where many specimens must be screened. Decontaminated and concentrated specimens should be inoculated onto appropriate media and examined weekly for up to 8 wk for visible colonies. Radiometric culture systems (BACTEC) detect $^{14}CO_2$ released from labeled substrate by replicating mycobacteria and decrease the time necessary to obtain positive cultures to 1–3 wk. Mycobacterial culture is essential as approximately 50% of pulmonary TB cases are sputum-smear negative. Detection of mycobacterial antigens or mycobacterial DNA in clinical specimens by enzyme immunoassay and polymerase chain reaction techniques is currently an area of intense research.

Fiberoptic bronchoscopy with brushing, washing, BAL, or transbronchial lung biopsy also has a high diagnostic yield in appropriately selected patients. Transbronchial biopsies demonstrating typical caseating granulomata allow rapid diagnosis and specific treatment. Most patients should be evaluated by smears on expectorated or induced sputum prior to bronchoscopy. It is inadvisable to expose medical staff to infection with TB during invasive diagnostic procedures when the diagnosis can be made by smears or the clinical and radiographic findings warrant empiric antituberculous treatment pending culture results. Bronchoscopic specimens are rarely the sole source of positive AFB smears and cultures. Institution of appropriate respiratory isolation procedures, notification of public health authorities to facilitate contact tracing, rapid examination of expectorated deep respiratory secretions, and consideration of empiric anti-TB therapy pending or in lieu of invasive diagnostic procedures are all important aspects of individualized patient management.

### Treatment

Modern treatment of TB is based on the use of multiple drug regimens to prevent the emergence of drug resistance given in appropriate dosages for adequate periods of time (see Chapter 37). The 1994 American Thoracic Society–Centers for Disease Control and Prevention guidelines for TB treatment are a comprehensive source of information about many aspects of TB chemotherapy. Adequate treatment of TB requires months of therapy; patient adherence with drug treatment is absolutely essential for good clinical outcome and the prevention of acquired drug resistance. Currently available drug susceptibility testing methods usually require several weeks to perform. Therefore, an initial treatment regimen should be selected based on available information about local drug resistance and patient demographics. Previous TB treatment, recent residence in or origin from countries with known high drug resistance rates such as Southeast Asia, or HIV infection or AIDS (particularly with exposure to known drug-resistant TB cases) are the strongest known predictors for drug resistance.

Due to recent increases in reported rates of drug resistance, it is recommended that initial treatment begin with four drugs unless the likelihood of primary drug resistance is negligible ($<2\%$) based on ongoing local drug susceptibility surveillance testing. Excellent cure rates have been obtained with modern short course regimens utilizing 2 mo of daily isoniazid, rifampin, ethambutol, and pyrazinamide followed by 4 mo of daily or two or three times weekly isoniazid and rifampin (if the patient's isolate is found to be susceptible to isoniazid and rifampin). A similar regimen of comparable efficacy that can be administered as directly supervised therapy in the clinic or patient's home consists of isoniazid, rifampin, pyrazinamide, and ethambutol daily for 2 wk followed by these same drugs twice a week for 6 wk and finally twice weekly isoniazid and rifampin for 16 wk. Ethambutol can be discontinued if the patient's isolate is found to be sensitive to isoniazid and rifampin. Nine months of combination therapy with isoniazid and rifampin has comparable efficacy to the 6-mo regimens listed above for the treatment of patients with susceptible organisms.

Major outbreaks of multiple-drug-resistant (MDR) TB recently have been reported in the United States. Drug resistance also appears to be common and may be increasing in other regions including Asia and South America, although data are less complete. MDR TB isolates by definition are resistant to at least isoniazid and rifampin; strains resistant to up to seven primary and secondary drugs have been reported. The clinical and radiographic manifestations of MDR TB are similar to disease caused by drug-susceptible organisms. Treatment of patients with suspected MDR TB is a complex and rapidly evolving area. Adequate respiratory isolation measures to prevent nosocomial spread of such pathogens is critical. Multiple-drug regimens containing older second-line agents such as para-amino salicylic acid and cycloserine, and newer drugs such as amikacin, fluoroquinolones, and $\beta$-lactam–$\beta$-lactamase inhibitor combinations are in clinical use; prolonged treatment is required, the incidence of serious side effects is high, and only limited data on short- and long-term efficacy are available. Cases of suspected MDR TB should be managed in conjunction with expert consultation from physicians skilled in this area.

### TB preventive therapy

Preventive drug therapy is highly beneficial for individuals infected with *M. tuberculosis* who are at significant risk for the development of active TB. Preventive therapy with 6 to 12 mo of isoniazid is approximately 85% effective against the development of active TB in HIV-noninfected individuals and also has been shown to be effective in PPD-positive, HIV-infected persons.

Debate concerning the widespread use of isoniazid preventive therapy has centered on the competing risks of morbidity and mortality from isoniazid (primarily hepatotoxicity) and the risks to the patient and the community from the development of active TB. The risk of hepatotoxicity is clearly age-related; this complication is rare before age 35. Young postpartum women also may be at increased risk for hepatotoxicity. High-risk groups of individuals with positive tuberculin skin tests who should receive preventive therapy regardless of age include known recent skin test converters, HIV-infected persons, and close contacts of newly diagnosed smear-positive TB cases. The effectiveness of preventive drug therapy using non-isoniazid-containing regimens for individuals exposed to MDR TB is unknown.

Comprehensive current recommendations regarding cutpoints for tuberculin skin testing, patient groups who should receive preventive therapy, skin testing and preventive therapy in HIV-infected individuals, and preventive therapy for persons exposed to MDR TB are contained in the 1994 ATS-CDCP guidelines. Three different criteria for defining a "positive" tuberculin skin test (5 TU PPD by intracutaneous [Mantoux] injection) are proposed in these guidelines based on the risk of tuberculous infection and the risk of progression to active TB once infected (Table

**Table 57.3** Definitions of a positive tuberculin skin test in different risk groups

| Risk group | Description | "Positive" PPD |
|---|---|---|
| High | HIV-infected individuals; close contacts of persons with infectious TB; individuals with fibrotic lesions consistent with healed TB on chest X-ray | ≥5 mm |
| Intermediate | Other at risk individuals (see Table 57.4) and infants and children < 4 years of age | ≥10 mm |
| Low | None of the above; persons not in any recognized high risk group or environment | ≥15 mm |

Adapted with permission from American Thoracic Society—Centers for Disease Control and Prevention. Am J Respir Crit Care Med 1994; 149:1359–1374.

57.3). These criteria also have been selected to minimize overtreatment due to false positive skin test reactions in otherwise healthy individuals.

Six to 12 months of daily isoniazid preventive therapy is recommended for PPD-positive individuals in the following groups (Table 57.4). Twelve months of treatment is recommended for HIV-infected individuals. Active tuberculosis must be excluded by clinical, chest radiographic, and sputum (when indicated) examination before initiating isoniazid preventive therapy.

## Pulmonary disease due to atypical mycobacteria

Many species of "atypical" mycobacteria other than *M. tuberculosis* can produce cavitary pulmonary disease in humans. These ubiquitous organisms have lower intrinsic virulence than *M. tuberculosis* and produce invasive disease in persons with underlying structural lung diseases such as bullous emphysema or in immunosuppressed individuals.

Atypical mycobacteria are usually classified based on the rapidity of growth on solid media and production of pigments when incubated in conditions of light or darkness. Atypical mycobacterial species cannot be reliably distinguished from *M. tuberculosis* by AFB smears. Speciation is performed by colonial morphology and biochemical testing of culture isolates; more recently, sensitive and specific rapid DNA probe tests have been developed to identify *M. tuberculosis* complex, *M. avium*, *M. intracellulare*, *M. kansasii*, and *M. gordonae*. Many species have been reported to cause necrotizing pulmonary disease, although a few species account for the bulk of cases. In addition to pulmonary disease, many atypical mycobacteria cause disseminated disease in patients with AIDS. Disease due to representative species will be discussed. The reader is referred to the excellent comprehensive review by Wolinsky for detailed information.

Despite retrospective series claiming subtle differences between the chest radiographic findings in atypical mycobacterial disease and TB, in day-to-day practice the common radiologic findings are indistinguishable. Apical fibrocavitary disease with volume loss is the most common radiographic manifestation of atypical mycobacterial disease.

Atypical mycobacteria may colonize the lower airway, especially in the presence of other chronic lung disease; therefore care must be taken to distinguish invasive disease due to these organisms from colonization. In addition, diagnostic equipment such as bronchoscopes may become contaminated with waterborne atypical mycobacteria if inadequate disinfection procedures are followed; recovery of atypical mycobacteria from

**Table 57.4** Persons for whom isoniazid preventive therapy against TB is recommended

1. HIV-infected individuals and persons suspected of being HIV-infected (actual HIV infection status unknown)
2. Close contacts of newly diagnosed infectious TB cases including PPD (−) children and adolescents who have had close contact with infectious TB cases during the previous 3 mo
3. Recent PPD skin test converters (≥10 mm increase in PPD size within a 2 yr time period in individuals <35 yr old or ≥15 mm increase in PPD size within a 2 yr time period in individuals ≥35 yr old)
4. Patients with medical conditions associated with an increased risk of developing active TB including diabetes mellitus, prolonged glucocorticosteroid or other immunosuppressive therapy, hematologic malignancy, intravenous drug abuse (without concomitant HIV infection), end stage renal disease, and conditions associated with rapid weight loss such as the postgastrectomy state or chronic alcoholism
5. Individuals <35 yr old with PPD ≥10 mm with the following characteristics:
   a. Immigrants from nations in Latin America, Asia, and Africa with a high prevalence of TB
   b. Medically underserved, low-income groups
   c. Residents of long-term care facilities such as prisons, nursing homes, and mental hospitals
6. Individuals <35 yr old with PPD ≥15 mm who have none of these risk factors

Adapted with permission from American Thoracic Society—Centers for Disease Control and Prevention. Am J Respir Crit Care Med 1994; 149:1359–1374.

bronchoscopic specimens must be carefully evaluated for clinical significance. Atypical mycobacteria are frequently resistant to many of the mycobacterial drugs commonly used in the treatment of TB. Drug treatment of pulmonary disease due to atypical mycobacteria is difficult and requires prolonged therapy. Diagnostic criteria for atypical mycobacterial disease in patients with cavitary pulmonary lesions proposed by the American Thoracic Society require the identification of the atypical mycobacterium in smears and moderately heavy growth in culture from *two or more* sputum or bronchoscopic specimens and the exclusion of other possible causes such as TB or the endemic mycoses.

### *M. avium-intracellulare* disease

*M. avium-intracellulare* complex (MAC) are a group of rapidly growing mycobacteria that produce chronic slowly progressive necrotizing pneumonitis in HIV-noninfected patients and disseminated disease in patients with AIDS in Europe and the United States.

Pre–HIV-era series emphasized the role of MAC as a cause of chronic necrotizing apical fibrocavitary disease similar to TB in elderly patients with chronic obstructive pulmonary disease. The prevalence of chronic MAC pulmonary disease among HIV-noninfected persons has been reported to be increasing in the United States. MAC also has been recently implicated as a cause of upper and midlung field non-cavitary disease in middle-aged women without other predisposing factors. Disseminated MAC disease in patients with advanced AIDS is notable for the relative rarity of pulmonary lesions despite the enormous bacillary burden in other tissues (see Chapter 100).

In HIV-noninfected individuals, cavitary disease due to MAC often is indolent; patients with noncavitary disease frequently achieve improvement or cure without treatment. Treatment of underlying pulmonary disease with antibiotics, bronchodilators, and smoking cessation should be optimized. MAC is highly resistant to most antibiotics. When treatment is necessary, regimens should be tailored according to sensitivity tests. Rifabutin or rifampin, ethambutol, amikacin, and clofazamine may be included in combination regimens; newer agents including the macrolides azithromycin and clarithromycin and fluoroquinolones will likely have an important role in treatment. The duration of treatment should be 18 to 24 mo.

### *M. kansasii* disease

*M. kansasii* produces chronic pulmonary disease similar to reactivation TB. Disease due to this pathogen occurs sporadically throughout the world but is most common in the central and southwestern United States and in England and Wales. Disseminated disease in AIDS patients is increasing in many areas. In HIV-noninfected patients with chronic obstructive disease, treatment with isoniazid, rifampin, and ethambutol is recommended for 18 mo.

## Deep Endemic and Opportunistic Pulmonary Mycoses

Solitary or multiple pulmonary cavities are common manifestations of the deep pulmonary mycoses. The endemic mycoses are caused by dimorphic fungi that appear as hyphal forms in the environment and as yeast forms in human tissues. The prevalence of the deep pulmonary mycoses shows marked geographical variation and is highest in endemic regions (Table 57.5). Several of these pathogens are found in abundance in warm, moist soils. The principal fungi causing cavitary lung disease will be discussed individually in subsequent sections. *Paracoccidioides brasiliensis* and less commonly *Sporothrix schenkii* also cause fibrocavitary pulmonary disease. The reader is referred to the references for additional information about these pathogens.

**Table 57.5** Epidemiology of deep endemic pulmonary mycoses

| Mycosis | Climatic, ecological and occupational factors | Geographic range |
|---|---|---|
| Blastomycosis | Moist soil; persons working outdoors (foresters, hunters, construction workers, campers) | Southeastern and south-central USA (Ohio and Mississippi River valleys); midwestern states and Canadian provinces bordering the Great Lakes and St. Lawrence River Valley. Sporadic cases in Central and South America and Africa |
| Coccidioidomycosis | Lower Sonoran life zone (arid and semiarid climates) | Western hemisphere in North (especially southwestern USA), Central (Guatemala, Honduras), and South America (Venezuela, Argentina, Paraguay, Bolivia, Colombia) |
| Cryptococcosis | Soils contaminated by bird droppings | Worldwide |
| Histoplasmosis | Warm, humid climates; areas contaminated by bird droppings | Most common in central USA (Ohio and Mississippi River Valleys); also Central and South America. Sporadic cases worldwide (Asia, Africa) |
| Paracoccidioidomycosis | Moist soil in tropical and subtropical forests | Western Hemisphere. Ranges from southern Mexico 23° N latitude to Argentina 35° S latitude, especially Brazil, Colombia and Venezuela |
| Sporotrichosis | Saprophyte of wood, plants and soil. Common among gardeners, florists, farm and construction workers | Worldwide, especially south-central USA (Mississippi and Missouri River valleys), Mexico, Central and South America |

## Histoplasmosis

Histoplasmosis is an invasive pulmonary infection due to the dimorphic fungus *Histoplasma capsulatum*, an organism endemic to the Ohio and Mississippi River valleys of the central United States. Endemic foci also exist in Central and South America and sporadic cases have been reported worldwide. The organism grows well in soil, especially soil contaminated by bird or bat feces. Infectious spores are aerosolized in massive numbers when such soil deposits are disrupted. Primary infection following exposure to moderate inocula in normal hosts usually is asymptomatic or manifested by an acute, self-limited influenza-like illness. Seventy-five percent of patients have normal chest radiographs during the acute illness; a few have patchy bronchopneumonia with or without hilar lymphadenopathy. Granulomatous inflammation and caseous necrosis may occur at sites of infection; these lesions heal with fibrosis and frequently calcify. Pleural effusion is rare and should suggest alternative diagnoses, especially acute tuberculous pleurisy. Massive inhalation of *H. capsulatum* spores can result in overwhelming diffuse pneumonia.

### Clinical manifestations

Chronic cavitary histoplasmosis occurs most commonly in elderly patients with severe underlying bullous emphysema or other underlying structural lung disease. This form of histoplasmosis is roentgenographically indistinguishable from reactivation TB but usually has a more indolent clinical course (Fig. 57.5). Fever (50%), malaise, cough productive of mucoid sputum, night sweats, and chest pain are present in most cases; 20% are asymptomatic.

### Diagnosis

The diagnosis of histoplasmosis is suggested by the appropriate clinical history and chest X-ray findings. A detailed travel and residence history is important in bringing histoplasmosis into the differential diagnosis in patients presenting with compatible symptoms outside endemic regions.

The diagnosis of histoplasmosis is confirmed by demonstrating the organism in smears and cultures of infected secretions or tissues. *H. capsulatum* is a small, thin-walled spherical or oval yeast 2 to 4 $\mu$m in diameter with a single, narrow-based bud. The organism may be difficult to identify in KOH-treated sputum preparations; Wright-stained sputum smears were positive in two-thirds of cases evaluated by one experienced laboratory.

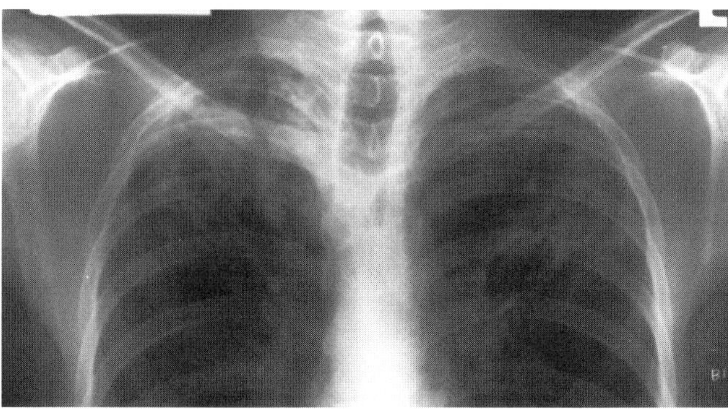

**Fig. 57.5** Pulmonary histoplasmosis.

The yeast forms are best demonstrated in tissue biopsies with the Gomori methenamine silver method. Cultures are positive in 10%–15% of cases of self-limited acute pulmonary histoplasmosis, 67%–85% of patients with chronic necrotizing pulmonary histoplasmosis, and 84%–90% of patients with disseminated disease. Cultures may require 2–4 wk to become positive. In disseminated histoplasmosis in HIV-noninfected individuals, bone marrow, lung, and lymph node biopsies each have an approximately 70% diagnostic yield.

Serological testing is sometimes useful to support the clinical diagnosis of histoplasmosis. Complement fixation antibody assays are more sensitive but less specific than immunodiffusion assays. Low levels of complement-fixing antibodies are present in 20%–30% of normal individuals residing in endemic areas; titers > 1:32 or a fourfold increase in titer comparing acute and convalescent serum specimens suggest recent or active disease. Serum immunodiffusion tests demonstrating both positive H and M bands are highly suggestive of active infection. Complement fixation antibody testing is negative in one-fourth, positive at low titer (<1:32) in one-fourth, and strongly positive in one-half of patient with chronic cavitary histoplasmosis. Histoplasmin skin testing is not useful for the diagnosis of clinical disease and may transiently elevate antibody titers against mycelial antigens, creating false-positive serological test results. Newer, highly specific enzyme immunoassay (EIA) tests detect glycoprotein antigens of *H. capsulatum* in serum and urine and are positive in 92% of patients with disseminated disease but in only 44% and 22% of cases of acute and chronic pulmonary disease, respectively. Unfortunately, all of these serological and antigen detection tests are less useful in severely immunocompromised patients, including HIV-infected individuals.

### Treatment

Acute pulmonary histoplasmosis is usually self-limited in immunocompetent individuals. Patchy pneumonic lesions and thin-walled cavities heal spontaneously in many patients. Thick-walled, enlarging cavities, progressive infiltrates, and patients with persistent symptoms require treatment. Based on accumulated clinical experience, initial therapy with ketoconazole is reasonable for chronic, non-life-threatening forms of pulmonary histoplasmosis in immunocompetent patients. Patients with AIDS frequently have poor ketoconazole absorption and itraconazole is the preferred triazole for the treatment of mild histoplasmosis in HIV-infected individuals. Amphotericin B (2–2.5 g total dose) is required in patients who fail ketoconazole or as initial therapy in normal or immunosuppressed patients with moderately severe or life-threatening pulmonary or disseminated histoplasmosis. Due to the high likelihood of relapse, chronic lifelong suppressive treatment with amphotericin B or a triazole is indicated in HIV-infected patients with histoplasmosis (see Chapter 102).

## Blastomycosis

Blastomycosis is a disseminated or focal granulomatous lung disease due to *Blastomyces dermatitidis*, a dimorphic fungus endemic to the central and southeastern United States, including the Ohio and Mississippi River valleys, the midwestern states, and Canadian provinces bordering the Great Lakes region and the St. Lawrence River Valley. Sporadic cases also have been reported from Central and South America and Africa. *B. dermatitidis* inhabits moist soil rich in decaying vegetable matter. Microepidemics of disease have been reported among forestry workers, hunters, and visitors to wet, wooded areas. Primary disease after inhalation of spores has an incubation period of 30 to 45 d. Acute blastomycosis may be asymptomatic (50% of cases) or present as a flu-like illness with chest X-ray abnormalities or acute bronchopneumonia. Self-limited infection probably is common. Early or late dissemination can occur to skin, bone, central nervous system, and the genitourinary tract. Approximately 20% of patients with disseminated blastomycosis develop characteristic papular ulcerating skin lesions resembling squamous cell skin cancers.

The most common chest radiographic finding is acute nonsegmental confluent bronchopneumonia. Single or multiple lung masses also occur and cavitation is present in 15% of cases. Intrathoracic lymphadenopathy and pleural effusion are infrequent. Contiguous rib destruction is occasionally present and mimics lung cancer.

### Diagnosis

Rapid diagnosis has been difficult due to the poor specificity of serological tests and the prolonged time required for growth in culture. Confirmation of the diagnosis requires demonstration of the organism or growth in culture. The organism is a round or oval yeast 5–18 $\mu$m in diameter with a refractile cell wall and a distinctive, single, broad-based bud in tissue and respiratory secretions and is best seen with Gomori methenamine silver or periodic acid Schiff (PAS) stains. *B. dermatitidis* also can be visualized after 10% KOH treatment or on Papanicolaou stains used routinely for sputum and bronchial cytologic examinations. Mucicarmine negativity and lack of multiple buds allow differentiation from *H. capsulatum*, *C. neoformans*, and *P. brasiliensis*. The presence of typical skin lesions should be actively sought; biopsy and culture of skin lesions can result in rapid and definitive diagnosis.

### Treatment

Acute pulmonary blastomycosis may resolve spontaneously; however, late endogenous reactivation with disseminated disease may occur. It currently is impossible to predict which patients will resolve their pneumonia without treatment and which will develop late dissemination with serious complications. For this reason many clinicians favor treatment of all patients with blastomycosis. Ketoconazole 400 mg/day for at least 6 mo has been found to be highly effective (89% cure rate) in limited forms of blastomycosis in immunocompetent patients. Amphotericin B in total doses of 30–35 mg/kg is the drug of choice for blastomycosis in immunocompromised patients and for the treatment of disseminated or CNS blastomycosis in all patients.

## Coccidioidomycosis

Coccidioidomycosis is caused by *Coccidioides immitis*, a dimorphic fungus endemic to the southwestern United States and scattered semiarid areas in central and western South America. *C. immitis* grows and sporulates in moist soil and is spread by aerosolization of arthrospores during the dry summer months. Primary infection in endemic areas frequently is asymptomatic but may result in a brief and usually self-limited influenza-like illness ("valley" or "desert fever") with cough, myalgias, and erythema nodosum. Disseminated disease with destructive bone and skin lesions or meningitis may occur and is more common among dark-skinned (particularly Filipino) and HIV-infected individuals.

Patchy focal air space or nodular infiltrates are the most common radiographic findings; these lesions have a high propensity to cavitate. Cavity formation is more common in patients with diabetes mellitus. The border zone between normal and infected pulmonary tissue is often sharply delineated in coccidioidomycosis resulting in a characteristic thin-walled cavitary lesion with little surrounding infiltrate (Fig. 57.6). Ninety percent of cavitary lesions are solitary and 70% are located in the upper lung fields. Twenty percent of patients have associated hilar lymphadenopathy. Peripheral blood eosinophilia is another important diagnostic clue.

### Diagnosis

*C. immitis* appears as a large 30–100 $\mu$m spherule containing multiple smaller 2 to 5 $\mu$m endospores and can be seen in KOH-treated or Papanicolaou smear preparations of sputum, bronchial washings, or BAL fluid. Calcofluor fluorescent white staining may improve the diagnostic yield. The organism can be demonstrated in tissue biopsies by silver staining methods. *C. immitis* can be readily cultured on selective media but is easily aerosolized, and definitive isolation can pose a significant nosocomial infection hazard to laboratory personnel if routine laboratory safety procedures are not followed. Coccidioidin skin testing has little diagnostic value due to limited specificity.

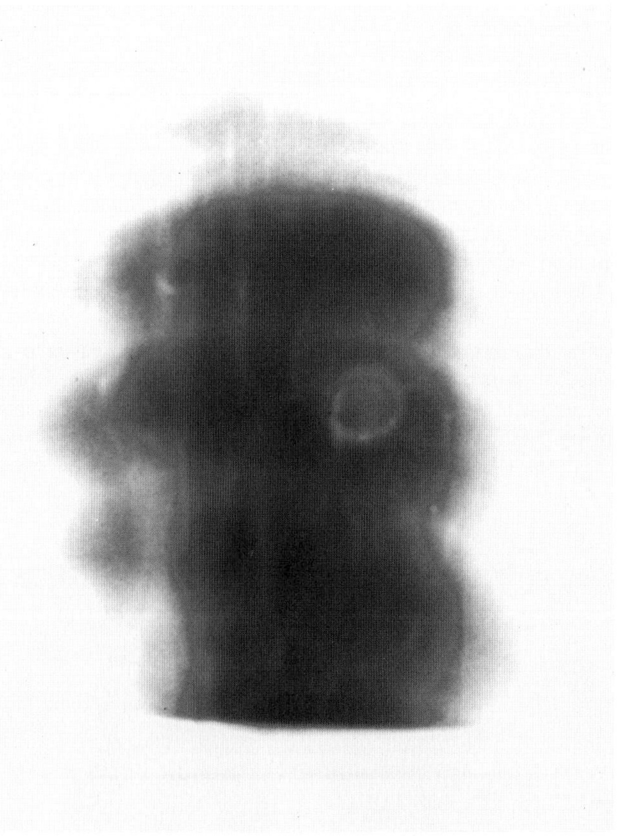

**Fig. 57.6** Plain tomogram of thin-walled upper lobe nodule due to coccidioidomycosis. Note lack of surrounding infiltrate, central lucency, and thin, calcified rim of lesion.

Serologic diagnosis is more useful for the diagnosis of coccidioidomycosis than other fungal lung infections. Tube precipitation IgM antibody tests are positive early in coccidioidal infection but become negative within 1–6 mo. Complement-fixing IgG antibody tests become positive later than tube precipitin tests and remain positive for years. Slightly more than one-half of patients with localized pulmonary disease have positive complement fixation antibody serology. Acute complement-fixation antibody titers greater than 1:32 or persistently rising titers suggest the presence of disseminated disease. A more specific agar-gel test has been developed that may be useful in cases in which coccidioidomycosis is a major diagnostic consideration and the complement-fixing antibody test is positive at low titer.

#### Treatment

Primary *C. immitis* infection usually is self-limited and does not require treatment. Ketoconazole and fluconazole have been used to treat acute disease in individuals with known risk factors for disseminated disease; their effectiveness in this setting is unknown. Disseminated disease should be treated with parenteral amphotericin B. Meningitis due to *C. immitis* is particularly difficult to treat even with the use of intrathecal amphotericin B. High dose fluconazole (at least 400 mg/d) has been effective in the therapy of meningitis in some patients.

### Cryptococcosis

The respiratory tract is the portal of entry for *Cryptococcus neoformans*, a ubiquitous 5–20 $\mu$m encapsulated monomorphic yeast with worldwide distribution causing pneumonia, cutaneous lesions, and meningitis, especially in immunosuppressed or HIV-infected individuals; *C. neoformans* also may colonize patients with lung cancer.

Cryptococcal pneumonia presents as a subacute or chronic pneumonia with weight loss, fever, nonproductive cough, and dyspnea. The most characteristic lesion is the "infiltrative mass"—a well-defined, peripheral lung lesion with little surrounding infiltrate; lobar and bronchopneumonia also may occur. Nodules and masses occasionally cavitate. Hilar lymphadenopathy and pleural effusion are unusual. AIDS patients with disseminated disease or cryptococcal meningitis may present with normal chest X-rays.

Cryptococcal pneumonia is diagnosed by visualizing the organism in deep respiratory secretions or lung tissue. The capsule of the organism stains well with PAS or mucicarmine stains. Focal endobronchial ulcerations sometimes are visible at bronchoscopy and contain abundant organisms. Detection of cryptococcal antigen in the serum or CSF or demonstration of the yeast forms on India ink preparations of CSF in patients with CNS symptoms are useful diagnostic procedures. Whereas cryptococcal pneumonia in immunocompetent patients may resolve spontaneously, about 90% of immunosuppressed and probably all patients with advanced AIDS will develop progressive disease. When pulmonary cryptococcosis is diagnosed in compromised hosts, lumbar puncture, biopsy of suspicious cutaneous lesions, and other investigations based on clinical symptoms should be performed to evaluate for disseminated disease. Prolonged treatment with amphotericin B, with or without 5-fluorocytosine, is indicated for all immunosuppressed individuals. Chronic lifelong maintenance therapy with intermittent amphotericin administration or fluconazole is necessary in HIV-infected patients due to the extremely high rate of relapse in the absence of chronic suppressive therapy.

### Cavitary Lung Disease Due to Other Opportunistic and Saprophytic Fungi

Saprophytic fungi may cause pneumonia or disseminated infection in immunocompromised hosts. These pathogens are monomorphic and appear in tissue and the environment as hyphal forms. These organisms can colonize the respiratory tract; colonization, therefore, must be distinguished from invasive disease when these organisms are isolated from respiratory secretions.

### Aspergillosis

*Aspergillus* species are ubiquitous saprophytic fungi that cause allergic bronchopulmonary aspergillosis, invasive pulmonary aspergillosis in immunocompromised hosts, chronic necrotizing pulmonary aspergillosis, and mycetoms ("fungus balls"). Aspergilli have septate hyphae with characteristic dichotomous branching at 45° angles and can be identified in tissue with PAS or Gomori methenamine silver stains.

#### Aspergilloms

Aspergilloms are interwoven masses of fungal mycelia that usually develop within cavities or cystic spaces secondary to TB, sarcoidosis, and other lung diseases. Most aspergilloms are due to *A. fumigatus*; other species are isolated only rarely.

Most patients with aspergilloms have few symptoms, although fever, weight loss, and malaise may occur. The most common and potentially most serious symptom is hemoptysis, which occurs in more than one-half of the patients at some time during their clinical course. Hemoptysis may be scanty and intermittent, or massive, resulting in death due to asphyxia.

The classical X-ray finding is the air-crescent sign, consisting of a homogenous mass at the base of the cavity with a crescent of air visible superior to the fungal mass (Fig. 57.7). The air-crescent sign is not pathognomonic of aspergilloma; pulmonary

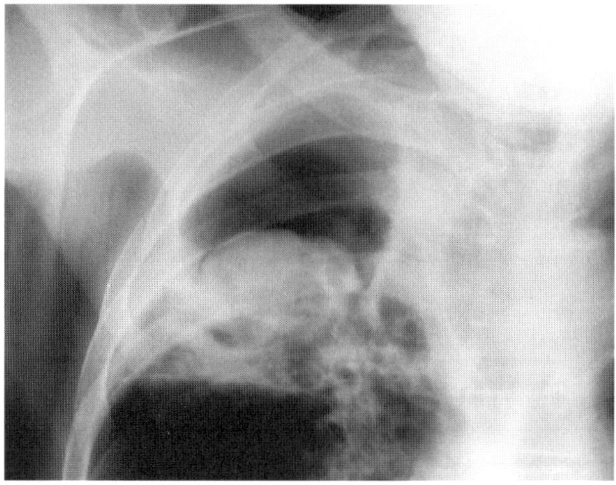

**Fig. 57.7** Aspergilloma in old tuberculous cavity with air-crescent sign.

gangrene, blood clots in old cavities, hydatid lung cysts, and lung abscesses may show similar findings. Serum aspergillus precipitins can be detected in more than 90% of nonimmunosuppressed patients with aspergilloms. Sputum cultures positive for *Aspergillus* are suggestive, but not diagnostic, as the organism may colonize patients with abnormal lung parenchyma without producing disease.

The management of pulmonary aspergilloma is controversial. Spontaneous lysis has been reported to occur in 10% of cases; clinical or radiographic features predictive of spontaneous resolution are unknown. Medical treatment of these lesions, including intracavitary instillation of amphotericin B, has been uniformly unsuccessful. Due to other underlying chronic lung diseases, many patients with aspergilloms have limited pulmonary function reserve and may not tolerate lung resection surgery. Surgical mortality in patients undergoing lung resection for massive or recurrent hemoptysis is approximately 10%; significant postoperative complications occur in 20%–25%. Surgical resection of the involved lobe (after bronchoscopic confirmation of the origin of bleeding) should be reserved for patients with massive hemoptysis with adequate pulmonary functional reserve. Hemoptysis in patients with aspergilloms usually is due to bleeding from hypertrophied bronchial arterial vessels in the cavity wall; hence, bronchial arterial embolization is a useful measure for acute control of massive hemoptysis or treatment of patients with inadequate lung function for lung resection surgery. Unfortunately, the rate of recurrent bleeding is high (10%–20% at 1 yr) in patients treated with bronchial arterial embolization.

### Invasive aspergillosis

*Aspergillus* species rarely cause invasive disease in normal hosts. Major known risk factors for invasive aspergillosis include neutropenia, glucocorticosteroid therapy, chronic alcoholism, and disorders of neutrophil function such as chronic granulomatous disease. In the absence of normal granulocyte function, mycelia invade small pulmonary blood vessels, leading to local thrombosis of small pulmonary arterioles with tissue infarction and cavitation. Invasive pulmonary aspergillosis also has been described in patients with advanced AIDS.

Clinical presentations of invasive pulmonary aspergillosis are highly variable. Persistent fever unresponsive to empiric antibiotic treatment for gram-negative pathogens and staphylococci, cough, pleuritic chest pain, and hemoptysis ("pseudopulmonary embolism") are frequent, although nonspecific, presenting manifestations in neutropenic patients.

Up to 25% of neutropenic patients may have a normal chest X-ray at the onset of symptoms. Nodular peripheral infiltrates are the most common early manifestation of invasive pulmonary aspergillosis (IPA). Cavitation is frequent and usually develops days to weeks later in the clinical course. The presence of a mass or nodule with a surrounding zone of low attenuation (the "halo sign") on chest CT scan in the appropriate clinical setting has been suggested as a useful early diagnostic clue to IPA. Pulmonary lesions due to IPA typically worsen or cavitate after resolution of neutropenia due to an influx of neutrophils and intense local inflammation.

Tissue biopsy with demonstration of tissue invasion is necessary for definitive diagnosis. Transbronchial or open lung biopsy is, however, not without risk in immunocompromised thrombocytopenic patients. Despite limited (13%–50%) sensitivity, the isolation of *A. fumigatus* or *A. flavus* from nasopharyngeal swabs, deep respiratory secretions, or BAL fluid in high-risk neutropenic patients is highly correlated with the presence of invasive pulmonary disease and warrants consideration or continuation of empiric antifungal therapy.

Treatment of invasive pulmonary aspergillosis requires prolonged therapy with amphotericin B. Rapid escalation to high daily doses of amphotericin B (1.0–1.5 mg/kg/d) may improve outcomes although nephrotoxicity may become a limiting factor. Newer imidazoles such as itraconazole have excellent in vitro activity against aspergilli and may have a useful role in later stages of therapy in less immunocompromised patients.

### Chronic necrotizing pulmonary aspergillosis

Chronic necrotizing pulmonary aspergillosis (CNPA) is a more indolent and less invasive form of aspergillosis, typically affecting middle-aged and elderly adults with milder host immunological abnormalities such as diabetes mellitus or structural lung disease such as COPD. Patients with CNPA generally present with several months of fever, night sweats, productive cough, weight loss, and leukocytosis. The most common radiographic manifestation is that of a slowly progressive upper lobe necrotizing pneumonia with adjoining pleural thickening. Eighty percent of patients have cavitation visible on plain chest X-ray. CNPA has also been called "semi-invasive" aspergillosis to emphasize that invasive disease with tissue destruction is present adjacent to cavitary lesions which also may contain mycetoms.

Serum aspergillus precipitins are usually positive in CNPA. Transbronchial or open lung biopsy with culture is diagnostic if limited tissue invasion with typical mycelia is present. Invasive disease may be patchy; therefore, a clinical diagnosis sufficient to indicate therapy may be made if *Aspergillus* is recovered on culture of deep respiratory secretions, no other significant respiratory pathogens are recovered, and consistent clinical and radiographic findings are present.

Parenteral amphotericin B is the treatment of choice for severe disease. Prolonged treatment with itraconazole appears promising in early multicenter trials. Surgical resection should be limited to patients with adequate pulmonary function reserve who cannot tolerate or fail medical therapy.

## Other fungal infections

Many other saprophytic fungi can cause invasive cavitary pulmonary disease in immunocompromised hosts. Zygomycetes of the order Mucorales may produce invasive sinopulmonary disease similar to invasive aspergillosis in patients with poorly controlled diabetes mellitus, diabetic ketoacidosis, or hematologic malignancies. The Zygomycetes are distinguished by broad, irregularly shaped hyphae with random branching and few septations. *Pseudoallescheria boydii* is another increasingly common pathogen in immunocompromised patients. *P. boydii* is highly resistant to amphotericin and treatment is difficult; surgical resection of infected necrotic tissue, when possible, and prolonged treatment with ketoconazole or itraconazole are current therapeutic approaches. Despite the high prevalence of oral thrush and severe candidal esophagitis in immunocompromised and HIV-infected patients, *Candida* species only rarely have been implicated as etiologic agents of invasive necrotizing pneumonia. This complication is most likely to occur in patients with neutropenia or disordered neutrophil function.

## Cavitary Lung Disease Due to Parasitic Infections

Cavitary pulmonary disease may occur in parasitic infections due to *Strongyloides stercoralis*, *Paragonimiasis westermanii*, and *Entamoeba histolytica*. These diagnoses are established by visualization of typical larvae, eggs, or amebae in appropriate clinical specimens (stool and/or sputum). Cavitary lung disease in amebiasis usually manifests as right lower lobe pneumonia or lung abscess due to transdiaphragmatic spread from a hepatic abscess. Echinococcal (hydatid) cysts occasionally present as isolated pulmonary cavities without surrounding infiltrates. A peculiar irregular, scalloped air-crescent sign, the "water lily sign," may be apparent in echinococcal lung abscesses due to the appearance of the membranes of the collapsed cyst floating on the liquid contents of the cavity. Detailed travel, recreational, and occupational histories are essential in the diagnosis of these uncommon causes of cavitary pulmonary disease.

## Summary

Necrotizing infectious pathogens are the most common causes of cavitary pulmonary disease. Drainage of infected necrotic material into the bronchial tree or pleural space is necessary to provide the air–tissue (fluid) interface required for the radiographic appearance of a cavity. Mycobacterial disease, deep fungal infections, and acute necrotizing pneumonia due to a limited number of pyogenic and anaerobic organisms are the most common infectious causes of cavitary lung disease. The presence of pulmonary cavitation should alert the clinician to the possibility of these etiologic agents. Differentiation of chronic from acute courses, extrapulmonary findings, and certain radiographic features provide important diagnostic clues. Many infectious etiologies have overlapping clinical and radiographic features or are associated with lower airway colonization as well as invasive disease. Demonstration of the etiologic organism by smear, culture, and, in some instances, tissue biopsy is required for definitive diagnosis and effective therapy. Ancillary laboratory testing such as serologies may be useful for the diagnosis of fungal infections. Finally, local epidemiological characteristics are of great help in establishing the list of putative pathogens to be considered.

### ANNOTATED BIBLIOGRAPHY


American Thoracic Society–Centers for Disease Control and Prevention. Treatment of tuberculosis and tuberculosis infection in adults and children. Am J Respir Crit Care Med 1994; 149:1359–1374.
*Most recent consensus statement regarding preventive therapy and treatment of tuberculosis in all age groups. Includes information about antimycobacterial drugs and potential side effects and describes approaches to management of TB in HIV-infected patients and MDR TB.*

Bartlett JG. Anaerobic bacterial infections of the lung and pleural space. Clin Infect Dis 1993; 16 (Suppl 4):S248–255.
*Broad review of the literature on anaerobic infections including findings in 193 bacteriologically proven cases evaluated by the author. Confirmation of the etiologic role of anaerobes in patients with pulmonary disease is rarely made today due to abandonment of techniques such as transtracheal aspiration to obtain uncontaminated lung specimens. Excellent review of clinical features, bacteriology, and treatment.*

Fox CW, George RB. Cavitary lung disease. Postgrad Med 1992; 91:313–331.
*Describes diagnostic approach to cavitary lung disease based on radiographic features and history.*

Fraser RG, Paré JAP, Paré PD, Fraser RS, Genereux GP. Diagnosis of Diseases of the Chest, 3rd ed. WB Saunders, Philadelphia, PA, 1990.
*The most comprehensive textbook of pulmonary disease. Organization utilizes a clinical-radiographic-pathological approach to diagnosis. Exhaustively referenced sections on infectious and cavitary pulmonary diseases.*

Gallant JE, Ko AH. Cavitary pulmonary lesions in patients infected with human immunodeficiency virus. Clin Infect Dis 1996; 22:671–682.
*Comprehensive review of the differential diagnosis of infectious and noninfectious causes of cavitary pulmonary lesions in HIV-infected individuals.*

Iseman MD. Treatment of multidrug-resistant tuberculosis. N Engl J Med 1993; 329:784–791.
*Comprehensive review of risk factors for drug resistance and treatment approaches to MDR TB.*

Palmer PES. Pulmonary tuberculosis—usual and unusual radiographic presentations. Semin Roentgenol 1979; 14:204–242.
*Well-illustrated review of the entire spectrum of radiographic lesions seen in pulmonary tuberculosis.*

Reed JC. Chest Radiology: Plain Film Patterns and Differential Diagnosis, 2nd ed. Year Book Medical, Chicago, pp 293–329, 1987.
*Reviews differential diagnostic features of solitary and multiple pulmonary cavitary disease.*

Sarosi GA, Davies SF. Fungal Diseases of the Lung, 2nd ed. Raven Press, New York, 1993.
*Comprehensive review of all major endemic and saprophytic fungal lung diseases. Up to date discussions of clinical and microbiological features, role of serologic tests, and treatment.*

Shlaes D, Lederman M, Chmielewski R, Tweardy D, Wolinsky E. Elastin fibers in the sputum of patients with necrotizing pneumonia. Chest 1983; 83:885–889.
*Describes a simple and rapid technique for examining sputum for the presence of potassium hydroxide (KOH)-resistant elastin fibers highly characteristic of necrotizing pneumonia. Illustrations of positive findings are included.*

Wolinsky E. Non-tuberculous mycobacteria and associated diseases. Am Rev Respir Dis 1979; 119: 107–159.
*Pre-HIV era review of the role of atypical mycobacteria in human disease.*

Woodring JH, Fried AM. Significance of wall thickness in solitary cavities of the lung. Am J Roentgenol 1983; 140:473–474.
*Prospective validation study confirming value of guidelines for using maximum cavity thickness as an indicator of the etiology of solitary pulmonary cavities.*

# 58

# Diffuse Pulmonary Infiltrates and Acute Respiratory Distress Syndrome

KENNETH P. STEINBERG

The development of acute respiratory failure in the presence of diffuse pulmonary infiltrates represents one of the most difficult diagnostic and therapeutic dilemmas in critical care medicine. Etiologies of this syndrome include a wide variety of diffuse pulmonary infections, direct physical or chemical lung injury, and noninfectious manifestations of extrapulmonary disease processes including severe sepsis. Although this presentation may be triggered by a wide variety of illnesses or injuries, the clinical picture and histopathology are remarkably uniform, creating what is referred to as the acute respiratory distress syndrome (ARDS). Despite the sophisticated monitoring and support systems now available in intensive care units, and recent reports of improving survival, only approximately half of all patients who develop ARDS will survive. Because many ARDS victims are young, previously healthy adults, the effect in terms of productive life lost is considerable. Therefore, in the management of ARDS, it is of paramount importance to exclude specific infectious and other treatable causes of diffuse lung disease.

This chapter will deal primarily with ARDS: its manifestations and its management. Many respiratory infections are mentioned, as are other acute intrinsic lung diseases, that need to be considered in a differential diagnosis of acute, diffuse lung disease. This chapter will not deal specifically with each of those processes since detailed discussions of specific infectious etiologies can be found elsewhere in this book. Similarly, this chapter will deal only with acute processes that lead to acute respiratory failure. Chronic, diffuse lung diseases, such as idiopathic pulmonary fibrosis, are not discussed.

## Pathogenesis and Pathology of ARDS

The pathologic changes in lung histology that characterize ARDS, known as *diffuse alveolar damage,* represent a relatively nonspecific response to injury. Not only are these changes found in other disease processes such as fibrosing alveolitis and drug-induced pulmonary disease, the pattern shows little variability, even among cases of ARDS associated with widely divergent causes. As ARDS develops and evolves, complex changes occur in the lung, which have been divided into three stages based on pathological and clinical findings. It is not clear that every case of ARDS evolves in such a stepwise fashion, passing from one stage to the next leading ultimately to resolution or death, and clinically, it can be difficult to distinguish one stage from another. Nevertheless, it may be helpful to understand this classification scheme, as therapy for ARDS might differ depending on the stage of the disease.

Early ARDS is frequently referred to as the *exudative phase,* given the outpouring of cells and proteinaceous material into the airspaces. Inflammatory cells, primarily neutrophils, accumulate within the alveolar space and contribute to the lung injury process through the release of granular enzymes and oxidants. Type I alveolar epithelial cells appear to be the most susceptible to injury, undergoing cytopathic changes extremely early, with resultant damage to the alveolar basement membrane. Pulmonary vascular endothelial cells are also affected, although the histologic changes are less striking and occur more slowly. Endothelial and epithelial cells undergo changes in permeability, allowing accumulation of interstitial and alveolar edema fluid. Hyaline membranes, identical to those seen in premature infants with respiratory distress syndrome, are caused by the aggregation of fibrin and other proteins in the alveolar space. Alveolar flooding, along with distortion of alveoli by septal edema and impairment of surfactant function, all contribute to the loss of functional lung units through microatelectasis. As the process continues, there is loss of pulmonary microvasculature associated with endothelial injury and intravascular thrombosis.

Although prior depletion of neutrophils in experimental animals has led to amelioration of the lung injury induced by various stimuli, there are now many clinical reports of patients with profound neutropenia who developed ARDS. Neutrophils may not be required for the development of lung injury, but they certainly represent at least one mechanism by which tissue damage is initiated or amplified during ARDS. Other inflammatory pathways and cell types are also involved. Proteins in the complement cascade, kinin system, and coagulation system are susceptible to the action of proteases, generating products with pro-inflammatory activity. Phospholipase products of arachidonic acid including platelet-activating factor, prostaglandins, and leukotrienes have also been identified as mediators of lung inflammation. Tumor necrosis factor (TNF) and other cytokines (e.g., interleukin [IL]-1, IL-6, IL-8) are likely to be important intermediates, particularly in cases of ARDS associated with sepsis and multiple trauma. In addition, the lipopolysaccharide (LPS) molecule itself appears to have direct cytotoxic effects, along with a multitude of other actions mediated indirectly through the activation or priming of inflammatory cells. The potential role of free fatty acids in the pathogenesis of lung injury after long-bone fractures has been implicated in the fat embolism syndrome (FES).

Patients may not survive this early phase of ARDS; they often succumb to their underlying illness. In others, the exudative phase may resolve spontaneously without further lung injury. In many patients, however, ARDS will persist for over a week. The *organizational phase* begins within 3–7 d of lung injury and is characterized by alveolar cell, endothelial cell, and fibroblast proliferation, perhaps an attempt by the lung to heal itself. During this time, much of the alveolar edema fluid resolves, although gas exchange, pulmonary mechanics, and chest radiographs can still be grossly abnormal.

If resolution still does not occur during this organizational phase, ARDS can progress to a fibrotic or *fibroproliferative phase*. Pulmonary fibrosis is well documented in patients with ARDS and appears to be associated both with fibroblast proliferation and increased collagen synthesis. Increased amounts of lung collagen have been documented as early as a few days after ARDS onset, and ongoing, disordered collagen deposition leads to an accumulation of extracellular matrix, alveolar and interstitial scarring, capillary obliteration, and architectural distortion. This fibroproliferation carries with it high risk that prolonged ventilatory support may be needed, and risk of death from respiratory and multiple organ failure. Importantly, the recovery of normal lung function in many survivors of ARDS has been taken as evidence that pulmonary fibrosis complicating ARDS is not necessarily a permanent, or fatal, process.

## Etiologies

The acute respiratory distress syndrome can be precipitated by diverse clinical events, the most common of which are listed in Table 58.1, that can cause lung injury via direct or indirect mechanisms. Direct causes of injury to the lung include pulmonary contusion from blunt chest trauma, aspiration of gastric contents, inhalational injuries such as smoke and other toxic gas inhalation, and diffuse pulmonary infection. Aspiration of gastric contents is a fairly common cause of ARDS in most hospitals while pulmonary contusion is common in centers that treat large numbers of patients with chest trauma.

### Infectious causes of diffuse pulmonary infiltrates and ARDS

In patients with pneumonia, the term ARDS is generally reserved for the process associated with systemic effects of infection in which the pathogenesis presumably is endothelial injury related to intravascular activation of inflammatory mediators. It is often difficult, however, to determine whether diffuse infiltration is directly due to generalized involvement of the lung by microorganisms or arises secondary to a more localized pulmonary process that may lead to sepsis with resultant widespread intravascular injury. Additionally, once

**Table 58.1** Clinical disorders associated with ARDS

| Direct lung injury | Indirect lung injury[a] |
|---|---|
| Aspiration of gastric contents | Severe sepsis |
| Pulmonary contusion | Major trauma<br>Multiple long bone fractures<br>Hypovolemic shock |
| Toxic gas (smoke) inhalation | Hypertransfusion |
| Near-drowning | Acute pancreatitis |
| Diffuse pulmonary infection | Drug overdose |
| | Reperfusion injury<br>Post–lung transplantation<br>Post–cardiopulmonary bypass |

[a]Due to activation of an acute, systemic inflammatory response with hematogenous delivery of inflammatory mediators to the lung.

diffuse infection occurs, whether related to viral pneumonia, diffuse bacterial pneumonia, or *Pneumocystis carinii* pneumonia, supportive measures such as the application of mechanical ventilation and PEEP are usually the same as for ARDS of other etiologies.

Almost any pneumonia can cause ARDS when it first causes overwhelming sepsis. There are, however, some important pulmonary infections that are associated with diffuse pulmonary infiltrates and respiratory failure that should be considered when managing a patient with ARDS of unknown etiology. Multilobar pneumonia from bacterial pathogens is probably the most common of these, although it is frequently accompanied by sepsis. A listing of potential pathogens is given in Table 58.2. While *Mycoplasma pneumonia* generally presents with mild, diffuse interstitial infiltrates and a benign course, fulminant pneumonia and ARDS can be an unusual manifestation of this illness. Even rarer, and harder to diagnose, is infection with *Mycoplasma fermentans*. This has been reported in small outbreaks on the mid-Atlantic coast of the United States, may not be diagnosed until autopsy, and requires treatment with tetracycline, not erythromycin. Pneumonia with other rare organisms such as *Yersinia pestis* (plague), *Francisella tularensis* (tularemia), *Chlamydia psittaci* (psittacosis), and *Coxiella burnetti* (Q fever) can cause diffuse pulmonary infiltrates and ARDS. Good history-taking is the key to suspecting these organisms.

There are three mechanisms by which *Mycobacterium tuberculosis* can present with diffuse pulmonary infiltrates. One presentation is diffuse tuberculous pneumonia, which generally occurs after a rupture of a cavity with resultant endobronchial spread throughout the lung. Hematogenous dissemination leads to miliary tuberculosis with its classic radiographic pattern. Miliary TB, however, does not necessarily result in acute respiratory failure, but full-blown ARDS, with pathologically confirmed diffuse alveolar damage, can complicate some of these cases. If ARDS develops before the diagnosis of TB is known, the radiographic and clinical pattern may be indistinguishable from other causes of ARDS and the diagnosis of TB delayed or even missed.

Adenoviruses and influenza viruses can cause viral pneumonia with diffuse pulmonary infiltrates but rarely cause fulminant respiratory failure. Varicella can cause pneumonia and ARDS, especially in adults, which can occasionally be quite severe. Herpes simplex virus and cytomegalovirus pneumonia are usually complications of immunosuppression. Finally, hantavirus infection leading to the hantavirus pulmonary syndrome is a newly recognized cause of severe respiratory failure with diffuse pulmonary infiltrates and non-cardiogenic pulmonary edema.

Fungal infections with *Histoplasma capsulatum, Coccidioides immitis,* and *Cryptococcus neoformans* can lead to diffuse pneumonias. Histoplasmosis and coccidioidomycosis can be hematogenously disseminated and therefore can present with a miliary pattern on chest radiograph. Cryptococcosis is rarely miliary in appearance. It usually presents as an extensive pneumonic process when it leads to respiratory failure. These disseminated or extensive fungal infections occur almost exclusively in immunocompromised hosts.

*Pneumocystis carinii* pneumonia (PCP) occurs in hosts with defective cellular immunity and has become one of the more common causes of diffuse pulmonary infection in the era of AIDS. Fulminant PCP, with its diffuse pulmonary infiltrates, severe respiratory distress, and profound hypoxemia, mimics ARDS and should be at the top of the differential diagnosis of diffuse pulmonary infections when one is confronted with a case of ARDS of unknown etiology. Disseminated toxoplasmosis is

**Table 58.2** Infectious agents associated with diffuse pulmonary infiltrates and respiratory failure

| |
|---|
| BACTERIA |
| *GRAM POSITIVE* |
| *Staphylococcus aureus* |
| *Streptococcus pneumoniae* |
| *GRAM NEGATIVE* |
| *Franciscella tularensis* |
| *Legionella* species |
| *L. pneumophila* |
| *L. micdadei* |
| *Pasteurella multocida* |
| *Salmonella* species |
| *Yersinia pestis* |
| *MYCOBACTERIUM TUBERCULOSIS* |
| Mycoplasma |
| *M. pneumoniae* |
| *M. fermentans* |
| *RICKETTSIA* |
| *Coxiella burnetti* |
| *CHLAMYDIA* |
| *C. psittaci* |
| *C. pneumoniae* |
| VIRUSES |
| Cytomegalovirus (CMV) |
| Respiratory syncytial virus (RSV) |
| Herpes simplex virus (HSV) |
| Varicella zoster virus (VZV) |
| Adenovirus |
| Influenza virus |
| Hantavirus |
| FUNGI |
| *Histoplasma capsulatum* |
| *Coccidioides immitis* |
| *Cryptococcus neoformans* |
| PARASITES |
| *Pneumocystis carinii* |
| *Toxoplasma gondii* |
| *Strongyloides stercoralis* |

another cause, albeit rare, of diffuse pulmonary infiltrates in patients with HIV infection.

## Extrapulmonary causes of ARDS

Despite this impressive array of infectious agents, indirect causes of lung injury make up the majority of cases of ARDS. Indirect lung injury refers to a process that occurs primarily outside the lung with secondary, usually blood-borne, damage to the lung. In this setting, activation of circulating mediators of inflammation, including cytokines, prostaglandins, leukotrienes, complement fragments, and platelet-activating factor, leads to damage of the pulmonary capillary endothelium and secondary lung injury. Severe sepsis, with or without documented infection, and severe trauma including multiple long-bone fractures, hemorrhagic shock, and massive transfusion (usually defined as more than 10–15 units of blood in a 24-h period) account for most cases of ARDS. Other etiologies of ARDS include pancreatitis, drug overdose (tricyclic antidepressants, narcotics, and aspirin are the most common), and cardiopulmonary bypass. Many other etiologies have been described in case reports but account for very few cases of ARDS.

There are specific pulmonary disorders that may have a fulminant course, presenting as acute respiratory failure with diffuse radiographic infiltrates (Table 58.3). Some of these processes can mimic ARDS, clinically and/or pathologically, but since they are associated with other known diagnoses they are often considered separately. Many of these diagnoses have unique treatments and should be thought of when evaluating a patient with ARDS of unknown etiology. Some of these processes have distinctive features or histories that suggest the diagnosis. Others, such as acute eosinophilic pneumonia, may be missed unless carefully thought about.

## Hantavirus pulmonary syndrome

In the spring of 1993, a cluster of patients with severe acute respiratory failure were identified in the Four Corners area of the southwestern United States. The etiologic agent was a newly identified virus of the hantavirus genus of the *Bunyviradae* family of enveloped RNA viruses. This virus has subsequently been called the Sin Nombre virus and is thought to be transmitted by aerosols of the infected feces and urine of the deer mouse. The disease has been named hantavirus pulmonary syndrome (HPS) and since 1993 has been sporadically diagnosed across the United States. Different animal vectors and different (but closely related) hantaviruses appear to be involved in different parts of the country. Hantaviruses are not unique to the United States. They have been identified around the world and are variably pathogenic. Some, for example, hantaan virus in Asia, are associated with hemorrhagic fever with renal syndrome.

The initial symptoms of hantavirus infection are virtually identical to those of other common acute viral syndromes. As the illness progresses, respiratory signs and symptoms become predominant with dyspnea, pleuritic chest pain, hemoptysis, and diffuse rales. Fever is common and hypotension often develops primarily due to profound volume depletion as highly proteinaceous fluid leaks into damaged lungs. The chest radiograph reveals diffuse alveolar edema. Thrombocytopenia, neutrophilia, and increased hematocrit (due to plasma volume depletion) are common. The progression of this noncardiogenic pulmonary edema and respiratory failure is rapid and dramatic, often leading to death within 48 h. The case fatality rate is approximately 60%. Autopsy studies have revealed diffuse alveolar damage with edema, hyaline membranes, and a marked, mononuclear, interstitial inflammatory infiltrate. Unlike ARDS, polymorphonuclear leukocytes are generally not seen.

Because of the unique clinical syndrome, viral etiology, and pathology [lack of polymorphonuclear leukocytes, or, neutrophils (PMN)], it is not clear that HPS should be considered a cause of ARDS. Nevertheless, it is a cause of noncardiogenic pulmonary edema secondary to epithelial and endothelial lung injury associated with a high mortality. Treatment currently consists of aggressive supportive care. For these reasons, it is similar to ARDS—hence, the inclusion of HPS in this chapter.

# Epidemiology/Host Factors

The incidence of ARDS has been variably estimated at 15,000–150,000 cases per year in the United States. In most series, infectious etiologies appear to be the most common precip-

**Table 58.3** Noninfectious etiologies of acute respiratory failure associated with diffuse pulmonary infiltrates

| | |
|---|---|
| CARDIOVASCULAR | Congestive heart failure |
| DRUGS/TOXINS | Paraquat<br>Aspirin<br>Heroin/narcotics<br>Toxic gas inhalation<br>Tricyclic antidepressants<br>Acute radiation pneumonitis |
| IDIOPATHIC | Nonspecific interstitial pneumonitis<br>Acute eosinophilic pneumonia<br>Sarcoidosis[a]<br>Rapidly progressive interstitial pulmonary fibrosis[a] (Hamman-Rich syndrome) |
| IMMUNOLOGIC | Acute lupus pneumonitis<br>Bronchiolitis obliterans organizing pneumonia[a]<br>Goodpasture's syndrome<br>Idiopathic pulmonary hemosiderosis[a]<br>Hypersensitivity pneumonitis<br>Leukoagglutinin reaction |
| METABOLIC | Alveolar proteinosis[a] |
| MISCELLANEOUS | Fat embolism syndrome<br>Amniotic fluid embolism<br>High altitude pulmonary edema<br>Neurogenic pulmonary edema |
| NEOPLASTIC | Lymphangitic carcinomatosis[a]<br>Leukemic infiltration<br>Lymphoma |

[a] Usually a subacute or chronic disorder that can progress rapidly or be far advanced on first presentation.

itants, with sepsis syndrome and bacterial or viral pneumonia leading the list. The majority of septic patients are not affected; however, approximately 35%–50% of patients with sepsis syndrome will develop ARDS. Major traumatic injury, often involving extensive soft tissue damage, is also a frequent cause with approximately 25% of victims developing ARDS. Aspiration of gastric contents is an etiology frequently encountered in patients with an altered level of consciousness. Other risk factors include massive transfusion, inhalation injury, pancreatitis, near-drowning, and drug overdose. Many other causes of ARDS have been described in case reports and small series.

Since ARDS occurs in less than 50% of patients at risk for developing lung injury, one might expect there to be specific host factors that play a role in the development of the syndrome. Nevertheless, very few factors have been identified that suggest individual patient susceptibility. As described above, some risk factors have a greater predisposition to the development of lung injury than others. Patients with severe sepsis, for example, are more likely than trauma patients to develop ARDS.

Within the subset of risk factors, however, there are some features that do increase the likelihood that ARDS will develop. Severity of illness appears to play an important role. It has been shown that more severely traumatized patients are more likely to develop ARDS than less severely injured patients, an observation that appears to be independent of the presence of shock. One explanation for this could be that the extent of soft-tissue or bone injury relates to the level of inflammatory mediators released into the bloodstream, resulting in a greater or lesser propensity to develop lung injury and multiorgan dysfunction.

Age is another factor that has been shown to be an independent risk factor for the development of ARDS. Patients over the age of 70 with sepsis are more likely than younger patients to develop ARDS. Perhaps more importantly, age is also a factor in outcome. There is a higher fatality rate in older patients than in younger patients that also appears to be independent of severity of illness. The effect of gender has not been well evaluated, but there is some suggestion that women with trauma are more likely than men to develop ARDS when corrected for severity of illness. It is not known if gender also affects outcome.

Once a patient develops ARDS, the course is highly variable, lasting from a few days to several months. The median time on mechanical ventilation is 10–14 d, but as many as 10%–20% of patients remain ventilator dependent for more than 3 wk. Even in patients who resolve their underlying illness or injury and respond readily to supportive therapy, the course usually lasts several days, in contrast to patients with cardiogenic pulmonary edema, who typically respond to therapy much more rapidly, improving over hours or 1 to 2 d.

Thus, the major factors linked to both the development and outcome of ARDS are age, the underlying risk factor, severity of illness, preexisting comorbidities, and the development of complications, especially infection and multiple organ failure. One-third of the deaths in ARDS patients are related to the underlying disease or injury—that is, death is caused by events occurring before the onset of ARDS. The remaining two-thirds of ARDS deaths are due to complications that have their onset either coincident with or after ARDS onset. The most common fatal course appears to be development of a nosocomial infection followed by development of systemic manifestations of sepsis syndrome and multiple organ system failure. Only a relatively small fraction of nonsurvivors (approximately 15%) die a respiratory death—that is, due to insupportable hypoxemia or respiratory acidosis that is refractory to treatment. Although the majority of patients do not die a respiratory death, most of them still meet the criteria for ARDS at the time of death and are still on mechanical ventilation.

## Clinical Manifestations

ARDS is a syndrome representing the abrupt onset of diffuse lung injury and characterized by severe hypoxemia and generalized pulmonary infiltrates in the absence of cardiac failure. The reason for using the term ARDS is that it denotes a common syndrome despite multiple etiologies or associated illnesses and implies similar if not identical pathophysiology. Once the diagnosis of ARDS is made the application of certain principles of supportive therapy is warranted regardless of etiology.

Awake patients become anxious, agitated, and dyspneic. Initially, dyspnea may be exertional but it progresses quickly to severe dyspnea at rest, tachypnea, and hypoxemia. Inflammatory changes in the lung lead to a reduction in lung compliance. This stiffening of the lungs, in turn, leads to small tidal volumes, rapid respiratory rates, and an increase in the work of breathing. Initially, patients may be able to compensate and maintain acceptable arterial blood gases, perhaps even generating a respiratory alkalosis. The vast majority of patients deteriorate over several hours, requiring intubation and mechanical ventilation. Mechanical ventilation, however, is not a necessary requirement for the diagnosis of ARDS: A few patients with mild lung injury and normal mentation can occasionally avoid extubation, either with high-flow oxygen therapy or the use of noninvasive respiratory support such as mask CPAP (continuous positive airway pressure).

While severity of illness varies, patients may be profoundly hypoxemic during the early, exudative phase of ARDS. Physiologically, hypoxemia at this time results from intrapulmonary shunting since alveoli are atelectatic or filled with exudate and hyaline membranes. Thirty-three to 50 percent of ARDS-related deaths occur within the first 3–7 d. These patients who die during this early stage of ARDS often succumb to their underlying illness and not to respiratory failure. Other patients improve and are extubated. Nevertheless, given the average time on a ventilator of 10–14 d, a significant number of patients continue to have severe respiratory failure at the end of 1 wk. The fatality rate of persistent, severe ARDS in patients who survive the first week of therapy is not well described, but some data suggest it may be similar to the 40% overall fatality rate of ARDS. Reasons for late deaths include progressive respiratory failure or, more commonly, nosocomial pneumonia, sepsis, multiple organ failure, and other complications of ICU care.

During the fibroproliferative phase of ARDS, gas exchange abnormalities persist due now to ventilation/perfusion abnormalities and increased dead-space ventilation rather than physiologic shunting. The lungs often become very stiff and fibrotic. Patients respond less well to the application of positive end-expiratory pressure (PEEP). Vascular occlusion and destruction is believed to be responsible for increased dead-space ventilation, pulmonary hypertension, and occasional right heart failure.

## Laboratory Studies

The chest radiograph usually reveals diffuse bilateral infiltrates consistent with pulmonary edema. These infiltrates may be mild or dense, interstitial or alveolar, patchy or confluent. They should, however, represent parenchymal disease and should not be explained by effusions, atelectasis, or masses. The chest X-ray can initially be misleading since there is no distinct pattern to the development of these infiltrates. They may develop quickly and symmetrically, even before hypoxemia occurs, or more gradually and asymmetrically. It can also be difficult radiographically to distinguish cardiogenic pulmonary edema from ARDS. It is not uncommon for the chest X-ray to have focal infiltrates early in the course of ARDS, interpreted at that time as pneumonia or segmental atelectasis, only to progress over a few hours or days to a complete "white-out." In the proper clinical setting, these radiographic conundrums should not exclude early ARDS as the cause of an at-risk patient's acute deterioration.

Arterial blood gas measurements are markedly abnormal in patients with ARDS. Initially, patients generally have a respiratory alkalosis along with hypoxemia. Because the $PaO_2$ is influenced by the fraction of inspired oxygen ($FIO_2$), most ARDS definitions have defined hypoxemia in terms of a $PaO_2/FIO_2$ ratio or an arterial-to-alveolar oxygen gradient ($PaO_2/PAO_2$ ratio). As dead-space ventilation and work of breathing increase, the ability to effectively clear carbon dioxide is compromised and the initial respiratory alkalosis gives way to respiratory acidosis.

There are few other laboratory abnormalities linked specifically to ARDS. While many abnormalities have been identified, a diagnostic test for lung injury does not exist at this time. Many of the laboratory abnormalities seen in patients with ARDS relate to the underlying illness. Because ARDS usually occurs in conjunction with systemic inflammation, abnormalities in other organ functions are also common. Hematologic abnormalities are very common, including leukocytosis or leukopenia and anemia. Thrombocytopenia is also common as a reflection of underlying systemic inflammation and endothelial injury. Full-blown disseminated intravascular coagulation (DIC) occurs less frequently and is usually due to sepsis, severe trauma, or head injury. Renal function may be abnormal due to decreased renal perfusion or acute tubular necrosis. Liver function tests can be elevated in either a hepatocellular or cholestatic pattern. These abnormalities reflecting multiorgan dysfunction are entirely related to the underlying systemic inflammation that accompanies ARDS.

Other laboratory abnormalities have been described that may be more specific for endothelial injury. Von Willebrand's factor antigen (VWF) is elevated in the serum of patients at risk for ARDS. Complement levels are abnormal in the serum of patients with ARDS. Other acute phase reactants, such as ceruloplasmin, have also been shown to be increased. Finally, multiple cytokine levels are increased in the serum of patients at risk for and with ARDS. Tumor necrosis factor, IL-1, IL-6, and IL-8 have all been shown to be present in increased amounts. Some authors have tried to correlate the level of these cytokines with the likelihood of developing ARDS or death. Unfortunately, at this time, none of these markers can be used clinically to predict individual outcomes or to help guide management.

Many investigators have explored the lungs of ARDS patients for biochemical and cellular abnormalities that might predict onset or outcome of ARDS. Inflammatory mediators such as cytokines, reactive oxygen species, leukotrienes, and activated complement fragments are some of the mediators found in the bronchoalveolar lavage (BAL) fluid of affected patients. Cellular analysis of BAL fluid reveals high neutrophil counts in patients at risk and with early ARDS. Neutrophils commonly make up more than 60% of the total cell population of BAL fluid. (Normal is <5%.) Interestingly, it appears that as ARDS resolves, neu-

**Table 58.4** Diagnostic criteria for acute lung injury (ALI) and ARDS*

| | Onset | Oxygenation[a] | Chest radiograph | PAOP[b] |
|---|---|---|---|---|
| ALI criteria | Acute | $PaO_2/FIO_2 \leq 300$ mm Hg | Bilateral interstitial or alveolar infiltrates | ≤ 18 mmHg if measured or no clinical evidence of left atrial hypertension |
| ARDS criteria | Acute | $PaO_2/FIO_2 \leq 200$ mm Hg | Bilateral interstitial or alveolar infiltrates | ≤ 18 mmHg if measured or no clinical evidence of left atrial hypertension |

*Adapted from Bernard GR, Artigas A, Brigham KL, et al. The American-European Concensus Conference on ARDS: definitions, mechanisms, relevant outcomes, and clinical trial coordination. Am J Respir Crit Care Med 1994;149:818–24.

[a]Regardless of level of positive end-expiratory pressure (PEEP).

[b]Pulmonary artery occlusion pressure.

trophils are replaced by alveolar macrophages. It is postulated that, while macrophages can certainly contribute to the acute inflammatory process, they also seem to be important in the resolution and healing of lung injury.

One interesting finding in BAL is a marker of pulmonary fibrosis known as *procollagen peptide III* (*PCPIII*). When fibroblasts are active in the lung, and secreting collagen, the type of collagen being made is type III collagen. It is secreted first as a procollagen, and then a fragment is cleaved off the procollagen molecule to create collagen. The fragment left after creating type III collagen is known as *PCPIII*. In a study of serial bronchoscopies done during the course of ARDS, the level of PCPIII in BAL correlated very strongly with mortality. High levels of PCPIII predicted a poor outcome in those patients. It has been thought that the severity of pulmonary fibrosis during ARDS correlates with outcome, and PCPIII probably reflects this process. This measurement is currently being used experimentally to determine if high-risk patients might respond to therapies designed to decrease the fibrotic response after lung injury.

## Diagnosis

The development of ARDS is usually rapid, occurring most often within 12 to 48 h of the predisposing event, although it may take up to 5 d in rare instances. Respiratory distress, severe hypoxemia, and generalized pulmonary infiltrates are all necessary for the diagnosis of ARDS. The specific definition of ARDS has varied depending on the author and the attempt to describe the severity of the disease. Recently, a joint American–European consensus statement was published suggesting a uniform defi-nition of acute lung injury (ALI) and ARDS (Table 58.4). Bilateral pulmonary infiltrates must be present although correlation between the roentgenographic abnormalities and the degree of hypoxemia can be variable. Hypoxemia with a $PaO_2/FIO_2$ ratio less than 300 defines acute lung injury while a lower ratio of less than 200 describes ARDS. If measured, pulmonary artery occlusion pressure is usually less than 18 mmHg. Total respiratory compliance is usually reduced, but this is generally not required for the diagnosis. Regardless of the definition applied, it is conceptually important to recognize that acute lung injury represents a spectrum of severity with definable ARDS at the far end of the spectrum. Thus, the term ARDS describes the most severe forms of acute lung injury but ALI can exist without ARDS.

To date, no specific laboratory findings of ARDS have been described other than those necessary to meet the criteria of the syndrome. As a syndrome, the diagnosis of ARDS requires a careful historical and physical examination and the exclusion of specific processes that require unique therapy. In most cases, the inciting event is obvious and the development of respiratory failure can be seen as a direct consequence of that event. In that setting, very little is generally required to make a clinical diagnosis. Whenever immunosuppression exists, as in AIDS, hematologic malignancy, or organ transplantation, the search for opportunistic infections becomes a high priority. Patients with severe thrombocytopenia can develop intrapulmonary hemorrhage. The likelihood of a drug-induced pneumonitis, from radiation or chemotherapy, also increases in this population.

Even more challenging can be the case for which no obvious etiology exists. Occasionally patients will walk into an emergency room with respiratory failure and diffuse pulmonary infiltrates. The patient may be a "normal" host with no evidence of injury, extrapulmonary infection, drug ingestion, or toxic exposure. In that setting, a diffuse pulmonary infection or primary pulmonary disorder becomes more probable. It is prudent to consider and rule out PCP and TB in patients presenting in such a fashion, even when no apparent risk for immunosuppression exists, in addition to considering more exotic diagnoses.

Bronchoscopy with bronchoalveolar lavage (BAL) is one of the mainstays of the evaluation of patients, immunocompromised or not, with ARDS of unclear etiology. This can be accomplished safely in most patients by experienced operators. While analysis of BAL fluid is not specific for ARDS, it is done to rule out other acute processes. The presence of high numbers of eosinophils (>15%–20% of the total cell count) suggests acute eosinophilic pneumonia. High lymphocyte counts suggest hypersensitivity pneumonitis, sarcoidosis, bronchiolitis obliterans organizing pneumonia (BOOP), and other acute forms of interstitial lung disease. Many erythrocytes, especially in the presence of hemosiderin-laden macrophages, suggests pulmonary hemorrhage of some etiology. Cultures should be sent for all likely infectious agents, depending on the clinical setting, and cytology should be performed for pneumocystis carinii (PCP), malignancy, and viral inclusion bodies. The urinalysis is helpful when considering pulmonary-renal syndromes such as Goodpasture's syndrome. Occasionally serologies are sent to rule out systemic lupus erythematosis. A search for malignancy, especially leukemia and lymphoma, should be considered. Transbronchial lung biopsies are generally contraindicated in a mechanically ventilated patient, yet it is very rare that an open lung biopsy is required. It is often nondiagnostic when the disease process has not already been identified by careful clinical evaluation and bronchoscopy.

ARDS may develop as a part of the fat embolism syndrome after long-bone fractures. Fat embolism syndrome is characterized by mental status changes, conjunctival and axillary petechiae, anemia, thrombocytopenia, and diffuse lung injury, with hypoxemia occurring 24–72 h after injury. The pathogenesis has not been clearly elucidated but is believed to be due to release of toxic free fatty acids from bone marrow fat after trauma. Acute lung injury follows long-bone fractures in 5%–10% of patients. The incidence of full-blown fat embolism syndrome has declined dramatically in recent years, however, because of earlier stabilization of fractures.

## Therapy

### Goals

The therapeutic goals in ARDS are twofold: (*1*) cardiorespiratory support and (*2*) treatment of the underlying precipitating event. It can not be overemphasized that identification and early, aggressive treatment directed at the inciting cause of ARDS is imperative for resolution of lung injury and respiratory failure. The reader is referred to the appropriate chapter for treatment of sepsis (Chapter 50) and the various infectious agents that can cause diffuse lung infection (Chapter 56). This section will deal primarily with support and treatment of the resultant lung injury.

Other than treatment of the underlying cause of ARDS in a given patient, there is no convincing evidence that any available treatments have a therapeutic effect in the sense of modifying or hastening resolution of ARDS. Therefore, therapy is directed at the correction of physiological abnormalities presenting a threat to life or organ function, especially hypoxemia and tissue hypoxia, while avoiding therapeutic complications. Although some patients respond to oxygen therapy alone, mechanical ventilation is usually required, along with PEEP. Newer modes of mechanical ventilation offer an alternative when conventional therapy is inadequate or associated with complications. Fluid management must balance the need for adequate cardiac output and prevention of renal failure against the potential for exacerbation of pulmonary edema.

Therapeutic controversy exists concerning: (*1*) what level of $FiO_2$ is nontoxic to the lung, (*2*) the risk/benefit ratio of higher PEEP and lower $FiO_2$ versus lower PEEP and higher $FiO_2$; (*3*) the risk/benefit ratio of high PEEP with maintenance of cardiac output by volume administration or vasoactive agents, (*4*) the preferred mode of mechanical ventilation, (*5*) the philosophy of fluid management (i.e., whether to "dry out" the patient and run the risk of reduced organ perfusion or to maintain euvolemia and organ perfusion or to maintain euvolemia and organ perfusion at the risk of increased lung water), and (*6*) the use of colloid versus crystalloid solutions in fluid management.

## Oxygen therapy, mechanical ventilation, and PEEP

The major physiological abnormality in ARDS is hypoxemia due to shunt. The work of breathing is substantially increased, not only by reduced lung compliance but also by the increased minute ventilation requirement imposed by hypermetabolic conditions and increased physiologic dead space. Most patients with ARDS require tracheal intubation and mechanical ventilation either to overcome hypoxemia or to alleviate discomfort due to excessive work of breathing. Although supplemental oxygen therapy alone is rarely adequate, the application of continuous positive airway pressure (CPAP) through a tight-fitting mask or endotracheal tube is sometimes sufficient to improve both oxygenation and patient comfort.

High concentrations of oxygen have been shown to be toxic, producing direct lung injury resembling ARDS. Although an $FiO_2$ of 0.8 or higher has been demonstrated to do this, especially when applied for prolonged periods of time, there is no clear agreement as to what level of $FiO_2$ is nontoxic. One common recommedation is to use the lowest $FiO_2$ achieving adequate oxygenation (arterial oxygen saturation above 90%), adding PEEP if this goal cannot be achieved with an $FiO_2$ less than 0.6.

If mechanical ventilatory support is used, important clinical decisions include the mode of ventilation and tidal volume ($V_T$). The conventional approach has been to use volume-controlled ventilation in either the assist/control (A/C) mode or the intermittent mandatory ventilation (IMV) mode. Both modes of ventilation have risks and benefits associated with their use, and there is no data to support the routine use of one over another. The use of pressure-controlled ventilation has been advocated in ARDS patients with very stiff lungs and high minute ventilation requirements. Inverse ratio ventilation (IRV) using the pressure control mode has also been used successfully in a few patients when conventional ventilation, even with high $FiO_2$ and PEEP, has been inadequate. Because of its potential adverse hemodynamic effects, IRV should be applied only with careful monitoring by experienced personnel. It is important to note that no specific mode of ventilation has proven to decrease mortality in ARDS, and, when applied properly, the vast majority of patients with ARDS can be managed with standard volume-controlled ventilation.

Until recent years, it was common practice to use relatively high tidal volumes of 12 to 15 ml/kg in all persons with acute respiratory failure, including ARDS. There is a growing body of evidence, however, to suggest that overdistension of damaged lung can lead to further lung injury and barotrauma. The available lung volume for ventilating an ARDS patient is reduced by nature of the disease itself, and thus, finding an appropriate and safe tidal volume can be difficult. I recommend starting at 10 ml/kg in most ARDS patients and adjusting downward as necessary. In patients with particularly stiff lungs, it may be useful to measure compliance at several different tidal volumes, creating a $V_T$-compliance curve. As tidal volume is increased, more compliant regions of lung may become relatively overdistended, causing total lung compliance to decrease. It may be more reasonable, in that setting, to select the lowest tidal volume associated with the peak compliance. Some have gone further, suggesting that the tidal volumes should be reduced in ARDS until the peak alveolar pressure (measured as a static, inspiratory hold pressure or plateau pressure) is less than 30–40 cm $H_2O$. This strategy, which is rapidly achieving wide acceptance, attempts to minimize ventilator-induced injury by limiting alveolar overdistension. While hypoventilation may result, the actual goal of therapy is not to create hypercapnia with respiratory acidosis but to limit stretching of the lungs by limiting $V_T$. If, in limiting excessive stretch, the $PaCO_2$ rises, it is accepted as a necessary side effect of the reduced volumes. Several anecdotal reports and case series have reported improved survival using this lung-protective strategy but, to date, no randomized controlled trials of limiting $V_T$ or of permissive hypercapnia have been done. Thus, while permissive hypercapnia is an attractive, theoretically sound hypothesis, it remains unproved in the management of ARDS.

Positive end-expiratory pressure remains a mainstay of ventilatory management in patients with ARDS. The improvement in arterial $PaO_2$ with PEEP is associated with an increase in lung volume measured as functional residual capacity. Presumably, this increase in functional residual capacity results from either opening of previously collapsed lung units or preventing alveolar collapse at end-expiration. PEEP does not decrease extravascular lung water; in fact, total lung water may increase somewhat with the application of PEEP.

Whenever added PEEP is applied, the resultant effects on the respiratory system and oxygen delivery must be carefully assessed. It should not be assumed that the cardiopulmonary response to PEEP will be beneficial, even in those generally considered to be excellent candidates. Since cardiopulmonary status may be changing rapidly in critically ill patients receiving PEEP therapy, the goal of PEEP therapy in ARDS is either to improve oxygen delivery (the product of cardiac output and arterial oxygen content) or to maintain the same oxygen delivery with an increase in $PaO_2$ that allows a reduction in the $FiO_2$. Arterial pressure, cardiac output (if available), lung compliance, and $PaO_2$ or oxygen saturation should be assessed just before application of PEEP.

## Pharmacologic therapy

ARDS has resisted pharmacologic manipulation for over 20 yr. Nevertheless, several therapeutic approaches have been attempted and many more will be studied in the near future. As more information becomes available, through the development of new agents and clinical trials, the pharmacologic approach to a patient with ARDS will hopefully improve. Some of the important potential therapies are considered here.

Corticosteroids clearly have multiple antiinflammatory properties. Despite this, several recent well-controlled clinical trials have failed to demonstrate any clear benefit either in the early treatment or in the prevention of ARDS. Randomized controlled trials have also failed to demonstrate a beneficial effect of corticosteroids in sepsis (Chapter 50). In fact, in some of these trials, the use of corticosteroids in early ARDS and sepsis increased the number of deleterious effects, including prolonged mechanical ventilation, nosocomial infection, and death.

In addition to reducing inflammation, corticosteroids may suppress collagen formation and facilitate collagen breakdown; they are used clinically in several fibrotic diseases of the lung. Consequently, it is conceivable that corticosteroids may have a beneficial effect on the fibroproliferative stage of ARDS, leading several researchers to attempt treatment of so-called "chronic" ARDS with high-dose corticosteroids. Three small case series, with a combined number of 45 patients, demonstrated a consistently high survival rate. Unfortunately, these studies are neither randomized nor controlled, and firm conclusions should not be made. The risks of prolonged use of corticosteroids in the ICU are high, and further investigation is necessary. Unless there are specific indications, generally related to the underlying illness, the routine use of corticosteroids is not currently recommended in patients with ARDS.

Prostaglandin $E_1$ is a vasodilator with antiinflammatory properties that has been shown to lower pulmonary artery pressures and increase cardiac output in ARDS. Because the drug is 95% metabolized during a single pass through the lung, vasodilatation of the systemic vasculature is usually minimal. Despite an earlier report of improved survival in ARDS patients treated with prostaglandin $E_1$, a recent multicenter, controlled trial showed no reduction in ARDS severity, duration, or mortality. Other modulators of the inflammatory response, including pentoxifylline, ibuprofen, antioxidants, and antibodies directed against endotoxin, complement fragments, and tumor necrosis factor, have recently been or are currently being studied.

Surfactant replacement, so successful in infant respiratory distress syndrome, is also being evaluated in ARDS. Pulmonary surfactant is grossly abnormal, quantitatively and qualitatively, in ARDS, and these surfactant abnormalities probably cause much of the syndrome's deranged pulmonary physiology. There are several anecdotal reports in the literature of successful treatment of ARDS using various surfactant products. Subsequently, a large trial of aerosolized surfactant replacement in sepsis-induced ARDS yielded no difference in outcome. Other surfactant products and delivery techniques are being studied, but so far, surfactant replacement can not be recommended for the treatment of ARDS.

Ketoconazole is a synthetic imidazole derivative approved for use as an antifungal agent. Interestingly, ketoconazole is also a potent *in vitro* inhibitor of several pro-inflammatory pathways. It is both a thromboxane synthetase inhibitor and a 5-lipoxygenase inhibitor, thereby blocking the synthesis of prostaglandins and leukotrienes that can promote lung inflammation. Two preliminary studies have suggested ketoconazole may be effective in reducing the incidence of ARDS in critically ill surgical patients. Despite these encouraging preliminary results, a large randomized controlled trial of ketoconazole in early ARDS revealed no benefit of ketoconazole compared to placebos.

Nitric oxide, when inhaled at low concentration, is a selective pulmonary vasodilator. It can lower pulmonary artery pressures, improve ventilation-perfusion matching within the lung, and improve oxygenation. Unfortunately, nitric oxide is very difficult to administer safely, as it requires specialized delivery and monitoring systems. Efficacy in ARDS, with regard to improved survival, is also lacking. For these reasons, nitric oxide should not be used at this time for the treatment of ARDS.

## ANNOTATED BIBLIOGRAPHY


Bernard GR, Artigas A, Brigham KL et al. The American-European Consensus Conference on ARDS: definitions, mechanisms, relevant outcomes, and clinical trial coordination. Am J Respir Crit Care Med 1994; 149:818–824.

*This article describes the recent internationl consensus conference definitions of ARDS and acute lung injury. It also summarizes the known mechanisms of lung injury and describes the current controversies involved in making the diagnosis of these syndromes.*

Craig KC, Pierson DJ, Carrico CJ. The clinical application of positive end-expiratory pressure (PEEP) in the adult respiratory distress syndrome (ARDS). Respir Care 1985; 30(3):184.

*An excellent and practical approach to the use of PEEP in the management of ARDS.*

Duchin JS, Koster FT, Peters CJ et al. Hantavirus pulmonary syndrome: a clinical description of 17 patients with a newly recognized disease. N Engl J Med 1994; 330:949–955.

*The original scientific article describing this newly recognized syndrome.*

Hudson LD, Milberg JA, Anardi D, Maunder RJ. Clinical risks for development of ARDS. Am J Respir Crit Care Med 1995; 151:293–301.

*One of the best studies describing the epidemiology of risk factors for ARDS.*

Kollef MH, Schuster DP. Medical progress: the acute respiratory distress syndrome. N Engl J Med 1995; 332:27–37.

*An excellent clinical review of contemporary ARDS management, emphasizing the techniques used to diagnosis and treat patients with this disorder.*

Marini JJ. New approaches to the ventilatory management of the adult respiratory distress syndrome. J Crit Care 1992; 7:256.

*A thorough and well-written description of the basis for most of the recent changes in management of mechanical ventilation for ARDS including permissive hypercapnia.*

Milberg JA, Davis DR, Steinberg KP, Hudson LD. Improved survival of patients with acute repsiratory distress syndrome (ARDS): 1983-1993. JAMA 1995; 273:306–309.

*This study desribes the recent changes in mortality of ARDS at one institution over the period of a decade.*

Montgomery AB, Stager MA, Carrico CJ et al. Causes of mortality in patients with the adult respiratory distress syndrome. Am Rev Respir Dis 1985; 132:485.

*This article identified sepsis and multiple organ failure as the primary causes of mortality in patients who died after onset of ARDS. Only 15% of patients actually died from unsupportable respiratory failure.*

Pingleton SK. Complications of acute respiratory failure. Am Rev Respir Dis 1988; 137:1463.

*A review of the various complications that can befall a patient in the ICU receiving mechanical ventilation.*

Tuxen DV. Permissive hypercapnic ventilation. Am J Respir Crit Care Med 1994; 150:870.

*A review of the clinical utility and adverse effects of permissive hypercapnia. Despite the lack of randomized, controlled trials, this article argues for the clinical use of this ventilatory approach.*

# 59

# Pleurisy and Empyema

HARTMUT LODE, TOM SCHABERG, AND J. ELLER

A variety of infectious or inflammatory processes can involve the pleural membranes that enclose the lung and thoracic cavity. These give rise to characteristic symptoms and signs that require recognition and specific management. This chapter focuses on infectious diseases causing *pleurisy*, *pleural effusions*, or *empyema*. Much of the discussion will revolve around distinguishing and managing uncomplicated effusions that accompany pneumonia (*parapneumonic effusions*) from those that lead to empyema.

## Definition of Terms

The pleura is the serous membrane that covers the lung parenchyma, the mediastinum, the diaphragm, and rib cage. The pleura is subdivided into the *visceral* pleura, which covers the entire surface of the lung, including the interlobar fissures, and the *parietal* pleura, which covers the inner surface of the thoracic cage, mediastinum, and diaphragm. Normally there is a thin (10–17 $\mu$m) layer of fluid between the visceral and parietal pleura. The pleural fluid is essentially an ultrafiltrate of serum with similar chemical composition but lower protein level. Normally the pleural fluid moves from the capillaries in the parietal pleura to the pleural space. In the absence of disease, pleural fluid does not accumulate because the rate of its removal to the parietal pleural lymphatics is equivalent to the low volume of liquid that is formed.

*Pleural effusions* have classically been divided into transudative and exudative effusions. A transudative pleural effusion occurs when abnormalities in the factors that influence pleural fluid movement result in its accumulation in the pleural space. In contrast, exudative pleural effusions occur when the pleural surfaces themselves are altered in such a way (e.g., by infection or inflammation) that an increased quantity of protein-rich fluid is formed.

The pleural space may become infected from the contiguous spread of pneumonia, from infection in the mediastinum or subdiaphragmatic space, or following a thoracic surgical procedure or penetrating chest trauma. Pleural infection is most frequently due to common bacterial respiratory pathogens, but can also be seen with tuberculosis and as a result infection transmitted by fungi, viruses, and parasites. With pleura-associated pneumonia, mediastinal infection, and subdiaphragmatic abscess, increased pleural capillary permeability can also cause the formation of noninfected "sympathetic" pleural effusions. With pneumonia, the sterile inflammatory fluid that results is termed an uncomplicated *parapneumonic effusion*. Such sympathetic effusions need not be mechanically removed; drainage needs to be performed only when *empyema* exists. The word "empyema" means suppuration; this disease has been known to the medical community since the fifth century B.C. when Hippocrates described in detail its symptomatology and management.

*Pleuritis* or *pleurisy* is inflammation of the pleural surfaces. Pleuritis is usually accompanied by sharp chest pain made worse on inhalation or movement and is often associated with the development of pleural effusions. Pleuritis can accompany pneumonias or pulmonary infarction or may be a primary event as in certain infections (e.g., Coxsackie B virus) or inflammatory processes (e.g., systemic lupus erythematosis).

## Epidemiology: Incidence and Etiologies of Pleural Effusion

Pleural effusion is a common diagnostic problem, and management. It has been estimated that up to 10% of all patients hospitalized in internal medicine wards may have some form of pleural effusion. The leading etiology is cardiac failure (30%–40% of all cases of pleural effusion). The incidence per year of diseases causing pleural effusions in the United States is listed in Table 59.1.

About half of exudative pleural effusions are parapneumonic; about three-quarters are bacterial and one-quarter viral in etiology. The next-most-frequent cause of exudative pleural effusion is malignancy; bronchial and breast carcinomas are the most common etiologies. Pleural effusion is also caused by pulmonary emboli (8%), by liver cirrhosis (6%), and by gastrointestinal diseases (especially pancreatitis) (3%).

The differential diagnosis of pleural effusions is displayed in Table 59.2. Generally only those cases that are accompanied by pleural inflammation or trauma cause pleuritic chest pain or pleurisy.

## Pathophysiology of Pleural Effusion Formation

A pleural effusion develops when the amount of pleural fluid that enters the pleural space exceeds the amount that is removed via the lymphatics. According to the current understanding of pathophysiology, pleural effusions can result from increased pleural fluid formation, decreased lymphatic clearance from the pleural space, or a combination of these two factors. Pleural effusions have classically been divided into transudative and exudative types.

### Transudative pleural effusion

Normally, the lymphatic flow from the pleural space is about 0.01 ml/kg/h or 15 ml per day, but the total capacity of the lymphatics is about 300 ml per day. Under normal conditions, the

**Table 59.1** Approximate annual incidence of various types of pleural effusions in the United States

| | |
|---|---|
| Congestive heart failure | 500,000 |
| Pneumonia (bacterial) | 300,000 |
| MALIGNANT DISEASE | 200,000 |
| Lung | 60,000 |
| Breast | 50,000 |
| Lymphoma | 40,000 |
| Other | 50,000 |
| Pulmonary embolization | 150,000 |
| Viral disease | 100,000 |
| Cirrhosis with ascites | 50,000 |
| Gastrointestinal disease | 25,000 |
| Collagen vascular disease | 6,000 |
| Tuberculosis | 2,500 |
| Asbestos exposure | 2,000 |
| Mesothelioma | 1,500 |

Adapted from Light R.W. Pleural diseases. 2nd ed. Philadelphia, Lea & Febiger (1990): 76

capacity of pleural lymphatics to clear fluid is approximately 20 times its formation rate with a net gradient of 6 cm $H_2O$. If the capillary pressure is elevated in either the visceral or parietal pleura, excess fluid can traverse the pleural membranes.

In the clinical situation, increased pressure in the systemic capillaries of the parietal pleura is rarely associated with pleural effusions. Furthermore, chronic pulmonary arterial hypertension does not lead to pleural effusion. In contrast, pleural effusions are common with left ventricular failure due to elevation of the pulmonary capillary wedge pressure. Experimentally it has been demonstrated that the increased rate of fluid formation is due to movement of lung interstitial fluid across the visceral pleura into the pleural space rather than due to direct hyperfiltration from the parietal capillaries in the visceral pleura.

Typically transudative pleural effusions have white cell counts $<1000/\mu l$, protein values of $<2.0$ g/l, glucose and lactate dehydrogenase (LDH) values equivalent to serum, and pH values of 7.40. They also develop without accompanying pleuritic chest pain. Most transudative effusions are not due to infectious diseases.

## Exudative pleural effusion

Disease of the pleura itself can lead to accumulation of pleural fluid by three different mechanisms: *First*, pleural surfaces can be altered in such a way that permeability increases and more protein and fluid enter the pleural space for a given net pressure difference between the capillaries, the interstitium, and the pleural space. This mechanism probably accounts for the majority of exudative pleural effusions seen with infections, primary pleural inflammatory conditions (e.g., systemic lupus erythematosus [SLE] or rheumatoid arthritis), and malignancies. *Second*, a pleural effusion may develop if the lymphatic flow from the pleural space is decreased. *Third*, the pleura may be altered such that the pleural pressure is negative. The most common situation in which this mechanism accounts for a pleural effusion is bronchial obstruction leading to atelectasis of a lower lobe or a complete lung. Each of these mechanisms can lead to the formation of exudative pleural effusions. With exudative effusions, the protein concentration typically exceeds 3.0 g/l (Fig. 59.1). The leukocyte count may be elevated in proportion to the degree of inflammation that accompanies the exudate.

While a number of diseases may be responsible for causing exudative effusions, these findings on pleural fluid analysis must first prompt a search for primary pleural space or contiguous infection. Pneumonia is initiated by the aspiration of microorganisms into subpleural alveoli with a failure of their removal by resident alveolar macrophages (see Chapter 56). Bacterial pneumonias may be associated with a 36%–57% incidence of pleural effusions. These "parapneumonic" effusions may be uncomplicated and characterized by free-flowing fluid, which resolves spontaneously with antibiotic therapy, or complicated and require pleural space drainage for resolution of pleural sepsis (Fig. 59.2). The natural course of a complicated parapneumonic effusion is to develop into single or multiple loculations that progress into empyema. "Primary" empyema can be initiated by direct deposition of organisms in the pleural space, either from an occult pneumonia or by hematogenous spread. In the latter situation transudative effusions caused by other diseases such as congestive heart failure (CHF) may become secondary infected.

**Table 59.2** Differential diagnosis of pleural effusions

TRANSUDATIVE PLEURAL EFFUSIONS

| | |
|---|---|
| Congestive Heart Failure | Urinothorax |
| Cirrhosis | Myxedema |
| Nephrotic syndrome | Pulmonary emboli |
| Superior vena cava obstruction | Sarcoidosis |
| Peritoneal dialysis | Malignancy atelectasis |

EXUDATIVE PLEURAL EFFUSIONS

| | |
|---|---|
| *NEOPLASTIC DISEASES* | *DRUG-INDUCED PLEURAL DISEASE* |
| Metastatic Disease (Carcinoma, lymphoma, leukemia) | *MISCELLANEOUS DISEASES AND CONDITIONS* |
| Mesothelioma | Asbestos exposure |
| *INFECTIOUS DISEASES* | Postpericardiectomy or postmyocardial infarction syndrome |
| Bacterial infections | Meig's syndrome |
| Tuberculous pleurisy | Sarcoidosis |
| Fungal infections | Pericardial disease |
| Parasitic infections (amebiasis, paragonimiasis, echinococcosis) | Uremia |
| Viral infections | Trapped lung |
| Nocardial infection | Radiation therapy |
| *PULMONARY EMBOLIZATION* | Postpartum pleural effusion |
| *GASTROINTESTINAL DISEASES* | Amyloidosis |
| Pancreatitis | Electrical burns |
| Subphrenic abscess | Iatrogenic injury |
| Intrahepatic abscess | *HEMOTHORAX* |
| Splenic abscess | *CHYLOTHORAX* |
| Esophageal perforation | |
| Abdominal surgical procedures | |
| Diaphragmatic hernia | |
| Endoscopic variceal sclerotherapy | |
| *COLLAGEN VASCULAR DISEASE* | |
| Rheumatoid pleuritis | |
| Systemic lupus erythematosus | |
| Immunoblastic lymphadenopathy | |
| Sjögren's syndrome | |
| Familial Mediterranean fever | |
| Churg-Strauss syndrome | |
| Wegner's granulomatosis | |

Following deposition of organisms, there is migration and adherence of polymorphonuclear granulocytes [PMNs] to the adjacent pleural endothelium.

Oxygen metabolites, PMN lysosomal constituents, arachidonic acid, and metabolites released by activated PMNs result in endothelial injury of the pulmonary, subpleural, and pleural vessels and cause increased capillary permeability. Interleukin-8 (IL-8) is a major chemotactic factor for PMNs in pneumonia and empyema and tumor necrosis factor (TNF)-$\alpha$ produced by macrophages during infection may play a role in the local production of IL-8. The resultant extravascular lung water increases the lung interstitial pleural pressure and drives more fluid from the interstitium across the mesothelium into the pleural space. If the rate of fluid production exceeds lung lymphatic clearance, the protein-rich fluid accumulates.

If the inflammatory process continues unabated, further endothelial injury occurs with increased localized permeability, edema, and formation of a greater volume of pleural fluid. The pleural fluid is then characterized by an increased number of polymorphonuclear granulocytes [PMNs], a fall in pH as well as in glucose, and an increase in LDH-features characteristic of an empyema. The pleural fluid/serum glucose ratio is often <0.5 with an absolute pleural fluid concentration of usually <40 mg/dl because of increased glycolysis from polymorphonuclear granulocyte [PMN] phagocytosis and bacterial metabolism. As the end products of glucose metabolism, $CO_2$, and lactate accumulate in the pleural space, the pH may fall to <7.10 and LDH increases, often to >1000 units per liter, due to cell lysis. When these events have been completed, the exudative fluid that results with its high polymorphonuclear granulocyte [PMN] content and other features is said to be an empyema.

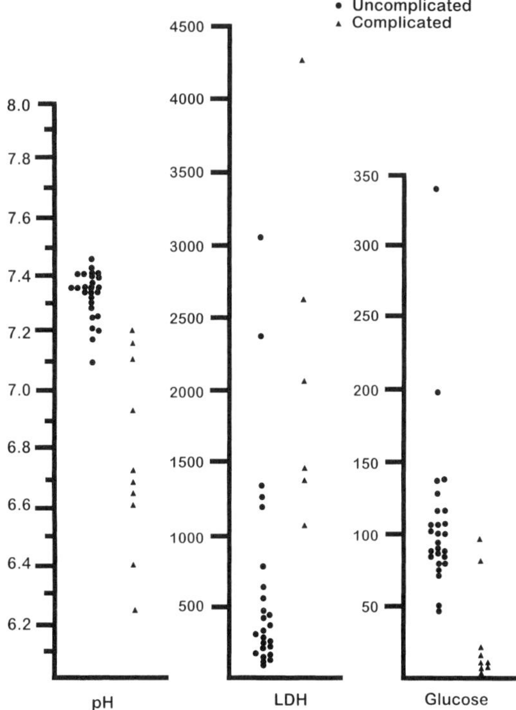


**Fig. 59.2** Distribution of pleural fluid pH, lactic dehydrogenase (LDH), and glucose levels in uncomplicated and complicated parapneumonic effusions. [Reprinted from Light RW, Girard WM, Jenkinson SG, George RB: Parapneumonic effusions. Am J Med 1980; 69:507–511, with permission from Excerpta Medica Inc.]

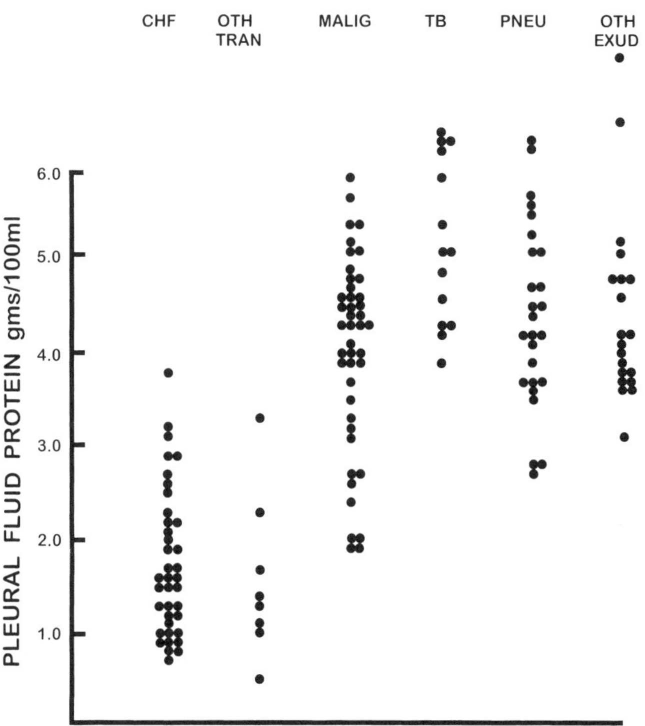


**Fig. 59.1** Pleural fluid protein levels in effusion secondary to congestive heart failure (CHF), other transudates (OTH,TRAN), malignant disease (MALIG), tuberculosis (TB), pneumonia (PNEU), and other exudates (OTH EXUD). Each point represents one pleural fluid. Note that the distribution of protein levels for all categories of exudative pleural effusions is similar. [Used with permission from Light RW, MacGregor MI, Luchsinger PC, Ball WC: Pleural effusions: the diagnostic separation of transudates and exudates. Ann Intern Med 1972; 77:507–513.]

## Clinical Manifestations

### Presentation

The clinical presentation will vary with the nature of the underlying disease process. Patients who have infectious causes for pleurisy or pleural effusion fall into several different categories. Patients with *bacterial pneumonia* and pleural effusion will usually present with an acute febrile illness consisting of pleuritic chest pain (pleurisy), sputum production, and leukocytosis (see Chapter 56). Pleurisy and pleural effusions are more characteristic of pneumococcal and streptococcal infections than those caused by other bacteria. Staphylococci may cause either primary bronchopneumonia or hematogenous pneumonia with cavitation and lead to bronchopleural fistula formation and empyema. "Atypical" pathogens such as *Chlamydia pneumoniae*, *Mycoplasma pneumoniae*, and *Legionella* can also cause effusions with pneumonia but only rarely empyema.

Patients with anaerobic bacterial infections involving the pleural space usually present with a subacute illness. In one series, the duration of symptoms before presentation averaged 10 d, with 70% of the patients having symptoms for more than 7 d. The majority of patients with anaerobic pleural pulmonary infections will have significant weight loss as well as leukocytosis and mild anemia. In addition, most have a history of alcoholism, an episode of unconsciousness, or some other factor that predisposes to aspiration. Poor dental hygiene and gingivitis with multiple carious teeth that harbor a high anaerobic bacterial population are other characteristic features.

Tuberculous pleurisy is an important cause of pleural exudate in young patients; it is being diagnosed with increasing frequency in the elderly patient as well. In the older patient tuberculosis may coexist with other diseases, such as congestive heart failure, malignancy, and pneumonia, causing diagnostic dilemmas. If hematogenous spread has occurred, patients may present with bilateral effusions. Most patients with tuberculous pleural effusions will have well-established delayed hypersensitivity to *Mycobacterium tuberculosis* protein antigens.

Community-wide episodic pleurisy, which in some patients is accompanied by pericarditis, is characteristic of coxsackie B infection. It typically occurs in the late summer or early fall in temperate countries. These patients are often young, are not very ill, and will have fever without cough and small pleural effusions without pneumonia on chest X-ray. The illness is self-limited and requires only symptomatic treatment. Other viral causes of pleurisy and pleural effusion include adenovirus species and herpes-group viruses (Epstein-Barr Virus [EBV], cytomegalovirus [CMV], varicella, *H. simplex*). The latter occur most frequently in patients who are immunosuppressed and have systemic infection with these agents.

## Physical findings

Physical findings vary with the cause of the disease process. With pneumonia or primary empyema 85% of patients have a temperature greater than 38° C. The chest examination varies in relation to the amount of the effusion and the presence of active inflammation. Dullness to percussion-diminished vocal fremitus, decreased breath sounds, and egophony above the area of dullness are characteristic findings with pleural effusions. Contralateral shift of the mediastinum can be seen with greater than 1500 ml of fluid in the pleural space. With pleural inflammation there is often "splinting" (decreased respiratory movement) of the affected side. There may also be superficial tenderness over the rib cage. A pleural rub may be present; such rubs are usually low-pitched and sound like two pieces of leather rubbing together. The remainder of the physical examination should focus on the sinuses, teeth and throat, the skin and joints, and the heart and abdomen, looking for systemic disorders or infections that might cause pleural effusion or pleurisy.

# Diagnosis

## Radiological investigation

The value of standard chest radiography in complex pleural pulmonary disease may be limited. Although the existence of a free-flowing effusion can be established, identification of loculation is often difficult. In parapneumonic effusions computerized tomography (CT) is helpful in differentiating parenchymal from pleural disease, evaluating the parenchymal disease, determining localization, characterizing the pleural surfaces, and guiding pleural drainage. A thin-section chest CT may reveal a pulmonary parenchymal process not readily seen on standard chest X-rays (see Chapter 12). The use of intravenous contrast medium provides localization of fluid collections and enhancement of the pleural membranes (Figs. 59.3, 59.4). If there is a possibility that the empyema or effusion is from a subdiaphragmatic source, the CT scan should be extended to include the abdomen.

## Thoracentesis

All patients who have substantial effusions > 300 ml with or without a pneumonic infiltrate should undergo a diagnostic thoracentesis. Generally, withdrawal of a sample of 50 ml fluid for

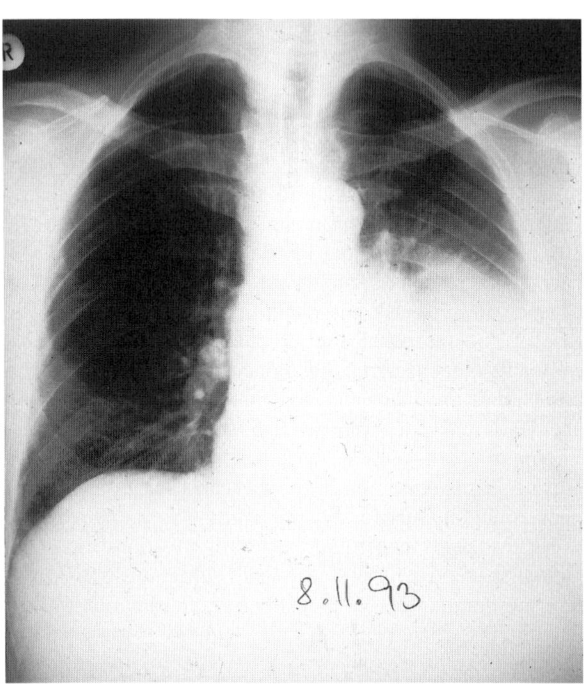


(a)

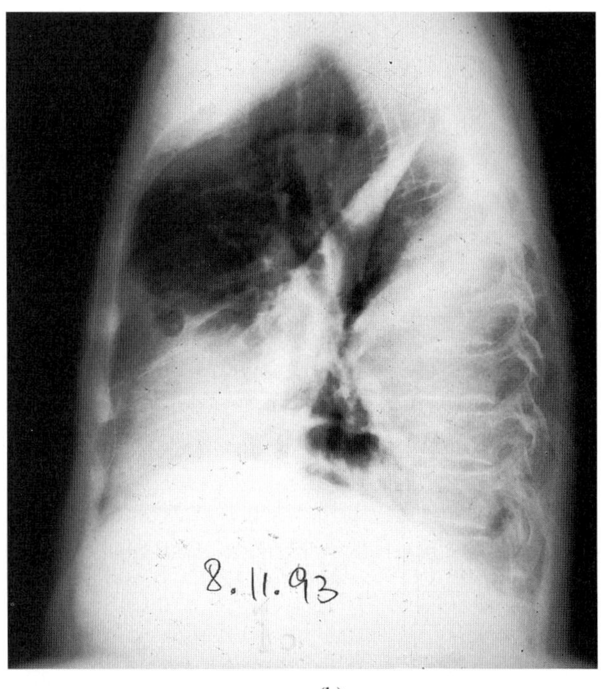


(b)

**Fig. 59.3** *A,B* PA and lateral chest X-rays of a patient with a left pleural effusion complicating left lower lobe pneumonia.

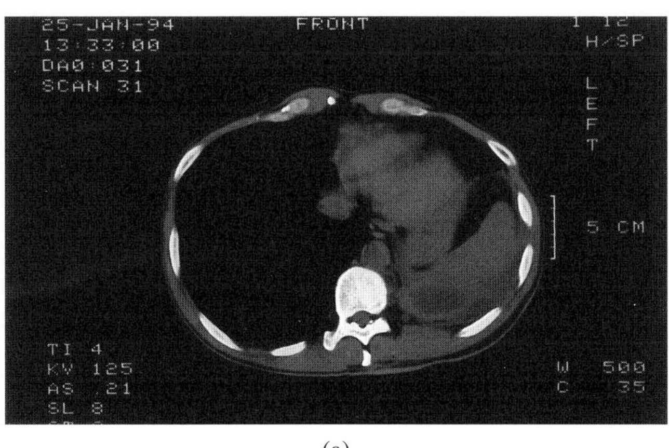


(a)

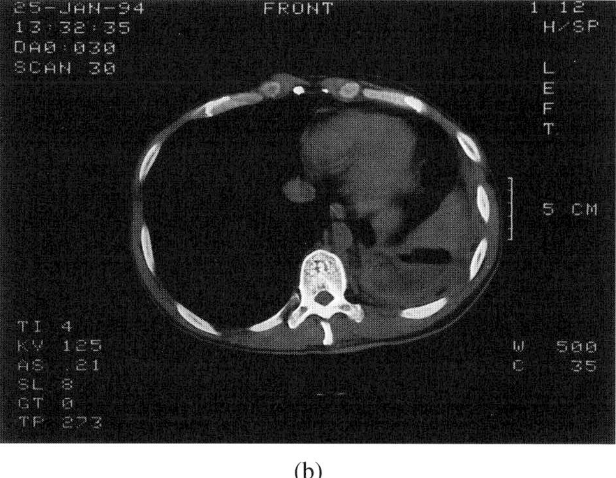


(b)

**Fig. 59.4** *A,B* CT scan of a patient with a left pleural effusion due to empyema. Note the air fluid level on *B*.

analysis is adequate. When TB or malignancy is suspected, thoracentesis should be accompanied by pleural biopsy. The fluid should routinely have the following determined: cell count with differential, protein, LDH, glucose, and amylase. If the pH is to be determined, the fluid must be aspirated into a syringe used for determining blood gases, which is then sealed to prevent escape of $CO_2$ and a falsely high reading. The fluid should be gram stained both aerobically and anaerobically. Although usually unrevealing, mycobacterial special stain and culture tests should be carried out on the fluid. Pleural biopsies, examination, and culture are much more likely to be positive; however, cytological exam should be performed on exudative fluids. Besides pleural fluid cultures, all patients with suspected pleural space infection should have blood cultures and, if possible, sputum cultures. An intermediate-strength purified protein derivate standard (PPD-S) should be placed intradermally along with several controls. Debate exists as to whether all patients with parapneumonic effusions should undergo thoracentesis, particularly if the effusions are small and if they appear on the second or third day of treatment in a patient who is doing well. Most such patients can be managed without the need for a diagnostic thoracentesis.

## Microbiology

In the prepenicillin era, the dominant agent of pneumonia and empyema was *Streptococcus pneumoniae*. While these organisms remain the leading cause of bacterial pneumonia, studies of empyema in the antibiotic era indicate prevalence of a wide variety of organisms. Beside *Streptococcus pneumoniae* and other streptococci, *staphylococcus aureus* and a variety of gram-negative aerobic pathogens have been isolated in recent studies (Table 59.3). These organisms are usually seen on gram stain or

**Table 59.3** Aerobic organisms isolated from infected pleural fluid

| | Series | | | |
|---|---|---|---|---|
| Organism | Bartlett[a] | Varkey[b] | Total | Percentage |
| GRAM-POSITIVE BACTERIA | | | | |
| *Staphylococcus aureus* | 17 | 7 | 24 | 20 |
| *Staphylococcus epidermidis* | 5 | 0 | 5 | 4 |
| *Streptococcus pneumoniae* | 5 | 6 | 11 | 9 |
| *Streptococcus faecalis* | 5 | 4 | 9 | 7 |
| *Streptococcus pyogenes* | 4 | 5 | 9 | 7 |
| *Streptococcus* (*other*) | 8 | 6 | 14 | 12 |
| | 44 | 28 | 72 | |
| GRAM-NEGATIVE BACTERIA | | | | |
| *Escherichia coli* | 11 | 4 | 15 | 12 |
| *Klebsiella* species | 6 | 1 | 7 | 6 |
| *Proteus* species | 2 | 1 | 3 | 2 |
| *Pseudomonas* species | 10 | 8 | 18 | 15 |
| *Enterobacter* species | 0 | 3 | 3 | 2 |
| Others | 1 | 2 | 3 | |
| | 30 | 19 | 49 | |

[a]Bartlett J.G., Gorbach S.L., Thadepalli H., Finegold S.M. Bacteriology of empyema. Lancet (1974) I: 338–340

[b]Varkey B., Rose H.D., Kutty C.P.K., Politis J. Empyema thoracis during a ten-year period. Arch Intern Med (1981) 141: 1771–1776

**Table 59.4** Bacteriological results for anaerobic bacterial infections of the lung

| | Bartlett[a] | Finegold et al.[b] |
|---|---|---|
| PERIOD REVIEWED | 1968–1975 | Early 1980s |
| NO. CASES | 193 | 196 |
| TOTAL ANAEROBIC STRAINS | 461 | 656 |
| AVERAGE NO./CASE | 2.4 | 3.3 |
| NO. MIXED AEROBIC-ANAEROBIC INFECTIONS | 51% | NS[c] |
| ISOLATES | | |
| Bacteroides sp. (Black pigmented strains) | 76 | 112 |
| B fragilis group | 38 | 14 |
| Bacteroides sp (other) | 37 | 160 |
| Fusobacterium nucleatum | 56 | 58 |
| Peptostreptococci | 130 | 66 |
| Clostridia | 18 | 20 |
| Eubacteria | 18 | 46 |
| Actinomyces | 5 | 28 |
| Non-sporulating gram-positive bacteria (other) | 27 | 52 |

[a]Bartlett J.G. Bacterial infections of the pleural space. Seminars in Respiratory Infections (1988) 3:308–21.

[b]Finegold S., George W., Mulligan M. Anaerobic infections. Disease-A-Month (1985) 31: 8–77.

[c]NS, not specified.

grow readily in aerobic cultures unless inhibited by prior antibiotic therapy. Blood cultures are often positive.

An anaerobic bacterial etiology should be suspected in pleural fluid yielding a polymicrobial flora (Table 59.4). The presence of putrid discharge, either of empyema fluid or sputum, is characteristic of anaerobic infection. With regard to specific bacteria, these infections usually involve multiple species derived from the upper airways where they represent the usual bacterial flora in the gingival crevices. The dominant isolates in cases associated with aspiration are *Bacteroides melaninogenicus*, anaerobic streptococci (*Peptostreptococci*), and *Fusobacterium nucleatum* (Table 59.5) Anaerobic empyemas may also result from a subphrenic abscess where the dominant organism usually reflects the colonic flora.

In the case of tuberculous pleural effusions or empyema the intermediate-strength tuberculin test will usually be reactive, but recovery of organisms on acid-fast stain or culture of the fluid is typically low (<20%—see Chapter 57). Pleural biopsy histology and culture can increase this yield to ~80%. In patients with reactivation disease as the cause for the tuberculous effusion apical infiltration or cavitation is common. In patients with primary progressive tuberculosis there may be little or no pulmonary infiltration; or, conversely, lobar infiltrates with hilar adenopathy may be present.

In patients with viral or mycoplasmal disease causing pleurisy or pleural effusions, the organism may be difficult to recover. Coxsackie B is usually isolated in stool cultures during active disease. *Mycoplasma* species may be isolated from the sputum or disease may be documented serologically (see Chapter 56).

**Table 59.5** Characteristics of complicated and uncomplicated parapneumonic effusions

| | Uncomplicated | Complicated |
|---|---|---|
| Appearence | Cloudy yellow | Cloudy yellow to thick pus |
| Odor | Odorless | Putrid (if anaerobic) |
| Glucose level | >50 mg/dl | Usually <50 mg/dl |
| Protein level | 2.0–6.0 mg/dl | 2.0–6.0 mg/dl |
| White cell count | 500–150,000 | 500–150,000 |
| pH | >7.20 | <7.00 |
| LDH | <1000 IU/l | >1000 IU/l |
| Graim's stain | Negative | Positive (sometimes) |
| Culture | Negative | Positive (sometimes) |

Adapted from Light RW. Parapneumonic effusions and empyema. Seminars in Respiratory Medicine (1987) 9:37–42.

## Management

### Antibiotics

Prompt antibiotic therapy of pneumonia should decrease the likelihood of development of a parapneumonic effusion and the progression of an uncomplicated to complicated effusion by decreasing the lung capillary leak, resulting in more rapid clearance of pleural space bacteria. There is little difference in penetration of the various penicillins and cephalosporins into empyemas and uninfected parapneumonic fluids; all provide high levels of activity with adequate serum drug concentrations. Other drugs showing excellent pleural penetration include clindamycin and ciprofloxacin, with pleural fluid/serum ratios of 79% to 167%, 1 to 4.5 h after single or multiple doses. With these antibiotics, the pleural fluid drug concentrations almost always exceed the accepted minimal inhibitory concentration (MIC) for organisms most likely to cause empyemas. In contrast to these antibiotics, aminoglycosides may be inactivated or penetrate less well into empyemas than into uncomplicated parapneumonic effusions. Inactivation occurs in the presence of purulent exudate, pleural fluid acidosis, or a hypoxic environment.

Comparative antibiotic trials in empyema have not been done. Based on the likely organisms that cause empyema, i.e., *S. pneumoniae*, anaerobes, and staphylococci, and also considering where the infection was acquired (community acquired or nosocomial), an optimal antibiotic treatment can usually be determined. In community-acquired infection, single-agent therapy with ampicillin and sulbactam or amoxicillin and clavulanic acid, and combined therapy with a second-generation cephalosporin together with clindamycin, are both reasonable initial empiric antibiotic choices. If the patient's illnesses have features suggestive of atypical pathogens, then a macrolide (erythromycin, clarithromycin, or azithromycin) should be added. In the nosocomial setting, with an increased risk of aerobic gram-negative pathogens causing pneumonia, initial single-agent therapy with imipenem, meropenem, ticarcillin-clavulanic acid, or piperacillin with tazobactam or a combined therapy with a third-generation cephalosporin together with clindamycin is acceptable. Empyemas that arise from an intraabdominal location can be treated as outlined for nosocomial infection. Definitive antibiotic therapy should be guided by the results of pleural and blood cultures and determination of antimicrobial susceptibilities on isolated organisms.

The duration of antibiotic therapy depends on the clinical setting. Patients with uncomplicated effusions accompanying pneumonia can be treated based on the etiology of the pneumonia without dose escalation or increased duration of therapy (see Chapter 56). Patients with empyemas should receive at least several weeks of therapy, similar to treating necrotizing pneumonia and lung abscess. Periodic evaluation of the chest X-ray or CT scan should be carried out along with measurements of the leukocyte count, the ESR or CRP, and the temperature as markers of therapeutic response. In treating empyemas caused by anaerobes, oral clindamycin, oral amoxicillin and clavulic acid, ampicillin and sulbactam should be continued for several weeks once parenteral antibiotics are discontinued. The precise duration of therapy will be determined by the therapeutic response both in terms of resolution of the signs of inflammation and fever and in improvement of the radiologic findings. Tuberculosis causing pleural disease is treated the same as other forms of pulmonary tuberculosis (see Chapters 37 and 57).

### Pleural space drainage

In addition to proper antibiotic treatment, drainage of the pleural space, usually by means of chest tube insertion, is necessary for all patients with complicated parapneumonic effusions or empyema. This is required to promote prompt resolution of the infection and to avoid complications such as pleural fibrosis or "trapped" nonfunctional lung. The rapid identification of patients who are likely to develop complicated parapneumonic effusions or empyema could improve clinical outcome by allowing early pleural space drainage. Unfortunately it is not always easy to differentiate clinically patients with complicated parapneumonic effusions from those with uncomplicated effusions. Pleural fluid analysis remains the most useful diagnostic test in identifying the stage of a parapneumonic effusion and guiding therapy. If frank pus is aspirated at thoracocentesis, consistent with an empyema, effective pleural space drainage should be accomplished without delay. Likewise, if organisms are seen on gram stain most clinicians favor prompt chest tube drainage in addition to antibiotic therapy.

With fluids that are not grossly purulent or infected, the pleural fluid protein concentration, leukocyte count, or percentage of PMNs cannot themselves differentiate complicated (i.e., needing drainage before loculation occurs) from uncomplicated effusion. Additional analysis of parapneumonic pleural fluid has suggested that a pH $< 7.00$, a glucose $< 40$ mg/dl, and an LDH $> 1000$ U/l indicate a complicated parapneumonic effusion. The combined pleural fluid pH data from several investigations, which used similar methods, indicate that a pH of $>7.30$ on initial thoracentesis virtually always predicts a good outcome with antibiotic treatment only. A pH of $<7.14$ predicts that pleural space drainage is necessary to control pleural infection and to avoid pleural fibrosis (Figs. 59.1, 59.2). While some clinicians have downplayed the critical importance of pleural fluid pH, additional pleural fluid biochemical parameters may provide helpful data to differentiate complicated from uncomplicated effusions (Table 59.5).

A chest tube is effective only if it can be placed properly into the parapneumonic fluid. A lateral decubitus radiograph or a CT scan can verify that the fluid is not loculated. With a free-flowing effusion, the chest tube can be placed at the bedside. Thoracoscopy may be helpful for a proper placement of a chest tube in complicated, loculated effusions. An optimally placed chest tube should rapidly and completely evacuate the pleural space and lead to expansion of the lung, essentially eliminating the subsequent development of an empyema cavity. The chest tube should be removed when drainage becomes serous and is $<50$ ml per day.

### Management of empyema

Additional approaches for management of empyema have included *intrapleural fibrinolytic administration* or *pleural lavage and drainage*.

With *intrapleural fibrinolytic therapy*, streptokinase (250,000–500,000 U/d) is administered to improve the drainage of the intrapleural fluid. This fibrinolytic agent is most effective if used early in the evolution of the parapneumonic effusion before significant fibrosis occurs in the pleural space. *Pleural lavage and drainage* may be accomplished following the implantation of two Monaldi catheters into the empyema cavity by continuously administering physiological saline or polyvidon-containing fluid.

While favorable results have been observed with both of these approaches, they need to be submitted to careful, controlled multicenter trials to definitively demonstrate their superiority to conventional drainage techniques.

Persistent pleural sepsis leads to a late organizational stage of a parapneumonic effusion and requires aggressive surgical drainage. This is usually the result of chest tube failure or delayed presentation before definitive management can be initiated. Controversy exists among thoracic surgeons concerning the preferred treatment procedure—that is, open drainage or empyemectomy/decortication. However, early fibronolytic therapy and double-spaced lavage have made major operations unnecessary in some hospitals, indicating their promise as generally indicated treatments for empyema.

## ANNOTATED BIBLIOGRAPHY

Alfageme I, Muñoz F, Peña N, Umbria S. Empyema of the thorax in adults. Chest 1993; 103:839–843.
*Report on etiology, microbiologic findings, and management of 82 episodes of empyema.*

Bartlett JG, Finegold SM. Anaerobic infections of the lung and pleural space. Am Rev Respir Dis 1974; 110:807–812.

Bryant RE, Salmon CJ. Pleural empyema. Clin Infect Dis 1996; 22:747–764.
*State of the art article. Anatomy, pathophysiology, clinical and radiological, and treatment of empyema.*

Heffner JE, Brown LK, Barbieri C, DeLeo JM. Pleural fluid analysis in parapneumonic effusions. Am J Respir Crit Care Med 1995; 151:1700–1708.
*A meta-analysis of 7 studies regarding the clinical utility of pleural fluid pH, LDH, and glucose for identifying complicated parapneumonic effusions that require drainage.*

Light RW. Management of parapneumonic effusions. Chest 1991; 100:892–893.

Light RW, Girard WM, Jenkinson SG, George RB. Parapneumonic effusions. Am J Med 1980; 69:507–512.

Light RW, ed. Pleural diseases, 3rd ed. Williams & Wilkins, Baltimore, MD, 1995.
*Review article about drainage-instrumentation, suction methods and surgery of pleural diseases.*

Light RW, Vargas FS. Pleural sclerosis for the treatment of pneumothorax and pleural effusions. Lung 1997; 175:213–223.
*Review of the different methods, indications, contraindications, and recommendations for pleural sclerosis.*

Loddenkemper R, Boutin C. Thorascopy: present diagnostic and therapeutic indications. Eur Respir J 1993; 5:1544–1555.
*Review article on the advances and indications in thorascopy.*

Miller KS, Shan SA. Chest tubes: indications, technique, management and complications. Chest 1987; 91:258–264.

Pots DE, Levins DC, Shan SA. Pleural fluid pH in parapneumonic effusions. Chest 1976; 70:328–331.

Sarosi GA. Infections of the pleural space. Seminars in Respiratory Infections 1988; 3.
*A complete volume on infections of the pleural space with articles about bacterial, tuberculous, fungal, parasitic, and pleuropulmonary manifestations of actinomycosis and nocardiosis.*

Shan SA. Disease of the pleura. Seminars in Respiratory Medicine 1987; 9.
*A complete volume on different aspects of pleural diseases (parapneumonic effusions, empyema, malignant effusions, pleural tuberculosis, and other causes of pleural effusions) including anatomy and pathophysiology.*

Shan SA. State of the art. Am Rev Respir Dis 1988; 138:184–234.

Shan SA. Management of complicated parapneumonic effusions. Am Rev Respir Dis 1993; 148:813–817.
*Review of definitions, pathophysiology, diagnosis, and management of parapneumonic effusions.*

Strange C, Shan SA. The clinician's perspective on parapneumonic effusions and empyema. Chest 1993; 103:259–261.
*Report of a interactive symposium on pleural space infections on personal management preferences for empyema.*

# 60

# Intraoral Infections

JOHN S. GREENSPAN AND DEBORAH GREENSPAN

Oral infections are so common and widespread as to be almost accepted as inevitable, yet most are both preventable and treatable. Some are infections found only in the mouth—for example, dental caries and periodontal diseases—while many are secondary reflections of infection elsewhere or are the oral tissue expressions of systemic processes. Oral infections can cause considerable morbidity while a few, if left untreated, may be fatal. The varied and tenacious oral flora are particularly adept at recognizing and taking advantage of any weakness in the host's immunological and other defense mechanisms. It is therefore common for oral infections to flourish in patients with immune deficiencies such as those induced by HIV infection, immunosuppressive therapy or lymphoproliferative disease; diabetes; xerostomia due to Sjogren's syndrome or drug therapy; and some forms of anemia.

## Bacterial Infections

Oral and dental bacterial infections can lead to bacteremia, depending on the location, severity, and bacterial virulence, so bacterial endocarditis and infection of cardiovascular and orthopedic grafts or implants are possible complications that must be avoided in those at risk by administering antibiotic prophylaxis before dental procedures.

### Caries

Dental caries was for centuries one of mankind's most common and debilitating afflictions (tooth decay); it is now far less common in the majority of the United States population. This is largely ascribed to community water fluoridation, fluoride toothpastes, and the contributions of fluoridated water to food, milk, and other ingested fluids. About 50% of those in the United States 17 years or younger are free of caries. However, in the developing world as well as among the economically underprivileged in developed countries, caries is as prevalent as ever. Similarly, aging individuals experience root caries, while those with reduced salivary secretion due to Sjögren's syndrome, cancer radiotherapy to the head and neck (Plate 22), and drug side effects, as well as diabetics, can experience severe and extensive caries. Baby bottle tooth decay is common among infants fed by bottle with fluids rich in sucrose or other fermentable carbohydrates. Dental caries is caused by *Streptococcus mutans* and is characterized by progressive destruction of the hard tissues of the teeth, first enamel in the case of crown caries, followed by dentine. Root caries attacks cementum and then dentine. The greater part of traditional dental practice focused on the treatment of caries by removal of the diseased tooth tissue, followed by replacement of the original tooth form with silver amalgam, resin composite, porcelain, or cast gold restorations. Increasingly, the emphasis on caries control is shifting to preventive approaches based on nutritional counseling, water fluoridation, and the use of fluoride applied topically by a dental professional or in toothpaste. Public health campaigns advocating fluoridation of water supplies continue to be needed, for many communities have yet to institute that most cost effective of disease-prevention measures.

### Pulpitis

Inflammation of the delicate connective tissue tooth pulp, which is closely confined within the unyielding hard tissue dentine of the surrounding tooth, may be caused by bacteria that enter through a carious lesion. Other causes include pulp exposure through trauma, abrasion, as with excessive use of toothbrush or dental floss, heavy wear or attrition, or chemical erosion from dietary or regurgitated acid. The organisms involved reflect the extensive and diverse bacteria found in dental plaque and include several gram-negative anaerobes. In acute pulpitis, there is an influx of polymorphs and macrophages, hyperemia and edema. The rigid hard tissue precludes expansion, so pressure within the pulp chamber rises. The tooth is at first sensitive to hot and cold, but pain soon follows, becoming continuous and throbbing, often worse at night. Irreversible tissue damage and pulp abscess formation ensue if the tooth is not treated. The pulp dies and infection may spread, eventually, to the periapical tissues. Occasionally, pulp inflammation is mild and confined to a portion of the pulp, usually a pulp horn located near a carious lesion, causing focal reversible pulpitis with mild and intermittent pain, which may be reversible on removal of the cause. Chronic pulpitis may occur with long-lasting or mild insult or can be the consequence of acute pulpitis. Again, symptoms may be mild, absent, or intermittent, and, rarely, severe. In children and teenagers, the exposed pulp of a molar may proliferate through a large and open carious exposure to form a granulation tissue mass or pulp polyp (chronic hyperplastic pulpitis). The symptoms of pulpitis, such as pain, may be poorly localized, may be referred to other sites, and should be investigated carefully to differentiate this condition from others, including sinusitis, periodontal abscess, and orofacial neuralgias. Pulpitis, unless early and mild, usually is treated by extirpation of the pulp followed by endodontic occlusion of the pulp cavity—a procedure commonly referred to as a "root canal." Alternatively, tooth extraction may be indicated.

### Periapical disease

Pulpal infection, unless adequately treated, usually spreads to the tissues adjoining the apical openings of the pulp canal, resulting in acute inflammation with painful periapical abscess if the infection is virulent, or periapical granuloma when the inflammation is chronic. This may be associated with mild pain and some tenderness or may evoke no symptoms. Small groups of odontogenic epithelial cells within the periodontal ligament, the cell rests of Mallassez, which are remnants of the epithelial root sheath of Hertwig that forms root dentine, may proliferate within and around a periapical granuloma to form a periapical (radicular) cyst. While the periapical abscess usually forms too rapidly for bone resorption and radiolucency to occur, both periapical granuloma and periapical cyst are associated with radiolucency at the tooth apex. However, infection within either of those two lesions may become more severe, leading to abscess formation. Pus, where present, may track through the alveolar bone to the gingiva as a parulis (gumboil) or may spread into adjoining soft tissues, causing cellulitis. Other paths of discharge include to the skin of the face or submandibular region, as well as into the maxillary sinus. Severe submandibular space cellulitis, Ludwig's angina, which can originate with caries and periapical infection of a mandibular molar, extends into the submandibular soft tissues and the floor of the mouth (see below). Treatment of periapical infection involves elimination of the cause, drainage of pus, and appropriate antibiotics. More severe infection may need "through and through" drainage, both intraoral and extraoral.

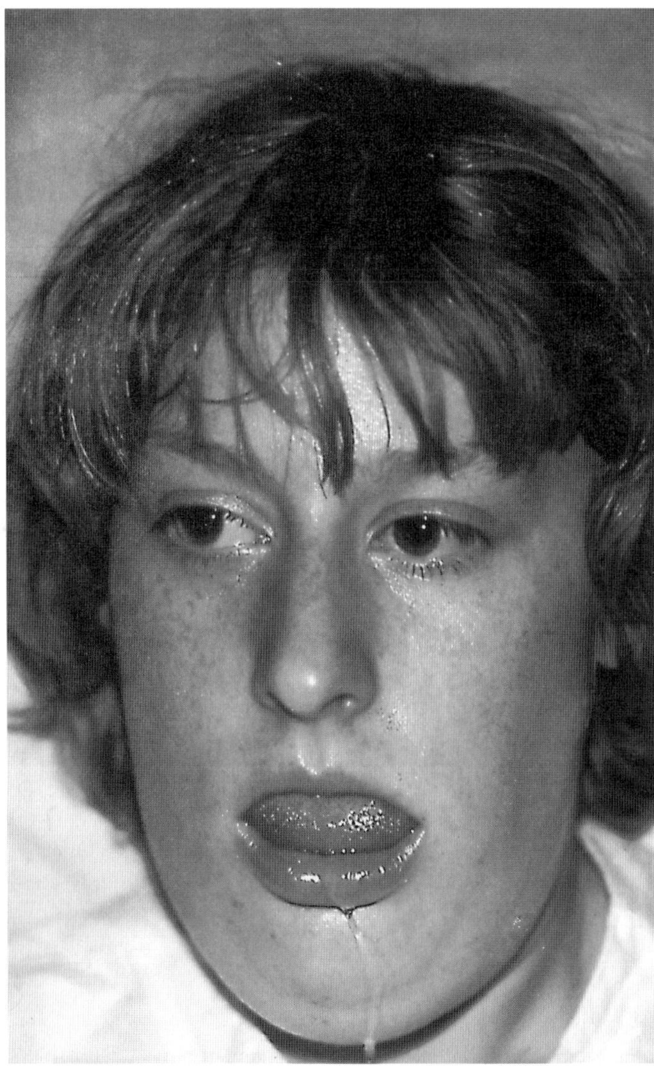

**Fig. 60.1** Ludwig's angina. [Courtesy of Dr M A Pogrel.]

## Ludwig's angina and related conditions

This acute cellulitis of the submandibular and sublingual spaces (Fig. 60.1) is a rare complication of dental infection and may follow tooth extraction. Immunocompromised individuals are at increased risk. Other forms of infection in and around the mandible or floor of the mouth are less frequently involved. Few modern microbiological studies have been reported but the flora appears to be mixed aerobic and anerobic and similar to that associated with periapical and periodontal disease, with the addition of coliform organisms and pseudomonads in some cases. Brawny edema without pus is present, causing dysphagia, tongue elevation, dyspnea, even life-threatening glottal edema, requiring in some cases tracheotomy. These changes can spread rapidly, with significant impairment occurring within a few hours. Disseminated intravascular coagulation as a complication has been reported. All cases require some form of airway maintenance. Additional measures include prolonged antibiotic therapy directed at the polymicrobial aerobic and anerobic flora (e.g., penicillin G and metronidazole or imipenem), extraction of teeth which are the origin of the infection, maintenance of fluid balance, and drainage. Other spreading infections seen as complications of oral infection include those of the face and related fascial spaces (Figs. 60.2, 60.3), lateral pharyngeal space, retropharyngeal space, and even the mediastinum. All of these have the potential to compromise the airway as well as to produce multiple septic complications. Management includes appropriate debridement and drainage and antimicrobial therapy as outlined for Ludwig's angina.

## Periodontal diseases

Most periodontal diseases are bacterial infections. While gingivitis is almost universal in the population, periodontitis is less common. Nevertheless, up to 75% of the population is likely to develop one of the forms of periodontitis at some time. Like dental caries, periodontal disease is one of the most common human afflictions. In addition, it also appears to be decreasing with better general dental hygiene. Periodontal disease is caused by groups of bacteria that form dental plaque, a complicated ecosystem which attaches to the tooth surface. Plaque is produced by complex combinations of aerobic and anaerobic microorganisms which vary among the different forms of periodontal disease. Many of the same organisms can be found in the mouth in the absence of disease. The establishment of the infectious nature of the common forms of periodontal disease has led to important improvements in technological and behavioral approaches to the prevention and control of periodontal diseases, and now one can expect to be free from tooth loss due to periodontal disease. However, despite these gains, many people are still at risk from such aggressive forms of periodontal infection as juvenile periodontitis, rapidly progressive periodontitis, refractory periodontitis, and necrotizing ulcerative periodontitis, or from the forms of periodontitis associated with systemic disease including diabetes, HIV infection, and other forms of immunodeficiency. Other groups who are at risk for periodontal diseases include the physically and mentally handicapped, the aged, and those who do not receive oral-health education or adequate care because of economic and social factors.

The most common form of periodontal disease, adult peri-

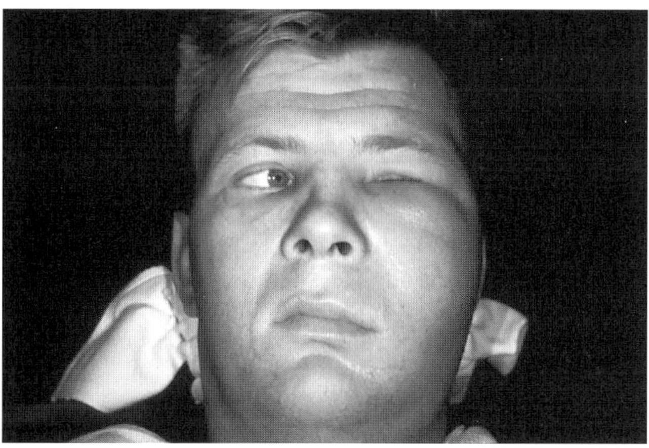

**Fig. 60.2** Periorbital abscess resulting from dentoalveolar infection arising in maxillary molar tooth. [Courtesy of Dr M A Pogrel.]

odontitis or chronic inflammatory periodontal disease, is usually asymptomatic unless bone loss has progressed to the stage when teeth become loose and even exfoliate, or unless acute episodes cause the formation of a periodontal abscess. There is separation of connective tissue from root surfaces and resorption of the bone supporting the teeth. Long viewed as a slow continuous process, it is now clear that many involved sites progress in brief episodic bursts. The opportunity to detect or predict these episodes of active destruction using clinical "chairside" tests will be of considerable value, perhaps leading to earlier, more effective treatment. There is evidence suggesting that neutrophil defects are factors in the development of both localized and generalized forms of juvenile periodontitis. It may become possible to interrupt the development of these rapidly progressive conditions with agents that modify neutrophil functions.

The very aggressive, destructive periodontal disease associated with HIV infection has features resembling necrotizing ulcerative gingivitis superimposed upon rapidly progressive periodontitis. This severe periodontal disease is now called *necrotizing ulcerative periodontitis* (Plate 23). Such lesions occasionally lead to exposure and sequestration of fragments of alveolar bone and may even extend beyond the tooth-supporting tissues to adjoining soft tissue and bone. Similarly, in diabetes, where severe and rapidly progressive periodontal disease may be

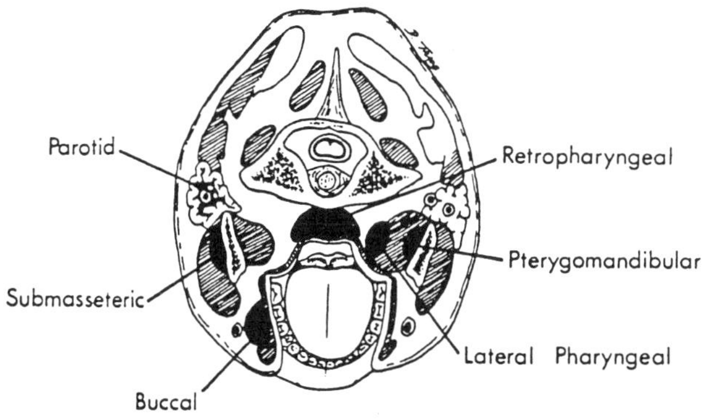


**Fig. 60.3** Fascial spaces around the jaw and face. [Reprinted with permission from Topazian RG, Goldberg MH. Oral and Maxillofacial Infections, W.B. Saunders, Philadelphia, PA, 1994.]

seen, the problems of cause, prevention, and treatment remain unsolved. These are two examples of systemic diseases, associated with severe periodontal disease, where the discomfort, functional loss, and disfigurement of oral disease may be a major cause of morbidity and even mortality.

### Microbiology

The colonization of the tooth surface by plaque microorganisms appears to involve bacterial adhesins that bind to tooth and tissue receptors and to similar molecules on other bacteria. It may become possible to interfere with bacterial adhesion by seeding the mouth with nonadherent mutants. At least 300 species of bacteria have been identified in dental plaque. The predominant periodontal pathogens include *Prevotella intermedia*, *Actinobacillus actinomycetemcomitans*, *Capnocytophaga sputigena*, *Bacteroides forsythus*, *Campylobacter rectus*, *Eikenella corrodens*, *Fusobacterium nucleatum*, *Eubacterium brachy*, *Haemophilus aphrophilus*, *Peptostreptococcus micros*, *Selenomonas* sp., *Streptococcus intermedius*, and several spirochetes, as well as others in specific periodontal infections. It is not clear how these anaerobes cause damage as regards whether bacteria invade the tooth-supporting tissues, what cytokines or other molecules cause damage, and whether the damage involves modification of or interference with host immunological or tissue cells or their products. Interactions between bacteria, both synergistic and inhibitory, are doubtless important.

The old idea of distant spread of oral pathogens causing local or generalized infectious or other inflammatory disease (the theory of "focal infection") has taken on new life with the observation that, just as periapical and periodontal infection can lead to bacterial endocarditis, so can they be the origin of the bacteria infecting bone and other prostheses, including artificial hips or knees. Links have been described with coronary artery disease and low birthweight offspring.

### Host response/immunology

The relative importance of destructive and protective host factors in periodontal disease is unclear, as are the relationships between microorganisms and the cellular and biochemical elements of the host response. The ability of periodontal fibroblasts to produce and degrade collagen appears to be an important factor in the degree of bone destruction. Investigations are underway to evaluate whether modification of osteoclast functions may be clinically useful.

### Treatment

In order to stop and even reverse periodontal disease, it is essential to remove or destroy the causative bacteria. Mechanical removal of soft plaque and mineralized calculus (scaling and root planing), surgical debridement, and antimicrobial agents are used, depending on the type, location, and severity of tissue damage and infection. Antibacterial rinses such as clorhexidine are increasingly used as one way to control infection, but more sophisticated local delivery systems for both antibacterial and antibiotic agents are becoming available. Antiinflammatory drugs have been tried; drugs that could interfere with harmful cells or cytokines while sparing the positive elements of the host response may also be useful. The use of membranes to protect reparative fibroblasts as they create new periodontal tissues and bone has been an important new therapy. This method of guided tissue regeneration can be supplemented with molecular biological products such as bone-inducing cytokines.

### Prevention

Most cases of periodontal infection can be prevented by a combination of effective personal oral hygiene (toothbrushing and flossing), which stops the accumulation of plaque that produces the pathogenic flora, supplemented by dental professional prophylactic measures. Cost-effective health education for the population must include instruction on how to maintain immaculate oral hygiene so as to prevent chronic inflammatory periodontal disease and certain forms of caries. The question of a vaccine for periodontal diseases is under active investigation as the identity of the microorganisms involved becomes clearer. However, this area of research is at an early stage. Problems include the large number of possible microorganims, the appropriate antigens from those bacteria thought to be important, the weakness of the evidence that immune activity can be protective, the best route of administration, safety, efficacy, and cost-effectiveness.

### Acute necrotizing ulcerative gingivitis (ANUG)

This painful and rapid-onset condition is seen in young people as well as older adults with underlying debilitation and/or immunosuppression, ANUG is probably an opportunistic infection associated with spirochetes and fusiform bacteria. Other host predisposing factors may include stress and smoking. There is pain, spontaneous gingival bleeding and distinctive halitosis. The tips of the gingival papillae, and subsequently the adjoining gingival soft tissues, show ulceration with a gray pseudomembrane, marked sensitivity, and bleeding with the slightest touch. The edge of the lesion shows a bright red margin. If untreated, the condition persists for several days to a week or 2 and usually subsides, leaving gingival cratering and deformity, although a chronic version sometimes persists. The deformity predisposes to chronic inflammatory periodontal disease. However, the acute phase of ANUG may occasionally progress to destruction of adjoining soft and hard tissues well beyond the alveolus (noma or cancrum oris—Fig. 60.4). Treatment of ANUG involves gentle cleaning of the affected sites using dental scalers and curettes, analgesics, saline or clorhexidine mouth rinsing, supplemented (not replaced) by systemic antibiotics such as penicillin 500 mg QID, 7 d, or metronizadole 250 mg QID, 7 d. Gingival and bone deformity, if present, should be corrected by periodontal surgery to prevent recurrence.

### Periodontal abscess

Abscess formation may complicate the course of many periodontal diseases. Usually, these arise as acute exacerbations of chronic disease. However, gingival abscess may be due to impaction of soft tissue by food or other hard material. Periodontal abscess presents with abrupt onset, mild to severe pain, swelling, and erythema of the gingiva and adjoining mucosa. The involved tooth may be loose, tender to percussion, and feel "high" on attempted biting. Pus may be seen exuding from the gingival crevice, marking its discharge from the opening of a periodontal pocket, or it may discharge through the alveolar bone and gingiva as a parulis. Distinction must be made between periodontal abscess, periapical abscess, and lesions of combined origin. Treatment involves drainage, antibiotics, and subsequent periodontal therapy to deal with the underlying periodontal disease.

### Pericoronitis

Partially erupted teeth, notably mandibular third molars that are impacted against the anterior border of the ramus, can be sites of infection due to accumulation of debris and plaque. Here, too, suppuration can occur, with swelling, proliferation of mucosa over the crown, occlusion of this soft tissue with the opposing maxillary teeth, and limitation of opening of the mouth. Pain may be severe and lymphadenopathy and fever may be seen. Cleaning and debridement, combined with irrigation using saline or povidone/iodine, may give immediate relief and should be followed by mouth rinsing with warm saline for several days. Systemic antibiotics are used when there are constitutional symptoms or lymphadenopathy. Penicillin, amoxicillin, or erythromycin for patients who show hypersensitivity to penicillin is effective and must be used for at least 5 d.

## Noma (Cancrum Oris)

Noma is mostly an infection of children, seen in association with severe malnutrition. It involves rapidly progressive necrosis of oral soft tissues and exposure of alveolar or facial bone. A similar lesion may be seen in adults with leukemia or agranulocytosis or who are on cytotoxic drugs. Noma resembles the severe necrotizing stomatitis seen in HIV infection, but noma affects the cheeks and face and heals with scarring and soft-tissue defects. Noma may be related to or even arise from ANUG or pericoronitis and may be caused by a similar fusospirochetal infection. Death may follow as the result of septicemia, diarrhea, or pneumonia. Treatment involves attention to predisposing malnutrition or disease, establishment of electrolyte and fluid balance, local debridement of necrotic tissue, and antibiotic therapy, usually intravenous penicillin.

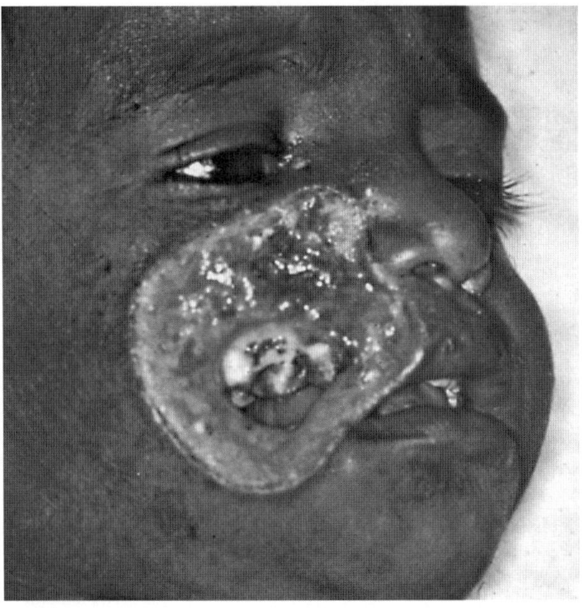

**Fig. 60.4** Noma. [Reprinted with permission from Pindborg JJ. Atlas of Diseases of the Oral Mucosa, Munksgaard Intl. Publishers, Copenhagen, Denmark, 1993.]

## Osteomyelitis

Infection of the jawbone, osteomyelitis, may be a rare complication of other oral infections, may be associated with underlying ischemia, or may arise spontaneously.

### Acute osteomyelitis

Acute osteomyelitis of the maxilla or mandible may be secondary to trauma such as fracture of the jaw or surgical procedures or may be due to spread of infection through bacteremia from a distant site or locally from a periapical abscess. There is significant pain, while other clinical features include fever, malaise, and enlarged lymph nodes which also may be painful. Occasionally, mandibular osteomyelitis may cause paresthesia of the lower lip. Symptomatic osteomyelitis may precede radiographic changes.

Treatment of acute osteomyelitis involves identification of the organism by culture of exudate, appropriate antibiotic therapy, and the institution of drainage, with removal of bony sequestra and bony recontouring when necessary. A common form of acute infection of the jaws is known as alveolar osteitis or "dry socket." In this complication of the extraction of teeth, the blood clot within the tooth socket disintegrates and there is infection of the adjoining bone. The condition is seen less frequently now because of the development of more effective protocols for tooth extraction.

### Chronic osteomyelitis

This may be a sequel of the acute form, or may present without the history of an acute episode. A notable example, osteoradionecrosis, is seen in some head and neck cancer patients as a complication of radiation therapy due to ischemia and death of bone cells. It may be triggered by spread of infection from carious teeth, by periodontal disease, or by surgical intervention, or it may occur without any detectable microorganism. Chronic osteomyelitis may be painful and there may be swelling. Radiographs show irregular loss of bone with a motheaten appearance. Antibiotics may be helpful in the case of osteoradionecrosis but may not alter the progression, which may involve sequestration or fracture. Other forms of chronic osteomyelitis include diffuse sclerosing osteomyelitis and Garre's osteomyelitis, in which there is proliferative periostitis. Focal sclerosing osteomyelitis produces a dense radiopaque mass of sclerotic bone at the apex of one or more teeth. This condition is not helped by antibiotics and surgical intervention is not indicated except for diagnosis.

## Intracranial spread

A rare complication of oral bacterial infections is intracranial spread, notably intracranial epidural abscess, subdural abscess, brain abscess, and cavernous sinus thrombosis. The clinical features are described elsewhere in this book (see Chapter 77), as are approaches to the management of these life-threatening complications.

## Bacterial sexually transmitted diseases (STDs)

Most if not all STDs can be transmitted through oral–genital or oral–anal contact (see Chapters 70–72).

### Syphilis

Primary syphilis (chancre) can present on the lip or intraoral sites as a painless indurated ulcer. There is enlargement of localized lymph nodes, which are, however, painless. Healing usually occurs spontaneously in 1 to 3 mo. Secondary syphilis may also produce oral lesions, including mucous patches or snail track ulcers (condylomata lata). These may occur on any mucosal surface (Plate 24) and may mimic aphthous ulcers but do not usually have an erythematous border. Finally, in tertiary syphilis the mouth may be the location of gummata, granulomatous inflammatory lesions which may cause palatal perforation. Syphilitic glossitis was also a common feature of tertiary syphilis prior to the antibiotic era. Congenital syphilis can produce tooth deformities, the most common of which are notched incisors (Hutchinsons incisors) and deformed (mulberry) molars. Mucocutaneous rashes may also be seen. While it is possible to identify *Treponema pallidum* using darkfield microscopy, it must be remembered that a number of other spirochetes that are part of the normal oral flora can readily be isolated from the mouth, making diagnosis using this technique inappropriate.

### Gonorrhea

Gonorrhea may produce pharyngeal ulcers and mucositis. Rarely, the oral mucosa may be involved. The diagnosis and treatment of gonorrhea are discussed in Chapter 71.

## Other oral bacterial infections

### Actinomycosis

Oral soft tissue, salivary gland, and bone infections due to *Actinomyces* species (cervicofacial actinomycosis) present as persistent swellings, very hard on palpation, with occasional pain and fever, red or purple changes in the overlying skin, and eventual perforation with discharge of pus that contains bacterial colonies ("sulfur granules"). The infection may arise as a complication of periapical disease. Lymph nodes and bone become involved, and the disease is both insidious and intractable. Nocardia infections (nocardiosis) produces similar lesions. Therapy involves surgical drainage and prolonged antibiotic use (see Chapter 38).

### Tuberculosis

*Mycobacterium* tuberculosis can cause oral lesions, notably ulcers and salivary gland swellings, in individuals with systemic disease. Rare cases of tuberculous abscesses, tooth socket infection, periapical granulomas, and jawbone osteomyelitis have been described in patients with long-standing active tuberculosis. Diagnosis involves biopsy and culture. The oral lesions resolve with appropriate systemic antituberculous therapy (see Chapter 37).

Other bacterial infections with occasional oral manifestations include bacillary angiomatosis (nodules), leprosy (nodules or lepromas), scarlet fever (glossitis and mucositis), diphtheria (mucositis with pseudomembrane), tularemia (ulcers and stomatitis resembling syphilis), and enterobacterial infections.

## Fungal Infections

### Candidiasis

Oral candidiasis is the most common oral fungal infection, with a prevalence in the general population of about 1%, which rises to over 50% in association with HIV infection. Other predisposing factors include diabetes, hypoparathyroidism. anemia, xerostomia, immunosuppressive diseases and treatments, systemic antibiotic therapy, pregnancy, infancy, and old age. It is not clear whether lesions are due simply to an overgrowth of the normally commensal fungus in response to host defects or whether particularly pathogenic strains emerge or are acquired. *Candida albicans* is the organism most frequently involved, with smaller numbers of cases yielding *C. tropicalis*, *C. torulopsis*, *C. glabrata*, *C. krusei*, and other species.

Clinical presentations have been classified in a number of ways, but the most useful at present is based on the appearances of oral candidiasis in association with HIV infection. Three forms are seen: pseudomembranous, erythematous, and angular cheilitis. A fourth form, hyperplastic candidiasis or candidal leukoplakia, is not seen in HIV infection but may occur in association with other predisposing factors. Severe oral involvement, a feature of mucocutaneous candidiasis, is often associated in a genetically determined syndrome with endocrinopathy, such as Addison's disease, hypoparathyroidism, hypothyroidism, and diabetes mellitus. Other forms involve cell-mediated immunodeficiency and iron metabolism defects.

#### Pseudomembranous candidiasis ("thrush")

White, soft, removable plaques of fungal hyphae, epithelial cells and keratin, inflammatory cells, fibrin, and debris may cover any portions of the oral and pharyngeal mucosa (Plate 25). There is often little if any pain in the early stages, although tenderness, pain, and dysphagia may follow. The plaques can by wiped away, leaving a red, bleeding, tender surface.

#### Erythematous candidiasis

Typically seen on the palatal (Plate 26) and dorsal tongue mucosa, this presents as painless, subtle red areas. The glossitis involves loss of papillae, leaving a smooth red surface. An associated condition is denture stomatitis, confined to the area covered by complete or partial dentures, especially the palate. The mucosa is bright red, smooth or slightly irregular, with neither pain nor bleeding.

#### Hyperplastic candidiasis

This rare form is seen on the buccal mucosa at the commissures and has been described on the tongue, although it is probable that some of those reports were confusing hairy leukoplakia with candidiasis. Median rhomboid glossitis is, however, usually due to *Candida* infection.

#### Angular cheilitis

Cracking and fissuring at the corners of the mouth may be due to candidal or bacterial infection (Plate 27). Distinction may be made using a potassium hydroxide preparation of a smear of the lesion to demonstrate fungal hyphae.

#### Treatment

Therapy for oral candidiasis is intended to alleviate the symptoms, which include burning pain, soreness, and dysguesia, and which may occur with all of the clinical presentations of oral candidiasis. Therapy involves the use of topical and systemic antifungals. Topical treatment for oral candidiasis includes mycostatin, as vaginal troches 100,000 U dissolved slowly in the mouth three to four times a day, or as mycostatin oral pastilles 200,000 U, one to two pastilles dissolved in the mouth five times a day. Other antifungals include mycelex oral troches 10 mg, one tablet dissolved in the mouth five times a day. With good compliance, each of these remedies usually clears the oral lesions. Unfortunately, compliance can be a problem because some of the preparations have unpleasant flavors and because of length of time the tablets must be used in the mouth each day.

Systemic antifungal therapy has the advantage of requiring only once-daily dosage. However, systemic antifungal drugs may interact with other medications (see Chapter 38). Ketoconazole is taken as one 200 mg tablet per day at the same time as food. Adverse effects of ketoconazole can include changes in liver function and in adrenal hormone metabolism, nausea, and skin rash. Ketoconazole may not be adequately absorbed in people with HIV infection because they often show changes in gastric pH, poor absorption, and other gastrointestinal problems associated with HIV infection. Fluconazole is frequently an effective agent for the treatment of oral candidiasis.

The dose is one 100 mg tablet per day. Interactions may occur between fluconazole and other drugs, such as rifampin, so the use of fluconazole should be avoided in these cases. Fluconazole is well absorbed and tolerated but its use may be associated with the emergence of resistance. Although true antifungal resistance, based on laboratory testing, appears to be rare and confined to the use of fluconazole, clinical lack of efficacy is seen and is often due to poor compliance or poor absorption of the antifungal. Relapses are common and, once an individual has had two episodes of oral candidiasis, maintenance therapy may be helpful. The value of long-term antifungal prophylaxis for oral candidiasis in HIV-positive individuals who have not yet experienced oral candidiasis is uncertain.

The oral lesions of penicillinosis due to *P. marneffei* resemble pseudomembranous candidiasis, as do rare examples of mucosal colonization by *Saccharomyces* sp., both seen in HIV-infected individuals. Geotrichosis is another rare superficial mycosis seen in association with HIV infection. Other superficial fungal infections which can produce oral lesions include sporotrichosis and rhinosporidiosis.

### Histoplasmosis and other fungal infections

Most cases of oral histoplasmosis now occur in association with HIV infection (Plate 28). The lesions present as painful ulcers on any oral mucosal surface which may mimic squamous cell carcinoma, and biopsy and culture or serological studies are required for diagnosis. Usually, seen as part of disseminated disease, a few cases have represented the initial or even only lesion of reactivated histoplasmosis. The oral lesions usually respond to systemic antifungals (see Chapter 42).

Other deep fungal infections which can involve the oral tissues include mucormycosis, cryptococcosis, aspergillosis, coccidioidomycosis, and blastomycosis. Most produce chronic nonhealing ulcers.

## Viral Infections

### Herpes simplex

Both primary and recurrent herpes simplex can involve the orofacial areas. Primary herpetic gingivostomatitis affects children, teenagers, and young adults, with vesicles on the gingiva, mucosa, and vermilion border of the lips which usually rupture, leaving painful, ragged ulcers. There is fever, malaise, and associated tender lymphadenopathy. Herpes virus can be identified by culture, immunofluorescence, or PCR testing in the fluid from the vesicles, ulcer exudate, or biopsied lesions. Recurrence on the border of the lip (cold sores) (Plate 29) or recurrent intraoral herpes of the gingiva and hard palate mucosa are common. Vesicles form then rupture. In HIV infection, herpes labialis and intraoral herpetic ulceration (Plate 30) may be nonhealing, and while most of such lesions respond to acyclovir, increasingly, acylovir-resistant lesions are being seen.

### Varicella/zoster virus (VZV)

Painful oropharyngeal vesicles and ulcers are a prominent feature of chicken pox, while a more diffuse stomatitis may be seen in severe cases. Reactivation of VZV infection in adults may involve one or more branches of the trigeminal nerve and be associated with oral lesions. Vague tooth-associated pain may be described, and there may be associated facial paralysis because of involvement of branches of the facial nerve (Ramsay Hunt syndrome). Healing usually follows in a few weeks but is often followed by prolonged neuralgia. For the immunosuppressed patient with zoster, high-dose acyclovir is indicated (see Chapter 43).

### Epstein-barr virus (EBV)

In patients with infectious mononucleosis, there is usually cervical lymphadenopathy, sore throat, and often pharyngitis, while gingivitis, stomatitis, oral ulcers, and palatal petechiae have been described (see Chapter 57).

Burkitt's lymphoma, nasopharyngeal carcinoma, and other upper aerodigestive tract carcinomas may involve EBV as an etiological agent, although evidence for such a role for the virus in Sjogren's syndrome and oral squamous cell carcinoma is, as yet, less convincing.

#### Hairy leukoplakia (HL)

Originally described among homosexual men in San Francisco in 1984, this white lesion of the tongue has been seen in the mouths of those infected with the human immunodeficiency virus worldwide (Plate 31). Its presence in HIV-positive individuals usually but not always indicates fairly rapid progression to acquired immunodeficiency syndrome in the absence of antiretroviral therapy. Although the lesion appears to be common in HIV-positive persons, it is also, albeit rarely, seen in other conditions associated with immunosuppression. Epstein-Barr virus is associated with and presumably causes hairy leukoplakia. The lesion presents as a white patch that is often corrugated or even hairy. It may be extensive, even covering the dorsal surface of the tongue. Its prevalence and incidence are not yet fully documented, but reports give a range of from 20% point prevalence in those with otherwise asymptomatic HIV infection in the United States to 36% in patients in Tanzania with full-blown AIDS. Hairy leukoplakia is also found in heart, kidney, and bone marrow transplant recipients. One study of kidney transplant patients found as high a prevalence as is usual among AIDS patients. Hairy leukoplakia is occasionally seen on parts of the oral mucosa other than the tongue but not at mucosal sites elsewhere. The histological features associated with HL include superficial folds or corrugations, thickening and acanthosis with groups or horizontal bands of ballooning cells resembling koilocytes, absence of atypia, and the lack of a connective tissue inflammatory cell infiltrate. Although these histological appearances are highly suggestive of the diagnosis of HL, they are not unique, as they are rarely seen in other forms of leukoplakia. A definite diagnosis is made by the discovery of EBV in the lesion. EBV is present in the epithelial cells of HL as a fully replicating infection with copious viral particles demonstrable by electron microscopy, viral antigen readily detected by immunocytochemistry, and EBV DNA in high copy number as the complete genome in linear virion form and demonstrable by Southern blot or in situ hybridization. The latter technique forms the basis for some fairly straightforward noninvasive approaches to the detection of EBV and hence to the diagnosis of HL. To date, neither severe dysplasia nor carcinoma has been seen in association with HL. However, with the lengthening of life expectancy of HIV-infected persons through better prophylaxis and treatment of opportunistic infections, the malignant potential of HL ultimately will be determined. HL is usually asymptomatic, although slight discomfort and concern about appearance are occasionally reported. HL responds dramatically to high doses of acyclovir. Single case reports of response to ganciclovir and retinoids require confirmation.

### Cytomegalovirus (CMV)

Oral ulcers are seen in some HIV-infected patients with disseminated CMV infection and in a few cases have been the first lesions of CMV disease.

There are as yet no accounts of oral lesions due to the recently described members of the herpesviridae, HHV6 and HHV7, although oral lesions of Kaposi's sarcoma, perhaps caused by a herpes virus, are common in AIDS.

### Human papillomavirus (HPV)

HPV is associated with papillomas and more subtle oral mucosal lesions. Oral warts are common, especially among immunosuppressed individuals. Clinical appearances include cauliflower, spiky and flat forms. The HPV types involved include HPV 2 and 7 for the papillomatous warts and HPV 13 and 32 for flat warts (focal epithelial hyperplasia or Heck's disease). Emerging evidence links HPV types with oral verrucous and squamous cell carcinomas as well as with oral precancerous lesions. Oral warts can be excised using surgery, laser, cryosurgery, and cautery. Among HIV-infected persons, recurrence is common.

### HIV

Many of the numerous and common oral complications of HIV infection have been mentioned in this discussion, including oral candidiasis, hairy leukoplakia, herpes simplex and zoster, cytomegalovirus ulcers, warts, periodontal disease, tuberculosis, histoplasmosis, and other rare mycoses. In addition, Kaposi's sarcoma and AIDS lymphoma, both non-Hodgkin's and Hodgkin's, are seen in the mouth, as are the lesions of thrombocytopenic purpura. Aphthous ulcers are more severe and prolonged in this population, while a CD8 lymphoinfiltrative condition involves the salivary glands, producing clinical features that resemble Sjogren's syndrome. Candidiasis, oral ulcers, and pharyngitis occur during the acute retroviral seroconversion syndrome. Aphthous ulcers and gingivitis have been reported also. Oral infections are often the first clinical sign of immune deficiency due to HIV and are often useful indicatiions for the initiation of antiretrovirfal therapy as well as anti-PCP prophylaxis.

## Other viral infections

### Herpangina

This cocksackievirus infection of childhood causes outbreaks of papules and red-rimmed vesicles on the posterior oral mucosa, including the soft palate, tongue and tonsils, and pharynx. These break down and the ensuing ulcers heal in a few days (see Chapter 57).

### Human hand-foot and mouth disease

This cocksackievirus disease affects children and young adults and is characterized by a maculopapular or vesicular skin rash predominantly on the palms and soles with similar lesions on the intraoral and oropharyngeal mucosae. These heal spontaneously after several days.

### Measles

The pathognomonic oral sign of this childhood paramyxovirus infection is the presence of Koplik's spots. These erythematous macules with central white spots appear on the buccal mucosa following the prodrome of malaise, fever, cough, photophobia, and conjunctivitis. The characteristic maculopapular skin rash follows in 2 d.

### Mumps

This paramyxovirus infection involves salivary glands, notably both parotids, which become swollen. Salivary gland duct orifices may become enlarged, swollen, and obstructed. There is severe pain on eating, salivation, and swallowing. Other viral infections which occasionally cause salivary gland inflammation include the parainfluenza group, CMV, enteroviruses, and choriomeningitis virus.

### Molluscum contagiosum

Rarely, intraoral lesions with the typical appearances of those of the skin have been reported, mostly in association with HIV infection. Nodules a with central depression and containing characteristic pox virus particles on electron microscopy are found.

## Parasitic Infections

Protozoal diseases with rare oral involvement include Chaga's disease, leishmaniasis, trichomoniasis, toxoplasmosis, and amebiasis. Helminth infection can also have oral involvement and include schistosomiasis, hydatid disease, ascariasis, cystercercosis, and trichinosis. Where any of these diseases are endemic, or in people who have spent time in such areas, they should be included in the differential diaporesis of oral ulcers and swellings.

## ANNOTATED BIBLIOGRAPHY

Greenspan JS, Greenspan D. Oral complications of HIV infection. In: Medical Management of AIDS, Fifth Edition. Sande M, Volberding PA, eds. WB Saunders, Philadelphia, PA, 1996.

*A brief practical approach to the diaporesis and management of these lesions.*

Regezi JA, Sciubba JS, eds. Oral Pathology, 2nd ed. WB Saunders, Philadelphia, PA, 1993.

*A detailed review of the clinical features and pathology of oral diseases.*

Topazian RG, Goldberg MH, eds. Oral and Maxillofacial Infections, 3rd ed. Philadelphia; WB Saunders, Philadelphia, PA, 1994.

*An in-depth discussion of the clinical features, diaporesis, and treatment of oral infections.*

# 61

# Diarrhea and Gastroenteritis

HERBERT L. DUPONT

Acute diarrhea and gastroenteritis are common medical complaints and can be serious health problems for certain well-defined populations. The frequency of diarrhea in the developing world varies according to region. In these areas, outside cholera endemic regions, diarrhea as a public health problem is primarily found in children <5 yr of age. The total number of estimated cases of acute diarrheal disease in this age group in the developing world may be as many as 1 billion cases annually. The number of bouts of diarrhea per child per year averages approximately six. In comparison, similar aged children in the United States have one to two bouts/child/yr. Not only are diarrhea rates three to six times higher in developing regions compared with the United States and western Europe, mortality is also impressively higher (see Chapter 93). In the United States, diarrhea-associated mortality is most common among the elderly.

In this chapter, we will review the high-risk groups for diarrhea in the industrialized regions of the world, the important causes of diarrhea, the host factors that relate to susceptibility or resistance to enteric infection, clinical features, laboratory studies, and procedures used in making an etiologic diagnosis and management strategy.

## Epidemiology: High-Risk Settings and Patient Groups

While diarrheal disease is an occasional complaint in all populations, certain groups of individuals more often suffer acute and chronic diarrhea. Population groups where diarrhea represents a major health problem include infants and young children living in developing regions; non-toilet-trained infants attending day care centers; persons residing in residential institutions for the mentally retarded; elderly persons living in nursing homes; gay males and persons with the acquired immune deficiency syndrome (AIDS); and travelers from industrialized regions entering tropical and semitropical regions of the developing world (see Chapter 93).

### Day care centers

In urban day care centers, conditions are favorable for transmission of enteric pathogens. A large number of non-toilet-trained infants are housed in settings where a limited number of persons change diapers and prepare and serve food and where objects such as toys are shared between children. The overall incidence of diarrhea identified in one study carried out in Houston day care centers was found to be 0.44 episodes/child/yr, which actually is lower than national projections for pediatric diarrhea. However, selected centers were shown in the study to have high rates (three to four episodes/child/yr).

When a child develops diarrhea in a day care setting, fecal organisms can be found in large numbers on shared objects and hands of the infants and employed staff. Risk factors for diarrhea occurrence include having multiple diaper change areas, a low staff-to-child ratio (more often seen in private than government-run centers), having the same staff perform both diaper change and meal service duties, low frequency of handwashing among staff, and failure to regularly clean toys and other shared objects. The major pathogens found in day care centers are those that cause infection following exposure to small numbers of organisms, including *Shigella*, *Giardia*, and *C. parvum*. Other agents frequently encountered in day care centers include rotavirus and *Salmonella* spp. Any enteric pathogen introduced into a day care center may be rapidly spread within the environment due to unhygienic conditions and the number of highly susceptible persons present.

### Residential institutions for the mentally retarded

In residential institutions for the mentally retarded, hygienic conditions are often substandard and rates of enteric infection are high. Diarrhea tends to be hyperendemic and outbreaks, particularly due to *Shigella*, are common. Immunity to prevalent microorganisms occurs with increasing time at the institution, presumably through prior exposure. Diarrhea is the most important problem among newly admitted infants and children.

### Gay males

Specific sexual practices in some homosexual men result in a high risk for fecal oral transmission of enteric pathogens in this population. The resulting diarrhea often is associated with enteric infection with more than one pathogen. Any organism showing a fecal oral route of transmission (especially those infective at low inocula) will be seen with high frequency in these patients. The gay male with diarrhea may have multiple pathogens found in stools if extensive laboratory studies are done.

Four organisms, *Neisseria gonorrhoea*, herpes simplex, *Chlamydia trachomatis*, and *Treponema pallidum*, may be transmitted through direct inoculation via receptive anal intercourse leading to proctitis. The resulting proctitis can be diagnosed clinically and through endoscopy where involvement will be confined to the distal 15 cm of colon.

### Acquired immune deficiency syndrome (AIDS)

Diarrhea is an important and frequent complaint of patients with AIDS. It occurs early and is especially common in the African form of the disease. AIDS patients in the United States and western Europe often complain of diarrhea with or without wasting, yet onset is later in the progression of the disease. A subset of gay males with HIV infection may acquire enteric infection as outlined above. Immunologic deficiency during AIDS involves intestinal immune factors and increases susceptibility to a broad array of pathogens, including those with normally low virulence. In addition, some AIDS patients will have diarrhea on a noninfectious basis.

## Multiple cases (food or beverage vehicle)

It is virtually never possible to implicate a food or beverage vehicle in the transmission of enteric disease when a single case of illness occurs. An exception to this is rarely seen in the setting where the agent identified in a diarrhea case is also found in a food item, a portion of which was earlier consumed. The incubation period of enteric infection may vary from 8 h to a week. Also, the number of potential sources of infection is great. On the other hand, when multiple cases are reported, the point of common exposure can often be determined. By then determining an incubation period and examining the specific clinical features, a preliminary etiology for the outbreak should be suspected.

Foodborne disease is becoming more common. This relates to the increasing distribution of food items on a worldwide basis and the growing trend to eat out of the home in public restaurants or in airplanes. Among high-risk subgroups, consumption of unpasteurized milk and untreated water is an important predisposing factor.

# Etiology of Diarrhea

Table 61.1 lists those organisms that can cause diarrhea, highlighting those that may be prominent pathogens in patients with AIDS. In nonimmunodeficient patients the microbial causes of diarrhea differ according to age, the season, and the geographic setting (Table 61.2). The age groups showing differences in frequency of pathogens are infants less than 1 yr of age, children 1 to 5 yr of age, and adults. Pathogens differ in nonindustrialized regions versus the highly industrialized areas. Finally, seasonal factors are important with certain pathogens occurring during cooler months while others are found more in the warmer seasons.

**Table 61.1** Etiologic agents of diarrhea

| | |
|---|---|
| PARASITES | *Microsporidia* (*Enterocytozoon bieneusi*)[a], *Cryptosporidium parvum*,[a] *Isospora belli*,[a] *Cyclospora*,[a] *Giardia lamblia* and *Entamoeba histolytica*, *Dientameba fragilis*, *Strongyloides stercoralis*, *Capillaria philippinensis*, *Fasciolopsis buski*, *Trichuris trichiuria*, *Schistosoma* spp., *Sarcocystis* spp. |
| BACTERIA | *Salmonella enteritidis*,[a] *Shigella* spp.,[a] *Campylobacter* spp.,[a] *Clostridium difficile*,[a] *Mycobacterium avium* complex,[a] diarrheagenic *Escherichia coli* (adherent *E. coli*,[a] enteropathogenic *E. coli*, enterotoxigenic *E. coli*, enteroinvasive *E. coli*, enterohemorrhagic *E. coli*), *Aeromonas* spp., *Plesiomonas shigelloides*, *Vibrio cholerae*, noncholera *Vibrios*, *Yersinia enterocolitica*, *Edwardsiella tarda*, enterotoxigenic *Klebsiella* spp., *Clostridium perfringens*, enterotoxigenic *Staphylococcus aureus*, and *Bacillus cereus* food poisoning |
| FUNGI | *Candida* spp.[a] |
| VIRUSES | Rotaviruses, Norwalk virus, enteric adenoviruses, coronaviruses, astroviruses, caliciviruses, cytomegalovirus,[a] HIV[a] |

[a]Pathogens prominent in AIDS patients although any of the pathogens may on occasion infect HIV-infected persons.

## Bacteria

Bacterial enteropathogens account for approximately 20% of acute diarrhea seen in most populations. The frequency varies by age and geography. In industrialized regions such as the United States and western Europe, the major definable bacterial agents are the invasive pathogens, *Shigella*, *Salmonella*, and *C. jejuni*. *Shigella* is infectious at low inocula, explaining the potential for the organism to be spread person to person as is seen in day care centers. When a child acquires shigellosis in a family, more than half of the siblings will become secondarily infected. In the developing world, enterotoxigenic *E. coli* is an important agent in the local children and in international visitors to these regions. *Vibrio parahemolyticus* and other noncholera *Vibrio*s are important causes of seafood-associated diarrhea in all regions. *Aeromonas* occurs everywhere but is particularly common in Southeast Asia. *Plesiomonas shigelloides* diarrhea is associated with international travel or exposure to seafood. An extensive outbreak of *Vibrio cholerae* 01 infection (cholera) has occurred in South and Central America since early 1991. In parts of Asia where cholera is endemic, *V. cholerae* 01 is being replaced by *V. cholerae* 0139 as the most important etiologic agent in this serious form of diarrhea. Additional microbiologic capability is required to establish the diagnosis.

Foodborne enteric diseases due to elaboration of preformed toxin of *Staphylococcus aureus* or *Bacillus cereus* results in vomiting shortly after consuming the contaminated food item. *Clostridium perfringens* causes foodborne infection which may involve many persons exposed to the contaminated food. *Yersinia enterocolitica* is a common cause of fever and dysenteric diarrhea in Canada, Scandinavia, and South Africa.

## Parasites

The parasitic agents are worldwide in distribution. They are major causes of endemic diarrhea in the United States, accounting for approximately 5% of cases of illness. *Cryptosporidium parvum* may be found in low levels in drinking water, which explains the potential for infection by the parasite in patients with AIDS. When the level of contamination in municipal water sources becomes high, extensive community outbreaks result. *Giardia lamblia* and *C. parvum* infect persons at very low inocula, explaining the epidemiologic observation of person-to-person spread for both.

## Viruses

Viruses cause one-third to one-half of diarrhea and gastroenteritis in virtually all settings. Infection by rotaviruses (usually group A and occasionally non–group A rotaviruses), enteric adenoviruses type 40 and 41, astroviruses, caliciviruses, and coronoviruses are particularly common in infants. Rotavirus is the most important cause of gastroenteritis in infants under the age

**Table 61.2** Potential etiology of diarrhea according to age of the host, geographic region, and season

| General factor | Specific relationship | Consideration of etiology[a] |
|---|---|---|
| Age of host | Infant (<1 yr of age) | A lower frequency of pathogen found; agents found more commonly are rotavirus, *Salmonella* spp., and EPEC |
| | Child | Viral and bacterial agents are common |
| | Adult | A low frequency of pathogen identification is seen in endemic diarrhea; bacterial agents are common in travelers |
| Geographic factors | Tropical and semitropical regions | Bacterial agents are common in children and among travelers to these areas (ETEC, *Shigella* spp., etc.) |
| Seasonal factors | Temperate climates | Viral agents more common in wintertime |
| | Tropical and semitropical regions | *C. jejuni* (autumn/winter) and ETEC (summer) often show different seasonal pattern |

[a]Abbreviations: EPEC = enteropathogenic *E. coli*; ETEC = enterotoxigenic *E. coli*.

of 1 yr in all world regions. In developing regions, the small round viruses, including Norwalk virus, often produce gastroenteritis in the same age group as rotavirus. In the United States, Norwalk and related viruses are more common causes of gastroenteritis in older children and adults. Common vehicles of transmission of Norwalk in the community are food and water. Extensive community outbreaks of Norwalk or other viral agents occur when municipal water systems become contaminated.

## Fungi

Although controversial and difficult to document, *Candida albicans* appears to rarely cause diarrhea in persons who are debilitated from HIV infection, diabetes mellitus, or malnutrition or have received a prolonged course of antimicrobial therapy. Although diarrhea may occur in patients with other systemic fungal infections such as histoplasmosis, the nature of the intestinal process is largely undefined.

## Pathogenesis

There exist at least three important mechanisms whereby diarrhea occurs. The first and undoubtedly the most important in acute diarrhea is intestinal fluid and electrolyte transport leading to watery diarrhea. A secretory enterotoxin working through cyclic nucleotide pathways often explains the abnormal intestinal fluid movement. The second most important mechanism is presence of unabsorbed solutes that serve as an osmotic drag, pulling water and electrolytes. The malabsorption may be specific, as seen in disaccharidase deficiency, often caused by a small-bowel viral infection, or it may be more general, as seen in patients with extensive mucosal disease (e.g., tropical and nontropical sprue). Ingestion of nonabsorbed sugars and other substances (e.g., magnesium-containing laxatives) may lead to the occurrence of diarrhea. Finally, intestinal motility abnormalities may result in diarrhea. In viral gastroenteritis, impaired gastric emptying probably explains the common occurrence of vomiting. Motility abnormalities probably are more important in patients with chronic diarrhea (e.g., irritable bowel syndrome, inflammatory bowel disease).

## Host Factors

### Age and hygienic problems

As a global public health problem, diarrhea is largely a pediatric disease, causing the biggest problem for children less than 5 yr of age. The vast majority of deaths occur in infants under 2 yr of age in developing regions. The high rates of diarrhea and fatality in the developing world underscore the relationship between enteric infection and general hygienic conditions. In the United States and western Europe, diarrhea has its most profound effect on the elderly living in nursing homes. More deaths occur in association with diarrhea in the elderly than in infants and young children.

### Hypochlorhydria

The stomach serves as a barrier for ingested microbes. The low pH found in the stomach is bactericidal for enteropathogens.

Patients with prior gastric surgery for peptic ulcer disease and those with achlorhydria or hypochlorhydria are more susceptible to enteric infection and diarrhea. Also, the resultant disease in these patients may be more severe clinically. Several studies have been carried out in cholera endemic areas showing the strong relationship between clinical cholera and preexistent hypochlorhydria. The role of the inhibitors of gastric acid production ($H_2$ blockers and the $H^+/K^+$ ATPase enzyme inhibitors) in predisposing persons to diarrhea is potentially important and poorly studied. It would appear from the lack of published reports that the common nocturnal use of $H_2$ blockers is not an important risk factor for diarrhea.

## Immunodeficiency

Immunodeficiency states involving the gastrointestinal tract often render the host more susceptible to enteric infection. Agamma-globulinemia, including IgA deficiency, makes persons more susceptible to parasitic infection (particularly *Giardia lamblia*). T cell deficiency as occurs in AIDS also renders the patient susceptible to a variety of enteric pathogens (see below).

## Genetic factors

Patients who are HLA B 27 positive may develop Reiter's syndrome following enteric infection with *Shigella flexneri*, *C. jejuni*, or *Y. enterocolitica*. Patients with blood group O are more susceptible to cholera and its complications. Certain strains of pigs are resistant to scours caused by porcine enterotoxigenic *E. coli* because they lack the small-bowel receptors for organism attachment. Patients with serum antibody to Norwalk virus are more susceptible to subsequent infection by the virus than a subset with no serologic evidence of prior infection, indicating that humoral immunity is not only not protective but those who develop serologic responses to this agent may be uniquely susceptible to infection. Additional studies of host genetic makeup in predisposing to enteric infectious diseases are needed.

## Clinical Manifestations

There are four important clinical presentations of enteric infection. The first is *diarrheal disease*, in which unformed or poorly formed stools are passed in greater than usual frequency when compared to the normal state. Associated symptoms such as nausea, vomiting, malaise, abdominal cramping and pain, fecal urgency, and tenesmus are commonly found as well. The second clinical syndrome is *gastroenteritis*. Here vomiting is a major feature of the illness. In the third, the patient has significant *fever* (>102° F) and exhibits variable degrees of systemic toxicity. A fourth syndrome is *febrile dysenteric diarrhea* in which the stools passed contain gross blood and mucus. Diarrhea can be further characterized according to duration as acute (<14 d), persistent (≥14 d), or chronic (≥30 d).

Clinical aspects of diarrheal illness provide important clues as to possible etiology, determine the extent of the workup, and may influence treatment. Diarrhea is best categorized by severity on a functional scale: *mild*—no alteration of activities occurs; *moderate*—a forced change in schedule occurs; and, *severe*—the patient is disabled for a period of time, usually confined to bed. Table 61.3 lists the above-noted clinical features along with the probable etiologic agents to consider when these findings are identified.

## Fever

When a patient with diarrhea has fever (oral temperature > 100.2° F), an invasive/inflammatory pathogen is often responsible. In these patients the major causes of a febrile illness are the invasive and inflammation-evoking bacteria, *Shigella*, *C. jejuni*, or *Salmonella*, as well as *Clostridium difficile*, *Aeromonas* spp, or the viruses, usually rotavirus in an infant or a small round virus (e.g., Norwalk virus) in an older child or adult.

## Vomiting

When vomiting is the major manifestation of the illness (e.g., ten episodes vomiting and passage of only one or two stools during a 24 h time period) there are usually two etiologic considera-

**Table 61.3** Potential causes of diarrhea according to clinical presentation

| Clinical presentation | Potential etiologic agents and conditions to consider |
|---|---|
| Acute watery diarrhea without fever/dysentery | Classically enterotoxigenic *E. coli* or *Vibrio cholerae*, can be caused by virutally all enteric pathogens (bacterial, viral, and parasitic) |
| Vomiting as the primary symptom (gastroenteritis) | Viral gastroenteritis (see specific viruses in Table 61.1) or food poisoning (due to preformed toxin produced by *Staphylococcus aureus* or *Bacillus cereus*) |
| Febrile dysentery (passage of grossly bloody stools) | *Shigella* or *C. jejuni*, occasionally *Salmonella*, *Aeromonas* spp., enteropathogenic *E. coli*, *C. difficile*, enterohemorrhagic *E. coli*, *Vibrio parahemolyticus*, *Entamoeba histolytica*, and idiopathic ulcerative colitis |
| Persistent diarrhea (lasting ≥14 days) | *Giardia*, *Cryptosporidium parvum*, small-bowel bacterial overgrowth, lactase deficiency, bacterial enteropathogen (e.g., *Shigella*, or adherent/enteropathogenic *E. coli*), Brainerd diarrhea |

tions. The first is food poisoning due to preformed toxin present in a food item consumed. The toxin may have been elaborated by *S. aureus* or *Bacillus cereus*. Here the incubation period will be less than 4 h in nearly all cases, and usually less than 2 h. The other consideration in the patient with a vomiting illness is viral gastroenteritis—most commonly rotavirus in an infant or a small round virus (e.g., Norwalk virus) in an older child or an adult where in both cases the incubation period usually is between 8 h and 48 h.

## Dysentery

Dysentery refers to the passage of bloody stools, often of small volume, with passage of mucus, cramping and tenesmus, and is indicative of invasion and or injury of the colonic mucosa by a pathogen or its toxin. When the previously healthy patient, not having recently received antimicrobial drugs, has diarrhea and is passing bloody stools, the two most important causes in the United States are *Shigella* and *C. jejuni*. Other considerations for the etiology of dysentery include *Salmonella*, *Aeromonas*, *Vibrio parahemolyticus*, *Yersinia enterocolitica*, invasive *E. coli*, enterohemorrhagic *E. coli* (O157:H7), and *Entamoeba histolytica*. Inflammatory bowel disease involving the colon or rectum can have a dysenteric presentation indistinguishable from infectious etiologies.

## Persistent diarrhea

When diarrhea lasts longer than 2 wk, the illness is classified as persistent. In this discussion we will consider the problem among persons living in industrialized regions and among persons from this part of the world traveling to the developing world. In Chapter 93, the problem of persistent endemic diarrhea occurring in the developing world is discussed.

Etiologies of persistent diarrhea in developed countries include: (*1*) *Infection with Giardia lamblia* explains no more than 2%–4% of acute diarrhea cases seen in most areas; however, it may explain 20%–30% of the cases of persistent diarrhea in many settings; (*2*) *C. parvum*; (*3*) *bacterial overgrowth* in the small bowel, where colonic flora grows in the small bowel secondary to intestinal stasis interfering with intestinal absorption resulting in steatorrhea and diarrhea; (*4*) *small-bowel mucosal injury* acquired during infection and causing intestinal lactase deficiency. This is particularly common in viral gastroenteritis and *Giardia* infection; (*5*) *bacterial agents* such as *Shigella* and enteropathogenic and enteroadherent *E. coli* may produce persistent diarrhea; (*6*) *host deficiencies* will lead to persistent diarrhea often associated with enteric infection by recognized pathogens. These conditions include AIDS and trace metal and vitamin deficiencies in children living in the developing world; (*7*) "*Brainerd diarrhea*." This is an idiopathic illness that follows consumption of unpasteurized milk or untreated water (surface or well water). The diarrhea may last for more than 1 yr. Intestinal biopsy often shows areas of focal mucosal inflammation, but Brainerd diarrhea is essentially a diagnosis of exclusion. The prognosis is usually good in this form of chronic diarrhea. In all patients with persistent diarrhea, idiopathic inflammatory bowel disease should be considered.

## Diagnosis

In approaching diagnosis and management, it is advisable to categorize patients into severity groups and to divide them into healthy hosts versus those with immunosuppression (especially AIDS). For mild diarrhea, no workup is required. Laboratory evaluation is advised only for moderate and severe disease (Table 61.4).

## General laboratory studies and procedures

### Complete blood count

The white blood count and white blood cell differential are not normally performed in the routine workup of diarrhea cases. However, in the toxic or febrile dysenteric patient, a leukocytosis and/or shift to the left of the differential suggests bacillary dysentery, due to *Shigella*, *C. jejuni*, or an invasive *E. coli*.

**Table 61.4** Use of diagnostic procedures in the evaluation of patients with diarrhea

| Diagnostic procedure | Indication |
|---|---|
| Fecal leukocyte test | In all patients with moderate and severe diarrhea if the test is readily available and inexpensive to perform |
| Stool culture | Patients with severe diarrhea, persistent diarrhea, patients with AIDS-related diarrhea, febrile and dysenteric patients, presence of fecal leukocytes, hamburger-associated diarrhea in an area known to have a problem with 0157:H7 *E. coli* diarrhea, or hemolytic uremic syndrome |
| Blood culture | Febrile and toxic patients |
| Parasite examination | Patients with persistent diarrhea, recent travel to mountainous areas of North America or to Russia, exposure to day care center; diarrhea in a gay male or in a patient with AIDS |
| *Clostridium difficile* toxin assay | Any patient who is on or has recently received antimicrobials |
| Rotavirus antigen | Hospitalized infant (<2 yr of age) with gastroenteritis |
| EnteroTest for small bowel fluid and flexible sigmoidoscopy | In areas where there has been some experience with the test in the workup of persistent diarrhea; gay male with moderate to severe diarrhea, or patient with AIDS not responsive to empiric antibacterial therapy and nonspecific drugs designed to improve symptoms |

#### Fecal leukocytes

The proper staining procedure for routine evaluation of diarrhea for fecal leukocytes is to employ dilute methylene blue stain. If mucus strands are present when moving a wood applicator stick through the fecal sample, a strand is placed on a glass slide. After adding the stain, a wet mount preparation may be evaluated using the high dry objective of the microscope after applying a coverslip. Alternatively, the sample may be allowed to dry, followed by heat fixing, staining with methylene blue, and then examining under oil. In evaluating the gay male with diarrhea, the gram stain is preferred to methylene blue since identification of intracellular diplococci will help establish the diagnosis of anorectal *Neisseria gonorrhoea* infection.

When many leukocytes are found in fecal samples, the patient has diffuse colonic inflammation. When there is focal colitis or the small bowel is the site of the inflammation, leukocytes will not be readily identified in stool samples because of dilution in the fecal stream. The major causes of diffuse colonic inflammation in the patient not having recently received antimicrobials are *Shigella*, *Salmonella*, and *C. jejuni*. In the case of patients who have recently received antimicrobial therapy, *Clostridium difficile* should be suspected as well. Other organisms/conditions which may on occasion produce colonic inflammation of a diffuse nature (hence positive fecal leukocytes) include *Aeromonas*, *V. parahemolyticus*, and *Y. enterocolitica*. Fecal leukocytes will be present in patients with colitis caused by inflammatory bowel disease and may be seen in persons with allergic gastroenteritis.

#### EnteroTest

A commercially available nylon string with a gelatin capsule affixed to the end (EnteroTest) may be useful to identify pathogens in the upper small bowel. The capsule is swallowed the night before coming to the clinic or in the early morning before breakfast and before the clinic visit. The string is then withdrawn followed by scraping of the adherent mucus into a sterile petri dish. The string is checked for pH to document that it reached the alkaline small bowel. The mucus collected may then be subjected to microscopic study for parasites (*Giardia*, *Crypto-sporidium*, or *Strongyloides*) and quantitative microbiology for bacterial overgrowth. Quantitation of bacterial growth can be obtained by treating the sample similar to a urine culture using selective and nonselective media (see Chapter 16). Aerobic growth of $\geq 10^5$ colony-forming units is consistent with bacterial overgrowth.

#### Endoscopy

Endoscopy should generally be reserved for patients with bloody or persistent diarrhea in whom stool cultures, ova and parasite exam, and measurements of *C. difficile* toxin are negative or unrevealing. Flexible sigmoidoscopy can be helpful in the gay male, where differentiation between proctitis (inflammation confined to the distal 15 cm of rectosigmoid) and proctocolitis (inflammation beyond 15 cm of distal colon) has important diagnostic and therapeutic significance (see above).

### Specific microbiologic tests

#### Stool and blood culture

Considering the relatively low frequency of identifying specific bacterial pathogens in patients with acute diarrhea (about 20%), it is not advisable to perform stool cultures in the majority of cases of illness. Clinical features should be used to direct the performance of a stool cultures in order to improve the chances for identification of a pathogen (Table 61.4). In brief, stool cultures are indicated if the patient is febrile or dysenteric, or if illness is clinically severe or persistent, when stools contain many leukocytes, and in geographic areas and settings where *E. coli* 0157:H7 infection is common (e.g., multiple symptomatic patients with a common source exposure and bloody diarrhea).

#### Parasite exam

In the patient with acute diarrhea, tests for parasites are positive in less than 10% of cases unless certain clinical or epidemiologic features are present. There are several indications for performing parasitic examination in the diarrhea patient (Table 61.4), the most important being persistence of symptoms. Other factors include well-defined risk factors including travel to mountainous areas of North America or to Russia or exposure to day care centers.

#### Virus antigen

Since there is no treatment for viral gastroenteritis other than support with fluid and electrolyte replacement, establishing an etiologic diagnosis is usually of little practical value. In infants admitted to the hospital with severe gastroenteritis, documentation of rotavirus infection may avoid useless administration of antimicrobial therapy. Similarly, type 40 and 41 enteric adenovirus may be sought by antigen testing of fecal samples, where specific identification is useful for epidemiological purposes.

## Management

### The otherwise-healthy host

The patient with mild diarrhea is best treated with fluids and electrolytes. *Oral fluid-electrolyte therapy* is important in infants and in the elderly, particularly when the diarrhea is intense or prolonged. Ideally, solutions with adequate electrolyte composition should be used in these patients (e.g., Pedialyte, Ricealyte). If not available, hypotonic soft drinks augmented with Saltine crackers should be suitable unless the patient has moderate to severe dehydration, profuse watery diarrhea, or persistent diarrhea. In Chapter 93 the use of oral rehydration solution for children with diarrhea and variable degrees of dehydration is described.

*Symptomatic treatment* may be given to patients with moderate to severe diarrhea to improve symptoms. Symptomatic treatment is useful in shifting illness to a less severe category and allowing a person to better function during an enteric illness. *Motility-inhibiting drugs* (e.g., loperamide) are the most effective and will reduce diarrhea (number of unformed stools passed) by 80%. The drugs work by slowing the movement of the intestinal fluid column (i.e., prolongation of intestinal transit), facilitating mucosal absorption of fluids and electrolytes. Loperamide is usually preferred to diphenoxylate. Although of equal efficacy in reducing diarrhea, diphenoxylate contains atropine sulfate, which may be associated with objectionable anticholinergic effects while providing no additional antidiarrheal benefit. Also, the overdose consequences (central opiate effects) are much more serious for diphenoxylate than loperamide, in case an infant inadvertently takes a parent's or older sibling's medication. The recommended dose of loperamide for adults is 4 mg initially, followed by 2 mg after each unformed stool not to exceed 8 mg/d (over-the-counter dose) or 16 mg/d (prescription dose). The drug is given for no more than 48 h. The antimotility drugs should *not* be used in febrile or dysenteric disease since invasive bacterial illness may be prolonged.

*Bismuth subsalicylate* (BSS) is probably the drug of choice for treatment of the vomiting associated with gastroenteritis. While of some value, BSS is less effective than the antimotility drugs in decreasing acute diarrhea. Its mode of action is through salicylate-dependent antisecretory pathways. The dose of BSS for therapy of acute diarrhea in adults is 30 ml (or two tablets) each 30 min for eight doses (total dose 240 ml or 16 tablets over 3 1/2 h). The drug may be given for up to 2 d. Acetylsalicylic acid may also favorably improve acute diarrhea; however, its toxicity to gastric mucosa precludes routine use.

Novel antisecretory drugs are being developed that may reduce diarrhea without motility changes. This may remove the threat of prolongation of disease in the face of infection by an invasive bacterial pathogen and eliminate the problem of post-treatment constipation seen with the antimotility agents.

*Antimicrobial therapy* may be employed in certain clinical settings on an empiric basis or when a treatable pathogen is identified (see Table 61.5). Moderate-to-severe travelers' diarrhea and febrile dysenteric diarrhea may be treated with antibacterial agents since bacterial agents explain a majority of cases of illness. Some clinicians would use metronidazole empirically in patients with persistent diarrhea in view of the importance of *Giardia* in this setting. When a bacterial enteropathogen is identified in diarrheal stools in a patient with moderate-to-severe illness antimicrobial therapy may be employed. Similarly, for patients with clinically important diarrhea in whom *Giardia* cysts or trophozoites or *E. histolytica* trophozoites with ingested red blood cells are identified, specific treatment may be given. In the patient with AIDS and diarrhea, curative or suppressive therapy may be indicated if an etiologic agent is identified. Use of antimicrobial drugs for other diarrhea cases on an empiric basis should be discouraged. The common use of antibacterial drugs in developing countries has led to the development of resistance among bacterial enteropathogens. This is a serious problem in certain areas for strains of *Shigella* (especially *S. dysenteriae* 1), *C. jejuni*, and *Salmonella*.

## The patient with AIDS

In the AIDS patient with diarrhea, ideally two freshly passed stools should be submitted to the laboratory to be examined for parasites and bacterial enteropathogens (listed in Table 61.1). The stools should be assayed for *C. difficile* toxin. One or two blood cultures should be obtained for enteric bacterial pathogens and *Mycobacterium-apium-intracellulare*. If an agent is identified, specific treatment is given. If not, an empiric course of a fluoroquinolone (norfloxacin 400 mg BID, ciprofloxacin 500 mg BID, ofloxacin 300 mg BID, or fleroxacin 400 mg QD) may be given for 7 to 10 d. With failure of a response, the patient may be given an empiric course of metronidazole 250 mg three or four times a day for 7 d. With good clinical response, metronidazole should probably be continued for 14 d. With no response, the agent can be discontinued after 7 d.

If symptoms continue or recur, it is advisable to treat the patient symptomatically with a motility-inhibiting drug such as loperamide for control of diarrhea. If symptoms are largely

**Table 61.5** Antimicrobial therapy in the adult patient with diarrheal disease

| Empiric treatment | Recommended drug and dosage |
|---|---|
| Travelers' diarrhea | Norfloxacin 400 mg BID, ciprofloxacin 500 mg BID, ofloxacin 200–300 mg BID, or fleroxacin 400 mg QD for 1–3 d |
| Febrile dysenteric diarrhea | Same drug and dose as travelers' diarrhea, drug given for 3–5 d |
| Persistent diarrhea | Metronidazole 250 mg QID for 7–10 d for healthy host. In the AIDS patient, the drug should be given for at least 14 d if an initial clinical response occurs |
| AGENT-SPECIFIC DIARRHEA | |
| Shigellosis | Treat as febrile dysenteric diarrhea (above) |
| Salmonellosis | No treatment unless toxic and febrile or patient is >70 yr of age or is immunosuppressed; then treat as travelers' diarrhea for 7–10 d |
| Campylobacteriosis | Erythromycin 250 mg QID for 5 d |
| *Aeromonas* or *Plesiomonas* diarrhea | Treat as shigellosis |
| *C. difficile* colitis | Metronidazole 250 mg QID for 10 d; for treatment failures vancomycin 125 mg QID for 10 d |
| Giardiasis | Metronidazole 250 mg QID for 7–10 d |
| Cryptosporidiosis | None or paromomycin 500 mg QID for 5–7 d. In the AIDS patient, the drug should be given for at least 14 d |
| Intestinal Amoebiasis | Metronidazole 750 mg TID for 5 d plus diiodohydroxyquin 650 mg TID for 20 d |
| Isosporiosis or *Cyclorspora* in an HIV+ patient | TMP/SMX 160 mg/800 mg qid for 10 d, then 160 mg/800 mg three times a week indefinitely |
| Microsporidiosis in an HIV+ patient | No therapy proven to be effective, metronidazole 500 mg TID, albendazole or atovaquone may be tried |

**Table 61.6** Symptomatic treatment of the patient with AIDS-associated diarrhea*

| Drug | Dosage | Comments—see text for dosages |
|---|---|---|
| Loperamide | 4 mg initially, then 2 mg after each unformed stool not to exceed 16 mg/d | Standard therapy if cost is not a critical issue |
| Diphenoxylate with atropine | 4 mg QID as needed | Least expensive, has overdose liability for young children, may have objectional anticholinergic side effects when taken in maxium doses |
| Tincture of opium | 0.3–1 ml/kg/dose every 3–4 h for a maximum of 6 doses/d | Has overdose liability, may cause weakness, hypotension, drowsiness, dizziness |
| Attapulgite | 1.2–1.5 g after each unformed stool or each 2 h, maximum daily dosage 9g | Safest preparation, will make stools more formed, not effective in severe disease |
| Octreotide | 50–100 mg each 8 h IV; increasing by 100 mg/dose at 48 h intervals with a maximum dose of 500 $\mu$g/d | Used when no other symptomatic treatment offers help, the parenteral route is inconvenient. Side effects include nausea, headache and dizziness, flushing, hyper- or hypoglycemia |

*All patients should be encouraged to drink fluids and take in salt to meet losses from diarrhea and vomiting; patients should not be treated with bismuth subsalicylate (to prevent bismuth encephalopathy).

controlled, this approach should be continued as the management plan.

Patients not responding to empiric treatment and poorly controlled with symptomatic treatment should undergo upper and lower intestinal endoscopy (Esophagogastroduodenoscopy [EGD] and flexible sigmoidoscopy) with biopsy of suspicious lesions for one of the agents listed in Table 61.1. Therapy at that point is dictated by findings from the endoscopy study.

Unfortunately, there remains an important fraction of patients with AIDS who fail to respond to symptomatic treatment and have a negative endoscopy evaluation. These patients should be tried on a variety of symptomatically acting drugs, and serial endoscopy procedures may be required to eventually establish the diagnosis.

Table 61.6 provides a list of available drugs and dosages used to treat diarrhea symptoms associated with diarrhea in patients with AIDS. For most cases, the patient is treated with loperamide. Patients failing to respond may be treated with two of the agents although the chance for drug toxicity will increase. Bismuth subsalicylate should *not* be used in these patients due to the potential for developing bismuth encephalopathy.

## ANNOTATED BIBLIOGRAPHY


Azalpurkar R, Schiller L, Little K, Santangelo W, Fordtran J. The self-limited nature of chronic idiopathic diarrhea. N Engl J Med 1992; 327:1849–1852.

*This study provides data to suggest that persons with persistent diarrhea without identifiable cause have a benign course. This justifies a conservative approach to workup and management of these patients.*

Blacklow N, Greenberg H. Viral gastroenteritis. New Engl J Med 1991; 325:252–264.

*A review of the important viral causes of diarrhea is provided.*

DuPont H. Review article: infectious diarrhoea. Aliment Pharmacol Ther 1994; 8:3–13.

*A review of the current pharmacologic strategies in managing acute diarrhea is provided.*

DuPont H, Ericsson C. Prevention and treatment of traveler's diarrhea. N Engl J Med 1993; 328:1821–1827.

*In this article one current approach to the management of travelers' diarrhea is provided.*

DuPont HL, Marshall GD. HIV-associated diarrhoea and wasting. Lancet 1995; 346:352–356.

*After presentation of a case of chronic diarrhea and biliary tract disease in a patient with AIDS, an approach to workup and management is provided.*

Guerrant R, Bobak D. Bacterial and protozoal gastroenteritis. N Engl J Med 1991; 325:327–340.

*A review of the important bacterial and parasitic causes of diarrhea is provided.*

Harris J, DuPont H, Hornick R. Fecal leukocytes in diarrheal illness. Ann Intern Med 1972; 76:696–703.

*This study indicates the value of the fecal leukocyte test in detecting enteric pathogens which cause diffuse inflammation of the colon. It indicates that the methylene blue stain in preferred for most patients.*

Osterholm M, MacDonald K, White K, et al. An outbreak of a newly recognized chronic diarrhea syndrome associated with raw milk consumption. JAMA 1986; 256:484–490.

*A potentially important cause of persistent diarrhea ("Brainerd diarrhea") of presumed infectious origin is described.*

Quinn T, Stamm W, Goodell S, et al. The polymicrobial origin of intestinal infections in homosexual men. N Engl J Med 1983; 309:576–582.

*The study outlines the current approach to evaluation of diarrhea in gay males where the anatomic site of intestinal involvement suggests specific etiologic agents. Demonstration of the value of flexible sigmoidoscopy in evaluating these patients is provided.*

Teasley D, Gerding D, Olson M, et al. Prospective randomized trial of metronidazole versus vancomycin for clostridium-difficile-associated diarrhoea and colitis. Lancet 1983; 2:1043–1046.

*In this study, metronidazole is established as the optimal initial treatment of antibiotic-associated colitis due to* C. difficile.

# 62

# Hepatitis

MARGARET C. SHUHART AND ROBERT L. CARITHERS, JR.

Viral hepatitis continues to be a significant cause of morbidity and mortality worldwide, and in recent years it was the third most frequently reported infectious disease in the United States. The focus of this chapter is the hepatotropic viruses, the most common cause of viral hepatitis in humans.

## Etiology: Hepatotropic Viruses

There are five recognized hepatotropic viruses, known as hepatitis viruses A, B, C, D, and E. Although the acute illness is similar regardless of etiologic agent, they have important differences in terms of virology, epidemiology, and chronic sequelae. Their defining characteristics are listed in Table 62.1 and are discussed in detail below. A number of other viruses can cause liver disease in humans. These are listed in Table 62.2 and will not be discussed further in this chapter.

Hepatitis G virus (HGV) recently has been described. This RNA virus, a member of the *Flaviviridae* family, is parenterally transmitted and appears to have a worldwide distribution. A recent U.S. blood bank study found that HGV has a higher prevalence among blood donors than HCV. However, HGV infection is equally prevalent in blood donors with and without elevated aminotransferases. Furthermore, multiple studies have found no association between HGV and liver disease, and recent data suggest that HGV is unlikely to be hepatotropic. HGV is not discussed further in this chapter.

## Epidemiology

Viral hepatitis is worldwide in distribution, but both the incidence and prevalence of infection have marked geographic differences. These differences are largely due to biologic and ecologic factors, but variations in case definitions, reporting practices, and access to medical care may also contribute. Furthermore, acute infections are often subclinical and therefore go undetected.

### Hepatitis A (HAV)

The seroprevalence of hepatitis A varies significantly, from 13% in Scandinavian countries, to 40% in the United States, to 95% in the South Pacific Islands. In developing countries in Asia and Africa, inapparent childhood infection is almost universal. With improved sanitation and hygiene, infection is delayed and increasing numbers of adults are susceptible to infection. In industrialized nations where childhood infection rates are low, HAV is a frequent cause of sporadic and epidemic hepatitis.

Hepatitis A is primarily transmitted by the fecal–oral route; the infected liver serves as the source for the virus in feces. Most infections are acquired just before or at the onset of symptoms, when fecal shedding is at its peak. Person-to-person contact is the primary mode of HAV transmission. Epidemics due to contaminated food or water also occur but play a minor role in the spread of hepatitis A. Blood-borne transmissions have been rarely reported and are due to the brief period of viremia which occurs during the incubation period and the early acute phase of illness.

### Hepatitis B

Hepatitis B is the most common cause of acute and chronic hepatitis worldwide. In the United States it is estimated that approximately 300,000 individuals contract hepatitis B each year. More than 300 million people worldwide and 1 million people in the United States are chronic carriers of HBV. The risk of developing chronic infection is inversely proportional to age (Table 62.1). The prevalence of chronic HBV infection varies widely, ranging from 0.3% to 1.5% in North America to as high as 5% to 20% in sub-Saharan Africa and Asia. A high prevalence has also been reported in native Alaskan villages. Individuals with chronic HBV infection may have no liver disease or may have chronic hepatitis with or without cirrhosis. Chronic HBV infection also carries a significant risk for hepatocellular carcinoma. In the United States approximately 15% to 25% of patients with chronic HBV die prematurely of cirrhosis.

Transmission of HBV is predominantly parenteral, sexual, or via maternal–neonatal transmission. Oral–oral contact spread also occurs, and is responsible for transmission to household members; there is no evidence for fecal–oral spread of HBV. Shared vehicles such as razor blades and toothbrushes and passive vectors such as tattoo needles may also contribute to the spread of HBV.

### Hepatitis C

Hepatitis C infection is also a common cause of acute and chronic hepatitis worldwide. The prevalence of antibody to HCV (anti-HCV) is approximately 1% in western countries and ranges from 1% to 6% in the East. In the United States, groups with high prevalence rates include injection drug users and hemophiliacs (60%–90%), hemodialysis patients (20%), and individuals with high-risk sexual behaviors (1%–10%). Similar prevalence rates have been reported among high-risk groups in Eastern countries. Approximately 80%–85% of individuals with exposure to hepatitis C develop chronic hepatitis and 20%–25% with chronic infection develop cirrhosis. The incidence of hepatocellular carcinoma in patients with chronic HCV infection is approximately 5% in western countries but is as high as 50% in Japan. The reasons for this are unclear but may be related to undetermined environmental factors, viral genotype, and/or genetic predisposition.

**Table 62.1** Viral, epidemiologic, and clinical characteristics of the hepatotropic viruses

| | Hepatitis | | | | |
|---|---|---|---|---|---|
| | A | B | C | D | E |
| Family | *Picornavirus* | *Hepadnavirus* | *Flavivirus* | Uncertain | *Calcivirus*[e] |
| Size (nm) | 27 | 42 | 30–60 | 30–38 | 27–32 |
| Genome | RNA | DNA | RNA | RNA | RNA |
| Transmission | Fecal–oral | Parenteral<br>Sexual<br>Perinatal<br>Oral–oral | Parenteral<br>Sexual<br>Perinatal | Parenteral<br>Sexual[b] | Fecal–oral |
| Mean incubation period in days (range) | 28 (15–50) | 120 (45–160) | 45–55 (12–160) | 35 (21–140) | 40 (14–54) |
| Case-fatality rate (%) | 0.1 | 0.2–1 | <1 | 2–20[c] | 0.5–4[f] |
| Rate of chronicity (%) | None | 3–5[a]<br>20–50<br>70–90 | 80–85 | 1–3[d]<br>70–80 | None |

[a]Perinatal infection, 70%–90%; children <5 yr, 20%–50%, older children and adults, 3–5%.

[b]Sexual transmission limited to endemic areas and among high-risk groups in developed countries.

[c]Risk for fulminant hepatitis highest in superinfection of chronic HBV.

[d]Rate 70%–80% in superinfection of chronic HBV.

[e]Tentative classification; genetic sequences of nonstructural proteins are similar to rubella virus and furoviruses.

[f]Averages 20% in pregnant women in their second or third trimester.

Hepatitis C is primarily transmitted parenterally. Since the onset of blood donor screening for HCV in 1990, there has been a dramatic reduction in transfusion associated hepatitis C infection. Nearly one-half of the reported cases of acute HCV in the United States are associated with injection drug use. Recently, intranasal cocaine use with sharing of straws has been associated with HCV transmission. Exposure to contaminated blood also occurs in health care workers and hemodialysis patients. Transmission of HCV in dialysis centers is believed to occur through poor infection control practices such as sharing medication vials and supplies between patients. Although tattooing, acupuncture, and body piercing represent other possible percutaneous exposures, they have not been proven to be associated with HCV infection in the U.S.

Case control and serologic studies have reported conflicting results with respect to sexual transmission. Nevertheless, approximately 10% of individuals with acute HCV report recent sexual contact with a known HCV-positive partner. The overall risk of sexual transmission is estimated to be 5%, but the overall importance of sexual transmission is unclear. However, sexual transmission from partner to partner in a stable monogamous relationship appears to be quite uncommon. Vertical transmission occurs in up to 6% of pregnancies, has been demonstrated in both HIV-infected and HIV-negative mothers, and is more likely when viral burden is high. There is no evidence for HCV transmission through breastfeeding. Household transmission accounts for fewer than 5% of cases of acute hepatitis; it likely occurs through sharing of razors and toothbrushes and other exposures to contaminated blood. Transmission via oral–oral contact has been suggested by serologic studies of family members in Asia and Europe, although other risk behaviors were not well characterized in these studies. There is no evidence that HCV is spread through casual contact in the United States.

**Table 62.2** Other human viruses associated with acute hepatitis

| Childhood and adult hepatitis | Neonatal hepatitis |
|---|---|
| Epstein-Barr virus[a] | Rubella |
| Coxsackie viruses A and B | Cytomegalovirus |
| Echoviruses | Herpes simplex virus |
| Yellow fever virus | |
| Cytomegalovirus[b] | |
| Measles virus | |
| Rubella | |
| Herpes simplex virus[c] | |
| Adenovirus[d] | |

[a]Biochemical hepatitis in 90%; jaundice and/or hepatomegaly in 10%–20%.

[b]Usually subclinical; may cause hepatomegaly and abnormal liver tests (cytomegalic mononucleosis); clinically mild hepatitis in the immunocompromised.

[c]Rarely causes fulminant hepatitis in immunocompetent and immunocompromised patients; fulminant hepatitis also reported in pregnancy.

[d]Rarely causes fulminant hepatitis in immunocompromised patients; causality not proven in immunocompetent patients.

## Hepatitis D

HDV is a defective RNA virus that causes hepatitis only in individuals who are concurrently infected with HBV, either as a coinfection with HBV or as a superinfection of chronic HBV carriers. The prevalence of HDV among HBsAg-positive blood donors is low (1.4% to 8%). As expected, the prevalence is highest among injection drug users (20% to 53%) and hemophiliacs (48%–80%). HDV is endemic in countries in southern Europe,

North Africa and the Middle East, where superinfection of chronic HBV carriers is common.

HDV is most efficiently transmitted by blood and blood products. However, in countries in which HDV is endemic, infection is believed to be spread by intimate person-to-person contact. In developed countries, spread to intimate contacts has been reported only in high-risk groups. Perinatal transmission of delta virus is rare.

### Hepatitis E

Hepatitis E virus (HEV) is a common cause of sporadic and epidemic hepatitis in developing countries of the Indian subcontinent, Asia, and Africa. While there have been no reported outbreaks in the United States, Canada, or the industrialized nations of Europe or Asia, sporadic cases have occurred in individuals visiting endemic areas. Sporadic cases not associated with travel to an endemic area have been reported in Europe. A single such case of sporadic HEV was recently reported in the United States. The isolated HEV strain in this case was highly homologous to a strain recently isolated from American swine. Using recently developed serological tests, 1% to 2% of blood donors in the United States test positive for anti-HEV. Whether this represents past infection with HEV or cross-reactivity with another agent is unclear. For reasons that are not clear, mortality is significantly higher in infected pregnant women, reaching 20% in the third trimester of pregnancy. HEV infection is not associated with chronic liver disease.

HEV is transmitted via the fecal–oral route; the source of infection is usually contaminated drinking water, and outbreaks often occur following floods in the rainy season. It is uncertain whether person-to-person spread is responsible for sporadic cases. Seroepidemiologic and virologic data suggest that HEV is less readily transmitted than HAV.

## Host Factors

The host immunologic response is likely the primary cause of hepatocellular injury due to viral hepatitis. This is discussed in detail below. Other host factors playing a role in viral acquisition and in manifestation of disease are discussed in the sections on epidemiology and pathogenesis.

## Pathogenesis

### Hepatitis A

The pathogenesis of hepatitis A is not fully understood. Classification of HAV as a picornavirus is indirect evidence for cytopathogenicity, as most picornaviruses are cytopathic and viral replication leads to cell death. However, there is more direct evidence for an immunopathogenic mechanism. Studies of both hepatic and peripheral blood lymphocytes from patients with acute HAV suggest that HLA class I–restricted cytotoxicity is responsible for hepatocellular necrosis in acute HAV infection.

### Hepatitis B

The pathogenesis of HBV is immune-mediated. Although a humoral response with immune-complex formation is noted during the prodrome and early phase of infection, there is no evidence that immune complexes play a role in hepatocellular injury. The cell-mediated immune response appears to be far more important, and likely controls hepatocellular injury either by the inhibition of viral replication or by the destruction of HBV-infected hepatocytes. Evidence to date suggests that HBV-infected hepatocytes expressing both HLA class I peptides and HBV nucleocapsid proteins (HBcAg and HBeAg) are recognized and destroyed by activated cytotoxic $CD8^+$ cells. It is likely that this cell-mediated immune response also determines the resolution or persistence of HBV infection.

### Hepatitis C

The pathogenesis of hepatitis C virus is not yet certain, but existing evidence supports both cytopathic and immune-mediated mechanisms. A cytopathic effect is seen in experimental flaviviral infections. Further indirect evidence for cytopathogenesis come from the response to $\alpha$-interferon, where the reduction in serum RNA levels is accompanied by normalization of aminotransferases. However, in most studies serum HCV RNA levels and intrahepatic antigen expression do not correlate with the severity of histologic disease. Immunopathogenesis is supported by the finding of $CD8^+$ and $CD4^+$ lymphocytes in portal, periportal, and lobular infiltrates. Furthermore, recent studies have demonstrated that HCV-specific intrahepatic cytotoxic T cells produce pro-inflammatory cytokines; these cytokines may be involved in hepatocellular injury. It is possible that both cytopathic and immune-mediated mechanisms play a role, and that host–viral interactions determine which predominates in a given individual.

### Hepatitis D

The pathogenesis of HDV is uncertain. Liver histology in acute HDV supports a cytopathic effect. However, in vitro studies have not consistently demonstrated cytotoxicity in association with either HDAg or HDV RNA. Findings in chronic HDV infection are more consistent with an immune-mediated pathogenesis. In chronic HDV, circulating immune complex levels correlate with aminotransferase levels. Furthermore, portal inflammation in chronic HDV correlates with liver expression of HDV antigen. Finally, intrahepatic mononuclear cells are predominantly T lymphocytes and cytotoxic T lymphocytes appear to be concentrated in areas of hepatocellular necrosis. Further studies are needed to confirm these findings.

### Hepatitis E

Work on the pathogenesis of hepatitis E virus is very preliminary. A possible cytotoxic effect is supported by the presence of relatively fewer lymphocytes and more polymorphonuclear cells in portal infiltrates. However, studies of tissue from experimentally infected monkeys suggest an immunopathogenesis: Lymphocyte and monocyte infiltrates are found in areas of hepatocyte dropout, and direct contact can be seen between the lymphocytes and hepatocytes.

## Clinical Manifestations

The vast majority of cases of acute viral hepatitis are asymptomatic. Symptomatic hepatitis may be icteric or anicteric and is occasionally responsible for significant morbidity. Fulminant hepatitis is rare but often is fatal unless urgent liver transplantation is possible.

The symptoms associated with all viral hepatitides are very similar. In the early phase of illness, patients experience a flu-like prodrome. A low-grade fever and chills are common; occasionally temperatures reach 39–40°C. One of the most frequently reported symptoms is a loss of appetite, usually with a frank aversion to food. Cigarette smoke and other strong odors are often offensive. Vomiting is usually mild and self-limited, and diarrhea is often reported. Within several days patients notice dark urine, pale stool, and right upper quadrant abdominal pain. Jaundice is usually noted several days after the onset of dark urine. Some patients with acute viral hepatitis may have a transient rash, most commonly macular erythema. Rarely infants and young children with acute HBV develop a skin lesion termed *infantile papular acrodermatitis* (*Gianotti-Crosti syndrome*), a nonpruritic papular erythematous eruption of the face and extremities with lymph-adenopathy. Arthralgias occur in 10%–20% of patients with acute hepatitis. Rare neurologic symptoms include Guillain-Barre syndrome, meningitis, encephalitis, cranial nerve involvement, myelitis, polyneuritis, and mononeuritis. Patients with acute HBV may develop an illness similar to serum sickness, with urticaria and other rashes, polyarthritis, and rarely glomerulonephritis. Only one or two components of the illness may be present. Symptoms are due to immune complex deposition in the skin, joints, and glomeruli.

In most patients with acute viral hepatitis, the physical examination is normal with the exception of liver enlargement and right upper quadrant tenderness. A small liver on exam predicts a poor outcome; this finding is consistent with either fulminant hepatitis and extensive hepatic necrosis, or acute hepatitis superimposed on preexisting cirrhosis. The spleen may be palpable and may be particularly enlarged in cases of HDV. Spider angiomas and palmar erythema may be transiently present. Encephalopathy, ranging from mild confusion to obtundation and coma, is absent unless fulminant hepatitis develops.

## Clinical Variants

### Fulminant hepatitis

Rarely, patients with acute viral hepatitis develop fulminant hepatitis. Fulminant hepatitis is particularly increased in frequency in HDV superinfection of chronic HBV carriers and in acute HEV infection in pregnancy. Case fatality rates are listed in Table 62.1. Fulminant hepatitis is associated with massive or submassive hepatic necrosis, and patients typically present with encephalopathy, coagulopathy, jaundice, and renal failure. Progression to cerebral edema and death is not uncommon.

### Cholestatic hepatitis

Cholestatic viral hepatitis is characterized by a prolonged illness with persistent, profound jaundice and pruritus, and is most commonly seen with acute HAV infection. Often this variant of acute viral hepatitis is confused with extrahepatic biliary obstruction. Since the most common cause of extrahepatic biliary obstruction is choledocholithiasis, and since the latter generally does not result in bilirubin levels much above 10 mg/dl, viral hepatitis should be considered in patients with bilirubin levels higher than 10 to 15 mg/dl.

### Relapsing hepatitis A

Approximately 10% of patients in apparent remission from acute HAV infection have one or more exacerbations of disease with recrudescence of symptoms and aminotransferase elevations and reappearance in serum of IgM anti-HAV. During the relapse phase, symptoms tend to be similar to or milder than those experienced during the initial phase, although fulminant relapses have been reported. Some patients may develop symptoms consistent with autoantibody or immune complex formation. With respect to symptoms, the duration of remissions and relapses vary, ranging from 2 to 18 wk. Aminotransferases may remain elevated for as long as 12 mo. The pathogenesis of relapsing HAV is uncertain but may be due to either persistent infection (as evidenced by persistent excretion of HAV in stool) or an altered immune response to the infection.

## Laboratory Studies

Within several days of the onset of prodromal symptoms, serum aminotransferase levels become elevated. The alanine aminotransferase (ALT) is typically greater than the aspartate aminotransferase (AST). Peak aminotransferase levels usually range from 500 to 5000 U/l. Peak levels do not correlate well with the degree of hepatocellular injury or the etiologic agent. In icteric hepatitis, the serum bilirubin begins to rise several days following the elevation in AST and ALT and usually peaks in 10–14 d at 5–15 mg/dl. However, in patients with preexisting liver disease, peak levels may be significantly higher. Alkaline phosphatase is usually normal or only mildly elevated. Serum proteins are usually normal, but decreased albumin and increased $\gamma$-globulin may be seen in more severe cases. Hypoalbuminemia may also signify preexisting chronic liver disease. The prothrombin time (PT) is usually within 5 s of control but may be markedly prolonged in patients with more severe disease.

The hemoglobin and hematocrit are usually normal or only mildly decreased. Occasionally hemolytic anemia occurs, usually in association with glucose-6-phosphate dehydrogenase deficiency. Typical of acute viral hepatitis is a mild leukopenia and granulocytopenia with relative lymphocytosis. A leukocytosis greater than 12,000 is uncommon in nonfulminant hepatitis. Agranulocytosis, thrombocytopenia, pancytopenia, and aplastic anemia are rare. Urinalysis may reveal a few red blood cells and mild proteinuria. Frank renal failure is rare unless in association with fulminant hepatitis. Abdominal ultrasound typically reveals hepatomegaly and a thickened gallbladder wall. Occasionally EKG changes such as bradycardia, P-R prolongation, and T-wave depression are seen.

## Diagnosis

The diagnosis of acute viral hepatitis is usually made according to typical clinical features, laboratory tests, and the course of illness. Determining the specific agent requires serologic testing, as discussed below. A liver biopsy is generally unnecessary. Rarely, acute hypotension, heart failure, or shock can mimic acute viral hepatitis. However, these conditions are readily recognized and are associated with recovery of aminotransferase elevations in only a few days. Features differentiating acute viral hepatitis from drug-induced hepatitis or alcoholic liver disease are discussed below.

Serologic assays for the different hepatotropic viruses are listed in Table 62.3. On the initial evaluation of a patient with acute hepatitis, four serologic assays should be obtained: IgM antibody to HAV (anti-HAV), IgM antibody to HBV core antigen (anti-HBc), HBV surface antigen (HBsAg), and antibody to HCV (anti-HCV).

The diagnosis of hepatitis E should be sought in the appropriate clinical and epidemiologic setting. A more detailed discussion of the serologic diagnosis of viral hepatitis follows.

## Hepatitis A

The diagnosis of acute hepatitis A can be made in an individual with acute hepatitis who is positive for IgM anti-HAV. IgM anti-HAV persists in serum for 3 to 12 mo, making it also possible to retrospectively diagnosis acute hepatitis A in patients who present following the resolution of biochemical hepatitis. Rarely, a positive rheumatoid factor results in a false-positive IgM anti-HAV. IgM levels decline during the convalescent phase, at which time serum IgG levels increase. IgG anti-HAV persists for life, conferring immunity.

## Hepatitis B

The diagnosis of acute hepatitis B can be made in the presence of HBsAg and IgM anti-HBc. A positive HBsAg alone is inadequate to make the diagnosis of acute HBV as its presence may indicate chronic HBV infection with a superimposed acute hepatitis of another etiology. Furthermore, at the time of testing, HBsAg may not be detected in up to 10% of cases of acute HBV: The level may be below the sensitivity threshold of the assay, clearance of HBsAg may have already occurred (the patient is in the "window period"), or anti-HBs may have already appeared by the time the patient presents. However, IgM anti-HBc is present in virtually all cases of acute HBV. Anti-HBc is present at the onset of symptoms and persists for life, while IgM anti-HBc persists for only 3 to 12 mo. IgM may be present at low levels in patients with chronic infection and active viral replication, but levels are generally below the sensitivity threshold of the assay.

Patients who have persistent HBsAg 6 mo following the onset of hepatitis are considered to have developed chronic infection. Supplemental testing at this time should include tests for either HBeAg, a secreted product of the nucleocapsid gene of HBV, or HBV DNA. Both indicate active viral replication. Antibody to HBeAg (anti-HBe) should also be tested, as its presence predicts eventual resolution of infection.

**Table 62.3** Serologic diagnosis of viral hepatitis

| Serologic test | Significance |
|---|---|
| HAV | |
| IgM anti-HAV | Acute or recent infection |
| IgG anti-HAV | Past infection; immune to reinfection |
| HBV | |
| HBsAg | Acute or chronic infection |
| Anti-HBs | Resolved infection; immune to reinfection |
| IgM anti-HBc | Acute infection |
| IgG anti-HBc | Resolved infection or chronic infection |
| HBeAg/HBV DNA | Active viral replication |
| Anti-HBe | No viral replication; if HBsAg-positive, at risk for disease relapse/flare. |
| HCV | |
| Anti-HCV (EIA-2) | Recent acute infection, chronic infection, or false-positive test[a] |
| Anti-HCV (RIBA-2) | Confirms positive EIA-2[a] |
| HCV RNA | Acute or chronic infection |
| HDV | |
| Anti-HDV | Acute or chronic infection[b] |
| HEV | |
| Anti-HEV | Acute or chronic infection |

[a]May indicate resolved infection if HCV RNA is negative.

[b]May be only transiently positive in HDV/HBV coinfection.

## Hepatitis C

Currently available diagnostic assays for anti-HCV include a second-generation enzyme immunoassay assay (EIA-2) and a more specific confirmatory recombinant immunoblot assay (RIBA-2). Because the period of time between acquisition of HCV and the development of antibodies to HCV may be several weeks, the diagnosis of acute hepatitis C infection may require the demonstration of serum HCV RNA. The EIA-2 is positive in approximately 50% of patients on initial presentation with acute hepatitis C and in 90% of patients at some time during the acute illness, but it may take as long as 6 mo to become positive. Furthermore, anti-HCV may persist for years or a lifetime following exposure whether or not chronic hepatitis has developed. Finally, although methods for detecting IgM anti-HCV have been developed, these have not been consistently helpful in the diagnosis of acute infection. For these reasons, a patient with acute hepatitis who has negative serologies for HAV and HBV should be tested for HCV RNA, regardless of anti-HCV results. HCV RNA is present in serum within 1 to 2 wk of exposure—thus, as early as 10–12 wk before the rise in ALT or the onset of symptoms. HCV RNA determination by polymerase chain reaction is available in many clinical virology laboratories. The most sensitive assays detect less than 100 copies per ml of serum. A branched DNA quantitative assay for HCV RNA is now commercially available but is sensitive only to HCV RNA levels of at least $2.0 \times 10^5$ Eq/ml.

## Hepatitis D

The only commercially available serologic test for hepatitis D infection in the United States tests for antibody to HDV (anti-HD) and does not differentiate between IgM and IgG. The diagnosis of acute HDV/HBV coinfection relies on the presence of both anti-HD and IgM anti-HBc. Confirming HDV infection in this setting can be difficult because anti-HDV may be only transiently present or present in low titers. In addition, the assay is less sensitive for IgM, which may predominate early in coinfection. Thus, if HDV/HBV coinfection is suspected, one may need to repeat testing for anti-HDV over the ensuing weeks to confirm the diagnosis. The retrospective diagnosis of acute resolved HDV is also difficult, as IgG levels are detectable for only a short duration. The diagnosis of HDV superinfection is usually easier to make; anti-HDV appears early, reaches high titers, and persists for life. Since HDV competes with HBV for replication, markers of HBV replication (HBV DNA and HBeAg) may be absent. However, HBsAg and anti-HBc (IgG) will be positive. Assays for HDV antigen (HDAg) are commercially available in Europe. Their utility in detecting acute infection is limited, as serum HDAg is short-lived and may require repeated testing for detection. The assay is not helpful in persistent infection because HDAg often cannot be detected due to complex formation with anti-HD.

### Hepatitis E

HEV infection can be diagnosed using an enzyme-linked immunoassay for detecting antibody or polymerase chain reaction for detecting viral RNA. The ELISA can detect both IgM and IgG antibodies and has been useful in the diagnosis and monitoring of acute HEV infection. However, there are currently no commercially available assays for anti-HEV.

## Monitoring and Treatment

In the majority of cases, symptomatic acute viral hepatitis can be managed in the outpatient setting. Patients should be seen weekly, with monitoring of liver biochemistries, albumin, and prothrombin time. They should also be counseled to present immediately for any signs of increased bruising or bleeding or change in mental status. It is rare for vomiting to be severe or protracted. However, patients who are unable to maintain hydration with oral intake should be admitted to the hospital for intravenous hydration.

Patients with encephalopathy, however mild, have fulminant hepatitis by definition and are at significant risk for poor outcome. All such patients should be admitted for observation. Patients with grade II encephalopathy (confused, but awake or arousable) should be in the intensive care unit. These patients need to be closely monitored as hepatic encephalopathy can progress rapidly. Patients who develop grade III encephalopathy (unarousable) should be intubated for airway protection and considered for urgent liver transplantation. Those who progress to grade IV encephalopathy (coma) require intracranial pressure monitoring. Clinical signs suggesting the development of cerebral edema appear at intracranial pressures greater than 30 mmHg. Pressures above this level should be treated with intravenous boluses of 20% mannitol in doses of 0.5 to 1 g/kg. Barbiturate-induced coma may be utilized in cases where intracranial pressure cannot be otherwise controlled. In patients who progress to grade IV encephalopathy the prognosis is grave; these patients rarely survive without urgent liver transplantation and often die awaiting a donor liver.

## Prevention and Immunoprophylaxis

Discussions regarding the prevention of viral hepatitis often focus on passive and active immunoprophylaxis strategies (Table 62.4), yet the efficacy of these strategies in controlling the spread of viral hepatitis remains uncertain. Clearly pre-exposure prophylaxis for HAV is effective. However, it is still too early to assess the effect of population-based vaccination strategies for both HAV and HBV. Furthermore, postexposure immunoprophylaxis for either HAV or HBV appears to suppress clinical illness but often does not prevent transmission. Regardless, passive immunoprophylaxis is advised in most cases of known exposure to viral hepatitis, and currently available vaccines are recommended for certain high-risk groups.

**Table 62.4** Immunoprophylaxis of viral hepatitis

| Hepatitis | Pre-exposure | Postexposure |
|---|---|---|
| A | *Passive (for travelers to endemic areas not desiring vaccine)*: Immune globulin 0.02 ml/kg IM as a single dose for visits ≤3 mo; 0.06 ml/kg, repeated every 4–6 mo for visits >3 mo. *Active*: Adults—1440 ELISA units (EL.U.) IM (single dose); children 2–18 yr—720 EL.U. IM in 2 doses given 1 mo apart; booster given at 6 mo–12 mo[a] (Havrix, SmithKline Beecham) | *Passive*: Immune globulin 0.02 ml/kg IM as a single dose, no later than 2 wk after exposure[b] |
| B | *Active*: Age >19 yr—10 μg IM; age 11–19—5 μg IM; age <11—2.5 μg IM; repeat dose at 1 and 6 mo (Recombivax HB, Merck Sharp and Dohme)[c] | *Passive*: HBV-specific immune globulin (HBIG), given within a few hours to a few days of exposure[d] *Active*: As listed for pre-exposure[d] |
| C | *Active*: None available | *Passive*: None recommended |
| D | None available[e] | None available[e] |
| E | *Passive*: None available for travelers (immune globulin from developed countries lacks antibodies to HEV) | *Passive*: Immune globulin from endemic areas has no proven efficacy in sporadic or epidemic infection |

[a]Recommended for: (1) individuals travelling to or living in endemic areas (complete initial vaccination at least 2 wk prior to exposure); (2) populations that experience cyclic epidemics (native Alaskans and American Indians); (3) individuals at increased risk due to employment (caretakers for the developmentally disabled, employees of daycare facilities, laboratory workers who handle HAV, handlers of primates that may harbor HAV); (4) individuals with high-risk behavior (homosexual males with multiple partners and intravenous drug users); (5) individuals with chronic liver disease.

[b]Household contacts, contacts in day-care centers and custodial care institutions, and people exposed to a common vehicle; not recommended for school, work, and casual contacts; hygiene practices in hospitals should be adequate prophylaxis for medical personnel.

[c]Health care workers, hemodialysis staff and patients, recipients of high-risk blood products and multiple blood transfusions, injection drug users, homosexual men/others with multiple sexual partners, household and sexual contacts of HBsAg-positive individuals, populations with high endemicity, all infants and children.

[d]*Passive*: for sexual contacts of individuals with acute HBV, preferably within 2 wk of last exposure, and after needle-stick or permucosal exposure to blood/body fluids; *passive/active*: for neonates born to HBsAg-positive mothers (give HBIG within 12 h of birth).

[e]Immunization against HBV prevents superinfection and coinfection; HBIG in post-exposure prophylaxis prevents against coinfection only.

Recommendations for prophylaxis against viral hepatitis in the United States are listed in Table 62.4.

Preventive measures are of paramount importance in reducing the spread of viral hepatitis and warrant brief mention. The person-to-person spread of enterically transmitted viruses can be reduced with proper personal hygiene, and food-borne epidemics can be halted if the source of infection is identified. Although shellfish sanitation practices have improved in the United States, shellfish-associated hepatitis continues to be a problem due to illegal harvesting of bivalves from contaminated waters. The use of condoms is recommended for the prevention of sexually transmitted hepatitis.

The rate of transfusion-associated hepatitis has been reduced with blood donor screening for HBV and HCV. Instrument-associated hepatitis can be prevented by placing disposable sharp instruments in the appropriate receptacles and by sterilizing reusable equipment with heat inactivation or an appropriate disinfectant. Transmission of HCV in dialysis centers can be prevented by improving infection control practices. Although the transmission of HBV and HCV from health care worker to patient has been documented, cases are few and usually involve staff performing major invasive procedures. However, health care workers who have acute hepatitis, or in whom transmission of hepatitis to a patient has been documented, should be removed from direct patient care. The spread of infection from patients to health care workers can be prevented by regular hand washing and by exercising universal precautions with all blood, body fluids, and excreta.

## Chronic Hepatitis

### Definition and diagnosis

The clinical diagnosis of chronic viral hepatitis is made when abnormal liver biochemistries persist for at least 6 mo. In the case of HBV, the diagnosis is confirmed by the persistence of HBsAg, and active viral replication is indicated by the presence of HBeAg and HBV DNA. In chronic HDV superinfection of HBV, anti-HDV persists and evidence for HBV replication may disappear. Patients with chronic HCV infection typically remain anti-HCV-positive and HCV RNA-positive, although severely immunocompromised patients may not have detectable antibody. Some patients with chronic HCV may be intermittently viremic.

### Therapeutic strategies

Alpha-interferon has been the primary agent in the treatment of chronic HBV and is currently the only approved agent for this use. The standard dose is 5 million units subcutaneously daily for 4 mo. Overall, approximately 40% have a sustained response with loss of serum viral replication markers. Those more likely to respond to $\alpha$-interferon include women, those who acquired the infection in adulthood, and those who have an ALT level over 200 u/L and HBV DNA level less than 100 pg/ml.

Other agents that are currently being studied include famcyclovir and lamivudine. In two recently published trials, a 6-mo course of lamivudine effectively reduced serum HBV DNA to undetectable levels in over 90% of patients taking 100 mg or 300 mg daily. However, this response was sustained in fewer than 20% in both studies, and fewer than 10% seroconverted to anti-HBe during treatment or follow-up. Recently presented data suggest that longer duration therapy may result in higher seroconversion rates.

Three interferons are now FDA-approved for the treatment of chronic hepatitis C: interferon $\alpha$-2b, interferon $\alpha$-2a, and consensus interferon, a synthetic recombinant type I interferon derived by assigning the most frequently observed amino acid in each position of several $\alpha$-interferon subtypes to generate a consensus sequence. The approved dose of interferon $\alpha$ is 3 million units subcutaneously 3 times a week for 12–24 mo. In earlier studies using 6 months of therapy, normalization of ALT at the end of treatment was seen in 40% of patients and sustained response off therapy occurred in 15%–20%. More recent studies using virological endpoints report sustained response rates of only 10%–15% using a 6-mo course of treatment. Virological sustained response rates increase to 25% when treatment is extended to 12 mo. Ribavirin, a nucleoside analogue, is ineffective when used alone. However, preliminary data suggest that treatment with ribavirin in combination with interferon-$\alpha$ results in sustained virological response rates of 25%–35%. Patients who have complete viral clearance at the end of therapy and who relapse after discontinuation of treatment have an excellent chance of achieving a sustained response to retreatment with higher dose and longer term treatment or combination therapy with interferon and ribavirin. In contrast, nonresponders to initial therapy have very low response rates to retreatment.

Treatment of chronic HDV infection with $\alpha$-interferon has been disappointing. Although biochemical and virologic responses have been reported, sustained responses are rare.

## Differentiating Viral Hepatitis from Drug-Induced Hepatitis and Alcoholic Hepatitis

Differentiating among viral, alcoholic, and drug-induced hepatitides is often possible based on the history alone. Occasionally, however, a patient presents with hepatic encephalopathy or gives a history containing more than one possible risk factor. In this setting there are few features which help to distinguish among the possible etiologies. Drug hepatotoxicity and acute viral hepatitis are usually clinically, biochemically, and histologically indistinguishable from each other, but often can be differentiated from alcoholic hepatitis based on aminotransferase levels. In alcoholic hepatitis, AST and ALT are always <500 U/l, and usually <200 U/l, while aminotransferase elevations in symptomatic viral or drug-induced hepatitis are usually at least ten times normal. An AST:ALT ratio greater than 2:1 is very suggestive of alcoholic hepatitis but is only seen in 60% of cases. Typically the ALT is greater than the AST in acute viral hepatitis, although this is not a specific finding; in fulminant hepatitis the AST may be greater than the ALT. Cholestasis with hyperbilirubinemia can be profound in all three situations. Very rarely a liver biopsy is needed to clarify the etiology of acute hepatitis, although it is of limited value unless steroid therapy is being considered for the treatment of severe alcoholic hepatitis.

## Granulomatous Liver Disease

Patients with granulomatous liver disease generally present with asymptomatic abnormal liver biochemistries, although nonspecific symptoms such as fever, malaise, and anorexia may be present. Aminotransferases are often mildly elevated, while the alkaline phosphatase may be moderately to markedly abnormal.

**Table 62.5** Causes of granulomas on liver biopsy

| INFECTIOUS CAUSES | |
|---|---|
| *BACTERIA* | *SPIROCHETES—TREPONEMA* |
| Brucella | *VIRUSES* |
| Cat-scratch disease | Cytomegalovirus |
| Tularemia | Epstein-Barr virus |
| Listeria | HIV |
| Yersinia | Influenza B |
| Syphilis | Varicella |
| Whipple's disease | |
| *FUNGI* | NONINFECTIOUS CAUSES |
| Aspergillus | *CHEMICALS* |
| Blastomyces | *DRUGS* |
| Candida | *PRIMARY HEPATOBILIARY DISEASE* |
| Coccidiomyces | *SYSTEMIC INFLAMMATORY DISORDERS* |
| Cryptococcus | Crohn's disease |
| Histoplasma | Hepatic granulomatous disease (idiopathic) |
| *HELMINTHS* | Hypogammaglobulinemia |
| Ascaris | Immune complex disease |
| Clonorchis | Polymyalgia rheumatica |
| Schistosoma | Sarcoid |
| Strongyloides | Systemic lupus erythematosis |
| *PROTOZOA* | Wegener's granulomatosis |
| Amoeba | *NEOPLASM* |
| Leishmania | Hepatocellular carcinoma |
| Toxoplasma | Lymphoma (Hodgkin's and non-Hodgkin's) |
| *RICKETTSIA—Q FEVER* | Renal cell carcinoma |
| *SCHISTOSOMA* | *MISCELLANEOUS—BCG VACCINE* |

Frank jaundice develops in a small percentage of individuals. Granulomatous liver disease is a histologic diagnosis, and multiple etiologies exist. The most common causes are sarcoidosis, tuberculosis, shistosomiasis, and primary liver disease (particularly primary biliary cirrhosis), although in up to 10% the etiology remains uncertain. Other causes of hepatic granulomas are listed in Table 62.5. Many drugs can cause granulomatous liver injury, and a complete list is beyond the scope of this chapter. Drugs should always be suspected, even if a reported association cannot be found. Features suggesting drug toxicity include granulomas which are rich in eosinophils. Clinical evaluation should include careful geographic and drug histories, a chest X-ray, skin tests, serum antibodies, and a slit-lamp examination of the eyes (sarcoid). Liver histologic examination should include a microbiologic evaluation for fungal, mycobacterial, and viral etiologies. It may also be necessary to perform CT scanning and to evaluate other tissues to reach a definitive diagnosis.

## ANNOTATED BIBLIOGRAPHY


Alter MJ. Epidemiology of hepatitis C in the West. Semin Liver Dis 1995; 15:5–14.
*A thorough review of the prevalence and modes of transmission of HCV in western countries.*

Alter MJ, Mast EE. The epidemiology of viral hepatitis in the United States. Gastro Clin North Am 1994; 23:437–453.
*A review of hepatitis viruses A through E.*

Dienstag JL, Perrillo RP, Schiff ER, Bartholomew M, Vicary C, Rubin M. A preliminary trial of lamivudine for chronic hepatitis B infection. New Engl J Med 1995; 333:1657–1661.
*A double-blind, randomized trial of lamivudine in 32 patients with chronic HBV infection.*

Glikson M, Galun E, Oren R, Tur-Kaspa R, Shouval D. Relapsing hepatitis A. Review of 14 cases and literature survey. Medicine 1992; 71:14–23.
*The authors describe several cases of HAV recrudescence, review the clinical and biochemical features reported in the literature, and discuss theories regarding the pathogenesis.*

Gonzalez-Peralta R, Lau JYN. Pathogenesis of hepatocellular damage in chronic hepatitis C virus infection. Semin Gastrointest Dis 1995; 6:28–34.
*A detailed review of published data regarding the pathogenesis of HCV.*

Krawczynski K. Hepatitis E. Hepatology 1993; 17:932–941.
*A review of the epidmiological, clinical, and pathological features of HEV. Molecular virology is also detailed.*

Lok ASF, Gunaratnam NT. Diagnosis of hepatitis C. Hepatology 1997; 26 (Suppl. 1):48S–56S.
*A recent publication reviewing the clinical utility of diagnostic tests for HCV.*

National Institutes of Health Consensus Development Conference Panel Statement: Management of Hepatitis C. Hepatology 1997; 26 (Suppl. 1):2S 10S.
*A recently published statement reviewing the epidemiology, natural history, diagnosis, and management of hepatitis C infection. Recommendations to patients regarding transmission of the virus are also addressed, and areas for future research are identified.*

Nevens F, Main J, Honkoop P, Tyrrell DL, Barber J, Sullivan MT, Fevery J, De-Man RA, Thomas HC. Lamivudine therapy for chronic hepatitis B: a six-month randomized dose-ranging study. Gastroenterology 1997; 113:1258–1263.
*A recent study of lamivudine therapy in 51 patients with chronic HBV.*

Pappas SC. Fulminant viral hepatitis. Gastroenterol Clin North Am 1995; 24:161–173.
*A recent review of the diagnosis and management of fulminant hepatitis.*

Sjogren MH. Serologic diagnosis of viral hepatitis. Gastroenterol Clin North Am 1994; 23:457–477.
*A review of serologic tests for the diagnosis of hepatitis A through E.*

# 63

# Pyogenic Biliary Tract and Hepatic Infections

JAN V. HIRSCHMANN

The liver normally remains sterile, even though it is a major site for removing organisms from the systemic and portal circulations. Systemic bacteremia is a common, transient event that attends such daily activities as brushing the teeth; much less often it occurs as a complication of established infections. The incidence of asymptomatic portal bacteremia arising from the intestinal tract is unknown, but blood cultures from the portal vein at laparotomy for noninflammatory intraabdominal processes are sometimes positive. The liver's potent reticuloendothelial system ordinarily eliminates this hematogenous contamination without difficulty, but may fail because of hepatic damage, impaired phagocytosis, or persistent, intense bacteremia.

The biliary tract is also normally sterile, although the liver may excrete into the bile some of the organisms removed during bacteremic episodes. The other major potential entry site of microbes into the biliary ducts is from reflux of duodenal contents through the sphincter of Oddi. Several factors limit the frequency of such ascending contamination. In most normal hosts the duodenum is sterile or contains a sparse flora. Furthermore, the high pressure of the sphincter acts as a potent mechanical barrier to microbial migration, and the average daily excretion of 800 to 1000 ml of bile helps to flush out whatever organisms enter the biliary tract. Other protective mechanisms include the inhibitory effects of bile salts and secretory IgA on bacterial growth. When these various defenses falter, especially because of ductal obstruction, infection may occur.

## Acute Cholecystitis

### Etiology

The initiating event in acute cholecystitis is almost always cystic duct obstruction. In 90%–95% of cases the cause is a gallstone. When cholelithiasis is absent (acute acalculous cholecystitis), the occlusion is usually from inspissated bile, typically in patients with serious underlying surgical or medical disorders. In about half of patients with acute cholecystitis, bacteria, primarily gram-negative bacilli are found in the bile or gallbladder wall, but their presence is nearly always a secondary phenomenon rather than the cause of the inflammation. Only rarely does primary infection of the gallbladder occur; occasionally, *Salmonella typhi* has been implicated, and in patients with human immunodeficiency virus (HIV) infection, cryptosporidia, microsporidia, and cytomegalovirus are sometimes responsible.

### Epidemiology

In western countries gallstones occur in about 10% of the adult population, with a female:male ratio of about 2–3:1. Their frequency rises with age: in those over age 60 about 10%–15% of males are affected, compared to 20%–40% of females. During their lifetime, only about one-third of patients with gallstones will develop symptoms from them, at a rate of about 1% to 2% per year. Most of these episodes are self-limited bouts of biliary colic; about 10% or less are attacks of acute cholecystitis.

In western countries cholesterol is the principal constituent of about 85%–90% of gallstones. When biliary cholesterol secretion is increased or bile acids diminished, cholesterol crystals can precipitate and combine with thick gallbladder mucoproteins to form sludge, which is the probable matrix on which calculi develop. Increased risk for such stone formation occurs with advancing age, obesity, northern European or Native American ethnic origin, estrogen therapy, marked weight loss, disorders of the terminal ileum (such as Crohn's disease), prolonged fasting, leanness, primary biliary cirrhosis, and chronic cholestasis. Other potential factors leading to cholesterol stones are increased biliary proteins, lipoproteins, calcium, pH, and gallbladder stasis.

In Africa and Asia, the prevalence of cholelithiasis is low, and most calculi consist of pigment, not cholesterol. Black pigment stones, formed by bilirubin polymers and large amounts of mucin glycoproteins, develop in patients with cirrhosis or chronic hemolysis, especially from the thalassemias, where bilirubin excretion is increased. Brown pigment stones, calcium salts of unconjugated bilirubin combined with various amounts of protein and cholesterol, tend to form when biliary stasis and infection coexist.

### Pathogenesis

In patients with gallstones, biliary pain occurs when a stone occludes the cystic duct, causing a markedly increased pressure within the gallbladder lumen. Transient obstruction leads to biliary colic, a self-limited episode of abdominal discomfort that usually lasts for a few hours or less. When the obstruction is more protracted, acute cholecystitis may develop, probably because concentrated bile causes chemical irritation of the gallbladder wall, perhaps made more susceptible because distension has impaired blood flow to it. Bacteria are present in the bile or gallbladder wall of about 40%–65% of cases, but complicate rather than initiate the inflammation. The most common isolates are *Escherichia coli*, *Klebsiella pneumoniae*, *Enterobacter* sp., *Enterococcus* sp., and various streptococci. Anaerobes are present in a small minority; *Clostridium perfringens* is the most common, but *Bacteroides* sp. are rare. How the organisms arrive in the gallbladder, which is normally sterile, is uncertain. They could ascend from the duodenum through the sphincter of Oddi and travel up the common bile duct, entering the gallbladder through the cystic duct. Alternatively, they could traverse the gut, journey via the portal vein to the liver, and enter the bile, which is then excreted into the biliary system and stored in the gallbladder.

Unlike acute cholecystitis with gallstones, which most commonly occurs in middle-aged women, acalculous cholecystitis typically develops in those with serious medical or surgical disorders, especially older men (average age about 65), although the young may be afflicted as well. When the attack occurs, many patients have already been hospitalized, usually for several weeks, because of major trauma, burns, sepsis, or operative procedures, and have commonly received narcotics and no recent oral feedings. Outpatients who develop acute acalculous cholecystitis frequently have significant atherosclerotic vascular disease. The pathogenesis of acute acalculous cholecystitis is uncertain. The factors of narcotic use, lack of oral intake (which ordinarily stimulates gallbladder emptying), and impaired blood flow because of hypotension, volume depletion, or vascular disease may lead to gallbladder stasis and distension. The viscid bile within could cause cystic duct obstruction and provoke inflammation of an ischemic gallbladder wall, which may be easily irritated by the constituents of inspissated bile. It is also more prone to gangrene and perforation, which are much more frequent in this disorder than in acute cholecystitis associated with gallstones.

Indeed, all the major complications of acute cholecystitis are most common in the elderly, especially males with vascular disease. Empyema of the gallbladder, the presence of pus within its lumen, usually occurs in older patients who have had pain for several days, although the reason for the development of suppuration is unclear. Gangrene and perforation most commonly involve the fundus of the gallbladder, where the vascular supply is poorest. Factors causing impaired circulation to that region include low cardiac output due to cardiac disorders, diminished flow through visceral vessels narrowed by atherosclerotic disease, and compression of the gallbladder's intrinsic vasculature from increased intraluminal pressure and inflammatory edema of the gallbladder wall. Perforation may occur directly into the peritoneal cavity, causing peritonitis, or, more commonly, it is confined by adjacent structures, leading to a pericholecystic abscess.

Emphysematous cholecystitis is also a disorder of older males, often with diabetes mellitus, and many cases occur as a complication of acute acalculous cholecystitis. Bacteria present in the bile or gallbladder wall, especially *C. perfringens* or facultative gram-negative bacilli such as *E. coli*, form gas in the anaerobic conditions that prevail when severe tissue ischemia develops from vascular compromise. The gases produced, hydrogen and nitrogen, are poorly soluble, and radiographic techniques may detect them in the gallbladder lumen or wall.

## Clinical features

Many patients with acute cholecystitis associated with cholelithiasis, but few of those with the acalculous variety, have had previous episodes of biliary colic, presumably from transient cystic duct occlusion by gallstones. These attacks may develop after a large meal and are often accompanied by nausea and sweating. The pain can have a dramatic beginning, reaching maximal severity at its onset or shortly afterward; in others, the intensity gradually increases. Once it reaches its peak, the pain is nearly always constant, not fluctuating, and typically occurs in the epigastrium, less commonly the right upper quadrant, and rarely in the left upper quadrant, precordium, or lower abdomen. It may radiate to the area just below the right scapula, or, occasionally, to the right shoulder tip. The pain usually begins to subside gradually after a few minutes to a few hours.

Acute cholecystitis commonly begins with pain identical to that of biliary colic, but it persists longer and eventually shifts to the right upper quadrant. Fever may develop, but it is usually mild. Physical examination commonly reveals right upper quadrant tenderness and sometimes a visible or palpable mass. Murphy's sign, the abrupt cessation of inhalation during palpation of the right upper quadrant, may be evident as the examiner's hand encounters the descending, inflamed, and painful gallbladder.

In acute acalculous cholecystitis occurring in hospitalized patients, the presence of preceding abdominal pain from trauma or surgery, alterations in mentation, and difficulties in communication because of mechanical ventilation often make the clinical diagnosis difficult. Most patients have right upper quadrant pain or tenderness, but in some, abdominal discomfort is diffuse or absent. Fever usually occurs and is sometimes the only sign. Other findings may be unexplained abdominal distension, loss of bowel sounds, and sepsis of unknown origin. Clinical evaluation cannot usually distinguish emphysematous cholecystitis, empyema of the gallbladder, or gallbladder perforation from uncomplicated cases of acute cholecystitis.

## Laboratory studies

Leukocytosis with an increased number of immature neutrophils is common. The serum bilirubin and liver enzymes are often normal, but may be elevated, even without a concurrent common duct stone, probably because edema and inflammation of the gallbladder neck causes partial obstruction of the adjacent common hepatic or common bile duct. Positive blood cultures are quite unusual in patients with gallstones, although they may occur more frequently in acalculous cholecystitis.

A plain film of the abdomen is typically unhelpful but may demonstrate gallstones, about 15%–20% of which contain enough calcium to be radiopaque; gas in the gallbladder lumen or wall, indicating emphysematous cholecystitis; or stones outside the gallbladder, betokening perforation.

## Diagnosis

Ultrasound examination of the abdomen is very sensitive and specific for gallstones, which are detectable as echogenic spots producing a shadow. Features suggesting acute cholecystitis include a thickened gallbladder wall, intramural gas, a pericholecystic fluid collection, and the exacerbation of pain when the examiner presses the transducer over the gallbladder ("sonographic Murphy's sign").

Intravenous technetium-99m bound to an iminodiacetic acid (such as hepatic iminodiacetic acid or diisopropyl iminodiacetic acid) is ordinarily excreted into the bile ducts and enters the gallbladder. Failure of the radionuclide to visualize the gallbladder suggests cystic duct obstruction; this technique has a sensitivity and specificity of about 95% in detecting acute cholecystitis, including the acalculous form, in patients examined for upper abdominal pain.

## Treatment

Although most episodes of acute cholecystitis resolve spontaneously, especially in younger patients, recurrence is common, and in the elderly, complications are frequent and sometimes fatal. Prompt surgery, therefore, is appropriate for most patients. The traditional technique has been open cholecystectomy, but a laparoscopic approach results in less pain, a shorter hospitalization, and a more rapid return to normal activities. About 30% of attempted laparoscopic cholecystectomies for acute cholecystitis, however, require conversion to an open procedure, most commonly because extensive inflammation or adhesions make dissection difficult and hazardous.

In patients considered too ill to undergo general anesthesia and abdominal surgery, cholecystostomy—tube drainage of the gallbladder—is an alternative. Options include radiographically guided transhepatic insertion of a catheter into the gallbladder or placement of a tube through a small abdominal incision performed under local anesthesia. For patients with acalculous cholecystitis, this treatment may suffice, since recurrence is rare, but in those with cholelithiasis, subsequent cholecystectomy may be necessary.

Clinicians commonly administer antibiotics for acute cholecystitis, but these agents have little effect on reducing or eliminating bacteria in infected gallbladders, in part because they do not enter an obstructed gallbladder in appreciable quantities. This failure of antibiotics to reach the site of infection explains why controlled trials have shown that agents that achieve high concentrations in the bile in *unobstructed* biliary tracts are no better in the treatment or prevention of infectious complications of acute cholecystitis than those that attain lower levels. The potential benefit of antibiotics, thus, is not to eradicate organisms present in the gallbladder but to control extraluminal extension of infection, such as bacteremia and intraperitoneal suppuration. Many studies have shown that antibiotics given prior to cholecystectomy also reduce the incidence of postoperative wound infections, which usually occur from the bacteria present in the bile. Unless an infectious complication, such as peritonitis or an abscess, is present at surgery, however, postoperative antimicrobial therapy is unnecessary. The antibiotics chosen should be active against enteric gram-negative bacilli, such as *E. coli* and *Klebsiella* sp. Whether their spectrum should include coverage for *Enterococcus* sp. and anaerobes is debated, but regimens without such activity are usually satisfactory. A reasonable approach is a first-generation cephalosporin, such as cefazolin, for most patients. In those who are critically ill or develop acute cholecystitis during hospitalization, an aminoglycoside, such as gentamicin or tobramycin, combined with ampicillin or mezlocillin represents one of many rational choices. Another effective regimen for severe disease is mezlocillin or piperacillin alone.

The mortality rate for surgical therapy of uncomplicated acute cholecystitis is about 2%. It is much higher for acute acalculous cholecystitis (10%–30%), perforation (15%), gallbladder empyema (15%–25%), and emphysematous cholecystitis (15%).

## Acute Cholangitis

### Etiology

Acute cholangitis usually occurs from bile duct occlusion complicated by infection and is apparently more frequent when the obstruction is partial rather than complete. The most common underlying cause is a gallstone that has migrated from the gallbladder. Other frequent sources of the biliary tract obstruction are benign bile duct stricture; extrinsic compression from pancreatitis, paraductal lymph node enlargement, or a cystic duct gallstone; and malignancies of the bile duct, gallbladder, ampulla of Vater, pancreas, or duodenum. Some cases occur as complications of diagnostic studies, such as transhepatic or endoscopic retrograde cholangiography, or following therapeutic procedures, such as stent placements to relieve biliary obstructions.

### Epidemiology

The average age of patients with acute cholangitis is about 60, reflecting the common time in life for cholelithiasis, malignancies, and biliary tract strictures. The risk factors for gallstones are the same as for acute cholecystitis; about 15% of patients with gallbladder stones have common duct stones, which often cause no symptoms for years, if at all. About 95% of those with calculi in the common duct have concurrent ones in the gallbladder, whence they presumably originate. Occasionally, stones, usually the brown pigment variety, *form* in the common duct, typically in the presence of chronic biliary tract obstruction and bacterial colonization with enteric organisms. This process is especially characteristic of the disorder known as recurrent pyogenic cholangitis, which occurs in China, Southeast Asia, and the Philippines. The cause is unclear, but parasitic infestation of the biles ducts with *Clonorchis sinensis* or *Ascaris lumbricoides* may lead to strictures, chronic biliary stasis, and bacterial colonization.

In patients with a biliary stent or drainage catheter, acute cholangitis tends to develop a few weeks after placement and is usually associated with obstruction of the device.

### Pathogenesis

In the absence of acute cholangitis, 75%–90% of bile cultures are positive in patients with common duct stones, where biliary tract obstruction is usually incomplete, compared to 25%–50% in those where it is total, which is most frequent with malignancies. The most common organisms are *E. coli*, *Klebsiella pneumoniae*, and enterococci. As in acute cholecystitis, the route by which these bacteria reach the biliary tract is unclear. Portal vein bacteremia, removal of the organisms by the liver, and excretion of them into the bile is one possibility. Ordinarily, these bacteria would pass into the duodenum, but with biliary tract obstruction the organisms could proliferate and cause inflammation. An alternative mechanism is reflux of duodenal contents into the common bile duct with migration proximal to the site of occlusion, bacterial multiplication, and inflammation of the bile ducts.

The pressure in the biliary tract is normally about 70 to 160 mm of water. With obstruction, it may exceed 200, frequently causing the bacteria present to reflux into the hepatic veins and perihepatic lymphatics, eventuating in systemic bacteremia.

### Clinical manifestations

Fever is present in almost all patients with acute cholangitis; chills and jaundice occur in about two-thirds. Abdominal pain, nearly always in the right upper quadrant, is present in about 40%–80%. In 1877 Charcot delineated a triad of clinical features indicative of acute cholangitis: fever, jaundice, and right upper quadrant pain. This combination exists in about 20% of cases. Nausea and vomiting occur in about 50%. On physical examination fever is usually greater than 38.5°C, jaundice is commonly evident, and mild right upper quadrant tenderness is present in about two-thirds of patients. Severe or generalized abdominal tenderness, marked peritoneal signs, or absent bowel sounds should suggest another diagnosis. Significant hypotension, indicative of septic shock, occurs in about 5%. In many patients, especially the elderly, unexplained fever may be the only clinical manifestation of acute cholangitis.

### Laboratory studies

Leukocytosis, often with an increase in immature forms, occurs in about 80% of patients; a few have leukopenia in response to severe sepsis. The serum bilirubin is elevated in over 90% of cases, as are the alkaline phosphatase and $\gamma$-glutamyltransferase. The transaminases are increased in about 70%–80%, usually to levels less than occur in viral hepatitis. The serum amylase is high in about 30%–40% of patients with cholangitis, but this finding does not necessarily indicate accompanying pancreatitis.

About 20%–40% of patients have positive blood cultures, usually with a single organism. The most common bacteria present are *E. coli* (about 50% of cases), *Klebsiella* sp. (10%), *Enterococcus* sp. (10%), *Proteus* sp. (5%), and *Enterobacter* sp (5%). *Pseudomonas* sp. are isolated in about 10%, usually those with nosocomial infections, especially associated with biliary tract manipulations, such as endoscopic retrograde cholangiography. Anaerobes are present in less than 5%. This same range of organisms is present in bile cultures, which are positive in nearly all patients with acute cholangitis, but grow more than one organism in about 50% of cases.

### Diagnosis

In over 90% of cases, abdominal ultrasound or CT will demonstrate dilatation of the proximal obstructed bile duct to a diameter greater than 1.5 cm. CT usually provides greater anatomic information when a pancreatic mass causes the obstruction. More definitive detail of the biliary tract requires cholangiography, which may be performed by transhepatic cannulation of a dilated duct or via an endoscopic retrograde approach through the ampulla of Vater.

### Treatment

With intravenous fluids and antimicrobial therapy, about 85% of patients will improve, usually within 24 h. Many antibiotic regimens are reasonable, none clearly superior. An aminoglycoside, such as gentamicin or tobramycin, combined with ampicillin is a good choice. Controlled trials have also demonstrated equivalent efficacy for mezlocillin or piperacillin alone. Coverage for anaerobes such as *Bacteroides fragilis* with the addition of an agent like metronidazole or clindamycin is usually unnecessary, but it may be prudent with severely ill patients and those with biliary stents or previous biliary tract surgery, especially biliary-enteric bypass procedures. Careful clinical studies have not convincingly demonstrated that agents that achieve very high biliary levels in the *absence* of obstruction, like cefoperazone, are superior in the treatment of acute cholangitis to those that attain considerably lower levels such a combined aminoglycoside-ampicillin regimen.

In patients with severe or worsening infection, emergency biliary decompression is necessary, usually via transhepatic or endoscopic retrograde catheter drainage. Endoscopic sphincterotomy with removal or fragmentation of stones is typically successful in common duct obstruction from cholelithiasis. In refractory cases, malignant causes, or other difficult circumstances, temporary drainage via a nasobiliary catheter is typically satisfactory. Transhepatic drainage with external catheters or stents placed by an endoscopic or transhepatic approach are other nonsurgical options. Emergent operative treatment is usually reserved for those who fail these procedures.

Once the acute episode has resolved, some patients require elective surgery, including cholecystectomy, choledochotomy, sphincteroplasty, major resection of obstructing lesions, or biliary-enteric bypass procedures.

Most patients with acute cholangitis complicating a biliary stent or biliary drainage catheters will respond to antibiotic therapy. Many will require replacement of the device because of malfunction, usually from obstruction.

The mortality rate from acute cholangitis is about 5%, the major complications being septic shock, acute renal failure, and hepatic abscesses.

## Hepatic Abscess

### Etiology

Hepatic abscesses may be bacterial (pyogenic), amebic, or fungal. Pyogenic abscesses may occur as complications of: (*1*) biliary tract obstruction and cholangitis from stones, strictures, or malignant diseases; (*2*) portal vein bacteremia arising from intraabdominal processes such as diverticulitis, perforated viscera (complicating such diseases as colonic carcinoma), appendicitis, and pancreatic abscesses; (*3*) systemic bacteremia from such disorders as infective endocarditis or pulmonary suppuration; (*4*) spread of infection from a contiguous site such as a subphrenic abscess; (*5*) penetrating or blunt hepatic trauma. Some bacterial hepatic abscesses are cryptogenic—that is, no predisposing factor is apparent (Fig. 63.1). Amebic liver abscesses are complications of intestinal infection with *Entamoeba histolytica*. Fungal abscesses are usually caused by *Candida* sp., most frequently *C. albicans*, but others, especially *C. tropicalis*, may also be responsible.

### Epidemiology

Pyogenic liver abscesses can occur at any age, but the average is about 60, reflecting the time of life when the major underlying diseases (cholelithiasis, biliary and pancreatic malignancies, diverticulitis, and colonic carcinomas) are most common. Males outnumber females in a ratio of about 1.5–2.0:1. Amebic abscesses typically occur in young adults, with about 90% being males. In the United States and many other industrialized nations, most people with amebic abscesses are immigrants from countries where amebiasis is endemic. Hepatic candidiasis occurs almost exclusively in patients with cancer, usually leukemia, who have had prolonged neutropenia and extended antibiotic therapy. Many have also recently received systemic corticosteroids. In this infection males and females are equally affected.

### Pathogenesis

About 70% of pyogenic liver abscesses are in the right lobe, partly because it is larger than the left lobe and partly because vascular factors favor flow to it. Whether these abscesses are solitary (approximately 60% of cases) or multiple depends primarily upon the underlying cause. In those complicating biliary tract obstruction, the process usually involves all intrahepatic ducts, and several abscesses in both lobes of the liver are common. The responsible organisms are typically the facultative gram-negative bacilli, such as *E. coli*, that cause cholangitis.

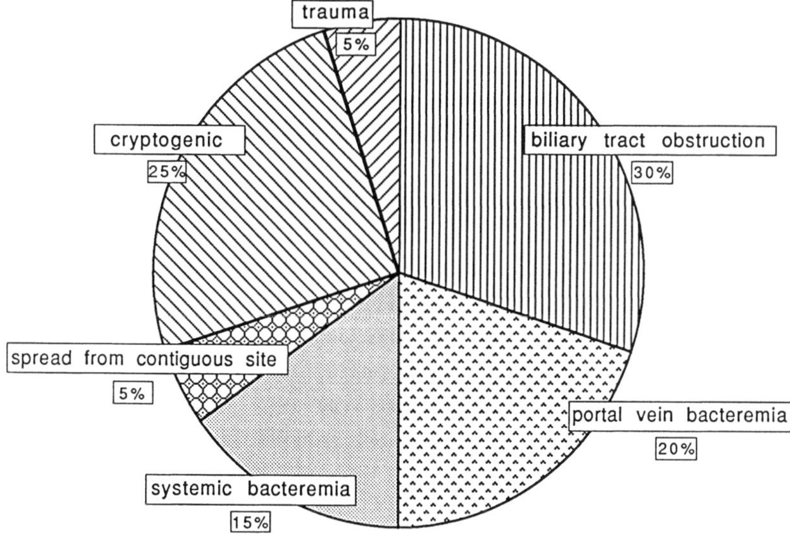


**Fig. 63.1** This diagram illustrates the approximate distribution of identifiable sources of pyogenic hepatic abscesses.

When portal bacteremia arising from intraabdominal infections causes abscesses, they are usually solitary lesions. A preceding event in many patients may be suppurative thrombophlebitis of the portal vein or one of its branches (pylephlebitis), which may cause areas of hepatic ischemia because of thrombosis of the vein or emboli from the infected clot. The bacteria causing this type of liver abscess are the bowel flora, including facultative gram-negative rods and anaerobes, both cocci and bacilli. Areas of hepatic ischemia may also occur with endocarditis, when septic emboli from the infected cardiac valve enter the hepatic artery, occlude vessels, and cause focal areas of liver damage. In systemic bacteremia without endocarditis the frequency, duration, or intensity of the bacteremia may overwhelm the liver's defenses. In these cases, the abscesses are commonly multiple and small, and the usual organisms are facultative or aerobic gram-positive cocci such as streptococci and staphylococci. In pyogenic abscesses arising from a contiguous focus of infection, the suppurative process probably invades the liver capsule and lodges in the adjacent parenchyma. A similar event occurs with penetrating trauma, which directly introduces organisms into the liver tissue. With blunt trauma, however, hemorrhage can occur in the liver parenchyma, and subsequent bacteremia may later cause infection in the damaged area. The frequent presence of enteric gram-negative bacilli in these abscesses suggests that the mechanism is more often portal, than systemic, bacteremia.

Amebic abscesses usually develop in previously asymptomatic intestinal carriers of *E. histolytica*. The organisms presumably travel via the portal vein to the liver, where they may produce focal necrosis and a relatively anaerobic environment that allows the parasites to proliferate. The young age of most of the patients may indicate recent acquisition of the protozoon and an inadequate immune response to prevent extraintestinal infection. The marked male predominance remains unexplained.

Candidal hepatic abscesses probably occur because the patients have white cells that are insufficient in number or function to ward off yeasts that reach the liver via the portal vein from the intestines, where they proliferate because protracted antibiotic therapy has markedly reduced the normal bacterial flora, allowing overgrowth of the resident fungi. Although the organisms invade the liver and produce symptoms of infection during the period of neutropenia, actual abscess formation occurs only when the granulocyte number returns to normal.

Hepatic abscess formation by catalase-positive bacteria (*S. aureus*, enteric gram-negative bacilli) or fungi (especially, *Candida* sp.) is a complication of chronic granulomatous disease or neutrophil myeloperoxidase deficiency. In both circumstances, oxidative killing mechanisms of neutrophils are impaired (see Chapter 11).

## Clinical manifestations

Whether the abscesses are pyogenic, amebic, or fungal, the clinical manifestations are similar. The duration of symptoms before the patient seeks medical attention may be a few days, when the onset is dramatic, or several weeks, when the manifestations are more muted. About 90% of patients have fever, and most have abdominal pain, usually localized to the right upper quadrant. Anorexia, nausea, vomiting, and weight loss are common. In an occasional patient, pleuritic chest pain, cough, dyspnea, or referred right shoulder pain is prominent because inflammation has spread to involve the diaphragm or pleura. Right upper quadrant tenderness is present in most patients. Jaundice is uncommon and usually reflects an underlying biliary tract obstruction rather than hepatic inflammation from the abscess. The chest examination may reveal dullness to percussion, decreased breath sounds, or crackles over the right lower lung field because of a raised right hemidiaphragm, pleural effusion, atelectasis, or pneumonia.

## Laboratory studies

Routine laboratory tests do not discriminate amebic from pyogenic abscesses. In both, leukocytosis and a raised alkaline phosphatase are present in about 80%, anemia in about 50%–60%, and elevated transaminases in about 60%. Hyperbilirubinemia occurs in less than 25% of cases. In hepatic candidiasis the neutrophil count is normal in most, but increased in some; the alkaline phosphatase is elevated in about 60; and the transaminases are high in about 15%.

In approximately 40% of patients with pyogenic or amebic abscesses the chest radiograph is abnormal, demonstrating changes in the right hemithorax, including lower lobe atelectasis or pneumonia, an elevated hemidiaphragm, or a pleural effusion.

## Diagnosis

An abdominal ultrasound examination is an excellent initial imaging technique for suspected hepatic abscesses, for it identifies the vast majority of patients with these infections, reliably differentiates solid from liquid masses, and demonstrates biliary tract obstruction. An alternative is abdominal CT, which may be somewhat more sensitive and can more accurately detect extrabiliary intraabdominal infections, such as diverticulitis, appendicitis, and pancreatic abscesses (Fig. 63.2). Both CT and ultrasound can identify pylephlebitis (thrombosis of the portal vein or its tributaries), which may be present in patients with hepatic abscesses originating from an intraabdominal suppurative focus. With hepatic candidiasis both imaging techniques are usually negative until the neutropenia has resolved and abscess formation has occurred.

In about 50% of patients with pyogenic abscesses, blood cultures are positive, usually with a single organism, which is most commonly *E. coli* or a streptococcus. *Streptococcus milleri* has a particular tendency to cause hepatic abscesses, which should be suspected in cases of bacteremia due to this organism. Cultures of abscess pus yield one organism in about 40% of patients, while 60% are polymicrobial. About 50%–70% grow facultative or aerobic gram-negative bacilli such as *E. coli*, *Klebsiella* sp., *Proteus* sp., or *Enterobacter* sp.; 25% have facultative gram-positive cocci such as *Enterococcus* sp., streptococci, or *Staphylococcus aureus*; and 40%–50% yield anaerobes such as *Fusobacterium nucleatum*, *Bacteroides* sp., and gram-positive cocci.

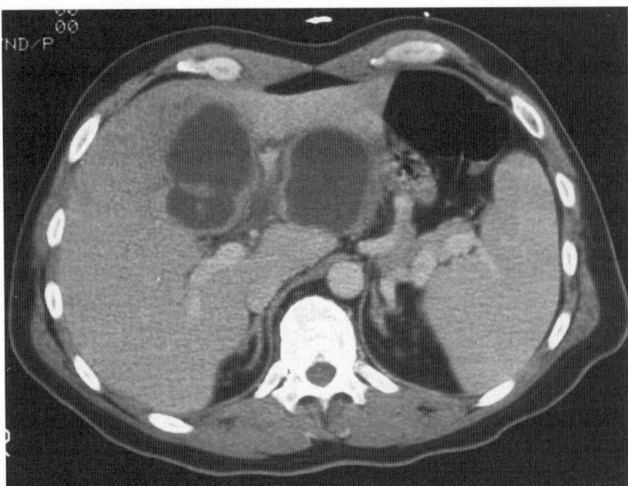

**Fig. 63.2** An abdominal CT scan demonstrates two large hepatic abscesses, one in each lobe of the liver. The infections occurred as a complication of a perforated colonic carcinoma.

In patients with amebic abscesses, stool examination demonstrates *E. histolytica* in only about 10%–15%, and, although fluid aspirated from the liver may have the characteristic anchovy paste appearance, the organism is usually not detectable there, either. The most helpful diagnostic technique is an amebic serologic test, such as indirect hemagglutination, counterimmunoelectrophoresis, ELISA, or agar gel diffusion. These studies are positive in about 95% of patients with amebic liver abscesses but may be negative early in the course of disease and should be repeated 5 to 7 d later in suspicious cases. They are reliable even in endemic areas because they are not positive in those with asymptomatic intestinal carriage of the parasite, but only in patients with invasive disease. The indirect hemagglutination serology, however, may remain positive for years; in patients with a history of previous invasive amebiasis, the other tests, which revert to negative 6 to 12 mo after treatment, are more helpful in evaluating the presence of active disease.

In hepatic candidiasis, blood cultures grow the organism in only a small number of patients. Definitive diagnosis usually requires a liver biopsy, which can reveal the fungus on culture or histologic examination.

## Treatment

For pyogenic abscesses, if the responsible organisms are unknown, a reasonable regimen is an aminoglycoside combined with clindamycin. Some patients are cured with antimicrobials alone, usually with treatment of 4–6 wk, but most seem to require drainage. One option, especially for small, solitary abscesses, is a single percutaneous needle aspiration; for many, this approach suffices, but others need repeated aspirations or another technique. The most successful has been percutaneous drainage with a catheter inserted under ultrasonic or CT guidance and left in place until the cavity has closed, which usually requires about 2 wk. Several catheters are necessary when multiple abscesses are present. Absolute contraindications to percutaneous catheter drainage are a severe bleeding disorder or a location that does not allow a safe approach. With successful drainage, antibiotics have usually been given for about 2 wk. Surgery now is usually reserved for patients who have failed catheter drainage or who have underlying conditions that themselves require operative intervention, such as resectable malignancies. The mortality rate for pyogenic liver abscesses is about 10%–20%.

Amebic abscesses usually respond to antimicrobial therapy alone. Metronidazole, given as 750 mg every 8 h by mouth or intravenously for those unable to take oral medication, is the drug of choice. Most patients respond quickly, and the recommended duration of therapy is 10 d. For those without improvement after 3–4 d an alternative treatment is dehydroemetine 1.0–1.5 mg/kg IM (maximum 90 mg) every day for 5 days and chloroquine 600 mg orally the first day followed by 300 mg on subsequent days for 2–3 weeks. Needle aspiration is appropriate if the abscess fails to improve, if the diagnosis is uncertain, or if there is suspected secondary bacterial infection (a rare complication). The mortality rate is less than 5%.

The treatment for hepatic candidiasis is amphotericin B with or without flucyosine. In those who fail or cannot tolerate this program, an alternate therapy is oral or intravenous fluconazole. The mortality rate for patients with this disorder is about 50%, although in some, death is from their underlying disease, rather than the infection.

## ANNOTATED BIBLIOGRAPHY


### Acute Cholangitis

Sinanan MN. Acute cholangitis. Infect Clin North Am 1992; 6:571–599.
*An excellent and thorough review of cholangitis with an extensive bibliography that includes all the major papers.*

### Acute Cholecystitis

Babb RR. Acute acalculous cholecystitis. A review. J Clin Gastroenterol 1992; 15:238–241.
*A succinct review, a bit sparse on details, but with an extensive bibliography.*

Zucker KA, Flowers JL, Bailey RW, Graham SM, Buell J, Imbembo AL. Laparoscopic management of acute cholecystitis. Am J Surg 1993; 165:508–514.
*A clinical series of 83 patients undergoing laparoscopic cholecystectomy for acute cholecystitis. This procedure seems safe and effective, so long as the threshold for conversion to an open procedure is low when problems occur.*

### General

Johnston DE, Kaplan MM. Pathogenesis and treatment of gallstones. N Engl J Med 1993; 328:412–421.
*A comprehensive overview of cholelithiasis that is especially good on the pathogenesis and epidemiology of gallstones, including the risks of complications in those with them.*

Sung JY, Costerton JW, Shaffer EA. Defense system in the biliary tract against bacterial infection. Dig Dis Sci 1992; 37:689–696.
*A review of the defense mechanisms that keep the liver and biliary tract normally sterile despite episodes of bacteremia from the systemic and portal circulations and reflux of duodenal contents into the bile ducts.*

### Liver Abscess

Barnes PF, De Cock KM, Reynolds TN, Ralls PW. A comparison of amebic and pyogenic abscesses of the liver. Medicine 1987; 66:472–483.
*A series from Los Angeles County–University of Southern California Medical Center. Most patients with amebic liver abscesses were young Hispanic males, while those with pyogenic abscesses were older and of various ethnic backgrounds. In amebic abscesses the symptoms were more often acute and localized to the right upper quadrant, while they were more chronic and nonspecific in pyogenic abscesses. The clinical features overlapped substantially, however, and the epidemiologic factors were more predictive. Amebic serology was very helpful in diagnosing amebic abscesses, being positive in 94% of cases.*

Frey CF, Zhu Y, Suzuki M, Isaji S: Liver abscesses. Surg Clin North Am 1989; 69:259–271.
*A review of both pyogenic and amebic liver abscesses that provides a good summary of the relevant literature.*

Li E, Stanley SL. Protozoa. Amebiasis. Gastroenterol Clin N Am 1996; 25:471–492.
*A thorough review of the intestinal and hepatic manifestations of infection with Entamoeba histolytica.*

Stain SC, Yellin AE, Donovan AJ, Brien HW. Pyogenic liver abscess. Modern treatment. Arch Surg 1991; 126:991–996.
*A clinical series of 54 patients treated at Los Angeles County–University of Southern California Medical Center from 1984 to 1990. All received antibiotics, and for some that therapy alone was satisfactory. Many were successfully treated with aspiration alone; others received percutaneous catheter drainage. Only 15% underwent operative drainage.*

Thaler M, Pastakia B, Shawker TH, O'Leary T, Pizzo PA. Hepatic candidiasis in cancer patients: the evolving picture of the syndrome. Ann Intern Med 1988; 108:88–100.
*A review of cases from the National Cancer Institute as well as previously published reports. This paper emphasizes the importance of liver biopsy in establishing the diagnosis.*

# 64

# Infectious Complications of Pancreatitis

E. PATCHEN DELLINGER

Acute pancreatitis frequently presents a diagnostic dilemma to the treating physician. The underlying pathophysiology of the disease is not infectious, but involves the activation of pancreatic enzymes in and around the pancreas itself with secondary inflammation and tissue destruction. The precise pathophysiological mechanisms underlying this inappropriate enzyme activation are not known; however, the clinical settings in which it occurs are well documented. The most common causes of pancreatitis in the United States are gallstone disease, presumably with passage of a common bile duct stone, and alcoholism. Other less frequent causes include severe hypertriglyceridemia, and medications, while a significant minority of cases are traumatic or idiopathic. The incidence of infectious complications of pancreatitis varies with the manner in which the patients are identified, but in general fewer than 5% of all patients with the diagnosis of pancreatitis develop a specific infectious complication. The risk of infection increases with the severity of the disease, and 15% to 40% of patients with "severe" pancreatitis may become infected. Since the manifestations of acute pancreatitis often include fever and leukocytosis it becomes important to distinguish sterile inflammation from complicating infection.

## Diagnosis of Pancreatitis

The initial management of a patient with acute pancreatitis should be directed toward confirming the diagnosis and beginning initial supportive treatment. The diagnosis of pancreatitis is supported by a clinical picture of abdominal pain and tenderness associated with an elevated serum amylase and lipase level. While occasional cases of pancreatitis have been reported without elevation of amylase, this is not common. Amylase levels do return to normal more quickly than lipase levels, so if lab tests are being obtained some time after the onset of the acute illness, lipase may be a more sensitive indicator. A mild case of pancreatitis may exhibit no more than mild abdominal pain and tenderness with an elevated serum level of amylase and lipase. In severe cases a patient may present with hypovolemic shock secondary to massive fluid sequestration in the area of retroperitoneal inflammation, and can rapidly manifest hemorrhage, hypoxemia, renal failure, and a variety of metabolic abnormalities that progress to multiple organ failure and death.

Mild cases demonstrate no changes on computerized tomography (CT) of the pancreas, while moderate and severe cases show increasing degrees of pancreatic swelling and edema with peripancreatic edema and fluid collections. The differential diagnosis of pancreatitis includes a perforated viscus with release of amylase-rich fluids into the peritoneal cavity and resulting elevation of serum amylase levels. The distinction is important because bowel perforation requires immediate operative intervention while pancreatitis rarely benefits from early operation, and most cases of pancreatitis need no operation at all. Early diagnostic efforts should attempt to identify the etiology of pancreatitis. In a patient who has not had a prior cholecystectomy, an ultrasound exam is the most sensitive and specific method of determining the presence of gallstones. Pancreatitis caused by gallstones should be followed by a cholecystectomy after the patient is stable, during the same hospitalization or shortly thereafter in most cases.

Traditionally, the severity of an episode of acute pancreatitis has been graded using a set of indicators determined during the first 48 h of the illness. These are called Ranson's prognostic indicators after the author of the paper (in 1974) describing them (Table 64.1). Patients with one or two of Ranson's criteria after 48 h have a mortality risk of less than 1%; those with three or four criteria, a mortality risk of 15%; and those with six or seven criteria, a 100% mortality. More recently the Acute Physiology and Chronic Health Evaluation (APACHE) II grading system, originally developed to estimate mortality in patients admitted to intensive care units, has been applied to patients with acute pancreatitis. This grading system is used and has been authenticated in a wide variety of illnesses including intraabdominal infection and can be applied immediately at the time of patient admission rather than waiting 48 h.

A diagnostic difficulty with these patients arises because the initial presentation of pancreatitis shares many elements with an acute infection. Pancreatitis causes retroperitoneal inflammation, and this stimulates an elevated white blood cell count, temperature, and pulse rate in many cases, even in the absence of any bacterial contamination. Mild to moderate cases of pancreatitis result in an infectious complication in fewer than 2% of cases, and patients with mild pancreatitis certainly do not need any antimicrobial treatment. The incidence of infectious complications rises as the severity of the disease increases. A patient with a mild case of pancreatitis can present with abdominal pain and elevated serum amylase but little or no alteration of vital signs. On the other hand, a very severe case of necrotizing pancreatitis with massive retroperitoneal peripancreatic and pancreatic necrosis may present with cardiovascular collapse, including tachycardia, hypotension, oliguria, and respiratory failure progressing rapidly to renal failure, cardiac failure, and death. While the clinical picture in these severe cases resembles that of sepsis and certainly does involve systemic cytokine release ("SIRS," see Chapter 50), bacteria are rarely involved during the first week. In one study of severe pancreatitis complicated by infected necrosis or abscess the average time of diagnosis for infected necrosis was 2 wk after the onset of disease, and for abscess, 5 wk. Rarely, infected necrosis has been diagnosed as early as 4 d.

**Table 64.1** Ranson's prognostic criteria*

| |
|---|
| PANCREATITIS NOT DUE TO GALLSTONES ON ADMISSION |
| Age > 55 yr |
| White blood cell count > 16,000/mm$^3$ |
| Glucose > 200 mg/dl |
| Lactic dehydrogenase > 350 U/l |
| Aspartate aminotransferase > 250 U/l |
| Within 48 h of Admission |
| Decrease in hematocrit > 10 points |
| Increase in blood urea nitrogen > 5 mg/dl |
| Calcium < 8 mg/dl |
| Partial pressure of oxygen < 60 torr |
| Base deficit > 4 mmol/l |
| Fluid deficit > 6 l |
| GALLSTONE-INDUCED PANCREATITIS |
| Age > 70 yr |
| White blood cell count > 18,000/mm$^3$ |
| Glucose > 220 mg/dl |
| Lactic dehydrogenase > 400 U/l |
| Aspartate aminotransferase > 250 U/l |
| Within 48 h of Admission |
| Decrease in hematocrit > 10 points |
| Increase in blood urea nitrogen > 2 mg/dl |
| Calcium < 8 mg/dl |
| Partial pressure of oxygen < 60 torr |
| Base deficit > 5 mmol/l |
| Fluid deficit > 4 l |

*Reprinted with permission from Steinberg W, Tenner S. Acute Pancreatitis. N Engl J Med. 1994; 330:1198–1210.

## Infections Complicating Pancreatitis

### Definitions

In discussing pancreatitis-associated infections, it is necessary to distinguish between different types of infections that follow and are specific to acute pancreatitis. Some discussions confuse this issue by lumping together all infections occurring after acute pancreatitis. The earliest type of infection that occurs after pancreatitis is infected pancreatic necrosis. This is characterized by bacterial growth and invasion of necrotic peripancreatic tissues that are found in the retroperitoneum in the most severe instances of acute pancreatitis. This is the most serious form of pancreatitis-related infection; it is difficult to treat effectively and exhibits a mortality of 5% to 50% in different series. It is characterized by unpredictable, but extensive spread in the retroperitoneum that is not limited by natural anatomic boundaries. Infected pancreatic necrosis can occur as early as 3 d and as late as 8 wk after the initial clinical presentation of pancreatitis. Typically, the majority of cases are diagnosed and treated within 2 wk.

*Pancreatic abscess* describes a more localized infection in the retroperitoneum, either in or adjacent to the pancreas. As with infected pancreatic necrosis, it is associated with necrotizing pancreatitis but is confined within a capsule of granulation tissue and adjacent organs. The contents are purulent and may contain small amounts of tissue debris. The distinction between abscess and infected necrosis is a matter of degree and there is a continuum between the two extremes. Pancreatic abscesses tend to occur later in the course of the disease than infected necrosis and after the acute inflammation has subsided. The average time of diagnosis and treatment in one report was 5 wk and 2 wk, respectively, for abscess and infected necrosis. The mortality of pancreatic abscesses tends to be about one-half that of infected necrosis.

A *pseudocyst* can become infected weeks to months after the onset of pancreatitis. The pseudocyst may exist for some time before becoming infected, and by definition it is relatively well walled-off from surrounding tissues. This tends to confine the infection anatomically. Although the existence of a pseudocyst implies that some tissue necrosis occurred during the acute attack, this is not always appreciated at the time, and the pseudocyst may not be recognized until later. Use of the term *infected pseudocyst* is now discouraged because of past misunderstandings. A pseudocyst with pus and systemic signs of infection should be called an *abscess* and should be treated like an abscess. If a pseudocyst with relatively clear fluid in a patient without obvious systemic signs of infection is found to contain bacteria at the time of a surgical procedure, it is considered colonized, and the procedure is a contaminated procedure. However, it can be managed in the same manner as uninfected pseudocysts, and successful pseudocyst-enterostomy can commonly be performed in this setting.

### Other nosocomial infections

Although this chapter focuses primarily on infections specific to pancreatitis, patients with this condition are at risk for the entire spectrum of nosocomial infections that may affect any seriously ill patient. The more severe the initial illness, the more interventions that are required, and the greater the risk for infections at other sites. These include intravenous device-related infections, urinary tract infections, respiratory tract infections *Clostridium difficile* colitis, and other less common nosocomial infections. The prevention and treatment of these infections is not distinct or unique in patients with pancreatitis.

### Differentiating infected from uninfected cases

During the early phases of an episode of acute necrotizing pancreatitis the clinical picture is not very different in a patient with severe uninfected pancreatitis and one with infected necrosis. In one report with significant numbers both of infected and uninfected patients, there were differences between these groups with respect to temperature, base excess, $pO_2$, and hypotension, but large numbers of patients who were not infected had abnormal findings in each area. In addition there was no difference in WBC count between the infected and noninfected patients (Table 64.2). Thus, these traditional markers of infection are relatively nonspecific in patients with acute necrotizing pancreatitis.

Important information can be obtained by performing CT of the pancreas with contrast infusion. This can detect areas of the pancreas and peripancreatic tissues that have impaired perfusion as indicated by lack of intravenous contrast enhancement. Percutaneous CT- or ultrasound-guided fine needle aspiration can provide gram stain and culture information for the tissues in these regions. Patients with greater impairment of perfusion have a higher likelihood of positive aspirates, indicating peripancreatic infected necrosis. The risk of infection increases directly with the increase in nonperfused tissue (Figs. 64.1–64.3).

**Table 64.2** Clinical differences between patients with infected and with sterile pancreatic necrosis*

| | Infected (41%) | Sterile (59%) |
|---|---|---|
| Temperature > 38.5° C | 58% | 17% |
| Base excess > −4 | 50% | 20% |
| $pO_2$ < 60 torr | 52% | 25% |
| White blood cell count > 10,000 | 83% | 74% |
| White blood cell count > 16,000 | 38% | 38% |
| Systolic blood pressure < 80 torr | 20% | 9% |

*Adapted with permission from Block, S., M. Buchler, et al. (1987). "Sepsis indicators in acute pancreatitis." *Pancreas* 2(5):499–505.

## Microbiology

The organisms recovered from patients with infectious complications of pancreatitis are similar regardless of the type of infection encountered and reflect predominantly enteric flora with some increased representation by *Pseudomonas aeruginosa*, *Candida* species, and staphylococci (Table 64.3). The apparent increased recovery of *Candida* species seen in these patients when compared to patients with other forms of intraabdominal infection appears to be due to patients who have already had one or more operations prior to the culture, or extensive prior antibiotic therapy. However, data in this regard are incomplete. While enteric anaerobic bacteria are commonly recovered, their incidence is noticeably lower than in other forms of intraabdominal infection.

The route by which microorganisms reach the area of infection is debated. The most frequently postulated routes are by intestinal translocation, bacteremia, or reflux from the bile duct or duodenum. Definitive data from humans are not available. Animal models are consistent with all routes of infection but support most strongly the likelihood of some form of translocation.

## Antimicrobial treatment

The timing and route of infection have potential relevance in guiding protocols for antibiotic administration in patients with severe pancreatitis. The prevalence of fever, leukocytosis, and abdominal tenderness at the onset of pancreatitis and the knowledge that patients who develop complications of pancreatitis tend to have infections have led many physicians to prescribe empirical antimicrobial agents during the initial phases of the illness. Early trials testing the utility of "prophylactic" antibiotic administration to patients with acute pancreatitis failed to provide useful information because the patients studied had such a low rate of infection (2%) that there was no chance to observe a difference even if an effective treatment had been used. These data, the small number of patients with pancreatitis who develop an infection, the delayed occurrence of infection, and the known ineffectiveness of prophylactic antibiotics in settings where the risk of infection is prolonged have led some to advise against the routine administration of prophylactic antibiotics for any patients with acute pancreatitis. Since all patients with identified infec-

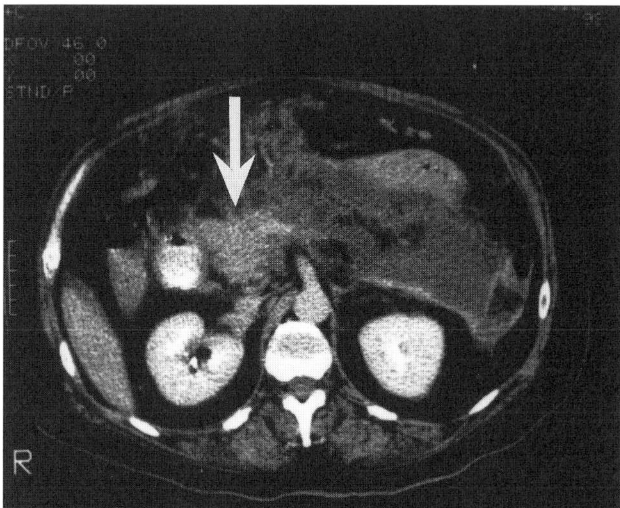


**Fig. 64.1** CT scan demonstrating perfusion of head of pancreas (arrow) and nonperfusion of much of body and tail of pancreas and surrounding tissues with extensive swelling and peripancreatic edema. Note heterogeneity of pancreatic and pancreatic tissues. This case was infected as demonstrated by fine needle aspirate. [Figure courtesy of Patrick C. Freeny, Professor of Radiology and Director, Abdominal Imaging, CT/MR, University of Washington Medical Center.]

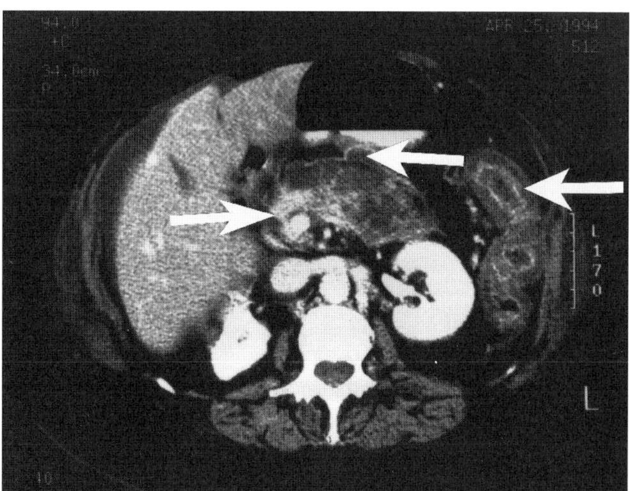


**Fig. 64.2** CT scan demonstrating noninfected pancreatic and peripancreatic necrosis. Only a small portion of the head of the pancreas adjacent to the superior mesenteric artery is perfused with contrast (arrow). Marked swelling of and heterogeneity of tissues between the pancreas and stomach (arrow) are present. Note also characteristic findings of pseudomembranous colitis of the splenic flexure of the colon (arrow). [Figure courtesy of Patrick C. Freeny, Professor of Radiology and Director, Abdominal Imaging, CT/MR, University of Washington Medical Center.]

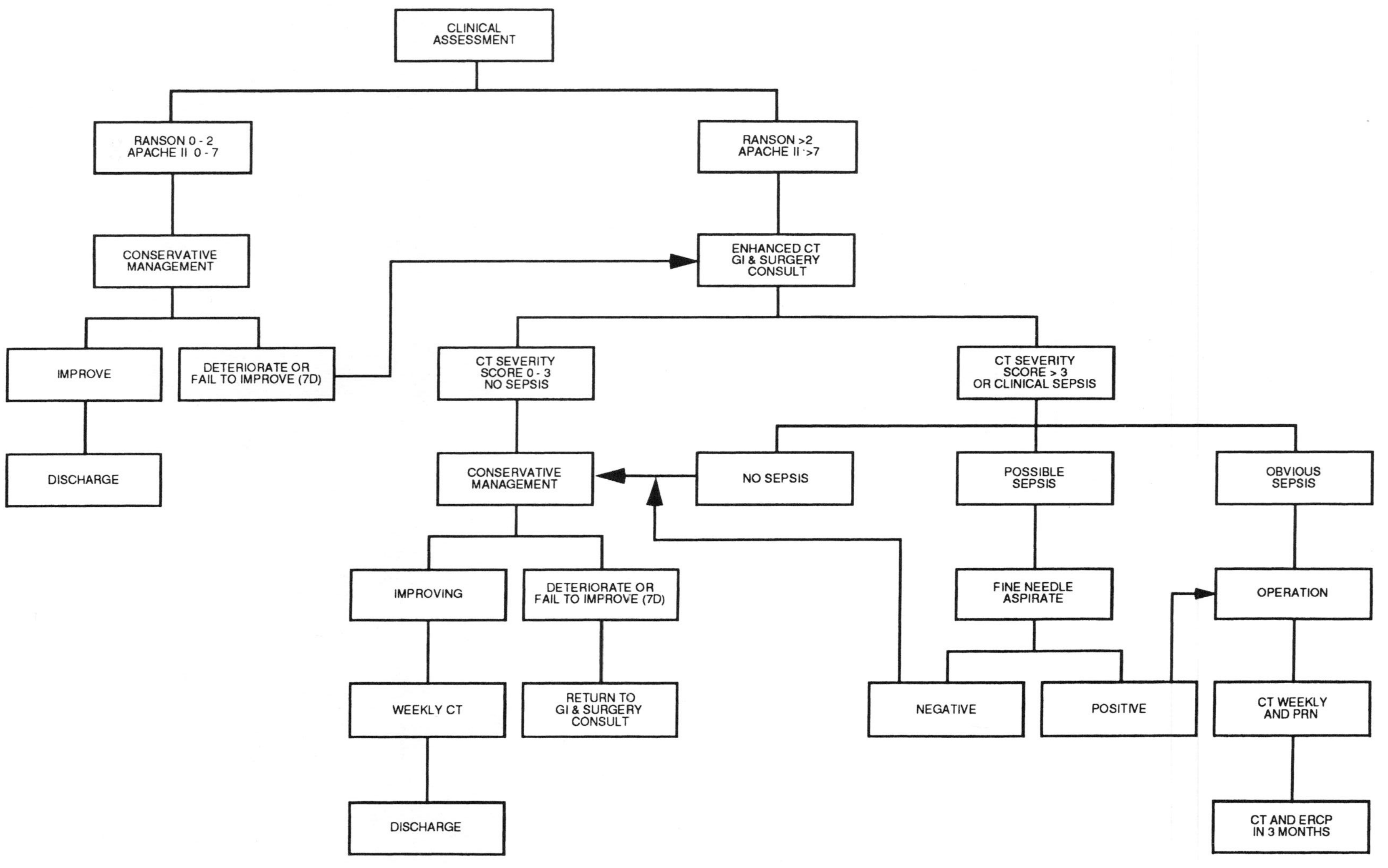


**Fig. 64.3** Pancreatitis management algorithm.

**Table 64.3** Microorganisms isolated from infections complicating acute necrotizing pancreatitis*

| Species | Approximate range of isolates (%) |
|---|---|
| *Escherichia coli* | 17–35 |
| *Pseudomonas aeruginosa* | 11–16 |
| *Enterococcus* species | 10–15 |
| *Staphylococcus aureus* | 10–15 |
| *Klebsiella pneumoniae* | 5–24 |
| Other enteric gram negative bacilli | 15–30 |
| *Candida* species | 5–15 |
| *Bacteroides* species and other anaerobes | 5–14 |
| Coagulase-negative staphylococci | 5–10 |
| *Streptococcus* species | 6–9 |

*The organisms are listed in descending order of their isolation. In many cases isolates are multiple. Thus, the sum of the ranges indicated is 89–183.

Data for this table were abstracted and summarized from Aloia et al (1994) and Bradley (1989) [please see Annotated Bibliography]; Calandra et al. Clinical significance of Candida isolated from peritoneum in surgical patients. Lancet. 1989; 2(8677):1437–1440; and Adams et al. Percutaneous catheter drainage of infected pancreatic and peripancreatic fluid collections. Arch Surg. 1990; 125:1554–1557.

tion in this setting require intervention, either by open operation or by percutaneous catheter placement, it may be prudent to withhold antibiotic administration until the diagnosis of infection has been made and operative plans have been formulated.

However, recent trials cast doubt on this approach and suggest that early administration of antibiotics to patients with necrotizing pancreatitis as demonstrated by contrast enhanced CT scans may prevent some episodes of infection. In a multicenter trial, 74 patients with necrotizing pancreatitis at six different centers were randomized to receive either imipenem/cilastatin or placebo for 14 d. An increasing incidence of infectious complications of pancreatitis was observed with increasing degrees of necrosis, and the incidence of infectious complications in the antibiotic-treated group was significantly lower than that in the placebo group (12% versus 30%, $P < 0.01$). Of note is the very high overall proportion of patients with infectious complications in this study, confirming that they represent a relatively high risk group. The difference in mortality (7% versus 12%) was not statistically significant. While this trial is very suggestive, recommendations based upon this high-risk patient group may not be applicable to other patient groups. The percentage of patients screened for this trial who were found to be eligible is not given in the paper, but in other trials with varying definitions of severe pancreatitis, the proportion of all admissions for pancreatitis that fall into this category varied from 5% to 28%. Some additional concerns regarding this study are that it was not blinded and that it was conducted at 6 different centers with different operative indications, possibly influenced by the unblinded nature of the study. Although numbers of infections were different, there were no differences study in numbers of operations, incidence of multiple organ failure, or mortality.

Another trial from Finland randomized 60 patients with necrotizing pancreatitis secondary to alcohol between intravenous cefuroxime or no antibiotics. Patients were admitted with an elevated C-reactive protein concentration (>120 mg/l within 48 hours of admission) and necrosis by dynamic CT scan. The nonantibiotic group developed more infections per patient (1.8 versus 1.0, $p = 0.01$), and had a higher mortality (seven versus one, $p = 0.03$), but the number of patients with pancreatic infection and the number of operations was the same in both groups. The majority of patients operated in this study had sterile cultures at the first operation. The incidence of positive central venous catheter cultures for *Staphylococcus epidermidis* was high, and the same organism was isolated from peripancreatic tissue subsequently in four of the patients who died. A major problem with line sepsis or catheter-management protocols may have biased the results of the study. This study also was not blinded.

A study in the Netherlands compared the effect of selective digestive decontamination with colistin sulfate, amphotericin B, and norfloxacin in addition to parenteral cefotaxime, given until the elimination of gram negative rods from the mouth and rectum, to a no-treatment control for the prevention of infection in patients with severe acute pancreatitis. This prospective randomized trial treated patients until they were being managed on a regular ward and had resumed a regular diet. One hundred and two patients with high Imrie scores and/or severe computed tomography findings were enrolled. There was no significant difference in mortality between groups unless a multivariate analysis was done to control for severity. Deaths during the first 2 weeks were the same in both groups, and there was no significant difference in total deaths or in the incidence of operative intervention. However, the treatment group experienced a significant reduction in late mortality, and there was also a reduction in pancreatic infections. This study also was not blinded.

While these trials are very suggestive, much of the information is inconclusive and/or contradictory. Definitive recommendations regarding early use of prophylactic antibiotics for this difficult patient group should await information from additional prospective trials. The choice of antimicrobial agents for patients with severe pancreatitis, either for treatment or prophylaxis, should depend primarily on the susceptibility spectrum of the organisms most commonly recovered from these infections. Although some have argued that the choice should depend on penetration of antibiotics into pancreatic duct secretions or into pancreatic tissue, there are no reports either from animal models or clinical trials that demonstrate a difference in efficacy on this basis. The areas of infection are all poorly perfused, and the effect of inflammation on drug penetration into these areas is unknown. Furthermore, all such infections require operative debridement and/or drainage. Thus the most important factor related to success is probably the relevant antimicrobial susceptibility spectrum. Logical and appropriate choices include imipenem alone; an aminoglycoside, a third-generation cephalosporin, or ciprofloxacin combined with metronidazole or clindamycin; aztreonam combined with clindamycin; or one of the advanced-generation penicillin/$\beta$-lactamase-inhibitor combinations.

## Operative treatment of infection

The treatment of infected necrosis requires open operative debridement of the involved retroperitoneal tissues. Opinions differ as to the optimal management after the initial operation. The spectrum includes one operation with subsequent operations as indicated by clinical condition; operation with postoperative catheter irrigation; scheduled reoperations; or leaving the abdomen open for subsequent dressing changes and debridement in the ICU. Mortality for all treatment strategies is high, and complications include secondary infections, enteric fistulas, and major bleeding from pseudo-aneurysms.

Abscesses, when diagnosed, should be drained, either in an open procedure or by percutaneous placement of a catheter. The contents of these abscesses tend to be complex and do not always permit successful catheter drainage. While initial treatment may be begun with a radiologically guided percutaneous catheter, this approach has a high rate of failure, and the clinician who elects this approach must follow the clinical response and be prepared to provide open exploration and drainage.

## Management plan

Clinicians at the University of Washington Medical Center with an interest in severe pancreatitis* have evolved the following algorithm for managing these patients (Fig. 64.3). Patients are initially assessed for severity of disease. Those with mild disease (Ranson score ≤ 2 [see Table 64.1] or APACHE II ≤ 7) are observed. They receive intravenous fluids and are kept NPO until resolution of abdominal pain and tenderness. A nasogastric tube is not used unless the patient is vomiting. Those who improve are discharged when well. Those who deteriorate or fail to improve over 7 d are evaluated in the same manner as patients with severe disease. Patients with severe disease are studied with a contrast-enhanced CT scan and receive consultation from the Gastroenterology and the GI Surgery services. Patients with mild disease by CT and without signs of sepsis are observed with conservative management as described above. Patients observed to improve are studied with a CT at weekly intervals and discharged when well. Those who deteriorate or fail to improve follow the next pathway.

A patient with an abnormal CT and equivocal signs of sepsis should undergo a CT-guided fine needle aspirate of the pancreatic and peripancreatic tissues. A patient with a negative aspirate should be observed, while a patient with an aspirate positive either by gram stain or culture for bacteria or yeast should be explored for debridement as described below. A patient with obvious worsening clinical sepsis such as SIRS with shock (see Chapter 50) should be operated upon for presumptive diagnosis of infection after initial resuscitation and attempts at stabilization. The operative procedure achieves debridement of the necrotic retroperitoneal tissues regardless of bacterial findings. Extensive intraoperative debridement is performed and soft drains and irrigation catheters are placed. The CT scan is used intraoperatively to ensure the complete exploration of all involved areas. Reoperation is guided by the adequacy of the initial procedure, the patient's condition, and findings on serial CT scans.

Antibiotic administration generally is withheld during the initial evaluation and during observation and conservative management unless a bacteriologically diagnosed infection is identified or a decision has been made to operate for known or presumed retroperitoneal infection or abscess. The antibiotic choice is guided initially by local sensitivity patterns and knowledge of the usual spectrum of the pathogens recovered in pancreatitis-related infections (Table 64.3). Subsequent antibiotic management is guided by results of culture and susceptibility studies. The presence of yeast in early smears or culture results is indication for specific treatment with fluconazole or amphotericin B (see Chapter 42).

*E. P. Dellinger, P. C. Freeny, W. S. Helton, M. B. Kimmey, M. N. Sinanan.

## ANNOTATED BIBLIOGRAPHY

Aloia T, Solomkin J, Fink AS, Nussbaum MS, Bjornson S, Bell RH, Sewak L, McFadden DW. Candida in pancreatic infection: a clinical experience. Am Surg 1994; 60(10):793–796.

*A recent examination of the incidence of* Candida *infections in patients with pancreatitis.*

Bittner R, Block S, Buchler M, Beger HG. Pancreatic abscess and infected pancreatic necrosis. Different local septic complications in acute pancreatitis. Dig Dis Sci 1987; 32(10):1082–1087.

*An examination of the difference between infected peripancreatic necrosis and pancreatic abscesses from a clinical team with vast experience in the treatment of these conditions.*

Block S, Buchler M, Bittner R, Beger HG. Sepsis indicators in acute pancreatitis. Pancreas 1987; 2(5):499–505.

*An examination of the clinical signs and symptoms compared between patients with uninfected pancreatitis and with infected pancreatitis.*

Bradley EL III. Antibiotics in acute pancreatitis. Current status and future directions. Am J Surg 1989; 158(5):472–477, and Dellinger EP. Antibiotics in acute pancreatitis—editorial comment. Am J Surg 1989; 158:477–478.

*A review examining penetration of various antibiotics into pancreatic tissue and secretions and speculating on the clinical relevance of this information in relation to the susceptibility patterns of pathogens frequently recovered from patients with infectious complications of pancreatitis. See also editorial comment.*

Bradley EL III. A clinically based classification system for acute pancreatitis. Summary of the International Symposium on Acute Pancreatitis, Atlanta, GA, September 11 through 13, 1992. Arch Surg 1993; 128(5):586–590.

*Report of a consensus conference on definitions for complications of pancreatitis emphasizing infectious complications.*

Fan ST, Choi TK, Fan FL, Lai EC, Wong J. Pancreatic phlegmon: what is it? Am J Surg 1989; 157(6):544–547.

*A clinical description of the course of patients with and without infected peri-pancreatic necrosis.*

Fedorak IJ, Ko TC, et al. Secondary pancreatic infections: are they distinct clinical entities? Surgery 1992; 112(4):824–830.

*An exploration of the clinical differences and microbiological similarities between different forms of infection complicating severe pancreatitis.*

Gerzof SG, Banks PA, Robbins AH, Johnson WC, Spechler SJ, Wefzner SM, Snider JM, Langevin RE, Jay ME. Early diagnosis of pancreatic infection by computed tomography-guided aspiration. Gastroenterology 1987; 93(6):1315–1320.

*A description of the technique and results of fine-needle, CT-guided aspiration of the pancreas and peri-pancreatic tissues for diagnosis of infectious complications of pancreatitis.*

Hariri M, Slivka A, Carr-Locke DL, Banks PA. Pseudocyst drainage predisposes to infection when pancreatic necrosis is unrecognized [see comments]. Am J Gastroenterol 1994; 89(10):1781–1784.

*An examination of potential complications and failure of percutaneous drainage of some pancreatic infections.*

Kazantsev GB, Hecht DW, Rao R, Fedorak LJ, Gaffuso P, Thompson K, Djuricin G, Prinz RA. Plasmid labeling confirms bacterial translocation in pancreatitis. Am J Surg 1994; 167(1):201–206.

*An experimental study demonstrating contamination of peri-pancreatic tissues by translocation in an animal model of pancreatitis and infection.*

Luiten EJ, Hop WC, Lange JF, Bruining HA. Controlled clinical trial of selective decontamination for the treatment of severe acute pancreatitis. Ann Surg 1995; 222(1):57–65.

*Selective digestive decontamination did not change overall mortality, but may have reduced late deaths in this study.*

Madry S, Fromm D. Infected retroperitoneal fat necrosis associated with acute pancreatitis. J Am Coll Surg 1994; 178(3):277–282.

*A description of the clinical course and treatment of infected peri-pancreatic tissue associated with severe pancreatitis including the observation that all patients in this series had necrosis and infection only of peri-pancreatic tissues and not of the pancreas itself.*

Medich DS, Lee TK, Melhem MF, Rowe MI, Schraut WH, Lee KK. Pathogenesis of pancreatic sepsis. Am J Surg 1993; 165(1):46–50.

*Another exploration of the route of infection in severe pancreatitis using an animal model that demonstrates the importance of translocation.*

Pederzoli P, Bassi C, Vesentini S, Campedelli A. A randomized multicenter clinical trial of antibiotic prophylaxis of septic complications in acute necrotizing pancreatitis with imipenem. Surg Gynecol Obstet 1993; 176(5):480–483.

*The first report to demonstrate a beneficial effect of prophylactic antibiotics administered at the onset of severe necrotizing pancreatitis.*

Rao R, Fedorak I, Prinz RA. Effect of failed computed tomography-guided and endoscopic drainage on pancreatic pseudocyst management. Surgery 1993; 114(4):843–847.

*An examination of the circumstances under which percutaneous drainage of pancreatic abscesses is likely to fail.*

Sainio V, Kamppainen E, Puolakkainen P, Taavitsainen M, Kivisaari L, Valtonen V, Haapiainen R, Schroder T, Kivilaakso E. Early antibiotic treatment in acute necrotising pancreatitis. Lancet 1995; 346(8976):663–667.

*This paper purports to find a benefit from early treatment of patients with severe pancreatitis with cefuroxime, but problems with venous line infections and early operations on patients without infection may have biased the results.*

Steinberg W, Tenner S. Acute Pancreatitis. N Engl J Med 1994; 330:1198–1210.

*An excellent recent general review of the topic of acute pancreatitis.*

# 65

# Peritonitis and Intraabdominal Abscesses

E. PATCHEN DELLINGER

Bacterial peritonitis and intraabdominal abscess are most conveniently discussed together, since one is frequently the cause of the other. They share a similar microbiological etiology, usually derived from the gastrointestinal tract, they are treated with the same selection of antibiotics, and they both usually have underlying causes that require surgical intervention. The word *peritonitis* indicates inflammation of the peritoneum, but the most common cause of this inflammation is bacterial infection. If the infection occurs "spontaneously," without a demonstrable anatomic source of bacteria, it is termed *primary* or *spontaneous peritonitis.* This is far less common than secondary peritonitis—that is, peritoneal infection secondary to an anatomic lesion such as bowel perforation, bowel obstruction, or contamination during an abdominal operation. Tertiary peritonitis describes a failure of host-defense mechanisms in the face of persistent or recurrent intraabdominal infection after initial treatment with operation and antimicrobial agents.

## Primary Peritonitis

### Pathogenesis

Primary peritonitis is much less common than secondary peritonitis, and although it can rarely occur in any patient, it tends to occur predominantly in specific patient risk groups. The majority of cases occur in patients with hepatic ascites. The other group of patients known to be at risk includes adults and children with nephrotic syndrome. Both of these groups of patients have accumulation of fluid that is deficient in opsonic proteins in the peritoneal cavity, and both have a number of systemic host-defense defects, perhaps putting them at increased risk for this infection. The source of the infection is thought to be bacteremia in many cases, and a significant number of patients with primary peritonitis have simultaneous bacteremia with the same organism. Another postulated source of infection is translocation across the wall of the intestinal tract, a route that can be demonstrated with ease in experimental animals and one that would explain the frequent recovery of enteric organisms from patients with primary peritonitis. A much smaller number of cases of primary peritonitis, presumably bacteremic in origin, occur in children without liver disease or nephrotic syndrome. These cases are usually due to organisms known to cause bacteremia such as *Streptococcus pneumoniae* and *S. pyogenes.*

### Clinical manifestations and treatment

Any patient with ascites who presents with an acute change in condition must be suspected of having primary peritonitis. Although most patients will have abdominal tenderness, fever, and leukocytosis, up to one-third may lack significant tenderness, and normothermia or hypothermia is not uncommon. The definitive diagnosis is made by sampling the ascites and obtaining a positive culture. A positive gram stain of the fluid is very specific for peritonitis, but the low numbers of bacteria found in the ascitic fluid in most cases make this a relatively insensitive test. Some white blood cells are normally found in uninfected ascites, but a WBC count greater than 500/$\mu$l or absolute polymorphonuclear cell count greater than 250/$\mu$l can be used to make the presumptive diagnosis of primary peritonitis and to begin empirical antimicrobial therapy while awaiting culture results. An antimicrobial agent active against both aerobic and facultative enteric gram-negative bacilli and streptococcal species should be used as initial empiric therapy. Good choices include a third-generation cephalosporin, imipenem/cilastatin, meropenem, ticarcillin/clavulanate, or piperacillin/tazobactam. The mortality associated with primary peritonitis exceeds 50% in many series, reflecting the severe underlying disease that forms the setting for this syndrome. The detection of two different organisms, either on gram stain or in culture, usually indicates secondary peritonitis rather than primary peritonitis and is nearly always associated with a specific gastrointestinal source requiring surgical intervention.

## Secondary Peritonitis and Intraabdominal Abscess

### Pathogenesis

Secondary peritonitis and intraabdominal abscess represent two ends of a continuum of responses to contamination of the peritoneal cavity caused by perforation of the gastrointestinal tract. When bacteria and other gastrointestinal substances are released into the peritoneal cavity, a typical inflammatory response results with recruitment of macrophages and polymorphonuclear leukocytes and release of humoral inflammatory mediators including elements of the complement and coagulation cascades with formation of fibrin. If the contamination is small and is not repeated, host defenses may succeed in clearing it entirely. In many cases this inflammatory response succeeds in localizing the infectious process to the immediate vicinity of the contamination, although some bacteria remain and eventually multiply. An abscess results, a partial victory for host defenses in limiting the spread of infection and segregating it from the rest of the peritoneal cavity. Some degree of peritoneal inflammation (peritonitis) is always present with an intraabdominal abscess unless it is entirely retroperitoneal. The progression of systemic responses to an abscess tends to be more gradual than for peritonitis.

If the gastrointestinal contamination is too great to be limited by the initial inflammatory response, peritonitis will result.

Because a greater surface area of peritoneum is involved, the immediate systemic consequences of the infection are usually greater, and the symptoms more severe. If bacteria and irritating gastrointestinal fluids are distributed throughout the peritoneal cavity, the resulting diffuse inflammatory response can cause fluid accumulation and consequent reduction in circulating blood volume equivalent to a 50% body surface area burn. Both the bacteria and the inflammatory mediators are partially cleared from the peritoneal space through diaphragmatic lymphatics that empty into the venous system, resulting in an early systemic response to the infection.

## Clinical manifestations and diagnosis

The diagnosis of peritonitis is made primarily on the basis of history and physical examination. The history often includes elements of nausea, abdominal pain, altered bowel habit, either diarrhea or constipation, fever, and chills. Initial pain may have been visceral, poorly localized, as in the periumbilical pain that often is the first sign of appendicitis, later localized as inflammation results, and then diffuse as the perforation occurs. An upright chest X-ray may demonstrate free air after a perforated peptic ulcer, but free air is uncommon in other forms of peritonitis. More complex examinations such as ultrasound or CT scan are seldom useful. While temperature and white blood cell count are usually elevated, neither is necessary to make the diagnosis of peritonitis. Physical exam will reveal abdominal tenderness, often with percussion tenderness, and may include involuntary abdominal-wall muscle spasm. The diffuse nature of the findings usually precludes an accurate determination of the etiology of the peritonitis prior to operation. The most important decision that must be made is that peritonitis exists and that operative intervention is required.

An intraabdominal abscess may be more difficult to diagnose than peritonitis because it is localized and walled off and may be situated in parts of the abdominal space that are less available to physical examination such as the subphrenic spaces or the pelvis. Evolution of symptoms is usually more gradual than with peritonitis. Historically, intraabdominal abscesses were most commonly the result of appendicitis, diverticulitis, or perforated peptic ulcers. In the second half of the 20th century the increasing number and complexity of intraabdominal procedures, performed on increasingly complicated patients, has led to an increasing incidence of postoperative intraabdominal infections, especially abscesses.

The incidence of intraabdominal infection within 30 d of an abdominal operation has been estimated at 2%. Looking at this relationship in the other direction, one notes that from 30% to 70% of serious intraabdominal infections are postoperative. Diagnosis in the postoperative period can be more difficult because fever, leukocytosis, and abdominal pain are part of the normal recovery process after most open abdominal operations. The best results are obtained through careful serial examinations conducted by the operating surgeon who is familiar with the details of the procedure and the elements of it that may predispose to postoperative infection. Temperature elevations, leukocytosis, or abdominal symptoms that persist or begin after the fourth postoperative day are more likely to reflect a genuine postoperative infection than those noted earlier. Radiological studies, especially CT scans and ultrasound exams, are more likely to be helpful for diagnosis in postoperative patients and in locating abscesses above the costal margin and in the pelvis. These exams are more helpful in the second week after operation than in the first since fluid collections are common in the early postoperative period without infection, and as time passes, the radiological features of abscess become more evident on CT scan (Fig. 65.1).

## Treatment

Since the great majority of intraabdominal infections are due to anatomic lesions that must be corrected, surgical intervention, either by celiotomy or by percutaneous drainage of an abscess, is always an essential part of the treatment plan. Only a small number of intraabdominal infections are treated appropriately without operative intervention, and all of those can usually be diagnosed presumptively in a short time and with minimal testing. They include pyelonephritis without obstruction, enteritis, mild cases of diverticulitis, mild cases of cholangitis that respond quickly to antimicrobial management, most cases of salpingitis, and primary peritonitis. If one of these conditions cannot be diagnosed, then the patient either has a condition requiring operative intervention or does not have an intraabdominal infection. Treatment of an intraabdominal abscess or secondary peritonitis with antimicrobial agents but without operative intervention delays definitive treatment and increases the morbidity and mortality of the underlying condition. It is for this reason that a patient with abdominal pain and tenderness, fever, and leukocytosis should not be treated with empirical antimicrobials unless a prompt operative intervention has been scheduled or an intraabdominal infection that does not require operative intervention has been convincingly diagnosed.

The spectrum of systemic illness associated with peritonitis or intraabdominal abscess can be quite wide. While cardiorespiratory disturbances can be mild in some early cases, profound instability may result as the illness progresses. Major fluid shifts into the abdomen can cause hypotension and tachycardia. The combination of altered respiratory dynamics associated with abdominal pain and distention and the systemic effects of cytokines and other inflammatory mediators can cause serious respiratory embarrassment. As time passes without definitive treatment, respiratory failure can be followed by renal and hepatic failure.

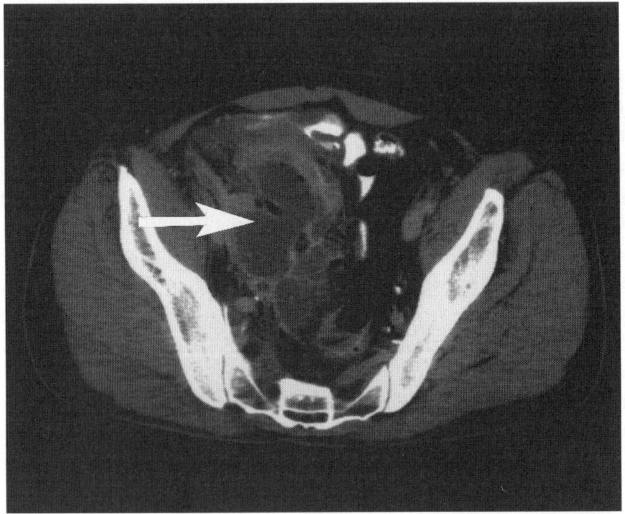

**Fig. 65.1** CT scan demonstrating bilobed multiloculated right lower quadrant abscess (arrow) following appendectomy for perforated appendicitis. Small gas bubbles can be seen within the abscess. Adjacent bowel contains contrast. [Figure courtesy of Patrick C. Freeny, Professor of Radiology and Director, Abdominal Imaging, CT/MR, University of Washington Medical Center.]

The cardiorespiratory status of any patient with the recent diagnosis of intraabdominal infection must be evaluated. Although operative intervention is necessary to reverse these complications, initial resuscitation must be accomplished before operation is attempted. Aggressive fluid resuscitation is usually required, and normalization of urine output, blood pressure, and pulse rate serve as endpoints. If response is delayed or volumes required are large then invasive hemodynamic monitoring may be needed. Volume resuscitation is usually the primary treatment required, and pressors should be used rarely and sparingly. Supplemental oxygen and/or intubation with mechanical ventilation is often necessary, if not in the preoperative period then during the initial postoperative period. The role of anticytokine antibodies, cytokine receptor antagonists, or other inflammatory response modifiers is unknown at this time but under active investigation.

### Operative intervention

Operative treatment of peritonitis requires an open celiotomy to determine the cause and to correct it. This may involve closure of a perforation, relief of bowel or duct obstruction, or removal of an inflamed or infarcted viscus. Although abscess formation in spontaneous disease represents a partial victory for host defenses in localizing the infectious process, after an operation for peritonitis, the development of an abscess represents a failure of the therapeutic effort to resolve the infection. Nonviable tissue, foreign materials from the bowel, and fibrin clots act as adjuvants that increase the local virulence of bacteria, decrease the effectiveness of host defenses, and increase the probability of postoperative abscess formation. Removal of these adjuvant substances at the time of the operation can be helpful, although techniques that greatly prolong the operation or result in increased bleeding or tissue injury are not recommended. Irrigation of the peritoneal cavity is useful for removing macroscopic adjuvant materials, but despite a voluminous literature discussing irrigation with and without antimicrobials added, there is no convincing evidence that irrigation removes bacteria or improves outcome.

Intraabdominal abscesses must be drained. This can be done at open operation through the peritoneal cavity, by local operation directly over the abscess without traversing the peritoneal cavity or by radiologically guided percutaneous catheter placement. The benefit of a transperitoneal operation is the opportunity to correct other anatomic problems or to locate other abscesses. The benefit of extraperitoneal drainage lies in preventing contamination of previously uninfected areas of the peritoneum. The benefit of percutaneous drainage is the same, as well as the potential avoidance of an anesthetic and a surgical incision. Despite the apparent differences of these approaches, series comparing them do not show any clinically important differences in outcome in patients with a similar degree of illness treated by these different approaches. Approximately 25% of intraabdominal abscesses will require a second procedure for complete resolution regardless of the initial technique employed. The decision regarding the best approach for a specific patient should be made by the surgeon who would be responsible for dealing with the problem if a radiological, percutaneous technique is attempted and is not successful.

### Antimicrobial treatment

The microbiology of intraabdominal infection is complex. The initial inoculum from a colonic injury can contain more than 400 different identifiable bacterial species. Competition between species and with host defenses results in elimination of most of this inoculum, but most intraabdominal infections still reveal from two to six different organisms, both anaerobic and facultative, on culture. Approximately 15 organisms account for 90% of the isolates reported in large series (Table 65.1). Because of this large number of organisms, and because a definitive culture of the infection cannot be obtained until the operative intervention (which is usually after antimicrobial agents have been started), initial treatment is always empirical. Even under ideal circumstances, the identity of the facultative species will not be known for 18–24 h, nor their antimicrobial sensitivities for 36–48 h. For anaerobes, initial growth is not known for 48 h and antimicrobial sensitivities for at least 2 d after that. One can see that the results of antimicrobial sensitivity testing of anaerobes frequently do not affect the treatment of the average patient.

It is preferable to begin treatment with an antimicrobial agent(s) that possesses activity against all organisms recovered. However, the large number of organisms that may be present and the variable sensitivities of these organisms make achievement of this goal in 100% of cases impractical. Many studies comparing different antimicrobial choices have led to a consensus that the regimen chosen should provide substantial activity

**Table 65.1** Bacteriology of intraabdominal infection*

| Aerobic species | Approximate percent of patients with species | Anaerobic species | Approximate percent of patients with species |
|---|---|---|---|
| *Escherichia coli* | 60 | *Bacteroides* species | 72 |
| *Streptococcus* | 28 | *Bacteroides fragilis* | 38 |
| *Enterobacter/Klebsiella* | 26 | *Eubacteria* | 24 |
| *Proteus* | 22 | *Clostridia* | 17 |
| *Enterococcus* | 17 | *Peptostreptococci* | 14 |
| *Pseudomonas* | 8 | *Peptococci* | 11 |
| *Staphylococcus* | 7 | *Propionibacterium* | 9 |
| *Candida* | 2 | *Fusobacteria* | 8 |

*Adapted with permission from Hau T et al. Current Problems in Surgery XVI, October 1979, Mosby YearBook Inc, St. Louis, MO.

against enteric gram-negative bacilli and gram-positive cocci and against enteric anaerobes. Controversy exists over whether every regimen should possess activity against enterococci and *Pseudomonas* species. A single report has indicated a higher rate of treatment failures due to *Pseudomonas* species in a treatment regimen for gangrenous and perforated appendicitis that did not possess activity against *Pseudomonas*. No report demonstrates a difference in outcome related to differences in antimicrobial activity against *Enterococcus* species.

A list of acceptable antimicrobial choices for intraabdominal infections is presented in Table 65.2. There appears to be no major advantage of any one of these regimens over another in clinical trials. There are not convincing data that determine the optimal duration of antimicrobial treatment for intraabdominal infection. Traditional practice has been to continue antimicrobial agents until the patient demonstrates general clinical improvement marked by decrease in tachycardia, pain, distention, and anorexia. In addition, antimicrobial agents are usually continued until the temperature has been under an arbitrary limit (often 37.6° C) for 24 or 48 h. These guidelines commonly result in an average duration of administration of antimicrobial agents of 7 to 10 d. The importance of the level of the absolute white blood cell (WBC) count when antimicrobial agents are stopped is debated. Certainly the probability of recurrent infection is higher if the WBC is elevated, but the value of continuing antimicrobial agents for a longer time when the WBC is elevated is unknown. If a patient is not exhibiting the desired clinical response 4 to 6 d after operative intervention, it is rare for a change or addition of antimicrobial agents to make an important difference. The most common intervention needed at that time is a reoperation or manipulation of percutaneous drains.

**Table 65.2** Acceptable antibiotic choices for initial, empirical treatment of peritonitis or intraabdominal abscess

| |
|---|
| COMMUNITY-ACQUIRED INFECTION OF MILD TO MODERATE SEVERITY |
| Ampicillin-sulbactam 3 g, i.v., q 6 h |
| or |
| Cefoxitin 1 g, i.v., q 4–6 h |
| or |
| Cefotetan 1 g, i.v., q 12 h |
| or |
| Ticarcillin-clavulanic acid 3.1 g, i.v., q 4–6 h |
| SEVERE AND HOSPITAL-ACQUIRED INFECTION |
| An antianaerobe[a] plus a third-generation cephalosporin[b] |
| or |
| An antianaerobe[a] plus ciprofloxacin, 400 mg, i.v., q 12 h |
| or |
| An antianaerobe[a] plus an aminoglycoside[c] |
| or |
| Aztreonam, 1–2 g, i.v., q 8 h, plus clindamycin, 900 mg, i.v., q 8 h |
| or |
| Imipenem-cilastatin, 500 mg, i.v., q 6 h |
| or |
| Meropenem 1 g, i.v., q 8 h |
| or |
| Piperacillin-tazobactam, 4.5 g, i.v., q 8 h |

[a]Clindamycin, 900 mg, i.v., q 8 h, or metronidazole, 1 g, i.v., q 12 h.

[b]Cefotaxime, ceftazidime, or ceftizoxime, 1 g, i.v., q 8 h; or ceftriaxone, 1–2 g, i.v., q 24 h.

[c]Amikacin, 15–20 mg/kg, q 24 h or gentamicin, netilmicin, or tobramycin, 7 mg/kg, q 24 h (increase interval between doses to 36 h for estimated creatinine clearance [Ccr] = 40–59 ml/min; 48 h for Ccr = 20–39 ml/min; and based on serum levels to achieve serum levels < 1 mg/l for at least 4 h before next dose when Ccr < 20 ml/min).

The value of cultures obtained during operation for intraabdominal infection and the utility of adjusting antimicrobial treatment based on those cultures are controversial. Retrospective reviews examining the care of patients with peritonitis have failed to demonstrate significant differences between patients with and without operative cultures, and more discouragingly, have demonstrated that changes in antimicrobial treatment regimens frequently fail to make use of the culture and sensitivity information that is available. In one study, among patients who had a change of antimicrobials, change to an inappropriate regimen was more common than change to an appropriate one. In this study also, the patients who had no change of antimicrobial fared the best. Nevertheless, although the most favorable group consisted of those patients who received an appropriate combination of antimicrobials initially, additional analysis of the data demonstrates that there was an advantage for those patients whose antibiotics were changed from an inappropriate to an appropriate combination (Table 65.3). Rather than abandoning the practice of culturing intraabdominal infections, we might achieve better outcomes for our patients if we more precisely identified the results of culture and antimicrobial sensitivity tests and acted upon them.

## Outcome

The prognosis for patients with intraabdominal infection varies considerably depending on the age of the patient, the underlying diseases and cause of infection, and the severity of illness at the time of diagnosis. A young adult with acute appendicitis has a mortality risk of less than 0.1% and a risk of subsequent complication of less than 5%. An elderly postoperative patient with underlying renal or pulmonary disease, on steroids, hypotensive, with a subphrenic abscess or anastomotic leak has an acute mortality risk greater than 80%. Most modern series of patients with intraabdominal infection, excluding appendicitis, treated with operation and antimicrobial agents report mortalities in the range of 10% to 35% depending on the patient mix and comorbid diseases. The probability that a second operation or drainage will be required to resolve the underlying problem ranges from 20% to 30%, and patients with severe underlying disease have a higher risk. A number of studies suggested that mortality risk was influenced by the organ of origin of infection (other than appendix), but careful examination of that hypothesis has failed to confirm this opinion. The most important factor is the severity of illness observed in the patient at the time of diagnosis. Patients receiving steroids at the time that intraabdominal infection develops and those who experience a delay in diagnosis also experience an increased mortality.

## Tertiary Peritonitis

Tertiary peritonitis is not actually a third type of peritonitis, but rather it describes the clinical circumstance of persistent peritonitis after initial operative and antimicrobial treatment. In this setting patients continue to demonstrate clinical signs and symp-

**Table 65.3** Consequences of changing antibiotic correctly, incorrectly, or not at all†

| | Antibiotic choice | | | |
|---|---|---|---|---|
| | No change | Appropriate change | Inappropriate change | *P** |
| No. of patients | 372 | 41 | 67 | |
| Length of stay | 10.9 d | 14.8 d | 19.0 days | n.a. |
| Wound infection | 13.2% | 14.6% | 16.4% | n.s. |
| All complications | 18.5% | 22.0% | 34.3% | <0.005 |
| Abscess | 7.5% | 19.5% | 23.9% | <0.0001 |
| Reoperations | 12.1% | 22.0% | 31.3% | <0.0001 |
| Death | 5.4% | 7.3% | 13.5% | <0.02 |

†Adapted with permission from Mosdell DM, Morris M et al. 1991. Antibiotic Treatment for Surgical Peritonitis, *Ann Surg* 214:543–552.

*Bartholomew's test for order (Barlow, Bartholomew et al. 1972; Fleiss 1981); n.a.—not available; n.s.—not significant.

toms of infection despite initial apparently appropriate treatment. CT scans are often unhelpful because abscess formation has not occurred. At reexploration continued inflammatory changes are noted without an anatomic focus such as an intestinal leak, and the organisms recovered tend to be resistant to prior antimicrobial agents employed, are characteristic of hospital-acquired flora, and are often thought of as not likely to be pathogens in the peritoneal cavity. Typical flora of tertiary peritonitis include coagulase negative staphylococci, enterococci, *Viridans* streptococci, *Pseudomonas* species, and *Candida* species. These patients have a very high mortality even with reoperation and administration of antimicrobial agents effective against all recovered organisms.

## Specific Causes of Intraabdominal Infection

### Appendicitis

Appendicitis is primarily due to obstruction of the appendiceal lumen and is best solved by removal of the appendix. It becomes an infectious disease problem only when the diagnosis is not made prior to full-thickness injury of the wall of the appendix with resulting contamination of the right lower quadrant by fecal organisms. The appendix may be obstructed either by a fecal concretion or by lymphoid tissue at its base. If complete obstruction occurs, continued mucus secretion results in increasing pressure that eventually exceeds the perfusion pressure of the mucosa leading to ulceration and bacterial invasion of the wall. The distention of the appendix stimulates visceral nerves with the resulting periumbilical pain and nausea that is characteristic of early appendicitis, and the wall invasion and resulting inflammation cause the typical localized right lower quadrant pain and tenderness. In patients where the appendix is in the pelvic or retrocecal position and thus does not contact parietal peritoneum, the physical examination is not as characteristic and the initial diagnosis may be delayed. Eventually, full-thickness gangrene of the appendix can occur (gangrenous appendicitis) and then macroscopic perforation (perforated appendicitis). If the preceding inflammatory process has caused adhesions that wall off the process from the rest of the peritoneal cavity then a localized infectious process will result. If inflammatory adhesions have not walled off the perforated appendix, then peritonitis will result. Gross fecal contamination of the peritoneal cavity or free air can occur, but this is unusual because the original obstructive process is usually still present between the perforation and the cecum.

The diagnosis of appendicitis should nearly always lead to operation and antibiotics as soon as is practical. If the process has been diagnosed and the appendix removed before gangrene or perforation, then the antibiotics used function as prophylactic antibiotics for the surgical incision, and postoperative antibiotics are not needed. If gangrene or perforation has occurred, then the antibiotics should be continued in the postoperative period until the patient has demonstrated a satisfactory clinical response just as in other cases of peritonitis or abscess. The choice of antimicrobial agents is not different from other causes of secondary intraabdominal infection.

Some patients present with a more indolent course of appendicitis, developing over several days, or occasionally more than a week, with the finding of a right lower quadrant mass. In these cases, if the patient does not have a severe systemic response to infection, an initial CT scan or ultrasound examination can be used to differentiate between a soft-tissue inflammatory mass and an abscess. If an abscess is found, some patients will respond well to percutaneous drainage followed by an interval appendectomy in 6–12 wk. If a clinical response to percutaneous drainage is not obvious within 48 to 72 h then operative drainage, with or without appendectomy, should be pursued. If abscess drainage is not followed by appendectomy, then the risk of recurrent appendicitis is greater than 25%. In patients with a mass but without a demonstrable abscess by CT, initial treatment with antimicrobial agents and observation can be attempted. Approximately a third of these patients will fail to respond and require early operative intervention. The patients whose symptoms improve with antimicrobial therapy should also have an interval appendectomy after the acute process has resolved.

### Diverticulitis

Diverticulitis is an infectious complication of diverticulosis, the condition marked by multiple herniations of the colonic mucosa through the muscular wall of the colon. These diverticula occur most commonly in the region of the sigmoid colon but can occur anywhere in the colon. They are increasingly common with age, being demonstrable by barium enema in approximately 50% of patients over the age of 50. Fewer than a third of patients with demonstrable diverticula will have diverticulitis, and the majority of patients with diverticulitis will not require an operation for treatment. Diverticulitis occurs when the mucosa of one or more diverticula is breached, resulting in bacterial invasion of the peridiverticular tissues. The exact cause of mucosal injury is not known, but is thought to be mechanical in nature, related to the increased colonic pressures that are believed to cause the diverticula in the first place. Because the diverticula are covered by pericolonic fat, either in the mesentery or in the appendices epiploicae, the initial mucosal breech usually causes local inflammation and induration without peritonitis or localized abscess. In this early phase, the symptoms are marked by localized pain, most common in the left lower quadrant with or without change in bowel habit, and the signs include fever, leukocytosis, and localized tenderness with or without a palpable mass. A CT obtained at this time will demonstrate thickening and edema of the pericolonic tissues.

A patient with mild, early diverticulitis can be treated with a low residue or clear liquid diet and oral antimicrobial agents active against both facultative and anaerobic colonic bacteria. Suitable choices include ampicillin with clavulanic acid, cotrimoxazole, or an oral flouroquinolone combined with metronidazole or clindamycin, or even an oral tetracycline. For patients with more significant systemic signs of infection or those with nausea and vomiting, hospital admission, intravenous fluids and antimicrobial agents, and NPO status are appropriate. Antimicrobial choices are the same as those discussed for peritonitis and intraabdominal abscess. Any patient ill enough to warrant hospital admission should probably have a CT scan within 24 to 48 h of admission unless complete remission of signs and symptoms has been achieved. This is necessary to rule out the presence of a well-defined intraabdominal abscess that requires percutaneous or operative drainage.

Advanced cases of diverticulitis are marked by formation of true abscesses adjacent to the colon in addition to the induration and inflammation in pericolonic tissues (Fig. 65.2). Percutaneous drainage of such an abscess may result in a colocutaneous fistula, but if this is well controlled, it can allow the patient to be prepared for an elective, one-stage operative intervention rather than an emergency procedure and the necessity for an additional operation in the future. A diverticular abscess, if allowed to persist, can cause small- or large-bowel obstruction and may eventually rupture, causing diffuse peritonitis. Patients who are operated upon for large abscesses or peritonitis may require an initial resection combined with colostomy followed by a second procedure for colostomy closure scheduled after several months of recovery.

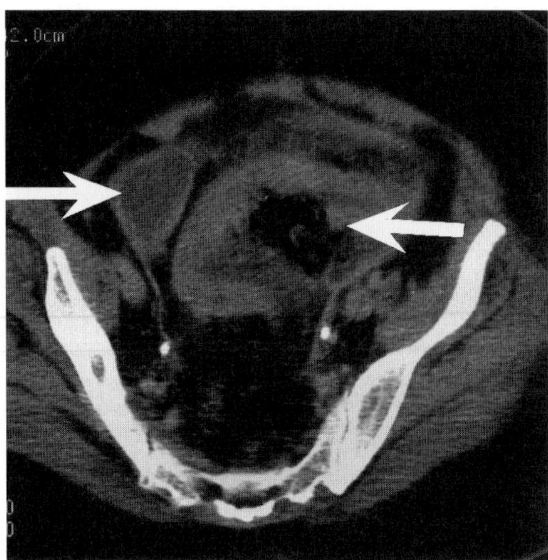

**Fig. 65.2** CT scan demonstrating diverticulitis. Thick-walled sigmoid colon surrounds complex area with soft tissue, fluid and gas (arrow). Fluid-filled structure in the right side of the abdomen is right colon (arrow). [Figure courtesy of Patrick C. Freeny, Professor of Radiology and Director, Abdominal Imaging, CT/MR, University of Washington Medical Center.]

## Perforated peptic ulcer

Patients with perforated peptic ulcer usually have an abrupt onset of signs and symptoms of diffuse peritonitis, and on radiological investigation frequently have evidence of free intraperitoneal air. A prior history of symptoms suggesting peptic ulcer disease may or may not be present. If the diagnosis is made early (within 48 h), infectious complications are rare, and a first-generation cephalosporin administered in a prophylactic manner at the time of operative closure of the perforation is usually sufficient. Fewer than 5% of patients operated upon within 48 h of perforation develop a postoperative infectious complication. Delay in diagnosis leads to an increase in the number and variety of intraabdominal infectious complications, and these patients require a course of antimicrobial therapy continued until a clinical response has been observed and tailored to the organisms recovered at the time of operation. The flora recovered after an early perforation are primarily gram-positive organisms consistent with oral flora and candida species. As time passes following the perforation, the number of species increases, perhaps due to overgrowth in the small intestine and reflux due to the resulting ileus, or due to bacterial translocation promoted by the inflammatory focus in the peritoneum.

## ANNOTATED BIBLIOGRAPHY

Boey J, Wong J, Ong GB. Bacteria and septic complications in patients with perforated duodenal ulcers. Am J Surg 1982; 143(5):635–639.

*This paper explores the risk factors for infection after treatment of perforated duodenal ulcers and demonstrates that early perforation rarely causes infectious complications.*

Bohnen JMA, Mustard RA, Schouten BD. Steroids, APACHE II score, and the outcome of abdominal infection. Arch Surg 1994; 129:33–38.

*This paper explores the risk factors for failure of initial therapeutic effort and for death following operation for intraabdominal infection.*

Bohnen JMA, Solomkin JS, Dellinger EP, Bjornson HS, Page CP. Guidelines for clinical care: anti-infective agents for intraabdominal infection. Arch Surg 1992; 127:83–89.

*A thorough discussion of options for antimicrobial agents in the treatment of intraabdominal infections and the rationale and evidence that supports the recommendations given. This is a policy statement of the Surgical Infection Society.*

Christou NV, Barie PS, Dellinger EP, Waymack JP, Stone HH. Surgical Infection Society intra-abdominal infection study. Prospective evaluation of management techniques and outcome. Arch Surg 1993; 128:193–199.

*A report of over 200 patients treated for intraabdominal infection. The authors formed a committee of the Surgical Infection Society which selected seriously ill patients with APACHE II score ≥ 10 with the intent of identifying factors that would predict the requirement for a second operation to resolve the intraabdominal infectious process.*

Dellinger EP, Wertz MJ, Meakins JL, Solomkin JS, Allo MD, Howard RJ, Simmons RL. Surgical infection stratification system for intra-abdominal infection. Arch Surg 1995; 120:21–29.

*A multicenter study examining risk factors for death following treatment of intraabdominal infection. This was the first study to validate the predictive value of the APACHE score for patients with intraabdominal infection.*

Doberneck RC, Mittelman J. Reappraisal of the problems of intra-abdominal abscess. Surg Gynecol Obstet 1982; 154:875–879.

*This paper describes a series of patients treated for intraabdominal abscess and describes the difference in clinical course for patients with and without successful initial drainage of the abscess.*

Dougherty SH, Saltzstein EC, Peacock JB, Mercer LC, Cano P. Perforated or gangrenous appendicitis treated with aminoglycosides. How do bacterial cultures influence management? Arch Surg 1989; 124(11):1280–1283.

*A paper that examines the actions taken by clinicians in response to culture and antimicrobial susceptibility data for patients with perforated or gangrenous appendicitis.*

Hau T, Ahrenholz DH, Simmons RL. Secondary bacterial peritonitis: the biologic basis of treatment. Curr Probl Surg 1979; XVI(10):1–65.

*A superb, comprehensive exploration of the pathophysiology, microbiology, and natural history of secondary peritonitis. This monograph is still very up-to-date except for discussion of specific antibiotics.*

Lennard ES, Dellinger EP, Minshew BH, Wertz MJ. Implications for leukocytosis and fever at conclusion of antibiotic therapy for intra-abdominal sepsis. Ann Surg 1982; 195:19–24.

*An examination of the outcome for patients who were treated for intraabdominal infection, and differences in outcome associated with differences in white blood cell count at the time that antibiotic treatment was stopped.*

Levison MA. Percutaneous versus open operative drainage of intra-abdominal abscesses. Infect Dis Clin North Am 1992; 6:525–544.

*A careful comparison of outcome in patients with intraabdominal abscess, treated either by percutaneous placement of drainage catheters or by open operative drainage.*

Mosdell DM, Morris DM, Voltura A, Pitcher DE, Twiest MW, Milne RL, Miscall BG, Fry DE. Antibiotic treatment for surgical peritonitis. Ann Surg 1991; 214:543–552.

*An examination of a community experience in the treatment of peritonitis. This report examines the influence of antimicrobial susceptibilities on outcome and the effect of changing antibiotics after susceptibilities are known.*

Pitcher WD, Musher DM. Critical importance of early diagnosis and treatment of intra-abdominal infection. Arch Surg 1982; 117(3):328–333.

*This paper examines the influence of delay in diagnosis and treatment of intraabdominal infection.*

Polk HC Jr, Fry DE. Radical peritoneal debridement for established peritonitis. The results of a prospective randomized clinical trial. Ann Surg 1980; 192(3):350–355.

*This paper examines the efficacy of extensive and meticulous debridement of all peritoneal surfaces at the time of treatment of intra-abdominal infection.*

Pusajo JF, Bumaschny E, Doglio GR, Cherjovsky MR, Lipinski AI, Hernandez MS, Egurrola MA. Postoperative intra-abdominal sepsis requiring reoperation. Value of a predictive index. Arch Surg 1993; 128:218–223.

*These authors examined the utility of an index and management algorithm to aid in the early diagnosis and treatment of postoperative intraabdominal infection.*

Rotstein OD, Pruett TL, Simmons RL. Microbiologic features and treatment of persistent peritonitis in patients in the intensive care unit. Can J Surg 1986; 29(4):247–250.

*This paper characterizes tertiary peritonitis and describes the typical microbiology and treatment outcome.*

# 66

# Infective Endocarditis

ADOLF W. KARCHMER

*Infective endocarditis* is the term applied to microbial infections involving the endothelial surface of the heart. This infection primarily occurs on the leaflets of heart valves, but occasionally on the low-pressure side of a ventricular septal defect, on chordae tendineae, or on the mural endocardium at the site of impact of a regurgitant jet of blood or an intracardiac foreign body such as an intravascular catheter or a pacer lead. The characteristic lesion of endocarditis is the *vegetation*, a variably sized platelet-fibrin mass that is attached to the underlying endothelium and in which are enmeshed the causative microorganisms. Because polymorphonuclear leukocytes are a scant component of the vegetation, this infection is considered to be located at the site of reduced host defenses. *Endarteritis*, which is clinically and pathologically similar to endocarditis, involves the endothelium of arterio-arterial shunts (patent ductus arteriosus), arteriovenous shunts, or a coarctation of the aorta.

The endothelium of the heart is in general resistant to infection by blood-borne organisms. Occasionally microorganisms, particularly *Staphylococcus aureus*, establish infection on structurally normal valves. More typically, however, endocarditis is engrafted on abnormal valves or at other endothelial sites where sterile platelet-fibrin thrombi (called *nonbacterial thrombotic endocarditis*, or *NBTE*) have formed. It is these lesions to which bacteria adhere during transient bacteremia and wherein bacteria multiply to cause infective endocarditis. Properties unique to specific bacteria facilitate their survival in the bloodstream, adherence to NBTE, and local multiplication. Consequently, although a vast array of microorganisms have been reported to cause endocarditis, the majority of cases are caused by a relatively narrow spectrum of bacteria with biologic properties that enhance their ability to cause this infection. The complex interaction between these microorganisms and the human host that results in endocarditis involves the endothelium, the coagulation system, the host immune system, the structural state of the heart, specific properties of bacteria, and events which generate bacteremia.

Although infective endocarditis was originally considered *acute* or *subacute* based upon the interval from onset of symptoms until death, today these terms are used to designate the toxicity of the illness and the tempo of disease progression. Patients with acute endocarditis experience marked constitutional symptoms and toxicity, and infection often progresses over days to cause valvular destruction and metastatic sites of infection. In contrast, those with subacute endocarditis experience mild toxicity and the illness evolves over weeks with more limited valve damage and rare instances of metastatic infection. *S. aureus* is the prototypic cause of acute endocarditis and viridans streptococci, enterococci, and the fastidious gram-negative coccobacilli that reside in the oral cavity and upper respiratory tract are the typical causes of the subacute presentation. It is more likely that the clinical presentations of endocarditis are a continuum with these presentations representing the ends of the spectrum. Similarly, although the microbial causes of endocarditis often cause a typical pattern of illness, a given organism can cause variable presentations ranging from acute to subacute.

## Etiology

The etiology of endocarditis can be considered in terms of the age of the infected patient (Table 66.1) or in terms of selected clinical settings which predispose to endocarditis (Table 66.2). The patients in these settings, in part, have unique age distributions which impact the age-related etiologic spectrum.

Endocarditis that occurs in children during the initial 2 mo of life is often the consequence of nosocomial infection, as is reflected in the spectrum of microbiologic causes. Occasional cases are caused by group B streptococci (*Streptococcus agalactiae*), an organism that is acquired during parturition and that frequently causes septicemia among neonates. Among older children viridans streptococci and *S. aureus* are the predominant organisms. These same organisms remain the major causes of endocarditis among adults, although enterococci become increasingly prominent as age increases beyond 60 yr.

Intravenous injection of drugs by addicts is associated with a high risk for endocarditis. *S. aureus* causes more than 50% of endocarditis occurring in intravenous drug abusers (IVDA) and more than 70% of those episodes which involve the right heart valves (Table 66.2). Viridans streptococci and enterococci primarily infect previously abnormal left heart valves in these patients as they do in non-IVDA. Lastly, intravenous injection of drugs is a major predisposition for polymicrobial endocarditis.

Nosocomial endocarditis is the consequence of intravascular device-related bacteremia in 45% to 65% of cases; genitourinary and gastrointestinal instrumentation and wound infections are other important sources for the initiating bacteremias in these cases. Central venous catheters and flow-directed pulmonary artery catheters have been associated with cryptic right-sided endocarditis. Endocarditis or other deep infections complicate 3% to 8% of *S. aureus* catheter-related bacteremias and 0.85% to 3% of nosocomial enterococcal bacteremias. A recent report notes that on transesophageal echocardiographic evaluation (TEE) of patients experiencing *S. aureus* catheter-related bacteremia, 16 of 69 (23%) had findings consistent with endocarditis. Among patients with a prosthetic valve, the risk of prosthetic valve endocarditis (PVE) as a consequence of nosocomial bacteremia may be 16%. Although the frequency of endocarditis as a consequence of nosocomial bacteremia is relatively low, the persistence of bacteremia for 3 or more days after removal of infected vascular devices and initiation of antibiotic treatment requires

**Table 66.1** Etiology of native valve endocarditis by age group of infected patients

| | Percent of cases | | | |
|---|---|---|---|---|
| | Children | | Adults | |
| Microorganism | Neonates | 2 mo–15 yr | 15–60 yr | >60 yr |
| STREPTOCOCCI | | | | |
| Viridans | | 40–47 | 45–65 | 30–45 |
| Group B | 15–20 | 3 | | |
| STAPHYLOCOCCI | | | | |
| *S. aureus* | 40–50 | 25 | 30–40 | 25–30 |
| Coagulase-negative | 10 | 5 | 3–5 | 5–8 |
| ENTEROCOCCI | | 4 | 5–8 | 15 |
| GRAM-NEGATIVE BACILLI | 10[a] | 5[b] | 4–8[b] | 5[b] |
| FUNGI | 10 | 1 | 1 | 1 |
| POLYMICROBIAL | 4 | | 1 | 1 |
| OTHER | | | 1 | 2 |
| CULTURE-NEGATIVE | 4 | 0–15 | 3–10 | 5 |

[a]Enterobacteriaceae.

[b]Predominantly *Hemophilus* species, *Actinobacillus actinomycetemcomitans*, *Cardiobacterium hominis*.

careful evaluation for endocarditis. Moreover, if the 23% rate of endocarditis among patients with *S. aureus* catheter-related bacteremia is confirmed, all patients experiencing this type of bacteremia should be assessed using TEE.

The microbiology of PVE reflects the nosocomial or community acquisition of infection which in turn is demonstrable in the time of onset of PVE after cardiac surgery (Table 66.2). More than 80% of the coagulase-negative staphylococci that cause PVE during the initial year after valve surgery are methicillin-resistant. This resistance pattern probably results from the nosocomial acquisition of these infections with delayed clinical onset accounting for cases between 2 and 12 mo. Less than 30% of co-

**Table 66.2** Microbiology of infective endocarditis developing in selected clinical settings*

| | Number of cases (%) | | | | | |
|---|---|---|---|---|---|---|
| | Intravenous drug abuse | | Prosthetic heart valves Time of onset after surgery | | | Nosocomial |
| Organisms | Right-sided (*N* = 346) | Left-sided (*N* = 204) | <2 mo (*N* = 73) | 2–12 mo (*N* = 38) | >12 mo (*N* = 94) | (*N* = 45) |
| *Staphylococcus aureus* | 265 (77) | 48 (23) | 10 (14) | 4 (11) | 12 (13) | 20 (44) |
| Coagulase-negative staphylococci | | | 28 (38) | 19 (50) | 14 (15) | 10 (22) |
| Streptococci | 19 (5) | 31 (15) | | | 31 (33) | 2 (4) |
| Enterococci | 6 (2) | 49 (24) | 5 (7) | | 10 (11) | 8 (18) |
| Gram-negative bacilli[a] | 18 (5) | 24 (12) | 8 (11) | 2 (5) | 1 (1) | 2 (4) |
| Fastidious gram-negative coccobacilli[b] | | | | 1 (3) | 11 (12) | |
| Diphtheroids | | | 9 (12) | 1 (3) | 2 (2) | |
| Fungi (*Candida* sp. primarily) | 0 | 25 (12) | 7 (10) | 2 (5) | 3 (3) | 2 (4) |
| Polymicrobial | 21 (6) | 14 (7) | | | | |
| Miscellaneous | 8 (2) | 6 (3) | 3 (4) | 2 (5) | 1 (1) | |
| Culture negative | 9 (3) | 7 (3) | 3 (4) | 4 (11) | 9 (10) | 1 (2) |

*Data from multiple sources documented in Karchmer, AW: "Infective Endocarditis." In: Heart Disease, 5th Edition, E. Braunwald (Ed.), Philadelphia: W.B. Saunders Co., 1997; pp. 1077–1103.

[a]Primarily *P. aeruginosa* and Enterobacteriaceae

[b]HACEK group (see text)

agulase-negative staphylococci causing PVE more than a year after valve implantation are methicillin-resistant. These cases are almost exclusively community acquired.

The microorganisms that frequently cause endocarditis share some biologic properties. In general they are relatively resistant to the complement-mediated bactericidal activity of serum and thus survive during bacteremia to reach the valve. They also possess extracellular carbohydrate surface elements that specifically facilitate adherence to the NBTE or valve endothelium. They also resist host defenses in the nascent infected vegetation, including platelet microbicidal proteins, and thus replicate to cause full endocarditis.

Viridans streptococci, which cause 30% to 65% of native valve endocarditis and late-onset PVE, are not a species but rather organisms from the oropharyngeal flora that are $\alpha$-hemolytic when grown on blood agar and nontypeable by the Lancefield method. These organisms are very susceptible to penicillin (the minimum inhibitory concentration (MIC) is $\leq 0.1$ $\mu$g penicillin/ml for $>80\%$) and are killed synergistically by penicillin plus gentamicin. The nutritionally variant viridans organisms, *Streptococcus adjacens* and *Streptococcus defectivus* (now included in the genus *Abiotrophia*) which cause 5% of streptococcal endocarditis, require media supplemented with pyridoxal hydrochloride or L-cysteine, and are more resistant to penicillin and penicillin-aminoglycoside synergy. *Streptococcus bovis*, which causes 25% of streptococcal endocarditis, is a component of gastrointestinal tract flora and when causing bacteremia or endocarditis is commonly associated with colonic polyps or malignancy. Although there is a superficial biochemical similarity between *S. bovis* and enterococci, *S. bovis* is highly susceptible to penicillin, as contrasted with the relative penicillin-resistance of enterococci. Lancefield groupable streptococci (groups A, B, C, G, and F) and *Streptococcus pneumoniae* cause endocarditis occasionally.

Enterococci, which are part of the gastrointestinal tract flora and cause occasional genitourinary tract infection, cause 5% to 15% of native valve and late-onset prosthetic valve endocarditis. *Enterococcus faecalis* and *Enterococcus faecium*, the predominant human pathogens in this genus, cause 85% and 10% of enterococcal endocarditis, respectively. Enterococci are resistant to cephalosporins, penicillinase-resistant penicillins, and therapeutic concentrations of aminoglycosides. Most strains are inhibited but not killed by the cell-wall active agents penicillin G, ampicillin, teicoplanin, and vancomycin, and can be killed by the synergistic interaction of one of these cell-wall active agents and either gentamicin or streptomycin. For clinically relevant bactericidal synergy to occur a strain must be able to be inhibited by achievable serum concentrations of one of the cell-wall active agents *and* must not have high-level resistance to the aminoglycoside (streptomycin MIC $\geq$ 2000 $\mu$g/ml or gentamicin MIC $\geq$ 500 to 2000 $\mu$g/ml). In very rare strains, synergy cannot be obtained with one of these aminoglycosides, even though high-level resistance to the aminoglycoside is not demonstrable. Emergence of enterococci with antibiotic resistance that precludes bactericidal synergy with some or all antibiotic combinations has increased the complexity of selecting therapy for patients with enterococcal endocarditis.

*Staphylococcus aureus* is a major etiologic agent of endocarditis in all settings. Over 90% of these organisms are resistant to penicillin G because of $\beta$-lactamase; the majority remain susceptible to penicillinase-resistant penicillins and first-generation cephalosporins. Strains which produce a penicillin-binding protein (called *2a* or *2'*) with decreased affinity for $\beta$-lactam antibiotics are resistant to methicillin and other available $\beta$-lactam antibiotics. Methicillin-resistant *S. aureus* (MRSA), which is an important cause of endocarditis that is acquired nosocomially or during intravenous drug abuse, is generally susceptible to vancomycin and teicoplanin.

Coagulase-negative staphylococci, an important cause of PVE, are implicated in 3% to 8% of cases involving native valves. Strains causing nosocomial PVE—that is, that which occurs in the year after valve implantation, are usually *S. epidermidis*, while nonepidermidis strains cause almost 50% of later-onset, community acquired cases. Place of acquisition has a similar impact upon the distribution of species of coagulase-negative staphylococci that cause native valve endocarditis. While coagulase-negative staphylococcal endocarditis generally presents in a subacute manner, *Staphyloccus lugdunensis* may cause an infection with systemic toxicity and frequent valve destruction that resembles *S. aureus* endocarditis.

Fastidious gram-negative coccobacilli, which are part of the upper respiratory tract and oropharyngeal flora, cause 5% to 10% of native valve and late-onset prosthetic valve endocarditis. These organisms, called the HACEK group, include *Hemophilus aphrophilus*, *Hemophilus parainfluenzae*, *Actinobacillus actinomycetemcomitans*, *Cardiobacterium hominis*, *Eikenella corrodens*, and *Kingella* species. Most strains are susceptible to ampicillin, aminoglycosides, quinolones, and third-generation cephalosporins. A few strains, however, produce $\beta$-lactamase and are resistant to penicillin G and ampicillin. *Pseudomonas aeruginosa*, Enterobacteriaceae (including *Salmonella* species and *Serratia marcescens*), *Neisseria gonorrheae*, and *Brucella* species cause endocarditis occasionally.

*Corynebacterium* species, called *diphtheroids*, infect prosthetic valves and infrequently also cause cases of native valve endocarditis. Recently, by using special blood culture techniques and serologic tests, *Bartonella quintana* and *Bartonella henselae* have been recognized as causes of subacute endocarditis in cases that otherwise would have remained culture negative. As many as 3% of cases of endocarditis may be caused by *Bartonella* species. The rickettsia *Coxiella burnetii*, which causes Q fever, is an important cause of endocarditis in Europe and the United Kingdom. *Candida* species and *Aspergillus* species are the major causes of fungal endocarditis.

Blood cultures remain negative in 3% to 14% of patients with clinically diagnosed endocarditis. In 35% to 50% of patients with culture-negative endocarditis, the failure to isolate an organism from blood can be attributed to recent antibiotic therapy. Other patients are infected with fastidious organisms which are difficult to isolate from blood (*Bartonella*, *Brucella*, nutritionally variant streptococci, some HACEK organisms, *Legionella* species), with organisms that are frequently not isolated from blood (fungi, *Aspergillus* species), and with organisms that are detected by serologic tests (*Coxiella burnetii*, *Chlamydia* species).

## Epidemiology and Host Factors

The overall incidence of endocarditis, which is similar in developed and developing countries, ranges from 1.7 to 4.2 cases/100,000 person yr and increases steadily after 30 yr of age. It exceeds 15 cases/100,000 person yr after 60 yr of age. Rheumatic heart disease, congenital heart disease, mitral valve prolapse, degenerative valve disease, asymmetric septal hypertrophy, and IVDA are noted as predisposing conditions in 55% to 75% of patients with native valve endocarditis. Prosthetic valves are infected in from 7% to 25% of endocarditis cases. Rheumatic heart disease, a major predisposing condition in developing countries, is less frequently encountered as a predisposition in developed countries. Neonatal endocarditis is frequently nosocomial. Endocarditis developing later in childhood is often community acquired and occurs in the setting of congenital aortic valve disease, ventricular septal defect, tetralogy of Fallot, or complex cyanotic heart disease, often after partial surgical correction. Mitral valve prolapse with associated regurgitation also predisposes to endocarditis in later childhood. Among adults, mitral valve prolapse with a murmur of mitral regurgitation is associated with 3.5 to 8.2 times increased risk for endocarditis. In the absence of audible mitral regurgitation the risk of endocarditis involving a prolapsed valve is reduced by a factor of ten. The risk of endocarditis among IVDA is estimated to be severalfold higher than that noted for patients with rheumatic heart disease or prosthetic valves. The cumulative incidence of PVE in four large studies ranges from 1.4% to 3.1% at 12 mo, 4.1% to 5.4% at 4 yr, and 3.2% to 5.7% at 60 mo. The risk of PVE is not uniform over time. It is greatest in the first 6 mo after valve surgery. With the exception of IVDA, the currently prominent endocarditis predispositions in developed countries occur with increased frequency as patients age. Not surprisingly, the median age of patients with endocarditis in developed countries has gradually increased from 30 to 40 yr in the preantibiotic and early antibiotic eras to 47 to 64 yr in recent decades.

## Clinical Manifestations

The clinical manifestations of endocarditis (Table 66.3) are the consequence of (*1*) intracardiac tissue destruction due to infection; (*2*) embolization of infected or bland material from vegetations; (*3*) bacteremic seeding of remote sites; and (*4*) immune tissue injury due to deposition of antigen–antibody complexes and local complement activation. In addition, constitutional symptoms are the result of the bacteremia itself.

Fever, the most common symptom and sign among patients with endocarditis, may be minimal or absent in the very elderly, those with chronic renal failure, and occasionally in those with heart failure. Among patients with a subacute presentation, fever is low grade (usually ≤39.4°C), intermittent, and not associated with rigors. This contrasts with the higher temperature and chills noted with acute endocarditis.

Murmurs, which are ultimately heard in 80% to 85% of patients, may be difficult to hear in those with tricuspid endocarditis and may develop late in the course of *S. aureus* endocarditis. Changing or new murmurs, not related to increased heart rate or cardiac output, are most likely noted in patients with acute disease or PVE and result from damage to valve leaflets, ruptured chordae tendinae, intracardiac fistulae, or dehiscence or dysfunction of a prosthetic valve.

The peripheral manifestations of endocarditis, which include Osler's nodes, splinter hemorrhages, petechiae, Janeway lesions, and Roth spots, are associated with prolonged courses of untreated endocarditis. As a consequence of early diagnosis and effective treatment, these manifestations are found infrequently. Additionally, they are not seen among patients with infection restricted to right heart valves. These findings are not pathognomonic for endocarditis. Splinter or subungual hemorrhages in the distal nail bed are likely the result of trauma as contrasted with the more proximal lesions. Roth spots, oval retinal hemorrhages with pale centers, are also seen with severe anemia or collagen vascular disease. Splenomegaly, another manifestation associated with prolonged infection, is seen in 15%–50% of endocarditis patients.

Musculoskeletal symptoms, including back pain, are not uncommon. These symptoms must be distinguished from the occasional episode of hematogenous skeletal infection, especially since the latter may require specific therapy.

Systemic emboli, which may be the presenting clinical event, are a common complication of endocarditis and may lead to local infarction or focal infection of various organs. Clinical findings are unique to the organ involved. A splenic embolus may cause left upper quadrant pain, left shoulder pain, and a pleural effusion. In contrast, emboli to the mesenteric vasculature may cause abdominal pain, ileus, and gastrointestinal bleeding. Splenic abscess formation, which occurs in 3% to 5% of patients with endocarditis, is clinically indistinguishable from splenic infarction. The frequency of emboli decreases rapidly with effective antimicrobial treatment.

Valve destruction, rupture of chordae tendineae, or dehiscence or dysfunction of prosthetic valves not only alters ausculatory findings but, if hemodynamically significant, also causes congestive heart failure. Infection which extends beyond the valve

**Table 66.3** The clinical manifestations of endocarditis

| Symptoms | % | Signs | % |
|---|---|---|---|
| Fever | 85 | Fever | 90 |
| Rigors | 45–75 | Murmur | 80–85 |
| Anorexia | 25–55 | New/changing murmur | 10–40 |
| Weight loss | 25–35 | Neurologic abnormalities | 30–40 |
| Malaise/fatigue | 25–40 | Arterial emboli | 20–40 |
| Dyspnea | 20–40 | Splenomegaly | 15–50 |
| Cough | 25 | Osler's nodes | 5–10 |
| Headache | 15–40 | Splinter hemorrhages | 5–15 |
| Myalgias/arthralgias | 15–30 | Petechiae | 10–40 |
| Chest pain | 10–35 | Janeway lesions | 5–10 |
| Abdominal pain | 5–15 | Roth spots | 5–10 |
| Back pain | 5–10 | | |

into the annulus and adjacent tissues occurs in 10% to 15% of patients with native valve infection and 45% to 60% of those with PVE. Invasive infection, which occurs most commonly with aortic valve infection, may be clinically silent or may present as persistent fever during appropriate antibiotic therapy, new abnormal cardiac rhythms, electrocardiographic conduction abnormalities, or evidence of pericarditis. Invasive infection, especially at an aortic site, is often associated with valve or prosthesis dysfunction. Renal dysfunction may occur as a consequence of deteriorated hemodynamics. In 15% of patients, diffuse immune-complex-mediated glomerulonephritis results in azotemia. This complication is usually noted early after diagnosis and initiation of therapy. It generally improves with effective antibiotic treatment.

Symptoms and signs of central nervous system injury occur in 30% to 40% of patients with endocarditis and are associated with increased mortality. Embolic stroke is the most common neurologic complication. Intracranial hemorrhage resulting from rupture of a mycotic aneurysm or hemorrhage into an infarct occurs in 5% of patients. Bacterial cerebritis and microabscess formation complicate acute endocarditis, especially that caused by *S. aureus*, and may be accompanied by a cerebrospinal fluid pleocytosis with polymorphonuclear leukocytes as the predominant cell type. More often the cerebrospinal fluid in subacute endocarditis has an aseptic profile. Occasional patients experience headaches, seizures, or confusion.

## Laboratory Studies

Many laboratory studies obtained from patients with active untreated endocarditis are abnormal, but only the direct culture and histological examination of the vegetation provide a definite diagnosis. That many tests are abnormal is not unexpected given the systemic aspects of the infection and the many potential extracardiac complications.

Blood cultures are the most important test to obtain in the evaluation of a patient with suspected endocarditis. Because bacteremia in patients with endocarditis is continuous, cultures can be drawn at any time. Organisms are isolated with similar frequency from venous and arterial blood. In patients who have not received antibiotics previously and who are not infected by an unusually fastidious organism, it is likely that blood cultures will be positive in virtually all patients, that the first or second culture will be positive in more than 98% of patients, and that ultimately multiple cultures (the majority of those obtained) will be positive. In fact, almost half of the 3% to 14% of patients with endocarditis reported to be blood culture-negative can be attributed to the administration of antibiotics prior to obtaining cultures. In the remainder of patients with culture-negative endocarditis, infection is caused by fastidious organisms or those not recoverable in broth media.

Three or four sets of blood cultures from separate venipunctures should be obtained over 24 h. For each set at least 10 ml of blood should be inoculated into an aerobic and anaerobic (thioglycollate broth) bottle. Cultures should be incubated for a minimum of 21 d and then be subcultured to solid media before being termed sterile (negative). Special subculture media and culture techniques are required when highly fastidious organisms are sought, and lysis-centrifugation blood cultures should be obtained if fungal endocarditis is suspected. When blood cultures are negative, serologic tests (antibody to *Legionella*, *Bartonella*, *C. burnetii*, *Brucella*, *Chlamydia* species) or antigen detection tests (cryptococci, histoplasma) may be helpful. If patients with blood-culture-negative endocarditis undergo valve replacement surgery, special studies of the resected vegetation should be performed. These include culture, routine microscopy, and fluorescent antibody staining for suspected pathogens. Polymerase chain reaction (PCR) to amplify the bacterial gene encoding 16S ribosomal RNA with subsequent sequencing of this gene and tracing of its bacterial origin have allowed an etiologic diagnosis of endocarditis from culture-negative vegetations.

Normochromic normocytic anemia, a mild leukocytosis, and an elevated erythrocyte sedimentation rate (average approximately 55 mm/h) are typically noted in subacute endocarditis. In patients with acute endocarditis the leukocytosis is more marked. High serum concentrations of circulating immune complexes are noted in patients with endocarditis that has persisted for longer periods. Rheumatoid factor is detected in the serum of 50% of patients who have been ill for 6 wk or more. In addition, other tests that reflect immune stimulation are abnormal (quantitative immune globulins, cryoglobulins, and C-reactive protein). The urine analysis reveals proteinuria and hematuria in 50% of patients, even when renal function remains normal. Studies evaluating specific organ systems may be abnormal if that system is involved by an extracardiac complication of endocarditis. For example, increased creatinine, blood urea nitrogen, and an active urine sediment are noted in patients with diffuse immune-complex-mediated glomerulonephritis. In 75% of patients with tricuspid valve endocarditis, chest roentgenograms will reveal abnormalities consistent with septic emboli.

Echocardiography, while not a sensitive screening test for endocarditis in unselected patients with positive blood cultures or unexplained fever, is a very sensitive and specific test in patients with active endocarditis. This test can provide not only anatomic evidence of the diagnosis but can also define intracardiac complications as well as the hemodynamic function of the heart. Transthoracic echocardiography (TTE) can adequately image the aortic and mitral valves in many patients with native valve endocarditis; nevertheless, transesophageal echocardiography (TEE) using biplane technology with color flow and continuous as well as pulsed Doppler is optimal. TEE allows very small vegetations to be imaged and is the procedure of choice for assessing the pulmonic valve, prosthetic valves (especially in the mitral position), and the perivalvular areas for abscesses. In patients with proven native valve endocarditis, the sensitivity of TEE for detection of vegetations ranges from 90% to 100% while that of TTE ranges from 58% to 65%. Among patients with PVE the sensitivity of TEE in detecting vegetation ranges from 82% to 96% while that of TTE is 16% to 36%. The sensitivity of TEE in detecting vegetations in patients with suspected endocarditis is 82% to 94% and increases if repeat studies are performed. Even with repeat TEE, persisting false-negative studies are noted in 4% to 13% of patients. Thus, TEE is useful to confirm the diagnosis in highly suspect patients and to exclude the diagnosis of endocarditis when the clinical suspicion is not high.

The detection of an apparent vegetation in a patient does not prove the diagnosis of endocarditis. Infected vegetations cannot be reliably distinguished from those that are the sterile residua of previously treated endocarditis, a marantic vegetation, or the NBTE associated with the antiphospholipid antibody syndrome. Additionally, thickened valves, valve calcifications, and ruptured chordae may be mistaken for vegetations. The evolution of vegetations on repeat echocardiogram after effective antimicrobial therapy is highly variable; in 3 wk to 3 mo after initiation of therapy 30% will have disappeared, 40% remain unchanged, 20% are smaller, and 10% are larger. Thus, in the context of effective antibiotic therapy, changes in vegetation size should be interpreted with caution. In contrast, when antimicrobial therapy appears ineffective, increasing vegetation size may serve to confirm that impression.

TEE is more sensitive and specific than TTE for detection of myocardial and perivalvular abscesses. The sensitivity and specificity for abscess identification were 28% and 98% for TTE compared with 87% and 95% for TEE. Multiple studies suggest that patients with a vegetation larger than 10 mm in greatest dimension are more likely to experience embolic events than are those with smaller vegetations. Although some studies propose echocardiographic vegetation criteria that indicate a high risk for failure of antimicrobial therapy and a need for surgery, these criteria are not sufficiently definitive. Decisions regarding surgical intervention as treatment of endocarditis require the integration of all echocardiographic findings and clinical events.

In patients with endocarditis the electrocardiogram may reveal nonspecific changes and rhythm disturbances. New-onset, persistent conduction system delays, especially in the context of aortic valve endocarditis, may indicate invasive infection. The sensitivity of the conduction abnormalities in detecting abscesses is 28%.

Magnetic resonance imaging is an effective technique with which to image paravalvular extension of infection and fistulous track formation. This technique has not shown more sensitivity than state-of-the-art TEE, however, Scintography is not a sufficiently sensitive technique for reliable imaging of vegetations or intracardiac abscesses.

## Diagnosis

The presentation of patients with endocarditis, whether the infection is acute or subacute, combines constitutional symptoms with localized signs and symptoms. Many of these represent complications of endocarditis rather than the endocardial infection itself. The auscultatory, hemodynamic, and cardiac rhythm findings may be the only direct manifestations of the endocardial infection. On occasion these direct manifestations of endocarditis may be absent or obscure. Consequently, the diagnosis of endocarditis must be considered when a patient presents with fever and one or more of the extracardiac features of endocarditis: persistent bacteremia, embolic phenomena, immune-complex-mediated disease. The occurrence of fever alone in a patient with an underlying cardiac valve lesion or a behavior pattern recognized to predispose to endocarditis raises the possibility of endocarditis. However, in patients with a heart murmur, the occurrence of other illnesses with fever may produce signs and symptoms that superficially mimic endocarditis. Other illnesses where fever and a heart murmur occur simultaneously may mimic culture-negative endocarditis: acute rheumatic fever, marantic endocarditis, systemic lupus erythematosus, carcinoid syndrome, antiphospholipid antibody syndrome, and atrial myxoma. Because of the varied clinical findings in endocarditis, positive blood cultures or positive cultures (or histopathology) from the vegetation are required to establish a definitive diagnosis. Occasionally serologic tests can be used to suggest the etiologic cause of endocarditis. Multiple positive blood cultures (evidence of a high-grade, persistent bacteremia) alone may serve as a clue to intravascular or endocardial infection, particularly when the organism recovered is one commonly associated with endocarditis or when focal infection giving rise to bacteremia is not evident.

Diagnostic criteria have been developed which embody the pathogenetic concepts of endocarditis, including microorganisms commonly associated with this infection, acute endothelial disease, embolic phenomena, and immune-mediated injury. (Tables 66.4, 66.5). When these criteria are used to assess the entire diagnostic evaluation, they provide a sensitive and specific approach to the diagnosis of endocarditis. Patients who, according to these criteria, have definite or possible endocarditis should be treated for endocarditis. Blood cultures yielding organisms that are either not typically associated with the infection or that are common contaminants must be positive persistently to support the diagnosis of endocarditis. Echocardiographic evidence of an endocardial process (vegetation) strengthens the diagnosis. However, a negative TEE, in spite of the sensitivity of the test, does not rule out endocarditis. The false-negative rate for TEE ranges from 6% to 18% and even with repeat examinations from 4% to 13%. Thus, echocardiography helps exclude the diagnosis of endocarditis only when the index of suspicion is low.

## Treatment

To effectively treat endocarditis therapy must eradicate the infecting organism as well as address complications such as valve rupture or abscess formation, hemodynamic deterioration, or focal extracardiac complications. This requires antimicrobial therapy which may need to be coupled with additional treatment including cardiac surgery. The selection of antimicrobial therapy is guided by the in vitro susceptibility of the causative microorganism and insights into treatment gained from experimental animal models and clinical studies of endocarditis caused by similar organisms. Unique characteristics of the infected vegetation are important determinants in achieving effective antimicrobial therapy. The vegetation is relatively devoid of host defenses. Consequently, the eradication of organisms is solely a function of antibiotic activity which must be bactericidal to be effective. However, bacteria in vegetations may reach densities of $10^9$ to $10^{10}$ organisms/g and become metabolically dormant and somewhat resistant to the bactericidal activity of $\beta$-lactam and glycopeptide antibiotics. Furthermore, antibiotics reach the deeper regions of avascular vegetations by passive diffusion. As a result, relatively high serum concentrations are required to insure that bactericidal vegetation levels are achieved. These considerations and clinical experience suggest that therapy must be bactericidal and should be delivered parenterally over relatively prolonged periods.

The bactericidal potency of antibiotics is estimated by measuring the minimum inhibitory concentration (MIC) and minimum bactericidal concentration (MBC) for an organism. The MIC is the lowest concentration that inhibits growth and the MBC is the lowest concentration that kills 99.9% of a standard inoculum during 24 h. The MIC and MBC of an antibiotic for an organism are usually the same or only differ by a factor of two or four. Occasionally the difference in the MIC and MBC of an organism for a $\beta$-lactam or glycopeptide antibiotic is tenfold or more. This phenomenon, which is called "tolerance," primarily reflects the slower killing of tolerant versus nontolerant strains. With a longer incubation time (48 h) these large differences in the MIC and MBC of tolerant organisms are eliminated. In clinical studies, the demonstration of tolerance in streptococci or staphylococci causing endocarditis has not been associated

**Table 66.4** Diagnostic criteria for infective endocarditis*

| |
|---|
| DEFINITIVE INFECTIVE ENDOCARDITIS |
| *PATHOLOGIC CRITERIA* |
| Microorganisms: demonstrated by culture or histology in a vegetation, *or* in a vegetation that has embolized, *or* in an intracardiac abscess, *or* |
| Pathologic lesions: vegetation or intracardiac abscess present, confirmed by histology showing active endocarditis |
| *CLINICAL CRITERIA, USING SPECIFIC DEFINITIONS LISTED IN TABLE 66.5* |
| 2 major criteria, *or* |
| 1 major and 3 minor criteria, *or* |
| 5 minor criteria |
| POSSIBLE INFECTIVE ENDOCARDITIS |
| Findings consistent with infective endocarditis that fall short of definite endocarditis but are not rejected |
| REJECTED |
| Firm alternative diagnosis accounting for manifestations of endocarditis, *or* |
| Sustained resolution of manifestations of endocarditis, with antibiotic therapy for 4 d or less, *or* |
| No pathologic evidence of infective endocarditis at surgery or autopsy, after antibiotic therapy for 4 d or less |

*Adapted from Durack DT, Lukes AS, Bright DK, and Duke Endocarditis Service. Am J Med 1994; 96:200–209, with permission.

with less than optimal response to treatment with penicillins, cephalosporins, or vancomycin. Consequently, the clinical relevance of tolerance has been questioned and the MIC of an organism, not the MBC, is used to plan treatment. Enterococci represent an exception since each strain has widely disparate MIC and MBC for penicillins and glycopeptides. Furthermore, enterococci are not killed by these antibiotics even with prolonged incubation. To kill enterococci, in fact, requires the combined ef-

**Table 66.5** Terminology used in the diagnosis of infective endocarditis*

| |
|---|
| MAJOR CRITERIA |
| *POSITIVE BLOOD CULTURE* |
| Typical microorganism for infective endocarditis from two separate blood cultures<br>(i) Viridans streptococci, *Streptococcus bovis*, HACEK group, *or*<br>(ii) Community-acquired *Staphylococcus aureus* or enterococci, in the absence of a primary focus, *or* |
| Persistently positive blood culture, defined as recovery of a microorganism consistent with infective endocarditis from:<br>(i) Blood cultures drawn more than 12 h apart, *or*<br>(ii) All of three or a majority of four or more separate blood cultures, with first and last drawn at least 1 h apart |
| *EVIDENCE OF ENDOCARDIAL INVOLVEMENT* |
| Positive echocardiogram<br>(i) Oscillating intracardiac mass, on valve or supporting structures, *or* in the path of regurgitant jets, *or* on implanted material, in the absence of an alternative anatomic explanation, *or*<br>(ii) Abscess, *or*<br>(iii) New partial dehiscence of prosthetic valve, *or* |
| New valvular regurgitation (increase or change in preexisting murmur not sufficient) |
| MINOR CRITERIA |
| Predisposition: predisposing heart condition *or* intravenous drug use |
| Fever ≥ 38.0°C (100.4°F) |
| Vascular phenomena: major arterial emboli, septic pulmonary infarcts, mycotic aneurysm, intracranial hemorrhage, conjunctival hemorrhages, Janeway lesions |
| Immunologic phenomena: glomerulonephritis, Osler's nodes, Roth spots, rheumatoid factor |
| Microbiologic evidence: positive blood culture but not meeting major criterion as noted previously[a] *or* serologic evidence of active infection with organism consistent with infective endocarditis |
| Echocardiogram: consistent with infective endocarditis but not meeting major criterion |

*Adapted from Durack DT, Lukes AS, Bright DK, and Duke Endocarditis Service, Am J Med 1994; 96:200–209, with permission.

[a]Excluding single positive cultures for coagulase-negative staphylococci and organisms that rarely cause endocarditis.

fect of an effective penicillin or glycopeptide plus an aminoglycoside to which the organism does not have high-level resistance. The enhanced antibacterial effect of the combination which results in killing is called *synergy* or a *synergistic bactericidal effect.* As a result of the relative resistance to antibiotics among enterococci, antibiotic combinations are required for optimal treatment of enterococcal endocarditis.

## Antimicrobial regimens

In selecting specific antimicrobial therapy for a patient with endocarditis, the potential for adverse reactions must be minimized. Doses of some agents must be adjusted for renal dysfunction. Similar antimicrobial regimens are recommended for treatment of native valve or prosthetic valve endocarditis caused by the same organism, with the exception of endocarditis caused by staphylococci. The duration of therapy for PVE, however, is generally longer than that for native valve infection.

### Streptococcal endocarditis

Four regimens are recommended for the treatment of patients with endocarditis caused by penicillin-susceptible (MIC $\leq$ 0.1 $\mu$g/ml) viridans streptococci or *S. bovis* (Table 66.6:1A–D). Bacteriologic cure rates with the penicillin G regimens exceed 98% among patients who complete therapy. Although clinical experience with the ceftriaxone and vancomycin regimens is more limited, similar cure rates have been noted. High cure rates with the 2-wk regimen are possible because of the bactericidal synergy that results from the penicillin–gentamicin combination. Although similar synergy usually results from combination therapy with penicillin and streptomycin, from 2% to 8% of viridans streptococci and *S. bovis* possess high-level resistance to streptomycin (MIC $\geq$ 2000 $\mu$g/ml) and are not killed synergistically with this combination. Consequently, streptomycin should not be substituted for gentamicin in this regimen (Table 66.6:1B) unless the absence of high-level streptomycin resistance in the causative strain has been proven. Teicoplanin has been used to effectively treat streptococcal endocarditis; however, published experience is limited. For patients with PVE caused by penicillin-susceptible streptococci, 6 wk of penicillin G with gentamicin during the initial 2 wk is recommended (Table 66.6:2A).

Patients with endocarditis caused by viridans streptococci with MICs ranging from $\geq$0.2 to $<$0.5 $\mu$g/ml have been cured with penicillin alone; nevertheless, combination therapy is generally recommended (Table 66.6:2A). Endocarditis caused by more penicillin-resistant streptococcal strains (MIC $>$ 0.5 $\mu$g/ml) and the nutritionally variant streptococci, *S. adjacens* and *S. defectivus*, are treated with the regimens recommended for therapy of enterococcal endocarditis (Table 66.6:3A or B). Endocarditis caused by Lancefield group G, C, or B streptococci appears to be associated with increased morbidity and mortality; accordingly combination therapy is recommended for patients with these forms of endocarditis (Table 66.6:2A).

For treatment of streptococcal endocarditis in patients who have had an urticarial or anaphylactic reaction to a penicillin or cephalosporin, vancomycin is recommended (Table 66.6:1D, 2B). Teicoplanin could be used as well. Among patients with milder forms of penicillin allergy (delayed maculopapular skin rash), ceftriaxone can be used cautiously to treat infection caused by penicillin-susceptible strains (Table 66.6:1C) or can be combined with gentamicin when strains are more resistant to penicillin (MIC $\geq$ 0.2 to $<$0.5 $\mu$g/ml). Penicillin-allergic patients with endocarditis caused by highly penicillin resistant strains (MIC $\geq$ 0.5 $\mu$g/ml) can be treated with ceftriaxone plus gentamicin, both for 4 to 6 wk, or with vancomycin plus gentamicin (Table 66.6:3C) as required by the severity of the allergic history.

### Enterococcal endocarditis

Three regimens designed to provide synergistic bactericidal therapy are recommended for treatment of enterococcal endocarditis (Table 66.6:3A–C). Treatment for 4 wk is generally adequate, although therapy for 6 wk is used in patients who have been symptomatic for 3 mo or more or who do not respond promptly after initiating therapy. These regimens result in cure rates of approximately 85% if the infecting organism does not have resistance that precludes synergy (see Etiology and Table 66.7). Higher doses of gentamicin (1.5 mg/kg every 8 h) are preferred in these regimens by some authorities. Also, streptomycin (9.5 mg/kg IM or IV every 12 h to achieve peak serum concentrations of 20 $\mu$g/ml) can be used instead of gentamicin if the strain does not possess high-level resistance to streptomycin. For patients allergic to penicillin, the vancomycin-gentamicin regimen is recommended (Table 66.6:3C) or a penicillin regimen can be used after appropriate desensitization. Teicoplanin is more active in vitro than vancomycin against enterococci. Limited clinical and laboratory data suggest it could be used in combination with an aminoglycoside in the treatment of enterococcal endocarditis. Cephalosporins combined with aminoglycosides do not result in bactericidal synergy and are not used in the treatment of enterococcal endocarditis.

Resistance to penicillin, ampicillin, vancomycin, teicoplanin, and the aminoglycosides sufficient to preclude bactericidal synergism, and in some instances even an inhibitory antibacterial effect, is increasingly being found among *E. faecalis* and *E. faecium.* As a result, it cannot be assumed that standard regimens for treatment of endocarditis (Table 66.6:3A–C) will provide synergistic therapy. The infecting strain must be tested in vitro so that the optimum standard or an alternate regimen can be identified (Table 66.7). Synergy requires the combination of an effective cell-wall active agent (penicillin, ampicillin, vancomycin, or teicoplanin) and an aminoglycoside (gentamicin or streptomycin) to which there is no high-level resistance. High-level resistance to gentamicin predicts loss of synergy for all other aminoglycosides except streptomycin. Organisms must be tested specifically for high-level resistance to streptomycin. If the strain possesses high-level resistance to gentamicin and streptomycin, synergistic therapy is not possible and a prolonged course (12 wk) of an effective cell wall agent is recommended. The cure rate with nonsynergistic therapy is 40%. Patients failing this therapy may benefit from excision and replacement of the infected valve (Table 66.7).

### Staphylococcal native valve endocarditis

A semisynthetic penicillinase-resistant penicillin is recommended for the treatment of endocarditis caused by methicillin-susceptible staphylococci (Table 66.6:4A). When treating patients who have a history of a penicillin allergy that is not associated with urticaria or anaphylaxis, a first-generation cephalosporin regimen may be used (Table 66.6:4B). Vancomycin is used when the history suggests that a penicillin or cephalosporin has caused an anaphylactic reaction. In an attempt to enhance $\beta$-lactam antibiotic therapy, the addition of gentamicin to the regimen

**Table 66.6** Antibiotic regimens for endocarditis caused by selected organisms*

| Infecting organism | Antibiotic | Dose and route[a] | Duration (wk) | Comments |
|---|---|---|---|---|
| 1. Penicillin-susceptible Viridans streptococci, *Streptococcus bovis*, and other streptococci (penicillin MIC ≤ 0.1 μg/ml) | A. Penicillin G | 12–18 million units IV daily either continuously or in equally divided doses q 4 h | 4 | |
| | B. Penicillin G plus | 12–18 million units IV daily continuously or in equally divided doses q 4 h | 2 | Avoid aminoglycoside containing regimen when potential for nephrotoxicity or ototoxicity is increased |
| | Gentamicin | 1 mg/kg IM or IV q 8 h | 2 | |
| | C. Ceftriaxone | 2 g IV or IM daily as single dose | 4 | Can be used in patients with nonanaphylactic, nonurticarial penicillin allergy; intramuscular ceftriaxone is painful |
| | D. Vancomycin[c] | 30 mg/kg IV daily in equally divided doses q 12 h | 4 | Use for patients with urticarial or anaphylactic penicillin or cephalosporin allergy |
| 2. Relatively penicillin-resistant streptococci (Penicillin MIC ≥ 0.2 to <0.5 μg/ml) | A. Penicillin G plus | 18–24 million units IV daily continuously or in equally divided doses q 4 h | 4 | |
| | Gentamicin | 1 mg/kg IM or IV q 8 h | 2 | |
| | B. Vancomycin[c] | See dose in regimen 1D | 4 | Use for treating penicillin allergic patients |
| 3. Enterococci—in vitro evaluation for susceptibility to ampicillin, penicillin, vancomycin, and teicoplanin; β-lactamase production; and high-level resistance to gentamicin and streptomycin required (see Table 66.7 and text for regimens used to treat markedly resistant strains) | A. Penicillin G plus | 18–30 million units IV daily continuously or in equally divided doses q 4 h | 4–6 | See text for use of streptomycin instead of gentamicin in these regimens. Four weeks of therapy recommended for patients with <3 mo of illness who respond promptly to treatment. Treatment for endocarditis caused by relatively penicillin resistant (MIC ≥ 0.5 μg/ml), *S. adjacens* and *S. defectivus* |
| | Gentamicin | 1 mg/kg IM or IV every 8 h | 4–6 | |
| | B. Ampicillin plus | 12 q IV daily continuously or in equally divided doses q 4 h | 4–6 | |
| | gentamicin | Same dose as regimen 3A | 4–6 | |
| | C. Vancomycin[c] plus | 30 mg/kg IV daily in divided doses q 12 h | 4–6 | Use for patients with penicillin allergy. Do not use cephalosporins |
| | gentamicin | Same dose as regimen 3A | 4–6 | |
| 4. Staphylococci infecting native valves (assume penicillin resistance); methicillin-susceptible | A. Nafcillin or oxacillin plus optional addition of | 12 q IV daily in divided doses q 4 h | 4–6 | Penicillin—18–24 million units daily in divided doses q 4 h can be used instead of nafcillin, oxacillin, or cefazolin if strains do not produce β-lactamase |
| | gentamicin | Same dose as regimen 3A | 3–5 d | |
| | B. Cefazolin plus optional addition of | 2 g IV q 8 h | 4–6 | Cephalothin or other first-generation cephalosporin in equivalent doses can be used; this regimen can be used for patient with nonanaphylactic penicillin allergy |
| | gentamicin | Same dose as regimen 3A | 3–5 d | |
| | C. Vancomycin[c] | 30 mg/kg IV in divided doses q 12 h | 4–6 | Use for patients with urticarial or anaphylactic reaction to penicillin or cephalosporin |
| 5. Staphylococci infecting native valves; methicillin-resistant | Vancomycin[c] | 30 mg/kg IV in divided doses q 12 h | 4–6 | |

(*continued*)

**Table 66.6** Antibiotic regimens for endocarditis caused by selected organisms* —*Continued*

| Infecting organism | Antibiotic | Dose and route[a] | Duration (wk) | Comments |
|---|---|---|---|---|
| 6. Staphylococci infecting prosthetic valves; methicillin-susceptible (assume penicillin resistance) | Nafcillin or oxacillin<br>plus<br>gentamicin<br>plus<br>rifampin[d] | 12 g IV daily in divided doses q 4 h<br><br>1 mg/kg IV or IM q 8 h<br><br>300 mg p.o. q 8 h | ≥6<br><br>2<br><br>≥6 | First-generation cephalosporin or vancomycin could be used in patients with nonanaphylactic penicillin reaction. Use gentamicin during initial 2 wk. See text for alternates for gentamicin. For patients with immediate penicillin allergy, use regimen 7 |
| 7. Staphylococci infecting prosthetic valves; methicillin-resistant | Vancomycin[c]<br>plus<br>gentamicin<br>plus<br>rifampin[d] | 30 mg/kg IV in divided doses q 12 h<br><br>1 mg/kg IV or IM q 8 h<br><br>300 mg p.o. q 8 h | ≥6<br><br>2<br><br>≥6 | Use gentamicin during the initial 2 wk of therapy. See text for alternatives to gentamicin. Do not substitute a cephalosporin or imipenem for vancomycin |
| 8. HACEK organisms[b] | A. Ceftriaxone | 2 g IV or IM daily as a single dose | 4 | Cefotaxime or other third-generation cephalosporin in comparable doses may be used |
| | B. Ampicillin<br>plus<br>gentamicin | 12 q IV daily continuously or in equally divided doses q 4 h<br>1 mg/kg IV or IM q 8 h | 4<br><br>4 | Test organism for $\beta$-lactamase production. Donot use this regimen if $\beta$-lactamase is produced |

*Adapted from Wilson WR, Karchmer AW, Bisno AL, et al., Antibiotic Treatment of Adults with Infective Endocarditis Due to Viridans Streptococci, Enterococci, Other Streptococci, and HACEK Microorganisms. JAMA 1995; 274:1706–1713.

[a]Recommended doses are for adults with normal renal and hepatic function. Doses of gentamicin, streptomycin, and vancomycin must be adjusted in patients with renal dysfunction. Use ideal body weight to calculate doses (men = 50 kg + 2.3 kg per inch over 5 feet; women = 45.5 kg plus 2.3 kg per inch over 5 feet).

[b]HACEK organisms include *Hemophilus parainfluenzae, Hemophilus aphrophilus, Actinobacillus actinomycetemcomitans, Cardiobacterium hominis, Eikenella corrodens, Kingella kingii.*

[c]Peak levels obtained 1 h after completion of the infusion should be 30 to 45 $\mu$g/ml; doses greater than 2 g/24 h should not be used unless serum concentration is monitored. Infuse over 1 h to avoid histamine-release reaction.

[d]Rifampin increases the dose of warfarin or dicumarol required for effective anticoagulation.

during the initial 3 to 5 d of treatment has been suggested (Table 66.6:4A,B). Longer periods of aminoglycoside therapy have resulted in renal dysfunction and consequently are not recommended. The combination of a $\beta$-lactam and an aminoglycoside results in enhanced killing of staphylococci in vitro; nevertheless, combination therapy has not resulted in higher cure rates than has $\beta$-lactam therapy alone. The addition of rifampin to the vancomycin regimen for *S. aureus* native valve endocarditis

**Table 66.7** Evaluation of resistance among enterococci and selection of therapy for enterococcal endocarditis

1. Determine the susceptibility (MIC) to candidate cell-wall active antimicrobials including penicillin (ampicillin), vancomycin, and teicoplanin and test for $\beta$-lactamase production (nitrocefin test)
   A. If penicillin, ampicillin, vancomycin, and teicoplanin[a] susceptible, use one
   B. If penicillin or ampicillin resistant (MIC ≥ 16 $\mu$g/ml) use vancomycin or teicoplanin
   C. If $\beta$-lactamase is produced, use vancomycin, teicoplanin, or ampicillin–$\beta$-lactamase inhibitor
   D. If vancomycin resistant (MIC ≥ 16 $\mu$g/ml) consider teicoplanin[a]
2. Determine whether high-level resistance to gentamicin and streptomycin is present
   A. No high-level resistance to either, use either aminoglycoside
   B. High-level resistance to either gentamicin or streptomycin, use the agent to which the organism doesn't possess high-level resistance
   C. If high-level resistance to both aminoglycosides is noted, omit the aminoglycoside from the regimen
3. Alternative regimens: concurrent surgical removal of the infected valve may be required
   A. No synergy possible (2,C), use an effective wall active agent for 12 wk
   B. If no effective cell-wall active agent, consider quinupristin-dalfopristin[a] if infection is due to a susceptible *E. faecium* or suppressive therapy with chloramphenicol or tetracycline

[a]Not approved by the Food and Drug Administration for use in the United States.

**Table 66.6** Antibiotic regimens for endocarditis caused by selected organisms*

| Infecting organism | Antibiotic | Dose and route[a] | Duration (wk) | Comments |
|---|---|---|---|---|
| 1. Penicillin-susceptible Viridans streptococci, *Streptococcus bovis*, and other streptococci (penicillin MIC $\leq 0.1$ $\mu$g/ml) | A. Penicillin G | 12–18 million units IV daily either continuously or in equally divided doses q 4 h | 4 | |
| | B. Penicillin G plus | 12–18 million units IV daily continuously or in equally divided doses q 4 h | 2 | Avoid aminoglycoside containing regimen when potential for nephrotoxicity or ototoxicity is increased |
| | Gentamicin | 1 mg/kg IM or IV q 8 h | 2 | |
| | C. Ceftriaxone | 2 g IV or IM daily as single dose | 4 | Can be used in patients with nonanaphylactic, nonurticarial penicillin allergy; intramuscular ceftriaxone is painful |
| | D. Vancomycin[c] | 30 mg/kg IV daily in equally divided doses q 12 h | 4 | Use for patients with urticarial or anaphylactic penicillin or cephalosporin allergy |
| 2. Relatively penicillin-resistant streptococci (Penicillin MIC $\geq 0.2$ to $<0.5$ $\mu$g/ml) | A. Penicillin G plus | 18–24 million units IV daily continuously or in equally divided doses q 4 h | 4 | |
| | Gentamicin | 1 mg/kg IM or IV q 8 h | 2 | |
| | B. Vancomycin[c] | See dose in regimen 1D | 4 | Use for treating penicillin allergic patients |
| 3. Enterococci—in vitro evaluation for susceptibility to ampicillin, penicillin, vancomycin, and teicoplanin; $\beta$-lactamase production; and high-level resistance to gentamicin and streptomycin required (see Table 66.7 and text for regimens used to treat markedly resistant strains) | A. Penicillin G plus | 18–30 million units IV daily continuously or in equally divided doses q 4 h | 4–6 | See text for use of streptomycin instead of gentamicin in these regimens. Four weeks of therapy recommended for patients with <3 mo of illness who respond promptly to treatment. Treatment for endocarditis caused by relatively penicillin resistant (MIC $\geq 0.5$ $\mu$g/ml), *S. adjacens* and *S. defectivus* |
| | Gentamicin | 1 mg/kg IM or IV every 8 h | 4–6 | |
| | B. Ampicillin plus | 12 q IV daily continuously or in equally divided doses q 4 h | 4–6 | |
| | gentamicin | Same dose as regimen 3A | 4–6 | |
| | C. Vancomycin[c] plus | 30 mg/kg IV daily in divided doses q 12 h | 4–6 | Use for patients with penicillin allergy. Do not use cephalosporins |
| | gentamicin | Same dose as regimen 3A | 4–6 | |
| 4. Staphylococci infecting native valves (assume penicillin resistance); methicillin-susceptible | A. Nafcillin or oxacillin plus optional addition of | 12 q IV daily in divided doses q 4 h | 4–6 | Penicillin—18–24 million units daily in divided doses q 4 h can be used instead of nafcillin, oxacillin, or cefazolin if strains do not produce $\beta$-lactamase |
| | gentamicin | Same dose as regimen 3A | 3–5 d | |
| | B. Cefazolin plus optional addition of | 2 g IV q 8 h | 4–6 | Cephalothin or other first-generation cephalosporin in equivalent doses can be used; this regimen can be used for patient with nonanaphylactic penicillin allergy |
| | gentamicin | Same dose as regimen 3A | 3–5 d | |
| | C. Vancomycin[c] | 30 mg/kg IV in divided doses q 12 h | 4–6 | Use for patients with urticarial or anaphylactic reaction to penicillin or cephalosporin |
| 5. Staphylococci infecting native valves; methicillin-resistant | Vancomycin[c] | 30 mg/kg IV in divided doses q 12 h | 4–6 | |

*(continued)*

**Table 66.6** Antibiotic regimens for endocarditis caused by selected organisms* —*Continued*

| Infecting organism | Antibiotic | Dose and route[a] | Duration (wk) | Comments |
|---|---|---|---|---|
| 6. Staphylococci infecting prosthetic valves; methicillin-susceptible (assume penicillin resistance) | Nafcillin or oxacillin plus | 12 g IV daily in divided doses q 4 h | ≥6 | First-generation cephalosporin or vancomycin could be used in patients with nonanaphylactic penicillin reaction. Use gentamicin during initial 2 wk. See text for alternates for gentamicin. For patients with immediate penicillin allergy, use regimen 7 |
| | gentamicin plus | 1 mg/kg IV or IM q 8 h | 2 | |
| | rifampin[d] | 300 mg p.o. q 8 h | ≥6 | |
| 7. Staphylococci infecting prosthetic valves; methicillin-resistant | Vancomycin[c] plus | 30 mg/kg IV in divided doses q 12 h | ≥6 | Use gentamicin during the initial 2 wk of therapy. See text for alternatives to gentamicin. Do not substitute a cephalosporin or imipenem for vancomycin |
| | gentamicin plus | 1 mg/kg IV or IM q 8 h | 2 | |
| | rifampin[d] | 300 mg p.o. q 8 h | ≥6 | |
| 8. HACEK organisms[b] | A. Ceftriaxone | 2 g IV or IM daily as a single dose | 4 | Cefotaxime or other third-generation cephalosporin in comparable doses may be used |
| | B. Ampicillin plus | 12 q IV daily continuously or in equally divided doses q 4 h | 4 | Test organism for β-lactamase production. Donot use this regimen if β-lactamase is produced |
| | gentamicin | 1 mg/kg IV or IM q 8 h | 4 | |

*Adapted from Wilson WR, Karchmer AW, Bisno AL, et al., Antibiotic Treatment of Adults with Infective Endocarditis Due to Viridans Streptococci, Enterococci, Other Streptococci, and HACEK Microorganisms. JAMA 1995; 274:1706–1713.

[a]Recommended doses are for adults with normal renal and hepatic function. Doses of gentamicin, streptomycin, and vancomycin must be adjusted in patients with renal dysfunction. Use ideal body weight to calculate doses (men = 50 kg + 2.3 kg per inch over 5 feet; women = 45.5 kg plus 2.3 kg per inch over 5 feet).

[b]HACEK organisms include *Hemophilus parainfluenzae*, *Hemophilus aphrophilus*, *Actinobacillus actinomycetemcomitans*, *Cardiobacterium hominis*, *Eikenella corrodens*, *Kingella kingii*.

[c]Peak levels obtained 1 h after completion of the infusion should be 30 to 45 μg/ml; doses greater than 2 g/24 h should not be used unless serum concentration is monitored. Infuse over 1 h to avoid histamine-release reaction.

[d]Rifampin increases the dose of warfarin or dicumarol required for effective anticoagulation.

during the initial 3 to 5 d of treatment has been suggested (Table 66.6:4A,B). Longer periods of aminoglycoside therapy have resulted in renal dysfunction and consequently are not recommended. The combination of a β-lactam and an aminoglycoside results in enhanced killing of staphylococci in vitro; nevertheless, combination therapy has not resulted in higher cure rates than has β-lactam therapy alone. The addition of rifampin to the vancomycin regimen for *S. aureus* native valve endocarditis

**Table 66.7** Evaluation of resistance among enterococci and selection of therapy for enterococcal endocarditis

1. Determine the susceptibility (MIC) to candidate cell-wall active antimicrobials including penicillin (ampicillin), vancomycin, and teicoplanin and test for β-lactamase production (nitrocefin test)
   A. If penicillin, ampicillin, vancomycin, and teicoplanin[a] susceptible, use one
   B. If penicillin or ampicillin resistant (MIC ≥ 16 μg/ml) use vancomycin or teicoplanin
   C. If β-lactamase is produced, use vancomycin, teicoplanin, or ampicillin–β-lactamase inhibitor
   D. If vancomycin resistant (MIC ≥ 16 μg/ml) consider teicoplanin[a]
2. Determine whether high-level resistance to gentamicin and streptomycin is present
   A. No high-level resistance to either, use either aminoglycoside
   B. High-level resistance to either gentamicin or streptomycin, use the agent to which the organism doesn't possess high-level resistance
   C. If high-level resistance to both aminoglycosides is noted, omit the aminoglycoside from the regimen
3. Alternative regimens: concurrent surgical removal of the infected valve may be required
   A. No synergy possible (2,C), use an effective wall active agent for 12 wk
   B. If no effective cell-wall active agent, consider quinupristin-dalfopristin[a] if infection is due to a susceptible *E. faecium* or suppressive therapy with chloramphenicol or tetracycline

[a]Not approved by the Food and Drug Administration for use in the United States.

**Table 66.6** Antibiotic regimens for endocarditis caused by selected organisms*

| Infecting organism | Antibiotic | Dose and route[a] | Duration (wk) | Comments |
|---|---|---|---|---|
| 1. Penicillin-susceptible Viridans streptococci, *Streptococcus bovis*, and other streptococci (penicillin MIC ≤ 0.1 μg/ml) | A. Penicillin G | 12–18 million units IV daily either continuously or in equally divided doses q 4 h | 4 | |
| | B. Penicillin G plus | 12–18 million units IV daily continuously or in equally divided doses q 4 h | 2 | Avoid aminoglycoside containing regimen when potential for nephrotoxicity or ototoxicity is increased |
| | Gentamicin | 1 mg/kg IM or IV q 8 h | 2 | |
| | C. Ceftriaxone | 2 g IV or IM daily as single dose | 4 | Can be used in patients with nonanaphylactic, nonurticarial penicillin allergy; intramuscular ceftriaxone is painful |
| | D. Vancomycin[c] | 30 mg/kg IV daily in equally divided doses q 12 h | 4 | Use for patients with urticarial or anaphylactic penicillin or cephalosporin allergy |
| 2. Relatively penicillin-resistant streptococci (Penicillin MIC ≥ 0.2 to <0.5 μg/ml) | A. Penicillin G plus | 18–24 million units IV daily continuously or in equally divided doses q 4 h | 4 | |
| | Gentamicin | 1 mg/kg IM or IV q 8 h | 2 | |
| | B. Vancomycin[c] | See dose in regimen 1D | 4 | Use for treating penicillin allergic patients |
| 3. Enterococci—in vitro evaluation for susceptibility to ampicillin, penicillin, vancomycin, and teicoplanin; β-lactamase production; and high-level resistance to gentamicin and streptomycin required (see Table 66.7 and text for regimens used to treat markedly resistant strains) | A. Penicillin G plus | 18–30 million units IV daily continuously or in equally divided doses q 4 h | 4–6 | See text for use of streptomycin instead of gentamicin in these regimens. Four weeks of therapy recommended for patients with <3 mo of illness who respond promptly to treatment. Treatment for endocarditis caused by relatively penicillin resistant (MIC ≥ 0.5 μg/ml), *S. adjacens* and *S. defectivus* |
| | Gentamicin | 1 mg/kg IM or IV every 8 h | 4–6 | |
| | B. Ampicillin plus | 12 q IV daily continuously or in equally divided doses q 4 h | 4–6 | |
| | gentamicin | Same dose as regimen 3A | 4–6 | |
| | C. Vancomycin[c] plus | 30 mg/kg IV daily in divided doses q 12 h | 4–6 | Use for patients with penicillin allergy. Do not use cephalosporins |
| | gentamicin | Same dose as regimen 3A | 4–6 | |
| 4. Staphylococci infecting native valves (assume penicillin resistance); methicillin-susceptible | A. Nafcillin or oxacillin plus optional addition of | 12 q IV daily in divided doses q 4 h | 4–6 | Penicillin—18–24 million units daily in divided doses q 4 h can be used instead of nafcillin, oxacillin, or cefazolin if strains do not produce β-lactamase |
| | gentamicin | Same dose as regimen 3A | 3–5 d | |
| | B. Cefazolin plus optional addition of | 2 g IV q 8 h | 4–6 | Cephalothin or other first-generation cephalosporin in equivalent doses can be used; this regimen can be used for patient with nonanaphylactic penicillin allergy |
| | gentamicin | Same dose as regimen 3A | 3–5 d | |
| | C. Vancomycin[c] | 30 mg/kg IV in divided doses q 12 h | 4–6 | Use for patients with urticarial or anaphylactic reaction to penicillin or cephalosporin |
| 5. Staphylococci infecting native valves; methicillin-resistant | Vancomycin[c] | 30 mg/kg IV in divided doses q 12 h | 4–6 | |

(*continued*)

**Table 66.6** Antibiotic regimens for endocarditis caused by selected organisms* —*Continued*

| Infecting organism | Antibiotic | Dose and route[a] | Duration (wk) | Comments |
|---|---|---|---|---|
| 6. Staphylococci infecting prosthetic valves; methicillin-susceptible (assume penicillin resistance) | Nafcillin or oxacillin plus | 12 g IV daily in divided doses q 4 h | ≥6 | First-generation cephalosporin or vancomycin could be used in patients with nonanaphylactic penicillin reaction. Use gentamicin during initial 2 wk. See text for alternates for gentamicin. For patients with immediate penicillin allergy, use regimen 7 |
| | gentamicin plus | 1 mg/kg IV or IM q 8 h | 2 | |
| | rifampin[d] | 300 mg p.o. q 8 h | ≥6 | |
| 7. Staphylococci infecting prosthetic valves; methicillin-resistant | Vancomycin[c] plus | 30 mg/kg IV in divided doses q 12 h | ≥6 | Use gentamicin during the initial 2 wk of therapy. See text for alternatives to gentamicin. Do not substitute a cephalosporin or imipenem for vancomycin |
| | gentamicin plus | 1 mg/kg IV or IM q 8 h | 2 | |
| | rifampin[d] | 300 mg p.o. q 8 h | ≥6 | |
| 8. HACEK organisms[b] | A. Ceftriaxone | 2 g IV or IM daily as a single dose | 4 | Cefotaxime or other third-generation cephalosporin in comparable doses may be used |
| | B. Ampicillin plus | 12 q IV daily continuously or in equally divided doses q 4 h | 4 | Test organism for β-lactamase production. Donot use this regimen if β-lactamase is produced |
| | gentamicin | 1 mg/kg IV or IM q 8 h | 4 | |

*Adapted from Wilson WR, Karchmer AW, Bisno AL, et al., Antibiotic Treatment of Adults with Infective Endocarditis Due to Viridans Streptococci, Enterococci, Other Streptococci, and HACEK Microorganisms. JAMA 1995; 274:1706–1713.

[a]Recommended doses are for adults with normal renal and hepatic function. Doses of gentamicin, streptomycin, and vancomycin must be adjusted in patients with renal dysfunction. Use ideal body weight to calculate doses (men = 50 kg + 2.3 kg per inch over 5 feet; women = 45.5 kg plus 2.3 kg per inch over 5 feet).

[b]HACEK organisms include *Hemophilus parainfluenzae, Hemophilus aphrophilus, Actinobacillus actinomycetemcomitans, Cardiobacterium hominis, Eikenella corrodens, Kingella kingii.*

[c]Peak levels obtained 1 h after completion of the infusion should be 30 to 45 μg/ml; doses greater than 2 g/24 h should not be used unless serum concentration is monitored. Infuse over 1 h to avoid histamine-release reaction.

[d]Rifampin increases the dose of warfarin or dicumarol required for effective anticoagulation.

during the initial 3 to 5 d of treatment has been suggested (Table 66.6:4A,B). Longer periods of aminoglycoside therapy have resulted in renal dysfunction and consequently are not recommended. The combination of a β-lactam and an aminoglycoside results in enhanced killing of staphylococci in vitro; nevertheless, combination therapy has not resulted in higher cure rates than has β-lactam therapy alone. The addition of rifampin to the vancomycin regimen for *S. aureus* native valve endocarditis

**Table 66.7** Evaluation of resistance among enterococci and selection of therapy for enterococcal endocarditis

1. Determine the susceptibility (MIC) to candidate cell-wall active antimicrobials including penicillin (ampicillin), vancomycin, and teicoplanin and test for β-lactamase production (nitrocefin test)
   A. If penicillin, ampicillin, vancomycin, and teicoplanin[a] susceptible, use one
   B. If penicillin or ampicillin resistant (MIC ≥ 16 μg/ml) use vancomycin or teicoplanin
   C. If β-lactamase is produced, use vancomycin, teicoplanin, or ampicillin–β-lactamase inhibitor
   D. If vancomycin resistant (MIC ≥ 16 μg/ml) consider teicoplanin[a]
2. Determine whether high-level resistance to gentamicin and streptomycin is present
   A. No high-level resistance to either, use either aminoglycoside
   B. High-level resistance to either gentamicin or streptomycin, use the agent to which the organism doesn't possess high-level resistance
   C. If high-level resistance to both aminoglycosides is noted, omit the aminoglycoside from the regimen
3. Alternative regimens: concurrent surgical removal of the infected valve may be required
   A. No synergy possible (2,C), use an effective wall active agent for 12 wk
   B. If no effective cell-wall active agent, consider quinupristin-dalfopristin[a] if infection is due to a susceptible *E. faecium* or suppressive therapy with chloramphenicol or tetracycline

[a]Not approved by the Food and Drug Administration for use in the United States.

has not improved the outcome and is not recommended for routine therapy. Among IVDA-, methicillin-susceptible *S. aureus* endocarditis that is confined to the right heart valves and is uncomplicated can be treated effectively using a semisynthetic penicillinase-resistant penicillin in combination with an aminoglycoside, each for 2 wk. A 2-wk regimen using vancomycin plus an aminoglycoside has not been shown to be effective in this population. In addition, some IVDA with right-sided *S. aureus* endocarditis remain febrile for prolonged periods during therapy and should not be treated with abbreviated antibiotic therapy.

Vancomycin is the only agent with established efficacy for the treatment of endocarditis caused by methicillin-resistant staphylococci (Table 66.6:5). Although methicillin-resistant staphylococci are susceptible in vitro to teicoplanin, the efficacy of teicoplanin treatment of staphylococcal endocarditis is not clear. Failure of teicoplanin has in part been related to pharmacodynamics. The efficacy of teicoplanin treatment of staphylococcal endocarditis is improved when trough serum concentrations are maintained at $\geq 25$ $\mu$g/ml. Nevertheless, concern remains regarding teicoplanin treatment of *S. aureus* endocarditis because of the potential emergence of staphylococci that are resistant to teicoplanin.

### Staphylococcal prosthetic valve endocarditis

Experimental and clinical evidence indicate that coagulase-negative staphylococcal prosthetic valve endocarditis, and probably that due to *S. aureus* as well, is optimally treated with combination antimicrobial therapy. Furthermore, rifampin, by virtue of an ability to kill staphylococci in the static phase of their growth cycle and those that are adherent to foreign bodies, is an essential component of the combination. Because rifampin-resistant staphylococci emerge rapidly and frequently during treatment with rifampin alone or rifampin plus one other agent, two effective antistaphylococcal agents are used in combination with rifampin for the treatment of staphylococcal PVE (Table 66.6:6, 7). The largest clinical experience is in the treatment of methicillin-resistant coagulase-negative staphylococcal PVE with vancomycin, rifampin, and gentamicin. However, the increased frequency of resistance to gentamicin among staphylococci has limited the utility of this regimen. Consequently, it is often necessary to identify an alternative aminoglycoside or a quinolone that is effective against the staphylococcal isolate to serve as the third antimicrobial in combination therapy. In treating staphylococcal PVE caused by a methicillin-susceptible strain a $\beta$-lactam antibiotic is substituted for vancomycin. The susceptibility of an infecting strain to rifampin must be determined before initial therapy and also when the bacteremia fails to clear or relapse occurs. If in vitro resistance to rifampin is noted, the agent should not be used. Because of the importance of rifampin in therapy and the ease with which staphylococci become rifampin-resistant, it is prudent to establish the in vitro susceptibility of the causative organism and treat the patient briefly to reduce the number of organisms at the site of infection before beginning rifampin.

### HACEK endocarditis

Ceftriaxone or another third-generation cephalosporin is recommended for the treatment of endocarditis involving native or prosthetic valves that is caused by this group of organisms. Ampicillin combined with gentamicin is an alternative regimen if the organism does not produce $\beta$-lactamase (Table 66.6:8A,B).

### Endocarditis caused by other organisms

A wide variety of organisms cause sporadic cases of endocarditis. Detailed regimens for the treatment of patients with these forms of endocarditis must be researched individually (see Kaye D., *Infective Endocarditis*, 2nd ed. Raven Press). When treating endocarditis in patients with negative blood cultures, clinical and epidemiologic clues to etiology should be considered, including a prior clinical response to antimicrobial therapy. If special tests do not suggest a fastidious cause of culture negative endocarditis (see Etiology), patients with infection of a native valve are treated with ampicillin plus gentamicin (Table 66.6:3A) and those with an infected prosthesis should receive this regimen plus vancomycin.

## Other considerations in antimicrobial therapy

### Initiation of therapy

In patients who present with either acute endocarditis or hemodynamic instability indicating a need for urgent surgery treatment must be initiated empirically immediately after three or four sets of blood cultures have been obtained. However, when hemodynamically stable patients with subacute endocarditis present for evaluation, particularly after having received brief periods of ineffective antibiotic therapy, it is prudent to obtain blood cultures and to briefly delay antibiotic therapy. If the initial cultures remain negative, the delaying of therapy allows additional blood cultures to be obtained without the confounding effect of empiric treatment.

### Monitoring antibiotic therapy

Patients being treated for endocarditis require continued careful evaluation during therapy. Failures of recommended regimens manifest by persistent fever or "breakthrough" bacteremia during therapy are likely the result of intracardiac or extracardiac complications or erroneous in vitro susceptibility studies. Early detection of failed therapy and initiation of adjunctive therapy or revision of antimicrobial therapy, as required by the clinical situation, can be life-saving. Monitoring therapy with a serum bactericidal titer, the highest dilution of the patient's serum during therapy that kills 99.9% of a standard inoculum of the infecting organism, is not recommended when endocarditis is being treated with an optimal regimen. This test may be useful when treating endocarditis caused by atypical organisms when optimal treatment has not been established or when treating patients with unconventional regimens. Serum concentrations of teicoplanin, vancomycin, and aminoglycosides should be measured periodically when these agents are used. This facilitates optimal dosing and may reduce the frequency of adverse events. Renal function and complete blood counts should be monitored when therapy can adversely impact these systems. Blood cultures should be obtained during the initial days of therapy or when fever persists or recurs. The need for blood cultures after completing therapy to confirm cure is controversial. Nevertheless, they should be obtained if cure is uncertain, fever recurs, or preoperatively if surgical intervention is to be undertaken within weeks to several months after completion of antibiotic therapy.

### Outpatient therapy for endocarditis

Patients with endocarditis who have responded to the early phase of antibiotic therapy, who clinically and echocardiographically do not seem at high risk for threatening complications of endocarditis, and who are reliable in complying with complex instructions can be considered for completion of antibiotic therapy outside of the hospital. Pharmacokinetic properties of some antimicrobials that allow administration as a single daily dose and technology that simplifies administering multiple doses of an antibiotic daily make outpatient therapy practical. Patients who are treated in an outpatient setting must be apprised of the potential complications of both endocarditis and therapy and must be followed carefully to detect promptly untoward events.

## Cardiac surgical intervention in endocarditis

Cardiac surgery can play an important role in the treatment of endocarditis. Unacceptably high mortality and morbidity are noted when endocarditis patients with intracardiac complications or with unresponsive infection are treated with antibiotics alone. The outcome of endocarditis in these settings is improved when treatment combines antimicrobial therapy and aggressive early cardiac surgical intervention.

Under selected circumstances, cardiac surgery is indicated during the course of antimicrobial therapy (Table 66.8). Moderate or severe congestive heart failure (New York Heart Association class III or IV) due to new or worsening valve dysfunction is associated with mortality rates ranging from 50% to 90% if patients are treated medically. In contrast, mortality rates are reduced to 20% to 40% when patients with similar complications undergo valve replacement. Similar improvement in outcome is effected when patients with PVE complicated by prosthesis dysfunction and heart failure are treated surgically. Aortic valve regurgitation is associated with more rapidly progressive heart failure and a need for earlier surgery than is mitral valve incompetence. Onset of PVE within the year after valve replacement surgery and infection of an aortic valve prosthesis are associated with an increased risk of perivalvular infection and subsequent dehiscence of the prosthesis. Dehiscence associated with hemodynamic deterioration or that which results in an overtly unstable hypermobile device (a finding indicative of dehiscence exceeding 40% of the valve circumference) regardless of hemodynamic status warrants surgical intervention.

Uncontrolled infection requires surgical intervention in an effort to excise the infected tissue. This situation is encountered when endocarditis is caused by antibiotic-resistant organisms—for example, *Candida* species, some gram-negative bacilli (*P. aeruginosa*, *Stenotrophomonas* species), and some enterococci (see Table 66.7). Some patients with uncomplicated endocarditis caused by *Candida* species appear to be cured with medical therapy. This therapy often includes years, if not lifelong, treatment with an imidazole orally. Cure of patients with complicated candida endocarditis requires cardiac surgery as well as prolonged oral imidazole therapy. Patients with PVE who relapse after optimal antimicrobial therapy are likely to have perivalvular invasive disease and are more likely to be cured if treated with antibiotics and replacement of the infected prosthesis.

Other clinical circumstances will often, although not always, warrant surgical intervention (Table 66.8). Although most patients with endocarditis that is complicated by perivalvular infection will usually require surgery, antibiotic therapy alone has been successful in selected instances. *Staphylococcus aureus* endocarditis involving native mitral or aortic valves or a prosthetic valve is associated with very high mortality rates. If patients with these forms of *S. aureus* endocarditis do not have a rapid and complete response to antibiotic therapy, particularly those with infected prosthetic valves, they may benefit from surgical intervention.

Systemic emboli occur in 35% of patients with an echocardiographically demonstrable vegetation larger than 10 mm and in 20% of those with smaller or no detectable vegetations. Although some authors have advocated surgery to prevent emboli when vegetations exceed 10 mm, it is not clear that surgery will reduce thromboembolic events or improve outcome. The frequency of systemic emboli decreases rapidly with effective antibiotic therapy and, furthermore, only emboli to the cerebral and coronary arteries result in severe morbidity or mortality. Vegetation size and mobility are in themselves rarely indications for valve replacement. These features, however, may combine with other clinical considerations to prompt earlier surgery. Additionally, the ability to excise vegetations and repair actively infected valves may decrease the risks of surgical intervention and make surgery to prevent embolic complications in patients with large vegetations more acceptable.

The timing of surgical intervention is a critical element in outcome. Because postoperative mortality increases in a direct relationship with the severity of hemodynamic disability at the time of surgery, it is essential that patients undergo surgery before the development of severe intractable congestive heart failure, regardless of the duration of preoperative antimicrobial therapy. Similarly, patients with uncontrolled infection who require surgery should undergo prompt surgical intervention. Only when both infection is controlled and hemodynamics are compensated and stable is it reasonable to delay surgery. It may be prudent to delay surgery for 10 to 14 d after embolic cerebral infarction and 21 to 28 d after intracranial hemorrhage in order to avoid perioperative exacerbation of these neurologic complications. The presence of a mycotic aneurysm requires careful timing of surgery and avoidance of a prosthesis that requires postoperative anticoagulation. A mycotic aneurysm should be repaired prior to cardiac surgery, when possible.

**Table 66.8** Reasons for cardiac surgical intervention during therapy of native or prosthetic valve endocarditis

| |
|---|
| INDICATIONS FOR SURGERY |
| Valve dysfunction resulting in moderate to severe congestive heart failure |
| Unstable hypermobile prosthetic valve |
| Uncontrolled infection: persistent bacteremia, ineffective antimicrobial therapy, most patients with fungal endocarditis |
| Relapse following optimal antibiotic treatment of PVE |
| RELATIVE INDICATIONS FOR SURGERY |
| Extension of infection into perivalvular tissue (myocardial abscess) |
| *Staphylococcus aureus* infection of an aortic, mitral, or prosthetic valve |
| Prosthetic valve endocarditis caused by *Pseudomonas aeruginosa* |
| Relapse after maximal antimicrobial therapy (native valves) |
| Large (>10 mm) hypermobile vegetations by echocardiogram |
| Persistent unexplained fever (≥10 d) during empiric therapy of culture negative endocarditis |
| Endocarditis caused by *C. burnetii* or *Brucella* species |

## Treatment of extracardiac complications

Antimicrobial therapy alone is rarely effective treatment for splenic abscess. In general, effective therapy requires either percutaneous catheter drainage or splenectomy. To avoid recrudescent infection and the risk of infecting a newly implanted prosthesis, splenic abscess should be effectively treated prior to cardiac surgery.

Cerebral angiography or possibly magnetic resonance angiography is indicated to evaluate endocarditis patients with intracranial hemorrhage or with persistent headache or focal neurologic symptoms. Cerebral mycotic aneurysms that have leaked should be repaired surgically when this is anatomically feasible. Unruptured mycotic aneurysms may resolve during antimicrobial therapy. Single cerebral aneurysms that persist or become larger during or after antibiotic therapy should be considered for surgical repair when this is feasible without serious neurologic injury.

Extracranial mycotic aneurysms that have leaked, expanded during antimicrobial therapy, or persist after therapy should be repaired. Aneurysms of intraabdominal arteries should be repaired because rupture may result in life-threatening hemorrhage.

## Anticoagulant therapy

Among patients with native valve endocarditis, anticoagulant therapy is used only when there is a clear indication independent of the underlying endocarditis and when the risk of intracranial hemorrhage is not increased. Among patients with PVE involving devices that usually require maintenance anticoagulant therapy, carefully monitored anticoagulation is continued. Anticoagulant therapy should not be initiated when PVE involves a prosthesis that does not usually require this therapy. If central nervous system complications occur in patients with endocarditis who are receiving anticoagulant therapy, anticoagulation should be reversed until the increased risk of intracranial hemorrhage has abated.

## Prevention of Endocarditis

Efforts to prevent endocarditis have been codified in recommendations for prophylactic antimicrobial use that are widely applied in developed countries. Although these recommendations vary somewhat from country to country, they are derived from an understanding of the pathogenesis, epidemiology, and microbiology of infective endocarditis. The excess frequency of cardiac valvular and structural abnormalities in patients with endocarditis compared with the general population identifies lesions with high, intermediate, and low or negligible risks for endocarditis (Table 66.9). Patients with lesions at relatively high and intermediate risk are targets for antibiotic prophylaxis for endocarditis. The organisms that frequently cause endocarditis have unique properties that facilitate their adherence to and survival on endothelial surfaces. Although the patients at risk for endocarditis may develop infection any time these organisms enter the bloodstream, it is practical to attempt chemoprophylaxis only in conjunction with procedures and events likely to cause bacteremia with these organisms (Table 66.10). This list of procedures is not all inclusive and the position on the list for some procedures is not absolute. Some physicians may elect to give prophylaxis to high-risk patients who are to undergo a procedure that usually does not justify prophylaxis. Infection at the target site for one of these procedures increases the risk of bacteremia and justification for prophylaxis. Ideally, infection at the target site should be eradicated before procedures are performed. Expert committees have designed regimens for chemoprophylaxis to be used with specific procedures (Tables 66.11, 66.12). These regimens are structured to prevent viridans streptococci and other streptococci from causing en-

**Table 66.9** Risk of endocarditis attributable to preexisting cardiac abnormalities*

| Relatively high risk | Intermediate risk | Very low or negligible risk[b] |
|---|---|---|
| Prosthetic heart valves[a] | Mitral-valve prolapse with regurgitation (murmur) | Mitral valve prolapse without regurgitation (murmur) |
| Previous infective endocarditis[a] | Pure mitral stenosis | Trivial valvular regurgitation on echocardiography without structural abnormality |
| Cyanotic congenital heart disease[a] | Tricuspid valve disease | Isolated atrial septal defect (secundum) |
| Patent ductus arteriosus | Pulmonary stenosis | Arteriosclerotic plaques |
| Aortic regurgitation | Asymmetric septal hypertrophy | Coronary artery disease |
| Aortic stenosis | Bicuspid aortic valve or calcific aortic sclerosis with minimal hemodynamic abnormality | Cardiac pacemaker, implanted defibrillators |
| Mitral regurgitation | Degenerative valvular disease in elderly patients | Surgically repaired intracardiac lesions, with minimal or no hemodynamic abnormality, more than 6 months after operation |
| Mitral stenosis and regurgitation | Surgically repaired intracardiac lesions with minimal or no hemodynamic abnormality, less than 6 mo after operation | Prior coronary bypass graft surgery |
| Ventricular septal defect | | Prior Kawasaki disease or rheumatic fever without valvular dysfunction |
| Coarctation of the aorta | | |
| Surgically repaired intracardiac lesion with residual hemodynamic abnormality | | |
| Surgically constructed systemic-pulmonary shunts[a] | | |

[a]Lesions considered at highest risk for endocarditis.

[b]Prophylaxis against endocarditis not recommended.

*Adapted from Durack DT, Prevention of Infective Endocarditis, N Engl J Med 1995; 332:38–44; and Dajani AS, et al., Prevention of Bacterial Endocarditis: Recommendations of the American Heart Association, JAMA 1997; 277:1794–1801, and Leport, C, et al., Antibiotic Prophylaxis for Infective Endocarditis, Eur Heart J 1995; 16(Suppl B):126–131.

**Table 66.10** Procedures for which prophylaxis is or is not recommended*

| Prophylaxis recommended | Prophylaxis not recommended |
|---|---|
| Dental procedures known to induce gingival or mucosal bleeding, including professional cleaning and scaling | Dental procedures not likely to cause bleeding, such as adjustment of orthodontic appliances and simple fillings above the gum line |
| Tonsillectomy or adenoidectomy | Intraoral injection of local anesthetic |
| Surgery involving gastrointestinal or upper respiratory mucosa | Shedding of primary teeth |
| Bronchoscopy with rigid bronchoscope | Tympanostomy tube insertion |
| Sclerotherapy for esophageal varices | Endotracheal tube insertion |
| Esophageal dilation | Bronchoscopy with flexible bronchoscope, with or without biopsy[a] |
| Gallbladder surgery | Transesophageal echocardiography[a] |
| Endoscopic retrograde cholangiography with biliary obstruction | Cardiac catheterization |
| Cystoscopy, urethral dilation | Gastrointestinal endoscopy, with or without biopsy[a] |
| Uretheral catheterization if urinary infection is present | Cesarean section |
| Urinary tract surgery, including prostate surgery | Vaginal hysterectomy[a] |
| Incision and drainage of infected tissue[b] | In the absence of infection: urethral catheterization, dilatation and curettage, uncomplicated vaginal delivery, therapeutic abortion, insertion or removal of intrauterine device, sterilization procedures, laparoscopy[a] |
| Vaginal hysterectomy complicated by infection | Incision or biopsy of surgically scrubbed skin |
| Vaginal delivery complicated by infection | |

*Adapted from Dajani AS, et al: Prevention of Bacterial Endocarditis: Recommendations of the American Heart Association, JAMA 1997; 277:1794–1801; Leport C, et al., Antibiotic Prophylaxis for Infective Endocarditis, European Heart J 1995; 16(Suppl B):126–131.

[a]In patients at highest risk, physicians may elect to use prophylaxis for these procedures.

[b]Antibiotic prophylaxis should be directed against the most likely endocarditis-associated pathogen(s), often staphylococci.

docarditis after dental and upper respiratory or upper gastrointestinal track procedures and to provide prophylaxis against potential enterococcal and streptococcal endocarditis after genitourinary procedures. When staphylococcal bacteremia is anticipated in association with a procedure, chemoprophylaxis should be modified accordingly.

The efficacy of chemoprophylaxis has not been established in clinical studies. Case-control studies draw widely discrepant conclusions regarding efficacy, cost–benefits, and risk–benefits. Although regimens that differ slightly from those outlined have been recommended by expert committees from various countries and a European consensus group (Leport C. et al., *European Heart J* 1995; 16[Suppl B]:126–131), the differences are minor and prophylaxis is accepted practice at this time. Accordingly, it is incumbent upon physicians to make patients aware of their risk for endocarditis, the procedures for which prophylaxis is advised, and the specifics of chemoprophylaxis. Additionally, since many cases of endocarditis occur in the absence of pre-

**Table 66.11** Antibiotic regimens for prophylaxis with oropharyngeal, respiratory, and upper gastrointestinal tract procedures*

| Setting | Regimen[a] |
|---|---|
| Standard regimen[b] | Amoxicillin, 2.0 or 3.0 g orally 1 h before procedure |
| Regimen for amoxicillin/penicillin-allergic patients | Cephalexin or cefadroxil 2.0 g orally 1 h before procedure |
| | *or* |
| | Clindamycin, 300–600 mg orally 1 h before procedure[c] |
| Regimen for patients unable to take oral medications | Ampicillin, 2.0 g IM or IV 30 min before procedure; then either ampicillin, 1.0 g IM or IV, or amoxicillin, 1.5 g orally 6 h after initial dose |
| Regimen for ampicillin/amoxicillin/penicillin-allergic patients unable to take oral medications | Clindamycin, 300 mg IV 30 min before procedure then 150 mg 6 h after initial dose |
| Regimen for patients considered at highest risk and not candidates for standard regimen | Use standard regimen for genitourinary and gastrointestinal procedures |
| Regimen for ampicillin/amoxicillin/penicillin-allergic patients considered at highest risk | Use regimen for allergic patients undergoing genitourinary and gastrointestinal procedures |

*Adapted from Dajani AS, et al: Prevention of Bacterial Endocarditis: Recommendations by the American Heart Association, JAMA 1997; 277:1794–1801 and Leport C, et al: Antibiotic prophylaxis for infective endocarditis. Eur Heart J 1995; 16(Suppl B):126–131.

[a]Doses for adults. Initial pediatric doses are as follows: ampicillin or amoxicillin, 50 mg/kg; clindamycin, 10 mg/kg; cephalexin or cefadroxil 50 mg/kg; gentamicin, 2.0 mg/kg; and vancomycin, 20 mg/kg. Follow-up doses should be one-half the initial dose. *Total pediatric dose should not exceed total adult dose.*

[b]Generally recommended for all patients, including those at highest risk; physician may elect more vigorous regimens.

[c]New macrolides—for example, clarithromycin 500 mg orally, have been recommended as an alternative to clindamycin.

**Table 66.12** Antibiotic regimens for prophylaxis with genitourinary/gastrointestinal procedures*

| Setting | Regimen[a] |
|---|---|
| Standard regimen | Ampicillin, 2.0 g IV plus gentamicin, 1.5 mg/kg (not to exceed 120 mg) IV or IM 30 min before procedure followed by ampicillin, 1.0 g IV, or amoxicillin, 1.5 g orally 6 h after initial dose |
| Regimen for ampicillin/amoxicillin/penicillin-allergic patients | Vancomycin, 1.0 g IV infused over 1 h plus gentamicin, 1.5 mg/kg (not to exceed 120 mg) IV or IM, 1 h before procedure. May repeat vancomycin 1.0 g IV 12 h after initial dose |
| Alternate regimen for intermediate-risk patient/ Low-risk procedure | Amoxicillin, 2.0 to 3.0 g orally 1 h before procedure, or ampixillin 2.0 g IV 30 min before the procedure or vancomycin 1.0 g IV infused over 1 h |

*Adapted from Dajani AS, et al: Prevention of Bacterial Endocarditis: Recommendations by the American Heart Association, JAMA 1997; 277:1794–1801, and Leport C, et al., Antibiotic prophylaxis for infective endocarditis. Eur Heart J 1995; 16(Suppl B):126–131.

[a]Doses for adults. Repeat doses of vancomycin or gentamicin require adjustment for renal dysfunction. Initial pediatric doses, see Table 66.11, footnote.

disposing procedures, patients at risk for endocarditis should be encouraged to minimize the risk of bacteremia—to maintain good oral hygiene, avoid oral irrigating devices, and seek prompt treatment for infections that are potentially associated with bacteremia.

## ANNOTATED BIBLIOGRAPHY


Croft CH, Woodward W, Elliott A, Commerford PJ, Barnard CN, Beck W. Analysis of surgical versus medical therapy in active complicated native valve infective endocarditis. Am J Cardiol 1983; 51:1650–1655.

*A carefully analyzed retrospective study of the impact of cardiac surgical intervention in the outcome of complicated native valve endocarditis. These data argue forcefully for early surgical intervention in complicated endocarditis.*

Dajani AS, Taubert KA, Wilson W et al. Prevention of bacterial endocarditis. Recommendations by the American Heart Association. JAMA 1997; 277:1794–1801.

*Those lesions at risk for endocarditis and the procedures warranting antimicrobial prophylaxis are identified. The specific antimicrobial regimens recommended by a multidisciplinary committee on behalf of the American Heart Association are provided. The rationale for each recommendation is clearly stated and well referenced. A thoughtful approach to mitral valve prolapse is provided.*

Dreyfus C, Serraf A, Jebara VA et al. Valve repair in acute endocarditis. Ann Thorac Surg 1990; 49:706–713.

*Repair of the mitral valve during active infective endocarditis, a new form of surgical intervention instead of valve replacement, allows resection of vegetations and restoration of valve function with low perioperative mortality.*

Durack DT. Prevention of infective endocarditis. N Engl J Med 1995; 332:38–44.

*A thoughtful, extensively referenced consideration of the rationale and justification for antimicrobial prophylaxis for endocarditis.*

Durack DT, Lukes AS, Bright DK. New Criteria for diagnosis of infective endocarditis: Utilization of specific echocardiographic findings. Am J Med 1994; 96:200–209.

*The extensive experience of a university hospital endocarditis service is analyzed to develop a clinically applicable, standardized approach to the diagnosis of infective endocarditis. The new criteria are very sensitive and specific.*

Goldenberger D, Kunzili A, Vogt P, Zbinden R, Altwegg M. Molecular diagnosis of bacterial endocarditis by broad-range PCR amplification and direct sequencing. J Clin Microbiol 1997; 2733–2739.

*This study demonstrates the utility of molecular techniques in recovering bacterial genes for 16S ribosomal RNA from surgically excised vegetations and the use of these genes to establish an etiologic diagnosis of culture-negative endocarditis.*

Karchmer AW. Infective endocarditis. In: Heart Disease, 5th ed. Braunwald E, ed. WB Saunders, Philadelphia, PA, pp 1097–1104, 1997.

*An extensively referenced chapter which examines diverse aspects of endocarditis in detail and documents many of the data supporting the recommendations contained in this chapter.*

Karchmer AW, Gibbons GW. Infections of prosthetic heart valves and vascular grafts. In: Infections Associated with Indwelling Devices, 2nd ed. Bisno AL, Waldvogel FA, eds. American Society for Microbiology, Washington, DC, pp 213–249, 1994.

*A detailed consideration of epidemiologic, microbiologic, and clinical aspects of prosthetic valve endocarditis is presented and detailed recommendations for antibiotic and surgical therapy are provided.*

Kaye D. Infective Endocarditis, 2nd ed. Raven Press, New York, 1992.

*Comprehensive multi-authored monograph with detailed considerations of virtually all aspects of infective endocarditis. Each chapter is extensively referenced.*

Leport C, Horstkotte D, Burckhardt D, Group of Experts of the International Society for Chemotherapy. Antibiotic prophylaxis for infective endocarditis from an international group of experts toward a European consensus. Eur Heart J 1995; 16(Suppl B):126–131.

*A review of indications, target procedures, and recommended regimens for antibiotic prophylaxis for endocarditis from European countries and the United States. While differences in approach in various countries exist, they are not great.*

Mugge A. Echocardiographic detection of cardiac valve vegetations and prognostic implications. Infect Dis Clin North Am 1993; 7:877–898.

*A thoughtful consideration of the role of echocardiography in the diagnosis and management of endocarditis based on the detection of vegetations and their prognostic implications.*

Stamboulian D. Outpatient treatment of endocarditis in a clinic-based program in Argentina. Eur J Clin Microbiol Infect Dis 1995; 14:648–654.

*A careful consideration of outpatient antimicrobial therapy for endocarditis including selection of patients, feasible regimens, and economic impact of this effective strategy for treatment.*

Steckelberg JM, Murphy JG, Ballard D et al. Emboli in infective endocarditis: the prognostic value of echocardiography. Ann Int Med 1991; 114:635–640.

*A careful prospective consideration of the relationship of echocardiographically demonstrated vegetations to subsequent embolic complications during therapy. The frequency of embolic complications decreases rapidly with therapy. These observations call into question the role of cardiac surgery to prevent systemic emboli.*

Wilson WR, Steckelberg JM, eds. Infective endocarditis. Infect Dis Clin North Am 1993; 7(1).

*This issue provides well-referenced, authoritative discussions of controversial or temporally relevant topics related to infective endocarditis.*

Wilson WR, Karchmer AW, Bisno AL et al. Antibiotic treatment of adults with infective endocarditis due to viridans streptococci, enterococci, other streptococci, and HACEK microorganisms. JAMA 1995; 274:1706–1713.

*Consensus antibiotic recommendations for the treatment of the common bacterial causes of infective endocarditis are presented. Selected references justifying the recommended regimens are included.*

# 67

# Intravenous Catheter-Related Infections, Suppurative Thrombophlebitis, and Mycotic Aneurysms

DANIEL P. LEW AND JACQUES SCHRENZEL

It is estimated that more than half of the patients admitted to hospitals, both in the United States and in Europe, require, at one time or another, intravenous infusions. The rates of use of intravenous devices increase up to 100% in critically ill patients, in particular when admitted to intensive care units. Although very useful for the therapy of hospitalized patients, intravenous catheters are associated with a significant risk for developing infectious and noninfectious complications.

## Epidemiology

Due to the lack of standard definitions, one has to be especially careful when discussing the rates of catheter-related infections. In this chapter, we consider a catheter as infected (or colonized) when rolling back and forth the tip of the catheter on an agar plate reveals ≥15 colony-forming units (cfu; semiquantitative method), or when >1000 cfu/ml are cultured by quantitative techniques. Conversely, the catheter is considered as contaminated when culture results are lower than these cutoff values. Finally, the diagnosis of a catheter-related bacteremia requires the isolation of the same microorganism from the catheter as in blood cultures, with no other potential source of infection.

The probability of developing a catheter-related bacteremia has been estimated to be between 1% and 3% for central venous catheters. The risk is much lower for peripheral venous catheters. In fact, the occurrence of multiple cases of peripheral venous catheter infections suggests a nosocomial outbreak. Several reviews have dealt with this problem in recent years.

A recent analysis of 18 well-defined articles published on the incidence and the consequences of central intravenous catheter infections in 4404 catheters in Intensive Care Unit (ICU) patients gave a rate of 13.4% microbial colonization and 3.0% bacteremia. Based on available data, the number of clinically significant central venous catheter infections is estimated to be higher than 1 million/yr in the western world.

The consequences of bacteremia associated with intravenous device infection can be multiple and serious. A recent review of 102 catheter-associated bacteremias over 45 mo, in one single institution, found a rate of 32% of major complications. These included septic shock, prolonged septicemia, and multiple infectious metastatic lesions (pneumonia, meningitis, epidural abscess, septic arthritis, endocarditis, and arteritis). The risk of major complications was highest in episodes caused by *Candida*, *Pseudomonas aeruginosa*, *Staphylococcus aureus*, or multiple pathogens, and the most severe complications were usually caused by *S. aureus*. In a meta-analysis of catheter-related *S. aureus* bacteremia, the pooled data of 11 published studies showed that 24% had associated complications and 15% associated mortality. In contrast to *S. aureus*, the consequences of coagulase-negative staphylococcal bacteremia have been more difficult to assess. Until the 1970s, this was considered to be a harmless microorganism. In uncontrolled studies, crude mortality (i.e., mortality without subtraction of other potentially lethal comorbidities) ranged from 18% to 57%. An early publication reported a mortality attributable to this microorganism in 13.6% of patients and an excess length of stay of 8.5 d when compared to controls. Several other studies have shown that coagulase-negative staphylococcus bacteremia associated with vascular catheters is an important cause of febrile morbidity in hospitalized patients. The economic impact of these infections is considerable: They cause a significant prolongation of the length of hospitalization. In 1993, costs directly attributable to these infections were estimated globally to be US$ 3707 per episode, reaching US$ 6064 when *S. aureus* was the causative microorganism.

## Pathogenesis

Bacteria usually colonize the catheter from the skin by migration along the external surface of the catheter into the subcutaneous tissues. As is the case in most foreign body infections, the presence of a biomaterial increases the risk of infection considerably even with a low inoculum of microorganisms that are often of low virulence, such as coagulase-negative staphylococci. Soon after insertion, catheters are selectively coated with tissue proteins which promote bacterial attachment. The most important of these are fibrinogen/fibrin, present in large amounts, and fibronectin. Although present in much lower amounts, fibronectin is a stronger promoter of staphylococcal adhesion than fibrinogen; fibronectin is also less susceptible to proteolytic cleavage by tissue or plasma proteases.

The material of which an intravascular catheter is made also plays an important role in the pathogenesis of device-related infections—namely, by promoting deposition of specific host proteins that stimulate bacterial adhesion (e.g., *S. aureus*). Catheters made of Teflon® are more resistant to adherence by coagulase-negative staphylococci than are catheters made of polyvinyl chloride, and polyurethane catheters appear to be far less likely to become colonized in clinical use than catheters made of polyvinyl chloride.

There appears to be a relationship between the thrombotic and infectious complications of central venous catheters. A recent pathological study in patients who died with a central intravenous device in place showed that 38% of patients had mural thrombi, 5.6% had right atrial mural thrombi, and 5.6% had nonbacterial thrombotic endocarditis. A highly significant statistical correlation between septicemia and thrombosis was found in the same study. This is not surprising since several of the proteins present in thrombi (thrombospondin in addition to fibrinogen and fibronectin) promote bacterial or fungal adherence.

Other important mechanisms of microbial colonization include contamination by microorganisms of the hub of the central venous perfusion by the hands of medical personnel, or sometimes contamination of the infusate or even disinfectants. This is followed by propagation of microorganisms within the lumen of the catheter. Finally, and more rarely, remote infection may lead to hematogenous seeding of the intravascular component of the catheter.

## Infection as a Function of the Type of Catheter

The three most commonly used approaches of IV therapy are central venous catheters, surgically implanted central venous catheters, or peripheral venous catheters:

### Central venous catheters

Central venous catheters inserted percutaneously into the subclavian, internal jugular, or femoral vein have come into wide use for the administration of fluids, blood products, total parenteral nutrition (TPN), hemodynamic monitoring, and especially for the prolonged administration of drugs, most frequently antibiotics. Central venous catheters are clearly the intravascular devices most likely to cause iatrogenic septicemia at present, probably because they are larger and remain in place for longer periods.

### Surgically implanted central venous catheters

Surgically implanted central venous catheters with an attached subcutaneous Dacron® cuff—the Hickman and Broviac catheters—have gained wide use as all-purpose vascular access for patients who have undergone bone marrow transplantation, who have leukemia, or who simply require prolonged administration of parenteral drugs. These catheters are used routinely in home TPN programs and by many centers for home IV antibiotic therapy. Used for drawing all blood specimens as well as the administration of all fluids, drugs, and blood products, these devices are a major advance in terms of patient comfort but are also associated with catheter-related bacteremia. Complicating infection rates do not vary significantly with the type of catheter used.

### Peripheral venous catheters

The small, percutaneously inserted Teflon® and polyurethane catheters now used for peripheral IV therapy are associated with a very low risk of catheter-related bacteremia (usually tenfold lower than central venous catheters). By contrast, phlebitis is much more frequent, reaching in some series an incidence of 30% (half of the phlebitis cases occur upon removal of the catheter). Risk factors associated with phlebitis are: underlying diseases (i.e., hematological malignancies, solid tumors, or immunodeficiency diseases), catheter length, contamination of hub, and pH of the solution $<5$. Peripheral catheters inserted by surgical cutdown have been associated with a very high risk of sepsis; presently there is rarely a need to perform such a procedure.

## Diagnosis of Intravenous Catheter Infections

Clinical criteria for the diagnosis of intravenous catheter infection have low sensitivity and specificity. In many instances bacteremia may occur without apparent local clinical infection or any sign of phlebitis.

The general clinical features of infusion-related sepsis are indiscernible from bloodstream infections arising from any other site (see Chapter 50). Infusion-related sepsis occurring in a critical care unit is particularly insidious. Sepsis associated with phlebitis, inflammation, or purulence of the cannula insertion site, with no apparent extravascular source of infection, should be considered highly suspicious of an infusion-related source. This is particularly true when infection occurs in a patient who is an unlikely candidate for sepsis or when the sepsis is refractory to antimicrobial therapy.

When infusion-related sepsis is suspected, blood cultures should be obtained from at least two separate peripheral venipunctures. The value of drawing standard blood cultures through the suspected catheter is unsettled, but it may increase the likelihood of a contaminated culture. It is recommended only if simultaneous percutaneously drawn blood cultures are also obtained and all of the blood cultures are processed quantitatively. In catheter-related sepsis, a marked increase in the concentration of organisms should be found in catheter-drawn specimens compared with percutaneously drawn cultures.

Local inflammation does not always mean infection and bacterial cultures are necessary to confirm a clinically suspected diagnosis of catheter acquired infection. For culturing catheters, the most commonly accepted bacteriological technique is the semiquantitative method developed by D. Maki. It requires rolling the intracutaneous segment of the catheter back and forth on an agar plate. Growth of $\geq 15$ colony-forming units of a microorganism is considered to represent colonization/infection. This technique has a low positive predictive value ($\leq 30\%$ in several studies) unless the catheter has remained in situ for prolonged periods of time. Other techniques have been developed, such as shaking a segment of the catheter with a vortex device followed by quantitation of the released bacteria. Alternatively, staining of the surface of the catheter followed by direct microscopy has been suggested as a rapid and reliable technique.

Most of these new tests are somewhat cumbersome to perform. Therefore, currently the most accepted definition of catheter-related infection is based on Maki's technique. The definition of catheter-associated bacteremia requires isolation of the same microorganism from the catheter and from concurrent blood cultures with no other potential source. In epidemiological studies, plasmid typing for coagulase-negative staphylococci (and thus demonstration that the same microorganism is present both in the blood and on the catheter) is required in order to rule out the possibility of a contamination (see Chapter 15).

## Microbiology of Catheter-Associated Infections

In most studies of catheter-acquired infections 30%–40% of colonizing microorganisms are coagulase-negative staphylococci and 5%–10% are *S. aureus*—that is, microorganisms which are part of the skin flora. Due to the higher pathogenicity of *S. aureus*, positive cultures for this microorganism have a higher predictive value. Nosocomially acquired pathogens are usually found at lower frequency and include enterococci, *Enterobacter* spp., *Pseudomonas aeruginosa* and *Candida* spp. at rates of around 5% for each one of these microorganisms. Table 67.1 compares the microbiology of catheter colonization with the microorganisms leading to catheter-related bacteremia. In Intensive Care Units, an increase in the incidence of gram-negative bacterial infection has been observed over the past decade; a higher proportion of catheter-related fungemia has also been observed. These differences may be due to the characteristics of the patients (underlying diseases, immunosuppression, systemic anti-infectious prophylaxis or therapy), the care to the catheter (frequency and type of dressing, antibacterial ointment, type of catheter), the definition of the catheter-related infections, or the local nosocomial epidemiology.

## Management of Central Venous Catheter Infections

As soon as infection of a central venous catheter is suspected, appropriate diagnostic and therapeutic measures must be performed. Microbiological diagnosis should include several blood cultures obtained both through the catheter and through a peripheral vein. Superficial cultures of the skin and the hub are usually not performed, unless there is a local purulent discharge or suspicion of purulent phlebitis, in which case a Gram stain and culture are valuable. Semi-quantitative or quantitative culture of the intracutaneous segment of the removed catheter itself is the approach of choice for the definitive diagnosis of central venous catheter infection. In some centers, in order to preserve the intravenous access, guidewire exchange is used and if a significant number of micro-organisms subsequently grows from the old catheter in culture, antibiotics are given. But in the authors' view, guidewire exchange should not be attempted if infection is suspected.

In the presence of catheter-associated bacteremia the standard practice has been to remove the catheter and to start intravenous therapy directed against staphylococci (Table 67.2). Cryptogenic bacteremias, particularly with coagulase-negative staphylococci, are common in the vulnerable patients with surgically implanted central venous catheters. These bacteremias can often be successfully treated without having to remove the catheter, possibly because they do not originate from the catheter or because they reflect transient luminal contaminants. If, however, septicemia in a patient with a cuffed, surgically implanted catheter is associated with clear-cut infection of the subcutaneous tunnel (tunnel infection), with evidence of septic thrombosis of the involved central vein, with septic pulmonary emboli, with right-sided endocarditis, or if it does not resolve within 2 to 3 d after the beginning of IV antimicrobial therapy, the catheter should be removed. Similarly, a catheter colonized by *Pseudomonas* spp. or *Candida* spp. is probably better managed by the immediate removal of the line, due to high risk of treatment failure.

Since up to 50% of coagulase-negative staphylococci are resistant to methicillin, vancomycin is the empiric antibiotic of choice. The therapy can be switched to a penicillin derivative if the antimicrobial sensitivity is appropriate. The length of recommended intravenous therapy is usually 7 d for coagulase-negative staphylococci and 2 wk or more for *S. aureus*. A recent meta-analysis has suggested that for *S. aureus* infections 2 wk of intravenous therapy may be too short because of the presence of a significant rate of septic complications requiring more prolonged therapy. Thus in the presence of *S. aureus* bacteremia, which is prolonged (>3 d) or if there is suspicion of a distal site of infection (osteomyelitis, endocarditis), therapy for 4 to 6 wk is more appropriate. Replacing vancomycin by teicoplanin offers the opportunity to treat methicillin-resistant staphylococci by using the intravenous or the intramuscular route in a single daily dose. In the authors' view, there are not enough data to consider teicoplanin as a mandatory alternative therapy to vancomycin; in fact, at the end of 1997, the drug had only been widely approved for use in Europe. Teicoplanin therefore should be restricted to specific situations where vancomycin cannot be safely administered. The new streptogramin combination quinupristin/dalfopristin appears to be a promising alternative. It has been available for compassionate use, particularly for the treatment of vancomycin-resistant enterococci. However, further clinical trials are necessary to assess its efficacy and indications.

**Table 67.1** Microbiology of catheter-related infections*

| | Pulmonary arterial catheters (Swan-Ganz):[a] | | Central and peripheral catheters:[b] |
|---|---|---|---|
| Microorganisms | Catheter colonization | Catheter-related bacteremia | Catheter colonization |
| Coagulase-negative staphylococci (CNS) | 56% | 37% | 30–40% |
| *S. aureus* | 5% | 26% | 5–10% |
| *P. aeruginosa* | 4% | 5% | 3–6% |
| Other gram-negative rods | 19% | 11% | 3–7% |
| *Streptococcus* and *Enterococcus* spp. | 6% | 5% | 4–6% |
| *Candida* spp. | 7% | 16% | 2–5% |
| Other | 3% | — | — |

*Data obtained from two meta-analyses of Widmer (1990) and Mermel and Maki (1994).

[a]Intensive care units.

[b]All wards.

**Table 67.2** Scheme for the management of central venous catheter infections (for surgically implanted catheters, refer to the discussion)*

| Conditions | Microorganisms | Therapy | Alternative therapy | Duration |
|---|---|---|---|---|
| CLINICAL SUSPICION | | Remove and culture the catheter, draw 2–3 pairs of blood cultures | | |
| No sepsis | | Clinical monitoring | | |
| Sepsis | | Vancomycin | | Until identification |
| Catheter colonization[a] | | Clinical monitoring | | |
| Catheter-related bacteremia (without any complication) | CNS | Vancomycin (MRCNS) or flucloxacillin[b] or nafcillin (MSCNS) | Teicoplanin[c] (MRCNS) or penicillin G or cefazolin (PSCNS) | 7 d |
| | GNR | 3rd generation cephalosporin | Quinolone | 14 d |
| | *P. aeruginosa* | Ceftazidime + aminoglycoside | Piperacillin/tazobactam or cefepime or imipenem/cilastatin | 14 d |
| | *S. aureus* | Vancomycin (MRSA) or flucloxacillin[b] or nafcillin (MSSA) | Teicoplanin[c] (MRSA) or penicillin G or cefazolin (PSSA) | 14 d |
| | *Candida* spp. | Ampho B (0.3–0.5 mg/kg/d) | Fluconazole[d] (400 then 200 mg/d) or liposomal ampho B (5 mg/kg/d) | Ampho B[e] or 2–4 wk fluconazole |
| Catheter-related bacteremia[f] with (possible) complication | | Same therapy as the uncomplicated catheter-related bacteremia, but with prolonged duration<br>Anticoagulation with heparin (if not contraindicated)<br>Consider surgery if evolution is not favorable | | 4–6 wk |
| Septic thrombophlebitis (large vessels) | | Same therapy as the uncomplicated catheter-related bacteremia, but with prolonged duration<br>Anticoagulation with heparin (if not contraindicated)<br>Consider surgery if evolution is not favorable | | 4–6 wk |

*CNS: Coagulase-negative staphylococci; GNR: gram-negative rods; MRCNS: methicillin-resistant CNS; MSCNS: methicillin-sensitive CNS, PSCNS: penicillin-sensitive CNS; MRSA: methicillin-resistant *S. aureus*; MSSA: methicillin-sensitive *S. aureus*; PSSA: penicillin-sensitive *S. aureas*; ampho B: amphotericin B.

[a]Colonization, determined by Maki's technique (or a quantitative culture), is predictive for bacteremia: treatment should be reserved for patients with clinical symptoms and/or positive blood cultures.

[b]Flucloxacillin is not available in the United States.

[c]Teicoplanin is currently not available in the United States; refer to the discussion for details.

[d]Fluconazole in this setting had a similar success rate as amphotericin B; however, the study did not include neutropenic or immunocompromised patients (Rex et al. 1994).

[e]The dosage of amphotericin B is dependent on the degree of candidemia; if a septic metastasis is proven (e.g. osteomyelitis) the usual dosage is 1–2 g.

[f]Prosthetic or damaged cardiac valve (CNS or *S. aureus*); sustained *S. aureus* bacteremia (>3 d); (suspected) endocarditis or infectious metastatic focus (all strains).

When antibiotics are given to high-risk patients for prolonged periods, *Candida* spp. are more likely to be the infecting pathogen. For catheter-related fungemia, amphotericin B remains the drug of choice; the liposomal formulation of amphotericin B and fluconazole need further comparative evaluation to be considered as first-choice therapy (see Chapters 38, 42).

## Optimal Intravenous Catheter Care: Prevention of Intravenous Catheter Infections

Considerable efforts have been devoted to assessing risk factors, establishing optimal care, and developing catheters made of new materials which may help to prevent intravenous catheter infections.

Hospitals with well-trained special IV catheter teams experience the lowest rates of central venous catheter-related sepsis (2% or less). Such teams provide more consistent attention to aseptic technique during central catheter insertion and in follow-up care of the site, and they assure careful monitoring of all infusions at least daily. Most home TPN and IV antibiotic therapy programs, which emphasize teaching the patient to care meticulously for his or her own catheter, report rates of complicating infection of less than one septicemia per five patient yr (<1/1800 catheter d).

The risk of central venous catheter infections is dependent on the site and on the duration of catheterization. Venous access by the internal jugular vein is considered to be associated with a higher risk of infection than the subclavian vein insertion site. The latter, however, has a higher rate of nonseptic complications upon insertion (pneumothorax, arterial puncture, etc.). By analysis of several studies, it is possible to calculate a cumulative risk of 10% of catheter-related bacteremia when the central venous catheter is left in place for 3 wk. This increase is linear with time and does not appear to change even with frequent removal of the catheter and insertion of a new IV line on another site. Thus the only recommendation that can be made is to shorten as much as possible the overall utilization time of central venous catheters for an individual patient. The catheter should be exchanged if there is an obvious malfunction (occlusion) or suspicion of infection.

Vigorous hand washing must always precede the insertion of a cannula. Persons inserting central venous catheters should exercise meticulous aseptic techniques, including wearing a sterile gown and gloves and draping the site with a large sterile sheet. Disinfection of the insertion site with a reliable antiseptic (recent studies suggest chlorhexidine 2% to 4% is more effective than iodophors) and meticulous attention to aseptic technique during insertion constitute the first line of defense against catheter-related infections. Limiting the duration of peripheral venous cannulation to no longer than 3 d and central venous catheter placement in ICU patients to no more than 5 d will greatly reduce the risk of infection. However, as yet there are no firm guidelines to recommend a specific time interval to change the IV line—and in many instances, central venous catheters are not changed and are left in place as long as needed, usually 1 to 2 wk, unless there is a suspicion of infection. Replacing the entire IV delivery system every 72 h will reduce the risk of sporadic sepsis from contaminated infusate.

A well designed prospective randomized study showed a higher risk for catheter infection if transparent dressings were used instead of gauze. Local moisture appears to be a risk factor in this situation. The importance of keeping the insertion site as clean and dry as possible is now accepted. Dressing changes every 48 h are currently recommended. Periodic site care, cleansing the skin about the insertion site with an antiseptic, and redressing the catheter with a sterile dressing are of value and recommended for arterial and central venous catheters. Changing central catheters over a guidewire is not recommended as a routine practice but can be done safely in special circumstances if a stringent aseptic protocol is followed.

### Catheter material

Several additional measures have been shown to decrease catheter-related infections. These include silver-impregnated cuffs, antimicrobial coating, and antiseptic-impregnated catheters. A silver-impregnated cuffed catheter was shown to lower the bacterial colonization (9.1% versus 28.9%) as well as to reduce the rate of bacteremia (1.0% versus 3.7%), but this has not been confirmed by another group. Similar results were obtained with antimicrobial-coating or antiseptic-bound catheters. However, to date, there is no consensus about the cost-effectiveness of such novel approaches and whether selected subgroups of patients might benefit from these preventive, more expensive measures.

## Suppurative Thrombophlebitis and Septic Thrombosis

### Intravenous catheter-related infections

The most serious form of intravascular catheter-related infection is suppurative phlebitis, and in the large central veins, septic thrombosis. With peripheral IV catheters, this infection invariably has originated from plastic catheters left in place for prolonged periods, particularly in burn patients. Septic thrombosis of the large central veins usually derives from percutaneously inserted central catheters used in burn patients or patients with other surgical infections and is characterized by high-grade septicemia and, often, septic pulmonary emboli. In any patient with an intravenous device who develops high-grade cryptogenic sepsis, suppurative thrombophlebitis or septic thrombosis of the large central veins should always be suspected.

Suppurative phlebitis is one of the most serious complications of peripheral catheterization. This purulent infection of the vein is a very severe disease. In suspected cases, the vein can be examined with a small cutdown and milked distally in an effort to express pus. Confirmed pus from the lumen of the vein calls for consideration of immediate surgical intervention.

With peripheral septic thrombophlebitis the involved vein segment should be resected surgically after withdrawal of the catheter. With septic thrombosis of the large central veins, the catheter should also be removed, and if there are no contraindications, the patient should be heparinized; high-dose bactericidal antimicrobial therapy, as would normally be used for endocarditis, should be given for at least 4 to 6 wk.

### Pelvic suppurative thrombophlebitis and pylephlebitis

*Pelvic suppurative thrombophlebitis* is related to pelvic tissue damage. It is therefore mainly encountered in women of childbearing age, in association with parturition or abortion. Patients with pelvic abscess or undergoing gynecological or pelvic surgery constitute another group at risk to develop a suppurative thrombophlebitis. The pathogenesis is poorly understood. Blood flow stasis and/or the hypercoagulable state of pregnancy may favor the development of a pelvic thrombus. This thrombus can then be seeded by bacteria gaining access to the site from another infectious focus (e.g., a gynecological infection). Typically, high fever with acute abdominal pain appear 1 to 2 wk after delivery or postoperatively. For anatomical reasons (right ovarian vein being more susceptible to compression), most cases are located in the lower right abdominal quadrant. Bacteremia is infrequent, usually making the microbiological etiology difficult to establish. Multiple small septic pulmonary emboli are often visible on the chest X-ray and represent useful diagnostic clues.

Anaerobes have been the most frequently isolated bacteria and treatment should include high doses of penicillin G combined with metronidazole or clindamycin. Valuable alternatives are ceftriaxone combined with metronidazole or imipenem. Surgical drainage must be performed when medical therapy is unsatisfactory.

*Pylephlebitis* is a suppurative thrombophlebitis of the portal vein. This rare complication of an abdominal infection is characterized by fever, acute abdominal pain, and signs of portal hypertension. Unlike ascending cholangitis, jaundice is rare in pylephlebitis except in cases complicated by multiple liver abscesses. The diagnosis requires angiography, but ultrasonography or CT scan can reveal thrombosis of the portal vein with possible hepatic abscesses. The management is essentially the same as described above, but with prolonged antimicrobial therapy. Anticoagulation may benefit some patients by preventing septic embolization to the liver. Surgical intervention should be reserved for cases that have not responded to antibiotics and heparin.

## Mycotic Aneurysms

Mycotic aneurysm is an old term defining a mushroom-shaped arterial aneurysm. Many bacteria and some fungi can cause mycotic aneurysms in the proper setting. *Treponema pallidum*, which causes syphilitic aneurysms, more often gives rise to a diffuse aortitis. Pathologically, a mycotic aneurysm is an inflammation of the arterial wall either causing—or less commonly arising on—an aneurysm. However, the pathogenesis differs between primary and secondary mycotic aneurysms. Primary mycotic aneurysms are related to a direct trauma of the artery or caused by an extension from a contiguous infected focus. Secondary mycotic aneurysms arise from intravascular sources of infection (infective endocarditis or any bacteremia) and lead to arterial wall infection by hematogenous contamination.

Most mycotic aneurysms result from hematogenous seeding of the intima during a bacteremia or a fungemia. They are predominantly located on damaged vascular intima: usually atherosclerotic plaques but also on preexisting anatomic abnormalities causing turbulent blood flow. The disease is typically encountered in older men since 70% of cases involve the aorta, the vessel most commonly and severely damaged by atherosclerosis. Interestingly, *Salmonella typhimurium* and *Salmonella choleraesuis* are more frequently recovered than *S. aureus* in these infections. The reason why *Salmonella* has a higher ability to infect abnormal arterial walls is not known. Infective endocarditis can lead to septic microemboli into the arterial nutrient vessels, the vasa vasorum. Mycotic aneurysms then typically develop in the proximal thoracic aorta and peripheral vessels, including cerebral arteries. In the latter location, they may present as a cause of intracranial hemorrhage or stroke complicating endocarditis (see Chapter 66).

In primary mycotic aneurysms, *S. aureus* is the most frequent pathogen if the infection arises from a direct arterial trauma. This situation is encountered in parenteral drug abusers, in gunshots wounds, as well as in iatrogenic lesions. Other causes include direct extension from an infection focus.

The diagnosis of secondary mycotic aneurysms may be difficult. Symptoms are usually nonspecific, including low-grade fever with an inflammatory syndrome. Focal pain, consequences of local impaired blood supply, and sepsis with positive blood cultures are suggestive of an arterial infection. Unfortunately, the diagnosis is often made as a consequence of rupture of the infected aneurysm. Localized symptoms in the presence of an infective endocarditis should prompt an extensive radiological workup including MRI and angiography to identify potential mycotic aneurysms that might be treated by surgery. In cerebral aneurysms, neuroradiological intervention can sometimes provide a satisfactory outcome. However, such radiological findings may be complicated by the possible presence of "bland" preexisting aneurysms. In a septic patient, the finding of a new aneurysm or the evidence for a recent enlargement suggest a mycotic aneurysm, as well as a perianeurysmal fluid collection. The only specific diagnostic sign is the presence of gas in the aortic wall, but it is rare.

Treatment involves a prolonged antimicrobial course (at least 4 wk) and often if possible a complete resection of the infected tissue. The long-term follow-up has to be especially careful, focusing on bleeding or reinfection of the graft site.

## ANNOTATED BIBLIOGRAPHY


Arnow PM, Quimosing EM, Beach M. Consequences of intravascular catheter sepsis. Clin Infect Dis 1993; 16:778–784.

*Cost analysis of catheter sepsis: very expensive disease even without lawsuit.*

Benezra D, Kiehn TE, Gold GWM, Brown AE, Turnbull ADM, Armstrong D. Prospective study of infections in indwelling central venous catheters using quantitative blood cultures. Am J Med 1988; 85:495–498.

Brun Buisson C, Abrouk F, Legrand P, Huet Y, Larabi S, Rapin M. Diagnosis of central venous catheter-related sepsis. Critical level of quantitative tip cultures. Arch Intern Med 1987; 147:873–877.

Groeger JS, Lucas AB, Coit D, Laquaglia M, Brown AE, Turnbull A, Exelby P. A prospective, randomized evaluation of the effect of silver impregnated subcutaneous cuffs for preventing tunneled chronic venous access catheter infections in cancer patients. Ann Surg 1993; 218:206–210.

Hulliger S, Pittet D. Incidence, morbidité et mortalité des infections dues aux cathéters veineux centraux en réanimation. Réan. Urg. 1994; 3 (3 bis): 365–369.

Jernigan JA, Farr BM. Short-course therapy of catheter-related *Staphylococcus aureus* bacteremia: a meta-analysis. Ann Intern Med 1993; 119: 304–311.

*Exhaustive meta-analysis focusing on ideal treatment duration and complications due to* S. aureus *catheter-related bacteremia.*

Kearney RA, Eisen HJ, Wolf JE. Nonvalvular infections of the cardiovascular system. Ann Intern Med 1994; 121:219–230.

*Recent and detailed review on infectious vascular complications, except those due to the catheters.*

Lecciones JA, Lee JW, Navarro EE, Witebsky FG, Marshall D, Steinberg SM, Pizzo PA, Walsh TJ. Vascular catheter-associated fungemia in patients with cancer: analysis of 155 episodes. Clin Infect Dis 1992; 14:875–883.

Linares J, Sitges Serra A, Garau J, Perez JL, Martin R. Pathogenesis of catheter sepsis: a prospective study with quantitative and semiquantitative cultures of catheter hub and segments. J Clin Microbiol 1985; 21:357–360.

*Comparison of two methods to culture the catheters in patients on total parenteral nutrition.*

Maki DG, Weise CE, Sarafin HW. A semiquantitative culture method for identifying intravenous-catheter-related infection. N Engl J Med 1977; 296:1305–1309.

Maki DG, Cobb L, Garman JK, Shapiro JM, Ringer M, Helgerson RB. An attachable silver-impregnated cuff for prevention of infection with central venous catheters: a prospective randomized multicenter trial. Am J Med 1988; 85:307–314.

Maki DG, Stolz SM, Wheeler S, Mermel LA. Prevention of central venous catheter-related bloodstream infection by use of an antiseptic-impregnated catheter. Ann Intern Med 1997; 127:257–266.

*A large randomized, controlled trial based on standardized definitions.*

Mermel LA, Maki DG. Infectious complications of Swan-Ganz pulmonary artery catheters: pathogenesis, epidemiology, prevention, and management. Am J Respir Crit Care Med 1994; 149:1020–1036.

*Excellent review of the problems related to Swan-Ganz catheters with a meta-analysis. Exhaustive bibliography.*

Pearson ML. Guidelines for prevention of intravascular device-related infections. Part I. Intravascular device-related infections: an overview. The Hospital Infection Control Practices Advisory Committee. Am J Infect Control 1996; 24:262–293.

Plemmons RM, Dooley DP, Longfield RN. Septic thrombophlebitis of the portal vein (pylephlebitis): diagnosis and management in the modern era. Clin Infect Dis 1995; 21:1114–1120.

Raad II, Bodey GP. Infectious complications of indwelling vascular catheters. Clin Infect Dis 1992; 15:197–208.

*Definitions of catheter-related infections, complications, and therapy discussed by experts in the field.*

Raad I, Darouiche R, Dupuis J et al. Central venous catheters coated with minocycline and rifampin for the prevention of catheter-related colonization and bloodstream infections. A randomized, double-blind trial. Ann Intern Med 1997; 127:267–274.

Rex JH, Bennett JE, Sugar AM et al. A randomized trial comparing fluconazole with amphotericin B for the treatment of candidemia in patients without neutropenia. N Engl J Med 1994; 331:1325–1330.

Vaudaux P, Pittet D, Haeberli A, Lerch PG, Morgenthaler JJ, Proctor RA, Waldvogel FA, Lew DP. Fibronectin is more active than fibrin or fibrinogen in promoting *Staphylococcus aureus* adherence to inserted intravascular catheters. J Infect Dis 1993; 167:633–641.

Widmer AF. IV-related infections. In: *Prevention and Control of Nosocomial Infections.* Wenzel RP, ed. Williams & Wilkins, Baltimore, MD, pp 771–805, 1997.

*Excellent review on prevention of catheter-related infections.*

# 68

# Myocarditis and Pericarditis

A. MARTIN LERNER

*Myocarditis* and *pericarditis* refer to inflammation of the heart muscle or pericardial membranes. They may be acute, subacute, or chronic in presentation and can be caused by direct invasion by a pathogenic bacterium, fungus, or virus, or represent an autoimmune response stimulated by these agents. Pericarditis is often accompanied by the development of a pericardial effusion which may in some cases acutely lead to *pericardial tamponade*. When the process of pericardial inflammation becomes chronic, the resulting fibrosis can lead to *pericardial constriction*. Myocarditis is usually manifest as cardiac myocyte and electrical dysfunction and may result in acute or chronic congestive heart failure. Myocarditis and pericarditis may occur simultaneously with infection by specific agents such as enterovirus or the spirochete of Lyme disease, *Borellia burgdorferi*.

The term *myocarditis* implies the presence of an associated inflammatory response in the heart; however, in some circumstances myocyte necrosis or dysfunction can cause myofiber dropout without an inflammatory response. The long-term consequence of this process may be a *cardiomyopathy*. Fibrosis follows if myocardial drop-out has occurred.

Pericarditis, pericardial effusion, and cardiomyopathy may be caused by a variety of disorders other than infection. This chapter will focus on the infectious causes of myocarditis and pericarditis, and on their etiologies, recognition, clinical consequences, and management.

## Cardiac Abnormalities in Pericarditis and Myocarditis

The pericardial sac normally contains 15 to 20 ml of clear pericardial fluid that arises from lymphatic flow. A fine capillary endomyocardial lymphatic system is found in the endocardial tissues and interstitial areas of the myocardium and extends into collecting channels subjacent to myocardial fibers. There, lymphatic channels coalesce, completing tertiary lymphatic vessels and lymphatic trunks which again join at the epicardium into a fine lymphatic system. The subepicardial tissues have a diffuse lymphatic network. Lymph flows from endocardial and interstitial myocardium to epicardial lymphatics and finally to the tracheal bronchial lymph nodes of the mediastinal lymphatic collecting system. The parietal pericardium has no lymphatics. Inflammation induced by the presence of infectious agents in the pericardium and/or myocardium can block lymphatic flow and lead to pericardial effusion. Mediastinal lymphatic obstruction produces lymphangiectasis and retrograde flow of lymph to the pleura. This leads to pleural effusion (Chapter 59). Blockage of the lymphatics in the mediastinum *and* in the epicardium can cause pericardial effusion. Pericardial inflammation may be accompanied by concomitant myocarditis, leading to a mixed clinical picture known as *myopericarditis*.

During myocarditis, the force of myocardial contraction is often diminished by myocyte destruction. Both myocarditis and pericarditis can cause loss in the power function of the heart and lead to diastolic restriction by different mechanisms. With pericarditis, effusion may impair cardiac filling during diastole and reduce cardiac output. The most severe manifestation of this phenomenon is *cardiac tamponade*, which can cause shock and death if not promptly recognized and treated. With myocarditis, besides diminished systolic function, ventricular dilation during diastole may be impaired.

The end stage of myocarditis may result in cardiomyopathy. Cardiomyopathies may be dilated or nondilated and hypertrophic. Hypertrophic cardiomyopathies are almost always due to mechanisms other than infection (e.g., idiopathic or hypertensive). Dilated cardiomyopathies can result from infection or other causes of myocyte injury and death (ischemic, toxic, etc.). In dilated cardiomyopathies mural thrombi are common and peripheral emboli to the lungs or systemic circulation may occur depending on whether the thrombi reside within the right ventricle or left ventricle. These may develop acutely during the acute inflammatory phase of myocarditis or later in the course when inflammation has subsided.

## Etiology

Enteroviruses, pyogenic bacteria, *B. burgdorferi*, *Mycobacterium tuberculosis*, and systemic fungi are the most frequent infectious causes of myocarditis and pericarditis (Table 68.1). Pericarditis may also develop in metabolic disorders, such as uremia, or in collagen vascular diseases, including systemic lupus erythematosis, dermatomyositis, and scleroderma. Patients with myocardial infarction may develop a postinfarction pericarditis. Pericardial effusions and myocardial injury can occur posttrauma or after cardiac surgery. Metastatic or cardiac malignancies may present with pericardial effusion. At times it will not be clear whether the etiology is infectious or noninfectious, so it becomes necessary to exclude a role for infection.

## Pathogenesis

### Viral myopericarditis

Recently, specific enterovirus RNA has been utilized as a probe in in situ hybridization assays to demonstrate virus in the myocardium. Group-specific RNA can recognize coxsackievirus A,

**Table 68.1** Clinical findings in pyogenic pericarditis and coxsackievirus B myopericarditis*

| Finding | Pyogenic (%) | Coxsackievirus B (%) |
|---|---|---|
| SYMPTOMS OR SIGNS | | |
| Acutely ill (toxic, fever, dyspnea) | 100 | 58 |
| Raised jugular venous pulse | 100 | 21 |
| Increased cardiac dullness | 100 | 74 |
| Adynamic pericardium | 100 | 11 |
| Muffled heart sounds | 94 | 11 |
| Hepatomegaly | 94 | 21 |
| Paradoxical pulse | 88 | 11 |
| Cardiac tamponade | 88 | 0 |
| Pleural effusion | 56 | 5 |
| Pericardial friction rub | 38 | 26 |
| Ascites | 31 | 0 |
| Pitting edema | 25 | 5 |
| Apical systolic murmur | 10 | 68 |
| LABORATORY FEATURES | | |
| Polymorphonuclear leukocytosis | 100 | 74 |
| Enlarged cardiac silhouette | 100 | 74 |
| Abnormal ECG (low voltage; Q ST, q ST segments) | 100 | 100 |
| Arrhythmia | Rare | Common |
| Pericardiocentesis with isolation of bacterium or virus from fluid | 100 | Rare |
| Pericardial fluid | Exudate | Usually exudate |

*Data taken from Klacsman, PG et al. Am J Med 1977; 63:666 and Sainani GS et al. Br Heart J 1975; 37: 819.

coxsackievirus B, and echovirus infection. Myocardial enterovirus infection is multifocal and random. In one study enterovirus RNA was found in 23 of 95 (24%) patients with a clinical suspicion of acute myocarditis including ten of 33 patients (30%) with dilated cardiomyopathy of recent origin. Persistence of enterovirus in the heart appears to be a central feature of chronic enteroviral heart disease. During persistent infection in murine myocarditis models, 100% of myocardial cells can be shown to be infected, sustaining myocardial inflammation. T lymphocytes and macrophages are crucial in limiting myocardial virus replication. A controversy exists as to whether myocardial injury is due to virus-induced pathobiological events or results from autoimmune processes initially triggered by viral infection.

Experimental evidence suggests that immunologically mediated mechanisms may be responsible for many cases of viral-induced myocardial injury. Cytotoxic monoclonal antibodies that recognize epitopes in both enteroviruses and the bacterium *Streptococcus pyogenes* have been identified. Monoclonal antibodies to streptococcal M protein can cross-react with human cardiac myosin and other $\alpha$-helical coiled molecules and neutralize coxsackieviruses B3 and B4 and poliovirus type 1. These data suggest an immunological similarity between poststreptococcal rheumatic myocarditis and enterovirus-induced primary myocardial disease. Another antibody that cross-reacts with the coxsackievirus B3 capsid viral protein 1 and myosin was recently identified. Epitopes of the cardiac sarcolemma also cross-react with enteroviral proteins, and this may be an etiologic trigger of autoreactive myocarditis. Finally, T cells may mediate lysis of cardiac myocytes in experimental models.

The clinical signs of myopericarditis are predominantly those of myocarditis or pericarditis. The pathological findings are as follows: In myocarditis the acute process may be interstitial with a mixed inflammatory infiltrate and very little or no myofiber necrosis. Inflammatory cells can be found between muscle bundles and surrounding coronary arteries with spread to the pericardial sac. Some cases of myopericarditis are associated with a diffuse asymmetric myofiber necrosis that involves the full thickness of the myocardium and is associated with Q waves in the resting electrocardiogram. The lesions may resemble those of coronary thrombosis with myocardial infarction by perfusion nuclear scan. However, coronary vessels remain open. Ventricular aneurysms may follow.

Endovascular spasm may be induced during acute infectious myocarditis. Myocardial lesions distal to the spastic artery may heal with permanent scars and sometimes even with myocardial calcification. In benign interstitial myopericarditis, recovery may be anatomically and physiologically complete. In other cases myocyte destruction may be replaced by scarring.

## Pyogenic pericarditis

Pyogenic bacteria may reach the pericardial sac hematogenously or from contiguous pulmonary infection, leading to a vigorous acute inflammatory response by polymorphonuclear leukocytes.

Acute purulent pericarditis often produces a thick 8 to 12 mm pericardium sometimes containing 500 to 2000 ml of a viscid fibrinous or yellow purulent exudate with varying amounts of granulation tissue. The left lower lobe of the lung may be adherent to the thoracic wall, and the pericardium may adhere to the myocardium and be covered by a cottage cheese-like material. A fibrinous granulomatous pericarditis with no free fluid may occur. Concomitant myocardial abscesses are often present, especially in cases of acute infective endocarditis associated with *Staphylococcus aureus*. Systemic fungal infections such as *Histoplasma capsulatum* or opportunistic *Candida* or *Aspergillus* species may complicate cancer chemotherapy and also produce myocardial abscesses.

Many patients with pyogenic pericarditis have an underlying disease such as recent thoracic surgery, chronic renal failure, cancer, myocardial infarction, diabetes mellitus, myeloproliferative disorders, or sickle cell anemia. Acute purulent pericarditis may be a complication of suppurative infections (in other locations) such as pneumonia, meningitis, infective endocarditis, skin infections, and endometritis. Direct pulmonary extension from left lower lobe pneumonias or infection following perforating injuries to the chest wall may occur. Myocardial abscesses may rupture into the pericardium, and a subdiaphragmatic suppurative lesion may occasionally be the source of purulent infection.

### Tuberculous pericarditis

This is a relatively rare complication of pulmonary or systemic tuberculosis (TB). It may develop during the course of active pulmonary tuberculosis or as a consequence of hematogenous spread during miliary TB or as an isolated occurrence. In some cases tuberculous involvement of mediastinal lymph nodes leads to direct extension into the pericardium. Rarely, tuberculous pericarditis may be purulent. Both pericardial tamponade and constriction are major complications.

## Epidemiology

### Enteroviruses

Enteroviruses appear to be the dominant cause of idiopathic myopericarditis. Coxsackieviruses belonging to group B probably account for most cases, although echoviruses and group A coxsackieviruses may be involved. Cases of enterovirus (coxsackievirus A or B or echoviruses) occur in all seasons of the year, but in the Northern Hemisphere the fewest cases are seen in the first quarter and the most in the second and third quarters, corresponding to the seasonal distribution of the prevalence of enteroviruses. At least half of the cases of coxsackievirus and echovirus infections are subclinical. Endemic sporadic infection with occasional brisk outbreaks of the coxsackieviruses and echoviruses have been documented. The clinical syndromes associated with each enterovirus are variable and include undifferentiated febrile illness, upper respiratory syndromes, exanthems, lymphadenitis, pleurodynia, orchitis, gastroenteritis or life-threatening meningoencephalitis, hepatitis, pneumonia, hemolytic uremic syndrome, or myopericarditis. About 5% of all symptomatic cases of coxsackievirus infections involve the heart. During infancy, mortality rates of acute infectious myocarditis may be as high as 50%.

Infections with coxsackieviruses and echoviruses are common throughout the world. By adult life most people have significant titers of neutralizing antibodies to many of these viruses. Neutralizing antibodies confer long-lasting, type-specific protection from infection and disease. Contagion among enteroviruses is from person to person by the fecal–oral route, but some spread can occur by the air-borne method. Virus excretion in feces peaks in late summer and fall and may persist for many weeks. Virus in the pharynx persists for a shorter period of time. Viremia is usual during incubation periods but is usually absent during the early days of clinical disease. Infectivity in households is high (76% of exposed susceptible persons).

### Other viruses

Pericarditis and myocarditis resulting from cytomegalovirus infections are usually complications in immunosuppressed patients. Acute Epstein-Barr virus (EBV) infections may rarely cause myopericarditis. The role of Epstein-Barr virus and/or cytomegalovirus in the cardiomyopathy of chronic fatigue syndrome is being explored. Rarely, pericarditis may complicate influenza or adenovirus infections.

### Bacteria

Significant changes in the bacterial pathogens of purulent pericarditis have occurred in the past 30 yr. Formerly, 80% of cases were caused by aerobic gram-positive cocci (*Streptococcus pneumoniae*, *Staphylococcus aureus*, or *Streptococcus pyogenes*). These organisms now account for about 40% of the cases. On the other hand, gram-negative bacilli (*Escherichia coli*, *Proteus* species, *Pseudomonas aeruginosa*, *Salmonella* and *Shigella* species, *Neisseria meningitidis*, and *Borrelia burgdorferi*) are more common today. Numbers and percentage of cases of tuberculous pericarditis vary with the prevalence of tuberculosis; TB pericarditis may occur in patients with AIDS (see Chapter 100).

### Parasites

American trypanosomiasis (Chagas disease), trichinosis, toxoplasmosis, amebiasis, and echinococcosis are systemic parasitic infections that sometimes produce myopericarditis. Chagas disease is endemic in South America and echinococcis is in highest prevalence in the Mid and Far East. Trichinosis, toxoplasmosis, and amebiasis are worldwide.

## Clinical Manifestations

Comparative signs and symptoms of viral and bacterial myo-pericarditis are shown in Table 68.1. In general, patients with pyogenic pericarditis are more acutely ill with anorexia, fever, chills, and chest pain than those with viral myopericarditis in which only chest pain or cardiac arrythmias or congestive heart failure may be the principal feature. Physical findings may help differentiate pyogenic pericarditis from viral myopericarditis. Raised jugular venous pulsations, an adynamic pericardium with impalpable apical pulses, muffled heart sounds, hepatomegaly, paradoxical pulses, and cardiac tamponade are among the striking physical findings of pyogenic pericarditis. Pleural effusions and pitting edema are also more common in purulent pericarditis. None of these signs is common in coxsackievirus B myopericarditis, unless sufficient pericardial fluid has accumulated to cause tamponade.

**Table 68.2** Treatment of pericarditis

| Agent | Medical | Surgical (for cardiac tamponade or constrictive pericarditis) |
|---|---|---|
| PERICARDITIS<br>(Enteroviruses, e.g., coxsackievirus, echoviruses, other viruses (Epstein-Barr virus, cytomegalovirus, human immunodeficiency virus) | Acute phase (first 14 d)<br>Avoid corticosteroids, alcohol, $\beta$-blockers, anticoagulants, nonsteroidal anti-inflammatory agents; give digitalis, diuretics, anti-arrhythmic agents as needed | Pericardiocentesis |
| | Chronic phase—supportive therapy with rest (no exercise) until stable | Pericardiocentesis or pericardiectomy |
| PURULENT PERICARDITIS<br>*GRAM-POSITIVE COCCI*<br>*Staphylococcus aureus*<br>*Staphylococcus epidermidis*<br>*Streptococcus pneumoniae*<br>*Streptococcus pyogenes* | For specifically sensitive organisms penicillin G (20–30 million units/d IV for 4–6 wk) or nafcillin (1.5–2.0 g IV, every 4 h for 4 wk).<br>For methicillin-resistant *Staphylococcus aureus* and all strains of *Staphylococcus epidermidis*, vancomycin IV: all antibiotics are continued for 4–6 wk. | Tube drainage, decortication, pericardiectomy as required |
| *GRAM-NEGATIVE BACILLI*<br>*Escherichia coli, Proteus, Enterobacter, Pseudomonas,* species | Two appropriate bactericidal antibiotics according to susceptibility studies, usually an extended spectrum penicillin (e.g., timentin) or 3rd-generation cephalosporin (ceftazidime) plus an aminoglycoside (e.g., gentamicin, tobramycin). All antibiotics are continued for 4–6 wk | Tube drainage, decortication, pericardiectomy |
| *FUNGI*<br>*Histoplasma, Aspergillus, Sporotrichosis, Mucormycosis, Blastomyces, Candida* species | The drug of choice remains amphotericin B, 0.4–0.6 mg/kg IV for 10 wk<br>Fluconazole and itraconazole have potential efficacy. Dosages have not been established. | Tube drainage, decortication, pericardiectomy |
| *Mycobacterium tuberculosis*, isoniazid-sensitive strain | A three-drug regimen, daily for 12 mo including isoniazid (INH), rifampin (RIF) and pyrazinamide (PZA) plus prednisone | Tube drainage, decortication, pericardiectomy |
| Isoniazid-resistant strains | A four-drug regimen including INH, RIF, PZA, and streptomycin (SM) or ethambutol (EMB) | |

Cardiac involvement in Lyme disease is predominantly a myocarditis that develops 6 to 9 wk after the primary infection. Besides a history of *erythema migrans*, an active arthritis involving large joints may be present. Conduction disturbances, including complete heart block, are common.

Pericardial friction rubs are best heard to the left of the midsternal border while the patient is sitting up, leaning forward, and not breathing. Pericardial rubs are accentuated during inspiration or expiration and may be mono-, di-, or triphasic, corresponding to atrial or ventricular systole or to early ventricular diastole. Pericardial or pleural pericardial friction rubs are often also palpable. Myocardial compromise may be manifest as softened heart sounds, an S3 gallop, a mitral regurgitant murmur (with ventricular dilation), and signs of hypotension or congestive heart failure.

## Laboratory Studies

A polymorphonuclear leukocytosis, an enlarged heart on chest radiogram, and an elevated erythrocyte sedimentation rate are frequent findings in both acute pyogenic *and* viral myopericarditis. Pleural effusions may accompany cardiomegaly on chest X-ray. The lack of pulmonary venous congestion coupled with cardiac enlargement is a clue to pericardial effusion.

## Electrocardiography

In either purulent or coxsackievirus B myopericarditis, electrocardiographs show low voltage and diffuse ST segment elevation (Figure 68.1) or depression or both. Left ventricular hypertrophy, systolic murmurs, and arrhythmias (sinus bradycardia, atrial fibrillation, complete heart block) are more frequent in viral myopericarditis but can also be seen in Lyme disease. In a patient with a systemic mycosis (candidiasis, aspergillosis) a new conduction disturbance suggests a diagnosis of fungal myocarditis.

## Echocardiography

Echocardiography evaluates wall motion, estimates ejection fractions, and validates the presence of significant pericardial effusion and whether pericardial tamponade dynamics are present. Two-dimensional (2D) transthoracic echocardiography is easy to perform, relatively inexpensive, and has largely replaced older methods employing angiocardiography or radioisotopic scanning of the intracardiac blood pool. A sonolucent space at echocardiography (ultrasonogram) separating the ventricular wall motion from a motionless pericardial echo indicates a pericardial effusion (Figure 68.2). False-negative examination does occur in a small percentage of patients with small effusions.

Recently, monoclonal antimyosin antibodies labeled with in-

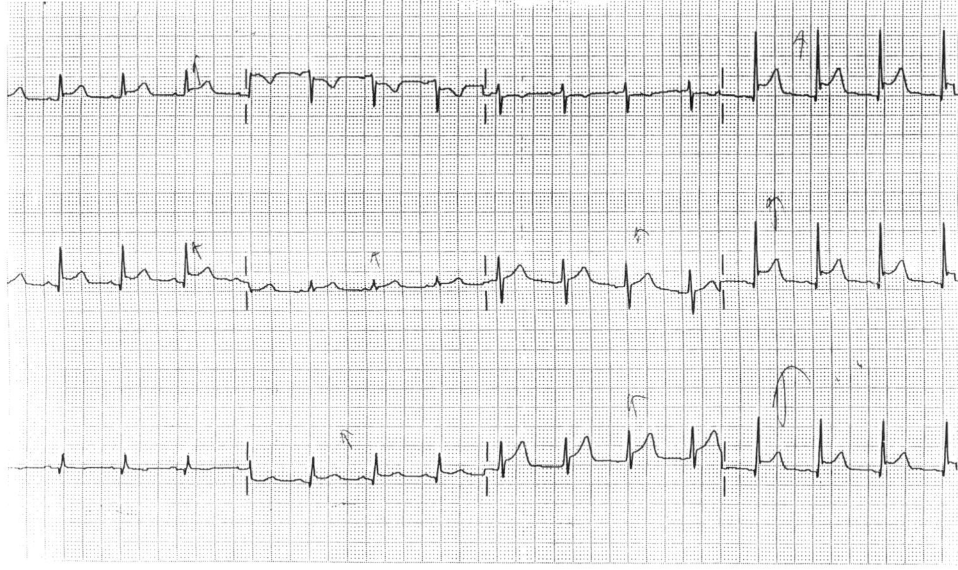

**Fig. 68.1** Electrocardiogram on a patient with acute pericarditis demonstrating diffuse ST segment elevation (I, II, AVL, AFV, $V_2$-$V_6$).

dium-111 have been utilized to detect myocardial injury. Diffuse labeling is seen in myopericarditis, while segmental involvement is found in myocardial infarction.

## Specific laboratory studies

Aspiration and analysis of pericardial fluid if present is often helpful in reaching an etiologic diagnosis. Pericardiocentesis carries with it, however, the risk of cardiac puncture, and as such is best performed by a skilled operator in an operating room or catheterization laboratory with simultaneous echocardiographic monitoring. Microbiological specimens should be processed promptly. Open pericardial biopsy may be indicated for the diagnosis of a chronic pericarditis such as that caused by tubercle bacilli.

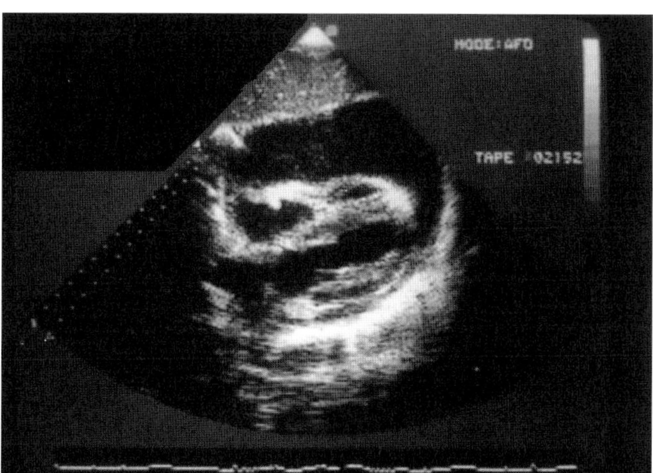


**Fig. 68.2** 2D Echocardiogram on a patient with a pericardial effusion demonstrating a broad sonoluscent region surrounding the ventricles in the center.

Appropriate tissue cultures and/or intraperitoneal inoculations of suckling mice may be used for the isolation of enteroviruses from throat or rectal swabs and from blood or pericardial fluid. Coxsackieviruses or other enteroviruses are rarely cultured from pericardial fluids. Viral nucleic acids may be recognized by polymerase chain reaction or in vitro hybridization techniques. Approximately 50% of cases of acute viral myopericarditis contain enterovirus RNA.

The etiology of pyogenic pericarditis is proved by isolation of the causative bacterium. Attempts should be made to isolate aerobic and anaerobic bacteria, fungi, and acid-fast bacilli. Gram, acid-fast, and methenamine silver stain preparations of pericardial exudates must be examined. Polymerase chain reactions may also be used to identify specific bacterial antigens.

Tubercle bacilli are isolated in about 40% of cases of *Mycobacterium tuberculosis* pericardial infections; the recovery rate is improved if biopsies are cultured. Nucleic acid hybridization methods using highly specific DNA probes, polymerase chain reaction (PCR), and molecular "DNA fingerprinting" techniques are rapidly increasing the accuracy and time until specific diagnosis to hours.

Right ventricular endomyocardial biopsies may be useful to evaluate cases of myocarditis. These can document myocardial necrosis, myofiber loss, the presence and type of inflammatory infiltrate, and T cell characterization. They can also be probed for the presence of specific viral nucleic acids. Langhans giant cells suggest tuberculosis. Special stains recognize bacteria, tubercle bacilli, or fungi. Interstitial or myonecrotic inflammation with a mixed lymphocytic infiltrate suggests viral myopericarditis. At electron microscopy, myofiberdisarray and hypertrophy *without* an inflammatory exudate indicates a cardiomyopathy.

Serologic diagnosis of specific causes of myocarditis/pericarditis is often difficult. IgM-neutralizing type-specific antibodies are usually found in serum in acute enteroviral invasions. However, there is considerable cross reaction between the serotypes of coxsackieviruses. As such, heterotypic neutralizing antibody responses may occur and obscure the interpretation of both IgM and Ig antibody titers.

Noninfectious etiologies for pericarditis and pericardial effusion should be considered, particularly in uremic patients or those with manifestations of collagen vascular disease. Malignancy metastatic to the pericardium commonly causes a bloody effusion and may be diagnosed by cytology or biopsy.

## Management (Table 68.2)

### Viral pericarditis

No specific therapy is yet available for enterovirus myopericarditis or most of the other viral infections of the heart. Ganciclovirus has not been systematically tested in the therapy of cytomegalovirus (CMV) myopericarditis but should be administered in proven cases (see Chapter 36).

Patients with a benign virus myopericarditis without significant cardiac muscle necrosis require rest for about 30 d. Strenuous exercise should be avoided during the convalescent period. (In murine models of coxsackievirus B3 myocarditis, exercise changes a benign nonlethal infection to one with a very high mortality. Virus titers per gram of myocardium are increased 500×.) Alcohol should be avoided. Patients with destruction of cardiac muscle must convalesce for at least 3 mo. Arrhythmias, angina-like pain, cardiomegaly, and congestive heart failure are poor prognostic signs.

Anticoagulants are contraindicated in viral myopericarditis because of the danger of inducing cardiac tamponade. Corticosteroids have been studied in controlled clinical trials of viral myopericarditis. No specific value has been found for these agents. Angiotensin-converting inhibitors and calcium channel blockers used in experimental animal models of myocarditis can decrease inflammatory infiltrates, diminish endovascular spasm, and ameliorate disease. However, no human clinical trials have been conducted.

### Pyogenic pericarditis

Surgical management along with intensive specific antibacterial therapy against the specific causative organism for 4 to 6 wk is often necessary. Local installation of antibiotics into the pericardial sac is not useful. In patients with pericarditis caused by pyogenic bacteria, relief of pressure by a simple pericardiocentesis may be insufficient. Decortication with resection may be required and may also be necessary to prevent the development of pericardial constriction.

In tuberculous pericarditis if antimicrobial therapy is begun promptly, drainage procedures may not be necessary (see Chapter 37). The concomitant use of prednisone (80 mg per day for 6 to 8 wk and then discontinued by slowly decreasing the dose over an additional 14 d) suppresses inflammation within the pericardium, enhances reabsorption of effusion, and retards pericardial constriction. Administration of glucocorticosteroids will not usually lead to worsening of the tuberculosis in the presence of effective antimicrobial therapy.

## Prognosis

The prognosis for both purulent or virus myopericarditis' depends upon the extent of disease at diagnosis and the appropriateness of therapy. Cardiac disability including heart failure, cardiomegaly, persistent precordial pain, and abnormal electrocardiograms may result. The larger the residual cardiac silhouette, after the resolution of pericardial effusion, the worse the prognosis. Arrhythmias, mural thrombi, and pulmonary emboli may follow.

The mortality rate in purulent pericarditis is high (over 50%). Mortality is highest in fungal myopericarditis in immunosuppressed patients and approaches 90%. Follow-up clinical studies include electrocardiograms, chest X-rays, echocardiograms, and exercise tests the frequency of which will be dictated by the severity of the disease. Studies with antimyosin antibody may be helpful in evaluating the extent and persistence of myocardial injury.

## Prevention

There are no vaccines available for enterovirus infections (other than polio, which is not a known cause of myopericarditis). Preventative measures for pyogenic or tuberculous pericarditis are those for bacterial or tuberculous infections in general.

## ANNOTATED BIBLIOGRAPHY

Aretz HT, Billingham ME, Edwards WD et al. Myocarditis (a histopathologic definition and classification). Am J Cardiovasc Pathol 1987; 1: 3–14.

*A simple morphologic classification ("the Dallas system") of myocarditis is outlined. This classification is based upon endomyocardial biopsy evaluation of inflammatory infiltrate, myocyte damage, and fibrosis.*

Cunningham MW, Antone SM, Guliza JM et al. Cytotoxic and viral neutralizing antibodies cross react with streptococcal M protein, enteroviruses and human cardiac myosin Proc. Natl Acad Sci USA 1992; 89:1320–1324.

*Evidence for an autoreactive commonality for immunologic injury to the heart between shared antigens in* Streptococcus pyogenes *and enteroviruses is presented.*

Herskowitz A, Campbell S, Deckers J et al. Demographic features and prevalence of idiopathic myocarditis in patients undergoing endomyocardial biopsy. Am J Cardiol 1993; 71:982–986.

*This is an excellent clinical description of patients with myocarditis.*

Kandolf R, Klingel K, Zell R et al. Molecular mechanisms in the pathogenesis of enteroviral heart disease: acute and persistent infections. Clin Immunol Immunopathol 1993; 68:153–158.

*Recognition of a group-specific common enteroviral RNA segment by in situ hybridization offers a sensitive means of diagnosis of coxsackievirus A, coxsackievirus B, and echovirus myocarditis/pericarditis and dilated cardiomyopathies.*

Klacsmann PG, Bulkley BH, Hutchins GM. The changed spectrum of purulent pericarditis. An 86-year autopsy experience in 200 patients. Am J Med 1977; 63:666–673.

*This is a good review of purulent pericarditis.*

Lekakis J, Nanas J, Athanassia M et al. Anti-myosin scintigraphy for detection of myocarditis. Chest 1993; 104:1427–1430.

*This method of detecting clinical myopericarditis offers advantages not previously available.*

Lerner AM, Zervos M, Dworkin HJ, Chang CH, O'Neill W. A unified theory of the cause of chronic fatigue syndrome. Infect Dis Clin Prac 1997; 6:239–243.

Rose NR, Herskowitz A, Newman DA. Auto-immunity in myocarditis: models and mechanisms. Clin Immunol Immunopathol 1993; 68:95–99.

*The role of virus infection of the heart in initiating an autoreactive myocarditis, genetic regulation in the host, and the interplay between virus persistence and auto-immunity are discussed.*

Sainani GS, Dekate MP, Rao CP. Heart disease caused by Coxsackievirus B infection. Br Heart J 1975; 37:819.

*This is a fine review of virus myopericarditis.*

# 69

# Urinary Tract Infections

WALTER E. STAMM

Urinary tract infections (UTI) are among the most common bacterial infections experienced by humans. On a worldwide basis, Harding and Ronald have estimated that 150 million UTIs occur annually, resulting in an estimated 6 billion dollars in health care costs. These infections range from asymptomatic bacteriuria on the one hand to acute pyelonephritis and gram-negative septicemia on the other. Urinary tract infections have been classified in a number of ways, including uncomplicated (occurring in the absence of predisposing conditions) or complicated (occurring in patients with abnormal urologic anatomy or function or immunosuppression); lower tract (involving the urethra or bladder) or upper tract (involving the ureters, kidneys, or prostate); and symptomatic or asymptomatic. This chapter will address the most common categories of UTI seen by clinicians—namely (*1*) acute uncomplicated cystitis in women, (*2*) recurrent UTI in women, (*3*) acute uncomplicated pyelonephritis in women, (*4*) complicated UTI in men and women, (*5*) asymptomatic bacteriuria, and (*6*) catheter-associated UTI.

## Etiology

The vast majority of UTIs are caused by bacteria. In selected patients (diabetics, catheterized patients or those with abnormal urinary tracts), candida may cause UTI. Adenoviruses are a recognized cause of acute hemorrhagic cystitis, mostly in children or young adults. Otherwise, however, symptomatic viral infections of the urinary tract are rare. Over 90% of UTIs are caused by a single bacterial species. In cases of uncomplicated cystitis and pyelonephritis, *Escherichia coli* accounts for more than 75% of infections (Table 69.1). In patients with recurrent or complicated UTIs, *E. coli* remains the most common organism but the proportion of cases due to other organisms (usually klebsiella, proteus, enterobacter, or enterococci) increases, as does the likelihood of isolating an organism with increased antibiotic resistance. In hospital-acquired UTIs, a much wider range of organisms is isolated (Table 69.1), and both antibiotic resistant isolates and candida are common pathogens, particularly if the patient has received prior courses of antimicrobial treatment.

Coagulase-negative staphylococci have often been considered urinary contaminants, but *Staphylococcus saprophyticus* has now clearly been demonstrated to be a urinary pathogen. In urine specimens, this species can be reliably identified as a coagulase-negative staphylococcus that is resistant to novobiocin. The vast majority of *S. saprophyticus* infections occur in young women (Table 69.1), most commonly in spring and summer.

Anaerobic bacteria, lactobacilli, corynebacteria, streptococci (other than enterococci), and *Staphylococcus epidermidis* constitute the normal flora of the perineum and distal urethra, and seldom cause UTI. When seen in cultures of voided urine these organisms are usually urinary contaminants.

*Staphylococcus aureus* bacteremia often causes metastatic infection of the kidney; ascending cystitis or pyelonephritis due to *S. aureus* is very unusual in patients who have not undergone instrumentation or catheterization. In men, enterococcal UTI frequently arises in the setting of urinary tract obstruction, catheterization, or instrumentation.

The role of other organisms as causes of urinary infection remains speculative. *Gardnerella vaqinalis* can be isolated from the urine of women with and without urinary symptoms but its pathogenic role is uncertain. *Ureaplasma urealyticum* and *Mycoplasma hominis* probably account for some cases of acute pyelonephritis, and perhaps some cases of cystourethritis as well. *Hemophilus influenzae* occasionally causes community-acquired urinary tract infection, including pyelonephritis.

## Epidemiology

The incidence of UTI varies dramatically with age and gender (Table 69.2). The prevalence of UTI in the neonatal period is approximately 1%, and infections during this period are often associated with bacteremia and/or functional or anatomic abnormalities of the urinary tract. In the first year of life, the incidence of UTI is higher in males than in females. In contrast, in early childhood (ages 1 to 5), the prevalence of bacteriuria in girls rises to 4.5% whereas in boys it falls to 0.5%. Infections in young boys are often associated with congenital abnormalities of the urinary tract or with lack of circumcision. Between one-third and one-half of UTIs in the first 5 years of life in young girls are associated with vesicoureteral (V-U)reflux. The prevalence of UTI in girls age 6–12 in the United States is approximately 1%, with 5% of girls experiencing UTI at some time. Bacteriuria and symptomatic UTI are rare in elementary school age boys.

During adolescence, the occurrence of UTI increases strikingly in young women. Approximately 20% of young women have at least one episode of UTI each year. By age 25, over 80% of women have experienced one or more UTIs. An estimated 7 million cases of acute cystitis occur in young women each year, making these among the most frequent of infections in this age group. In addition, this figure probably underestimates the true incidence of these infections, since some studies suggest that at least half of all UTIs resolve without coming to medical attention. During this period of life, UTI are 50-fold more common in women than in men. The major risk factors contributing to UTI in women of this age group appear to be sexual intercourse, diaphragm–spermicide use, exposure to spermicide alone, failure to void after intercourse, delayed voiding, and possibly prior

**Table 69.1** Microbial species most commonly associated with specific types of UTI*

| | Acute uncomplicated cystitis | Acute uncomplicated pyelonephritis | Complicated UTI | Catheter-associated UTI |
|---|---|---|---|---|
| *E. coli* | 79 | 89 | 32 | 24 |
| *S. saprophyticus* | 11 | 0 | 1 | 0 |
| *Proteus* | 2 | 4 | 4 | 6 |
| *Klebsiella* | 3 | 4 | 5 | 8 |
| Enterococci | 2 | 0 | 22 | 7 |
| *Pseudomonas* | 0 | 0 | 20 | 9 |
| Mixed | 3 | 5 | 10 | 11 |
| Other | 0 | 2 | 5 | 10 |
| Yeast | 0 | 0 | 1 | 28 |
| *S. epidermidis* | 0 | 0 | 15 | 8 |

*Data in columns 1 and 2 are from 607 episodes of cystitis and 84 episodes of pyelonephritis in Seattle; data from columns 3 and 4 are from Platt et al., Am J Epid 1986; 124:977–985 and from Gasser et al., Am J Med 1987; 82 (Suppl 44):278–279. Columns add to more than 100% due to polymicrobial infections.

Table reproduced with permission from Stamm WE, Urinary Tract Infection in *Infectious Diseases*, Saunders, 1992.

antibiotic use. Nearly all UTIs among young women are uncomplicated; that is, these patients have no anatomic or functional abnormalities in the urinary tract. Although traditional teaching has been that all UTIs in men should be considered complicated, recent studies suggest that uncomplicated infections do occur in some young men. Such uncomplicated UTIs among young men are uncommon, but risk factors associated with them include homosexuality, HIV infection, and lack of circumcision.

In the later years of life, the incidence of UTI sharply increases in both sexes with a progressive reduction in the female:male ratio. Lack of estrogenic hormones, uterine or bladder prolapse, reduced bladder tone, incontinence, and postvoid residual urine

**Table 69.2** Overview of the epidemiology of UTI by age group*

| | Females | | Males | |
|---|---|---|---|---|
| Age group | Prevalence (%) | Risk factors | Prevalence (%) | Risk factors |
| Neonate | 1 | Anatomic or functional urologic abnormalities | 1 | Anatomic or functional urologic abnormalities |
| 1–5 | 4–5 | Congenital abnormalities<br>V-U reflux | 0.5 | Vaginal or rectal intercourse<br>Lack of circumcision<br>HIV infection |
| 5–15 | 4–5 | V-U reflux | 0.5 | None |
| 16–35 | 20 | Sexual intercourse, spermicide exposure, antimicrobials, past history of UTI | 0.5 | |
| 35–65 | 35 | Gynecologic surgery<br>Bladder prolapse<br>Estrogen lack<br>Incontinence<br>Residual urine<br>nonsecretor | 20 | Prostatic hypertrophy<br>Obstruction,<br>Catheterization,<br>Surgery |
| Over 65 | 40 | As above, plus incontinence, chronic catheterization | 35 | As above, plus incontinence, chronic catheterization |

*Reproduced with permission from Stamm WE, Urinary Tract Infection, in *Infectious Diseases*, Saunders, 1992.

appear to be important risk factors in women. Most of these infections in men occur in the setting of urinary catheterization, instrumentation, and bladder outlet obstruction due to prostatic hypertrophy.

## Pathogenesis

In community-acquired UTI, ascending infection usually results from the entry of bacteria colonizing the anterior urethra and/or the vaginal introitus into the bladder. Bloodborne spread of pathogens from distant sites of infection occurs occasionally, most commonly with *S. aureus*. Relapsing infection from unresolved foci in the prostate, kidney, or in calculi may seed other parts of the urinary tract.

The pathogenesis of community-acquired UTI has been most carefully studied in young women, in whom most infections arise. The short female urethra allows bacteria colonizing its distal end to enter the bladder. In addition, the proximity of the urethral meatus to the rectum in women facilitates colonization of the periurethral area with coliform bacteria. It has been repeatedly observed that the organisms which eventually cause UTI usually colonize the vagina and the periurethral area beforehand. Factors that promote colonization of the vaginal introitus are poorly understood but appear to include diaphragm–spermicide use, spermicide exposure, and exposure to selected types of antimicrobials, especially beta-lactams.

Bacterial adherence to vaginal and uroepithelial cells is the initial step in colonization of the lower urinary tract. Several studies have demonstrated that uroepithelial cells from women prone to recurrent UTI bind more bacteria than cells from women with no history of UTI. These data could suggest a genetic predisposition to UTI in some women. This hypothesis is further supported by the fact that women who are nonsecretors of blood group antigens have an apparent increased risk of UTI and their epithelial cells bind *E. coli* in greater numbers than do cells from secretors. Other factors such as estrogenic hormones, spermicides, and antibiotics also influence bacterial binding to epithelial cells and may alter risk of UTI.

### Bacterial factors

In contrast to most *E. coli* found in the normal fecal flora, those *E. coli* that cause community-acquired UTI (called uropathogenic *E. coli*) belong to distinct clones that possess specific virulence factors, including pili that mediate adherence to vaginal and uroepithelial cells, resistance to the bactericidal activity of human serum, production of hemolysin and cytotoxic necrotizing factor, presence of chromosomal aerobactin, and increased amounts of K capsular antigen. These organisms belong to a limited number of O, K, and H serogroups. The adhesive properties of these organisms are important determinants not only of infectivity but in some cases also of a propensity to develop upper tract infections. Adhesion is mediated by specific bacterial ligands which attach as lectins to host cell-wall carbohydrate residues that serve as receptors. These ligands are usually small proteins located at the tips of bacterial fimbriae.

Once attachment to uroepithelial cells occurs, bacterial virulence factors other than adhesins become important. Most uropathogenic strains produce hemolysin, which may be important in initiating tissue invasion and cell damage, in making iron available to invading *E. coli*, and in lysing leukocytes. Siderophores, such as aerobactin, are iron-scavenging proteins which are found with increased frequency in uropathogenic strains. The presence of K-antigen protects bacteria from complement-mediated killing and from phagocytosis by leukocytes. Endotoxin derived from the *E. coli* cell wall may be an important initiator of the inflammatory process in the kidney.

Many or all of these virulence factors are characteristically found in *E. coli* strains isolated from infections in urologically normal patients, especially those infections involving the kidney. Thus, these factors appear necessary for such strains to infect the intact host and overcome normal defense mechanisms. However, they are less important in patients with structural or functional abnormalities of the urinary tract. *E. coli* strains infecting the upper tracts of children with vesicoureteric reflux or adults with urologic abnormalities do not usually exhibit the typical virulence factors found in the uropathogenic *E. coli*–infecting nonimpaired hosts.

### Host factors

Small numbers of bacteria enter the female bladder frequently but infection rarely ensues. A variety of host factors act in concert to prevent infection. The flushing and diluting effects of urine accumulation and voiding help to clear infection. Factors obstructing urine flow, altering normal voiding mechanisms, or causing postvoid residual urine markedly increase the risk of UTI. The acidity, high urea concentration, and extremes of osmolality in urine make it a poor culture medium for many anaerobic and fastidious bacteria and inhibit the growth of many other organisms. Bacteria grow less well in urine collected from men than from women, probably because of the inhibitory activity of prostatic secretions. Tamm-Horsfall protein (normally produced by renal epithelial cells) may act as a barrier to infection with enterobacteriaciae because it possesses large numbers of mannose residues which bind bacterial adhesins and competitively inhibit attachment to epithelial cells. Taken together, these factors often successfully defend the bladder against small bacterial inocula but they may be overcome by larger inocula or by more virulent bacteria. Urinary catheters, urinary stones, and structural abnormalities often provide a refuge for bacteria that may be extremely difficult or impossible to eradicate with antimicrobials.

Once urinary infection has been established, a local inflammatory response develops characterized by an influx of polymorphonuclear leukocytes (PMNs) and macrophages which ingest and destroy bacteria. This response is mediated by cytokines (particularly interleukin [IL]-6 and IL-8) produced by urinary epithelial cells in response to bacterial attachment. Subsequently, PMNs recruited into the urine also produce IL-6 and IL-8. Urine inhibits the phagocytic functions of PMNs, including migration, aggregation, and killing. The inflammatory response itself is in part responsible for the symptoms of cystitis. Cystitis is seldom associated with a marked systemic response to infection and levels of IL-6 and IL-8 in the blood are not elevated. In contrast, most patients with pyelonephritis have elevated serum levels of cytokines (IL-6, IL-8, tissue necrosis factor [TNF]) and manifest systemic symptoms.

## Clinical Manifestations

The symptoms of UTI in young children are often nonspecific: fever, poor feeding, and vomiting usually are the major manifestations. Abdominal discomfort may be present. UTI should always be excluded in children with unexplained fever. After early childhood, the classical symptoms of dysuria, urgency, and frequency generally are present in patients with UTI. Adult women with cystitis usually have frequent and urgent voiding of small volumes of urine and often experience lower abdominal heaviness or lower back pain. The urine may be foul smelling or turbid and is bloody in one-third of cases. The onset of symptoms is usually abrupt. Some patients progress over several days to develop signs and symptoms of upper tract involvement, including fever, rigors, nausea, vomiting, abdominal pain, and flank pain. However, studies comparing clinical signs and symptoms with the localization of bacteria to the upper or lower urinary tract by laboratory techniques have demonstrated a poor correlation between clinical manifestations and localization results.

In the elderly, UTIs are often asymptomatic; further, as in childhood, symptoms and signs are frequently nonspecific when present. In addition, frequency, urgency, nocturia, and incontinence may have multiple causes in this age group. One should have a low threshold for culture of the urine in elderly patients with an unexplained increase in urinary frequency, incontinence, or lower abdominal discomfort. Patients with neurogenic bladders or an indwelling catheter typically have few or no symptoms referable to the bladder when they develop UTI; signs and symptoms of pyelonephritis and unexplained fever or septicemia are more commonly seen.

## Acute uncomplicated cystitis

Acute uncomplicated cystitis occurs most commonly in young women but may also be seen in young men, older men and women, and children. Typical symptoms include dysuria, urinary frequency, urgency, voiding of small urine volumes, and suprapubic or pelvic pain. Suprapubic tenderness is present in only about 10%–20% of patients with cystitis, and gross hematuria in about 20%–30%, but both are relatively specific findings for cystitis in young women when present.

Acute cystitis must be differentiated from other conditions in which dysuria may be a prominent symptom, especially vaginitis and urethral infections caused by sexually transmitted pathogens. Table 69.3 summarizes the features useful in assigning a patient with dysuria to one of these diagnostic categories. Approximately 10%–15% of patients with characteristic symptoms of acute uncomplicated cystitis have unrecognized infection of the upper urinary tract (occult renal infection) when localization studies such as the bladder washout test are done. The likelihood of occult renal infection is increased in women with a lengthy (>7 d) duration of symptoms, a history of recent UTI, and in lower socioeconomic groups.

## Acute pyelonephritis

Acute pyelonephritis characteristically presents with localized flank, low back, or abdominal pain, and systemic symptoms such as fever, rigors, sweats, headache, nausea, vomiting, malaise, and prostration. Antecedent or concomitant symptoms of cystitis may or may not be present. Fever and flank pain are relatively specific indicators of acute renal infection.

A wide spectrum of illness is encountered among patients with acute pyelonephritis, ranging from mild disease to full-blown gram-negative sepsis. Volume loss from recurrent vomiting may necessitate intravenous administration of fluids and antimicrobial agents. A minority of patients with acute pyelonephritis develop necrotizing intrarenal and perinephric abscesses or gram-negative sepsis. These manifestations occur more frequently in patients with associated urinary tract obstruction or diabetes and necessitate aggressive diagnostic and therapeutic efforts, including ultrasonography or computed tomography and urological surgery.

## Complicated urinary tract infections

Urinary tract infections are often categorized as "complicated" or "uncomplicated" depending upon the presence or absence of host conditions known to promote infection, account for persistence of infection, or lead to recurrence. Generally, uncomplicated cystitis or pyelonephritis occurs in young women who have no structural or functional urologic abnormalities. Among females, complicated infections occur mainly in premenarchal girls or postmenopausal women. All urinary infections in males should probably be considered complicated until proven otherwise. As discussed above, the clinical manifestations of complicated UTI are more often atypical and nonspecific than in uncomplicated UTI. When complicating host factors are present, antimicrobial resistance is more common, response to therapy (even with agents active against the patient's pathogen) may be delayed or absent, complications of infection are more frequently encountered, and recurrences are more common.

**Table 69.3** Major infectious causes of acute dysuria in women

| Condition | Pathogen | Pyuria | Hematuria | Urine culture[a] cfu/ml | Symptoms, signs, and factors |
|---|---|---|---|---|---|
| Cystitis | *E. coli*, *S. saprophyticus*, *Proteus* species, klebsiella species | Usually | Sometimes | $10^2$ to $\geq 10^5$ | Abrupt onset, severe symptoms, multiple symptoms (dysuria, increased frequency, and urgency), suprapubic or low back pain; suprapubic tenderness on examination |
| Urethritis | *C. trachomatis*, *N. gonorrhoeae*, herpes simplex virus | Usually | Rarely | $<10^2$ | Gradual onset, mild symptoms, vaginal discharge or bleeding (due to concomitant cervicitis), lower abdominal pain, new sexual partner; cervicitis or vulvovaginal herpetic lesions on examination |
| Vaginitis | *Candida* species, *Trichomonas vaginalis* | Rarely | Rarely | $<10^2$ | Vaginal discharge or odor, pruritus, dyspareunia, external dysuria, no increased frequency or urgency; vulvovaginitis on examination |

[a]Values indicate colony-forming units (cfu) per milliliter or urine.

## Diagnosis

Confirmation of UTI requires documentation of bacteriuria by appropriate culture. Suprapubic aspiration avoids contamination of the urine during collection but is rarely used in practice except in pediatric or selected adult patients. Urethral catheterization can also be used to collect a specimen for urine culture: contamination of specimens collected by "in and out" catheterization is infrequent as compared with contamination of voided specimens. However, it is mildly uncomfortable for the patient, time consuming, and thus infrequently used. In the patient with an indwelling catheter, however, specimens for culture should be obtained from the specimen collection port on the catheter.

In clinical practice, urine cultures from the noncatheterized patient are usually performed on voided urine specimens which in women are readily contaminated with perineal bacteria. Quantitative cultures and specific identification of the type of organisms in the urine are used to distinguish culture contamination (usually low bacterial counts and usually nonpathogenic species, often with several species present) from true infection (usually higher counts of typical uropathogens only). The concentration of microorganisms in urine is usually determined by culturing a known volume of urine ($10^{-2}$ or $10^{-3}$ ml) or can be estimated using a dipslide method. The finding of $>10^5$ bacteria/ml of voided urine was shown by Kass, Sanford, and others to differentiate infected from contaminated urines in women with asymptomatic bacteriuria or acute pyelonephritis. Since these studies, many physicians have considered $\geq 10^5$ cfu (colony-forming units)/ml a specific criterion for the diagnosis of all UTIs. However, 30%–40% of women with acute cystitis caused by *E. coli*, *S. saprophyticus*, and *Proteus* have colony counts in midstream urine between $10^2$ and $10^4$ cfu/ml. Similarly, low bacterial counts in voided urine may be seen in patients with acute pyelonephritis. Thus, in acutely symptomatic women, a more appropriate threshold value for defining "significant bacteriuria" is $\geq 10^2$ colonies/ml of a known uropathogen. Failure to use this criterion in these patient groups seriously compromises the sensitivity of the urine culture. Since many microbiology laboratories use culture techniques that accurately detect $10^3$ but not $10^2$ cfu/ml, a $10^3$ cfu/ml criterion may be more practical for many clinicians and laboratorians. Clinicians should request that their clinical laboratory utilize techniques which allow detection of $10^3$ cfu/ml in symptomatic patients and report the results of cultures with $10^3$–$10^5$ cfu/ml of a uropathogen,

As alternatives to culture methods, several more rapid techniques for the detection of bacteriuria have been developed in recent years. These methods detect bacterial growth using photometry or bioluminescence and can provide results in as few as 2 h. In general, these methods achieve a sensitivity of 95%–98% and >99% negative predictive value compared with conventional cultures when bacteriuria is defined as $\geq 10^5$ cfu/ml. Thus, they are excellent for "screening out" negative cultures using this definition of bacteriuria. However, the sensitivity of these tests falls to 50%–60% or less when detecting bacteriuria between $10^2$ and $10^4$ cfu/ml, which is necessary in acutely symptomatic patients.

Tests for detecting urinary leukocytes, erythrocytes, or bacteria allow presumptive confirmation of UTI at the time of initial patient evaluation without the expense and delays associated with urine culture. Among women with uncomplicated infection, pyuria is a highly sensitive indicator of urinary tract infection when accurately determined using a hemocytometer chamber. In fact, its absence should cause the diagnosis of UTI to be questioned in this patient group. However, assessment of pyuria using the centrifuged urine sediment method that is employed in many laboratories is far less accurate and reproducible than counting leukocytes in uncentrifuged urine using a chamber method. The leukocyte esterase "dipstick" method is somewhat less sensitive in identifying pyuria than the hemocytometer method, but it can serve as an alternative approach where microscopy isn't available. In complicated UTI and catheter-associated UTI, both the sensitivity and specificity of pyuria as an indicator of UTI decrease as compared with patients who have uncomplicated infection.

Microscopic hematuria is found in 40%–60% of patients with acute cystitis and is uncommon in other dysuric syndromes in young women. Thus, among young women with possible UTI, its presence is a highly specific indicator of cystitis. Urinary calculi or tumors must be considered in elderly patients with hematuria. Microscopic bacteriuria, best assessed using gram-stained, uncentrifuged urine, is found in over 90% of UTIs with colony counts of $\geq 10^5$ cfu/ml, and is a highly specific finding. However, bacteria are not readily detected microscopically with lower colony count infections ($10^2$–$10^4$ cfu/ml). Therefore, microscopic hematuria and bacteriuria lack sensitivity but are reasonably specific for UTI in most patient groups.

Until recently, most authorities have recommended that urine culture and antimicrobial susceptibility testing be performed in any patient with a suspected urinary tract infection. However, the expected spectrum of infecting bacterial species and their antimicrobial susceptibility profile are highly predictable in women with acute uncomplicated cystitis. Further, treatment decisions are usually made and therapy is often completed before culture results are known. Thus, it may be reasonable and certainly more cost-effective to manage women who have typical symptoms of acute, uncomplicated cystitis without an initial urine culture. While this approach has not been extensively studied, what data are available suggest that empiric treatment of women with suspected uncomplicated UTI is safe, effective, and cost-effective. Two approaches have been suggested—namely, empiric treatment based on typical symptoms and signs alone, and empiric treatment based on symptoms and signs and the presence of pyuria. There are as yet insufficient data to differentiate the effectiveness, safety, and cost of these two approaches. Women with symptoms and signs suggestive of acute cystitis in whom no complicating factors are present should either be treated empirically or have a urinalysis or a leukocyte esterase test performed. If positive for pyuria, these tests provide sufficient documentation of UTI such that a urine culture and susceptibility testing can be omitted. Urine culture should be obtained, however, in women in whom symptoms and urine microscopy leave the diagnosis of cystitis in question. Pretherapy cultures and susceptibility testing are also essential in the management of patients with suspected upper tract infections, in patients in whom complicating factors are present, and in all male patients, since in these situations a variety of pathogens may be present and their antibiotic susceptibility profile is not readily predictable.

## Treatment

In general, all symptomatic UTI should be treated with antimicrobials. The antibacterial spectrum of the agent should cover the likely infecting organisms but should minimally disrupt the normal gut and perineal flora. Successful treatment of uncomplicated lower tract infections correlates with inhibitory concentrations of antimicrobial achieved in the urine, not with tissue concentrations. Some antimicrobials that are successfully used to treat cystitis (nitrofurantoin, for example) do not achieve microbicidal serum or tissue levels but are present in high concentrations in the urine. Urinary concentrations of many antibiotics are much higher than corresponding serum levels and may exceed the minimum inhibitory concentration of some "resistant" organisms. This may account for the clinical observation that some patients with cystitis are cured by antibiotics to which their infecting organism was "resistant."

## Acute uncomplicated cystitis

The traditional approach to treatment of acute uncomplicated cystitis recommended 7–10 d of therapy with an oral antibiotic. However, single-dose therapy is effective in treating the majority of such women, is less costly, and is associated with fewer side effects than longer therapy. In studies with adequate sample size to detect 15%–20% differences in efficacy, however, single-dose therapy has been less effective than 7–10 d therapy. In addition, selected patients such as pregnant women; those with diabetes, immunosuppressive conditions, or urinary tract abnormalities; and those with >7 d of symptoms before starting therapy are more likely to fail single-dose therapy.

Cure rates with single-dose therapy are in part related to the drug used. Thus, higher cure rates have generally been observed with trimethoprim, trimethoprim-sulfamethoxazole, and fluoroquinolones; lower cure rates have been seen with ampicillin, amoxicillin, and other $\beta$-lactam agents. This probably results mainly from the very rapid urinary excretion of the latter compounds and the prolonged urinary excretion of the former. The 30%–40% incidence of resistance to ampicillin among *E. coli* causing community-acquired urinary tract infections also contributes substantially to the decreased efficacy of ampicillin and amoxicillin.

Recent studies have evaluated the use of a 3-d course of therapy for treatment of acute uncomplicated cystitis. On theoretical grounds, 3-d therapy can be expected to be more effective than single-dose therapy, especially in patients with unrecognized complicating factors, and it may be more effective than single-dose therapy in eradicating *E. coli* from the vaginal reservoir. Three-day regimens of trimethoprim, trimethoprim-sulfamethoxazole, or fluoroquinolones have been associated with an incidence of adverse effects as low as that seen with single-dose therapy and with cure rates which appear comparable to those achieved with 7–10 d courses of therapy. Thus, 3-d therapy currently appears to be the preferred short-course regimen in treating acute uncomplicated lower UTI. Short-course therapy (Table 69.4) should be reserved for women with presumed acute uncomplicated cystitis who have no known complicating factors. When complicating factors are present in a patient with presumed acute lower urinary tract infection, therapy should be continued for at least 7 d (Table 69.4).

## Acute pyelonephritis

Patients with acute pyelonephritis (Table 69.4) can be subdivided into those with mild disease that can be managed in the outpatient setting; those who are sufficiently ill to require hospitalization for parenteral therapy; and those with complicated infection occurring in the setting of prior catheterization, hospitalization, urologic surgery, or known urological abnormalities. The first group can be treated successfully and at lesser expense with oral antibiotics in the outpatient setting, assuming adequate compliance and follow-up can be assured.

Therapy for the majority of patients with acute pyelonephritis requires hospital admission, intravenous fluids, and parenteral antibiotics. The combination of ampicillin and an aminoglycoside has traditionally been recommended as empiric therapy for patients hospitalized with uncomplicated acute pyelonephritis, with ampicillin being continued alone if the infecting organism proves susceptible. However, because of the increasing frequency of resistance to ampicillin, among even community-acquired *E.coli* strains, the attractiveness of ampicillin as part of an empiric regimen for gram-negative infections is much diminished. The major advantage of the traditional ampicillin/gentamicin regimen is its effectiveness against both *Enterococcus* and *Pseudomonas*, in addition to the more common causative agents—namely, aerobic gram-negative bacilli. However, in uncomplicated acute pyelonephritis, such coverage is usually unnecessary since the vast majority of cases are due to *E. coli*, *Klebsiella*, or *Proteus*. Given the availability of a number of alternative intravenous antibiotics with activity against most Enterobacteriaciae, and the capability of excluding enterococcal infection with the urine gram stain, it may be preferable to initiate therapy with one of these single agents. A number of different antimicrobials can be used for empiric treatment of acute uncomplicated pyelonephritis, including a parenteral fluoroquinolone, a third-generation cephalosporin, or an aminoglycoside alone (Table 69.4). The selection of which of these drugs to use depends upon local antimicrobial sensitivity patterns, the patient's prior history of infecting organisms, and the likelihood of unusual pathogens such as enterococci or pseudomonas. Therapy can be modified after 24–48 h when susceptibility testing results are available. Parenteral therapy should be used until the patient is able to take fluids by mouth, is symptomatically improved, and has become afebrile. The total duration of therapy for acute uncomplicated pyelonephritis in women should generally be 10–14 d.

The presence of complicating factors in patients with upper urinary tract infection requires more aggressive management, closer follow-up, and in some cases a longer duration of therapy. Urologic consultation should be considered as part of the initial management of such patients. Similarly, patients with suspected pyelonephritis who have symptoms of renal colic or a stone on their admission abdominal X-ray, or who fail to improve after 3 d of appropriate antibiotic therapy, should be suspected of harboring a stone, an underlying anatomic abnormality, a urinary tract obstruction, or an acquired complication of infection, such as an intrarenal or perinephric abscess. In such cases, ultrasonography, computed tomography, or an excretory urogram should be performed and urologic consultation should be obtained.

## Prophylaxis of recurrent infection in women

Many women have occasional episodes of cystitis, but in 20%–25%, recurrent episodes occur with such frequency (>3 per year) that antimicrobial prophylaxis is justified. The vast majority of these women have normal urinary tract anatomy and function, have infections confined to the lower urinary tract, and experience repeated reinfections with different bacterial strains. In some women, UTIs can be temporally related to sexual intercourse or diaphragm use, but in the majority no specific predisposing factors are apparent.

Simple measures such as voiding immediately after sexual in-

**Table 69.4** Treatment regimens for bacterial urinary tract infections*

| Condition | Characteristic pathogens | Mitigating circumstances | Recommended empirical treatment |
|---|---|---|---|
| Acute uncomplicated cystitis in women | *E. coli, S. saprophyticus, P. mirabilis, Klebsiella pneumoniae* | None | 3-day regimens: oral trimethoprim-sulfamethoxazole, trimethoprim, norfloxacin, ciprofloxacin, ofloxacin, lomefloxacin, or enoxacin[a] |
| | | Diabetes, symptoms for >7 d, recent urinary tract infection, use of diaphragm, age >65 yr | Consider 7-d regimen: oral trimethoprim-sulfamethoxazole, trimethoprim, norfloxacin, ciprofloxacin, ofloxacin, lomefloxacin or enoxacin[a] |
| | | Pregnancy | Consider 7-d regimen: oral amoxicillin, macrocrystalline nitrofurantoin, cefpodoxime proxetil, or trimethoprim-sulfamethoxazole[a] |
| Acute uncomplicated pyelonephritis in women | *E. coli, P. mirabilis, K. pneumoniae, S. saprophyticus* | Mild-to-moderate illness, no nausea or vomiting—outpatient therapy | Oral[b] ciprofloxacin, ofloxacin, lomefloxacin, or enoxacin for 10–14 d |
| | | Severe illness or possible urosepsis—hospitalization required | Parenteral[c], ceftriaxone, ciprofloxacin, ofloxacin, or gentamicin (with or without ampicillin) until fever gone; then oral[b] trimethoprim-sulfamethoxazole, norfloxacin, ciprofloxacin, ofloxacin, lomefloxacin, or enoxacin for 14 d |
| Complicated urinary tract infection | *E. coli*, proteus species, klebsiella species, pseudomonas species, serratia species, enterococci, staphylococci | Mild-to-moderate illness, no nausea or vomiting—outpatient therapy | Oral[b] norfloxacin, ciprofloxacin, ofloxacin, lomefloxacin, or enoxacin for 10–14 d |
| | | Severe illness or possible urosepsis—hospitalization required | Parenteral[c] ampicillin and gentamicin, ciprofloxacin, ofloxacin, ceftriaxone, aztreonam, ticarcillin-clavulanate, or imipenem-cilastatin until fever gone; then oral[b] trimethoprim-sulfamethoxazole, norfloxacin, ciprofloxacin, oflaxacin, lomefloxacin, or enoxacin for 14–21 d |

*Treatments listed are those to be prescribed before the etiologic agent is known (gram staining can be helpful); they can be modified once the agent has been identified. The recommendations are the authors' and are limited to drugs currently approved by the Food and Drug Administration, although not all the regimens listed are approved for these indications. Fluoroquinolones should not be used in pregnancy. Trimethoprim-sulfamethoxazole, although not approved for use in pregnancy, has been widely used. Gentamicin should be used with caution in pregnancy because of its possible toxicity to eighth-nerve development in the fetus.

[a]Multiday oral regimens for cystitis are as follows: trimethoprim-sulfamethoxazole, 160–800 mg every 12 h; trimethoprim, 100 mg every 12 h; norfloxacin 400 mg every 12 h; ciprofloxacin, 250 mg every 12 h, ofloxacin, 200 mg every 12 h; lomefloxacin 400 mg every day; enoxacin 400 mg every 12 h; macrocrystaline nitrofurantoin, 100 mg four times a day; amoxicillin, 250 mg every 8 h; and cefpodoxime proxetiil, 100 mg every 12 h.

[b]Oral regimes for pyelonephritis and complicated urinary tract infection are as follows: trimethoprim-sulfamethoxazole, 160–800 mg every 12 h, norfloxacin 400 mg every 12 h; ciprofloxacin, 500 mg every 12 h, ofloxacin, 200–300 mg every 12 h; lomefloxacin, 400 mg every day; enoxacin, 400 mg every 12 h; amoxicillin, 500 mg every 8 h; and cefpodoxime proxetil, 200 mg every 12 h.

[c]Parenteral regimens are as follows: trimethoprim-sulfamethoxazole, 160–800 mg every 12 h; cirrofloxacin, 200–400 mg every 12 h; ofloxacin, 200–400 mg every 12 h; gentamicin, 1 mg per kilogram of body weight every 8 h; ceftriaxone, 1–2 g every 8 h; and aztreonam, 1 g every 8–12 h.

tercourse or using a form of contraception other than the diaphragm may be effective in those women in whom these factors are related to recurrent infection. If such measures are not successful, three antimicrobial strategies can be employed: (*1*) continuous low-dose prophylaxis, (*2*) postcoital single-dose prophylaxis, or (*3*) self-administered single-dose treatment. The choice of management strategy depends upon the factors predisposing to recurrent infection, the number of infections per year, and the patient's preference. In general, continuous prophylaxis is preferred in women experiencing three or more infections per year; patient-administered 3 d therapy should be reserved for women with one or two infections per year; and postintercourse prophylaxis should be used for women who clearly relate their infections to sexual activity. There are no clear guidelines as to when to stop prophylaxis, but most often at least 6 mo is given initially. Low-dose prophylaxis and postcoital prophylaxis have both been demonstrated to be highly effective, safe, and well tolerated, even over periods of 5 yr. Emergence of resistant strains while on prophylaxis have been infrequent.

## Asymptomatic bacteriuria

Bacteriuria (defined as $>10^5$ bacteria/ml) in pregnancy is associated with a markedly increased risk of developing acute pyelonephritis and may jeopardize the pregnancy. Women should be screened for bacteriuria during the first trimester of pregnancy and promptly treated. In adults who are not pregnant, there is little convincing evidence that treatment of asymptomatic bacteriuria is beneficial. Exceptions may include selected high-risk patients such as those with neutropenia or a renal transplant. At present, there is no reason to treat asymptomatic bacteriuria in elderly patients or in most patients with catheter-associated UTI.

## Catheter-Associated Urinary Tract Infections

Catheter-associated UTI constitutes 35%–40% of all hospital-acquired infections. While most of these infections are asymptomatic, some cause cystitis or pyelonephritis; catheter-associated bacteriuria is the most common source of gram-negative bacteremia in hospitalized patients and has been associated with a threefold increase in mortality, prolonged hospital stay, and increased hospital costs.

Bacteria gain entry to the catheterized bladder in several ways. They may be introduced at the time of catheterization; they may enter on the external surface of the catheter in the urethral mucus sheath (periurethral route); or they may enter the drainage system by contamination of the collecting bag or disconnection of the junction between the catheter and collecting tube and ascend through the lumen of the catheter (intraluminal route). The importance of the last is illustrated by the marked reduction in the incidence of catheter-associated UTI since the introduction of sterile closed-drainage systems. Currently, the periurethral route appears to be the most frequent route of bacterial entry, especially in women. Antecedent rectal and periurethral colonization plays an important role in the subsequent development of catheter-associated bacteriuria.

The overall risk of infection increases with the length of time that the catheter is in place. About 50% of men and women catheterized for 2 wk become bacteriuric, and all patients with permanent indwelling catheters eventually become infected. Risk of catheter-associated UTI is greater in women, in patients whose sterile closed-drainage system is disconnected, and in patients not receiving systemic antibiotics. Patients with neurogenic bladders typically have very frequent episodes of asymptomatic bacteria and in prospective studies are bacteriuric 40%–60% of the time. The infecting organisms often cycle, and polymicrobial infections are common.

Providing that the system is not breached, bacteriuria can be prevented in the majority of patients for up to 10 d with modern sterile closed collecting systems and catheters. A variety of additional preventive approaches to further reduce the occurrence of bacteriuria have been evaluated, but none has been highly effective or widely used. In general, for example, antibiotic ointments applied to the urethral meatus have not been protective. Silver-impregnated catheters have been developed recently and may prevent bacteriuria, especially in chronically catheterized patients. The use of systemic antibiotics has a definite short-term effect in reducing the prevalence of UTI in catheterized patients, but in the long term it predisposes to infection with resistant strains. This approach may be appropriate for the short-term prevention of infection in high-risk patients, but it is probably unwise for periods of catheterization longer than 1 wk.

In general, catheter-associated bacteriuria should be treated only in patients with symptomatic infection. When treatment is to be started, it is preferable to remove the catheter, start appropriate therapy, and then reintroduce a new catheter and drainage system if indwelling catheterization is still required. Concretions (biofilms) on the internal surface of the catheter often serve as a reservoir for bacteria in which they are protected from antimicrobials. If such "infected" catheters are left in place, relapsing infection will occur when antimicrobial therapy is stopped. If there is fever and flank pain, parenteral treatment should be started immediately. There is insufficient evidence to cite an optimum length of treatment for catheter-associated UTI; 7 d of therapy is usually given. Resistant bacteria and fungi (candida, torulopsis) are often isolated in catheterized patients receiving multiple courses of broad spectrum antimicrobials. Thus, symptomatic bacterial infections should be treated on the basis of antimicrobial sensitivities. Yeast isolation does not necessarily require treatment, since many episodes will clear without treatment, but repeated isolations or symptomatic infections should be treated with oral fluconazole therapy or amphotericin B irrigation of the bladder.

## ANNOTATED BIBLIOGRAPHY


International Journal of Antimicrobial Agents. Special issue: Urinary Tract Infections. Edited by I.M. Hoepelman. 1994; 4:81–139.
*A series of state-of-the-art articles presenting concise but complete overviews of current knowledge on the pathogenesis, host response, and clinical management of urinary tract infections.*

Kunin CM. Urinary tract infections in females. Clin Infect Dis 1994; 18:1–12.
*An excellent overview of all aspects of urinary tract infection in women, including therapeutic approaches.*

Norrby SR. Short-term treatment of uncomplicated lower urinary tract infections in women. Rev Infect Dis 1990; 12:458–467.
*A metaanalysis and summary of trials addressing treatment of lower urinary tract infection in women.*

Stamm WE. Catheter-associated urinary tract infections: epidemiology, pathogenesis and prevention. Am J Med 1991; 91 (Suppl 3B):3B-65S-71S.
*Complete discussion of catheter-associated urinary tract infections, including epidemiology, pathogenesis, and prevention but also addressing clinical management.*

Stamm WE, Hooton TM. Management of urinary tract infections in adults. N Engl J Med 1993; 329:1328–1334.
*Comprehensive overview of management approaches and treatment regimens for management of urinary tract infections.*

Urinary tract infections. In: *Infectious Disease Clinics of North American*, Andriole VT, ed. 11:499–751, 1997.
*This monograph contains 14 excellent articles written by experts in the field addressing the epidemiology, pathogenesis, diagnosis, treatment, and prevention of UTI. An excellent up-to-date resource.*

# 70

# Genital Herpes, Syphilis, and Genital Ulcer Disease

H. HUNTER HANDSFIELD

Of the five classical venereal diseases—gonorrhea, syphilis, chancroid, lymphogranuloma venereum (LGV), and granuloma inguinale (donovanosis)—four are characterized by genital ulceration, often with inguinal lymphadenopathy. In addition, genital herpes has become recognized in the past two decades as one of the most common sexually transmitted diseases (STD) in industrialized countries. Beyond the immediate local and occasional systemic manifestations of genital ulcer disease (GUD), serious long-term sequelae are common. As for most STDs, these complications selectively affect women and their children. In addition, GUD has emerged as a potent risk factor for sexual transmission of human immunodeficiency virus (HIV).

A genital ulcer can be defined as a discrete mucosal or cutaneous discontinuity involving the genitals, perineum, or surrounding tissues in the presence of otherwise normal skin and mucous membranes. This chapter emphasizes the clinical approach to diagnosis and treatment of the common infective causes of GUD in sexually active young persons in the United States and industrialized countries. Conditions not addressed in detail include those that are rare in young adults, such as cancer; disorders characterized by skin or mucosal disruption as a component of diffuse genital dermatitis, such as superficial fissures in yeast vulvovaginitis; and conditions that may involve but are not specific to the genitals, such as psoriasis, erythema multiforme, and impetigo.

## Etiology

### Herpes simplex viruses

Herpes simplex virus type 2 (HSV-2) is the predominant cause of genital herpes, although the type 1 virus (HSV-1) is responsible for a substantial and apparently growing minority of cases. The herpesviridae are double-stranded DNA viruses with an icosahedral capsid and an outer lipid-containing envelope. Other members of the herpesviridae are addressed in Chapter 4. HSV-1 and -2 have numerous genetically stable antigenic differences, notably among several outer membrane glycoproteins, the basis of type-specific antibody tests.

#### *Treponema pallidum*

*Treponema pallidum*, the cause of syphilis, is a member of the bacterial order Spirochaetales and one of only a few treponemes known to be pathogenic for man. Sustained cultivation of *T. pallidum* has not been accomplished, which has limited the development of knowledge about the organism and the pathogenesis of syphilis. The treponeme that causes sexually transmitted syphilis is indistinguishable from those responsible for yaws (*T. pallidum* subsp. *pertenue*), pinta (*T. carateum*), or endemic syphilis (*T. pallidum* var. *Bosnia*). Individual organisms typically are 10–13 $\mu$m in length and have about one spiral turn for each micron of length. The 0.15 $\mu$m diameter of *T. pallidum* is below the resolution of light microscopes, so that indirect methods, such as darkfield or phase microscopy, are required to visualize the organism.

#### *Haemophilus ducreyi*

*Haemophilus ducreyi*, the cause of chancroid, is a small gram-negative bacillus. Ribosomal RNA typing suggests a closer relationship of the organism to *Actinobacillus* than to other *Haemophilus* species, although *H. ducreyi* remains the accepted name. The organism is nutritionally fastidious, slow to grow, and often difficult to isolate, even when experienced laboratories use highly enriched media.

#### *Chlamydia trachomatis*

Lymphogranuloma venereum is caused by *C. trachomatis* serovars $L_1$, $L_2$, and $L_3$. Compared to the more prevalent oculogenital strains, these serovars grow rapidly, are more cytolytic in cell culture, and are lethal to mice following intracerebral inoculation.

#### *Calymmatobacterium granulomatis*

*Calymmatobacterium granulomatis*, the cause of granuloma inguinale, is a small, pleomorphic gram-negative coccobacillus that in pathological material typically appears intracellularly in macrophages ("Donovan bodies"). *Cal. granulomatis* recently has been sustained in culture for the first time, which will lead to improved characterization of the organism in the near future.

## Epidemiology

Few published studies in the past two decades have addressed the etiology of GUD in sexually active patients in industrialized countries, and recently reported studies described highly selected populations in settings where syphilis or chancroid were known to be especially common. Table 70.1 summarizes the spectrum of GUD in populations attending STD clinics, based on older reports, unpublished data, and recent studies in developing countries. The proportion of cases attributed to herpes has risen over the past two decades in both developing and industrialized countries as the atypical nature of many herpetic lesions has been increasingly appreciated and as improved methods to detect HSV infection have been employed.

**Table 70.1** Etiology of genital ulcer disease in patients attending STD clinics*

| | % | |
|---|---|---|
| | North America | Tropical developing countries |
| Genital herpes | 60–70 | 0–20 |
| Syphilis | 0–20 | 10–20 |
| Chancroid | 0–10 | 50–60 |
| Other/unknown | 10–20 | 20–30 |

*Based on published and unpublished studies and the author's clinical experience. The epidemiology of the genital ulcer diseases varies widely; the table is only a rough guide.

## Genital herpes

Genital herpes is by far the most common cause of GUD in sexually active young adults in North America. Annual first visits to health care providers in the United States for genital herpes rose from an estimated 20,000 in the late 1960s to about 250,000 visits in the mid 1990s, reflecting both rising incidence and increased recognition. Seroepidemiologic studies showed that by the early 1990s an estimated 22% percent of the U.S. population ≥12 yr old was seropositive for antibody to HSV-2, compared with an estimated 17% a decade earlier (Figure 70.1). The same studies confirmed the role of sexual transmission by showing that few patients <15 years old are seropositive and that the prevalence rises most rapidly from age 15 to age 40. Most HSV-2–seropositive persons lack histories of genital herpes or unexplained genital lesions, indicating that many cases of genital herpes, perhaps a majority, are subclinical. Most new cases of genital herpes are acquired from sex partners with subclinical viral shedding. In contrast to industrialized countries, genital herpes has been infrequently recognized as a cause of GUD in most developing countries. However, recent studies using polymerase chain reaction (PCR) to detect HSV DNA have demonstrated that in some developing countries a substantial portion of GUD is due to genital herpes.

## Syphilis

Although the causes of GUD are highly variable between different geographic areas and over time, syphilis has been the second most common cause of GUD in patients at risk for STDs in developing countries and probably in most industrialized countries as well (Table 70.1). Most cases in the United States occur in settings of poverty, prostitution, substance abuse, or social disruption. Figure 70.2 shows the reported incidence of primary and secondary syphilis in the United States from 1981 to 1996. About 11,400 cases (4.3 per 100,000 population) were reported in the United States in 1996, compared with the modern peak of 50,500 cases (16.6 per 100,000) in 1990. The declining case rates in the early 1980s were due primarily to falling rates in homosexual and bisexual men, but from 1986 to 1990 there was a remarkable resurgence of the infection in heterosexual men and women and of neonatal congenital syphilis, associated with increasing rates of crack cocaine addiction and related social factors. The subsequent decline probably is attributable to a combination of public health control measures and social and behavioral changes. The steady convergence of the reported case rates in women and men partly reflects a continuing decline in syphilis in homosexual and bisexual men. The rapidly declining rates in the 1990s and the increasing concentration of cases in relatively few geographic areas, primarily in the southeast, may create an opportunity to eliminate endogenous syphilis in the United States.

## Chancroid

As shown in Table 70.1, chancroid is the predominant cause of GUD in many developing countries, especially in tropical climates. There was a remarkable rise in reported chancroid cases in the United States in the mid-1980s, with a peak of about 5,000 reported cases in 1987. As for syphilis, this trend appeared to be fueled by the epidemic of crack cocaine abuse, which in turn fos-

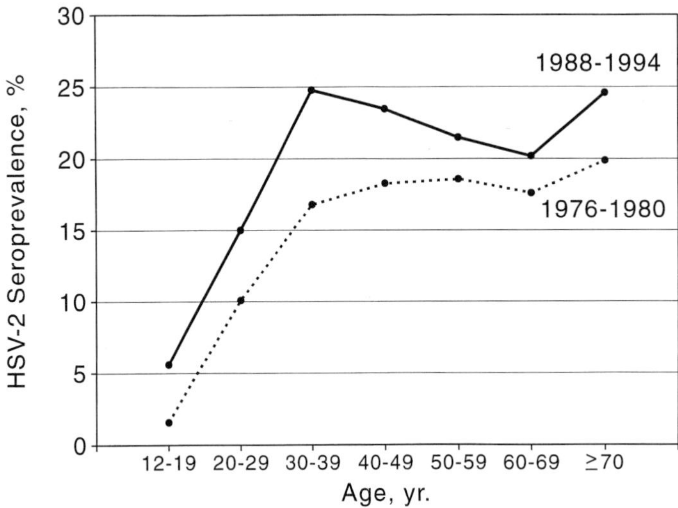


**Fig. 70.1** Prevalence of type-specific antibody to type 2 herpes simplex virus in the United States according to age, from the National Health and Nutrition Examination Survey 1976–1980 (mid-point 1978) and 1988–1994 (mid-point 1991). [Adapted from Fleming DT, McQuillan GM, Johnson RE, et al. N Engl J Med 1997; 337:1105–1111.]

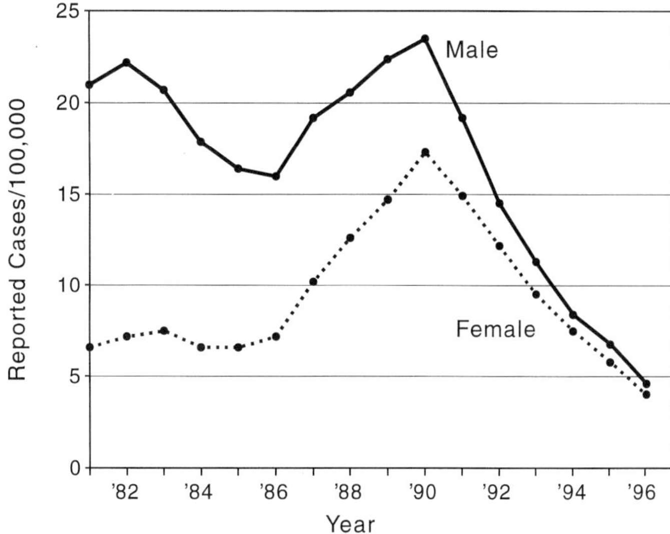


**Fig. 70.2** Incidence of reported primary and secondary syphilis according to sex, United States, 1981–1996 (from the Centers for Disease Control and Prevention, U.S. Public Health Service).

tered both overt and "opportunistic" commercial sex. In industrialized countries chancroid tends to occur in localized epidemics, and it persists as an occasional cause of GUD in only a few cities in the United States. Chancroid declined dramatically in the United States after 1990, and only 386 cases were reported in 1996. However, reported cases underestimate the true burden of disease, partly because bacteriologic confirmation is difficult and often not attempted. Throughout the world, chancroid appears to be more closely linked than any other STD with prostitution, substance abuse, and economic deprivation. This may occur because asymptomatic infection is uncommon, and maintenance of a chancroid outbreak may require a population of persons who continue sexual exposure despite painful genital lesions; addiction and economic pressures may provide the necessary incentives.

## Other conditions

In the United States LGV is rare, with a mean of 260 cases reported each year in the 1990s; only 75 cases were recognized in 1996. The primary lesion of LGV is an evanescent papule or ulcer that usually resolves before the patient seeks care, and inguinal lymphadenopathy is the main clinical manifestation. LGV occasionally presents as acute proctocolitis, especially in homosexually active men who are the receptive partners in rectal intercourse.

Granuloma inguinale is rare even in most developing countries; in the United States, a mean of only 11 cases were reported annually in the 1990s. The infection is most commonly recognized in the Indian subcontinent, Papua New Guinea, isolated areas of Australia, and parts of the Caribbean, and most cases in the United States probably are imported from such endemic areas.

Uncommon causes of GUD in sexually active young persons include fixed drug eruptions (often due to tetracycline therapy for STD), carcinoma, immunologic diseases such as Behçet's syndrome, and pyogenic infection, which occasionally complicates other, primary causes of GUD. Trauma is an uncommon cause; it is likely that many patients who attribute genital lesions to injury actually are providing presumed explanations. For example, patients sometimes attribute genital ulcers to inadequate lubrication during intercourse or to zipper injury. Trauma is a likely explanation of GUD only if there is a clear history of a traumatic event, usually with bleeding, and when other diagnoses have been excluded.

## Host Factors

The dominant host determinants of acquisition of GUD are those associated with all STDs—multiple sex partners, intercourse with a new partner, selection of high-risk partners, and failure to use condoms. Several demographic, behavioral, and socioeconomic markers influence these behaviors, and all STDs are most common in poor, nonwhite, unmarried persons between 15 and 30 yr of age. However, these markers and risk factors do not apply equally for all STDs. For example, chancroid and syphilis are largely limited to poor, minority populations in urban environments, whereas genital herpes is common in all socioeconomic strata. A partial explanation for these differences lies in the duration of infection: The clinical course of infectious syphilis or chancroid is measured in weeks, whereas genital herpes and other viral STDs are transmissible for many years, perhaps for the life of the infected person. As a result, low rates of sexual partner change are sufficient to sustain transmission of HSV-2 in a population, but syphilis and chancroid are sustained only in populations with especially high rates of partner change.

Uncircumcised men are at increased risk for chancroid, and perhaps for syphilis and herpes, probably because the preputial sac provides a reservoir that prolongs exposure to the partner's genital secretions, and because the skin of the glans penis is less cornified than in circumcised men. The association of an intact foreskin with HIV infection also is well documented. Infection with HIV has an adverse effect on the natural course of HSV infection and probably syphilis, and also impairs the response of herpes, chancroid, and perhaps syphilis to therapy.

## Pathogenesis

### Genital herpes

After inoculation, HSV penetrates epithelial cells, followed by ballooning degeneration, focal necrosis, an initial polymorphonuclear leukocytic response, and production of multinucleated giant cells. The virus migrates along sensory nerve axons toward the dorsal root ganglia, where latent infection is established. Healing of the initial mucocutaneous lesions is associated with development of neutralizing antibody and a cellular immune response. Prior infection with either virus type reduces susceptibility among persons reexposed to HSV and ameliorates the clinical course of infection with the opposite type. Up to 40% of symptomatic initial episodes of genital herpes are due to HSV-1, but the clinical recurrence rate is lower than for genital HSV-2 infection. Therefore, ≥90% of clinically recognized outbreaks of recurrent genital herpes are due to HSV-2.

The mechanisms of reactivation, migration of HSV virions from the dorsal root ganglia along sensory nerve axons, and recurrent mucocutaneous lesions are incompletely understood. Local trauma or inflammation (e.g., sunburn) commonly results in recurrent orolabial herpes due to HSV-1, but such triggers have not been clearly documented for genital herpes. Reports that menstruation, sexual intercourse, stress, fatigue, or other factors stimulate symptomatic recurrences of genital HSV-2 infection have not been corroborated by controlled studies.

### Syphilis

The pathogenesis of syphilis is similar to that of tuberculosis. Both diseases are caused by slowly replicating pathogens whose natural containment depends on cell-mediated immunity and are characterized by a primary infection that usually is mild or asymptomatic, accompanied by silent bacteremia and establishment of quiescent infection in various organs, probably in intracellular loci. Low-grade infection usually persists indefinitely without further clinical manifestations, but destructive granulomatous inflammation results if the infection reactivates, sometimes as the result of acquired immunodeficiency.

As for many cutaneous or mucosal infections, the first step in pathogenesis is attachment of *T. pallidum* to epithelial cells. Replication of the organism initially occurs without visible inflammation, although a polymorphonuclear leukocytic response eventually ensues. The extent of localized tissue necrosis and thus development of the initial genital ulcer, the chancre, is directly correlated with the concentration of treponemes at the site of inoculation; in experimental syphilis, there is a linear relationship between inoculum size and time to development of the chancre. Silent bacteremia and local lymphatic spread begin soon after local inoculation and before appearance of the chancre. The clinical signs of secondary syphilis, like the chancre, develop when the concentration of treponemes reaches an "inflammatory threshold" in the infected tissues. Local and systemic cellular immune responses eventually result in clearing of the large majority of organisms, healing of the chancre, and resolution of the clinical manifestations of secondary syphilis. However, infection persists in numerous organs, perhaps especially in immunologically privileged sites such as the central nervous system. Several antibodies are produced, primarily to components of the *T. pallidum* outer membrane, but their role in clearing the infection and on protective immunity are uncertain. "Reaginic" antibody, the basis of the Venereal Disease Research Laboratory (VDRL) and rapid plasma reagin (RPR) tests, probably develops to lipid components of the organism's outer membrane, or perhaps to components of the host's cell membranes; it may have a role in opsonization.

### Chancroid

Knowledge of the pathogenesis of chancroid is limited. Initial attachment of *H. ducreyi* to epithelial cells, which may be mediated in part by specific adhesins, is followed by cell penetration and necrosis, probably mediated by lipooligosaccharide. The initial inflammatory papule rapidly evolves into a pustule and then an ulcer. Despite the locally aggressive nature of the infection, fever and disseminated infection occur rarely, if ever. Antibodies are produced to several outer membrane proteins, but their contribution to acquired immunity is unknown; repeated infections are common in endemic areas.

### Lymphogranuloma venereum

The classical primary lesion of LGV is an evanescent papule, pustule, or ulcer, but such lesions are observed uncommonly. Instead, it is possible that the primary infection often is manifested by urethritis or cervicitis, as for infection with other *C. trachomatis* serovars. Primary LGV proctitis is well documented. Lymphatic spread results in regional lymphadenopathy, with central necrosis and liquefaction that typically evolves over 2–4 wk. Both humoral and cellular immune responses occur, and it is likely that delayed hypersensitivity is largely responsible for the chronic, relapsing lymphadenopathy and lymphatic obstruction that are the classical hallmarks of untreated infection.

### Granuloma inguinale

Little is known of the molecular pathogenesis of *Cal. granulomatis* infections. The organism appears to replicate intracellularly within macrophages, and the histological picture and course suggest that the clinical manifestations are due largely to a cell-mediated immune response. Contiguous spread of subcutaneous infection results in satellite regional masses and ulcers, typically in the inguinal region. Although systemic symptoms do not occur, disseminated osteolytic lesions have been described.

## Clinical Manifestations and Differential Diagnosis

As implied by the relative frequencies of the causes of GUD (Table 70.1), the differential diagnosis in young, sexually active patients in much of the United States is primarily genital herpes versus syphilis, and almost all patients should be evaluated for both of these infections. Patients with lesions suggestive of chancroid should be evaluated for this disease, as should persons sexually exposed in chancroid-endemic areas. In most settings in industrialized countries, however, it is necessary to evaluate young, sexually active patients for other causes of GUD only after herpes, syphilis, and chancroid have been excluded.

### Genital herpes

The clinical characteristics of genital herpes are summarized in Table 70.2. Primary genital herpes, by definition, is the patient's first infection with either HSV type and typically is the most symptomatic form of the disease. Primary herpes can be severe,

**Table 70.2** Characteristics of symptomatic genital herpes

| | Type of infection | | |
|---|---|---|---|
| | Primary | Initial nonprimary | Recurrent |
| Lesions | Many, bilateral | Fewer | Few, unilateral |
| Cervicitis or urethritis | Common | Occasional | Uncommon |
| Neuropathic complications | Common | Uncommon | Rare |
| Regional lymphadenopathy | Usual | Occasional | Uncommon |
| Systemic manifestations | Usual | Occasional | Rare |
| Usual duration | 2–6 wk | 1–3 wk | 5–10 d |

with multiple crops of extensive lesions, often with urethritis, cervicitis, regional lymphadenopathy, neuropathy, or aseptic meningitis. Nonprimary initial herpes is the first clinically recognized infection, generally with HSV-2, in a patient previously infected with HSV, usually orolabial HSV-1; it is intermediate in severity. Recurrent herpes is the second or subsequent clinically recognized genital outbreak. Symptomatic recurrences of genital herpes usually are mild and brief, without mucosal involvement or systemic symptoms, but some patients with recurrent herpes experience a neuropathic prodrome, such as paresthesias that begin from a few hours to 2 d before overt cutaneous lesions appear. Subclinical infection is superimposed on this scheme. Most primary and initial, nonprimary infections are unrecognized because they cause atypical, mild or nonspecific symptoms or are entirely asymptomatic. Many of these patients, as well as some who have symptomatic first episodes, have subclinical rather than overt recurrences. Most cases of the rare syndrome of recurrent benign lymphocytic meningitis (Molleret's meningitis) are due to reactivation of central nervous system HSV-2 infection.

Classical herpetic lesions typically appear in clusters. The individual lesion evolves over 2–3 d from an erythematous papule to a vesicle containing clear fluid, then to a pustule. The epithelial surface may be shed at any time, resulting in burning pain and superficial, tender ulcerations. Early ulceration is the rule on moist surfaces, such as the vulva, partly explaining the more severe course in women than in most men. On dry surfaces, lesions develop crusts after several days, with rapid subsequent healing. The time from papule to encrustation and healing is substantially longer in primary and initial than recurrent herpes (Table 70.2).

Plates 32 and 33 illustrate classical lesions of genital herpes. Clusters of vesicles, pustules, or grouped superficial ulcers involving the genitals, anus, perineum, or surrounding areas are sufficiently typical to warrant a clinical diagnosis, although the diagnosis normally should be confirmed with a test for HSV. When lymphadenopathy is present, the nodes are firm and mildly to moderately tender; they do not become fluctuant and the overlying skin usually is not inflamed, which helps to distinguish herpes from chancroid, LGV, and pyogenic infection. Primary infection is accompanied by herpetic cervicitis in 70% of women and urethritis in 20%–30% of men. Urethritis in men usually causes scant discharge but severe dysuria, often with localized tenderness along the penile shaft at the sites of intraurethral herpetic lesions.

Although such classical presentations are frequent, "atypical" ulcers may be more common; many lesions are so trivial they are not recognized. However, if patients or clinicians are alerted to the possibility of herpes, such as by serological testing or following diagnosis of the infection in a sex partner, they often recognize previously unknown lesions. Plates 34 and 35 illustrate the broad range of lesions that genital herpes can cause. They demonstrate the importance of testing for HSV infection in patients who present with "nonspecific" genital ulcers or whose lesions resemble those of chancroid, syphilis, or other diseases.

During the first year following symptomatic initial or primary genital herpes due to HSV-2, the mean frequency of symptomatic recurrences is 4 per year in women and 5 per year in men; about 40% of patients have at least 6 and 20% have 10 or more outbreaks. The rate of recurrences may decline slightly thereafter, but most patients continue to have symptomatic outbreaks for several years. However, persons with genital HSV-1 infection experience an average of only one symptomatic outbreak per year, and many patients have no recurrences. Among persons with recognized recurrences, HSV can be isolated from the genitals or anus up to 7% of the days between symptomatic outbreaks, although the frequency of subclinical viral shedding probably declines after 1–2 years following the initial infection. The prevalence of subclinical shedding in HSV-2 seropositive persons who never had clinically recognized genital herpes is unknown, but the virus can be detected in about 1% of asymptomatic HSV-2-seropositive STD clinic patients or pregnant women.

## Syphilis

Primary syphilis usually presents with a genital ulcer, the chancre, which appears 3–6 wk after inoculation. The classical chancre is indurated, has a clean, nonpurulent base, and is only mildly tender (Plate 36), but atypical lesions are common. Inguinal lymphadenopathy, usually bilateral, often is present. The involved nodes usually are mildly tender and nonfluctuant and the overlying skin is not erythematous, features that distinguish syphilis (and genital herpes) from chancroid and LGV.

The chancre and regional lymphadenopathy resolve spontaneously after several weeks. Secondary syphilis typically develops 2–4 mo after infection but sometimes overlaps with primary syphilis. The most consistent manifestation is a generalized papulosquamous skin rash that typically involves the trunk and the palms and soles (Fig. 70.3). However, the appearance is highly variable and the rash can mimic psoriasis, eczema, scabies, erythema multiforme, and a wide variety of other dermatoses. Although the rash of secondary syphilis usually is nonpruritic, a complaint of itching does not exclude the diagnosis. Patchy alopecia of the scalp, painless mucous membrane lesions called "mucous patches," and wart-like condylomata lata of the genitalia or perineum may be present (Plate 37). Numerous other systemic or neurological manifestations also may occur, sometimes without cutaneous lesions.

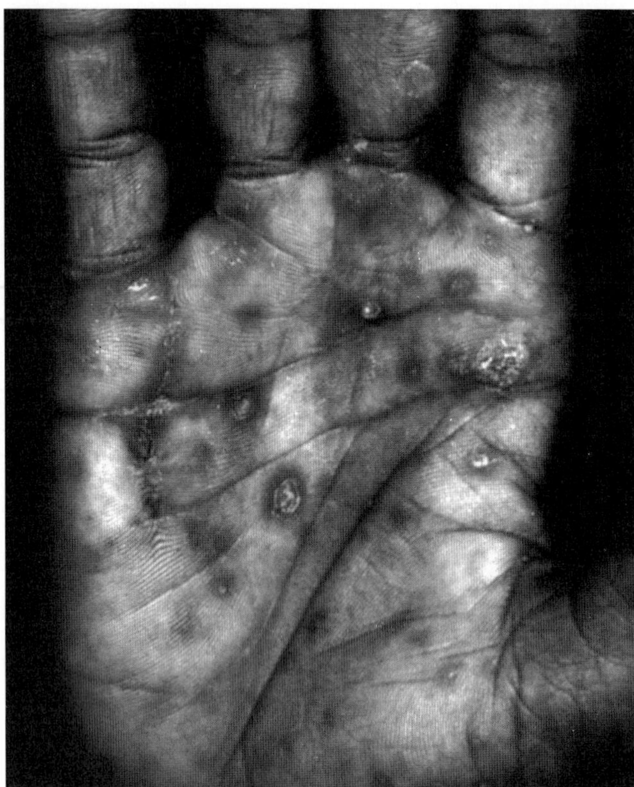

**Fig. 70.3** Papulosquamous lesions of the palms in a patient with secondary syphilis.

Like the chancre, the clinical manifestations of secondary syphilis resolve spontaneously, usually after 2–3 mo, although the skin rash and other features sometimes reappear within the first year of infection. The secondary stage is followed by latent syphilis. By definition, the patient is asymptomatic and infection is detected only by serological reactivity. True resolution ("biological cure") may sometimes follow, but viable treponemes persist in most cases, perhaps within macrophages or other cells in the liver, spleen, lymph nodes, central nervous system, and other sites. In the preantibiotic era, overt tertiary syphilis eventually developed in 10%–20% of patients, usually 5–20 yr after the primary infection, and involved the central nervous system, heart, bones, skin, or other organ systems. However, classical late syphilis is now very rare in the United States, perhaps because most persons receive antibiotics for intercurrent infections. Today the most common serious outcome of syphilis is congenital infection, resulting from placental transmission from an infected mother to the fetus; most cases occur when the mother has syphilis less than a year in duration. Neurosyphilis is the most common recognized complication in adults, but most cases now are diagnosed in persons with syphilis of 1 to 4 yr in duration, and the usual manifestations are those of meningeal or meningovascular syphilis—which usually pres-ent with signs of meningitis, cranial nerve dysfunction, or stroke—rather than tabes dorsalis or general paresis, the classical syndromes of late neurosyphilis.

## Chancroid

Chancroid was historically called "soft chancre," reflecting the lesion's nonindurated nature compared with syphilis. Most ulcers occur on the penis, especially under the foreskin in uncircumcised men, and near the introitus in women. Typically one to three lesions are present, but there may be several, especially in women. The shape may be round, oval, or irregular (Plate 38, Fig. 70.4). The edges are erythematous and may be undermined, the base typically is covered with purulent exudate, and the lesion usually is very tender. However, some cases are mild with nonspecific-appearing lesions. Up to two-thirds of patients with chancroid have inguinal lymphadenopathy, which may be unilateral or bilateral. Overlying cutaneous erythema and fluctuance are the rule (the "bubo"), helping to distinguish chancroid from syphilis or herpes (Plate 38). Untreated, and sometimes despite effective antibiotic therapy, fluctuant lymph nodes rupture and drain spontaneously. Despite the highly inflammatory nature of the local manifestations, fever and other systemic manifestations occur rarely, if ever.

## Lymphogranuloma venereum

The classical presentation of LGV is bilateral inguinal lymphadenopathy, and the primary genital ulceration rarely is seen. Initially the lymph nodes are moderately tender, often with overlying erythema, and may be fluctuant. Untreated, there may be repeated cycles of spontaneous rupture and drainage, and patients with chronic infection may present with indurated, matted nodes, often with sinus tracts and secondary pyogenic infection. Rarely, lymphatic obstruction supervenes, with elephantiasis involving the genitals or lower extremities; such presentations are now very rare. Acute proctocolitis was a frequent manifestation of LGV in homosexually active men in the late 1970s but now is uncommon. Fever and malaise are seen occasionally, especially in proctocolitis, and aseptic meningitis occasionally occurs.

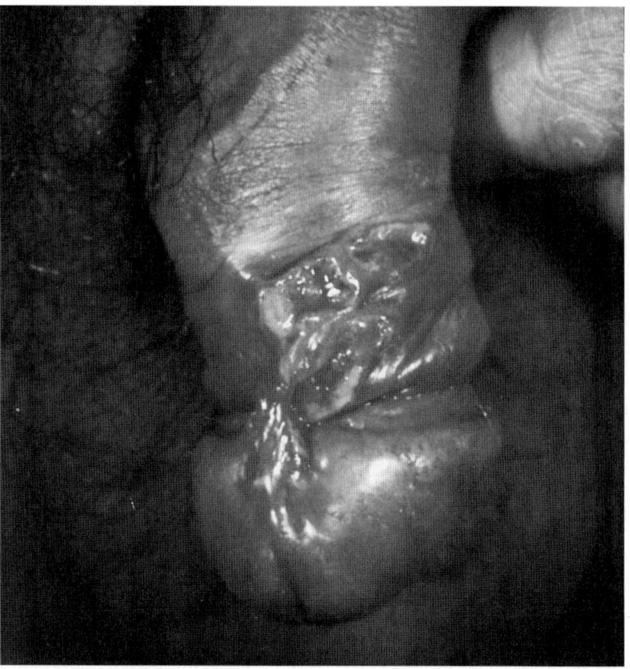

**Fig. 70.4** Large, irregularly shaped penile ulcer due to chancroid; the lesion had eroded through the frenulum, under which a probe could be passed.

### Granuloma inguinale

Granuloma inguinale presents with one or more indolent, mildly tender ulcerative lesions, typically with hypertrophic granulation-like tissue. Sometimes the lesions spread inexorably, rarely leading to penile autoamputation, and the appearance may be similar to that of squamous cell carcinoma. Inguinal masses are common, due more frequently to subcutaneous extension of inflammatory tissue than to lymphadenopathy per se.

### Other conditions

A large number of other conditions can cause genital ulceration, irrespective of the patient's risk for STD. Injury is often implicated by patients but, as discussed above, trauma should be accepted as the diagnosis only if the history of injury is clear and other, more common causes of GUD are excluded. Fixed drug eruptions are seen occasionally in STD clinics, because the tetracyclines are a common cause and are often used in STD management. These reactions typically begin 7–10 d after starting the offending drug (sometimes after it has been discontinued). The clinical picture is similar to that of a second-degree burn, with initial erythema and tenderness followed by sloughing of the superficial epithelium. Secondary pyogenic infection of scabies or other initial inflammatory conditions occasionally presents with pustules or ulcerative lesions. Behçet's syndrome typically causes deep, painful, necrotic genital ulcers, usually with a history of recurrent oral ulceration.

Virtually any dermatosis can affect the genitals, occasionally with ulceration. For example, psoriasis of the penis may present with ulceration, especially in patients who vigorously cleanse the lesion in an attempt to remove the typical scale. Contact dermatitis, sometimes due to detergents or other chemicals, occasionally involves the genitals and can present with genital ulceration in combination with a more diffuse, characteristic dermatitis. Squamous cell cancer of the penis or vulva may present as GUD. Stevens Johnson syndrome presents with genital or oral mucosal ulceration plus the typical skin rash of erythema multiforme; this diagnosis can be confusing, because genital herpes is a common trigger of erythema multiforme. Cat scratch disease (Chapter 53) is among the most common diagnoses in patients who present with prominent inflammatory inguinal lymphadenopathy without GUD. The correct diagnosis usually can be suspected or confirmed by history and physical examination, although special methods, such as biopsy, sometimes are required.

## Diagnosis

### History and examination

The clinical evaluation of patients with GUD is straightforward; an accurate presumptive or confirmed diagnosis usually can be determined quickly and inexpensively. The most common errors in the diagnosis of GUD probably are failure to test for HSV infection and failure to perform a syphilis serology, often because the ulcer lacks the classical appearance of the common STDs or because the clinician does not assess the patient's behavioral risks or is unaware of the varied manifestations of herpes.

The history should stress the onset and clinical course of the ulcer(s). For example, did the ulcer begin as a blister-like or pimple-like lesion? Is it painful? Other local symptoms and systemic manifestations should be solicited, as should diagnoses or symptoms in the patient's sexual partner(s). The history should encompass sexual exposures and the settings in which they occurred, substance abuse, and recent travel. A careful physical examination is essential, including inspection of the lesion, characterization of inguinal lymphadenopathy, a complete genital examination, and a general physical examination, with emphasis on the skin, mucous membranes, and lymph nodes.

Patients with established or suspected syphilis, regardless of clinical staging, also require careful cardiovascular and neurological examinations, especially assessment of the cranial nerves, deep tendon reflexes, posterior spinal column signs (e.g., position and vibration sense), mental status, and signs of meningitis (which may be subtle). Because of potential effects on the response to therapy, assessment for HIV infection is a high priority. Examination of the cerebrospinal fluid (cell count, protein, and VDRL) is indicated for all patients with neurological signs or symptoms, regardless of clinical staging; for patients with latent syphilis of $\geq$1 yr duration or unknown duration, especially for younger patients (e.g., <50 yr old) or if the VDRL or RPR titer is $\geq$1:8; and for patients in whom the serum VDRL or RPR titer does not decline as expected following treatment of syphilis of any stage. Some experts advise routine cerebrospinal fluid examination for all HIV-infected patients with any stage of syphilis, but recent studies suggest this is unnecessary unless a specific indication is present.

### Approach to laboratory diagnosis

Although the history and physical examination often will lead to a highly probable diagnosis, laboratory assessment is recommended. Table 70.3 summarizes a succinct, practical approach to the assessment of patients who present with genital ulceration. A test for HSV usually should be done, but it may be considered optional if there are classical signs of genital herpes, such as a cluster of vesicles or tender superficial ulcers. Even in these cases, however, a positive test often will help convince a doubting patient about the diagnosis. In addition, the virus type provides prognostic information; persons with genital HSV-1 infection are less likely to have symptomatic recurrence than

**Table 70.3** Laboratory evaluation of sexually active patients with genital ulcer disease

| |
|---|
| LESIONS TYPICAL OF GENITAL HERPES[a] |
| Culture or direct FA[b] test for HSV (recommended but optional; see text) |
| Screening tests for other STD (syphilis, HIV, chlamydia, and gonorrhea) |
| OTHER GENITAL ULCERS |
| Culture or direct FA test for HSV (or PCR, if available)[c] |
| Darkfield microscopy or direct FA test for *T. pallidum* |
| Syphilis serology |
| SELECTED CASES |
| Culture for *H. ducreyi* |
| Culture for pyogenic bacteria |
| Biopsy |
| Type-specific HSV serology[d] |

[a]For example, a cluster of superficial ulcers or vesiculopustular lesions.

[b]FA denotes fluorescent antibody.

[c]PCR denotes polymerase chain reaction.

[d]Type-specific HSV serology may have value as a routine diagnostic test in all patients with GUD when inexpensive assays become available.

those infected with HIV-2. Definitive diagnosis of herpes also is recommended before beginning long-term suppressive therapy. All patients with first-episode genital herpes should be tested for other common STDs, such as syphilis, chlamydial infection, gonorrhea, and HIV infection. In this setting, the syphilis serology may be viewed as a screening test (because the patient is at risk for STD) rather than part of the diagnostic workup for GUD. Culture for HSV is recommended, but the direct fluorescent antibody test can be used. The Tzanck test—staining lesion scrapings by the Wright-Giemsa or Papanicoulaou method for cytologic examination—has poor sensitivity, especially in ulcerated lesions, and usually is not useful. The sensitivity of culture is maximal for intact vesicles and early, moist, tender ulcers; in recurrent herpes in particular, cultures obtained more than 48 h after onset usually are negative. Diagnostic tests using the polymerase chain reaction appear to be highly sensitive and may soon be commercially available.

Complete evaluation for both HSV infection and syphilis is always indicated for sexually active patients who present with GUD that does not have the classical appearance of genital herpes (Table 70.3). At a minimum this should include a culture or other sensitive test for HSV and a serological test for syphilis. Because herpes is the most common cause of GUD, regardless of the appearance of the lesion, failure to test for HSV often will lead to misdiagnosis. Darkfield microscopy also is indicated but is not always readily available; as an alternative, most public health laboratories offer the direct fluorescent antibody test for *T. pallidum*. If the clinical appearance or history suggests chancroid, a culture for *H. ducreyi* should be done on the lesion and, if there is fluctuant lymphadenopathy, on a needle aspirate from the lymph node. Sensitive polymerase chain reaction tests for *H. ducreyi* and *T. pallidum* have been developed but are not widely available.

If the diagnosis remains elusive following the initial evaluation, follow-up and repeat laboratory tests, especially syphilis serology, often are helpful. An acute and/or convalescent type-specific HSV serological test using Western blot or enzyme immunoassay may be helpful, if available. Serological tests for HSV antibody using other methods offered by most commercial laboratories in recent years do not accurately distinguish HSV-1 from HSV-2 antibody. However, accurate type-specific serological tests will be widely available in the near future. If regional lymphadenopathy is prominent, LGV should be assessed by testing the lymph node aspirate or lesion for *C. trachomatis* and performing an LGV complement fixation test; if available, type-specific chlamydia serology with the microimmunofluorescence test is recommended. If granuloma inguinale is suspected, a scraping of the lesion should be crushed between two microscope slides, stained with the Wright-Giemsa method, and examined for intracellular Donovan bodies; culture tests for *Cal. granulomatis* may be available soon. Some cases may require biopsy, culture of the ulcer or lymph node aspirate for pyogenic bacteria, or other special tests.

## Serological tests for syphilis

The interpretation of serological tests for syphilis is less complex than sometimes believed. The nontreponemal tests, including the VDRL and RPR tests, detect "reaginic" antibody and are sensitive and inexpensive, making them useful for screening. They become reactive within the first 4–6 wk of infection and are positive at presentation in about 70% of patients with primary infection and virtually all persons with later stages of syphilis. The nontreponemal tests are easily quantitated and the titer is correlated with disease activity, so the VDRL and RPR tests are useful in assessing the response to treatment and in judging the likelihood of active disease in seropositive patients. However, reaginic antibody is nonspecific, and the first reactive nontreponemal test in a particular patient always requires confirmation with a *T. pallidum*–specific antibody test, such as the fluorescent treponemal antibody-absorbed (FTA-ABS) test or the microhemaggulutination test for treponemal antibody (MHA-TP). Because of their cost and procedural complexity, these assays are not generally considered suitable for screening.

The VDRL or RPR antibody titers typically decline by two to three dilutions within 3 mo of successful treatment of primary or secondary syphilis, and usually become negative within 12 mo. However, the decline is less rapid after treatment of later stages of syphilis, and detectable antibody—usually in titers ≤1:4—may persist indefinitely. It is commonly believed that the FTA-ABS, MHA-TP, and other treponemal antibody tests remain reactive for life, regardless of successful cure or disease activity, but in fact these tests become negative within 3 yr of successful treatment in at least 25% of patients with primary syphilis. However, almost all patients treated at the secondary stage or later will have reactive treponemal tests for life. Performance of a *T. pallidum*–specific antibody test is rarely indicated in a patient with a negative RPR or VDRL test; regardless of past therapy, such patients rarely have active syphilis and most are at very low risk for future reactivation. The effects of cellular immune deficiency in general and HIV infection in particular on the serological tests for syphilis are poorly understood. Reports suggest both enhanced serological responses in some patients and an increased frequency of false-negative tests in others, but both effects appear to be infrequent; in most HIV-infected patients both the treponemal and nontreponemal tests can be interpreted normally.

## Treatment

Although treatment ideally should be based on a definitive diagnosis, most patients with sexually acquired GUD should be treated empirically while awaiting test results. Amelioration of first-episode genital herpes with antiviral drugs is largely dependent on early treatment, and syphilis and chancroid often occur in patients who may be unavailable for follow-up or who may continue sexual activity despite advice to the contrary.

## Genital herpes

Acyclovir has been the mainstay of therapy. Penciclovir, another recently developed thymidine kinase inhibitor, also is active against HSV. Famciclovir is an orally administered prodrug of penciclovir, and valacyclovir is a prodrug of acyclovir. Both valacyclovir and famciclovir offer substantial improvement in bioavailability compared with acyclovir and are highly effective. (see Chapter 39).

Table 70.4 shows the recommended acyclovir, valacyclovir, and famciclovir regimens for genital herpes. Intravenous acyclovir is indicated for severe primary herpes, especially if aseptic meningitis is present or severe sacral neuropathy causes transient bladder paralysis, but most patients are treated orally. Blood and intracellular levels of acyclovir are modest in some patients, and valacyclovir or famciclovir orally may benefit patients with slow clinical responses to oral acyclovir. Episodic

**Table 70.4** Treatment of genital herpes simplex virus infection*

| |
|---|
| FIRST-EPISODE GENITAL HERPES |
| Acyclovir 400 mg orally 3 times daily (or 200 mg 5 times daily) for 7–10 d |
| Valacyclovir 1.0 g orally 3 times daily for 7–10 d |
| Famciclovir 250 mg orally 3 times daily for 7–10 d |
| SEVERE INFECTION THAT REQUIRES PARENTERAL THERAPY |
| Acyclovir 5–10 mg/kg body weight intravenously every 8 hr until clinical resolution is attained, followed by acyclovir, valacyclovir, or famciclovir orally to complete 7–10 d total therapy |
| EPISODIC TREATMENT OF RECURRENT OUTBREAKS |
| Acyclovir 400 mg orally 3 times daily (or 800 mg twice daily, or 200 mg 5 times daily) for 5 d |
| Valacyclovir 500 mg orally twice daily for 5 d |
| Famciclovir 125 mg orally twice daily for 5 d |
| SUPPRESSIVE THERAPY[a] |
| Acyclovir 400 mg orally twice daily |
| Valacyclovir 500–1,000 mg orally once daily |
| Famciclovir 250 mg orally twice daily |

*Author's recommendations, modified from the 1998 guidelines of the Centers for Disease Control and Prevention

[a]Suppressive therapy should be interrupted at 1-year intervals to reassess the frequency of symptomatic recurrences. Treatment reduces the frequency and severity of recurrences but does not entirely prevent them, nor does it completely suppress subclinical shedding of herpes simplex virus.

treatment of symptomatic recurrences is clinically beneficial only if begun promptly, ideally when prodromal symptoms appear or within 24 h of lesion onset. Topical acyclovir has little clinical effect for either initial or recurrent herpes and is rarely indicated. Continuous suppressive therapy is highly effective in reducing the frequency and severity of symptomatic recurrences of genital herpes; it is indicated primarily for patients with ≥6 episodes per year, persons with particularly severe recurrences, and patients who are psychologically distressed. Suppressive therapy markedly reduces subclinical viral shedding as well as symptomatic outbreaks, and in the future suppressive therapy may prove to have a role in preventing transmission.

Resistance of HSV to acyclovir and other thymidine kinase inhibitors is an occasional problem in immunodeficient patients on chronic treatment but is observed rarely in immunocompetent persons. HSV isolates from patients with genital herpes that persists or progresses on maximal doses of acyclovir, penciclovir, famciclovir, or valacyclovir should be tested for resistance.

## Syphilis

Penicillin remains the drug of choice for treatment of all stages of syphilis. Penicillin therapy has reduced efficacy in HIV-infected patients, even when high-dose therapy is administered in-

**Table 70.5** Treatment of adults with syphilis*

| |
|---|
| PRIMARY, SECONDARY, AND LATENT SYPHILIS <1 YR IN DURATION |
| Regimen of choice: benzathine penicillin G 2.4 million units intramuscularly in a single dose[a] |
| Penicillin-allergic patients: doxycycline 100 mg orally twice daily for 2 wk or tetracycline 500 mg orally 4 times daily for 2 wk |
| TERTIARY SYPHILIS (EXCEPT NEUROSYPHILIS) AND LATENT SYPHILIS ≥1 YR IN DURATION |
| Regimen of choice: benzathine penicillin G 2.4 million units intramuscularly once weekly for 3 doses |
| Penicillin-allergic patients: doxycycline 100 mg orally twice daily for 4 wk or tetracycline 500 mg orally 4 times daily for 4 wk |
| NEUROSYPHILIS |
| Regimen of choice: aqueous penicillin G 3–4 million units intravenously every 4 h for 10–14 d |
| Alternative: procaine penicillin G 2.4 million units intramuscularly once daily, plus probenecid 500 mg orally 4 times daily, for 10–14 d |
| Penicillin-allergic patients: densensitize and treat with penicillin |
| Additional therapy: some experts recommend following either of the above regimens with up to 3 doses of benzathine penicillin G, 2.4 million units intramuscularly, at weekly intervals |

*Based on the 1998 guidelines of the Centers for Disease Control and Prevention.

[a]Some experts recommend that in HIV-infected patients this regimen be repeated twice at weekly intervals.

travenously for neurosyphilis. Few data exist on the efficacy of oral penicillins or other $\beta$-lactam antibiotics, such as cephalosporins, and only parenteral therapy is recommended. Oral doxycycline is the primary option for patients with well-documented penicillin allergy, but is less effective, in part because of reduced compliance. Penicillin is the only recommended drug for the treatment of neurosyphilis; persons with documented allergy should be desensitized and treated with penicillin. The recommendations for treatment of syphilis are shown in Table 70.5.

### Chancroid

Several studies in the past decade have documented the efficacy of single-dose treatment of chancroid with ceftriaxone or azithromycin and with 3-d regimens of ciprofloxacin or other fluoroquinolones. Erythromycin is effective but requires compliance for 7 d. All regimens have somewhat reduced efficacy in the presence of HIV infection, a common problem in persons with chancroid. Fluctuant lymph nodes should be aspirated as often as necessary to prevent spontaneous rupture. The 1998 CDC recommendations are shown in Table 70.6.

### Other conditions

Doxycycline 100 mg orally twice daily for 3 wk is the recommended regimen for both LGV and donovanosis. Patients with nonsexually transmitted genital ulcers should be managed according to the specific diagnosis.

## Prevention and Control

The principles of prevention and control of GUD are not materially different than for other STDs. Personal prevention is accomplished by sexual abstention or by selection of partners at low risk, and by use of condoms for sexual exposure in other than committed, permanent, mutually monogamous relationships. The clinician has an important role in educating patients accordingly. Other elements of prevention and control include community-based education and reporting of cases to enhance the epidemiologic data that are crucial to public health prevention efforts. Partner notification and treatment, using full therapeutic doses of appropriate antibiotics, are central to the control of syphilis and chancroid; most local or state health departments are willing to assume this responsibility. Any patient at risk for STD should be screened for syphilis and HIV infection.

The risk of HSV transmission in herpes-discordant couples is reduced but not eliminated by avoiding sexual contact in the presence of symptomatic episodes. Therefore, counseling patients about the frequency of subclinical viral shedding and educating them to recognize subtle clinical manifestations may help to prevent transmission to their sex partners. Subclinical shedding of HSV-2 is most frequent in the first 6–12 mo following primary infection; patients who have sexual partners without known genital herpes should use condoms for all sexual encounters during this interval. Because the risk of neonatal herpes is maximal when primary herpes occurs near term, it is especially important for pregnant women without herpes to avoid sexual exposure to an infected partner and to have no new sexual partners in the third trimester. Type-specific HSV serological tests will be useful in counseling patients and thus in preventing herpes when they become available. Research is in progress toward developing vaccines against HSV-2.

**Table 70.6** Recommended regimens for treatment of chancroid*

| |
|---|
| Azithromycin 1.0 g orally in a single dose |
| Ceftriaxone 250 mg intramuscularly in a single dose |
| Ciprofloxacin 500 mg orally twice daily for 3 d |
| Erythromycin 500 mg orally 4 times daily for 7 d |

*Based on the 1998 guidelines of the Centers for Disease Control and Prevention.

### ANNOTATED BIBLIOGRAPHY

Centers for Disease Control and Prevention. 1998 guidelines for treatment of sexually transmitted diseases. Morbid Mortal Weekly Rep 1998;47 (No. RR-1).
*CDC's evidence-based recommendations for treatment of STDs.*

Eng TR, Butler WR, eds. The Hidden Epidemic: Confronting Sexually Transmitted Diseases. National Academy Press, Washington, DC, 1997.
*A comprehensive review of STD epidemiology and the inadequacy of STD prevention in the United States by the Institute of Medicine, National Academy of Sciences.*

Fleming DT, McQuillan GM, Johnson RE, et al. Herpes simplex virus type 2 in the United States, 1976 to 1994. N Engl J Med 1997; 337:1105–1111.
*The results of national population-based surveys of HSV-2 seroprevalence, showing a 30% increase from the late 1970s to the early 1990s.*

Gordon SM, Eaton ME, George R et al. The response of symptomatic neurosyphilis to high-dose intravenous penicillin G in patients with human immunodeficiency virus infection. N Engl J Med 1994; 331:1469–1473.
*Five of 11 HIV-infected patients with neurosyphilis had been treated recently with benzathine penicillin G for early syphilis, and high-dose IV penicillin G failed to cure three of seven patients followed for 6 months.*

Handsfield HH. Color Atlas and Synopsis of Sexually Transmitted Diseases. McGraw-Hill, New York, 203 pp, 1992.
*An extensively illustrated practical approach to diagnosis and management of the common STDs.*

Holmes KK, Sparling PF, Mårdh P-A, Lemon SM, Stamm WE, Piot P, Wasserheit JN, eds. Sexually Transmitted Diseases, 3rd ed. McGraw-Hill, New York, 1998.
*The definitive textbook on sexually transmitted diseases.*

Hook EW III, Marra CM. Acquired syphilis in adults. N Engl J Med 1992; 326:1060–1069.
*A well-written, comprehensive review of the pathogenesis, epidemiology, clinical manifestations, and treatment of syphilis.*

Kaplowitz LG, Baker D, Gelb L et al. Prolonged continuous acyclovir treatment of normal adults with frequently recurring genital herpes simplex virus infection. JAMA 1991; 265:747–751.
*Documentation of the safety and efficacy of acyclovir in suppressing symptomatic recurrent genital herpes.*

Koutsky LA, Stevens CE, Holmes KK et al. Underdiagnosis of genital herpes by current clinical and viral-isolation procedures. N Engl J Med 1992; 326:1533–1599.
*Using the polymerase chain reaction to detect HSV in genital lesions and type-specific serology, this study shows that HSV causes most cases of "nonspecific" genital ulcerations.*

Lynch PJ, Edwards L. Genital Dermatoses. Churchill Livingstone, New York, 292 pp, 1994.
*A comprehensive text that addresses both infective and noninfective dermatologic conditions that involve the genitals.*

Marrazzo JM, Handsfield HH. Chancroid: new developments in an old disease. Curr Clin Top Infect Dis 1995; 15:129–152.
*A comprehensive review of* Haemophilus ducreyi *and chancroid.*

Morse SA, Trees DL, Htun Y, et al. Comparison of clinical diagnosis and standard laboratory and molecular methods for the diagnosis of genital ulcer disease in Lesotho: association with human immunodeficiency virus infection. J Infect Dis 1997; 175:583–589.
*The polymerase chain reaction was superior to traditional methods to detect* Haemophilus decreyi, Treponema pallidum, *and herpes simplex virus; HSV was an unexpectedly common cause of genital ulceration; and all causes of genital ulcer were associated with HIV infection.*

Rolfs RT, Joesoef MR, Hendershot EF, et al. A randomized trial of enhanced therapy for early syphilis in patients with and without human immunodeficiency virus infection. N Engl J Med 1997; 337:307–314.

*Among 541 patients with early syphilis, those with HIV infection responded less well serologically, but there were no differences in the clinical response to therapy; addition of high-dose oral amoxicillin to the standard benzathine penicillin regimen offered no incremental benefit.*

Romanowski B, Sutherland R, Fick GH et al. Serologic response to treatment of infectious syphilis. Ann Intern Med 1991; 114:1005–1009.

*A careful analysis of the long-term response of serological tests for syphilis following treatment, which confirmed earlier data showing that treponemal tests revert to negative in many patients treated for primary syphilis.*

Wald A, Zeh J, Barnum G et al. Suppression of subclinical shedding of herpes simplex virus type 2 with acyclovir. Ann Intern Med 1996; 124:8–15.

*A well-done study that documents both the high frequency of subclinical shedding of HSV-2 in women with recurrent genital herpes and the substantial (but incomplete) reduction of shedding in response to antiviral therapy.*

# 71

# Urethritis, Epidydimitis, Orchitis, Prostatitis

KIMBERLEY K. FOX, SUSAN F. ISBEY, MYRON S. COHEN, AND CULLEY C. CARSON III

Urethritis is a clinical syndrome generally characterized by urethral discharge and dysuria. It may be complicated by epididymitis and orchitis, which are also discussed in this chapter. The pathognomonic laboratory finding in urethritis is an increased number of polymorphonuclear leukocytes (PMN) on the gram stain of a urethral smear. Some patients have increased PMNs on urethral smear but lack symptoms of infection, so some cases are considered asymptomatic. Urethritis is almost always sexually acquired, but occasionally it derives from coliform bacteria or noninfectious causes.

## Urethritis

Urethritis is generally divided into gonococcal and nongonococcal disease, which denotes the historical importance of *Neisseria gonorrhoeae* and the relative lack of understanding of other causes of urethral inflammation until recent years. Nongonococcal urethritis (NGU) is a heterogeneous group of disorders caused by a multitude of pathogens. Treatment is directed at the likely etiologic agents.

## Etiologies

The most common causes of urethritis are *Neisseria gonorrhoeae* and *Chlamydia trachomatis* (Table 71.1) *Neisseria gonorrhoeae* is a gram-negative diplococcus which has a kidney-bean shape on gram stain. Humans are the only host of *N. gonorrhoeae*, and the bacteria is highly adapted for growth on the mucosal membranes. Infectivity has been estimated from studies of partners of people with identified infection. The infectivity of an infected male for his female sexual partners is around 70%; the infectivity of the female for her sexual partners approaches 60%–80% with multiple episodes of vaginal intercourse. The incubation period for gonococcal urethritis is short: three-quarters of men develop symptoms within 4 d, and 90% within 14 d. The use of subcurative doses of antibiotics during this time will prolong the incubation period. The urethral discharge caused by gonococcal infection is generally purulent and copious, and large numbers of PMN and gram-negative intracellular diplococci are seen on gram stain. A small number of men develop asymptomatic gonococcal infection after exposure, particularly those infected with strains having certain serotypes and auxotypes. Asymptomatic infections may play a disproportionate role in the spread of *N. gonorrhoeae*. A growing number of isolates of *N. gonorrhoeae* are resistant to the penicillins and tetracyclines, antibiotics traditionally used for therapy. More recently, strains resistant to the fluoroquinolones have been described.

*Chlamydia trachomatis* is the single most common cause of NGU, accounting for 30%–50% of cases. Recent studies suggest the proportion of NGU cases due to *C. trachomatis* may be declining in many areas. *Chlamydia trachomatis* is an obligate intracellular pathogen too small to see on gram stain. Humans are the only natural host of *C. trachomatis*, except for a murine biovar. The infectivity of the male for the female is around 30%, while the infectivity of female for male is around 45%–70%. *Chlamydia trachomatis* has a longer incubation period and produces more subtle symptoms than *N. gonorrhoeae*. Many cases remain asymptomatic. As many as 25% of men with gonococcal urethritis have coexistent chlamydial infection. *Chlamydia trachomatis* does not respond to most of the antibiotic regimens generally used for gonococcal infection.

*Ureaplasma urealyticum* is probably the most frequent cause of nonchlamydial NGU, though its role as a pathogen has been controversial. It clearly causes symptomatic urethral infection which responds to specific therapy in some men, but it has also been found to colonize as many as 60% of asymptomatic men attending sexually transmitted disease clinics. *Ureaplasma urealyticum* likely accounts for 10%–40% of NGU. *Mycoplasma hominis* was long thought to be a cause of NGU but recent studies have failed to confirm its role as a genital pathogen. More recently, *Mycoplasma genitalium* has been implicated as a cause of urethritis.

At least 20% of NGU cases are caused by agents other than *C. trachomatis* and *U. urealyticum*. Herpes simplex virus can produce urethritis, especially during primary infection. Typical herpetic lesions are generally seen on the penis, suggesting the diagnosis. Yeast balanitis can be associated with a concomitant distal urethritis. A small number of men may have symptoms of urethritis caused by infection with *Trichomonas vaginalis*. Coliform bacteria occasionally cause urethritis, especially in the setting of phimosis or urethral stricture, or following urethral instrumentation, and may cause an associated periurethral abscess. Syphilis may cause a urethral discharge without dysuria when the chancre is endourethral. Similarly, intraurethral condyloma acuminata may cause urethral discharge that is painless. Limited evidence suggests that adenovirus, *Hemophilus influenzae*, *Clostridium difficile*, *Neisseria meningitidis*, and anaerobic bacteria cause some cases of urethritis.

Noninfectious etiologies are found in a very small percent of cases of urethritis. Alcohol ingestion has long been known to cause a mild dysuria and in fact was thought to be the cause of postgonococcal urethritis before the recognition of *Chlamydia* and *Ureaplasma*. Other forms of chemical irritation include spermicides and occasionally bath products. More unusual causes include endourethral tumor, Stevens-Johnson syndrome, and

**Table 71.1** Causes of urethral discharge

| Infections | Noninfectious causes |
|---|---|
| *Neisseria gonorrhoeae* | Chemical irritants (spermicides, bath products) |
| *Chlamydia trachomatis* | Foreign bodies |
| *Ureaplasma urealyticum* | Endourethral neoplasm |
| *Mycoplasma genitalium* | Stevens-Johnson syndrome |
| Herpes simplex virus | Wegener's granulomatosis |
| *Trichomonas vaginalis* | |
| *Candida* species | |
| Coliform bacteria | |
| *Treponema pallidum* | |
| Condyloma acuminata | |

Wegener's granulomatosis. Repeated vigorous urethral stripping may eventually cause the production of a clear urethral discharge. A foreign body in the urethra will cause a mucoid or bloody discharge and may become secondarily infected. Heavy crystalluria or calculous gravel in the urine can produce dysuria and may have the appearance of a urethral discharge. Finally, the remnants of semen at the meatus or urinary incontinence may be misinterpreted by the patient as urethral discharge.

## Epidemiology

Like other sexually transmitted diseases, urethritis occurs most commonly in young sexually active persons. The peak age group is 20–24 yr, followed by 15–19 and 25–29 yr. Urethritis occurring in older persons should prompt consideration of alternative etiologies in addition to sexually transmitted pathogens.

The incidence of reported gonorrhea in the United States has been falling since 1975, while the incidence of reported NGU has risen rapidly in recent years and is currently about twice that of gonococcal urethritis. Some of the increase in reported NGU is likely due to increased awareness and reporting of the syndrome rather than actual increases in occurrence. Epidemiologic studies have shown NGU to be more common than gonococcal urethritis in whites, college students, those belonging to higher educational and socioeconomic levels, and in people with fewer total sexual partners. However, there is enough overlap between the groups to make differentiation by these factors alone impossible.

## Host factors

Immunity to pathogens causing urethritis is poorly understood. Recurrent infections caused by gonorrhea and chlamydia argue against a long-lived protective effect after infection. However, there is some evidence for strain-dependent immunity for both pathogens among commercial sex workers in Africa. No special racial or genetic factors predispose to mucosal sexually transmitted diseases causing urethritis. However, environmental factors such as mucosal trauma, oral contraceptive use, and spermicide use may alter susceptibility to infection. In addition, there is evidence for an increased rate of cervicitis among younger as compared with older women, and this may be true for urethritis as well.

## Pathogenesis

Urethral infection requires that the pathogen be able to attach to the epithelium and evade host defenses well enough to survive and multiply. The gonococcus accomplishes this by a set of complex mechanisms which has been elucidated over several decades of research. At least two outer membrane proteins, pilin and Opa, are important in adherence. Lipooligosaccharride (LOS) may stimulate an inflammatory response. Gonococci must have mechanisms to evade ingestion by polymorphonuclear leukocytes, and these appear to include the antioxidant catalase, DNA repair mechanisms, and competition for molecular oxygen. Gonococci that cause disseminated infection must also possess the ability to invade the mucosa and survive humoral defenses, including a complement-mediated bactericidal attack.

The pathogenesis of chlamydial infection is less well understood. *C. trachomatis* has a unique life cycle in which the infectious particle, the elementary body, attaches to and enters an epithelial cell, and then reorganizes into the metabolically active reticulate body, which multiplies; the resultant reticulate bodies then condense into elementary bodies. These are released when the host cell ruptures, completing the cycle. Direct cytoxicity, along with the host immune response to selected chlamydial antigens, creates the clinical manifestations of infection. There is no evidence that *C. trachomatis* can persist in a truly latent state in epithelial cells, but long-lived, slowly replicating infection is probably common. Such chronic infections stimulate a long-lived humoral and cell-mediated response which may explain some of the long-term complications of *C. trachomatis* infection, including Reiter's syndrome and pelvic inflammatory disease.

## Clinical manifestations

The classic clinical features of urethritis are dysuria and discharge. Either one or both may be present, and the pattern of symptoms may provide a clue to diagnosis. Dysuria may be felt along the shaft of the penis or only at the meatus. The latter suggests a process extending from the external skin (i.e., yeast infection) rather than a primary urethritis. Patients may report minor penile discomfort unrelated to urination, but frequency and urgency are not generally part of this clinical syndrome and should suggest bacterial urinary tract infection. The discharge may be mucoid or purulent, ranging in color from clear to white, yellow or green. It may be profuse or present only before the first void in the morning.

Gonococcal urethritis classically produces a profuse yellow-green discharge and dysuria, with acute onset of symptoms. NGU conversely produces a mucopurulent or mucoid discharge which may be seen only after urethral stripping or in the morning before voiding. A small crust at the meatus may be the only manifestation of discharge in NGU. Dysuria is also present, though somewhat less frequently than with gonorrhea, and the onset of symptoms is insidious. Unfortunately, many cases of urethritis do not fit either of the classic descriptions precisely, so differentiation based on clinical grounds is accurate in only three-quarters of cases. However, the presence of dysuria without urethral discharge is a very good (90%) predictor of NGU. Chlamydial NGU and nonchlamydial NGU produce similar signs and symptoms.

Gonococcal and nongonococcal urethral infection are often asymptomatic. Fifty percent of infected partners of women with gonorrhea or chlamydial infection are asymptomatic. Asymptomatic carriage of *N. gonorrhoeae* develops in a small proportion of newly infected men. One-quarter to one-half of men infected with *C. trachomatis* are asymptomatic. If these men are not identified by contact tracing or screening of high risk populations, they remain untreated and thus serve as a reservoir for infecting others. Asymptomatic urethral carriage is common in men who develop disseminated gonococcal infection, which is discussed further in Chapter 80. Untreated symptomatic infection usually becomes asymptomatic over months, although infectiousness may persist. *Trichomonas vaginalis* urethral carriage is usually asymptomatic in men, allowing them to serve as efficient vectors of the infection.

Urethritis in primary herpes simplex virus infection causes severe dysuria and a profuse mucoid discharge, often with localized urethral tenderness at the site of ulceration. External genital ulcers are also usually present, along with regional lymphadenopathy.

Several symptoms raise the possibility of alternative diagnoses. Frequency and urgency, especially in association with hematuria, suggest acute cystitis or infection higher in the urinary tract. Painless hematuria usually originates in the bladder or kidney from a variety of largely noninfectious causes. Hesitancy, dribbling, and nocturia mandate evaluation for urologic disorders. Prostate tenderness is generally not associated with simple urethritis, although rarely urethritis may accompany prostatitis. Painful ejaculation without dysuria, blood in the ejaculate, and pain radiating from the urethra to the pelvis or back are not seen in urethritis and should prompt evaluation for other disorders.

Untreated gonococcal or nongonococcal urethritis can lead to a variety of complications. Conjunctivitis is acquired in 1%–2% of patients by self-inoculation. Epididymitis occurs in another 1%–2% of patients, with equal risk from *N. gonorrhoeae* and *C. trachomatis*. Reiter's syndrome (urethritis, conjunctivitis, and arthritis in addition to other manifestations) occurs in a small proportion of patients following infectious urethritis (see Chapter 80). Gonococcal urethral infection sets the stage for disseminated gonococcal infection. The relationship of acute NGU to chronic urethritis or to subacute or chronic prostatitis remains unclear; prostatic secretions in men with NGU may contain increased PMN in a modest percentage of cases. Rarely, lymphadenopathy accompanies simple urethritis, but this finding should prompt consideration of other diagnoses. Prolonged untreated gonococcal infection is still a common cause of urethral stricture in the developing world.

The clinical manifestations of urethritis in women are similar to those in men, though they are usually overshadowed by symptoms related to concomitant cervicitis. Dysuria in women is most often caused by cystitis or vulvovaginitis. Cystitis produces internal dysuria characterized by a deep burning sensation, along with frequency and urgency, whereas vulvovaginitis produces external dysuria due to the irritant effect of urine on the inflamed perineum. Acute urethral syndrome is the name given to a clinical syndrome in which women have symptoms resembling cystitis, pyuria, and less than $10^5$ bacteria/ml of urine. When bacteriuria is present, the etiology is likely the coliform organisms typical of cystitis; when bacteriuria is absent, *C. trachomatis* is often found and the symptoms respond to appropriate therapy.

Physical examination in a patient with symptoms of urethritis should include a complete evaluation for sexually transmitted diseases, including genital ulcer disease. Preferably, the patient should not urinate for at least 2 h preceding the exam as this will remove the discharge from the urethra. The examiner should first look for spontaneous discharge, and then for more subtle evidence of discharge such as crusting on the head of the penis or irritation of the meatus. If no discharge is found, the urethra should be stripped by applying gentle pressure along the penis from base to head. This often produces a small amount of discharge which is extremely useful for diagnosis. Discharge should be applied immediately to a microscope slide for gram stain. Subsequently, a calcium alginate endourethral swab should be inserted at least 2 cm into the urethra to collect the specimen for culture and other laboratory tests. The exam should include evaluation for complications of urethritis such as epididymitis.

Women with urethritis should have a complete pelvic exam with cervical cultures as described in Chapter 72. Urethral stripping may be accomplished by compressing the urethra against the symphysis pubis. A urethral swab should only be inserted into the most superficial part of the female urethra.

## Laboratory studies

The urethral discharge should be subjected to a gram stain. The presence of greater than four PMNs per oil-immersion field averaged over five fields in the maximally dense part of the slide is usually considered objective evidence of urethritis, although the exact number of PMN required is debated. Time since last micturition as well as observer bias may account for the variation seen in different studies. The presence of gram-negative intracellular diplococci indicates gonococcal urethritis with 95% sensitivity and 98% specificity and is adequate justification for therapy. When atypical intracellular or typical extracellular gram-negative diplococci are seen, the gonorrhea culture is positive only 20%–30% of the time. Some of these patients with negative cultures may indeed have gonococcal urethritis, as the sensitivity of the culture is less than 100%.

Culture or another test for *N. gonorrhoeae* should be performed if the gram stain is negative or equivocal. Culture must be performed on selective media such as modified Thayer-Martin to provide proper nutrients and inhibit growth of genital flora. For optimal sensitivity it should be plated at the bedside and processed immediately. Occasionally *N. gonorrhoeae* may be sensitive to the concentrations of vancomycin used in the media, producing a false-negative culture.

Other useful laboratory tests for *N. gonorrhoeae* include DNA probe and DNA amplification tests. These tests offer no sensitivity advantage over culture except in settings where optimal culture quality cannot be maintained. However, DNA amplification tests can be applied to urine without loss in performance (see below).

*Chlamydia trachomatis* can be cultured, but the expense and complexity of this technique limit its clinical utility. Several nonculture methods, including a DNA probe, enzyme immunoassay, and direct fluorescent antibody tests, have become the mainstay of *C. trachomatis* diagnostics. These tests have limited sensitivity (60%–80%) but good specificity (97%–99%), especially when confirmatory testing is performed. Rapid antigen tests which can be performed in the physician's office in less than 30 min have also become available but are largely unsatisfactory due to their very low sensitivity. The performance of all nonculture tests depends on several factors, including presence of symptoms and the sampling technique used. Since chlamydial urethritis is frequently asymptomatic, a positive test for *C. trachomatis* should be considered evidence of infection despite lack of symptoms. It should be recognized, however, that the use of even a highly specific test for screening a low-prevalence population will lead to some false positive results. However, with use of amplification techniques such as polymerase chain reaction (PCR) and ligase chain reaction (LCR), it is clear that the sensitivity of other methods for detection of *C. trachomatis* (including culture) is limited, so a negative test does not exclude the possibility of a chlamydial infection.

Urine may be used for diagnosis of urethritis, and the newer diagnostic tests utilizing urine have begun to revolutionize management of this disease. The sediment of the first 10 cc of voided urine may be gram stained and examined for PMN and bacteria. If the first-voided urine contains PMN and mucous threads while the remainder is clear, urethritis is likely; if PMN are equal in both parts, the source of infection is more likely in the bladder or upper urinary tract. The presence of at least 10 PMN per high-power field in first-voided urine is 90% predictive of gonococcal or chlamydial infection. Culture of midstream urine identifies cystitis or upper tract infection.

PCR and LCR are amplification techniques which can be used to detect DNA in urine as well as other genital specimens. These tests are more than 98% sensitive and specific for *N. gonorrhoeae* and *C. trachomatis* infections in urine specimens. Detection of *N. gonorrhoeae* in urine by these techniques is equal to urethral culture in terms of sensitivity and specificity. These techniques for detection of *C. trachomatis* are better than all other methods. In addition, testing of urine in women predicts endocervical *C. trachomatis* as accurately as testing of an endocervical specimen. Urine testing offers the possibility of collecting specimens in nonclinical settings.

*Ureaplasma urealyticum* testing is not widely available and is seldom clinically useful since the organism is often present without being pathogenic. *Trichomonas vaginalis* may be identified on the gram stain, although it is better seen on a wet mount in which motility can be appreciated. Both of these methods are insensitive compared to culture, which is not generally available. Wet mount of a urethral smear taken prior to the first morning void has a sensitivity of approximately 80% for diagnosis of *T. vaginalis*.

## Diagnosis of symptomatic urethritis

A simplified approach to diagnosis and treatment in the symptomatic patient with urethritis is outlined in Figure 71.1. On the initial visit, a gram stain of the urethral smear will determine whether the patient has gonococcal urethritis, NGU, or no evidence for urethritis. A urethral smear positive for *N. gonorrhoeae* is considered diagnostic, and the patient should be treated for gonorrhea along with adjunctive therapy for possible concomitant NGU. If the smear has PMN, but no typical intracellular gram-negative diplococci, a tentative diagnosis of NGU is made and the patient should begin NGU therapy while the test for *N. gonorrhea* is pending.

If the smear does not show evidence of urethritis, a second examination may be necessary. If possible, the patient should be examined before the first morning void or after a prolonged period without micturition; urethral stripping should then be performed. If this fails to produce discharge, microscopy of the first 10 cc of the first void urine or an endourethral swab smear may yield a diagnosis. In sexually active men empiric therapy for NGU should be given. Alternatively, if the history is not suggestive of a sexually transmitted disease, other diagnoses including cystitis and prostatitis should be considered.

If no microbiologic diagnosis is made and the patient fails to respond to empiric therapy for NGU, or has recurrence of symptoms after therapy, reevaluation is necessary. Common causes of recurrence or persistence include an untreated partner, tetracycline-resistant *U. urealyticum*, and *T. vaginalis* infection. Less common causes are yeast balanitis, herpes simplex infection, and prostatitis. If the partner was treated, it is reasonable to initiate empiric erythromycin for *U. urealyticum* with or without metronidazole for *T. vaginalis*. If symptoms persist, evaluation for prostatitis and urologic disorders is recommended (see section below). If no cause can be found, a 4–6 wk course of a tetracycline or erythromycin can be tried, although the long-term effectiveness of this is unknown.

## Diagnosis of asymptomatic urethritis

As indicated above, a small percentage of patients with *N. gonorrhoeae* and one-quarter to one-half of men with *C. trachomatis* urethritis will be asymptomatic. Historically, it has been difficult if not impossible to identify these patients: cost-effectiveness studies evaluating leukocyte esterase testing of first void urine and/or specific testing for *C. trachomatis* have demonstrated great expense per case identified. However, the availability of urine PCR and LCR testing simplifies identification of such patients with chlamydial infection. It seems likely that sexual history algorithms will be developed to justify blind screening for *N. gonorrhoeae* and *C. trachomatis*.

## Treatment

Treatment of urethritis is directed at the likely etiologic agents. Uncomplicated gonococcal urethritis should be treated with single-dose curative therapy. The Centers for Disease Control and Prevention in 1993 recommended either ceftriaxone 125 mg IM, cefixime 400 mg orally once, ciprofloxacin 500 mg orally once, ofloxacin 400 mg orally once, or spectinomycin 2 gm IM; the last drug is especially useful in patients intolerant of cephalosporins and quinolones, including pregnant women. The cephalosporins have the advantage of activity against incubating *T. pallidum*, though it is not known whether the doses of oral cephalosporins used for *N. gonorrhoeae* are adequate to abort incubating syphilis. Penicillin and tetracycline are no longer appropriate due to high levels of resistance. The recommended regimens cure more than 95% of uncomplicated genital infections with *N. gonorrhoeae*. It should be noted, however, that pharyngeal infection is best treated with ceftriaxone or ciprofloxacin.

Patients with gonorrhea require adjunctive therapy for NGU with doxycycline 100 mg orally twice daily for 7 d or azithromycin 1 g orally in a single dose. This therapy prevents the development of postgonococcal urethritis due to *C. trachomatis* or *U. urealyticum*, a common syndrome prior to the use of such therapy. Erythromycin 500 mg orally four times daily for 7 d may be substituted in patients intolerant of tetracyclines or pregnant women. The risk of azithromycin in pregnancy is believed to be similar to that of erythromycin. Amoxicillin 500 mg orally three times daily for 7 d can be useful in pregnant women with gastrointestinal intolerance to erythromycin, though it may not be equally effective. Minocycline 100 mg orally at bedtime for 7 d has also been shown to be effective, but has the disadvantage of vestibular toxicity.

Persistent or recurrent urethritis may be treated with erythromycin 500 mg orally four times daily for tetracycline-resistant *U. urealyticum* and/or metronidazole 2 g orally once for

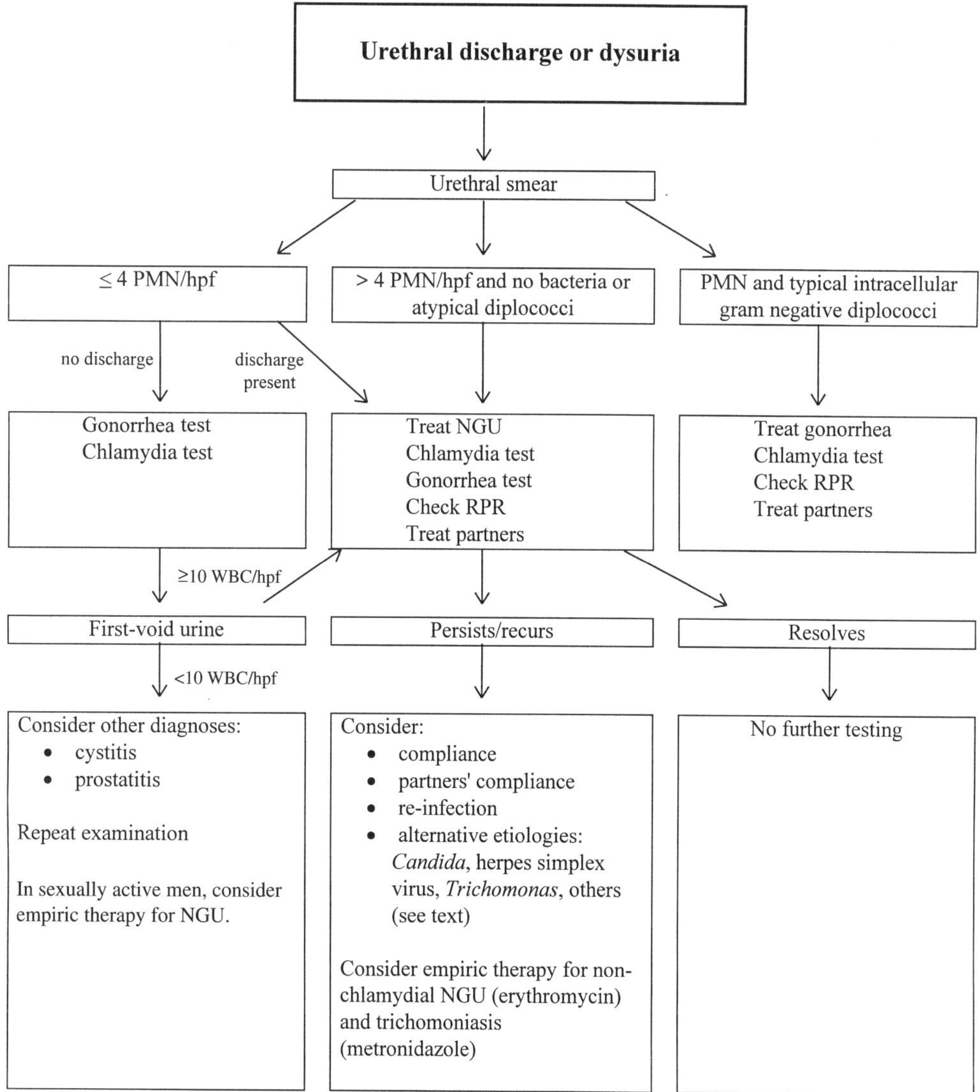


**Fig. 71.1** Algorithm for management of urethritis. PMN, polymorphonuclear leukocyte; hpf, high-power field; NGU, nongonococcal urethritis; RPR, rapid plasma reagin test. [Adapted from Fox KK, Kohen MS. Gonococcal and chlamydial urethritis. In Infectious Diseases, Armstrong D, Cohen J, eds. Mosby International, 1999.]

trichomoniasis. A prostatic focus of infection may be responsible for recurrence of NGU which occurs days to weeks after therapy. If this is suspected, a 3–6 wk course of doxycycline or erythromycin can be tried. Therapies for other specific organisms may be found in Chapter 38.

Treatment of the sexual partner is critical. Any sexual partner in the previous 60 d should receive treatment, even if signs and symptoms of infection are lacking. The likelihood of infection and risk of transmission justify this treatment on epidemiologic grounds.

Urethritis is a marker of risk for other sexually transmitted diseases. It is not known whether therapy for *N. gonorrhoeae* or *C. trachomatis* aborts incubating syphilis. Accordingly, patients with urethritis need a serologic test for syphilis. In addition, tests for HIV and hepatitis B are appropriate. Patients without immunity to hepatitis B should be vaccinated. All patients with sexually transmitted diseases (STD) should also receive counseling on STD and HIV prevention, including abstinence and condom use. Abstinence should be recommended until the patient and partner have completed their treatment regimens.

Current therapy for gonococcal infection is highly effective, with rapid resolution of symptoms. Most regimens for NGU are somewhat less effective, and the symptoms of NGU occasionally persist for several days beyond the end of therapy. Tests of cure for *N.gonorrhoeae* and *C. trachomatis* are not necessary.

## Epididymitis and Orchitis

Acute inflammation of the epididymis usually occurs as a complication of urethritis or cystitis. Epididymitis is unilateral except when it occurs as a part of systemic infection. Most cases of orchitis result from the extension of an infectious process in the epididymis. It is critical to rapidly differentiate epididymitis and orchitis from testicular torsion, which is a surgical emergency.

## Etiologies and epidemiology

The most common pathogens associated with epididymitis vary by age and the presence of urinary tract disorders (Table 71.2). In prepubertal children, epididymitis is usually associated with urinary tract anomalies and is caused by enteric organisms, including *Escherichia coli*, *Klebsiella*, *Proteus*, and *Pseudomonas aeruginosa*. In men under the age of 35, epididymitis is usually a sexually acquired infection caused by *N. gonorrhoeae* or *C. trachomatis*; however, homosexual men who practice anal insertive intercourse may develop urethritis and epididymitis due to gram-negative bacilli. In older men, epididymitis is usually caused by enteric organisms, generally in association with a urinary tract infection and/or acquired urinary tract disorder.

Occasionally epididymitis is part of a systemic infection caused by *Mycobacterium tuberculosis*, *Streptococcus pneumoniae*, *Brucella* species, *Neisseria meningitidis*, or *T. pallidum*. *Histoplasma capsulatum*, *Coccidioides immitis*, and *Cryptococcus neoformans* have also been reported to cause epididymitis as a part of disseminated infection. In such cases it is frequently bilateral. Amiodarone causes lymphocytic infiltration and fibrosis of the epididymis which responds to dose reduction.

Epididymo-orchitis results from contiguous spread of the infectious process from epididymis to testis. Orchitis occurs without epididymal involvement primarily in mumps orchitis in postpubertal males and much less commonly with Coxsackie B virus infection.

## Host factors

Children with epididymitis usually have urinary tract anomalies causing recurrent urinary tract infections which are complicated by epididymal involvement. In adults under age 35, epididymitis commonly occurs as a complication of sexually transmitted urethritis, with no underlying urinary tract abnormality. Over age 35, the predisposing host factor is more likely to be an acquired urinary tract disorder that increases the risk of urinary tract infection, such as benign prostatic hypertrophy, prostatic calculi, urinary retention due to neurogenic bladder, recent urinary tract instrumentation, chronic urethral catheterization, or prostatitis.

## Pathogenesis

Epididymitis related to urethral or urinary tract infection is thought to be caused by the reflux of infected urine or seminal vesicle secretions into the vas deferens and the epididymis. This reflux may be caused by straining. Other possible routes of spread to the epididymis include the lymphatics and the sheath of the vas deferens. Epididymitis related to systemic infection results from hematogenous seeding of the epididymis.

## Clinical manifestations

Epididymitis presents with acute scrotal and often inguinal pain, frequently with a history of straining or lifting prior to the onset of pain. Symptoms of the underlying urinary tract infection or urethritis may also be present, although as few as 50% of patients with gonococcal epididymitis have urethral discharge. In the hospitalized patient with recent urinary tract instrumentation, epididymitis may present as unexplained fever. Systemic symptoms other than fever are generally not seen unless the epididymitis is a complication of systemic infection.

On physical exam, the epididymis is swollen and tender, and the affected side of the scrotum is red and edematous. The swelling occurs first in the tail of the epididymis, which lies against the lower pole of the testis, then progresses to include the head along the upper pole of the testis. All patients with epididymitis should be examined for urethral discharge and prostate tenderness. An acquired hydrocele may be present due to inflammatory fluid within the tunica vaginalis.

Complications of epididymitis are unusual but may occur more commonly in homosexual men with coliform infection. Untreated epididymitis may progress to involve the ipsilateral testis, producing epididymo-orchitis; in this case, tenderness and swelling of the testis are noted, and fever is more prominent. Infarction of the testicle due to thrombosis of the spermatic vessels or scrotal abscess may occur. Infertility results from bilateral epididymitis with occlusion of the vas deferens or epididymis. Chronic epididymal pain following epididymitis is poorly understood and unresponsive to antimicrobials.

Mumps orchitis produces testicular pain and swelling along with fever and malaise. Preceding parotitis provides a clue to the diagnosis but is subclinical in 30%–40% of cases. Testicular at-

**Table 71.2** Causes of epididymitis in adults

| Age group | Risk factors | Etiologies | Therapy |
|---|---|---|---|
| Under 35 yr | Sexual contact | *Neisseria gonorrhoeae*, *Chlamydia trachomatis* | Ceftriaxone plus doxycycline |
| Over 35 yr | Urinary tract disorders or instrumentation | Enteric gram-negative bacilli | Oral quinolone (ofloxacin) or cotrimoxazole if mildly ill; intravenous antibiotics active against enteric gram-negative bacilli if severely ill |
| Any | Disseminated infection with organism | *Mycobacterium tuberculosis*, *Brucella* species, *Streptococcus pneumoniae*, *Histoplasma*, other fungi | Directed against specific organism |

rophy follows 50% of cases but only results in sterility when bilateral involvement is present.

## Laboratory studies

Laboratory testing should include a urethral smear, urethral or urine tests for *N. gonorrhoeae* and *C. trachomatis*, urinalysis, and urine culture. If prostate tenderness is present, culture of prostatic secretions should be undertaken. In some cases, epididymal aspiration culture may be necessary to make a microbiologic diagnosis.

## Diagnosis

Epididymitis is generally a clinical diagnosis which must be differentiated from other causes of acute scrotal pain, including testicular torsion. Torsion is common in boys and young men and may be recurrent. Factors which suggest torsion are history of recurrent scrotal pain, acute onset of pain and swelling with rapid progression, elevation or rotation of the testis, and swelling of both epididymis and testis. In the presence of any of these factors, the patient should be emergently referred for urologic evaluation. Doppler or radionuclide scan may be used to assess blood flow to the testis, but these studies should not delay surgical exploration since infarction may occur within hours.

Testicular tumor may also present with scrotal pain and swelling, and this diagnosis must be considered in any patient who fails to respond to antimicrobial therapy. An ultrasound examination is useful to identify a testicular mass. Simple hydrocele and spermatocele usually cause painless swelling of the scrotum and can be identified by transillumination. Varicocele likewise is usually painless and disappears in the supine position. A hernia may be more difficult to diagnose, but it usually causes mild pain of gradual onset and a mass superior to the testes, and it may be reducible or have bowel sounds.

## Treatment

Management of epididymitis and orchitis requires bed rest with scrotal elevation to increase lymphatic drainage until scrotal tenderness resolves. Antimicrobial therapy is directed at the likely pathogens pending results of laboratory tests. If urethritis is present, the patient should receive ceftriaxone 250 mg IM plus doxycycline 100 mg orally twice daily for 10 d. Alternatively, ofloxacin 300 mg orally twice daily for 10 d is effective but cannot be used in children under 18 years of age. Ofloxacin is effective against *N. gonorrhoeae*, *C. trachomatis*, and many gram-negative organisms. As with other sexually transmitted diseases, the partner should be treated and the patient evaluated for syphilis, HIV infection, and immunity to hepatitis B.

If underlying urinary tract infection is present, the mildly ill patient may be treated with cotrimoxazole or an oral quinolone; ofloxacin has the advantage of activity against *N. gonorrhoeae* and *C. trachomatis* in addition to the gram-negative bacilli likely to cause urinary tract infection. Broad-spectrum intravenous antibiotics effective against aerobic gram-negative bacteria, including *Pseudomonas*, are necessary if the patient is more severely ill. Therapy should continue for at least 2 wk and be modified according to urine or epididymal culture results. Patients with epididymitis complicating urinary tract infection require evaluation for chronic prostatitis and functional or anatomic abnormalities of the urinary tract.

# Prostatitis

As many as 50% of men will develop symptoms referable to the prostate gland at some point in their lives. For therapeutic and prognostic reasons, it is important to identify specific subgroups of symptomatic males with bacteria in urine or prostatic secretions from the larger group of men with symptoms but without bacteriuria. Inflammatory disorders of the prostate fall into four distinct syndromes (Table 71.3). Acute bacterial prostatitis (ABP) is recognized easily in the patient who has a systemic illness, localizing signs, and urine cultures positive for a causative organism. Chronic bacterial prostatitis (CBP) is characterized by vague urinary symptoms or no symptoms, a history of recurrent urinary tract infections (UTIs), an unremarkable physical exam, and negative urinalysis and culture between acute episodes of cystitis. Inflammatory cells and typical organisms may be recovered on culture of prostatic secretions. Patients with nonbacterial prostatitis (NBP) have no history of urinary tract infections and negative urine and prostatic fluid analysis and cultures, but inflammatory cells are present in expressed prostatic secretions. Prostatodynia is a nonspecific descriptive diagnosis applied to patients with symptoms referable to the prostate but no history of recurrent UTIs or abnormalities in prostatic secretions.

## Host factors and pathogenesis

The prostate gland, which surrounds the male urethra, is a tubuloalveolar gland with dorsal, median, and lateral lobes. These lobes communicate with the urethra through multiple ducts without sphincters near the verumontanum in the prostatic urethra. Under androgenic stimulation, the prostate gland secretes 30%–40% of the ejaculate fluid volume. Normal prostatic secretions contain lysozyme, prostatic antibacterial factor (PAF, a bactericidal zinc-containing polypeptide), prostate specific antigen (PSA, a serine protease with kallikrein-like activity), proteolytic enzymes, other divalent cations, citric acid, spermine, and immunoglobulins. Prostatic fluid is slightly acidic (pH 6.4 to 7.3), but with increasing age or infection, secretions become more alkaline.

In CBP, levels of zinc, other divalent cations, citric acid, enzymes, and PAF in prostate secretions are reduced while their serum levels remain normal. Whether this generalized prostatic secretory defect precedes or follows the development of chronic infection is not clear. Antigen-specific mucosal antibody responses have been observed in the setting of prostatic infection resulting in increased levels of immunoglobulins, especially IgA and IgG, and polymorphonuclear leukocytes in prostatic fluid.

Microorganisms most likely gain entry to the prostate through the urethra via ascending infection, intraurethral reflux of infected urine, lymphatic dissemination from the rectum, or direct introduction by instrumentation. Indirect evidence in support of urinary reflux comes from crystallographic studies of prostatic calculi which contain compounds found in urine but not in prostatic fluid. More direct evidence comes from a study in which instillation of suspensions containing carbon particles into the bladder prior to transurethral resection of the prostate resulted in intraductal carbon particles in the prostate glands on microscopic exam of resected prostate specimens in seven of ten patients. Other mechanisms of microbial access to the prostate include urethral instrumentation, indwelling urethral catheterization, and prostatic surgery. Bacterial urethritis secondary to *Neisseria gonorrhoeae* or *Chlamydia trachomatis* may precede prostatic infection although gonococcal prostatitis is seen infrequently today.

**Table 71.3** Selected disorders of the prostate

| | Acute prostatitis | Chronic prostatitis | Nonbacterial prostatitis | Prostatodynia |
|---|---|---|---|---|
| Symptoms | Dysuria, urgency, frequency, nocturia, lower abdominal pain, fever, chills | History of recurrent cystitis, asymptomatic between episodes | Perineal or pelvic discomfort, urinary or ejaculatory discomfort | Perineal or pelvic discomfort, urinary or ejaculatory discomfort |
| Signs | Prostate very tender, swollen | Exam unremarkable | Exam unremarkable | Exam unremarkable |
| Etiologies | Enterobacteriaceae, *Pseudomonas*, *Enterococcus* | Enterobacteriaceae, *Pseudomonas*, *Enterococcus* | Unknown; neuromuscular dysfunction and autoimmune processes have been hypothesized | Unknown; neuromuscular dysfunction and psychosocial factors have been hypothesized |
| Laboratory tests | Urinalysis abnormal, increased WBC in EPS,[a] urine and EPS cultures positive | Urinalysis and culture negative between episodes of cystitis; increased WBC in EPS, EPS culture positive | Urinalysis and culture negative, increased WBC in EPS, EPS culture negative | Urine and EPS normal, cultures negative |
| Treatment | Fluoroquinolones, trimethoprim-sulfamethoxazole | Fluoroquinolones, trimethoprim-sulfamethoxazole | Doxycycline, symptomatic therapy (see text) | Symptomatic therapy (see text) |

[a]EPS = expressed prostatic secretions; see text for method of collecting secretions.

Pathogens isolated in cultures of urethral and prostatic secretions from males with CBP have occasionally been isolated from vaginal cultures of sexual partners, suggesting that sexual transmission may play a role in infection of the prostate. Hematogenous dissemination may lead to fungal and mycobacterial infections of the prostate.

## Acute bacterial prostatitis

Acute bacterial prostatitis (ABP) is characterized by symptoms of lower urinary tract infection including dysuria, frequency, nocturia, and urgency. Low-back pain, perineal pain, and lower abdominal or suprapubic discomfort may be prominent and patients are systemically ill with fever, chills, and myalgias. Patients may present with urinary retention secondary to acute prostatic edema and compression of the prostatic urethra. On physical exam, the prostate is warm, diffusely swollen, tender, and sometimes tense. Expressed prostatic fluid contains many polymorphonuclear leukocytes and bacteria, but *prostatic massage should be avoided in the setting of ABP* because of the possibility of precipitating bacteremia. The urinalysis contains numerous white blood cells and urine cultures are positive for the infecting organism. While 80% of ABP is caused by *E. coli*, other gram-negative organisms (such as *Proteus*, *Klebsiella*, *Enterobacter*, *Pseudomonas*, and *Serratia*) and *Enterococcus* are also isolated.

Examination of biopsy specimens in the setting of ABP reveals inflammation of part or all of the prostate gland with a predominantly polymorphonuclear cellular infiltrate, diffuse edema, and stromal hyperemia. Microabscesses may be present early in infection while later in untreated infection large collections of pus may be seen. Complications of ABP include abscess formation, bacteremia, epididymitis, seminal vesiculitis, pyelonephritis, prostatic infarction, chronic bacterial prostatitis, and granulomatous prostatitis.

Evaluation of the patient with ABP should include blood and urine cultures prior to the initiation of antibiotic therapy; a complete blood count; an electrolyte panel with blood urea nitrogen (BUN), creatinine, and glucose; a urinalysis and urine gram stain; and evaluation of volume status. Treatment of ABP includes antibiotics, hydration, analgesics and bedrest. In the hemodynamically stable patient who can tolerate oral medication and who is unobstructed, it is not usually necessary to give intravenous antibiotics for ABP. Patients with bladder outlet obstruction and ABP frequently require temporary suprapubic catheterization.

Studies comparing antibiotic regimens in the treatment of acute bacterial prostatitis are lacking, but pharmacokinetics considerations favor selected classes of drugs. Under normal circumstances, drug diffusion from the plasma and accumulation in the prostate gland favors lipid-soluble, basic drugs with a high pKa. These predictions have been borne out experimentally in elegant studies of antibiotic levels in prostate secretions of healthy dogs where basic compounds such as macrolides, azalides, fluoroquinolones, clindamycin, and trimethoprim achieved high levels in prostate fluid relative to plasma. Drugs which did not diffuse well into the prostate fluid under normal conditions included penicillins, cephalosporins, tetracycline, nitrofurantoin, and vancomycin. How the alteration in pH of prostatic secretions in the setting of infection or advanced age affects prostate drug levels is not known at the present time. Based on clinical experience, it is felt that inflammation increases the diffusion of many drugs in the prostate gland.

Unless the urinary gram stain shows gram-positive cocci, empiric antibiotic therapy is directed primarily against enteric gram-negative rods and modified based on subsequent culture and sensitivity results. Oral regimens commonly employed in the treatment of ABP include trimethoprim-sulfamethoxazole (160 mg TMP and 800 mg SMX by mouth twice a day), and the fluoroquinolones (norfloxacin 400 mg, ciprofloxacin 500 mg, or ofloxacin 300 mg by mouth twice a day) for a minimum of 4 wk. Trimethoprim-sulfamethoxazole is used for intravenous therapy as well in doses of 8–10 mg of the trimethoprim component per kg body weight divided in two to four doses per day. Another parenteral regimen is ampicillin (2 g every 6 h) and gentamicin (2 mg/kg loading dose followed by 3–5 mg/kg/d divided in three doses). This regimen should be used if enterococcal infection is suspected. Drug doses should be adjusted for renal function and aminoglycoside levels should be monitored during therapy. Clinical response is generally rapid and oral regimens can usually be employed after 1 wk of parenteral therapy or 48 h after the patient is afebrile. Lack of improvement should prompt evaluation for complications of ABP and other causes of fever. Transrectal ultrasound of the prostate is recommended if prostatic abscess is suspected. With the decreasing incidence of gonococcal prostatitis, the incidence of prostatic abscess is declining as well.

## Chronic bacterial prostatitis

True chronic bacterial infection of the prostate (CBP) is now a rare clinical entity (accounting for approximately 5% of prostatitis cases) but is a frequent clinical diagnosis. Many patients with CBP are asymptomatic. Some patients present with vague complaints of perineal pressure or discomfort, low back pain, difficulty voiding, dysuria, frequency, urgency, postejaculatory pain, or hemospermia. However, the hallmark of CBP is recurrent UTIs with the same organism, and CBP is the most common cause of recurrent UTIs in men. For this reason, men with recurrent UTIs should be evaluated for CBP.

On physical exam, the typical patient with CBP is afebrile, and exam of the prostate is unremarkable unless there is coexistent prostatic hypertrophy or nodularity suggestive of malignancy. The urinalysis and blood count are frequently normal. Radiologic studies, cystoscopy, and biopsy may identify coexisting problems or complications of prostatitis but do not establish the diagnosis. The diagnosis of CBP is based on the results of quantitative bacterial cultures of urine and prostatic secretions and microscopic examination of expressed prostatic secretions (EPS) using the localizing techniques first described by Meares and Stamey in 1968. The patient with a full bladder is asked to void and the first 10 ml is collected and labeled voided bladder urine-1 ($VB_1$). This urine volume represents the urethral specimen. The patient is asked to void again and 10 ml of a midstream urine specimen is collected as $VB_2$. This specimen represents the bladder specimen. With the patient in the knee–chest position, the prostate is massaged and expressed prostatic secretions (EPS) from the urethral meatus are collected in a sterile container. If no prostate secretions can be expressed from the urethra with prostate massage alone, then pressure on the penile urethra from proximal to distal may be required. The first 10 ml of urine after prostate massage ($VB_3$) is collected as well. All four specimens are sent to the microbiology laboratory for quantitative cultures and for microscopic examination of the EPS and spun sediments of the urine specimens for WBCs and microorganisms.

Although there is some disagreement on the number of WBCs in normal prostatic secretions, the smear of the prostatic fluid is generally considered abnormal if it contains ≥10–15 WBCs per high-power field (HPF) (when the urethral and midstream specimens contain insignificant pyuria). If the patient has significant bacteriuria prior to obtaining the EPS ($\geq 10^5$ colony-forming units [cfu] per ml) then the infection cannot be localized. Pretreatment for 2–3 d with an antibiotic such as penicillin, ampicillin, or nitrofurantoin, which achieve good levels in the urine but have poor prostate penetration, will sterilize the urine but not affect bacterial counts from the EPS. The localization study can then be repeated in 4–5 d.

An increased number of WBCs in the EPS is not limited to prostatitis but can also be seen in conditions such as anterior urethritis, urethral stricture, urethral diverticula, and in normal males after sexual stimulation or activity. The finding of aggregates or casts of WBCs in the EPS supports a diagnosis of prostatic inflammation. A more specific predictor of prostatitis may be the finding of macrophages containing oval fat bodies in the EPS. There is evidence that these fat-laden macrophages are not seen in the EPS of normal men, are increased in the EPS of men with nonbacterial prostatitis (NBP), and are prominent in the EPS of patients with bacterial prostatitis. These cells are not seen in anterior urethritis.

Localization of inflammation may also be accomplished by comparison of the quantitative cultures of $VB_1$, $VB_2$, EPS, and $VB_3$. If the bacterial counts in quantitative cultures from $VB_1$ and $VB_2$ exceed those from EPS and $VB_3$, then the anterior urethra or bladder is presumed to be the focus of inflammation. If numbers of organisms isolated from EPS and/or $VB_3$ are greater than those from $VB_1$ or $VB_2$ by an order of magnitude or more, then the prostate is presumed to be the source of infection. Although suggestive, the validity of these criteria has never been established in clinical studies.

On biopsy, the inflammation seen in CBP is less marked than in ABP and is more focal. These inflammatory changes can be seen in patients without prostatitis and are therefore not diagnostic of CBP. With increasing age, prostatic calculi are seen more frequently. In one series, prostatic calculi were noted as incidental findings on pelvic radiographs in 13% of adult males. These are most often asymptomatic, but in the setting of recurrent bacterial infection involving the posterior genitourinary tract, they may become colonized and serve as a nidus of recurrent urinary and prostatic infection.

As in ABP, the organisms most commonly isolated in CBP are the enteric gram-negative rods (especially *E. coli*, other Enterobacteriaceae and pseudomonads) and *Enterococcus*. The role of other gram positive organisms in CBP is less clear; *S. saprophyticus* has been implicated as a pathogen in some series, but not in others. No role has been clearly identified for the gram-positive organisms commonly found in the anterior urethra such as coagulase-negative staphylococci, micrococci, diphtheroids, or streptococci. Treatment of CBP is directed against the same pathogens as in ABP but duration of therapy is much longer. Trimethoprim-sulfamethoxazole (160 mg TMP, 800 mg SMX) given orally twice a day for a minimum of 4 and as long as 16 wk has been an effective treatment regimen for many years. More recently, the fluoroquinolones such as ciprofloxacin and ofloxacin have become available. These are probably the most effective drugs currently available for treatment of CBP. Other antibiotics which have been used to treat CBP, including carbenicillin indanyl sodium, erythromycin, minocycline, doxycycline, and cephalexin, are generally less effective than the fluroquinolones and TMP-SMX.

Even with prolonged therapy there is a high rate of relapse of

CBP. Thus, long-term cure rates for CBP even with prolonged regimens may be only 30%–40%, while symptomatic improvement may be seen in another 30% of patients. This is seldom due to the development of microbial resistance on antibiotic therapy. In patients who relapse after a full course of therapy for CBP, suppressive therapy with TMP-SMX (160 mg TMP, 800 mg SMX once a day) or nitrofurantoin (100 mg once or twice a day) decreases symptoms and the frequency of recurrence of UTIs.

Rare causes of infection of the prostate include the deep mycoses (aspergillosis, candidiasis, histoplasmosis, blastomycosis, coccidioidomycosis, cryptococcosis, and paracoccidiodomycosis) and *Mycobacterium tuberculosis*, as well as some of the atypical mycobacteria, actinomycosis, brucellosis, syphilis, and herpes. Fungal prostatitis is uncommon and the presentation may be similar to benign prostatic hypertrophy. A fungal infection of the prostate should be considered in the differential diagnosis of the elderly or immunocompromised patient with genitourinary symptoms including those patients with AIDS, diabetes mellitus, or neutropenia or on chronic steroid therapy. In urogenital tuberculosis, mycobacteria can often be isolated from semen or EPS, and in 20% of cases, these fluids may be the only source of positive cultures. Gonococcal prostatitis is rarely seen today, but it is more common in men less than 35 yr old. Virtually all men with gonococcal prostatitis have a history of antecedent urethritis, during which time it is hypothesized that the accessory sex glands become infected. Treatment for uncomplicated anterior urethritis may be inadequate to clear the posterior infection, leading to the development of prostatitis.

## Nonbacterial prostatitis

Approximately 90% of men with symptoms of prostatitis have nonbacterial prostatitis (NBP) or prostatodynia (see next section). NBP is the most common inflammatory disorder of the prostate, occurring about eight times as frequently as bacterial prostatitis. Patients with NBP complain of dysuria, nocturia, urgency, frequency, and pain or discomfort referable to the suprapubic, perineal or genital region and postejaculatory pain. The physical exam of the prostate is unremarkable. However, there is objective evidence of prostatic inflammation with an increase in WBCs and macrophages with oval fat bodies in the EPS. The cause of the inflammation in NBP is not clear but may involve infectious organisms and/or mechanical factors leading to reflux of urine into the prostate, neuromuscular dysfunction, or an autoimmune process.

Routine bacterial cultures of urine and prostatic secretions are negative or contain commensal organisms such as *S. epidermidis*, which is not felt to be a significant pathogen. Fungi, anaerobes, and various viruses have been excluded as causal in NBP. However, there is evidence from EPS culture studies that *Ureaplasma urealyticum* may be associated with some cases of NBP and that treatment directed against this organism may be effective. Of 82 men with chronic prostatitis symptoms and *U. urealyticum* isolated in significantly greater numbers from the EPS than the urethra, 71 (86%) had a favorable response to tetracycline. Several of the organisms associated with NBP are commensals or frequently isolated from the genitourinary tract in the absence of clinical disease. The finding of antigen-specific IgA or IgG in the EPS, while seldom practical, supports the etiologic role of some of these organisms in NBP.

Therapy of NBP is unsatisfactory because the etiology of this inflammatory condition is unknown. In the symptomatic patient with negative bacterial cultures and evidence of prostatic inflammation, a trial of therapy with doxycycline (100 mg orally, twice a day) or erythromycin base (500 mg orally, four times a day) for 3 wk may be beneficial with regard to symptoms, secretory function, and urodynamic parameters. Consideration should also be given to treatment of sexual partners. The decision to retreat with further courses of antibiotics should be based on response to initial therapy. For patients with flares of this often-chronic, recurrent process, sitz baths, nonsteroidal anti-inflammatory drugs, and bed rest may provide symptomatic relief. In general, patients should be encouraged to eat a well-balanced diet, exercise regularly, and engage in their usual level of sexual activity. For patients in whom urinary symptoms predominate, anticholinergic agents may be useful for urgency, and $\alpha$-receptor blocking agents for obstructive symptoms. Repeated prostatic massage should be avoided as it can precipitate bouts of synovitis, iridocyclitis, and conjunctivitis in patients with prior episodes of these complications. There is no proven benefit to vitamin therapy or oral zinc preparations.

## Prostatodynia

Patients with symptoms referable to the genitourinary tract but no history of antecedent urinary tract infections, no evidence of infection in urine and prostate fluid cultures, and no evidence of inflammation on examination of the EPS are given a diagnosis of prostatodynia or prostatosis. The etiology of these symptoms is unclear. Various hypotheses have been advanced including tension myalgia of the pelvic floor, urodynamic abnormalities such as internal sphincter dyssynergia, and psychological factors. Mild bladder outlet obstruction leading to reflux of urine into the prostate has been suggested by some authors based on the observation of mild to moderate bladder trabeculation on cystoscopy and narrowing of the prostatic urethra in the area of the external urethral sphincter (EUS) in the absence of EUS electrical activity. Treatment of this frequently chronic condition includes reassurance, emotional support, and control of symptoms with $\alpha$-blockers and low doses of muscle relaxants.

### ANNOTATED BIBLIOGRAPHY


Berger RE. Acute epididymitis. In: Sexually Transmitted Diseases, 2nd ed. Holmes KK, Mardh PA, Sparling PF et al. eds. McGraw-Hill, New York, pp 641–651, 1990.

*This chapter provides thorough coverage of epididymitis, including diagnosis, management, and complications.*

Bowie WR. Urethritis in males. In: Sexually Transmitted Diseases, 2nd ed. Holmes KK, Mardh PA, Sparling PF et al. eds. McGraw-Hill, New York, pp 641–651, 1990.

*This chapter is a comprehensive review of the etiology, epidemiology, clinical manifestations, differential diagnosis, and treatment of urethritis.*

Centers for Disease Control and Prevention. Recommendations for the prevention and management of *Chlamydia trachomatis* infections, 1993. MMWR Morb Mortal Wkly Rep 1993; 42(No. RR-12).

*This issue of the MMWR summarizes current knowledge about infections caused by* C. trachomatis *and provides practical management recommendations.*

Centers for Disease Control and Prevention, 1998. Guidelines for treatment of sexually transmitted diseases. MMWR Morb Mortal Wkly Rep 1998; 47 (No. RR-1).

*Recommendations for treatment of sexually transmitted infections in the United States, based on review of recent literature.*

Colleen S, Mardh P-A. Prostatitis. In: Sexually Transmitted Diseases. 2nd ed. Holmes KK, Mardh P-A, Sparling PF et al. eds. McGraw-Hill, New York, pp 652–662, 1990.

*A detailed treatment of prostatitis including inflammation caused by sexually transmitted agents. 93 references.*

Doble A. Chronic prostatitis. Br J Urol 1994; 74:537–541.

*A concise review of scientific knowledge about prostatitis and delineation of the areas in which knowledge is incomplete.*

Hay PE, Thomas BJ, Gilchrist C et al. A reappraisal of chlamydial and nonchlamydia acute nongonococcal urethritis. Int J STD AIDS 1992; 3:191–195.
*Comparison of clinical history and response to therapy in 112 men with chlamydial and nonchlamydial NGU.*

Krieger JN. Prostatitis, epididymitis, and orchitis. In: Principles and Practice of Infectious Diseases, 4th ed. Mandell GL, Benett JE, Dolin R, eds. Churchill Livingstone, New York, pp 1098–1102, 1995.
*A brief overview of prostatitis from an infectious disease point of view. This chapter contains sections on epididymitis and orchitis as well.*

Krieger JN, Jenny C, Verdon M et al. Clinical manifestations of trichomoniasis in men. Ann Intern Med 1993; 118:844–849.
*In this study of men attending a sexually transmitted disease clinic, trichomoniasis was a common diagnosis and was associated with symptoms and signs of urethritis.*

Meares EM. Prostatitis and related disorders, In: Campbell's Urology, 7th ed. Walsh PC, Retik AB, Vaughan ED, Wein AJ. eds. WB Saunders, Philadelphia, 1998; 615–630.
*An extensive review of prostatic physiology, pathology and the pathogenesis and treatment of the various forms of prostatitis; 83 references.*

Meares EM, Stamey TA. Bacteriologic localization patterns in bacterial prostatitis and urethritis. Invest Urol 1968; 5:492–518.
*Original reference describing methods of collecting urine and prostatic massage specimens for localizing inflammation in the male lower urinary tract.*

Wong ES, Hooton TM, Hill CC, McKevitt M, Stamm WE. Clinical and microbiological features of persistent or recurrent nongonococcal urethritis in men. J Infect Dis 1988; 158:1098–1101.
*This study of 70 men with persistent or recurrent NGU assesses clinical and laboratory features of the disease and response to therapy.*

# 72

# Vulvovaginitis, Cervicitis, and Pelvic Inflammatory Disease

JOANNE E. EMBREE AND ROBERT C. BRUNHAM

Vulvovaginitis, cervicitis, and pelvic inflammatory disease (PID) are generally caused by infections of the lower and upper female genital tract. Although the etiological agents of vulvovaginitis generally differ from those of cervicitis and PID, these syndromes frequently occur concurrently. Together, these infections are of major public health concern because of the frequency of doctor visits associated with vulvovaginitis and cervicitis and due to the impact that PID exerts on the reproductive health of women.

## Vulvovaginitis

### Etiology and epidemiology

The etiologic agents associated with vulvovaginitis are *Candida* species, *Trichomonas vaginalis*, and polymicrobial overgrowth of bacteria (*Gardnerella vaginalis*, *Mycoplasma hominis*, *Ureaplasma urealyticum*, *Mobiluncus*, *Bacteroides bivius* and *disidens*) leading to bacterial vaginosis. Occasionally, vulvovaginitis may be caused by other aerobic bacterial pathogens such as group A $\beta$ hemolytic *Streptococcus*, *Staphylococcus aureus*, and *Hemophilus influenzae*, *Salmonella*, or *Shigella*. Children are more likely than adults to be affected with these organisms. As well, prepubertal children develop vaginitis but not cervicitis with infection by *Neiserria gonorrhoeae* and *Chlamydia trachomatis*. Additionally, vulvovaginitis may be associated with pinworm, herples simplex virus (HSV), or cytomegalovirus (CMV) infection. Especially in prepubertal girls, noninfectious causes of vulvovaginal inflammation are commonly identified—that is, chemical irritation due to bubble baths, perfumes, or detergents; physiological discharge associated with hormonal changes; atrophic vaginitis; foreign body; or trauma.

### Host factors, pathogenesis, pathology

Acquisition of *T. vaginalis* is generally associated with conditions which predispose to the acquisition of sexually transmitted diseases; these are discussed in more detail in the section of cervicitis. Bacterial vaginosis results from the overgrowth of anaerobic bacteria which may be sexually transmitted, since it is more common among women attending sexually transmitted disease (STD) clinics. Alternatively, it may be the result of selective pressure secondary to antibiotic use for aerobic pathogens. Candidal overgrowth is associated with high levels of estrogen, which in part explains the extremely high rates (35%–50%) of symptomatic candidal vaginitis seen in pregnant women and the observation that recurrent disease tends to be associated with onset of the menstrual cycle. Vaginal candidiasis can also be associated with immunosuppression, as it occurs in women on immunosuppressive therapy or who are infected with the human immunodeficiency virus (HIV). Women with diabetes also are prone to recurrent candidal vaginal infections. Antibiotic use is also frequently complicated with candidal vaginal overgrowth. Predisposing factors for vaginal infections with other aerobic bacterial or viral infections are primarily related to exposure. Infrequent changing of tampons can predispose to some of these vaginal infections—in particular, *S. aureus*.

With the exception of vaginitis due to anaerobic organisms, there is generally an acute, intense, inflammatory response in the vaginal mucosa and large numbers of leukocytes in the vaginal fluid. With bacterial vaginosis, the inflammation is much milder or is not present at all. The odor associated with this condition is due to the aromatic amines putrescine and cadaverine produced by the anaerobic bacteria. These are volatilized when in contact with basic solutions such as KOH. (Addition of the latter to vaginal fluid constitutes the "whiff test," resulting in the distinctive fishy odor in patients with bacterial vaginosis).

### Clinical manifestations

The clinical manifestations of vulvovaginitis are classically considered to be reflective of the causative agent involved; however, considerable overlap occurs, and the positive predictive value of diagnosis based only on the characteristics of the discharge is less than 40% even with highly trained observers. With candidal vaginitis, the vaginal walls are reddened; the discharge is white, thick, of a cheesy consistency, and adherent to the vaginal walls. There is often associated intense vulvovaginal pruritus. The vulvar area may be reddened and satellite fungal patches and excoriations may be observed. The pH of the vagina is usually normal ($<4.5$). Often, the symptoms worsen or appear shortly before the onset of menses. Trichomonal vaginitis usually presents with vaginal inflammation and a copious, thin yellow- or green-tinged discharge which has a pH $> 4.5$. These may be associated foul odor, abdominal pain, urinary frequency, dysuria, and perineal soreness. Frequently, the symptoms worsen at the time of menses onset. Trichomonas is usually sexually transmitted, and symptoms usually first appear between 1 to 3 wk after contact with an infected partner. Bacterial vaginosis may frequently be asymptomatic, but a thin, homogenous, gray, foul-smelling discharge associated with minimal vaginal wall inflammation may be present on physical examination. Women may complain of a foul-smelling odor after intercourse. Vaginitis due to staphylococcal or streptococcal infection is usually accompanied by intense inflammation and tenderness. That due to HSV is often accompanied by small ulcerative lesions on the cervix or perineal area which may be missed if a thorough examination is not done.

There is no distinctive syndrome associated with vaginal infections with CMV or the genital mycoplasma.

### Laboratory studies and diagnosis

Diagnosis is partially based on the appearance of the vaginal discharge and vaginal walls during a speculum examination, but testing the pH and performing a microscopic examination of the vaginal secretions (wet prep) with and without added KOH should also be done. The diagnosis of candidal vaginitis can be made when the vaginal walls and discharge have a typical appearance, the secretions have a normal pH, and yeast are seen in the wet prep. Trichomonal vaginitis is also diagnosed when the vagina and discharge are typical and is confirmed if trichomonads are demonstrated on the wet prep examination. Bacterial vaginosis is diagnosed if two or more of the following are present: homogeneous gray discharge, pH > 4.5, fishy odor from the vaginal secretions when KOH is added (whiff test), and the presence of "clue cells," which are bacteria coated vaginal epithelial cells on microscopic examination. For postpubertal women, if the diagnosis is not clear after examination of the patient and the wet prep, culture of the vaginal secretions for aerobic bacteria, HSV, candida, and trichomonas should be done. For young children, culture of the secretions should always be done for *N. gonorrhoeae*, *C. trachomatis*, *Streptococcus*, other aerobic bacteria, and HSV. Also, depending upon the circumstances, examination for pin worms should be considered. The examination for the etiologic agents of vaginitis in postpubertal women should also include diagnostic tests for cervicitis and a bimanual examination for evidence of PID.

### Therapy and management

Therapy should be directed at the specific pathogens identified as described in Chapter 38. Generally, if the symptoms resolve, a repeat physical examination is not required. For women with unexplained candidal vaginal infections which are recurrent or refractory to treatment, investigations for an underlying cause such as diabetes or HIV infection should be considered. In children, if an STD is identified, an investigation for sexual abuse is warranted.

## Cervicitis

### Etiology

Cervicitis can be divided into two distinct clinical syndromes: endocervicitis (or mucopurulent cervicitis), which is inflammation of the mucous membranes of the cervical canal, and ectocervicitis, which is inflammation of the stratified squamous epithelium of the cervix. Endocervicitis is most frequently associated with *C. trachomatis* and *N. gonorrhoeae* infection and occasionally with infections such as HSV and *H. influenzae*. Ectocervicitis is found in association with vulvovaginitis caused by *T. vaginitis*, *Candida albicans*, CMV, or HSV.

Cervicitis is a surprisingly confusing clinical entity to diagnose. Signs of cervical inflammation may be clinically evident or may only be apparent on colposcopy or histological examination. Cervical inflammation is not invariably associated with the recovery of etiological agents; and in contrast, *C. trachomatis* and *N. gonorrhoeae* may infect the cervix without any accompanying inflammation at all.

### Epidemiology

The prevalence of clinically apparent cervicitis has not been extensively studied, but mucopurulent cervicitis has been noted in 19%–26% of women attending STD clinics in the United States. The populations "at risk" for cervicitis are primarily the same populations at risk for STDs in general: young women who have unprotected vaginal intercourse in nonmutually monogamous relationships. While pregnant women or those on the birth control pill may also be at greater risk of developing infection upon exposure, prepubertal girls rarely, if ever, develop cervicitis or cervical infection due to STD pathogens.

*C. trachomatis* and *N. gonorrhoeae* infection are the most common clinically significant organisms detected in association with mucopurulent cervicitis. The prevalence of *C. trachomatis* infections ranges from 4.5% to 32% while that of *N. gonorrhoeae* is lower, ranging from 0.2% to 14%. Cervical infection with these two organisms is also frequently found in association with the diagnosis of acute PID: Rates of *C. trachomatis* cervical isolation vary from 5% to 51%, while of rates of *N. gonorrhoeae* isolation from the cervix are reported to vary from 0% to 80%.

There is little information concerning the relative frequencies of cervical infection attributable to the other reported causative organisms: HSV, CMV, and trichomonad cervicitis may be responsible for up to 15% of cases. In a proportion of cases of diagnosed cervicitis, no pathogenic organism is identified. The capacity of the genital mycoplasmas or the anaerobic organisms responsible for bacterial vaginosis to produce cervicitis has not been determined, although mucopurulent cervicitis frequently accompanies bacterial vaginosis. The frequency of noninfectious causes of cervical inflammation is also unknown.

### Host factors, pathogenesis, pathology

Cervical infection due to the STD pathogens follows exposure from an infected partner. Although controlled studies have not been done, the risk of establishment of infection following exposure is thought to be approximately 30%–50% and is probably somewhat higher for gonococci than for chlamydia. The presence of cervical ectopy may facilitate the establishment of infection following exposure: Thus women who are young, nulliparous, taking the birth control pill, or who are pregnant may be at higher risk of developing cervicitis, as they have a relatively larger area of cervical ectopy. Cervicitis due to *Candida* or in association with bacterial vaginosis follows overgrowth of organisms in the vagina following a change in the vaginal flora and pH.

While the natural history of infection due to these organisms has not been well studied, in the absence of treatment they may remain persistent for months to years (particulary chlamydia). With the exception of HSV and syphilis, the STD pathogens associated with cervicitis generally cause disease localized to the epithelial surfaces, and systemic invasion does not take place. Why some women develop clinically apparent cervicitis with infection by these organisms while others do not is unknown.

There are subtle differences in the appearance of cervicitis due to different agents, which is best appreciated by colposcopic examination. Distinctions on biopsy tissue are also possible. With chlamydial infections, focal micro-ulcerations, reactive cellular changes, edema, dilatation and proliferation of capillaries, and plasma cell infiltration are seen. The pathological features associated with *N. gonorrhoeae* infections have not been well described; however, the clinical manifestations are similar to that of *C. trachomatis*. HSV infections show deep ulceration and lymphocytic infiltration and *T. vaginalis* classically produces punctate hemorrhages on the cervical epithelium, giving the cervix a "strawberry" appearance. Both *C. trachomatis* and CMV infection are associated with immature metaplasia seen on colposcopic examination.

## Clinical manifestations

Classically, endocervicitis due to *C. trachomatis* and/or *N. gonorrhoeae* is associated with a mucopurulent endocervical discharge which appears yellow when collected on a white cotton swab. Microscopic examination reveals ≥30 neutrophils per 400× microscopic field. The cervix appears inflamed with edema and erythema and bleeding may easily be induced. Cervicitis due to HSV may show ulcerative lesions involving both the endocervix and ectocervix as well as other areas of the external genitalia. Primary chancre due to *T. pallidum* may be visualized on the cervix and usually involves a rounded ulcer with a well defined margin and a thickened base. The base of the ulcer may be red initially but eventually becomes covered with a gray exudate. Cervicitis due to *T. vaginitis* is usually associated with a yellow frothy vaginal discharge and the cervix itself may have a punctate strawberry-like appearance. This may be more apparent when women are examined with the use of colposcopy. Cervicitis secondary to candidal vaginitis is usually seen with a typical vaginal cheesy discharge which is also apparent on the surface of the cervix. Clinically apparent cervicitis in association with CMV infection, bacterial vaginosis, or genital mycoplasma infection has not been well delineated but is similar to that seen in association with chlamydial infections.

As stated previously, cervicitis is not invariably associated with the isolation or detection of pathogenic organisms, and in a number of cases STD pathogens may be recovered from the cervix with no associated clinical findings.

## Laboratory studies and diagnosis

The diagnosis of cervical infections caused by STD pathogens based upon the clinical diagnosis of cervicitis is neither sensitive nor specific. Thus, the presence of yellow endocervical discharge was only 54% sensitive and 82% specific and provided a positive predictive value for STD pathogens of only 45% in one study. The sensitivity and positive predictive value of this clinical sign decreases significantly when an inexperienced physician conducts the examination or when the prevalence of STD is low. However, use of the presence of two or more of the following—young age (≤24 yr), recent change in sexual partner within the preceding 2 mo, nonuse of barrier protection during intercourse, yellow mucopurulent cervical discharge, and easily induced cervical bleeding—could be used to predict more than 90% of chlamydial infections in a family practice clinic setting in Seattle. Therefore, historical factors associated with risk behavior coupled with physical findings of cervicitis may be clinically useful in predicting the presence of STD pathogens in some populations.

Clinically, physicians must decide whether to screen all patients for STD cervical pathogens, only those whose symptoms or signs of cervicitis, and/or those with identifiable risk factors for STD acquisition. Physicians practicing in STD clinics or other settings with high disease prevalence will need to screen all patients for these agents. Those in family practice clinics likely should screen only those with risk factors and those who have compatible signs and symptoms. Pregnant women comprise a special group of patients for whom routine screening for STD cervical pathogens should be considered, particularly for those patients who are young and unmarried. Colposcopic examination may increase the physician's diagnostic ability, and the use of colposcopy in STD, Gynaecology, and Obstetric clinics to aid in the diagnosis of cervicitis deserves further study. The benefits of increasing the sensitivity and specificity of the clinical diagnosis and therefore the cost saving in more directed testing for pathogens and specific treatment must be balanced against the need for available facilities, trained colposcopists, and the additional time needed to do the procedure.

Specific diagnosic methods for cervical infection due to various agents are shown in Table 72.1. Currently used antigen detection tests are felt to be specific but not highly sensitive for detecting cervical infection by *C. trachomatis* and *N. gonorrhoeae* in postpubertal women. Recently, diagnostic tests for *C. trachomatis* have been developed using polymerase chain reaction (PCR) and ligase chain reaction (LCR) to detect chlamydial DNA in clinical specimens which are considerably more sensitive than antigen detection methods. LCR, in particular, has been shown to reliably detect *C. trachomatis* in urine in both men and women. When these test systems become commercially available, they will considerably improve our ability to diagnose this infection. However, no test, including culture LCR or PCR, detects 100% of infected patients.

## Therapy and management

Therapy for cervicitis should ideally be directed by the results of etiological testing. In instances of cervicitis and association with exposure to an individual known to be infected with a STD, presumptive therapy can be given. In circumstances where determination of the infective agent is not possible, treatment may have to be given based on the patient's clinical presentation. Using this approach, patients less than 25 yr of age or with a new sexual partner who present with mucopurulent cervicitis should be treated presumptively for *C. trachomatis* and *N. gonorrhoeae* and followed for resolution of signs of infection.

Therapies for specific pathogens are found in Chapter 38. Management also includes notification and treatment of recent sexual contacts when *C. trachomatis*, *N. gonorrhoeae*, and/or *T. pallidum* is detected. Also, since individuals who acquire these infections are at higher risk of also acquiring HIV infection, counselling and offering HIV testing are appropriate for these patients. Generally, if *N. gonorrhoeae* is identified, treatment for both *N. gonorrhoeae* and *C. trachomatis* should be given. For cervical infections with *C. trachomatis* and *N. gonorrhoeae*, there is generally no need to obtain specimens for "test-of cure" if signs and symptoms resolve, if the patient is felt to be reliable, and if contacts have been notified and treated. However, repeat testing of infected pregnant women following treatment is advisable. Patients with primarily syphilis will need follow-up serological testing to ensure that the infection has been successfully eradicated.

# Pelvic Inflammatory Disease (Salpingitis)

## Etiology and epidemiology

Acute salpingitis is not a reportable disease, and therefore accurate data on incidence is lacking. Salpingitis is almost always a

**Table 72.1** Recommended laboratory tests for the etiological diagnosis of cervicitis

| Organism | Test | Comment |
|---|---|---|
| *Chlamydia trachomatis* | Culture<br>Antigen detection<br>PCR/LCR[a] | Culture is considered the "gold standard" but is not readily available. Antigen detection tests now have reasonable sensitivity and high specificity for the diagnosis of cervical infection. PCR or LCR offers very high sensitivity and specificity |
| *Neisseria gonorrhoea* | Culture<br>Antigen detection<br>Gram stain | Culture is preferred if available to monitor for drug resistance. Antigen detection is a suitable alternative for cervical infection. Gram stain showing intracellular diplococci has low sensitivity and specificity in women. LCR is still experimental but has high sensitivity and specificity |
| *Trichomonas vaginalis* | Direct exam<br>Culture | Direct examination of "wet prep" specimen for motile trichomonads is often adequate. Culture may increase sensitivity |
| Cytomegalo virus | Culture | Not routinely done |
| Herpes simplex virus | Culture | Not routinely done |
| *Treponema pallidum* | Direct<br>Microscopic<br>Exam of exudate | Must be processed immediately. Serology should also be done but may not be positive at this stage |
| *Candida* spp. | Direct<br>Culture exam | Direct examination of "wet prep" specimen for yeast after addition of KOH is usually adequate. Culture results can be difficult to interpret |
| Bacterial vaginosis | Direct<br>Exam of vaginal exudate | 2 of 4 criteria for diagnosis: homogeneous discharge, pH ≥4.5, clue cells, fishy odor with addition of KOH to wet prep slide |
| Genital mycoplasmas | Culture | Not routinely done |
| Other bacteria | Culture | Consider if heavy growth or pure growth |

[a]PCR, polymerase chain reaction; LCR, ligase chain reaction.

bacterial infection, although rare cases due to HSV have been reported. Earlier studies of microbial etiology were based on cervical, endometrial, and cul-de-sac cultures and were of limited value in determining the microbial etiology due to contamination with colonizing flora. In those studies, about 80% of patients yielded a picture of complex polymicrobial etiology. With laparoscopic sampling, less than 30% of women were found to have polymicrobial tubal infection. The sexually transmitted organisms *N. gonorrhoeae* and *C. trachomatis* are implicated in approximately one-half of the cases while a variety of facultative and obligate anaerobes are involved in one-quarter of cases and the remainder are etiologically undefined. Serological studies suggest that approximately 50% of etiologically undefined cases may be due to chlamydial infection. Culture of the cervix may be more sensitive than tubal culture in detecting salpingitis since only 40%–50% of women with cervical gonococcal or chlamydial infection and visual evidence of salpingitis on laparoscopy have the organism recovered from the upper genital tract. In addition, recent studies using LCR on upper genital tract tissues have demonstrated more frequent positives with this technique than with culture for chlamydia. Over 85% of women with gonococcal and/or chlamydial cervicitis and lower abdominal pain clinically suggestive of salpingitis have had visual confirmation of salpingitis during laparoscopy. The usefulness of cervical or vaginal cultures in the identification of nongonococcal nonchlamydial salpingitis is unclear.

The majority of studies have been performed among women judged ill enough to require hospitalization and laposcopic examination, and thus the etiology of acute salpingitis seen among women who are managed as outpatients is less well defined. As many as 50% may not actually have PID, and many of the confirmed cases are culture negative. However, of those cases in which an etiological agent is identified, *C. trachomatis* was the most common organism found.

## Host factors and pathogenesis

Salpingitis results from ascending microbial infection of the fallopian tubes which almost always arises in the lower genital tract and passes through the cervix and the endometrium to involve the tubes. *Mycobacterium tuberculosis* is the principle exception to the rule as it spreads to the serosal surface of the fallopian tubes via the bloodstream. As the majority of women with acute salpingitis have histological evidence of endometritis and as endometritis also frequently complicates mucopurulent cervicitis, it is reasonable to suppose that microbes initially infecting the lower genital tract can pass through the cervix to infect the endometrium and subsequently the fallopian tubes. Infected exudate leaving the tubal ostia is the source of peritoneal infection.

Since both gonococci and chlamydia are nonmotile, questions remain as to how they spread to the fallopian tubes. Further, the tempo of ascending spread is largely undefined. Local contiguous spread along the mucosal surface in a canalicular fashion from the cervix to the fallopian tube is the most likely explanation. However, some cases of salpingitis are not accompanied by endometritis and occur too soon after acquisition of cervical infection to be adequately explained by this mechanism. In these cases, rapid spread to the salpinx by "piggy-backing" on motile sperm or other motile microbes has been postulated. As both gonococci and chlamydia can attach to sperm and bacteria-laden sperm remain motile, this mechanism is biologically feasible. However, as radiolabeled microspheres or carbon particles can be rapidly transported by an unknown mechanism from the cervix to the fallopian tubes, these bacteria may reach to the upper genital tract by this same unknown mechanism.

The pathogenesis of salpingitis due to nonsexually transmitted pathogens is unstudied. Limited data suggests that these women have distinct epidemiological characteristics that differ from women with STD-related salpingitis. Compared to women with gonococcal or chlamydial salpingitis, women with non-STD pathogens are older, less often have a history of gonorrhea, and lack other risk markers for STD infection. The mechanism through which they acquire their infection is unclear, but multiple transmission and pathogenetic mechanisms are probable. Intrauterine device (IUD)-associated salpingitis is more commonly due to nongonococcal nonchlamydial infection than is spontaneous salpingitis; IUDs may act to increase the risk of salpingitis by breaching cervical uterine defense mechanisms. Current data suggests that IUDs of the types presently manufactured have a small incremental risk of salpingitis (risk ratios < 2.0) and that the risk is restricted to a short interval (4 mo) after IUD insertion. Thus the reproductive tract defense mechanism compromise induced by IUDs seems transient.

Since most gonococcal and chlamydial infections do not result in salpingitis, host defense mechanisms must limit the infection to the cervix. Menses is a potential risk factor for gonococcal and to a lesser extent, chlamydial salpingitis. Most cases of gonococcal salpingitis begin within 2 wk of the onset of the menstrual cycle, and thus loss of cervical defense mechanisms during menses may be the most reasonable explanation for this association. The exact nature of these defenses is unknown, but cervical tissue is a source of secretory immunoglobulins, and cervical mucous contains a variety of antimicrobial factors including lactoferrin, complement components, and peroxidase.

Production of antibodies may be more important than previously thought in reducing the risk of salpingitis following cervical infection. Antibodies to gonococcal opacity proteins have been found to substantially reduce the risk of salpingitis complicating cervical gonococcal infection. Women with high antibody titers to chlamydia have a lower risk of salpingitis following therapeutic abortion. Both those observations were based on study of serum antibodies, and it seems probable that cervical antibodies would be even more important in limiting infection to the lower genital tract.

$H_2O_2$-producing lactobacilli found in the vagina, together with host-derived peroxidase and chloride ion, may be a nonspecific defense mechanism preventing vaginal and cervical infections with STD agents. This system may also limit infection to the cervix and prevent salpingitis by reducing pathogen multiplication within the lower genital tract. IUD use may substantially reduce this protective mechanism since lactobacilli are noticeably absent from the vaginal flora of women using IUDs, and this may in part explain the mechanism by which IUDs cause salpingitis.

Women with a previous episode of salpingitis are at increased risk of ectopic pregnancy and tubal infertility. Among women who have had salpingitis, approximately 15%–20% become infertile due to tubal occlusion and 5%–10% will have an ectopic pregnancy, despite receiving appropriate diagnostic services and antimicrobial therapies. Older age, multiple episodes of salpingitis, and nongonococcal etiology are the principle risk factors for salpingitis sequelae. Among women with salpingitis, those with nongonococcal nonchlamydial tubal infections (often complicated by tubal abscess) or with chlamydial infection have the poorest reproductive outcome.

The extensive tubal damage associated with tubal abscess due to *H. influenzae* or anaerobic infection is a sufficient explanation for the high rate of postsalpingitis tubal obstruction seen in this circumstance. The mechanism by which *C. trachomatis* results in postsalpingitis tubal damage is less clear. However, emerging data suggest that immunopathologic responses to a chlamydial heat shock protein may be important. Women with *C. trachomatis*-associated tubal infertility or ectopic pregnancies often have antibodies to this protein antigen, whereas women with uncomplicated chlamydial infection do not. As the immune responses to heat-shock proteins are determined in part by immune response genes in the major histocompatibility complex, genetic factors may be important in the pathogenesis of chlamydial salpingitis sequelae.

## Clinical features and diagnostic criteria

In general, salpingitis has a wide clinical spectrum ranging from silent to atypical to cases with typical features. Typical salpingitis is characterized by abrupt onset of lower abdominal pain shortly following menstruation in a young sexually active woman. Examination shows fever, marked lower abdominal pain with guarding, with or without an adnexal mass, and mucopurulent cervical discharge. However, approximately 50% of women with acute salpingitis present with more subtle manifestations. Unfortunately, a simple and perfectly accurate diagnostic algorithm for the diagnosis of salpingitis does not yet exist. A reasonable approach for clinicians is to clinically diagnose salpingitis in a sexually active woman who is found to have cervical and uterine motion tenderness with adnexal tenderness and who has one or more of the following: (*1*) elevated C-reactive protein or erythrocyte sedimentation rate (ESR) ≥25, (*2*) palpable adnexal mass, (*3*) temperature ≥38°C, and (*4*) positive gonococcal or chlamydial test. These criteria represent a tradeoff between common sense, tests commonly available to clinicians that yield objective data, and the absence of a well-tested clinical algorithm. However, these guidelines do need to be objectively validated.

Laparoscopy for the routine diagnosis of salpingitis is probably not indicated. In addition to the attendant risk of general anesthesia and cost, laparoscopy has been found to be only 50% sensitive for the diagnosis of tubal infection (as determined by fimbrial histology) and is only 80% specific. Laparoscopy should be reserved as a fallback test when the diagnosis of salpingitis remains uncertain, when alternative serious diagnoses seem probable, or where laposcopic drainage of a tubal abscess is required. All women who are suspected to have salpingitis should have a serum pregnancy test to exclude ectopic pregnancy unless pregnancy risk is deemed negligible.

## Treatment and management

Antimicrobials have improved the natural history of acute salpingitis. In the pre-antibiotic era, women with salpingitis had a mortality rate of 1.3%, were ill for an average of 3 mo, and had a postinfection infertility rate of 80%. With antimicrobial therapy, mortality has virtually been eliminated and most (80%) women are clinically well within 2 wk of treatment. However, 10%–30% of women treated with antimicrobials still have postinfection tubal infertility.

Table 72.2 shows the recent Centers for Disease Control (CDC) recommendations for ambulatory and in-hospital treatment of acute salpingitis. Hospitalization is recommended for

**Table 72.2** Recommended antimicrobial therapy for women with salpingitis

1. INPATIENT TREATMENT

One of the following:

*RECOMMENDED REGIMEN A*

**Cefoxitin** 2 g IV every 6 h **or cefotetan** IV 2 g every 12 h

**plus**

**Doxycycline**[a] 100 mg PO or IV every 12 h

The above regimen is continued for at least 48 h after the patient improves clinically. After discharge from hospital, doxycycline 100 mg PO, every 12 h, should be continued for 10–14 d

*RECOMMENDED REGIMEN B*

Clindamycin 900 mg IV every 8 h

**plus**

**Gentamicin** loading dose IV or IM (2 mg/kg of body weight) followed by a maintenance dose (1.5 mg/kg) every 8 h

The above regimen is continued for at least 48 h after the patient improves. After discharge from hospital, doxycycline 100 mg PO, every 12 h, should be continued for 10–14 d. Continuation of clindamycin 450 mg PO, every 6 h, for 10–14 d may be considered as an alternative.

2. OUTPATIENT MANAGEMENT

*RECOMMENDED REGIMEN A*

**Cefoxitin** 2 g IM **plus probenecid** 1 g PO, concurrently **or ceftriaxone** 250 mg IM **or** an equivalent **cephalosporin**

**plus**

**Doxycycline** 100 mg PO, every 12 h, for 10–14 d **or**

**Tetracycline** 500 mg PO, every 6 h, for 10–14 d

*RECOMMENDED REGIMEN B*

**Ofloxacin** 400 mg PO, every 12 h, for 14 d

**plus**

**Clindamycin** 450 mg PO, every 6 h for 14 d **or**

**Metronidazole** 500 mg PO, every 12 h for 14 d

[a]Alternative regimen for patients who do not tolerate doxycycline/tetracycline. Substitute **erythromycin** 500 mg PO, every 6 h, for 10–14 d.

women with severe disease who are unable to tolerate oral medication, for women with adnexal mass(es), and for women in whom the diagnosis is uncertain and in whom laparoscopy may be necessary. Hospitalization is recommended for adolescents because of potential noncompliance with oral medication. Adnexal masses are best treated in hospital with IV therapy because of the poor fertility prognosis and because of the potential need for surgical drainage of abscesses. An approach to rationally selecting a specific antimicrobial regime is given in Table 72.3, which classifies salpingitis as typical, atypical, polymicrobic, or chronic. Clinical classification of the PID syndrome allows rational choice from among the many regimes recommended by the CDC. This approach, while practical, has yet to be rigorously evaluated.

The type of antimicrobial treatment chosen has only a limited effect on the postinfection infertility rate, and the currently observed rate of infertility (10%–30%) likely represents the occurrence of irreversible tubal damage before the patient presents for treatment. Whether modulation of the host inflammatory response with biologic response modifiers (such as steroids and nonsteroidal anti-inflammatory agents) together with appropriate antimicrobial treatment will improve postinfection infertility rate is the subject of current clinical trials. The immunopathologic process resulting in chlamydial infertility may be responsive to immunomodulators.

HIV infection increases the incidence of a variety of other infections, including salpingitis. Emerging data from Nairobi, Kenya, suggests that HIV-infected commercial sex workers have a twofold increased incident rate of salpingitis. The increased risk is seen for both gonococcal and chlamydial salpingitis; U.S. data show that women with salpingitis have an increased prevalence of HIV and that HIV-infected women with salpingitis appear to respond more slowly to antimicrobial therapy. Thus, the available data suggests that HIV substantially alters the natural history of salpingitis. Based on these observations, women with salpingitis should be offered HIV testing; if positive, they likely will require hospitalization for parenteral antimicrobial therapy of the illness.

## Control of Salpingitis, Cervicitis, and Vulvovaginitis

Control strategies for salpingitis should be viewed within the context of the salpingitis causal pathway. Salpingitis and its seque-

**Table 72.3** Clinical classification of salpingitis as an approach to empiric management

| | Typical | Atypical | Polymicrobic | Chronic |
|---|---|---|---|---|
| Onset | Acute (<72 h) | Subacute (>3 d <3 wk) | Variable | Chronic (>3 wk) |
| Age | <20–25 yr | <20–25 yr | 25–29 yr | >30 yr |
| Manifestations | Pain/fever | Pain or menometrorrhagia | Pain/fever | Bleeding/mass |
| Onset with menstruation | ++ | +/− | +/− | − |
| Predisposition | − | − | IUD/prior damage | − |
| Abscess | − | − | ++ | +/− |
| Etiologic agents* | *Neisseria gonorrhoea*<br>*Streptococcus pyogenes*<br>*Staphylococcus aureus* | *Chlamydia trachomatis*<br>*Neisseria gonorrhoea*<br>*Mycoplasma* spp. | Anaerobes<br>*Escherichia coli*<br>*Hemophilus influenzae* | Actinomyces<br>*Mycobacterium tuberculosis* |
| Empiric therapy | Cefoxitin and doxycycline | | Clindamycin and gentamicin | Requires invasive diagnosis prior to therapy |

lae are the outcome of complex behaviorial and biologic attributes of women and the social environment in which women live. Over 20% of women with one episode of salpingitis subsequently develop another episode. This suggest that many women with salpingitis are found in a social matrix which puts them at continuing high risk for reinfection.

Since most cases of salpingitis result from cervical infection with STD agents, STD control in the population will have a substantial impact in reducing the incidence of PID and subsequent infertility. The main strategies to control gonococcal and chlamydial infection include the laboratory diagnosis of infection among women with cervicitis, screening for subclinical infection, contact tracing from test-positive individuals, and appropriate treatment and follow-up of infected persons. Contact tracing of male partners of women with gonococcal and chlamydial salpingitis is particularly important since salpingitis seems to be an early complication of infection, and many source-male contacts are "super spreaders" who have asymptomatic and unrecognized urethral infection.

Women can reduce the risk of salpingitis and its sequelae by delaying the initiation of sexual intercourse, limiting their number of sexual partners, and using STD barrier methods such as condoms, diaphragms, and spermicides.

Clinicians can assist in the control of salpingitis by correctly recognizing and treating clinical cervicitis and salpingitis, by screening for asymptomatic chlamydial and gonococcal infections among at-risk individuals, and by providing appropriate treatment for gonococcal and chlamydial infection. Only with the concerted efforts of public health authorities and clinicians in the community can the salpingitis pathway be interrupted.

## ANNOTATED BIBLIOGRAPHY


Brunham RB, Embree JE. Cervicitis, endometritis, and salpingo-oophoritis. In: Infectious Diseases. A Treatise of Infectious Process, 5th ed. Hoeprich PD, Jordan MC, Ronald AR, eds. JB Lippincott, Philadelphia, PA, pp. 582–593, 1994.

*A general reference reviewing the relationship of these three disease entities.*

Brunham RC, Paavonen J, Stevens CE, Kiviat N, Kuo C-C, Critchlow CW, Holmes KK. Mucopurulent cervicitis: the ignored counterpart in women of urethritis in men. N Engl J Med 1984; 11:1–6.

*This article describes the clinical findings associated with cervicitis.*

Centers for Disease Control. Sexually transmitted diseases treatment guidelines. MMWR Morb Mortal Wkly Rep 1993; 42(RR-14):75–81.

*These are recent guidelines developed for treatment of pelvic inflammatory disease.*

Handsfield HH, Jasman LL, Roberts PL, Hanson VW, Kothenbeutel RL, Stamm WE. Criteria for selective screening for *Chlamydia trachomatis* infection in women attending family planning clinics. JAMA 1986; 255:1730–1734.

*This article defines the sensitivity and specificity of signs of chlamydial cervicitis in a relatively low-risk population.*

Health and Welfare Canada. Canadian STD guidelines for the prevention, diagnosis, management and treatment of sexually transmitted diseases in neonates, children, adolescents and adults. 1995 update. Can Communicable Dis Rep 1995; 21S4:1–215.

*This is another set of guidelines for the treatment of pelvic inflammatory disease.*

Plummer FA, Chubb H, Simonsen JN, Bosire M, Slaney L, Nagelkerke NJD, Maclean I, Ndinya-Achola JO, Waiyaki P, Brunham RC. Antibody to opacity proteins (Opa) correlate with a reduced risk of gonococcal salpingitis. J Clin Invest 1994; 93:1748–1755.

*A new study showing that gonococcal immunity can prevent ascending infection.*

Potteratt JJ, Philips L, Rothenberg RB, Darrow WW. Gonococcal pelvic inflammatory disease: case-finding observations. Am J Obstet Gynecol 1980; 138:1101–1104.

*These epidemiologists report that source male contacts of women with gonococcal pelvic inflammatory disease frequently have asymptomatic urethral infection.*

Sellors J, Mahony J, Goldsmith C, Rath D, Mander R, Hunter B, Taylor C, Groves D, Richardson H, Chernesky M. The accuracy of clinical findings and laparoscopy in pelvic inflammatory disease. Am J Obstet Gynecol 1991; 164:113–120.

*This is another classic paper on pelvic inflammatory disease which compares clinical findings with those from laparoscopic examination.*

Soper DE, Brockwell NJ, Dalton HP. False-positive cultures of the cul-de-sac associated with culdocentesis in patients undergoing elective laparoscopy. Obstet Gynecol 1991; 77:134–138.

*This study argues against the use of culdocentesis for the etiologic diagnosis of pelvic inflammatory disease because of frequent false-positive results.*

Sweet RL, Blankfort-Doyle M, Robbie MO, Schacter J. The occurrence of chlamydial and gonoccal salpingitis during the menstrual cycle. JAMA 1986; 255:2062–2064.

*This study demonstrates that the first 2 wk of the menstrual cycle are associated with an elevated risk for both gonococcal and chlamydial pelvic inflammatory disease.*

Washington AE, Cates W, Wasserheit JN. Preventing pelvic inflammatory disease. JAMA 1991; 266:2574–2580.

*This review comprehensively reviews individual and population measures to reduce the risk of pelvic inflammatory disease.*

Westrom L. Incidence, prevalence, and trends of acute pelvic inflammatory disease and its consequence in industrialized countries. Am J Obstet Gynecol 1980; 138:880–892.

*This is a complete review of the epidemiology of pelvic inflammatory disease.*

Westrom L, Joesoef R, Reynolds G, Hagdu A, Thompson SE. Pelvic inflammatory disease and fertility. A cohort study of 1,844 women with laparoscopically verified disease and 657 control women with normal laparosopic results. Sex Trans Dis 1992; 19:185–192.

*This is the classic paper which describes the symptoms, signs and clinical consequences of pelvic inflammatory disease.*

# 73

# Meningitis

YOUNG S. KIM AND MARTIN G. TAÜBER

Bacterial meningitis is most frequently caused by a limited number of encapsulated bacteria. It is an often devastating infection localized in the subarachnoid space that can severely affect the functioning and structural integrity of the brain. Because of the marked polymorphonuclear pleocytosis in the cerebrospinal fluid (CSF), bacterial meningitis is commonly referred to as pyogenic meningitis. Rarely, organisms other than bacteria (fungi, ameba) cause pyogenic meningitis (see aseptic and chronic meningitis). Young children and older adults are at highest risk for developing bacterial meningitis. While appropriate antibiotic therapy has dramatically reduced the morbidity and mortality of the disease compared to the pre-antibiotic era, many patients still suffer from severe sequelae. Clinicians therefore must institute empiric therapy quickly in patients with symptoms or signs compatible with bacterial meningitis.

## Bacterial Meningitis

### Etiology

A limited number of pyogenic bacteria cause the vast majority of cases of bacterial meningitis (Table 73.1), while many other bacteria, including anaerobes, have caused occasional cases of meningitis. There is a close association between the age of the patient and the spectrum of organisms responsible for meningitis. In infants less than 1 mo of age, three types of pathogens (*Streptococcus agalactiae* [group B streptococcus], gram-negative enteric organisms [*Escherichia coli, Klebsiella pneumoniae*], and *Listeria monocytogenes*) account for the vast majority of cases. Beyond the neonatal period, three organisms are responsible for at least 75% of all cases: *Hemophilus influenzae* type b, *Neisseria meningitidis* (serotypes A, B, C, occasionally Y), and *Streptococcus pneumoniae*. *Hemophilus influenzae* is the most common organism in young children aged 1 mo to approximately 4 yr. In older children and adults, pneumococci and meningococci make up the majority of cases; meningococci typically are seen in children and younger adults, while pneumococci are most prevalent in older people. In addition to age, other host-specific factors predispose to the development of meningitis caused by certain microorganisms (Table 73.1)

### Epidemiology

The incidence of bacterial meningitis varies greatly in different areas of the world. This variability is accounted for primarily by the epidemiology of *N. meningitidis*, which causes epidemics of meningitis. Small outbreaks typically occur in populations of young adults living in close quarters, such as dormitories or military camps, or among schoolchildren, and their occurrence is not restricted to particular geographic locations. Major epidemics, which dramatically affect the incidence of the disease, have periodically occurred in certain parts of the world, including sub-Saharan Africa ("meningitis belt"), Europe (particularly Scandinavia), Asia, and South America. During these epidemics, attack rates can reach several hundred per 100,000 population, with devastating consequences particularly in areas with limited medical resources. Independent of the occurrence of epidemics, meningococcal meningitis shows a peak incidence worldwide in winter and early spring. Other causes of meningitis also tend to be clustered in the winter months.

In the United States, 15,000 to 25,000 cases of bacterial meningitis are estimated to occur annually (approximate annual incidence: 5 to 10 cases/100,000 population). The extremes of age are preferentially affected by meningitis. Young children 1 mo to 2 yr of age have until recently been the age group predominantly affected by bacterial meningitis, *H. influenzae* being the most common organism. The use of new conjugate *H. influenzae* type b vaccines, which are much more immunogenic in young children than the older polysaccharide vaccines, have profoundly reduced the incidence of invasive *H. influenzae* infection, including meningitis, in the United States and some European countries. Elimination of the most important cause of meningitis in these young children has reduced the overall incidence of bacterial meningitis in this age group.

### Pathogenesis

Colonization of the upper respiratory tract mucosa by the pathogen generally is the first step in the pathogenesis of meningitis (Fig. 73.1). Meningeal pathogens—for example, pneumococci or meningococci—spread within population units, such as families or schools, and nasopharyngeal carrier states can persist for weeks to months. Viral infections of the upper respiratory tract may also facilitate the colonization of the oropharyngeal mucosa with pathogenic bacteria, such as *H. influenzae* and pneumococci. Colonization of neonates occurs during birth.

Following colonization, the major route resulting in meningitis involves invasion of the local mucous membrane and transient bacteremia with subsequent infection of the central nervous system. Occurrence of bacteremia is favored by inadequate humoral immunity, hence the increased risk for meningitis in young children; and by anatomical or functional asplenic states (sickle cell disease, thalassemia, others). Pneumonia can also lead to bacteremia and subsequent meningitis, particularly in the case of pneumococcal pneumonia. In contrast, sinusitis and otitis are believed to cause meningitis by direct invasion of the subarachnoid space from the adjacent cranial structures.

In a minority of patients, microorganisms invade the CNS and

**Table 73.1** Bacterial causes of acute meningitis

| Pathogen | Conditions favoring infection with specific pathogen |
|---|---|
| *Streptococcus pneumoniae* | Extremes of age; sinusitis; otitis media, pneumonia, endocarditis; blunt head trauma; CSF leak |
| *Neisseria meningitidis* | Older children–young adults; epidemics; terminal complement deficiencies |
| *Hemophilus influenzae* | Age 1 month to 4 years; sinusitis; otitis media; CSF leak |
| *Listeria monocytogenes* | Neonates; pregnancy; alcoholism; diabetes mellitus; corticosteroid or immunosuppressive therapy |
| *Streptococcus agalactiae* (group B streptococci) | Neonates |
| *Escherichia coli* | Neonates; neurosurgery; penetrating head trauma (nosocomial meningitis), neutropenia, bacteremia |
| Enterobacteriaceae (*Klebsiella* sp., *Serratia* sp.) | Neurosurgery; head trauma (nosocomial meningitis) neutropenia, bacteremia |
| *Enterobacter* sp., *Citrobacter* sp. | Neonates (meningitis/brain abscess), elderly neutropenia, bacteremia |
| *Pseudomonas aeruginosa* | Neurosurgery, penetrating head trauma, neutropenia, bacteremia |
| *Staphylococcus aureus* | Neurosurgery; penetrating head trauma; CSF shunts; chronic CSF leak, endocarditis, epidural abscess |
| *Enterococcus* sp. | Neonates; neurosurgery, endocarditis |
| *Propionibacterium acnes* | CSF shunts; neurosurgery; dermal sinus |
| Coagulase-negative staphylococci | CSF shunts |

cause meningitis as a direct result of disruption of the cranial integrity. This occurs most commonly following trauma or neurosurgical procedures. Rarely, focal infections of structures adjacent to the CSF space, such as osteomyelitis of the skull or vertebrae, or epidural abscess, can lead to meningitis when bacteria gain access to the CSF space. The pathogens leading to meningitis in these patients include staphylococci and gram negative enteric organisms. The latter (including coagulase-negative staphylococci) represent important pathogens in the setting of ventricular shunts. Chronic CSF fistulas, either congenital or acquired following trauma, also increase the risk of meningitis resulting from direct microbial invasion.

Concentrations of complement and anticapsular antibodies in CSF are low. The resulting deficiency in opsonization of encapsulated meningeal pathogens greatly reduces the effectiveness of granulocytes in the CSF and allows for rapid multiplication of the meningeal pathogen once they have reached the CSF space. Bacterial multiplication is associated with the release of bacterial products (cell wall fragments, lipopolysaccharides) that trigger the inflammatory response in the subarachnoid space, upregulate adhesion molecules on brain vascular endothelial cells, and promote the recruitment of granulocytes into the CSF. It is this granulocytic inflammation that appears primarily responsible for inducing the complex pathophysiologic CNS alterations associated with bacterial meningitis. These include changes in cerebral blood flow, the development of intracranial hypertension and brain edema, alterations in the hydrodynamics of CSF flow and of brain metabolism, and ultimately the development of functional and structural damage to the brain. The detailed mechanisms responsible for the development of brain injury during meningitis are incompletely understood, but it appears that adjunctive therapies of meningitis aimed at down-regulating the inflammatory response have beneficial effects on neurologic outcome (see below).

## Clinical manifestation

Meningitis is the most likely diagnosis in patients who present with the classical triad of fever, headache, and a stiff neck. Other signs and symptoms reflecting consequences of the inflammatory process within the central nervous system occur less frequently (Table 73.2). All patients complaining of headache or presenting with altered mental status must be carefully examined for evidence of meningeal irritation (i.e., meningism, Kernig's or Brudzinski's sign). Bacterial meningitis can be present in patients in whom the clinical diagnosis is not obvious. This is particularly true at the extremes of age, in infants, and in the elderly. In children under 2 yr of age, signs of meningeal inflammation are frequently absent, and the most common clinical presentations include only fever and alteration of level of consciousness (irritability, lethargy), which are present in over 90% of patients. Similarly, in elderly patients fever may be minimal, headache may not be a prominent complaint, signs of meningeal irritation may be difficult to elicit, and mental status changes may be the only symptoms that bring the patient to medical attention. In patients with suspected meningitis, a careful skin examination for the characteristic purpuric or petechial skin rash of *N. meningitidis* should be performed (see Chapter 51).

Untreated meningitis is characterized by progressive loss of consciousness, commonly associated with other neurologic signs including seizures and focal deficits, and leads to coma and death. Patients presenting in coma have a very high mortality (up to 50%). Systemic complications of the infectious process include septic shock, disseminated intravascular coagulation (particularly

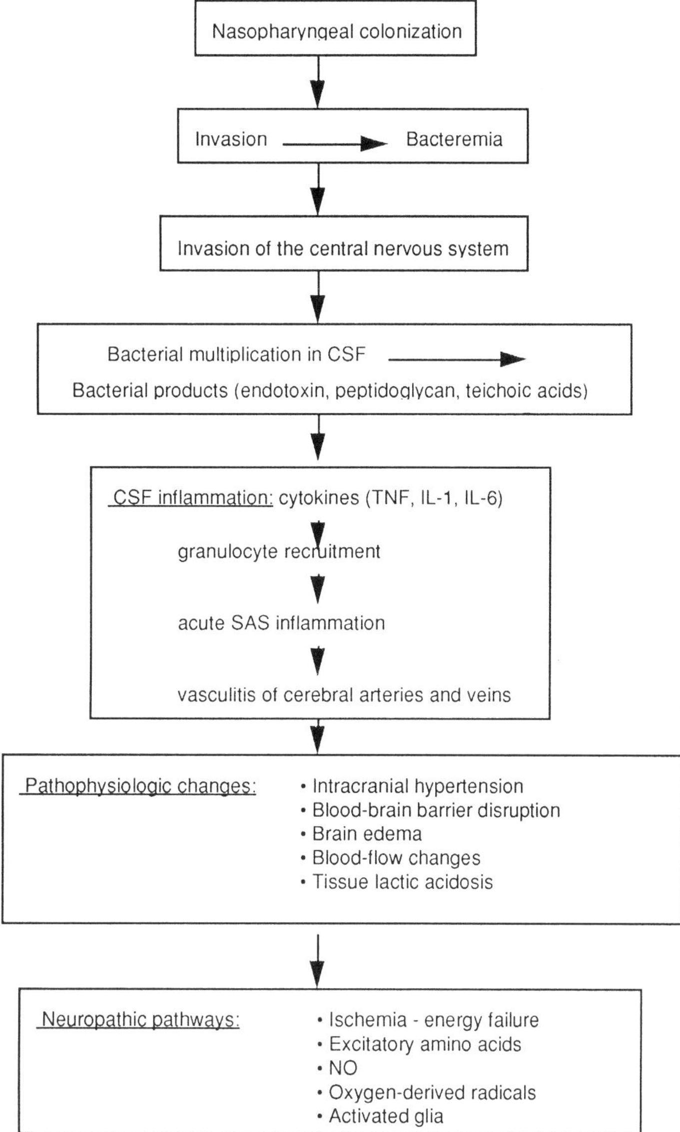


**Fig. 73.1** Pathogenesis of bacterial meningitis. NO, nitric oxide; SAS, subarachnoid space.

with meningococcal infections), and acute respiratory distress syndrome (ARDS) (see Chapter 50).

## General laboratory studies

While the diagnosis of bacterial meningitis is made by examination of the cerebrospinal fluid (see below), systemic abnormalities are commonly also present. These can include:

1. *Acute inflammation*: Differential blood count will frequently show a leukocytosis with left shift. Erythrocyte sedimentation rate and other acute phase reactants are typically elevated (see Chapter 14).
2. *Bacteremia*: Blood cultures should always be performed prior to initiation of antibiotic therapy. Blood cultures reveal the infecting organism in >50% of cases.
3. *Syndrome of inappropriate antidiuretic hormone (ADH) secretion (SIADH)*: Patients should be examined for evidence of electrolyte imbalance. Hyponatremia is common and may indicate dehydration (low urine sodium concentration) or SIADH (high urine sodium concentration) (see Chapter 14).
4. *Disseminated intravascular coagulation (DIC)*: This systemic complication is most commonly seen in patients with meningococcal meningitis. Platelet count, prothrombin time (PT)/partial thromboplastin time (PTT), fibrinogen, fibrin d-dimers should be measured in patients with suspected DIC (see Chapter 13).

## Diagnosis of bacterial meningitis

The diagnosis of bacterial meningitis is established by examination of cerebrospinal fluid (CSF), which shows a characteristic pattern of abnormalities (Table 73.3). However, none of these abnormalities is 100% sensitive or specific for the diagnosis of bacterial meningitis. While performing the lumbar puncture, CSF pressure should always be recorded. Immediate examination of the CSF provides valuable information. A gram stain of uncentrifuged (in the case of turbid CSF) or centrifuged CSF indicates the presence of white blood cells, their approximate type distribution (mononuclear versus polymorphonuclear), and whether organisms are present. The gram stain should be repeated in the

**Table 73.2** Symptoms and signs of acute bacterial meningitis

| Symptoms | Signs |
|---|---|
| Headache | Fever |
| Photophobia | Meningismus |
| Nausea and vomiting | Kernig's sign[a] |
| | Brudzinski's sign[b] |
| | Altered mental status |
| | Cranial nerve palsies |
| | Seizures |
| | Focal neurologic deficits |
| | Papilledema |

[a]Patient in supine position with leg flexed at hip and knee will resist extension of the leg at the knee due to back/neck pain.

[b]Passive neck flexion induces flexion of hip and knee.

microbiology laboratory, where an experienced technician carefully searches for scarce organisms. Cultures for bacteria and fungi should always be performed, even in patients already treated with antibiotics. Many laboratories will also offer tests for the detection of bacterial antigens by immunological methods, such as counterimmunoelectrophoresis (CIE) or latex particle agglutination (LPA). These tests can be particularly helpful in patients who have partially treated bacterial meningitis (i.e., the patient who presents while taking oral antibiotics), but their sensitivity does not exceed approximately 90%.

## Therapy

### Initial management

Bacterial meningitis represents a medical emergency, particularly in patients with rapidly progressive disease and severely impaired CNS function. In these patients, we recommend initiation of empiric therapy without the delay almost invariably associated with diagnostic procedures such as lumbar puncture or CT scan (Fig. 73.2). One or two blood cultures should be obtained before administering the first antibiotic dose (for guidance of empiric antibiotic therapy, see below). We also administer adjunctive therapy with dexamethasone in patients with rapidly progressive disease concomitantly with the first antibiotic dose (for more detail, see below). Once empiric therapy has been initiated, further diagnostic workup is performed. In patients with focal neurologic signs and clinical evidence of increased intracranial pressure, such as impaired mental status or papilledema, a head CT scan should be performed prior to the lumbar puncture to rule out mass lesions that may lead to cerebral herniation. In all other patients, a lumbar puncture can usually be safely performed. Further therapy will depend on the findings in CSF. In patients who are clinically stable and are unlikely to be adversely affected if antibiotics are not administered immediately, a lumbar puncture represents the first step, unless there is clinical suspicion of a mass lesion (see above, and Fig. 73.2). If performing a head CT first is deemed safer, antibiotic therapy should be instituted after blood cultures are taken, and the patient should be closely watched while in the scanning room or waiting in a hallway for the examination. Findings in the CSF, and on CT, if performed, will guide the further diagnostic workup and therapy in all patients.

### Empiric antibiotic therapy

Empiric antibiotic therapy generally must be instituted before a causative organism is identified. Table 73.4 summarizes possible choices for empiric therapy in different patient populations, designed to cover the likely pathogens in these patients. Doses of antibiotics recommended in the therapy of meningitis are listed in Table 73.5. It is recommended that antibiotics be administered intravenously by bolus infusion at high doses. High doses are needed because only a small fraction of the serum concentration (between 3% and 15% for most $\beta$-lactam antibiotics) penetrates into the CSF and because only antibiotic concentrations that exceed the minimal bactericidal concentration (MBC) ten- to 30-fold are rapidly bactericidal in the CSF.

Empiric therapy is primarily based on the age of the patient, with possible modifications if there are positive findings on CSF gram stain or special risk factors present (Table 73.4). If there is uncertainty, it is safer to choose regimens with broad coverage, as they can usually be modified within 24–48 h when antibiotic sensitivities of the infecting organism become available. An important factor in the choice of empiric antibiotic therapy is the emergence of organisms with increasing resistance to antibiotics. Most importantly, pneumococci that are relatively resistant (minimal inhibitory concentration [MIC] 0.1–1.0 $\mu$g/ml) or highly re-

**Table 73.3** Typical findings in the CSF of patients with bacterial meningitis, aseptic meningitis, and chronic meningitis

| Parameter | Bacterial meningitis | Aseptic meningitis | Chronic meningitis |
|---|---|---|---|
| Opening pressure | >180 mm water | <180 mm water | Normal to increased |
| CSF WBC count | >1000/mm$^3$ | 100–1000/mm$^3$ | 20–500/mm$^3$ |
| % neutrophils | >80% | <20%[a] | 10%–50% |
| Protein concentration | >100 mg/dl | 50–100 mg/dl | Usually >100 mg/dl |
| Glucose concentration | <40 mg/dl | Normal | Normal to low |
| CSF/serum glucose ratio | <0.6 | >0.6 | Normal to low |
| Gram stain | Positive (~70%)[b] | Negative | Negative |
| Culture | Positive (70–90%)[b] | Negative | Depending on etiology |

[a]May be higher very early in the course.

[b]Pretreatment with antibiotics is the most important reason for negative result.

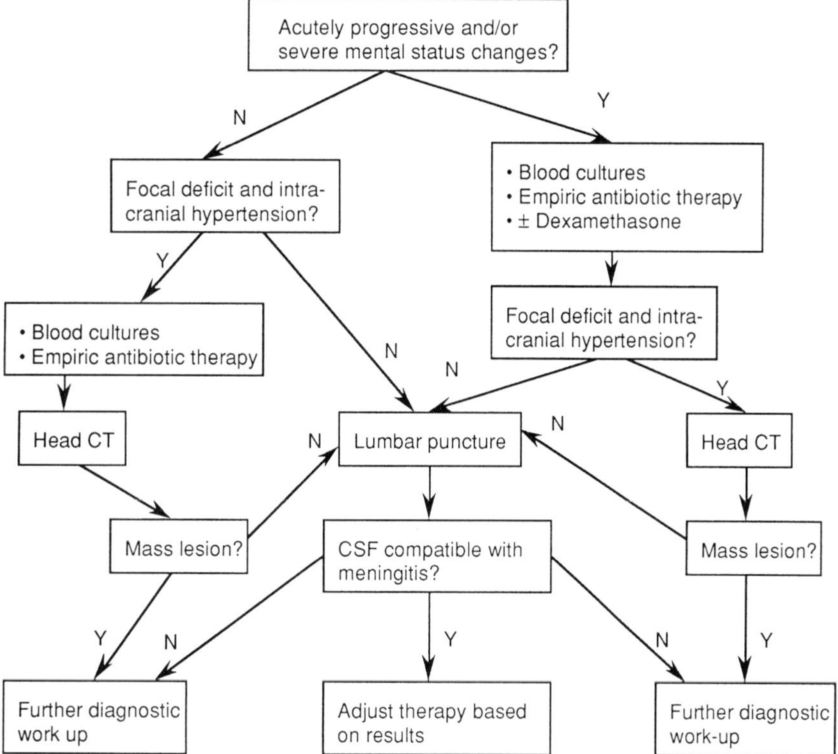


**Fig. 73.2** Algorithm for the approach to patients with suspected bacterial meningitis. N, no; Y, yes.

sistant (MIC > 1.0 μg/ml) to penicillin have become increasingly prevalent, including in many areas in Europe and the United States. Many of the penicillin-resistant organisms also have reduced sensitivity to cephalosporins, and failure of these drugs in the treatment of pneumococcal meningitis due to resistant organisms has occurred. Empiric therapy with dual antibiotic coverage effective against β-lactam resistant pneumococci may therefore be prudent unless a patient is unlikely to have pneumococcal meningitis (e.g., gram stain indicates other etiology) or the incidence of highly resistant pneumococci is very low in a particular area of the world. If a patient is at risk for infection with *L. monocytogenes*, ampicillin or penicillin should be part of the empiric therapy. In patients at risk for infections caused by difficult to treat gram-negative bacilli with a high likelihood of resistance to many β-lactam drugs, inclusion of an aminoglycoside in the empiric therapy regimen is recommended until the or-

**Table 73.4** Empiric antibiotic therapy of bacterial meningitis*

| Patient group | Antibiotic |
|---|---|
| Neonates | Ampicillin plus aminoglycoside or Ampicillin plus cefotaxime |
| Infants (1–3 mo) | Ampicillin plus cefotaxime |
| Children (3 mo to 6 yr) | 3rd-generation cephalosporin (plus rifampin or vancomycin)[a] |
| Older children, adults (no specific risk factors) | Penicillin G or 3rd-generation cephalosporin (plus rifampin or vancomycin)[a] |
| Immunocompromised patients | 3rd-generation cephalosporin plus ampicillin (plus aminoglycoside) |
| Neurosurgery, head trauma | 3rd-generation cephalosporin plus nafcillin (plus aminoglycoside) |
| Chronic CSF fistula | 3rd-generation cephalosporin plus nafcillin or vancomycin |

*Third-generation cephalosporins: cefotaxime, ceftriaxone, ceftizoxime.

[a]To cover for β-lactam-resistant pneumococci; select regimen based on the likelihood of these organisms in your patient.

**Table 73.5** Dosage of antibiotics commonly used in the therapy of bacterial meningitis

| | Dose and dosing interval | |
|---|---|---|
| Antibiotic | Children (>1 mo) | Adults |
| Penicillin G | 50,000 U/kg q4h | 3–4 M U q4h |
| Ampicillin | 75–100 mg/kg q6h | 2 g q4h |
| Cefotaxime | 50 mg/kg q6h | 2–3 g q6h |
| Ceftriaxone | 50 mg/kg q12h | 2–3 g qd |
| Ceftizoxime | 50 mg/kg q6h | 4 g q8h |
| Nafcillin | 50 mg/kg q6h | 1.5 g q4h |
| Chloramphenicol | 25 mg/kg q6h | 1.5 g q6h |
| Vancomycin | 10 mg/kg q6h | 0.5–0.75 g q6h |
| TMP/SMX | 5/20 mg/kg q6h | 5/20 mg/kg q6h |

ganism has been identified and its antibiotic sensitivities are known.

### Definitive antibiotic therapy

Identification and sensitivity testing of the causative organism is followed by adjustment of antibiotic therapy to provide optimal but narrow coverage (Table 73.6). Information on antibiotic sensitivities is crucial in the cases of the pneumococcus (see above), *H. influenzae*, and enterobacteriaceae or staphylococci commonly causing bacterial meningitis in neurosurgical patients. In the vast majority of organisms, including the gram-negative enteric rods, sensitivity patterns allow the use of systemic antibiotics alone (third-generation cephalosporins with or without aminoglycosides, quinolone). Only very rarely, intrathecal therapy with aminoglycosides has to be considered, if the organism is only sensitive to members of this antibiotic class. Routine antibiotic testing of *Neisseria*, streptococci other than pneumococci, and *L. monocytogenes* is usually not required for guidance of antibiotic therapy. Optimal duration of treatment of bacterial meningitis has not been carefully studied, but a total of 7 d appears adequate if the disease is caused by *H. influenzae* or *N. meningitidis*, while treatment should be extended to 10–14 d when any of the other common organisms, including pneumococci, are responsible, and to 21 d for neonatal meningitis. Staphylococcal meningitis should be treated at least for 2 wk, but more prolonged therapy is necessary whenever there is the possibility of infection of adjacent structures, such as osteomyelitis.

**Table 73.6** Antibiotic therapy for specific bacterial pathogens*

| Organism | Antibiotics |
|---|---|
| *HEMOPHILUS INFLUENZAE* | 3rd generation cephalosporin; ampicillin (if sensitive); chloramphenicol[a] |
| *STREPTOCOCCUS PNEUMONIAE* | Penicillin G; 3rd-generation cephalosporin; chloramphenicol[a] |
| Reduced penicillin sensitivity | 3rd-generation cephalosporin |
| Penicillin resistant | 3rd-generation cephalosporin plus vancomycin or rifampin |
| *NEISSERIA MENINGITIDIS* | Penicillin G; Chloramphenicol[a] |
| *STREPTOCOCCUS AGALACTIAE* | Penicillin G or ampicillin (plus aminoglycoside) |
| *LISTERIA MONOCYTOGENES* | Ampicillin (plus aminoglycoside) or trimethoprim/sulfamethoxazole |
| *ENTEROBACTERIACEAE* | 3rd-generation cephalosporin ± aminoglycoside |
| *PSEUDOMONAS AERUGINOSA* | Ceftazidime plus aminoglycoside or fluoroquinolone (e.g., ciprofloxacin) |
| *STAPHYLOCOCCUS AUREUS* | Nafcillin, flucloxacillin, cloxacillin |
| Methicillin-resistant *Staphyloccus aureus* | Vancomycin |

*Third-generation cephalosporins: cefotaxime, ceftriaxone, ceftizoxime.

[a]In penicillin allergic patients.

### Adjunctive therapy

Several recent clinical trials have indicated that adjunctive therapy with dexamethasone improves the neurologic and audiologic outcome in bacterial meningitis. This has been shown primarily in children with *H. influenzae* meningitis, while the data are more limited for children with pneumococcal and meningococcal meningitis, and only scant for adults with bacterial meningitis. It should also be noted that both experimental and clinical data suggest that the maximal benefit of dexamethasone is achieved when the drug is given either shortly before or at the same time as the first antibiotic dose. This is probably related to the fact that corticosteroids reduce the release of proinflammatory cytokines that are stimulated by bacterial products liberated from the pathogen by the bactericidal action of antibiotics.

Based on the available data, dexamethasone is recommended in all children over 6 wk of age with bacterial meningitis, beginning, if possible, 10 to 15 min prior to the first antibiotic dose. The recommended dose is 0.15 mg/kg IV every 6 h for a duration of 2 to maximally 4 d. The role of dexamethasone in the newborn is presently unclear. Dexamethasone therapy should not be restricted to children with severe disease, since prevention of hearing loss was also achieved in children with relatively mild disease. In the absence of controlled data for adult patients, a conservative approach could consist of giving dexamethasone (same dose as in children) to patients who have clinical evidence of impaired central nervous system physiology with altered mental status, high CSF pressure, signs of brain edema on CT scan, hearing impairment, or rapidly progressive disease. When instituting dexamethasone therapy, it is mandatory to confirm the bacterial etiology of meningitis. If this cannot be achieved within 24 to 48 h, it is safer to stop the antiinflammatory drug and to reassess the appropriateness of the chosen antimicrobial therapy. At present, there is no evidence that treatment with dexamethasone for 1 to 2 d has any adverse effects on outcome of viral meningitis. It is important that patients who are given dexamethasone be closely monitored for evidence of gastrointestinal blood loss.

There is no recognized benefit to either prophylactic or full anticoagulation in the management of patients with bacterial meningitis, and the recognized involvement of the cerebral vasculature by the inflammation is likely to increase the risk of cerebral hemorrhage in anticoagulated patients with bacterial meningitis.

### Supportive care

In critically ill patients with bacterial meningitis, aspects of supportive care can become complex and may mandate admission to a critical care unit. Patients with severe meningitis are frequently neurologically depressed and prone to seizures and may need intubation for airway protection or assisted ventilation. In addition, children may have complex requirements for fluid therapy, with the need for a careful clinical assessment of fluid status, repletion of fluid deficits, and monitoring of patients for SIADH. If SIADH is present (normal intravascular volume, falling serum sodium, reduced urine output with urine sodium concentration >50 mEq/l), water should be restricted as guided by monitoring the serum sodium and volume status until the SIADH has resolved, usually within 1–2 d. In addition, attempts to actively reduce intracranial hypertension should be undertaken in patients with clinical evidence of markedly increased intracranial pressure and severely impaired CNS function, and intracranial pressure should be monitored invasively during the acute phase of the disease, when possible. While there is minimal controlled experience in reduction of intracranial pressure in meningitis, several means have been used successfully in some patients: elevation of the end of the bed at an angle of ~30°; hyperventilation (with $PaCO_2$ to 25–30 mmHg); dexamethasone (if not already part of therapy); CSF removal if an intraventricular catheter is in place for intracranial pressure monitoring; and possibly intravenous bolus infusions with mannitol (0.25 g/kg).

### Monitoring during therapy

If a patient responds clinically to therapy, repeat CSF examination appears unnecessary. This should be reserved for patients in whom there is doubt about the accuracy of the initial diagnosis or the efficacy of therapy (for example, because of marginal sensitivity of the infecting organism to the chosen antibiotics). Secondary fever after an initial response to therapy is a common problem in patients with meningitis, particularly in children, and is most commonly due to infected intravenous lines, secondary infections which require drainage (septic arthritis, purulent pericarditis, pleural or intracranial empyema), or drug fever. Sterile subdural effusions, which occur in approximately one-third of children with meningitis, usually do not require drainage, unless symptoms or signs of intracranial hypertension are present. Obstructive hydrocephalus, which occurs in less than 5% of patients, usually manifests within the first few weeks after infection and should be treated with ventriculoperitoneal shunting. Audiologic assessment of patients can be reserved for those clinically suspected of hearing impairment resulting from the disease. Neurologic sequelae, including hearing impairment, cranial nerve palsies, and motor deficits can improve for several months after the acute illness and appropriate, individually tailored supportive therapies should be arranged for patients who are left with sequelae from the disease.

## Aseptic Meningitis

Aseptic meningitis refers to a clinical syndrome of meningitis that is usually associated with a lymphocytic pleocytosis in the CSF and in which no microorganism can be readily identified on gram stain and by bacterial cultures of the CSF. Viruses are the most common cause of aseptic meningitis, and viral meningitis is sometimes used synonymously with aseptic meningitis. While viral meningitis is usually a self-limiting, benign condition, there are numerous nonviral and noninfectious etiologies of aseptic meningitis, some of which require specific therapy.

## Etiologies

### Viruses

Viruses are the most common cause of aseptic meningitis and enteroviruses account for >80% of cases with identified causes. Among these, coxsackievirus A and B, echovirus, other enteroviruses, and poliovirus most commonly cause meningitis. Enteroviruses are transmitted by the fecal–oral route and are spread through close contact such as in households and day care centers, thus mostly affecting infants, young children, and their caretakers. Many of these viruses have associated clinical findings which may point to the diagnosis (Table 73.7). Patients with agammaglobulinemia or hypogammaglobulinemia may develop a severe or chronic meningoencephalitis when infected with enteroviruses.

Mumps is spread by respiratory droplets and causes neurologic complications ranging from meningitis to severe encephalitis. Young children are most commonly affected, boys two to five times more frequently than girls. Mumps meningitis typically follows mumps parotitis, and salivary gland swelling has resolved when aseptic meningitis develops.

Lymphochoriomeningitis (LCM) virus infections used to be most prevalent in young adults and in impoverished populations but have become uncommon, sometimes occurring in laboratory workers and pet owners. Patients present with symptoms typical for acute meningitis. After initial improvement, some may relapse in a second phase of meningitis that is believed to be immune mediated.

Arbovirus infections (St. Louis encephalitis, western equine encephalitis, California encephalitis, and eastern equine encephalitis viruses) are transmitted by mosquitos and usually present with encephalitis (see Chapter 74), but a minority of patients have meningitis with a paucity of symptoms suggestive of encephalitis. Children and young adults, who generally have milder infections, are the most likely to present with aseptic meningitis.

Herpesviruses, particularly herpes simplex virus (HSV), cause numerous neurologic complications, including aseptic meningitis. Primary genital herpes caused by HSV type 2 is the most

**Table 73.7** Characteristic features of aseptic meningitis by etiology

| Agent | Season | Clinical signs | Comments |
|---|---|---|---|
| Enteroviruses | Summer/fall | Nonspecific | Children and young adults; culture throat and stool |
| Coxsackievirus | Summer/fall | Petechial rash, pleurodynia, herpangina, myopericarditis, conjunctivitis | Children and young adults; culture throat and stool |
| Echovirus | Summer/fall | Dermatomyositis | Children and young adults; culture throat and stool |
| Western equine encephalitis | Summer/fall | | Infants and older adults |
| California encephalitis | Summer/fall | May localize to temporal lobes | Children |
| Eastern equine encephalitis | Summer/fall | Mortality 50% | Children and older adults; CSF WBC often $>1000/mm^3$ |
| St. Louis encephalitis | Summer/fall | Urinary frequency and dysuria | Adults >35yr |
| Herpes simplex virus | No seasonal pattern | Occurs with primary genital herpes | CSF glucose may be low |
| Cytomegalovirus | No seasonal pattern | Very rare complication | |
| Ebstein-Barr virus | No seasonal pattern | Complication of mononucleosis | |
| Mumps | Spring | Orchitis, oophritis, pancreatitis | Children and young adults; CSF glucose may be low |
| Lymphocytic choriomeningitis (LCM) | Fall/winter | Exposure to rodents; alopecia, orchitis, arthritis, myopericarditis | CSF glucose may be low; CSF pleocytosis may be $>1000/mm^3$ |
| Human immunodeficiency virus (HIV) | Any | Mononucleosis-like syndrome in a high-risk group for HIV | Check serology; if negative, recheck in 3 mo |
| Syphilis | Any | In the acute infection and in neurosyphillis | CSF VDRL positive |
| Lyme disease | Summer/fall | History of tick bite or erythema migrans | Check blood serology |
| Leptosporosis | Summer/fall | Biphasic illness after water exposure | First phase check blood and CSF cultures; second phase check urine cultures and serology |

common syndrome in which aseptic meningitis develops. By recent estimates, one-third of women and one-eighth of men had herpetic meningitis with the primary infection. Urinary retention and local autonomic symptoms are commonly associated. Aseptic meningitis is much less likely with recurrent herpes. Herpetic aseptic meningitis is a benign and self-limited illness, in contrast to encephalitis, which may lead to devastating neurologic sequelae and death (Chapter 74). Varicella zoster virus, cytomegalovirus, and Epstein-Barr virus (EBV) have also been reported to cause aseptic meningitis. Mollaret's meningitis is a benign, lymphocytic, recurrent meningitis; recent data suggest that some cases of Mollaret's meningitis may be a consequence of HSV-1 or EBV.

Acute infection with HIV-1 causes a mononucleosis-like illness with fever, malaise, rash, myalgias, and arthralgias which can be associated with aseptic meningitis, and the possibility of acute HIV infection should be entertained in patients with aseptic meningitis, particularly when associated with other symptoms (rash).

Other viruses rarely causing aseptic meningitis include adenovirus, measles, and rubella.

### Bacteria

While bacterial meningitis typically presents as acute pyogenic meningitis, some bacterial infections can cause an aseptic meningitis syndrome. Patients with bacterial meningitis partially treated with antibiotics may have progressive symptoms of meningitis with a CSF profile very similar to aseptic viral meningitis. A careful history regarding the use of antibiotics should be obtained in patients with aseptic meningitis, and CSF counterimmunoelectrophoresis or latex agglutination against the common meningeal pathogens should be performed if partially treated meningitis is suspected. Parameningeal bacterial infections such as ostoeomyelitis of the vertebral body or skull and epidural empyema are associated with an aseptic meningitis. The CSF pleocytosis that accompanies these infections usually shows polymorphonuclear leukocytes (PMNs) as the predominant cell type. Symptoms of meningitis are generally mild, if present at all. Bacterial endocarditis can cause a cerebritis, characterized by vasculitis of the small cerebral vessels, which can also be associated with aseptic meningitis.

Spirochetes commonly cause brain infections with meningeal inflammation and a CSF profile similar to viral meningitis. Early (most commonly 2°) syphilis rarely (~1% of all cases) causes acute, aseptic meningitis that can be associated with hydrocephalus, cranial nerve palsies, and encephalitic changes; CSF changes include a monocytic pleocytosis, positive Venereal Disease Research Laboratory (VDRL), increasing protein (most patients), and reduced glucose concentrations (~50% of cases). Aseptic meningitis is a manifestation of early Lyme disease and is frequently associated with cranial and peripheral neuropathies. Symptoms are usually quite mild and the meningitis subsides without any specific therapy, although the disease progresses. Both the early and second phase of leptospirosis cause an aseptic meningitis. In the first phase, symptoms are typical for meningitis. Although the CSF is acellular at this stage, the spirochetes may be recovered in the CSF. After remission of symptoms, the second phase of the disease, mediated by an immune response to the spirochetes, causes very intense headaches with signs of encephalitis. The CSF shows a moderate lymphocytic pleocytosis and is sterile. The meningitis resolves without specific therapy over the course of a few weeks.

### Ameba

*Naegleria fowleri* (rarely *Acanthamoeba* spp.) can cause a rare, acute amebic meningoencephalitis that occurs most commonly in children and young adults. The organism is acquired by swimming in freshwater. The clinical picture is very acute, similar to bacterial meningitis with frequent signs indicating brain involvement. The CSF shows a polymorphonucear pleocytosis with increased protein and decreased glucose concentrations, blood, and a negative gram stain. A fresh sample of CSF should be examined for ameba directly under the microscope in suspected cases. The disease is fatal in 95% of cases.

### Noninfectious etiologies

Neurosurgery in the posterior fossa can result in an aseptic meningitis (*posterior fossa syndrome*). The cause of this syndrome is unknown. Patients typically have had a neurosurgical procedure in the days preceding the onset of meningitis and postoperative glucocorticoids are being tapered. Signs of meningitis appear rapidly, but patients often do not look very ill. The CSF has a polymorphonuclear pleocytosis with elevated protein and low glucose mimmicking bacterial meningitis, but cultures remain negative even if patients have not received antibiotics. The syndrome is diagnosed after excluding infectious causes (particularly bacteria) and is treated by increasing glucocorticoids for several days before restarting a slow taper.

Other noninfectious diseases causing aseptic meningitis include carcinomatous meningitis, sarcoidosis, systemic lupus erythematosis, and Behçet's disease. Many drugs have been linked to aseptic meningitis, most importantly trimethoprim-sulfamethoxazole, nonsteroidal antiinflammatory drugs, and the antibody directed against T cells, OKT3.

## Epidemiology

A recent report noted 8000–13,000 cases of aseptic meningits over a 7 yr period in the United States. The true incidence rate is likely to be higher since aseptic meningitis is often not reported. There is marked seasonal variation, with peaks in the summer and fall that lead to a four- to sevenfold increase over the rates in winter. The seasonal variation is a direct reflection of the acquisition of viral infections associated with aseptic meningitis (see above for specific viruses).

Aseptic meningitis is most commonly seen in children and young adults. Children often come in contact with enteroviruses in day care centers and school. Similarly, their caretakers and other young adults are the populations most frequently infected with enteroviruses. Younger adults are also most likely to come in contact with other agents causing aseptic meningitis, such as sexually transmitted infections (HIV, HSV, syphilis). Finally, outdoors activities can lead to aseptic meningitis by exposure to mosquitos (arboviruses), ticks (Colorado tick fever, Lyme disease), and animals or animal products (LCM, brucella).

## Clinical manifestations

The clinical manifestations of aseptic meningitis are often indistinguishable from bacterial meningitis. Fever, headache, photophobia, nausea with vomiting, and meningismus—all with acute onset—are most common. Severe neurologic findings, including seizures, on the other hand, are very uncommon in most forms of aseptic meningitis. Overall, symptoms are generally milder than those of pyogenic meningitis. Most cases of aspetic meningitis represent a self-limited disease that does not lead to sequelae, even though constitutional symptoms can persist for several weeks. Other clinical findings associated with specific etiologies are shown in Table 73.7.

### Laboratory studies

Laboratory tests routinely performed in the evaluation of febrile patients, including complete blood count (CBC), electrolytes, liver function tests, blood cultures, chest radiograph, and urinalysis show no or only nonspecific abnormalities in patients with aseptic meningitis. The most important laboratory study is the examination of the CSF. Cell counts with differential, glucose and protein concentrations, bacterial and fungal cultures, and CSF-VDRL should be performed routinely in all patients with suspected meningitis. Viral cultures of the CSF can be positive for some viruses, but the yield is generally low. To isolate enteroviruses, throat and stool should be sent for viral cultures, since after the first 3 d of symptoms, enteroviruses are only recovered in the stool and throat.

The remainder of the evaluation is guided by clinical judgment. CIE or LA against bacterial pathogens should be performed in the CSF if partially treated bacterial meningitis is suspected. Appropriate cultures and serologies should be preformed if brucellosis is a concern. Serologies for HIV, Lyme disease, and acute and convalescent LCM or mumps titers should be obtained based on clinical suspicions.

### Diagnosis

The diagnosis of aseptic meningitis is made based on the history, physical examination, and laboratory findings. The CSF profile characteristically shows a lymphocytic pleocytosis (>80% lymphocytes) with counts typically less than 1000 white blood cells/mm$^3$ (Table 73.3). Early in the course, the CSF may have a polymorphonuclear pleocytosis, suggesting bacterial meningitis. The pleocytosis, however, becomes lymphocytic over the first 48 h of illness. Thus, a follow-up lumbar puncture may help to establish the diagnosis. The glucose is typically normal, although there are some exceptions (e.g., mumps, LCM, herpes simplex) (see Table 73.7). CSF protein concentration is typically normal or mildly elevated. Bacterial and fungal cultures of the CSF are sterile (barring contamination). Other laboratory tests outlined above may assist in the identification of the causative agent. In at least 30% of cases, no etiology can be identified.

### Treatment

Typically, the clinician is confronted with a febrile patient with signs of meningeal irritation. After a lumbar puncture, patients are often started on antibiotics to cover possible bacterial infection (see empiric therapy of bacterial meningitis, Table 73.4). Antibiotics can be stopped if the CSF formula is more compatible with aseptic than pyogenic meningitis and if CSF cultures remain negative. Viral meningitis is a benign illness and resolves without specific therapy in most patients. In patients who have hypo- or agammaglobulinemia and severe meningoencephalitis, intravenous and intrathecal immunoglobulin may be helpful. Supportive measures such as intravenous hydration and analgesia may offer patients symptomatic relief. If a causative agent is identified, treatment must be tailored accordingly.

## Chronic Meningitis

Chronic meningitis is a syndrome characterized by signs and symptoms of meningitis, often accompanied by signs of encephalitis, and CSF inflammation with a lymphocytic predominance. There are many infectious and noninfectious etiologies of this syndrome, a number of which lead to substantial morbidity and mortality. Clinical presentation, laboratory tests, and CSF findings have few distinguishing features and cultures are frequently negative, thus challenging the clinician's skills in evaluating and treating patients with chronic meningitis.

Chronic meningitis must be distinguished from recurrent meningitis. Patients with chronic meningitis have progressive symptoms with persistent CSF abnormalities over days to months without disease free periods. Patients with recurrent meningitis, in contrast, have recurrent acute periods of disease interspersed with disease-free intervals.

### Etiologies

#### Bacteria

##### *Tuberculosis*

Tuberculous meningitis is the most common cause of chronic meningitis. The presentation is typical for chronic meningitis, with slowly progressive headache and signs of meningeal irritation with or without fever. Abducens nerve (lateral rectus) palsy and other cranial nerve palsies as well as hydrocephalus are common complications. Untreated, the disease progresses to severe encephalopathy, with mental status changes, coma, and ultimately death. In younger patients, tuberculous meningitis often occurs during active primary infection at extraneural sites, while in older patients, it often represents reactivated disease limited to the central nervous system. PPD skin tests are negative in up to 50% of patients presenting with tuberculous meningitis. The diagnosis is confirmed by a positive CSF culture; however, tubercle bacilli are recovered in only 38%–88% of cases. The CSF smears for acid-fast bacilli are positive in a minority of cases (10%–20%). CSF typically shows a moderate pleocytosis with several hundred cells and predominance of lymphocytes. The glucose concentration is often low; protein concentration is usually markedly elevated.

##### *Syphilis*

All forms of neurosyphilis are associated with a chronic meningitis. Cranial nerve palsies are common, with facial and acoustic nerves most frequently affected. Hypoglycorrachia is seen in half of all cases. The diagnosis is made by a positive CSF-VDRL associated with mild, lymphocytic CSF inflammation.

##### *Lyme Disease*

*Borrelia burgdorferi* infection should be considered in patients with meningitis who had a possible tick exposure in endemic regions. Many do not recall the tick bite, but the rash of Lyme disease, erythema migrans, is often noticed. Meningitis may persist for weeks and may be associated with cranial and peripheral neuropathies (see Chapter 95).

#### *Brucella*

Chronic meningitis is an unusual complication of brucellosis. Symptoms of brucella meningitis tend to progress over months to years. The diagnosis should be entertained when there is a history of exposure to farm animals or their unpasterized products in endemic regions (Mediterranean, Central America). Transient hemianesthesias and paresthesias are prominent; CSF cultures are positive in less than half of all cases, but antibody tests in serum are highly sensitive and specific.

### Fungi

#### *Cryptococcus*

Meningitis caused by *Cryptococcus neoformans*, a ubiquitous fungus, presents with symptoms ranging from subacute meningoencephalitis to fever of unknown origin. Defects in cellular immunity, such as AIDS, Hodgkin's disease, lymphosarcoma, and prolonged use of high dose steroids represent a high risk for the infection, but in the pre-AIDS era, half of all cases of cryptococcal meningitis occurred in patients who had no identified immune defect. Cerebrospinal fluid usually shows a moderate lymphocytic pleocytosis, but in AIDS patients inflammation may be absent. The glucose concentration is usually slightly reduced and protein concentration elevated. Examination of the CSF with India ink can quickly alert the clinician to the diagnosis, but is insensitive. Cryptococcal antigen latex agglutination is more sensitive (>85% sensitivity); it should also be performed on the patients serum. A false-positive cryptococcal antigen may be caused by infection with *Trichosporon beigii*; CSF fungal cultures confirm the diagnosis.

#### *Coccidioidomycosis*

*Coccidioides immitis* grows in the dry, sandy soils of the southwestern United States and Central and South America. Infection is acquired by inhalation of the spores. Meningitis may present during disseminated disease or as an isolated syndrome following primary, subclinical infection. High-risk groups for disseminated disease include Filipinos, blacks, Native Americans, Hispanics, Asians, and pregnant women. There are few distinguishing features of the disease; some patients with generalized disease have erythema nodosum, and hydrocephalus is a common complication of meningitis. Cerebrospinal fluid eosinophilia in patients with a compatible exposure history should alert the clinician to the possibility of coccidioidal meningitis. Complement-fixing antibodies are present in the CSF in 75%–95% of cases. The diagnosis may also be made with a serum complement-fixing antibody titer of ≥1:16. Cerebrospinal fluid cultures are positive in one-third to one-half of patients. The laboratory should be alerted to the possible presence of *Coccidioides* in clinical specimens to allow for measures to protect personnel from exposure.

#### *Histoplasmosis*

Chronic meningitis is a rare complication of histoplasmosis. The diagnosis should be entertained in patients from the endemic regions—Ohio River Valley of the United States, the Caribbean, and South America. In normal hosts, oral mucosal lesions of histoplasma are seen in ~15% of patients and may be diagnostic. Cerebrospinal fluid cultures are positive in 27%–65% of cases. Histoplasma polysaccharide antigen is found in the urine, blood, or CSF in the majority of patients.

#### *Opportunistic fungi*

Candida and aspergillus rarely cause meningitis as a result of disseminated infection or intracranial placement of a shunt or drain. Risk factors for fungemia by these opportunistic pathogens are severe granulocytopenia, prolonged use of antibiotics or steroids, hyperalimentation, abdominal surgery, intravenous drug use and intravenous catheter use. Neonates are particularly prone to disseminated candidal infection. A neutrophilic pleocytosis and hypoglycorrachia are typically present and may initially suggest the diagnosis of bacterial meningitis. CSF cultures are diagnostic.

### Parasites

#### *Neurocysticercosis*

Cysticercosis is endemic in Mexico, South America, and Asia. Infection is acquired by eating food contaminated with eggs of *Taenia solium* (pork tapeworm). Larvae traverse the intestines and disseminate into tissue where they encyst and remain largely quiescent. Symptomatic disease develops as the larvae degenerate, presumably by inciting an immune response. Seizures are the most common presentation. Intraventricular cysts and basilar cysts (racemose cysticercosis) may present with signs of obstructive hydrocephalus and lead to CSF alterations, including a lymphocytic pleocytosis with eosinophils. Head CT scans showing multiple, partially calcified lesions, and serologies provide support for the diagnosis.

#### *Acanthamoeba*

*Acanthamoeba* spp. are a rare cause of a chronic, granulomatous meningoencephalitis occurring in immunosuppressed patients. Patients often have seizures and other focal neurologic deficits and the disease progresses to death over weeks to months. The CSF shows a mild to moderate mononuclear pleocytosis.

#### *Angiostrongylus cantonensi*

The rat lung worm is most prevalent in Asia and the Pacific Islands and is acquired most often by ingestion of raw or inadequately cooked shellfish or snails. Symptoms are typical for chronic meningitis; rash with pruritus is also common. Infection results in peripheral eosinophilia and chronic eosinophilic meningitis. Worldwide, it is the most common cause of eosinophilic meningitis. It resolves spontaneously within 2 mo.

### Other infections

Other less common infectious causes of chronic meningitis are organisms that usually cause abscesses but may leak into the subarachnoid space, such as blastomycosis, paracoccidioidomycosis, phaeohyphomycoses, *mucor* spp., actinomycosis, nocardia, and toxoplasmosis. Less common fungi causing this syndrome include *Sporothrix schenckii* and chromoblastomycoses.

### Noninfectious

#### *Neoplastic disease*

Meningeal carcinomatosis may cause a chronic meningitis which is difficult to distinguish from infectious etiologies. Subacute onset of intractable headache and altered mental status, often associated with cranial nerve palsies, represent the typical clinical presentation. While the CSF pleocytosis is mild, the glucose is frequently disproportionately low. Examination of the CSF cytology may show atypical cells. Cancers of the breast, lung, stomach, pancreas, malignant melanoma, and primary brain tumors commonly cause meningeal carcinomatosis. Hematologic cancers such as leukemias and lymphomas may also cause this syndrome.

#### *Sarcoidosis*

Neurosarcoidosis is an uncommon complication of sarcoid. Basilar inflammation is a prominent feature of the disease resulting in cranial nerve palsies. Peripheral neuropathies, long tract signs, cerebellar abnormalities, and diabetes insipidus have also been reported. The CSF shows a lymphocytic pleocytosis and usually a normal glucose. Signs of the systemic disease lead to the diagnosis, while isolated neurosarcoidosis can be very difficult to diagnose, even with invasive tissue biopsies.

#### *Others*

Less common noninfectious causes include granulomatous angiitis, Behçet syndrome, and Vogt-Koyanagi-Harada syndrome.

## Clinical manifestations

Symptoms of chronic meningitis show few characteristic features that would allow clues as to the underlying etiology. Headache usually is of gradual onset; signs of overt meningeal irritation are often subtle in the early stages of disease. Left to progress untreated, signs of encephalitis may follow, resulting in a picture of subacute meningoencephalitis. Associated symptoms include malaise, fatigue, nausea with vomiting, and progressive intellectual decline. Fever may be variable or consistently absent. Neurologic findings depend on the involved areas of the brain, but there are some distinguishing features of the neurologic syndrome associated with specific etiologies of chronic meningitis (Table 73.8).

The general exam is critical in patients with chronic meningitis and may give clues to the diagnosis. The skin may show evidence of secondary syphilis, cryptococcal disease, erythema nodosum (coccidioidomycosis, sarcoidosis), or histoplasmosis. Lymphadenopathy and hepatosplenomegaly may suggest systemic illnesses such as sarcoidosis, cancer, or disseminated infections. Lung exam, including chest radiographs, can provide important findings in many systemic diseases, including tuberculosis, coccidioidomycosis, histoplasmosis, and sarcoidosis. Many causes of chronic meningitis may be associated with uveitis or retinal lesions that can be identified on an eye exam.

**Table 73.8** Chronic meningitis associated with basilar localization and cranial nerve palsies*

| Etiology | Cranial nerve palsy |
|---|---|
| Tuberculosis | VI |
| Lyme disease | VII[a] |
| Sarcoidosis | VII |
| Syphilis | VII, VIII |
| Carcinomatous meningitis | VI, VII |

*Basilar meningitis may lead to neuropathies of many cranial nerves. The most common associations are shown.

[a]Often bilateral.

## Laboratory studies

Many systemic diseases can be associated with chronic meningitis, and general laboratory studies, including complete blood cell count and WBC differential, liver and kidney function, etc., should be performed, even though they rarely identify specific etiologies of meningitis. Blood cultures for fungi, mycobacteria, and, if indicated, brucella, should be obtained; WBC buffy coat should be examined, if histoplasmosis is suspected. Serologies can provide supportive evidence for many of the infectious causes of chronic meningitis (cryptococcosis, syphilis, histoplasma, coccidioides, cysticercosis [*Taenia solium*], brucella).

Examination of the CSF should include cell counts with differential, glucose and protein concentration, CSF-VDRL, cytology, and cryptococcal antigen test. Cerebrospinal fluid should be cultured for bacteria, fungi, mycobacteria and, if indicated, brucella.

Brain imaging studies can be very helpful in patients with chronic meningitis. Many of the etiologies of chronic meningitis cause a basilar meningitis that can be visualized on MRI scan with its excellent resolution of the brainstem and posterior fossa. Calcified lesions such as those of neurocysticercosis or tuberculomas are best seen on CT scan.

## Diagnosis

A careful history is indispensable in the evaluation of patients with chronic meningitis. Many cases of chronic meningitis defy diagnosis by culture, serology, or cytology, and a presumptive diagnosis is based on clues from the history, unique clinical features, supportive laboratory findings, and response to empiric therapy (e.g., tuberculosis). A history of residence in or travel to areas of the world with endemic infections or exposure to animals or animal vectors (ticks) must be carefully obtained.

Important clues may be present on physical examination (see above). The CSF profile, although similar for many causes of chronic meningitis, can have some unique features (Tables 73.3, 73.9); MRI or CT scan of the brain may support the diagnosis of cysticercosis, toxoplasmosis, or lymphoma. They can also document evidence of brain involvement (encephalitis).

**Table 73.9** Cellular characteristics of CSF pleocytosis in chronic meningitis

| Neutrophilic | Eosinophilic |
|---|---|
| *Actinomycosis* | *Coccidioides* |
| *Nocardia* | Neurocysticercosis |
| *Brucella* | Schistosomiasis |
| *Aspergillus* | *Angiostrongylus* |
| *Pseudallescheria* | *Gnathostoma* |
| *Candida* | Lymphoma |
| Cytomegalovirus in HIV patients | |

## Treatment

Tuberculous meningitis is treated with standard antituberculous regimens, unless dictated otherwise by known resistance (see Chapter 37). Initial therapy includes isoniazid, rifampin, ethambutol, and in cases of increased likelihood of isoniazid (INH) resistance pyrazinamide; all these drugs appear to cross the blood-brain barrier sufficiently to achieve adequate concentration in the CSF. The daily dose of INH should be increased to 10 mg/kg until clinical improvement is seen. The duration of therapy is the same as for pulmonary tuberculosis (Chapter 57). Prednisone at a dose 60–80 mg per day is advocated by many authorities. Steroids are tapered once there is clinical improvement. Patients should be followed for the development of hydrocephalus, which is a common complication of tuberculous meningitis and may require shunting.

Neurosyphilis is best treated with 12–24 million units per day of intravenous aqueous crystalline penicillin for 10–14 d. Daily procaine penicillin (2.4 million units intramuscularly) with probenecid for 10–14 d may be an alternative regimen. Because other antibiotics have not been adequately studied, patients who are penicillin allergic should be considered for desensitization. CSF should be examined every 6 mo until the inflammation has subsided to assess the adequacy of treatment. HIV-infected patients may have a increased risk for treatment failures and should be followed more frequently (every 3 mo).

Facial nerve palsies from Lyme disease may be treated with doxycycline 100 mg orally twice daily for 21 d as in early Lyme disease; amoxicillin may be used as an alternative agent. Active meningitis should be treated with ceftriaxone, 2 g/d intravenously, for 21 d.

Brucella meningitis is treated with doxycycline plus one or two other antibiotics. Most authorities recommend trimethoprim/sulfamethoxazole with or without rifampin in addition to doxycycline. Therapy should be continued until there is resolution of symptoms and normalization of the CSF.

In patients not infected with HIV, standard therapy for cryptococcal meningitis consists of amphotericin B combined with 5-flucytosine. Amphotericin is dosed at 0.3 mg/kg/d to achieve a total dose of 2.5 g; 5-flucytosine is given at a dose of 37.5 mg/kg every 6 h orally for 6 wk. Fluconazole may be used after clinical improvement. In AIDS patients, mild disease (defined as an absence of mental status changes and CSF cryptococcal antigen titers $<$1:1028) may be treated with fluconazole, 400 mg daily, for 6–10 wk. For more severe disease, amphotericin B (0.6–0.9 mg/kg daily) is recommended for at least the first 2 wk of therapy. If the patient is clinically improved after 2 wk, therapy can be switched to fluconazole. HIV-infected patients are rarely cured and require permanent suppression of the disease (see Chapter 102). Fluconazole, 100–200 mg daily, is the chronic suppressive therapy of choice.

*Coccidioides* meningitis may have to be treated with intrathecal amphotericin B, even though limited experience suggests that fluconazole may be effective in some patients. The amphotericin dose is 0.1–0.3 mg intrathecally and may be administered daily in patients who tolerate the medication or thrice weekly in those who are less tolerant. Intrathecal amphotericin may cause an arachnoiditis with worsening of symptoms. Therapy should be continued until the CSF WBC is less than ten; then amphotericin should be reduced to once or twice weekly until the CSF is normal for 1 yr. Systemic amphotericin is also administered to treat any extraneural sites of infection (total dose 0.5 to 1.0 g). Relapse rates are high despite aggressive therapy.

CNS histoplasmosis is treated with amphotericin B, 0.7 mg/kg daily, for 2 wk, followed by 50 mg every other day to achieve a total dose of 10–15 mg/kg. In severe cases, intrathecal amphotericin B may be required. Relapse rates are very high, despite maximal therapy.

Cysticercosis is treated traditionally with praziquantel, 50 mg/kg/d, in three doses, for 2 wk, combined with prednisone to reduce the risk of CNS side effects caused by heightened inflammation from the dying parasite. Some experts advocate the use of albendazole, which achieves similar response rates with a lower incidence of seizures. Seizures require antiepileptic therapy (phenytoin or pentobarbital). Shunts should be placed in patients with hydrocephalus.

### ANNOTATED BIBLIOGRAPHY


Ellner JJ, Bennett JE. Chronic meningitis. Medicine 1976; 55:341–369.
*Review of cases with comments and notations of the salient clinical features of the various etiologies.*

Gripshover BM, Ellner JJ. Chronic meningitis. In: Principles and Practice of Infectious Diseases. Mandell GL, Bennett JE, Dolin R, eds. Churchill Livingstone, New York, 1995.
*Excellent general overview of chronic meningitis.*

Leonard JM, Des Pres RM. Tuberculous meningitis. Infect Dis Clin North Am 1990; 4:769–787.
*An excellent review of the literature covering a difficult topic. It addresses all important aspects of clinical presentation, diagnostic approach, and therapy, including the role of corticosteroids.*

Odio CM, Faingezicht I, Paris M et al. The beneficial effects of early dexamethasone administration in infants and children with bacterial meningitis. N Engl J Med 1991; 324:1525–1531.
*Dexamethasone as adjunctive therapy to antibiotics may be beneficial, particularly in children with* Hemophilus meningitis. *One important effect of dexamethasone is blockage of cytokines (TNF-α, IL-1, IL-6) that are released when bacteria are lysed following their encounter with antibiotics. The optimal time point for the administration of dexamethasone seems to be just prior to or simultaneously with the first antibiotic dose.*

Rotbart HA. Viral meningitis and the aseptic meningitis syndrome. In: Infections in the Central Nervous System. Scheld WM, Whitley RJ, Durack DT, eds. Raven Press, New York, 1991.
*A thorough and comprehensive review of the topic, with all the necessary practical information for the management of patients with aseptic meningitis.*

Spanos A, Harrell FE, Durack DT. Differential diagnosis of acute meningitis—an analysis of the predictive value of initial observation. JAMA 1989; 262:2700–2707.
*CSF examination is still the most important diagnostic test; CSF culture is most sensitive, gram stain has a sensitivity of 70%–80%, and detection of antigens is generally not more sensitive than gram stain. When markedly*

*abnormal, CSF neutrophil count and CSF glucose and protein concentrations are all highly predictive of bacterial meningitis.*

Täuber MG, Sande MA. General principles of therapy of pyogenic meningitis. Infect Dis Clin North Am 1990; 4:661–676.

*A summary of the principles that guide antimicrobial therapy of bacterial meningitis. High doses of antibiotics that are bactericidal against the infecting organism and achieve CSF levels at least ten to 30 times the minimal bactericidal concentration (MBC) usually can sterilize the CSF within 12 h. Release of proinflammatory bacterial products may be a problem.*

Tunkel AR, Wispelwey B, Scheld WM. Bacterial meningitis: recent advances in pathophysiology and treatment. Ann Intern Med 1990; 112:610–623.

*Experimental work over the last decade has provided us with a much better understanding of the molecular aspects of inflammation and the pathophysiology of bacterial meningitis. This review summarizes these findings and discusses practical aspects of the management of meningitis.*

Wenger JD, Hightower AW, Facklam RR et al. Bacterial meningitis in the United States, 1986: report of a multistate surveillance study. J Infect Dis 1990; 162:1316–1323.

*The most recent study on the epidemiology of bacterial meningitis in the United States performed by the CDC.* Hemophilus influenzae *was the most frequent pathogen, followed by* N. meningitidis *and* S. pneumoniae. *With the new* H. influenzae *type b vaccines, this has changed dramatically.*

# 74

# Encephalitis

R. TYLER FRIZZELL AND RICHARD J. WHITLEY

The term *encephalitis* refers to acute or subacute infection of brain tissue. This infection is frequently accompanied by altered mentation, fever, and neurological signs such as seizures. Whatever the etiologic agent, encephalitis can result in significant neurological morbidity and mortality and remains a major public health problem worldwide. The loss of life and productivity is especially tragic because its victims are often young and otherwise healthy individuals. Worldwide, measles and Japanese B encephalitis account for tens of thousands of cases of central nervous system (CNS) infection. In the United States, approximately 20,000 cases of encephalitis occur yearly, most of which are clinically mild. Herpes simplex virus (HSV) is the principal cause of sporadic encephalitis and is associated with significant morbidity and mortality in spite of available treatment (Fig. 74.1). While the list of organisms that can infect brain tissue is long, ranging from protozoans such as *Toxoplasma gondii* to spirochetes (*Treponema pallidum*, *Borrelia burgdorferi*) and pyogenic bacteria that cause meningitis (Chapter 73), this chapter focuses on acute viral and postinfectious encephalitis.

## Etiology

Many viruses can cause infection of the CNS, resulting in either encephalitis or meningitis; however, rabies and B virus cause encephalitis only. Table 74.1 summarizes the most important etiologic agents associated with encephalitis, according to viral classification. Viruses that cause encephalitis can be broadly classified as among either the DNA or RNA families of viruses. Among the DNA viruses, herpesviruses (HSV-1, HSV-2, cytomegalovirus (CMV), varicella-zoster virus [VZV], Epstein-Barr virus [EBV], human herpesvirus-6 [HHV-6], and B virus), especially HSV, are the leading causes of human disease both in the United States as well as worldwide. The RNA viruses are a more heterogeneous group that cause CNS disease and include arboviruses, enteroviruses, paramyxoviruses (measles and mumps), rhabdovirus (rabies), arenaviruses (lymphocytic choriomeningitis), and retroviruses.

## General Pathogenesis and Host Response

This chapter excludes chronic CNS viral diseases, including HIV encephalopathy (see Chapter 97). Most CNS viral infections present with similar histopathological findings, but disease pathogenesis is quite different. Viremia and retrograde neuronal transport are both important mechanisms involved in the pathogenesis of encephalitis. Postinfectious encephalitis appears to be an autoimmune response as evidenced by the absence of viral antigen in the brain and associated characteristic CNS and systemic immune responses.

Viral infection of the CNS may be a manifestation of either primary and/or secondary viremia. Viral replication at the site of entry is followed by primary viremia and spread to regional lymph nodes as well as other portions of the reticuloendothelial system (RES); secondary viremia may ensue. The development of encephalitis is determined in part by the magnitude of viremia. Capillary endothelial cells in the brain support the replication of some viruses, including enteroviruses, togaviruses, and bunyaviruses. Arenaviruses infect choroid plexus epithelial cells.

In another mechanism of CNS entry, mononuclear cells, such as mumps-infected T cells, may invade the CNS by diapedesis at portions of the nervous system having fenestrations in the capillaries. Once virus enters the CNS, specific *neurovirulence* factors influence the development of disease. Neurovirulence is the ability of the virus to cause CNS disease and is determined by both viral growth in the brain and neuroinvasiveness. Growth in the CNS is the most common measure of virulence. Neuroinvasiveness reflects the capacity of the virus to enter the CNS from a portal of entry.

Man possesses complex host defenses against viral infections in general, especially those leading to encephalitis. Natural barriers to infection include the skin, gastric pH, respiratory cilia, and the blood-brain barrier. This last barrier comprises endothelial cells with interspersing tight junctions, a continuous basement membrane, and glial cells with foot processes.

Humoral and cellular immune defenses of the CNS include responses of T and B lymphocytes, monocyte/macrophages, and the extracellular proteins produced by these cells (Chapter 11). $CD4^+$ helper cells of the CNS produce cytokines which are important for T- and B-cell regulation and monocyte/macrophage activation. Antigen recognition by $CD4^+$ T cells is MHC class II restricted. The $CD8^+$ T cell is a cytotoxic suppressor which is MHC class I restricted. These cells also produce cytokines that may lead to local inflammation. Macrophages influence activation of T and B cells and are important in the development of immune-mediated demyelination. Host genetic differences are likely to influence defense against viruses causing encephalitis. The relevant host defenses involved in CNS infections are considered with each pathogen.

## Postinfectious and Postvaccination Encephalitis

The pathogenesis of encephalitis following infection with influenza, measles, acute hemorrhagic leukoencephalitis virus, or Semple rabies vaccination appears to be immune regulated. Demyelination and perivenular inflammation are characteristic

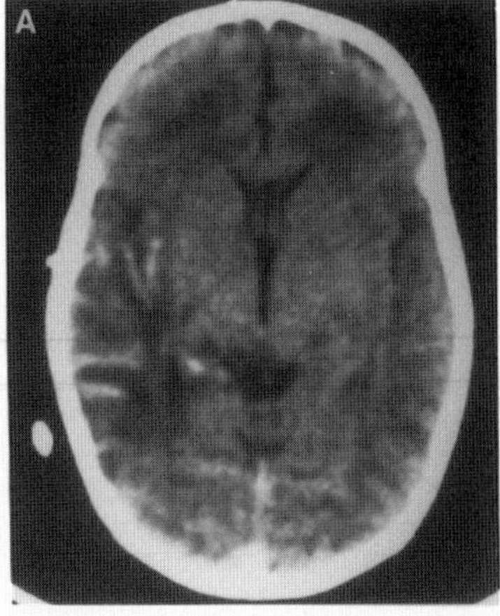

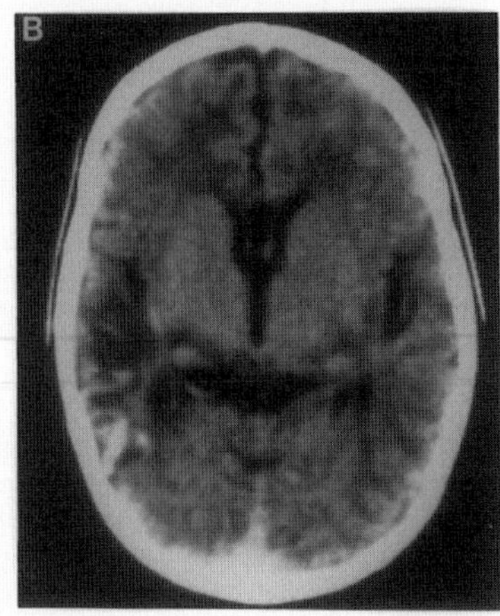

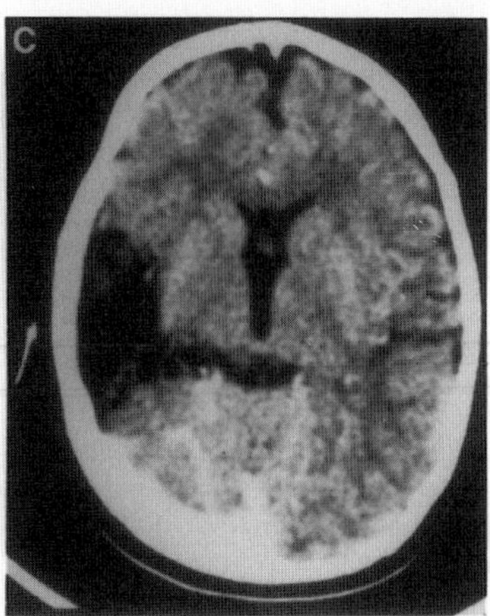


**Fig. 74.1** Serial CT scanning (24 h intervals) of a patient with confirmed HSE.

features as observed in experimental allergic encephalitis. This disorder is a cell-mediated autoimmune disease in animals following myelin/adjuvant administration. Soluble factors released by the $CD4^+$ cells, including interleukin [IL]-2 and $\gamma$-interferon, are increased locally in the affected brain tissue. With disease resolution, local levels of IL-4, IL-10, and transforming growth factor-beta (TGF-$\beta$) increase. These cytokines are thought to be downregulators of the immune response (Chapter 12). Oral administration of myelin basic protein to immunized animals results in an increase in these cytokines systemically as well as the suppression of the encephalitis in animal models.

In measles, cytotoxic lymphocytes directed against myelin basic protein have been identified in 47% of encephalitis cases but also in 15% of individuals without encephalitis. No measles antibodies are recovered from the cerebrospinal fluid (CSF) and no viral antigen can be visualized. On the other hand, evidence of measles infection of the CNS can be detected by polymerase chain reaction (PCR) of the CSF. Activation of T cells follows measles infection, but the mechanisms which lead to encephalitis remain unclear. Most patients (75%) with post-Sample rabies vaccine encephalitis demonstrate antibody against myelin basic protein.

## Epidemiology, Clinical Presentation, and Treatment

### Herpes virus infections

#### Herpes simplex virus

*Epidemiology*

Herpes simplex encephalitis (HSE) occurs worldwide and throughout the year. Human to human contact is responsible for transmission of HSV. The spread of HSV-1 is usually by saliva or lesion vesicular fluid (labial or genital). HSV-2 is spread by direct contact with infectious genital secretions.

Brain infection attributed to HSV can be caused by either HSV-1 or HSV-2, differing primarily according to age. During the newborn period, HSV-2 is the usual cause of CNS infection, but HSV-1 can also infect the brain. Neonatal HSV infection occurs at an incidence of approximately one in 3500 live births yearly. Over 50% of neonates with HSV infection have CNS disease. In contrast, individuals over 6 mo of age with HSE have disease primarily caused by HSV-1. The incidence of HSE in older individuals is about one in 200,000 in the United States, resulting in approximately 1250 cases yearly. One-third of the cases of HSE occur in individuals less than 20 yr of age while one-half occur in patients greater than 50 yr old.

Significant morbidity occurs in survivors of HSV infections of the CNS, even with treatment, irrespective of age. For example, following neonatal HSE, less than 50% of surviving children develop normally. For older children and adults, only approximately 30% of survivors return to normal function.

*Pathogenesis*

Encephalitis which occurs in the newborn differs from that in older individuals. Intrapartum infection is the most common mode of transmission of neonatal HSV infection, accounting for over 85% of cases. Risk factors for the acquisition of neonatal HSV infection include application of a fetal scalp monitor, type of maternal infection (primary versus recurrent), and duration of ruptured membranes (>6 h). Infection of the newborn brain can either localize to the temporal lobes or result in diffuse gray matter disease.

In older children and adults, cranial nerves I and V have been defined as portals of HSV entry into the CNS, although direct evidence is lacking. Classically, a necrotizing process affects the inferior medial portion of the temporal lobe. Approximately 30% of HSE cases are caused by primary infection and the remainder by recurrent infection. Once in the CNS, HSV infects the cell and shuts off cellular DNA, RNA, and protein synthesis after initiating transcription of $\alpha$ (immediate early), $\beta$ (early), and $\gamma$ (late) genes. The cell is lysed, and newly formed virus is released.

The neuroinvasive properties of HSV have been studied. Mutant viruses (thymidine kinase mutants or genetically engineered viruses), as a rule, are at least 10,000-fold less likely to cause encephalitis when inoculated intracerebrally in animal models. Similarly, glycoprotein (g)E and gI mutants do not cause encephalitis in animals. Importantly, an HSV neurovirulence gene, the $\gamma_1$ 34.5 gene, has been defined in experimental systems. The deletion of this gene renders HSV avirulent in animal models of CNS disease.

**Table 74.1** Causes of viral encephalitis

| | Approximate incidence | Comments |
|---|---|---|
| HERPES VIRUSES | | |
| HSV | 1250 cases/year in USA | Most common cause of sporadic fatal encephalitis in USA |
| VZV | 1/1000 patients with chicken pox develop CNS disease | Mortality low except in immunosuppressed patients |
| CMV | 1/1000 live births | Rare cause of encephalitis in healthy adults |
| EBV | Increasingly recognized as diagnostic techniques improve | Low mortality |
| B viruses | 30 cases responded in literature | Severe encephalitis, mortality high |
| ARBOVIRUSES | | |
| *ALPHAVIRUSES* | | |
| EKE | Low but outbreaks occur | Mortality 50%–75% |
| WEE | | Mortality 3%–9% |
| VEE | | Mortality 1% |
| *FLAVIVIRUSES* | | |
| SLE | Low but outbreaks occur | Mortality 2%–20% |
| Japanese B | Several epidemics documented | Mortality 20%–50% |
| *BUNYEVIRUSES* | | |
| LaCrosse | Most common cause arbovirus infection in USA | Mortality low |
| California | Low but outbreaks occur | Mortality low |
| RHABDOVIRUSES | | |
| Rabies | High in certain regions of the world | Uniformally fatal |
| ARENAVIRUSES | | |
| LCMV | Low | |
| Lassa Fever | Low | Cause of hemorrhagic fever |
| PARAMYXOVIRUSES | | |
| Mumps | Uncommon where vaccine is routine | Common cause of meningoencephalitis in unvaccinated |
| Measles | 1.5 million/yr mortality in world | Most deaths associated with opportunistic infections |
| ENTEROVIRUSES | | |
| Polioviruses | Common where vaccination is not routine | |
| Echovirus | | Usually causes aseptic meningitis; mortality low |
| Coxsackievirus | | |
| ORTHOMYXOVIRUSES | | Follows postinfluenza encephalitis; mortality low |

### *Clinical presentation*

Neonatal HSV infection of the CNS is characterized by seizures, tremors, bulging fontanelle, and long-tract signs. Skin lesions are absent in at least 40% of cases; thus, CNS infection must be considered in neonates with fever even in the absence of skin lesions. Most cases (75%) of disseminated HSV infection have associated encephalitis. The morbidity associated with brain infection is high. Many survivors have neurological deficits such as spasticity, blindness, and mental retardation, in spite of early intervention with antiviral therapy. Imaging studies show devastating brain changes such as porencephaly and encephalomalacia.

Herpes simplex encephalitis in older children and adults presents with a history of fever, headache, and altered consciousness (all occur in over 90% of patients), although these findings are not specific. The patient's level of consciousness varies from alert to comatose and usually continues downward with little evidence of improvement in the absence of therapy. Focal neurological signs, including aphasia or dysphasia, anosmia, and focal seizures, are common (about 50% of cases). Papilledema is a less common finding and, certainly, a poor prognostic sign, warranting rapid intervention. A focal seizure in the presence of the acute onset of fever and CSF pleiocytosis should alert the physician to the possibility of HSE. Since HSE is a treatable disease, its inclusion in the differential diagnosis and the initiation of acyclovir therapy are essential.

Many other CNS diseases can mimic HSE (Table 74.2). In one study of 432 patients undergoing brain biopsy for presumptive HSE, HSV was the cause of encephalitis in only 45% of cases.

**Table 74.2** Diseases that mimic herpes simplex encephalitis*

| Disease | No. of patients |
|---|---|
| TREATABLE (38) | |
| *ABSCESS OR SUBDURAL EMPYEMA* | |
| Bacterial | 5 |
| Listeria | 1 |
| Fungal | 2 |
| Mycoplasmal | 2 |
| Tuberculosis | 6 |
| Cryptococcal | 3 |
| Rickettsial | 2 |
| Toxoplasmosis | 1 |
| Mucormycosis | 1 |
| Meningococcal meningitis | 1 |
| Tumor | 5 |
| Subdural hematoma | 2 |
| Systemic lupus erythematosus | 1 |
| Adrenal leukodystrophy | 6 |
| NONTREATABLE (57) | |
| *NONVIRAL* | |
| Vascular disease | 11 |
| Toxic encephalopathy | 5 |
| Reye's syndrome | 1 |
| *VIRAL* | |
| Togavirus infections | |
| St. Louis encephalitis | 7 |
| Western equine encephalomyelitis | 3 |
| California encephalitis | 4 |
| Eastern equine encephalitis | 2 |
| *OTHER HERPESVIRUSES* | |
| Epstein Barr virus | 8 |
| Cytomegalovirus | 1 |
| *OTHERS* | |
| Echovirus infection | 3 |
| Influenza A | 4 |
| Mumps | 3 |
| Adenovirus infection | 1 |
| Progressive multifocal leukoencephalopathy | 1 |
| Lymphocytic choriomeningitis | 1 |
| Subacute sclerosing panencephalitis | 2 |

*Data drawn from 432 patients: 195 (45%) had HSV; 142 (33%) had no diagnosis; 95 (22%) had *other* diagnosis, which is tabulated here.

In 22% of cases, alternative diagnoses were established, including infections of bacterial, fungal, and parasitic origin. Other identified disease processes included vascular disease, subdural hematoma, tumor, and adrenal leukodystrophy. In 33% of cases, however, no diagnosis could be made.

### *Host response*

Antibody responses in HSE correlate with disease severity. Cytotoxic T-lymphocyte responses are depressed in HSE, at least in adults; but, the contribution of cell-mediated immune responses to the disease pathogenesis is unknown.

Humoral immune responses in the newborn are not totally protective against neonatal HSV encephalitis. The presence of antibody at the onset of the disease appears to restrict disease to the skin or CNS. Neonates with encephalitis demonstrate delayed T-cell proliferative responses to HSV as compared to older children with disease. Disease progression may be more extensive in neonates with severely impaired T-cell responses. Levels of interferon $\alpha$ and $\gamma$ are depressed in neonates with encephalitis whereas tumor necrosis factor (TNF)-$\alpha$ levels are unchanged.

The detection of antibodies in the CSF of older children and adults has been used for diagnostic purposes (seroconversion in the CSF). However, humoral immune responses do not occur promptly enough to assist in making decisions on the institution of antiviral therapy. At present, infection of the central nervous system by herpes simplex virus is best detected by PCR of CSF or viral isolation and/or antigen detection of brain tissue.

## Varicella-zoster virus

### *Epidemiology*

Varicella-zoster virus (VZV) infection occurs worldwide and humans are the only reservoir. Virus is spread by respiratory secretions, and disease appears most prevalent in the winter and spring. Most children experience varicella in the preschool years; the annualized incidence of chickenpox is equivalent to the birth rate. The incidence of CNS complications of varicella is approximately 1 in 1000 cases. Yearly, there are approximately 300,000 to 500,000 cases of shingles in the United States. Following herpes zoster, 1%–5% of patients develop paresis in regions adjacent to the affected dermatome. The paresis usually occurs within 2 wk of the rash onset. In those who develop CNS symptoms, the neurological signs suggest a diffuse encephalitis without focal localization. Patients who develop encephalitis usually recover completely except for some who are immunosuppressed.

### *Pathogenesis*

Varicella-zoster virus replicates in the mucosa of the upper respiratory tract and produces a primary viremia. Virus seeds the reticuloendothelial system (RES) and replicates at that site; secondary viremia develops with the subsequent appearance of typical cutaneous lesions of chickenpox. Infection of capillary endothelial cells, including those of the CNS, and mononuclear cells occurs. In some patients, particularly those with AIDS, electron microscopy demonstrates the presence of herpes virus–like particles; in situ hybridization has been employed to confirm VZV antigen in the brain. Varicella CNS disease may also be postinfectious. In these cases, signs of CNS disease occur weeks after infection, and CNS pathology reveals demyelination.

### *Clinical presentation*

Brain infection following varicella occurs about 5 to 20 d following the onset of rash. The most common manifestation is cerebellar ataxia; encephalitis is much less common. Delirium is common, but seizures are unusual. Cerebellar ataxia usually resolves fully.

## Cytomegalovirus

### *Epidemiology*

Man is the only host of cytomegalovirus (CMV) infection. In the United States and western Europe, between 50% and 90% of adults have antibodies to CMV, depending upon socioeconomic status. Immune compromised patients (transplant recipients and individuals with HIV infection) are more likely to develop clinically apparent CMV infection. Modes of transmission include contact with infected secretions (saliva, breast milk, urine, semen, and vaginal secretions) and blood. Congenital infection with CMV occurs in 1% of all live births with one of 10 infected children suffering severe CNS disease. Clinical disease is common in immune-compromised patients and may be due to either relapse or primary infection. Patients with AIDS appear at highest risk for CMV disease of the CNS (see Chapter 97).

#### *Pathogenesis*

Disease attributed to CMV is determined largely by host responses of MHC II–restricted cytotoxic T lymphocytes, natural killer (NK) cells, or antibody-dependent killer (K) cells. The virus can bind $\beta$-2 microglobulin, protecting it from neutralization by antibody. Cytomegalovirus infection can also induce the synthesis of a cellular protein which acts as an Fc receptor and can bind immunoglobulin, allowing CMV to evade immune attack. Antigen-bearing cells can be found in CNS capillary endothelium, suggesting direct blood-borne spread to the brain. The virus can infect glia and neurons; the ependymal and subependymal regions are preferred. Pathological changes include the presence of microglial nodules, perivascular infiltration, hemorrhage, and necrosis.

#### *Clinical presentation*

An immunocompromised patient with a progressive and diffuse encephalitis should be considered as having possible CMV infection. In a retrospective review of 14 autopsy confirmed cases of CMV encephalitis in patients with AIDS, the onset was subacute. These patients manifested widespread systemic disease including pneumonitis, adrenalitis, and retinitis, all attributed to CMV infection. In these patients the clinical decline is rapid, and mean survival time for patients with CMV encephalitis is about 5 wk. A polyradiculopathy and associated CSF pleocytosis have also been identified in patients with CMV infection and AIDS (Chapter 97).

#### *Host response*

The role of antibody responses in affecting the progression of CMV disease progression is unclear. Cell-mediated immune responses are depressed with symptomatic primary infections leading to diminished cytotoxic T-lymphocyte responses. In the mouse, cytotoxic T Iymphocytes can protect the host from lethal CMV infection; a cell-mediated immune response to a 72 kDa nonstructural viral protein has been described. Recovery from CMV disease in transplant recipients is associated with the elaboration of NK and K cell immune responses and an effective cytotoxic T-cell response.

### Epstein-barr virus

#### *Epidemiology*

Infection with Epstein Barr-virus occurs worldwide. In developing countries, infection occurs at an early age, wheras in the United States, approximately 50% of people are infected by college age. Acquisition of infection is from human saliva. No seasonal variation exists in the occurrence of EBV infection. While EBV infection has been shown to be an occasional cause of acute encephalitis, recognition is infrequent because the diagnosis is difflcult. The advent of PCR techniques to demonstrate EBV DNA in CSF may, however, reveal CNS EBV disease to occur more frequently than currently is appreciated.

#### *Pathogenesis*

Epstein-Barr virus infects and transforms human B lymphocytes. Infection of the B lymphocytes is mediated by envelope glycoproteins gp220 and gp350. CR2, the receptor for the C3d component of complement, serves as the receptor on B lymphocytes for EBV. These lymphocytes can adhere to cerebral blood vessels and cause vasculitis. Infected Iymphocytes can also enter the brain, and EBV DNA can be detected by PCR in brain tissue. The control of the infected cell population is determined by class I MHC restricted cytotoxic T lymphocytes. The number of EBV-infected cells is inversely related to the magnitude of the cytotoxic T-lymphocyte (CTL) response. The role of CTL responses in CNS EBV infection is unclear.

#### *Clinical presentation*

Encephalitis is often mild, and recovery is complete unless the patient is immune compromised. Another manifestation of EBV infection, the infectious mononucleosis syndrome (Chapter 53), is often present. An IgM response to EBV proteins develops early. IgG responses occur to several antigens but their overall importance for recovery from EBV infection is unclear.

### B virus

#### *Epidemiology*

Herpes B virus, a common infection of macaques, has been recognized as a pathogen in humans since 1933. Overall, there are approximately 30 cases in the world's literature. This virus is indigenous to Old World monkeys such as the rhesus (*Macaca mulatta*) and the cynomolgus (*Macaca fascicularis*). Transmission of virus has been documented in technicians who handle monkey ceIls for preparation of polio vaccine. Human to human transmission also has occurred. An outbreak of B virus encephalitis occurred in Pensacola in 1987 and, subsequently, in Michigan a few years later.

#### *Pathogenesis*

Following a monkey bite, B virus viral replication occurs at the site and is followed by spread to local lymphatics and draining lymph nodes. In the human, spread to the CNS, including the spinal cord, is via retrograde neuronai transport. Viremia does not appear to be important in the pathogenesis of B virus encephalitis. Atthough rhesus monkeys suffer little morbidity from B virus, inoculation of the hind limb of a rabbit results in paralysis in 7 to 8 d followed by fatal encephalitis.

#### *Clinical presentation*

A vesicular eruption occurs at the bite site resulting in erythema and Iymphangitis. Neurological signs appear 3 to 7 d later. Long-tract signs, particularly transverse myelitis, can occur. Altered consciousness and seizures leading to coma are common. Neurological impairment in survivors is expected.

## Arboviruses

Arthropod-borne viruses include the alphaviruses, flaviviruses, bunyaviruses, and, in at least one case, a reovirus. Arthropods (mosquitoes and ticks) transmit infection from animal hosts to humans, leading to encephalitis in rare instances.

*Alphaviruses* are small, positive (+), single-stranded RNA-enveloped viruses. Eastern equine encephalitis (EKE) virus was isolated in 1933 from horses. The Centers for Disease Control and Prevention (CDC) reported five cases in 1993. Mortality is high, ranging from 50% to 75%. Western equine encephalitis (WEE) virus was first isolated in 1930. In 1993 the CDC reported 13 cases of WEE. Unlike the mortality associated with EKE, WEE has an associated mortality of 3%–9%. Venezuelan equine encephalitis (VEE) virus was isolated in 1938. In 1971 there were 19 nonfatal cases of VEE in Texas, occurring concomitantly with equine fatalities. Mortality associated with VEE is reported to be 1% but is higher in children less than 5 yr of age. Everglades virus has also been associated with encephalitis.

*Flaviviruses* are + single stranded RNA viruses which have similar morphology to alphaviruses but with a distinctive genomic structure and replication cycle. St. Louis encephalitis (SLE) virus was isolated from humans in 1933. It occurs throughout the United States but outside the New England region. A widespread outbreak occurred in the Orlando, Florida. In 1993, 18 cases were reported in the United States. The mortality from the disease is 2%–20%, depending upon the patient's age. Japanese B encephalitis was described in 1871 but the virus was not isolated until 1935. From 1871 to 1919, several epidemics were documented. Mortality associated with Japanese B encephalitis is between 20% and 50%. Murray Valley (Australian X) encephalitis was identified in 1951 from the Murray Darling River Basin. Encephalitis epidemics occurred in 1917 and 1918 in New South Wales, Australia, at which time the mortality was 70%. Other encephalitic flaviviruses include Rocio, West Nile, Kyasnur, Forest, Powassan, Ilheus, Negishi, Russian Spring-Summer, Louping Ill, and Central European.

*Bunyoviruses* are negative single-stranded RNA viruses. LaCrosse encephalitis virus, a bunyavirus, is the most common cause of arbovirus infection in the United States. A closely related but distinct virus is California encephalitis virus. Other causes of encephalitis in this group include Jamestown Canyon, Snowshoe Hare, and Tahyna viruses. These viruses collectively comprise the California serogroup of bunyaviruses.

*Reoviruses* are double stranded RNA viruses without an envelope. Colorado tick virus is the most common member of this family which causes encephalitis in humans.

### Epidemiology

Table 74.3 denotes the location, vectors, and hosts of arboviruses which cause encephalitis in humans. The most important is Japanese B encephalitis, which is responsible for tens of thousands of cases per year. A recently developed vaccine will hopefully reduce the frequency of this disease. Late summer is the peak time for acquisition oúencephalitis. California virus is the most common cause of arbovirus encephalitis in the United States. Epidemics of California encephalitis have not been reported. In addition to the viruses listed in Table 74.3, there are two flaviviruses which have unknown vectors. Rocio virus, for which birds are the host, causes encephalitis in Brazil. Rio Bravo virus encephalitis, for which bats are the host, occurs in Central and South America. The hosts for Colorado tick virus are squirrels and chipmunks and the vector is the dermacentor tick.

### Clinical presentation

The EKE virus causes the most severe disease of the alphaviruses. Seizures and focal neurological signs lead to stupor and coma with about 80% of survivors having significant neurological sequelae. Seizures and lethargy may accompany WEE but focal signs and coma are usually absent. Severe disease is also more common in infants and young children. Myalgia and pharyngitis associated with encephalitis are clues to VEE, which causes disease most commonly in the young. St. Louis encephalitis can cause stupor, and about 20% of survivors have neurological deficits. Japanese B virus and Murray Valley encephalitis virus affect children most often. Virus spreads hematogenously to the basal ganglia and movement disorders are present in 90% of patients. A temperature of >104° F is common. Russian spring–summer encephalitis may manifest with bulbar signs and paralysis. Epilepsy partialis continua occurs in some survivors. About 30%–60% of survivors have neurological deficits.

California encephalitis is usually mild. This summer encephalitis may present with a more severe course, particularly in children. Seizures are common (50%), and 10% have subsequent epilepsy; other complications include cognitive dysfunction and paresis.

### Host response

Humoral immune responses develop early in the course of infection and, in the case of certain flaviviruses, are protective. For example, patients with good IgM and IgG antibody responses survive whereas fatal outcomes are related to poor humoral immune responses. Antibody persistence confers immunity to the same but not different strains of virus. Cytotoxic T lymphocytes are not required for recovery from alphavirus encephalitides. Modest immunosuppression does not influence the clinical course of disease.

## Rabies

### Epidemiology

Rabies exists worldwide. The Philippines has the highest incidence of disease. In the United States, the number of cases of rabies is generally below five annually. They usually represent imported cases with the exception of one case in the Northeast in 1993. In the United States dogs, raccoons, skunks, foxes, and bats harbor rabies. In South and Central America, Africa, and Asia, rabies remains a major public health problem. Dogs and cats are infected in South and Central America. In North Africa, the dog is the major reservoir for the transmission of rabies to humans. In sub-Saharan Africa, both the jackal and the dog are infected. In Europe, the fox transmits rabies. Rabies appears to be more prevalent in the winter and spring, although exposure in summer occurs as well.

The location of the bite of an infected animal influences the development of the disease. Bites on the head lead to clinical rabies in up to 80% of cases whereas upper and lower extremity bites lead less frequently and more slowly to disease.

**Table 74.3** Encephalitis attributed to arbovirus infections

| Arbovirus | Location | Vector(s) | Host(s) |
|---|---|---|---|
| ALPHAVIRUSES | | | |
| Eastern equine birds, encephalitis | US—East, Gulf Coast; South and Central America, Caribbean | Mosquitoes (Culiseta + *Aedes* | Various species of Wood tick |
| Western equine birds, encephalitis | US—West, Midwest; Canada | Mosquitoes (*Culiseta* + *Culex* | Various species of Wood tick |
| Venezuela equine encephalitis | US—Southwest; Central and South America | Mosquitoes (*Aedes* + *Culex*) | Rodents, equines |
| Everglades | Florida | Mosquitoes | Rodents |
| FLAVIVIRUSES | | | |
| SLE | US—Central, Southern; West Caribbean | Mosquitoes (*Culex*) | Birds |
| Japanese B | Northern and Southeast Asia, India | Mosquitoes (*Culex*) | Birds, pigs |
| Murray Valley | Australia, New Guinea | Mosquitoes (*Culex*) | Birds |
| West Nile | Africa, Middle East, Europe | Mosquitoes (*Culex*) | Birds |
| Ilheus | South America | Mosquitoes (*Psorophora*) | Birds |
| Ishi birds | Japan | Ticks (?) | Small mammals |
| Louping ill | Great Britain | Ticks (*Ixodes*) | Rodents, sheep |
| Powassan birds | Russia | Ticks (*Ixodes*) | Small mammals |
| Kyasnur Forest chipmunks | India | Ticks (*Hemophysalis*) | Goats, squirrels, birds |
| BUNYAVIRUSES | | | |
| Lacrosse mammals | US—Midwest, Eastern | Mosquitoes (*Aedes*) | Squirrels, |
| Tahyna animals, | Eastern Europe, Italy, South France | Mosquitoes (*Aedes* + *Culiseta*) | Domestic, Rabbits |
| Jamestown Canyon | US including Alaska | Mosquitoes (*Aedes* + *Culiseta*) | White-tailed deer |
| Snowshoe hare other | Nova Scotia, Quebec, Ontario | Mosquitoes (*Aedes* + *Culiseta*) | Snowshoe hare, Mammals |

### Pathogenesis

In the 18th century, Morgagni postulated that rabies spread via nerves to the brain; Pasteur later demonstrated neuronal spread of the virus; and the presence of mature virions and naked nucleocapsids were visualized in peripheral nerves. Rabies localizes in the neuromuscular junction and travels to the spinal cord or brain at a rate of approximately 3 mm/day. The role of the acetylcholine (ACh) receptor, functioning as a receptor for rabies, is still disputed, as rabies can infect cells which do not express ACh receptors. Rabies neurovirulence is mediated by the envelope G glycoprotein; infectivity is nearly totally lost following its removal from the virus. Similarly, antibodies to free G protein decrease neurovirulence. Pathogenicity is also associated with the amino acid arginine at position 333 (antigenic site III) of the G protein. Site III mutants spread more slowly within the CNS, infecting host cells more slowly.

### Clinical presentation

Prior to behavioral changes characteristic of rabies, pain occurs at the bite site. Pharyngeal spasm, opisthotonos, and excessive salivation precede paralysis and death, which is in almost all cases inevitable, even within modern means of intensive care support.

### Host responses

The administration of antibody following rabies exposure lengthens the time until disease develops. Resistance to infection is conferred by the production of neutralizing antibodies following vaccination. IgG antibodies neutralize rabies virus and cooperate in antibody-dependent cell-mediated cytotoxicity. Antibody responses occur within 1 wk following infection and are directed against the N protein. Cell-mediated responses involve cytotoxic T lymphocyte responses to the G glycoprotein.

## Arenaviruses

### Epidemiology

Lymphocytic choriomeningitis (LCMV) virus causes disease in Europe as well as North America. Both the field mouse, *Mus musculus*, and hamsters transmit infection to humans. The mouse acquires infection by a transovarian route or during early fetal life. Humans become infected by mouse feces or other secretions. Transmission occurs most frequently in winter. Lassa virus is present in West Africa and is transmitted by the *Mastomys* genus of rats. Human to human transmission in the hospital has resulted in deaths.

### Pathogenesis

Neurovirulence of LCMV appears related to the viral polymerase and is determined by a gene that does not encode envelope glycoproteins. Lassa virus infection leads to disturbances in endothelial and platelet function.

### Clinical presentation

Meningitis attributable to LCMV occurs more commonly than encephalitis. Encephalitis is associated with bulbar and ascending paralysis. Lassa fever virus infection of the CNS is associated with diffuse systemic viral infection. Tremors and seizures are common; cranial nerve deficits are usually absent. Deafness occurs in 5% of survivors.

### Host response

Cytotoxic T-lymphocyte responses are critical host defenses to LCMV; impaired responses can lead to fatal infection.

## Paramyxoviruses

Paramyxoviruses are negative, single-stranded, enveloped RNA viruses. Two members of the genus cause CNS disease: mumps and measles. In 1927, mumps virus proved to have neurotropic properties, commonly causing meningoencephalitis until universal vaccination began in 1967 in the United States. Approximately 0.5%–2.3% of cases of mumps encephalitis are fatal. In the early 20th century, the pathological findings of postmeasles encephalitis were reported, suggesting a postinfectious encephalomyelitis. Measles remains a major public health problem in many areas of the world where infection continues unabated and has an associated mortality of 1.5 million people annually. Most deaths attributed to measles are not the consequence of encephalitis but rather of opportunistic respiratory infections occurring as a consequence of the immune deficiency associated with infection. Measles encephalitis has a mortality of about 20%.

## Mumps virus

### Epidemiology

Mumps is transmitted by respiratory secretions. Approximately 95% of adults in the United States and western Europe are immune to mumps through vaccination or natural infection. Mumps encephalitis develops in approximately 1% of naturally acquired mumps infection and is most common in males between the ages of 5 and 9 yr of age. The severity of encephalitis is less morbid than that which follows measles.

### Pathogenesis

Mumps infects the CNS in about 50% of all cases. The virus infects mononuclear cells which then cross into the CNS where the blood-brain barrier is fenestrated. Infection of choroid plexus and ependymal cells occurs. In primates, more virulent strains of mumps invade the brain parenchyma. Neurovirulence varies according to virus strain, but molecular mechanisms responsible for mumps encephalitis have not been clarified. Antibodies directed against the hemagglutinin or neuraminidase glycoproteins correlate with decreased neurovirulence in vivo. Demyelination in addition to perivascular infiltrates is sometimes observed, suggesting the possibility of an autoimmune response.

### Clinical presentation

Although meningitis is the most common CNS manifestation, encephalomyelitis may complicate mumps infection, resulting in deafness and polyneuritis. Hydrocephalus following mumps encephalitis of the newborn has been reported. Virus may also cause unusual focal neurological signs, including cortical blindness. Typically, mumps meningitis develops about 5 d after the onset of parotitis. Asymptomatic CNS involvement is common. Seizures occur in 20%–30% of symptomatic patients, and a small percentage of patients become obtunded. Almost all patients eventually recover.

### Host response

Antibodies protect against mumps infection; thus, seropositivity correlates with protection. Hamsters can be protected from mumps by administration of neutralizing antibodies within several days of the virus inoculation. Cell-mediated immune responses may influence the clinical course of the disease in that mumps-specific cytotoxic T lymphocytes ameliorate the severity of the infection in cyclophosphamide immune-suppressed hamsters.

## Measles virus

### Epidemiology

In Third World countries, the incidence of measles essentially equals the number of surviving children since almost all children develop disease. Encephalitis follows the onset of the rash typically by 4 to 5 d in one in 800 to 2000 cases. Of children with encephalitis, 10%–20% of the survivors develop significant neurological sequelae.

### Clinical presentation

There is an abrupt decline in consciousness with sudden obtundation or confusion; focal neurological signs, especially seizures, are common. Encephalitis is usually severe. Survivors have neurological deficits, which include blindness, paraplegia, and/or ataxia.

### Host response

The administration of immune globulin modifies the clinical course of the disease, implying a role for antibody foundation in disease resolution. Most patients develop lymphopenia in response to measles with falls in $CD4^+$ and $CD8^+$ cells but no change in the $CD4^+/CD8^+$ ratio. T-cell unresponsiveness to mitogen stimulation is common. Postmeasles encephalitis is associated with increased "trafficking" of lymphocytes to the brain and is independent of the virus replication in the CNS. Levels of soluble IL-2 and $\gamma$-interferon are elevated.

## Picornaviruses

Members of the picornavirus family are small, single-stranded RNA viruses without an envelope and include rhino-, polio-, echo-, and coxsackieviruses. The latter three families of viruses cause encephalitis in man and other primates. In the United States, symptomatic poliomyelitis may occur following the administration of the attenuated oral polio vaccine (OPV) to individuals who are not recognized as immune-compromised. Rarely, secondary spread of OPV to nonimmune individuals may cause mild disease. Cases are more common elsewhere around the world where vaccination is not routine. Both echovirus and coxsackievirus usually cause aseptic meningitis but can also result in encephalitis. Infection with these viruses is usually associated with a low mortality except in patients with X-linked agammaglobulinemia. In these patients CNS echovirus infection may persist for months, despite therapy with immunoglobulin.

## Enteroviruses

### Epidemiology

Poliovirus causes disease worldwide but has been essentially eradicated from the United States by childhood vaccination. Polio is the prototype enteroviral disease of the CNS. Virus transmission is by a fecal–oral route. Coxsackie- and echoviruses are likewise transmitted by fecal–oral routes; spread among small children is common. The peak incidence of enteroviral diseases is late summer and early fall.

### Pathogenesis

Poliovirus replicates in gastrointestinal associated lymphoid tissue (GALT). Although poliovirus can spread experimentally through the sciatic nerve, conventionally it is thought to spread to the CNS system by viremia. Neurovirulence of poliovirus is determined in part by a 5′ noncoding region, localized to nucleotide 472. Substitution of cytosine with uracil results in an avirulent virus. The capsid proteins VP1 and VP3 also influence neurovirulence. Substitution of lysine for arginine at amino acid position 3333 in VP1 and of phenylalanine for serine at amino acid position 2034 in VP3 both reduce neurovirulence.

### Clinical presentation

Most cases of polio present as aseptic meningitis, but progression to frank encephalitis with resulting paralysis occurs in one in 1000 cases. Occasional brainstem encephalitis (bulbar polio) is associated with high mortality. Infants are at highest risk for encephalitis. Echo- and coxsackieviruses usually present as an aseptic meningitis; morbidity and mortality are common following in utero infections or in the immune-compromised host.

## Orthomyxoviruses

The prototype member of this family is influenza which causes a postinfluenza syndrome. Encephalitis following influenza was recognized as a complication of the Asian influenza epidemics in the 1950s. Children are usually afflicted and the mortality is low.

## Miscellaneous agents

Acute hemorrhagic leukoencephalitis usually follows an upper respiratory tract infection. While it is presumed to be of viral etiology, no agent has been identified. Focal neurologic signs predominate the clinical picture. Surviving patients usually have significant neurological impairment. The computed tomograph has a characteristic appearance with widespread, bilateral white matter involvement.

## Diagnostic Studies

### Cerebrospinal fluid evaluation

The evaluation of CSF is mandatory, obtained either by lumbar puncture or by ventriculostomy. Pleocytosis, with a polymorphonuclear leukocytosis progressing to a monocytosis, is often present in patients with encephalitis. Elevation of the protein concentration is common. In the case of HSE, the protein concentration increases as disease progresses. There is usually an elevation of the RBCs as well. Approximately 3%–5% of patients with HSE have a normal CSF formula. In patients with postmeasles encephalitis, myelin basic protein may be present, but one-third of patients have a normal CSF formula. Although the CSF traditionally has not been helpful in making a diagnosis of any specific encephalitis, including HSE, the introduction of PCR will assist in defining the specific etiology, as can be achieved in diagnosing HSE.

### Neurologic imaging

Computed tomography (CT) of the head, preferably with and without contrast, is mandatory since surgical emergencies must be identified. The CT scan may appear normal; however, a normal scan does not exclude viral encephalitis. Magnetic resonance imaging (MRI) is the study of choice when possible, as it provides a more detailed examination of the anatomy and physiology. However, this study is difficult in patients with altered mental status and should not be considered mandatory. In the case of HSE, there may be significant edema and hemorrhage in the temporal regions. Other common CT findings in HSE are a hypodense area and nonhomogeneous contrast enhancement. Bilateral temporal lobe involvement is nearly pathognomonic for HSE. Cytomegalovirus encephalitis can result in ventriculomegaly and, by MRI, increased signal intensity in the surrounding white matter and diffuse subependymal gadolinium enhancement. Findings by CT and MRI are not necessarily pathognomic for any viral encephalitides other than HSE.

### Electroencephalography

Periodic spike wave activity with high voltage and slow wave complexes are observed by electroencephalography (EEG) in patients with HSE but may occur in other conditions as well. An EEG is mandatory in patients with suspected status epilepticus to rule out the presence of subclinical epilepsy.

## Specific Diagnostic Approaches

### Herpesvirus infections

The greatest diagnostic experience has been accumulated with HSV infection of the CNS. Antibodies are found to HSV in the CSF but usually occur late in the disease course and are helpful only for retrospective analysis. Antibodies are present in 85%–90% of cases but 15%–20% false positives occur 4 wk after the onset of infection.

Polymerase chain reaction utilizes primers from HSV DNA sequences and has become the diagnostic approach to HSE. In a recent study, cerebrospinal fluids from 43 consecutive patients with HSE diagnosed by virus isolation (13) or by CSF antibody detection (30) were PCR positive in all of 42 cases. Sixty patients with a febrile illness, who were HSE negative, served as controls and none had a positive PCR result. Multiple groups have reported the utility of PCR assays for the diagnosis of HSE, and to date, the sensitivity and specificity are greater than 95% and 99%, respectively. False negatives occur in the presence of hemoglobin in the CSF or when inhibitors are present. Polymerase chain reaction assays can also identify HSE from postmortem samples which have been fixed in formalin.

In spite of the apparent utility of PCR, brain biopsy will continue to play a role, albeit limited, in the diagnosis of some patients with encephalitis. At this time it appears prudent to proceed with biopsy in patients with an encephalitis of unknown etiology (specifically those HSV DNA negative by PCR) who deteriorate neurologically on acyclovir therapy. The importance of biopsy is reflected by the National Institute of Allergy and Infectious Diseases and Collaborative Antiviral Study Group (NIAID CASG), which demonstrated that 43% of patients with suspected HSE had other diagnoses (Table 74.2). The biopsy complication rate was less than 3% (usually local hemorrhage or edema). Persistent epilepsy attributed to the biopsy has not been established. Unless the CT is helpful in guiding the neurosurgeon to a specific brain region, the anterior inferior temporal lobe should be biopsied, and at least a 1 $cm^3$ portion of tissue should be obtained. Careful consideration should be given by the neurosurgeon to the performance of a temporal lobectomy in cases where temporal lobe edema and/or hemorrhage may result in uncal herniation. The tissue sample should not be placed in formalin. One portion is placed immediately on ice and sent for virus isolation, immunofluorescence, and electron microscopic studies. A second portion should be sent to the microbiology laboratory for culture of suspected pathogens, and a third portion sent for routine histopathological examination. The pathological findings of various encephalitides are listed in Table 74.4.

As stated earlier, VZV is usually not isolated from the CSF. Utilizing PCR technology, VZV DNA is detected in CSF early in the course of encephalitis following varicella but then disappears. Virus can be recovered from vesicles by aspirating fluid with a tuberculin syringe and directly inoculating this fluid onto susceptible cell lines. Serologic assessment for VZV traditionally has employed a complement-fixation (CF) antibody assay, although more sensitive antibody assays are now available. The fluorescent antibody membrane antigen (FAMA) assay allows seroconversion to be promptly detected and is associated with a fourfold or greater rise in titer. The test is used extensively, and the antibodies persist much longer than with other assays.

Regarding the diagnosis of CMV in patients with CNS symptoms, CMV early antigen has been demonstrated in patients with clinical evidence of CMV encephalitis but not in control patients. Polymerase chain reaction assessment of CSF will detect CMV DNA. This assay is applicable to the detection of EBV DNA in CSF samples, as well.

B virus can usually be retrieved from vesicles at the site of the bite. The CSF culture is usually negative for B virus.

## Arbovirus infections

Hemagglutination inhibition (HI) and complement fixation (CF) have been replaced by detection of IgM antibodies in most cases using EIA and IFA and, more recently, by a PCR assay for viral DNA. With Japanese B encephalitis, Ig antibody is present early; its detection is sensitive and specific for the diagnosis of disease. The IgM-capture ELISA is well suited for early detection of local synthesis of antibodies to Japanese B encephalitis in the CSF.

## Rabies

The diagnosis of rabies can be accomplished by several methods. First, identification of rabies in the brain (immunofluorescence or histopathology) of the attacking animal will define exposure of a patient. Second, full-thickness skin biopsy from the nape of the neck and examination of sensory neurons using immunofluorescence antibodies has a sensitivity of between 50% and 94% and a specificity which approaches 100%. Third, fluorescence staining of brain-biopsy specimens from the patient can be helpful. The best region for biopsy is the cerebellum. Negri

**Table 74.4** Histopathologic findings in encephalitis

| Agent | Perivascular cuffing | Hemorrhage | Neuronophagia | Demyelination | Comments |
|---|---|---|---|---|---|
| HSV | + | + | + | − | Intranuclear inclusions in 50% |
| EBV | + | − | − | − | |
| Herpes B | + | + | + | − | Extensive hemorrhage |
| Alphavirus | + | +/− | +/− | − | More severe in EEF |
| Flavivirus | + | + | + | − | Japanese B may involve cord |
| Bunyavirus | + | − | − | − | California viruses |
| Rabies virus | + | − | + | − | Negri bodies not always present |
| Lassa virus | + | − | − | − | Pathological studies in man limited |
| Mumps virus | + | − | − | +/− | May demonstrate immune-mediated changes |
| Post Semple vaccine | + | − | − | + | |
| Post varicella | + | − | − | + | |
| Post measles | + | − | − | + | |
| Hemorrhagic leukencephalitis | + | + | − | + | Arteriolar and venular involvement |

bodies, which are eosinophilic intracytoplasmic inclusions, are composed of viral antigens and are pathognomonic for rabies. Negri bodies are found postmortem in nearly 60% of cerebellar specimens and 40%–76% of hippocampal specimens. Immunofiuorescence staining of corneal cells from a touch impression (the inner canthus) is rarely used to diagnose rabies today because of its low sensitivity. Inoculation of brain tissue from an animal with suspected rabies into a susceptible animal's brain is still performed for diagnostic purposes.

### Arenaviruses

Lymphocytic choriomeningitis may be isolated from the CSF throughout the acute illness. The IFA test is useful in the diagnosis of both LCMV and Lassa fever since serum antibodies appear early. About 50% of patients with Lassa fever have IgG or IgM antibodies by d 5 and almost all patients develop antibodies by d 5 of illness.

### Paramyxoviruses

Mumps virus can be recovered from the CSF in cases of CNS infection in 17%–58% of cases. The presence of an elevated CSF/serum mumps antibody ratio is considered evidence of mumps infection ofthe CNS. Measles antigen or antibodies are generally not present in the CSF except as discussed earlier. Virus from throat or stool cultures are positive for measles early in the disease. Polymerase chain reaction testing for measles is available.

### Enteroviruses

Stool cultures are positive for the various enteroviruses early in the disease. More recently, PCR evaluation of CSF has been established to be of diagnostic value.

## Treatment

### General management

Table 74.5 outlines the treatment for patients with suspected viral encephalitis. Besides administration of antiviral therapy, if available, management includes reduction of intracranial pressure. Hyperventilation and hyperosmolar fluid administration to reduce increased intracranial pressure have not been shown to be effective; however, improved outcomes in patients with traumatic encephalopathies are observed when attention is focused on the maintenance of adequate hydration and cerebral perfusion: Data that demonstrate that encephalitic patients have an improved outcome with such management are lacking. If patients have elevated intracranial pressures (ICP) then pressure monitoring and maintenance of ICP at 15 mmHg is indicated.

### Antiviral therapy

#### Herpesvirus infections

Herpesvirus encephalitides are the only conditions for which there are established therapies. Several nucleoside inhibitors including vidarabine and acyclovir have been used to treat HSE. Acyclovir is the treatment of choice for HSV, VZV, and B virus infections of the CNS. Data comparing survival of patients with biopsy-proven HSE who received acyclovir or vidarabine are displayed in Figure 74.2. Mortality at 18 mo was 28% for those who received acyclovir but 50% for those who received vidarabine; 62% of the survivors had moderate or severe neurological deficits. Thus, the combined overall significant morbidity and mortality of HSE in this study (even with acyclovir therapy) was greater than 70%. Mortality decreased to 8% if therapy was started less than 4 d after the onset of clinical symptoms, but the outcome was uniformly poor in patients with a Glasgow Coma Score of less than 6.

The dosage of acyclovir in the treatment of HSE is 10 mg/kg/every 8 h for 14–21 d but clinical circumstances should dictate the duration of treatment. Newborns with HSV infections should also be treated with acyclovir at this dose. Therapy should be reinstituted for clinical relapses which occur in 5%–10% of cases of HSE.

Acyclovir is recommended in the treatment of encephalitis or myelitis which may complicate varicella zoster virus infection.

**Table 74.5** Guidelines for the management of the encephalopathic patient

| |
|---|
| STUDIES |
| CT of the head to identify surgical lesions |
| EEG if indicated to rule out subclinical status epilepticus<br>or<br>identify focal epilepsy |
| INTERVENTIONS |
| Swan-Ganz Catheter |
| Arterial line catheter |
| Foley catheter |
| Ventriculostomy—CSF analysis |
| CEREBRAL PERFUSION PRESSURE MANAGEMENT (CPP = MAP − ICP) |
| Maintenance CPP > 80 mmHg vasopressor usage occasionally required |
| Adequate hydration using Swan-Ganz Parameters |
| Normocapnea |
| Avoid excessive diuretics and hyperosmolar state |

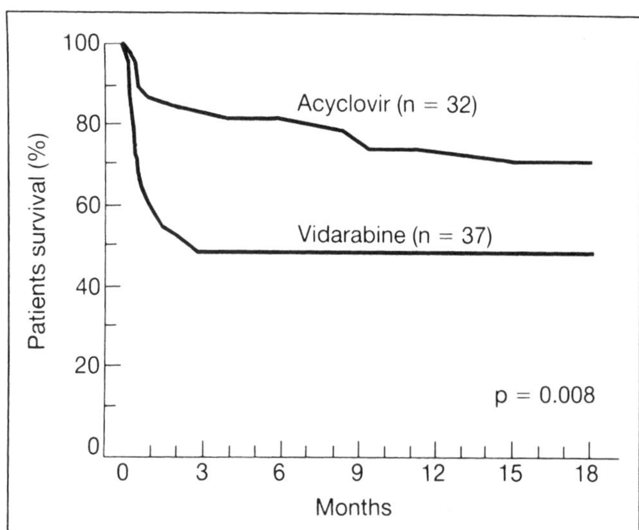


**Fig. 74.2** Mortality following treatment of herpes simplex encephalitis: Acyclovir versus vidarabine.

The effect of acyclovir on CNS complications of VZV infection is unknown. The dose is 10 mg/kg IV over 1 h q 8 h.

Ganciclovir is the treatment of choice for CMV infections of the CNS in individuals with HIV infection. Therapy is administered at 10 mg/kg d (divided BID) for 2 to 3 wk. Therapeutic failures are common.

For possible B virus infection, prophylactic acyclovir therapy is recommended by most experts if a monkey bite occurs, at least until cultures of the animal and wound site are available. Acyclovir is recommended for acute infection, and the dosage schedule is the same as for HSE. The efficacy of acyclovir in the treatment of B virus infection has not been systematically examined; however, case reports document patients who have made full recovery from B virus infection.

### Other CNS viral infections

Management of other viral infections of the CNS, including those caused by arboviruses, rabies, and enteroviruses, remains supportive care with the following exceptions.

For Lassa fever, ribavirin, a broad-spectrum antiviral drug, is reported to be effective therapy, and a 10 d course decreased mortality from 76% to 9%. A 2 g IV loading dose is given, followed by 1 g every 6 h for 4 d and then 0.5 g every 6 h for 6 d.

While no controlled trials are available and case reports are suspect, ribavirin therapy may decrease the severity and duration of measles both in normal adults and immunosuppressed children with life-threatening disease. Therapy is not routinely recommended but, if elected, it should be continued for 2–3 wk.

In children with x-linked agammaglobulinemia, $\gamma$-globulin therapy (0.2 ml/kg body weight, IM) is a consideration for the treatment of enteroviral disease, attributable to coxsackie or echoviruses, although it is unproven.

## Prevention

### Herpesvirus infections

At the present there are no established therapies for the prevention of HSV infections, let alone HSE, although two candidate subunit vaccines are in clinical trials. Varicella-zoster immune serum globulin (VZIG administered after exposure) is effective in the prevention or amelioration of varicella in individuals at high risk, but it is of no value in the treatment of established disease. Recently, the United States Food and Drug Administration licensed a live VZV vaccine for both healthy and immunocompromised individuals. The impact of this vaccine on the prevention of VZV complications of the CNS is unknown. At this time, no vaccines are of established value for the prevention of EBV, CMV, or HHV-6. Monkeys should be screened for B virus infection before use. Gloves and other protection against bites are mandatory.

### Arbovirus infections

Prevention of Japanese B encephalitis is accomplished with the Biken vaccine which requires three doses administered subcutaneously 1 wk apart followed by a booster at 1 yr. Vaccines are available for several of the other arbovirus infections and are recommended for personnel at high risk. Vector control is important as there is no specific therapy for any of the arbovirus encephalitides.

### Rabies

A vaccine is available for people at risk for rabies; the human diploid cell vaccine (HDCV) is given intradermally or intramuscularly in 0.1 ml doses for a total of three injections. Rabies immune globulin is also administered; 10 IU/kg into the wound and 10 IU administered IM. The Semple vaccine should be avoided if possible. A vaccine administered to wild animals, in a bait, has been considered.

### Paramyxovirus infections

A live attenuated vaccine is available for mumps and measles. Postexposure protection for measles should consist of 0.25 ml/kg of immunoglobulin up to 15 ml, if exposure is less than 6 d previously. The vaccine should be given 3 mo later.

### Enterovirus infections

Among the greatest successes in the prevention of viral disease of the CNS is the universal deployment of the poliovirus vaccine (see Chapter 45). Prior to the introduction of vaccination in the United States, there were nearly 20,000 cases of paralytic polio annually. Today, there are less than ten cases annually, all related to vaccination in the unsuspected immune-compromised host. The risk of paralytic polio following immunization is one case in 2.6 million doses of vaccine.

## ANNOTATED BIBLIOGRAPHY


Aurelius E, Johansson B, Skoldenberg B, Staland A, Forsgren M. Rapid diagnosis of herpes simplex encephalitis by nested polymerase chain reaction assay of cerebrospinal fluid. Lancet 1991; 337:189.
*This paper summarizes the utility of PCR for diagnosis of herpes simplex encephalitis.*

Baer GM, Fishbein DB. Rabies post-exposure prophylaxis. N Engl J Med 1987; 316:1270.
*An excellent review of utilization of vaccine and rabies immune globulin for prevention of rabies after animal bites.*

Eldridge BR. Strategies for surveillance, prevention, and control of arbovirus diseases in Western North America. Am J Trop Med Hyg 1987; 37:77.
*Review of arbovirus infections and their control.*

Fishbein DB, Robinson LE. Rabies. N Engl J Med 1993; 329:1632–1638.
*An excellent review of rabies.*
*Johnson RT. The pathogenesis of acute viral encephalitis and postinfectious encephalitis. J Infect Dis 1987; 155:359.*
*Summary of an Infectious Diseases Society of America lecture.*

Johnson RT. The virology of demyelinating diseases. Ann Neurol 1994; 36:554.
*Basic review of the pathogenesis of demyelination following viral infection.*

Lakeman A, Whitley R, the NIAID CASG. Diagnosis of herpes simplex encephalitis: Application of polymerase chain reaction to cerebrospinal fluid from brain biopsied patients and correlation with disease. J Infect Dis 1995; 171:857–863.

Rosen L. The natural history of Japanese encephalitis virus. Annu Rev Microbiol 1986; 40:395.
*Basic review of a significant cause of CNS disease in Pacific Rim countries.*

Whitley R. Viral encephalitis. N Engl J Med 1990; 323:242–250.
*An overview of viral encephalitis.*

Whitley RJ, Cobbs CG, Alford CA et al. Diseases that mimic herpes simplex encephalitis: diagnosis, presentation and outcome. JAMA 1989; 262:234.
*Causes of focal encephalopathic changes are delineated.*

Whitley R, Gnann J. Acyclovir: a decade later. N Engl J Med 1992; 327:782.
*An overview of the use of acyclovir in the treatment of herpesvirus infections.*

Whitley RJ, Tilles J, Linneman C et al. Herpes simplex encephalitis: clinical assessment. JAMA 1982; 247:317.
*This paper defines the presentation of HSE, including laboratory findings.*

# 75

# Infections Associated with Myelopathy, Radiculopathy, and Neuropathy

CHRISTINA M. MARRA

*Myelopathy* refers to a disorder of the spinal cord, *radiculopathy* to disorders of the motor or sensory nerve roots as they exit the spinal cord, and *neuropathy* to disorders of peripheral nerves. These entities are often distinguishable based on clinical findings (Table 75.1). With the exception of poliomyelitis, patients with acute myelopathy develop rapid onset of symmetrical, flaccid lower extremity weakness; a sensory level; bowel and bladder dysfunction; and neck, back, or radicular pain. The upper extremities may also be involved, particularly in ascending myelopathy. With time, upper motor neuron signs such as increased extremity tone, exaggerated deep tendon reflexes, and upgoing toes may be evident; patients with slowly evolving, chronic myelopathy may have these upper motor signs when first examined. Patients with radiculopathy develop pain and sensory deficits or weakness in the distribution of spinal roots. Radiculopathy may be localized (segmental) or diffuse. Deep tendon reflexes are diminished or lost, and bowel and bladder dysfunction is rare unless sacral roots are affected. Patients with neuropathy complain of pain, dysesthesia, or weakness in the distribution of one or more peripheral or cranial nerves. Radiculopathy and neuropathy may be difficult to distinguish. In some cases, such as Guillain-Barré syndrome, the spinal roots and peripheral nerves may be affected by the same pathological process.

The focus of this chapter is on infectious agents that are associated with myelopathy, radiculopathy and neuropathy. In some instances, such as poliomyelitis, direct infection of neural structures causes the clinical syndrome. In other cases, the clinical neurologic syndrome is seen following other manifestations of an infectious disease. Such instances are often termed *parainfectious*, and they are assumed to be autoimmune. Myelopathy associated with encephalitis (encephalomyelitis) will not be covered in this chapter; it is discussed in Chapter 74.

## Myelopathy

The syndrome of acute myelopathy can be due to a variety of causes, including spinal cord compression by abscess or tumor; intramedullary tumor or vascular malformation; effects of irradiation; vascular compromise; paraneoplastic syndrome; systemic lupus erythematosus; neurosarcoidosis; multiple sclerosis; parainfectious processes; and direct infection of the cord.

### Parainfectious syndromes: transverse myelopathy

Transverse myelopathy (also termed *transverse myelitis*) is a clinical description, defined as "an acute intramedullary dysfunction of the spinal cord, either ascending or static, involving both halves of the cord, often over a considerable length, and appearing without any history of previous neurological disease." It is uncommon, with an estimated annual incidence of 1.34 per million in Israel and 4.6 per million in the United States. Transverse myelopathy most commonly affects older children and young adults.

Although the clinical syndrome of transverse myelopathy may be due to direct infection of the spinal cord, it is most often attributed to a parainfectious process. Transverse myelopathy follows an upper respiratory tract infection in about 40% of cases. Associated infections include influenza, varicella, measles, mumps, and *Mycoplasma*. Onset of symptoms of spinal cord dysfunction usually develop between 9 and 21 d after resolution of the acute infectious disease. Transverse myelopathy may also occur after immunizations, including hepatitis B, tetanus, and rabies vaccinations. The disorder is thus thought to be autoimmune, particularly because peripheral blood lymphocytes from patients with transverse myelopathy proliferate in response to myelin antigens. In support of this hypothesis, neuropathological changes range from demyelination to necrosis (Fig. 75.1).

The most common initial *symptoms* of transverse myelopathy are paresthesias, back pain, and leg weakness. Bowel and bladder dysfunction and a well-demarcated sensory level ensue. The majority of patients have a progressive course that evolves over 1 to 14 d, followed by stabilization and complete or partial neurologic recovery. A slower, stuttering course that evolves over several weeks may be seen in a minority of patients. A subset of patients (about 20% in one study) have rapid onset of symptoms, usually within an hour, but ranging from 1 to 12 h; these patients have the poorest neurologic recovery.

*Diagnostic studies* to exclude compressive or vascular lesions should be performed. The study of choice is contrast enhanced magnetic resonance imaging (MR) centered at the level of involvement of the spinal cord, or myelography if MR is not available. In one report 82 (50%) of 164 patients initially diagnosed with myelopathy or myelitis were found to have a compressive lesion. If signs are consistent with cord infarction (intact vibration and position sense), spinal angiography may be considered to assess patency of the radicular arteries and of the anterior spinal artery.

In transverse myelopathy, MR and myelography may show diffuse cord swelling, most commonly in the thoracic region. Increased T2 signal over several cord levels may be seen on MR, sometimes with enhancement (Fig. 75.2). Cerebrospinal fluid (CSF) may show mild mononuclear pleocytosis, with counts usually less than 200 white blood cells (WBC)/$\mu$L, and mildly elevated protein concentration, with values usually less than

**Table 75.1** Clinical features of myelopathy, radiculopathy and neuropathy

| | Myelopathy | Radiculopathy | Neuropathy |
|---|---|---|---|
| Pain | Neck, back, or radicular distribution | Radicular distribution | May be present in distribution of affected nerve |
| Weakness | Usually symmetrical, with lower extremities involved more than upper extremities | Weakness in distribution of affected spinal roots | Weakness in distribution of affected motor nerves |
| Sensory loss | Sensory level may be present | Sensory deficits in distribution of affected spinal roots | Sensory deficits in distribution of affected sensory nerves |
| Bowel or bladder dysfunction | Present | Rare, unless sacral roots involved | Absent |
| Reflexes | May be absent initially, then brisk, with upgoing toes | Diminished or lost | Diminished or lost |

100 mg/dl. Cerebrospinal fluid glucose concentration is usually normal. Because direct infection of the spinal cord may cause a clinical syndrome similar to parainfectious or autoimmune transverse myelopathy, CSF evaluation should include studies to exclude infectious etiologies that are potentially treatable (see below).

*Treatment* of autoimmune transverse myelopathy is controversial. Use of high-dose steroids has been advocated but has not been shown to be of clear benefit.

## Infectious myelopathy

The most common causes of infectious myelopathy are enteroviruses, particularly polioviruses; herpes viruses, including varicella zoster and herpes simplex viruses; and the human retrovirus, human T-cell lymphotropic virus type I (HTLV-I, Table 75.2).

### Poliomyelitis

Wild-type poliovirus infection remains a significant public health problem in the developing world, where vaccination rates may be low and the efficacy of oral attenuated poliovirus vaccine (OPV) is diminished. The World Health Organization estimates that 140,000 cases of paralytic disease occurred in 1992. Poliomyelitis is primarily seen in children less than 3 yr of age. The incubation period is 4 to 35 d, and most cases occur 1 to 3 wk after exposure. As with other enteroviruses, the disease is seasonal, with peaks in summer and fall in temperate climates and less seasonal predominance in tropical climates.

Wild-type poliovirus transmission has been essentially eradicated from the Americas by widespread vaccination programs. Nonetheless, certain groups in the developing world such as

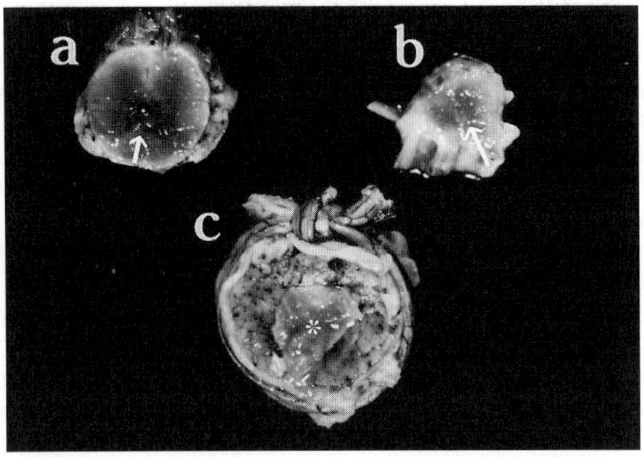

**Fig. 75.1** Spinal cord from a patient with transverse myelopathy. Horizontal sections of thoracic spinal cord (a), lumbar spinal cord (b), and conus medullaris with cauda equina (c) are shown from upper left to lower right. On gross inspection, there is darkening (necrosis) of the central portion of the spinal cord. Microscopic examination showed necrosis and vacuolization of white matter of the entire cord distal to the midcervical region, without evidence of inflammation.

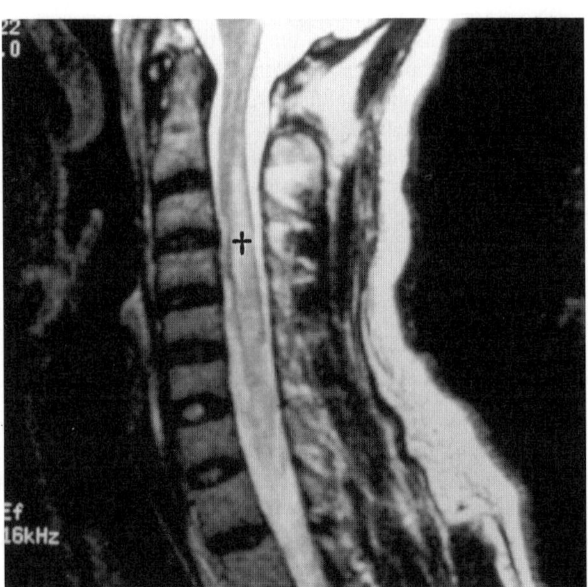

**Fig. 75.2** Sagittal T2-weighted magnetic resonance image of the cervical spinal cord from the patient shown in Fig. 75.1. There is diffuse enlargement, and increased signal intensity of the spinal cord over several segments.

**Table 75.2** Infectious causes of myelopathy

| Agent | Key features |
|---|---|
| ENTEROVIRUSES | |
| Polio<br>Coxsackie<br>Echo<br>Hepatitis A<br>Other enteroviruses | Although common in the developing world, wild-type polio rarely occurs in the United States. Most cases are oral vaccine recipients, or persons exposed to recipients. Coxsackie A7 and enterovirus 71 are associated with outbreaks of paralysis. Weakness due to nonpolio enteroviruses is usually milder than in poliomyelitis. Diagnosis is established by culture of virus from CSF, throat swab, or stool, or by identification of antibody in CSF. Polymerase chain reaction may supplant these studies in the future |
| HERPESVIRUSES | |
| Varicella<br>Human cytomegalovirus<br>Herpes simplex types 1 and 2<br>Epstein Barr virus<br>Herpes simiae | Myelopathy due to varicella most common with reactivation (shingles), and may be seen in the absence of rash. Myelopathy due to human cytomegalovirus and herpes simplex viruses may coexist with radiculopathy. Epstein-Barr and herpes simiae viruses are rare causes of myelopathy. Detection of viral DNA in CSF by polymerase chain reaction is more often positive than CSF viral cultures. Appropriate antiviral therapy is indicated |
| RETROVIRUSES | |
| HTLV-I and HTLV-II<br>HIV | Myelopathy due to HTLV or HIV has a more subacute, chronic course than for above agents. Examination rarely shows a sensory level. Diagnosis is usually based on clinical findings and serology. In HTLV infections, CSF cytology may be abnormal. Patients with HTLV-I or HTLV-II may improve with steroids. Some patients with HIV-related myelopathy improve with zidovudine |
| OTHER VIRUSES | |
| Rabies<br>Hepatitis B | In about 20% of rabies cases, myelopathic symptoms and signs predominate<br>Hepatitis B is a very rare cause of myelopathy |
| BACTERIA | |
| Lyme Disease<br>Syphilis<br>Tuberculosis | Myelopathy due to Lyme disease usually coexists with radiculopathy, cranial neuropathy, or encephalitis. Myelopathy due to syphilis is uncommon. Diagnosis of both spirochetal diseases is supported by identification of antibody or DNA in CSF. Myelopathy due to tuberculosis may be caused by intramedullary abscess or granuloma or by adhesive arachnoiditis |
| FUNGI | |
| Cryptococcosis | Myelopathy may be due to intramedullary granuloma |
| PARASITES | |
| Schistosomiasis<br>Toxoplasmosis | Myelopathy is an uncommon complication of both infections and is caused by intramedullary granuloma or abscess. Diagnosis is confirmed by tissue examination; a presumptive diagnosis is made by response to empiric therapy |

members of religious groups that generally do not accept vaccination remain at high risk for wild-type polio. A recent outbreak of paralytic poliomyelitis in 71 members of an unvaccinated religious community in the Netherlands, where vaccination rates of 1 yr olds in the general population has been about 97%, underscores this point. The last cases of wild-type paralytic poliomyelitis in the United States were reported in 1979. Between 1980 and 1989, 80 cases of vaccine-associated and five cases of imported wild-type poliomyelitis were reported in the United States. Those at risk for vaccine-related disease include OPV recipients and their contacts, and immunologically abnormal individuals, particularly those with hypo- or agammaglobulinemia. The risk of vaccine-related polio is estimated at one case per 2.5 million doses distributed. Approximately three-quarters of cases are associated with administration of the first or second vaccination.

Poliovirus is a picornavirus in the genus *Enterovirus*. There are three types; type 1 is the most frequent cause of epidemics and type 2 is the least frequent cause of epidemics. Overall, one in 200 patients infected with polioviruses develop paralysis. Paralysis rates are highest with type 1 and lowest with type 3. Susceptibility to paralysis increases with age; adolescents and adults are greater than ten times more likely to become paralyzed than children.

Vaccine-associated paralytic poliomyelitis is usually due to type 3 virus in immunocompetent individuals and to type 2 virus in immunodeficient individuals. Type 3 is the most genetically unstable of the three vaccine viruses and is more likely to revert to a neurovirulent form. Type 2 may also revert to a neurovirulent form but is thought to cause disease in immunodeficient individuals because it is the most likely of the three to cause viremia.

In most cases, poliovirus infection causes a mild and nonspecific illness characterized by low-grade fever, malaise, headache, sore throat, and gastrointestinal complaints. A small proportion of infected individuals go on to develop aseptic meningitis, and even fewer develop paralysis of the limbs without sensory changes. The legs are more commonly involved than the arms, and proximal muscles generally are more involved than distal. Muscle pain and tenderness are usually present, particularly in older patients. Physical examination shows flaccid paralysis with areflexia. The pattern of paralysis is typically asymmetrical, in contrast to that of transverse myelopathy or Guillain-Barré syndrome. Atrophy of the affected limbs begins quickly, usually within a week of onset. The nuclei of the lower cranial nerves may be involved, leading to dysarthria, dysphagia, and sometimes dyspnea. Respiratory compromise may result from brainstem involvement or from weakness of the diaphragm and intercostal muscles. Autonomic instability and dysfunction may also result from brainstem involvement, leading to cardiac dysrhythmias and hyper- or hypotension.

The CSF is almost always abnormal, with 20–300 WBC/$\mu$l. Polymorphonuclear leukocytes may be seen early, but mononuclear cells usually predominate. The protein concentration is mildly elevated, but is usually less than 200 mg/dl. CSF glucose concentration is normal. Unlike for other enteroviruses, CSF cultures for poliovirus are rarely positive. Virus may be cultured from pharyngeal secretions for 2 to 4 wk after disease onset, and more commonly from stool specimens, where viral excretion persists for 2 to over 6 wk. Serologic testing of acute and convalescent sera can confirm the diagnosis.

The differential diagnosis includes parainfectious transverse myelopathy, Guillain-Barré syndrome, acute intermittent porphyria, other enteroviral infections, pseudoparalysis due to osteomyelitis in children, botulism, diphtheria, tick paralysis, and encephalomyelitis. The constellation of symptoms and signs, including fever, flaccid asymmetrical weakness, little or no sensory symptoms, and inflammatory CSF distinguish poliomyelitis from the other entities.

With appropriate attention to respiratory function, the mortality from poliomyelitis is low, but about 30% of survivors have residual weakness. Treatment is supportive.

### Varicella-zoster virus

As noted above, transverse myelopathy may occur in patients with primary varicella infection, and it is assumed to be due to a parainfectious process. A recent report that identified varicella DNA in CSF from an individual with primary varicella infection and myelopathy suggests that direct infection of the spinal cord may also occur in some cases.

Myelopathy is an uncommon complication of reactivation of varicella infection (herpes zoster) and is more common in immunocompromised individuals. In one series, it was estimated to occur in 0.8% of such patients. Onset is characteristically 2 wk after the appearance of rash but may occur before the rash or in the absence of rash (zoster sine herpete). Initially, weakness and loss of vibratory sensation (if present) are ipsilateral to the rash, and loss of pain and temperature sensation are contralateral, consistent with unilateral cord involvement (Brown-Sequard syndrome). Symptoms and signs progress subacutely to a clinical picture similar to transverse myelopathy. A relapsing and remitting course has also been described. CSF examination shows mild to moderate mononuclear pleocytosis and normal or mildly elevated protein concentration. Varicella virus is uncommonly recovered from CSF; evidence of virus in CSF by polymerase chain reaction has been more frequently reported. Pathological examination reveals evidence of viral infection of the cord, with typical viral inclusions or immunohistochemical detection of viral antigens. Outcome of zoster myelopathy is variable. In one series that included patients treated with corticosteroids, antivirals (vidaribine or acyclovir), or both, three (12%) of 25 patients recovered completely, six (24%) had little or no improvement, and 16 (64%) showed partial improvement. A rapidly progressive, fatal course has also been described. Patients with zoster myelopathy should be treated with intravenous acyclovir or penciclovir (see Chapter 39).

### HTLV-I and HTLV-II

The etiologic agent of adult T-cell leukemia/lymphoma, HTLV-I, has recently been identified as the cause of a chronic progressive myelopathy identical to tropical spastic paraparesis. Infection with this virus is endemic in the Caribbean, southern Japan, equatorial Africa, and the Seychelles, with endemic foci in Central and South America, Melanesia, and South Africa. Sporadic cases have been reported in the United States and in Europe. The virus is transmitted by blood transfusion, sharing of infected paraphernalia by injection drug users, sexual contact, and breast feeding. Only a small proportion of infected individuals develop myelopathy; the estimated lifetime risk is 0.25%.

Myelopathy usually becomes evident in adulthood and is more common in women. The underlying pathophysiology appears to be a chronic meningomyelitis. Patients complain of insidious onset of stiffness or weakness in one or both legs, often with distal paresthesia, back pain, and bowel and bladder dysfunction. Neurological examination shows increased lower extremity tone and weakness of the proximal muscles. The gait may be slow and scissoring. Sensory symptoms are more striking than signs, but vibration sense is frequently impaired. Reflexes are hyperactive in arms and legs, with ankle clonus and upgoing toes. Less often, cerebellar signs, optic neuropathy and other cranial nerve deficits, and absent or depressed ankle reflexes are evident. Rarely, uveitis may coexist with HTLV-I associated myelopathy. The course of HTLV-1–associated myelopathy is usually slowly progressive; 10 yr after onset, 30% of individuals are bedridden and 45% are unable to ambulate without assistance. Progression is more rapid in patients with onset at a young age and in those who acquire infection via blood transfusion.

Magnetic resonance imaging of the spinal cord may be normal; diffuse high signal on T2-weighted images or thoracic atrophy may also be seen. In 60%–75% of patients, T2-weighted brain MR shows patchy nonspecific high signal intensity in the deep white matter or in the periventricular regions. The CSF may show mild lymphocytosis with atypical T cells resembling adult T-cell leukemia cells. CSF protein may be elevated, with increased intrathecal IgG synthesis. Antibody to HTLV-I is demonstrated in both CSF and serum, and peripheral blood $CD4^+$ T cell numbers may be elevated with an increased CD4/CD8 ratio.

As many as 50% of patients with HTLV-I-associated myelopathy improve with high-dose oral prednisone, although benefit may not be sustained. Small, unblinded studies suggest that improvement may be observed with high-dose intravenous immunoglobulin or with danazol, an anabolic steroid.

A myelopathy clinically similar to that caused by HTLV-I has been described in patients infected with HTLV-II. Myelopathy in HIV-infected patients coinfected with HTLV-I or HTLV-II has also been described.

### HIV

A steadily progressive spastic–ataxic myelopathy is seen in patients infected with HIV. In an AIDS autopsy series, 22% of consecutive studies revealed abnormalities in the lateral and posterior columns of the thoracic cord. This complication of HIV usually occurs in the setting of advanced immunosuppression and is often seen in patients with dementia.

## Radiculopathy and Neuropathy

## Parainfectious syndromes

### Guillain-Barré syndrome

Acute inflammatory demyelinating polyradiculoneuritis, or Guillain-Barré syndrome, is the most frequent cause of acute flaccid paralysis in children and adults in the United States and Europe. It is nonepidemic and nonseasonal, with median age of onset in the fifth decade. The annual incidence ranges from 0.75 to two cases per 100,000 population throughout the world. The pathogenesis of the syndrome is unknown. It is thought to be an inflammatory peripheral neuropathy that causes demyelination, especially of nerve roots. Axonal degeneration may be a consequence of demyelination, although a purely axonal form of Guillain-Barré likely occurs.

Guillain-Barré syndrome may develop after vaccination, general surgery, anesthesia, and treatment with thrombolytics. It is seen more frequently in patients with systemic disorders such as sarcoid, Hodgkin's disease and other lymphomas, and systemic lupus erythematosus. The syndrome is believed to be postinfectious, developing in 50%–75% of cases 2 to 4 wk after symptoms of an acute infectious disease. Typically implicated are HIV, human cytomegalovirus, Epstein-Barr virus, and *Mycoplasma pneumoniae*. In the last few years, *Campylobacter jejuni* enteritis has been identified as the most common antecedent infection in patients with Guillain-Barré syndrome, occurring in about 30% of cases. Onset of neuropathy is typically about 10 d after *Campylobacter* infection. Although typical Guillain-Barré may follow *Campylobacter* infection, this infection may be associated with more severe clinical manifestations and poorer neurologic recovery than other infections, perhaps because it is more often associated with a primary axonal neuropathy.

Presenting symptoms of Guillain-Barré syndrome include paresthesia in the distal extremities, followed by leg weakness and variable weakness of the arms, face, and oropharyngeal muscles. Patients commonly complain of pain in the back, flanks, or legs. Physical examination shows symmetric limb weakness and absent or diminished deep tendon reflexes. Facial weakness is present in about one-half of patients. Sensory abnormalities are minimal, and transient bowel and bladder dysfunction may be present early in the course. Weakness progresses for 1 to 4 wk, plateaus for 2 to 4 wk (but sometimes for months), and then slowly improves. About one-quarter of patients initially require mechanical ventilation.

The CSF may be normal in the first few days of weakness, but it usually becomes abnormal after the first week. The CSF WBC is usually less than 10 mononuclear cells/$\mu$l but can be as high as 50/$\mu$l; CSF protein concentration is generally above 55 mg/dl. This "albuminocytologic dissociation" is characteristic. Abnormalities of motor nerve conduction, including slowing of conduction velocities, prolonged distal latencies, and dispersion of evoked responses, are characteristic of demyelination and are seen in up to 90% of patients in the first 2 wk of illness. Conduction block, characterized by a decrease in the amplitude of the muscle action potential elicited distally compared to proximally, is a frequent finding.

The differential diagnosis of Guillain-Barré syndrome includes spinal cord compression and transverse myelopathy, vasculitic neuropathy, poliomyelitis and other enteroviral infections, Lyme disease, diphtheria, botulism, acute intermittent porphyria, tick paralysis, hexacarbon abuse, and toxin or heavy metal poisoning.

Plasma exchange is the best-studied treatment for Guillain-Barré. This modality shortens the time to unassisted ambulation and duration of mechanical ventilation, particularly if started within the first 1 to 2 wk of illness. A recent randomized trial suggests that IV Ig is as effective as plasma exchange for the treatment of Guillain-Barré syndrome. The combination of the two modalities offers no additional benefit compared to each alone.

Outcome in Guillain-Barré syndrome is good in the majority of patients: 15% have no residual deficit and 65% have minor neurologic sequelae such as numbness or foot drop that do not impair activities of daily living. About 5% die from autonomic instability, cardiac arrhythmias, sepsis, or pulmonary embolism; 5% to 10% have permanent disabling neurologic deficits. A poor prognosis is associated with a severe, rapidly progressive course, older age, need for assisted ventilation, and severely reduced muscle action potential amplitudes on nerve conduction studies.

### Bell's Palsy

Bell's palsy, or idiopathic facial nerve paralysis, is a common disorder, with an annual incidence of 20 to 25 persons per 100,000. The etiology of this disorder is unknown. About 40% of patients report a recent upper respiratory infection prior to the onset of facial weakness, implicating a parainfectious process. A recent study identified HSV-1 DNA in facial nerve endoneurial fluid from 11 out of 14 patients with Bell's palsy who had failed medical therapy, compared with 0 out of 21 controls. Enhancement of the facial nerve in the fallopian canal by MR and increased prevalence or increased mean serum IgG titers to herpes simplex virus have also been identified in patients with Bell's palsy. Taken together, these data support the contention that Bell's palsy is due to reactivation of HSV infection leading to inflammation and compression of the nerve in some patients with the disorder. Additional infectious diseases associated with facial weakness include HIV, Lyme disease, syphilis, varicella zoster virus, polio, leprosy, tetanus, diphtheria, and middle ear or mastoid infection. Noninfectious etiologies include temporal bone fracture, sarcoid, tumors in the cerebellopontine angle or temporal bone, tumor or infection of the parotid gland, diabetes, hypertension, pregnancy, multiple sclerosis, and Guillain-Barré syndrome.

Patients with Bell's palsy complain of abrupt onset of unilateral facial weakness that includes the forehead. Pain in the face or behind the ear is present in 50%–60% of affected individuals. Abnormal taste, hyperacusis, and decreased tearing may also be noted. Physical examination shows unilateral weakness of the muscles of facial expression. Although many patients complain of facial numbness, objective abnormalities are uncommon. Decreased taste sensation can be demonstrated at the bedside, as can decreased lacrimation by Schirmer test, and abnormal stapedial reflex by impedance test if the pathology is proximal in the nerve.

Many authorities recommend treatment with oral prednisone,

1 mg/kg/d for at least 5 d, followed by a 5 d taper. Although several studies have failed to show an improvement in time to recovery or in degree of recovery with steroid treatment, some have shown that this therapy decreases pain and protects against denervation. Results of a recent trial suggest that acyclovir may improve functional outcome of patients with Bell's palsy. Ideally, therapy would be reserved for patients who are most likely to have HSV-1 infection of the facial nerve and are therefore most likely to benefit from treatment with acyclovir; further study is required to establish methods for identifying such individuals.

Fifty to 80% of patients with Bell's palsy make a full recovery, but those with the most severe weakness are less likely to return to normal. Speed and extent of recovery are correlated. Complete recovery is usually seen by 12 wk after onset; incomplete recovery may not be evident until 2 mo and usually stabilizes by 9 mo. There may be facial synkinesis secondary to aberrant axonal regrowth.

## Infectious radiculopathy and neuropathy

The most common causes of infectious radiculopathy and neuropathy are herpesviruses, including varicella-zoster virus, human cytomegalovirus, and herpes simplex type 2 virus; and bacterial diseases, particularly Lyme disease, syphilis, and leprosy (Tables 75.3, 75.4).

### Varicella-zoster virus

Pain, dysesthesia, and objective sensory abnormalities in the dermatome affected by the rash are hallmarks of herpes zoster, or shingles. In addition, symptomatic weakness of extremities occurs in about 3% of patients. Segmental weakness of thoracic musculature is probably much more common but is clinically unrecognized. Whether muscle weakness is the result of involvement of the anterior horn cells or the anterior nerve roots is unknown.

Weakness is usually noted in the first 2 wk after appearance of rash and most commonly occurs in myotomes corresponding to affected dermatomes. However, in up to 10% of cases, muscle weakness may be distant from the affected dermatome. Too few patients with muscle weakness secondary to zoster have been treated with antivirals to comment on its utility. Nonetheless, the prognosis of limb weakness is generally good; 55% recover completely and 25% improve significantly. Proximal muscle weakness generally recovers more fully than distal weakness.

Ramsay Hunt syndrome classically refers to herpes zoster involving the external auditory canal accompanied by facial weakness or auditory and vestibular symptoms. More widespread involvement is now appreciated, and the syndrome is synonymous with cephalic zoster accompanying a variety of cranial nerve abnormalities. The rash of zoster can be seen on the palate, uvula, buccal mucosa, tonsils, tongue, face, or neck. Involvement of any combination of cranial nerves has been described, resulting in facial weakness, hearing loss, vertigo, weakness of the palate or tongue, and ophthalmoplegia or visual loss. Cranial nerve deficits can be unilateral or bilateral. Vesicles usually appear at the same time as paresis but may occur before or after weakness. Pain may precede the onset of rash by several days. Only a few vesicles may be seen, or in some cases none are evident (zoster sine herpete). The syndrome is believed to be due to direct viral infection of nerves, ganglia, or brainstem, but some authors contend that the syndrome is parainfectious.

Complete facial nerve recovery is less likely to occur in Ramsay Hunt syndrome than in "idiopathic" Bell's palsy. In a Dutch study, motor recovery defined as normal strength or residual mild weakness was seen in 97% with incomplete facial paralysis at presentation and in 52% with initially complete paralysis. However, complete recovery without sequelae was seen in only 66% and 10%, respectively. Case reports suggest that recovery may be improved by treatment with intravenous acyclovir and

**Table 75.3** Infectious causes of radiculopathy

| Agent | Key features |
|---|---|
| HERPESVIRUSES | |
| Herpes simplex type 2 | Sacral radiculitis is an uncommon complication of primary or recurrent genital infection. Therapy with acyclovir may be beneficial |
| Varicella | As in myelopathy, radiculopathy due to varicella is seen with reactivation (shingles). While sensory changes in the distribution of the affected spinal root or cranial nerve are the rule, weakness in corresponding myotomes may also occur. Therapy with acyclovir, often with steroids, has been beneficial in some patients with cephalic zoster with cranial nerve abnormalities (Ramsay Hunt syndrome) |
| Human cytomegalovirus | Radiculopathy, often with myelopathy, is seen in patients with HIV, and may have a rapidly progressive course. Early therapy with ganciclovir or foscarnet may lead to clinical improvement |
| BACTERIA | |
| Lyme disease | Triad of meningitis, cranial neuritis, and painful radiculitis is the most common early neurologic complication of Lyme disease. |
| Syphilis | Radiculopathy is a rare complication of syphilis. Cerebrospinal fluid profile is similar to that seen in syphilitic meningitis |

**Table 75.4** Bacterial infections that cause neuropathy

| Agent | Key features |
|---|---|
| Leprosy | May cause mononeuritis multiplex or symmetrical distal neuropathy. Nerve injury may occur during reversal reactions |
| Botulism | Toxin-mediated. Typical clinical findings include cranial neuropathies, symmetrical descending weakness, and normal sensation. Paresthesias and asymmetric weakness are seen in some patients |
| Diphtheria | Toxin-mediated. Characterized by cranial neuropathy, followed by peripheral neuropathy involving motor more than sensory nerves |

oral prednisone, but no large controlled study has been performed.

### Herpes simplex type 2 sacral radiculitis

Genital herpes simplex type 2 (HSV-2) infection may be accompanied by symptoms of sacral radiculitis, including back and leg pain, sacral-distribution sensory loss or paresthesia, urinary retention, constipation and impotence. This is an uncommon complication of primary (and occasionally recurrent) genital infection, occurring in 2%–5% of patients, but may be seen in up to 50% of men with HSV-2 proctitis. Physical examination demonstrates sacral sensory abnormalities, loss of rectal sphincter tone, and diminished bulbocavernosus reflex. Cystometry shows a hypotonic bladder. Most reported patients have mild lymphocytic CSF pleocytosis with normal or slightly elevated protein. Symptoms usually resolve over days to weeks. Although controlled clinical trials have not been performed, patients who present early in the course of disease may benefit from therapy with acyclovir.

### Human cytomegalovirus polyradiculitis

An inflammatory lumbosacral polyradiculopathy due to human cytomegalovirus (CMV) is an uncommon complication in patients also infected with HIV. It is seen in individuals with advanced immunosuppression and is characterized by rapid progression of leg weakness that may lead to paraplegia within days. Most affected individuals have urinary retention or constipation, and about half have severe back pain. Physical examination shows bilateral, sometimes asymmetrical, proximal and distal lower extremity weakness, depressed or absent lower extremity deep tendon reflexes, and sacral sensory loss. Occasionally there may be concomitant evidence of cord involvement, with hyperreflexia and upgoing toes. Cerebrospinal fluid is remarkable for a profile characteristic of bacterial meningitis: polymorphonuclear pleocytosis with counts often above 1000/$\mu$l, low glucose, and high protein. CSF cultures yield CMV about half the time; CMV PCR may be more sensitive.

Treatment with ganciclovir or foscarnet may result in improvement in strength if therapy is instituted within the first 1 to 2 wk of illness, but improvement may be delayed for several months in some cases. Dosing regimens have been identical to those for CMV retinitis, with initial induction followed by maintenance doses (see Chapter 39). Response to therapy is predicted by improvement in CSF abnormalities. Failure of the CSF to improve after 2 wk of treatment should prompt consideration of change in therapy or of continuing high-dose induction doses rather than switching to maintenance doses. Development of CMV radiculitis in a patient already being treated for CMV disease of other organ systems has a poor prognosis.

### Lyme radiculitis

The triad of meningitis, cranial neuritis, and painful radiculitis (Bannwarth's syndrome) is the most common early neurological complication of Lyme disease and is particularly common in Europe. In a study of 187 patients with well-documented Lyme disease in Denmark, 86% had radicular pain and 12% had muscle weakness involving multiple motor roots. Pain was more common in older patients and usually began in the region of previous erythema migrans rash. Despite the observation that radiculitis may improve spontaneously, antibiotic therapy is indicated to hasten clinical recovery and prevent other complications of Lyme disease; treatment is discussed in Chapter 96.

### Leprosy

Leprosy, or Hansen's disease, is a chronic infection due to *Mycobacterium leprae* that primarily affects skin and peripheral nerves. It is prevalent in Africa, Asia, India, and Latin America. Leprosy affects as many as 5.5 million persons worldwide. In the United States, 150–200 cases are reported per year.

Disease manifestations of leprosy are determined by host immune response. At one polar extreme, patients with tuberculoid (paucibacillary) leprosy demonstrate mononeuritis multiplex early in their course, with enlarged nerves associated with hypopigmented, anesthetic skin lesions. Weakness, with claw hand deformity or foot drop, is common. At the other end of the spectrum, patients with lepromatous (multibacillary) leprosy develop a more symmetrical distal sensory neuropathy later in the course of disease. Patients with borderline states are at particular risk of nerve injury during reversal reactions, which may occur in as many as 50% of patients within 6 to 12 mo of initiating therapy with dapsone. Multidrug therapy with rifampin, clofazimine, and dapsone is recommended for multibacillary disease, and dapsone with rifampin for paucibacillary disease. However, exact regimens and duration of therapy remain controversial.

## ANNOTATED BIBLIOGRAPHY

Adour KK, Ruboyianes JM, Von Doersten PG, Byl FM, Trent CS, Quesenberry CP Jr, Hitchcock T. Bell's palsy treatment with acyclovir and prednisone compared with prednisone alone: a double-blind, randomized, controlled trial. Ann Otol Rhinol Laryngol 1996; 105:371–378.

*Randomized double-blind trial of acyclovir 400 mg by mouth five times per day for 10 days versus placebo in combination with open-label prednisone 1 mg/kg by mouth in two equal divided doses per day (minimum*

*60 mg per day) for treatment of Bell's palsy. Functional recovery was significantly better in acyclovir-treated subjects and significantly fewer acyclovir-treated subjects experienced moderate to severe contracture with synkinesis.*

Case records of the Massachusetts General Hospital (case 42–1994). N Engl J Med 1994; 331:1437–1444.
*Excellent discussion of differential diagnosis of acute transverse myelopathy.*

Devinsky O, Cho E-S, Petito CK, Price RW. Herpes zoster myelitis. Brain 1991; 114:1181–1196.
*Clinical and pathologic review of 13 patients with rigorously defined herpes zoster myelitis, and review of reported cases. Documents viral infection of the spinal cord, supporting role of antiviral therapy.*

Gelber RH. Hansen's disease. West J Med 1993; 158:583–590.
*Excellent review, with focus on drug regimens other than those recommended by the World Health Organization.*

Gessain A, Gout O. Chronic myelopathy associated with human T-lymphotropic virus type I (HTLV-I). Ann Intern Med 1992; 117:933–946.
*Review of clinical, epidemiologic, immunologic and virologic aspects of HTLV-1 associated myelopathy.*

Gilden DH, Beinlich BR, Rubinstien EM, Stommel E, Swenson R, Rubinstein D, Mahalingam R. Varicella-zoster virus myelitis: an expanding spectrum. Neurology 1994; 44:1818–1823.
*Report of four cases of varicella zoster associated myelopathy, two of whom had a relapsing and remitting course. Varicella DNA was identified in CSF from all three patients with CSF pleocytosis.*

Jeffery DR, Mandler RN, Davis LE. Transverse myelitis. Retrospective analysis of 33 cases, with differentiation of cases associated with multiple sclerosis and parainfectious events. Arch Neurol 1993; 50:532–535.
*Only study providing annual incidence of transverse myelopathy in the United States, estimated at 4.6 per million. The authors conclude that parainfectious transverse myelopathy may be distinguishable from multiple-sclerosis-associated transverse myelopathy based on clinical, neuroimaging, and cerebrospinal fluid findings.*

Plasma Exchange/Sandoglobulin Guillain-Barré Syndrome Trial Group. Randomised trial of plasma exchange, intravenous immunoglobulin, and combined treatments in Guillain-Barré syndrome. Lancet 1997; 349:225–230.
*Randomized trial of plasma exchange, IV Ig, or plasma exchange immediately followed by IV Ig for patients with severe Guillain-Barré syndrome. Plasma exchange and IV Ig had equivalent efficacy; there was no additional benefit of the combination of the two treatment modalities.*

Price RW, Plum F. Poliomyelitis. In: Handbook of Clinical Neurology, vol 34. Vinken PJ, Bruyn GW, eds. Elsevier/North Holland Biomedical Press, Amsterdam, pp 93–132, 1978.
*Clearly written, comprehensive review of poliovirus infection.*

Ropper AH, Poskanzer DC. The prognosis of acute and subacute transverse myelopathy based on early signs and symptoms. Ann Neurol 1978; 4:51–59.
*Retrospective study of 52 patients seen at the Massachusetts General Hospital with a diagnosis of transverse myelitis from 1955 to 1975. Uses a broader definition of transverse myelopathy than other studies, which enables the authors to provide a description of the spectrum of initial clinical presentation and correlate with outcome.*

Ropper AH. The Guillain-Barré syndrome. N Engl J Med 1992; 326:1130–1136.
*Succinct review of the syndrome.*

Strebel PM, Sutter RW, Cochi SL, Biellik RJ, Brink EW, Kew OM, Pallansch MA, Orenstein WA, Hinman AR. Epidemiology of poliomyelitis in the United States one decade after the last reported case of indigenous wild virus-associated disease. Clin Infect Dis 1992; 14:568–579.
*Establishes risk of vaccine associated poliomyelitis as approximately one case per 2.5 million OPV doses distributed, and documents increased risk with first or second vaccine administration.*

Thomas JE, Howard FM. Segmental zoster paresis—a disease profile. Neurology 1972; 22:459–466.
*Retrospective review of 1,210 patients with herpes zoster. Sixty-one patients had segmental muscle weakness, 28 of whom had cranial nerve palsies. Complete functional recovery was seen in 55%, and partial recovery in 30%.*

# 76

# Focal Central Nervous System Infections

ALLAN R. TUNKEL AND W. MICHAEL SCHELD

Focal infections of the central nervous system (CNS) are frequently devastating, with most of the serious consequences occurring as a result of mass effect with compression of important CNS structures. The CNS possesses several defense mechanisms (e.g., an intact cranium and the blood-brain barrier) to prevent entry of various microorganisms, but once organisms have gained entry into the CNS, host defense mechanisms are often inadequate to control the infection. In addition, the effectiveness of antimicrobial therapy is limited by the poor penetration of many agents into the CNS. Therefore, concomitant surgical therapy is often needed. The following sections review the common focal infections of the CNS, with emphasis on approach to diagnosis and management.

## Brain Abscess

### Epidemiology, etiology, and pathogenesis

Brain abscess is one of the most serious focal CNS infections. It is generally regarded as a rare disease, with large autopsy series reporting occurrence rates of 0.18%–1.3%. The incidence varies depending upon geographic locale, accounting for ~1 in 10,000 general hospital admissions. The median age of patients is 30–45 yr; most series report a male predominance (~2:1). Mortality rates for brain abscess in the preantibiotic era ranged from 40% to 60%, although these rates have recently decreased to about 5%–20%, likely a result of recent developments in diagnosis and treatment (see below). One study reported that the prognosis of brain abscess appears to be primarily determined by the rapidity of progression of disease before hospitalization and the patient's mental status on admission.

#### Pathogenesis

The etiologic agents that are responsible for causing brain abscesses vary depending upon the pathogenesis of infection and the underlying condition of the host. The most common pathogenic mechanism of brain abscess formation is *spread* from *a contiguous focus* of infection, usually from the middle ear, mastoid cells, or paranasal sinuses. Most cases of brain abscess secondary to otitis media occur in the temporal lobe and cerebellum; etiologic agents include streptococci, *Bacteroides fragilis*, and members of the Enterobacteriaceae family. The frontal lobe is the predominant site of abscess localization as a result of paranasal sinusitis. When brain abscess complicates sphenoid sinusitis, the temporal lobe or sella turcica is usually involved; streptococci are the predominant species isolated, although anaerobes, *Staphylococcus aureus*, and gram-negative bacilli have also been recovered.

A second mechanism of brain abscess formation is *hematogenous dissemination* to the brain from a distant focus of infection. These abscesses are usually multiple and multiloculated, and they carry a higher mortality rate than abscesses that arise from contiguous foci of infection. The most common initial source of infection is chronic pyogenic lung disease (i.e., lung abscess, bronchiectasis, and empyema). The most likely infecting organisms are anaerobes (*Fusobacterium* and *Bacteroides* species) and streptococci. Hematogenous dissemination may also occur from wound and skin infections, osteomyelitis, pelvic infections, cholecystitis, and other intraabdominal infections; acute bacterial endocarditis, due to *S. aureus*, may also cause multiple brain abscesses. Other predisposing conditions are cyanotic congenital heart disease, hereditary hemorrhagic telangiectasia, and esophageal dilatation and sclerosing therapy for esophageal varices.

*Trauma* is a third pathogenic mechanism of brain abscess formation. This may occur secondary to an open cranial fracture with dural breech, after neurosurgery, or as a result of a foreign body injury. Contaminated retained bone fragments and debris provide a nidus of infection that subsequently evolves into an abscess. Likely infecting microorganisms after trauma include staphylococci, streptococci, gram-negative bacilli, and anaerobes. Finally, brain abscess is *cryptogenic* in about 20% of patients, although many of these cases most likely occur secondary to unrecognized dental foci of infection.

#### Etiologic agents

The most commonly isolated *bacterial species* in brain abscesses are streptococci (aerobic, anaerobic, and microaerophilic) in 60%–70% of cases; these organisms usually reside in the oral cavity, appendix, and female genital tract and have a proclivity for abscess formation. *Staphylococcus aureus* is currently isolated in 10%–15% of cases (compared to 25%–30% in the preantibiotic era), although the frequency of its isolation is increased in patients with cranial trauma and infective endocarditis. Isolation of anaerobes has increased with attention to proper isolation techniques, with *Bacteroides* species isolated in 20%–40% of cases, often in mixed culture. The enteric gram-negative bacilli (*Proteus* species, *Escherichia coli*, *Klebsiella* species, and *Pseudomonas* species) are isolated in 23%–33% of cases. Less commonly (<1% of cases) other bacterial species may be isolated; these include *Hemophilus influenzae*, *Streptococcus pneumoniae*, *Listeria monocytogenes*, and *Nocardia asteroides*. *Nocardia* is isolated more often in patients with deficiencies in cell-mediated immunity and probably spreads to the brain via hematogenous dissemination from distant foci of infection (e.g., the lung). *Actinomyces* species are more commonly isolated in patients with pulmonary and odontogenic infections. Space-occupying lesions caused by *Mycobacterium tuberculosis* were thought to be rare, but tuberculomas have been observed in a minority of cases of tuberculous meningitis.

*Fungi* are being increasingly recognized as causes of brain abscess due to increased numbers of immunocompromised patients. Patients with neutropenia or neutrophil defects are at increased risk for infection caused by *Candida*, *Aspergillus*, and *Rhizopus* species. Patients with diabetes mellitus and ketoacidosis are predisposed to the development of rhinocerebral mucormycosis; cerebral mucomycosis with abscess formation also occurs in injection drug abusers. *Pseudallescheria boydii* may enter the CNS by direct trauma, hematogenous dissemination from a pulmonary source, through an intravenous catheter, or by direct extension from infected sinuses. Although *Cryptococcus neoformans* usually causes meningitis, CNS mass lesions caused by this organism have also been reported.

Brain abscesses may also occur as a result of infection by various *protozoa* and *helminths*, depending upon the geographic locale and the patient's underlying condition. With the advent of the acquired immunodeficiency syndrome (AIDS), infection caused by *Toxoplasma gondii* has become an important cause of focal CNS disease; estimates of the prevalence of toxoplasmic encephalitis in patients with AIDS have ranged from 2.6% to 30.8%. Other risk groups for CNS toxoplasmosis include patients with reticuloendothelial malignancies (due either to the malignancy itself or to associated immunosuppressive or cytotoxic drug therapy) and following immunosuppressive therapy after organ transplantation. Cysticercosis caused by *Taenia solium* is a major cause of brain lesions in the developing world, accounting for 85% of all brain infections in Mexico City.

## Clinical manifestations

Most of the clinical manifestations of brain abscess occur as a result of the presence of a space-occupying lesion within the brain (Table 76.1). Only about one-half of patients with bacterial brain abscess present with the classic triad of fever, headache, and a focal neurologic deficit. It is also important to note that the clinical presentation of brain abscess in immunosuppressed patients may be masked by the diminished inflammatory response.

Other clinical manifestations depend upon brain abscess location. Patients with a frontal lobe abscess often present with headache, drowsiness, inattention, and deterioration of mental status; the most common focal neurologic signs are hemiparesis (with unilateral motor signs) and a motor speech disorder. Patients with cerebellar abscesses may present with ataxia, nystagmus, vomiting, and dysmetria. The presentation of a temporal lobe abscess may include ipsilateral headache and aphasia if the lesion is in the dominant hemisphere; a visual field defect (e.g., an upper homonymous quadrantanopia) may be the only presenting sign. Abscesses localized to the brainstem usually present with facial weakness, fever, headache, hemiparesis, dysphagia, and vomiting.

**Table 76.1** Common symptoms and signs in patients with brain abscess

| Symptom or sign | Frequency (%) |
|---|---|
| Headache | ~70 |
| Mental status changes | ≤70 |
| Focal neurologic deficits | >60 |
| Fever | 45–50 |
| Seizures | 25–35 |
| Nausea and vomiting | 25–50 |
| Nuchal rigidity | ~25 |
| Papilledema | ~25 |

Patients with brain abscess caused by certain fungal pathogens may present with specific clinical characteristics. Patients with *Aspergillus* brain abscess most commonly manifest signs of a stroke referable to the involved area of brain; evidence of aspergillosis in other organ systems is common. Patients with rhinocerebral mucormycosis initally present with complaints referable to the eyes or sinuses, including headache, facial pain, diplopia, lacrimation, and nasal stuffiness or discharge. As the infection spreads posteriorly, patients may develop proptosis and external ophthalmoplegia. Cranial nerve abnormalities (II–VII, IX, and X) and blindness may occur as a result of vascular compromise; thrombosis is a striking feature of this disease because the organisms have a proclivity for blood vessel invasion.

The clinical manifestations of CNS toxoplasmosis may be variable, ranging from an acute onset with a confusional state to an insidious process evolving over several weeks; the initial symptoms and signs may be focal, nonfocal, or both. Focal abnormalities depend upon the intracranial location; there is a predilection to localize in the basal ganglia and brainstem, producing extrapyramidal symptoms resembling Parkinson's disease. Nonfocal symptoms and signs may predominate and include generalized weakness, seizures, headache, confusion, lethargy, alteration of mental status, personality changes, and coma.

## Diagnosis

The diagnosis of brain abscess has been revolutionized by the availability of computed tomography (CT), and more recently MR imaging, which have rendered other diagnostic tests such as angiography, ventriculography, pneumoencephalography, and radionuclide brain scanning virtually obsolete. CT is an excellent means to examine the brain parenchyma, paranasal sinuses, mastoid cells, and middle ear, and it also yields information concerning the extent of surrounding edema, presence or absence of a midline shift, presence of hydrocephalus, and the possibility of imminent ventricular rupture. The sensitivity of CT for brain abscess ranges from 95% to 99% (see Chapter 12). The characteristic CT picture is a lesion with a hypodense center and a peripheral uniform ring enhancement following the injection of contrast material; this is surrounded by a variable hypodense area of brain edema; CT may also reveal nodular enhancement and areas of low attenuation without enhancement; this finding is seen during the early cerebritis stage prior to abscess formation, although once the abscess progresses, contrast enhancement is observed. In the later stages as the abscess becomes encapsulated, contrast no longer differentiates the lucent center and the CT appearance is similar to the early cerebritis stage.

CT scanning also has the major advantage of permitting stereotactic CT-guided aspiration of the abscess to facilitate bacteriologic diagnosis and determine organism susceptibility to antimicrobial agents; if the lesion appears encapsulated by CT scan criteria, aspiration for diagnosis and drainage can be performed without delay. In several series, there was no associated mortality and low morbidity (4%–6%) by use of this technique. Specimens obtained at the time of aspiration should be sent for gram stain and other special stains (e.g., Ziehl-Neelson, modified acid-fast, and silver stains) which may give a clue to likely etiologic diagnosis. Routine aerobic and anaerobic cultures should also be sent, as well as cultures for *Nocardia*, mycobacteria, and fungi. Histopathologic examination may also be indicated, particularly for evaluation of brain abscesses in the immunocompromised host (e.g., for identification of *T. gondii* and *Aspergillus* species).

The data on the role of magnetic resonance (MR) imaging in the diagnosis of brain abscess are very encouraging; MR imaging appears to offer advantages over CT in the early detection of cerebritis, cerebral edema, and satellite lesions. T1-weighted images (Fig. 76.1) characteristically demonstrate a peripheral zone of mild hypointensity (representative of edema formation) related to adjacent brain, which surrounds a central zone of more marked signal hypointensity (indicative of the necrotic center of the abscess); these two regions are separated by a capsule that appears as a discrete rim which is isointense to mildly hyperintense. On T2-weighted images, there is a markedly increased area of signal intensity in the zone of edema when compared to adjacent brain, whereas the central core is isointense to hyperintense compared to gray matter; the capsule appears as a well-defined hypointense rim at the margin of the abscess. Contrast-enhanced scans, using the paramagnetic agent gadolinium diethylenetriamine penta-acetic acid (Gd-DTPA), have the advantage of clearly differentiating the central abscess, the surrounding contrast-enhancing rim, and the cerebral edema surrounding the abscess. Its lack of ionizing radiation, greater tissue characterization, lack of bone artifact (which improves its sensitivity in posterior fossa lesions), and the decreased toxicity of Gd-DTPA as compared with CT contrast agents make MR imaging the procedure of choice in evaluation of brain abscesses.

In the diagnosis of brain abscess, $^{111}$indium-labeled scintigraphy is a diagnostic modality that may prove to be complementary to CT or MR imaging. Although the sensitivity of this test is high, false-negative scans do occur.

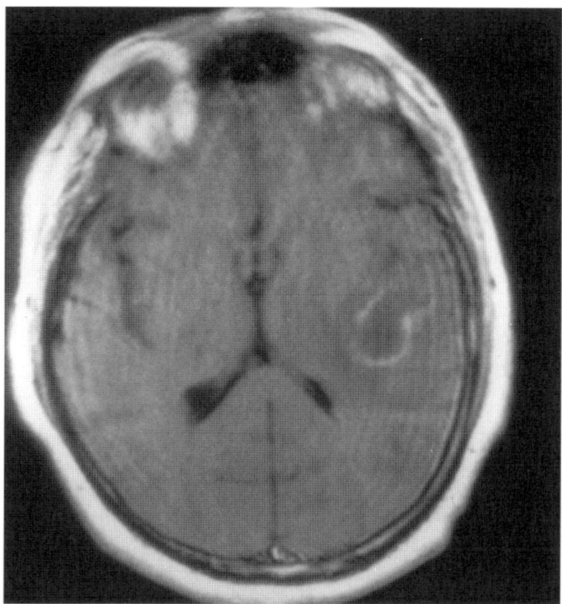

**Fig. 76.1** T1-weighted axial MR of the brain with gadolinium enhancement revealing a hypodense mass in the left temporal lobe with ring enhancement and surrounding edema.

## Treatment

### Antimicrobial therapy

When a diagnosis of brain abscess is made, either presumptively by radiographic studies or definitively by aspiration of the abscess, antimicrobial therapy should be initiated. The choice of antimicrobial agent is dependent upon its ability to penetrate into brain abscess pus. For bacterial brain abscess, empiric therapy (based on predisposing condition) should be initiated if aspiration is impractical or delayed (Table 76.2). In human immunodeficiency virus (HIV)-infected patients, toxoplasmosis is the most common cause of brain abscess, especially if multiple enhancing lesions are observed on CT or MR imaging. In HIV-infected patients who are serologically positive for *T. gondii* and have a consistent radiographic picture, empiric therapy for toxoplasmic encephalitis (i.e., pyrimethamine plus sulfadiazine) is often employed. A clinical and radiographic response is usually observed within 10 and 14 d, respectively, of initiation of therapy.

Once an infecting microorganism is identified, either by microbiologic or histopathologic means, antimicrobial therapy can be modified for optimal treatment (Table 76.3); recommended dosages of antimicrobial agents for CNS infections are shown in Table 76.4. Most authorities recommend that antimicrobial therapy for bacterial brain abscess be continued for 4–8 wk, although the time duration is uncertain and may relate to the initial surgical procedure (see below). Shorter antimicrobial courses (3–4 wk) may be appropriate for patients undergoing excision of the abscess. Although surgery is often required for optimal therapy of bacterial brain abscess (see below), certain subgroups of patients can be managed with antimicrobial therapy alone. These include patients with medical conditions that increase the risk of surgery, multiples abscesses, abscesses in a deep or dominant location, concomitant meningitis or ependymitis, early abscess reduction with clinical improvement after antimicrobial therapy, and abscess size under 3 cm. In patients treated nonoperatively, contrast-enhanced CT or MR scans (maximum slice thickness of 5 mm) should be obtained weekly for the first 4 wk or until definite abscess shrinkage is observed, followed by monthly scans until lesions no longer exhibit contrast enhancement and antimicrobial agents have been discontinued at least 2 wk. Surgery is indicated for an increase in abscess size at any time or if there is no change after 4 wk of antimicrobial therapy. Complete resolution of the abscess cavity, mass effect, and contrast enhancement may not occur for up to 6 mo after completion of successful therapy. Antimicrobial therapy for nocardial brain abscess has ranged from 3 to 12 mo, although therapy for immunosuppressed patients should probably be continued for up to 1 yr, with careful follow-up to monitor for response.

### Surgical therapy

Most patients with a brain abscess require surgical therapy for optimal management. The two procedures judged to be equivalent by outcome are aspiration of the abscess after burr hole placement and complete excision after craniotomy. The procedure of choice must be individualized. Aspiration may be performed by sterotactic CT or intraoperative ultrasound guidance, which af-

**Table 76.2** Empiric antimicrobial therapy of bacterial brain abscess

| Predisposing condition | Usual bacterial isolates | Antimicrobial regimen |
|---|---|---|
| Otitis media or mastoiditis | Streptococci (anaerobic or aerobic), *Bacteroides* species, Enterobacteriaceae | Penicillin + metronidazole + a third-generation cephalosporin[a] |
| Sinusitis (frontoethmoidal or sphenoidal) | Streptococci, *Bacteroides* species, Enterobacteriaceae, *Staphylococcus aureus*, *Hemophilus* species | Vancomycin + metronidazole + a third-generation cephalosporin[a] |
| Dental sepsis | Mixed *Fusobacterium* and *Bacteroides* species, streptococci | Penicillin + metronidazole |
| Penetrating trauma or postneurosurgical | *Staphylococcus aureus*, streptococci, Enterobacteriaceae, *Clostridium* | Vancomycin + a third-generation cephalosporin[a] |
| Lung abscess, empyema, bronchiectasis | *Fusobacterium*, *Actinomyces*, *Bacteroides* species, streptococci, *Nocardia asteroides* | Penicillin + metronidazole + a sulfonamide[b] |
| Bacterial endocarditis | *Staphylococcus aureus*, streptococci | Vancomycin + gentamicin |

[a]Cefotaxime or ceftriaxone; ceftazidime is used if *Pseudomonas aeruginosa* is suspected.

[b]Sulfadiazine or trimethoprim-sulfamethoxazole; include if *Nocardia asteroides* is suspected.

**Table 76.3** Antimicrobial therapy of brain abscess

| Organism | Standard therapy | Alternative therapies |
|---|---|---|
| *ACTINOMYCES* SPECIES | Penicillin G | Clindamycin |
| *ASPERGILLUS* SPECIES | Amphotericin B[a] | Itraconazole[b] |
| *BACTEROIDES FRAGILIS* | Metronidazole | Chloramphenicol, clindamycin |
| *CANDIDA* SPECIES | Amphotericin B[a] | Fluconazole |
| *CRYPTOCOCCUS NEOFORMANS* | Amphotericin B[a] | Fluconazole |
| ENTEROBACTERIACEAE | Third-generation cephalosporin[c] | Aztreonam, trimethoprim-sulfamethoxazole, fluoroquinolone |
| *FUSOBACTERIUM* SPECIES | Penicillin G | Metronidazole |
| *HEMOPHILUS* SPECIES | Third generation cephalosporin[c] | Aztreonam, trimethoprim-sulfamethoxazole |
| *LISTERIA MONOCYTOGENES* | Ampicillin or penicillin G[d] | Trimethoprim-sulfamethoxazole |
| *MYCOBACTERIUM TUBERCULOSIS* | Isoniazid + rifampin + pyrazinamide ± ethambutol | |
| *NOCARDIA ASTEROIDES* | Trimethoprim-sulfamethoxazole or sulfadiazine | Minocycline, imipenem, a third-generation cephalosporin,[c] fluoroquinolone |
| *PSEUDALLESCHERIA BOYDII* | Miconazole | Fluconazole[b] |
| *PSEUDOMONAS AERUGINOSA* | Ceftazidime[d] | Aztreonam,[d] fluoroquinolone[d] |
| *STAPHYLOCOCCUS AUREUS* | | |
| Methicillin-sensitive | Nafcillin or oxacillin | Vancomycin |
| Methicillin-resistant | Vancomycin | |
| *STREPTOCOCCUS MILLERI*, OTHER STREPTOCOCCI | Penicillin G | Third-generation cephalosporin,[c] vancomycin |
| *TOXOPLASMA GONDII* | Pyrimethamine + sulfadiazine | Pyrimethamine + clindamycin, azithromycin,[b] atovaquone[b] |

[a]Addition of flucytosine should be considered.

[b]Efficacy not yet proven in brain abscess due to this organism.

[c]Cefotaxime or ceftriaxone.

[d]Addition of an aminoglycoside should be considered.

**Table 76.4** Recommended dosages of antimicrobial agents for central nervous system infections in adults*

| Antimicrobial agent | Total daily dosage | Dosing interval (hours) |
|---|---|---|
| Amikacin[a] | 15 mg/kg | 8 |
| Amphotericin B | 0.6–1.0 mg/kg[b] | 24 |
| Ampicillin | 12 g | 4 |
| Atovaquone | 3000 mg | 6–12 |
| Azithromycin | 1200 mg | 24 |
| Aztreonam | 6–8 g | 6–8 |
| Cefotaxime | 8–12 g | 4–6 |
| Ceftazidime | 6 g | 8 |
| Ceftriaxone | 4 g | 12 |
| Chloramphenicol | 4–6 g | 6 |
| Ciprofloxacin | 800 mg | 12 |
| Clindamycin | 1200–2400 mg[c] | 6 |
| Ethambutol[d] | 15 mg/kg | 24 |
| Fluconazole | 400 mg | 24 |
| Flucytosine[d] | 150 mg/kg | 6 |
| Gentamicin[a] | 3–5 mg/kg | 8 |
| Isoniazid[d] | 300 mg | 24 |
| Itraconazole | 400 mg | 12 |
| Metronidazole | 30 mg/kg | 6 |
| Miconazole | 1.5–3.0 g | 8 |
| Nafcillin | 9–12 g | 4 |
| Oxacillin | 9–12 g | 4 |
| Penicillin | 24 million units | 4 |
| Pyrazinamide[d] | 15–30 mg/kg | 24 |
| Pyrimethamine[d] | 25–100 mg[c] | 24 |
| Rifampin[d] | 600 mg | 24 |
| Sulfadiazine[d] | 4–6 g | 6 |
| Tobramycin[a] | 3–5 mg/kg | 8 |
| Trimethoprim-sulfamethoxazole | 10 mg/kg[e] | 12 |
| Vancomycin[a] | 2–3 g | 8–12 |

*Patients with normal renal and hepatic function. Unless indicated, the intravenous mode of administration is used.

[a]Need to monitor peak and trough serum concentrations.

[b]Dosages up to 1.5 mg/kg/d may be used for aspergillosis or mucormycosis.

[c]Higher dosages utilized in AIDS patients with toxoplasmic encephalitis.

[d]Oral administration.

[e]Dosage based on trimethoprim component.

fords the surgeon rapid, accurate, and safe access to virtually any intracranial point; aspiration can also be used for rapid relief of increased intracranial pressure. Excision is frequently required when there is incomplete drainage by aspiration of multiloculated lesions, for abscesses exhibiting gas on radiologic evaluation, for traumatic abscesses that may contain retained foreign bodies, and for abscesses located in the posterior fossa. In patients with worsening neurologic deficits, including deterioration of consciousness or signs of increased intracranial pressure, surgery should be performed emergently. Brain abscess excision is contraindicated in the early stages before a capsule is formed. The optimal therapy of fungal brain abscess usually requires a combined medical and surgical approach.

#### Adjunctive therapy

Corticosteroid therapy has been utilized as one method to manage increased intracranial pressure in patients with brain abscesses, although its use remains controversial. Corticosteroids may retard the encapsulation process, reduce antimicrobial entry into the CNS, increase necrosis, and alter the appearance of ring enhancement on CT as inflammation subsides; this latter factor obscures information from sequential studies. Corticosteroids are most useful, however, in the patient with deteriorating neurologic status and increased intracranial pressure, where they may prove to be life-saving. When used, corticosteroids should be administered for the shortest time possible and withdrawn when the mass effect no longer poses significant danger to the patient.

## Subdural Empyema

### Epidemiology, etiology, and pathogenesis

The term *subdural empyema* refers to a collection of pus in the space between the dura and arachnoid. Subdural empyema accounts for about 20% of all localized intracranial infections. This disease was essentially lethal prior to the advent of antimicrobial therapy, but with current modalities of diagnosis and treatment, mortality rates now range from 10% to 20%, but may be higher in patients presenting in stupor or coma. Subdural empyema may develop at any age but is most common in the second and third decades of life; males are affected four times more frequently than females.

#### Pathogenesis

The most common predisposing conditions to subdural empyema are *otorhinologic infections*, especially of the paranasal sinuses (50%–80% of cases). Infection spreads to the subdural space via valveless emissary veins in association with thrombophlebitis or via extension of an osteomyelitis of the skull with an accompanying epidural abscess. The mastoid cells and middle ear are the source in 10%–20% of cases. Other predisposing conditions include skull trauma, neurosurgical procedures, and infection of a preexisting subdural hematoma. Hematogenous dissemination (e.g., from the pulmonary system) occurs in a minority of cases (~5%). In adults, bacterial meningitis is a very unusual cause of subdural empyema. However, in infants, meningitis is an important predisposing condition for the development of subdural empyema, occurring in about 2% of infants with bacterial meningitis.

#### Etiologic agents

A number of bacterial species have been isolated from cranial subdural empyema; these include streptococci (~35%–40%), staphylococci (~15%), and aerobic gram-negative bacilli (~3%). In addition, anaerobic organisms (including anaerobic and microaerophilic streptococci and *Bacterodes fragilis*) are recovered in up to 100% of cases; polymicrobial infections are common.

These organisms make up the microbial flora frequently isolated from patients with chronic sinusitis or cranial abscesses. Spinal subdural empyema is a rare condition occurring secondary to metastatic infection from a distant site; *S. aureus* is the most frequent isolate, whereas streptococci are found less frequently.

## Clinical manifestations

Subdural empyema can present as a rapidly progressive, life-threatening condition. Symptoms and signs relate to the presence of increased intracranial pressure, meningeal irritation, and/or focal cortical inflammation; 60%–90% of patients have evidence of an antecedent infection (e.g., sinusitis or otitis media). A prominent complaint is headache (initially localized to the infected sinus or ear) which becomes generalized as the infection progresses. With increases in intracranial pressure, vomiting is a common complaint. About one-half of patients have an altered mental status early in infection, with progression to obtundation if treatment is not initiated. Fever is present in most cases. Focal neurologic signs appear within 24–48 h and progress rapidly, with eventual involvement of the entire cerebral hemisphere. The most common focal signs are hemiparesis and hemiplegia, but ocular palsies, dysphasia, homonymous hemianopsia, dilated pupils, and cerebellar signs have all been described. More than 50% of patients present with seizures, which may be either focal or generalized. About 80% of patients have signs of meningeal irritation (i.e., meningismus), although fewer have Kernig's or Brudzinski's sign. Papilledema is seen in <50% of cases. Without treatment, there is rapid neurologic deterioration with signs of increased intracranial pressure and cerebral herniation. It is also important to note that this fulminant picture may not be seen in patients with subdural empyema following cranial surgery or trauma, in those who have received prior antimicrobial therapy, in those with infected subdural hematomas, or in patients with infections metastatic to the subdural space.

Spinal subdural empyema usually manifests clinically as fever, radicular pain, and symptoms of spinal cord compression which may occur at multiple levels. Clinical distinction from spinal epidural abscess is difficult (see below).

## Diagnosis

The diagnosis of subdural empyema should be considered in any patient with meningeal signs and a focal neurologic examination. The diagnostic procedure of choice is either CT with contrast enhancement or MR imaging (Fig. 76.2). On CT scanning, there is typically a crescentic or elliptically shaped area of hypodensity below the cranial vault or adjacent to the falx cerebri. Depending on the extent of disease, there is often associated mass effect. With administration of intravenous contrast, there is a fine, intense line of enhancement which can be seen between the subdural collection and the cerebral cortex. Extensive mass effect on the ipsilateral cerebral hemisphere, which is out of proportion to the small size of the extra-axial collection, is invariably present, manifested as ventricular compression, sulcal effacement, and midline shift. Unfortunately, false-negative CT scans have been described. MR imaging provides greater clarity of morphologic detail, may detect an empyema not seen on CT, and is particularly valuable in detecting subdural empyemas located at the base of the brain, along the falx cerebri, or in the posterior fossa. On the basis of signal intensity, MR imaging can also differentiate empyema from most sterile effusions and chronic hematomas. Based on these findings, MR imaging is considered the diagnostic modality of choice for subdural empyema.

## Treatment

The therapy of subdural empyema requires a combined medical and surgical approach. Surgical therapy is essential because antimicrobial agents alone do not reliably sterilize these lesions, and surgical decompression is needed to control increased intracranial pressure. In addition, cultures of purulent material are useful to guide antimicrobial therapy.

### Antimicrobial therapy

Once purulent material is aspirated, antimicrobial therapy should be initiated. Therapy is based on results of the gram stain and the bacteria likely to be present at the site of primary infection (see above). If the primary infection is paranasal sinusitis, otitis media, or mastoiditis, empiric therapy with vancomycin, metronidazole, and a third-generation cephalosporin (cefotaxime or ceftriaxone, or ceftazidime if *Pseudomonas aeruginosa* is suspected) is recommended pending organism identification and susceptibility studies. Parenteral therapy should be continued for 3–6 wk, depending upon the patient's clinical response. If an associated osteomyelitis is present, longer periods of intravenous, and perhaps oral, therapy may be required.

### Surgical therapy

The optimal surgical approach for subdural empyema (i.e., craniotomy versus burr hole drainage) is controversial. Previous studies documented a lower mortality rate in patients undergoing craniotomy, although this may be because a larger percentage of gravely ill patients underwent drainage via burr holes because of the greater surgical risk. Drainage via burr hole placement may

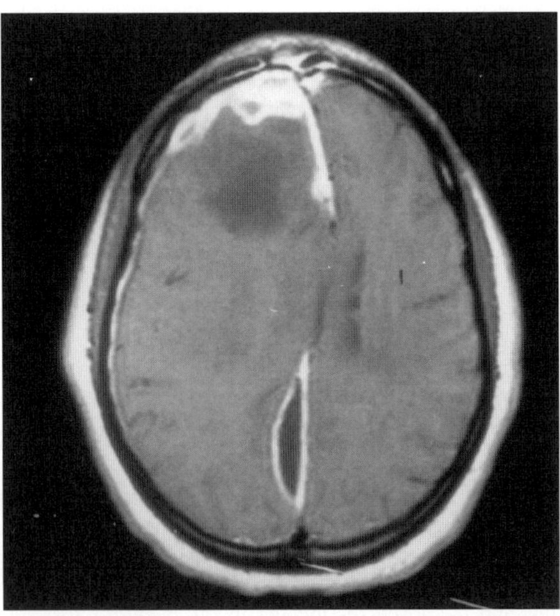

**Fig. 76.2** T1-weighted axial MR of the brain with gadolinium enhancement revealing a hypodense mass in the right frontal region with marked meningeal thickening, abnormal enhancement, and midline shift. Posteriorly, there is an elliptically shaped density in the interhemispheric fissure.

be more efficacious in the early stages of subdural empyema when the pus is liquid; aspiration is more difficult as the fluid becomes thicker with disease progression. If burr hole drainage is to be used, multiple burr holes should be placed, permitting extensive irrigation. It is important to note, however, that this mode of drainage, even with catheter irrigation, may not be adequate in about 10%–20% of patients. Craniotomy may also be essential for posterior fossa subdural empyema. In patients undergoing craniotomy, a wide exposure should be afforded to allow adequate exploration of all areas where infection is suspected. In addition, surgical correction of an antecedent otorhinologic infection may be necessary.

## Epidural Abscess

### Epidemiology, etiology, and pathogenesis

The term *epidural abscess* refers to a localized infection between the dura mater and the overlying skull or vertebral column. Cranial epidural abscess is rare, with an incidence of 5% in relation to all forms of intracranial suppuration. Cranial epidural abscess can cross the cranial dura along emissary veins, so subdural empyema is often present. Therefore, the etiologies of cranial epidural abscess are usually the same as those described for subdural empyema (see above).

Spinal epidural abscess is also rare, with an incidence rate of ~0.2–2.8 cases/10,000 hospital admissions; mortality rates have been as high as 23%–32% in surgically treated patients.

#### Pathogenesis

Spinal epidural abscess follows hematogenous dissemination from foci elsewhere to the epidural space (25%–50% of cases) or by extension from vertebral osteomyelitis. Hematogenous spread occurs as a result of infections of the skin (furuncles, cellulitis, infected acne), urinary tract, periodontal area, pharynx, lung, or mastoids; no source is identified in ~40% of cases. Blunt spinal trauma may also provide a devitalized site that is susceptible to infection following transient bacteremia; a history of spinal trauma is obtained in ~30% of patients. Other predisposing conditions for spinal epidural abscess include penetrating injuries, extension of decubitus ulcers or paraspinal abscesses, back surgery, lumbar puncture, and epidural anesthesia. Bacteremia may be an important predisposing factor since the incidence of spinal epidural abscess is increased in patients who abuse intravenous drugs. The likely infecting organisms in spinal epidural abscess are staphylococci (~65%), streptococci (~8%), and aerobic gram-negative bacilli (~17%).

### Clinical manifestations

Patients with *cranial epidural abscess* may present insidiously with the clinical presentation overshadowed by the primary focus of infection (e.g., sinusitis or otitis media). The usual complaint is headache, although the patient may otherwise feel well unless the clinical course is complicated by development of a subdural empyema or involvement of deeper intracranial structures. Since the dura is closely apposed to the inner surface of the cranium, the abscess usually enlarges too slowly to produce sudden major neurologic deficits unless there is deeper intracranial extension. Eventually focal neurologic signs may develop and either focal or generalized seizures. Without appropriate treatment, papilledema and other signs of increased intracranial pressure may develop. If the abscess is localized near the petrous bone, patients may present with Gradenigo's syndrome, manifested clinically by involvement of cranial nerves V and VI with unilateral facial pain and weakness in the lateral rectus muscle.

*Spinal epidural abscess* may develop rapidly within hours (following hematogenous dissemination) or may pursue a chronic course over months (associated with vertebral osteomyelitis). As the abscess increases in size, it follows the path of least resistance and extends laterally along the dural sheath; it can stretch the entire length of the spinal cord. Patients initially have focal vertebral pain, followed by root pain, defects of motor, sensory, or sphincter function, and finally paralysis. The most consistent symptom is pain which is accompanied by local tenderness in over 90% of cases. Fever is present in most patients during the course of their illness; headache and neck stiffness may also occur. With involvement of the cervical spinal cord, respiratory function may be impaired. When patients present with muscle weakness, sensory deficits, and disturbances of sphincter control, there may be a rapid transition to paralysis, indicating the need for emergent evaluation, diagnosis, and treatment.

### Diagnosis

Computed tomography and MR imaging are the diagnostic procedures of choice for cranial epidural abscess, demonstrating a superficial, circumscribed area of diminished intensity. The possibility of adjacent subdural empyema or other intracranial involvement can also be assessed. Magnetic resonance imaging or CT should also be performed in cases of suspected spinal epidural abscess, although MR imaging is recommended since it can visualize the spinal cord and epidural space in both sagittal and transverse sections and can also identify accompanying osteomyelitis, intramedullary spinal cord lesions, and joint space infection (Fig. 76.3). Furthermore, assessment of response to therapy is readily performed with these techniques.

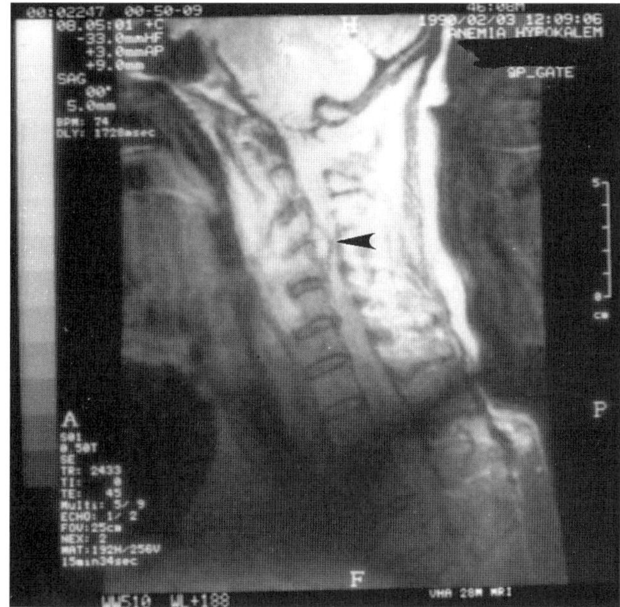

**Fig. 76.3** Proton-weighted sagittal MR of the cervical spine revealing an epidural collection at the C3–C4 level compressing the spinal cord ventrally (arrowhead).

## Treatment

### Antimicrobial therapy

Recommendations for antimicrobial therapy of cranial epidural abscess are the same as for cranial subdural empyema (see above). Presumptive antimicrobial therapy for spinal epidural abscess must include an antistaphylococcal agent (either nafcillin or vancomycin). Coverage for gram-negative bacilli (e.g., ceftazidime) must also be included for any patient with a history of spinal procedure or injection drug abuse. In patients who have undergone a spinal procedure, empiric therapy should include vancomycin for presumed *Staphylococcus epidermidis* infection. Antimicrobial therapy for uncomplicated spinal epidural abscess should be continued for 3–4 wk and for 6–8 wk if osteomyelitis is present.

### Surgical therapy

The surgical therapy of cranial epidural abscess is primarily aimed at drainage of the collection to prevent further accumulation and neurologic changes. In patients with spinal epidural abscess, laminectomy with decompression and drainage may need to be performed as a surgical emergency to minimize the likelihood of permanent neurologic sequelae. A delay in the diagnosis following development of neurologic dysfunction appears to be largely responsible for poor outcome associated with spinal epidural abscess. Some patients have been treated with antimicrobial therapy alone (i.e., those with an unacceptably high surgical risk or those without neurologic deficits), although these patients must be carefully followed for clinical deterioration and for progression by radiologic studies. In a recent literature review (from 1970 to 1990) of 38 patients with spinal epidural abscess, 23 recovered with nonsurgical treatment, two died, and one worsened; the rest either remained the same or improved. However, there have been no prospective, randomized trials comparing the efficacy of antimicrobials plus surgery to antimicrobial therapy alone. Rapid surgical decompression should be performed in patients with increasing neurologic deficit, persistent severe pain, or increasing temperature or peripheral white blood cell count.

# Septic Thrombophlebitis

## Epidemiology, etiology, and pathogenesis

### Pathogenesis

Septic intracranial thrombophlebitis refers to both venous thrombosis and suppuration. This process may begin within the veins and venous sinuses or may follow infection of the paranasal sinuses, middle ear, mastoid, face, or oropharynx. Conditions that increase blood viscosity or coagulability such as dehydration, polycythemia, pregnancy, oral contraceptive use, sickle cell disease, malignancy, and trauma increase the likelihood of thrombosis. Septic thrombophlebitis may also occur in association with bacterial meningitis, subdural empyema, or epidural abscess. Occasionally, infection may result from metastatic spread from distant sites of infection.

The antecedent conditions that predispose to septic intracranial thrombophlebitis depend upon the close proximity of various structures to the dural venous sinus system. The usual predisposing conditions to cavenous sinus thrombosis are paranasal sinusitis (especially frontal, ethmoidal, and sphenoidal) or infection of the face or mouth.

### Etiologic agents

*Staphylococcus aureus* is the most important infecting pathogen in cavernous sinus thrombosis (isolated in over two-thirds of cases) because of the importance of this organism in infections of the face, scalp, and in acute sphenoid sinusitis. Less common isolates include streptococci (~17%), pneumococci (~5%), gram-negative bacilli (~5%), and *Bacteroides* species (~2%). Otitis media and mastoiditis are associated with lateral sinus thrombosis and infection of the superior and inferior petrosal sinuses. Infections of the face, scalp, subdural and epidural spaces, and meningitis are associated with infection of the superior sagittal sinus.

## Clinical manifestations

The clinical manifestations of septic intracranial thrombophlebitis depend upon the location of involvement. Patients with inadequate collateral flow of the cortical venous system present with impaired consciousness, focal or generalized seizures, symptoms of increased intracranial pressure, and focal neurologic signs such as hemiparesis; if the dominant hemisphere is involved, aphasia is also common.

Location is also important in infections of the dural venous sinuses. The most common complaints in cavernous sinus thrombosis are periorbital swelling (73% of cases) and headache (52% of cases); headache is more common if the antecedent condition is sinusitis rather than facial infection. Other symptoms include drowsiness, diplopia, lacrimation, photophobia, and ptosis. On examination, fever is present in 90% of cases. Other signs include proptosis, chemosis, periorbital edema, and weakness of extraocular muscles due to involvement of cranial nerves III, IV, and VI. A lateral gaze palsy may be an early neurologic finding in cavernous sinus thrombosis, since the abducens nerve is the only cranial nerve traversing the interior of the cavernous sinus. Other findings include papilledema or venous engorgement (65% of cases), change in mental status (55% of cases), and meningismus (40%) which is secondary to retrograde spread of the thrombophlebitis. About 25% of patients have dilated or sluggishly reactive pupils, decreased visual acuity which frequently progresses to blindness, and dysfunction of cranial nerve V. Duplicate findings may also occur in the opposite eye as the infection spreads through the intercavernous sinuses. Patients with septic cavernous sinus thrombosis may present either acutely or chronically. Acute infection is generally secondary to facial infection, with onset less than 1 wk; the patient appears toxic with rapid development of symptoms and signs and rapid progression to bilateral findings. Chronic infection is usually secondary to dental infection, otitis media, or paranasal sinusitis, in which orbital manifestations are usually unimpressive; involvement of the contralateral eye is a late and inconsistent finding.

Patients with septic lateral sinus thrombosis most often complain of headache (80% of cases). Since otitis media is a common predisposing condition to this location, earache, vomiting, and vertigo may also occur. Signs include fever (79%) and ear findings (98%); there may also be palsy of cranial nerve VI, facial pain, altered facial sensation, papilledema, and mild nuchal rigidity. Septic thrombophlebitis of the superior sagittal sinus leads to abnormal mental status, motor deficits, nuchal rigidity, and papilledema; seizures occur in over half of the patients. Involvement of the inferior petrosal sinus may produce Gradenigo's syndrome, consisting of ipsilateral facial pain and lateral rectus muscle weakness.

## Diagnosis

Magnetic resonance imaging is the noninvasive procedure of choice for the diagnosis of septic intracranial thrombophlebitis; CT is considerably less sensitive and reliable than MR imaging. MR imaging visualizes blood vessels and can differentiate between thrombus and normally flowing blood; the evolution and resolution of the entire process can be followed. The paranasal sinuses can also be fully evaluated by MR imaging, providing information concerning subdural and epidural infection, cerebral infarction, cerebritis, hemorrhage, and cerebral edema. When MR imaging or CT is negative, but the suspicion of septic intracranial thrombophlebitis remains high, carotid arteriography with venous phase studies should be performed. In cavernous sinus thrombosis, narrowing of the intracavernous segments of the carotid artery is revealed. Orbital venography may also be useful and is the most definitive method of demonstrating cavernous sinus thrombosis.

## Treatment

### Antimicrobial therapy

The choice of antimicrobial therapy for septic intracranial thrombophlebitis depends upon the antecedent clinical condition; likely organisms are similar to those observed in cranial subdural empyema and epidural abscess (see above). For example, if the antecedent condition is paranasal sinusitis, empiric therapy should be directed toward staphylococci, streptococci, aerobic gram-negative bacilli, and anaerobes. In cavernous sinus thrombosis, an antistaphylococcal agent (e.g., nafcillin or vancomycin) should always be included in empiric therapeutic regimens because of the high incidence of isolation of *S. aureus* in this infection.

### Surgical therapy

Optimal management of septic intracranial thrombophlebitis may require surgical therapy. Drainage of infected sinuses may be needed when antimicrobial therapy alone is ineffective; this is especially true in patients with cavernous sinus thrombosis secondary to sphenoid sinusitis. For lateral sinus thrombosis, internal jugular vein ligation has been utilized as has thrombectomy, although the efficacy of these procedures is poorly defined.

### Adjunctive therapy

Anticoagulation therapy (i.e., heparin) for septic intracranial thrombophlebitis is controversial, although there are data to support its use to prevent spread of the thrombus from the cavernous sinus to other dural venous sinuses and cerebral veins. There is also evidence to suggest that the combination of anticoagulation and antimicrobial therapy reduces mortality if utilized early in the treatment of cavernous sinus thrombosis, although the hazards of intracranial hemorrhage (bleeding from sites of cortical venous infarction or from sites on the intracavernous walls of the carotid artery) must be recognized. Anticoagulation is not recommended for lateral sinus vein thrombophlebitis because cortical veins overlying the infected mastoid may become occluded, resulting in small venous hemorrhagic infarcts, making the risk of intracerebral hemorrhage prohibitively high.

## ANNOTATED BIBLIOGRAPHY


Baker AS, Ojemann RG, Baker RA. To decompress or not to decompress—spinal epidural abscess. Clin Infect Dis 1992; 15:28–29.

*Editorial and critical literature review of the paper by Wheeler et al.*

Danner RL, Hartman BJ. Update of spinal epidural abscess: 35 cases and review of the literature. Rev Infect Dis 1987; 9:265–274.

*Retrospective review of 35 cases of spinal epidural abscess compared to 153 cases in the literature. The authors recommend a combined approach to management with antibiotics and surgical drainage.*

Kaufman DM, Miller MH, Steigbigel NH. Subdural empyema: analysis of 17 recent cases and review of the literature. Medicine 1975; 54:485–98.

*Review of 17 cases of subdural empyema seen at their institution with a critical analysis of other reported cases up to that time.*

Krauss WE, McCormick PC. Infections of the dural spaces. Neurosurg Clin North Am 1992; 3:421–433.

Silverberg AL, DiNubile MJ. Subdural empyema and cranial epidural abscess. Med Clin North Am 1985; 69:361–374.

Southwick FS, Richardson EP Jr, Swartz MN. Septic thrombophlebitis of the dural venous sinuses. Medicine 1985; 65:82–106.

*Review of all cases of septic dural venous thrombosis at the Massachusetts General Hospital from 1948 to 1984.*

Tunkel AR, Scheld WM. Central nervous system infection in the compromised host. In: Clinical Approach to Infection the the Compromised Host, 3rd ed. Rubin RH, Young LS, eds. New York: Plenum, pp 163–210, 1994.

Wheeler D, Keiser P, Rigamonti D, Keay S. Medical management of spinal epidural abscess: case report and review. Clin Infect Dis 1992; 15: 22–27.

*Case report and review of 37 cases in the literature of medical management of spinal epidural abscess.*

Wispelwey B, Scheld WM. Brain abscess. In: Principles and Practice of Infectious Diseases, 4th ed. Mandell GL, Bennett JE, Dolin R, eds. Churchill-Livingstone, New York, pp 887–900, 1995.

# 77

# Ocular and Periocular Infections

ANNABELLE A. OKADA AND ANN SULLIVAN BAKER

A systematic approach to any presumed infection of the eye allows the physician to most effectively select first-line antimicrobial therapy before an etiological agent is actually identified. The systematic approach presented in this chapter is based on location of infection, or other easily discernible clinical characteristics, in order to provide a framework for thinking about eye infections for the ophthalmologist and nonophthalmologist alike.

## Infections of the Eyelids and Adnexa

### Localized infections

#### Hordeolum, chalazion

A localized inflammatory swelling in the eyelid usually represents either a hordeolum or a chalazion, depending on the chronicity and in part on the type of gland involved. A *hordeolum* (L. "barley," also commonly referred to as a "sty") is an acute infection, usually accompanied by tenderness, originating in the gland of either Zeiss or Moll, both adjacent to the eyelash follicles in the external layers of the eyelid (external hordeolum), or in the meibomian glands within the tarsus of the eyelid (internal hordeolum). On the other hand, a *chalazion* (Gr. "hailstone") is a chronic, lipogranulomatous inflammation, usually without tenderness, that occurs due to blockage of one or more of the meibomian glands. A chalazion will commonly evolve from an internal hordeolum.

In either case, the pathogen is usually *Staphylococcus aureus*, and the infection will generally respond to warm compresses and local application of appropriate antibiotic ointment (e.g., erythromycin four times a day). However large hordeola, and infections that are threatening to spread throughout the eyelid, may require judicious treatment with a short course of oral antibiotics. Persistent abscesses also often require incision and drainage, a conjunctival approach being the most appropriate in order to avoid visible scarring. Unfortunately the condition tends to recur, although usually not in the exact same location, and some measure of prophylaxis may be accomplished with good eyelid hygiene. In an older person, multiple recurrences in the same location or persistence of inflammation despite appropriate treatment should alert the physician to the possibility of malignancy, either basal cell carcinoma or sebaceous gland carcinoma.

#### Dacryoadenitis

When inflammation involves the temporal portion of the upper eyelid, infection of the lacrimal gland, or *dacryoadenitis*, should be considered, although this is not a very common entity. The swelling and tenderness are usually deep within the superior eyelid, often producing mechanical ptosis and an S-shaped curvature to the eyelid. Edema may extend into the temporal fossa and preauricular nodes may be palpable. Tension on the upper eyelid up and outward may easily induce herniation of the inflamed palpebral lobe of the lacrimal gland from beneath. The orbital lobe of the lacrimal gland is much less frequently involved. The causative organism is usually either *Neisseria gonorrhoeae* (young adults) or the mumps virus (children). Actinomycetic infection may be indicative of calculus formation within ducts of the gland. The differential diagnosis should include noninfectious causes such as sarcoidosis, Sjögren's syndrome, and thyroid-associated ophthalmopathy when in the absence of pain, and idiopathic inflammatory pseudotumor when acute pain is present. In addition, tumors of the lacrimal gland can also present with pain and swelling, particularly adenoid cystic carcinoma.

#### Dacryocystitis

When the inflammation is located in the nasal portion of the lower eyelid, particularly in the presence of a darkly discolored, tender mass in the medial canthal region which when palpated causes extrusion of pus from the lacrimal punctum, infection of the lacrimal sac or dacryocystitis is likely. The pathogenesis involves blockage of the nasolacrimal duct and generally occurs only in infants and older adults. In acute cases, the causative organism is commonly *S. aureus*, *Streptococcus pyogenes*, or *Streptococcus pneumoniae*, while *Actinomyces* or fungi, such as *Aspergillus* or *Candida albicans*, can often be isolated in chronic cases. Gram stain and culture of any expressed pus can aid in directing treatment, which should include systemic antibiotics directed toward penicillin-resistant staphylococci (e.g., nafcillin) given orally or intravenously. Surgical drainage is frequently required and recurrences are not uncommon unless the physical blockage is corrected. Noninfectious dacryocystocele, granulomatous processes such as Wegener's granulomatosis, and lacrimal sac tumors can also present with swelling in the medial canthal region although these are less likely to produce pain.

### Diffuse infections

#### Blepharitis

*Blepharitis* is a generalized, inflammation of the eyelid margins and can cause burning, itching, scaling, crusting, lid swelling, eye redness, and/or matting of the eyelashes particularly upon awakening (Plate 39). An acute, transient form occurs in neonates in association with seborrheic dermatitis of the face and scalp (cradle cap). However, the common form of blepharitis is chronic, often difficult to eradicate, and may occur in association with atopic dermatitis in children or rosacea in adults. *Staphylococcus aureus* or *Staphylococcus epidermidis* is usually implicated in the disease process, although it is unclear whether the pathogenesis is one of a true infection or an inflammatory response to certain bacterial toxins.

First-line therapy should include a routine of gentle lid scrubbings, warm compresses, and antibiotic ointment (bacitracin or erythromycin). Children with atopic dermatitis may occasionally need the short term addition of topical corticosteroid eyedrops (with careful monitoring of intraocular pressure because of the possibility of steroid-induced glaucoma). Finally, adults with rosacea often benefit from long term treatment with low-dose tetracycline or one of its derivatives (minocycline or doxycycline), although the mechanism of its action is not fully understood since nearly 75% of *S. epidermidis* strains are resistant to tetracycline. One important caveat is that blepharitis in children and adults is always bilateral. A unilateral inflammation of the eyelids should prompt consideration of other causes—particularly malignancy, if the patient is an older adult.

#### Preseptal cellulitis

Cellulitis of the periocular tissues is traditionally divided into *preseptal cellulitis* (confined to the eyelids in front of the orbital septum) and *periorbital cellulitis* (involving both the eyelids and the orbital tissues behind the septum) (Fig. 77.1). The latter is discussed in more detail in the orbit section. A patient presenting with unilateral, generalized swelling of the eyelids, with or without fever and peripheral leukocytosis, must be deftly categorized as having one or the other because of the difference in treatment and possible complications. To make a diagnosis of preseptal cellulitis there must be no proptosis, no decrease in vision, no ocular motility disturbance, and no pain with eye movement (Table 77.1). Frequently the infection results from a penetrating wound to the eyelid, and the causative organism is usually either *S. aureus* or *S. pyogenes*. In children under the age of 5, however, *Hemophilus influenzae* is most common, often in association with otitis media or sinusitis. Occasionally, an unattended hordeolum will evolve into preseptal cellulitis.

In evaluating the severity of infection, peripheral blood count and orbital CT scan should be considered. In addition, gram stain and culture of discharge from the eye may be helpful. Mild cases in adults can be treated on an outpatient basis with oral antibiotics (such as dicloxacillin or amoxicillin/clavulanate) for 7 to 10 d, antibiotic ointment applied to the eyelids, and daily follow-up until resolution. Severe cases in adults, and almost all cases in infants and children, should prompt hospitalization and treatment with intravenous antibiotics (ampicillin/sulbactam, cefuroxime, or nafcillin *and* ceftazidime is recommended). With improvement, the antibiotics can be switched to an oral regimen for a total treatment course of 10 to 14 d.

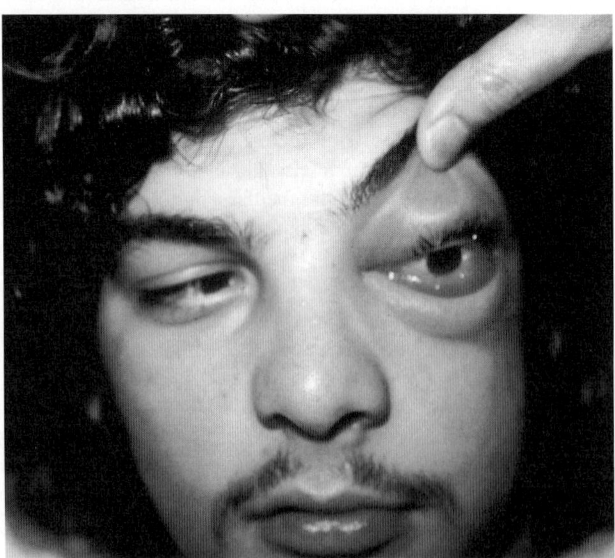

**Fig. 77.1** Orbital cellulitis. Lid edema, erythema, and slight limitation of lateral gaze due to edema, note sixth nerve palsy.

## Conjunctival Infections

The clinical signs and symptoms associated with common causes of conjunctivitis in adults are listed in Table 77.2.

### Purulent conjunctivitis

Purulent discharge is usually indicative of a *bacterial conjunctivitis* although moderate-to-severe cases of viral epidemic keratoconjunctivitis can sometimes also be quite purulent. In bacterial conjunctivitis, patients present with acute onset of unilateral or bilateral conjunctival injection and edema, often in association with conjunctival papillae. The most common causes are *S. aureus*, *S. pyogenes*, *S. pneumoniae*, and *Hemophilus* spp.; however, the most destructive pathogens are gonococcus and *Pseudomonas aeruginosa*. Gonococcus in particular is often said to have a hyperacute presentation with severe inflammation and discharge developing over 12 h.

Pretreatment gram stain and cultures should be performed. In the child, pharyngeal and/or middle ear drainage should also be evaluated. For first-line antibiotic therapy, erythromycin ointment applied 4 times a day for 1 to 2 wk is recommended, except when gonococcus or *Pseudomonas* is suspected. The latter cases should be treated with systemic antibiotics. An inadequately treated infection can lead to corneal ulceration, corneal perforation, and ultimately loss of vision. Patients with documented gonococcal infection should, of course, also have workup and treatment for other sexually transmitted diseases.

### Nonpurulent conjunctivitis

#### Viral conjunctivitis

In contrast to bacterial conjunctivitis, viral conjunctivitis tends to have a more watery discharge and is typically associated with tarsal conjunctival follicles and preauricular lymphadenopathy. The most common type is the easily transmissible *epidemic keratoconjunctivitis (EKC)*, usually caused by adenovirus type 8 or 19, while an acute hemorrhagic conjunctivitis is often seen with infections by enterovirus type 70 or coxsackievirus type A24. The conjunctivitis may be preceded by an upper respiratory infection or by contact with someone with a "pink eye"—particularly among school-age children. The onset is acute and may initially be predominantly unilateral, although virtually all cases eventually become bilateral via self-contamination. In the hospital setting, transmission by contamination is a constant worry, and health care personnel should always take great care in washing hands and disinfecting eye examination instruments. Furthermore, patients with viral conjunctivitis are urged to avoid close contact with others, especially in schools and hospitals, dur-

**Table 77.1** Clinical signs and symptoms of preseptal cellulitis and orbital cellulitis

| Signs and symptoms | Preseptal | Orbital |
|---|---|---|
| Vision | No significant change | May be decreased |
| Ocular motility | No significant change | Varying degrees of ophthalmoplegia |
| Proptosis | Absent | Present |
| Eyelid swelling and redness | Present | Present |
| Conjunctival edema and injection | Present | Present |
| Fever | Mild if any | Often present |
| Meningeal signs | Absent | May be present |
| Lethargy | Absent | Common in children |
| Peripheral leukocytosis | Absent | Common |
| CT scan | Preseptal swelling | Proptosis, mottling of orbital fat, preseptal swelling |
| History | Puncture wound, hordeolum | Puncture wound, upper respiratory infection, sinusitis, dental abscess, recent surgery, diabetes mellitus or other chronic disease |

ing the contagious period of the initial 2 wk after onset of symptoms.

The process is self-limited, and treatment is generally symptomatic with cool compresses and occasionally cycloplegic eye drops. Erythromycin ointment is also administered to prevent a superimposed bacterial infection, since severe cases have been known to lead to corneal ulceration and subsequent bacterial co-infection. When the diagnosis is in doubt, gram stain and cultures of conjunctival swabbings should be performed to rule out bacterial and chlamydial infection. In addition, although the acute infection will resolve in about 2 wk, persistent subepithelial opacities within the cornea can sometimes lead to a mild decrease in visual acuity. These opacities will respond to topical corticosteroid eyedrops. However, they tend to recur with tapering of the steroids, often making treatment difficult in light of the possible side effects of cataract and glaucoma.

### Adult chlamydial conjunctivitis

*Chlamydia trachomatis* is a common cause of subacute or chronic conjunctivitis in teenagers and young adults and occurs as a sexually transmitted disease. Typically the discharge is watery, with the presence of inferior tarsal conjunctival follicles and preauricular lymphadenopathy. The patient or his or her sexual partner may have a history of vaginitis, cervicitis, or urethritis. The diagnosis can be made by identifying inclusion bodies in a Giemsa stain of conjunctival scrapings or by direct immunofluorescent staining of the same. Culture or polymerase chain reaction assay can also establish the diagnosis. In addition, the patient and any sexual partners should be evaluated for genital chlamydia and other sexually transmitted diseases. Recommended treatment involves a 2 wk course of either oral tetracycline or doxycycline or erythromycin.

### Trachoma

*Chlamydia trachomatis* is also the etiological agent in *trachoma*. This disease is a major public health problem in developing countries where large portions of the population live under unsanitary and crowded living conditions. In particular, severity of disease appears to be associated with the lack of face washing of children and the lack of clean water and toilet facilities. Transmission by flies that cluster on the eyes is also a well-known association. Trachoma starts as a bilateral, nonpurulent, follicular conjunctivitis in young children living in endemic areas, usually by the age of 2 yr. Chronic inflammatory thickening of the tarsal con-

**Table 77.2** Differential diagnosis of common causes of conjunctivitis

| Signs and symptoms | Viral[a] | Bacterial | Chlamydial | Allergic |
|---|---|---|---|---|
| Discharge | Minimal, watery | Profuse, purulent | Profuse, watery | Minimal |
| Tearing | Profuse | Moderate | Moderate | Moderate |
| Itching | Minimal | Minimal | Minimal | Marked |
| Preauricular node | Common | Uncommon | Common | None |
| Gram/Giemsa stain | Monocytes | Bacteria, PMNs | PMNs, cytoplasmic inclusion bodies | Eosinophils |
| Associated sore throat or fever | Occasionally | Seldom | None | None |

[a]Adenovirus or enterovirus.

junctiva with papillary hypertrophy evolves thereafter, and gradually cicatrization of the eyelids, trichiasis (misdirected eyelashes), and permament corneal scarring lead to blindness. The diagnosis can be confirmed using the same laboratory tests as in adult inclusion conjunctivitis. Treatment consists of topical tetracycline or erythromycin, with oral tetracycline or doxycycline used in severe disease. Prevention by education to encourage facial cleaning and fly control is of equal importance in endemic areas.

#### Ophthalmia neonatorum

*Ophthalmia neonatorum* is the purulent conjunctivitis that occurs in newborns within the first month of life with a reported incidence of as low as 1.6% of newborns in the United States to as high as 7% to 12% of newborns elsewhere in the world. The disease presents clinically with bilateral purulent discharge, eyelid edema, conjunctival injection, and occasionally preauricular lymphadenopathy. The time course of presentation can often aid in determining an etiological diagnosis. Conjunctivitis occurring within the first few days of life is commonly associated with toxicity from silver nitrate prophylaxis administered at birth. Gonococcal conjunctivitis also generally occurs within the first week of birth and can be a particularly aggressive infection leading to severe keratitis if inadequately treated. Chlamydial conjunctivitis, the most common cause of ophthalmia neonatorum in developed countries, usually presents with a somewhat delayed onset of 1 or more wk, particularly when erythromycin ointment prophylaxis had been administered at birth. Both gonococcal and chlamydial conjunctivitis occur as a result of direct inoculation during passage through the birth canal in an infected mother. Gram stain, Giemsa stain, direct immunofluorescence staining, and culture of conjunctival scrapings may allow proper identification of the organism, although a high percentage of cultures are known to be unrevealing.

With the exception of chemical conjunctivitis, antibacterial treatment should be administered systemically for 7 to 10 d. Currently, a third-generation cephalosporin (e.g., ceftriaxone) is recommended for gonococcal conjunctivitis in order to cover penicillin-resistant strains. *Chlamydia trachomatis* conjunctivitis should be treated with oral erythromycin at a dose of 50 mg/kg/d, which will also cover any concomitant systemic infection, such as chlamydial pneumonitis. In both gonococcal and chlamydial disease, the infant's parents should be evaluated and treated for sexually transmitted diseases. Other causes of neonatal conjunctivitis include bacteria such as *Staphylococcus aureus*, *S. pneumonia*, and *H. influenza*, as well as herpes simplex virus. The last should be treated with systemic acyclovir in order to reduce the risk of disseminated infection.

## Corneal Infections (Keratitis)

### Trauma or debilitated patients

Corneal ulceration due to trauma should always arouse suspicion of fungal infection, particularly when the trauma involved organic matter such as a tree branch or soil. Depending on the region of the world, the most common fungal pathogens include *Candida* and *Aspergillus* (both prevalent in northern climates) and *Fusarium* (prevalent in southern climates). In addition, intensive care unit patients can often develop infection in association with exposure keratitis, *Pseudomonas aeruginosa* being the most common organism. Other patients at risk for bacterial or fungal ulcers include those with a history of cocaine abuse, advanced malignancy, and AIDS. Clinical signs and symptoms include acute loss of vision, pain, photophobia, conjunctival injection, and focal whitening and edema of the cornea (Plate 40). Less frequently, a hypopyon may accompany corneal infiltrate. All patients should undergo a careful slit lamp examination to rule-out a foreign body, possible corneal perforation, and associated anterior segment trauma or inflammation. Gram and Giemsa stains and culture of corneal scrapings should be performed prior to initiation of antibiotic therapy. In addition, a Calcofluor white smear or Gomori stain can aid in making a diagnosis of fungus.

If perforation and fungal infection have been ruled out, treatment can be initiated with topical cycloplegia (e.g., 0.25% scopolamine two to three times a day) and topical antibiotics. (We prefer a broad-spectrum combination of 14 mg/ml tobramycin and 133 mg/ml cefazolin given alternately every hour.) The duration of treatment and choice of antibiotics are then tailored to the size of the ulcer, the culture results, and the clinical course. If fungal infection is suspected, initial treatment may include topical 0.15% amphotericin B given once an hour, as well as oral ketoconazole (when *Candida* is involved) or itraconazole (when *Aspergillus* is involved). Oral fluconozole achieves excellent levels in the cornea, as opposed to most systemic antibiotics. Admission to the hospital and systemic antibiotics should be considered for particularly large or aggressive ulcers, most fungal ulcers, and cases in which follow-up or medical compliance is in doubt.

### Contact lens-related

A history of contact lens wear in a patient who presents with a corneal ulcer should automatically initiate a routine of stains and culture of contact lenses and lens cases in use, in addition to that of corneal scrapings. Severe pain and photophobia, seemingly disproportionate to the clinical presentation, is often said to accompany *Acanthomoeba* infection, particularly dreaded because of the difficulty in diagnosis (often requiring corneal biopsy) and notorious unresponsiveness to treatment. Patients often have a history of swimming with their contact lenses, overnight or extended wear use, lack of nightly contact lens sterilization, or of use of tap water or homemade saline solution to clean their lenses. The *Acanthomoeba* corneal ulcer itself often takes on a ring-like opacification with relative central clearing (Plate 41). Treatment for *Acanthomoeba* should include a combination of topical polymyxin-neomycin gramicidine (e.g., Neosporin), 0.1% propamidine isethionate (e.g., Brolene), 1% clotrimazole, and/or oral ketoconazole. Medical failures often require corneal transplantation in order to eradicate the infection.

### Herpes virus

The commonly seen *Herpes simplex virus (HSV) keratitis* in adults usually represents a recurrent infection, and patients typically present with a unilateral dendritic corneal ulcer (the dendrites have no true terminal bulbs and stain poorly with fluorescein) in association with photophobia and decrease in vision. Pain may not be prominent, due to the loss in corneal sensation that commonly occurs with HSV infection. Diagnosis is based on the clinical presentation, and treatment by an eye specialist should include one of the topical antiviral agents (usually 1% trifluorothymidine or 3% vidarabine); HSV keratitis may evolve into either a disciform keratitis or a necrotizing interstitial keratitis, both of which require the addition of corticosteroids to suppress the component of autoimmune inflammation and sometimes corneal transplantation if perforation occurs.

*Herpes zoster ophthalmicus (HZO)* refers to "shingles" or a vesicular rash in the distribution of the ophthalmic branch of the trigeminal nerve, caused by the varicella-zoster virus (VZV). The eye has a higher risk of involvement when vesicles are present at the tip of the nose, indicative of the nasociliary branch being affected. In contrast to HSV dendrites, the corneal dendrites seen in HZO keratitis typically have well-delineated terminal bulbs that stain well with fluorescein. There may be concomitant uveitis, retinitis, optic neuritis, scleritis, glaucoma, or cranial nerve palsy. Current treatment involves 800 mg of acyclovir administered orally 5 times a day, or 500 mg of fanciclovir given orally 3 times a day, for a 5 to 10 d course. The immunocompromised host should be treated with intravenous acyclovir. A short course of topical or oral corticosteroids may also be considered to treat the keratitis and/or uveitis and to try to reduce the possibility of postherpetic neuralgia which is believed to occur due to inflammation and scarring of the trigeminal nerve. Because of the increased chance of systemic VZV dissemination with the use of oral corticosteroids, antiviral therapy should be administered concomitantly.

## Intraocular Infections

## Focal (uveitis, retinitis)

### Toxoplasmosis

In immunocompetent patients, retinitis due to *Toxoplasma gondii* usually presents as reactivation of a congenital (intrauterine) infection; acquired toxoplasmosis rarely involves the eye. The natural host for the organism is the cat, and disease is transmitted to humans via ingestion of tissue cysts in animal meats or eggs or by contact with oocysts in cat feces, sand, or soil. Reactivation of a congenital lesion can occur at any age, and it must be remembered that ocular toxoplasmosis is a fairly common cause of leukocoria (the observation of a white pupil) in children. Examination of the ocular fundus will reveal a white, fluffy, focal, necrotizing retinitis adjacent to an old chorioretinal scar, with varying degrees of vitritis and anterior chamber inflammation (Plate 42). Possible complications include chronic iridocyclitis, cataract, glaucoma, and retinal detachment. Usually the diagnosis is based on a combination of clinical findings and presence of a rise in the specific anti–*T. gondii* IgG and IgM titers by immunofluorescence assay. Therapy is suggested only when (*1*) the lesion is near the macula or optic nerve, (*2*) the lesion is associated with heavy hemorrhage or inflammation, or (*3*) the patient is immunocompromised. In these cases, the currently recommended regimen includes pyrimethamine (with folinic acid), sulfadiazine, and prednisone, with or without the addition of clindamycin. However, since the process is generally self-limited, a lesion in the periphery of the retina can be merely followed without treatment.

### Toxocariasis

Infection by the ascarid worm *Toxocara canis* is associated with pica, or with contact with puppies and dogs. Human infection occurs after ingestion of the organism's eggs and takes one of two forms: either the systemic disease of visceral larval migrans that most prominently causes hepatosplenomegaly and pulmonary disease (toddlers 2 to 4 yr of age) or ocular toxocariasis (older children and young adults). Toxocariasis must of course be included in the differential diagnosis for leukocoria in any child. Live larvae characteristically do not elicit much inflammation in the retina but, on their death, a severe uveitis can result. The typical presentation is a whitish, raised granuloma in the posterior pole or periphery of the retina, frequently associated with an intense vitritis. Diagnosis is based on the clinical presentation and a concomitant rise in anti–*T. canis* antibody titers. Periocular and systemic corticosteroid therapy assists in controlling the eye inflammation, but attempts to treat with antihelminthic agents, such as thiabendazole and diethylcarbamazine, have not been met with success. A newer, possibly more effective compound, levamisole hydrochloride, is currently under evaluation. Prognosis depends on location of the granuloma and degree of associated inflammation.

### Viral retinitis

Because of the increase in patients with acquired immunodeficiency syndrome (AIDS), patients with organ transplants on immunosuppression, and the use of chemotherapy in the treatment of malignancies, the most commonly encountered viral retinitis among adults today is *cytomegalovirus (CMV) retinitis* that occurs as an acquired, opportunistic infection. More than one-half of these cases manifest as ocular disease alone, without any evidence of systemic infection. The classic presentation is a unilateral or bilateral necrotizing retinitis with varying degrees of hemorrhage and vitreous inflammation (Plate 43). The most common site is in the midperiphery of the fundus. Thus sometimes an active lesion is not noticed by the patient until central vision decreases and the macula is involved. Diagnosis is based on the characteristic fundus appearance. Treatment may involve either intravenous ganciclovir or foscarnet. Despite long term maintenance therapy, reactivation occurs in up to 50% of patients. Recently, intravitreal ganciclovir (injections or implant) and oral ganciclovir have been useful in treating relapses.

*Acute retinal necrosis* is also a relatively newly described disease, but unlike CMV retinitis, it may occur in otherwise healthy adults. Early on in the disease course, a mild anterior uveitis is common, accompanied by keratic precipitates and presence of vitreous cells. This is then followed within days to weeks by a necrotizing retinitis in the periphery of the retina, with prominent vasculitis and areas of hemorrhage and vascular occlusion (Plate 44). The etiological agent in most cases has been identified as being either varicella-zoster virus (VZV) or herpes simplex virus (HSV). Diagnosis is usually based on clinical appearance, although definitive identification of the pathogenic virus can be made by use of polymerase chain reaction assay on aqueous or vitreous humor samples. Therapy consists initially of intravenous acyclovir for 14 d followed with an oral regimen for a total course of 4 to 8 wk. Prognosis of patients depends upon quick institution of appropriate therapy such that the complications of macular involvement and retinal detachment can be avoided.

## Diffuse (endophthalmitis)

Endophthalmitis is the diffuse infection of the vitreous body and retinal and uveal layers of the eye. Exogenous endophthalmitis, the most common form of the disease, results from either surgical or traumatic penetration of the eye. The majority of cases of acute postoperative endophthalmitis occur within days to weeks after surgery and are due to gram-positive cocci, particularly coagulase negative staphylococci, *S. aureus*, or *Streptococcus* spp. A subacute and insidious form of postoperative endophthalmitis can occur with *Propionibacterium acnes*. Traumatic endophthalmitis is also frequently associated with gram-positive cocci although the proportion is smaller, due to a higher percentage of cases attributed to *Bacillus cereus*, gram-negative bacteria, and fungi.

Endogenous endophthalmitis (also called *metastatic endophthalmitis*), on the other hand, is a rare type of endophthalmitis that occurs in patients debilitated with chronic diseases such as diabetes mellitus and malignancy or in association with surgical procedures or intravenous hyperalimentation. The pathogenic mechanism involves hematogenous spread of blood-borne microbes from a site distant to the eye. Staphylococcal and streptococcal organisms are the most common bacteria; approximately two-thirds of cases of endogenous endophthalmitis are caused by *Candida albicans* and other fungi. Systemic workup is mandatory in these patients, as this will often reveal an occult endocarditis or bowel carcinoma. *Bacillus cereus* causing endogenous infection is reportedly associated with intravenous drug abuse. Symptoms include pain and decreased vision. On examination, opacified vitreous, loss of red reflex, and hypopyon (white blood cells layered in the inferior anterior chamber) are observed.

Determination of the etiological agent should be attempted by stains and cultures of vitreous aspirates, for both bacteria and fungi, prior to the institution of antibiotic treatment. For bacterial infections, initial therapy should include intravitreous administration of vancomycin in combination with an aminoglycoside (for intravitreal injection, amikacin is recommended because of its lower retinal toxicity compared to other aminoglycosides) or ceftazidime. Empiric intravenous therapy with vancomycin and ceftazadine will provide broad-spectrum coverage until vitreal cultures are available. Oral quinolones such as ofloxacin may also be useful. Medical therapy for fungal infections should include intravitreal and intravenous amphotericin B, with possible oral fluconazole therapy as a later supplement. Surgical vitrectomy may be required to clear the eye of vitreous debris and and reduce the number of infectious organisms and can be conducted in conjunction with initial vitreous sampling for culture purposes prior to starting antibiotics. In general, the prognosis can be fairly good for postoperative endophthalmitis but is almost uniformly poor in cases of traumatic and endogenous endophthlamitis unless recognized and treated early.

## Orbital Infections

### Cellulitis

As opposed to preseptal cellulitis, *orbital cellulitis* is a more generalized, usually unilateral infection of the postseptal orbit and periorbital tissues. Clues that can aid in distinguishing preseptal from orbital cellulitis are listed in Table 77.1. The pathogenesis of orbital cellulitis can involve either contiguous spread of infection from sinusitis (most common) or a dental abscess, implantation via a puncture wound, or hematogenous spread from one of a multiple number of sites. The local clinical signs and symptoms include unilateral pain and inflammatory swelling of the periorbital tissues, proptosis, ophthalmoplegia, conjunctival edema, and decrease in vision (Fig. 77.1). In addition, in children fever, lethargy, and elevation of the white blood cell count are typical. The most likely pathogens are bacteria, *S. aureus* and *Streptococcus* spp. being common among all age groups, and *Hemophilus influenzae* is associated with infections in young children. In immunocompromised patients, *Pseudomonas aeruginosa* or fungi should be ruled out. The diagnostic workup in any patient should include full ophthalmological and otolaryngological examinations and cultures, orbital CT scan and/or ultrasound, peripheral blood count, and blood cultures. Lumbar puncture should be considered in children with meningeal signs. Orbital cellulitis requires hospital admission for intravenous antibiotics, a penicillinase-resistant penicillin such as nafcillin with third-generation cephalosporins being the antiobiotics of choice. Other options include cefuroxime or ampicillin/sulbactam. Completion of therapy with oral antibiotics, such as cefuroxime, dicloxacillin, or amoxicillin-clavulanate, is reasonable. An abscess found on CT scan requires surgical drainage. Possible complications include development of an orbital abscess or less commonly, cavernous sinus thrombosis (Fig. 77.2).

### Phycomycosis

Fungal infection of the orbit can be a particularly devastating disease and occurs primarily in patients with diabetic ketoacidosis or in patients on immunosuppressive therapy. Infection by one of the *Phycomycetes*, either *Mucor* or *Rhizopus* spp., is most common although other fungi such as *Aspergillus* can be involved.

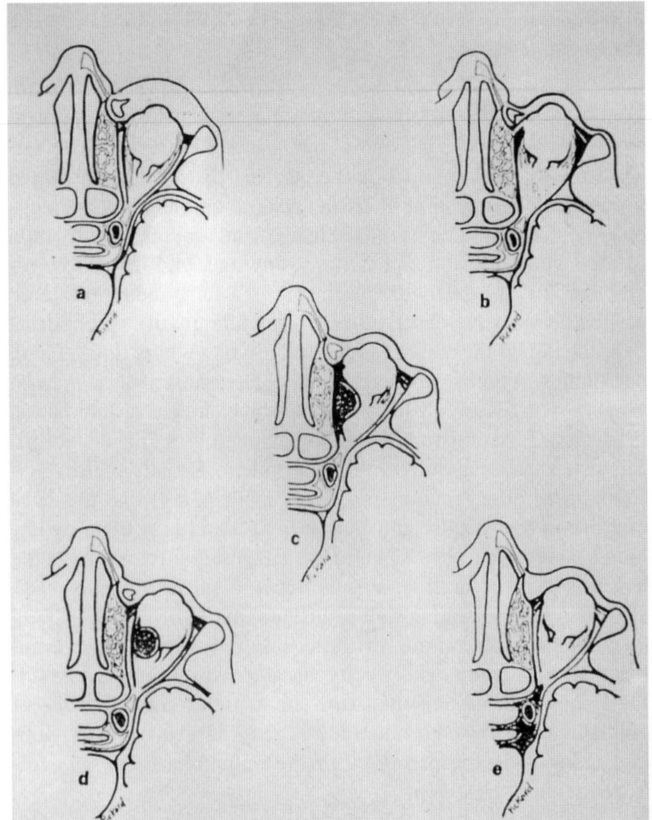


**Fig. 77.2** Orbital infections (Chandler). Orbital inflammation (*a*), orbital cellulitis (*b*), superiosteal abscess (*c*), orbital abscess (*d*), cavernous sinus thrombophlebitis (*e*). [Used with permission from J.R. Chandler, O.J. Langenbrunner, F.R. Stevens, The pathogenesis of orbital complications in sinusitis Laryngoscope 80:1414, 1970.]

The pathogenesis of *Phycomycetes* infection involves vascular invasion, resulting in a process of thrombotic necrosis. Clinically, a foul-smelling seropurulent discharge is typical, with dark, necrotic discoloration of the periorbital tissues. Development of a black eschar is a late finding and is generally indicative of advanced disease. The infection is often an extension from the paranasal sinuses, and involvement of the orbital apex, cavernous sinus, and central nervous system is a well-known complication. The diagnosis usually requires examination of biopsied tissue for fungi. Tissue cultures, CT scan, and MRI are also essential to the workup. Treatment must be instituted promptly and aggressively with local debridement to clean margins, drainage of necrotic areas, and systemic administration of amphotericin B and possibly flucytosine. In addition, any metabolic imbalance in patients should be corrected. The infection can be successfully managed if caught early on; however, exenteration of the orbit is sometimes necessary in severe cases.

## Special Clinical Situations

### Syphilis

The ocular manifestations of congenital syphilis can include an anterior uveitis or a chorioretinitis in the early stages of disease. However, the classic finding of interstitial keratitis, which along with deafness and malformed incisors forms Hutchinson's triad, does not occur until late in the disease course. Ten to 40 percent of children with untreated congenital syphilis will develop such an interstitial keratitis between the ages of 5 and 20. Eighty percent of cases are bilateral, with vascular infiltration and edema of the cornea observed acutely upon clinical examination. Ultimately, visual loss secondary to corneal scarring is common, with or without concomitant optic atrophy due to posterior uveitis. Treatment 14 d of intravenous penicillin is usually adequate, followed by procaine penicillin weekly for 3 wk. In adults, areas of pigment mottling in the fundus, at times severe enough to resemble retinitis pigmentosa, can be indicative of congenital syphilis.

In acquired syphilis, the extreme variation in possible ocular manifestations has prompted a reputation for syphilis as being the "great masquerader." Eye involvement, although not very common, usually occurs in the secondary or tertiary stages. Clinical findings can include ocular surface inflammation (scleritis, interstitial keratitis), anterior uveitis (iridocyclitis), posterior uveitis (multifocal choroiditis, neuroretinitis), or one of number of different neuro-ophthalmic disorders (Argyll-Robertson pupil, ocular motor palsy, etc.). In addition, visual field defects may develop due to lesions in the visual pathways of the central nervous system. Because of the wide variation in possible presentations, syphilis serological testing should be a routine part of any workup for unexplained ocular inflammation. Furthermore, patients with suspected ocular syphilis should also undergo lumbar puncture in order to look for evidence of neurosyphilis. If neurosyphilis is documented, treatment should include intravenous penicillin (e.g., 24 million units of penicillin G over 10 d) followed by procaine penicillin weekly for 3 wk (see Chapter 70). Topical corticosteroids are often utilized to aid in control of the local ocular inflammation. Prognosis is dependent on early detection of disease and adequate treatment.

### Acquired immunodeficiency syndrome (AIDS)

There are a wide variety of ocular manifestations, both noninfectious and infectious, observed in association with HIV-1 infection as summarized in Table 77.3. (Most of the infectious manifestations have already been covered elsewhere within this chapter; see also Chapter 100.) The most common eye manifestation by far is the cotton wool spot, reportedly observed in approximately 50% of patients and believed to result from focal axoplasmic ischemia in the retinal nerve fiber layer. A single spot or cluster will often appear and disappear within the course of a couple of months, occasionally with small hemorrhages. They are not known to cause any visual disturbances, and importantly, their transient and nonprogressive nature distinguishes them from early stages of CMV retinitis. No treatment is necessary. Human immunodeficiency virus itself has also been shown to be present in the retina of AIDS patients by polymerase chain reaction studies, and although its presence may be contributing to the pathogenesis of cotton wool spots, it does not cause a retinitis.

Cytomegalovirus retinitis, the most common ocular infection associated with AIDS, occurs in up to 45% of patients. Toxoplasmic retinitis is the next most common infectious manifestation, and in AIDS it appears to occur in the course of newly acquired primary infection or dissemination to the retina from latent extraocular sites, rather than as a reactivation of congenitally acquired cysts. More than one-half of patients with ocular toxoplasmosis also have toxoplasmic encephalitis.

Herpes zoster ophthalmicus (HZO), caused by the varicella-

**Table 77.3** Ocular manifestations of AIDS

| Noninfectious | Infectious |
|---|---|
| Kaposi's sarcoma of eyelid, conjunctiva or orbit | Herpes zoster ophthalmicus |
| Lymphoma of eyelid or orbit | Herpes simplex keratitis |
| Conjunctival microvasculopathy | Fungal or bacterial keratitis |
| Keratoconjunctivitis sicca | Molluscum contagiosum |
| Subconjunctival hemorrhage | Cytomegalovirus retinitis |
| Corneal ulceration | Acute retinal necrosis |
| Acute angle-closure glaucoma | Toxoplasmic retinitis |
| Ocular motor nerve palsy | Syphilitic retinitis |
| Papilledema | *Pneumocystitis carinii* choroiditis |
| Retinal microvasculopathy and cotton wool spots | Fungal or bacterial endophthalmitis |

zoster virus, is typically a disease of the elderly, and thus its development in a young person should immediately arouse suspicion of HIV infection. In fact, HZO may be the first manifestation of HIV infection, and it has been shown to be associated with an increased risk for progression to full-blown AIDS. In HIV patients, the disease course is often more severe and prolonged, and it may be associated with CNS and/or systemically disseminated viral infection. Therapy includes intravenous acyclovir (10 mg/kg every 8 h for 10 to 14 d) followed by oral acyclovir.

### Lyme disease

First described in 1975, Lyme disease is a multisystem illness caused by the spirochete *Borrelia burgdorferi* and is transmitted to humans via tick bites of *Ixodes* species in temperate wooded areas of the United States, Europe, and Japan (see Chapter 95). Stage I of the disease is characterized by a localized erythema migrans that develops within 1 to 3 wk following the initial tick bite. Stage II represents hematogenous dissemination of the spirochete, usually with erythema chronica migrans and often central nervous system disturbances such as cranial neuritis and meningitis. Finally, stage III is believed to be a state of persistent infection and/or autoimmune-mediated disease, with chronic arthritis and nervous system disease such as demyelination syndrome.

The ocular manifestations of Lyme disease include conjunctivitis, reportedly observed in 11% of stage I patients. However, most of the eye involvement takes place in stages II and III, as an extension of CNS involvement, and usually consists of either intraocular inflammations such as pars planitis, vitritis and retinal vasculitis, or neuro-ophthalmic disorders such as optic neuritis, ocular motility dysfunction, and Horner's syndrome. An interstitial keratitis similar to that seen in tertiary syphilis has also been reported in stage III patients. All of these clinical presentations are diagnostically nonspecific. Therefore, in general, any uveitic or neuro-ophthalmic disease in a patient who is living or has been in an endemic area for Lyme disease, particularly when there are systemic findings of rash or arthritis, should prompt a rule out of the disease using appropriate serological testing. Lyme uveitis can be quite resistent to oral antibiotics, often requiring intravenous penicillin G or ceftriaxone.

## General Principles of Antibiotic Administration in Eye Infections

In contrast to infections at other sites of the body, there are structural barriers to the eye that can prevent the adequate penetration of antimicrobial agents administered either topically or intravenously. In the front of the eye, the avascular cornea has an epithelial layer (and a precorneal tear film) that serves as a barrier against non-lipid-soluble compounds. However, in the inflamed or ulcerous cornea this barrier is effectively broken down, and with frequent and high concentrations of topical antibiotic administration, effective penetration into the corneal stroma and the anterior chamber can be achieved. Unfortunately, topical administration of antibiotics does not produce adequate drug levels in the posterior part of the eye. Occasionally subconjunctival antibiotic injections are used for severe corneal ulcers or infections associated with anterior perforation of the eye (such as in traumatic endophthalmitis or postsurgical endophthalmitis). The choice of antimicrobial agents should be determined using the same principles that govern antibiotic use for other parts of the body.

In the back of the eye, the retina and choroid are easily accessed via their respective vasculatures, allowing for good penetration with intravenous antibiotics. However, the blood-ocular barrier that exists at the nonfenestrated retinal vessel level does not allow much penetration of compounds into the vitreous body, the area infected in endophthalmitis. Here again inflammation plays a role in breaking down this barrier into the eye. However loculation of infections within the vitreous add to the difficulty in achieving adequate antibiotic levels via the intravenous route. Thus, the most effective manner in which consistently high levels of drugs can be achieved in the vitreous is by direct, intravitreal injection. The one caveat is that too high a drug concentration, particularly of the aminoglycosides, is toxic to the retina (may cause sudden necrosis). Therefore, strict guidelines regarding the concentrations used and mixing of antibiotics for intravitreal injections must be followed. Finally, certain antibiotics penetrate the vitreous more effectively, such as vancomycin, penicillins, and ceftazidime, and more recently some of the newer oral quinolones.

## ANNOTATED BIBLIOGRAPHY


### Textbooks for general information

Albert DA, Jakobiec FA, eds. Principles and Practice of Ophthalmology. WB Saunders, Philadelphia, PA, 1994.
*An encyclopedic resource, but with in-depth coverage, on virtually all topics related to the eye and visual sciences.*

Ciulla TA, Baker AS, eds. Massachusetts Eye & Ear Infirmary Residents' Guide to Ocular Antimicrobial Therapy. AK Peters, Boston, 1996.
*A pocket-size useful guide for ocular antibiotic doses for eye infections.*

Durand M, Riley GJ, Baker AS. Eye infections. In: A Practical Approach to Infectious Diseases, 3rd ed. Reese RE, Betts RF, eds. Little, Brown, Boston, pp 184–210, 1996.
*An informative, easy-to-use, guide to eye infections.*

Kanski JJ, Thomas DJ. The Eye in Systemic Disease. Butterworth-Heinemann, London, pp 110–116, 1990.
*An excellent review of the eye complications that are associated with systemic infections.*

O'Brien TP, Green WR. Eye infections. In: Principles and Practice of Infectious Disease, 3rd ed. Mandell GL, Douglas RG, Bennett JE, eds. Churchill-Livingstone, New York, pp. 975–1001, 1994.
*A summary of the topic, with good guidelines to follow.*

### References for selected clinical situations

*AIDS*: Holland GN. Acquired immunodeficiency syndrome and ophthalmology. The first decade. Am J Ophthalmol 1992; 114:86–95.
*Provides a comprehensive view of the ocular manifestations of AIDS.*

*Contact Lens Wear*: Schein OD, Glynn RJ, Poggio EC, Seddon, Kenyon KR, Microbial Keratitis Study Group. The relative risk of ulcerative keratitis among users of daily-wear and extended-wear soft contact lenses. A case-control study. N Engl J Med 1989; 321:773–778.
*The definitive study on corneal infections with contact lens use.*

*Endogenous endophthalmitis*: Okada AA, Johnson RP, Liles C, D'Amico DJ, Baker AS. Endogenous endophthalmitis: a 10 year retrospective study. Ophthalmol 1994; 101:832–838.
*Largest reported series on the clinical and microbiological profile, and prognosis, of patients with this rare disease.*

*Lyme disease*: Smith JL. Ocular lyme borreliosis—1991. Int Ophthalmol Clin 1991; 31:17–38.
*An excellent summary of the various presentations and treatment considerations in this disease.*

# 78

## Osteomyelitis

JON T. MADER, MAURO ORTIZ, AND JASON H. CALHOUN

*Osteomyelitis* is a term to describe infection in bone. The root word *osteon* (bone) and *myelo* (marrow) are combined with *-itis* to define the clinical state in which bone is infected with microorganisms. Osteomyelitis can be classified by duration (acute, chronic), by pathogenesis (trauma, hematogenous, surgery, true contiguous spread), by site (spine, hip, tibia, foot), by extent (size of defect), and by type of patient (infant, child, adult, compromised host). Bone infections are currently classified etiologically by the Waldvogel system as being either hematogenous osteomyelitis or osteomyelitis secondary to a contiguous focus of infection. Contiguous focus osteomyelitis has been further subdivided into osteomyelitis with or without vascular insufficiency.

In the Waldvogel classification, osteomyelitis may be acute or chronic. Acute disease is characterized by a suppurative infection accompanied by edema, vascular congestion, and small-vessel thrombosis. The vascular supply to the bone is compromised as the infection extends into the surrounding soft tissue. Large areas of dead bone or sequestra may be formed when both the medullary and periosteal blood supplies are reduced. Reactive new bone may form around infected bone and is termed *involucrum.* Established or chronic infection is comprised of a nidus of infected dead bone or scar tissue and an ischemic soft tissue envelope. If established osteomyelitis is not medically and surgically treated, it leads to an indolent refractory infection.

An alternative classification system to the Waldvogel classification has been developed by Cierny and Mader. The Cierny-Mader staging system (Table 78.1) is based on the anatomy of the bone infection and the physiology of the host. The classification is determined by the status of the disease process regardless of its etiology, regionality, or chronicity. The anatomic types of osteomyelitis are medullary, superficial, localized, and diffuse. Stage 1 or *medullary osteomyelitis* denotes infection confined to the intramedullary surfaces of the bone. Hematogenous osteomyelitis and infected intramedullary rods are examples of this anatomic type. Stage 2 or *superficial osteomyelitis*, a true contiguous focus infection of bone, occurs when an exposed infected necrotic surface of bone lies at the base of a soft-tissue wound. Stage 3 or *localized osteomyelitis* is usually characterized by a full thickness, cortical sequestration which can be removed surgically without compromising bony stability. Stage 4 or *diffuse osteomyelitis* is a through-and-through process that usually requires an intercalary resection of the bone to arrest the disease process. Diffuse osteomyelitis includes those infections with a loss of bony stability either before or after debridement surgery.

The patient is classified as an A, B, or C host (Table 78.1). An A host represents a patient with normal physiologic, metabolic, and immunologic capabilities. The B host is either systemically compromised or locally compromised or both. When the morbidity of treatment is worse than that imposed by the disease itself, the patient is given the C host classification. The terms *acute* and *chronic osteomyelitis* are not used in this staging system since areas of macronecrosis must be removed regardless of the acuity or chronicity of an uncontrolled infection. The stages are dynamic and interact according to the pathophysiology of the disease. They may be altered by successful therapy, host alteration, or treatment. This classification system aids in the understanding, diagnosis, and treatment of bone infections in children and adults.

### Etiology

In hematogenous osteomyelitis, a single pathogenic organism is almost always recovered from the bone (Table 78.2). In infants, *Staphylococcus aureus*, *Streptococcus agalactia*, and *Escherichia coli* are most frequently isolated from blood or bones, whereas in children over 1 yr of age, *Staphylococcus aureus*, *Streptococcus pyogenes*, and *Hemophilus influenzae* are most commonly isolated. The incidence of *Hemophilus influenzae* infection decreases after age 4. In adults, *Staphylococcus aureus* is the most common organism isolated.

Multiple organisms are usually isolated from the infected bone in contiguous focus osteomyelitis (Table 78.2). *Staphylococcus aureus* remains the most commonly isolated pathogen. However, gram-negative bacilli and anaerobic organisms are also frequently isolated.

### Source of Infection

Osteomyelitis may be caused from hematogenous spread or from a contiguous focus of infection. Contiguous-focus osteomyelitis has been further subdivided into osteomyelitis with or without vascular disease. Hematogenous osteomyelitis usually involves the metaphysis of long bones in children or the vertebral bodies in adults. The most common causes of contiguous-focus osteomyelitis are trauma, perioperative infections, nonsurgically induced contiguous infections, and infected foreign bodies. Contiguous-focus osteomyelitis with vascular disease commonly occurs in the bones of the feet in patients with severe ischemic or neuropathic disease such as diabetes mellitus.

Skeletal tuberculosis is the result of hematogenous spread of the *Mycobacterium tuberculosis* early in the course of a primary infection. Rarely, skeletal tuberculosis may be a contiguous infection from an adjacent caseating lymph node. Atypical mycobacteria including *M. marinum*, *M. avium-intracellulare*, *M. fortuitum*, and *M. gordonae* have all been associated with osteoarticular infections. Bone infections may also be caused by a variety of fungal organisms including coccidioidomycosis, blastomycosis, cryptococcus, and sporotrichosis.

**Table 78.1** Cierny and Mader staging system

| | |
|---|---|
| ANATOMIC TYPE | |
| Stage 1 | Medullary osteomyelitis |
| Stage 2 | Superficial osteomyelitis |
| Stage 3 | Localized osteomyelitis |
| Stage 4 | Diffuse osteomyelitis |
| PHYSIOLOGIC CLASS | |
| A Host | Normal host |
| B Host | Systemic compromise (Bs) |
| | Local compromise (Bl) |
| | Systemic & local compromise (Bls) |
| C Host | Treatment worse than the disease |
| SYSTEMIC OR LOCAL FACTORS THAT AFFECT IMMUNE SURVEILLANCE, METABOLISM, AND LOCAL VASCULARITY | |
| *SYSTEMIC (BS)* | *LOCAL (BL)* |
| Malnutrition | Chronic lymphedema |
| Renal, hepatic failure | Venous stasis |
| Diabetes mellitus | Major vessel compromise |
| Chronic hypoxia | Arteritis |
| Immune disease | Extensive scarring |
| Malignancy | Radiation fibrosis |
| Extremes of age | Small-vessel disease |
| Immunosuppression or immune deficiency | Neuropathy |
| | Tobacco abuse |

## Epidemiology

The epidemiology of osteomyelitis shows several broad trends. The incidence of hematogenous osteomyelitis is decreasing in many populations. In Glasgow, Scotland, 275 cases of acute hematogenous osteomyelitis in children under 13 yr were reviewed from 1970 to 1990. During the same period of time the population of children under 13 in Glasgow, Scotland, fell by an average of 2% per year. When comparing 1970 to 1990, there was a fall from 64 to 19 cases of acute hematogenous osteomyelitis. The number of cases of osteomyelitis involving long bones decreased while osteomyelitis from all other sites remained the same. The incidence of *Staphylococcus aureus* infections decreased from 55% to 31% over the 20 yr time period. In contrast to hematogenous osteomyelitis, the incidence of contiguous-focus osteomyelitis is increasing, probably due to motor vehicle accidents and the increasing use of orthopedic hardware and total joint arthroplasties. There is an increased incidence of hematogenous and contiguous-focus osteomyelitis in males versus females. Finally, osteomyelitis occurs with a higher frequency in immunocompromised patients.

**Table 78.2** Osteomyelitis: commonly isolated organisms

| Hematogenous osteomyelitis (monomicrobic infection) Cierny-Mader stage 1 | | |
|---|---|---|
| Infant (<1 yr) | Childhood (1–16 yr) | Adults (>16 yr) |
| Group B streptococcus | *Staphylococcus aureus* | *Staphylococcus aureus* |
| *Staphylococcus aureus* | *Streptococcus pyogenes* | *Staphylococcus epidermidis* |
| *Escherichia coli* | *Haemophilus influenzae* | Gram-negative bacilli |
| | | *Pseudomonas aeruginosa* |
| | | *Serratia marcescens* |
| | | *Escherichia coli* |
| Contiguous focus osteomyelitis (polymicrobic infection) Cierny-Mader stages 2, 3, and 4 | | |
| | *Staphylococcus aureus* | |
| | *Staphylococcus epidermidis* | |
| | *Streptococcus pyogenes* | |
| | *Enterococcus species* | |
| | Gram-negative bacilli | |
| | Anaerobes | |

## Host Factors

Host factors are primarily involved with containment of the infection once it is introduced adjacent to or into the bone. On occasion, host factors may predispose the host to the development of osteomyelitis. Thus, host deficiencies that lead to bacteremia favor the development of hematogenous osteomyelitis. Host deficiencies involved with direct inoculation of organisms and/or contiguous spread of infection from an adjacent area of soft-tissue infection are primarily involved with the lack of containment of the initial infection. Three patient groups with an unusual susceptibility to acute skeletal infections are those with sickle cell anemia, chronic granulomatous disease, and diabetes mellitus. Many systemic and local factors influence the ability of the host to elicit an effective response to infection and treatment (Table 78.1).

The functional impairment caused by the disease, reconstruction operations, and metabolic consequences of aggressive therapy influence the selection of candidates for treatment. A draining sinus with minimal pain and/or dysfunction is not itself an indication for surgical treatment. At times, the procedures required to arrest or palliate the disease are of such magnitude for the compromised host that treatment can lead to loss of function, limb, or life. The condition of the host and the relative disability caused by osteomyelitis are contained in the Cierny-Mader classification (Table 78.1).

## Pathophysiology

Primary hematogenous osteomyelitis occurs mainly in infants and children. The most common site of hematogenous seeding is the metaphysis, particularly in the hip, because of the anatomy of the growing metaphysis. The growth plate separates the epiphyseal blood supply from the metaphyseal vessels. The metaphyseal arteries end at the growth plate by connecting with large sinusoidal veins. The blood flow slows here, allowing bacteria to proliferate, especially if there has been slight trauma with resultant hematoma formation. In infants, medullary infection may spread to the epiphysis and joint surfaces through capillaries which cross the growth plate. The adjacent joint is usually infected in infants with osteomyelitis. In children the infection is confined to the metaphysis and diaphysis. The joint is spared unless the metaphysis is intracapsular. Cortical perforation at the proximal radius, humerus, or femur can lead to infection of the elbow, shoulder, or hip joint, respectively, regardless of the age of the patient. The infection can also cause elevation of the periosteum (Fig. 78.1) and the formation of a so-called Brodie's abscess (Fig. 78.2A–C).

Hematogenous long bone osteomyelitis is rarely found in the adult population. When it occurs, adult hematogenous osteomyelitis may be a primary or a secondary infection (reactivation). Primary infections are usually found in compromised hosts. The infection begins in the diaphysis but may spread to involve the entire medullary canal. Extension into the joint may occur since the growth plate has matured and once again shares vessels with the metaphysis. As the periosteum is firmly adherent to the bone in adults, cortical penetration usually leads to a soft-tissue abscess. In time sinus tracts may form which connect the sequestered nidus of infection to the skin via soft tissue extension.

Secondary hematogenous infections in adults are more common and represent reactivation of a quiescent focus of hematogenous osteomyelitis initially developed in infancy or childhood.

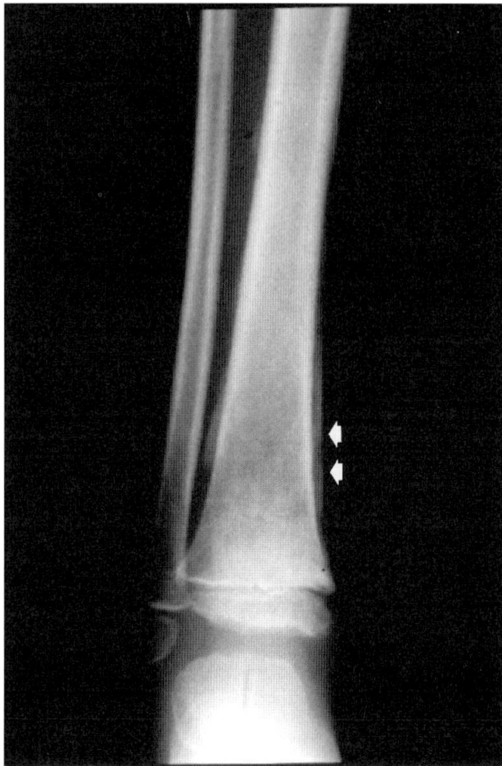

**Fig. 78.1** Anterior–posterior radiograph of the lower leg of a 10 yr-old girl with acute hematogenous osteomyelitis. There is generalized osteopenia and a small lytic lesion in the distal medial tibia. Periosteal elevation (**arrows**) is present in the distal tibial shaft. The surgical bone culture was positive for methicillin sensitive *Staphylococcus aureus*.

Secondary hematogenous osteomyelitis in adults generally has a metaphyseal localization.

Contiguous-focus osteomyelitis in adults is usually caused by trauma, nosocomial infection from surgery, and true contiguous infection from an adjacent infected wound. In the trauma patient additional factors that contribute to the subsequent development of osteomyelitis are the presence of hypotension, inadequate debridement of a fracture site, malnutrition, alcoholism, and smoking. Because they cannot contain the initial infection, patients with systemic or metabolic disorders that impair their ability to fight infection are prone to the development and progression of osteomyelitis.

Finally experimental studies indicate that an important factor in prolonging a focus of osteomyelitis is the formation of an impregnable glycocalyx surrounding the infecting organisms. This glycocalyx protects the organisms from the action of phagocytes as well as access by most antimicrobials. Evidence indicates that a surface negative change of devitalized bone or metal implants promotes glycocalyx formation.

## Clinical Manifestations

### Signs and symptoms

Neonatal osteomyelitis is characterized by a paucity of systemic and local findings. Local findings include edema and decreased motion of a limb. An infected joint effusion adja-

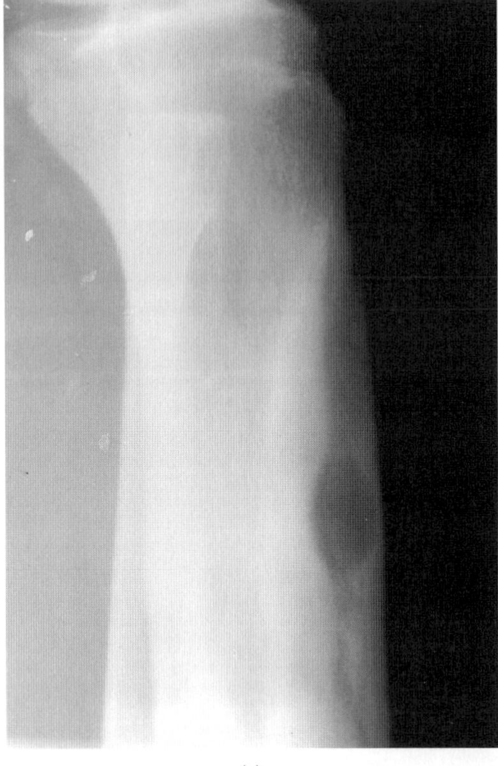

(a)

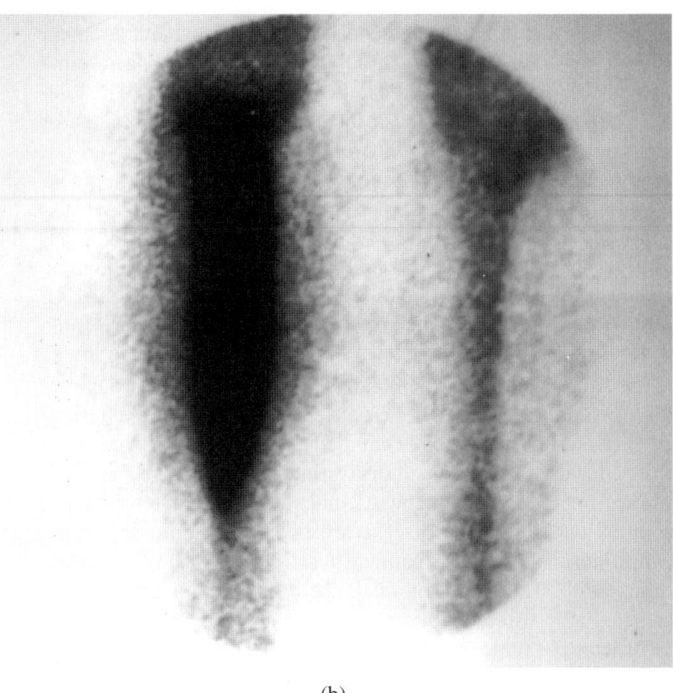

(b)

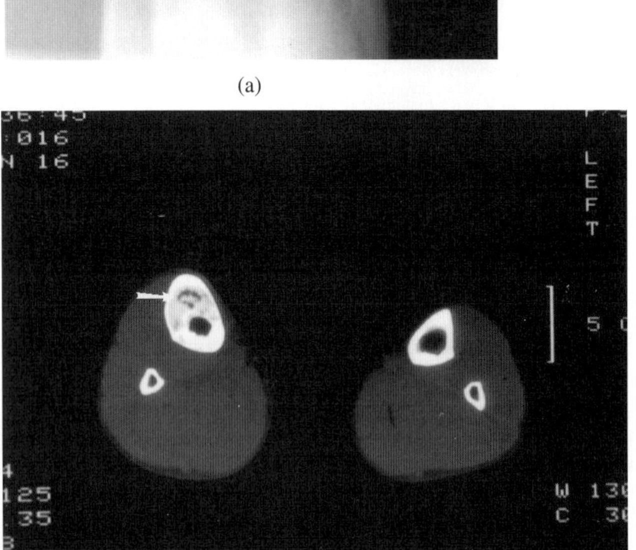


(c)

**Fig. 78.2** *(a)* Lateral radiograph of the proximal right tibia in a 17 yr-old boy with a Brodie's abscess. The radiograph shows a single lucent lesion located in the tibial metaphysis. The surgical bone culture was positive for methicillin sensitive *Staphylococcus aureus*. Brodie's abscess is the name given to a chronic localized bone abscess. The patient presented with a 8 wk history of knee pain and low-grade fever. Subacute cases usually present with fever, pain, and periosteal elevation, while chronic cases are often afebrile and present with longstanding dull pain. The lesion is typically single and located near the metaphysis. Seventy-five percent of these patients are less than 25 yr of age.
*(b)* Technetium$^{99m}$ methyldiphosphonate scan (3 hr scan) shows increased radiotracer uptake in the proximal right tibia.
*(c)* The CT scan through both proximal legs shows a lytic lesion (**arrow**) in the right proximal tibia with a well-defined, sclerotic border. There is some necrotic bone in the middle of the lytic lesion.

cent to the bone infection is present in approximately 60% of the cases.

Children with hematogenous osteomyelitis may present with acute signs of infection including abrupt fever, irritability, lethargy, and local signs of inflammation. However, 50% of children present with vague complaints, including pain of the involved limb of 1 to 3 mo in duration and minimal if any temperature elevation. Children with hematogenous osteomyelitis usually have normal soft tissue enveloping the infected bone and are capable of a very effective response to infection. Thus, children have the potential to resorb large sequestra and generate a significant periosteal response to the infection. This latter feature leads to substantial formation of bone formed at the margin of the infection (involucrum) (Fig. 78.3). The involucrum provides skeletal continuity and lessens the development of nonunion and pathologic fractures. In children the joint is usually spared from infection unless the metaphysis is intracapsular as is found at the proximal radius, humerus, or femur.

Adults with primary or secondary hematogenous osteomyelitis usually present with vague complaints consisting of nonspecific pain and few constitutional symptoms of 1 to 3 mo in duration. However, acute clinical presentations with fever, chills, swelling, and erythema over the involved bone(s) are occasionally seen. The source of bacteremia may be a trivial skin infection or a more serious infection such as acute or subacute bacterial endocarditis. Hematogenous osteomyelitis that involves either long bones or vertebrae is an important complicaton of injection drug abuse.

Patients with contiguous focus osteomyelitis often present with localized bone and joint pain, erythema, swelling, and drainage around the area of trauma, surgery, or wound infection. Signs of bacteremia such as fever, chills, and night sweats may be

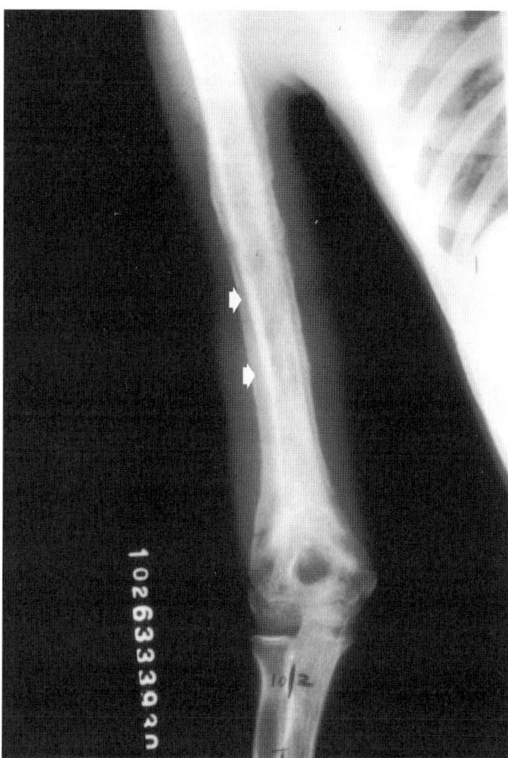

**Fig. 78.3** A radiograph of the right humerus of a 16 yr-old girl with hematogenous osteomyelitis. There are lytic changes, periosteal elevation, and involucrum (**arrows**) in the middle and distal humeral shaft. Extensive involucrum lends stability to osteomyelitic bone in the pediatric age group.

present in the acute phase of osteomyelitis, but not in the chronic phases.

Both hematogenous and contiguous-focus osteomyelitis can progress to a chronic condition. Local bone loss, areas of dead necrotic bone (sequestrum), and bony sclerosis are common. Persistent drainage and/or sinus tracts are often found adjacent to the area of infection. The patient usually presents with chronic pain and drainage. If present, fever is low grade. The sedimentation rate is usually elevated reflecting chronic inflammation, but the leukocyte count is usually normal. The chronic disease is usually not or slowly progressive. If a sinus tract becomes obstructed, the patient may present with a localized abscess and or a soft-tissue infection.

Any bone may be involved in skeletal tuberculosis, but the infection usually involves one site. In children or adolescents, the metaphyses of the long bones are most frequently infected. In the adult, the most often involved are the axial skeleton, followed by the proximal femur, knee, and small bones of the hands and feet. In the axial skeleton or long bone, pyogenic osteomyelitis evolves much more quickly and initially produces an acute or subacute infection. In contrast, tuberculosus spondylitis or osteomyelitis is subacute to chronic in presentation and progresses slowly over a period of months to years. Sixty percent of the patients with skeletal tuberculosis have evidence of extraosseous tuberculosis.

The most common clinical presentation of a fungal bone infection is a cold abscess overlying an osteolytic lesion. Joint space extension may occur in coccidioidomycosis and blastomycosis.

## History and physical exam

A thorough history—a review of systems, past medical history, and physical examination—must be obtained to identify systemic disease and to evaluate the integrity and condition of the musculoskeletal component involved. The patient must be able to tolerate rigorous surgical, medical, and rehabilitation protocols. Underlying disease may render the patient a poor surgical risk. The symptom complex assessment is carefully documented for future reference. Any history of allergies or drug toxicity is obtained.

In patients with hematogenous osteomyelitis, the general exam evaluates potential entry sites of the infecting organisms including endocarditis. In patients with contiguous-focus osteomyelitis, the wound is closely examined. In patients with contiguous-focus osteomyelitis with generalized vascular disease the blood supply and sensation are carefully evaluated

On examination of the limb, any previous operations must be noted, including scars, previous flap designs and the remaining options for local flap coverage. Local signs of stasis, hypoxia, and induration are noted. Range of motion above and below the disease segment is recorded.

On history and physical examination, the physician must assess whether the patient is a surgical candidate, the degree of bone necrosis, the extent of bone and soft-tissue involvement, and the rehabilitation potential. If the patient is a systemically or locally compromised, methods of host improvement are discussed with the patient (Table 78.3).

## Laboratory Studies

Although hematological studies do not confirm the diagnosis of osteomyelitis, they may be useful in assessing the response to treatment. The leukocyte count may be elevated in acute osteomyelitis, but it is often normal in more chronic cases. The sedimentation rate is usually elevated in both acute and chronic osteomyelitis. Elevated sedimentation rates and leukocyte counts generally fall with appropriate therapy, but both may increase acutely following debridement surgery. A sedimentation rate that returns to normal during the course of therapy is a favorable prognostic sign. Laboratory studies to monitor the nutritional status

**Table 78.3** Patient management: methods of host alteration

| |
|---|
| PATIENT EDUCATION—NO SMOKING |
| NUTRITIONAL SUPPLEMENTATION |
| Malnutrition |
| Alcohol abuse |
| Immune compromise |
| Renal/hepatic failure |
| Diabetes |
| HYPERBARIC OXYGEN: CIERNY-MADER BL, EXTENSIVE GRANULATION BEDS, REFRACTORY OSTEOMYELITIS |
| SPECIAL CONSIDERATIONS |
| Local compromise: pressure garments, local or microvascular tissue transfers |
| Pressure sores: force distribution |
| Diabetes: blood glucose control |
| Major vessel disease: arterial bypass surgery |
| Chemical suppression: discontinue or alter medications |
| Sepsis—toxicity: emergency decompression or drainage |

of the patient as well as any toxic effects from antibiotic treatment regimens are also necessary. Baseline laboratory studies including a complete blood count, Chem 10 blood chemistry panel, erythrocyte sedimentation rate, urinalysis, serum albumin, and a total iron binding capacity should be initially obtained and monitored regularly while the patient is on antibiotic therapy. Total iron binding capacity and albumin are markers of the nutritional status of the patient with osteomyelitis.

## Diagnosis

### Radiographs and scans

Radiographs are important for the diagnosis, staging, and evaluation of the progression of osteomyelitis. Common radiographic changes include osteopenia, scalloping, thinning of cortical bone, and loss of the trabecular architecture in cancellous bone. A sequestrum is radiodense relative to normal bone (Fig. 78.2C). Periosteal elevation may be present as well as soft-tissue swelling when an abscess or cellulitis is present.

Radionuclide scans, computerized tomography, or magnetic resonance imaging may be obtained when the diagnosis of osteomyelitis is ambiguous or to help gauge the extent of bone and soft tissue infection. In general, it is not usually necessary to obtain these scans for long bone and diabetic foot osteomyelitis. However, in suspected vertebral osteomyelitis the technetium$^{99m}$ methyldiphosphonate and magnetic resonance imaging scans are useful (Fig. 78.4B,C).

The technetium$^{99m}$ methyldiphosphonate scan demonstrates increased isotope accumulation in areas of increased blood flow and reactive new bone formation (Figs. 78.2B, 78.4B). However, it does not distinguish between osteoblastic changes caused by a healing fracture from those due to infection. A second class of radiopharmaceuticals used for the evaluation of osteomyelitis includes gallium$^{67}$ citrate and indium$^{111}$ chloride. Gallium$^{67}$ citrate and indium$^{111}$ chloride attach to transferrin, which leaks from the bloodstream into areas of inflammation. Gallium and indium scans also show increased isotope uptake in areas concentrating polymorphonuclear leukocytes, macrophages, and malignant tumors. Since these scans do not show bone detail well, it is often difficult to distinguish between bone and soft tissue inflammation. A comparison with a technetium$^{99m}$ methyldiphosphonate scan helps resolve this problem and can distinguish between increased technetium$^{99m}$ uptake due to a fracture from infection induced osteoblastic activity (Chapter 12).

Indium-labeled leukocyte scans are less useful in the evaluation of osteomyelitis. Indium-labeled leukocyte scans are positive in approximately 40% of patients with acute osteomyelitis and 60% of patients with septic arthritis. In most cases it is wise to couple indium$^{111}$ with technetium$^{99m}$ scans. Patients who have chronic osteomyelitis, bony metastases, and degenerative arthritis often have negative indium$^{111}$ scans.

Computerized axial tomography (CAT) may play a role in the diagnosis of osteomyelitis. Increased marrow density occurs early in the infection (Fig. 78.2C). The CAT scan can also help identify areas of necrotic bone and assess the involvement of the surrounding soft tissues. In a difficult infection, the computerized axial tomography scan may assist in selecting the surgical approach.

Magnetic resonance imaging (MRI) has been recognized as a useful modality for diagnosing the presence and extent of musculoskeletal sepsis (Fig. 78.4C). (see Chapter 12). The spatial resolution of MRI makes it useful in differentiating between bone and soft-tissue infection. Metallic implants in the region of interest may produce focal artifacts, thereby decreasing the utility of the image. Initial MRI screening usually consists of a T1-weighted and a T2-weighted spin-echo pulse sequence. In a T1-weighted study, edema and fluid is dark while fat including the fatty marrow of bone is bright. In a T2-weighted study, the reverse is true. The typical appearance of osteomyelitis is a localized area of abnormal marrow with decreased signal intensity on T1-weighted images and increased signal intensity on T2-weighted images. On occasion there may be decreased signal intensity on T2-weighted images. Post-traumatic or surgical scarring of the marrow is seen as a region of decreased signal intensity on T1-weighted images with no change of the T2-weighted image. Sinus tracts are seen as areas of high signal intensity on the T2-weighted image extending from the marrow and bone through the soft tissues and out of the skin. Cellulitis is seen as diffuse areas of intermediate signal in the T1-weighted images of the soft tissues, with increased signal on the T2-weighted images of the same area. Since differentiation of infection from neoplasm on the basis of the MRI may be difficult, clinical and radiographic confirmation is necessary. This is particularly true in trauma patients where the utility of MRI in evaluation of long bone osteomyelitis is not as well established.

### Microbiologic documentation

The diagnosis and determination of the etiology of long bone osteomyelitis rests on the isolation of the pathogen(s) from the bone lesion or blood or joint culture. In Cierny-Mader stage 1 or hematogenous osteomyelitis, positive blood or joint cultures can often obviate the need for a bone biopsy when there is radiographic or radionuclide scan evidence of osteomyelitis.

Except in hematogenous osteomyelitis where positive blood or joint fluid cultures may suffice, antibiotic treatment of osteomyelitis should be based on meticulous cultures of bone taken at debridement surgery or from deep bone biopsies. If possible, cultures should be obtained before antibiotics are initiated. Sinus tract cultures are not reliable for predicting which or if gram-negative organisms will be isolated from infected bone. However, sinus tract cultures growing *S. aureus* show a positive correlation with bone cultures.

## Treatment

Appropriate therapy of osteomyelitis includes adequate drainage, thorough debridement, obliteration of dead space, wound protection, and specific antimicrobial coverage. If the patient is a compromised host, an effort is made to correct or improve the host defect(s) (Table 78.3). In particular, attention should be paid to good nutrition and to a smoking cessation program, besides dealing with specific abnormalities such as control of diabetes. Thus, an attempt is made to improve the nutritional, medical, and vascular status of the patient and to provide optimal care for any underlying disease.

### Antibiotic management

After cultures are obtained, a parenteral antimicrobial regimen is begun to cover the clinically suspected pathogens (Table 78.4).

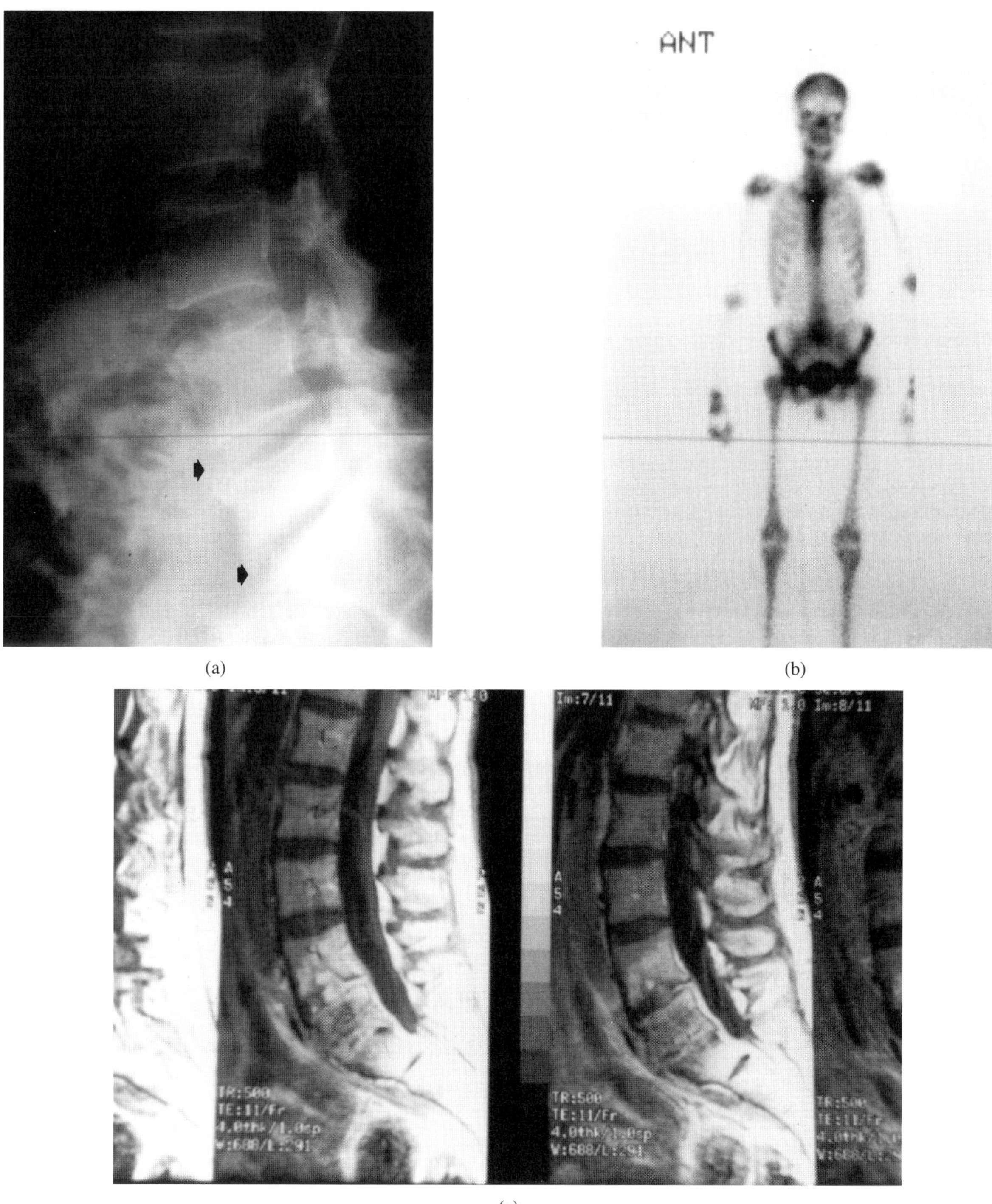


**Fig. 78.4** *(a)* Lateral radiograph of vertebral osteomyelitis in this 35 yr-old woman. A lateral view of the lumbar spine shows joint space narrowing of the L4–L5 and L5–S1 disc spaces (**arrows**). There is loss of the adjacent vertebral end plates with accompanying sclerosis. *(b)* The technetium$^{99m}$ methyldiphosphonate scan shows increased radiotracer uptake at the L4–S1 levels. The technetium scan displays increased isotope accumulation in areas of increased blood flow and reactive new bone formation. *(c)* The T1-weighted (TR/TE 500/11 ms) MR image shows irregularities of the vertebral end-plates at L4–L5 and L5–S1. There is increased signal demonstrated throughout the entire body of L4 consistent with osteomyelitis and/or bone marrow edema.

Once the organism is identified, specific antibiotics can be selected by appropriate sensitivity methods.

Stage 1 or hematogenous osteomyelitis in children (Fig. 78.5) usually can be treated with antibiotics alone. Antibiotic therapy alone is possible because children's bone is very vascular and they have a very effective response to infection. Stage 1 osteomyelitis in adults (Fig. 78.5) is more refractory to therapy and is usually treated with antibiotics and surgery. The patient is treated for 4 wk with appropriate parenteral antimicrobial therapy, dated from the initiation of therapy or after the last major debridement surgery. If the initial medical management fails and the patient is clinically compromised by a recurrent infection, medullary and/or soft tissue debridement will be necessary in conjunction with another 4 wk course of antibiotics.

Oral antibiotic therapy can be utilized for treatment of pediatric stage 1 osteomyelitis. However, it is recommended that the child initially receive 2 wk of parenteral antibiotic therapy prior to changing to an oral regimen. High doses of the quinolone class of antibiotics have been reported to cause articular cartilage damage in young animals, generating some concern regarding the long-term use of these agents in infants and children. Therefore, in most circumstances, pediatric patients should not be given the quinolone class of antibiotics.

In stage 2 osteomyelitis (Fig. 78.6) the patient may be treated with a 2 wk course of antibiotics following superficial debridement and soft-tissue coverage. The arrest rate is approximately 80%.

In stages 3 (Fig. 78.7) and 4 (Fig. 78.8) osteomyelitis the patient is treated with 4 to 6 wk of parenteral antimicrobial therapy dated from the last major debridement surgery. Without adequate debridement most antibiotic regimens fail no matter what the duration of therapy. Even when all necrotic tissue has been adequately debrided, the remaining bed of tissue must be considered contaminated with the responsible pathogen(s). Therefore it is important to treat the patient for at least 4 wk with antibiotics.* The arrest rate is approximately 90%. Outpatient intravenous therapy using long-term intravenous access catheters, such as Hickman or Groshong catheters, decreases hospitalization time. Oral therapy using the quinolone class of antibiotics for gram-negative organisms is currently being utilized in adult patients with osteomyelitis. The currently available quinolones have relatively poor activity against *Streptococcus* sp., *Enterococcus* sp., and anaerobes. The quinolones have modest activity against *Staphylococcus aureus* and *epidermidis*, and resistance is increasing. Coverage of aerobic gram-positive organisms should be obtained with other antibiotics such as clindamycin or ampicillin and a $\beta$-lactamase inhibitor. Before changing to an oral regimen, it is recommended that the patient initially receive 2 wk of parenteral antibiotic therapy. The patient must be compliant and agree to close outpatient follow-up.

Due to the need for prolonged therapy, antibiotics employed in the treatment of bone and joint infection must be nontoxic, convenient to administer, and cost-effective. Bone concentration of the treatment antibiotic may be an important factor in eradicating the organism from the bone. Using a rabbit model for *Staphylococcus aureus* osteomyelitis we found clindamycin to have the greatest bone-to-serum ratio followed by vancomycin, nafcillin, moxalactam, tobramycin, cefazolin, and cephalothin. The significance of bone antibiotic concentrations is unclear but clindamycin gave the best treatment results in experimental *Staphylococcus aureus* osteomyelitis.

*Some recent studies indicate that the combination of careful debridement and restoration of a blood supply using myocutaneous flaps can permit a shorter duration of antibiotics.

## Surgical management

Surgical management of osteomyelitis can be very challenging. The principles of treating any infection are equally applicable to the treatment of infection in bone. These include adequate drainage, extensive debridement of all necrotic tissue, obliteration of dead spaces, adequate soft-tissue coverage, and restoration of an effective blood supply. The goal of debridement is to leave healthy, viable tissue. However, even when all necrotic tissue has been adequately debrided, the remaining bed of tissue must be considered contaminated with the responsible organism.

The challenge in treating osteomyelitis, as compared to infection of soft tissue alone, involves bone debridement. Adequate debridement may leave a large bony defect termed *dead space.* Appropriate management of dead space created by debridement surgery is mandatory in order to arrest the disease and maintain the integrity of the skeletal part. The goal of dead-space management is to replace dead bone and scar tissue with durable vascularized tissue. Secondary intention healing is discouraged since the scar tissue that fills the defect may later become avascular. Complete wound closure should be attained whenever possible. Local tissue flaps or free flaps may be used to fill dead space. They have the advantage of increasing blood supply to the affected area. An alternative technique places cancellous bone grafts beneath local or transferred tissues where structural augmentation is necessary. Careful preoperative planning is critical

**Table 78.4** Osteomyelitis: initial antibiotic therapy

| | |
|---|---|
| HEMATOGENOUS OSTEOMYELITIS (MONOMICROBIC INFECTION) CIERNY-MADER STAGE 1 | |
| Long Bone | |
| Children | Nafcillin ([a]) or Clindamycin ([a]) |
| Adults | Nafcillin ([a]) or Clindamycin ([a]) + Ofloxacin |
| Vertebral | Nafcillin ([a]) + Cefotaxime |
| CONTIGUOUS FOCUS OSTEOMYELITIS (POLYMICROBIC INFECTION) CIERNY-MADER STAGES 2A,B, 3A,B, 4A,B | |
| Long Bone | Clindamycin ([a]) + Ofloxacin |
| Mandibular | Clindamycin |
| Pelvic | Ampicillin/sulbactam + Ciprofloxacin |
| CONTIGUOUS FOCUS OSTEOMYELITIS WITH VASCULAR DISEASES (POLYMICROBIC INFECTION) CIERNY-MADER STAGES 2B, 3B, 4B | |
| Diabetic Foot Osteomyelitis | Clindamycin or ampicillin/sulbactam + ciprofloxacin |

[a]Vancomycin when methicillin-resistant *Staphylococcus aureus* (MRSA), methicillin-resistant *Staphylococcus epidermidis* (MRSE) or *Enterococcus* sp. suspected.

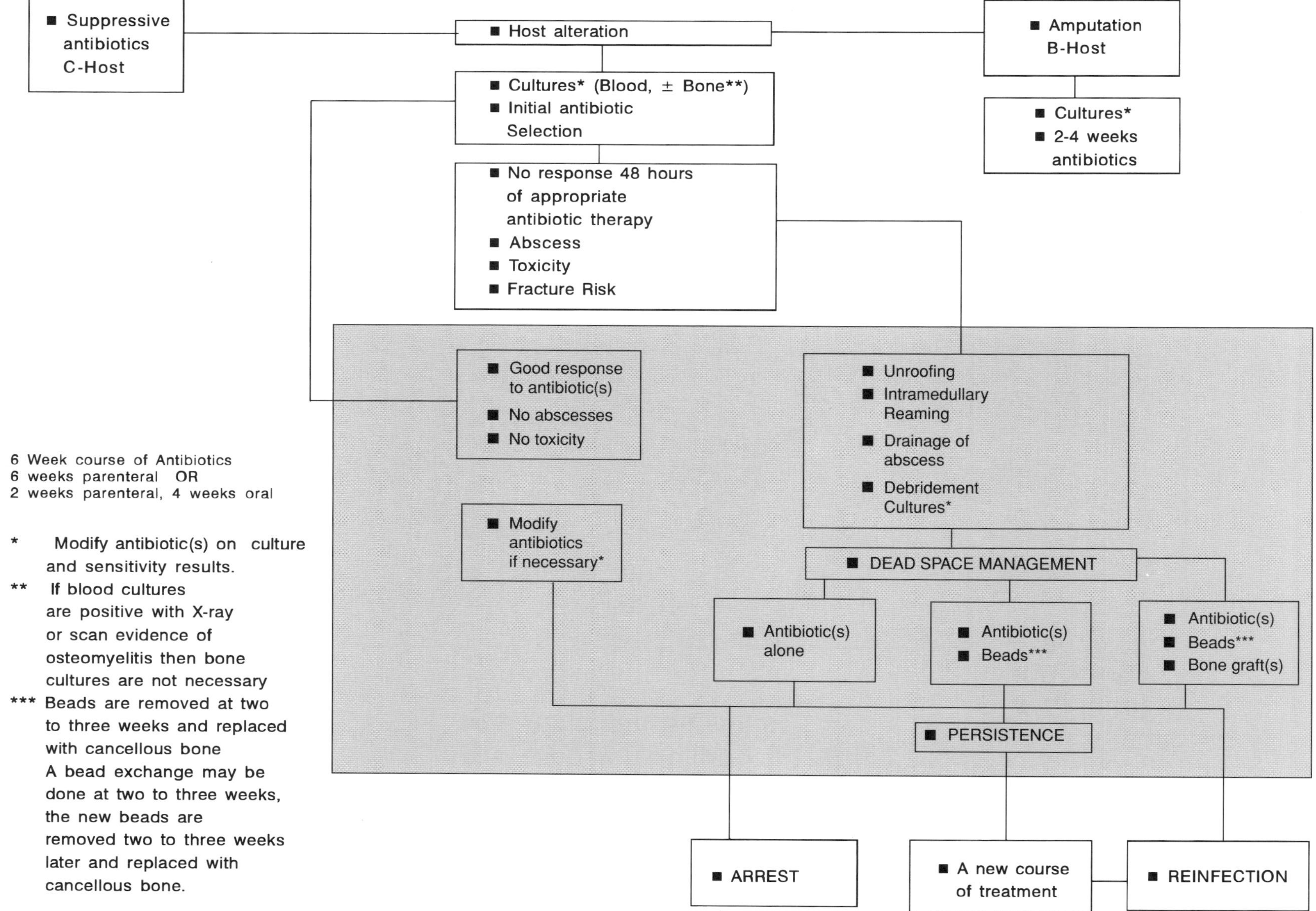
■ Suppressive antibiotics C-Host
■ Host alteration
■ Amputation B-Host
■ Cultures* ■ 2-4 weeks antibiotics
■ Cultures* (Blood, ± Bone**) ■ Initial antibiotic Selection
■ No response 48 hours of appropriate antibiotic therapy ■ Abscess ■ Toxicity ■ Fracture Risk
■ Good response to antibiotic(s) ■ No abscesses ■ No toxicity
■ Unroofing ■ Intramedullary Reaming ■ Drainage of abscess ■ Debridement Cultures*
■ Modify antibiotics if necessary*
■ DEAD SPACE MANAGEMENT
■ Antibiotic(s) alone
■ Antibiotic(s) ■ Beads***
■ Antibiotic(s) ■ Beads*** ■ Bone graft(s)
■ PERSISTENCE
■ ARREST
■ A new course of treatment
■ REINFECTION
6 Week course of Antibiotics
6 weeks parenteral OR
2 weeks parenteral, 4 weeks oral
* Modify antibiotic(s) on culture and sensitivity results.
** If blood cultures are positive with X-ray or scan evidence of osteomyelitis then bone cultures are not necessary
*** Beads are removed at two to three weeks and replaced with cancellous bone
A bead exchange may be done at two to three weeks, the new beads are removed two to three weeks later and replaced with cancellous bone.

**Fig. 78.5** Treatment algorithm: Cierny-Mader stage 1 long bone osteomyelitis.

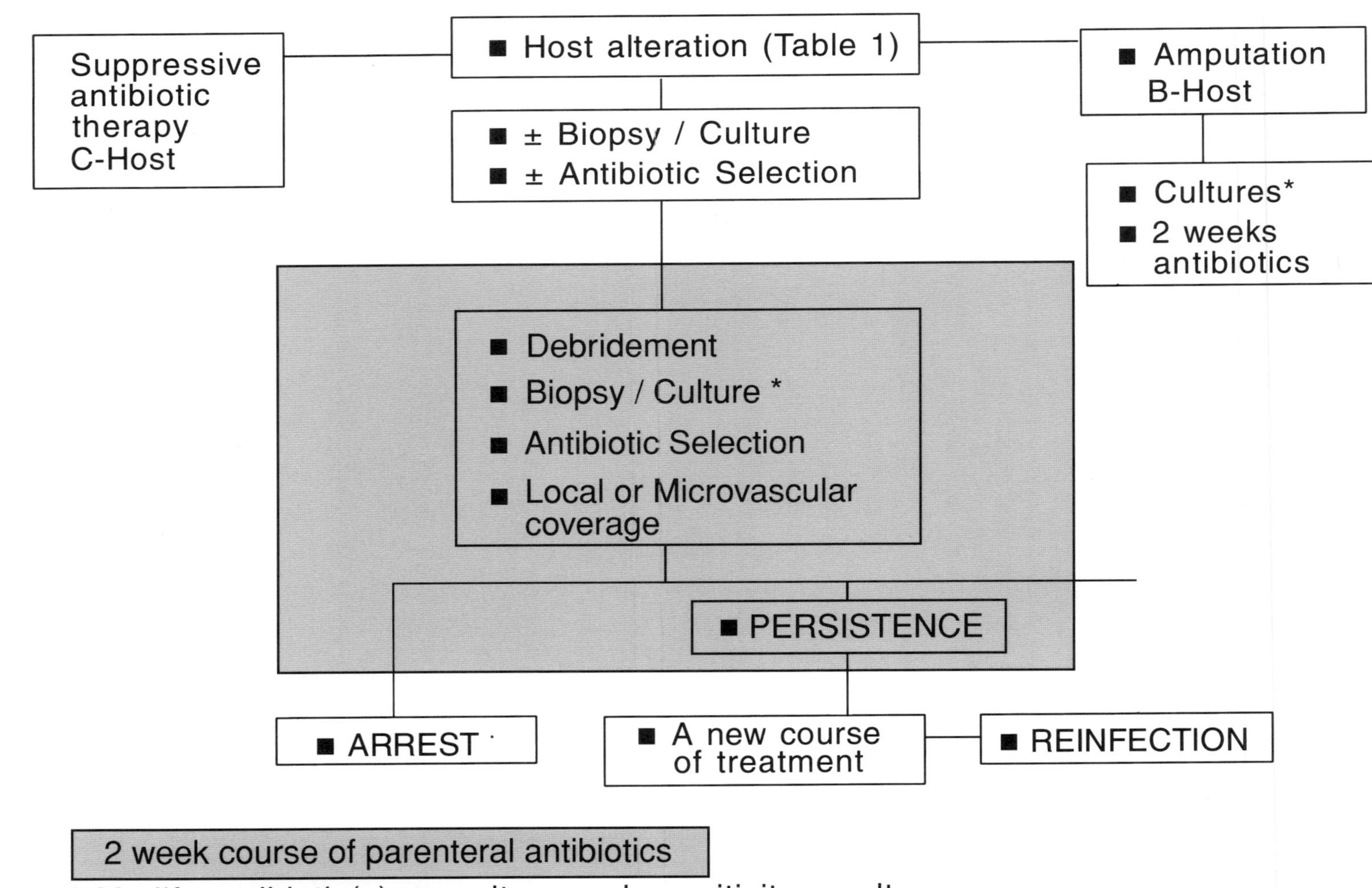


**Fig. 78.6** Treatment algorithm: Cierny-Mader stage 2 long bone osteomyelitis.

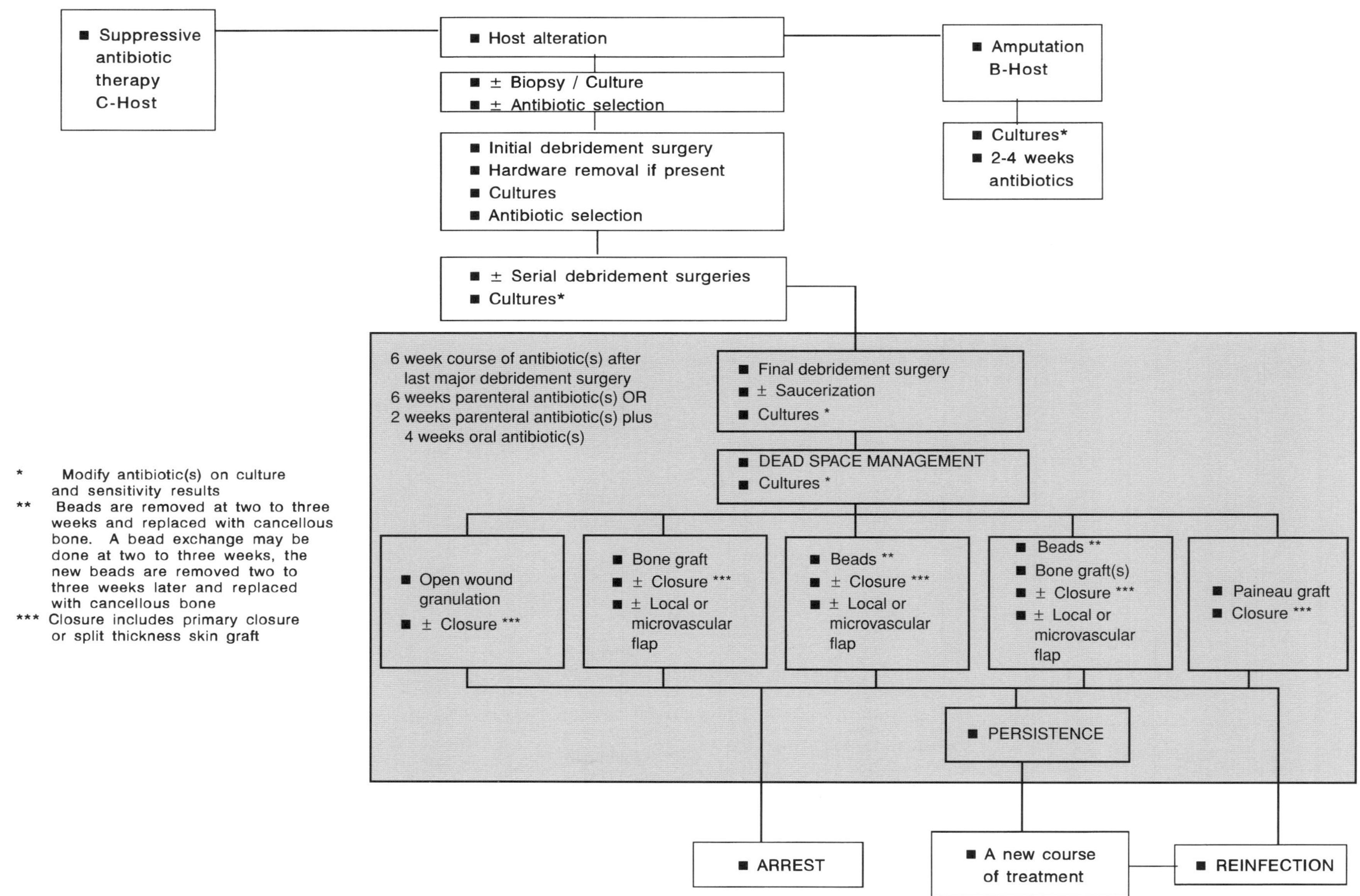
■ Suppressive antibiotic therapy C-Host
■ Host alteration
■ Amputation B-Host
■ ± Biopsy / Culture
■ ± Antibiotic selection
■ Cultures*
■ 2-4 weeks antibiotics
■ Initial debridement surgery
■ Hardware removal if present
■ Cultures
■ Antibiotic selection
■ ± Serial debridement surgeries
■ Cultures*
6 week course of antibiotic(s) after last major debridement surgery
6 weeks parenteral antibiotic(s) OR
2 weeks parenteral antibiotic(s) plus 4 weeks oral antibiotic(s)
■ Final debridement surgery
■ ± Saucerization
■ Cultures *
■ DEAD SPACE MANAGEMENT
■ Cultures *
■ Open wound granulation
■ ± Closure ***
■ Bone graft
■ ± Closure ***
■ ± Local or microvascular flap
■ Beads **
■ ± Closure ***
■ ± Local or microvascular flap
■ Beads **
■ Bone graft(s)
■ ± Closure ***
■ ± Local or microvascular flap
■ Paineau graft
■ Closure ***
■ PERSISTENCE
■ ARREST
■ A new course of treatment
■ REINFECTION
* Modify antibiotic(s) on culture and sensitivity results
** Beads are removed at two to three weeks and replaced with cancellous bone. A bead exchange may be done at two to three weeks, the new beads are removed two to three weeks later and replaced with cancellous bone
*** Closure includes primary closure or split thickness skin graft

**Fig. 78.7** Treatment algorithm: Cierny-Mader stage 3 long bone osteomyelitis.

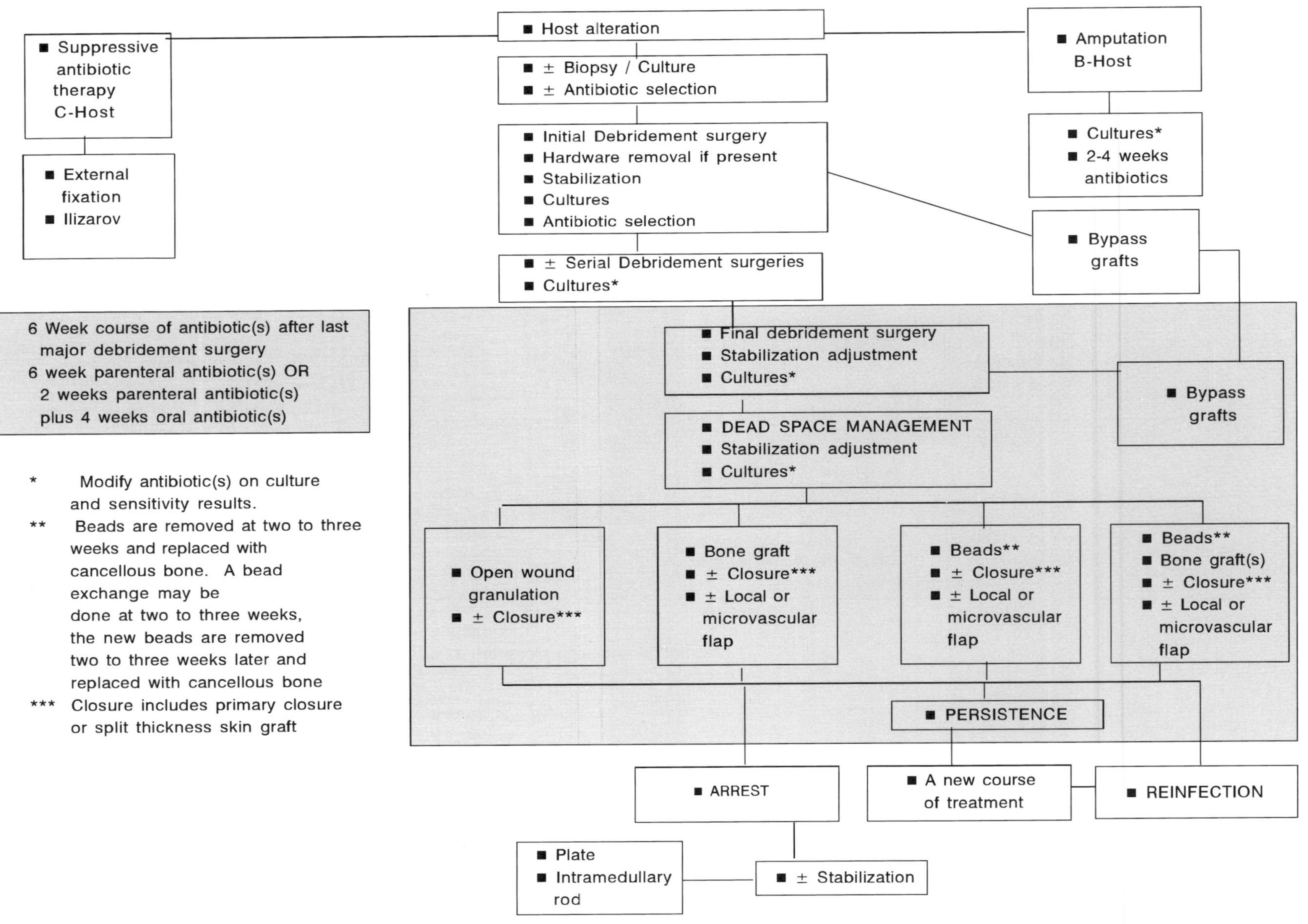


**Fig. 78.8** Treatment algorithm: Cierny-Mader stage 4 long bone osteomyelitis.

to the conservation of the patient's limited cancellous bone reserves. Open cancellous grafts without soft tissue coverage are useful when a free tissue transfer is not a treatment option and local tissue flaps are inadequate. Antibiotic-impregnated acrylic beads may be used to sterilize and temporarily maintain dead space. The beads are usually removed within 2 to 4 wk and replaced with a cancellous bone graft. The most commonly used antibiotics in beads are vancomycin, tobramycin, and gentamicin.

If movement is present at the site of infection, measures must be taken to achieve permanent stability of the skeletal unit. Stability may be achieved with plates, screws, rods, and/or an external fixator. External fixation is preferred over internal because of the tendency of medullary rods to become secondarily infected and to spread the extent of the infection. A new type of external fixator allows bone reconstruction of segmental defects and difficult infected nonunions. The Ilizarov external fixation method utilizes the theory of distraction histogenesis whereby bone is fractured in the metaphyseal region and slowly lengthened. The growth of new bone in the metaphyseal region pushes a segment of healthy bone into the defect left by surgery. The Ilizarov technique is used for difficult cases of osteomyelitis when stabilization and bone lengthening is necessary. The method may also be used to compress nonunions and correct malunions. The technique is labor intensive and requires an extended period of treatment averaging 8.5 mo in the device. The Ilizarov pins usually become infected and the device is painful. The Ilizarov is commonly used in a small group of patients for reconstruction of difficult deformities that results from osteomyelitis. The Ilizarov external fixation method is utilized by most tertiary care hospitals.

Adequate soft-tissue coverage of the bone is necessary to arrest osteomyelitis. Small soft tissue defects may be covered with a split thickness skin graft. In the presence of a large soft tissue defect or with an inadequate soft-tissue envelope, local muscle flaps and free vascularized muscle flaps may be placed in a one or two stage procedure. Local and free muscle flaps, when combined with antibiotics and surgical debridement of all nonviable osseous and soft tissue for chronic osteomyelitis, have a success rate ranging from 66% to 100%. Local muscle flaps and free vascularized muscle transfers improve the local biological environment by bringing in a blood supply important in host defense mechanisms, antibiotic delivery, and osseous and soft-tissue healing.

The Cierny-Mader classification of osteomyelitis not only stratifies the disease and host condition but also provides guidelines for the surgical management of the disease. In stage 1 osteomyelitis or medullary osteomyelitis (Fig. 78.5) the nidus of infection is entirely within the medullary canal of the bone. It usually is caused by blood-borne bacteria or the introduction of surgical hardware such as an intramedullary nail. Because of the location, surgical treatment is usually more straightforward than in other types of bone involvement. In pediatric patients without hardware, surgical therapy is usually not necessary. In adults with primary or secondary stage 1 osteomyelitis, a thorough intramedullary reaming and unroofing is usually done with or without bone grafting. Soft tissues are reapproximated and the limb is protected by external means (brace or cast) until structural integrity of the bone is reestablished by normal remodeling.

In stage 2 or superficial osteomyelitis (Fig. 78.6), the surface of the bone is exposed because of an overlying soft-tissue defect. The superficial cortex becomes involved with the infection and eventually becomes sequestered (stage 3 progression) if treatment is delayed. The most important aspect of treatment is soft-tissue coverage after adequate debridement to bleeding cortex. This may be a simple problem involving local tissue, or it may require free tissue transfer.

Stage 3 or localized osteomyelitis (Fig. 78.7), combines the problems of both stages 1 and 2. The treatment involves the modalities employed for both of these categories of disease. Bone is sequestered, medullary extension of the infection is common, and major soft-tissue defects may be present as well. These patients may require external fixation for structural support while the bone graft incorporates. Complex reconstruction of both the bone and soft tissue is frequently necessary.

Stage 4 or diffuse osteomyelitis (Fig. 78.8), combines problems of stages 1, 2, and 3. Instability is a problem before or after surgery. Therefore treatment often must be directed toward establishing structural stability and obliterating debridement gaps by means of cancellous bone grafts or the Ilizarov technique. Free flaps and vascularized bone grafts are other possible treatment modalities. All of the modalities previously discussed may have a place in the treatment of diffuse osteomyelitis.

## Therapy of osteomyelitis secondary to contiguous focus infection with vascular diseases

Because of the relative inability of the host to participate in the eradication of the infectious process, this type of osteomyelitis is difficult to treat. These infections are insidious and are often beyond simple salvage by the time the patient seeks medical therapy.

Determination of the vascular status of the tissue at the infection site is crucial in the evaluation of these patients. Although several methods can be used to determine the vascular status, measurements of cutaneous oxygen tensions and pulse pressures are the most commonly employed. Cutaneous oxygen tensions are obtained using a modified Clark electrode applied to the skin surface. Cutaneous oxygen tensions provide guidelines for determining the location of adequately perfused tissue. The values are also helpful in predicting the benefit of local debridement surgery and in selecting surgical margins where healing can be expected to occur. Hyperbaric oxygen therapy may facilitate healing in areas where borderline oxygen tensions are present.

The patient may be managed with suppressive antibiotic therapy, local debridement surgery, or ablative surgery. The decision regarding treatment options used is based on tissue oxygen perfusion at the infection site, extent of the osteomyelitis, and patient preference.

The patient can be offered long-term suppressive antibiotic therapy when a definitive surgical procedure would lead to unacceptable patient morbidity or disability, or in cases in which the patient refuses local debridement or ablative surgery. Even with suppressive antibiotic therapy, in time, most of these patients will require an amputation of the involved bone.

Local debridement surgery and a 4 wk course of antibiotics may be employed in the patient who has localized osteomyelitis and good tissue oxygen perfusion. Unless good tissue oxygen tensions are present, the wound will fail to heal and ultimately require an ablative procedure. Installation of antibiotic-impregnated methyl-methacrylate beads to obliterate dead space may improve therapeutic responses.

The patient with extensive osteomyelitis and poor tissue oxygen perfusion usually requires some type of ablative surgery. Digital and ray resections, transmetatarsal amputations, midfoot disarticulations, and Chopart, Lisfranc, and Syme amputations (amputation of the foot with retention of the heel pad) permit the patient to ambulate without a prosthesis. The amputation level is determined by the vascularity and potential viability of the tissues proximal to the site of infection and the requirements of a thorough debridement. The patient is given 4 wk of antibiotics when infected bone is surgically transected. Two weeks of antibiotics are given when the infected bone is completely excised, but some residual soft-tissue infection remains. When the amputation is performed proximal to the bone and soft-tissue infection, the patient is given 1 to 3 d of antibiotic therapy.

### Adjunctive hyperbaric oxygen therapy

The results of several open clinical trials have shown that adjunctive hyperbaric oxygen (HBO) therapy may be useful in the treatment of chronic osteomyelitis. Morrey reported on 40 patients with chronic osteomyelitis who met all of the following criteria: the infection had persisted longer than 1 mo; at least one surgical debridement had been performed; at least 2 wk of parenteral antibiotics had been administered; and the patients had been followed for at least 1 yr after treatment. All patients had chronic refractory osteomyelitis with a recurrence of this infection despite previous aggressive antibiotics and surgical treatment. After HBO therapy, appropriate surgery, and treatment with antibiotics, 34 patients (85%) remained clinically free of disease, and six experienced recurrences of their osteomyelitis. Using the same criteria, Davis evaluated 38 patients who were treated with adjunctive HBO. Of these 38 patients, 34 remained free of clinical signs of osteomyelitis. While the results of these clinical trials are encouraging, the specific role of HBO in the treatment of osteomyelitis is difficult to assess because of the many other patient-, surgical-, organism-, bone-, and antibiotic-related variables that may be of importance

Animal studies performed in an experimental *Staphylococcus aureus* osteomyelitis model have shown that hyperbaric oxygen administered under standard treatment conditions is effective in eradicating *Staphylococcus aureus* from infected bone. Osteomyelitic bone in this experimental model has decreased blood flow and a greatly decreased partial pressure of oxygen. HBO was effective in *Staphylococcus aureus* osteomyelitis because it increased intramedullary oxygen to tensions at which phagocytic killing may proceed more efficiently. In a *Pseudomonas aeruginosa* osteomyelitis model, HBO potentiated the aminoglycoside tobramycin.

Wound healing is a dynamic process which requires an adequate oxygen tension to proceed. In the ischemic or infected wound, HBO provides oxygen to promote collagen production, angiogenesis, and ultimately wound healing.

### Therapy for *Mycobacterium tuberculosis*, atypical mycobacterial, and fungal skeletal infection

Therapy for skeletal *M. tuberculosis* involves prolonged antibacterial chemotherapy (see Chapter 37) and in some cases surgical debridement. Atypical mycobacterial infections involving bone include *M. marinum*, *M. avium-intracellulare*, *M. fortuitum*, and *M. gordonae*. These infections seem to respond well to surgery alone. The role of antituberculous therapy, particularly with organisms like *M. avium-intracellulare*, is not clear. Therapy for fungal osteomyelitis involves surgical debridement and antifungal chemotherapy (see Chapter 42).

## Prevention

Decreasing the known risk factors for the development of osteomyelitis should decrease the incidence of osteomyelitis. The basic mechanisms for the development of osteomyelitis include hematogenous dissemination, direct inoculation, and contiguous spread from an adjacent infection. The major risk factors for acute hematogenous osteomyelitis include circumstances that predispose to bacteremias. The major circumstances include infections of indwelling intravascular catheters, distant foci of infection, and intravenous drug abuse. Infection of the skin, respiratory tract, and urinary tract represent the distant sites of focal infection most commonly associated with acute osteomyelitis. The second major mechanism for the development of osteomyelitis is direct inoculation. The major direct inoculation injuries include animal and human bites and puncture wounds. Diagnostic procedures may also inadvertently result in the inoculation of a neighboring osseous structures. Surgical procedures such as internal fixation of long bones and skeletal traction may lead to an infection of the bone. Osteomyelitis may develop as a consequence of contiguous spread of infection from an adjacent soft-tissue infection particularly if vascular insufficiency is present. The major risk factors for the development of chronic infection of bone include inadequate or delayed management of acute osteomyelitis or an unrecognized bone infection. Two groups of patients with an increased susceptibility to acute skeletal infections are those with sickle cell anemia and chronic granulomatous disease. Prevention of osteomyelitis includes decreasing the incidence of bacteremias, inoculation injuries, and wound infections. Since none of these reductions is currently possible, osteomyelitis will remain a major problem for the foreseeable future.

Prophylactic antibiotics are recommended for total joint arthroplasties. To be effective, adequate concentrations of the antibiotic have to be present in the tissue at the time of incision. Cefazolin is the most commonly used antibiotic for prophylaxis. Prophylactic antibiotics alone have lowered the incidence of infection of prosthetic joint infection from an average of 3.4% to 0.85%.

Total joint arthroplasties may be infected from a hematogenous source. Prophylactic antibiotics have been advocated for the prevention of prosthetic joint infections in patients undergoing procedures that are associated with transient bacteremias. Although the use of prophylaxis in this stetting is controversial, its use is widely accepted in patients undergoing dental manipulation who have gingival or periodontal infection.

## Vertebral Osteomyelitis

Pyogenic vertebral osteomyelitis is usually hematogenous in origin. In contrast to hematogenous long bone osteomyelitis, vertebral osteomyelitis occurs more frequently in adults than children. An arterial route rather than via Batson's venous plexus is believed to be the most likely route of infection. The segmental arteries supplying the vertebrae usually bifurcate to supply two adjacent bony segments. Therefore, the disease usually involves two adjacent vertebrae and the intervertebral disc. In the normal host, *Staphylococcus aureus* remains the most commonly isolated organism. However, in intravenous drug users, *Pseudomonas aeruginosa* is the most commonly isolated organism. Other sources of infection include the genitourinary tract, skin and soft tissue, respiratory tract, infected IV sites, endocarditis, dental infection, and unknown sources.

### Diagnosis

Anteroposterior and lateral radiographic views of the spine will reveal intervertebral disc space narrowing, with destruction and new bone formation at the anterior edge of the vertebral disc (Fig. 78.4A). A CT or MRI scan can demonstrate evidence of osteomyelitis before X-ray changes occur with evidence of paravertebral soft tissue swelling and bone destruction (Fig. 78.4C). The technetium polyphosphate $^{99m}$Tc scan also can detect spinal abnormalities in the early stages of infection, even before radiographic changes are seen. The technetium scan is a useful screening test for vertebral osteomyelitis if the X-ray is equivocal (Fig. 78.4B). Gallium/indium scans are difficult to interpret due to the high concentration of hematopoietic tissue in vertebral bodies.

A definitive diagnosis of vertebral osteomyelitis rests on the isolation of the organism from bone. A bone biopsy is generally required, since blood cultures are usually sterile. The biopsy should be performed under fluoroscopy or CT scan for guidance into the infected areas. In addition to aerobic and anaerobic bacterial cultures, the specimens should be sent for fungal and mycobacterial stains and cultures, as well as histology. If the original cultures are negative, an open surgical biopsy should be performed before starting empiric antibiotic therapy.

## Therapy

Biopsy and debridement cultures dictate the choice of antibiotic(s). The antibiotics are given for 4 to 6 wk and are dated from the initiation of therapy or from the last major debridement surgery. Surgical therapy is usually not necessary, except in cases where the patient develops an extension of the infection, such as paravertebral or epidural abscesses, when medical management fails, or where instability is pending. The neurological status of the patient must be closely monitored. Surgical fusion of the involved vertebrae is usually not required as spontaneous bony fusion occurs in 1 to 12 mo following appropriate antibiotic therapy. The success of treatment of patients treated with bed rest alone is not substantially different from those who are ambulatory and stabilized with a cast, a corset, or a brace.

## Vertebral tuberculosis

Skeletal tuberculosis is the result of hematogenous spread of the tuberculous bacillus early in the course of a primary infection. Rarely, vertebral tuberculosis develops as a contiguous infection from an adjacent caseating lymph node or from lymphatic spread from the pleural space. Either the primary bone infection or a reactivated quiescent primary bone infection elicits an inflammatory reaction, followed by the development of granulation tissue. The granulation tissues erodes and destroys the cartilage and cancellous bone. Eventually the infection causes bone demineralization and necrosis. Cartilage is destroyed slowly by granulation tissue, and the disc space is preserved for considerable periods. Proteolytic enzymes that can destroy cartilage are not produced in skeletal tuberculosis. Healing involves deposition of fibrous tissue. Pain is the most frequent clinical complaint.

In vertebral tuberculosis, the thoracic vertebral bodies are most frequently infected, followed by the lumbar and cervical vertebral bodies. Vertebral infection usually begins in the anterior portion of a vertebral body adjacent to an intervertebral disc. The infections spreads into the intervertebral disc and adjacent vertebrae. A paravertebral abscess develops in 50% of patients. Sixty percent of patients with vertebral tuberculosis have evidence of extraosseous tuberculosis.

Tissue for culture and histology is almost always required for the diagnosis of skeletal tuberculosis. Cultures for *Mycobacterium tuberculosis* are positive in approximately 60% of the cases, but 6 wk may be required for growth and identification of the organism. Histology showing granulomatous tissue compatible with tuberculosis and a positive tuberculin test are sufficient to begin tuberculosis therapy. However, a negative skin test does not rule out skeletal tuberculosis. Antimicrobial therapy is as described for pulmonary disease (see Chapter 37) except the duration of treatment is 1 yr or longer. In most cases antimicrobial therapy alone is adequate for treatment. However, advanced neurologic defects and severe anatomic instability require aggressive orthopaedic debridement and/or stabilization.

*Acknowledgments*—The authors wish to thank Diane Asmuth and Donna Milner-Mader for manuscript research and preparation.

## ANNOTATED BIBLIOGRAPHY

Calhoun JH, Mader JT. Antibiotic beads in the management of surgical infection. Am J Surg 1989; 157:443–449.
*Antibiotic beads have been used for successful treatment of dead space created by debridement surgery. Antibiotic beads provide high seroma antibiotic concentrations (dead space) and negligible systemic concentrations.*

Calhoun JH, Cantrell J, Lacy J et al. Treatment of diabetic foot infection: Wagner classification, and outcome. Foot Ankle 1988; 9:101–106.
*In 850 patients with diabetic foot infections, the Wagner's classification system allowed the development of rational therapy algorithms. Morbidity and mortality form diabetic foot infections can be decreased by intensive care of early infections and aggressive local care, antibiotics, and surgical treatment for more advanced infections.*

Calhoun JH, Anger DM, Mader JT. The Ilizarov technique in the treatment of osteomyelitis. Tex Med 1991; 87:56–59.
*The Ilizarov fixator was successfully used to reconstruct large segmental defects created to arrest osteomyelitis. Infected nonunions and angulation problems in infected bone were also successfully reconstructed.*

Cierny G, Mader, JT. Adult chronic osteomyelitis. Orthopedics 1984; 7:1557–1564.
*A review of the medical and surgical treatment of adult chronic osteomyelitis based on the Cierny-Mader staging system.*

Cierny G, Mader JT, Pennick H. A clinical staging system of adult osteomyelitis. Contemp Orthop 1985; 10:17–37.
*A new staging system for the stratification of osteomyelitis is described. The staging system is based on anatomic localization of the infection, the status of the host, and the degree of disability. Treatment algorithms have been developed for each stage.*

Couch L, Cierny G, Mader JT. Inpatient and outpatient use of the Hickman catheter for adults with osteomyelitis. Clin Orthop 1987; 219:226–235.
*Patients with osteomyelitis and their families were trained to give intravenous antibiotics through a Hickman catheter. There were very few infectious or noninfectious complications. The Hickman catheter was a safe catheter for giving inpatient and outpatient antibiotics to patients with osteomyelitis. Safe outpatient intravenous antibiotic(s) administration decreases the cost of osteomyelitis.*

Lisbona R, Rosenthall L. Observations of the sequential use of $^{99m}$Tc phosphate complex and $^{67}$Ga imaging in osteomyelitis, cellulitis, and septic arthritis. Radiology 1977; 123:123–129.
*Technetium localizes to bone and gallium is tagged on to transferrin and goes to areas of inflammation. The gallium scan is smudged and localization of the inflammation is often difficult. Sequential scanning with technetium and gallium allows a better anatomic localization and diagnosis osteomyelitis.*

Mackowiak PA, Jones SR, Smith JW. Diagnostic value of sinus tract cultures in chronic osteomyelitis. JAMA 1978; 239:2772.
*With the exception of* Staphylococcus aureus, *there is poor correlation of sinus tract cultures with bone cultures in patients with osteomyelitis. Sinus tract cultures should not be relied on for determining which pathogens are causing osteomyelitis.*

Mader JT, Adams KR, Wallace WH et al. Hyperbaric oxygen as adjunctive therapy for osteomyelitis. Infect Dis Clin North Am 1990; 4:433–440.
*Hyperbaric oxygen is used for the treatment of difficult stages of osteomyelitis (Cierny-Mader 3B and 4B). Mechanistically, HBO increases the oxygen tension in infected tissues including bone. An adequate oxygen tension is necessary for oxygen-dependent killing of organisms by the PMNs and for fibroblast activity leading to angiogenesis and wound heal-*

*ing. There is a direct killing effect of oxygen on fastidious anaerobic organisms.*

Mader JT, Cantrell JS, Calhoun JH. Oral ciprofloxacin compared with standard parenteral antibiotic therapy for chronic osteomyelitis in adults. J Bone Joint Surg 1990; 72(A):104–110.
*In a small randomized study oral ciprofloxacin was as effective and as safe as parenteral antibiotic therapy for the treatment of post-traumatic bacterial osteomyelitis in adults.*

May JW Jr, Jupiter JB, Gallico GG 3d et al. Treatment of chronic traumatic bone wounds. Microvascular free tissue transfer: a 13-year experience in 96 patients. Ann Surg 1991; 214:241–250.
*A high incidence of long-term successful management of long bone contiguous focus osteomyelitis can be obtained with appropriate antibiotics, debridement surgery and adequate soft-tissue coverage.*

Patzakis MJ, Abdollahi K, Sherman R et al. Treatment of chronic osteomyelitis with muscle flaps. Ortho Clin North Am 1993; 24:505–509.
*Successful results in the treatment of chronic osteomyelitis were obtained by giving specific antibiotic therapy, debridement of all nonviable tissues, stabilization with an external fixator, and local or free tissue transfers followed by bone grafting if necessary.*

Sapico FL, Montgomerie JZ. Pyogenic vertebral osteomyelitis: report of nine cases and review of the literature. Rev Infect Dis 1979; 1:754–776.
*Nine patients with pyogenic vertebral osteomyelitis and 309 patients in the medical literature were reviewed. Parenteral antibiotic therapy for 4 wk or longer resulted in a good response, but shorter courses resulted in higher rates of failure. Early diagnosis and prompt, aggressive therapy resulted in minimal complications, residual neurologic deficits, and a low mortality.*

Sayle B, Cierny G, Mader JT. Indium-111 chloride imaging in the detection of osteomyelitis. J Nuc Med 1983; 24:72.
*Indium$^{111}$ chloride is tagged to transferrin which goes to inflamed bone marrow caused by infection. Indium$^{111}$ chloride scans are negative in healed fractures but are positive in acute and chronic osteomyelitis. Indium$^{111}$ chloride scans are also positive in tumors and bony nonunions (inflammation from motion).*

Unger E, Moldofsky P, Gatenby R et al. Diagnosis of osteomyelitis by MR imaging. Am J Roentgenol 1988; 150:605–610.
*Because of its ability to separate soft-tissue diseases from underlying bone marrow. MR may be used to evaluate patients with positive bone scintigraphy to improve the specificity and accuracy of diagnosis for osteomyelitis. MR reveals bone marrow abnormalities.*

Waldvogel FA, Medoff G, Swartz MN. Osteomyelitis: a review of clinical features, therapeutic considerations, and unusual aspect. N Engl J Med 1970; 282:198–206,260–266,316–322.
*The most complete review of the clinical features and therapeutic options for osteomyelitis. The manuscript presents the most commonly used staging system for osteomyelitis.*

# 79

# Infectious and Postinfectious Arthritis

MEKONNEN ABEBE, LEE D. KAUFMAN, AND BENJAMIN J. LUFT

Infectious arthritis is a potentially serious condition with significant morbidity and disability if not detected and treated early. *Staphylococcus aureus* remains the most common cause of infectious arthritis in adults and children over the age of 2 yr, while *Hemophilus influenzae* type b is the most frequent cause between the ages of 6 mo and 2 yr, although the incidence of *H. influenzae* disease is declining in the United States since the introduction of the conjugate vaccine. A number of bacterial, viral, fungal, and parasitic agents cause acute or chronic infectious arthritis. Mycobacterial and fungal infections commonly cause chronic monarthritis, while *Neisseria gonorrhoeae* and certain viruses cause acute polyarthritis. Postinfectious arthritis, an aseptic inflammatory joint disease, has been associated with many different bacterial and certain viral agents. We will review the etiology, pathogenesis, clinical manifestations, and management of infectious and postinfectious arthritis.

## Epidemiology

There are two peak age groups for septic arthritis. The first occurs in children who are less than 3 yr of age (40%) and the second peak is in individuals over the age of 60 yr.

Infectious arthritis appears to be more common in males except for that caused by *Neisseria gonorrhoeae*, which is more common in females. Disseminated gonococcal infection (DGI) is a common cause of acute septic arthritis in young, healthy, sexually active adults. DGI is also the most common cause of newly diagnosed arthritis requiring hospitalization, while gram positive cocci make up the overall majority of causes of infectious arthritis.

The most commonly involved joints in adults are the knee (40%–54%) and hip (15%–20%) followed by shoulder, wrist, ankle, and elbow in decreasing frequency. In children the hip joint is most affected (60%), followed by the knee joint (35%).

## Host Factors

The most important host factor that predisposes adult patients to infectious arthritis is underlying chronic joint disease (40%–50%), particularly rheumatoid arthritis and osteoarthritis. In children and adults with no chronic joint diseases there is often a history of preceding minor trauma or prodromal upper respiratory tract infection and/or otitis media (e.g., *H. influenzae*). Intra-articular corticosteroid injections in patients with chronic joint disease, prosthetic joint surgery, repeated joint aspirations, and arthroscopic examination may predispose to infectious arthritis by interruption of capillary integrity.

Other conditions that predispose to infectious arthritis include immunosuppression, diabetes mellitus, malignancy, intravenous drug use, and extra-articular infections such as urinary tract infection and bacterial endocarditis. The deficiency of terminal complement components is an important host factor in susceptibility to infection with *N. gonorrheae* and *N. meningitidis*.

Reactive arthritis (Reiter's syndrome) following extra-articular infections of the genitourinary and gastrointestinal tracts has been associated with many different species of microorganisms. Some recent investigations using polymerase chain reaction (PCR) have demonstrated chlamydia DNA but not viable organisms in the synovium of some patients with nondysentric Reiter's syndrome, suggesting a direct pathogenic role for the organism. Others have not corroborated these findings and were unable to identify chlamydial antigen or DNA in joint fluid or synovium from patients with Reiter's syndrome. In reactive arthritis following infection with several organisms including *Chlamydia trachomatis*, *Shigella flexneri*, *Yersinia enterocolitica*, and certain *Salmonella* species, the presence of the specific histocompatibility antigen HLA-B27 and related groups is an important predisposing host factor.

## Pathogenesis

Most cases of infectious arthritis occur due to hematogenous spread of an infectious agent to a synovial surface already damaged from coexisting arthritis or trauma. Other routes include contiguous spread from osteomyelitis, cellulitis, septic bursitis, tenosynovitis and local abscess, or direct introduction during arthrocentesis (rare) or arthroscopy.

The synovium is extremely vascular and contains no limiting basement membrane, thus promoting easy access of blood contents to the synovial space. Following introduction of bacteria, which multiply in the subsynovial space, migrating polymorphonuclear leukocyte (PMNs) fill the articular cavity. Potential factors contributing to cartilage and bone destruction are the interplay of the direct effect of the microorganisms and their toxic products and the host response factors such as the intense PMN infiltration, release of cytokines such as interleukin-1 and tumor necrosis factor, as well as the resultant rise of pressure in the joint space. The extent of damage to articular cartilage, synovium, and bone likely depends on the size of the inoculum and the virulence of the organism in relationship to the host response. If it remains untreated, permanent loss of joint function develops.

*Staphylococcus aureus*, the most common cause of infectious arthritis, binds to bone sialoprotein, a glycoprotein known to be specifically localized to bone tissue. Binding leads to production and activation of a chondrocyte protease that contributes to the articular cartilage degradation noted in staphylococcal infectious arthritis.

In the pathogenesis of DGI, the attachment of the gonococcus to mucosal and possibly synovial cells is facilitated through pili-mediated adhesion. The pili also confer resistance to killing by neutrophils and to phagocytosis by mononuclear cells. Additional factors felt to be important in the dissemination of some strains of *N. gonorrhoeae* include outer membrane components such as low molecular weight protein I (IA) and gonococcal peptidoglycans.

Immune mechanisms rather than direct infection appear to be more likely in chronic inflammation such as Lyme arthritis. A cell mediated immune response develops early during the course of Lyme infection, accompanied by potent humoral immune responses to 41 kDa flagella protein. This is followed by antibody response to antigen with molecular mass of 66 to 73 kDa. During the chronic phase of the disease which is characterized by prolonged episodes of arthritis, antibody production to lower molecular weight antigens including outer surface proteins A and B (Osp A and B) occurs. *Borrelia burgdorferi* can be detected in synovial fluid by PCR early in the course of Lyme arthritis but is rarely found in synovial fluid in those patients who have joint inflammation for more than 1 yr and who have received multiple courses of antibiotics. This indicates continued inflammation after the spirochetes are successfully eradicated from the joint. The prolonged inflammatory response may be related to antigen mimicry that arises from the similarity of synovial and spirochaetal proteins such as Osp A and B in genetically susceptible individuals. Similar pathogenetic mechanisms may apply in other postinfectious arthridites such as Reiter's syndrome.

## Etiology

### Bacterial arthritis

*Staphylococcus aureus* is the most common cause of acute monarticular and polyarticular infectious arthritis in adults and children over the age of 2 yr (Table 79.1). Methicillin resistant *Staphylococcus aureus* (MRSA) is becoming an important causative agent in adults hospitalized in institutions with MRSA outbreaks. *Staphylococcus epidermidis* is the most common cause of prosthetic-joint infections (40%), followed by *S. aureus* (20%). *Hemophilus influenzae* type b is the most frequent cause of infectious arthritis between the ages of 6 mo and 2 yr but it is a rare cause of arthritis after 5 yr of age.

In neonates and infants, bacterial arthritis is most commonly caused by *S. aureus*, group B streptococci, and aerobic gram-negative bacilli. In hospital-acquired cases, staphylococci are the predominant cause (62%) , followed by candida (17%) and gram-negative bacilli (15%). The portal of entry includes umbilical catheters, central lines, and femoral venipuncture.

Streptococci cause infectious arthritis in a similar frequency of both adults and children. Group A $\beta$-hemolytic streptococcus is the most common, while group B streptococcus is an important cause of bacteremia and arthritis in neonates, adults with diabetes mellitus, and patients with prosthetic devices. Group G and rarely group C streptococci have been implicated in infectious arthritis mainly in patients with underlying joint diseases or prosthetic joints; *S. pneumoniae* is uncommon except in children with sickle cell disease.

*Neisseria gonorrhoeae* is the most frequent cause of septic arthritis in adults below the age of 30 yr. The serotype most commonly associated with disseminated gonococcal infection (DGI) is serotype IA, which is resistant to the complement mediated bactericidal activity of normal human sera. *Neisseria meningitidis* may also rarely cause an arthritis-dermatitis syndrome that can mimic DGI. Typically, affected patients have many more skin lesions, ranging from macules, and petechiae to purpura and vesiculopustules (see Chapter 51).

Gram negative bacillary arthritis occurs most frequently in the elderly with underlying chronic illnesses such as diabetes mellitus, renal failure, chronic joint disease such as osteoarthritis and rheumatoid arthritis, or previous trauma. The source of bacteremia in these patients is urinary tract infection in about 50% of cases. *Escherichia coli* is the most frequent isolate. *Salmonella* has been implicated in causing septic arthritis in patients with sickle cell disease and human immunodeficiency virus and in infants from developing countries. In intravenous drug abusers, the predominant organisms are *S. aureus* (including methicillin-resistant strains) and group A and D streptococci. A high prevalence of gram-negative bacilli, including *Pseudomonas aeruginosa*, *Serratia marcescens*, *Klebsiella*, and *Enterobacter* species have been reported as causes of arthritis in these patients with a predilection for the sternoclavicular and sacroiliac joints.

Anaerobic organisms are considered uncommon causes of infectious arthritis, but a recent review of a 10-yr experience at a military hospital indicates that anaerobic bacteria are of importance in bone and joint infections, particularly in patients with a history of trauma, prior surgery, presence of a prosthetic joint, contiguous infection, prior needle aspiration, diabetes mellitus, and malignancy. The organisms commonly isolated from infected joints were *Bacteroides* species, *Propionibacterium acnes*, anaerobic cocci, and *Clostridium* species. *Escherichia coli* has been associated with anaerobic septic arthritis.

Lyme arthritis caused by *Borrelia burgdorferi* is an important etiologic consideration in individuals who live in or have traveled to endemic areas and have had tick bites, particularly when the characteristic erythema migrans rash is present. Although the natural history of untreated early Lyme disease is variable, it is estimated that about 20% of those infected develop transient arthralgia, while about 60% develop arthritis, most with intermittent episodes. Only a small minority develop chronic erosive arthritis. The late phase of Lyme disease, which occurs weeks to years after the characteristic rash, is dominated by Lyme arthritis and neurologic abnormalities. Generally, the arthritis is self-limited and spontaneously remits within months to years after its initial onset.

Infected bite wounds can be complicated by septic arthritis. Human bites can lead to infectious arthritis with both mouth and skin flora including viridans streptococcus, *S. epidemidis*, *Eikenella corrodens* (a gram-negative bacillus), and anaerobes such as fusobacterium. *Eikenella corrodens* is resistant to clindamycin; metronidazole; and penicillinase-resistant synthetic penicillins. Dog or cat bites can lead to contiguous infection of a joint by organisms such as *Pasteurella multocida*. Rat bite fever caused by *Streptobacillus moniliformis* (a pleomorphic gram-negative bacillus) is associated with chills, rash and arthralgia, and, rarely, septic arthritis of large joints.

Secondary syphilis can lead to arthralgia, symmetric synovitis of knees and ankles, and sacroiliitis in association with periostitis, osteitis, and spondylitis. During tertiary syphilis, chronic synovitis of large joints may occur.

Mycobacterial infections usually cause chronic monarthritis.

**Table 79.1** Etiologic causes of infectious arthritis[a]

| Organism | Newborn | 1 mo–5 yr | >5 yr | >15 yr/adults |
|---|---|---|---|---|
| *Staphylococcus aureus* | 11–36 | 11–42 | 33–58 | 37–55 |
| *Staphylococcus epidermidis* | 0 | <1 | <1 | 3 |
| *Hemophilus influenzae* type b | 7 | 31–55 | 1 | <1 |
| Streptococci | 21 | 12 | 13–21 | 14–27 |
| *Neisseria gonorrhoeae* | 7 | 2 | 7 | N/A |
| *Neisseria meningitidis* | 0 | 3 | 1 | N/A |
| Gram-negative bacilli | 21 | 5 | 6 | 14–23 |
| Others | 7 | 3 | 5 | 4–8 |
| Unknown | 0–26 | 35 | 34 | 3–19 |

[a]Numbers represent reported percentages.
N/A—data not available in most series.

Tuberculous infection commonly involves single weight-bearing joints, but in patients over the age of 60 yr peripheral joints can be involved with a polyarticular pattern. *Mycobacterium kansasii* is the most common nontuberculous mycobacterium to cause arthritis, and it usually involves the wrist and hand, leading to carpal tunnel syndrome. *Mycobacterium marinum* is an unusual cause of septic arthritis but should be suspected if monarthritis occurs in the hands or wrists of patients who had contact with marine life, fish tanks, or swimming pools. Other atypical mycobacteria such as *M. avium*, *M. fortuitum*, *M. chelonei*, and *M. gordonae* can cause granulomatous synovitis, mainly in the hands or wrists in individuals who had nonpenetrating trauma. Lepromatous leprosy with erythema nodosum leprosum may be associated with symmetric inflammatory polyarthritis which resembles rheumatoid arthritis.

## Fungal arthritis

Fungal arthritis usually follows a chronic indolent course of several months that leads to delays in diagnosis and to inappropriate treatment such as intra-articular and systemic corticosteroids. Infectious arthritis caused by *Candida* species is not common. It presents either as a monarthritis following intra-articular inoculation during joint aspiration, corticosteroid injection or surgery, or more commonly as pauciarthritis following disseminated candidemia. *Candida albicans* is responsible for more than 80% of reported cases. The joint most commonly affected is the knee, although most patients develop polyarthritis. *Coccidioides immitis* can cause acute arthritis in a minority of patients following the hypersensitivity syndrome that occurs during primary infection known as "valley fever" or "desert rheumatism." Coccidioidal arthritis may be suspected when a patient, especially a non-Caucasian, immunocompromised man, presents with chronic progressive mono- or polyarthritis and a history of being in an endemic area such as the southwestern deserts of the United States, northern Mexico, and parts of Central and South America. Blastomycosis (caused by *Blastomyces dermatitidis*) is often found in the Mississippi and Ohio river valleys, southeastern United States, Canada, Central and South America, and Africa. Blastomycotic arthritis is usually monarticular and may occur by spread of adjacent osteomyelitis or by a hematogenous route. Patients often have evidence of pulmonary and cutaneous blastomycosis. Arthritis is a rare manifestation of disseminated histoplasmosis and cryptococcosis and is usually secondary to extension of adjacent osteomyelitis. *Sporothrix schenckii* causes a lymphocutaneous infection which usually occurs after cutaneous inoculation during outdoor work such as farming. Arthritis, bursitis, and tenosynovitis can follow sporotrichosis. The arthritis is usually chronic and commonly affects the knee, wrist, elbow, and small joints of the hands and feet.

## Viral arthritis

Viral arthritis is generally of acute onset and short lived, but chronic or recurrent arthropathy has been associated with persistent or latent infection with viruses which cause acute arthritis and human retroviruses such as human immunodeficiency virus 1 (HIV-1) and human T-cell lymphotropic virus 1 (HTLV-1) (Table 79.2).

Parvovirus $B_{19}$ infection is associated with clinical syndromes which include febrile illness and "slapped cheek" rash, erythema infectiosum (fifth disease) in children, or aplastic crisis in patients with hemoglobinopathy or hemolytic anemia. Intrauterine infection can result in spontaneous abortion or stillbirth, cutaneous vasculitis and arthritis. Arthritis caused by parvovirus $B_{19}$ occurs mainly in young adult women and it typically manifests as an acute symmetric polyarthritis. The clinical and laboratory findings of parvovirus $B_{19}$ may mimic systemic lupus erythematosus.

Hepatitis B arthritis is often accompanied with a urticarial rash and tends to resolve before the onset of jaundice. The arthritis is of sudden onset, associated with morning stiffness in some patients, and frequently involves small joints of the hands, knees, and ankles symmetrically. The hepatitis B surface antigen is positive and the aminotransferases are abnormal in most patients at the time of the arthritis.

**Table 79.2** Clinical features of viral infections often associated with arthritis*

| Virus | Frequency of arthritis | Joint involvement | Duration |
|---|---|---|---|
| Parvovirus $B_{19}$ | 50% adults (women 60%, men 30%)<br>Children 5% | Symmetric polyarthritis, small & large Joints | Arthritis <2 wk, arthralgia <4 wk<br>Recurrence or persistence 10% |
| Hepatitis B virus | Arthritis 10%,<br>Arthralgia 21% | Symmetric, usually migratory in some small & large joints | 1–3 wk<br>improves with onset of jaundice |
| Rubella virus | 15%–30% adult women<br>Children & men less often | Symmetric polyarticular, small & large joints, tenosynovitis, carpal tunnel syndrome | 1–28 d |
| Rubella Vaccine | 15% adult women,<br>1–5% children | Symmetric polyarticular, small & large joints, tenosynovitis | 1–46 d<br>chronicity or recurrence may occur |
| Mumps | 0.4%, males > females | Arthralgia, migratory polyarticular, monoarticular, large joints | <1–4 wk |
| Alphavirus (arthropod-borne) (Ross River virus, chikungunya, O'nyong-nyong, ockelbo, Sindibis, Mayaro) | Most adults | Symmetric, oligo or polyarticular small & large joints | 7–28 d,<br>may persist |

*Data from: Ytterberg, 1993, McCarthy DJ, Koopman WD, eds. Arthritis and allied conditions. 12Th ed. Vol 2, 2047–65. Smith, 1995, CID, 20: 225–31.

Rubella virus arthritis is most common in adult females and occurs 2–3 d after the eruption of rash. The arthritis is usually self-limited and is associated with tenosynovitis. Administration of rubella vaccine, an attenuated live virus, may rarely lead to an arthritis, chronic or recurrent.

Mumps arthritis affects predominantly men, and there is a higher prevalence of mumps orchitis among postpubertal men with arthritis (60%–70%) than among those without arthritis.

Several arthropod-borne alphaviruses are known to cause arthritis. Ross river virus causes epidemic polyarthritis in Australia and Pacific Islands and commonly affects adults between the ages of 20 and 40 yr. Chikungunya ("that which bends up") and O'nyong-nyong fever are members of the togavirus family with similar manifestations of fever, chills, rash, and multiple joint pains and occur in epidemic form in East Africa. Ockelbo disease, a viral illness of the alphavirus family, occurs in central Sweden annually and causes low-grade fever, rash, and joint pain.

A variety of rheumatologic manifestations have been described in patients with human immunodeficiency virus (HIV) infection: It has been associated with severe arthralgia and transient or persistent symmetric polyarthritis. The human T lymphotropic virus type 1 (HTLV-1) is noted to lead to a unique arthropathy characterized by chronic persistent oligoarthritis associated with proliferative synovitis in large joints. Synovial fluid and tissue from patients infected with HTLV-1 show atypical lymphocytes and HTLV-1 proviral DNA integrated into the DNA of synovial fluid cells and tissue cells.

## Parasites

Arthritis related to parasitic infections such as *Giardia lamblia*, *Crytosporidium*, and *Endolimax nana* has mostly been reactive arthritis. Occasionally direct joint infection has been noted with *Strongyloides stercorales*, *Onchocerca volvulus*, *Wuchereria bancrofti*, and schistosomiasis.

## Clinical Presentation

The majority of patients with acute infectious arthritis are febrile; about a third of the patients have only mild elevation in temperature. Most patients have pain and limitation of motion at the joint involved, but severely ill, bed-ridden elderly patients may not complain of joint pain. Children may present with fever, irritability, and impairment of ambulation. When the hip joint is involved, pain may be in the thigh or knee and may lead to diagnostic difficulty. The child will assume a position of comfort with the hip flexed, externally rotated, and abducted.

Most patients with infectious arthritis have visible joint swelling. This may be difficult to demonstrate in the hip and shoulder and lead to delay in diagnosis. It may be difficult to distinguish infectious arthritis from bursitis, cellulitis around a joint, or tendinitis. However, if there is painful limitation of movement it usually indicates joint involvement.

The etiologic agent influences the clinical presentation. Thus, the presentation is typically acute in most patients with infectious arthritis caused by staphylococci or streptococci, while those with mycobacterial and fungal arthritis as well as those with prosthetic joint septic arthritis often have a subacute or chronic presentation. Tenosynovitis with inflammation of multiple tendon sheaths occurs in about two-thirds of patients with DGI. This also occurs with rubella, sporotrichosis, and infections with *Moraxella* and nontuberculous mycobacteria. Characteristic skin lesions that accompany DGI (or meningococcemia with arthritis) are discussed in Chapter 51.

In a small number of patients with acute infectious arthritis (10%) multiple joints are involved, especially in those with rheumatoid, gonococcal, and viral arthritis.

## Laboratory Findings

The erythrocyte sedimentation rate (ESR) is nonspecific and is elevated in all causes of infectious arthritis. Although valuable, it may be difficult to interpret in the setting of preexisting inflammatory joint disease or coexisting infections at other sites. The peripheral blood leukocyte count is generally normal or minimally elevated in adults, while it is usually significantly raised in children with pyogenic arthritis.

The most important examination is the synovial fluid analysis. The synovial fluid leukocyte count is normally fewer than 180 cells per cubic millimeter and is generally considered inflammatory if it exceeds 2000. In acute infectious arthritis, the leukocyte count is often over 50,000 with predominant polymorphonuclear leukocytes. However, leukocyte counts up to 50,000 may be seen in acute rheumatoid arthritis or crystal arthropathy. In patients with septic arthritis and associated malignant neoplasm, corticosteroid use, or intravenous drug abuse, the initial leukocyte count is often below 50,000, probably due to compromised immune response. Synovial fluid protein or lactate dehydrogenase is of little value, possibly due to compromised immune response. A low synovial fluid glucose may suggest infectious arthritis, but this occurs in only about 50% of patients. Gram stain smears are positive in 75%–80% of patients with gram-positive organisms, 40%–50% with gram-negative bacilli, and less than 25% of those with *N. gonorrhoeae* infection.

Synovial fluid and blood should be cultured aerobically and anaerobically. Blood cultures are positive in about 30%–50% of patients with nongonococcal arthritis and 20% of patients with gonococcal arthritis. The yield is higher in polyarticular infection. If there is evidence for DGI, pharyngeal, rectal, cervical, and urethral specimens (as well as CSF if there are neurologic manifestations) should be plated on gonococcal media. Selective media supplemented with antibiotics (Thayer-Martin, Martin Lewis, and New York Media) are needed for isolation of gonococci from locations where competing bacteria are likely to be present such as pharynx, endocervix, urethra, and rectum (see Chapter 71). Nonselective media such as enriched chocolate agar is sufficient to isolate gonococci or meningococci from otherwise-sterile sites such as blood, synovial, and cerebrospinal fluids.

Crystals should be sought in the synovial fluid, but their presence does not completely exclude infection as septic and crystal arthritis occasionally coexist.

Diagnosis of mycobacterial and fungal arthritis require synovial fluid and tissue culture of synovial biopsy specimens.

Though not yet widely available, PCR has been shown to confirm the clinical diagnosis of gonococcal arthritis in patients whose synovial fluid culture is negative by standard culture techniques. PCR testing has also been shown to detect *B. burgdorferi* DNA and may become the gold standard as serologic diagnosis is problematic, particularly in the absence of characteristic erythema migrans.

Routine radiographs are not generally helpful in determining the cause of infectious arthritis. Common findings include periarticular soft-tissue swelling and widening of the joint space due to joint effusion or late-stage narrowing if there is cartilage destruction with an infected prosthetic radiograph. It may show loosening, abnormal lucency greater than 2 mm in width at the bone–cement interphase, and periosteal reaction. Ultrasound helps to demonstrate and facilitate the aspiration of hip effusions in children presenting with a painful joint. Computed tomographic imaging is more sensitive than radiograph in detecting effusion and associated osteomyelitis. MRI, on the other hand, is superior to plain radiographs, computed tomography, and radionuclide imaging in detecting pyogenic sacroiliitis and extra-articular spread of infection and is useful for the diagnosis of joint infection in pregnancy. Radionuclide imaging is not particularly helpful in the diagnosis of infectious arthritis except to exclude osteomyelitis.

## Approach to Diagnosis

The differential diagnosis of acute monarthritis includes infectious arthritis, acute rheumatoid arthritis, gout, chondrocalcinosis (pseudogout), and reactive arthritis. The history of rash, tick exposure, animal or human bite, sexual risk factors, intravenous drug use, menstruation or pregnancy, trauma, and travel gives important diagnostic clues.

Signs which suggest specific causes should be carefully evaluated. In an otherwise-healthy, sexually active young adult, findings such as five to 15 skin lesions, polyarticular involvement, and tenosynovitis strongly suggest gonococcal arthritis. Skin lesions in meningococcemia are more likely to be petechia and large in number (>100). Other conditions to be considered in patients with fever, multiple joint involvement, and skin lesions include Reiter's syndrome, Lyme disease, and acute rheumatic fever, each associated with typical cutaneous lesions (see Chapter 51).

Oral ulcers may suggest Reiter's syndrome, Behçet's syndrome, systemic lupus erythematosus, or HIV arthropathy. In patients with polyarthritis and systemic clinical features consistent with viral infection serologic tests must be obtained to confirm the diagnosis.

In a patient with a history of tick exposure and erythema migrans, the diagnosis of Lyme arthritis can be supported by elevated serum IgG antibodies. The wider use of PCR testing to detect *B. burgdorferi* DNA in the synovial fluid may help overcome the difficulty of interpreting serologic tests for Lyme disease.

A number of agents can cause chronic monarthritis. In individuals with history of ingestion of unpasteurized dairy products and those who work as butchers and veterinarians, a diagnosis of brucellosis should be considered. Mycobacterial infection causes progressive chronic arthritis which involves tendon sheaths, particularly at the wrist joints, leading to carpal tunnel syndrome. Various fungal agents cause chronic arthritis that varies with the geographic region, as previously described.

The final diagnosis depends on the synovial fluid analysis, gram stain, and cultures of the synovial fluid, blood, and other relevant sites. In suspected prosthetic joint infection, synovial biopsy may be helpful to confirm or refute the diagnosis of septic arthritis.

## Treatment

The initial antibiotic choice should be based on the synovial fluid leukocyte count, gram stain, age of the patient, and associated historical and physical features. Suggestions of antibiotics based on gram stain and the most likely organisms are given in Table 79.3.

If the gram stain is consistent with staphylococcus (gram-positive cocci in clusters) the initial treatment is either penicillinase-resistant synthetic penicillins (nafcillin or oxacillin) or a first-generation cephalosporin. Vancomycin should be substituted if methicillin-resistant *S. aureus* is highly likely (i.e., in institutions with a high prevalence of methicillin-resistant *S. aureus*). Ciprofloxacin with rifampin is a reasonable alternative in the adult patient). If the gram stain is suggestive of streptococcus (gram-positive cocci in chains), penicillin G or a first-generation cephalosporin is the choice, and if the patient is allergic to penicillin, vancomycin or clindamycin can be substituted.

Gram-negative organisms are well covered by a third-generation cephalosporin alone or with an aminoglycoside. Alternatives to the third-generation cephalosporins include extended-spectrum penicillins or carbapenems (i.e., piperacillin) or imipenem, with or without aminoglycosides.

In children (especially in the age group of 2 mo–3 yr), the presence of gram-negative cocci suggests *H. influenzae* and the treatment of choice is ceftriaxone 75–100 mg/kg/OD or in divided doses every 12 h; 20%–40% of isolates of *H. influenzae* type b causing invasive disease have been reported to be resistant to ampicillin.

The recommended antibiotic for disseminated gonococcal infection is ceftriaxone 1 g IV or IM every 24 h for 7–10 d. If symptoms improve after 3 d, patients can be given cefixime 400 mg BID for the remainder of the course.

If the synovial fluid analysis shows a highly inflammatory process and the gram stain is negative the antibiotic coverage should include both gram-negative and gram-positive organisms (see Table 79.3).

The usual duration of therapy of acute arthritis caused by *H. influenzae*, streptococci, or gram-negative cocci is 2 wk; for arthritis caused by staphylococci or gram-negative bacilli it is 3 wk.

Because antibiotic concentrations in joint fluid are usually high enough to insure inhibitory activity, only rarely is monitoring of serum drug activity indicated when treating a case of septic arthritis with parental antibiotics. Instillation of antibiotics during arthroscopic surgery or open drainage is not recommended as they may cause chemical synovitis.

Most patients with infectious arthritis respond to antibiotics alone and do not require further drainage procedures. Repeated needle aspiration is recommended if there is recurrent joint effusion during the first 5–7 d of treatment. If the joint effusion persists beyond 7 d surgical drainage may be necessary. In contrast to other infected joints, suppurative arthritis of the hip and shoulder generally requires radiographically guided aspiration and/or surgical drainage. Drainage of a septic joint reduces the intra-articular pressure and removes proteolytic enzymes, thereby protecting the articular cartilage.

In children with septic arthritis of the hip, prompt intervention is required. At the hip joint, the proximal end of the growing bone lies in the joint space and an increase in the intra-articular pressure leads to compromise of the intra-articular blood supply. This may cause necrosis, dislocation, and eventually growth arrest.

Early surgical drainage is also recommended for septic arthritis of the sternoclavicular joint because of frequent adjacent osteomyelitis and the extension of the infection posteriorly into the mediastinum. The other conditions under which early drainage is indicated include loculated effusion and septic arthritis in patients with rheumatoid arthritis. Anecdotal evidence suggests that in the properly selected patients, arthroscopic surgery may be an effective procedure for drainage and debridement with less morbidity than open arthrotomy.

## Prognosis and Outcome

Prognosis generally depends on age, comorbidity, the joint(s) affected, number and type of organisms involved, and host–microbial interactions.

In infants and neonates, involvement of the hip joint may lead to functional impairment and leg length discrepancy. The poor prognosticators in children include age below 6 mo, osteomyelitis with contiguous joint effusion, hip involvement, and delay in treatment over 4 d.

In older children and adults with no underlying disease, prognosis for survival and joint function preservation is excellent if treatment is given promptly. Elderly patients with polyarticular and polymicrobial bacterial arthritis may do poorly or develop residual joint problems, particularly if the hip or shoulder joints are involved. Other predictors of poor outcome are prolonged duration of symptoms before treatment (>1 wk), preexisting (rheumatoid) arthritis, use of immunosuppressant drugs, and persistence of positive cultures after a 7 d course of appropriate treatment. The overall mortality is about 10%, but it is more than three times greater with polyarticular than that with monarticular infection (23% versus 7%).

## Postinfectious Reactive Arthritis or Reiter's Syndrome

Postinfectious or reactive arthritis is an inflammatory poly- or oligoarticular arthritis in a genetically susceptible individual following infection initiated by many different species of microorganisms. The link has been established by demonstrating bacteria, bacterial fragments, DNA, RNA, and bacterial lipopolysaccharide in joints of patients with reactive arthritis, but how the infectious agent reaches the joint from the primary site of infection is not clearly determined. The genetic predisposition in reactive arthritis has been shown to be due to an interplay between an infectious agent and a major histocompatibility antigen gene product. About 80% of Caucasians presenting with reactive arthritis will be HLA-B27 positive. The HLA-B27 is believed to be directly involved in the immunopathogenic response to certain infectious agents (e.g., *Chlamydia*, *Shigella*). In the small percentage of patients who are HLA-B27 negative other susceptibility factors of environment or genetic origin may be operative. In 1981, an American Rheumatism Association ( now the American College of Rheumatology) subcommittee established preliminary criteria for the diagnosis of Reiter's syndrome as an

**Table 79.3** Suggested initial antibiotic choice for the treatment of infectious arthritis*

| Gram stain of synovial fluid | Likely organisms | Treatment regimen | | Comment |
|---|---|---|---|---|
| | | Primary | Alternative | |
| GRAM-POSITIVE COCCI | | | | |
| Neonate | *S. aureus*, group B streptococci, *S. pneumoniae* | Nafcillin or oxacillin | Vancomycin | |
| Child or adult | *S. aureus*, strept. | Nafcillin or oxacillin, ceph-1 | Vancomycin | If culture positive for streptococcus treat with penicillin or clindamycin. If allergies to penicillin use vancomycin or clindamycin |
| Adult with prosthetic joint | *S. epidermidis*, *S. aureus* | Vancomycin | Ciprofloxacin (if not *S. epidermidis*) | Increasing reports of methicillin-resistant *S. epidermidis*. Cure depends on surgical removal of joint devices |
| GRAM-NEGATIVE COCCI | | | | |
| child, esp. 3 mo–2 yr | *H. influenzae* | Ceftriaxone, cefotaxime, cefuroxime | Chloramphenicol, ampicillin/sulbactam | There are recent reports of *H. influenzae* arthritis resistant to ampicillin |
| Young adult | *N. gonorrhoeae* | Ceftriaxone, cefotaxime, or ceftizoxime | Spectinomycin, ciprofloxacin, ofloxacin | Ceftriaxone 1 g IV/IM (7–10 d), can be on cefixime 400 mg BID if improves after 3 d. If allergic to penicillin spectinomycin 2 g IM 2× daily, ciprofloxacin or ofloxacin 400 mg IV 2× daily can be used |
| GRAM-NEGATIVE BACILLI | | | | |
| Neonate | Enterobacteriaceae, *Pseudomonas* sp. | Ceph-3, aminoglycosides | | |
| Child, esp. 3 mo–2 yr | *H. influenzae*, Enterobacteriaceae | Ceftriaxone, cefotaxime | Ampicillin/sulbactam | |
| Adult | Enterobacteriaceae, *Pseudomonas* sp. | Ceph-3, Ap-Pen, & aminogycoside | Aztreonam, imipenem/cilastatin, ciprofloxacin | |
| NO ORGANISM SEEN | | | | |
| Neonate | *S. aureus* group B streptococci, Enterobacteriaceae | Nafcillin or oxacillin & ceph-3 | Nafcillin or oxacillin & aminoglycosides | If MRSA is prevelant vancomycin replaces nafcillin or oxacillin |
| Child, esp. 3 mo–6 yr | *H. influenzae*, *S. aureus*, streptococci | Nafcillin or oxacillin & ceph-3 | Vancomycin & ceph-3 | |
| >6 yr | *S. aureus*, streptococci | Ceph-1 or nafcillin or oxacillin | Vancomycin | |
| Young adult | *N. gonorrhoeae* *S. aureus* | Ceph-3 & nafcillin or oxacillin | Ceph-3 & vancomycin | *N. gonorrhaeae* resistant to penicillin or tetracycline has increased dramatically |
| Prosthetic joint, postoperative intrarticular injection | *S. epidemidus*, *S. aureus*, Enterobacteriaceae *Pseudomonas* sp. | Vancomycin & ciprofloxacin or aminogycoside or aztreonam | Imipenem/cilastatin | May require removal of prosthesis, drainage, and debridement arthroscopically or by open drainage |
| ANIMAL BITE | | | | |
| Human | Viridans strept., *S. epidermidis*, *E. corrodens*, *P. multocida*; *S. aureus* *Bacteroides* Peptosteptococcus | Ampicillin/sulbactam, ticarcillin/clavulanate | Cefoxitin, amoxicillin/ clavulanate | Wound care and debridment is most important |

(*continued*)

**Table 79.3** Suggested initial antibiotic choice for the treatment of infectious arthritis—*Continued*

| Gram stain of synovial fluid | Likely organisms | Treatment regimen: Primary | Treatment regimen: Alternative | Comment |
|---|---|---|---|---|
| Dog | Viridans strep, *E. corrodens* *P. multocida*; *S. aureus*, *Bacteroides* sp., *Fusobacterium* | Ampicillin/sulbactam, ticarcillin/clavulanate | Amoxicillin/ clavulanate or Cefoxitin or Clindamycin & FQ (adult) or Clindamycin & TMP/SMX/ (children) | Consider antirabies treatment. For penicillin-allergic patients doxycycline or ceftriaxone may be substituted |
| Cat | *P. multocida*, *S. aureus* | Ampicillin/sulbactam | Ceftriaxone | |
| LYME ARTHRITIS | *B. burgdoferi* | Ceftriaxone | Doxycycline | Lyme arthritis is usually treated with ceftriaxone 2 g IV/IM for 14 d. Doxycycline 100 mg BID for one mo has been successful. |
| MYCOBACTERIAL ARTHRITIS | *M. marinum* | Rifampin & ethambutol | Rifampin & minocycline or TMP/SMX | Treat for 6–12 wk. Some suggest treatment for up to 6 mo |
| | *M. kansasi* | INH & rifampin | | Treat for 6–12 wk |
| | *M. leprae* with erythema nodosum | Rifampin & clofazimine | | |
| FUNGAL ARTHRITIS | *Candida* Coccidiomycosis Sporotrichosis Pseudollescheria | Amphotericin B | Fluconazole, Itraconazole | Ampho. B is the drug of choice for fungal arthritis. 6–10 wk treatment may be successful (dose 2 g). Oral fluconazole and itraconazole have been successful for coccidiodal, sporotrichosis and pseudoallercheria infections |

*Data from: Steigbigel, 1983 Current Clinical Topics in Infectious Diseases, 4:1–29; Smith, 1995 CID, 20: 225–31.; Shaw, 1990, Clin Orthoped Rel Res, 257:212–225; Alloway, 1995, Semin Arthritis Rheum, 24: 382–90. Abbreviations: Ceph—cephalosporin (1 = first generation, 3 = third generation), TMP/SMX = trimethoprim/sulfamethoxazole, AP-Pen = antipseudomonal penicillin, FQ = fluoroquinolone.

episode of peripheral arthritis of more than 1 mo duration occurring in association with urethritis and/or cervicitis. The triggering event in Reiter's syndrome is usually a sexually transmitted infection (endemic or venereal form) or an episode of bacterial gastroenteritis (epidemic or dysenteric form).

*Chlamydia trachomatis* is the most common organism found in patients with Reiter's syndrome. *Clamydia trachomatis* has been isolated from the urethra of about 36%–69% of patients with sexually acquired Reiter's syndrome who have not been given antibiotics previously, and in at least 50% of patients with the syndrome, a high antibody titer to *C. trachomatis* has been found, suggesting recent infection. Recent evidence suggests a direct pathogenetic role for *C. trachomatis* in Reiter's syndrome. Although the infecting organism cannot be cultured from the joint fluid, direct immunofluorescence studies have demonstrated elementary bodies of *C. trachomatis*, and using PCR, *C. trachomatis* DNA has been detected in joints from patients with reactive arthritis. However, not all studies agree on this issue. *Ureaplasma urealyticum* has also been associated with Reiter's syndrome. The postenteric form of Reiter's syndrome has been described with *Shigella flexneri*, several species of *Salmonella*, *Campylobacter*, and *Yersinia*. The association between HIV infection and Reiter's syndrome remains unsettled. Some reports have indicated HIV infection as an independent risk factor, while others dispute the direct etiologic role of HIV.

Reiter's syndrome occurs principally in young men. The classic triad of arthritis, conjunctivitis, and urethritis is present in fewer than one-third of patients and the diagnosis may be missed. The arthritis is characterized by polyarticular joint disease predominantly involving the knees, ankle, hips, metatarsophalangeal, and wrist joints. A significantly distinct finding in Reiter's syndrome is local enthesopathy—inflammation at the bony insertions of tendons and ligaments. Ocular involvement commonly occurs as conjunctivitis and anterior uveitis. Mucocutaneous manifestations include painless oral ulcers, circinate balanitis, and keratoderma blennorrhagicum involving the palms, soles, extremities, and trunk.

The laboratory findings in patients with Reiter's syndrome are nonspecific. Urethral, cervical, and stool cultures should be done in an attempt to identify the infectious agent. If *C. trachomatis* infection is suspected, cervical or urethral specimens should be tested utilizing newer techniques that employ amplification of chlamydial DNA using PCR or LCR (ligase chain reaction). These appear to be the most sensitive and specific tests available for chlamydia diagnosis.

The basic approach to therapy is with nonsteroidal anti-inflammatory drugs (NSAIDs), physical therapy, and emotional support. In view of recent studies linking *C . trachomatis* to exacerbating flares of Reiter's syndrome, recommendation for several months of antibiotic therapy has been made (doxycycline 100 mg BID for 3–6 mo). Sulfasalazine and methotrexate may be useful for patients with polyarticular disease who fail to respond to NSAIDs.

## Enteropathic Arthritis

Various types of gastrointestinal diseases are associated with joint inflammation. These conditions include inflammatory bowel disease (IBD) (i.e., Crohn's disease and ulcerative colitis [UC]), reactive arthritis due to enteric pathogens, Whipple's disease, and postintestinal bypass surgery.

The oligoarthritis of IBD affects primarily large peripheral joints in about 10%–20% of patients, usually during periods of active gastrointestinal disease. The pathogenesis of the arthritis is speculated to be due to alterations in bowel flora and permeability which facilitate the entry of complexes containing bacteria, bacterial proteins, and other bacterial byproducts into the circulation. Surgical treatment of the bowel disease is associated with marked improvement in peripheral, but not axial, arthropathy of UC.

In Whipple's disease peripheral arthritis even without diarrhea is observed in about 50% of cases. The arthritis can be transient or chronic and is usually polyarticular and symmetric, involving large joints more than small ones. Electron microscopy shows bacilliform bodies in macrophages of lamina propria of the small intestine of patients with Whipple's disease. These bacilliform bodies are considered the etiologic agents because they disappear in patients successfully treated with antibiotics. Utilizing DNA hybridization and amplification techniques, a bacterium associated with Whipple's disease has been identified and given the proposed name *Tropheryma whippelli*. It is a gram-positive actinomycete not closely related to any known genus.

Following intestinal bypass surgery for obesity, polyarthritis develops in 20%–80% of patients 2–30 mo following the surgery. This is often accompanied by episodic fever and vesiculopustular skin lesions which resemble disseminated gonococcal infection. The pathogenetic mechanism is considered to be bacterial overgrowth and mucosal alterations in the blind loop.

## Acute Rheumatic Fever (ARF)

Acute rheumatic fever is a multisystem nonsuppurative inflammatory disease of children and young adults. It may involve the heart, joints, central nervous system, and subcutaneous tissue following untreated group A streptococcal pharyngitis. There are reports of a resurgence of ARF in some communities of the United States since the mid 1980s. The link between ARF and a prior group A streptococcal pharyngitis is well established, although the exact mechanism by which the organism leads to ARF is not known.

Acute rheumatic fever has diverse manifestations. Adults commonly present with sudden onset of fever and polyarthritis, while carditis occurs most frequently in young children. Subcutaneous nodules, erythema marginatum, and chorea are mainly seen in children.

In most patients with ARF, the attack starts with polyarthritis (75%), which is migratory and involves multiple joints (>6) in overlapping manner. The joints most involved are the knees, ankles, elbows, and wrists. In most cases, the polyarthritis subsides in about 4 wk without residual damage except for what is called *Jaccoud's arthropathy*. This is a rare sequela of protracted episodes of rheumatic fever manifested as reversible metacarpophalangeal subluxation and painless ulnar deviation without inflammation.

The diagnosis of ARF remains primarily clinical as there is no specific diagnostic test. The correct diagnosis depends on stringent use of the revised Jones Criteria supported by evidence of recent streptococcal infection either by serologic studies or throat culture. The response to salicylates is usually dramatic.

## Rheumatoid Arthritis

The cause of rheumatoid arthritis (RA) is considered multifactorial. In only 30% of patients with RA is the cause attributed to genetic factors (MHC and non-MHC) and in the rest it remains unexplained. Infectious agents have been considered to be involved in the pathogenesis of RA associated with chronic arthritis in children. Persistent rubella virus infection has been associated with juvenile rheumatoid arthritis. The demonstration of antibodies to bacterial peptidoglycan in children with pauciarticular arthritis and uveitis strongly suggests the etiologic role of bacterial infection in this disease. Other organisms associated with rheumatoid-like chronic arthritis include *Mycoplasma*, *B. burgdorferi* and parvovirus $B_{19}$.

There is renewed interest in the use of antibiotics for the treatment of RA. Minocycline (a semisynthetic tetracycline) 100 mg twice a day given for a period of 6 mo has been shown to be efficacious in the treatment of RA.

### ANNOTATED BIBLIOGRAPHY

Baker DG, Schumacher HR. Acute monarthritis. N Engl J Med 1993; 329:1013–1020.

*An overview of the causes of acute monarthritis and an approach to diagnosis and treatment.*

Bolanegra TS, Vasey FB. Musculoskeletal syndromes in parasitic diseases. Rheum Dis Clin North Am 1993; 19:505–513.

*The article describes the articular manifestations and management of parasitic diseases.*

Cuellar ML, Silveira LH, Espinola LR. Fungal arthritis. Ann Rheum Dis 1992; 51:690–694.

*A comprehensive review of fungal arthritis with exhaustive references.*

Dagan R. Management of acute hematogenous osteomyelitis and septic arthritis in the pediatric patient. Pediatr Infect Dis J 1993; 12:88–93.

*The article assesses the relative importance of the medical and surgical approaches to the treatment of pediatric osteomyelitis and septic arthritis.*

Gardner GC, Weisman MH. Pyarthritis in patients with rheumatoid arthritis. A report of 13 cases and a review of the literature from the past 40 years. Am J Med 1990; 88:503–511.

*A review of the features and diagnostic and therapeutic aspects of septic arthritis occurring in the setting of rheumatoid arthritis.*

Hughes RA, Keat AC. Reiter's syndrome and reactive arthritis: a current view. Semin Arthritis Rheum 1994; 24:190–210.

*A review of current understanding of the pathogenesis of reactive arthritis.*

Pinals RS. Polyarthritis and fever. N Engl J Med 1994; 330:769–774.

*A current review of the causes, diagnostic approach and management of polyarthritis and fever.*

Shaw BA, Kasser JR. Acute septic arthritis in infancy and childhood. Clin Orthop 1990; 257:212–215.

*The article emphasizes the need for early diagnosis, urgent drainage, and antibiotic therapy in children with septic arthritis.*

Shmerling RH, Delbanco TL, Tosteson AN et al. Synovial fluid tests. What should be ordered? JAMA 1990; 264:1009–1014.

*The study analyzes the clinical utility of synovial fluid tests in identifying infectious arthritis.*

Smith JW, Piercey EA. Infectious arthritis. CID 1995; 20:225–231.

*An excellent review of the pathogenesis, clinical manifestations, etiologic agents, and management of infectious arthritis.*

Wise CM, Morris CR, Wasilaukas BL et al. Gonococcal arthritis in an era of increasing penicillin resistance. Arch Intern Med 1994; 154:2690–2695.

*Overview of the features, clinical course, and treatment outcome of gonococcal arthritis with emphasis on the emergence of penicillin-resistant organism.*

Ytterberg SR. Viral arthritis. In: Arthritis and Allied Conditions: A Textbook of Rheumatology, vol, 119. McCarthy DJ, Koopman WJ, eds. Lea & Febiger, Philadelphia, PA, pp 2047–2065, 1993.

*A comprehensive reference on viral arthritis.*

# 80

# Myositis and Fasciitis

DENNIS L. STEVENS

Infections of the deep soft tissues are uncommon; they are often life-threatening processes, which require intense efforts to establish a diagnosis and begin aggressive surgical and medical treatment. Pyomyositis is usually caused by *Staphylococcus aureus*. It generally remains localized and is rarely associated with bacteremia, shock, and organ failure. In contrast, necrotizing fasciitis and myonecrosis are associated with toxic systemic effects including bacteremia, shock, and organ failure. This chapter will emphasize the clinical clues necessary to make an early diagnosis.

## Pyomyositis

Almost all such cases occur in the tropical geographical areas of the world. Infection occurs within a single muscle group in most cases and symptoms are localized pain, tenderness, and fever. Fever and chills are common, but bacteremia and cardiovascular collapse are unusual. Localized trauma is a predisposing factor in most cases. Diagnosis is usually made by needle aspiration, and patients respond to surgical drainage and appropriate antibiotics promptly. Pyomyositis has been recognized more commonly in North America among HIV+ patients. Though *Staphylococcus aureus* is still the most common organism isolated even in HIV+ patients, in 20% of cases unusual organisms have been recovered. Immunocompromised patients who are HIV− may be predisposed to gram-negative pyomyositis.

## Myalgia

In general, myalgia refers to muscle aches or pains which involve numerous muscle groups, and it is most commonly associated with systemic infection. Thus, myalgia may occur with any febrile illness, though in certain infectious diseases, myalgias are an important clinical clue. For example, diffuse myalgia is a cardinal manifestation of influenza.

Patients with epidemic pleurodynia have fever and chills with the sudden onset of severe, stabbing pain over the lower ribs or sternum. Pain may be intractable, and terms such as "devil's grip" have been coined to describe it. Patients with pleurodynia may be misdiagnosed as having pulmonary infarction or an acute myocardial infarction. Patients with toxoplasmosis may have either generalized or localized myalgia. In contrast, patients with trichinosis have very intense, but localized pain associated with encystment of trichinella larvae within the muscle. These patients usually do not have fever but may have periorbital edema and marked eosinophilia. In this sense it may be confused with eosinophilic fasciitis (Shulman's syndrome).

## Necrotizing Infections of the Soft Tissues

Necrotizing infections of the skin and underlying soft tissues have the common feature of fulminant destruction of tissue and systemic signs of toxicity associated with high mortality. Few infectious disease areas have a more confusing array of terms that describe these processes. Though many different terms have been used to describe clinical entities, necrotizing fasciitis is largely a surgical/anatomical/pathological diagnosis. Thus, patients with local evidence of an aggressive soft-tissue infection or patients with an innocuous local appearance of soft-tissue infection but with systemic toxicity should have surgical exploration of that site to determine if a necrotizing process is beginning. Though the clinical entity referred to as necrotizing fasciitis may occur alone, commonly there is also evidence of necrosis of the dermis and sometimes of the underlying muscle. The common pathologic features are extensive tissue destruction, thrombosis of blood vessels, abundant bacteria spreading along fascial planes, and an unimpressive presence of acute inflammatory cells, though small collections of PMNL or microabscesses may be described. Sometimes, muscle alone may be involved, without the underlying skin (e.g., *Clostridial myonecrosis*). Several clinical associations are well described in the medical and surgical literature and these are important because they may provide clues which may provide an earlier diagnosis.

## Meleney's Synergistic Gangrene

Infection is usually confined to the superficial fascia, usually occurs in postsurgical patients, and presents as a slowly expanding indolent ulceration. It results from a synergistic interaction between *Staphylococcus aureus* and microaerophilic streptococci and appears to be an extremely rare occurrence. Antibiotic therapy together with surgical debridement are the main courses of treatment.

## Clostridial Cellulitis

Infection is usually associated with local trauma or recent surgery. *Clostridium perfringens* is the most common strain associated with this entity. Gas is invariably found in the skin; the fascia and deep muscle are spared. Though this entity differs from clostridial myonecrosis because of less systemic toxicity, it is mandatory that thorough surgical exploration and debridement be the main objective means of distinguishing these entities. Magnetic resonance imaging (MRI) techniques or CT scans as well as a serum creatine phosphokinase assay (CPK) may be useful to determine if muscle is involved. Treatment is discussed under Gas Gangrene.

## Nonclostridial Anaerobic Cellulitis

Infection is associated with mixed anaerobic and aerobic organisms which also produce gas in tissues. Unlike clostridial cellulitis, this type of infection is usually associated with diabetes mellitus and often produces a foul odor. This must be distinguished from necrotizing cellulitis by surgical exploration.

## Necrotizing Fasciitis

Necrotizing fasciitis is a deep seated infection of the subcutaneous tissue that results in progressive destruction of fascia and fat but may spare the skin itself. Two clinical types exist. Type I necrotizing fasciitis is a *mixed infection* caused by aerobic and anaerobic bacteria and occurs most commonly after surgical procedures, in diabetic patients, or in those with peripheral vascular disease. Nonclostridial anaerobic cellulitis and synergistic necrotizing cellulitis are both variants of the same syndrome. It may not be important to distinguish these entities from one another, because all occur in diabetic patients and are caused by mixed anaerobic–aerobic bacteria. In addition to its spontaneous occurrence in diabetic patients, type I necrotizing fasciitis may also develop as a result of breach of the integrity of mucous membranes from surgery or instrumentation. In the head and neck region, bacterial penetration into the fascial compartments can result in a syndrome known as *Ludwig's angina* or may develop into necrotizing fasciitis. Both conditions are caused by mouth anaerobes such as *Fusobacteria*, anaerobic streptococci, *Bacteroides*, and spirochetes. Because of the proximity to vital structures of the neck, surgical exploration is important to prevent airway obstruction, to determine the level of soft-tissue involvement, and to establish which bacteria are involved. In the perineal area, penetration of the gastrointestinal or urethral mucosa may cause *Fournier's gangrene*, an aggressive infection caused by a mixture of aerobic gram-negative bacteria, enterococci, and anaerobic bacteria such as *Bacteroides* and peptostreptococcus. These infections may spread rapidly onto the anterior abdominal wall, into the gluteal muscles and, in males, frequently extend onto the scrotum and penis.

Type II necrotizing fasciitis is caused by group A streptococcus and was previously called *streptococcal gangrene*. In contrast to patients with type I necrotizing fasciitis, patients with type II are usually younger, do not have complicated medical illnesses, and have a history of blunt trauma or penetrating injury such as laceration, surgical procedures, etc. In such cases, it is the skin rather than mucous membranes that serve as the portal of entry for the streptococci. In recent years there has been a dramatic increase in the number of invasive infections such as necrotizing fasciitis caused by group A streptococcus.

### Clinical course of necrotizing fasciitis

Necrotizing fasciitis exhibits a remarkably rapid progression from an inapparent process to one associated with extensive destruction of tissue, systemic toxicity, loss of limb, or death. The early stages of infection may not be apparent, particularly in patients with postsurgical infection, gunshot or knife wounds, or with diabetes. In the last case, this may be related to neuropathy and anesthesia at the site of infection. Unexplained pain which increases rapidly over time may be the first manifestation. In patients with a preexisting reason for pain (surgical patients, trauma patients), the disease may progress to later stages before clinical evidence of infection is manifest. Similarly, diabetic patients may be unaware of the process; they tend to present late for medical care.

In most cases of necrotizing fasciitis caused by group A streptococcus, infection occurs deep in the tissues at a site of minor trauma such as a bruise, muscle strain, etc. Frequently there is no break in the skin. Within 24 h pain is apparent; malaise, myalgias, and anorexia may also be present. In some cases there may be mild overlying erythema. In other cases, excruciating pain in the absence of any cutaneous findings may be the only clue of infection. Within 24 to 48 h, erythema may darken to a reddish-purple color, with overlying blisters and bullae. Conversely, erythema may be absent and the characteristic bullae develop in normal appearing skin. The bullae are initially filled with clear fluid and rapidly take on a blue or maroon appearance (see Fig. 80.1A). When the bullous stage is observed, there is already extensive necrotizing fasciitis (see Fig. 80.1B) and patients usually exhibit fever and systemic toxicity.

Though many different M types of group A streptococcus have been associated with necrotizing fasciitis in the past, M types 1 and 3 have been the strains most commonly isolated from patients throughout the world. These strains can produce one or more of the pyrogenic exotoxins A, B, or C. Necrotizing fasciitis caused by these strains is frequently associated with *streptococcal toxic shock syndrome* (*Strep TSS*). The hallmarks of this syndrome are the early onset of shock and multiorgan failure.

Pyrogenic exotoxins possess the unique ability to simultaneously bind to the MHC class II portion of antigen-presenting cells, such as macrophage and specific $V_B$ segments of the T-lymphocyte receptor in the absence of classical antigen processing by the macrophage. Thus, pyrogenic exotoxins are superantigens and cause rapid proliferation of T cells bearing specific $V_B$ repertoires. Such stimulation of the host's immune cells is associated with production of both monokines (tumor necrosis factor [TNF]$\alpha$, interleukin [IL]-1, and IL-6) as well as the lymphokines (IL-2, $\gamma$ interferon, and TNF$\beta$). Expression of these cytokines in vivo likely contributes to shock and organ failure.

The pathogenesis of tissue destruction associated with streptococcal necrotizing fasciitis is less well defined, though we hypothesize that streptococcal toxins induce vascular damage resulting in tissue anoxia and rapid and extensive necrosis of fascia and muscle.

Laboratory tests such as CPK, SGOT, and serum creatinine are usually elevated and, together with leukocytosis with marked left shift, should be of sufficient concern to prompt surgical exploration. Some have advocated punch biopsy and frozen section to establish the diagnosis; however, they may be false negatives if the deep tissue is not adequately sampled. Bleeding and introduction of organisms from the skin or subcutaneous areas into the muscle should be of major concern. Much is to be said for direct exploration and visualization of the fascia. Debriding necrotic tissue, visualizing the underlying musculature, and obtaining material suitable for gram stains and culture are mandatory.

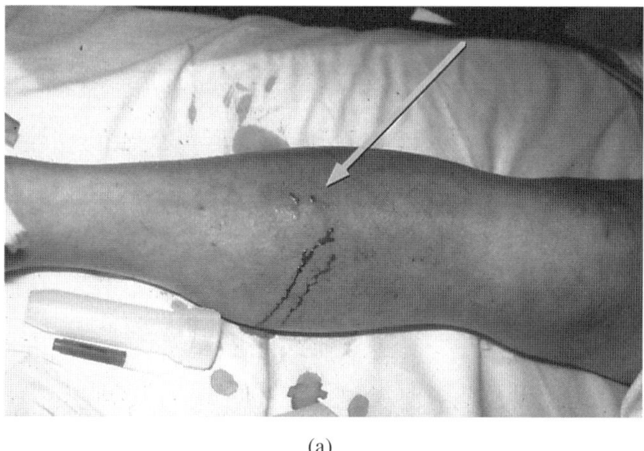

(a)

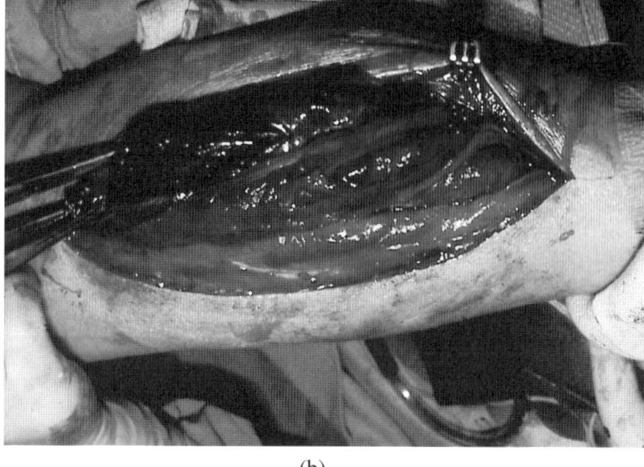

(b)

**Fig. 80.1** Bullous lesion associated with streptococcal toxic shock syndrome. A 45 yr-old male developed diffuse myalgia and fever. He was admitted for observation. Nine hours later, he complained of excruciating pain in the lower right leg. This small bullous lesion (*a*, see arrow) was apparent on the anterior skin. The skin was tight, but otherwise unremarkable. Anterior compartment pressures were measured by percutaneous needle placement, and manometry and pressures were high (hence the blood). Surgical exploration (*b*) revealed extensive necrotizing fasciitis and myositis. Intractable hypotension, ARDS, and renal impairment developed and he died less than 30 h after admission. Group A streptococci were grown from fascia, muscle, and blood.

## Myonecrosis

Clostridial gas gangrene or myonecrosis occurs in three different settings: "post-traumatic," spontaneous, and recurrent. First, and most commonly, post-traumatic gas gangrene develops after deep, penetrating injury that compromises the blood supply (e.g., knife or gunshot wound, crush injury), creating an anaerobic environment ideal for clostridial proliferation; *C. perfringens* accounts for 80% of such infections. The remaining cases are caused by *C. septicum*, *C. novyii*, *C. histolyticum*, *C. bifermentans*, and *C. fallax*. Other conditions associated with post-traumatic gas gangrene are bowel and biliary tract surgery, criminal abortion, retained placenta, prolonged rupture of the membranes, and intrauterine fetal demise. Spontaneous or nontraumatic gas gangrene is most commonly caused by the more aerotolerant *C. septicum*. Finally, recurrent gas gangrene caused by *C. perfringens* has been described in individuals with nonpenetrating injuries at sites of previous gas gangrene where spores of *C. perfringens* remain quiescent in tissue for periods of 10 to 20 yr and then germinate when minor trauma provides conditions suitable for growth.

## Post-traumatic gas gangrene

### Clinical manifestations

The first symptom is usually sudden and severe pain at the site of surgery or trauma. The mean incubation period is less than 24 h, but ranges from 6 to 8 h up to several days, probably depending on the amount of soil contamination or bowel spillage and degree of vascular compromise. The skin may initially appear pale but quickly changes to bronze, and then purplish red, and becomes tense and exquisitely tender. Bullae develop; they may be clear, red, blue, or purple. Gas present in tissue may be obvious by physical examination, soft-tissue radiographs, or computerized tomographic (CT) scan. Signs of systemic toxicity develop rapidly including tachycardia, low-grade fever, diaphoresis, followed by shock and multiorgan failure. Bacteremia occurs in 15% of patients and is often associated with brisk hemolysis. Patients have been described with hematocrits of 0 for as long as 24 h. Complications include jaundice, renal failure, hypotension, and liver necrosis. Renal failure is largely due to hemoglobinuria and myoglobinuria but complicated by acute tubular necrosis following hypotension. Renal tubular cells are likely directly affected by toxins, but this has not been proven.

### Pathogenesis

The initiating trauma introduces organisms (either vegetative forms or spores) into the deep tissues and produces an anaerobic niche with a sufficiently low redox potential and acid pH for optimal clostridial growth and toxin production. Necrosis progresses within hours. At the junction of necrotic and normal tissues no polymorphonuclear leukocytes (PMNLs) are present, yet pavementing of PMNL is apparent within capillaries and in small arterioles and postcapillary venules, followed later in the course by leukostasis within larger vessels. Thus, the histopathology of clostridial gas gangrene is completely opposite that seen in soft-tissue infections caused by organisms such as *Staphylococcus aureus*, in which an early luxuriant influx of PMNL localizes the infection without adjacent tissue or vascular destruction.

Theta toxin, a thiol-activated cytolysin, and alpha toxin, a phospholipase C, are the major lethal factors of *C. perfringens*. Both toxins are cytotoxic to PMNL in high concentration. Even at low concentrations, each toxin, singly and in combination, can delay PMNL influx into tissue, cause loss of vascular integrity, and induce shock in animals. Cardiovascular collapse may also be related to direct suppression of myocardial contractility by alpha toxin.

### Diagnosis

Increasing pain at the site of prior injury or surgery together with signs of systemic toxicity and gas in the tissue support the diagnosis. Definitive diagnosis rests on demonstrating large, gram-variable rods at the injury site. It should be noted that although clostridia stain gram-positive when obtained from bacteriologic media, when visualized from infected tissues, they appear both gram-positive and gram-negative. Surgical exploration is essential and demonstrates muscle that does not bleed or contract when stimulated. Grossly, muscle tissue is edematous and may have a reddish-blue to black coloration. Usually, necrotizing fasciitis and cutaneous necrosis are also present. Microscopic evaluation of biopsy material invariably demonstrates organisms among degenerating muscle bundles, and characteristically, an absence of acute inflammatory cells.

Blood cultures are usually positive in patients with myonecrosis, shock, and intravascular hemolysis. In contrast, some patients who are not ill may have positive blood cultures for *C. perfringens*, probably due to transient bacteremia from a gastrointestinal source. Positive blood cultures for the more aerotolerant *C. septicum* are more likely to be related to significant gastrointestinal pathology, such as carcinoma, and such cases are at greater risk for spontaneous gas gangrene, as described below.

## Treatment

Penicillin, clindamycin, tetracycline, chloramphenicol, metronidazole, and a number of cephalosporins have excellent in vitro activity against *C. perfringens* and other clostridia. No clinical trials have been conducted to compare the efficacy of these agents in humans. Experimental studies in mice suggest that clindamycin has the greatest efficacy and penicillin the least. Slightly greater survival was observed in animals receiving both clindamycin and penicillin; in contrast, antagonism was observed with penicillin plus metronidazole. Resistance of some strains to clindamycin suggests a combination of penicillin and clindamycin is warranted. The efficacy of clindamycin is related to its ability to suppress synthesis of toxins by *C. perfringens*.

Aggressive surgical debridement is mandatory to improve survival and prevent complications. The use of hyperbaric oxygen (HBO) is controversial though some nonrandomized studies have reported excellent results with HBO therapy when combined with antibiotics and surgical debridement. Experimental studies demonstrate slight benefit of HBO when combined with penicillin, though survivals were greater with clindamycin alone.

Therapeutic strategies directed against toxin expression in vivo, such as neutralization with specific antitoxin antibody or inhibiting toxin synthesis, may be valuable adjuncts to traditional antimicrobial regimens. Future strategies may target endogenous proadhesive molecules—that is, vascular integrins and platelet activating factor—such that toxin-induced vascular leukostasis and resultant tissue injury are attenuated.

### Prognosis

Patients presenting with gas gangrene of an extremity have a better prognosis than those with truncal or intra-abdominal gas gangrene, largely because it is difficult to adequately debride such lesions. HBO could be useful in such patients, yet there is little data on this subject. In addition to truncal gangrene, patients with associated bacteremia and intravascular hemolysis have the greatest likelihood of progressing to shock and death.

### Prevention

Aggressive debridement of devitalized tissue, as well as rapid repair of compromised vascular supply, greatly reduces the frequency of gas gangrene in contaminated deep wounds. Intramuscular epinephrine, prolonged application of tourniquets, and surgical closure of traumatic wounds should be avoided. Patients with contaminated wounds should receive prophylactic antibiotics.

## Spontaneous, nontraumatic gas gangrene due to *Clostridium septicum*

### Clinical manifestations

The onset of disease is abrupt, often with excruciating pain, although the patient may sense only heaviness or numbness. The first symptom may be confusion or malaise. Extremely rapid progression of gangrene follows. Swelling advances and blisters appear filled with clear, cloudy, hemorrhagic, or purplish fluid. The skin around such bullae also has a purple hue, perhaps reflecting vascular compromise resulting from bacterial toxins diffusing into surrounding tissues. Crepitus is apparent on palpation and gas in tissue is easily substantiated by routine soft-tissue radiographs (see Fig. 80.2). Histopathology of muscle and connective tissues includes cell lysis and gas formation; inflammatory cells are remarkably absent.

Predisposing factors include colonic carcinoma, diverticulitis, gastrointestinal surgery, leukemia, lymphoproliferative disorders, and either chemotherapy or radiation therapy. Cyclic neutrope-

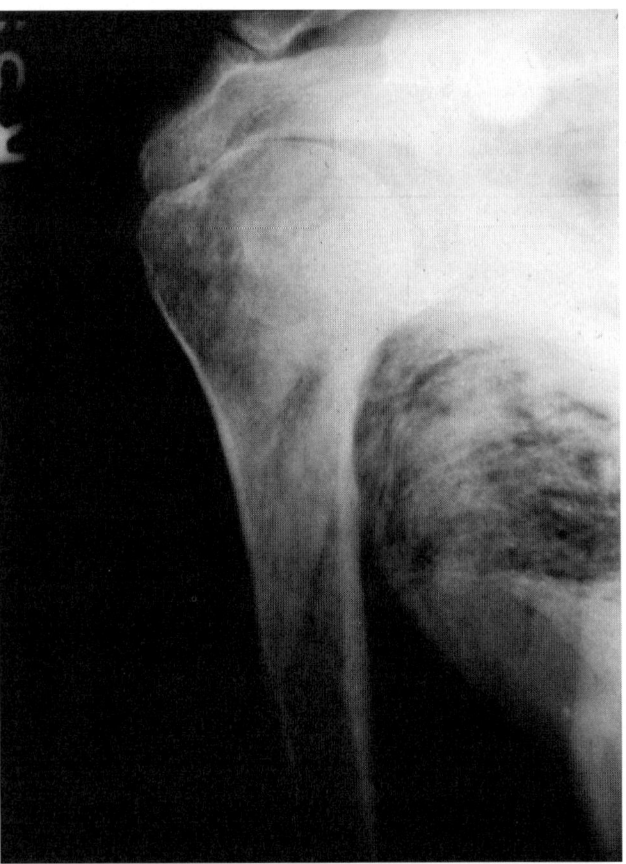

**Fig. 80.2** X-ray of shoulder showing gas in tissue. This patient developed spontaneous gas gangrene of the hand which spread rapidly up the arm and onto the thorax. *Clostridium septicum* was grown from blood and necrotic tissue of the arm. After receiving hyperbaric oxygen, antibiotics, and aggressive surgical debridement including disarticulation of the shoulder, the patient recovered. Two months later, barium enema demonstrated carcinoma of the colon.

nia is also associated with spontaneous gas gangrene due to *C. septicum*, and in such cases necrotizing enterocolitis, cecitis, or distal ileitis is commonly found. These gastrointestinal pathologies permit bacterial access to the bloodstream; consequently, the aerotolerant *C. septicum* can become established in normal tissues. Patients surviving bacteremia or spontaneous gangrene due to *C. septicum* should have appropriate diagnostic studies of the gastrointestinal tract to rule out pathology in this area.

### Diagnosis

Unlike traumatic gas gangrene, bacteremia in spontaneous gangrene precedes cutaneous manifestations by several hours, causing delays in the appropriate diagnosis and, as a consequence, an increase in the mortality rate. Thus, clinical recognition of bullous lesions in a patient with risk factors (see Clinical Manifestations) should trigger an aggressive diagnostic workup which should include blood culture, soft-tissue X-rays, aspiration of bullae, and surgical exploration for cultures and histopathology.

### Pathogenesis

*Clostridium septicum* produces four toxins: alpha toxin ($\alpha$, lethal, hemolytic, necrotizing activity); beta toxin ($\beta$, DNase); gamma toxin ($\gamma$, hyaluronidase); and delta toxin ($\Delta$, septicolysin, an oxygen labile hemolysin); as well as a protease and a neuraminidase. This alpha toxin does not possess phospholipase activity and is thus distinct from the alpha toxin of *C. perfringens*. Active immunization against alpha toxin significantly protects against challenge with viable *C. septicum*. The mechanism by which alpha toxin contributes to *C. septicum* pathogenesis is unknown; however, the recent cloning and sequencing of this toxin should facilitate studies in this area.

### Treatment

Though no comparative human trials have evaluated the efficacy of antibiotics or HBO for treating clinical cases of spontaneous gas gangrene, in vitro data suggests that *C. septicum* is uniformly susceptible to penicillin, tetracycline, erythromycin, clindamycin, chloramphenicol, and metronidazole. The aerotolerance of *C. septicum* may reduce the efficacy of HBO therapy.

### Prognosis

The mortality of spontaneous clinical gangrene ranges from 67% to 100% with the majority of deaths occurring within 24 h of onset. Risk factors include underlying malignancy and compromised immune status.

## ANNOTATED BIBLIOGRAPHY


Bryant AE, Bergstrom R, Zimmerman GA, Salyer JL, Hill HR, Tweten RK, Sato H, Stevens DL. *Clostridium perfringens* invasiveness is enhanced by effects of theta toxin upon PMNL structure and function: the roles of leukocytotoxicity and expression of CD11/CD18 adherence glycoprotein. FEMS Immunol Med Microbiol 1993; 7:321–336.

*This paper demonstrates that theta toxin contributes to pathogenesis by inhibition of PMNL function in high concentrations and that at lower concentrations induces upregulation of PMNL adherence molecules such as CD11/CD18 as well as endothelial adherence molecules such as platelet activating factor.*

Hook EW, Hooton TM, Horton CA, Coyle MB, Ramsey PG, Turck M. Microbiologic evaluation of cutaneous cellulitis in adults. Arch Intern Med 1986; 146:295.

Simmons RL, Ahrenholz DH. Infections of the skin and soft tissue. In: Surgical Infectious Diseases, 2nd ed. RJ Howard, RL Simmons, eds. Appleton & Lange, Norwalk, Ct, pp 377–441, 1988.

*A well-written, comprehensive textbook chapter on soft-tissue infections including necrotizing fasciitis and clostridium myonecrosis. Written from the perspective of a surgeon, the indications for surgical intervention and the importance of early and aggressive debridement are particularly valuable.*

Stevens DL. Invasive group A streptococcus infections. Clin Infect Dis 1992; 14:2.

*An article that reviews invasive group A streptococcal infections including bacteremia, necrotizing fasciitis, myositis, scarlet fever, and the Streptococcal Toxic Shock Syndrome (Strep TSS). The current epidemiology, clinical characteristics, laboratory features, and pathogenesis of Strep TSS are presented. The characteristics of strains of* Streptococcus pyogenes *associated with these infections such as M-type and pyrogenic exotoxin profiles are presented. A model to explain why the same strain of streptococcus may cause pharyngitis, scarlet fever, bacteremia, and Strep TSS is proposed.*

Stevens DL. *Streptococcus pyogenes* infections. In: Internal Medicine, JH Stein, ed. Mosby-Yearbook, St. Louis, MO., pp 2078–2086, 1994.

Stevens DL, Bryant AE, Adams K, Mader JT. Evaluation of hyperbaric oxygen therapy for treatment of experimental *Clostridium perfringens* infection. Clin Infect Dis 1993; 17:231–237.

*Using an experimental model of gas gangrene caused by* Clostridium perfringens, *the efficacy of penicillin, metronidazole, and clindamycin with or without hyperbaric oxygen was assessed. Hyperbaric oxygen alone did not improve survival time or survival. A modest additive effect was observed with penicillin and hyperbaric oxygen. No additive effects were observed with hyperbaric oxygen and clindamycin; however, the efficacy of clindamycin alone was greater than any other treatment evaluated.*

*Accompanying this article are two editorials that discuss the pros and cons of hyperbaric oxygen treatment in human cases of gas gangrene.*

Stevens DL, Gibbons AE, Bergstrom R, Winn V. The Eagle effect revisited: efficacy of clindamycin, erythromycin, and penicillin in the treatment of streptococcal myositis. J Infect Dis 1988; 158:23–28.

*This paper provides reconfirmation of the work of Harry Eagle, demonstrating that penicillin fails in experimental group A streptococcal infections associated with high inocula or delays in treatment. In contrast, erythromycin and clindamycin in particular were dramatically more efficacious.*

Stevens DL, Musher DM, Watson DA, Eddy H, Hamill RJ, Gyorkey F, Rosen H, Mader J. Spontaneous, nontraumatic gangrene due to *Clostridium septicum*. Rev Infect Dis 1990; 12(2):286.

*This paper reviews the literature and presents eight additional cases of spontaneous, nontraumatic gas gangrene cause by* Clostridium septicum. *The paper also demonstrates that blister fluid from patients with gas gangrene caused by this organism causes dose-dependent stimulation of PMNL chemiluminescence and causes profound ultrastructural changes of PMNL. These results may in part explain the paucity of leukocytes found at the site of infection in such patients.*

Stevens DL, Troyer B, Merrick D, Mitten JE, Olson R. Lethal and cardiovascular effects of crude and purified toxins from *Clostridium perfringens*. J Infect Dis 1988; 157:272–278.

*Purified alpha toxin and theta toxin each cause profound hypotension when infused into anesthetized rabbits. Alpha toxin suppressed myocardial contractility in ex vivo preparations in a dose-dependent manner, whereas theta toxin did not. Thus hypotension induced by alpha toxin is related at least in part by direct effects on the heart. These data also suggest that theta-toxin-induced hypotension may be related to the induction of endogenous factors such as platelet activating factor and prostacyclin.*

Weinstein L, Barza M. Gas gangrene. N Engl J Med 1972; 289:1129.

*This review article is a classic that describes the clinical features of gas gangrene.*

# 81

# Chronic Fatigue Syndrome

DEDRA S. BUCHWALD

Fatigue is a universal experience. Surveys in the developed world have found that between 10%–50% of people report currently experiencing fatigue, usually of an unspecified severity and limited duration. Fatigue is also a common complaint in primary care settings where the prevalence of fatigue is at least 20%. In most cases, such fatigue is transient, explained by prevailing circumstances, relieved by rest, and of little cause for medical concern. In both community and clinical settings, fatigue is often more frequent among women than men.

Fatigue can, however, be both persistent and disabling. In some cases, it may be the result of a recognized medical and psychological condition such as thyroid disease or depression. Less commonly, persistent fatigue may be the hallmark of chronic fatigue syndrome (CFS), an illness characterized by profound fatigue often accompanied by sleep disturbances, neurocognitive complaints, myalgias, and mood changes. Chronic fatigue syndrome has been reported worldwide and case definitions have been developed by the Centers for Disease Control and Prevention (CDC) and British and Australian researchers.

## Definition

Although diagnostic criteria only recently have been formulated, CFS is unlikely to be a new entity. Several clinical syndromes, both sporadic and epidemic, have been described previously that, in retrospect, appear to share key clinical features. These include neurasthenia, benign myalgic encephalomyelitis, and "chronic Epstein-Barr virus (EBV) infection." The original CDC case definition for CFS grew out of the controversy arising from publications in the medical literature and popular press describing an epidemic attributed to "chronic EBV infection" in Lake Tahoe, Nevada. In 1987, a group of epidemiologists, researchers, and clinicians convened by the CDC developed a consensus statement on the salient clinical characteristics of the syndrome. The proposed working case definition was designed to improve the comparability and reproducibility of clinical research and epidemiological studies and to provide guidelines for evaluating patients with chronic fatigue of unknown cause. "Chronic EBV infection" was renamed *CFS*, thus removing the implication that EBV is the etiologic agent and emphasizing the syndrome's most striking feature.

This original CDC case definition consisted of two major criteria, 11 symptom and three physical examination minor criteria. A case of CFS was required to have at least 6 mo of unexplained debilitating fatigue and a combination of eight minor symptom or physical examination criteria. In 1994, the CDC directed the formulation of a new international case definition which incorporated the major components of the original criteria. This new case definition eliminated the physical examination criteria (which have no diagnostic value), reduced the number of required concurrent symptoms, and clarified exclusionary conditions (Table 81.1). These criteria are not empirically based and have never been subjected to rigorous scrutiny. There are no diagnostic laboratory studies for CFS.

One of the first problems encountered in using the CDC criteria was distinguishing CFS from psychiatric disorders. This difficulty results from the substantial overlap between the symptoms of CFS and those of affective and somatization disorders. For example, a patient reporting fatigue, obviously a prerequisite for CFS, also is endorsing a symptom of major depression. Thus, when patients report symptoms of CFS, they are often simultaneously endorsing symptoms of psychiatric disorders. In fact, the similarity of CFS symptoms to those of major depression, and the high rate of pre-existing psychiatric disorders in patients with CFS, have led to the suggestion that CFS is simply depression or the modern reincarnation of neurasthenia.

There also has been confusion regarding the psychiatric exclusion criterion of the original CDC case definition as it does not clearly specify which patients and which disorders should be excluded. In 1991, the National Institutes of Health and the National Institute of Mental Health jointly recommended that patients with major depression, panic, generalized anxiety, and somatization disorder, who otherwise meet the CDC case definition, should not be excluded. The 1994 CDC criteria developed by international consensus excludes only those with schizophrenia, bipolar or psychotic depression, and substance-related and eating disorders (Table 81.1).

## Etiology and Pathophysiology

Many theories on the etiology and pathophysiology of CFS have been postulated; however, strong evidence to support any single one is lacking. Most researchers believe that no single factor will prove to be the cause in all, or even most, cases. However, up to 80% of patients report the onset of CFS was preceded by an acute viral illness. Previous work has shown that viruses can alter neuroendocrine function, as well as reset sleep mechanisms, either directly or through intermediary factors such as cytokines. These observations have lead to speculation that in CFS, a triggering event (e.g., a viral infection) leads to the continual production of cytokines such as those elaborated as part of the acute phase response (Fig. 81.1). These cytokines, in turn, disrupt sleep both directly and indirectly through their effects on the normal functioning of the hypothalamic-pituitary-adrenal (HPA) axis. Dysregulation of the HPA axis also may result from the infection itself or through the effects of cytokines. In any case, disruption of sleep occurs and, eventually, a condition of chronic fatigue results. In this regard, cytokines are known to cause the

**Table 81.1** 1994 Centers for Disease Control criteria for CFS

To meet criteria a case is required to fulfill all fatigue criteria in the absence of any exclusionary conditions. In addition, 4 of 8 symptom criteria must be present

FATIGUE CRITERIA

To meet criteria the fatigue must:
1. Be of at least 6 months duration
2. Not be "lifelong" (that is, the person can't ever remember feeling normal)
3. Result in a substantial reduction of occupational, educational, social, or personal activities compared to before illness onset
4. Not be the result of ongoing exertion or be relieved by rest

SYMPTOM CRITERIA

Symptoms must have started at the same time or after the onset of fatigue and be present simultaneously for at least 6 months during the illness
1. Impairment of short-term memory or concentration severe enough to cause a substantial reduction in previous levels of occupational, educational, social, or personal activities
2. Sore throat
3. Tender lymph glands in the neck or arm pits
4. Muscle pain
5. Joint pain involving more than one joint without swelling or redness
6. Headaches of a new type, pattern, or severity
7. Unrefreshing sleep
8. Malaise or fatigue lasting more than 24 hours after exertion

EXCLUSIONARY CRITERIA

1. Any other medical conditions that could mimic CFS such as malignancies, chronic infection, neuromuscular disease, etc.
2. Bipolar affective disorders, psychotic or melancholic depression, schizophrenia and dementia
3. Anorexia nervosa and bulimia
4. Alcohol or substance abuse within two years of the onset of fatigue or any time thereafter
5. Severe obesity (body mass index ≥45)

flu-like symptoms often associated with acute infections and also may induce a CFS-like syndrome when administered for therapeutic purposes. As with any chronic illness, symptoms lead to disability that is both due to, and results in, psychological distress.

## Epidemiology

There have been several studies of CFS among patients in general medical settings. A survey of 611 British ambulatory patients found only one subject had a CFS-like illness with at least 6 mo of significant fatigue. In a subsequent investigation in which patients underwent a comprehensive medical and psychological evaluation, 17 cases of CFS were detected among 686 patients attending a primary care practice. More recently, a prospective study in a primary care practice in the United States identified three cases of CFS among 1000 patients seeking care for any reason. Thus, by extrapolation to standardized rates, in these investigations the point prevalence of CFS ranged from 164 to 2500 per 100,000 persons among general medical patients.

Many previous population-based studies have examined the frequency of fatigue, but few have attempted to evaluate the prevalence of CFS in the community. Three studies in the United States, Australia, and Britain have indirectly approximated the prevalence of CFS in the community by identifying cases seeking care for fatigue through sentinel physicians. The prevalence of CFS reported in these studies ranged from 3.4 to 130 per 100,000 persons. Other estimates of the prevalence of CFS have relied on self-report for the diagnosis of CFS, used data from an epidemiological study of psychiatric illness, or information from viral serology request forms, none of which contained the specific items required to assess whether individuals met the CFS case definition. Finally, in a community study, enrollees in a health maintenance organization were surveyed by mail for the presence of chronic fatigue. Those with chronic fatigue underwent a medical and psychological evaluation. It was found that unexplained, debilitating fatigue of at least 6 mo duration had a point prevalence of 1,775 to 6321 per 100,000 persons. CFS was considerably less common, with an estimated point prevalence of 75 to 267 per 100,000 persons. Of interest, the population-based nature of this study resulted in the representation of a broader spectrum of illness. For example, only 14% of the chron-

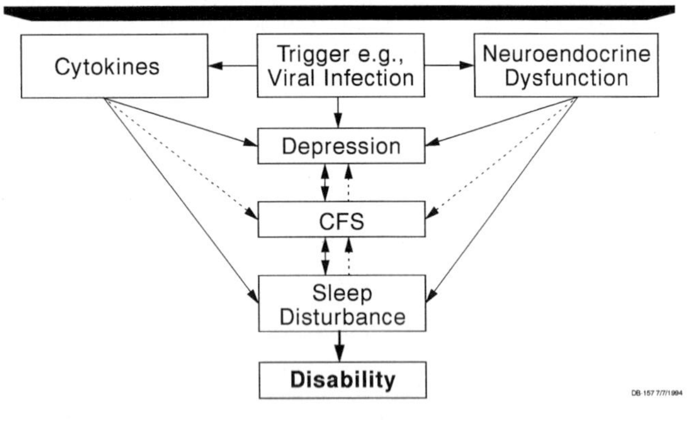

**Fig. 81.1** Postulated pathophysiological mechanism.

ically fatigued subjects in this study and none of those with CFS were unemployed, in contrast to 35%–45% in clinics specializing in CFS.

## Host Factors

### Gender, race, and ethnicity

Early reports in the lay press about the "yuppie flu," as well as findings published in the medical literature, suggested that CFS primarily affected young, successful, Caucasian women. An inspection of 30 articles published in peer-reviewed journals and symposium proceedings on CFS-like illnesses from 1985 to 1993 found that only five studies even addressed subjects' ethnicity/racial status. Of these five studies, three reported no minority participants and two found a marked preponderance of Caucasians. However, a growing body of evidence suggests that CFS affects persons from all socioeconomic classes, racial/ethnic groups, and both genders. In this regard, a clinic-based study found the spectrum of illness, including the demographic, clinical, laboratory, functional, or psychosocial features, is similar in white and nonwhite patients. In one community study of chronic fatigue (defined as 6 mo of disabling fatigue), nonwhites were actually underrepresented and African Americans were overrepresented compared to both the local and United States population.

It seems likely, then, that the paucity of minority patients with CFS seen in referral settings is, in part, a function of health care seeking. However, other factors—such as the affordability and accessibility of care, the perceived need for and acceptability and desirability of mainstream medical services, and cultural dynamics that influence the degree to which symptoms are perceived as problems—may be equally important.

### Psychiatric disorders

Many investigations have found considerable psychiatric illness in CFS. Rates for any current and any lifetime psychiatric diagnoses are 21%–72% and 26%–86%, respectively, among patients with CFS. Similarly, the prevalence of current (15%–54%) and lifetime (40%–76%) major depression is strikingly above that observed in the general population. Panic and somatization disorder are also not unusual. Studies which examined the temporal sequence of CFS and psychiatric disorder found that the psychiatric disorder often preceded the onset of fatigue. In fact, the high rate of pre-existing psychiatric illness, as well as the phenomenological similarity of CFS to major depression, has led to suggestions that CFS is a form of depression or neurasthenia. This, however, is an insufficient explanation, since at least 25% of CFS patients have no lifetime psychiatric illness, and even among those with major depression, the classical biological accompaniments appear to be absent.

There are several lines of evidence that argue against the contention that CFS is a form of depression and suggest a potentially different mechanism for the associated affective symptoms. For example, the polysomnographic findings characteristic of major depression, such as increases in sleep latency, number of awakenings, and rapid eye movement (REM) density, as well as decreases in REM sleep latency and slow wave sleep, are not observed in CFS. Another line of evidence is that the pattern of HPA axis dysregulation in CFS differs dramatically from the classical neuroendocrine findings of major depression. In the latter, resistance to pituitary–adrenal suppression has been clinically utilized in the form of the Dexamethasone Suppression Test. In contrast to the nonsuppression or hypercortisolemia seen in many severely depressed patients, nonsuppression is rare in CFS. Similarly, the changes in monoamine metabolism characteristic of major depression are not observed in CFS. Finally, antidepressants do not appear to be particularly effective in CFS, even among the subgroup of depressed patients. Taken together, these studies raise the possibility that different mechanisms are responsible for the depressive symptoms of major depression and CFS.

## Clinical Manifestations

### Symptoms

A prominent historical feature of CFS is its sudden onset in up to 85% of patients. Many patients recall that their illness began on a particular day with an upper respiratory or gastrointestinal "flu-like" syndrome often accompanied by fever. However, unlike the course of a usual viral syndrome, the illness lingered and patients never fully recovered. Subsequently, symptoms are present the majority of the time and are of sufficient severity to impair normal functioning.

The hallmark of CFS is overwhelming fatigue. Approximately 25% of CFS patients describe themselves as regularly bedridden or shut-in and unable to work, and one-third can work only part-time. Prior to the onset of CFS, patients were typically very physically active; however, since becoming ill even modest physical exertion results in an exacerbation of many of their symptoms. Although the exertion itself may be reasonably well tolerated, 6–24 h later, most patients report a marked worsening of the fatigue, cognitive function, and "flu-like" symptoms such as lymphadenopathy, pharyngitis, and fevers.

Sleep and neurocognitive disturbances are the other frequent and debilitating symptoms. In fact, impaired sleep may be the most frequent complaint in CFS, reported by up to 95% of patients, and includes hypersomnia, inability to fall or stay asleep, inadequate sleep time, and feeling unrested on rising. In addition, symptoms suggestive of sleep pathology such as sleepiness, drowsiness, and snoring with apnea are surprisingly common among CFS patients and should trigger the search for a concurrent sleep disorder. Neuropsychiatric symptoms such as word groping, decreased concentrating ability, and impaired short-term memory are also frequent. Several studies have found subtle information processing deficits on neuropsychological testing in patients with CFS.

Other persistent symptoms include myalgias, headaches, and pharyngitis (Table 81.2). In addition to the symptoms characteristic of CFS, many symptoms not typically associated with CFS and not required by the case definition, such as dizziness and nausea, are common.

### Physical examination findings

Abnormalities in the physical examination at any one visit are found in a minority of CFS patients. The presence of tender points is the most common abnormality on physical examination, found in 33%–70% of patients. Temperature >37.5°C (10%–20%), posterior and anterior cervical lymphadenopathy (20%–40%),

**Table 81.2** Commonly reported symptoms in CFS

| Symptom | Frequency (%) |
|---|---|
| Aching muscles | 93 |
| Awaken most mornings unrested | 91 |
| Muscle weakness | 91 |
| Difficulty concentrating | 90 |
| "Stress makes me worse" | 89 |
| Aching joints | 86 |
| Forgetfulness | 85 |
| Difficulty thinking | 82 |
| Weight gain | 78 |
| Need daily nap | 76 |
| Headaches | 75 |
| Shortness of breath | 72 |
| Unsteadiness | 69 |
| Morning stiffness | 69 |
| Blurred vision | 66 |
| Dizzy | 64 |
| Dry throat or mouth | 63 |
| Frequent nausea | 62 |
| Decreased sexual function | 61 |
| Rapid heartbeat | 55 |
| Tinnitus | 54 |

and pharyngeal inflammation (40%–60%) have all been described. Other findings such as hepatosplenomegaly are unusual.

## Laboratory Findings

Many laboratory abnormalities have been reported in CFS. However, these findings are diverse, often conflicting, and frequently modest in degree. In addition, it has not been shown that these findings explain the clinical features of CFS or correlate with changes in status over time.

### Routine studies

Serum hematological tests are generally normal. Although not usual, atypical lymphocytes have been reported in up to 30% of selected patients. Slightly elevated erythrocyte sedimentation rates are an occasional finding; values over 50 should alert clinicians to other causes of fatigue. In individual patients, routine chemistry tests are also generally unremarkable. However, in a study comparing routine laboratory tests obtained in approximately 600 patients with a chronically fatiguing illness and 150 control subjects, patients were significantly more likely to have increased levels of cholesterol (54% versus 33%) and alkaline phosphatase (18% versus 5%).

### Immunological tests

Patients with CFS may have circulating autoantibodies more frequently than healthy individuals. In particular, antinuclear antibodies are found in as many as 20% and rheumatoid factor in up to 10% of patients, typically in low concentrations without other evidence for connective tissue disorders. Antibodies to thyroid gland and other tissues may be occasionally found. Another report suggested that rheumatoid factor, antinuclear antibodies of ≥1:80, and anti-Ro are present in some patients with CFS and a Sjogren's syndrome–like clinical presentation.

Many studies have examined humoral immunity in CFS with conflicting results. Most commonly, immunoglobulin levels have been normal or mildly diminished. IgG subclass deficiencies, usually $IgG_1$ or $IgG_3$, also have been reported by some investigators. Several studies have found low levels of circulating immune complexes in CFS patients in up to a third of patients. Despite this abnormality, few patients have depressed complement, and none have clinical manifestations of immune complex-mediated disease.

The symptoms of CFS have been postulated, at least in part, to result from the inappropriate production of cytokines. However, the search for objective evidence of circulating cytokines has yielded mixed results. Although the assays used may have been insensitive, the medical literature suggests that interferons are infrequently, if ever, present. Other markers of immune activation including interleukin-1, interleukin 4, soluble interleukin-2 receptor, tumor necrosis factor, and $\beta$2 microglobulin have not been detected in CFS. In contrast, higher levels of interleukin-2, transforming growth factor $\beta$, neopterin, and interleukin-6 have been reported in some patients. These abnormalities have not, however, been reliably replicated. In an intriguing study using a functional assay of cytokine production, mitogen-stimulated release of interleukin-1 $\beta$ and tumor necrosis factor-$\alpha$ from peripheral lymphocytes was shown to be significantly greater, and release of transforming growth factor-$\beta$ lower, in CFS patients than in healthy individuals.

The numbers of $CD4^+$ and $CD8^+$ lymphocytes and the CD4/CD8 ratio are usually normal in CFS although both increases and decreases have been reported. A more uniform finding has been deranged T cell function. Patients may be anergic, have significant impairment of delayed hypersensitivity to multiple antigens, or decreased responsiveness to standard mitogen stimulation assays.

More recently, extensive analyses of lymphocyte cell surface markers among patients with CFS-like illnesses consistently have demonstrated an increase in the expression of activation markers, lending support to the theory of an underlying immune dysregulation. The most consistent findings have been a significant reduction in the suppressor subset, $CD8^+$ $CD11b^-$, a decrease in the CD4 $CD45RA^+$ suppressor inducer subset, and increases in the expression or density of the ICAM (CD54) on CD4 cells.

As with T cells, both increased and decreased numbers of B lymphocytes have been reported. Increases in $CD20^+$ and $CD21^+$ cells, particularly those coexpressing CD20 and CD5, and among CD19-staining B cells, with an expansion of the subpopulation of CD5 CD19 lymphocytes have been described but not confirmed by other investigators. Likewise, although abnormalities of natural killer cell number and function have been reported, findings have been inconsistent. Most studies have found a diminution in the absolute number, percentage, and cytolytic activity of natural killer cells. These findings are interesting given the important role of these cells in the host defense against viral infections.

### Virological assays

CFS-like illnesses have been attributed, either directly or indirectly, to a variety of infectious agents. The viruses that have been the object of the greatest scientific inquiry are the herpes viruses, including EBV and human herpes virus 6, as well as the enteroviruses and a putative novel retrovirus. However, despite the often postinfectious onset of CFS, objective evidence of viral involvement is, at present, inconclusive.

Early studies in the United States found elevated levels of antibodies to EBV in patients with a CFS-like illness. Subsequent investigations did not find evidence of a chronic EBV infection in blood or throat cultures, or in lymphocytes using in situ hybridization techniques. A substantial overlap in antibody titers between patients and healthy individuals also was documented, indicating that EBV is unlikely to be the etiologic agent in most cases. In a well-publicized outbreak of a chronically fatiguing illness in the Lake Tahoe area of Nevada, active replication of human herpes virus 6 was observed in lymphocyte cell cultures from 70% of patients compared to 20% of control subjects. These findings were felt to be manifestations of an underlying biological mechanism, and not as causative of CFS. In general, serological abnormalities (e.g., higher titers of antibodies to the early antigens of EBV or human herpes virus 6) have been interpreted as reflecting a defect in T cell function rather than a primary viral infection or clinically significant viral reactivation.

Several serological surveys in the United Kingdom found abnormal coxsackie B serologies among individuals with "myalgic encephalitis." Circulating complexes of coxsackie viral antigen and IgM have been inconsistently found in CFS patients, with isolation of enterovirus from stool in almost a quarter. Other support for an enteroviral infection comes from the demonstration of enteroviral nucleic acid in muscle cells of chronically fatigued patients more often than in those of control subjects. However, these techniques did not detect virus in many patients and are not routinely available in most clinical settings. Moreover, attempts at replication have not been successful.

Lastly, an initial report of a novel retrovirus in CFS patients that shares some nucleic acid sequence homology with human T lymphotropic virus II has not been confirmed. Infection with other known retroviruses such as human T lymphotropic virus I or II is also not associated with CFS. CFS has not been found to be caused by many other infectious agents including hepatitis C virus, *Chlamydia pneumoniae*, toxoplasma infection, and the Lyme disease spirochete, although it has been known to develop subsequent to acute infection with the latter.

### Allergy

An exacerbation of preexisting allergies or the development of new ones is reported by over half of patients with CFS. In addition to this clinical manifestation, increased cutaneous reactivity to allergens, increased levels of circulating IgE and IgE-bearing T and B cells, and greater lymphocyte responsiveness to allergens are present in CFS. The mechanisms linking allergy and CFS remain unknown, but it has been speculated that individuals who respond with unusual vigor to infectious antigens may also have a heightened reactivity to allergens.

### Neuroendocrine abnormalities

Recent investigations have highlighted the importance of factors other than the immune system, such as neuroendocrine function, in the pathophysiology of CFS. For example, a novel pattern of HPA axis dysfunction has been described, characterized by significant reductions in plasma and urinary glucocorticoid levels, elevated basal evening ACTH, an enhanced adrenocortical sensitivity to ACTH with a reduced maximal response, and normal cerebrospinal corticotropin-releasing hormone levels. Although not definitive, these findings are most compatible with a failure of corticotropin-releasing hormone production or release by the hypothalamus. Chronic fatigue syndrome patients also show significant reductions in basal plasma levels of 3-methoxy-4-hydroxyphenylglycol and increases in 5-hydroxyindoleacetic acid—a pattern quite different than that seen in depression. Additional evidence of perturbation of neuroendocrine function is the demonstration of low baseline levels and erratic secretion of arginine-vasopressin, and possible upregulation of hypothalamic 5-hydroxytryptamine receptors.

In conclusion, while some laboratory findings have been consistently found, most of the abnormalities observed in CFS are in tests performed only in research settings. As systematic, blinded studies using healthy control subjects resulted in the disappearance of many "abnormalities" initially thought to be characteristic of CFS, new evidence of immunological and neuroendocrine dysfunction has surfaced. It remains to be confirmed whether these findings reproducibly distinguish CFS patients from those with other illnesses.

## Diagnosis and Comorbid Conditions

Although it is uncommon for systemic disorders to present solely with fatigue, many recognized conditions such as multiple sclerosis and connective tissue diseases are associated with fatigue. All patients should be evaluated to exclude other causes of fatigue. More specifically, a detailed history, physical examination, and selected laboratory studies are indicated in any individual presenting with chronic fatigue that significantly affects daily activity. Equal emphasis must be placed upon the psychosocial evaluation, in particular, systematically screening for anxiety and mood disorders. Although no diagnostic studies exist for CFS, a reasonable initial laboratory test battery in evaluating patients with possible CFS consists of a complete blood count, erythrocyte sedimentation rate, chemistry panel, liver and thyroid function tests, and urinalysis. Other studies such as antinuclear antibodies, immune complexes, or lymphocyte subsets may be appropriate in some patients or in certain settings. Taken together, these tests may be helpful in supporting a diagnosis of CFS or in ruling out other conditions that can produce fatigue.

### Fibromyalgia

Several conditions such as fibromyalgia, sleep disorders, and Sjogren's syndrome frequently coexist with CFS. Although these conditions have a large number of demographic and clinical features in common with CFS, and may represent overlapping clinical syndromes, their exact relationship to CFS is not clear.

Fibromyalgia is a common rheumatic condition characterized by myalgias, fatigue, and disrupted sleep often associated with headache, irritable bowel syndrome, and a variety of other signs and symptoms. It occurs most commonly in women and may follow a viral illness or trauma. The diagnosis requires the presence of widespread musculoskeletal pain in conjunction with tenderness at a minimum of 11 of 18 specified musculoskeletal sites. Up to 70% of patients with CFS simultaneously meet criteria for fibromyalgia. The presence of fibromyalgia does not preclude a diagnosis of CFS.

## Disturbances of sleep

Well-documented sleep disorders are surprisingly common in CFS. Between 33% and 85% of chronically fatigued patients have concurrent sleep disorders such as sleep apnea, nocturnal myoclonus, periodic limb movements, and narcolepsy. Of note, in studies using measures of depression, sleep disorders occurred with at least equal frequency in depressed and nondepressed CFS patients.Perturbations in sleep duration and architecture in the absence of overt sleep disorders also may be important in CFS. Compared to healthy subjects, for example, those with CFS have significant decreases in sleep efficiency and time spent in REM sleep, and increases in onset latency to stage 2 sleep and a greater proportion of stage 4 sleep and delta sleep.

It is not known whether sleep disorders and changes in sleep architecture are causative or comorbid conditions in CFS. However, direct and indirect support for the hypothesis that sleep disruption is a manifestation of CFS comes from several observations. First, many patients who meet criteria for CFS do not have a primary sleep disorder on polysomnography. Second, there is a striking disparity between the severity of objective sleep pathology (usually mild) and the degree of fatigue reported by patients. Third, treatment meets with only limited success. Unlike the striking improvement typical of patients treated for primary sleep disorders not associated with CFS, those with CFS rarely recover entirely and most report only moderate improvement.

## Sjogren's syndrome

Many patients with CFS endorse sicca symptoms typical of Sjogren's syndrome. Moreover, approximately up to 60% of such patients will have a positive Schirmer's test. On laboratory testing, a positive ANA may be found in over 50%, rheumatoid factor in 14%, and anti-Ro in 5%. In comparing CFS patients with a Sjogren's syndrome–like condition to those with only CFS, the former group was found to be significantly more likely to have recurrent fever and a positive ANA but less likely to have an acute onset. At present, it is unclear if this subset of patients has unrecognized Sjogren's syndrome, a Sjogren's syndrome–like variant, or if sicca symptoms characterize a subset of CFS patients. The relatively low prevalence of autoantibodies, particularly anti-Ro, suggests that this condition, occurring with CFS, is not likely to represent primary Sjogren's syndrome. It is not known whether the natural history of sicca syndrome in the context of CFS differs from that of CFS alone.

## Treatment

There are no pharmacological treatments of proven efficacy for CFS; hence, interventions should be directed at relief of specific symptoms and reintegration into the individual's social and occupational network. Anecdotal reports have found that antidepressants benefit patients with CFS although clinical trials have come to a different conclusion. In particular, a combination of low doses of a serotonin reuptake inhibitor in the morning and a tricyclic antidepressant at bedtime is often used. Tricyclic antidepressants may improve sleep and reduce pain, particularly in patients with concurrent fibromyalgia. Nonsteroidal anti-inflammatory agents may provide additional relief. The choice of therapeutic agents should be guided by the profile of action of the individual drug (e.g., using a sedative drug in patients with insomnia). An adequate trial of an antidepressant with a standard therapeutic dosage for an adequate period of time may be required in some cases, although many patients may gain considerable symptom relief from low doses of medication (e.g., 5–10 mg of amitriptyline). In patients requiring therapeutic doses of antidepressants, either for specific CFS symptoms or concurrent psychiatric disorders, it is usually necessary to begin with a low dose and increase gradually.

Other therapies evaluated and found to be of little or no effectiveness in randomized controlled trials include the antiviral agent acyclovir, immunoglobulin infusions, leucocyte extract, and $B_{12}$–folic acid–liver extract. Nystatin was not useful in "chronic candidiasis," a similar, if not identical, condition. Magnesium injections, essential fatty acids and anti-viral agents have been reported to be helpful. Of importance, recent randomized, controlled trials of cognitive behavioral therapy and a structured exercise program were both of substantial benefit in patients with CFS.

Physical activities previously enjoyed should be gradually increased in a structured manner, often with the assistance of a physical therapist, as complete inactivity appears to promote fatigue. Continuity of care coupled with education, instruction in coping skills, and counseling are often neglected but important aspects of treatment for CFS. Reassessment for organic and psychiatric disorders should be performed at regular intervals; however, extensive laboratory testing without additional indications is not indicated.

## Course of Illness and Prognosis

CFS is not a progressive disease. In most cases, symptoms are most severe during the first 6 mo of illness, plateau relatively early, and recur with varying degrees of severity. Although detailed longitudinal studies are lacking, it appears most patients report a gradual recovery, usually punctuated with relapses precipitated by overexertion, stress, or infection. Moderate to complete recovery has been found in 26% to 57% of patients with CFS-like illnesses over varying periods of follow-up. Among such patients, predictors of return to work and clinical improvement include younger age, shorter duration of illness, and the absence of affective disorders. With the exception of suicide, death resulting directly from CFS has not been reported.

### ANNOTATED BIBLIOGRAPHY

Buchwald D, Cheney PR, Peterson DL, Henry B, Wormsley SB, Geiger A, Ablaski DV, Salahuddin SZ, Saxinger C, Biddle R, Kikinis R, Jolesz FA, Folks T, Balachandran N, Gallo RC, Komaroff AL. A chronic illness characterized by fatigue, neurologic and immunologic disorders, and active human herpes type 6 infection. Ann Intern Med. 1992; 116:103–113.
*Description of an illness cluster.*

Buchwald D, Pascualy R, Bombardier C, Kim P. Sleep disorders in patients with chronic fatigue. Clin Infect Dis. 1994; 18 Suppl 1:S68–72.
*Highly selected patients with chronic fatigue frequently have sleep disorders.*

Demitrack MA, Dale JK, Straus SE, Lau L, Listwak SJ, Kruesi MJ, Chrousos GP, Gold PW. Evidence for impaired activation of the hypothalamic-pituitary-adrenal axis in patients with chronic fatigue syndrome. J Clin Endocrinol Metab 1991; 73:1224–1234.
*Evidence is presented for a mild central adrenal insufficiency.*

Goldenberg DL, Simms RW, Geiger A, Komaroff AL. High frequency of fibromyalgia in patients with chronic fatigue seen in a primary care practice. Arthritis Rheum 1990; 33:381–387.

*Demonstration of high frequency of fibromyalgia in chronically fatigued patients.*

Fukuda K, Straus SE, Hickie I, Sharpe MC, Dobbins JG, Komaroff AL. The chronic fatigue syndrome. A comprehensive approach to its definition and study. International Chronic Fatigue Syndrome Study Group. Ann Intern Med 1994: 121.

*New case definition developed by international group of researchers and clinicians.*

Katon WJ, Buchwald DS, Simon GE, Russo JE, Mease PJ. Psychiatric illness in patients with chronic fatigue and rheumatoid arthritis. J Gen Intern Med 1991; 6:277–285.

*Describes frequency of psychiatric diagnoses.*

Komaroff AL, Buchwald DS. Chronic fatigue syndrome: an update. In: Coggins CH, Hancock EW, Levitt LJ, eds. Annual Review of Medicine, vol 49, Palo Alto, CA: Annual Reviews, 1998, 1–13.

*Review of clinical features.*

Schluederberg A, Straus SE, Peterson P, Blumenthal S, Komaroff AL, Spring SB, Lauday A, Buchwald D. Chronic fatigue syndrome research: definition and medical outcome assessment. Ann Intern Med 1992; 117:325–331.

*Overview of original case definition and discussion of general issues.*

Straus SE, Fritz S, Dale JK, Gould B, Strober W. Lymphocyte phenotype and function in the chronic fatigue syndrome. J Clin Immunol 1992; 13:30–40.

*Extensive analysis of lymphocyte subsets demonstrating immune activation.*

Vercoulen JH, Swanink CM, Zitman FG, Vreden SG, Hoofs MP, Fennis JF, Galama JM, van der Meer JW, Bleijenberg G. Randomized, double-blind placebo-controlled study of fluoxetine in chronic fatigue syndrome. Lancet 1996; 347:858–61.

*Documents lack of effectiveness of fluoxetine.*

# VI

## INFECTIONS IN SPECIAL PATIENT/RISK GROUPS

# 82

# Postsurgical Wound Infections

RONALD LEE NICHOLS

Postoperative wound infections remain a major source of morbidity and a less frequent source of mortality in the surgical patient. In a nationwide study occurring within a 12-month period in 1975–1976, it was estimated that wound infections accounted for about 24% of the total number of nosocomial (hospital acquired) infections. This figure represented more than 500,000 wound infections, or about 2.8 per 100 operations performed.

The incidence of wound infection varies from surgeon to surgeon, from hospital to hospital, from one surgical procedure to another, and most importantly from one patient to another. The average hospital stay was noted to double and the cost of hospitalizations was correspondingly increased when postoperative wound infection developed following six commonly performed operations during the mid-1970s. These figures of real cost and length of hospital stay are undoubtedly lower today for most of the surgical procedures that are done as outpatient procedures or require only a short duration of postoperative stay. In these cases, most of the wound infections are diagnosed and treated in the outpatient clinic or in the patient's home. However, major complications such as deep sternal wound infections continue to have a grave impact, increasing the duration of hospitalization as much as 20-fold and the cost of hospitalization fivefold. The development of any surgical wound infection following open-heart surgery has also been shown to result in a significant net loss of reimbursement to the hospital compared with uninfected cases, a factor that should serve as a potent incentive to hospitals to minimize the incidence of postoperative wound infections.

## Description of Clinical Wound Infections

The Hospital Infections Program, Center for Infectious Diseases of the Centers for Disease Control (CDC), has developed a set of definitions which are currently being utilized for the surveillance of nosocomial infections in the hospitals participating in the CDC National Nosocomial Infections Surveillance (NNIS) System. Surgical wound infections are divided into incisional and deep, and are only considered to be nosocomial if there is no evidence that the infection was present or incubating at the time of hospital admission.

### Definition of incisional surgical wound infection

Infection occurs at the incision site within 30 days after surgery and involves skin, subcutaneous tissue, or muscle located above the fascial layer; in addition, any of the following:

1. Purulent drainage from the incision or a drain located above the fascial layer
2. Organism isolated from culture of fluid from wound closed primarily
3. Surgeon deliberately opens wound, unless wound is culture negative
4. Surgeon's or attending physician's diagnosis of infection

### Definition of deep surgical wound infection

Infection occurs at operative site within 30 days after surgery if no implant is left in place or within one year if implant is in place. Implant is defined as a nonhuman-derived implantable foreign body (e.g. prosthetic heart valve, nonhuman vascular graft, mechanical heart, or hip prosthesis) that is permanently placed in a patient during surgery. Such an infection should also appear related to surgery and the infection involves tissues or spaces at or beneath the fascial layer; in addition, any of the following:

1. Purulent drainage from a drain placed beneath the fascial layer
2. Wound spontaneously dehisces or is deliberately opened by the surgeon when the patient has fever (>38°C) or localized pain or tenderness, unless wound is culture negative
3. An abscess or other evidence of infection seen on direct examination, during surgery, or by histopathologic examination
4. Surgeon's diagnosis of infection

Most superficial wound infections are diagnosed somewhere between the fourth and eighth postoperative day (late). When infection occurs during the first 48 hours after operation (early), it is characteristically a rapidly moving gangrenous infection caused by a single type of microorganism, most commonly either a *Clostridium* or beta-hemolytic *Streptococcus*. In these rare cases the dramatic clinical presentation may include profound systemic toxicity and rapid local advance of the infection, often involving all layers of the body wall.

## Pathogens Causing Surgical Wound Infections

The pathogens that are isolated from surgical wound infections vary, primarily based on the type of surgical procedure undertaken. In clean surgical procedures in which the gastrointestinal, gynecologic, and respiratory tracts have not been entered, *Staphylococcus aureus* from the exogenous environment or the patient's skin flora is the usual cause of infection. Less common organisms include *Staphylococcus epidermidis*, corynebacteria, and enterobacteriaceae. In the other categories of surgical procedures, including clean-contaminated, contaminated, and dirty, the polymicrobial aerobic-anaerobic flora closely resembling the normal endogenous microflora of the surgically resected organ are the most frequently isolated pathogens (see Table 82.1).

The importance of thoughtfully carried out epidemiologic and

**Table 82.1** Important microbiologic agents of infection following surgical procedures

| Type of surgical procedure | Common infecting bacteria |
|---|---|
| Clean (e.g., elective; nontraumatic; uninfected) | Gram-positive aerobic (streptococci, staphylococci) |
| Clean-Contaminated (e.g., nontraumatic; early trauma without foreign bodies, devitalized tissue, or fecal contamination; respiratory, or genitourinary tracts entered without gross spillage) | Polymicrobial aerobic and anaerobic (streptococci, staphylococci, enterobacteriaceae, pseudomonas, bacteroides and other anaerobes, enterococci) |
| Contaminated, Dirty (e.g., traumatic wounds with delayed treatment, foreign bodies, devitalized tissue, or fecal contamination; infection present; gastrointestinal spillage) | Polymicrobial aerobic and anaerobic (streptococci, staphylococci, enterobacteriaceae, pseudomonas, bacteroides and other anaerobes, enterococci) |

microbiologic investigations of the changing patterns of nosocomial pathogens in both outbreak investigations and in national surveillance data has been stressed since the early 1960s. Recently, the number of nosocomial infections caused by gram-positive cocci is again increasing with the emergence of enterococci and coagulase-negative staphylococci as important nosocomial pathogens. It has been observed that the majority of prosthetic vascular graft infections are now caused by mucin-producing strains of *Staphylococcus epidermidis*, which express varying degrees of adherence to the synthetic substrates. A rapid increase in the incidence of infection and colonization with vancomycin-resistant enterococci has also been reported in the last five years, resulting in a series of recommendations concerning the limitation of the use of vancomycin in several clinical settings.

Antibiotic-resistant strains of both gram-positive and gram-negative microorganisms and fungi are being increasingly isolated from infections in postoperative patients and from the hospital environment. Rapidly growing mycobacteria, *Rhodococcus bronchialis*, and *Candida tropicalis* have all been implicated in outbreaks of both deep and superficial wound infections following open-heart surgery. In the case of the mycobacteria infections, about 80% of the cardiac isolates were from the southern coastal states and the heterogeneity of the isolates suggests that most are unrelated but are derived from local environmental sources rather than from contaminated commercial surgical materials or devices. The outbreaks of wound infection due to both *R. bronchialis* and *C. tropicalis* were found to be common-source cluster epidemics with the removal of the sources from the cardiac team terminating the outbreaks.

## General Risk Considerations: Preventative Techniques

The most critical factors in the prevention of postoperative wound infection, although difficult to quantitate, appear to be the sound judgment and proper operative technique of the responsible surgeon and team as well as the general health and stage of disease of the individual patient. Many other factors have been proven to have a significant influence on the development of postoperative wound infection, especially in clean surgical procedures, where a generally low infection rate (<3%) is expected due solely to airborne exogenous microorganisms. These risk factors include the following:

### Non-antibiotic factors

#### Preoperative stay

A most striking correlation is seen in the relation between the duration of preoperative hospitalization and the development of postoperative wound infections. Cruse and Foord in 1973 reported that the overall infection rate was 1.1% for patients whose preoperative stay was one day; this infection rate doubled with each week that the patient remained in the hospital before surgery.

Today, most patients who undergo elective operation are admitted to the hospital on the morning of surgery or on the day prior to operation. This greatly decreases the chance for colonization with hospital bacteria and the chance of subsequent infection. However, those patients who develop surgical emergencies while hospitalized for other reasons and those with lengthy stays in the intensive care units have a significant chance of developing multiple nosocomial infections. Patients admitted for other medical problems should not have elective operations done later in the same hospital course because of the increased risk of infection due to hospital-acquired bacteria.

#### Preoperative shave

Preoperative razor shaving one day before surgery is associated with significantly higher wound infection rates. The use of a depilatory agent was associated with a 0.6% infection rate, contrasted to a 5.6% rate with razor preparations the day before surgery. Although the lowest infection rate found was in those patients who had received no shave, all surgeons prefer to operate in a "deforested" field. Therefore, the alternative method of hair clipping has been proposed, with an acceptably low infection rate of 1.7%, because the use of a depilatory agent is sometimes following by pain and skin reactions.

#### Abdominal drains

On the basis of experimental and clinical studies, it appears safe to conclude that the prophylactic use of abdominal drains is unwarranted and, indeed, may be a dangerous practice. Closed suction drainage is the method of choice when therapeutic abdominal drainage is indicated.

#### Preoperative showering

Preoperative showering or bathing with hexachlorophene-containing antiseptics on the evening before surgery decreases the postoperative wound infection rate. Today, many other antiseptic soaps are available that appear to offer similar protection. For patients going to the hospital from home on the morning of surgery (outpatient surgery) it appears to be a wise practice to also shower or bathe just prior to leaving the home.

#### Presence of remote infections

The presence of an active remote infection at the time of elective operation has been shown to greatly influence the development of subsequent postoperative wound infections. These infections, in order of frequency, occur in the urinary tract, skin, and respiratory tract. Antibiotic prophylaxis or surgical incision of a skin abscess on the night prior to surgery does not decrease the incidence of subsequent wound infections. However, preoperative treatment (>24 hours before surgery) has been shown to reduce the wound infection rate significantly, to a level similar to those patients without remote infections.

## Antibiotic Prophylaxis

Great strides have been made in the last decade concerning the rational use of antibiotic prophylaxis.

### Principles of antibiotic prophylaxis

Authoritative reviews of countless clinical studies concerning surgical prophylaxis have classified those patients who may be expected to benefit from perioperative antibiotics. Up to the present time prophylactic antibiotics are clearly indicated in patients undergoing *clean* operations utilizing a foreign body implant and in all *clean-contaminated* procedures. However, recent data suggest that prophylactic antibiotics may be of value in patients undergoing clean procedures *without* foreign implants. The use of antibiotics in patients with established infection (*dirty* cases) is considered to be therapeutic and will not be discussed in this chapter.

### Choice of antibiotics

No single antibiotic agent or combination should be relied on for effective prophylaxis in all operations. The agent or agents should be chosen primarily on the basis of their efficacy against the exogenous and endogenous microorganisms usually known to cause infectious complications in each clinical setting, as well as their pharmacokinetic properties, safety profile, and cost. Specific recommendations for agents of choice in each operative procedure have been offered by *The Medical Letter* and the American Medical Association in the *Drug Evaluations Annual—1995*.

### Timing of antibiotic prophylaxis

The effective use of prophylactic antibiotics depends to a great extent on the appropriate timing of their administration. Historically, the most common errors in prophylaxis, which undoubtedly dulled the luster of this approach, were the faulty timing of the initial administration and the common practice of continuing the antibiotic beyond 72 hours.

Current recommendations indicate that the parenteral antibiotic used in prophylaxis should be given in sufficient dosage within 30 minutes of incision. This can be facilitated by having the anesthesiologist give the antibiotic in the operating room shortly before operative incision when the intravenous lines are started. This timing replaces the former approach of giving the antibiotic "on-call" to the operating room, a technique that frequently resulted in low or absent serum and tissue levels of antibiotic at the actual time of operation if the patient's surgery was delayed. Evidence from clinical trials is mounting that this single preoperative dose of antibiotic results in the same efficacy as multiple doses of prophylactic antibiotics given during the perioperative course. Those that advocate single-dose prophylaxis generally recommend that another dose be given in operations lasting over three hours. It now appears that no additional benefit can be achieved from longer courses of antibiotic prophylaxis (over 24 hours) even in immunosuppressed patients.

When orally administered antibiotics are used for prophylaxis, as frequently practiced in elective colon resection, the agents should be given during the 24 hours before operation. Longer periods of preoperative preparation are not necessary and have been associated with the isolation of resistant organisms within the colonic lumen at the time of resection.

#### Route of administration of prophylactic antibiotics

Intravenous administration of the prophylactic antibiotic is preferred in most patients undergoing abdominal surgery. When this is accomplished in a relatively small volume over a short period of time (20–30 minutes), one can expect high serum and tissue levels. Oral administration of antibiotics at this time plays a major role only in the elective preparation of patients before elective colon operations.

## Patient-Related Factors Influencing Risk of Infection

Patient-related factors strongly influence the risk of postoperative infection. Until the late 1980s most infection control officers, operating room nurses, and surgeons thought that the type of operative procedure was the most critical factor in predicting the postoperative wound infection rate. The often quoted infection rates for the different types of operative procedures were as follows: clean (<2%), clean-contaminated (5%–15%), contaminated (15%–30%) and dirty (30%). Haley and colleagues (1985) were the first to stress the importance of identifying individual patients who are at high risk of surgical wound infection in each category of operative procedure, in the hope that this approach would result in an increase in the efficiency of routine surgical wound infection surveillance and control. Analyzing ten possible risk factors by stepwise multiple logistic regression techniques, they developed a model containing four risk factors (abdominal operations; operations lasting longer than two hours; contaminated or dirty-infected operation by traditional wound classification system; and patients having three or more comorbid diseases). They utilized the resultant formula in order to predict an individual patient's probability of developing a postoperative wound infection. This approach was then retrospectively examined on another group of 59,352 surgical patients admitted in 1975–1976 and was found to be a valid predictor of surgical wound infection. The authors concluded that their simplified index predicts surgical wound infection risk about twice as well as the traditional classification of wound contamination. Utilizing this model, low-, medium-, and high-risk levels of developing wound infection were identified in each of the categories of traditional wound classification. The overall wound infection rate in this study did progressively increase from clean (2.9%), to clean-contaminated (3.9%), to contaminated (8.5%) to dirty-infected (12.6%). However, there was noted to be a wide range of infection risk in patients in each category: in clean operations, 1.1% in low risk to 15.8% in high risk; in clean-contaminated operations, 0.6% in low risk to 17.7% in high risk; in contaminated operations, 4.5% in medium risk to 23.9% in high risk; and in dirty-infected operations, 6.7% in medium risk to 27.4% in high risk. It should be noted that no low-risk patients were identified in contaminated and dirty-infected operations.

More recently, the investigators at the CDC have evolved a new risk index based on the study of 84,691 surgical patients who developed 2376 surgical wound infections during the period of surveillance (January 1987–December 1990 ). The risk index score, ranging from 0 to 3 is the number of risk factors present among the following: (*1*) a patient with an American Society of Anesthesiologists (ASA) preoperative assessment score of 3, 4, or 5; (*2*) an operation classified as contaminated or dirty-infected; and (*3*) an operation lasting over "T" hours, where "T" depends upon the operational procedure being performed. The surgical wound infection rates for patients with scores of 0, 1, 2 and 3 were 1.5%, 2.9%, 6.8%, and 13.0%, respectively. The authors feel that the risk index (the statistical probability of a surgical wound infection developing in a patient) is a significantly better predictor of surgical wound infection than the traditional wound classification system and performs well across a broad range of operative procedures.

## Treatment of Surgical Wound Infections

Most surgical site infections are localized and are not highly invasive. Once identified by observing the local signs of inflammation, including rubor (redness), calor (heat), dolor (pain), tumor (swelling), and loss of function, the localized infection is surgically drained and debrided as indicated. Local care, including the frequent repacking of the wound with antiseptic-soaked gauze or sponges, is standard. The use of oral or systemic antibiotics is not routine and should be reserved for aggressive or deep infections in patients with evidence of systemic toxicity.

The treatment of the rarer more aggressive surgical wound infections, including the gas-forming gangrenous and necrotizing infections, requires a combination of effective parenterally administered antibiotics (see Table 82.2) as well as prompt aggressive surgical debridement of all involved tissue. Additionally, daily surgical debridements are required for 3–5 days in most of these patients. The use of hyperbaric oxygen treatments should be considered in all extensive clostridial infections.

## Wound Infections: Perspectives for the 1990s

The number of patients admitted to hospitals for inpatient surgery will continue to decrease while the number of outpatient surgical procedures will continue to increase. The severity of patient illness and risk for postoperative wound infection and other septic events in hospitalized patients will increase. These trends will require effective infection surveillance in both the hospital and the outpatient setting in order to collect meaningful data.

Specific patient risk factors for each operative procedure will be identified, and these risk factors will be utilized to plan prospective alterations in therapy studies with the intention of doing less for the low-risk patient and increasing the preventive and therapeutic modalities in the high-risk patient.

Further progress in the area of chemotherapeutic development will occur, with the emphasis placed on the use of oral or local regimens. The use of antibiotic prophylaxis before operative procedures will continue to be streamlined, based largely on further pharmacokinetic data which will influence administration techniques and limit the total dosage. Operative procedures that utilize foreign body implants will be done with implants that have been commercially bonded or prepared with antibiotics or antiseptics or that have surfaces to which bacteria cannot readily attach. Immunomodulators will be utilized to help prevent infectious complications in the immunosuppressed

**Table 82.2** Empiric antibiotic treatment regimens for commonly encountered surgical wound infections

| Type of infection | Common infecting bacteria | Antibiotic therapy[a] |
|---|---|---|
| Superficial-wound infections | Streptococci, staphylococci | Not employed as a routine. If needed: first-generation cephalosporin (e.g., cefazolin, IV or cephalexin, PO); penicillinase-resistant penicillin (e.g., methicillin, IV or oxacillin, PO) |
| Deep-wound infections, other than after gastrointestinal, female genital tract, or oropharyngeal surgery | Streptococci, staphylococci[b] (rarely enterobacteriaceae) | First-generation cephalosporin, IV or methicillin, IV. *Mixed infection*, suspected or seen in gram stain: second- or third-generation cephalosporin (e.g., cefoxitin, IV or ceftizoxime, IV); ampicillin/sulbactam, IV; ticarcillin/clavulanate, IV; piperacillin/tazobactam, IV[c] |
| Deep-wound infections after gastrointestinal, female genital tract, or oropharyngeal surgery | As above, plus bacteroides and other anaerobes, enterococci | Same as mixed infection, above |
| Gangrenous infections | $\beta$-streptococci; clostridia | Penicillin-G (high doses) |
| Necrotizing infections[d] | Polymicrobial aerobic and anaerobic | Same as mixed infection, above |

[a]Initial prompt surgical treatment, including drainage and debridement, is of primary importance in the management of surgical wound infections, and should be repeated as needed during hospital stay.

[b]Vancomycin should be used if methicillin-resistant *Staphylococcus aureus* or *S. epidermidis* (MRSA, MRSE) are isolated, especially when associated with prosthetic implants.

[c]In cases of nosocomial infections or primary antibiotic regimen failure, the use of imipenem/cilistatin should be considered.

[d]Includes Fournier's gangrene.

host. Infection control committees will ideally pay more attention to proper surveillance of the surgical wound than to the discussion of the relative merits of sacred cows!

## ANNOTATED BIBLIOGRAPHY


Antimicrobial chemoprophylaxis for surgical patients. In: American Medical Association. Drug Evaluations Annual 1995. pp 1369–1376. AMA, Chicago, Il 1995.

*A critical review and recommended antibiotic prophylactic regimens for various surgical procedures.*

Antimicrobial prophylaxis in surgery. Med Lett Drugs Ther 1997; 39:97–102.

*An authoritative discussion and recommendations on the appropriate use of antimicrobial prophylaxis in surgery.*

Centers for Disease Control and Prevention (CDC). Preventing the spread of vancomycin resistance: a report from the Hospital Infections Control Practices Advisory Committee. Federal Register 1994; 59:25758.

*Recommendations for the prevention and control of the spread of vancomycin resistance, with special focus on vancomycin-resistant enterococci.*

Gorbach SL, Condon RE, Conte JE Jr, et al. Evaluation of new anti-infective drugs for surgical prophylaxis. Clin Infect Dis 1992; 15(Suppl 1): 313–338.

*Guidelines and recommendations for the conduct of clinical trials of anti-infective drugs for surgical prophylaxis.*

Haley RW, Culver DH, Morgan WM, et al. Identifying patients at high risk of surgical wound infection. Am J Epidemiol 1985; 121:206–215.

*The first CDC-NNIS study of >65,000 patients which identified four risk factors for surgical wound infections (abdominal surgery, traditional surgical class 3 or 4, >3 diagnoses in chart, surgical duration >2 hours).*

Horan TC, Gaynes RP, Martone WJ, Jarvis WR, Emori TG. CDC definitions of nosocomial surgical site infections, 1992: A modification of CDC definitions of surgical wound infections. Infect Control Hosp Epidemiol 1992; 13:606–608.

*This article provides standardized definitions to be used for the surveillance, prevention, and control of nosocomial infections.*

Nichols RL. Surgical wound infection. Am J Med 1991; 91(Suppl 3B): 54–64.

*An analysis of the prevalence of surgical wound infections and the appropriate use of perioperative antibiotics in their prevention.*

Nichols RL, Smith JW. Anaerobes from a surgical perspective. Clin Inf Dis 1994; 18(Suppl 4): S280–286.

*The importance of anaerobic bacteria in surgical wound infections and recommended treatment regimens.*

Nichols RL. Bowel preparation. In: Surgical Infections Diagnosis and Treatment. Meakins JL, ed. Scientific America, New York, 1995.

*Review of the world literature of the efficacy of various mechanical and antibiotic regimens for the prophylaxis of infection following gastrointestinal surgery.*

Platt R, Zucker JR, Zalenik DF, et al. Perioperative antibiotic prophylaxis and wound infection following breast surgery. J Antimicrob Chemother 1993; 31(Suppl B): 43–48.

*A study which suggests that a single perioperative antibiotic administration will reduce the incidence of wound infections following clean (breast) surgery.*

# 83

# Burn Infections

ROBERTA MANN, BAIBA J. GRUBE, AND DAVID M. HEIMBACH

Systemic infection is the most common cause of death in the burn patient when all sites of infection are combined (lung, wound, and other). This is likely due to a combination of immune suppression, lung parenchymal damage from smoke inhalation, and the fact that, while massive burns can be excised, there is still no way to provide a clean, closed wound that provides an effective infection barrier. The best management of infection is to prevent it. If infection does occur, however, there must be a critical understanding of the sources of infection, the unique clinical signs and symptoms of sepsis in the burn patient, the specific organisms, and the specific treatment options in the burn patient. Although burned patients suffer the same nosocomial infections found in other hospitalized patients, the most common sites of infection in burned patients are the burn wound, the lungs, and intravascular sepsis from indwelling catheters. The major approaches to prevention of fatal infection in burned patients are vigilant daily physical examinations, meticulous adherence to isolation techniques, knowledge of the common sources of infection, and intense diagnostic evaluation at the first sign of sepsis.

The most common infection seen in burn patients in the 1990s is pneumonia, most often as part of the sequelae of smoke inhalation injury. Damage to respiratory epithelium, loss of cilia resulting in impaired mucous transport, periods of mechanical ventilation, and mucosal damage from toxic products of combustion from smoke contribute to the severity of pulmonary injury. The injured mucosa predisposes the lung to invasion by microorganisms and provides an excellent culture medium for further proliferation of bacteria. Management of pneumonia after smoke inhalation is similar to management of other nosocomial pneumonias and will not be discussed in detail here.

## Epidemiology

Thermal injury results in an acute and chronic inflammatory response. The incidence and extent of immunologic impairment are burn size related and predispose the burn patient to opportunistic nosocomial infections of bacterial, fungal, and viral origin. The source of bacterial invasion can be from endogenous and/or exogenous sources. Prevention of infection begins with control of the environment by modular isolation with unidirectional (from room to hall) airflow. Specially designed self contained laminar airflow units were recommended at one time, but they are very expensive, cause claustrophobia, and significant improvement in mortality justifying their cost and inconvenience has yet to be demonstrated. Patients maintained in strict isolation, as compared to an open ward environment, have significantly less cross-contamination. Autocontamination is not altered by mechanical barriers, but the probability of developing an invasive burn wound infection following bacterial autocontamination is significantly less (39%) than from cross-contamination (65%). Presumably, host resistance factors are more effective in protecting against strains of bacteria that make up a patient's normal flora than against exogenous organisms. In addition, normal flora often contains organisms of lesser intrinsic virulence than those acquired from the environment. Cultures may be taken of patients' wounds, anterior nares, and sputum at the time of admission to identify the endogenous flora and follow subsequent nosocomial colonization, particularly in intubated patients.

Prevention of infection also requires special techniques for direct patient care. Recommendations have included barriers such as caps, masks, shoe covers, sterile/nonsterile gloves, gowns, and aprons in some combination to be used by the personnel providing care. Since 1984 we have practiced a simplified isolation technique that has reduced unit-acquired colonization, delayed the time to onset of colonization when it does occur, and dramatically reduced cost. This protocol only requires handwashing between patients and mandatory use of gloves and disposable plastic aprons for direct patient contact. Isolation gowns, caps, and masks are no longer required for entry into patient rooms.

Much has been written about alterations in the immune system of burned individuals. B-cell function, T-cell function, and lymphokine production have all been shown to be altered after thermal injury. Abraham divides these host defense abnormalities into two groups: (*1*) deficiencies in the inflammatory response and neutrophil function provide bacteria with easier access to the host through damaged epithelial and endothelial barriers; and (*2*) once bacteria have gained access to the system, alterations in T- and B-cell function hinder the containment of the bacteremia. It should be noted that much of the original work on alterations of the host immune system following thermal injury was written prior to the popularization of the method of early excision and grafting. Given the dramatic decrease in the incidence of burn wound sepsis following this clinical advance, it would be interesting to know if the host immune alterations persist despite early removal of the eschar.

## Etiology

In the 1950s, *Staphylococcus* and *Streptococcus* were predominant pathogens in burn patients. In the 1960s, topical antimicrobial agents better contained bacterial wound flora, decreasing the incidence of early burn wound sepsis. With the arrival of effective antibiotics for gram-positive bacteria, gram-negative rods—particularly *Pseudomonas* and *Klebsiella*—became the most often reported pathogens. These organisms were subsequently replaced by hitherto unreported organisms such as *Serratia* and *Acinetobacter*, and finally by *Candida* and other fungi. Since the mid-1980s there has been a worldwide resurgence of *Staphylococcus*.

Since the institution of early excision and grafting, the predominant site of infection has changed from the burn wound to the lung, with pneumonia now being the most common site of infection in burned patients. Larger burns and older patients (>60 years of age) are associated with a higher incidence of burn wound infection than is seen in smaller burns or younger patients. Nutritional and medical status also bear directly on the host's ability to stave off an invasive burn wound infection.

## Pathophysiology

All burn wounds become colonized with microorganisms. Burn eschar is composed of dead and denatured dermis in which a wide variety of microbes can flourish. The quantity of organisms present, their intrinsic virulence, and the degree to which they invade host tissues determine their significance. Whereas microbial colonization should be expected, invasion of surrounding tissue is an ominous sign. Aggressive wound care and extreme vigilance are required to control the concentration of organisms in the burn wound in an effort to protect patients from invasive burn wound sepsis.

Burn wound infections are generally classified as invasive or noninvasive. If a burn wound is allowed to remain *in situ* and is treated with adequate debridement and topical antibiotics, after two to three weeks the naturally occurring microorganisms that colonize the wound will promote separation of the eschar-utilizing collagenases which they themselves produce. A layer of granulation tissue forms where the eschar separates and the improved blood supply and wound hypermetabolism help to limit the proliferation of microbes. As a result, the formation of granulation tissue is enhanced and the wound bed becames highly vascular and contains a low concentration of microorganisms, making it ideal for receiving skin grafts or biologic dressings. There may be little or no systemic response to separation of the eschar, depending on the size of the wound involved. Mildly elevated temperatures and leukocytoses may occur and may be a result of this localized inflammatory response. Quantitative cultures of eschar may contain >100,000 organisms/gram tissue, but biopsies of adjacent tissue (subeschar) will contain <100,000 organisms/gram tissue in noninvasive wound infections.

When burn wound infections become invasive, the concentration of microorganisms rises to greater than one million per gram of tissue. Developing granulation tissue becomes edematous and pale, with subsequent occlusion and thrombosis of new blood vessels. Lack of bleeding is evident on surgical exploration of the wound. As the infection advances, the surface becomes frankly necrotic and the infection spreads rapidly. At this stage, partial-thickness injuries will progress to full-thickness injuries, since the wound's blood supply is destroyed in the infection process. Patients with invasive burn wound infections may initially manifest symptoms consistent with mild infection, but will generally develop spiking fevers and leukocytosis as the infection progresses. However, signs of sepsis may be muted in burn patients, and the astute clinician must be wary even when a worsening clinical appearance of burn wounds has little apparent systemic response accompanying it. Invasive burn wound sepsis requires a very low threshold of suspicion, aggressive attempts at early detection, and extremely vigorous therapy to contain. Fortunately, the advent of aggressive surgical removal of the burn wound has made burn wound sepsis a rare event.

## Clinical Features

Due to the presence of microorganisms in wounds and ongoing tissue necrosis in the burn eschar, fever is often present in patients with burns. The continuous elaboration of endogenous pyrogens accounts for the frequent presence of fever. However, body temperature may be increased or normal with both invasive and noninvasive infections. Hypothermia can be an ominous sign, and may herald the onset of severe gram-negative septicemia. The white blood cell count is extremely variable and can be influenced by medication and immunosuppression as well as by early sepsis. An isolated white blood cell count will not help determine whether an invasive burn infection is present. However, sudden increases or decreases in white count or marked leftward shifts may be clues to serious infections. Advanced cases of burn wound sepsis may cause prolonged hypotensive episodes, large crystalloid fluid requirements, ileus, respiratory failure, and loss of mental acuity.

In the 1960s and 1970s systemic sepsis originating in the burn wound was the most dreaded complication for the burn patient because it was not only common but was generally fatal. Without preventive management, systemic sepsis inevitably occurs in the second or third week, leading to multisystem organ failure and death. Systemic antibiotics play little role in the prophylaxis of infections confined to the burn wound, since the avascular wound prevents adequate delivery of antibiotics to the bacteria. Fortunately, early burn excision has greatly diminished, although not eliminated, this problem. In our burn center, mortality due to sepsis thought to originate in the burn wound has decreased from 36% of deaths to 5% of deaths since early excision became usual practice. Once burn wound sepsis is established, if there is a necrotic eschar, the patient is unlikely to survive unless the dead, infected tissue is surgically removed, and even then only about 60% will survive.

## Diagnosis

Burn wound monitoring is essential, both for the individual patient and to keep track of the ecology of the burn unit. The best method for bacteriologic monitoring of the burn wound remains controversial. Surface cultures are easy to do and inexpensive, but do not accurately predict burn wound invasion in any individual patient. Quantitative biopsies of the burn wound have predictive ability when bacterial counts are greater than 100,000/gm of tissue, but they are more expensive and have less meaning later in the burn course after the burn eschar begins to separate. Histologic sections are useful to some, and histologic culture techniques have been described to show the depth of bacterial growth, but these techniques are expensive and cumbersome. Most centers rely on quantitative wound biopsies or surface swabs. While biopsy cultures are meaningless at the time of eschar separation, and are not predictive in patients with burns of less than 20% (who often have high bacterial levels without sepsis), most patients (87% in one study), with >100,000 organisms/gm do go on to develop sepsis.

In a study of 397 burn patients over a ten-year period, there was a 20% mortality in those patients with positive blood cultures. Positive blood cultures predict high mortality with gram-negative organisms, intermediate mortality with candida, and low mortality with gram-positive organisms. The progression of bacteremia to septicemia with the development of multisystem organ failure has a dismal prognosis.

Even minor thermal injury causes the liver to synthesize acute phase proteins by up-regulation of mRNA. These acute-phase reactants reach a plateau at six to seven days. The increased synthesis of alpha-one-antichymotrypsin and C-reactive protein is highest during and before the episode of sepsis is clinically evident. These may be markers to monitor as an early aid for diagnosis of sepsis. Serum levels of tumor necrosis factor (TNF) have been followed in critically ill burn patients with and without sepsis. TNF levels were elevated in septic burn patients and in 71% of those who died compared to only 31% of those who survived.

The burn patient manifests signs of sepsis as do other critically ill patients, except that the burn patient's "normal" hyperdynamic state mimics some of the typical signs of sepsis. Changes in status, rather than specific abnormalities must be sought in the burn patient.

Diagnosis of burn wound sepsis should be made in the presence of clinical deterioration, two or more signs of sepsis (listed in Table 83.1), and the presence of greater than 100,000 organisms/gm of tissue on quantitative culture. Blood cultures are often negative despite a septic picture and high bacterial counts in the wound.

In children, fever is not a reliable predictor of infection. At the first suspicion of sepsis, the wound must be inspected. Discoloration of the eschar, cellulitis of surrounding tissue, progressive separation of eschar, purulent drainage, and pain in the wound are worrisome signs. Black spots occurring within the wound or in unburned areas *(ecythyma gangrenosum)* are characteristic features of *Pseudomonas* burn wound sepsis.

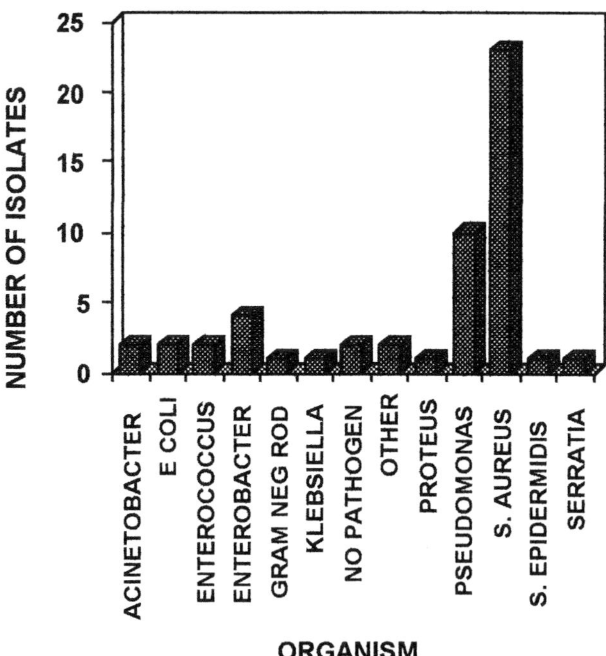


**Fig. 83.1** Nosocomial infections at University of Washington Burn Center, 1 January 1992–31 December 1992.

## Treatment

Successful treatment of burn wound infections is extremely difficult. Appropriate systemic antibiotics may ameliorate some systemic manifestations, but do little to treat the primary infection in the burn wound. Direct injection of antibiotics beneath the burn eschar has historical significance as an effective treatment but the size of the burned areas usually involved make this treatment technically difficult and clinically dubious. Emergent excision of infected burn eschar may be the only effective treatment. Excision removes the source of infection, but may massively seed the patient's vasculature during the operation. Operations performed in patients with a deteriorating cardiovascular status and pulmonary function are extremely hazardous.

**Table 83.1** Signs of sepsis in the burn patient

| |
|---|
| Hypo- or hyperthermia |
| Increasing or decreasing white blood cell count |
| Decreasing platelet count |
| Glucose intolerance |
| Increased gastric residuals |
| Disorientation |
| Tachycardia |
| Tachypnea |
| Falling $PaO_2$ |
| Increasing fluid requirements |
| Decreasing urine output |
| Increasing cardiac index |
| Decreasing peripheral resistance |

Infections originating in excised wounds may respond to antibiotics if there is adequate blood supply to the area. The choice of antibiotics is in part determined by available culture results. Often aminoglycosides and vancomycin are given in increased dosages and peak and trough levels must then be measured. Combinations of antibiotics, including third-generation cephalosporins, may be as effective and less toxic.

A recent review of antibiotic treatment in the burn patient outlines a general philosophy of management of infection and develops guidelines for systemic antibiotic administration. First, the burn patient will be exposed to microorganisms despite strict isolation techniques; therefore, constant surveillance of the patient's microflora and the unit's pattern is essential. Second, no single antibiotic or combination of agents will eliminate all microorganisms; in fact, if inappropriately administered, the emergence of resistant strains or opportunistic strains may result. Third, the responsible organism should be identified before administration of antimicrobial agents. While we generally adhere to this concept, assessment of the individual case must dictate appropriate treatment. Fourth, combination agents should only be used if they result in increased activity against the pathogen. Fifth, multiple agents create a greater risk of superinfection from resistant strains. Sixth, antibiotics should be administered only as long as are needed to eliminate the disease, but not for such a brief period that reemergence will occur when the drug is withdrawn. Seventh, serum levels must be followed for selected antibiotics, but additional variables must also be taken into account, such as local wound factors and the general immune state of the individual. It must be noted that antibiotics are metabolized differently in the burn patient. Serum antibiotic levels have been demonstrated to be consistently low in burn patients and thus daily antibiotic dosage must be regulated by following serum levels. The half-life of aminoglycosides is very significantly decreased in children with burns.

## Specific Organisms in Burn Patients

### Bacterial infections

Burn patients are at risk for infection by the same organisms that threaten any critically ill patient. Extensive review of all the types of bacterial infection they may acquire is beyond the scope of this chapter. Selected organisms that are especially problematic in today's intensive care environment will be discussed.

#### Gram-positive infections

##### *Streptococcus*

Outbreaks of *streptococcal* infections can occur from endogenous and exogenous sources. The *enterococci* are normal host flora residing in the gastrointestinal tract and female genitourinary tract and have recently emerged as more frequent pathogens. The increased incidence of enterococcal nosocomial infections is in part related to their resistance to many antibiotics, especially aminoglycosides and more recently to vancomycin. Enterococcal bacteremia alone may be fairly indolent, but when in association with polymicrobial infections, especially with gram-negative bacilli, shock occurs in 50% of the cases. Enterococcal burn wound infections are rare but should prompt aggressive therapy to prevent sepsis, which is associated with a significant mortality rate.

##### *Methicillin-resistant Staphylococcus aureus (MRSA)*

The occurrence of methicillin-resistant *Staphylococcus aureus* infections in burn units used to invoke special isolation, separate patient assignments, closure of a unit to admission and discharge, and systemic treatment of carriers. Recent longitudinal studies on the epidemiology and the mortality and morbidity of MRSA question the necessity of added control practices. In 14 patients with burns larger than 30% TBSA who developed MRSA, 57% had MRSA on admission by antibiogram analysis. The remaining 43% had methicillin-sensitive SA on admission. The authors suggest that MRSA may often arise from the endogenous flora. However, cross-infection within intensive care units clearly occurs as well. In two major epidemics of MRSA among burn patients, the mortality rate was 5%. Similar findings were observed in 1100 patients, where approximately half developed *S. aureus* infection, and half of those with *S. aureus* developed MRSA colonization with no apparent increase in mortality after using multiple regression analysis to control for burn size and age.

#### Gram-negative infections

Opportunistic infection with gram-negative organisms still cause increased mortality in bacteremic burn patients. The origin of these organisms can be endogenous or exogenous and they can readily colonize and invade the immune-compromised host.

The release of lipopolysaccharide (LPS) from the cell wall of gram-negative bacteria produces an acute inflammatory response, which in the worst clinical scenario presents as the syndrome known as multiple organ failure (MOF). One of the central mediators of the host immune response to LPS is tumor necrosis factor/cachectin (TNF), which is released from the activated macrophage. Regulation of the macrophage response is essential to preserve host defense and minimize cytokine-mediated, especially TNF-mediated, tissue injury. The pathophysiologic response to sepsis and/or LPS appears to escalate after 12–24 hours. The heightened response to a second-challenge dose of LPS may be due to the formation of lipopolysaccharide binding protein (LBP), a high-affinity glycoprotein. LPS–LBP complex stimulates binding to the monocyte/macrophage cellular receptor, CD14. Soluble CD14 levels have been found to be elevated in severely burned patients when clinical signs of sepsis were present. The LPS–LBP complex is 10,000-fold more active in stimulating production of TNF-alpha by the macrophage than is LPS alone (see Chapter 53).

##### *Pseudomonas*

The effective treatment of septicemia from a *Pseudomonas* wound infection and/or bacteremia requires vigilant surveillance of burn wounds for invasion, prompt initiation of appropriate antibiotic therapy, and rapid wound excision. Patients with *Pseudomonas aeruginosa* bacteremia tend to have a larger burn size and have a 28% increase in mortality over patients with sepsis involving less virulent organisms. The standard treatment approach is to use operative debridement (burn wound excision, if not done previously) and two synergistic antimicrobials.

#### Anaerobic bacteria

Anaerobic infections, although not a common finding in the burn unit, must be considered in certain wounds such as electrical injuries or certain locations such as perioral and perianal wounds. The most commonly isolated anaerobes include *Bacteroides melaninogenicus*, *Peptococcus*, and *Bacteroides fragilis.*

#### Unusual organisms

Outbreaks of *Acinetobacter calcoaceticus* have been reported in several burn units. The reservoir in one report was identified as the patients' mattresses. Risk factors included larger burns and Foley catheter use. It is important to identify the organism, which can be confused with *Neisseria*, because of its multiple drug resistances.

### Fungal infections

These devastating infections usually occur after the seemingly successful treatment of bacterial infection with multiple antibiotics. Fungal infections most often occur during the third to sixth week postburn. The use of multiple systemic antibiotics, and the use of topical agents that have little effect on fungi, combined with the severely compromised host defenses of the burned patient lead to opportunistic infections of the burn wound with fungi, especially *Candida* species.

#### *Candida* sepsis

Reports in the early 1980s suggested a mortality of 90%–100% with *Candida* sepsis in burn patients, whether treated or not. By 1986, *Candida* had risen to epidemic proportion in some burn centers, but early treatment with amphotericin B decreased mortality to about 32%, more in keeping with results in critically ill surgical patients. With increasingly selective use of antibiotics and less burn eschar to become infected (due to the practice of early excision), the incidence of positive *Candida* cultures in our burn ICU in 1987 included 13% of patients in the ICU more than seven days, but only 2% developed full-blown sepsis. Those who developed *Candida* sepsis had a mortality of 33%. *Candida* is an endogenous colonizer of the patient's skin, nasopharynx, gastrointestinal tract, and vagina. For this reason, many units administer prophylactic mycostatin orally and vaginally. The practice of early excision and grafting, aggressive nutritional support and early removal of invasive monitors, has reduced the incidence of *Candida* infection at the University of Washington Burn Center. Similarly, an aggressive wound excision plan and routine use of topical and enteral nystatin during an 11-year period has entirely prevented *Candida* sepsis at the Shriners Burns Institute in Galveston, Texas, eliminating the need for toxic systemic antifungal agents.

Sepsis caused by *Candida* species is diagnosed by positive cultures from three separate sites (e.g. bladder, wound, blood), and has been a dreaded complication in the immune-compromised patient with a major burn. The signs and symptoms of *Candida* septicemia are similar to those of bacterial sepsis, but *Candida* species will usually be recovered from multiple culture sites. The presence of a septic picture and positive cultures for *Candida* from the blood and one other source are considered by many to be sufficient indication for systemic treatment with amphotericin B. Any burn wound culture positive for *Candida* is reason to add nystatin to the topical agent already employed. The addition of nystatin in a 1:1 mixture with silver sulfadiazine or polymyxin B/bacitracin plus oral "swish-and-swallow" nystatin has nearly eliminated *Candida* wound infection and sepsis.

## Filamentous fungal infections

Other fungal infections are uncommon, but when they occur they are associated with a high degree of morbidity and are frequently fatal. Filamentous fungal spores are found in the environment and are spread via the airborne route. Patients who sustained their injuries in association with exposure to the ground or untreated water are also at risk for environmentally acquired filamentous spores.

Improved isolation techniques, better topical therapy, and early excision and grafting have significantly reduced the incidence of bacterial infections without substantial impact on fungal infections at the U.S. Army Institute of Surgical Research. The frequency of distribution of organisms was *Aspergillus* and *Fusarium* 68%, *Candida* 18%, *Mucor* and *Rhizopus* 9.1%, *Microspora* and *Alternaria* 5% each. The diagnosis can be suspected in a patient who becomes extremely toxic, with burn wounds that turn black, eschar that separates rapidly, subeschar tissue that converts to full-thickness necrosis, and unburned skin that develops necrotic lesions (ecthyma gangrenosum). The diagnosis is confirmed by histologic identification of the organism on emergency biopsy of the blackened wound. Cultures require one to two weeks to grow and are not very useful in the clinical setting. Emergent radical debridement of all involved tissue in association with rapid administration of antifungal chemotherapeutic agents has reduced the incidence of disseminated fungal infection and the need for amputations. Subfascial and muscular involvement may require amputation due to recurrence of disease along vascular channels. Depending upon the species present, systemic administration of amphotericin B (0.5 mg/kg body weight/day), alone or in conjunction with other antifungals, should be given. Investigation of environmental factors such as air ducts, ventilation systems, and false ceilings may be critical to eliminate spores from the modules in those units where there is a high incidence of filamentous fungal infection.

## Viral infection

Viral infections are diagnosed infrequently and are rarely fatal, but they may result in considerable morbidity. *Herpes simplex* virus (HSV) infections occur in an older population and are associated with tracheal intubation, facial burns, inhalation injury, prolonged hospitalization, and full-thickness burns. Cluster cases of HSV have occurred, but genetic analysis of the HSV isolates have shown them to be genetically unrelated. *Herpes* virus causes typical vesicular lesions within a healing burn. Once diagnosed, the patient should be isolated from all other burned patients. The lesions appear to be relatively self-limiting. Intravenous administration of acyclovir is used in the treatment of HSV infections.

The overall rate of primary *cytomegalovirus* (CMV) infection is 22.5%, while the reactivation rate is 56%. The data suggests that primary infections may be causally related to transfusion of CMV-positive blood products. In general the outcome from CMV is good, although there are some cases describing serious morbidity and mortality.

Children with clinical manifestations or even a history of exposure to viral exanthem (*Varicella, Rubella, Rubeola*) should be isolated from other patients during the clinical course or the incubation period. While these diseases are benign in normal individuals, they can have a fatal outcome in patients with severe burns.

## Prophylaxis

There is widespread controversy regarding the prophylactic use of antibiotics in burn patients. Meticulous wound care and topical agents are adequate for wounds that do not demonstrate invasion or clinical sepsis. Broad-spectrum antibiotics may affect normal microbial flora and directly influence the appearance of antibiotic-resistant bacteria. We performed a randomized prospective blinded study comparing the incidence of wound infection in patients treated with and without penicillin and were unable to demonstrate any difference in the rate of total infections, burn wound sepsis, or cellulitis. The short course, however, did not lead to the development of antibiotic-resistant bacteria.

In large burns, although efficacy remains unconfirmed, we generally provide perioperative (single dose at induction of anesthesia) *staphylococcal* coverage during the first week and then both gram-negative and gram-positive coverage beyond one week. Although there is a transient bacteremia during burn wound debridement, it has been demonstrated in burns less than 60% TBSA that a positive blood culture obtained intraoperatively is not associated with postoperative sepsis.

## Tetanus

Full-thickness burns are tetanus prone wounds. The need for tetanus prophylaxis is determined by the patient's current immunization status. The treating physician should follow the standard guidelines suggested by the American College of Surgeons (see Chapter 45).

## Antibiotics

Prior to the discovery of penicillin, 30% of burn patients died during the first week postburn from overwhelming $\beta$ hemolytic *streptococcal* sepsis. The availability of penicillin decreased *streptococcal* infections but did not influence mortality or the incidence of bacterial sepsis. Patients then survived the first postburn week only to die of penicillin-resistant, gram-negative bacteria during the second and third postburn week. The arrival of effective topical chemotherapeutic agents applied to the burn wounds adequately controlled *Streptococcus* and other gram positive bacterial colonization of the burn wound. Although some burn surgeons persist in giving prophylactic penicillin for several days postburn, prophylactic antibiotics have not been shown to be useful in the initial care of the burn patient when effective topical antimicrobial agents are used.

## Summary

Burn wound sepsis is rarely seen today in major burn centers due to an aggressive approach to wound care and the practice of early excision and grafting. Burn patients remain highly susceptible to infections due to injury-induced immunosuppression, but extreme vigilance and aggressive early treatment can substantially reduce the infectious complications commonly seen with large burns. Although the incidence of burn wound sepsis has decreased dramatically, systemic infections, particularly pneumonia, continue to be the major cause of mortality after extensive burns.

### ANNOTATED BIBLIOGRAPHY


Abraham E. Host defense abnormalities after hemorrhage, trauma, and burns. Crit Care Med 1989; 17(9):934–939.
*A summary of clinical and laboratory data documenting alterations in the host immune system following hemorrhage, trauma, and burns (74 references).*

Becker WK, Cioffi WG, McManus AT, et al. Fungal burn wound infection: a ten-year experience. Arch Surg 1991; 126:44–48.
*Ten-year review of experience with fungal burn wound infection. Factors that appear to have markedly reduced bacterial burn wound infection, including patient isolation, topical chemotherapeutic agents, and burn wound excision do not appear to have had a similar effect on fungal wound infection.*

Burke JF, Quinby WC, Bondoc CC, et al. The contribution of a bacterially isolated environment to the prevention of infection in seriously burned patients. Ann Surg 1977; 186:377–87.
*A comparison between three different styles of infection control in burn patients. Describes an environmentally controlled patient isolation unit (which proved superior in preventing infection) to both single room isolation on a burn isolation ward and conventional isolation techniques on an open burn ward.*

Dasco CC, Luterman A, Curreri PW. Systemic antibiotic treatment in burned patients. Surg Clin North Am 1987; 67:57–68.
*A comprehensive review.*

Durtschi MB, Orgain C, Counts GW, Heimbach DM. A prospective study of prophylactic penicillin in acutely burned hospitalized patients. J Trauma 1982; 22:11.
*Concludes that the routine administration of prophylactic penicillin neither protects against cellulitis and burn wound sepsis, nor promotes selection of antibiotic-resistant bacteria in hospitalized patients with acute thermal injury.*

Jones WG, Barie PS, Yurt RW, et al. Enterococcal burn sepsis: a highly lethal complication in severely burned patients. Arch Surg 1986; 121:649–653.
*Discussion of a burn unit's experience with enterococcal burn wound infections. Emphasis on prompt aggressive therapy to prevent the development of enterococcal sepsis with its associated high mortality.*

Lee JJ, Marvin JA, Heimbach DM, et al. Infection control in a burn center. J Burn Care Rehabil 1990; 11:575–580.
*Describes a simplified isolation technique for burn intensive care units which decreased unit-acquired microbial colonization from 63% to 33% and led to a significant delay in inception, from 7.8 to 21 days, in those colonized with* Pseudomonas aeruginosa. *Isolation costs dropped from $53,000 to $30,000 for a six-month period.*

Luterman A, Dasco CC, Curreri PW. Infections in burn patients. Am J Med 1986; 81:45.
*Describes the current management of infection and infection control in burn patients.*

Marano MA, Fong Y, Moldawer LL, et al. Serum cachectin/tumor necrosis factor in critically ill patients with burns correlates with infection and mortality. Surg Gynecol Obstet 1990; 170:32–38.
*Measured serum cachectin/TNF in 43 critically ill burn patients with and without sepsis. TNF detectable with greater frequency and in higher concentrations in patients with sepsis and in those who die of their burn injury.*

Mathison J, Tobias P, Wolfson E, et al. Regulatory mechanisms of host responsiveness to endotoxin/lipopolysaccharide. Pathobiol 1991; 59:185–188.
*Discusses regulation of LPS–monocyte/macrophage interactions by LPS-binding plasma proteins and by LPS-induced changes in monocyte/macrophage responsiveness.*

McManus AT, Mason AD, McManus WF, et al. What's in a name? Is methicillin-resistant *Staphylococcus aureus* just another *S. aureus* when treated with vancomycin? Arch Surg 1989; 123:1456–1459.
*Examines the significance of MRSA colonization and infection in 1100 consecutively admitted, seriously burned patients in whom vancomycin was used to treat all staphylococcal infections. Demonstrates no measurable increase in mortality attributable to MRSA in this population of burned, SA-infected patients.*

Shirani KZ, McManus AT, Vaughan GM, et al. Effects of environment on infection in burn patients. Arch Surg 1986; 121:31–36.
*Study showing that environmental manipulation can reduce infection rates and improve survival in burn patients.*

Yi-Ping Z. Clinical evaluation of extensive excision of burn escharectomy in the presence of septicaemia: analysis of 32 cases. Burns Incl Therm Inj 1984; 10:200.
*Discusses the therapeutic value of extensive escharectomy in 32 cases of burn septicemia.*

# 84

# Infections Complicating Traumatic Injury

WAYNE N. CAMPBELL

Blunt and penetrating injury represents the leading cause of death for individuals under 44 years of age in both industrialized Europe and the United States. Mortality rates due to unintentional injury from the early 1990s are as follows: United States—38.3 deaths/100,000 population; Germany—36.9/100,000; United Kingdom—26.9/100,000; France—59.8/100,000; Finland—55.7/100,000; and Japan—26.9/100,000. The vast majority of deaths occur in the first hours following injury, due primarily to exsanguination, respiratory failure, or devastating head injury. Rapid emergency transport systems and improved acute resuscitation measures have resulted in more early survivors. The potion of health care expenditures devoted to the acute care and rehabilitation of survivors is large, and infections contribute substantially to the cost in terms of both expenditures and mortality.

Seriously injured survivors are at extremely high risk for infections, which are often multiple. The incidence of infection after injury ranges from 20% to 63%, with the likelihood commensurate with the severity of the injuries. The cause of infectious complications can be roughly divided into (*1*) those resulting from the injuries or their surgical repair, and (*2*) the sequelae of invasive techniques of resuscitation and support, particularly ventilatory assistance and hemodynamic monitoring. Practically every supportive measure is associated with an increased risk of infection—the consequence of breaching intact skin and bypassing mucosal defenses. Infectious complications in the days immediately following injury are from the surgical and traumatic wounds or are pulmonary infections, as a result of aspiration during injury or intubation. Less commonly, an early infection will be caused by the emergent insertion of a vascular or urinary catheter without proper preparation. Several days to weeks into the hospital course, the predominant infections are nosocomial, with single or multiple occurrences of pneumonia, bacteremia, and urinary tract infection. At this time, intra-abdominal, intrathoracic, or prosthetic device infections may also be identified. The risk of late nosocomial infection is related to prolonged invasive catheterization, multiple surgeries, organ dysfunction, prolonged immobilization, suboptimal nutrition, blood transfusions, and medications, which may have obvious (steroids) or subtle (dopamine) effects on host resistance.

This chapter will briefly address trauma victims' predisposition to infection because of altered immunity, point out measures to prevent infections, review the guidelines for selection of prophylactic and empiric preemptive antibiotics, consider the difficulty of diagnosing infection in patients whose common indicators of infection are distorted by injury, and describe several specific post-trauma infections.

## Altered Host Immunity with Severe Trauma

Severe trauma or hemorrhage imparts a degree of temporary immunosuppression. The magnitude of immunologic impairment is not sufficient to result in infections often associated with immunodeficiency, such as cytomegalovirus and herpes zoster virus, *Aspergillus*, *Cryptococcus*, *Pneumocystic carinii*, or mycobacteria. It does, however, predispose to the development of bacterial and *Candida* infections, and shedding with possible clinically apparent reactivation of herpes simplex virus. A substantial amount of literature describes specific in vivo and in vitro immunologic abnormalities of trauma victims. Understanding or measuring the exact impact of these abnormalities for an individual patient is very difficult.

Practically every arm of immune defense demonstrates one or more abnormalities after trauma. Leukocyte superoxide production is increased and chemotaxis and adherence are reduced. Serum levels of complement are reduced. Antibody production, particularly IgM, is reduced, the result of B-lymphocyte dysfunction. Circulating T-lymphocyte subset ratios are altered, and multiple functional abnormalities have been described. T-lymphocyte dysfunction seems to correlate with an increased incidence of bacterial infection. This has been observed in trauma patients who demonstrate absent delayed hypersensitivity.

Impaired macrophage and T-lymphocyte communication after injury may be central to the immunosuppressed state. Macrophages fail to present antigen normally and produce increased $PGE_2$ and decreased interleukin-1 (IL-1). T-lymphocyte dysfunction manifests as abnormal quantities of circulating cytokines and failure of the delayed-hypersensitivity response. Severely injured patients may demonstrate abnormal in vitro lymphocyte responses for up to 20 days. Tumor necrosis factor (TNF) and interleukins 6 and 8 are increased. TNF increases may be transient, while IL-6 may remain elevated as long as 14–21 days. Interferon gamma levels are reduced, and IL-2 may remain suppressed for up to three weeks. An intriguing hypothesis for cytokine dysregulation centers on a monocyte subset that expresses a specific immunoglobulin receptor (FcR1). Its abnormal function, the consequence of an aberrant feedback loop, can result in the overproduction of inflammatory cytokines and prostaglandins. A substantial body of literature is developing about the rule of immunosuppressive cytokines. The possibility of manipulating specific host cytokines to affect the altered immune state following trauma is intriguing. Some preliminary investigations have been performed (Faist 1996) (see Chapter 46).

Beyond immunologic abnormalities that increase the risk of infection, the trauma victim's premorbid state is also important. Advanced age is a risk factor for more numerous and severe infectious complications, as are, likewise, structural and functional pulmonary abnormalities, morbid obesity, renal insufficiency, vascular insufficiency, and diabetes mellitus. Trauma victims infected with the human immunodeficiency virus (HIV) (approximately 4% of admissions to our institution) always cause heightened concern. While these patients are at increased risk for multiple opportunistic pathogens, because of their potentially immune-impaired state (see Chapter 100), post-trauma infections are typically caused by common bacterial pathogens such as *Staphylococcus aureus*, *Haemophilus influenzae*, and *Streptococcus pneumoniae*. HIV-infected trauma victims respond appropriately to proper antibiotic therapy. It is quite unlikely that, immediately following injury, they will develop opportunistic infections such as pneumocystis, toxoplasmosis, or cryptococcosis unless these were present before the injury. However, physicians must remain vigilant for the atypical presentations of active pulmonary and extrapulmonary tuberculosis that may accompany the HIV-infected trauma victim.

## Prevention of Infection in Trauma Patients

The most fundamental of all preventative measures is handwashing. Drug-resistant pathogens spread rapidly in intensive care units (ICUs) and substantially complicate the management of patients, as well as considerably increase the cost of care. The simple mechanical action of washing with soap and water is the most important measure to reduce the spread of nosocomial organisms (see Chapter 8). During outbreaks of nosocomial pathogens, use of a chlorhexidine solution rather than a bland soap is warranted. Senior physicians, nurses, and other health care providers *must* inculcate this practice in trainees. Used properly, body substance isolation (BSI) precautions also reduce the risk of transmission of infection both from patient to health care workers and from patient to patient. Strict adherence to appropriate gloving practices can be of great value in reducing cross-infection in ICUs.

Devices that bypass mucosal and skin barriers directly contribute to infection, and thus attention to the presence of and necessity for all catheters and drains is mandatory. Vascular and urinary catheters must be removed the moment they are not required. The same holds for postsurgical drains and chest tubes. Extubation, or if indicated, tracheostomy, as soon as possible decreases the risk of pneumonia. Changing from a nasogastric or nasotracheal tube to an oral gastric or endotracheal tube reduces the incidence of sinusitis. Possibly less obvious, but no less important, is early mobilization of the patient and aggressive nutritional support. Enteral feeding may be preferential to parenteral feeding.

Vascular catheters are common vehicles for nosocomial bacteremia (see Chapter 67). Their risk to the patient must be respected, and this risk demands that they be inserted with meticulous attention to sterility. Insertion sites must be visually examined daily, and removal of a central catheter should be strongly considered when there is any sign of local infection or unexplained systemic infection or even unexplained fever. Recently, silver-impregnated collagen cuffs became available for use at the skin–catheter interface. They are designed to provide an antiseptic mechanical barrier to microorganisms. They can be placed over standard catheters or on newly marketed central catheters, which have surfaces impregnated with silver sulfadiazine and chlorhexidine. A recently published randomized controlled trial indicates that antiseptic impregnated catheters may safely remain in place longer than standard central venous catheters before they become colonized with bacteria (Maki 1997). This is of particular value in the trauma victim. Trauma patients frequently have extremely limited sites of vascular access as a result of limb injury, vascular injury or thrombosis, severe coagulopathy, or anasarca. Routine changing of sites of catheterization may not be possible. Antiseptic-impregnated triple-lumen catheter use in such patients or placement of collagen cuffs on catheters used for hemodialysis may reduce catheter infection rates. Chlorhexidine-impregnated circular patches can be placed around the huge and essentially nonremovable extracorporeal oxygenation catheters for the same purposes. Such practices still need definitive studies to prove their worth, however.

A limited number of vaccines are of value in the trauma patient. Along with wound debridement, tetanus toxoid (with diphtheria toxoid) is administered if more than five years have elapsed since the patient's last booster. Patients with unknown or incomplete histories of tetanus vaccination require the combined use of adsorbed tetanus toxoid and tetanus immune globulin (see Chapter 48). Patients requiring splenectomy should receive pneumococcal vaccine at the time of spleen removal. Consideration should be given to administering *Haemophilus influenzae* type B conjugate and meningococcal vaccines to splenectomized patients.

## Antibiotic Prophylaxis and Preemptive Therapy

Strictly defined, antibiotic prophylaxis is the administration of antibiotics before tissues are disrupted or contaminated. This is the correct description of antibiotic use in trauma for surgeries such as open reduction and internal fixation of closed fractures, fasciotomies, and exploratory surgery where no hollow viscus injury is found. Preemptive empiric antibiotic therapy refers to the use of antibiotics during and after surgical repair of open fractures, repair of disrupted mucosal surfaces, debridement of devitalized soft tissue, or for hollow viscus rents with soiling of body cavities. Both prophylactic and preemptive, antibiotics administered to trauma victims reduce infections. A general discussion of specific surgical prophylaxis regimens is beyond the scope of this chapter, but an excellent review is available. Table 84.1 describes several commonly encountered traumatic injuries and recommended prophylactic or preemptive antibiotic regimens. The fundamentals of prophylactic antibiotic use are discussed in Chapter 45. Knowledge of these principles is valuable when faced with the unusual situations trauma often presents.

When tissues are grossly contaminated prior to surgery, longer courses of antibiotic therapy directed at likely bacterial pathogens are appropriate. Injuries such as high-grade open fractures, left colon injuries with soiling of the peritoneum and associated solid organ injury, or grossly contaminated open spine or open head injuries are examples. Antifungal therapy in these situations is almost never needed and should not be routinely employed. A critical aspect in dealing with dirty wounds is less the use of antibiotics, and more the practice of aggressive and frequent surgical debridement. When the surgeon feels that the tissues are clean and require no further debridement or irrigation, it is usually safe to stop antibiotics. Using this practice, we seldom exceed three to five days of preemptive antibiotics. Daily review of antibiotic selection and duration by the infectious-disease or critical-care physician with the surgeon is an effective approach.

A controversial use of prophylactic antibiotics that was pio-

**Table 84.1** Recommendations for prophylactic/preemptive antibiotics following traumatic injury

| Injury/surgery | Bacteria | Antibiotic | Dose/duration |
|---|---|---|---|
| Penetrating head injury | *S. aureus*, coagulase-negative staphylococci | Nafcillin | 2 gm IV q4h × 3–5 days |
| Otorrhea/rhinorrhea | *H. influenzae*, *N. meningitidis*, *S. pneumoniae*, *S. aureus* | None routinely, if infection clinically suspected, cefotaxime | 2 gm IV q4–6h 7–10 days |
| | | or ceftriaxone | 1–2 gm IV q12h 7–10 d |
| Open facial fractures | *S. aureus*, aerobic and anaerobic streptococci | Clindamycin or | 600 IV q8h × 24–48 hrs |
| | | ampicillin/sulbactam | 3.0 gm IV q6h × 24–48 hrs |
| Penetrating chest injury | *S. aureus*, aerobic streptococci | Cefazolin | 1–2 gm IV preinduction |
| Penetrating or blunt abdominal trauma requiring exploratory laparotomy | Gram-negative enterics and anaerobes | Cefoxitin or | 2 gm IV preinduction |
| | | beta-lactam/beta-lactamase inhibitor | Postoperative duration dependant on intra-abdominal injuries |
| Closed orthopedic fractures requiring internal fixation | *S. aureus*, coagulase-negative staphylococci | Cefazolin | 1–2 gm IV preinduction |
| Grade-III open orthopedic fractures | *S. aureus*, coagulase-negative staphylococci, gram-negative rods | Cefazolin, with or without gentamicin | 1–2 gm IV q8h and 1.9 mg/kg IV q8h respectively for 48–72 hrs |

neered in the trauma patient involves selective decontamination of the oropharynx and upper gastrointestinal tract with a suspension of broad-spectrum, usually nonabsorbable antibiotics. Typically, these are applied orally and instilled into the stomach. Studies of selective decontamination are very difficult to assess and compare because of great variability in design. We are not convinced that the possible reduction in lower respiratory tract infections achieved by using these antimicrobials improves patient survival sufficiently to justify the cost. However, this approach may have value if applied selectively to well-defined high-risk patients. Several large controlled trials have recently examined selective decontamination in multiple trauma patients (Quinio 1996).

The prophylactic use of immunoglobulin has been evaluated in both multitrauma and high-risk surgical ICU patients (see Chapter 47). Treated groups had a reduced incidence of infection compared with patients who received placebo, however there was no significant reduction in mortality. Since immunoglobulin synthesis may be reduced in these patients, administration of IVIG has a rationale, but further studies are needed with this expensive therapy before this practice can be routinely recommended.

## Diagnosis of Infection in the Trauma Victim

Perhaps the most difficult problem related to infection in the trauma victim is simply deciding when an infection is present. Fever is nearly universal in severely injured people, particularly those with head or spine injury, extensive blunt-tissue trauma, or large soft-tissue hematomas. Leukocytosis, thrombocytosis, or thrombocytopenia and coagulopathy may manifest as part of the host inflammatory response to tissue injury rather than infection (see Chapter 53). These physical and laboratory abnormalities may be present within hours of injury and last for days to weeks. This picture can be further complicated by a persistent hypermetabolic state, adult respiratory distress syndrome (ARDS), renal failure, and hepatopathy, which are not caused by an identifiable infection but result solely from the injury. The diagnostic value of inflammatory markers used to identify infection, fever, leukocytosis, and organ dysfunction, is often useless in the trauma patient. Trends or individual measurements that occur out of the patient's own established range become very important. Meticulous monitoring and recording of temperature, white blood cell count, lactate, bilirubin, blood urea nitrogen, creatinine, and coagulation parameters can be of great value in defining trends toward improvement or decline. Likewise, persistent changes in the hemodynamic state, increases in the requirement for respiratory support, or a positive fluid balance can provide subtle, valuable indicators of a developing infection.

Bacteriologic monitoring of patients may be useful. Surveillance cultures per se are not required, but we obtain two sets of blood cultures, a sputum culture and gram stain, a urinalysis, and complete blood count (CBC) for every temperature that exceeds 102.5 °F (39.8 °C), during a 24-hour period. Strict criteria should be used to define infections for both patient care and epidemiologic purposes (see below). Since colonization with pathogens is common, it is not appropriate to initiate antibiotic therapy for a tracheal aspirate or a urine or a wound culture simply because it grows a potential pathogen. Use of culture data must be always closely coupled with a detailed evaluation of the patient's current clinical condition and overall trends. This type of conscious effort will lead to more judicious use of empiric and therapeutic antibiotics.

## Specific Infections in Trauma Patients

### Surgical wound infections

Infections of surgical and trauma wounds account for approximately 10% of trauma infections. The majority of wound infections become evident only 48 hours or more after the surgical procedure (see Chapter 82). Although often not microbiologically proven, the majority of these are caused by *Staphylococcus aureus*, and *Streptococcus* species. A few may be caused by staphylococcus coagulase-negative species. Some surgical wound infections, especially streptococcal, or clostridial infections, occur more rapidly and may be fulminant within 24 hours. Gram-negative rods may also cause wound infections, which are usually polymicrobial. Polymicrobial infections involving gram-negative rods, enterococci, and anaerobes are often present in abdominal and perineal wounds. Promptly recognized and treated, bacteremia should rarely complicate wound infections in a trauma center.

Purulent material obtained from the wound should be gram-stained and cultured. The deeper the specimen (as for instance during debridement) the better, as superficial wound cultures often identify organisms that may not be causing the infection. Simply recovering bacteria from a wound, particularly an open wound, is not an indication for antibiotics. Superficial infections of wounds without substantial spreading cellulitis may often be treated by simply opening the wound and permitting drainage. Infections that involve deeper tissues, that have a substantial component of cellulitis, or that are accompanied by systemic evidence of infection should be treated aggressively with opening, debridement, and antibiotics. Daily inspection of all surgical wounds for swelling, warmth, erythema, and discharge is mandatory (see Chapter 82).

Traumatic wounds must be considered contaminated with microbes. Debridement of these wounds is the critical element in preventing infections. Repeated debridements and irrigations may be necessary over several days to completely remove devitalized/infected tissue and foreign bodies. Although uncommon, several pathogens that would be unusual in any other clinical setting may cause infection following trauma. When the patient has been exposed to brackish or salt water, *Aeromonas hydrophilia* or *Vibrio vulnificus* may cause rapidly progressive, tissue-destroying infections. Also, when soil or plant tissue has been inoculated into a wound, and the wound has not been debrided adequately, infections with *Escherichia coli* and *Pseudomonas aeruginosa*, and with soil fungi and mycobacteria such as *Mycobacterium fortuitum*, *M. chelonae*, or *M. marinum* are possible. These must be suspected and specific cultures obtained; otherwise the organisms will not be identified. Traumatic wounds caused by human or animal bites may also have unique pathogens. These injuries and antimicrobial requirements are discussed in Chapter 95.

### Intra-abdominal infections

If the abdominal CT scan and/or diagnostic peritoneal lavage on admission are negative, the likelihood of a blunt trauma victim developing an intra-abdominal infection is quite small. However, severe blunt trauma that requires laparotomy is associated with a 4% to 5% incidence of intra-abdominal infection. If bowel injury with intra-abdominal soiling has occurred, there is a substantial increase in risk for peritonitis or a complicated intra-abdominal infection. The risk of postoperative infection is increased in patients with blunt abdominal trauma who have kidney, liver, or pancreas injury, have undergone splenectomy, have sustained multiple extra-abdominal injuries, and require multiple blood transfusions.

Penetrating abdominal wounds are often complicated by postoperative peritonitis or intra-abdominal abscess. In one large series an overall abscess rate of 1% (stab) to 6% (gunshot) was found. The risk of infection is increased if the victim is older, has a left colon injury requiring colectomy, requires multiple blood transfusions, or has associated injury to other intra-abdominal organs (Chapter 65). Whether the initial injury is blunt or penetrating, the surgeons must vigorously lavage the abdominal cavity. It has not been resolved whether antiseptics or antibiotics should be part of the lavage fluid. A preemptive antibiotic regimen that covers both gram-negative aerobic organisms and both gram-negative and gram-positive anaerobic organisms is recommended (see Table 84.1). In most cases, antibiotics are not administered for longer than 24 to 48 hours. If the peritoneal soiling is particularly severe, second or third attempts to lavage and debride the abdominal cavity are warranted. In these cases, antibiotics may be continued for up to five to seven days. Infections which may occasionally develop in these patients can be extremely complicated. Difficult cases may involve multiple small collections in the pelvis or between loops of bowel, or infected retroperitoneal hematomas, or involvement of liver or pancreas. Without extensive sampling and culturing of these collections, it is often impossible to determine if any or all are infected. Serial abdominal CT scans may be the best means of noninvasively evaluating the importance of these collections.

Collections are usually drained via percutaneous catheter when clinically indicated. In the seriously ill patient sometimes the only way to resolve this issue is with repeat exploratory laparotomy. However, if the patient is improving on antibiotics and has intra-abdominal collections that cannot be sampled easily by percutaneous techniques, empirical treatment for 10 to 14 days, followed by close observation, is reasonable. Close cooperation among the surgical team, the critical-care physicians, and the infectious-disease specialist is the best approach to the management of these complicated patients (see Chapter 65).

### Post-traumatic CNS infections

Despite the large number of patients with head and spine injuries who are seen in a trauma unit, central nervous system infections are surprisingly uncommon, amounting to less than 4% of infections in head- and spine-injured patients. Three-quarters of those that occur are meningitis. Ventriculitis accounts for most of the rest and is related to the placement of a ventriculostomy catheter.

The possibility that a radiographically undocumented or clinically unrecognized dural tear has occurred in a patient with severe head injury must be considered. As many as 40% of patients with severe fractures of the middle third of the facial skeleton will have an unrecognized cerebrospinal fluid (CSF) fistula. Rhinorrhea and otorrhea are often not identified because the patient is intubated and recumbent and the tympanic membranes may be intact. Remarkably, even with the high number of potential dural tears, very few of these patients develop meningitis; the CSF fistulas close spontaneously. Nevertheless, all should be followed carefully for signs of developing meningitis. If fever or leukocytosis is present, or if an unexplained change in mental status occurs, an emergent CT scan and lumbar puncture are in order.

Head trauma is one situation in which the CT scan is usually indicated prior to lumbar puncture. If meningitis is strongly suspected, antibiotic therapy should not be delayed until after the CT scan. Cerebrospinal fluid should be sent for culture, cell count, protein, glucose, and latex agglutination studies. The gram stain should be done immediately and read by an experienced physician or technician (see Chapter 73). The patient who has severe head injury in whom a lumbar puncture cannot be performed because of brain edema and is clinically suspected of having meningitis, presents a difficult management problem. This dilemma is further complicated as the mental status cannot be assessed because of the injury or sedatives and paralytics. In these patients empirical administration of antibiotics for 7 to 14 days is unavoidable.

The bacteria most likely to be CNS pathogens in the trauma patient who has not had cranial-facial surgery are the upper respiratory flora: *Streptococcus pneumoniae*, *Neisseria meningitidis*, and *Haemophilus influenzae*. When surgical intervention of the face or head has occurred, nosocomial pathogens such as *Staphylococcus aureus*, coagulase-negative staphylococci, and gram-negative rods become potential pathogens. These must be considered when selecting an antibiotic regimen. Bactericidal antibiotics which cross the blood–brain barrier, administered in high doses frequently and intravenously, are essential for management (see Chapter 73).

Prophylactic antibiotics are not used routinely in open CNS injuries, as the risk of infection is low. Although antibiotics may prevent the uncommon occurrence of an early post-traumatic meningitis, the selection for and development of gram-negative meningitis is considered a potential problem of greater magnitude. Due to multiple antibiotic resistance in nosocomial gram-negative bacteria the treatment of meningitis is much more difficult. If brain tissue was grossly exposed or heavily contaminated with foreign material at the time of trauma, both debridement of the tissues by neurosurgeons and preemptive antibiotic therapy are warranted.

Penetrating wounds of the spine may disrupt the dura and increase the risk of meningitis, particularly if the penetrating missile or knife crossed mucosal barriers prior to entering the subarachnoid space. Like patients with open head injuries, those with penetrating spine injuries must be watched very closely; they may first develop a localized meningitis without generalized cerebral manifestations.

Patients with the intraventricular monitoring devices commonly required after severe head injury are at increased risk for CNS infections. Ventriculostomy catheters have been associated with infection rates as high as 10% to 20%. The risk of infection is increased if more than one catheter is required or if prolonged duration of monitoring is necessary. Manipulation and irrigation should be kept at a minimum. Subcutaneous tunneling of the catheter may lower the risk of infection. Prophylactic antibiotics are not indicated for the placement of ventriculostomy catheters in the setting of closed head injury. Daily CSF cultures *and* cell counts provide the most timely and useful means of monitoring for possible infectious complications. Treatment involves removal or replacement of the catheter and administration of antibiotics for either the identified or suspected nosocomial pathogen(s).

## Pneumonia

Pneumonia is a frequent complication of multiple traumatic injuries. Mechanical ventilation bypasses all airway defense mechanisms and exposes the alveoli directly to the upper respiratory flora. The diagnosis of pneumonia requires multiple criteria, including fever, leukocytosis, purulent sputum with a predominant pathogen(s), impaired respiratory function, and a pulmonary infiltrate that does not clear with aggressive physical therapy. Aggressive chest physical therapy and early mobilization are important measures to reduce the incidence of pneumonia.

In the trauma care setting, pneumonia can be broadly separated into early-onset or community-acquired and late-onset or nosocomially acquired infections. Pneumonias developing within two to seven days of the injury are often caused by aspiration at the time of injury or during emergent intubation. The most common pathogens are *Hemophilus* species, *Streptococcus pneumonia*, *Staphylococcus aureus*, and upper-respiratory anaerobes (see Chapter 56). Besides effective chest physical therapy antibiotic therapy which covers the likely pathogens is indicated. Appropriate initial antibiotic choices include either second or third-generation cephalosporin or a beta-lactam combined with a beta-lactamase inhibitor. Definitive therapy can be tailored to the results of sputum culture and sensitivities. Early institution of antibiotics for a suspected pulmonary infection is warranted in patients with pulmonary contusions; pneumonias develop quickly and are often caused by *Staphylococcus aureus* or *Haemophilus influenzae*. *S. aureus* infections in these patients can rapidly evolve into a complicated necrotizing pneumonia, commonly with bacteremia. In patients with pulmonary contusion or hemothoraces, daily sputum gram stains for several days following admission should be obtained. Purulent sputum that grows *S. aureus*, and slow resolution of the contusion on X ray, are indications for antistaphylococcal antibiotic therapy.

Nosocomial pneumonias typically develop after seven days of hospitalization. If they are caused by a gram-negative bacteria the mortality rate is high. Major chest injury, development of ARDS necessitating prolonged intubation, and the prior use of multiple antibiotics are but a few of the factors that predispose trauma patients to nosocomial gram-negative pneumonia. The diagnosis and management of gram-negative pneumonias is discussed in Chapter 56.

## Splenectomy

Patients who have undergone splenectomy may have an impaired ability to produce antibodies in response to infection. They also have reduced ability to clear bacteria from the bloodstream (see Chapter 86). It is not clear that there are more frequently or more severe infections immediately following splenectomy in the trauma patient. However, postsplenectomy leukocytosis and thrombocytosis make it difficult to assess for infectious complications.

Although the long-term risk of postsplenectomy sepsis appears to be quite low for those who have their spleen removed secondary to trauma, efforts to salvage the spleen rather than to remove it have been considered worthwhile. When splenectomy is necessary, pneumococcal vaccine should be administered. Trauma patients' immune response to the vaccine is usually preserved. Although there are no current recommendations regarding the use of *Neisseria meningitidis* or *Haemophilus influenzae* type B conjugate vaccine, both may be considered and are of low potential toxicity. Prophylactic antibiotics are not recommended routinely following splenectomy for trauma because of the low risk of acute and delayed infection.

## ANNOTATED BIBLIOGRAPHY


Caplan ES, Boltansky H, Snyder MS, et al. Response of traumatized splenectomized patients to immediate vaccination with polyvalent pneumococcal vaccine. J Trauma 1983; 23:801–805.

*Documents serologic response to pneumococcal vaccine in blunt-trauma victims.*

Cheadle WG. Immunology of surgical infection. J R Coll Surg Edinb 1992; 37:1–6.

*Overview of immune dysfunction in surgical patients.*

Clark RA, Hyslop NE Jr. Posttraumatic meningitis. In: Infections of the Nervous System. D. Schlossberg, ed. Springer-Verlag, New York, pp 50–63, 1990.

*Excellent review of post-traumatic meningitis.*

Classen DC, Evans RS, Pestotnik SL, et al. The timing of prophylactic administration of antibiotics and the risk of surgical-wound infection. N Engl J Med 1992; 326:281–339.

*Establishes that an optimal window exists for the administration of preoperative antibiotics.*

Cullingford GL, Watkins DN, Watts ADJ, Mallon DF. Severe late postsplenectomy infection. Br J Surg 1991; 78:716–721.

*Reviews the occurrence and timing of severe infections following splenectomy.*

Cushing D, Elliott S, Caplan ES, et al. Herpes Simplex Virus and Cytomegalovirus Excretions Associated with Increased Ventilatory Days in Trauma Patients. Abstract 22. American Association Surgery of Trauma, New Orleans, 1993.

*Describes increased shedding of HSV and CMV following blunt trauma. Mean ventilator days and bacterial pneumonias were increased in patients who excreted virus.*

Faist E, Schinkel C, Zimmer S. Update on the mechanisms of immune suppression of injury and immune modulation. World J Surg. 1996; 20:454.

*Discusses cellular, humoral and cytokine pertubation following trauma. Mentions possibilities for pharmacologic interventions.*

Intravenous Immunoglobulin Collaborative Study Group. Prophylactic intravenous administration of standard immunoglobulin as compared with core-lipopolysaccharide immunoglobulin in patients at high risk of postsurgical infection. N Engl J Med 1992; 327:234–241.

*Double-blind study indicating a benefit to prophylactic administration of immunoglobulin, but not with core-lipopolysaccharide, in reducing postsurgical infection.*

Invatury RR, Zubowski R, Psarras P, et al. Intra-abdominal abscess after penetrating abdominal trauma. J Trauma 1988; 28:1238.

*Twenty-nine patients developed intra-abdominal abscesses following 872 laparotomies for penetrating trauma. Abscesses were more common after gunshot wounds versus stab wounds. Fourteen patients developed multiple organ failure. Anatomic and physiologic scores were useful predictors of these complications.*

Kuchanek KD, Hudson BL. Advance report of final mortality statistics, 1992. Mortality Vital Statistics Report 1994; 43:1.

Maki D, Stolz S, Wheeler S, et al. Prevention of central venous-catheter related bloodstream infection by use of an antiseptic impregnated catheter. Ann Int Med 1997; 127:257.

*Chlorhexidine-silver sulfadiazine catheters were studied in 158 adult medical-surgical ICU patients. Antiseptic catheters were less likely to be colonized when removed. There were fewer catheter associated bacteremias in the treatment group, but the total number of blood stream infections were small.*

Miller-Graziano CL, Gyongyi S, Kodys K, Griffey K. Aberrations in posttrauma monocyte (MO) subpopulation: role in septic shock syndrome. J Trauma 1990; 30:S86–96.

*An aberrant monocyte population produced IL-6, $TNF_{\alpha}$, $TGF_{\beta}$, and $PGE_2$ in substantial quantities post-trauma and after bacterial challenge.*

Page CP, Bohnen JM, Fletcher R, McManus AT, et al. Antimicrobial prophylaxis for surgical wounds. Arch Surg 1993; 128:79–88.

*Good review of the general principles of antibiotic prophylaxis, and site-specific considerations and recommendations.*

Quinio B, Albanese J, Bues-Charbit M, et al. Selective decontamination of the digestive tract in multiple trauma patients. A prospective double-blind, randomized, placebo-controlled study. Chest 1996; 109:765.

*SDD reduced the incidence of broncho pneumonia and total antibiotic costs, but mortality and length of stay in the ICU were not changed.*

Reed RL, Ericsson CD, Wu A, et al. The pharmacokinetics of prophylactic antibiotics in trauma. J Trauma 1992; 32:21–26.

*The study specifically looked at amikacin kinetics post-abdominal trauma, but clearly points out how we may underdose prophylactic antibiotics in severely injured young people.*

Stillwell M, Caplan ES. The septic multiple-trauma patient. Crit Care Clin 1988; 4:345–373.

*Excellent review of trauma-related infections in general and specifically, ten years of experience in one trauma-center.*

Waydhas C, Nast-Kolb D, Jochum M, et al. Inflammatory mediators, infection, sepsis, and multiple organ failure after severe trauma. Arch Surg 1992; 127:460–467.

*Early-onset multiple organ failure may result from severe trauma without any obvious contribution from infection.*

# 85

## Prosthetic Device Infections

WERNER ZIMMERLI

In this chapter the problem of implant-associated infection is described. The most frequent infections and those with a complex management are presented in more detail. Prosthetic valve endocarditis is discussed in Chapter 66, and catheter-related infections in Chapter 67.

The presence of foreign material increases the pathogenic potential of bacteria. Many foreign devices transect cutaneous barriers, and thus provide a direct route of bacterial invasion. Implants are coated by a film of proteins such as fibronectin, fibrin, and laminin. Fibronectin plays a crucial role in promoting initial staphylococcal attachment. In addition, subcutaneous implants have been shown to impair the phagocytic-bactericidal capacity of local granulocytes. Device-related infections persist without treatment. This may be due to resistance of adherent bacteria to phagocytosis. Bacteria involved in device-related infections have a slow growth rate and adhere to surfaces. Many antibiotics are not bactericidal against staphylococci in the stationary phase of growth. Rifampin is an exception and only regimens including rifampin are efficacious against experimental *Staphylococcus aureus* foreign-body infections. The role of rifampin is now established in a controlled clinical study.

### Infections Associated with Cerebrospinal Fluid (CSF) Prosthetic Devices

Neurosurgical devices are used for the management of clinical conditions involving the CSF fluid dynamics. The main indications for CSF devices are the obstruction of the CSF flow, and occasionally the need for administration of drugs. Since the first use of internal CSF shunts in the early 1960s, different techniques have been used. Ventriculoperitoneal shunts are now the most common devices. In emergency surgery a temporary external ventricular drainage is preferred.

#### Etiology and epidemiology

Coagulase-negative staphylococci, especially *S. epidermidis*, cause more than 50% of the CSF shunt infections. These microorganisms predominate not only in early (<30 days), but also in late infections. *S. aureus* accounts for about 20%, streptococci for 10%, and gram-negative bacilli for 5%–15% of the shunt-associated infections. Skin microorganisms of low virulence, such as anaerobic diphtheroids, cause 5%–10% of CSF infections related to devices. The prevalence of infection has been highly variable, from <3% up to >30% of implanted shunts, due to the heterogenous patient groups and variable follow-up periods. Main risk factors for infection are extreme age (<1 and >60 years), revision surgery, and previous external drainage. During the last 20 years, the incidence of shunt infection has gradually decreased to 5% in internal CSF devices and to 5%–10% in ventriculostomy with external drainage.

#### Pathophysiology and clinical features

Shunts are infected by four different mechanisms: (*1*) colonization during surgery, (*2*) wound infection, (*3*) ascending infection from the distal end, and (*4*) hematogenous infection. The first mechanism is probably the most important, since microorganisms from skin flora are frequently implicated. Retrograde infection is a rare consequence of gut or bladder perforation by the peritoneal part of the shunt. The hematogenous route is not well documented.

One-third of the shunt-associated infections occur during initial hospitalization. Initial diagnosis may be difficult due to nonspecific fever in neurosurgical patients after trauma or surgery. The main symptoms are fever, irritability, anorexia, and behavioral changes. In case of shunt obstruction, signs of intracranial hypertension (e.g. headache and vomiting) predominate. In patients with ventriculoatrial shunts, tricuspid endocarditis has to be considered. If the infection becomes chronic, systemic signs of immune complex disease ("shunt nephritis") are occasionally observed.

#### Diagnosis

A CT scan that reveals hydrocephalus, or abdominal ultrasound that discloses a peritoneal cyst, indicates shunt dysfunction suggesting infection. The clinician should strive for a microbiological diagnosis. The lumbar puncture does not necessarily reveal shunt infection, whereas CSF from the shunt reservoir has been shown to be positive in >95% of the cases. This procedure must be performed under optimal sterile conditions. In the CSF, cell number and type, glucose, lactate, protein, gram stain, and culture should be performed. In normal ventricular CSF, the cell number is $<5 \times 10^6$/l without polymorphonuclear leukocytes, the CSF/serum glucose ratio >50%, the lactate concentration <3.5 mmol/l, and protein concentrations <150 mg/l. Blood cultures are often positive (>90%) in ventriculoatrial, but seldom (<25%) in ventriculoperitoneal shunt infection. In a typical clinical situation, or if CSF abnormalities are present, positive blood or CSF cultures for diphtheroids or coagulase-negative staphylococci should never be considered as contaminants.

#### Treatment and prophylaxis

If shunt infection is suspected, empirical antibiotic treatment has to be started immediately after sampling for microbiological tests. Since no recent prospective, randomized study has been performed to evaluate the best treatment option, no uncontroversial recommendations for the choice of the antimicrobial agents and the duration of treatment can be given. The therapeutic objectives are cure of infection and the maintenance of device function. These two goals are somewhat contradictory, since cure often requires removal of the foreign material. For empirical antibiotic therapy the following properties of the drugs are required: (*1*) A spectrum against the most frequent etiologic agents, (*2*) good penetration into CSF, and (*3*) activity on adherent microorganisms. No single agent fulfills all these criteria. A rational option, which however cannot be based on published clinical data, is the triple combination of vancomycin (1 g BID IV) or teicoplanin (800 mg QD IV) plus rifampin (600 mg BID IV) plus ceftriaxone (2 g BID IV). Rifampin and ceftriaxone have a good penetration into CSF, and vancomycin or teicoplanin should be added in order to prevent emergence of rifampin-resistent staphylococci. If shunt infection is microbiologically proven, and the neurosurgical device still required, various options have to be considered: (*1*) one-stage exchange of the shunt system and high-dose antibiotic therapy guided by the drug susceptibility testing, (*2*) removal of the device, ventriculostomy with temporary external drainage, reshunting after CSF sterilization (three to seven days) and a two- to three-week course of systemic antibiotic therapy, and (*3*) three to six weeks of IV antibiotic treatment without exchange of the device. Intraventricular therapy should be reserved for cases which do not respond to systemic antibiotics. In case of infection with gram-positive microorganisms, local treatment with teicoplanin (20 mg every 24–48 h) guarantees excellent bactericidal titers in the CSF. With a one-stage device replacement combined with high-dose antibiotics, roughly 70% of the infections can be eliminated. Delayed replacement with temporary ventriculostomy has a cure rate of >90%. Systemic treatment without removal of the infected shunt is successful in <40%. However, it can be tried in infections due to coagulase-negative staphylococci susceptible to rifampin. Antibiotic prophylaxis is recommended for shunt implantation. In a randomized double-blind trial, a two-day course of cotrimoxazole has proven its efficacy.

## Infections in Continuous Ambulatory Peritoneal Dialysis (CAPD)

Permanent indwelling peritoneal access devices for peritoneal dialysis have been used since the mid-1960s. CAPD is now a widely accepted treatment modality in chronic renal failure. The peritoneal access device (Tenckhoff catheter) is frequently complicated by infection.

### Etiology and epidemiology

*S. aureus* and coagulase-negative staphylococci are the predominant etiologic agents causing 50%–80% of the peritonitis episodes. Roughly 10% are caused by streptococci, and 20% by gram-negative bacilli. Rare isolates include fungi and mycobacteria.

The rate of peritonitis has markedly decreased over the past 10 years. Between 1979 and 1989 a decrease from 2.4 to 0.8 episodes per year has been reported in a U.S. study. The decrease of infective episodes is mainly due to better instruction of the patient, technical improvement of the device (e.g. titanium adapter), and especially to the elimination of *S. aureus* nasal carriage by local mupirocin ointment. With continuous mupirocin calcium ointment (2%) prophylaxis applied to the exit site, *S. aureus* catheter infection and peritonitis are as low as 0.13 and 0.04 episodes/dialysis year.

### Pathophysiology and clinical features

Four main sources of microbial contamination involved in CAPD-related infection can be recognized: (*1*) catheter contamination during implantation, (*2*) contamination of dialysis tubing during manipulation, (*3*) contaminated dialysate, and (*4*) bowel perforation. It is well documented that ascending infection during manipulation is the most important mechanism in exit site infection, since the rate of infection is fourfold higher in *S. aureus* carriers compared to noncarriers. Peritonitis is characterized by abdominal pain, nausea, vomiting, fever, and cloudy effluent after dialysis. Only a few patients manifest all these symptoms, and often in a mild form. Exit site and tunnel infections show local erythema, tenderness, and drainage.

### Diagnosis

The diagnosis of CAPD-associated infection is based on the triad of fever, abdominal pain, and cloudy drainage, and substantiated by dialysate analysis. The normal cell count in the effluent is below $5 \times 10^7$/l. During peritonitis a rise above $10^8$/l with a shift from mononuclear cells to granulocytes is observed. The centrifuged effluent reveals microorganisms in the gram stain in only 10%–40% of the cases. The most sensitive technique for culturing of peritoneal fluid is its injection in a blood culture system. Alternatively, a centrifugation lysis technique can be used. Ultrasound examination may reveal pericatheter fluid collection under some circumstances, e.g. in case of tunnel infection, which usually cannot be diagnosed by clinical criteria only.

### Treatment and prophylaxis

The treatment should be started as soon as a tentative diagnosis has been established. In general, the intraperitoneal (IP) route is recommended. The most important regimens are summarized in Table 85.1. Prolonged or repeated use of aminoglycosides should be avoided because of ototoxicity. The treatment of CAPD-related peritonitis has been reviewed by an advisory committee. The following management was proposed: If the gram stain reveals gram-positive or no bacteria, IP cefazolin plus aminoglycoside should be started. In centers with a high prevalence of methicillin-resistant *S. aureus*, vancomycin instead of cefazolin should be used. If gram-negative microorganisms are seen, treatment should be started with a third-generation cephalosporin (e.g., ceftazidime). In case of yeast, oral fluconazole (50–100 mg/day PO) can be tried. However, sometimes systemic amphotericin B is required. The presence of mixed flora suggests the possibility of a perforated viscus, and prompt surgical evaluation is warranted. In general, peritonitis due to gram-positive bacteria is treated for 10 days. In peritonitis due to gram-negative bacilli a 14-day course is suggested, with the exception of *Pseudomonas* or *Stenotrophomonas*, which are treated for at least three weeks. In patients with persistent symptoms after five to seven days of adequate antibiotic treatment, catheter removal should be considered. This is also necessary in fungal, mycobacterial, and *Pseudomonas* peritonitis, and in cases of three or more episodes of peritonitis with the same microorganism.

The most important measure to prevent peritonitis is the practice of meticulous aseptic techniques by patients and staff. Since *S. aureus* carriers have an increased risk of peritonitis, eradication of *S. aureus* from the nares and the skin is important. Mupirocin effectively decreases *S. aureus* nasal carriage, peri-

**Table 85.1** Antibiotic regimens for continuous intraperitoneal dosing of drugs in patients with CAPD-associated peritonitis (per 60–80 kg adult)*

| Drug | Initial loading dose (mg/L) | Maintenance dose (mg/L) |
|---|---|---|
| Cefazolin | 500 | 125 |
| Cefamandole | 500 | 250 |
| Ceftazidime | 250 | 125 |
| Imipenem | 500 | 200 |
| Vancomycin | 1000 | 25 |
| Teicoplanin | 400 | 40 |
| Amikacin | 25 | 12 |
| Gentamicin | 8 | 4 |
| Netilmicin | 8 | 4 |
| Tobramycin | 8 | 4 |

*According to Keane et al, p. 569; see Annotated Bibliography.

*Note*: Fluconazole, metronidazole, nafcillin, flucloxacillin, rifampin, trimethoprim-sulfamethoxazole, and quinolones should be given orally, and amphotericin B, piperacillin, and ticarcillin by the IV route.

tonitis, and exit site infection. It can be applied either monthly for 5 days in both nares or continuously to the exit site.

## Infections Associated with Orthopedic Devices

Orthopedic devices are used for bone fixation or joint replacement. Infection is frequent after internal fixation of open bone fractures, but rare after joint replacement. Infections associated with such devices are difficult to treat. Multiple surgical interventions are often required.

### Etiology and epidemiology

In all large series, *S. aureus* and coagulase-negative staphylococci are the most important microorganisms, accounting for about 50% of the infections. Other microorganisms such as enterobacteriaceae, streptococci, or anaerobes are less frequent. After stabilization of open fractures, mixed infections are common. The infection rate varies according to the type of surgery. After internal fixation of closed fractures or hip replacement it should be <1%–1.5%, after knee replacement <2%, and after elbow replacement <7%–9%. A high infection rate is observed after internal fixation of open fractures, namely 1%–5% after first degree, 5%–8% after second degree, and >10% after third degree. The latter type of fractures have to be considered as infected a priori.

### Pathophysiology and clinical features

As in other types of device-related infections, a local defect of host defense, and microbial adherence to the implant are important pathogenetic factors. Infections after joint replacement are classified as early, delayed, or hematogenous: Early infections are diagnosed during the first three months after surgery. They usually develop after wound infection or from an infected hematoma. Delayed or low-grade infections are characterized by subtle signs of inflammation, chronic persistent postoperative pain, or early loosening of the implant during the first two years after surgery. Hematogenous infections occur at any time after surgery. They are characterized by an acute onset with signs of infection (fever, local pain and inflammation), either with a primary focus or without detectable focus. Early hematogenous infection occurs after urinary tract infection; later on, skin infection, enterocolitis, and pneumonia are the most important sources.

The clinical picture of infection after internal fixation is characterized by local signs of inflammation, sinus tracts and fever. Due to the superficial localization of most internal fixation devices, the clinical diagnosis is easy.

### Diagnosis

There is no specific laboratory test for the diagnosis of device-related infection. Leukocytosis with increased band forms is typical, but not specific and may even be absent. The same applies for the C-reactive protein. Infection has to be considered if the C-reactive protein does not adequately decrease after surgery. The $^{99m}$technetium scan alone is not useful during several months after surgery. Its interpretation is improved by a simultaneous leukocyte scan. With plain radiographs, loosening can be diagnosed. Arthrography or fistulography allow judgement of the bone–cement interphase. For the optimal antimicrobial treatment, deep-tissue specimens or fluid aspirates should be cultured. If revision surgery is required, multiple tissue samples, not swab specimens, should be gained.

### Treatment and prophylaxis

Infections associated with internal fixation devices should be treated at least two weeks with intravenous antibiotics followed by three months of oral therapy according to Table 85.2. Revision surgery for microbiological diagnosis and debridement is usually required. The internal fixation device should be kept in place if it is still required and efficacious for stability. In case of instability, all foreign material should be explanted. In such cases, external fixation is a satisfactory method to stabilize bone fragments.

In infections associated with joint replacement, the type of surgical treatment of infection is based on consideration of various prognostic indicators. Figure 85.1 shows an algorithm of the

**Table 85.2** Systemic antimicrobial treatment of the most frequent infective agents in orthopedic device-associated infection

| Infective agent | Drug regimen | Dose[a] | Route |
|---|---|---|---|
| *Staphylococcus aureus* or coagulase-negative staphylococci | | | |
| Methicillin-sensitive | Nafcillin or flucloxacillin | 8 g/d | IV |
| | + rifampin | 900 mg/d | p.os |
| | × 2 weeks, followed by | | |
| | Ciprofloxacin | 1500 mg/d | p.os* |
| | + rifampin | 900 mg/d | p.os* |
| Methicillin-resistant | Vancomycin | 2 g/d | IV |
| | + rifampin | 900 mg/d | p.os |
| | × 2 weeks, followed by | | |
| | Ciprofloxacin[b] | 1500 mg/d | p.os* |
| | or fusidic acid | 500 mg/d | p.os* |
| | or teicoplanin | 400 mg/d | IV |
| | or cotrimoxazole | 2 ds tablets/d | p.os* |
| | + rifampin | 900 mg/d | p.os* |
| *Streptococcus* spp. | Penicillin G | 20 Mio U/d | IV |
| | × 4 weeks, followed by | | |
| | Amoxicillin | 2250 mg/d | p.os* |
| Anaerobes | Clindamycin | 2400 mg/d | IV |
| | × 2–4 weeks, followed by | | |
| | Clindamycin | 1200 mg/d | p.os* |
| Quinolone-sensitive gram-negative bacilli (except *Pseudomonas aeruginosa*) | Ciprofloxacin | 1500 mg/d | p.os* |
| *Pseudomonas aeruginosa* | Ceftazidim or cefepime | 6 g/d | IV |
| | + tobramycin × 2–4 weeks, followed by | | |
| | Ciprofloxacin | 1500 mg/d | p.os* |
| Mixed infection | Imipenem | 1500 mg/d | IV |
| | × 2–4 weeks, followed by individual regimens according to the susceptibility tests | | |

*Note*: susceptibility has to be confirmed.

*Duration: at least 3 months, or until 1 month after normalization of laboratory and clinical signs of infection.

[a]Dosages are shown for patients with normal renal and hepatic function; for dose modification in renal failure see Chapter 22.

[b]Quinolones should not be used in infections due to methicillin-resistant *S. aureus* because emergence of resistance frequently occurs.

management of suspected or confirmed hip arthroplasty. An infection of short duration in a patient with stable prosthesis can be treated by antibiotics alone, if there is no collection of fluid, otherwise revision surgery is required. An infection of long duration (≥1 year) or with loose prosthesis should always be treated by exchange of the implant. In case of microorganisms of low virulence and good bone and tissue conditions, an one-stage exchange is proposed by most authors. In all other cases, a two-stage exchange is required. Antibiotic treatment should be guided according to Table 85.2.

Perioperative antibiotic prophylaxis with a cephalosporin (cefazolin, cefamandole) had proved its efficacy. Especially in revision surgery, antibiotic-impregnated cement is used by most orthopedic surgeons. However, the definite proof of its efficacy is still lacking. In case of open fractures, an empirical short-term treatment of one to two weeks with a broad-spectrum antibiotic (cephalosporin or amoxicillin/clavulanic acid) is more appropriate than prophylaxis.

## Infections Associated with Pacemakers and Implantable Cardioverter Defibrillators (ICDs)

Permanent pacemakers are being increasingly used due to the aging of the population and broader indications. Since 1980 the automatic ICD has evolved as effective therapy for prevention of sudden cardiac death. Erosion of the generator pocket is more frequent with these devices than with pacemakers. Therefore, the risk for infection is higher in ICD. Pacemaker- and ICD-associated infections involve either the pulse-generator pocket, the electrode or both.

### Etiology and epidemiology

Most pacemaker- and ICD-associated infections are caused by staphylococci. During the first month after surgery *S. aureus* predominates. Delayed infections are generally caused by skin microorganisms of low virulence such as coagulase-negative staphylococci. In late hematogenous infection any microorganism can colonize the electrode. Infections with *Candida* spp., *Salmonella* spp. and other gram-negative microorganisms have been occasionally described. The rate of pacemaker infections varies from 0.13% to >10%. Nowadays it should not exceed 1%. The infection rate of ICD varies from 2%–11%.

### Pathophysiology and clinical features

Early infection (<2 weeks after surgery) is mainly caused by perioperative contamination of the device. Later infections are due to delayed infection with microorganisms of low virulence ac-

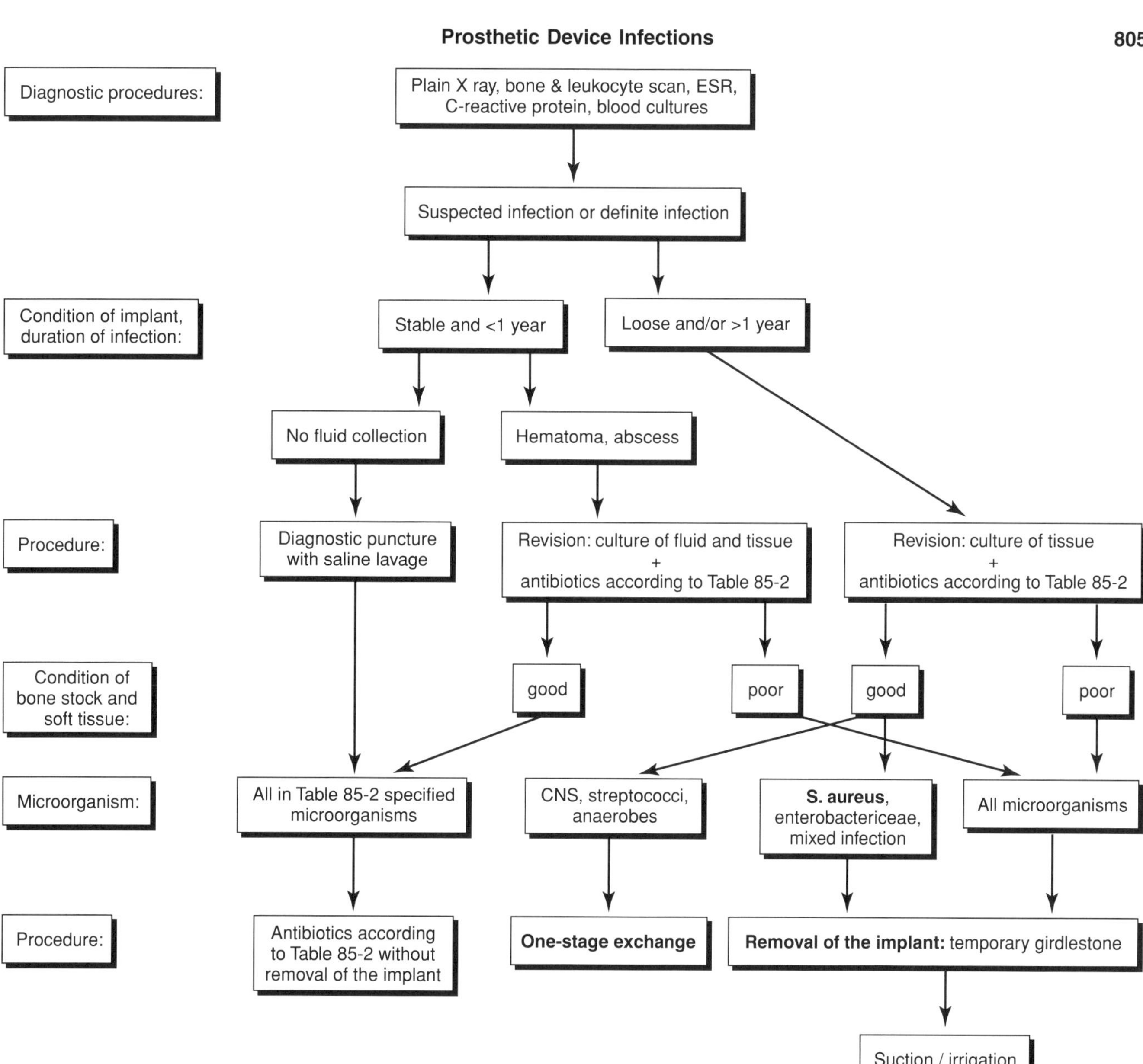


**Fig. 85.1** Management of infected hip arthroplasty.

quired during surgery, late wound infection following skin erosion over the pocket, or, rarely, hematogenous seeding to the pacemaker lead. Predisposing factors favoring infection include multiple revisions, pocket hematoma, skin erosion, diabetes mellitus, and steroid use.

The clinical presentation of pacemaker- and ICD-associated infection depends on which part of the system is infected. Pocket infection is more common than electrode infection. This is especially true for ICD, which may erode the generator pocket by pressure leading to infection after breaking of the skin. Most early infections are localized in the generator pocket, but can progress to clinical sepsis. Electrode infection may appear only months after implantation. About 15% are early-onset infections (<2 weeks), 40% are intermediate (2–26 weeks), and 45% are late onset (>6 months). The clinical picture varies from local signs of inflammation of the pocket or the tunnel, to systemic sepsis or endocarditis. In case of local necrosis, the diagnosis is obvious. However, if a patient has only fever and/or positive blood cultures, pacemaker-associated infection must be actively looked for, despite the lack of local manifestations.

## Diagnosis

Pocket infection can be suspected clinically, and confirmed by a laboratory work-up including differential white cell counts, C-reactive protein, several sets of blood cultures, and pocket aspiration if the ultrasound examination reveals an exudate. Electrode-associated infection is suspected in case of continuous bacteremia or unexplained increase of the pacing threshold. Transesophageal echocardiography may demonstrate vegetations on the tricuspid valve or on the electrode.

### Treatment and prophylaxis

The management of pacemaker- and ICD-associated infection is not standardized. A conservative treatment without removal of the device has a high failure rate. Therefore, all foreign material should generally be removed if blood or wound cultures are positive. Later than two months after surgery, manual lead removal is rarely successful. Entrapped electrodes can be removed by different techniques such as weighted traction, grasping with a Dotter basket, or an endomyocardial biopsy forceps. All these procedures are potentially dangerous, and have to be performed by an experienced person with a surgical backup. Appropriate empirical antibiotic treatment consists of high-dose nafcillin or flucloxacillin (2 g IV Q6h) combined with an aminoglycoside. In centers with endemic methicillin-resistent *S. aureus*, vancomycin (1 g BID IV) instead of nafcillin should be used. This regimen must be adapted according to the microbiological results. If endocarditis is excluded, and the device completely removed or exchanged, high-dose treatment should be continued for at least two weeks, or according to the clinical and laboratory (e.g., C-reactive protein) response. The pacemaker or ICD can be replaced with one-stage or two-stage surgery. In both cases, the anatomical position should be changed.

The risk of infection can be minimized if implantation is performed in the operating theater, the generator is placed submuscularly, and meticulous hemostasis is applied. There is no controlled study on antimicrobial prophylaxis with a timely regimen. However, as in other implant surgery, 1 g cefazolin as a single dose before surgery or continued every 6 hours after surgery for 24 hours is suggested.

## Infections Associated with Intrauterine Contraceptive Devices (IUDs)

IUDs were first described in 1909 and have been increasingly used during the last 60 years. During the late 1970s and early 1980s, an association between IUDs and pelvic inflammatory disease (PID) was shown in case-control studies. In a recent WHO-trial survey it was shown that PID among IUD users was most strongly related to the insertion process and to a background risk of sexually transmissible disease. During the first 20 days after insertion the incidence was 9.7 per 1000 years, and then dropped to a stable incidence of 1.4 per 1000 years. It was therefore concluded that IUDs should be left in place up to their maximum lifespan and should not routinely be replaced earlier. The risk of PID was 4.7 times higher in Africa than in the United States. A special problem in patients with IUDs is colonization with *Actinomyces*. *Actinomyces israelii* is part of the endogenous flora of humans and is found in the female reproductive tract. The spectrum of infection attributable to this organism extends from asymptomatic colonization to life-threatening disseminated pelvic actinomycosis mimicking metastatic carcinoma. The diagnosis of actinomycosis is difficult and requires a high degree of suspicion. Colonization with *Actinomyces* is detected by the use of Papanicolaou smears. Invasive actinomycosis is suspected when a pelvic mass is detected by clinical examination, ultrasound, or CT scan. Confirmation requires a guided biopsy for histology and anaerobic culture. Asymptomatic colonization with *Actinomyces* cannot be eradicated without removing the IUD. Symptomatic infection must be treated by removal of the IUD and high-dose penicillin (24 Mio U/day IV). Clindamycin (600 mg TID) combined with a quinolone is an alternative, since actinomycosis is most often a mixed infection. Surgical treatment is required in case of large abscesses with fistulous tracts.

## Infections Associated with Vascular Grafts

Infection of vascular grafts is the most serious complication of reconstructive vascular surgery, endangering not only the limb but also the life of the patient. Infection may occur immediately after surgery or develop at any time later.

### Etiology and epidemiology

According to 10 large series, 32% of the infections are due to *S. aureus*, 18% to coagulase-negative staphylococci, 13% to *E. coli*, 9% to streptococci and enterococci, 17% to different gram-negative bacilli, 3% to anaerobes, and 8% to miscellaneous microorganisms.

The true incidence of vascular graft-associated infection is unknown, because many infections occur late after surgery. In eight large series published during the last 30 years, the mean rate of graft infection was 2.7% (range 1.3%–6%). In the more recent series the incidence rate was at the lower limit of this range. The risk varies according to the site of implantation, and is highest with femoropopliteal protheses, and with the groin access. Other risk factors are diabetes mellitus, preoperative skin infection, postoperative urinary tract infection, prolonged ileus after surgery, and transient bacteremia. Aortic graft infection carries a mortality rate of 25%–75%. Peripheral grafts have a lower mortality rate of 5%–10%, but the amputation rate is between 30% and 60%.

### Pathophysiology and clinical features

Vascular graft infections are classified as early (within 2 months) and late (>2 months) after surgery. In two-thirds of the infections, the first symptoms occur immediately after surgery. In these cases, bacterial inoculation is thought to arise by contamination of the graft, by a contaminated wound after traumatic lesion, by the skin surface or nonsterile lymph in case of a peripheral skin infection, or by an intraoperatively opened viscus. Late infection may result from perioperative graft contamination with a microorganism of low virulence (e.g., *S. epidermidis*), or from bacteremia. The risk for hematogenous seeding decreases with time, and depends on the integrity of the neointima, as shown in animal studies.

The main signs are fever and wound infection, including hematoma and abscess formation, cellulitis, fistula, or graft exposure. If an aortic graft is inserted for a ruptured aortic aneurysm, postoperative fever is difficult to interpret. If the fever starts with a delay after surgery, graft infection must be suspected. Prolonged ileus after aortic graft surgery is frequent and reflects enteric ischemia. If late infection is suspected, the patient must be examined for recurrent inguinal wound infection, sinus drainage, gastrointestinal bleeding, and unexplained fever. Signs of peripheral septic emboli, thrombosis, new murmur, fistula, and wound discharge must be looked for. Finally, vascular graft infection may have unusual manifestations such as gastrointestinal bleeding, due to graft-enteric erosions or fistula. Other symptoms of this complication are fever, malaise, septic shock, and abdominal pain.

## Diagnosis

Laboratory signs of graft infection include increased C-reactive protein, and leukocytosis with a left shift. Microbiological identification should be attempted by blood cultures and/or needle aspiration of the perigraft space. CT scan or ultrasound detects gas, soft-tissue swelling, false aneurysm, or fluid surrounding the prothesis. CT-guided aspiration may confirm diagnosis. Bowel wall thickening >5 mm suggests graft-enteric fistula. The role of leukocyte scanning is controversial. This techniques has a high sensitivity (>80%) but a low specificity. The $^{111}$In-labeled human immunoglobulin G scan has an improved sensitivity and specificity. Magnetic resonance imaging can give precise extent of graft inflammation. However, periprosthetic fluid collection is physiologically present in 90% of the patients during the first week, and disappears only within 24 weeks. Angiography provides little help in confirming graft infection but may reveal graft thrombosis or a false aneurysm.

## Treatment and prophylaxis

The goals of the management of vascular graft infection include arresting hemorrhage, preservation of blood circulation and eradication of the microorganisms. The treatment depends on whether an aortic graft or an infrainguinal graft is infected. Surgical management of aortic graft infection includes an extra-anatomic bypass through a noninfected field. If the anastomosis is involved in infection, or in case of infected thrombosis, the graft has to be exchanged. In selected cases, revision surgery with suction/irrigation and muscle flap coverage is successful. In any case, surgery should be combined with a high-dose antibiotic regimen. Imipenem (0.5 g Q6h IV) is a reasonable empirical choice, and definitive treatment should be optimized according to the microbiological results. In case of *S. aureus* or *S. epidermidis*, the combination of flucloxacillin, nafcillin (2 g Q6h IV), or vancomycin (1 g BID IV) with rifampin (450 mg BID p.os or IV) may be advantageous; however, the role of rifampin has not been studied in clinical trials. For long-term treatment, an oral combination of a quinolone plus rifampin is reasonable. If the infected graft is left in place, treatment should be continued for about three months.

In infrainguinal graft infection, the surgical management depends on the patency of the distal vessels, and their suitability for a bypass. It involves either excision and revascularization with autologous material, continuous suction/irrigation combined with muscle flaps to cover the infected groin, or amputation. The antibiotic treatment is the same as described above. Perioperative antibiotic prophylaxis with a cephalosporin has proved its efficacy in randomized trials and is mandatory. Since the groin is the area most prone to infection, it should be avoided as the main incision site. Hematoma and lymphocele are strongly associated with wound and graft infection. Prevention includes meticulous hemostasis. The potential value of antibiotic prophylaxis during potential episodes of bacteremia (dental work, genitourinary or gastrointestinal tract manipulation) is unknown but usually advised.

## ANNOTATED BIBLIOGRAPHY


Bernardini J, Holley JL, Johnston JR, et al. An analysis of ten-year trends in infection in adults on continuous ambulatory peritoneal dialysis (CAPD). Clin Nephrol 1991; 36:29–34.

*Analysis of 303 episodes of CAPD-related infections over a 10-year period (1979–1989).*

Bernardini J, Piraino B, Holley J, et al. A randomized trial of *Staphylococcus aureus* prophylaxis in peritoneal dialysis patients: Mupirocin calcium ointment 2% applied to the exit site versus cyclic oral rifampin. Am J Kid Dis 1996; 27:695–700.

*Trial showing that mupirocin at the exit site provides an excellent prophylaxis for S. aureus peritonitis and exit site infection.*

Brodman R, Frame R, Andrews C, Furman S. Removal of infected transvenous leads requiring cardiopulmonary bypass or inflow occlusion. J Thorac Cardiovasc Surg 1992; 103:649–654.

*Restrospective study of 42 patients infected with transvenous leads in a 17-year observation of 7435 patients. Discussion of the management.*

Cruciani M, Navarra A, Di Perri G, et al. Evaluation of intraventricular teicoplanin for the treatment of neurosurgical shunt infections. Clin Infect Dis 1992; 15:285–289.

*Successful treatment of seven patients with CSF shunt infections with intraventricular teicoplanin. Excellent bactericidal activity of the CSF after intraventricular teicoplanin.*

Drancourt M, Stein A, Argenson JN, et al. Oral treatment of *Staphylococcus spp.* infected orthopaedic implants with fusidic acid or ofloxacin in combination with rifampicin. J Antimicrob Chemother 1997; 39:235–249.

*Rifampin plus ofloxacin and rifampin plus fusidic acid are equally effective in staphylococcal implant infections. Relatively low efficacy (50% vs 55%) because revision surgery was not performed, and part of the implants were unstable.*

Farley TMM, Rosenberg MJ, Rowe PJ, et al. Intrauterine devices and pelvic inflammatory disease: an international perspective. Lancet 1992; 339:785–788.

*This review of the WHO IUD clinical trial data explores the incidence and patterns of pelvic inflammatory disease (PID) risk with the use of IUD. The authors conclude that PID among IUD users is most strongly related to the insertion process and to the risk of sexually transmissible disease.*

Hannon RJ, Wolfe JHN, Mansfield AO. Aortic prosthetic infection: 50 patients treated by radical or local surgery. Br J Surg 1996; 83:654–658.

*Radical graft excision remains the preferred treatment in aortic prosthetic infection.*

Keane WF, Alexander SR, Bailie GR, et al. Peritoneal dialysis-related peritonitis treatment recommendations: 1996 update. Perit Dial Int 1996; 16:557–573.

*Recommendation of an advisory committee on peritonitis management. Diagnostic and therapeutic aspects are covered.*

Luzar MA, Coles GA, Faller B, et al. Staphylococcus aureus nasal carriage and infection in patients on continuous ambulatory peritoneal dialysis. N Engl J Med 1990; 322:505–509.

*In a study of 140 consecutive patients with CAPD, the relation of the nasal carriage of* S. aureus *to subsequent catheter exit-site infection or peritonitis is analyzed. The authors conclude that the nasal carriage of* S. aureus *is associated with increased risk of infection.*

Malone JM, Moore WS. Bacteremic infectability of vascular grafts: the influence of pseudointimal integrity and duration of graft function. Surgery 1975; 78:211–216.

*Animal model which illustrates the protective effect of the neointima during experimental bacteremia.*

Morissette I, Gourdeau M, Francoeur J. CSF shunt infections: a fifteen-year experience with emphasis on management and outcome. Can J Neurol Sci 1993; 20:118–122.

*Retrospective study of 44 episodes of CSF shunt infections in 38 patients. Analysis of different treatment options.*

O'Brien T, Collin J. Prosthetic vascular graft infection. Br J Surg 1992; 79:1262–1267.

*A review of the etiology, diagnosis, and management of prosthetic vascular graft infection.*

Pfeiffer D, Jung W, Fehske W, et al. Complications of pacemaker-defibrillator devices: diagnosis and management. Am Heart J 1994; 127:1073–1080.

*Retrospective study of 140 patients with pacemaker-defibrillator devices. Analysis of infections and other complications.*

Steckelberg JM, Osmon DR. Prosthetic joint infections. In: Infections Associated with Indwelling Medical Devices, 2nd ed. Bisno AL, Waldvogel FA, eds. American Society of Microbiologists, Washington, DC, pp 259–290, 1994.

*An excellent review of the various aspects of prosthetic joint infections and an analysis of 1033 cases of total hip and knee arthroplasty infections.*

Vaudaux PE, Lew DP, Waldvogel FA. Host factors predisposing to and influencing therapy of foreign body infections. In: Infections Associated with Indwelling Medical Devices, 2nd ed. Bisno AL, Waldvogel FA, eds. American Society of Microbiologists, Washington, DC, pp 1–29, 1994.

*A comprehensive review of different aspects of the pathogenesis of implant-associated infections.*

Von Graevenitz A, Amsterdam D. Microbiological aspects of peritonitis associated with continuous ambulatory peritoneal dialysis. Clin Microbiol Rev 1992; 5:36–48.

*An excellent review of pathogenesis, diagnostic features, epidemiology, and prevention of peritonitis in CAPD patients.*

Zimmerli W, Lew PD, Waldvogel FA. Pathogenesis of foreign body infection: evidence for a local granulocyte defect. J Clin Invest 1984; 73:1191–1200.

*Experimental guinea pig model showing that the interaction of exudate granulocytes with a nonphagocytosable implant results in a local granulocyte defect.*

Zimmerli W, Widmer AF, Blatter M, et al, for the Foreign-Body Infection Study Group. Role of rifampin for treatment of orthopedic implant-related staphylococcal infections. A randomized controlled trial. JAMA 1998; 279: 1537–1541.

*Placebo-controlled trial showing that implant-associated infections due to rifampin- and ciprofloxacin-susceptible staphylococci can be cured without removal of the device, given the implant is stable and the patient tolerates long-term (3–6 months) antimicrobial therapy.*

# 86

## Infection in the Immunodeficient Patient

MICHEL AOUN AND JEAN KLASTERSKY

The basic mechanisms involved in the acute inflammatory response (Chapter 10) and specific immunity (Chapter 11) are summarized in Table 86.1. Patients may have either genetic deficiencies of these mechanisms (primary immunodeficiency), usually expressing the consequences early in life, or they may develop acquired disorders of inflammation or immunity (acquired immunodeficiency) as a consequence of specific diseases or immunosuppressive therapy. Both primary and acquired immunodeficiencies are usually clinically expressed as an enhanced susceptibility to infection or an inability to contain certain infections. The pattern of infections is often specific for the given immunodeficiency. This chapter will review the general approaches to the diagnosis and evaluation of suspected immunodeficiencies. The nature of infecting agents that complicate specific immunodeficiencies, the empiric treatment of common infectious syndromes in these patient groups, and strategies to prevent infection will also be discussed. Detailed discussions of immunodeficiency and its consequences in HIV infection (Chapters 96, 97) and bone marrow and solid organ transplantation (Chapters 91, 92) are covered elsewhere.

### Pathogenesis of Immunodeficiency

### Primary immunodeficiency

Primary immunodeficiency is the consequence of a genetic defect that can involve any component of the inflammatory or immune system, such as phagocytes, complement, and B and T lymphocytes. The fundamental biologic disorder remains unknown for the majority of congenital immunodeficiencies, with the exception of a few diseases in which deficient enzymes were identified: adenosine deaminase (ADA) and purine nucleoside phosphorylase (PNP) deficiencies. In many instances, the genetic defect has been localized to the X chromosome.

#### Primary antibody deficiency disorders

These disorders, which are listed in Table 86.2, are characterized by recurrent respiratory infections—mainly pneumonia and sinusitis with encapsulated pyogenic bacteria. Few opportunistic fungal or viral infections result with the exception of enterovirus. Giardiasis is also a common infection, especially in immunoglobulin A (IgA) deficiency.

#### Primary cell-mediated immunodeficiencies

Primary cell-mediated immunodeficiencies (CMI), which are listed in Table 86.2, result from genetic defects that alter partially or completely T-cell functions. T-cell activation defects in a group of patients with T cells that fail to respond to mitogens have been identified. Although they appear to be phenotypically normal, T cells do not proliferate or produce cytokines upon T-cell receptor (TCR) stimulation. The defects may interfere with the surface expression of TCR on T cells, with signal transduction from TCR to intracellular molecules, or with interleukin-2 (Il-2) production.

Chronic mucocutaneous candidiasis has been associated with primary CMI deficiency. Interestingly, enhanced susceptibility to infection with a variety of intracellular pathogens as seen in acquired cellular immunodeficiency is not pronounced in this patient population.

#### Severe combined immunodeficiency disorders

Severe combined immunodeficiency disorders (SCID) have broad humoral and cellular immune defects (Table 86.2) and they have a poor prognosis. They can be transmitted as X-linked recessive or as an autosomal recessive disease. In the latter, ADA deficiency is present in 40% of the cases. Partial combined immunodeficiency disorders include Wiskott-Aldrich syndrome, which is an X-linked recessive disease associated with eczema, thrombocytopenic purpura, and combined humoral and cellular immune deficiency. Patients with these disorders fail to respond to polysaccharide antigens and develop infections with encapsulated bacteria. Ataxia-telangiectasia is characterized by a selective defect in B-cell IgA synthesis that is associated with decreased but not absent T cell–mediated immunity. Initially, these patients are susceptible to encapsulated bacteria, and progressively, they become susceptible to intracellular microorganisms. Job's syndrome is characterized by recurrent staphylococcal cutaneous and lung abscesses and elevated IgE concentrations. Abnormal lymphocyte response to mitogens and alterations of neutrophil chemotaxis have been described. Another defect with a similar infection profile is cartilage-hair hypoplasia disease. Leukocyte adhesion deficiency, which is due to a mutation of the CD18 encoding gene, interferes predominantly with adhesion of lymphocytes and phagocytes, but predisposes patients to severe infections with pyogenic bacteria only. The redundancy of other adhesion mechanisms on lymphocytes allows an escape from lymphocyte-mediated immunosuppression.

#### Complement

Primary deficiencies of the complement system, C2, C3, C5, are associated with infection by encapsulated bacteria, whereas deficiencies of C6 and C7 are complicated by disseminated *Neisseria* infections.

**Table 86.1** The major inflammatory and immune mechanisms

| |
|---|
| INFLAMMATORY |
| *PHAGOCYTES* |
| Polymorphonuclear phagocytes |
| Mononuclear phagocytes<br>Lungs<br>Liver<br>Spleen<br>Other tissues |
| *THE COMPLEMENT SYSTEM* |
| SPECIFIC IMMUNITY |
| *HUMORAL* |
| B cells and antibody production |
| Regulation by T cells and their cytokines |
| *CELLULAR* |
| Regulation by T cells and their cytokines |
| Cytotoxic T lymphocytes |
| Activation of macrophages |
| Natural killer cell enhancement |

**Table 86.2** Primary immunodeficiency disorders

| |
|---|
| ANTIBODY DEFICIENCIES |
| *ALL IMMUNOGLOBULINS* |
| X-linked hypogammaglobulinemia |
| Common variable hypogammaglobulinemia |
| Transient hypogammaglobulinemia of infancy |
| *SELECTIVE IMMUNOGLOBULINS* |
| IgG subclass deficiency |
| IgA deficiency |
| IgM deficiency |
| CELLULAR IMMUNE DEFICIENCIES |
| Thymic hypoplasia (DiGeorge syndrome) |
| Nezelof's syndrome |
| T-cell activation defects |
| Chronic mucocutaneous candidiasis |
| COMBINED IMMUNODEFICIENCIES |
| Severe combined immunodeficiency (SCID)<br>Adenosine deaminase deficiency |
| Wiskott-Aldrisch syndrome |
| Ataxia-telangectasia |
| Job's syndrome |
| COMPLEMENT DEFICIENCIES |
| Early components: C1, 4, 2, 3 |
| Alternate pathway components (P, B, I) |
| Late components: C5, 6, 7, 8, 9 |
| PHAGOCYTE DEFECTS |
| Congenital neutropenias |
| Functional neutrophil defects<br>Leukocyte A deficiency (LAD)<br>Chronic granulomatous disease (CGD)<br>Myelo defects<br>Chediak Hyashi syndrome |

### Phagocytes

Primary disorders of phagocyte functions include leukocyte adhesion deficiency, chronic granulomatous disease (CGD), Chediak-Higashi syndrome, and myeloperoxidase deficiency. Infection with pyogenic bacteria (Staphylococci, aerobic gram-negative rods) and opportunistic fungi (*Candida* sp., *Aspergillus* sp.) characterizes these disorders.

## Acquired Immunodeficiency

This may be a feature of some underlying diseases or it may be secondary to immunosuppressive therapy. Three major categories have been described: phagocyte defects, hypogammaglobulinemia, and cell-mediated deficiency (Table 86.3).

## Phagocyte defects

Polymorphonuclear (PMN) and mononuclear phagocytes play a major role in the defense against bacteria and opportunistic fungi. Therefore, granulocytopenia constitutes the most important risk factor for infection with these organisms. It is defined as an absolute neutrophil count below 1000 cells/ml. Chemotherapy-induced granulocytopenia is the most frequent situation encountered. However, in hematological malignancies, granulocytopenia may be due to marrow involvement by the malignant cells that displaces normal myelopoiesis. Less frequently, it can be the consequence of bone marrow invasion by solid tumor cells. Myelofibrosis and bone marrow necrosis are rare causes of granulocytopenia, usually in Hodgkin's disease and acute lymphoblastic leukemia. Drug-induced agranulocytosis, cyclic neutropenia, Felty's syndrome, and acquired immunodeficiency syndrome (AIDS) are additional causes of granulocytopenia. Radiation therapy, in which the fields are large enough to include a substantial volume of bone marrow, can be associated with transient neutropenia. There is a correlation between the granulocyte count and the risk for infection, which increases significantly when the granulocyte count drops below 500 cells/ml; almost all bacteremias complicating neutropenia occur at less than 100 granulocytes/ml.

Patients with qualitative abnormalities of phagocytes are also at increased risk of infection. Alterations in chemotaxis, phagocytosis, and microbial killing have been documented in patients with acute and chronic leukemia. The real impact of these abnormalities on the frequency of infection is often hard to assess because of the common simultaneous granulocytopenia. In fact, during a chronic or stable phase of granulocytic leukemias, infectious complications are rare. Other hematological disorders, such as myelodysplasia and preleukemic syndromes, can also lead to defective neutrophil functions. Paroxysmal nocturnal hemoglobinuria (PNH) patients have defective neutrophil chemotaxis and may also have neutropenia. In sickle cell anemia, impairment of phagocytosis has been described in addition to other immune defects, such as functional hyposplenism, decreased complement activation, and reduced serum opsonizing capacity.

Many other conditions, such as diabetes mellitus, uremia, cirrhosis, severe burns, and some infections including leprosy, mycobacterial infections, and leishmania, may be complicated by abnormal neutrophil function.

**Table 86.3** Acquired immunodeficiency disorders

| |
|---|
| ANTIBODY DEFICIENCIES |
| Multiple myeloma |
| Chronic lymphocytic leukemia |
| Waldenstrom's macroglobulinemia |
| Nephrotic syndrome |
| Cytotoxic chemotherapy |
| CELLULAR IMMUNE DEFICIENCIES |
| HIV infection |
| T-cell leukemias |
| Viral infections |
| Epstein-Barr virus (EBV) |
| Cytomegalovirus (CMV) |
| *THERAPEUTIC AGENTS* |
| Cytotoxic therapy |
| Cyclosporin A |
| Glucocorticosteroids |
| PHAGOCYTE DEFICIENCIES |
| Neutropenias |
| Metbolic disorders |
| Uremia |
| Diabetes |
| Ethanolism |
| Myelodysplastic syndromes |
| Splenectomy or splenic dysfunction |

## Hypogammaglobulinemia

Immunoglobulins and complement are essential for opsonization and phagocytosis of encapsulated pyogenic bacteria. In addition, neutralizing immunoglobulins play a major role in the defense against cytopathogenic viruses such as enteroviruses. Upon complement fixation, immunoglobulins can induce lysis of susceptible microbes and cells (see Chapter 11).

Hypogammaglobulinemia is present in 30% to 40% of patients with chronic lymphocytic leukemia (CLL). Antibody levels decrease proportionally to the stage of disease. In this disease, hypogammaglobulinemia is the result of unbalanced clonal immunoglobulin chain synthesis, which may not be reverted by chemotherapy.

Decreased production and increased catabolism are responsible for functional hypogammaglobulinemia in multiple myeloma and Waldenstrom's macroglobulinemia (despite the presence of increased monoclonal immunoglobulins). Inhibition of residual normal B lymphocytes by the activated suppressor regulatory cells in addition to clonal expansion of plasma cells are responsible for the defective immunoglobulin production. Some types of lymphoma and thymoma may be associated with hypogammaglobulinemia. Patients with allogeneic bone marrow transplantation have a decrease in immunoglobulin production 1 month after the procedure (see Chapter 88). Chronic graft-versus-host disease (CGVHD) results in defective B-cell help induced by donor T-suppressor cells. The consequence is a decrease in immunoglobulin production and a characteristic low serum level of IgA. Immunoglobulin loss secondary to nephrotic syndrome, exudative enteropathy, or burns may lead to hypogammaglobulinemia and increased risk of infection.

## Splenectomy

The spleen plays an important role in the clearance from the blood of encapsulated bacteria not opsonized efficiently by complement. Serious infections with pneumococci, streptococci, and *Hemophilus* sp. have been reported with an estimated risk of 3% during a 5-year follow-up period after splenectomy for Hodgkin's disease staging. The mortality rate can be as high as 88%. Functional asplenia secondary to either radiation therapy or to altered vascularization of the spleen, as in some hematological disorders, carries a similar risk of infection.

## Cell-mediated immunity

T lymphocytes control and mediate cellular immunity which constitutes an effective mechanism for the elimination of intracellular microorganisms. Acquired cellular immunity defects may be seen with hematological malignancies such as Hodgkin's disease, other lymphomas, hairy cell leukemia, and acute lymphocytic leukemia. Some viral agents can induce cellular immunodeficiency, the most prominent being HIV. Depressed CMI may be seen with infection by other viruses, such as cytomegalovirus (CMV), Epstein-Barr virus (EBV), respiratory syncitial virus (RSV), influenza, and hepatitis B, although with these latter agents, it is of low degree and transient. Tuberculosis, leprosy, leishmaniasis, typhoid fever, syphilis, and brucellosis may also alter cellular immunity during acute infection. Some chemotherapeutic agents, mainly cyclophosphamide, methotrexate, and azathioprine, can suppress T-lymphocyte functions.

## Complicating Infections

Because of impairment of host defenses, infection with conventional pathogens can lead to more severe disease than usual, while saprophytes, which are usually handled easily by the immune system, can result in disseminated opportunistic infections. The type of immunodeficiency markedly influences the nature of infection, and specific microorganisms are associated with specific immune defects (Table 86.4).

## Phagocyte disorders

In phagocyte dysfunction or granulocytopenia, the severity and duration of cell defects and breaches in anatomical barriers such as mucositis or indwelling catheters are additive in promoting infection with colonizing bacteria or opportunistic fungi. About 60% of febrile episodes in granulocytopenic patients are associated with infection; 20% of these are bacteremias, 20% are clinically documented infections, and 20% are microbiologically documented infections.

The most common sites of infection are the following:

1. The alimentary tract including oral cavity, esophagus, colon, and rectum. Oral mucositis is a major source for bacteremia due to viridans streptococci and other bacteria of the oral flora, including *Capnocytophaga* spp., *Eikenella corrodens*, *Stomatococcus mucilaginosus*, and *Rothia dentocariosa*. Necrotizing gingivitis is associated with *Bacteroides* spp. and esophagitis is mainly due to *Candida* spp. or herpes simplex virus. Necrotizing enterocolitis (typhlitis) is facilitated by previous mucosal damage of the bowel. *Clostridium septicum* and less frequently other clostridia are the causative agents. Ulcerations, emorrhagic necrosis, and transmural inflammation with marked thickening of the bowel wall are the main pathological findings. Enterocolitis is characterized by fever, acute abdominal pain, and diarrhea. Surgical resec-

**Table 86.4** Distribution of pathogens according to type of immunodeficiency

| NEUTROPENIA (PMN < 1000 CELLS/$\mu$L) | CELL-MEDIATED IMMUNODEFICIENCY | HUMORAL IMMUNODEFICIENCY |
|---|---|---|
| *PRIMARY BACTEREMIA* | *GASTROINTESTINAL INFECTIONS* | *RESPIRATORY AND SYSTEMIC INFECTION* |
| Conventional bacteria | *Salmonella sp.* | *Streptococcus pneumoniae* |
| *Streptococci viridans* | *Microsporidium* | *Hemophilus influenzae* |
| Enterobacteriacae: *E. coli*, *Klebsiella* spp. | *Cryptosporidium* | *GASTROINTESTINAL INFECTIONS* |
| *Pseudomonas aeruginosa* | *Strongyloides stercoralis* | *Giardia lamblia* |
| *PNEUMONIA OR SINUSITIS* | *RESPIRATORY INFECTIONS* | *CENTRAL NERVOUS SYSTEM INFECTIONS* |
| Conventional bacteria (frequent concomitant bacteremia) | *Fungi* | *Neisseria meningitidis* |
| *Aspergillus* spp. | *Coccidioides immitis* | Enterovirus |
| *Zygomycetes* spp. | *Histoplasma capsulatum* | |
| *Fusarium* spp. | *Cryptococcus neoformans* | |
| *Penicillin boydii* | *Bacteria* | |
| *Candida* spp. | *Mycobacterium tuberculosis* | |
| *SKIN AND SOFT TISSUE (INCLUDING CATHETER SITE)* | *Legionella* spp. | |
| Coagulase negative staphylococci | *Nocardia* spp. | |
| *Bacillus* spp. | *Rhodococcus equi* | |
| *Corynebacterium jeikeium* | *Parasites* | |
| *Pseudomonas aeruginosa* (ecthyma gangrenosum) | *Pneumocystis carinii* | |
| *Candida* spp., *Trichosporon* spp., *Malassezia furfur* | *Strongyloides stercoralis* | |
| *ORAL MUCOSITIS* | *Toxoplasma gondii* | |
| HSV | *Viruses* | |
| Oral bacterial flora | Cytomegalovirus (CMV) | |
| *Bacteroides* spp. (necrotizing gingivitis) | Herpes simplex virus (HSV) and varicella-zoster virus (VZV) | |
| *PERIANAL ABSCESS* | Adenovirus | |
| Polymicrobial (gram-positive cocci, gram-negative bacilli and anaerobes) | Respiratory syncitial virus (RSV) | |
| *TYPHLITIS* | Measles | |
| *Clostridium septicum* | *CENTRAL NERVOUS SYSTEM INFECTIONS* | |
| Other *Clostridia* | *Toxoplasma gondii* | |
| | *Cryptococcus neoformans* | |
| | *Listeria monocytogenes* | |
| | *Mycobacterium tuberculosis* | |
| | CMV | |
| | Polyomavirus JC | |

tion may be indicated. Perirectal abscess is usually polymicrobial, including anaerobes, predominantly *Bacteroides fragilis*, which are associated with facultatively anerobic gram-negative bacteria and gram-positive cocci.

2. The respiratory tract—mainly sinuses and lungs. During a short period of neutropenia (<5 days), pneumonia and sinusitis are usually caused by conventional pathogens, such as *Streptococcus pneumoniae* and *Hemophilus influenzae*, and less frequently, by *Enterobacteriacae* and *Pseudomonas aeruginosa*. However, the risk for fungal pneumonia or sinusitis, mainly aspergillosis and mucormycosis, increases proportionally to the duration of neutropenia.

3. The skin, including catheter-site, scrotum, inguinal, and axillary areas. "Tunnelitis" and catheter-site cellulitis are usually due to *S. aureus*, coagulase-negative Staphylococci, *Bacillus* spp., *Corynebacterium jeikeium*, *Candida* spp. *Fusarium* spp., *Hansenula anomala*, *Rhodotorula*, and *Malassezia furfur*, especially with total parenteral nutrition (see Chapter 85). *Ecthyma gangrenosum* in moisture-laden regions areas, such as the scrotum and inguinal or axillary areas, is most often due to *P. aeruginosa* and very rarely, to other gram-negative bacteria, such as *Enterobacter* spp. and *Aeromonas* spp. (see Chapter 52). Secondary skin lesions may be the only manifestation of many disseminated infections (Chapter 51).

In summary, bacteria originating from the colonizing flora already present in patients are responsible for initial episodes of infection during granulocytopenia. These include viridans streptococci, staphylococci, *Enterobacteriaceae*, and *P. aeruginosa*. Multiresistant nosocomial bacteria, selected by previous antibiotic therapy, as well as *Candida* spp. and *Aspergillus* spp., are more commonly encountered during secondary episodes.

A fundamental change in the distribution of microorganisms causing infection during granulocytopenia has occurred in the last two decades. The incidence of gram-negative bacilli, especially *P. aeruginosa*, has declined in many institutions while infections caused by gram-positive bacteria has increased dramatically. Reasons for this change include more frequent use of indwelling catheters, oral mucositis, prophylaxis with fluoroquinolones, and empiric treatment directed specifically against gram-negative bacteria.

### Cellular immune deficiency

T-cell immunodeficiency is associated with uncommon microorganisms, the majority of which are intracellular parasites. The major clinical syndromes that can be distinguished in these patients involve infections of gastrointestinal, respiratory, or central nervous systems.

Respiratory infections are by far the most frequent and involve various microorganisms, including bacteria such as *Legionella* spp., *Nocardia* spp., *Rhodococcus equi*, and mycobacteria; fungi such as *Coccidioides* spp., *Histoplasma capsulatum*, and *Cryptococcus* spp.; parasites such as *Pneumocystis carinii*, *Strongyloides stercoralis*, and *Toxoplasma gondii*; and viruses such as cytomegalovirus (CMV), herpes simplex virus (HSV), herpes zoster virus (HZV), adenovirus, respiratory syncitial virus (RSV), and measles.

Infections of the central nervous system are the most serious and life threatening in T-cell immundeficiency. Meningitis, meningoencephalitis, and brain abscesses are caused by relatively few specific pathogens. These include *Listeria monocytogenes*, *T. gondii*, *Cryptococcus neoformans*, CMV, *Mycobacterium tuberculosis*, and *Treponema pallidum*. Progressive multifocal leukoencephalopathy is due to the polyomavirus JC.

Gastrointestinal infections complicating cellular immune deficiency are caused by *Salmonella* spp., Cryptosporidum, Microsporidium, and *Isospora belli*. Bacillary angiomatosis due to *Bartonella quintana* is also recognized.

Humoral immunodeficiency, splenectomy, and deficiency of complement components C8, H, I, or P predispose patients to recurrent respiratory or bloodstream infections with *S. pneumoniae*, and to *H. influenzae* and *Neisseria* infections, especially *Neisseria meningitidis*. Enteroviruses, primarily echoviruses, have been responsible for a syndrome of chronic meningoencephalitis in patients with hypogammaglobulinemia.

Gastrointestinal infection due to *Giardia lamblia* has been reported frequently in hypogammaglobulinemia.

## Diagnostic Studies to Evaluate Immunodeficiency

The choice of tests will be determined by the nature of the infecting organisms or the suspicion of specific deficiencies resulting from certain diseases or therapy. Not all patients need evaluation with all tests.

The different tests used in diagnosing a patient with a suspected immundeficiency are described in Table 86.5. Complete and differential blood counts are indicated in all patients. Absolute neutrophil count is essential to detect neutropenia and its severity. A severe T-cell defect can be eliminated if the absolute lymphocyte count is normal. Ocassionally, determination of the platelet count is useful; for instance, Wiskott-Aldrich syndrome is always associated with thrombocytopenia purpura, and a normal platelet count eliminates this diagnosis. The presence of Howell-Jolly bodies in red blood cells is suggestive of asplenia, and examination of phagocytes for the presence of abnormal lysosomes is helpful for Chediak-Higashi diagnosis.

The evaluation of B-lymphocyte function relies mainly on the determination of quantitative immunoglobulins, serum protein electrophoresis, and measurement of antibody titers after immunization. Skin anergy to a common antigen such as candidin 1:1000 is the hallmark of T-cell immunodeficiency.

## Approaches to Treatment of Infectious Syndromes

A difficulty in the management of a febrile immunocompromised host resides in the distinction between infection and other noninfectious causes of fever, including underlying malignancy, chemotherapy, blood transfusion, pulmonary emboli, and drug fever. Nevertheless, fever remains the most constant and often the only indicator of infection, as immunocompromised patients, especially those with neutropenia, may lack an inflammatory reaction at the site of infection until myeloid recovery occurs.

The array of potential pathogens is very wide. In addition to

**Table 86.5** Evaluation of host defense

| |
|---|
| EVALUATION OF IMMUNE FUNCTION |
| Complete and differential blood counts |
| INNATE IMMUNITY |
| NK cell enumeration |
| NK cell function |
| Antibody-dependent cellular toxicity (ADCC) |
| MBP |
| ANTIBODY DEFICIENCY |
| Serum immunoglobulin levels of IgG, IgA, IgM, IgE |
| Natural antibody titers to blood group antigens (isohemagglutinims) |
| Antibody titers to previous or repeat immunization with protein antigens (tetanus, diphtheria) |
| Antibody titers to polysaccharide antigens (previous infections): *H. influenzae* and *S. pneumoniae* |
| IGG SUBCLASSES: IGG1, IGG2, IGG3, IGG4 |
| In vivo antibody response to antigen challenge: protein antigen and polysacharride antigen |
| B-cell enumeration: surface immunoglobulin and B cell–specific antigen |
| T-CELL DEFICIENCY |
| Absolute lymphocyte count, CD3, CD4, CD8 counts |
| Delayed hypersensitivity skin tests (PPD, candida, other) |
| T-cell function evaluation |
| Proliferation to mitogens |
| Proliferation to specific antigens |
| T-cell help |
| T-cell suppression |
| T-cell cytotoxicity |
| NEUTROPHIL FUNCTION DEFICIENCY |
| Rebuck skin window test |
| Nitroblue tetrazolium test (NBT) pr luminol-enhanced chemiluminescense |
| Special stains for myeloperoxidase phosphatase |
| Microbial and phagocytic assays |
| Chemotactic assays |

conventional microorganisms, many opportunistic agents should also be taken into account. Initial therapy should be directed against the most likely pathogens in patients documented to have specific immunodeficiencies (see Table 86.4).

## Empiric therapy in febrile neutropenia

### Initial episodes of fever

The optimal management of febrile neutropenic patients consists of rapid evaluation and initiation of empiric antibiotic therapy. Attributes of selected antibiotics should include (*1*) a broad spectrum of activity against gram-positive and gram-negative bacilli, including *P. aeruginosa*; (*2*) achievement of high serum bactericidal levels; and (*3*) low potential for emergence of resistance. Combination therapy consisting of an antipseudomonal $\beta$-lactam antibiotic and an aminoglycoside complies best with these criteria. However, the potential for renal and auditory toxicity and the necessity of close monitoring of blood levels of the aminoglycoside have led to other therapeutic choices.

Choosing antibiotics with synergistic activity appears to be important in patients with documented gram-negative bacteremia who remain profoundly neutropenic. As reported by De Jongh et al., in 75 neutropenic patients with gram-negative bacteremia, no favorable responses were observed in the absence of antibiotic synergy, whereas 64% of the patients responded in presence of synergy. Among the available $\beta$-lactam antibiotics, the selection should be determined by the local epidemiology of each institution. It is important to know which organisms are predominant and their pattern of susceptibility. For example, in one recent trial of the European Organization for Research and Treatment of Cancer—International Antimicrobial Therapy Cooperative Group (E.O.R.T.C.–I.A.T.C.G.), which compared piperacillin-tazobactam plus amikacin with ceftazidime plus amikacin, the former regimen was superior because of better coverage against gram-positive bacteria.

When using these combinations how long should treatment with the aminoglycoside be maintained? This question has been addressed in trial IV of the E.O.R.T.C.–I.A.T.C.G., which compared a short course versus a long course of aminoglycoside therapy and showed that a long course was superior only in patients with documented gram-negative bacteremia. Therefore, in all remaining situations other than when gram-negative bacteremia is present, the aminoglycoside can be discontinued after 48 h in order to avoid unnecessary toxicity. Alternatives to the combination of a $\beta$-lactam plus aminoglycoside have included double $\beta$-lactam combination and $\beta$-lactam monotherapy. Concern about antagonism and increased potential for emergence of resistance among gram-negative bacilli have contributed to make the double $\beta$-lactam choice unpopular. Monotherapy with ceftazidime or imipenem has been used successfully in several trials.

Should vancomycin be included in the initial regimen? In 1988, Rubin showed that administration of vancomycin can be delayed until gram-positive organisms are recovered from blood, without any excess in morbidity or mortality. In another study from the E.O.R.T.C.–I.A.T.C.G., the proportion of patients with gram-positive bacteremia who remain febrile was identical, regardless of whether they received vancomycin in initial therapy. However, there are some specific indications for initial treatment with vancomycin in addition to the other antibiotics: (*1*) patients with catheter-site cellulitis or tunnelitis should receive this treatment because of the high recovery of coagulase-negative staphylococci, methicillin-resistant staphylococci, or *Corynebacterium jeikeium*; and (*2*) there is a high proportion of penicillin-resistant staphylococci and methicillin-resistant *S. aureus* within the institution. If the initial regimen includes a third-generation cephalosporin, specific anti-anaerobic coverage should be added in cases of patients with necrotizing gingivitis or rectal tenderness, suggesting perirectal infection.

### Secondary episodes of fever

A secondary episode of fever refers to that which either persists or recurs after 5 days of primary therapy.

Modification of initial empiric therapy during a secondary episode of fever consists in shifting to a non-cross-resistant antibiotic in order to cover the multiresistant bacteria and addition of amphotericin B in order to cover possible *Candida* or *Aspergillus* infection. The incidence of candidiasis in immunocompromised patients is not well established. Two studies have reported 11 and 12 cases of candidiasis per 100 admissions for leukemia, while candidemia accounts for 5%–7% of all positive blood cultures in cancer centers. Laboratory tests are not often helpful. Blood cultures are positive in only one-third of autopsy-proven cases of candidiasis. Serological tests have low sensitivity. The non-albicans species have increased concomitantly with the use of fluconazole in many institutions. Clinical manifestations include relapse or persistence of fever despite broad-spectrum antibiotics, myalgia, hypotension, and maculopapular skin lesions. Endophthalmitis and chronic disseminated candidiasis are two important complications (see Chapter 6). Intravenous amphotericin B at a daily dose ranging from 0.5 to 1 mg/kg is the therapy of choice. Trichosporonosis, which is mainly due to *Trichosporon beigelii*, can present clinically in a manner very similar to that of candidiasis, with fever and papular skin lesions. In trichosporonois, cutaneous lesions often evolve into necrotic ulcers. Renal involvement with subsequent rapid renal failure is more frequent in trichosporonosis. Tests for serum cryptococcal antigen may be positive at a low titer ($<$1/32). Most cases in neutropenic patients have been fatal and *Trichosporon* is frequently resistant in vitro to amphotericin B.

Cases of unusual opportunistic yeasts causing fungemia in neutropenic patients have become more common. These include *Geotrichum candidum*, *Hansenula anomala*, *Rhodotorula*, and *Malassezia furfur*. The epidemiological, clinical, and prognostic factors have not been well defined. Most cases respond to removing the infected catheters and treatment with amphotericin B. In a patient with a long duration of neutropenia (exceeding 10 days), a recurring or persisting fever, despite the use of broad-spectrum antibiotics, pleuritic chest pain, dry cough, consolidation, or nodular lesion on chest X-ray or computerized tomography (CT) scan, the probability of pulmonary aspergillosis or mucormycosis is very high. Nasal discharge, epistaxis, and facial swelling and tenderness can indicate sinus involvement by either of these two opportunistic agents. Intravenous amphotericin B at 1 mg/kg daily dose is the therapy of choice. Surgical debridement of sinusitis is usually necessary (see Chapter 54).

## Pneumonia in patients with T-cell immunodeficiency

Diagnosis of etiologic agents pneumonia in the immunodeficient patient remains a challenge. About one-third of the immunocompromised patients who develop fever and pulmonary infiltrates have noninfectious diseases. A chest CT scan is superior to a standard X-ray for diagnosis. Bronchoalveolar lavage (BAL) constitutes the cornerstone for specific etiologic diagnosis, although the distinction between colonization and infection remains a problem. The histological demonstration of microorganisms in lung tissue is the reliable proof of infection by opportunistic agents. Transbronchial biopsy and transthoracic needle aspiration are highly dependant on the experience of the physician performing the procedure and may be complicated by pneumothorax and hemorrhage. Open lung biopsy provides the highest yield of specific etiology, but increases the morbidity of the critically ill patient. The decision to proceed with such invasive techniques and the timing of the procedure are very difficult to standardize and should be based on a careful analysis of each case.

Immunocompromised patients often fail to develop an antibody response to new antigens; furthermore, the detection of antibodies is not usually helpful for early diagnosis of infection. When performed, seroconversion has more value than isolated antibody levels. One of the major indications for detection of certain antibodies is to evaluate infection risk before giving immunosuppressive therapy. For example, CMV serology status of bone marrow transplant recipient and donor predicts the likelihood of post-transplant CMV infection (see Chapter 92). Conversely, detection of antigens in blood or other fluids is independent on the immunological status of the patient and has been very useful for the diagnosis of cryptococcal and CMV infections. Many methods are being developed to detect *Candida* and *Aspergillus* antigens. Slow-growing microorganisms such as *Mycobacteria*, *Toxoplasma gondii*, and CMV can be detected early by polymerase chain reaction (PCR).

Despite constant improvement of diagnostic methodologies, the specific etiology for febrile illnesses often remains unknown. Recognition of epidemiological and clinical features and definition of the type of the underlying immunodeficiency and radiological findings are important elements for the presumed diagnosis and the selection of empiric therapy. It is imperative to inquire about the past history of long dormant diseases, such as tuberculosis, and about travel or a stay in an endemic area of geographically well-defined diseases, such as coccidioidomycosis, histoplasmosis, or blastomycosis. Hospital contacts of the patient should be determined and the local epidemiology of a given hospital should be recognized; for example, it is essential to determine the most frequent microorganisms causing pneumonia and their susceptibility patterns. The clinical features associated with pneumonia, such as the mode of onset, the presence of chest pain or dyspnea, and the extrapulmonary manifestations, are also very helpful.

### Pulmonary infiltrates and specific pathogens

The type of pulmonary infiltrate may be indicative of the underlying pathogen, but it is not always pathognomonic (Fig. 86.1). Localized pulmonary consolidation is highly suggestive of bacterial pneumonia, aspergillosis, or mycormycosis. Diffuse alveolar infiltrates are highly suggestive of legionellosis, toxoplasmosis, strongyloidosis, and on rare occasions, of fulminant aspergillosis or mucormycosis.

Nodular lesions, with or without cavities, indicate the following fungal infections: aspergillosis, mucormycosis, coccidioidomycosis, histoplasmosis, or cryptococcosis. Cavitary lesions suggest tuberculosis, nocardiosis, infection by *Rhodococcus equi*, all the fungal infections, and necrotizing pneumonia due to anaerobes or gram-negative bacilli. Interstitial infiltrates suggest infection by *P. carinii* or viruses such as CMV, HSV, varicella zoster virus (VZV), or RSV. Miliary infiltrates indicate tuberculosis, coccidioidomycosis, and histoplasmosis. It should be stressed that these radiological patterns correspond to the early stage of the diseases and the radiological picture may be different if the patient is seen at a later stage. Furthermore, there are many exceptions to the typical descriptions given here. Consequently, only the integration of the epidemiological features, type of immunodeficiency, the clinical signs associated with the pneumonia, and the radiological patterns will allow the algorithms described below to be successful in predicting the responsible pathogen with a high degree of accuracy.

### Cavitary lesions

Figure 86.2 outlines an approach to a patient with T-cell immunodeficiency and cavitary lesions of upper lobes. A history of previous pulmonary tuberculosis or positive skin tuberculin test make the probability of tuberculosis very high. Since 1985, the incidence of tuberculosis is again increasing in many countries. Clusters of multidrug-resistant tuberculosis are reported increasingly among HIV patients and their contacts with a high mortality (see Chapter 100). If the patient had a previous history of coccidioidomycosis or histoplasmosis or a history of travel or stay in an endemic area, then amphotericin B therapy should be considered. A history of contact with farm animals is suggestive of *R. equi* infection. This is an intracellular bacterium and the antibiotics chosen should penetrate effectively into the cells. The therapy of choice is a combination of erythromycin and rifampicin and a long duration of therapy is required. A patient with nodular subcutaneous lesions and/or cerebral abscesses is likely to have nocardiosis and should be treated with trimethoprim-sulfamethoxazole (TMP/SMX) or sulfonamides until a definitive diagnosis can be made.

### Diffuse infiltrates

Figure 86.3 outlines the approach to a patient with T-cell immunodeficiency and diffuse alveolar infiltrates. If the patient has an acute onset with extrapulmonary manifestations such as diarrhea, headache, confusion, and abnormal liver function tests, then the possibility of *Legionella* pneumonia increases. The therapy of choice is a fluoroquinolone, such as ciprofloxacin, or a macrolide, such as erythromycin or azithromycin. Urticaria, pruritus, or gastrointestinal symptoms in a patient with a previous history of infection or who has stayed or traveled to an endemic area suggest *Strongyloïdes stercoralis* infection. Eosinophilia may be lacking in 50% of the cases. Thiabendazole (25 mg/kg/day) given intravenously for 15 days is the therapy of choice (see Chapter 40).

Finally, patients with T-cell immunodeficiency and subacute onset of pneumonia, dyspnea, hypoxia, and interstitial infiltrates are most likely to have *Pneumocystis carinii* pneumonia (PCP) (Fig. 86.4). The incidence of PCP in immunocompromised non-AIDS patients, particularly those treated with glucocorticosteroids, has increased recently, but the real significance of this observation still remains unknown. A combination of TMP/SMX at a dose of 20 and 100 mg/kg body weight, respectively, in four equally-divided daily doses given intravenously constitutes the therapy of choice. If the interstitial pneumonia is preceded by mucocutaneous lesions, then the possibility of HSV or VZV should be considered, although the current extensive use of acyclovir as a prophylaxis in patients on potent immunosuppressive therapy has made this a very uncommon situation.

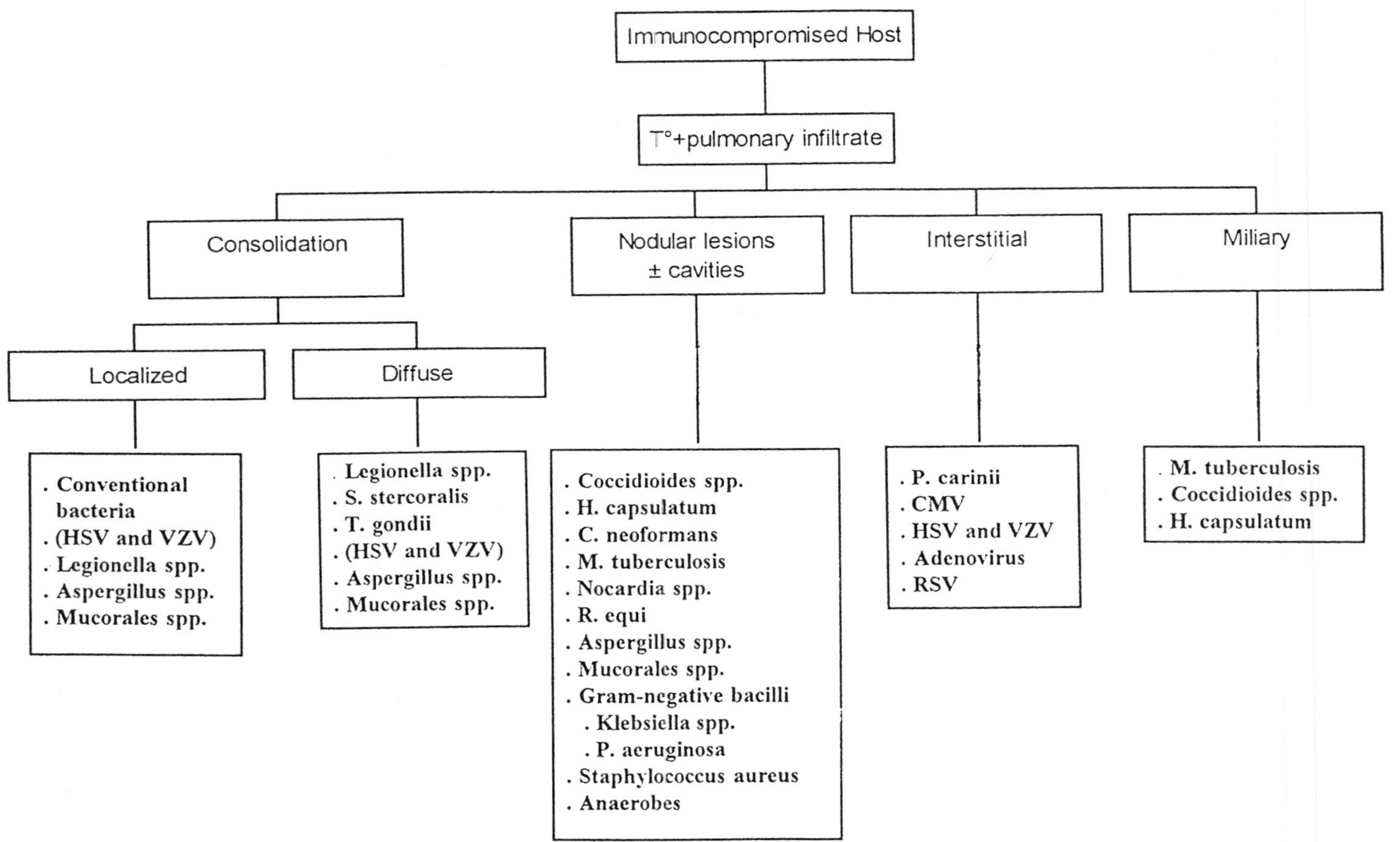


**Fig. 86.1** Relationship between pulmonary infiltrates and pathogens in immunocompromised host.

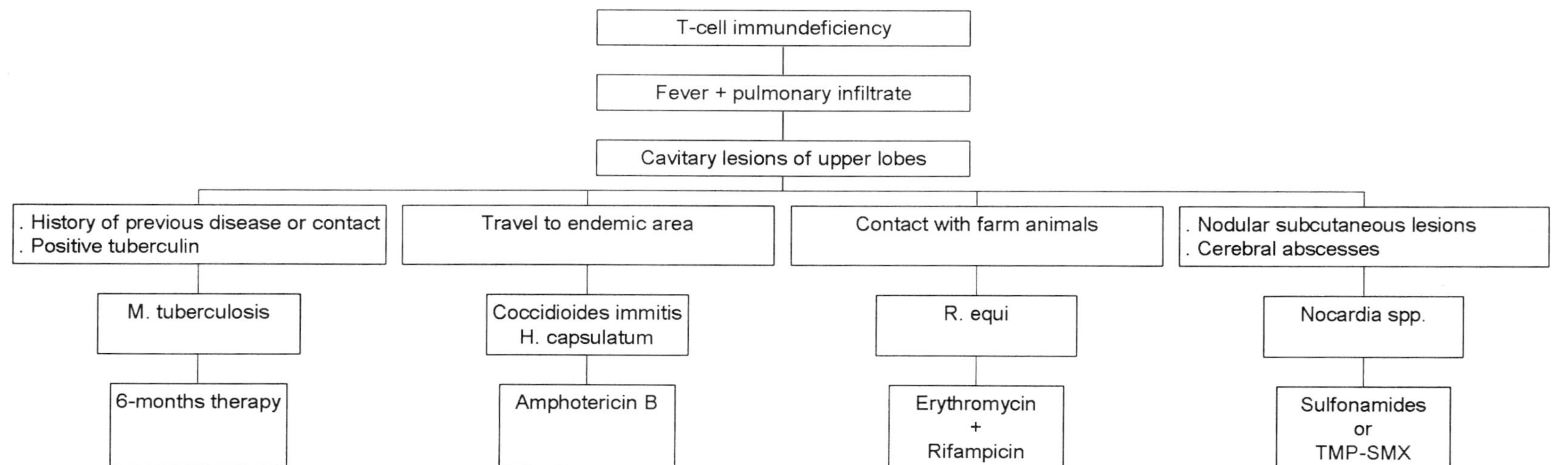


**Fig. 86.2** Algorithm in cavitary lesions according to epidemiological and clinical features.

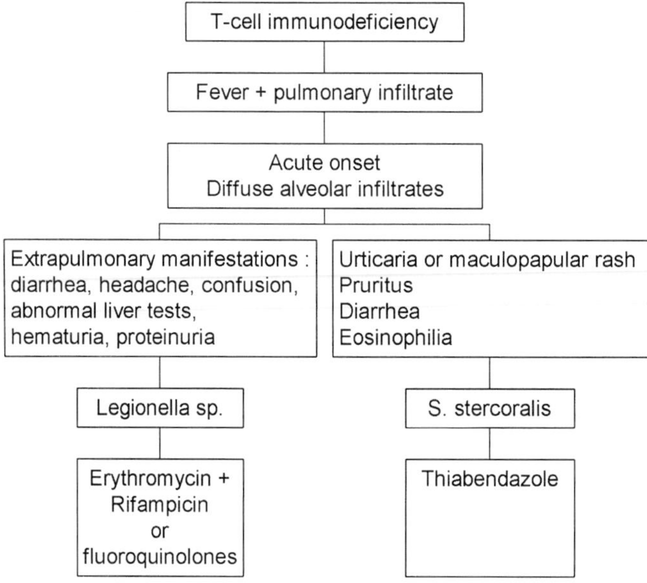


**Fig. 86.3** Algorithm in diffuse pulmonary infiltrate according to onset and extrapulmonary manifestations.

Patients with bone marrow transplantation (BMT), organ transplantation, or AIDS are at high risk of CMV interstitial pneumonia, which constitutes the principal differential diagnosis to PCP in this population. In general, adequate examination of the BAL fluid can easily differentiate the two diseases, although in AIDS patients, the two pathogens may coexist in 80% of patients. The response rate to ganciclovir is high in AIDS patients (60%–80%), whereas in BMT patients the response is 10%–40%, despite the suppression of viral replication. Addition of high-titered CMV immunoglobulins to ganciclovir has increased the response rate, but the major benefit has come from the early treatment of patients excreting the virus but who are not yet ill. Interstitial pneumonia may be the main feature of disseminated toxoplasmosis in patients with T-cell immunodeficiency. The transplanted organ may be the vehicle of contamination, although reactivation of long-dormant disease is the most frequent mode of infection.

Direct visualization of tachyzoites of *T. gondii* in BAL fluid constitutes the method of choice for early diagnosis. This necessitates a high degree of experience in recognition of the organisms by the person who is reading the slides. The therapy of choice is the combination of pyrimethamine with sulfadiazine.

## Prevention of infection

Prevention of infection in the immunodeficient patient involves reducing the acquisition of new pathogens from the environment, decreasing the risk of translocation from the endogenous flora, and enhancement of the host defenses.

Isolation of granulocytopenic patients in single rooms with

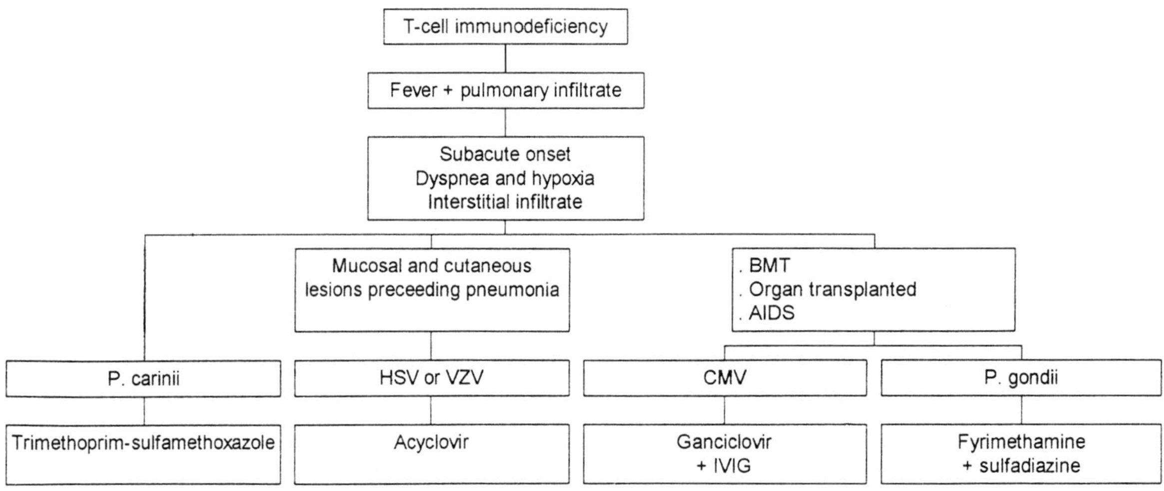


**Fig. 86.4** Algorithm in interstitial pulmonary infiltrates according to onset, clinical features and underlying conditions.

gowns, masks, and gloves is used in many institutions and helps mainly against nosocomial transmission of pathogens, but it does not prevent infection from endogenous sources. Fresh fruits and vegetables should be avoided and cooked food provided in order to decrease the acquisition of gram-negative bacteria such as *P. aeruginosa*. Allograft bone marrow recipients are often isolated in rooms with HEPA-filtered laminar airflow in order to prevent airborne acquisition of *Aspergillus*. Some controversy has developed over the actual efficacy of this highly expensive equipment because *Aspergillus* colonization may occur in patients before they enter the HEPA-filtered laminar airflow room. Prophylaxis with oral antibiotics, mainly oral fluoroquinolones, has decreased the incidence of gram-negative bacteremia in several randomized trials. However, resistant *E. coli* have been documented in patients who received fluoroquinolone prophylaxis. Fluconazole at a high dose of 400 mg daily has been shown to decrease systemic fungal infections in bone marrow transplant patients.

Intravenous acyclovir has been successfully administered prophylactically to allogeneic bone marrow–transplanted patients for prevention of herpetic and cytomegalovirus reactivation. *P. carinii* pneumonia in high-risk patients is prevented by the oral administration of trimethoprim-sulfamethoxazole in a dosage of one tablet per day, 3 days per week. Aerosolized pentamidine at 300 mg monthly constitutes an alternative for allergic patients, but it is less effective than dapsone (see Chapter 102).

In granulocytopenic patients, many investigators have tried to enhance the number and function of neutrophils. Granulocyte transfusion was the first applied treatment, but many factors have diminished efficacy, including high number of granulocytes required daily, questionable functional effectiveness of these cells, risk of alloimmunization and cytomegalovirus transmission, leukoagglutinin reaction with pulmonary edema, and lack of controlled studies. Recently, the use of the colony-stimulating factor (CSF) and granulocyte (G)-CSF to increase the yield of donor cells has circumvented the quantitative problems and has made it possible to administer as many as $10^{16}$ polymorphonuclear neutrophils (PMN) from a single donor. Consequently, there is a renewed interest in therapeutic granulocyte transfusions, especially in fungal infections with high mortality, such as aspergillosis. Enhancement of phagocytosis and shortening the period of neutropenia should result in a better outcome of fungal infections in neutropenic patients and controlled trials are ongoing in this field. Administration of either G-CSF or granulocyte-macrophage (GM) CSF during myelosuppressive therapy has shortened the period of neutropenia and reduced infectious complications in many patients (see Chapter 46).

Interferon-$\gamma$ as prophylaxis or adjunctive therapy to prevent bacterial infections in CGD patients has showed promising results. Unless patients are severely hypogammaglobulinemic, the administration of immunoglobulin to prevent infections in immunosuppressed patients has largely been unsuccessful.

## ANNOTATED BIBLIOGRAPHY

Aoun M, Klastersky J. Opportunistic infections in patients with cancer (Part I). Oncol Pract 1993; 2:6–11.

Aoun M, Klastersky J. Opportunistic infections in patients with cancer (Part II). Oncol Pract 1993; 3:5–11.

Buckley RH. Immunodeficiency diseases. JAMA 1992; 268:2797–2806.

*A concise review of ontogeny of the normal human immune system as well as the primary immunodeficiency disorders.*

De Jongh CA, Joshi JH, NewMan KA, Moody MR, Wharton R, Standiford HC, Schimpff SC. Antibiotic synergism and response in gram-negative bacteremia in granulocytopenic cancer patients. Am J Med 1986 May 30:80 (suppl. 5C): 96–100.

Fearon DT, Locksley RM. The instructive role of innate immunity in the acquired immune response. Science 1996; 272:1–164.

Hill HR. Infectious complicating congenital immunodeficiency syndromes. In: Clinical Approach to Infection in the Compromised Host. Rubin RH, Young LS, eds. Plenum Medical Book Company, New York, pp. 407–438, 1988.

*Practical overview of the serious infectious complications that occur in children with congenital immune deficiency diseases.*

Rubin RH, Young LS, eds. Clinical Approach to Infection in the Compromised Host. Plenum Medical Book Company, New York, 1988.

# 87

# Infection in the Organ Transplant Recipient

ROBERT H. RUBIN AND NINA E. TOLKOFF-RUBIN

Solid-organ transplantation has been an important approach to the treatment of failure of kidneys, liver, heart, lung, and pancreas over the past three decades. Initially the immunosuppressive regimens used to prevent allograft rejection were broad in their effects (high-dose glucocorticosteroids and azathioprine) and frequently complicated by infections which could culminate in either the death of the transplant recipient, or because of the need to reduce immunosuppression, sacrifice of the transplanted organ through rejection. More recent years have witnessed more sophisticated approaches to selective suppression of the cellular immune response and a better understanding of the role that infection by different organisms plays in modulating immunity as well as representing a threat to the patients. This chapter reviews the major aspects in the pathogenesis of infection in these patients, the role that infection by certain organisms plays in altering the immune responses, and the recognition, management, and prevention of the principal infections complicating allogeneic solid organ transplantation in the present time.

## Pathogenesis of Immunosuppression in Organ Transplantation

The two major barriers to successful organ transplantation, allograft rejection and life-threatening infection, are closely linked by the nature and intensity of the immunosuppressive therapy that is administered. An important truism of transplant practice is that any intervention that decreases the risk of infection will permit the more aggressive treatment of rejection; conversely, any intervention that decreases the risk of rejection, thus permitting the use of lesser amounts of immunosuppressive therapy, will decrease the risk of infection. Thus, the therapeutic prescription for the transplant patient has two components: an immunosuppressive strategy to prevent and treat rejection, and an antimicrobial strategy to make it safe.

The risk of infection in the transplant patient is determined by the interaction of two factors, the patient's net state of immunosuppression and the epidemiologic exposures he or she encounters. The net state of immunosuppression is a complex function to which a number of factors contribute (Table 87.1). The most important of these are the dose, duration, and temporal sequence of immunosuppressive drugs prescribed and whether immunomodulating infection is present.

Careful studies in both humans and animal models have shown that the various components of the immunosuppressive regimen have differing effects on the risk of important infections. Drugs such as cyclosporine, prednisone, FK-506 (tacrolimus), and rapamycin have a major inhibitory effect on the ability of the transplant recipient to develop a microbial-specific cytotoxic T-lymphocyte response, the critical host defense against such important infections in the transplant patient as the herpes group viruses (most importantly, cytomegalovirus and Epstein-Barr virus), fungi, and mycobacteria. In contrast, the antilymphocyte antibodies (both polyclonal and monoclonal), while they have an acute inhibiting effect on T-lymphocyte function, have an additional major effect in reactivating latent viral infection. The cytotoxic drugs, azathioprine and cyclophosphamide, have moderate effects on both these functions. Recently, it has been shown that such cytokines as tumor necrosis factor (TNF), liberated in response to the administration of the antilymphocyte antibodies, play an important role in this viral reactivation process. The greatest risk of clinical infection related to immunosuppressive therapy, then, occurs when antilymphocyte antibody therapy is administered when cytokine elaboration is greatest (in the treatment of acute rejection), and this is followed by cyclosporine- or FK-506-based maintenance immunosuppression. This sequence of events not only reactivates latent infection, it also then permits the virus to replicate unhampered by a key host response, thus amplifying the extent of the infection.

Such viruses as cytomegalovirus (CMV), Epstein-Barr virus (EBV), the hepatitis viruses, and the human immunodeficiency virus (HIV), in addition to causing directly a variety of infectious disease syndromes, contribute significantly to the net state of immunosuppression. This indirect effect predisposes the transplant patient to opportunistic infection with such organisms as *Pneumocystis carinii*, *Listeria monocytogenes*, and a variety of fungi. One measure of this is found in the following statistic: at Massachusetts General Hospital more than 90% of the opportunistic infections occur in individuals with immunomodulating viral infection; the remainder have turned out to be due to specific epidemiologic exposures. In addition, cytokines elaborated in response to one infection may play a role in promoting clinical disease due to another agent. Thus, CMV is a risk factor for EBV-related lymphoproliferative disease, and herpes group virus infection is promoted by urosepsis. Since these same cytokines are both elaborated in the rejection process and can modulate the display of histocompatibility antigens that may trigger the rejection process, the linkage between infection, rejection, and immunosuppressive therapy is even closer than first imagined. It is also apparent from this description that the nature of immunosuppressive therapy contributes to the net state of immunosuppression not only directly, but also indirectly, through its effects on the immunomodulating viruses. Indeed, as will be discussed below, this indirect effect is so important that antimicrobial strategies directed against immunosuppression-driven viral infection, particularly CMV, also offer protection against opportunistic infection with such other pathogens as fungi.

**Table 87.1** Factors contributing to the net state of immunosuppression in the organ transplant recipient

| |
|---|
| Dose, duration, and temporal sequence in which immunosuppressive drugs are prescribed |
| Presence of leukopenia, defects in the mucocutaneous surfaces of the body, or indwelling foreign bodies |
| Presence of metabolic derangements |
| Protein-calorie malnutrition |
| Uremia |
| Diabetes mellitus |
| Presence of infection with immunomodulatory viruses |
| Cytomegalovirus |
| Epstein-Barr virus |
| Human immunodeficiency virus |
| Hepatitis B virus |
| Hepatitis C virus |

## Epidemiology of Infection in the Organ Transplant Recipient

The epidemiologic exposures of importance for the transplant patient may occur in the community or within the hospital setting (Table 87.2). In the community, it has long been recognized that the geographically restricted systemic mycoses (blastomycosis, coccidioidomycosis, and histoplasmosis), *Mycobacterium tuberculosis*, and *Strongyloides stercoralis* can have a special impact on the transplant patient. The most common clinical pattern with these infections is reactivation of dormant infection followed by systemic dissemination, although both progressive primary infection and reinfection can also occur. In recent years as the numbers of successful transplant patients returning to the community have increased, it has become apparent that community-acquired respiratory infections such as influenza, parainfluenza, and adenovirus have a particular impact on this population. The incidence of both viral pneumonia and secondary bacterial and fungal pneumonias in transplant patients following community-acquired respiratory virus infection is far higher than in the general population, and efforts at protecting transplant patients from such infections need to be increased.

The transplant patient, like other immunosuppressed hosts, is particularly susceptible to nosocomial exposure to such organisms as *Aspergillus* spp.; *Legionella* spp.; such gram-negative bacilli as *Pseudomonas aeruginosa*; and other organisms. Most commonly, aerosols of organisms, often associated with hospital construction, result in pulmonary infection, although wound and nasal sinus infection can also occur. Two epidemiologic patterns of infection are noted: in the domiciliary, exposure occurs on the ward where the patient resides, cases cluster in time and space, and cases are prevented by insuring that the air supply is subjected to HEPA filters; in the nondomiciliary, exposure occurs when the patient is taken to such sites as the radiology suite or operating room for an essential procedure. Nondomiciliary outbreaks are far more difficult to detect because of lack of clustering, and are more difficult to prevent because of the difficulty of providing filtered air throughout the hospital environment. An important clue to the presence of a nondomiciliary hazard is the occurrence of infection with one of these organisms at a time when the patient's net state of immunosuppression should not normally permit such infections to occur. In terms of prevention, avoidance of areas of construction and the wearing of high-efficiency masks should be considered.

## Timetable of Infection Following Organ Transplantation

The general protocol for immunosuppressive therapy for organ transplant patients is relatively standardized (Table 87.3). As a result, the point in the post-transplant course at which different infections occur has become predictable. It is now possible to define a timetable of infection after organ transplantation (Fig. 87.1). Such a timetable is useful in three ways: first, it allows the clinician to design preventative strategies for particular infections that are targeted to periods of maximal risk and thus optimize cost-benefit ratios; second, it assists the clinician in determining the differential diagnosis when a transplant patient presents with such problems as pneumonia or fever of unknown origin; and third, it provides an important clue to the clinician of an excessive environmental hazard when an infection occurs at a time point when the net state of immunosuppression should not have been great enough to permit microbial invasion with this organism under normal circumstances. The post-transplant course can be divided into three time periods:

1. *First month post-transplant*: In the first month post-transplant, more than 95% of the infections that occur are the same bacterial and candidal infections of the wound, urinary and respiratory tracts, intravenous access devices, and drainage catheters that occur in nonimmunosuppressed individuals undergoing comparable forms of surgery. In such cases, the etiology is usually the same as in nontransplant patients, although the impact can be greater in the transplant patient. The major determinant of this form of infection is the technical skill with which the surgery is accomplished, and the manner in which the vascular access, drainage catheters, and endotracheal tubes are managed. Uncommon causes of infection during this time period include transplantation of a contaminated allograft (with the disastrous occurrence of

**Table 87.2** Epidemiologic exposures of importance in the organ transplant recipient

| |
|---|
| COMMUNITY EXPOSURES |
| Geographically restricted systemic mycoses (blastomycosis, coccidioidomycosis, histoplasmosis) |
| *Mycobacterium tuberculosis* |
| *Strongyloides stercoralis* |
| Respiratory viruses |
| Influenza |
| Parainfluenza |
| Respiratory syncytial virus |
| Adenovirus |
| Infections acquired through the ingestion of contaminated food or Water |
| *Salmonella species* |
| *Campylobacter jejuni* |
| *Listeria monocytogenes* |
| NOSOCOMIAL EXPOSURES[A] |
| *Aspergillus* spp. |
| *Legionella* spp. |
| *Pseudomonas aeruginosa* and other gram-negative bacilli |
| ? Pneumocystis carinii[b] |

[a]These exposures to contaminated air or potable water may occur on the ward ("domiciliary" exposure) or while traveling in the hospital for a procedure ("nondomiciliary" exposure).

[b]It is our belief that person-to-person spread of *Pneumocystis carinii* can occur between immunosuppressed individuals, and care must be take to protect against the nosocomial spread of this infection among transplant patients.

**Table 87.3** Standard immunosuppressive therapy protocol employed at Massachusetts General Hospital*

| Time post-transplant | Avg. daily prednisone dose (mg)[a] | Avg. daily cyclosporine dose, PO (mg/kg)[b] | Avg. daily azathioprine dose, PO (mg/kg)[c] |
|---|---|---|---|
| Day −1 | —— | 6 | 3 |
| Day 0 | 200 | 6 BID | 1.5–3 |
| Day 1 | 160 | 6 BID | 1.5–3 |
| Day 2 | 120 | 6 BID | 1.5–3 |
| Day 3 | 80 | 6 BID | 1.5–3 |
| Day 4 | 40 | 6 BID | 1.5–3 |
| Day 5 | 20 | 6 BID | 1.5–3 |
| Days 6–180 | 15–20 | 6 BID | 1.5–3 |
| After 6 months | 10–15 | Gradually decrease to 200–300/day | 1.5–3 |

*From Rubin (1994). If rejection occurs, then 500 mg methylprednisolone is administered IV daily × 2 (*in addition to usual immunosuppression*). If rejection continues, OKT3 (5 mg/kg daily × 10–14 days) or antithymocyte globulin (ATG; 750 mg IV day 1, then 1000–1250 mg daily × 10–14 days) is initiated. When this occurs, the cyclosporine dose is reduced by at least 50% (until 3 days prior to discontinuing the OKT3 or ATG) and azathioprine is reduced to 50 mg/day.

[a]May be administered as IV methylprednisolone or oral prednisone, depending on GI function.

[b]In the first 6 months posttransplant, the cyclosporine dose is adjusted to maintain a whole blood cyclosporine trough level of 250–400 ng/ml. In the special case of liver transplantation, IV cyclosporine 2.5 mg/kg BID is added to the oral regimen until the T-tube is clamped, when the IV therapy is discontinued. If oliguric renal failure develops in the peritransplant period, cyclosporine is discontinued and OKT3 or ATG, in the dosages outlined previously, are substituted.

[c]The dose of azathioprine is adjusted to maintain the WBC at a level of 4–10,000/mm$^3$; the usual adult dose of azathioprine is 100 mg/day.

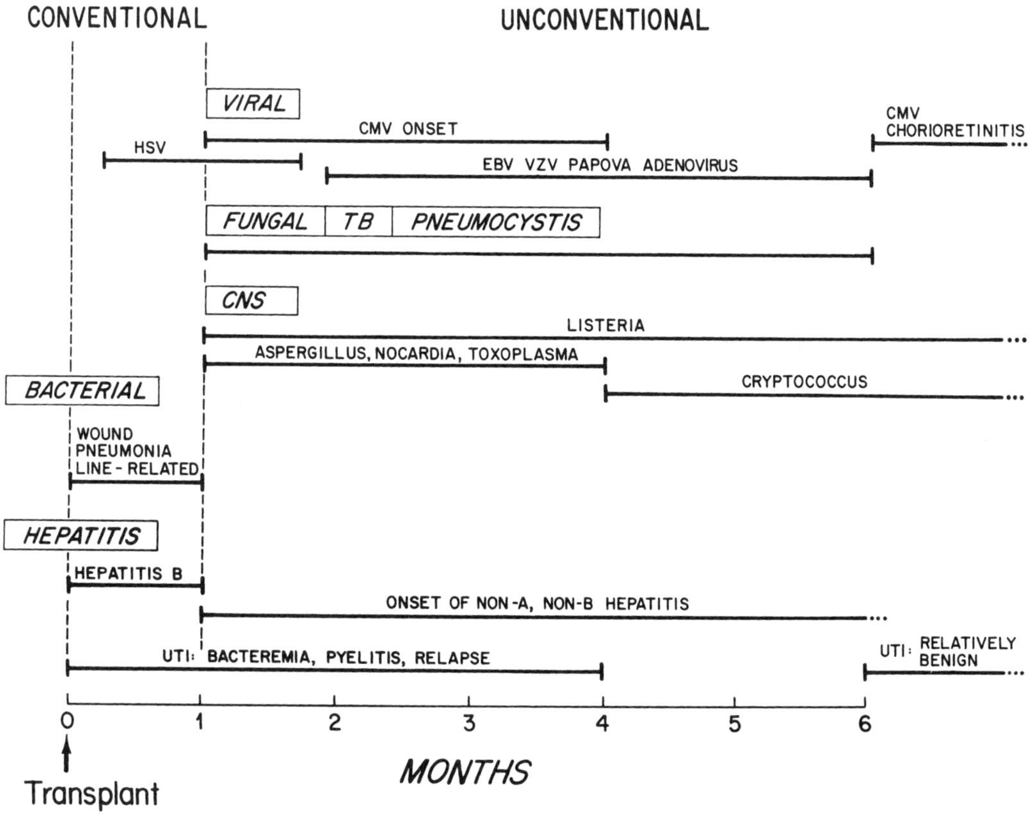


**Fig. 87.1** Timetable of infection following organ transplantation. [From Rubin, 1994.]

vascular suture line infection, mycotic aneurysm, and vascular rupture) and progression of infection that had been present prior to transplant. The last is a particular concern in liver and heart allograft recipients, who not infrequently come to transplantation critically ill and at risk for pneumonia, vascular access, and peritoneal infection. Active pulmonary infection is a strong contraindication to transplantation. Notable by their absence during this first month are opportunistic infections, even though the daily dose of immunosuppressive drugs is at its greatest during this period. This observation has led to the concept that it is the sustained administration of immunosuppressive therapy, "the area under the curve," rather than acute, high-dose therapy, that is the major determinant of the net state of immunosuppression.

2. *One to six months post-transplant*: The two major causes of infection during this time period include the immunomodulating viruses, cytomegalovirus (CMV) and Epstein-Barr virus (EBV); the hepatitis viruses (hepatitis B virus, HBV, and hepatitis C virus, HCV); and human immunodeficiency virus (HIV). These viruses exert their direct clinical manifestations during this period. In addition, the immunomodulatory effects of these viruses, in combination with the sustained administration of immunosuppression, now create a net state of immunosuppression that permits the occurrence of such opportunistic infections as those caused by *Pneumocystis carinii*, *Listeria monocytogenes*, and *Aspergillus* spp. without requiring an excessive epidemiologic exposure.

3. *More than six months Post-transplant*: Organ transplant patients who are more than six months post-transplant can be divided into three categories according to their infectious disease problems. Approximately 80% of the patients who have good allograft function and are receiving only maintenance immunosuppression are at risk for the same infections that affect the general community. These include influenza and the other community-acquired respiratory viruses, pneumococcal pneumonia, and urinary tract infection, with minimal risk of opportunistic infection. Approximately 10% of patients who have chronic viral infection (hepatitis B or C, CMV, HIV, EBV, papillomavirus, etc.) will develop inexorably progressive organ failure (e.g., cirrhosis from the hepatitis viruses or chorioretinitis from CMV), malignancy (e.g., hepatocellular carcinoma due to HBV and HCV, EBV-associated lymphoproliferative disease, and squamous cell carcinoma due to the papillomaviruses), and AIDS due to HIV infection. Finally, approximately 10% of patients, the "chronic n'er-do-wells," have relatively poor allograft function, have received too much acute and chronic immunosuppressive therapy, and frequently have chronic viral infection. These patients are at the highest risk of any organ transplant recipient for opportunistic infection with such pathogens as *Pneumocystis carinii*, *Cryptococcus neoformans*, *Listeria monocytogenes*, and *Aspergillus* spp.

**Table 87.4** Effects of viral infection on transplant recipients

| |
|---|
| DIRECT CAUSATION OF INFECTIOUS DISEASE SYNDROMES |
| Cytomegalovirus |
| Mononucleosis, hepatitis, pneumonia, GI ulcerations, chorioretinitis |
| Epstein-Barr Virus |
| Mononucleosis, hepatitis |
| Hepatitis B and C |
| Acute and chronic hepatitis |
| Human immunodeficiency virus |
| Mononucleosis, AIDS |
| INDIRECT EFFECTS OF VIRUSES |
| Immunosuppression leading to opportunistic superinfection |
| Cytomegalovirus, Epstein-Barr virus, hepatitis viruses, human immunodeficiency virus |
| Contribution to the pathogenesis of allograft injury |
| cytomegalovirus, ? others |
| Viral-associated oncogenesis |
| Epstein-Barr-virus-related post-transplant lymphoproliferative disorder, hepatitis-B- and C-related hepatocellular carcinoma, papillomavirus-related squamous cell carcinoma |

## Infections of Particular Importance in the Organ Transplant Recipient

### Viral infections

No other class of microorganisms has such a great an impact on organ transplant recipients as does the herpes group viruses, the hepatitis viruses, and the human immunodeficiency virus. The effects of these viruses include both the direct causation of clinical infectious disease syndromes and some indirect effects, such as contribution to the net state of immunosuppression, possible role in the pathogenesis of allograft injury, and role in the development of certain malignancies (Table 87.4).

#### Herpes viruses

By far the most important causes of infection in transplant patients are the herpes viruses. These agents have three properties—latency, cell association, and the potential for oncogenicity (demonstrated only for EBV virus, in the pathogenesis of EBV-associated lymphoproliferative disease)—that make them ideally suited for causing disease in this patient population. The term *latency* refers to the fact that once infected with one of these viruses (CMV, EBV, HSV-1, and HSV-2, and varicella zoster virus or VZV) infection is lifelong, but frequently without clinical manifestation. The same applies to HHV-6; although the consequences of this infection in transplant patients are not clear. An individual remains infected for life, even after demonstrable viral replication ceases. A number of factors, but in the context of transplantation particularly antirejection therapy with anti-T-cell antibodies (either monoclonal or polyclonal), will cause reactivation of latent virus. Seropositivity is the laboratory marker for the presence of virus. Once viral replication occurs, transmission between individuals and dissemination within an individual requires intimate cell-to-cell contact, thus rendering humoral immunity inefficient in controlling viral spread, and cell-mediated immunity the critical host defense. In particular, the key host defense is the development of viral-specific, MHC (major histocompatibility complex) -restricted cytotoxic T-cells—just that aspect of host defense most inhibited by current cyclosporine- or FK-506-based immunosuppressive programs. Thus, once virus is reactivated (as during treatment with antilymphocyte antibodies), its effects are amplified by the immunosuppressive program.

#### *CMV*

CMV continues to be the most important single pathogen in transplant patients, causing both important direct and indirect effects (Table 87.4). Three different patterns of transmission of CMV occur in transplant recipients, each with a different risk of causing clinical disease. In primary infection, a CMV-seronegative individual receives latently infected cells from a seropositive donor, with subsequent reactivation and dissemination. In over 90% of such instances, the infected cells are in the allograft, although viable leukocyte-containing blood products from seropositive donors can convey CMV infection in a similar fashion. In reactivation of infection, a CMV-seropositive individual reactivates endogenous virus. Finally, in superinfection, a seropositive individual receives latently infected cells from a seropositive donor, and the virus that reactivates and disseminates is of donor rather than recipient origin. The direct clinical effects of CMV infection in all the forms of organ transplantation are essentially identical, with one notable exception: the organ transplanted is affected far more than the native organ. Thus, CMV hepatitis is a clinical problem seen almost exclusively in liver transplant recipients, myocarditis in heart transplant recipients, and pneumonia has its highest attack rate in lung transplant recipients.

Approximately 60% of those at risk of primary infection, 10%–20% of those at risk of reactivation infection, and 20%–40% of those at risk of superinfection become clinically ill. However, these latter two statistics can be vastly changed by the form of immunosuppression that is administered. If seropositive recipients are immunosuppressed with cyclosporine, prednisone, and azathioprine, the incidence of clinical CMV disease is approximately 10%. If in addition prophylactic antilymphocyte antibody therapy is used the first five to seven days post-transplant, this risk doubles to approximately 20%. If antirejection antilymphocyte antibody therapy is needed, in addition to the basic immunosuppressive program, the risk of clinical disease rises to 65%. There is increasing evidence that cytokines, particularly tumor necrosis factor, elaborated as a result of antilymphocyte antibody therapy and allograft rejection, are the driving force behind these differences in the incidence of clinical disease.

Treatment of CMV clinical disease in organ transplant patients is with intravenous ganciclovir at a dose of 5 mg/kg twice daily (with dose modification in the face of renal dysfunction) for two to three weeks. Relapsing disease with such a regimen is observed in 10%–20% of seropositive individuals, but in more than 60% of those with primary disease. More prolonged courses of therapy, the addition of CMV hyperimmune globulin, and/or prolonged high-dose oral acyclovir therapy (e.g., 800 mg four times daily) are some of the strategies utilized to control relapsing disease. A variety of preventative regimens have been employed with moderate success (Table 87.5), with perhaps the most important new concept that has emerged is that the intensity of the preventative program must be linked to the intensity of the immunosuppressive program. Thus, if 5 mg/kg/day of ganciclovir is administered for the duration of antilymphocyte antibody therapy (so-called preemptive therapy), the incidence of symptomatic CMV disease is decreased by over 60%.

### EBV

Although EBV can cause a mononucleosis syndrome in transplant patients identical to that caused by CMV, the most important clinical effect of this virus in this patient population is its role in the pathogenesis of EBV-associated lymphoproliferative disease. Four risk factors have been identified for the occurrence of this entity: EBV seronegativity, and hence the risk of primary infection; high-dose immunosuppression, particularly with cyclosporine and antilymphocyte antibody treatment; a high level of EBV replication in the nasopharynx; and, possibly, preceding symptomatic CMV disease. The spectrum of clinical illness encompassed by the term *lymphoproliferative disease* is quite broad, ranging from a polyclonal lymphadenopathic process that disappears with a decrease in immunosuppression and high-dose antiviral therapy to a frankly malignant, monoclonal lymphoma. Optimal therapy for each of these forms of disease is still being established.

### VZV

Reactivation of HSV and VZV infection in seropositive transplant patients is quite common, with localized infections responsive to acyclovir therapy without systemic dissemination being the result. Disseminated primary infection, particularly with VZV, is a life-threatening process and requires prompt recognition and aggressive therapy with high-dose intravenous acyclovir (10 mg/kg every eight hours) to prevent visceral dissemination and death. All transplant candidates and patients should have their VZV serologic status checked, with seronegative individuals receiving zoster-immune globulin following exposures to the virus. Once the VZV vaccine becomes available, a high priority should be given to immunizing seronegative transplant patients and candidates.

**Table 87.5** Estimated efficacies of different prophylactic antiviral strategies against cytomegalovirus infection in different forms of organ transplantation*

| Type of transplant | Form of CMV infection[a] | Antimicrobial strategy used | Estimated efficacy |
|---|---|---|---|
| Kidney | Primary | CMV hyperimmune globulin | 2+ |
| | | High-dose acyclovir | 2+ |
| | | CMV hyperimmune globulin + moderate-dose acyclovir | 3+ |
| | Secondary | High-dose acyclovir | 3+ |
| | | CMV hyperimmune globulin + moderate-dose acyclovir | 3+ |
| Heart and/or lung | Primary | High-dose ganciclovir (1 month) | 0 |
| | Secondary | High-dose ganciclovir (1 month) | 4+ |
| Liver | Primary | CMV hyperimmune globulin | 0 |
| | Secondary | CMV hyperimmune globulin | 3+ |

*Modified from Rubin (1993). Unless otherwise noted, the regimens outlined were administered for a minimum of 3 months. Only semiquantitative assessments of efficacy are given, because of the recognition that the type of immunosuppression used will have a major effect on the efficacy of each of these regimens.

[a]Patients were not differentiated in the studies as to whether they had reactivation or superinfection; all patients seropositive for CMV prior to transplantation are grouped together.

### Hepatitis viruses

Transplantation of an organ from an HBV- or an HCV-infected individual into a seronegative recipient has an efficiency of transmission of the virus that approaches 100%. In the case of HBV, this is associated with the occurrence of fulminant hepatitis in the first few months post-transplant in many patients, as well as chronic hepatitis with a relatively short course in the remainder of individuals. Thus, there is universal agreement that all potential donors should be screened for HBSAg, and a positive result would rule out a potential donor. More controversial is the appropriate approach to hepatitis C. Approximately 5% of potential organ donors are anti-HCV positive; 50% of these harbor infectious virus, as shown by polymerase chain reaction assay for HCV RNA, with all of these being infectious. Unlike HBV, symptomatic HCV infection is very unusual in the first few years post-transplant, although chronic liver disease (and occasionally, hepatocellular carcinoma) starts becoming manifest after that point, with approximately 25% of transplant recipients with HCV infection having significant morbidity and/or mortality by 10 years post-transplant. Because of the shortage of organ donors, there is now considerable debate as to whether organs from HCV-positive donors should not be used for recipients with a pressing need for transplant, and for those, such as the elderly, for whom a more limited lifespan is likely. The strategy of only giving such organs to patients already anti-HCV positive is not helpful, as superinfection with consequences identical to those of primary infection appears to be the rule with this virus.

A second area of controversy is the management of patients already infected with HBV or HCV. The immunosuppressive therapy required to maintain allograft function will increase the level of replication of both these viruses, and a more accelerated course is to be expected, even though, for a time, liver function test abnormalities and even histologic evidence of disease activity may be blunted by the immunosuppression. Thus, the presence of chronic HBV or HCV infection prior to transplant should be regarded as a relative contraindication to transplantation, with liver biopsy to assess the status of the liver before the decision to proceed being seriously considered. In the special case of liver transplantation, patients with HBV infection are best served by an intensive and continuing course of hyperimmune globulin to prevent rapid destruction of the allograft. Unfortunately, therapy with interferon has been less effective in transplant patients than in nonimmunosuppressed individuals.

### Human immunodeficiency virus

Transplantation of an organ from an HIV-infected individual has a transmission efficiency that approaches 100%. Fortunately, with currently available serologic techniques, the risk of acquiring HIV infection by this route is vanishingly small, provided an appropriate donor blood sample is tested. Several instances in which a cadaveric donor's organs have transmitted the virus have occurred when the blood sample tested has been drawn only after many units of blood products had been administered following trauma.

A bigger issue is whether an HIV-infected individual is an appropriate candidate to receive an allograft. Data currently available suggest that among HIV-infected individuals receiving a transplant, approximately one-third do very poorly, dying in the first six months post-transplant; another third do very well, remaining asymptomatic six to eight years post-transplant with functioning allografts; and the remaining third have an intermediate result, developing overt AIDS approximately three years post-transplant. Whether these results can be improved upon with antiretroviral therapy in addition to *Pneumocystis* prophylaxis is unclear.

## Fungal infections

In addition to the previously discussed geographically restricted systemic mycoses, transplant patients are at risk for opportunistic infection with fungal species that rarely cause invasive infection in the normal host. *Candida* spp., *Pneumocystis carinii*, *Aspergillus* spp., *Cryptococcus neoformans*, and the Mucoraceae are the most important examples. Three patterns of infection are observed: primary infection, usually of the lungs, occasionally of the nasal sinuses, most commonly with *P. carinii*, *C. neoformans*, or *A. fumigatus*; sequential or concurrent secondary infection of lungs damaged by a previous process, or of vascular-access devices with *Aspergillus* spp., *Candida* spp., or *Torulopsis glabrata*; and primary cutaneous infection following a break in the integrity of the skin caused by *Aspergillus* spp., Mucoraceae, *Paecilomyces*, *Pseudallescheria boydii*, and a variety of dermatophytes.

### Candida

The most common fungal isolate from transplant patients is *Candida* spp. and the closely related *Torulopsis glabrata*, with the most frequent clinical manifestation being a mucocutaneous overgrowth syndrome: oropharyngeal thrush, esophagitis, vaginitis, intertrigo, and/or paronychia or onychomycosis. Topical therapy with nystatin or clotrimazole in conjunction with the correction of other contributing factors (e.g., correction of hyperglycemia and cessation of broad-spectrum antibacterial therapy) is usually adequate to control these problems, although fluconazole (in a dose of 200–400 mg/day) can be used if necessary. Bloodstream invasion, even if only transient, carries a risk of greater than 50% for visceral seeding; thus, there is an absolute requirement for systemic therapy with either fluconazole or amphotericin in all such individuals. Although fluconazole is a significant advance in the management of these infections, it is important to recognize that whereas *C. albicans* and *C. tropicalis* are susceptible, such yeast strains as *C. krusei* and *T. glabrata* are resistant.

### *Pneumocystis carinii*

The incidence of *P. carinii* pneumonia in the organ transplant recipient in the first six months post-transplant is approximately 10% unless effective prophylaxis is administered. The incidence is even higher in the "chronic n'er do wells," discussed above, for as long as they are maintained on immunosuppression. Low-dose (one single-strength tablet each day) trimethoprim-sulfamethoxazole therapy effectively eliminates the risk of not only *Pneumocystis*, but also listeriosis, nocardiosis, urosepsis, and, possibly, toxoplasmosis. When *Pneumocystis* pneumonia does occur in transplant recipients, it resembles that in other immunosuppressed patients—with subacute onset of fever, nonproductive cough, radiographic evidence of interstitial pneumonia, and hypoxemia out of proportion to either physical or radiographic findings.

### Aspergillus

The pathologic hallmark of *Aspergillus* infection in the transplant patient is blood vessel invasion, resulting in tissue infarction, hemorrhage, and metastases. In approximately 85% of cases the portal of entry is the lung, with the nasal sinuses accounting for 10%, and such sites as injured cutaneous surfaces accounting for the remainder. Metastatic infection is the rule, and the bases of clinical management are prevention, early recognition and prompt therapy when prevention fails, and therapy with amphotericin B—with the duration of therapy being linked with control of all sites of active infection.

## Bacterial infections

Bacterial infections in the transplant patient can be divided into three categories: conventional, with a particular susceptibility for infection of the lungs, the skin, and gastrointestinal tract; opportunistic, due to *Listeria monocytogenes* or *Nocardia asteroides*; and mycobacterial. As far as conventional bacterial infection is concerned, community-acquired bacterial pneumonia, usually following viral respiratory infection, occurs more commonly in the transplant patient than in nonimmunosuppressed individuals; that is, the attack rate for secondary bacterial pneumonia due to such organisms as *Streptococcus pneumoniae*, *Hemophilus influenzae*, and *Staphylococcus aureus* is higher than in the general population, particularly following influenza infection. The incidence of cellulitis, due to conventional gram-positive organisms is higher in transplant patients as well. In this instance, the increased prevalence is not so much due to the immunosuppressing effects of the treatment regimen, but rather because of breaks in skin integrity due to the effects of corticosteroids on skin tensile strength, as well as an increased incidence and severity of dermatophyte infection, thus providing a portal of entry for *Streptococcus pyogenes* and *Staphylococcus aureus*. Finally, two forms of gastrointestinal bacterial infection are observed: bacterial gastroenteritis due to such organisms as nontyphoidal salmonellae and *Campylobacter jejuni*; and an increased incidence of diverticulitis and gut perforation in this patient group. In general, the attack rate for these infections is higher than for the general population, and the rate of bacteremia and other complications is higher.

*Listeria monocytogenes* has as a portal of entry the gastrointestinal tract. Indeed, a not uncommon clinical syndrome is a febrile gastroenteritis syndrome caused by this organism. More commonly, bacteremia (with or without overt endocarditis), and/or central nervous system infection are the major clinical manifestations of infection with this organism. The effects of *Listeria* on the central nervous system may take one or two forms: a purulent meningitis or a focal cerebritis, with a particular propensity for involving the brain stem (in this instance, causing a bulbar polio-like syndrome).

The portal of entry for *Nocardia asteroides* is the lung, with this organism causing isolated pulmonary nodules or a subacute pneumonia. Early in its course, bloodstream invasion occurs, with metastases to other sites, particularly the skin and brain (usually causing focal parenchymal disease, occasionally a subacute–chronic meningitis). Manifestations of metastatic disease may be the first clinical clue to the presence of this infection. Both listeriosis and nocardiosis are most common one to four months post-transplant or in the "chronic n'er do well" population. Both are effectively prevented by low-dose trimethoprim-sulfamethoxazole prophylaxis.

Although atypical mycobacterial infection of skin damaged by some other process is not uncommon in transplant patients, the major mycobacterial problem in this patient population is infection due to *Mycobacterium tuberculosis*. Active tuberculosis, with a higher incidence of extrapulmonary disease than for non-immunosuppressed individuals, is more common in transplant patients than in the general population. Active tuberculosis is treated in these patients similarly to the way it is managed in the general population (with a preference for the use of isoniazid and rifampin therapy for approximately one year). The major issue here is to remember that rifampin (and perhaps isoniazid) will up-regulate hepatic cyclosporine metabolism, requiring increased doses in order to maintain adequate levels of immunosuppression. Therefore, close attention to cyclosporine blood levels is necessary in patients being treated with these drugs.

A more controversial question is the appropriate use of isoniazid prophylaxis in tuberculin positive individuals. Because of the complexities of using this drug in a patient population with an already high incidence of hepatic dysfunction, and because of the low risk of active tuberculosis if the patient does not have other risk factors for tuberculosis, for the majority of patients close surveillance rather than prophylaxis may be the better course of action. We reserve isoniazid prophylaxis for individuals who have a positive tuberculin skin test (see Chapter 63) and one or more of the following risk factors: recent tuberculin conversion, history of active disease, non-Caucasian racial status, the presence of other immunosuppressing conditions, the presence of significant abnormalities on chest X-ray, and the presence of protein-calorie malnutrition.

## General Approach to Antimicrobial Therapy in the Transplant Patient

There are three modes in which antimicrobial therapy can be administered: therapeutic, prophylactic, and preemptive. Therapeutic antimicrobial therapy is designed to treat established clinical infection. Prophylactic therapy involves the administration of antimicrobial agents to the entire susceptible population prior to an event in order to prevent clinical disease. This approach requires a condition important enough to justify prophylaxis, as well as a nontoxic therapy that can be shown to be cost-effective. Perhaps the most successful prophylactic regimen in transplantation is the aforementioned low-dose trimethoprim-sulfamethoxazole regimen. Preemptive therapy involves the prescription of antimicrobial therapy to a subgroup of individuals prior to onset of clinical disease, on the basis of a clinical or epidemiologic characteristic or a laboratory marker. Thus, the use of ganciclovir when antilymphocyte antibody therapy is required is an example of effective preemptive therapy, as is the eradication of asymptomatic candiduria with fluconazole prior to the development of an obstructing fungal ball. Increasingly in transplantation, the emphasis is on prevention of infection, and hence the increasing emphasis on cost-effective prophylactic and preemptive strategies.

The emphasis on infection prevention in transplant patients is made even more important by the possibility of drug interaction with cyclosporine. The key step in the metabolism of cyclosporine is a hepatic cytochrome P450 enzymatic function, which can be modulated by many drugs. Drugs that increase cyclosporine metabolism, and hence could lead to reduced immunosuppression and allograft rejection, include rifampin. Drugs that decrease cyclosporine metabolism, hence leading to higher cyclosporine blood levels, increased nephrotoxicity, and the potential for increased immunosuppression, include erythromycin (and presumably the newer macrolides) and the azoles (ketoconazole > itraconazole > fluconazole). Both of these forms of interaction can be dealt with by modification of cyclosporine dosages based on close monitoring of blood levels. Of greater concern is the occurrence of synergistic nephrotoxicity, which is not related to cyclosporine blood levels. This is most commonly seen with amphotericin, aminoglycosides, high-dose trimethoprim-sulfamethoxazole and fluoroquinolone therapy, and vancomycin. In addition, a useful general rule is that if unexplained renal dysfunction occurs, then a drug interaction with cyclosporine should be suspected, with antimicrobial agents being common culprits.

## Summary

A great deal of progress has been made in the delineation of the pathogenesis and the principles of infection management in transplant patients. It is apparent that the occurrence of infection is largely determined by the interaction of two factors, the patient's net state of immunosuppression and the epidemiologic exposures he encounters. These factors can be translated into an expected timetable according to which certain infections tend to occur, with this timetable then serving as the basis of cost-effective preventative strategies. In this regard, perhaps the most important lesson that has been learned is that the therapeutic prescription for the transplant patient has two components: an immunosuppressive strategy to prevent and treat rejection, and an antimicrobial strategy to make it safe. Thus, just as immunosuppressive regimens must be individualized for each patient, antimicrobial strategies, linked to these adjustments, must be individualized. As new immunosuppressive strategies are deployed, the obligation of the infectious-disease clinician is to define the etiology and timing of the associated infectious-disease risks, and then design appropriate antimicrobial responses. With the advent of new antiviral and antifungal agents, our ability to accomplish this task will be significantly increased, but the general principles will remain unchanged.

### ANNOTATED BIBLIOGRAPHY

Balfour HH Jr, Chace BA, Stapleton JT, et al. A randomized, placebo-controlled trial of oral acyclovir for the prevention of cytomegalovirus disease in recipients of renal allografts. N Engl J Med 1989; 320:1381–1387.

*The study that demonstrated the clearest benefits of high dose acyclovir prophylaxis in organ transplantation.*

Grattan MT, Moreno-Cabral CE, Starnes VA, et al. Cytomegalovirus infection is associated with cardia allograft rejection and atherosclerosis. JAMA 1989; 261:3561–3566.

*The study that demonstrates the clearest relationship between cytomegalovirus infection and allograft injury.*

Katkov WN, Rubin RH. Liver disease in the organ transplant recipient: etiology, clinical impact, and clinical management. Transplant Rev 1991; 5:200–208.

*A complete review of liver disease, both drug and induced, in the organ transplant recipient.*

Kusne S, Dummer JS, Singh N, et al. Infections after liver transplantation: An analysis of 101 consecutive cases. Medicine 1988; 67:132–143.

*A large series of liver transplant patients carefully analyzed for infection that demonstrates the importance of technical factors in the pathogenesis of these infections.*

Merigan TC, Reylund DG, Keay S, et al. A controlled trial of ganciclovir to prevent cytomegalovirus disease after heart transplantation. N Engl J Med 1992; 326:1182–1186.

*A careful study of ganciclovir prophylaxis in organ transplant recipients that demonstrates the importance of extended duration therapy, particularly in those patients at risk for primary CMV disease.*

Paya CV, Hermans PE, Washington JA II, et al. Incidence, distribution, and outcome of episodes of infection in 100 orthotopic liver transplantations. Mayo Clin Proc 1989; 64:555–564.

*A careful study of infection pathogenesis and prevention from a large, successful liver transplant program.*

Pereira BJG, Milford EL, Kirkman RL, et al. Prevalence of hepatitis C virus RNA in organ donors positive for hepatitis C antibody and in the recipients of their organs. N Engl J Med 1992; 327:910–915.

*A careful study of the transmission of hepatitis C virus via infected allografts.*

Pohl C, Green M, Wald ER, et al. Respiratory syncytial virus infection in pediatric liver transplant recipients. J Infect Dis 1992; 165:166–169.

*As more transplant patients return to normal lives the threat of community acquired respiratory virus infection increases. In this example, the impact of the respiratory syncytial virus is carefully delineated.*

Preiskaitis JK, Diaz-Mitoma F, Mirzayans F, et al. Quantitative oropharyngeal Epstein-Barr virus shedding in renal and cardiac transplant recipients: relationship to immunosuppressive therapy, serologic responses, and the risk of posttransplant lymphoproliferative disorder. J Infect Dis 1992; 166:986–994.

*An important study that delineates the effects of immunosuppression and antiviral therapy, on Epstein-Barr virus replication and subsequent risk of lymphoma.*

Rubin RH. The indirect effects of cytomegalovirus infection on the outcome of organ transplantation. JAMA 1989; 261:3607–3609.

*A careful study of the indirect effects of CMV infection on organ transplant recipients, including allograft injury and predisposition to opportunistic infection.*

Rubin RH. Infectious disease complications of renal transplantation. Kidney Int 1993; 44:221–236.

*A complete review of the infectious diseases complications of renal transplantation, their pathogenesis, and their clinical management.*

Rubin RH, Tolkoff-Rubin NE. Antimicrobial strategies in the care of organ transplant recipients. Antimicrob Agents Chemother 1993; 37:619–624.

*Principles of antimicrobial therapy in organ transplant recipients.*

Rubin RH. Infection in the organ transplant recipient. In Clinical Approach to Infection in the Compromised Host, 3rd ed. Rubin RH, Young LS, eds. Plenum Medical Book Company, New York, pp 629–705, 1994.

*A detailed review of all aspects of infection in organ transplantation.*

Samuel D, Bismuth A, Mathieu D, et al. Passive immunoprophylaxis after liver transplantation in HBsAg-positive patients. Lancet 1991; 1:813–815.

*The report that led to the current management of hepatitis B virus infection in liver transplant candidates.*

Snydman DR, Werner BG, Heinze-Lacey B, et al. Use of cytomegalovirus immune globulin to prevent cytomegalovirus disease in renal transplant recipients. N Engl J Med 1987; 317:1049–1054.

*The clearest demonstration of the prophylactic efficacy of CMV hyperimmune globulin prophylaxis against CMV infection.*

# 88

# Hematopoietic Stem Cell Transplantation

RALEIGH A. BOWDEN

Infections continue to be the major impediment to successful hematopoietic stem cell (HCT) transplantation, although major progress has been made in recent years in the prevention of viral and, more recently, candidal infections. Knowledge of the natural history of acquisition and/or reactivation of prior infection can assist the clinician in developing a likely differential diagnosis and distinguishing infectious from noninfectious complications in these often critically ill patients. The following chapter will review recent changes in the epidemiologic patterns of the various infections after HCT, the influence that prevention strategies has had on the timing of infection, and current treatment approaches in these patients.

## Nature and Mechanisms of Immunosuppression

Following HCT, patients experience a predictable pattern of immunosuppression. This is a result of both the conditioning therapy given to reduce the burden of underlying malignancy and ablate existing marrow/host defense in preparation for the transplanted marrow or peripheral blood stem cells, and, for patients undergoing allogeneic transplant, the development of acute graft-versus-host disease (GVHD). Both GVHD and the immunosuppressive therapy used to prevent or treat it result in ongoing immunosuppression that can persist for months or even years in some patients.

The techniques for HCT are undergoing a number of changes which may influence the timing and severity of infection. First, an increasing number of unrelated marrow donor transplants are being performed where the incidence of acute and chronic GVHD and concomitant risk and infection remain ongoing risks. In addition, it has been recently demonstrated that stem cells required for the establishment of the new immune system can be obtained from peripheral blood rather than marrow. These transplants, termed peripheral blood stem cell (PBSC) transplants, are becoming quite routine for patients undergoing autologous transplant, particularly for breast cancer, and PBSC transplants are being used increasingly for allogeneic transplants as well.

The impact of these procedural changes on the changing risk of transplant-associated infections needs to be carefully examined. At the present time, patients undergoing autologous transplants continue to have a similar risk for bacterial infection as patients undergoing allogeneic transplants, but have only about one-tenth the risk for development of life-threatening viral or fungal infections. PBSCs, plus the use of growth factors, may decrease the risk for bacterial infections by shortening the duration of neutropenia. A change in the risk for viral or fungal infections has not yet been shown to depend on the source of stem cells and at the present time the risk continues to correlate with the type of marrow donor, with patients undergoing allogeneic transplant at the highest risk.

## Epidemiology of Infections in Marrow Transplant Patients

Figure 88.1 outlines the natural history of the common infectious pathogens and associated host defense abnormalities that HCT patients experience during the first year after transplant prior to the availability of effective antiviral and antifungal prophylaxis. Patients who do not develop GVHD or are successfully treated are usually able to discontinue immunosuppressive therapy by the third and sixth month after transplant with a return to "normal immunity" by one and a half to two years following the marrow transplant.

### Bacterial infections

The timing of infection after HCT is specific to the type of organism. Bacterial infections continue to be the most common during the neutropenic period, resulting from invasion of the patient's endogenous flora, usually from the gastrointestinal tract or skin surface. The exception is infection with coagulase-negative *Staphylococcus*, which continues to occur as long as the central venous catheter remains in place. This pattern of bacterial infection has remained relatively constant over the past decade.

### Viral infections

In contrast, the most dramatic change in the frequency and timing of infection has been as a result of the introduction of viral and fungal prophylaxis. Viral infections result either from (*1*) reactivation of latent virus, as is the case of the herpesvirus group of infections, the most common viral infections after HCT or (*2*) acquisition of virus from blood products, as is seen with cytomegalovirus (CMV) and Epstein-Barr virus, or (*3*) less commonly, contact with infected individuals during this period of immunodeficiency. This latter mode of transmission is particularly common with respiratory viruses during the fall and winter months.

Figure 88.2 shows how the frequency and timing of herpes simplex virus (HSV) infection has changed with the use of acyclovir prophylaxis. The open bars relate the incidence prior to the availability of acyclovir. The solid bars show the incidence from the time when acyclovir prophylaxis (250 mg/m$^2$ every 12 hours) is given from the time at conditioning until day 30 after transplant. Once the cause of an oral infection occurring during

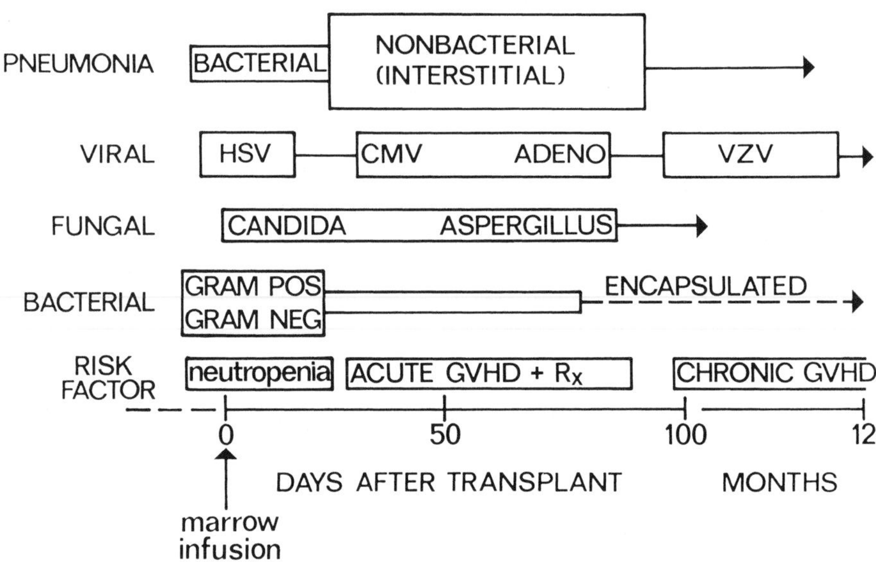


**Fig. 88.1** Predisposing risk factors and common infections by time after hematopoietic stem cell transplant (HCT). [From Meyers JD, Infections in marrow transplant. In: Principles and Practices of Infectious Diseases, 3rd ed., Churchill Livingstone, London, pp. 2291–2294, 1990, with permission.]

the first month after transplant in 80% of hosts, the incidence of HSV has been reduced by approximately 50%, and severity is now limited to the more typical oral or perineal lesions seen in normal hosts. The timing of HSV infection, however, has shifted to the 1–2 months after prophylaxis is discontinued. Because 80% of HSV-seropositive patients will reactivate HSV during the first month after transplant, acyclovir prophylaxis is now given routinely to all HSV-seropositive patients during the period of conditioning-related mucositis. Patients are then subsequently allowed to reactivate HSV to facilitate immune reconstitution at a time when morbidity is reduced.

Figure 88.3 shows the incidence of CMV infection in CMV-seropositive patients, comparing the pattern observed in the late 1970s before ganciclovir (open bars) was available with the pattern now seen in patients receiving ganciclovir prophylaxis (5 mg/kg/day) from the time of first positive culture or engraftment until day 80 after transplant (solid bars). Ganciclovir has markedly reduced the incidence of CMV disease early in the post-transplant period; however, the risk for CMV disease has been shifted to a later post-transplant time, after the ganciclovir prophylaxis has been discontinued. Currently, approximately 15% of patients receiving prophylaxis now develop CMV disease by day 180, a 50% reduction compared to what was seen by day 180 in the days before ganciclovir was available. Ganciclovir, when given for CMV prophylaxis, also effectively suppresses clinical infection with HSV and varicella zoster virus (VZV).

### Fungal infections

Fungal infection, and specifically that caused by *Candida* spp. and *Aspergillus* spp. has become the leading infectious cause of death in many centers with the successful prevention of CMV. While the incidence of *Candida albicans* has been virtually eliminated with fluconazole prophylaxis (Table 88.1), fluconazole does not prevent fluconozole-resistant *C. krusei*, *Aspergillus* spp., or other mold infections.

## Specific Complications by Organ Systems and Organism

### Blood stream infection

Bacteremia is the most frequently documented cause of bacterial infection after HCT. Over the past decade, gram-positive bacteria, and specifically coagulase-negative *Staphylococci* have replaced enteric gram-negative organisms as the leading causes of bacteremia. Bacteremia may present without fever when corticosteroids are given for prevention and treatment of GVHD. Coagulase-negative staphylococcal infections have been associated with the increased use of indwelling catheters and occur throughout the early post-transplant period irrespective of neutropenia. Because there remains no reliable way to distinguish true bacteremia from "catheter" contamination in these patients, a single blood culture should be considered an indication for treatment with antibiotics.

Gram-negative enteric organisms, particularly Enterobacteriaceae, *Klebsiella*, and *E. coli*, continue to be the second leading causes of bacteremia in most centers. While the incidence of *Pseudomonas* infection has decreased in recent years, presumably due to the increased use of empiric antibiotics with anti-*Pseudomonas* activity, empiric coverage for this organism during febrile neutropenia may still be necessary in centers where *Pseudomonas* continues to be prevalent.

*Candida* spp have become the fourth most common cause of bloodstream infection in seriously ill patients overall, including HCT patients. Fungemia occurs in approximately 10% of patients in marrow transplant centers where prophylactic fluconazole is not used. *Candida* spp. usually enter the portal bloodstream from the gastrointestinal tract, which is often heavily colonized in pa-

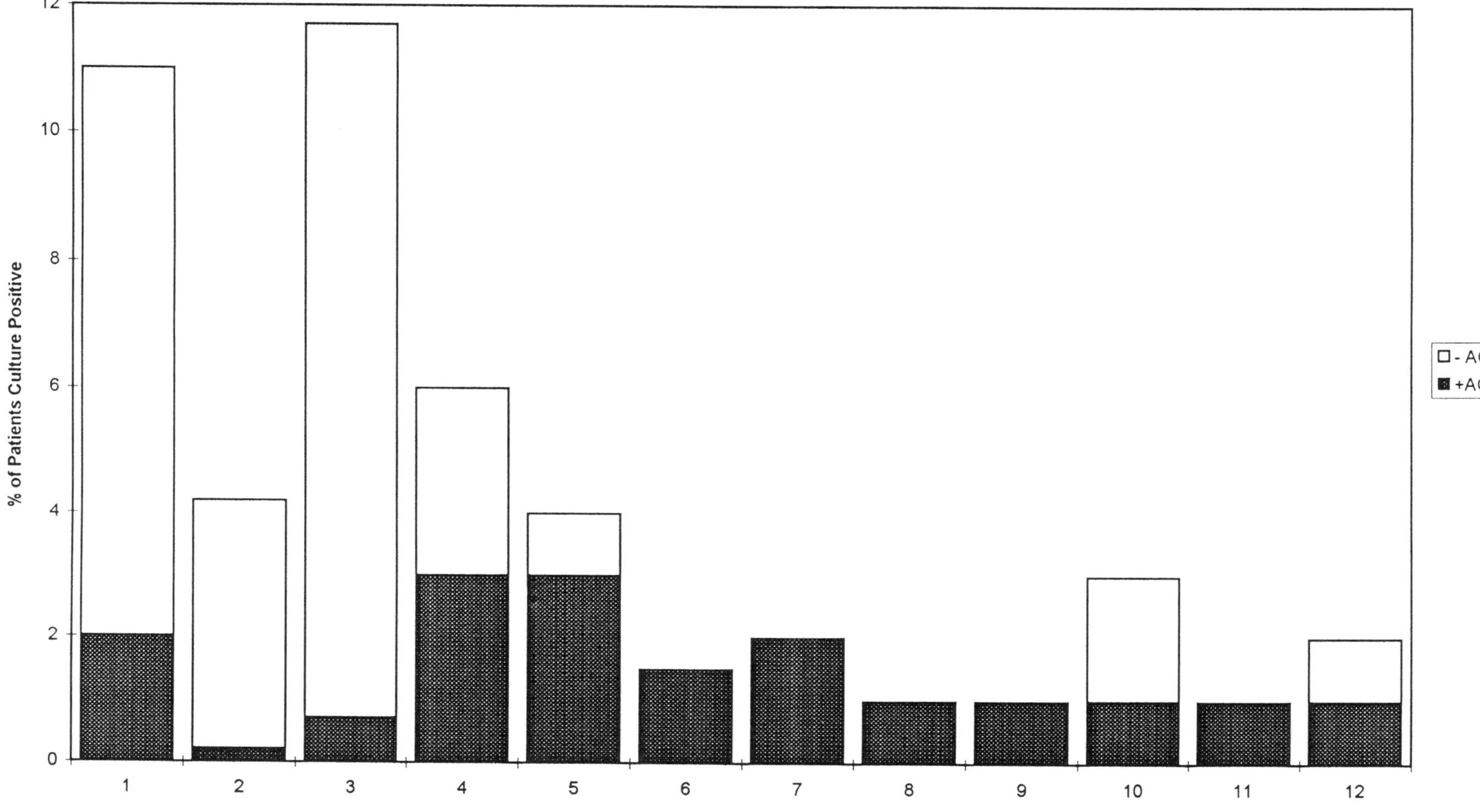


**Fig. 88.2** Percentage of all HCT patients developing herpes simplex virus during two separate time periods—one with and one without acyclovir prophylaxis for first positive culture after marrow transplant.

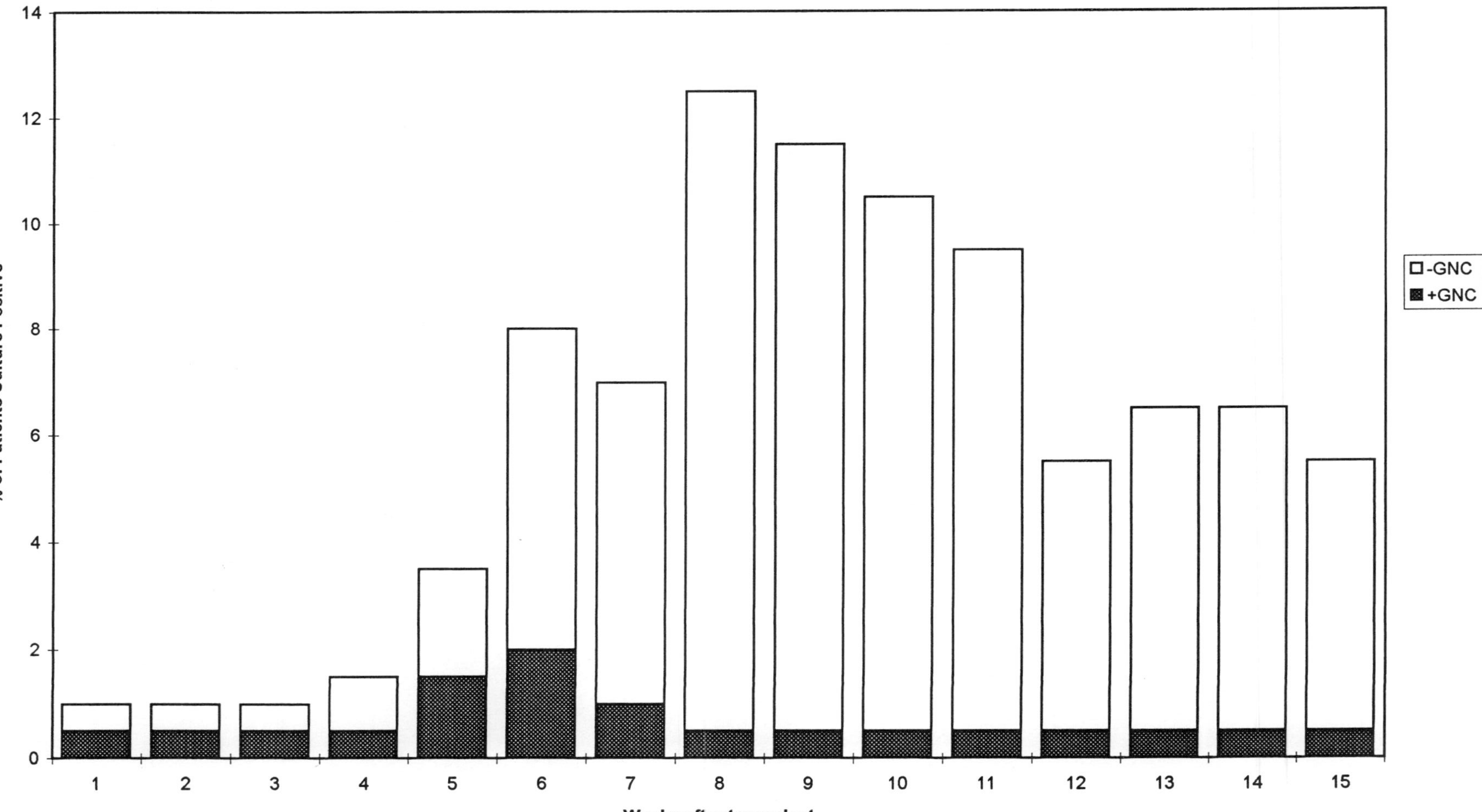


**Fig. 88.3** Percentage of CMV-seropositive HCT patients with positive blood cultures by week after transplant during two separate time periods—one with and one without ganciclovir prophylaxis.

**Table 88.1** Effect of prophylaxis of fungal infections with fluconazole in HCT or hematopoietic stem cell transplant patients*

| Fungus | Fluconazole (N = 142) | Placebo (N = 148) | *p* value |
|---|---|---|---|
| *Candida albicans* | 0 | 18 | .001 |
| *C. glabrata* | 3 | 6 | |
| *C. tropicalis* | 0 | 2 | |
| *C. guilliermondii* | 1 | 0 | |
| *C. parapsilopsis* | 0 | 1 | |
| *C. pseudotropicalis* | 0 | 1 | |
| Yeasts, unspecified | 0 | 1 | |
| *Aspergillus fumigatus* | 3 | 2 | |
| *Fusarium* spp. | 1 | 1 | |
| Unknown | 2 | 0 | |
| Total | 10 | 32 | 0.003 |

*Adapted from Slavin MA, Osborne B, Adams R, Levenstein MJ, Schoch HG, Feldman AR, Meyers JD, Bowden RA. Efficacy and safety of fluconazole prophylaxis for fungal infections after marrow transplantation—a prospective, randomized, double-blind study. J Infect Dis 1995; 171:1545–1552, with permission.

tients on broad-spectrum antibiotics. Even in the absence of gastrointestinal colonization, particular species of *Candida*, for example *C. parapsilosis*, have been observed in association with catheter infections, and epidemics have been reported from contaminated hyperalimentation fluid.

Candidal infection generally occurs early after transplant, with a median time of onset for fungemia of three weeks after transplant (Fig. 1). Centers which use fluconazole prophylaxis have seen a virtual elimination of *Candida albicans* infection (Table 88.1), but an increase in infections with non-*albicans Candida* spp., specifically *C. krusei*, *C. tropicalis*, and *C. parapsilosis* has occurred. Fluconazole, given at a dose of 400 mg/day, either through engraftment or until day 75, has virtually eliminated infections with *C. albicans*. Furthermore, fluconazole has reduced the incidence of invasive fungal infection, superficial fungal infection, and colonization; it has reduced the use of empiric amphotericin B; and if continued through day 75, it has reduced mortality. Resistance to fluconazole in this setting is of theoretical concern, but has not been experienced in larger HCT centers where fluconazole has now been used routinely for several years.

## Pneumonia

Pneumonia continues to be a common problem after marrow transplant, although with the availability of ganciclovir, the spectrum of agents causing pneumonia has changed dramatically. Bacterial infection continues to be the major cause of pneumonia during the neutropenic period, although the specific organism is often difficult to recover. Noninfectious pneumonia, termed "idiopathic pneumonia," which results from toxicity related to conditioning, occurs in approximately 30% of patients. The timing of idiopathic pneumonia can either be early, during the first few weeks after the transplant, or it may occur later, during the second to third month following transplant.

### Viruses

CMV pneumonia, once the leading infectious cause of death in the first 100 days after transplant, now occurs in less than 5% of patients during the first three months after transplant when routine ganciclovir prophylaxis is used. Other viral etiologies of pneumonia, particularly the respiratory viruses have taken on a relatively new importance with the successful prevention of CMV. Respiratory syncytial virus (RSV) continues to be the most common respiratory virus infection, followed by parainfluenza, rhinovirus, and influenza. The occurrence of respiratory viruses varies from year to year and only parainfluenza is seen with any frequency outside of the winter months. The onset of infection is either early post-transplant in patients who are already infected at the time of transplant, or after discharge from the hospital when patients may acquire it from infected family members or health-care givers. RSV progresses from upper respiratory to lower respiratory tract infection in approximately 50% of cases. The mortality rate with RSV pneumonia is approximately 80%, regardless of whether the infection occurred before or after engraftment.

Pulmonary infection with parainfluenza, particularly type 3, also leads to a high morbidity and mortality. Influenza infection is less frequent, and as with the other respiratory viruses, reflects the epidemiology in the community for any particular season. Influenza in the HCT patient often presents without the typical myalgias seen in normal hosts. Rhinovirus infection in transplants is usually confined to the upper respiratory tract. In a recent review at the FHCRC, only 1 of 32 respiratory-tract rhinovirus isolates was identified as coming from the lower respiratory tract.

### Fungi

Fungi are another important cause of pneumonia, with the predominant organism being *Aspergillus fumigatus*. Typically, *Aspergillus* spp. infection presents as either pneumonia or sinusitis, and has increased in some centers in recent years. While historically most common a median of six weeks after transplantation, more recent data show a bimodal distribution for *Aspergillus* spp. infection, with the earlier peak a median 16 days after transplant and a second, larger peak a median of 96 days after transplant. Patients undergoing allogeneic transplant are most likely to develop aspergillosis after engraftment in association with GVHD; autologous patients are at highest risk for the development of aspergillosis during the early peak. The organism enters through the upper respiratory tract and causes infection in the lungs with or without sinus involvement and can lead to dissemination to brain, skin, and, rarely, other organs. The early peak is likely due to infection acquired prior to transplant and may be increasing as more patients are coming to transplant with more prolonged courses or cycles of chemotherapy and associated neutropenia for their underlying refractory malignancy.

Other infectious causes of pneumonia are rare in marrow transplant patients. Primary candidal pneumonia is seen almost exclusively in the early post-transplant period in the presence of fungemia. Rarely, it occurs later after transplant in the critically ill, intubated patient who is heavily colonized with *Candida* spp. and has other risk factors, including glucocorticoid administration and prolonged usage of broad-spectrum antibiotics.

#### Other agents

Pneumocystis pneumonia is very uncommon in the setting of routine prophylaxis with trimethoprim-sulfamethoxazole (TMP-SMX). A recent review has shown that the major risk for this infection today is the patient who fails to take TMP-SMX prophylaxis because of a history of allergy. Other causes of community acquired pneumonia, including chlamydia and mycoplasma are also rare. In a recent study at the FHCRC, looking for these organisms by culture or PCR failed to reveal even a single positive in 84 consecutive BALs performed for diagnosis of an infiltrate on chest radiograph (unpublished data, R. Bowden). *Legionella* remains an infrequent but serious cause of nosocomial pneumonia in some centers.

### Sinusitis

Sinus disease after HCT is common, and begins as part of the generalized mucositis that follows conditioning radiation and chemotherapy. During the early post-transplant period, normal sinus drainage is altered and secondary infection can result. The etiology varies, and includes bacterial, fungal, and/or viral agents. Air/fluid levels on sinus CT scan are associated with a higher likelihood of recovering of infectious etiologies. Respiratory viruses, specifically RSV and parainfluenza, should be considered in the differential diagnosis during the respiratory virus season. Fungal sinusitis is particularly common in patients with GVHD and/or receiving glucocorticoid therapy. *Aspergillus* spp. can involve the sinuses and is often seen in conjunction with *Aspergillus* spp. pneumonia. Mold infections in the sinuses may less commonly lead to direct infection of the orbital tissues with or without direct extension to the brain. This is particularly common with the *Mucorales* order of Zygomyces.

### Gastrointestinal tract disorders

While diarrhea and abdominal pain are frequent complications in the weeks following HCT, infectious etiologies are rare. In a recent study at the FHCRC, diarrhea specimens were cultured for a variety of infectious agents and in only 10% was an infectious etiology defined. Astrovirus was the most common, followed by *Clostridium difficile*, adenovirus, and CMV. Diarrhea in the early post-transplant period is most commonly nonbloody with crampy abdominal pain and is associated with other signs of a regimen-related toxicity, which may include skin rash similar to a severe burn or diffuse erythema. Busulfan is one chemotherapeutic agent used for conditioning that may be particularly likely to cause diarrhea. After engraftment, diarrhea is most likely due to acute GVHD and is characteristically bloody, resembling sloughed tissue, and is often associated with fever, liver enzyme or bilirubin elevation, or the classic maculopapular rash of skin GVHD. Colitis due to *C. difficile* is seen after the use of systemic antibiotics and is common in marrow transplant patients. Because the organism can be a normal part of the intestinal flora, the presence of *C. difficile* toxin, not merely the presence of the organisms, should be the trigger to initiate therapy (see Chapter 64). Periodic outbreaks of diarrhea have been reported in institutions caring for HCT patients, particularly with enterovirus, and are associated with a high fatality rate.

A rare but important presentation of varicella zoster virus (VZV) reactivation is the occurrence of severe abdominal pain. Typically presenting in a patient on glucocorticosteroids with GVHD, the abdominal pain usually precedes the development of skin lesions by five to seven days and therefore can be quite difficult to diagnosis. A concomitant sudden rise in liver function tests may be another associated finding. A high index of suspicion and early institution of acyclovir may be life saving.

### Hepatobiliary disorders

The multiple causes of jaundice and liver enzyme elevation after HCT create an unusual challenge in distinguishing the infectious from the noninfectious causes of liver disease. The two major causes of hyperbilirubinemia in this setting are noninfectious and include veno-occlusive disease (VOD) and GVHD of the liver. VOD occurs early after transplant and is due to regimen-related damage of the liver. VOD is characterized by weight gain, hepatic tenderness, and an increase in conjugated bilirubin *without* concomitant liver enzyme elevation. It can progress to severe liver dysfunction resulting in hepatorenal syndrome, or it can remain mild and slowly resolve over the first one to two months after transplant. VOD is rarely confused with infection.

In contrast, elevated liver enzymes can occur for a variety of reasons, including noninfectious causes such as acute GVHD. The infectious differential diagnosis includes viral hepatitis with hepatitis C, B, and A, in that order of frequency. Other less common causes of viral hepatitis include CMV or adenovirus. Herpesviruses such as VZV or HSV can result in infection in the liver as part of disseminated infection, but occur rarely since the availability of effective antiviral prophylaxis. Table 88.2 shows the differential diagnosis, including infectious and noninfectious etiologies of elevated transaminases by degree of elevation of alanine aminotransferase (ALT) and aspartase aminotransferase (AST). An isolated elevation of alkaline phosphatase may indicate hepatic involvement with *Candida*, rare now in centers where fluconazole prophylaxis is used.

### Cutaneous disorders

Marrow transplant patients commonly experience skin rashes, which can be either infectious or noninfectious in etiology. Noninfectious causes of skin rashes include conditioning-related

**Table 88.2** Differential diagnosis of elevated hepatic transaminitis after marrow transplant

| |
|---|
| HIGHEST LEVELS OF AST/ALT (I.E. >150 UNITS/ML) |
| Viral hepatitis (to >1000 units/ml): HSV, VZV, adenovirus |
| Hepatitis B and C: varies with immune reconstitution |
| Graft-versus-host disease (70–350 units/ml) |
| Drug/TPN liver disease (to 500) |
| MODEST ELEVATION FOR AST/ALT: (I.E. <150 UNITS/ML) |
| Fungi (e.g. *Candida*) or bacterial (to 150 units/ml) |
| Tumor infiltration (including EBV-related (to 100 units/ml) |
| *Cholangitis lenta* (to 100 units/ml) |
| Venocclusive disease (to 100 units/ml) |

Abbreviations—AST: aspartase aminotransferase; ALT: alanine aminotransferase; HSV: herpes simplex virus; VZV: varicella zoster virus; TPN: total parenteral nutrition; EBV: Epstein-Barr virus.

toxicity, such rashes usually present during the first two weeks after transplant and are characterized by a diffuse erythroderma and can be associated with blistering of the digits of the hands and feet. Another cause of a diffuse skin rash is acute GVHD, which may begin initially as a faint erythroderma and later become maculopapular, and is often associated with fever and diarrhea shortly before or coincident with engraftment. Finally, drug eruptions, most commonly due to semisynthetic penicillins or cephalosporins used for empiric treatment of febrile neutropenia, may be indistinguishable from other forms of diffuse erythroderma after transplant. Specific diagnoses of diffuse skin rashes are best made by skin biopsy if treatment for GVHD and/or empiric change of antibiotics does not result in improvement of the rash.

Cutaneous infectious disorders in the transplant patient are often focal in nature. They include bacterial, viral, and fungal etiologies. Bacterial skin infections are often located at the central catheter exit site and may include the catheter tunnel tract. Cellulitis other than at intravenous line sites is uncommon. Less frequently, systemic gram-negative bacteremia can present with cutaneous manifestations including sparse, discrete scattered papules, often darkened or purpuric, usually on the trunk or extremities in association with other clinical signs of bacterial sepsis. Diagnosis is made by recovery of the organism in the blood or by culture of biopsy of the skin lesions (see Chapter 55).

The skin lesions associated with systemic fungal infection are often indistinguishable from bacterial emboli. In contrast to the bacteremia, where the blood culture is positive, the biopsy of the skin lesion in the patient with disseminated fungal infection may provide the only evidence for the fungal etiology diagnosis. Focal fungal dermatitis, particularly of the perineal area, is common during the period of neutropenia and is caused by *Candida* spp. or superficial dermatophytes.

Viral skin infections are usually caused by herpesviruses and typically present as a crop (or crops) of localized vesicles. VZV is the most common cause, and 84% of VZV develops as localized infection. This localized presentation can include the classic dermatomal distribution or may present atypically with a few clustered nonvesicular-appearing papules. Disseminated HSV infection often presents with only a few atypically distributed vesicles. Unless vesicular skin lesions present with the classic dermatomal presentation, the base of the lesions should be scraped and the cells examined by fluorescent antibody stain to confirm the diagnosis and to rule out the less usual occurrences of HSV. Rarely, skin GVHD can present as "dewdrop" vesicles, which can be distinguished from viral lesions because they lack the erythematous bases. They typically are bilaterally distributed on the shoulders or chest, break open with minimal trauma, and are not painful. Disseminated infection with HSV is extremely rare compared to VZV.

## Central nervous system (CNS) infections

While CNS dysfunction is relatively common after HCT, it is usually related to metabolic complications or complications of drug therapy and is rarely due to infection. Bacterial meningitis is very rarely seen, presumably due to the routine use of empiric antibiotics with good CNS penetration. Parameningeal infection such as ethmoiditis may rarely lead to bacterial meningitis. Viral encephalitis, again most commonly due to either HSV or VZV infection can occur but usually in the setting of disseminated infection and are rare now in the setting of antiviral prophylaxis.

A recent review of brain abscesses from an autopsy series in HCT patients showed that 58% were due to *Aspergillus* spp., typically presenting as a single or several large, discrete masses on CT scan and often associated with simultaneous infection in the lung or sinuses. Candidal brain infection was the second most common etiology, causing 33% of CNS abscesses. Candidal CNS abscesses were typically multiple, small, and in a miliary distribution. Less than 10% of CNS infections were caused by anaerobic or other typical bacteria seen as the major causes of brain abscesses outside the marrow transplant setting (see Chapter 76). Toxoplasmosis can also present as a brain abscess in patients known to be seropositive prior to transplant but is rare in the post-transplant setting.

## Diagnosis

Diagnostic approaches in evaluating infection after marrow transplant are guided by the knowledge of which organisms are likely pathogens for the specific time period. Fever is usually present, but may be absent in patients on glucocorticoids or with invasive mold infections. The most important diagnostic evaluation is the physical exam, because it may identify an obvious site of infection that may not be identified in blood or other cultures. Sites deserving particular attention include the sinuses, looking for tenderness or symptoms of post-nasal drainage; the oral cavity looking for focal ulcers, candidiasis, or black necrotic lesions suggestive of invasive mold infection; the chest; the perirectal area; and the skin. All suspicious lesions should be cultured immediately.

Blood cultures should be obtained for any fever of 38.0 °C or greater, and in some cases should be routinely performed in patients on high doses of corticosteroids who may not be able to develop a fever. Additional work-up of the febrile neutropenic patient should include a chest X ray. A urinalysis or culture may be helpful, especially in women or in patients with a history of previous urinary tract abnormalities, although, in general, urinary tract infections as a cause of fever are in these patients relatively uncommon. CSF evaluation is rarely helpful, as bacterial meningitis is very unusual in the setting of ongoing broad-spectrum antibiotic therapy. During the respiratory virus season, fever can be a sign of a potentially life-threatening respiratory virus infection. Nasopharyngeal swabs are useful for identifying respiratory viruses by culture or antigen detections in the appropriate symptomatic patient.

Aggressive diagnosis of suspected invasive infection is imperative in HCT patients. Committing patients to prolonged therapy with potentially toxic agents such as amphotericin B, ganciclovir, or other medications should only be done in conjunction with establishing a firm diagnosis. Furthermore, the spectrum of disorders causing fever in HCT patients compared to less immunocompromised patients is broad, and infections can progress rapidly if appropriate treatment is not instituted. Invasive diagnostic techniques such as biopsies of skin lesions or focal lesions of the lung or abdominal organs are critical in this patient population where infections must be treated aggressively and early in their course to optimize chances of a successful outcome. Other diagnostic procedures, such as bronchoalveolar lavage and needle or open biopsies should be encouraged.

Early diagnostic markers, including antigen detection and PCR, have now been developed (see Chapter 15); an increasing number of these are being pursued to address their role in identifying patients who might benefit from earlier treatment or prophylaxis. For example, a positive CMV culture from blood or BAL has been traditionally used to guide prophylactic or therapeutic ganciclovir to seropositive patients during the high-risk period. Culture is being rapidly being replaced by either CMV antigen detection in leukocytes or PCR of leukocytes or plasma.

The use of most early diagnostic markers for invasive fungal infection is still experimental. Metabolic markers for *Candida* spp., including D-Arabinotol or enolase, hold promise for predicting invasive candidal infection but require frequent sampling. Current areas of investigation are focusing on PCR detection of both *Candida* spp. and *Aspergillus* spp. and antigen detection for *Aspergillus* spp. Diagnosis and evaluation of treatment of these infections may benefit from the newer approaches and hopefully will result in an improvement in survival in patients with invasive fungal infections.

## Treatment

Treatment of specific infections is covered in Chapters 41–44 and will not be discussed in detail here. A few general comments will be made, however.

### Treatment of established bacterial infection

Proven bacterial infection should be treated with the antibiotics to which they are shown to be susceptible. The duration of therapy for bacteremia and other proven bacterial infections has not been completely defined, although two weeks from the time of the last positive blood culture will eradicate most uncomplicated episodes of bacteremia. An exception may be in patients with *Staphylococcus aureus* bacteremia, who should be evaluated for evidence of endocarditis before discontinuation of therapy at two weeks.

### Empiric therapy during the neutropenic period

It was first shown by Pizzo and coworkers that the institution of empiric therapy and its continuation until resolution of neutropenia could reduce infectious mortality. The use of antibiotics for empiric treatment of fever during the neutropenic period remains the accepted standard of care. The choice of antibiotics is determined by the institution-specific organisms and their susceptibility patterns. If the patient is neutropenic and develops a fever, empiric broad-spectrum coverage is always instituted before the culture results are known (see Chapter 90 for suggested regimens).

### Growth factors and granulocyte transfusions

The use of growth factors, including G-CSF and GM-CSF have clearly had their impact on shortening the duration of neutropenia after HCT (see Chapter 46). However, their role in reducing documented invasive infection remains controversial. There has been a reemergence of interest in using granulocyte transfusion for proven infection during the neutropenic period with the availability of growth factors which can be used to stimulate the donor prior to granulocyte collection. This technique often yields granulocyte numbers which are 10-fold higher than what has been seen with the more traditional methods of collection, resulting in measurable levels of circulating granulocytes in the adult recipient post-transfusion.

### Treatment of viral disease

Treatment of viral disease, including tissue-documented CMV or other herpesviruses has been well defined. Acyclovir (250 mg/m$^2$ every 8 hours for 7 days) is the recommended treatment of HSV infection. A dose of 500 mg/m$^2$ every 8 hours is recommended for treatment of VZV infection. Newer formulations using a prodrug of acyclovir offers the potential advantages of higher serum levels of acyclovir requiring less frequent administration. Studies defining their role in HCT patients are needed.

Treatment of CMV disease has been less well defined. While the combination of intravenous immunoglobulin (IVIG) (500 mg/kg every other day) plus ganciclovir (5 mg/kg BID) for two weeks has become standard treatment for CMV pneumonia, the mortality rate remains 50%–70% and the duration of required maintenance therapy remains unclear. Optimal therapy of CMV enteritis has not been established; the single published placebo-controlled study in HCT patients showed that two weeks of ganciclovir, while it reduced the viral load, did not improve clinical symptoms. Perhaps longer therapy or combination therapy with IVIG, as is given for pneumonia, would improve the outcome. There is not yet established effective therapy for adenovirus or for the respiratory viruses, including RSV. While aerosolized ribavirin is sometimes used to treat patients with RSV pneumonia, it is very costly and toxic, and its efficacy in the HCT setting has not been established. Acyclovir-resistant HSV or ganciclovir-resistant CMV has been successfully treated with foscarnet.

### Treatment of fungal infection

Systemic yeast infections (most *Candida* spp., cryptococcosis, histoplasmosis, or coccidioidomycosis) can be effectively treated with amphotericin B, fluconozole, or itraconazole (see Chapter 42). The outcome in patients with invasive mold infections remains poor, however, despite the use of amphotericin B. Treatment is limited by the paucity of available agents and the failure to recognize infection sufficiently early to effect a successful outcome. Combination therapy, including combining amphotericin with rifampin or one of the azoles may be of potential benefit, but the efficacy of any of these combinations has not been established.

At present, in patients with localized mold infection, surgical excision may give the patient the best chance for long-term survival. Patients with single nodules due to *Aspergillus* spp. or other molds may be cured with complete resection, followed by amphotericin therapy for presumed residual infection. HCT patient with sinusitis, as in other settings, may benefit as much from surgical drainage and debridement during acute infection as they do from appropriate antimicrobials.

## Prevention of Infection

### Antimicrobial prophylaxis

In general, prevention of infection in the HCT transplant patient has always been more successful than waiting until infection is documented before initiating treatment. The ability to successfully treat established CMV or fungal pneumonia remains limited, despite the availability of "effective" agents. The disadvantage of prophylaxis is that more patients will be given prophylaxis than will ultimately get infected, with associated cost and potential toxicity, which depend on the type of prophylaxis used. Increasing economic pressures to reduce health care costs, including hospital stay, and to eliminate "unnecessary preventative measures" in all patients will likely contribute to further definition of patients at highest risk for a particular infection in whom prophylaxis may be most cost-effective. For example, laminar airflow protection (LAF) while effective in some studies, is being replaced with effective antibiotic strategies that are significantly less expensive and may not require hospitalization.

Prophylaxis against bacterial infection during neutropenia with oral antibiotics such as ciprofloxacin, is being increasingly employed as outpatient therapy. The concern remains that the increased usage of quinolone antibiotics may lead to the emergence of resistance, especially with resistant streptococcal species. Studies in this area are clearly needed. Prolonged antibacterial prophylaxis is routinely used in patients with chronic GVHD and consists of daily penicillin or TMP-SMX. Prophylaxis with TMP-SMX against pneumocystis infection is standard for the first four months after transplant and can be given conveniently twice a week orally (e.g. double-strength tablet BID, for two consecutive days/week).

Antiviral prophylaxis focuses on the prevention of the herpesviruses during high-risk periods. Acyclovir prophylaxis (250 mg/m$^2$ BID) is given to all HSV-seropositive patients from the time of conditioning until day 30 after transplant. After that, patients are encouraged to tolerate mild reactivations without treatment to facilitate necessary immune reconstitution. Prophylaxis for CMV infection with ganciclovir (5 mg/kg for one week followed by once daily maintenance until day 100) is used routinely in most centers for the CMV-positive allogeneic patient, starting either at engraftment, at the time of first positive blood or BAL culture, or more recently for a positive antigenemia or PCR blood test. Prophylaxis is generally given for 80–120 days after transplant, although up to 15% of such patients remain at risk for late CMV disease (between days 100 and 180) following discontinuation of prophylaxis. VZV infection, which occurs in up to 40% of patients during the first year after transplant, is effectively prevented by the use of acyclovir, either 800 mg BID or 400 mg TID but requires prophylaxis for the entire first year after transplant to cover the high-risk period. Some centers use this form of prophylaxis in patients with ongoing chronic GVHD, or those who have undergone a mismatched transplant, since they have been shown to be at higher risk for developing VZV.

### Other preventative measures

#### Isolation techniques

Isolation techniques have become relatively less critical than in the past in the armentarium of infectious prevention measure with the availability of more convenient, efficacious, and cost-effective means of preventing infection. For example, since the protective (LAF) environment was first instituted, the major bacterial and fungal pathogens that are acquired during the neutropenic period can be controlled or prevented with oral or intravenous antibiotics. LAF is expensive to maintain and patients are often unable to tolerate the oral decontamination regimens required to sterilize the gastrointestinal tract. With increasing awareness that the major source of infection during the early post-transplant period is from the patient's own endogenous flora, many centers have abandoned the practice of wearing masks for health care workers, patients, and their families, even during there critical neutropenic period.

The major need for isolation procedures continues for patients colonized with resistant bacteria (e.g. vancomycin-resistant enterococci) and for patients with disseminated VZV, who may be excreting virus from their respiratory tract. Apart from these measures, assiduous handwashing remains the best "isolation technique" that we have for prevention of the infections marrow transplant patients are at risk for.

#### Immunoglobulin

As with isolation techniques, immunoglobulin has become a relatively costly mode of infection prevention that has been supplanted in many centers by more specific forms of preventative therapy. For example, the use of CMV-specific globulin or standard IVIG has been studied for over a decade with mixed results regarding its ability to prevent CMV infection or serious CMV disease in the marrow transplant setting. At best, infection or disease is reduced by as much as 50%. With the availability of ganciclovir for prevention of CMV and emphasis on cost containment, many centers have discontinued the use of routine IVIG administration for viral and/or bacterial infection prophylaxis. While of theoretical benefit, the use of routine IVIG administration appears best reserved for patients with demonstrated hypogammaglobulinemia after transplant, often seen in association with GVHD. Infection-specific monoclonal antibody usage (e.g. CMV monoclonal antibodies with high neutralizing titers to CMV) remain of investigational interest.

#### Vaccines

Vaccines have received little attention as a means of prevention in the early post-transplant period, presumably because patients' abilities to mount a sufficient immune response to vaccination is unlikely. One to two years after transplant, patients may require reimmunization to tetanus, diphtheria, polio, and hepatitis B (series of 3 injections, polio and hepatitis only), regardless of GVHD status. Vaccination with pneumococcus (7 and 24 months after transplant) and *Hemophilus influenza* (3 doses 6 months apart, starting at 7 months after transplant) should be considered after 6 months, since they are safe and patients are at high risk for these infections until their immune status has returned to normal, usually by the end of the first 12–18 months after transplant for patients without GVHD). Patients should be considered for influenza vaccination each fall. Revaccination with the mumps-measles-rubella vaccine may also be appropriate and is safe by two years following transplant. The recently available VZV vaccine, which is prepared from live-attenuated virus, should be used with extreme caution in the post-transplant period, including with family members, until more safety data are available in this setting.

## ANNOTATED BIBLIOGRAPHY

Cox GJ, Matsui SM, Lo RS, et al. Etiology and outcome of diarrhea after marrow transplantation: a prospective study. Gastroenterology 1994; 107:1398–1407.

*Largest published study of the etiology and outcomes of diarrhea after marrow transplant; includes data describing the incidence and etiology of infectious agents in the post-transplant complication.*

Gentile G, Micozzi A, Girmenia C, et al. Pneumonia in allogenic and autologous bone marrow recipients: a retrospective study. Chest 1993; 104:371–375.

*The most comprehensive publication to date describing pneumonia and its causes after marrow transplant.*

Goodrich J, Boeckh M, Bowden RA. Strategies for the prevention of cytomegalovirus disease after marrow transplant. Clin Infect Dis 1994; 19:287–298.

*A paper summarizing the current options of prevention of CMV after marrow transplant with antiviral therapy. The discussion focuses on the risks and benefits of each published approach.*

Hagensee ME, Bauwens JE, Kjos B, Bowden RA. Brain abscess following marrow transplantation: experience at the Fred Hutchinson Cancer Research Center, 1984–1992. Clin Infect Dis 1994; 19:402–408.

*The largest review of brain abscesses after marrow transplant; describes the clinical features of the presentation as it relates to the etiology of infection.*

Walter EA, Bowden RA. Infection in the bone marrow transplant recipient. In: Infectious Diseases Clinics of North America. Rubin RH, ed. 1995; 9: 823–848.

*This is a general review of the common infections after marrow transplant with focus on new developments in diagnosis and treatment.*

# 89

# Infection in the Malnourished Patient

PHILIPPE LEPAGE, ACHIM SCHWENK, PATRICK DE MOL, AND JEAN-PAUL BUTZLER

Among the host factors predisposing to infectious disease, protein-energy malnutrition (PEM) is probably the most frequent worldwide. PEM is defined as protein and calorie intake that is inadequate for meeting a person's metabolic needs.

In developing countries, up to 20% of children suffer from severe PEM, and the prevalence of moderate PEM is estimated between 3% and 46% of children. Inadequate diets, poverty, lack of education, poor environmental conditions, and recurrent infectious diseases are involved in the pathogenesis of PEM. Children under five years of age are the most affected, particularly during the weaning period. Severe PEM contributes to the high childhood mortality in developing countries. Furthermore, it has long-term consequences on the survivors, including growth deficiency and retarded mental development. The most commonly used anthropometric definitions of PEM for developing countries are summarized in Table 89.1.

In industrialized countries, protein-energy malnutrition is rare in the general population. In chronically ill patients, however, it often complicates the clinical course and has a measurable impact on treatment complications and outcome.

## Interaction between Nutrition, Infection, and the Immune System

Thirty years ago, Scrimshaw, Taylor, and Gordon published a classic monograph summarizing and clarifying the relations between infection, the host defenses and the nutritional status. At that time, it was widely recognized that starvation increases susceptibility to infectious disease. However, the interaction between inadequate food intake, infection, and immune defense is now regarded as more complex:

- protein-energy malnutrition is immunosuppressive;
- some infections are transmitted or promoted by inadequate food and water supply;
- recurrent and chronic infections lead to malnutrition, partly mediated by pathogenic immune reactions.

### Impact of infection and immune response on nutritional status

Severe infections such as sepsis are frequently associated with anorexia and diminished food intake. At the same time, physiological energy-saving mechanisms that allow healthy organisms to adapt even to longer periods of inadequate food supply are impaired in the infected organism. The difference between the healthy starvation response and the metabolic reaction to infection and trauma is described in Figure 89.1.

In a noninfected starving person, glucose levels are maintained by gluconeogenesis, using protein and lipid stores as sources for acetyl coenzyme A complex. After some days, energy-saving mechanisms are activated. Acetyl coenzyme A is preferentially metabolized to ketone bodies, an alternative energy source for the brain. Their production costs less energy than gluconeogenesis. This permits an economic use of lipid stores, maintaining both organ function and protein stores. Resting energy expenditure is reduced by 5% to 10%.

If the organism suffers from acute stress, such as in infection or trauma, food intake is reduced and energy costs of metabolism are increased at the same time. Muscle protein is preferentially metabolized for gluconeogenesis and for acute-phase proteins (see also Chapters 82 and 84). Lipolysis and liponeogenesis are both activated, resulting in relatively well-maintained fat stores, even in undernourished organisms. Resting energy expenditure may be increased by 15% to 40% in sepsis. In chronic infections, such as in AIDS, these metabolic patterns seem to be modified.

Intestinal infections may lead to considerable nutrient and energy loss from the intestines. In children with acute diarrhea, up to 30% of protein intake and up to 40% of fat intake may be lost in the stool.

In normal hosts, the nutritional consequences of infection are compensated for during convalescence. A period of rapid catch-up growth occurs in children as soon as food of high quality is available. It is often recommended that rehabilitation diets for young children should contain 30% more energy and 100% more protein than a usual diet. This increase in energy and protein is, however, often difficult to achieve in developing countries. Therefore, catch-up growth is frequently impaired in third-world countries and new infections may frequently happen, again deteriorating the state of nutrition of these children.

Inflammatory cytokines such as interleukin-1 (IL-1), interferon-$\alpha$ (IFN$\alpha$) and tumor necrosis factor $\alpha$ (TNF$\alpha$) seem to be the central regulators of the metabolic response to infection. Multiple interactions between one cytokine and its circulating receptor, as well as between different cytokines, have been found. Fever is caused by the hypothalamic action of IL-1, IL-6, TNF$\alpha$, and other cytokines, but hypothermia in sepsis may also result from TNF$\alpha$ release (see Chapter 50). Muscle proteolysis, lipolysis, gluconeogenesis, and reduced albumin synthesis are regulated by IL-1, TNF$\alpha$, their receptors, and prostaglandins. IFN$\alpha$ enhances the action of IL-1 and TNF$\alpha$ and induces fatty-acid synthesis. The hypertriglyceridemia seen in sepsis and in chronic infections may represent futile cycles of concurrent lipolysis and liponeogenesis but may also protect the organism by binding endotoxin.

Appetite is acutely suppressed by injection of IL-1 and TNF$\alpha$ into rodents, but the animals adapt to repeated injections. In man,

**Table 89.1** Anthropometric assessment of PEM in children in developing countries

| WEIGHT-FOR-AGE<br>Percentage of expected weight for age (%) | Edema | Nutritional status |
|---|---|---|
| 60–80 | 0 | Undernutrition |
| <60 | 0 | Marasmus |
| 60–80 | + | Kwashiorkor |
| <60 | + | Marasmic kwashiorkor |

| HEIGHT FOR AGE<br>Percentage of expected height for age (%) | Nutritional status |
|---|---|
| <90 | Stunting |

| WEIGHT FOR HEIGHT[a]<br>Percentage of expected weight for height (%) | Nutritional status |
|---|---|
| <80 | Wasting |

| MID-UPPER ARM CIRCUMFERENCE[b]<br>Circumference (cm) | Nutritional status |
|---|---|
| 12.5–14.0 | Mild to moderate malnutrition |
| <12.5 | Severe malnutrition |

a. Relatively age-independent indexes.

b. Relatively age-independent index.

a relation between cytokines and anorexia is not proven. On the other hand, severe PEM in children is associated with reduced production of IL-1 and other cytokines, as a part of the impaired immune response in malnutrition outlined below. More studies on the role of cytokines in the pathophysiology of malnutrition are needed.

## Impact of malnutrition on immune function

Severe PEM affects most elements of the specific immune response. Nonspecific defense functions, including the integrity of the intestinal mucosa, are also impaired. The cell-mediated immune response is most affected by PEM.

### Cell-mediated dysfunctions

Postmortem studies have revealed that thymus atrophy as well as atrophy of other lymphoid tissues such as the tonsils or adenoids—is frequently seen after severe or prolonged malnutrition and is often referred to as "nutritional thymectomy". Indeed, the cellular organization of the thymus is modified with depletion of lymphocytes in the cortex, loss of cortico-medullar differentiation and infiltration by fibroblasts. Thus, the most dramatic changes appear in regions of the thymus where T-cells predominate. The same modifications can be observed in T-cell-dependent areas of lymph nodes and the spleen.

In the peripheral blood, the total number of lymphocytes may be normal in moderate PEM, but a decrease to <800 $\mu$l is often

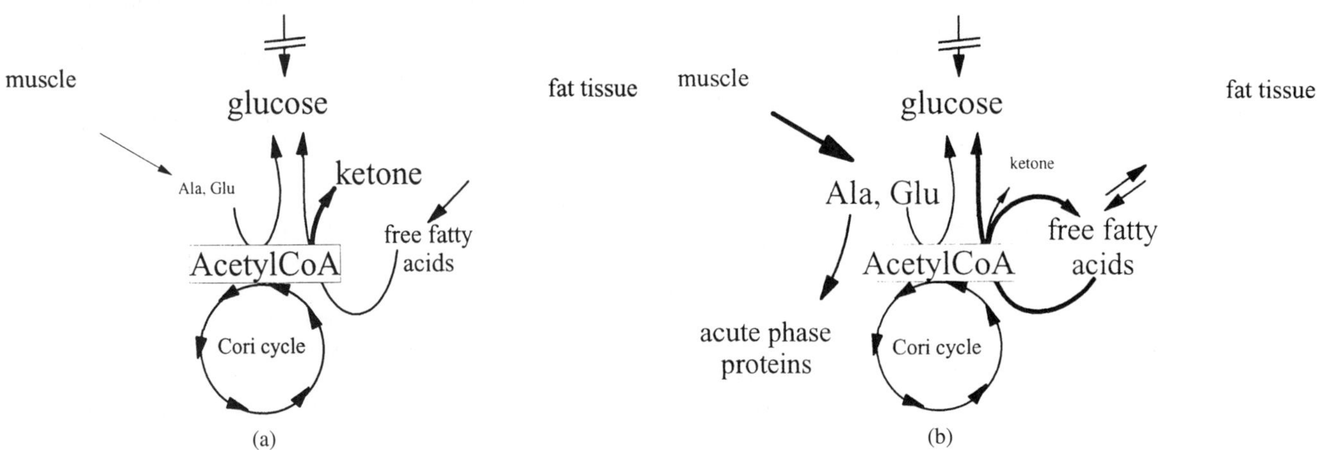


**Fig. 89.1** *A*: Normal metabolic adaption to starvation (simplified). *B*: Metabolic reaction to infection or other stress (simplified). Key: Ala = alanine, Glu = glutamine, AcetylCoA = acetyl coenzyme A complex.

used as a diagnostic sign of severe malnutrition. Even in moderate cases, the proportion of immature lymphocytes is increased, and helper cells (CD4+) are relatively decreased. Thereby, functional activity of these cells is impaired, demonstrated by reduced proliferative response to T-lymphocyte antigens or mitogens. Tuberculin skin tests reactions after bacillus Calmette-Guerin (BCG) vaccination are often negative in malnourished children. In the individual malnourished patient, however, the proliferative response may sometimes remain normal, or the number of mature T-cells may not increase despite adequate nutritional treatment. The significant depression of cell-mediated immunity may partly explain the high occurrence of viral, fungal, and gram-negative bacterial infections observed in children with PEM (see below).

#### Humoral immunity

Malnourished patients usually have normal or elevated serum immunoglobulin levels. However, functional tests may demonstrate impairment of some specific antibody activities. Moreover, because some vaccine antigens are T-cell dependent, impaired seroconversion may be anticipated. However, the results of immunogenicity studies to vaccination in malnourished subjects are sometimes unexpected. Some T-independent antigens (such as typhoid 0-antigen) may be nonimmunogenic, whereas some T-dependent ones (such as tetanus toxoid) may stimulate a specific response. Live virus vaccines may also induce unexpected results. The immunogenicity of measles vaccine is frequently normal but that of polio vaccine is usually reduced.

Secretory immunoglobulin A (s-IgA) plays a key role in the protection of mucosal surfaces against many infectious pathogens (see Chapter 11). There is a consistently depressed response of s-IgA in patients with severe malnutrition, involving both the concentration of s-IgA and the volume of secretions. Depression of the mucosal defense system can explain the increased prevalence of mucosal infections in malnourished children.

High levels of serum IgE are frequently noted. The most likely explanation for this abnormality is that PEM affects the immunoregulation of T-cells subsets and leads to overproduction of IgE.

#### Influence of malnutrition on other defense factors

Complement activity of both the classic and alternative pathway is reduced in severely malnourished patients. Synthesis is impaired, and the consumption of complement factors in the circulation is accelerated, the latter being due to increased levels of circulating immune complexes. The major consequence of these complement abnormalities is reduced phagocytosis of bacteria that are opsonized by the complement system (see Chapter 11).

Impaired migration of polymorphonuclear leukocytes to the sites of inflammation, reduced phagocytosis, and defective intracellular bacterial killing by leukocytes have been repeatedly described in severe PEM. Studies in malnourished children have shown that the lysozyme content of polymorphonuclear leukocytes is significantly reduced.

Wound healing is impaired in PEM, particularly in protein and/or zinc deficiency. This is due to decreased synthesis and deposition of collagen and results in a higher frequency of postoperative complications in malnourished patients.

Several aspects of the barrier function of the intestinal mucosa are affected by nutritional status. Proliferation of the mucosa is decreased, and s-IgA levels are decreased. The impact of nutrition on the resident intestinal flora requires further investigation; bacterial overgrowth may occur in the small bowel, facilitated by achlorhydria and s-IgA deficiency. This leads to malabsorption and to further deterioration of the nutritional status.

#### Special aspects of micronutrient deficiency

PEM is often associated with deficiencies of micronutrients such as vitamin A, zinc, riboflavin, and iron. These nutrients have a profound influence on the host's immunological status and its response to infection.

The role of vitamin A deficiency on immunity has been particularly well investigated in recent years. The cell-mediated immune system is impaired with a decrease in cytotoxic activities and natural killer cell numbers. Secretory immunoglobulins are also depressed and the integrity of cell membranes is disturbed. As a result, children with low vitamin A status show increased binding of infectious agents to the respiratory epithelial cells.

High-dose vitamin A supplements have been shown to decrease childhood mortality by about one quarter in communities where the prevalence of PEM is high. The observed death reduction was principally due to a fall in diarrhea- and measles-related deaths in supplemented children. Little or no impact on deaths due to respiratory infections or malaria was observed. Reviews of recent field trials found that vitamin A supplementation does not lower the risk of becoming infected. However, improvement of vitamin A status leads to less severe infections with, for example, reduced incidence of severe diarrhea or severe measles and lower rates of hospitalization.

## Epidemiology and Prognosis of Malnutrition

### Children in developing countries

The risk of infection and mortality associated with malnutrition has been the subject of several studies in the last two decades. In some regions the relation between anthropometric indices and infections or death was found to be linear; other studies suggest a nutritional threshold below which the infectious risk is markedly increased. For example, in a cohort study of children aged 15 to 26 months in Bangladesh, a clear threshold effect was shown for weight-for-age, height-for-age, and weight-for-height, with an increased risk of death only obvious among those children with severe PEM. In others, a weak relation between nutrition and outcome was found. The public-health implications of these studies are important because they may target special subgroups of children at particularly high risk of death.

Most studies have strongly suggested that PEM assessed by anthropometric measurements is highly associated with increased mortality. The predictive value of the different anthropometric indices on mortality has been further compared. In Bangladeshi children, the mid–upper arm circumference (a measure of muscle mass) was the best predictor of death. Interestingly, the prediction of death in young children by arm circumference has also been shown to be independent of age.

### Malnutrition in chronically ill adults in industrialized countries

Weight loss is a common manifestation of various infectious and other diseases (Table 89.2). In a general hospital in an industrialized country, about 40% of patients admitted to general surgery

**Table 89.2** Diseases commonly associated with malnutrition

| | |
|---|---|
| Infectious | Tuberculosis<br>AIDS<br>Measles<br>Pneumonia (nosocomial)<br>Upper respiratory infections (children)<br>Visceral leishmaniasis<br>Infectious diarrhea<br>Schistosomiasis |
| Malignant | Carcinoma of oropharynx, esophagus, and stomach<br>Other carcinoma<br>Malignant lymphoma |
| Endocrine | Diabetes mellitus<br>Hyperthyreosis<br>Hypophyseal insufficiency<br>Addison's disease |
| Renal | Chronic renal failure<br>Chronic pyelonephritis |
| Cardiovascular and pulmonary | Chronic heart failure<br>Hereditary valvular disorders<br>Cor pulmonale and emphysema<br>Cystic fibrosis |
| Gastrointestinal | Chronic diarrhea<br>Chronic pancreatitis<br>Malassimilation/malabsorption of other origin<br>Duodenal/gastric ulcer<br>Gastrectomy<br>Crohn's disease<br>Cystic fibrosis |
| Psychiatric | Depression<br>Psychosis<br>Anorexia nervosa<br>Alcohol and drug dependency<br>Dementia |
| Iatrogenic | Drug-induced nausea<br>Repeated diagnostic procedures requiring fasting |

and internal medicine are underweight. Moreover, weight is an insensitive marker of malnutrition because protein deficiency and loss of body cell mass are usually masked by an increase of extracellular mass. If body cell mass and albumin are measured, more than 50% of patients meet definitions of malnutrition. Even in the general U.S. population with its high rate of obesity, mortality is increased in those who have lost weight for whatever reason. In hospitalized patients, malnutrition is associated with a higher frequency of nosocomial pneumonia, bacteremia, and pressure sores, with longer hospitalization time and costs, and with higher mortality. One cannot distinguish whether malnutrition itself increases mortality in this population or is merely a marker of underlying disease. Prognostic data are more consistent for hypoalbuminemia than for other indices of malnutrition. However, circulating albumin levels are a function not only of protein nutrition but also of liver and kidney function, acute phase reaction, and vascular permeability. Artificial nutrition can reduce the rate of complications in malnourished patients with some diseases, such as gastrointestinal carcinoma, Crohn's disease, and enterocutaneous fistulae.

Complications of treatment can play a major role in contributing to malnutrition of chronically ill patients. Nausea and vomiting may result from various drugs, including oral antibiotics and antivirals. Antineoplastic chemotherapy causes severe nausea, which often is only partly controlled by serotonin antagonists or other antiemetics. Next to the hematopoietic system, the intestinal mucosa is most sensitive to the side effects of chemotherapy. Increased dose intensity is a widely used strategy to enhance the efficacy of chemotherapy, but this results in a higher incidence of nausea, diarrhea, and mucositis.

## Etiology and Epidemiology of Infectious Complications

### Gastrointestinal diseases

#### Acute diarrhea

Acute diarrhea is the most common cause of severe illness in developing countries. Based on the analysis of 22 recent active surveillance studies of diarrheal diseases in developing countries, it has been estimated that 2.6 episodes of diarrhea per child occur each year. Moreover, 3.3 million deaths per year are ascribed to diarrhea among children less than five years old in Africa, Asia, and Latin America. Mortality rates vary widely according to the region, from very high values in some studies in Africa and Asia to low values in most Latin America surveys.

Various studies have also observed that diarrhea is more frequent and fatal in severely malnourished children than in well-nourished subjects. For example, in one study from Nigeria, diarrhea occurred more frequently among malnourished children and these children were ill for longer periods than well-nourished subjects. The diarrheal case fatality rate may be 11 times higher in marasmic children than in well-nourished ones. With mild to moderate PEM, the relation between nutrition and the incidence and mortality of diarrhea is less obvious. However, a recent meta-analysis of longitudinal studies suggests a causal relation between nutritional status and diarrheal morbidity.

In many developing countries, fecal contamination of drinking water and food is the major reason for the increased incidence of diarrheal diseases in children. Ideally, drinking water should contain less than 10 coliforms and no fecal coliforms per deciliter. Environmental studies in different third-world communities have found the number of fecal coliforms in drinking water to vary from $10^3$ to more than $10^6$ per deciliter. Moreover, enteropathogens such as *Salmonella* are frequently cultured from drinking water in developing nations. Fecal bacteria are also more commonly recovered from the oropharynx of children living in poor environments than among those from affluent nations. Malnourished children have to cope with their highly contaminated environments by means of a disturbed local defense system, as outlined above.

The mechanisms by which enteropathogens produce diarrhea are discussed in Chapter 61. The relative frequency of enteric pathogens may vary widely from one region to another. Some of these agents are ubiquitous (e.g., rotavirus), others are much more common in the third world (e.g., enterotoxigenic *E. coli* or *Vibrio cholerae*). Few studies have compared the causes of diarrhea in well-nourished and malnourished children from the same community. The results of these investigations are inconsistent, with some studies showing an increased frequency of some pathogens (e.g., *Salmonella*) while in the others the prevalence of major enteropathogens was similar in well-nourished and malnourished children.

### Persistent diarrhea

Persistent diarrhea (defined as a diarrhea lasting 14 days or more) occurs in 3% to 20% of the episodes of diarrhea. Persistent diarrhea is frequently associated with malnutrition, either preceding nutritional deterioration or following established PEM. It is estimated that about 50% of diarrhea-associated deaths are due to persistent diarrhea.

Many causes have been found for this syndrome. Enteropathogens, such as enteroadhesive *E. coli* or *Shigella* have sometimes been found, but in most instances no organism has been isolated. An increasing number of children with persistent diarrhea are found to be HIV seropositive, and opportunistic intestinal pathogens (such as *Cryptosporidium* spp.) may be found. Other infections not primarily involving the gastrointestinal tract (such as measles) are sometimes associated with persistent diarrhea. Food allergy, for example allergy to cow's milk, is an important contributor to persistent diarrhea in some regions of the world. Likewise, carbohydrate intolerance, principally secondary lactase deficiency, may also be an important cause of persistent diarrhea, according to the mode of feeding. Low birth weight is also an important risk factor for the subsequent development of persistent diarrhea, especially if contaminated food and/or dietary allergens are introduced early in life.

### Intestinal parasites

Chronic and recurrent infections with intestinal parasites may contribute to PEM. In children with severe PEM, a heavy intestinal load of *Ascaris*, decreases protein and fat absorption reversibly. The effect of *Ascaris* on nutrition in mild and moderate PEM is less obvious. *Ascaris* infestation may also cause anorexia and lactase deficiency. The nutritional impact of *Schistosoma* species may be severe, especially during *Schistosoma mansoni* infection. Children chronically infected by *S. mansoni* are often wasted and short. Infestation with the *Trichuris* parasite may be associated with weight loss, short stature, edema, and anemia. Hookworm infestation is a well-recognized cause of anemia, protein deficiency, and nutritional edema. *Giardia lamblia* is a ubiquitous agent responsible for acute and persistent diarrhea. Its importance in the etiology of diarrhea seems to vary widely from one region to another. *Giardia* is also a well-known cause of malabsorption and therefore may aggravate the nutritional status (see Chapter 5).

## Respiratory infections

Infectious diseases of the respiratory tract are associated with malnutrition in both developing and industrialized countries. In 18th-century London, mortality from whooping cough followed the cycles of wheat prices. In our century each year, more than four million children in the developing world die of pneumonia and other acute respiratory infections (ARIs). ARI is one of the most common causes of hospital admissions in the third world. Again, ARIs are more frequent and more severe among malnourished children.

Clinical studies—using blood cultures and needle aspirations of the lung—have recently been carried out in several developing countries to determine the etiology of childhood pneumonia (1). These studies have consistently shown that *Streptococcus pneumoniae* and *Haemophilus influenzae* were, by far, the most important causes of bacterial pneumonias. *Staphylococcus aureus* and gram-negative bacilli were much less frequently cultured. Thus, the etiologies of bacterial pneumonias are similar in developing and developed countries (see Chapter 56).

Few studies have been published on the causes of ARI in malnourished children. From the limited data available, it can be concluded that *Streptococcus pneumoniae* and *Haemophilus influenzae* are also the prevalent bacterial pathogens causing pneumonia in PEM. However, malnourished children have a higher incidence of pneumonia caused by gram-negative bacilli, probably as a consequence of the frequent colonization of the oropharynx of these children by fecal bacteria.

Hospital-acquired pneumonia in industrialized countries is also influenced by the nutritional status of patients. Hypoalbuminemia and prior weight loss are potent risk factors for nosocomial pneumonia, together with neurological disease and nasotracheal intubation. Their influence is even higher in the elderly. Weaning from respirators is prolonged in malnourished patients. Immunological impairment, general malaise, increased colonization of the upper airways with pathogenic bacteria, and loss of respiratory muscle strength may be responsible for this association.

## Tuberculosis

The impact of poverty, overcrowding, and poor nutrition on the incidence of tuberculosis is well known from history. However, few studies have examined the incidence of tuberculosis in malnourished children. It is often difficult to differentiate the role in children of malnutrition per se from other potential risk factors associated with poverty, such as overcrowding. TNF$\alpha$ release by infected macrophages, although an important defense mechanism, may contribute to cachexia in tuberculosis patients. As may any severe chronic illness, tuberculosis may further deteriorate the nutritional status of children, and it is well recognized that affected patients fail to thrive despite adequate feeding. It is very difficult to diagnose tuberculosis in young malnourished children in developing nations because, first, affected children may present very few signs and symptoms and chest X-ray findings are often nonspecific; second, there is a high frequency of anergy to tuberculin skin test due to cell-mediated depression; third, sputum is often impossible to obtain and gastric washings have a poor yield; finally, the diagnostic technology available in most third-world nations is limited. Therefore, the diagnosis is frequently clinical, and antituberculous chemotherapy is often attempted if nutritional management fails after a few weeks. Once tuberculosis is established in children with overt malnutrition, it is more likely to be complicated by severe clinical features such as meningitis or miliary spread.

## Bacteremia

It is now recognized that the incidence of bacteremia is increased among children living in developing countries, although information is only available from a limited number of studies. The incidence of community-acquired bacteremia among febrile children in a study from Rwanda was 12% (as against 4% in most studies from industrialized countries). In a study from South Africa, bacteremia was twice as frequent among severely malnourished as among normal children or children with nutritional growth retardation.

*Salmonella* spp. are the most common bacterial pathogens isolated from blood cultures of children from developing nations. This is probably due to a high contamination of the environment with these organisms. However, common pathogens such as *Streptococcus pneumoniae* and *Haemophilus influenzae* are also frequently isolated in these children and are frequently associated with a poor outcome.

The case fatality rate of bacteremia is increased two- to fivefold in children with PEM, compared to normally nourished children.

## Measles

Despite the existence of an effective vaccine, measles remains a major cause of morbidity and mortality in many developing nations. In various regions of the third world, children with PEM have an increased risk of mortality from measles. However, factors other than nutrition, such as overcrowding, may explain the high case fatality rate associated with this disease in some poor communities where malnutrition is not prevalent.

The impact of measles on the nutritional status of children from developing countries is particularly severe and prolonged. In Africa measles is often reported in the weeks preceding kwashiorkor and significant weight loss is frequent during the acute phase of illness. Following measles, the incidence of serious infectious complications such as pneumonia or shigellosis may be increased for several months.

The acute and chronic negative consequences of measles on nutrition can be explained by various factors and are summarized in Figure 89.2. The severe and prolonged depression of cell-mediated immunity needs to be emphasized.

Pneumonia is the most frequent cause of mortality in measles. Fatal pneumonia can be a direct consequence of infection with the measles virus (giant cell pneumonia). It may also be secondary to bacterial (e.g., *Staphylococcus aureus*, *Klebsiella pneumoniae*) or viral (e.g., herpes simplex virus, adenovirus) infections. These secondary infections are frequently hospital acquired. Death can also be a consequence of measles-associated persistent diarrhea.

## Malaria

Malaria is one of the most frequent diseases observed in tropical countries. One species of *Plasmodium*, *P. falciparum*, responsible for the life-threatening form of malaria, causes more important nutritional consequences than the other plasmodia (*P. vivax*, *malariae*, and *ovale*—see Chapter 5). As in other chronic infections, malaria may induce muscle protein breakdown and loss of body nitrogen. Chronic malaria also interferes with placental function. Therefore, the birth weight of newborns from infected mothers is often reduced. Moreover, *Plasmodium falciparum* malaria is an important cause of severe hemolytic anemia in young children.

In contrast to most other infections, there is no evidence that malaria is more severe or difficult to treat in PEM. Nevertheless, *Plasmodium falciparum* infection induces cell-mediated immunosuppression and infected patients have been shown to be at increased risk for severe secondary infections such as diarrheal diseases or salmonellosis.

## HIV-1 infection

Weight loss occurs in about 90% of patients with symptomatic HIV disease (see Chapter 100). Multiple nutritional risk factors may be present in the same patient. Food intake is often reduced, due to oral and esophageal ulcerations, encephalopathy, drug-induced nausea, poverty, social isolation, or more frequently to unexplained anorexia. From animal studies, cytokines are presumed to be involved in the pathogenesis of anorexia, but this has not been proven in man. Metabolic consequences of HIV infection are similar to those in other infectious diseases with some im-

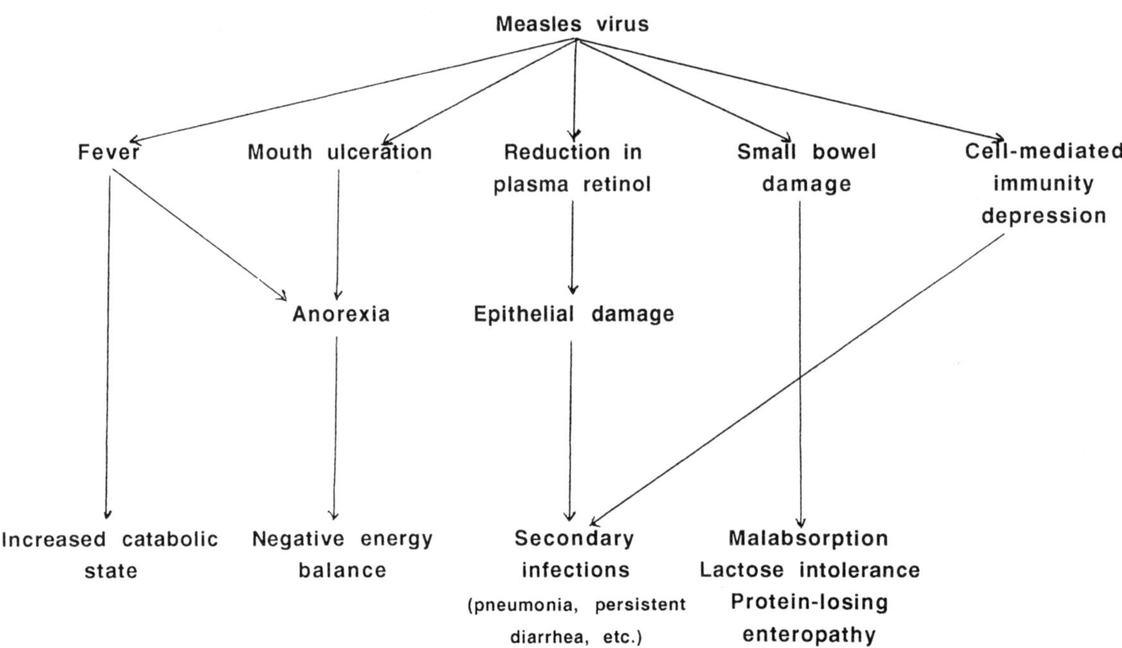


**Fig. 89.2** How measles infection affects the nutritional status of children.

portant exceptions. Even though resting energy expenditure may sometimes be increased, this does not drive weight loss; total energy expenditure is reduced rather than increased in weight-losing patients. They partly compensate their reduced food intake by reduced physical activity.

Malabsorption and diarrhea are frequent symptoms of HIV infection, suggesting that intestinal nutrient loss contributes to malnutrition. An infectious agent may be identified in two-thirds of diarrhea cases (see Chapters 61, 100). Inflammatory diarrhea, as in cytomegalovirus colitis, probably has fewer nutritional consequences than malabsorptive diarrhea, as in cryptosporidiosis. The functional disorders during HIV enteropathy have only partly been characterized. Malabsorption of carbohydrates, fat, and protein were found, but their role in the pathogenesis of malnutrition is unclear. Overt malabsorption will occur only if more than 90% of the resorptive function has been destroyed.

In Africa, the emerging HIV epidemic was first recognized as "slim disease." This demonstrates the particular interaction of malnutrition and HIV infection in developing countries. Poverty, chronic diarrhea, and tuberculosis are important cofactors in the African type of the Wasting Syndrome. The higher childhood morbidity and mortality in comparison to industrialized regions may also in part be attributed to the interaction between poverty, malnutrition, and HIV infection. Vitamin A deficiency is a major risk factor for perinatal HIV transmission studies in resource-poor countries and is now the target of ongoing intervention studies.

## Diagnosis and Management

### Basic nutritional assessment

The main obstacle to an adequate nutritional support in industrialized countries is the failure to measure the patient's weight. Indeed, more than half of malnourished patients are not recognized as such. Weight loss is often globally attributed to the disease the patient is hospitalized for, without any assessment of nutritional problems and the potential for nutritional intervention. Measurement of actual weight and height is inexpensive and may yield useful information on the general course of chronic disease. In bedridden patients, height may be inferred from knee height using reference tables. Most patients remember their usual body weight reliably enough for an estimate of weight loss.

Albumin is another readily available parameter of nutritional status. Its impact on prognosis, discussed above, makes it useful in identifying patients at risk of malnutrition. However, it is influenced by many nonnutritional parameters, such as vascular permeability and the acute phase reaction. Clinical judgment of physicians and nurses, including data on albumin and weight, is more accurate than many more elaborate techniques in identifying patients at risk for malnutrition.

Further methods of assessment, particularly for monitoring of treatment effects, are measuring short-lived serum proteins such as prealbumin, body composition analysis by bioelectrical impedance or anthropometry, and food intake assessments.

### Diagnosis and management in children from developing countries

#### Diagnosis

The diagnosis of infection is often difficult in malnourished children because clinical and biological perturbations may be discrete. Pyrexia and leukocytosis are frequently lacking. Malaria may be present without fever. Clinical signs may be unreliable; for example, estimating the level of dehydration is not easy, particularly in children with edema. Moreover, in spite ot active tuberculosis, the skin test to tuberculin is frequently negative.

#### Management site

Hospital and community care both play important roles in management of childhood malnutrition. Hospital care should be restricted to complicated and severe PEM cases (Table 89.3), given its cost, risk of nosocomial infections and emotional deprivation. High death rates after discharge from hospital have been repeatedly observed. Community-based nutritional rehabilitation centers have been very popular for 20 years, but the results obtained in terms of nutritional improvement and child survival have been disappointing. At-home management can be an effective and cost-effective intervention after one week of inpatient care when supervised by trained health workers.

#### Treatment

Table 89.4 summarizes the principal causes of death in severely malnourished children. Electrolyte and water imbalance and infections are important complications of PEM. A complete description of the nutritional management of severe PEM in developing countries is beyond the scope of this review but relies on the following points: At the initiation of care, energy is usually provided by oil and sugar; high-quality proteins, by dried skimmed milk powder. Rice-based salt-free meals are sometimes added. During the first week, children usually receive 80 to 100 ml/kg/day of a diet containing 70 to 80 Kcal/100 ml in 6 to 12 feeds per day. After one week, the volumes and caloric intakes are increased. Potassium, magnesium, zinc, copper, selenium, folic acid, multivitamins, and high-dose vitamin A are frequently added during the hospital stay. Ferrous sulfate is recommended after the first week of treatment.

#### Dehydration

The intravenous route should be avoided as far as possible because of the risk of cardiac failure. Nasogastric drip is the rec-

**Table 89.3** Criteria for hospitalization in children with severe PEM*

| In addition to a significant deficit in weight (e.g., <60% of standard weight for age or <70% height for weight), patient should have one or more of the following: |
|---|
| Edema (marasmic kwashiokor) |
| Severe dehydration |
| Persistent diarrhea and/or severe vomiting |
| Hypothermia |
| Clinical signs of shock |
| Signs of severe systemic or localized infection |
| Severe anemia (hemoglobin <5 gm/dl) |
| Jaundice |
| Purpura |
| Persistent anorexia |
| Young age (<1 year) |

*Adapted from Waterlow.

**Table 89.4** Principal causes of death in children with severe PEM*

| |
|---|
| Dehydration and electrolyte disturbances |
| Cardiac failure |
| Infections |
| Anemia |
| Hypothermia |
| Hypoglycemia |
| Liver failure |

*Adapted from Waterlow.

ommended method of rehydration if the child is too weak to drink. Children with severe PEM have a sodium overload and are deficient in both potassium and magnesium; the concentration of these electrolytes should therefore be adapted in the oral rehydration solution. The importance of early feeding with a caloric diet needs to be reemphasized. Because of the frequency of bacterial colonization of the small intestine and of the high prevalence of giardiasis, metronidazole is systematically added during rehydration therapy in some hospitals.

### Infections

The choice of antibiotic therapy during an infectious episode will depend on localization, severity, patient age, and local epidemiology of antimicrobial resistance. The problem of drug resistance is particularly troublesome in developing countries where multiresistant bacterial strains are recognized with increasing frequency among malnourished children. This high level of resistance sometimes requires therapy with antibiotics such as vancomycin (for *Streptococcus pneumoniae*) or by third-generation cephalosporins or quinolones (for nontyphoid *salmonellas*). The cost of these antibiotics is prohibitive for many hospitals in developing countries. Because of the difficulties in diagnosis and the severity of infections in these patients, routine empiric therapy with broad spectrum antibiotics has been adopted in many hospitals. These centers usually report encouraging results with antibiotics ranging from parenteral ampicillin alone to the combination of a beta-lactam with an aminoglycoside.

The metabolism of antibiotics and other drugs is altered in PEM. With chloramphenicol, for instance, pharmacokinetic studies have shown slow biotransformation in the liver of affected patients resulting in increased serum levels; therefore this drug should be used with caution in malnourished children. There is no evidence to support reduced dosage of other antibiotics or antituberculous drugs during malnutrition.

Tuberculosis must be suspected if the child does not improve following adequate therapy; empiric therapy is often required. Malaria is frequently overlooked and the signs may be very nonspecific during PEM. Therefore, in endemic areas, a blood film should be examined. Therapy will depend on the severity of clinical presentation and on the prevalence of chloroquine resistance. Appropriate deworming should be applied after the first week of therapy.

The clinical features of HIV infection and of malnutrition frequently overlap; therefore HIV antibody testing should be routinely performed in hospitals where HIV infection is common.

## Diagnosis and management in industrialized countries

It is beyond the scope of this chapter to describe the methods of nutritional treatment in detail (see Howard for review). However, some general rules apply to patients with malnutrition related to chronic disease.

The most efficient therapy of disease-associated malnutrition is to treat the underlying disease. Control of dysphagia, fever, or diarrhea will result in increased appetite and recovery. In most chronic diseases, however, only a partial control of the disease and its symptoms may be achieved. Moreover, the side effects of medical treatment may outweigh its beneficial effect on the nutritional status. If the reasons for weight loss are unclear, nutritional treatment should not be postponed until the diagnostic procedure is finished; this often leads to further weight loss. The decision to initiate artificial nutrition should be done in consensus with the patient and/or his relatives, taking into account the expected quality and length of survival.

Outside of intensive care units, nutritional treatment should be escalated stepwise. Counseling and nutritional assessment can clarify the specific reasons for malnutrition, lead to simple ways to increase food intake (e.g., pureed energy-dense food for a dysphagic patient), and identify those patients who need enteral or parenteral nutrition. These invasive methods should be used only if a trial of oral food intake either has failed or is contraindicated.

Enteral nutrition should be used instead of parenteral nutrition if feasible. Infectious complications are more frequent and more dangerous with parenteral feeding. The risk of catheter-related bloodstream infections is increased. The intestinal barrier against invasive bacteria, consisting of physical integrity of the mucosa, local immune reaction, and resident anaerobic flora, is impaired. Experimental data suggest a pivotal role for the intestinal barrier in the defense against sepsis.

Infectious complications of enteral tube feeding are usually less dangerous. Diarrhea is a frequent complication of enteral feeding, often caused by mistakes in application or triggered by concurrent antibiotic treatment . Nasoenteral feeding increases the risk of aspiration pneumonia. Percutaneous endoscopic gastrostomy may lead to wound infection, but this can usually be managed without removal of the tube.

The well-documented impact of malnutrition on postoperative infections and wound healing has led to the use of perioperative artificial nutrition. Most experts now agree that this should be given to patients presenting with moderate-to-severe malnutrition but not to every patient. In a large study in unselected patients, most of them with cancer, short-term perioperative parenteral nutrition did not improve prognosis. Infectious complications were more frequent with parenteral nutrition, and noninfectious complications were reduced only in malnourished patients.

Several nutrients are under investigation for a pharmacological influence on sepsis and critical illness. Immune-modulating properties of arginine, nucleotides, glutamine, branched-chain amino acids, $\omega$-3 fatty acids, and dietary fiber have been found in animal studies. Branched-chain amino acids may modulate the metabolic stress response. Nucleotides, arginine, and glutamine may become essential nutrients for the activated immune system. Glutamine is also an important fuel for the intestinal mucosa. The relation of $\omega$-3 to $\omega$-6 fatty acids regulates the formation and activity of prostaglandins and leukotrienes. Dietary fiber is digested by intestinal anaerobes to short-chain fatty acids, which are an important nutrient for the colonic mucosa. However, clinical studies in humans do not provide unequivocal evidence that any of these nutrients improve infectious morbidity and mortality in critically ill patients.

Glutamine is a semi-essential amino acid providing fuel to enterocytes and lymphocytes in metabolic stress. For technical reasons it is not contained in current standard solutions for parenteral nutrition. In patients after bone marrow transplantation, the addition of glutamine to parenteral nutrition reduced colonization and clinical infection with *Candida* spp. In a heterogenous population of intensive care patients, glutamine supplementation improved long-term survival. At present it is unclear whether these findings can be generalized to other patient populations.

## Public Health and Protein-Energy Malnutrition

To promote child survival and prevent PEM, several sustainable technologies have been identified in recent years. They have become known under the abbreviation GOBI-FFF given by UNICEF (Table 89.5).

Maternal education has been shown to be a major factor in child survival. Improvement in the water supply is another factor associated with a reduction in diarrheal morbidity and mortality. Introduction of sanitation and health education in poor communities has also improved survival. Improvement in personal hygiene practice is also very important; handwashing, for instance, seems a particularly cost-effective prevention against shigellosis and trachoma.

The case management of diarrheal diseases has been much improved by the introduction of oral rehydration therapy. The rapid correction of dehydration by oral rehydration makes early reintroduction of high-energy food possible, hence preventing further nutritional deterioration. Oral rehydration therapy is very effective in the management of established dehydration but it has no impact on the incidence of diarrhea. Therefore, it must be accompanied by other public-health interventions such as the improvement of food and water supplies and the use of latrines.

Immunization is another important public-health intervention that has been successfully implemented in many developing countries during the past 15 years. The World Health Organization's Expanded Program of Immunization (EPI) covers seven diseases: tuberculosis, diphtheria, pertussis, tetanus, poliomyelitis, measles and hepatitis B. The most lethal disease covered by the EPI is measles, with more than one million deaths per year in the third world. High immunization rates with measles vaccine can dramatically decrease the mortality and the severe nutritional morbidity associated with measles. In addition, a successful measles vaccine campaign may decrease the diarrhea-associated death. It should be noted that immunization offers no danger to subjects with PEM and that the vast majority of these children are able to respond to routine vaccination.

**Table 89.5** Appropriate technologies to improve child survival in developing countries: The UNICEF GOBI-FFF

| |
|---|
| **G**rowth monitoring |
| **O**ral rehydration therapy |
| **B**reast-feeding promotion |
| **I**mmunization |
| **F**emale education |
| **F**amily planning |
| **F**ood |

The advantages of breast feeding, both in industrialized and developing countries, are now well recognized. In developing countries, there is strong evidence from hospital- and community-based studies to support an inverse relation between breast feeding and overall mortality, mortality due to diarrheal diseases, respiratory infections, and mortality in high-risk neonates. Moreover, the protective effect of breast feeding may enhance child survival up to three years of age in communities with a high rate of malnutrition. Breast milk remains well tolerated during infection even when the appetite of children is reduced, so breast feeding may play an important role in nutritional support during infectious episodes. Similarly, morbidity due to diarrheal diseases and respiratory infections, and consequently hospital admissions, are reduced in breast-fed versus bottle-fed infants, in both developing and industrialized countries. In the developing world, another advantage of breast feeding is the inhibitory impact of lactation on fecundity and, consequently, its positive effects on birth spacing and child health. In poor urban women, however, prolonged breast feeding may be difficult to maintain. In areas of high HIV prevalence, decisions about breast-feeding policy must weigh the risks of infection and death from HIV with the risk of death from other common causes of infant mortality.

Supplementary feeding is a controversial issue. Food supplements given to pregnant women may increase the weight of their newborns. In small programs, supplementary feeding may in some instances improve growth of young children. In very large supplementary programs, however, the benefits of supplementary feeding seem limited. More benefit could be anticipated from food supplements targeted to malnourished children with the help of community-health workers. Several studies have shown that vitamin A megadoses every 3 to 4 months may significantly reduce mortality of young children from developing countries. The megadoses consist of 100,000 international units (IU) at 6–11 months of age and 200,000 IU at 12 months or older. Vitamin-rich foods and food fortification (eg, vitamin A-fortified sugar) have been successful in improving vitamin A status of children in some countries. Growth monitoring alone is not an effective strategy in preventing PEM. Finally, birth spacing is accompanied by a strong reduction in infant mortality in developing countries.

## Conclusion

Protein-energy and vitamin A deficiencies have a worldwide major impact on susceptibilty to infectious disease. Their treatment and prevention is one of the most cost-efficient public health strategies available. In turn, malnutrition is a feature of many chronic infectious diseases. Given in addition to causal treatment, nutritional support may improve symptoms, and perhaps outcome, of these diseases.

## ANNOTATED BIBLIOGRAPHY

Berkowitz FE. Infections in children with severe protein-energy malnutrition. Pediatr Infect Dis J 1992; 11:750–759.

*This review article examines the major infectious diseases occurring in children with protein-energy malnutrition. An attempt is made to compare the frequencies, fatality rates and specific etiologic agents found in malnourished and well-nourished children living in the same community.*

Bern C, Martines J, de Zoysa I, Glass RI. The magnitude of the global problem of diarrheal disease: a ten-year update. Bull World Health Organ 1992; 70:705–714.
*This article is based on the analysis of 22 recent active surveillance studies of diseases in developing countries. It is estimated that 2.6 episodes of diarrhea per child occur each year and that more than 3 million deaths per year are ascribed to diarrhea among children less than 5 years old in Africa, Asia and Latin America.*

Briend A, Woityniak B, Rowland MGM. Arm circumference and other factors in children at risk of death in rural Bangladesh. Lancet 1987; 2:725–758.
*Another study from rural Bangladesh of about 5,000 children aged 6 to 36 months were studied. It demonstrates that children at high risk of death can be detected by monthly measurement of mid upper arm circumference, which may be used in poor communities where interventions have to be selected.*

Chen LC, Chowdurhy AKMA, Huffman SL. Anthropometric assessment of energy-protein malnutrition and subsequent risk of mortality among preschool aged children. Am J Clin Nutr 1980; 33:1836–1845.
*This study, carried out among 2,019 children aged 13 to 23 months old in Bangladesh, shows that severely malnourished children, assessed by various anthropometric measurements, experienced substantially higher mortality than children with mild or moderate malnutrition.*

De Mol P, Brasseur D, Hemelhof W, et al. Enteropathogenic agents in children with diarrhea in rural Zaire. Lancet 1983; 516–518.
*A systematic study of enteropathogenic agents in the stools of children with diarrhea from a rural area of Kivu province in Zaire.* Campylobacter jejuni *and enterotoxigenic* Escherichia coli *were the most frequently recovered pathogens.*

Duncan CJ, Duncan SR, Scott S. Whooping cough epidemics in London, 1701–1812: infection dynamics, seasonal forcing and the effects of malnutrition. Proc R Soc Lond B Biol Sci 1996; 263:445–450.

Griffiths RD, Jones C, Palmer TEA. Six-month outcome of critically ill patients given glutamine-supplemented parenteral nutrition. Nutrition 1997; 13:295–302.

Grunfeld C, Feingold KR. Metabolic disturbances and wasting in the acquired immunodeficiency syndrome. N Engl J Med 1992; 327:329–337.
*A comprehensive review of the metabolic disorder and anorexia in AIDS cachexia. The putative role of cytokines in the pathogenesis is discussed.*

Hanson LC, Weber DJ, Rutala WA, Samsa GP. Risk factors for nosocomial pneumonia in the elderly. Am J Med 1992; 92:161–166.

Howard L. Parenteral and enteral nutrition therapy. In: Harrison's Principles of Internal Medicine, 13th ed. Isselbacher KJ, Braunwald E, Wilson JD, Martin JB, Fauci AS, Kasper DL, eds. New York, chap. 76, pp 464–471, 1995.
*A textbook review about artificial nutritional support via the enteral and parenteral route.*

Keusch GGT. Malnutrition, infection, and immune function. In: The Malnourished Child. Suskind R and Lewinter-Suskind L, eds. Raven Press, New York, pp 37–59, 1990.
*An excellent state-of-the-art summary on what is currently known on the impact of infection on the nutritional status and the impact of malnutrition on the immune function.*

Khanum S, Ashworth A, Huttly SRA. Controlled trial of three approaches to the treatment of severe malnutrition. Lancet 1994; 344:1728–1732.
*This controlled study demonstrates that at-home management of malnourished children can be an effective and cost-effective intervention after one week of inpatient care when supervised by trained health workers.*

Klausner JD, Makonkawkeyoon S, Akarasewi P, et al. The effect of thalidomide on the pathogenesis of human immunodeficiency virus type 1 and *M. tuberculosis* infection. J Acquir Immune Defic Syndr Hum Retrovirol 1996; 11:247–257.

Lepage P, Bogaerts J, Van Goethem C, et al. Community-acquired bacteremia in African children. Lancet 1987; 1:1458–1461.
*This prospective study shows that community-acquired bacteremia is common in children in Rwanda and is mainly caused by* Salmonella *species. Severe malnutrition and age under one year were associated with increased risk of death due to bacteremia.*

Macallan DC, Noble C, Baldwin C, et al. Energy expenditure and wasting in human immunodeficiency virus infection. New Engl J Med 1995; 333:83–88.

Pamuk ER, Williamson DF, Serdula MK, et al. Weight loss and subsequent death in a cohort of U.S. adults. Ann Intern Med 1993; 119:744–748.
*In this large epidemiological study weight loss was associated with an increased 5-year mortality, even in persons who were previously overweight.*

Schwenk A, Bürger B, Wessel D, et al. Clinical risk factors for malnutrition in HIV-1 infected patients. AIDS 1993; 7:1213–1219.
*In this descriptive study, anorexia, chronic fever, chronic diarrhea, and opportunistic infections were the major risk factors for weight loss in HIV-infected adults.*

Scrimshaw NS, Taylor CE, Gordon E. Interaction of nutrition and infection. WHO Monogr Ser 57. World Health Organization, Geneva, 1968.
*The first book entirely devoted to the interaction of nutrition and infection. This classical monograph also contains many interesting historical references.*

Semba RD, Miotti PG, Chiphangwi JD, et al. Maternal vitamin A deficiency and mother-to-child transmission of HIV-1. Lancet 1994; 343:1593–1597.

Thea DM, St. Louis ME, Atido U, et al. A prospective study of diarrhea and HIV-1 infection among 429 Zairian infants. N Engl J Med 1993; 329:1696–1702.

UNAIDS. HIV and infant feeding: an interim statement. Wkly Epidemiol Rec 1996; 71:289–291.

Underwood BA, Arthur P. The contribution of vitamin A to public health. FASEB J 1996; 10:1040–1048.

Van de Perre P, Simonon A, Msellati P, et al. Postnatal transmission of human immunodeficiency virus type 1 from mother to infant. A prospective cohort study in Kigali, Rwanda, N Engl J Med 1991; 325:593–598.

Waterlow JC. Protein Energy Malnutrition. London, Edward Arnold, 1992.
*A comprehensive textbook on childhood malnutrition in developing countries.*

Ziegler TR, Young LS, Benfell K, et al. Clinical and metabolic efficacy of glutamine supplemented parenteral nutrition after bone marrow transplantation. A randomized, double-blind, controlled study. Ann Intern Med 1992; 116:821–828.

# 90

# Intravenous Drug Abuse and Infection

CHRISTIAN RUEF

A wide variety of infectious diseases have been associated with intravenous drug abuse and these infections are in most cases directly related to the circumstances in which drugs are injected intravenously. Intravenous drug use remains a socially stigmatizing habit and is illegal in most countries. Negative public opinion of intravenous drug users (IDUs), together with law enforcement efforts, contributes to the marginalization of these patients in society. Dismal living conditions, homelessness, and inadequate nutrition, together with needle sharing under horrific hygienic conditions in "shooting galleries," abandoned houses, or railroad yards, have wrought havoc on thousands of young people throughout the world.

Many IDUs lack health insurance and depend on the public welfare system. Consequently, access to medical care is often difficult. Frequently the patients present with acute medical problems in emergency rooms of public hospitals. A comprehensive and continuous approach to evaluate the problems of these patients is often made very difficult by their erratic compliance with both treatment and keeping of appointments. This chapter will focus on issues, which are relevant to infections in IDUs. It will deal with infectious diseases which present as emergencies but will also address issues, which should be dealt with and goals which should be set in the long-term follow-up of IDU patients.

## Host Defense Alterations

Several studies have focused on the effects of intravenous drug use on humoral and cellular components of the host defense. No clear-cut, common, and typical defect can be ascribed to the use of parenteral drugs. The clinically relevant defects in host defense mechanisms are frequently the result of several coexisting disturbances, such as inadequate nutrition and abuse of alcohol, which contribute to the negative impact on health observed in patients with a long history of drug use. The most significant alteration of host defense in IDUs is caused by infection with HIV. The consequences of advanced HIV infection on the immune system are described in Chapter 99.

## Infectious Complications: Clinical Manifestations

### Initial approach to the febrile patient

Many IDUs seek medical help irregularly and typically present with acute problems. Fever is often the leading symptom, albeit a nonspecific one. The evaluation of the febrile IDU needs to be comprehensive and should be guided by knowledge of common as well as rare infectious problems presenting acutely in IDUs. Key elements of the history and physical examination of these patients are summarized in Table 90.1, together with appropriate diagnostic studies. Detailed information on the time and circumstances of the most recent injection of drugs, including information on the method used to solubilize the drug may provide some clues regarding possible microorganisms involved. *Staphylococcus aureus*, as part of the normal flora of the skin, causes most local or disseminated bacterial infections in users of intravenous heroin. However, if heating of the solution to solubilize the drugs is not necessary, as is the case for pentazocine and tripelennamine, live microorganisms that contaminate the solution may be introduced into the bloodstream. This particular scenario has led to clusters of *Pseudomonas aeruginosa* endocarditis. Additional outbreaks have been reported for *Serratia marcescens*, enterococci, *Pseudomonas cepacia* and methicillin-resistant *Staphylococcus aureus*.

### Local infections

Local bacterial infections at or near the injection site are the most common infectious problem in IDUs. This is not surprising given the prevalence of the unfortunate triad of nonsterile preparation of the drug, absent or insufficient disinfection of the skin, and poor injection technique. Infections either begin as superficial cellulitis or subcutaneous abscesses, which are typically observed after futile attempts to find patent veins for injection. The clinical course of soft-tissue infections is quite variable and depends on the pathogen involved. Superficial infections, frequently caused by *S. aureus* or streptococci, may spread rapidly and result in cellulitis or erysipelas (see Chapter 52). Subcutaneous infections are either caused by *S. aureus* or are mixed infections involving gram positive organisms as well as aerobic and anaerobic gram-negative bacteria, sometimes including such unusual bacteria as *Eikenella*, *Kingella*, and others. Rapidly progressive infections caused by group A streptococci may result in necrotizing fasciitis (see Chapter 80).

Some patients present with advanced local infections with destruction of soft tissue, or with spread to adjacent bone or articular structures. While these infections are typically on the forearm or antecubital area, longstanding intravenous drug use renders these sites inaccessible as a result of thrombosis and sclerosis of superficial veins. Subsequently other sites such as the neck, axilla, feet, and dorsal vein of the penis are used for drug injection. Consequently infections at these sites need to be sought in IDUs with fever.

#### Treatment of localized infections

Treatment of localized soft-tissue infections in IDUs frequently requires a combined surgical and medical approach. Incision and drainage of abscesses is key to the successfull management of

**Table 90.1** Evaluation of the febrile intravenous drug user

| |
|---|
| HISTORY |
| Time and site of most recent injection (needle sharing?) |
| Symptoms indicating organ disease (skin, soft tissue, respiratory tract, musculoskeletal system, central nervous system) |
| HIV status (known or unknown?) |
| Exposure to persons with tuberculosis or compatible respiratory symptoms |
| PHYSICAL EXAMINATION |
| Skin: phlebitis, cellulitis, abscesses, cutaneous signs of endocarditis |
| Mucous membranes: petechiae, *Candida* stomatitis |
| Signs compatible with HIV infection: *Candida* stomatitis, generalized lymphadenopathy, kachexia |
| Signs of cardiopulmonary disease: heart murmurs, tachycardia, tachypnea, rales, dullness |
| Signs of osteoarticular disease: swelling, tenderness, warmth |
| Signs of CNS disease: level of consciousness, focal neurological deficits |
| Evidence of hepatitis |
| Fundoscopic examination: signs of disseminated infection |
| LABORATORY STUDIES |
| *INDICATED IN EVERY PATIENT* |
| complete blood count with differential, blood cultures, HIV antibody test if unknown or negative test older than 3 months |
| *INDICATED IF HISTORY AND PHYSICAL EXAMINATION SUGGEST INVOLVEMENT* |
| Lungs: chest X-ray, sputum gram stain, acid-fast stain, cultures for bacteria, mycobacteria, stains for *Pneumocystis carinii* |
| CNS: CT scan, lumbar puncture for cultures, cryptococcal antigen, PCR (CMV) |
| Heart, abdomen: echocardiography, abdominal ultrasound, liver function tests |

many patients. Antibiotic therapy should be directed against gram-positive cocci and usually is modified once the culture results of the drained abscess are known. A short course of oral antibiotics following incision and drainage is sufficient for treatment of many abscesses, whereas cellulitis and soft-tissue phlegmon are often severe and require a course of parenteral antibiotic therapy.

Rapid surgical intervention is critical in cases with necrotizing fasciitis. This syndrome should be suspected in patients who develop local hyposensibility of the skin overlying the infection and in patients with systemic signs of sepsis, which appear to be out of proportion to the local appearance of the infection. While an elevated creatine kinase level may indicate muscle involvement and the demonstration of gas in soft tissue suggests the presence of anaerobes, these parameters are either nonspecific or relatively late signs. A high index of suspicion needs to be maintained in order to make this important diagnosis.

## Systemic bacterial or fungal infections

Bacteremic infections should be sought in every IDU patient with fever, regardless of the presence or absence of localized infections. Although bacteremia may occasionally be transient following intravenous injection of contaminated drugs, bacterial endocarditis is common in intravenous drug users. It is responsible for 8%–16% of hospital admissions in this population and caused 1.9%–8% of all deaths in IDU in New York City in the 1960s and '70s. Bacteria colonizing the skin are frequent causes, most often *S. aureus*. The drugs themselves or associated adulterants may be contaminated. Frequently, tap water or saliva is used to dissolve heroin or other substances. This explains the isolation of bacteria, such as *Neisseria sicca*, *N. subflavus*, *Stomatococcus mucilaginosus*, and others, which are part of the normal flora of the mouth, in blood cultures of patients with bacterial endocarditis. Not infrequently bacterial endocarditis in IDUs is polymicrobial (Table 90.2).

### Endocarditis

In contrast to endocarditis in nonaddicts, 60%–80% of cases of bacterial endocarditis associated with intravenous drug use are located on the tricuspid valve. The diagnosis of bacterial endocarditis in IDUs may be difficult based on clinical findings alone, since clinical signs such as petechiae, hemorrhages, CNS emboli, and heart failure are less commonly observed with right-sided endocarditis. This may explain the observation that up to 30% of febrile patients in which endocarditis was not initially suspected were found to have this infection. Fever, chills, and arthralgia are found in equal frequency in right-sided and left-sided endocarditis, whereas pulmonary signs such as chest pain and cough are more frequently reported by patients with tricuspid valve endocarditis. The diagnosis of bacterial endocarditis rests on the documentation of sustained bacteremia. Cardiac murmurs may be absent. Since vegetations on the tricuspid valve may usually be visualized by transthoracic echocardiography, transesophageal echocardiography is in most cases not needed to make the diagnosis.

Recommendations for treatment of bacterial endocarditis in IDUs are summarized in Chapter 66. Uncomplicated bacterial endocarditis involving the tricuspid valve can be successfully treated with a two-week course of combination therapy for many pathogens, including *S. aureus*.

The prognosis of right-sided endocarditis is good, with a mortality rate of 7% in one series. While vegetations greater than 2.0 cm are associated with a higher mortality, the presence of vegetations does not predict failure of medical therapy. Many patients with large vegetations and prolonged fever will ultimately respond to antibiotic therapy. Surgical intervention is rarely nec-

**Table 90.2** Pathogens causing infective endocarditis in intravenous drug users

| |
|---|
| COMMON |
| *Staphylococcus aureus*, coagulase-negative staphylococci |
| *Viridans* streptococci, group A streptococci, group D streptococci |
| LESS COMMON |
| *Neisseria subflava*, *Neisseria sicca* |
| *Corynebacterium* spp. |
| *Stomatococcus mucilaginosus* |
| HACEK group |
| Gram-negative rods: *Pseudomonas aeruginosa*, *Serratia*, *Klebsiella* |
| *Candida* |
| Polymicrobial infections |

essary and carries its own risk. The indication for surgical intervention should be reserved for patients with persistent or recurrent infection, which is refractory to optimal antibotic therapy. Valve excision rather than replacement with a prosthetic valve is preferred, since recurrent bacterial endocarditis and continued drug use are negative prognostic factors regarding the life expectancy of such a prosthetic valve. Septic pulmonary emboli occur frequently in patients with right-sided endocarditis and may complicate the clinical course if lung abscesses or pneumonia develop. However, since they are not associated with an adverse outcome, this complication also does not constitute an indication for surgical intervention.

If treatment is adequate, mortality from endocarditis is very low. However, in a substantial number of patients successful completion of treatment may be difficult to achieve because of poor patient compliance. In spite of the optimistic assessment above regarding a high cure rate, recurrences are common. Recurrences may be the result of insufficient compliance with antibiotic therapy, but in many patients reinfection is the consequence of continued drug use after discharge.

### Bacteremia and metastatic infections

Bacteremia may cause metastatic foci of infection in various organs. Septic pulmonary emboli and splenic or perinephric abscesses are typical complications of bacterial endocarditis. Infections of the sternoclavicular, sacroiliac, or other joints by *S. aureus* are well known in IDUs. Less commonly, large joints such as knee, hip, and the intervertebral disc space may be infected. Furthermore brain or epidural abscesses should be sought in patients with fever and localizing symptoms or findings. The diagnostic work-up of patients with suspected foci should always include blood cultures and, if technically feasible an attempt to aspirate or biopsy the involved area to obtain representative material for culture. Antibiotic therapy should be targeted against the known or suspected bacteria. Surgical intervention is frequently necessary to treat joint infections and preferably includes open drainage of the involved joint. The outcome of osteoarticular infections is usually good. Chronic osteomyelitis in IDUs has however been reported. It may occasionally be caused by unusual pathogens such as fungi.

## Viral infections

Viral infections may also present acutely in IDUs. Viral hepatitis is one of the most prevalent infectious complications of intravenous drug use. The seroprevalence for hepatitis B virus increases steadily during the years of drug use and reaches 60% to 80% in most series. Approximately 7% of drug users were found to have persistance of hepatitis B surface antigen (HBsAg). Serological evidence for hepatitis C virus infection was found in 48% of IDUs in Zurich. Some of these patients will develop chronic hepatitis. Delta virus hepatitis has caused small epidemics in IDUs and may result in fulminant hepatitis in the presence of hepatitis B virus infection. In addition to the two blood-borne hepatitis viruses, the seroprevalence for hepatitis A is also high in many populations of drug users. Among Zurich's IDUs 50% had evidence of hepatitis A infection, both past and acute. Acute viral hepatitis in IDUs presents with typical signs and symptoms including jaundice, loss of appetite, nausea, and fever. Supportive therapy and appropriate precautions to prevent disease transmission especially in the case of hepatitis A should be instituted. No specific antiviral therapy is available (see Chapter 62).

### Impact of HIV infection

The role of HIV infection in IDUs cannot be overstated. The consequences of HIV infection on host defense mechanisms have been detailed (Chapters 99, 100). Despite the knowledge of most IDUs of the risks for transmission of HIV, needle sharing and unprotected sexual intercourse still cause new infections. Thus, primary HIV infection should be considered in the febrile IDU, especially if mucocutaneous signs such as ulcers or a rash are present. However, infectious complications as a result of advanced immunosuppression are distinctly more frequent. These complications—including *Pneumocystis carinii* pneumonia, central nervous system toxoplasmosis, cytomegalovirus retinitis, disseminated *Mycobacterium avium-intracellulare* infection, and chronic diarrhea caused by *cryptosporidia*, Microsporidia, *Isospora belli*, or cytomegalovirus—are described in Chapter 100.

In addition to these well-known complications of AIDS, tuberculosis is observed relatively frequently in IDUs. Reactivation of old infection occurs as cellular host defenses deteriorate. However, the crowded living conditions of some IDUs have resulted in the spread of new infections among groups of homeless IDUs and clients of public shelters. Tuberculosis may present with atypical pulmonary symptoms or at extrapulmonary sites in patients with advanced HIV infection. A 12-month course of isoniazid chemoprophylaxis should be prescribed in all IDUs with positive PPD skin test after exclusion of active tuberculosis. As with other therapeutic strategies, compliance may be a significant obstacle to completion of the 12-month course.

Active tuberculosis in IDUs should empirically be treated with at least four drugs. A frequently used regimen includes isoniazid, rifampicin, pyrazinamide, and ethambutol. This combination should be continued until the results of susceptibility testing are known. In locations such as New York City, with a high rate of multi-drug-resistant tuberculosis cases, a pragmatic approach emphasizing the need for at least four drugs and the reinforcement of compliance is warranted. Whenever possible, directly observed therapy is preferred. The homeless and users of intravenous drugs are an important target population for epidemiological measures to prevent the further spread of multi-drug-resistant tuberculosis (MDR-TB).

## Pneumonia and sexually transmitted diseases

Bacterial pneumonias are also frequent problems in IDUs. Some patients may experience recurrent episodes, which may occasionally be caused by aspiration. Pneumococcal pneumonia is frequent in HIV-infected patients and may take a very aggressive course resulting in bacteremia, endocarditis, or meningitis. Penicillin-resistant pneumococci are endemic in many countries and treatment becomes more difficult.

Sexually transmitted diseases (STDs) are relatively common in IDUs, especially in persons engaging in prostitution in order to finance their addiction to drugs. Some reports describe an especially high prevalence of STDs in users of crack cocaine. While the rate of new syphilis infections is generally declining, this infection is still relatively common in drug users.

## Long-term Medical Care and Preventive Measures in IDUs

The cessation of intravenous drug use and ultimately a drug-free existence are the overriding goals of most physicians for their patients. Although these goals may be difficult to achieve, the patients' needs for urgent care of acute medical problems, and for long-term management of diverse medical and social problems should be addressed. Strategies to prevent or reduce future complications should be included. Some of these strategies are simple and straightforward, consisting of single injections to vaccinate IDUs against influenza and pneumococcal infections, respectively. These vaccinations should be offered to every IDU. Other efforts require a more elaborate organization and depend on the collaboration of the patient. All IDUs should be screened for the presence of hepatitis B infection. Based on the high risk for acquisition of hepatitis B the CDC recommends that seronegative drug users be vaccinated against hepatitis B. This may reduce the risk of severe delta infection. Completion of hepatitis B vaccination requires three injections given over the course of six months. Compliance with this schedule may be a problem.

Prevention of HIV infection should be the primary goal of all HIV-negative IDUs. This goal is achievable, if the patient adheres to recommendations and makes use of available resources. Avoidance of needle sharing is made possible in many cities through public syringe and needle exchange programs, which have been successful without increasing the number of IDUs or the number of injections per drug user. Other public-support programs, including accessible medical care, shelter, and food, are crucial for the prevention of major deterioration in health. Distribution of heroin to drug users by physicians as part of a government-sponsored program with the aim to reduce the rate of drug-related crimes is currently being evaluated in various cities. In order to achieve the goal of abstinence from drugs, substance abuse treatment centers and prescription of methadone have been successfully used. Unfortunately the number of treatment centers is too small to accommodate all prospective candidates for treatment. Another important strategy to prevent infectious complications of IDU including the risk of HIV infection is to discourage the switch from intranasal drug use to intravenous use. The comprehensive strategy to decrease the infectious risk associated with intravenous drug use further includes efforts to reduce the risk of HIV infection in sexual partners of HIV-infected IDUs and to provide adequate counseling to sexually active women to prevent pregnancies in HIV-infected women with ongoing intravenous drug use.

Many of these preventive strategies, especially chemoprophylaxis and vaccination, are relatively straightforward. Unfortunately, difficult access to medical care and poor compliance undermine these important measures. While difficult and often frustrating interactions with individual IDUs may at times prompt us to feel resentful against individual patients, we should keep in mind that addiction to intravenous drugs will be overcome by some. We should do all we can to help them cross that treacherous passage in their lives.

## ANNOTATED BIBLIOGRAPHY


Bernaldo de Quiros JC, Moreno S, Cercenado E et al. Group A streptococcal bacteremia. A 10-year prospective study. Medicine 1997; 76:238–248.
*Comprehensive review of this important infection in a sizable population of intravenous drug users. The study compares risk factors and clinical course in non-IV-drug users and IV-drug users.*

Des Jarlais DC, Friedman SR, Sotheran JL, et al. Continuity and change within an HIV epidemic: injecting drug users in New York City, 1984 through 1992. JAMA 1994; 271:121–127.
*Information on the seroprevalence of HIV infection in patients attending detoxification programs in New York City. Study illustrates that the seroprevalence has remained stable and that intravenous drug users have reduced behaviors with risks for transmission of HIV.*

Haverkos HW, Lange WR. Serious infections other than human immunodeficiency virus among intravenous drug abusers. J Infect Dis 1990; 161:894–902.
*Summary of a review meeting of experts in the field. Well-referenced overview of the major infections encountered in intravenous drug users.*

Hecht SR, Berger M. Right-sided endocarditis in intravenous drug users: prognostic features in 102 episodes. Ann Intern Med 1992; 117:560–566.
*Detailed description of clinical presentation, microbiology, course, and outcome of bacterial endocarditis in 121 intravenous drug users.*

O'Connor PG, Selwyn PA, Schottenfeld RS. Medical care for injection-drug users with human immunodeficiency virus infection. N Engl J Med 1994; 331: 450–459.
*Current review of the important issues to be addressed in the medical care of these patients. While focusing on patients with HIV infection, it provides a comprehensive discussion of clinical as well as psychosocial issues.*

Ribera E, Gomez Jimenez J, Cortes E et al. Effectiveness of cloxacillin with and without gentamicin in short-term therapy for right-sided *Staphylococcus aureus* endocarditis. A randomized, controlled trial. Ann Intern Med 1996; 125:969–974.
*This prospective study demonstrates that a short 2-week course of parenteral antibiotic therapy results in a high cure rate for right-sided endocarditis caused by* Staphylococcus aureus *in intravenous drug users.*

Samet JH, Shevitz A, Fowle J, Singer DE. Hospitalization decision in febrile intravenous drug users. Am J Med 1990; 89:53–57.
*This study establishes that clinical judgment is insufficient to distinguish reliably between minor and major illness in febrile intravenous drug users. A prudent approach remains to hospitalize patients when in doubt about follow-up.*

Szabo S, Lieberman JP, Lue YA. Unusual pathogens in narcotic-associated endocarditis. Rev Infect Dis 1990; 12:412–415.
*Bacterial endocarditis may be caused by a variety of usual and unusual pathogens, rendering the initial empiric antibiotic choice difficult.*

Tumbarello M, Tacconelli E, Lucia MB et al. Predictors of *Staphylococcus aureus* pneumonia associated with human immunodeficiency virus infection. Respir Med 1996; 90:531–537.
*Intravenous drug abuse and prior* Pneumocystic carinii *pneumonia were independent risk factors for the development of* Staphylococcus aureus *pneumonia. The study demonstrates that* S. aureus *is an important etiologic agent of bacterial pneumonia in drug abusers with HIV infection.*

Watters JK, Estilo MJ, Clark GL, Lorvick J. Syringe and needle exchange as HIV/AIDS prevention for injection drug users. JAMA 1994; 271:115–120.
*Needle exchange programs are both rapidly accepted by intravenous drug users and do not result in increased drug use.*

# 91

# Alcohol Abuse, Host Defenses, and Infection

ROB ROY MACGREGOR

The fact that drunkenness and chronic overuse of alcoholic beverages put the user at increased jeopardy for ill health in general and infections in particular has been a folk observation and self-evident fact for as long as alcohol has been used. One of the first learned treatises on the subject was written by Dr. Benjamin Rush, signer of the Declaration of Independence. Entitled "An Inquiry into the Effects of Ardent Spirits upon the Human Body and Mind," it listed tuberculosis, pneumonia, and yellow fever as complications of alcoholism. Koch showed that intoxicated rats had increased susceptibility to cholera, and Osler called alcoholism "the most potent predisposing factor to lobar pneumonia." The precise manner in which alcohol consumption puts the user at risk has been argued, with proponents favoring the effects of the user's neglect of his own health, the secondary effects of alcoholism such as malnutrition and impaired consciousness, or the direct effects of alcohol upon the body's defense mechanisms against infection. The answer, of course, is that all are important components of alcohol's negative impact on the incidence and severity of infectious diseases. This chapter will first address the known effects of alcohol exposure on the body's various arms of defense, including both immune and nonspecific defense mechanisms. Specific immunity will be further subdivided into the acute inflammatory reaction, cell-mediated immunity, humoral immunity, and the reticuloendothelial system. Then will follow a review of major infectious syndromes associated with alcoholism, including their methods of diagnosis and treatment.

## Host Defense Alterations

Host defense mechanisms can be divided into two general groups, nonspecific and specific (see Chapters 9, 10, 11). The former include general barriers to microbial invasion such as intact skin and mucosal surfaces, gag and cough reflexes, sensitivity to pain, and neurological alertness and coordination. Other nonspecific factors include the host's nutritional state, and the type of organisms colonizing nonsterile body surfaces. The specific defenses include the acute inflammatory reaction; cell-mediated immunity (CMI); humoral immunity, composed of antibodies and the complement system; and fixed tissue macrophages in the so-called reticuloendothelial system (RES), located in liver, spleen, lungs, and lymph nodes. Both acute and chronic alcohol consumption may variably alter each of these arms of defense. To understand these effects it is convenient to categorize them according to the predominant varieties of alcohol syndromes: acute intoxication, chronic persistent drinking (alcoholism), and alcoholic cirrhosis of the liver (Table 91.1).

### Acute intoxication

The anesthetic effects of alcohol produce a disinhibition of judgment, slowing of reaction time, inhibition of gag and cough reflexes, and ultimately a state of general anesthesia at sufficient blood alcohol levels. All of these influences increase the likelihood of acute bacterial infection, particularly pneumonia secondary to aspiration.

Acute intoxication has an anti-inflammatory effect, inhibiting the migration of polymorphonuclear leukocytes (PMNs) into sites of bacterial invasion; the higher the blood alcohol level, the poorer the PMN-exudative response into sites of experimental inflammation in animals and humans. This inhibition is caused by a reduced capacity of PMNs to marginate, adhere to endothelium, and leave the circulation. This in turn results from a failure to increase PMN surface membrane adherence molecules in response to activation signals generated by inflammatory mediators. This cell delivery defect also expresses itself as poor PMN and macrophage mobilization into bronchial lavage fluid, and depressed rates of bacterial clearing from lungs of experimentally intoxicated animals. Interestingly, other PMN functions, such as marrow production and release, chemotaxis, phagocytosis, degranulation, and intracellular killing, are unaffected by intoxicating concentrations of ethanol.

Cell-mediated immune and humoral functions do not appear to be affected adversely by acute inebriation, although this issue has not been addressed with modern techniques. RES clearance of aggregated albumin, a test of phagocytic capacity and perfusion, is unaffected by acute alcohol administration.

### Chronic persistent alcohol exposure (alcoholism)

Individuals in this category ingest alcohol on a daily basis, usually to a degree that interferes with the tasks of daily living. Owing to the induction of detoxifying liver enzymes, they metabolize ethanol more rapidly and often have a lower blood alcohol level than an alcohol-naive person would consuming the same volume. In addition, a shift in their cell membrane lipid composition toward a higher cholesterol content offsets the increased membrane fluidity caused by alcohol so that they may show fewer of its neurodepressant effects.

These adaptive responses allow chronic alcohol ingesters to function, but the effects on host defense mechanisms are wide-ranging. During times of relatively low blood alcohol levels, nonspecific effects include promotion of malnutrition and the colonization of the upper airway with gram-negative bacilli. However, when sufficiently intoxicated, these patients expose skin and mucous-membrane barriers to invasion and markedly

**Table 91.1** Alcohol effects on components of antimicrobial defense

ACUTE INTOXICATION

*SPECIFIC IMMUNITY*

*PMNs:*
- Depressed adhesion
- Decreased local delivery

*Humoral:*
- None known

*CMI:*
- Conflicting data

*RES:*
- Reduced pulmonary bacterial clearance

*NONSPECIFIC IMMUNITY*

Depressed cough and gag

Depressed consciousness

CHRONIC PERSISTENT ALCOHOL EXPOSURE (ALCOHOLISM)

*SPECIFIC IMMUNITY*

*PMNs:*
- Marrow maturation arrest
- Neutropenic response to infection
- Poor delivery when blood ethanol concentration is high

*Humoral:*
- Increased immunoglobulin concentrations
- Poor response to new antigens

*CMI:*
- Depressed delayed hypersensitivity
- Poor response to new antigens
- Lymphocyte blastogenesis poor in presence of alcohol
- Reduced lymphocyte response to IL-2

*RES:*
- Reduced intravenous clearance

*NONSPECIFIC IMMUNITY*

Increased colonization of upper airway by gram-negative bacilli

Malnutrition

ALCOHOLIC CIRRHOSIS OF THE LIVER

*SPECIFIC IMMUNITY*

*PMNs*:
- Marrow maturation arrest
- Neutropenic response to infection
- Poor delivery when blood ethanol concentration is high
- IgA chemotactic factor inhibitor

*Humoral:*
- Increased immunoglobulin concentrations

*CMI:*
- Poor response to new antigens
- Serum inhibitor of lymphocyte blastogenesis
- Reduced NK-cell activity

*RES:*
- Blood shunting past liver and spleen
- Fewer hepatic macrophages
- Reduced intravenous bacterial clearance

*NONSPECIFIC IMMUNITY*

Increased colonization of upper airway by gram-negative bacilli

Malnutrition

Hepatic encephalopathy

Hypoproteinemia/edema

*Key: PMNs: polymorphonuclear leukocytes; CMI: cell-mediated immunity; RES: reticuloendothelial system

increase the risk of aspirating bacteria into the lower respiratory tract.

Chronic alcohol exposure causes different effects on the acute inflammatory response than does acute intoxication. Chronic alcohol consumption can cause a maturation arrest in marrow PMN precursors both in vivo and in vitro. While this is not usually sufficient to cause neutropenia in the steady state, it may result in a sluggish or even neutropenic response to acute infection. The latter is reversible after several days free of alcohol. Decreased production of colony-stimulating factor and a direct marrow-toxic effect of alcohol both have been implicated. Once in the circulation, PMNs appear to adhere, diapedese, and move into the extravascular compartment normally, as long as blood alcohol levels are relatively low (<100 mg/dl). Higher levels can inhibit egress from the intravascular compartment just as in acute intoxication. Data on in vitro chemotactic functions are mixed, although the only controlled study showed that half of the subjects tested before and after extended drinking developed significant inhibition. PMN phagocytosis and killing of bacteria in vitro remains normal in these chronically exposed patients. The summation of these nonspecific and specific effects of chronic ethanol ingestion creates the alcoholic's markedly increased risk of developing bacterial pneumonia and cellulitis.

Cell-mediated immunity (CMI) is also profoundly affected by chronic alcohol intake. The high incidence of head and neck cancers (indicative of decreased tumor surveillance by CMI as well as reactivation of EB virus) and increased relapse of tuberculosis in chronic alcoholics are both strong epidemiological indicators of CMI dysfunction. Delayed hypersensitivity (DH) reactions have been reported to be smaller and less frequently positive among alcoholics than in normal populations. Rats fed high-alcohol diets for two weeks have shown reversible depression of DH to phytohemagglutinin. Short-term studies (four weeks) in humans have failed to demonstrate inhibition of established DH in alcoholics on a steady intake of alcohol and good nutrition. In contrast, these subjects were unable to establish new DH to antigens with which they were inexperienced. In vitro studies show an inhibition of CMI by alcohol; mitogenesis of lymphocytes from normal volunteers is suppressed by incubation with alcohol in a dose-dependent manner, apparently through the blocking of IL-2 stimulation. Mitogenesis of lymphocytes from alcoholics is also reported by some groups to be abnormal. Data on natural killer and cytotoxic T-cell activity are scanty and conflicting. Malnutrition is an independent suppresser of CMI as is liver injury, and both are likely to be inhibitory cofactors with alcohol itself in chronic alcoholism.

Humoral immunity has not been examined carefully in chronic alcoholics. As a group, those admitted for detoxification have higher concentrations of the various immunoglobulin classes than normal controls, and they do not have as good responses to pneumococcal and hepatitis B vaccines. In one study alcoholics failed to make antibody to a new sensitizing antigen although responses to recall antigens were normal. Complement levels have been found to be normal or slightly elevated.

The RES is also impaired by chronic drinking. Clearance of aggregated albumin was found to be slower in a group of alcoholics admitted for detoxification than in controls, and normalized four to seven days later. Livers taken from animals fed an alcohol diet for three weeks demonstrated reduced clearance and killing of bacteria when perfused ex vivo. Macrophages/monocytes (effector cells of the RES) exposed to alcohol chronically in vivo showed reduced phagocytic function when tested in vitro.

### Alcoholic liver cirrhosis

This clinical condition is rightfully a *complication* of alcohol ingestion rather than a clinical exposure category, but warrants highlighting as one of the alcohol syndromes that can impair host defense and lead to increased risk of infection. Once alcoholism has produced this severe complication, it becomes almost impossible to separate the immunosuppressive effects of alcohol itself from those of liver dysfunction and malnutrition. Nonetheless, a number of defects in defense have been described. Nonspecific factors which promote infection include hepatic encephalopathy, which can extend from mild confusion and somnolence to frank coma. The same shunting of portal blood around the liver that causes encephalopathy also allows bacteria to escape phagocytosis by the liver's fixed macrophages, promoting "spontaneous" bacteremia. Hypoproteinemia and tissue edema reduce the integrity of the skin barrier, promoting the development of bacterial cellulitis. Malnutrition is a chronic problem even in nondrinking patients with cirrhosis, and acts as a negative influence on all arms of host defense. Surprisingly, the in vivo inflammatory response to infection remains vigorous in spite of in vitro evidence of poor PMN chemotaxis in patients with alcoholic cirrhosis. Adherence, phagocytosis, and intracellular bacterial and fungal killing is normal in PMNs taken from patients with cirrhosis. In vivo assessment of splenic macrophage function has found it to be impaired; the degree of impairment was proportional to the extent of liver disease and correlated with the incidence of serious infections.

Cell-mediated immunity has been found to be defective in alcoholic cirrhosis. Responses to new sensitizing antigens are diminished significantly, whereas reactions to recall antigens are normal or only modestly depressed relative to results in normal control patients. Systematic enumeration and analysis of surface markers of the various T-cell subpopulations has not been reported. A serum factor that inhibits lymphocyte mitogenesis has been described in cirrhotics, along with reduced suppressor cell and natural killer cell activities. These effects can be enhanced by associated malnutrition. The significance of these in vitro abnormalities needs to be confirmed by in vivo tests wherever possible.

Immunoglobulin levels are usually increased in patients with cirrhosis. Evidence supports chronic stimulation by antigens shunting around the liver as the primary cause, although altered regulation of B-cell responses by T-cells may also contribute. Immunization with new or recall antigens elicits normal antibody responses in stable nondrinking patients with cirrhosis. No consistent or convincing abnormality of complement concentration or function has been shown in these patients.

RES clearance of iodinated aggregated albumin is impaired by cirrhosis, due to decreased perfusion of the liver and reduced functionally active sinusoidal macrophages. This phenomenon may explain the increased incidence of "spontaneous" bacteremia caused by pneumococcus and enteric bacilli (see next page) in cirrhotic patients.

## Infectious Complications

Alcohol ingestion, through impairment of both nonspecific and specific host defenses, predisposes drinkers to increased rates and severity of infections of many types and varieties. This section will discuss some of the most striking examples, note the settings in which they occur, and suggest empirical approaches to therapy.

### Pulmonary infections

These include bacterial pneumonia, lung abscess, and anaerobic empyema. Bacterial pneumonia is the most common serious infectious complication of alcohol abuse. This epidemiological association was clearly established well before the advent of modern medicine. During the 20th century, large population-based observational studies in Norway and Canada have demonstrated that alcoholics have a death rate from pneumonia three to seven times greater than for nonalcoholics, and hospital-based studies of pneumonia have shown alcoholics to be overrepresented both among the admissions and those with fatal outcome. *Streptococcus pneumoniae*, *Staphylococcus aureus*, *Hemophilus influenzae*, *Legionella* species, *Klebsiella pneumoniae*, and other gram-negative enteric bacilli all have been identified as major causes of alcohol-associated pneumonia. Many studies of pneumococcal disease emphasize the contribution of alcoholism to the development of infection and note that alcoholics are more prone to develop complications such as empyema, protracted fever, and slow resolution than are nonalcoholics. It is not clear how much influence the association of alcoholism and smoking-induced chronic obstructive pulmonary disease has on the overrepresentation of alcoholics among collected cases of *H. influenzae* pneumonia. Similarly, heavy alcohol intake and smoking have been major risk factors for both the development and severity of pneumonia in several outbreaks caused by *Legionella* species. Community-acquired gram-negative bacillary pneumonia is an uncommon event but must always be considered, particularly among chronic alcoholics. Pneumococcal pneumonia is common in all stages of alcohol abuse, whereas the others are predominately found among subjects who have been heavy drinkers for an extended period. Because of the range of potential pathogens, examination of the gram-stained morphology of sputum is particularly important for directing empirical antimicrobial therapy. In the absence of sputum, ceftriaxone is often recommended for its antibacterial spectrum, which includes pneumococci, *Haemophilus*, most staphylococci, and gram-negative bacilli. Erythromycin or one of the new macrolides should be added when infection with *Legionella* is suspected (see Chapter 56). Anaerobic lung abscess and empyema are additional bacterial pulmonary infections caused by the alcoholism (Chapter 59), with aspiration of mixed aerobic and anaerobic mouth flora usually occurring during an alcoholic stupor.

### Tuberculosis

The association between chronic alcohol abuse and tuberculosis has been noted since medieval times. The suppression of cell-mediated immune defenses by alcohol, discussed in the previous section, provides a likely mechanism, because intact CMI is critical for first controlling primary TB infection and then holding it in remission. Additional key risk factors for tuberculous disease include the self-abuse which accompanies alcoholism (malnutrition, hygiene neglect) recurrent exposure to contagious cases, and crowded living conditions such as result from homelessness and use of public shelters. Acting in concert, these risks create a tuberculosis attack rate among alcoholics living in the industrialized world which is more than 10 times that for nonalcoholics. Moreover, poor compliance with therapy programs and failure to keep appointments for monitoring result in rates of relapse 10–20 times that of nonalcoholics and leads to the selection of resistant organisms. The unfortunate dismantling of public health TB programs in the United States during the 1980s often prevented the aggressive follow-up of these difficult patients and helped create the recent problems with multi-drug-resistant (MDR) tuberculosis. For example, in 1992, 85% of patients diagnosed with pulmonary TB in one New York hospital left against medical advice and were lost to follow-up. To counteract these problems, the United States Public Health Service recommends that all treatment of alcoholics and others likely to have problems with compliance be administered as directly observed therapy; when this is done, cure rates are as good as those obtained in nonalcoholics. The current approved regimen uses initial four-drug therapy (INH/rif/PZA/EMB) until susceptibility tests are available (usually eight weeks), followed by four months of INH/rif (see Chapter 37). Close observation with periodic monitoring of liver chemistries is also recommended, because the frequency of drug-induced hepatitis is increased in the alcoholic population.

## Spontaneous bacteremia/peritonitis

These two syndromes are variants of the same phenomenon, namely, the failure of the RES in patients with alcoholic cirrhosis of the liver to clear effectively organisms in the bloodstream that usually only cause transient bacteremia from respiratory or gastrointestinal tract sources. When the infection remains in the bloodstream without clinical seeding of organs, it is referred to as spontaneous bacteremia; however, in the presence of ascitic fluid, this reservoir often becomes infected, leading to "spontaneous bacterial peritonitis" (SBP). In roughly two-thirds of cases the organism originates in the gut, leading to gram-negative bacillary or enterococcal peritonitis; the remaining third are due to pneumococci, group A streptococci, and staphylococci, thought to originate in the skin and respiratory tract. In three-quarters of cases, peritonitis is associated with bacteremia with the same organism. Perhaps owing to the advanced stage of the underlying cirrhosis necessary to produce SBP, mortality rates of 50%–75% have been described. Diagnostic suspicion should be high in febrile patients with ascites; examination of ascitic fluid will usually demonstrate >300 leukocytes (mostly PMNs)/$\mu$l in >90% of cases, with positive gram stains in 35%–50%. Because of the range of potential infecting organisms, empirical therapy should be broad-spectrum; reasonable choices include ceftriaxone (recognizing its inactivity against enterococci), a broad-spectrum penicillin plus an aminoglycoside (e.g., piperacillin and gentamicin), or vancomycin plus gentamicin. Therapy can usually be modified within 48 hours on the basis of blood and ascites culture results.

## Diphtheria

Although this once formidable disease has virtually disappeared from the U.S., it is still encountered in small clusters, usually among homeless urban alcoholics. Most infections are cutaneous, and are often associated with streptococcal pyoderma, poor hygiene, fomite spread, and significant frequencies of asymptomatic carriage. The 15% of cases which are in the upper airway can cause severe symptomatic illness and death. The association with alcoholism is thought to result from the poor hygienic habits of alcoholics. Diphtheria should be considered as a possible cause of any severe sore throat in an urban alcoholic, particularly if associated with a membrane. Therapy with erythromycin should be initiated on suspicion, and patients should be isolated.

## Other infections

Pancreatic abscess can complicate the frequent incidence of alcohol-induced pancreatitis, and usually requires combined antibiotic treatment for fecal organisms plus surgical drainage. Bacterial cellulitis, particularly of the lower legs, is a common problem among chronic alcoholics, and increases in the face of edema associated with cirrhosis. Gram-positive cocci are usually responsible, although enteric organisms may occasionally be found. Treatment with a first generation cephalosporin is usually effective. Meningitis does not have an increased incidence among alcoholics, although there appears to be a significant association with listeria meningitis (further evidence of alcohol suppression of macrophage function). Initial therapy for presumed bacterial meningitis in an alcoholic patient should take this into account if a specific diagnosis cannot be made by gram stain. Endocarditis has been reported to be increased among alcoholics with cirrhosis, with a higher proportion caused by gram-negative bacilli than in normal patients. An extended epidemiological study of HIV-infected men (the MACS Cohort) failed to detect any deleterious effect of alcohol consumption on the rate of progression to severe immunosuppression and AIDS.

In summary, there is extensive evidence for the potentiation of infections by alcohol abuse. Table 91.2 lists only those for which a causal relationship is clear.

**Table 91.2** Alcohol-associated infections

| |
|---|
| ACUTE INTOXICATION |
| Bacterial pneumonia |
| Pneumococcal, *Haemophilus influenzae*, staphylococcal, *klebsiella* |
| Lung abscess |
| Anaerobic empyema |
| Cellulitis |
| Pancreatic abscess |
| CHRONIC PERSISTENT DRINKING |
| *ALL OF THE ABOVE, PLUS* |
| Gram-negative bacillary pneumonias |
| Legionnaire's disease |
| Tuberculosis and the development of multidrug resistance |
| Diphtheria |
| *Listeria meningitis* |
| ALCOHOLIC CIRRHOSIS OF THE LIVER |
| *ALL OF THE ABOVE, PLUS* |
| Spontaneous bacteremia |
| Spontaneous bacterial peritonitis |

## ANNOTATED BIBLIOGRAPHY


Adams HG, Jordan C. Infections in the alcoholic. *Med Clin North Am* 1984; 68:179–200.
*This article briefly reviews data on host defense defects and then details infectious disease syndromes known or thought to be potentiated by alcoholism.*

Austrian R, Gold J. Pneumococcal bacteremia with especial reference to bacteremic pneumococcal pneumonia. *Ann Intern Med* 1964; 60:759–776.
*This is a classic review of cases of bacteremic pneumococcal pneumonia, from which comes much of our current understanding of incidence, natural history, and complications of the disease, including its behavior in alcoholics.*

Brudney K, Dobkin J. Resurgent tuberculosis in New York City. *Am Rev Respir Dis* 1991; 144:745–749.
*This article details the alarming increased incidence of tuberculosis in New York City, as well as the depressing results of attempts to have patients complete prescribed therapy.*

Gomez F, Ruiz P, Schreiber AD. Impaired function of macrophage Fc$\gamma$ receptors and bacterial infection in alcoholic cirrhosis. *N Engl J Med* 1994; 331:1122–1128.
*In in vivo clearance of IgG-coated erythrocytes, an assessment of splenic macrophage function was found to be impaired in cirrhotic patients. The degree of impairment was predictive of subsequent serious bacterial infections.*

Harnisch JP, Tronca E, Nolan CM, et al. Diphtheria among alcoholic urban adults: a decade of experience in Seattle. *Ann Intern Med 1989*; 111:71–82.
*Describes three outbreaks of diphtheria between 1972 and 1982. Of 1100 total infections, 86% were cutaneous and carried a 3% complication rate, in contrast to 21% for symptomatic nasopharyngeal infection. Most cutaneous infection was associated with streptococcal pyoderma.*

Kaslow RA, Blackwelder WC, Ostrow DG, et al. No evidence for a role of alcohol or other psychoactive drugs in accelerating immunodeficiency in HIV-1-positive individuals. *JAMA* 1989; 261:3424–3429.
*A review of men in the Multicenter AIDS Cohort Study showed that the risk of progressing to AIDS among HIV-seropositive men did not vary by their reported amount of daily alcohol consumption prior to reaching this stage.*

MacGregor RR. Alcohol and immune defense. *JAMA* 1986; 256:1474–1479.
*Written for an NIAAA review committee, this is an encyclopedic compilation of data available as of 1985.*

MacGregor RR, Louria DB. Alcohol and infection. In: Current Clinical Topics in Infectious Diseases. Remington and Swartz, ed. Blackwell Science. Malden MA, Vol 17, pp 291–315, 1997.
*A review that updates the 1986 JAMA article and adds a section on HIV infection.*

MacGregor RR, Safford M, Shalit M. Effect of ethanol on functions required for the delivery of neutrophils to sites of infection. *J Infect Dis* 1988; 157:682–689.
*PMN adherence to endothelial cells in vitro is increased by activating them with FMLP and other substances; in parallel, the adhesion molecule Mac-1 is enhanced on PMN surfaces. Incubation with ethanol prevents this increase.*

MacGregor RR. In vivo neutrophil delivery in men with alcoholic cirrhosis is normal despite depressed in vitro chemotaxis. *Alcohol Clin Exp Res* 1990; 14:195–199.
*Endotoxin-activated serum is powerfully chemotactic for PMNs in vitro; patients with cirrhosis often have a serum factor (IgA-associated) which inhibits this CF. Patients with this serum inhibitor were nonetheless able to mount brisk inflammatory responses to experimental skin abrasions, indicating that the in vitro factor did not prevent in vivo PMN chemotaxis and delivery.*

Smith FE, Palmer DL. Alcoholism, infection and altered host defenses: a review of clinical and experimental observations. *J Chronic Dis* 1976; 29:35–49.
*This article begins with infections associated with alcoholism and then reviews evidence for alcohol-induced immunosuppression.*

Tillotson JR, Lerner AM. Pneumonias caused by gram-negative bacilli. *Medicine* 1966; 45:65–76.
*Similarly, this review of cases of gram-negative rod bacterial pneumonia is responsible for much of our knowledge about this disease.*

Watson RR, ed. Alcohol, Drugs of Abuse, and Immune Function. CRC Press, Boca Raton, FL, 1995.
*A multiauthored volume with numerous monographs reviewing research data relating to alcohol and the different arms of host defense.*

Weinstein MP, Iannini PB, Stratton CW, Eickhoff TC. Spontaneous bacterial peritonitis. *Am J Med* 1978; 64:592–598.
*A review of 28 cases found a 57% mortality, with poor prognosis associated with encephalopathy, albumin ≤2.5g/dl, and bilirubin ≥8mg/dl. Enteric organisms were more deadly than those from the respiratory tract. They recommend empirical therapy for any patient whose ascitic fluid contains ≥1000 WBC/ml with >85% PMNs.*

Young CL, MacGregor RR. Alcohol and host defenses: infectious disease consequences. *Infect Med* 1989; 6:163–175.
*This article is written for the practicing clinician, and describes host defense defects and common infection syndromes associated with alcohol abuse.*

# 92

## Fever in Travelers to Tropical Countries

W. CONRAD LILES AND WESLEY C. VAN VOORHIS

Fever in travelers poses a diagnostic challenge to clinicians. Among the myriad of possible causes, many are geographically localized and, thus, unfamiliar (Table 92.1). In addition, some febrile illnesses in travelers to tropical countries are caused by infections that are potentially fatal if not recognized and treated expediently (Table 92.2). Furthermore, some of these infectious agents are highly communicable (Table 92.3), thereby posing significant risks to public health. Most febrile illnesses in travelers, however, are self-limited (e.g., viral upper respiratory infections and gastrointestinal infections). Thus, the challenge facing clinicians in the evaluation of fever in travelers is the detection of serious treatable or communicable infections while not submitting the majority of travelers with benign, self-limited causes of fever to expensive or invasive diagnostic evaluations. To succeed in this endeavor, clinicians must be aware of the epidemiology, distribution, mechanism of transmission, and clinical manifestations of the causes of fever in travelers.

### Epidemiology of Fever in Travelers

Retrospective surveys have documented a 1%–2% incidence of "high fever over several days" in short term (<3 months) travelers. Of these prolonged febrile illnesses, 35%–40% occurred only while the traveler was abroad, 35%–40% occurred during travel abroad and upon return to home, and 24% occurred at home only. Prolonged fever was significantly associated with longer stays (>4 weeks) in the tropics. Although the specific etiology is not established in most causes of travel-related fever, the most common illnesses are associated with severe diarrhea and acute respiratory tract infections (Table 92.1). Malaria and hepatitis are the most common documented cause of illnesses associated with persistent fevers that prompt the patient to seek medical evaluation. Typhoid fever and arboviral disease are examples of rarer causes of fever acquired in the tropics.

### History

History is of paramount importance in focusing the differential diagnosis of fever in travelers. Initially, it is important to establish the vaccination status of a patient. One must bear in mind that vaccinations vary in their efficacy to prevent infections. For example, efficacy ranges from the near complete ten-year protection provided by yellow fever vaccine to the approximate 50% six-month protection provided by cholera vaccine. The efficacy of the current hepatitis B vaccine series is greater than 90%, and the oral typhoid vaccine series is 70%–90% efficacious against *Salmonella typhi*, though less so against *S. paratyphi*. When a dose of oral polio vaccine is repeated in adult life as recommended, vaccine efficacy approaches 90%–100%. Thus, a documented history of recent vaccination administered appropriately renders the diagnosis of yellow fever, hepatitis B, polio, or typhoid fever unlikely. Appropriate administration of gamma globulin within three months of exposure or vaccination with the hepatitis A vaccine greatly reduces the possibility of hepatitis A. Similarly, a history of compliance with prophylaxis for malaria or diarrhea is helpful. However, one should bear in mind that prophylaxis for malaria is not 100% effective. It is also important to inquire as to previous diagnostic tests and treatment, some of which may have been performed abroad during travel.

### Exposures

One of the most important clues to evaluate in travelers with fever is the degree and types of exposures encountered by the traveler (Table 92.4). The risk of contracting a serious infection correlates with the duration of travel or residence in the tropics. Moreover, pathogens and clinical presentations of infection can vary significantly between short-term travelers and immigrants. For example, tuberculosis and filariasis may be relatively common causes of fever in immigrants from the third world, but these illnesses are extremely rare in short-term travelers. Schistosomiasis may present as Katayama fever (acute schistosomiasis) among travelers, but this syndrome is rarely observed in natives of endemic areas.

Because many diseases are limited in their geographic distribution, the travel itinerary is important to ascertain. Travel style can be associated with an increased risk of serious illness, especially if an individual resided with natives or participated in an "adventure tour," as opposed to a sojourn to urban, first-class hotels. Younger age and being a student are also associated with increased risk. Thus, it is important to learn the itinerary, duration of travel, style of travel, and activities during travel to ascertain the risk of serious disease presenting as fever.

Various exposures may be clues to define the differential diagnosis (Table 92.4). It is important to inquire specifically about bathing in fresh or salt water, animal contact, sexual contact, insect bites, injections, transfusions, caring for ill individuals (re: risk of nosocomial transmission, Table 92.3), and ingestion of possibly unclean water, unpeeled raw fruits, raw vegetables, raw or undercooked meat/seafood, or unpasteurized dairy products. One should be aware to inquire about bathing in fresh water in areas where schistosomiasis is prevalent, as cercariae penetrate the skin in fresh water, thereby establishing the infection. Given that travelers may be reluctant to volunteer information regarding sexual contact abroad, a complete sexual history is always important.

**Table 92.1** Relative risk of contracting certain infectious diseases by travelers to developing countries*

| High risk | Moderate risk | Low risk | Very low risk |
|---|---|---|---|
| Campylobacter enteritis | Chlamydia | Amebiasis | Anisakiasis |
| *E. coli* enteritis | Dengue | Ascariasis | Anthrax |
| Viral upper respiratory infection | Epstein-Barr virus | Chancroid | Chagas' disease |
| Viral gastroenteritis | Giardiasis | Cholera | Chikungunya |
| | Gonorrhea | Enterobiasis | Clonorchiasis |
| | Hepatitis A | Hepatitis B | Congo-Crimean hemorrhagic fever |
| | Hepatitis E | HIV | Diphtheria |
| | Herpes simplex | Leptospirosis | Ebola-Marburg hemorrhagic fever |
| | Malaria w/o prophylaxis | Polio | Echinococcus |
| | Salmonellosis | Rubella | Filariasis |
| | Shigellosis | Rubeola | Gnathostomiasis |
| | | Schistosomiasis | Lassa fever |
| | | Strongyloidiasis | Legionellosis |
| | | Syphilis | LGV |
| | | Trichuriasis | Malaria with prophylaxis |
| | | Tropical sprue | Melioidosis |
| | | Tuberculosis | Paragonimiasis |
| | | Typhoid fever | Pinta |
| | | | Plague |
| | | | Psittacosis |
| | | | Q fever |
| | | | Rabies |
| | | | Relapsing fever |
| | | | Rickettsial spotted fevers |
| | | | Toxocariasis |
| | | | Trichinosis |
| | | | Trypanosomiasis |
| | | | Tularemia |
| | | | Typhus |
| | | | Yaws |
| | | | Yellow fever |

*Reprinted with permission from Liles WC, Van Voorhis WC: Travel-acquired illnesses associated with fever. *In* Jong EC, McMullen R, eds., *The Travel and Tropical Medicine Manual*, 2nd ed., W. B. Saunders Co., Philadelphia, 1995, p. 203–234.

## Clinical characteristics

Knowledge of the apparent incubation period of illness in a specific case can narrow the diagnostic possibilities (Table 92.5). Likewise, it is important to establish the onset of fever in relation to exposures. Certain diseases may present very long after the period of exposure, such as amoebic abscess, malaria (especially *Plasmodium vivax* and *P. ovale*), echinococcus, and filariasis. It is also helpful to note whether the course of illness has been acute or chronic as outlined in Table 92.5. This table is helpful as a guide, but many of the chronic illnesses listed, such as American and African trypanosomiasis, may present as acute febrile syndromes during primary infection.

Fever patterns are usually of limited diagnostic utility in the evaluation of patients following travel to tropical countries. Fevers of primary malaria rarely exhibit the intermittent pattern characteristic of tertian or quartan fevers (every two or three days, respectively) experienced by native individuals with partial immunity. "Saddle-back fever," which refers to the phenomenon in which fever lysis is followed within several days by the resumption of high fevers, is found in 60% of cases of dengue fever, but can also be seen in other arboviral diseases, relapsing fever due to *Borrelia* spp., or *Plasmodium malariae* (quartan malaria) infection. Continuous fever with temperature/pulse dissociation, while characteristic of typhoid and typhus fever, is also common in arboviral infections. Remittent fevers, in which the body temperature fluctuates greater than 2 °C but does not completely return to normal, can occur in pulmonary TB, but may also be seen with bacterial sepsis and bacterial abscesses.

Specific symptoms may be very helpful in the diagnostic analysis. Severe myalgias, while characteristic of many febrile illnesses, are particularly prominent in arboviral infections such as chikungunya and dengue. Severe migratory arthralgias which persist following the resolution of fever are characteristic of chikungunya. Chills, though present in many febrile syndromes, are especially prominent in malaria, bacterial infections or sepsis, and dengue. Spontaneous bleeding suggests the possibility of infection with one of the hemorrhagic fever viruses (e.g., Lassa fever, yellow fever, dengue hemorrhagic fever) but may also occur with various bacterial and rickettsial diseases (Table 92.6).

Diarrhea associated with fever is typically caused by *Campylobacter* spp., *Salmonella* spp., *Shigella* spp., *Entamoeba histolytica*, or intestinal viruses. However, it is important to remember that many systemic illnesses can present with diarrhea. For example, diarrhea and/or nausea/vomiting were reported in 43% of cases of malaria in one series.

Respiratory symptoms suggest viral URIs but may be manifestations of TB, bacterial pneumonia, Q fever, melioidosis, or the pulmonary migration phase of helminths such as *Ascaris lumbricoides* and *Strongyloides stercoralis*. Hepatosplenomegaly

**Table 92.2** Selected potentially fatal febrile tropical infections with established treatments*

| Infection | Treatment |
|---|---|
| VIRUSES | |
| Congo-Crimean hemorrhagic fever | Ribavirin |
| Lassa fever | Ribavirin |
| BACTERIA | |
| Anthrax | Penicillin |
| Bartonellosis | Penicillin, tetracycline, chloramphenicol, or streptomycin |
| Brazilian purpuric fever | Ampicillin or chloramphenicol |
| Brucellosis | Tetracycline plus aminoglycoside, TMP-SMX or rifampin |
| Leptospirosis | Penicillin or ampicillin |
| Melioidosis | Ceftazidime |
| Plague | Streptomycin |
| Rickettsial spotted fevers | Tetracycline or chloramphenicol |
| Tuberculosis | Isoniazid, rifampin, ethambutol, plus pyrazinamide |
| Tularemia | Streptomycin or gentamicin |
| Typhoid fever | Ciprofloxacin, TMP-SMX, chloramphenicol, or ampicillin |
| Typhus | Tetracycline or chloramphenicol |
| PARASITES | |
| Amebiasis (liver abscess) | Metronidazole (followed by iodoquinol) |
| African trypanosomiasis | Suramin or pentamidine; melarsopol or DFMO for CNS infection |
| Malaria | Quinine or quinidine, plus tetracycline |
| Schistosomiasis | Praziquantel (consider corticosteroids) |
| Visceral leishmaniasis | Stibogluconate sodium or pentamidine |

*Reprinted with permission from Liles WC, Van Voorhis WC: Travel-acquired illnesses associated with fever. *In* Jong EC, McMullen R, eds., *The Travel and Tropical Medicine Manual*, 2nd ed., W. B. Saunders Co., Philadelphia, 1995, p. 203–234.

suggests malaria, hepatic amebiasis, acute schistosomiasis (Katayama fever), disseminated leishmaniasis, Epstein-Barr virus infection, or typhoid fever, among other infectious diseases (Table 92.7). The presence of lymphadenopathy should alert the clinician to the possibility of Epstein-Barr virus, HIV, acute schistosomiasis, plague, tularemia, trypanosomiasis, dengue, and other possible pathogens (Table 92.7). Meningismus, confusion, and other signs of CNS dysfunction may be caused by a variety of viral, parasitic, and bacterial agents (Table 92.8). Because many of these pathogens are restricted to certain ecological niches, the likelihood of infection with a given pathogen can often be estimated from the patient's geographic itinerary, season of travel, and exposure history. For example, Japanese encephalitis virus is limited to the Far East, is a disease of summer, and is transmitted by mosquitoes (see Chapter 74). Spinal-cord disease associated with fever can result from chistosomiasis, HTLV-1 infection, or poliovirus infection (see Chapter 75). Eosinophilic meningitis caused by the nematode *Angiostrongylus cantonensis* occurs widely in the humid tropics, especially in Oceania and Southeast Asia. Infection of the central nervous system by either *Gnathostoma spiningensus* or *Taenia solium* (i.e., neurocysticercosis) may also produce an eosinophilic pleocytosis in the cerebrospinal fluid.

Cutaneous manifestations of disease are very common, but seldom specific (Table 92.9). Erythema migrans in acute Lyme disease and rose spots in typhoid fever are examples of unique, specific rashes. Nonetheless, cutaneous manifestations can serve to refine a differential diagnosis considerably. As an example, an eschar at the site of inoculation is typical of typhus, anthrax, and Boutonneuse fever (*Rickettsia conorii*). Cutaneous ulcers are seen in leishmaniasis, tropical ulcers, Buruli ulcer (*Mycobacterium ulcerans*), cutaneous amebiasis, insect bites, syphilis, yaws, tuberculosis, and leprosy. When evaluating a patient who has received previous treatment, it is important to recall that rash and fever can be caused by reactions to drugs, such as sulfa drugs, antimalarials, and antibiotics. Rickettsial diseases are frequently associated with rash, but the absence of rash may be misleading and does not exclude the possibility of rickettsial disease.

## Specific Infectious Diseases to Consider in Evaluating Fever in Travelers to Tropical Countries

### Malaria

Fever in a traveler from a malarious area should be evaluated carefully with multiple blood smears for malaria. Four species

**Table 92.3** Selected tropical diseases with documented potential for nosocomial transmission*

| |
|---|
| Argentine hemorrhagic fever (Junin) |
| Bolivian hemorrhagic fever (Machupo) |
| Congo-Crimean hemorrhagic fever |
| Ebola virus disease |
| Lassa fever |
| Marburg virus disease |
| Meningococcemia |
| Plague |
| Rubella |
| Rubeola |
| Tuberculosis |
| Varicella |

*Reprinted with permission from Liles WC, Van Voorhis WC: Travel-acquired illnesses associated with fever. *In* Jong EC, McMullen R, eds., *The Travel and Tropical Medicine Manual*, 2nd ed., W. B. Saunders Co., Philadelphia, 1995, p. 203–234.

**Table 92.4** Exposures suggesting specific infections*

ANIMAL CONTACT
Anthrax
Babesiosis
Brucellosis
Hantavirus respiratory syndrome
Lassa fever
Leptospirosis
Plague
Psittacosis
Q fever
Rabies
Rat-bite fever
Toxoplasmosis
Viral hemorrhagic fevers
All tick-borne diseases

TICKS, FLEAS, LICE, MITES
Babesiosis
Colorado tick fever
Crimean-Congo hemorrhagic fever
Ehrlichiosis
Kyasanur Forest disease
Lyme disease
Murine typhus
Omsk hemorrhagic fever
Plague
Q fever
Relapsing fever
Rickettsialpox
Rickettsial spotted fevers
Scrub typhus
Tick-borne encephalitis
Tularemia
Typhus

TRANSFUSIONS OR INJECTIONS
Babesiosis
Bartonellosis
Chagas' disease
Ebola virus
Hepatitis B and C
HIV
HTLV-1
Leishmaniasis
Malaria
Q fever
Toxoplasmosis

RAW/UNDERCOOKED MEAT OR SEAFOOD
Cholera
Hepatitis A
Toxoplasmosis
Trichinosis
Vibrio parahemolyticus and vulnificus
Viral gastroenteritis

SEXUAL CONTACT
Chancroid
Chlamydia (PID and LGV)
Gonorrhea (PID and disseminated infection)
Granuloma inguinale
Hepatitis B (and possibly C)
Herpes simplex
HIV
HTLV-1
Syphilis

MOSQUITOES
Bancroftian filariasis
Alphavirus diseases
  Chikungunya
  Eastern equine encephalitis
  Mayaro fever
  O'nyong-nyong
  Ross River
  Sindbis
  Venezuelan equine encephalitis
  Western equine encephalitis
Flavivirus diseases
  Dengue
  Japanese encephalitis
  St. Louis encephalitis
  Yellow fever
  Others
Bunyavirus diseases
  LaCrosse
  Oropouche
Rift Valley fever

FRESH WATER (OR UNPEELED FRUITS/VEGETABLES)
Amcbiasis
Campylobacter enteritis
Dracontiasis
Enteric fever
Hepatitis A and E
Leptospirosis
Salmonellosis
Schistosomiasis
Shigellosis
Viral gastroenteritis

INGESTION OF UNPASTEURIZED MILK
Brucellosis
Listeriosis
Q fever
Salmonellosis
Tuberculosis

*Adapted in part and reprinted with permission from Liles WC, Van Voorhis WC: Travel-acquired illnesses associated with fever. *In* Jong EC, McMullen R, eds., *The Travel and Tropical Medicine Manual*, 2nd ed., W. B. Saunders Co., Philadelphia, 1995, p. 203–234.

of protozoa cause human malaria: (*1*) *Plasmodium falciparum*; (*2*) *P. vivax*; (*3*) *P. ovale*; and (*4*) *P. malariae*. These protozoa are transmitted to humans via bites of infected anopheline mosquitoes, which generally feed after dusk. Following inoculation, the organisms invade erythrocytes. *P. falciparum* is responsible for the most severe forms of malaria, due to its ability to infect erythrocytes of all ages and, thereby, induce high parasitemia. In contrast, *P. vivax* and *P. ovale* infect only young erythrocytes, and *P. malariae* infection is restricted to old, senescent erythrocytes. *P. falciparum* infection can be life threatening when associated with high parasitemia, blackwater fever, cerebral malaria, or the acute respiratory distress syndrome (ARDS). Drug resis-

**Table 92.5** Selected febrile illnesses of travelers classified by incubation period and typical clinical course*

| Short incubation (<28 days) | | Long incubation (>28 days) | |
|---|---|---|---|
| Acute course | Prolonged or relapsing course | Acute course | Prolonged or relapsing course |
| Arbovirus infection | Brucellosis | African trypanosomiasis | African trypanosomiasis |
| Bacterial dysentery | Epstein-Barr virus | Amebiasis | Amebiasis |
| Childhood viruses | Q fever | Hepatitis B | American trypanosomiasis |
| Dengue | Relapsing fever | Leptospirosis | Brucellosis |
| Hepatitis A | Schistosomiasis | Malaria | Filariasis |
| Influenza | Typhoid fever | Rabies | Leishmaniasis |
| Malaria | | | Melioidosis |
| Plague | | | Paragonimiasis |
| Rickettsial spotted fevers | | | Schistosomiasis |
| Rubella | | | Strongyloidiasis |
| Rubeola | | | Tuberculosis |
| Tularemia | | | |
| Typhus | | | |
| Yellow fever | | | |

*Adapted in part from Salata, RA, Olds RG: Infectious diseases in travelers and immigrants. *In* Warren KS, Mahmoud AAF, eds., *Tropical and Geographic Medicine*, 2nd ed., Mc-Graw-Hill Inc., New York, 1990, p.228–242. Reprinted with permission from Liles WC, Van Voorhis WC: Travel-acquired illnesses associated with fever. *In* Jong EC, McMullen R, eds., *The Travel and Tropical Medicine Manual*, 2nd ed., W. B. Saunders Co., Philadelphia, 1995, p. 203–234.

**Table 92.6** Important tropical infections associated with spontaneous bleeding*

| Infection | Geographic distribution |
|---|---|
| VIRUSES | |
| Argentine hemorrhagic fever (Junin) | South America |
| Bolivian hemorrhagic fever (Machupo) | South America |
| Chikungunya | Africa Asia (especially southeast Asia) |
| Crimean-Congo hemorrhagic fever | Africa, Asia, and eastern Europe |
| Dengue | Tropical regions of Africa, South America, Central America and the Caribbean, Asia, and Oceania |
| Ebola virus | Africa |
| Hantaan virus (Hemorrhagic fever with renal syndrome) | Asia, Africa, Oceania, the Americas, Europe |
| Kyasanur Forest disease | India |
| Lassa fever | Africa |
| Marburg virus | Africa |
| Omsk hemorrhagic fever | Asia (the former USSR) |
| Rift Valley fever | Africa |
| Yellow fever | Africa, South and Central America |
| BACTERIA | |
| Brazilian purpuric fever | South America |
| *Capnocytophaga canimorsus* | Widespread |
| Leptospirosis | Widespread |
| Meningococcemia | Widespread |
| Melioidosis | Asia, Oceania, Africa, and focal spots in the Americas |
| Plague | Asia, Africa, Europe, and the Americas |
| Rocky Mountain spotted fever | North and South America |
| Typhus | Widespread |
| *Vibrio vulnificus* | Widespread in coastal regions |

*Adapted in part from Wilson ME. *A World Guide to Infections: Diseases, Distribution, Diagnosis*, Oxford University Press, New York, 1991. Reprinted with permission from Liles WC, Van Voorhis WC: Travel-acquired illnesses associated with fever. *In* Jong EC, McMullen R, eds., *The Travel and Tropical Medicine Manual*, 2nd ed., W. B. Saunders Co., Philadelphia, 1995, p. 203–234.

**Table 92.7** Selected febrile illnesses causing organomegaly and/or lymphadenopathy*

| | Hepatomegaly | Splenomegaly | Generalized adenopathy | Localized adenopathy |
|---|---|---|---|---|
| VIRUSES | | | | |
| Cytomegalovirus | +/− | + | +/− | +/− |
| Dengue | +/− | +/− | + | − |
| Epstein-Barr virus | +/− | ++ | ++ | + |
| Hepatitis A and B | ++ | +/− | +/− | − |
| HIV | +/− | +/− | ++ | + |
| HTLV-I | ++ | ++ | ++ | +/− |
| BACTERIA | | | | |
| Anthrax | − | − | − | + |
| Brucellosis | + | ++ | + | +/− |
| Ehrlichiosis | + | + | − | − |
| Endocarditis | − | + | +/− | − |
| Enteric fever | ++ | ++ | +/− | − |
| Leptospirosis | +/− | + | + | − |
| Melioidosis | +/− | +/− | + | + |
| Plague | + | + | − | ++ |
| Q fever | ++ | ++ | − | − |
| Relapsing fever | ++ | ++ | +/− | +/− |
| Spotted fevers | + | + | +/− | +/− |
| Tuberculosis | +/− | +/− | +/− | ++ |
| Tularemia | +/− | +/− | +/− | ++ |
| Typhus | +/− | ++ | +/− | − |
| PARASITES | | | | |
| Acute schistosomiasis | ++ | ++ | ++ | +/− |
| African trypanosomiasis | +/− | + | ++ | + |
| Amebiasis (hepatic) | ++ | +/− | − | − |
| Babesiosis | ++ | ++ | +/− | +/− |
| Fascioliasis | ++ | +/− | − | − |
| Filariasis | − | − | + | ++ |
| Malaria | + | ++ | − | − |
| Toxocariasis (visceral larva migrans) | ++ | +/− | − | − |
| Toxoplasmosis | +/− | +/− | + | + |
| Visceral leishmaniasis | ++ | ++ | + | ++ |

Key to Table 92.7: Approximate frequency of physical finding in specified infection:

++: common

+: frequent

+/−: infrequent

−: rare/absent

*Reprinted with permission from Liles WC, Van Voorhis WC: Travel-acquired illnesses associated with fever. *In* Jong EC, McMullen R, eds., *The Travel and Tropical Medicine Manual*, 2nd ed., W. B. Saunders Co., Philadelphia, 1995, p. 203–234.

tance is most often associated with *P. falciparum*, such that one cannot exclude the diagnosis even when the patient received "adequate" malaria prophylaxis. Although patients usually develop symptoms of malaria within two weeks of exposure, clinical manifestations of *P. vivax*, *P. ovale*, and *P. malariae* infections can develop up to five years following exposure.

### Clinical manifestations

Typically, illness begins abruptly with intense rigors, fever, headache, malaise, and myalgias, sometimes associated with abdominal symptoms. Physical examination usually demonstrates fever, tachycardia, and orthostatic hypotension; hepatosplenomegaly is common. Laboratory studies typically reveal anemia, leukopenia, thrombocytopenia, and elevations in liver function tests (ALT, AST, and bilirubin). In primary attacks, fever is irregular and intermittent. A pattern of recurrent, periodic fevers may develop within 7 days in *P. vivax*, *P. ovale*, and *P. malariae* infections, while persistent hectic fevers are more characteristic of infection with *P. falciparum*.

### Diagnosis

Definitive diagnosis depends upon the demonstration of organisms on thin or thick blood smears stained with Giemsa stain (Fig. 92.1). The diagnosis of malaria in partially immune individuals or in those who have received prophylaxis or partial treatment may be complicated by low parasitemia. Multiple blood smears or serologies may be helpful when the patient is not likely to have been previously infected with malaria. Proper identifi-

**Table 92.8** Important tropical infections causing meningitis and encephalitis*

| Infection | Geographic distribution |
|---|---|
| VIRUSES | |
| California group encephalitis | America, Asia |
| Chikungunya | Africa, Asia |
| Crimean-Congo hemorrhagic fever | Africa, Asia, Europe |
| Japanese encephalitis | Asia, Oceania |
| Kyasanur Forest disease | Asia (India) |
| Lymphocytic choriomeningitis | Widespread |
| Murray Valley encephalitis | Oceania (Australia) |
| Omsk hemorrhagic fever | Europe (former USSR) |
| Oropouche | America |
| Poliomyelitis | Widespread |
| Rabies | Africa, America, Asia, Europe |
| Rift Valley fever | Africa |
| Rocio virus disease | America |
| Thogoto virus disease | Africa, Asia, Europe |
| Tick-borne encephalitis | Asia, Europe |
| Venezuelan equine encephalitis | America |
| West Nile fever | Africa, Asia, Europe, Oceania |
| BACTERIA | |
| Bartonellosis | America (Andes) |
| Brucellosis | Widespread |
| Leptospirosis | Widespread |
| Listeriosis | Widespread |
| Lyme disease | Widespread (especially America and Europe) |
| Meningococcal infection | Widespread (especially subSaharan Africa) |
| Rickettsioses | Widespread |
| Salmonnelosis | Widespread |
| Syphilis | Widespread |
| Tuberculosis | Widespread |
| FUNGI | |
| Blastomycosis | Africa, America, Asia, Europe |
| Coccidiomycosis | America |
| Cryptococcosis | Widespread |
| Histoplasmosis | Widespread |
| Sporotrichosis | Widespread |
| PROTOZOA | |
| African trypanosomiasis | Africa |
| Malaria | Widespread |
| Primary amebic meningoencephalitis | Widespread |
| Toxoplasmosis | Widespread |
| HELMINTHS | |
| Cysticercosis (*Taenia solium*) | Widespread |
| Eosinophilic meningitis (*Angiostrongylus cantonensis*) | Africa, America, Asia, Oceania |
| Gnathostomiasis | Africa, America, Asia, Oceania |
| Paragonimiasis | Africa, Asia |
| Strongyloidiasis (in immunocompromised hosts) | Widespread |
| Toxocariasis | Widespread |
| Trichinellosis | Widespread |

*Adapted in part from Wilson ME: *A World Guide to Infections: Diseases, Distribution, Diagnosis*. Oxford University Press, New York, 1991. Reprinted with permission from Liles WC, Van Voorhis WC: Travel-acquired illnesses associated with fever. *In* Jong EC, McMullen R, eds., *The Travel and Tropical Medicine Manual*, 2nd ed., W. B. Saunders Co., Philadelphia, 1995, p. 203–234.

cation of the *Plasmodium* species causing a given infection is important to define whether or not primaquine therapy will be necessary for definitive, radical cure.

## Treatment

Recommended treatment regimens for malaria are outlined below:

1. *P. vivax*, *P. ovale*—chloroquine phosphate: 1 gm (600 mg base) PO × 1 dose, then 0.5 gm in 6 hrs, then 0.5 gm daily for 2 days; plus primaquine: 26.3 mg (15 mg base) PO qd × 14 days. (Parenteral chloroquine [10 mg base/kg by rate-controlled IV infusion over 8 hrs, followed by 15 mg/kg over 24 hrs] can be employed for the treatment of patients unable to take oral medication.)
2. *P. malariae*, chloroquine-sensitive *P. falciparum*—chloroquine as above; primaquine not required.
3. Chloroquine-resistant *P. falciparum*—quinine: 2 capsules (300 mg salt, 250 mg base per capsule) PO TID × 3–7 days, plus doxycycline: 100 mg PO BID × 7 days. Quinidine should be employed if intravenous therapy is required—quinidine gluconate: 10 mg/kg IV over 1–4 hrs as loading dose, followed by 0.02 mg/kg/min IV × 72 hrs or until patient can swallow to complete course of therapy with oral quinine.

**Table 92.9** Selected infections characteristically associated with fever and cutaneous signs*

| Infection | Typical skin manifestations/rash |
|---|---|
| VIRUSES | |
| Dengue | Diffuse scarletiniform or macular rash; occasional petechiae or ecchymoses |
| Ebola/Marburg viruses | Maculopapular rash on trunk |
| Herpes simplex virus | Grouped vesicles |
| HIV (acute) | Morbilliform rash |
| Rubella | Maculopapular rash |
| Rubeola | Maculopapular rash |
| Varicella | Grouped vesicles or pustules |
| Viral hemorrhagic fevers | Petechiae, ecchymoses |
| Yellow fever | Jaundice |
| BACTERIA | |
| Anthrax | Eschar |
| Bartonellosis | Erythematous papules and nodules |
| Leptospirosis | Possible pretibial maculopapular rash |
| Lyme disease | Large, annular erythematous macule(s) |
| Meningococcemia | Petechiae and purpura—may involve palms/soles |
| Rickettsial spotted fevers | Diffuse macular or maculopapular rash—may involve palsm/soles; possible petechiae and eschar at primary inoculation site |
| Scarlet fever | Diffuse maculopaular rash |
| Scrub typhus | Eschar; diffuse macular or maculopapular rash |
| Syphilis (secondary) | Papular rash, possibly involving palms/soles |
| Tularemia | Ulcerated papulae at inoculation site |
| Typhoid fever | Rose-colored papules on trunk ("rose spots") |
| Typhus | Diffuse macular or maculopapular rash—occasional petechiae |
| PARASITES | |
| Acute schistosomiasis (Katayama fever) | Urticaria |
| African trypanosomiasis | Chancre, followed by generalized erythematous rash; possible erythema nodosum |
| American trypanosomiasis | Erythematous nodule at inoculation site—may be associated with periorbital edema |
| Cutaneous larva migrans | Migratory, serpingenous subcutaneous nodule(s) |
| Leishmaniasis | Ulcers, nodules |
| Onchocerciasis | Subcutaneous nodule(s), dermatitis |
| Strongyloidiasis | Larval currens (erythematous, serpingenous subcutaneous papules, often perirectal, associated with pruritis) |
| FUNGI | |
| Coccidioidomycosis | Macular or maculopapular rash; erythema nodosum |
| Histoplasmosis | Occasional erythema nodosum |
| Paracoccidioidomycosis | Papules and nodules, progressing to ulcers, often associated with extensive vegetations |
| Blastomycosis | Verrucous, ulcerated nodules; occasional erythema nodosum |

*Reprinted with permission from Liles WC, Van Voorhis WC: Travel-acquired illnesses associated with fever. *In* Jong EC, McMullen R, eds., *The Travel and Tropical Medicine Manual*, 2nd ed., W. B. Saunders Co., Philadelphia, 1995, p. 203–234.

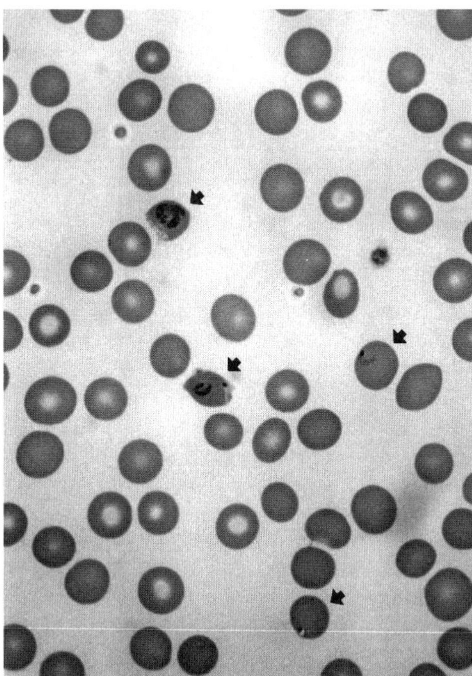

**Fig. 92.1** Wright stain of a thin blood smear from a patient with clinical malaria showing multiple erythrocytes infected with *Plasmodium falciparum* trophozoites at various stages of development (*arrows*).

*Notes:*

a. Corticosteroids are contraindicated for the treatment of cerebral malaria.

b. Exchange transfusion should be considered to achieve rapid reduction in parasite load in *P. falciparum* infections associated with parasitemia >10%, especially if symptoms of cerebral malaria (e.g., convulsions, obtundation, coma) are present.

c. All patients with severe malaria should initially be treated for *P. falciparum* if definitive identification of the infecting species is not available.

d. *P. falciparum* contracted in most regions of the world should be considered potentially resistant to chloroquine. "Chloroquine-sensitive" *P. fal-ciparum* is confined to Central America north of the Panama Canal, the Caribbean, the Middle East, and northern China. If the status of chloroquine resistance is in doubt, then patients with *P. falciparum* infection should be treated for chloroquine-resistant malaria.

e. Primaquine induces hemolysis in patients with underlying G6PD deficiency. Therefore, screening should be employed for most patients prior to initiation of this therapy.

f. In the United States, intravenous quinine is no longer available from the CDC. Quinidine gluconate should be employed in its place.

## Typhoid and paratyphoid fever (enteric fevers)

Enteric fever occurs following blood invasion with *Salmonella typhi* or *S. paratyphi*. Persistently rising fever, relative bradycardia, rose spots, and normal WBC counts are all clues to the diagnosis; however, some or all of these characteristics are not present in many cases. Complications include intestinal perforation, intestinal hemorrhage, coma, myocarditis, and disseminated intravascular coagulation (DIC). The organism can be cultured from blood and stool in 90% of documented cases, but culture of bone marrow and rose spots improves the diagnostic yield. Serology may be helpful if the patient has not been immunized. Neither the oral nor the parenteral vaccine provides complete immunity. In immunized patients, however, a higher percentage of individuals with enteric fever will have disease due to *S. paratyphi*. Students were more likely to acquire imported typhoid than any other occupational group. Major sources of imported typhoid in the United States include Mexico (40%) and India (15%). The relative risk of contracting typhoid fever appears to be greatest for travel to Peru, India, Pakistan, Chile, and Haiti. Resistance to antimicrobials has been reported for *S. typhi* isolates in many countries, though chloramphenicol, trimethoprim-sulfamethoxazole, and quinolones are usually effective.

## Arboviral diseases

Arboviral diseases are caused by arthropod-borne viruses; most are zoonoses. Greater than 400 arboviruses, classified into many families and genera, have been described. Some form of arboviral disease is present in all tropical regions. However, some arboviruses, such as O'nyong-nyong, Mayaro, Ross River, Oropouche, and Rift Valley fever viruses, are limited in geographic distribution (Table 92.10). Diagnosis usually depends on clinical suspicion with serologic confirmation, which generally requires acute and convalescent serum samples. The arboviral diseases can be divided into five syndromes based on clinical presentation: (*1*) undifferentiated fever; (*2*) dengue fever; (*3*) hemorrhagic fever; (*4*) encephalitis (see Chapter 74); and (*5*) pneumonitis. Undifferentiated fever (e.g., Oropouche, Mayaro, and sand fly fever) is generally characterized by one or more of the following: fever, headache, myalgias, pharyngitis, coryza, nausea, vomiting, and diarrhea. Dengue fever syndrome (dengue, chikungunya, o'nyong-nyong, Sindbis, West Nile, Ross River viruses) is characterized by fever, rash, and leukopenia. The spectrum of hemorrhagic fevers (Lassa fever, Ebola, Marburg, Congo-Crimean hemorrhagic fever, Argentine hemorrhagic fever, Bolivian hemorrhagic fever, dengue, yellow fever viruses) ranges from mild petechiae to severe purpura and a bleeding diathesis. Signs and symptoms of central nervous system dysfunction predominate in the encephalitis syndrome. Hantavirus respiratory syndrome, usually acquired following aerosol exposure to rodent droppings in the southwestern United States, presents as fever with pneumonia, progressing rapidly to distress ARDS and death.

Dengue is the most common and widespread arbovirus, with a worldwide distribution throughout the tropics and in many temperate zones. Dengue virus is a single-stranded RNA flavivirus transmitted by the day-biting urban mosquito, *Aedes aegypti*, or the jungle mosquito, *Aedes albopictus*. Four serotypes, 1, 2, 3, and 4, are recognized. Infection with one serotype results in immunity to that particular serotype; however, following a short period of protection, individuals are susceptible to infection with another serotype. The incubation period of dengue is five to eight days. Clinical infection ranges from a mild, self-limited febrile syndrome (classic dengue) to a hemorrhagic fever/shock syndrome (dengue hemorrhagic fever syndrome), defined by the presence of a platelet count less than 100,000/mm$^3$ and a hematocrit drop of 20%, with or without cardiovascular shock. A viral prodrome of nausea and vomiting is common, followed by high fever for a mean of five days, which often lyses abruptly. Myalgias are particularly prominent, giving rise to the common name of "breakbone fever." Headache (especially retroorbital), lymphadenopathy (usually cervical), and/or rash (scarletiniform, maculopapular, or petechial) frequently develop. The rash may occur late during the course of illness, and fever may reappear after several days (the "saddleback" fever pattern, present in about 60%). Evidence suggests that previous infection with one serotype of virus may predispose an individual to more severe disease upon infection with another serotype. This immune enhancement of viral pathogenesis is thought to result from immunoglobulin-mediated dengue virus uptake into monocyte/macrophages where viral growth is favored. This process may also exacerbate the clinical manifestations of dengue by potentiating monokine synthesis and release. Thus, development of the hemorrhagic fever/shock syndrome is almost exclusively restricted to long-term residents of endemic areas, not casual visitors like most travelers. Prolonged malaise and fatigue may complicate the convalescence period for months following resolution of other dengue symptoms.

Yellow fever is transmitted by both *Haemagogus* mosquitoes in the jungle environment and *Aedes aegypti* in urban settings. All recent cases of American yellow fever (approximately 50–200/year) were acquired in the jungle environment, but sporadic urban transmission still occurs in large African outbreaks. Despite the widespread distribution of *Aedes aegypti* in the Far East, yellow fever virus transmission has never been reported from this region. The spectrum of clinical disease ranges from a dengue-fever-like illness to a severe hemorrhagic illness associated with hepatic and renal failure. The disease is almost 100% preventable by vaccination with live attenuated 17D-strain vaccine.

Chikungunya virus infection has been noted in a number of travelers from Southeast Asia, especially Thailand. This disease presents in a similar fashion to classic dengue fever but is frequently complicated by prolonged migratory arthralgias, especially in females.

Viruses causing hemorrhagic fever syndromes, such as Lassa fever virus, Ebola virus, Marburg virus, and Machupo virus, have been associated with life-threatening infections that can be spread nosocomially (Tables 92.3 and 92.10). Patients who are suspected of having one of these viruses should be immediately placed in respiratory isolation. Laboratory studies should be limited, and personnel alerted to the possibility of contagious virus in patient specimens. In the United States, the Centers for Disease Control and Prevention (CDC) and the state health department should be contacted immediately. Early symptoms of both Ebola and Lassa fever include fever, malaise, weakness, and myalgias followed later by cough, pharyngitis, chest, and epigastric pain. Vomiting and diarrhea occur about day five, associated with fever to 39–40 °C. By the sixth day, respiratory distress, cardiac instability, hepatic and renal failure, and hemorrhagic phenomena begin to appear. Diagnosis is based on either isolation of the virus or demonstration of a four-fold rise in specific antibody titer. Early treatment with ribavirin may improve outcome with Lassa fever virus, Hantaan virus causing hemorrhagic fever with renal syndrome, and Congo-Crimean hemorrhagic fever. Other viruses of medical importance are listed in Table 92.10.

## Rickettsial diseases

Rickettsial diseases are acute, usually self-limited, febrile illnesses caused by obligate intracellular gram-negative bacteria of the family *Rickettsiaceae*. Rickettsial diseases can be divided into five major groups: typhus, scrub typhus, spotted fevers, Q fever, and trench fever. All are transmitted by ticks, fleas, lice, or mites, except Q fever, which is acquired by inhalation of aerosolized organisms. Infectious vasculitis is responsible for the typical pathologic manifestations of rickettsial disease. Incubation periods for the rickettsial diseases vary widely (2–30 days). Clinical illness is generally characterized by an abrupt onset of fever, chills, and sweats frequently associated with rash, headache, conjunctivitis, pharyngitis, epistaxis, myalgias, arthralgias, and hepatosplenomegaly. An eschar often develops at the site of the bite of the mite or tick in the spotted fever group and scrub typhus. Complications are rare, but include encephalitis, renal failure, and shock. The spectrum of illness ranges widely and includes subclinical infection. Most rickettsial disease reported in the United States is acquired domestically and represents Rocky Mountain spotted fever or ehrlichiosis. Tick typhus (Mediterranean spotted fever, Boutonneuse fever, and others) is the most commonly reported rickettsial disease of travelers. Tick typhus is endemic to areas of southern Europe, Africa, and the Middle East, though most cases were reported in travelers to Africa. Murine typhus and scrub typhus were the other rickettsial diseases diagnosed in travelers and reported to the CDC. Diagnosis generally depends on clinical suspicion (often mandating empiric antibiotic therapy), Weil-Felix reaction (rickettsiae share antigens with *Proteus mirabilis* strains), and specific serology. Therapy consists of tetracycline (2 gm/day) or chlor-amphenicol (1.5–2 gm/day), divided 4 times daily, generally for 3–4 days following defervescence and a minimum of one week. Recent evidence suggests that the fluoroquinolones may be acceptable alternatives for the therapy of rickettsial spotted fevers other than Rocky Mountain spotted fever.

## Helminths

### Schistosomiasis

This is a disease transmitted by cutaneous fresh water exposure in endemic regions. Katayama fever, or acute schistosomiasis, develops about 2–10 weeks following exposure. This serum-sickness-like illness is likely to represent a reaction against antigen-antibody complexes formed as a result of egg deposition. Characteristic clinical manifestations include fevers, chills, sweating, headache, cough, lymphadenopathy, hepatosplenomegaly, and eosinophilia. Most patients with Katayama fever experience a self-limited illness which is commonly undiagnosed. Travelers appear to be more likely to develop this syndrome than natives. Serologic studies are helpful in the diagnosis. Recommended treatment involves the administration of praziquantel and corticosteroids.

### Filariasis

The filariasis syndromes associated with fever include onchocerciasis (river blindness), lymphatic filariasis (lymphangitis, often complicated by bacterial superinfection), and nocturnal fever with or without pulmonary symptoms due to circulating microfilariae. Eosinophilia is common in patients with filariasis. The diagnosis is usually established by the demonstration of microfilariae in skin snips (onchocerciasis) or in blood (note that in lymphatic filariasis, the microfilariae often circulate nocturnally). Serologic studies can be helpful in suspected cases.

### Paragonimiasis

This is a pulmonary illness caused by a lung fluke that induces a febrile response either during its migration to the lungs or by

**Table 92.10** Epidemiology and clinical characteristics of viral hemorrhagic fevers

| Disease | Clinical syndrome | Geographic distribution | Vector |
|---|---|---|---|
| Yellow fever | Ranges from mild febrile illness to severe hepatitis and renal failure (with albuminura); biphasic course of illness may be noted | Tropical South America and subSaharan Africa | *Aedes aegypti* mosquito |
| Dengue | Classic dengue—fever, severe myalgias, and morbilliform rash<br>Dengue hemorrhagic fever—shock and DIC | Tropical and subtropical regions of the Americas, Africa, Asia, and Australia | *Aedes aegypti* mosquito |
| Chikungunya | Classic dengue-like illness, associated with severe arthralgias which often persist following resolution of fever | SubSaharan Africa, Southeast Asia, India, and the Philippines | *Aedes aegypti* mosquito |
| Oropouche | Fever, headache, malaise, and myalgias | Amazon region of Brazil and Trinidad; possibly Colombia | Various mosquito species |
| Lassa fever | Fever, severe headache, lumbar pain, chest pain, and thrombocytopenia; possible encephalitis, pneumonitis, and myocarditis | SubSaharan Africa | None<br>(High potential for person-to-person transmission) |
| Argentine hemorrhagic fever (Junin virus) | Insidious onset of fever, myalgia, headache, conjunctivitis, epigastric pain, nausea, and vomiting; possible shock. | Argentina (especially Buenos Aires province) | None |
| Bolivian hemorrhagic fever (Machupo virus) | Similar to Argentine hemorrhagic fever | Bolivia (department of Beni) | None |
| Marburg virus | Abrupt onset of fever, headache, conjunctivitis, myalgia, nausea, and vomiting; severe hemorrhagic complications and shock are common | Laboratory outbreaks involved with handling infected monkey tissues/cells; Uganda | None<br>(High potential for person-to-person transmission) |
| Ebola virus | Similar to Marburg virus | Isolated and nosocomial outbreaks in Zaire and Sudan | None<br>(High potential for person-to-person transmission) |
| Crimean-Congo hemorrhagic fever | Abrupt onset of fever, headache, arthralgia, myalgia, conjunctivitis, and abdominal pain; purpura and ecchymoses are common | Africa, Middle East, Eastern Europe | *Hyalomma* spp. (ticks)<br>(Potential for nosocomial transmission) |
| Hemorrhagic fever with renal syndrome (Hantavirus) | Abrupt onset of fever, headache, lethargy, abdominal pain associated with oliguria and acute renal failure; | Former Soviet Union, Korea, and China | None |
| Crimean-Congo hemorrhagic fever | Abrupt onset of fever, headache, arthralgia, myalgia, conjunctivitis, and abdominal pain; purpura and ecchymoses are common | Africa, Middle East, Eastern Europe | *Hyalomma* spp. (ticks)<br>(Potential for nosocomial transmission) |
| Hemorrhagic fever with renal syndrome (Hantavirus) | Abrupt onset of fever, headache, lethargy, abdominal pain associated with oliguria and acute renal failure; petechiae are common | Former Soviet Union, Korea, and China | None |
| Hantavirus respiratory syndrome | Abrupt onset of fever, cough and dyspnea, rapidly progressing to ARDS and death | Four corners region of southwestern USA; sporadic cases elsewhere in North America | None |

*Adapted in part from with permission from Liles WC, Van Voorhis WC: Travel-acquired illnesses associated with fever. *In* Jong EC, McMullen R, eds., *The Travel and Tropical Medicine Manual*, 2nd ed., W. B. Saunders Co., Philadelphia, 1995, p. 203–234.

its obstruction or destruction of lung parenchyma. Hemoptysis can occur, thereby mimicking pulmonary tuberculosis. The disease is acquired by ingestion of raw freshwater crustaceans or plants in Asia, Africa, and South America. Diagnosis can be established by examination of the sputum and stool for ova. Serologic studies are available. Treatment is with praziquantel (see Chapter 40).

#### Trichinosis

This systemic illness is usually associated with eosinophilia, muscle pain, fever, and often periorbital edema. It is acquired by the ingestion of undercooked meat, usually pork or sausage. Diagnosis is based on histopathologic demonstration of the organism in tissue from muscle biopsy or serologic confirmation.

### Protozoa

#### Amebiasis

*Entamoeba histolytica* is usually acquired by ingesting cysts in contaminated water or food, but may be transmitted sexually. Both amoebic dysentery and amoebic liver abscess may cause fever. Amoebic liver abscess is associated with right upper-quadrant discomfort, hepatomegaly, an elevated right hemidiaphragm, and markedly elevated antibody titers to *E. histolytica* antigens. Often, *E. histolytica* cannot be identified in the stool at the time of presentation of amoebic abscess. Treatment is with metronidazole plus another agent to clear luminal amoebae and cysts, such as iodoquinol (see Chapters 40 and 63).

#### Chagas' disease (American trypanosomiasis)

This disease is caused by infection with *Trypanosoma cruzi* acquired in mud or thatched-roof housing in endemic areas of South America via the bite of the reduviid bug. It is also transmitted by blood transfusion frequently in endemic countries and occasionally in the United States. Following an incubation period of 1–2 weeks, *T. cruzi* causes a febrile illness during the acute stage of infection which persists for 2–4 weeks. The illness is accompanied by local swelling at the site of inoculation of trypanosomes, lymphadenopathy, hepatosplenomegaly, petechial rash, and influenza-like symptoms. Treatment of the acute infection with benznidazole (Brazilian strains) or nifurtimox (Chilean and Argentine strains) may be beneficial (see Chapter 40). This disease is rare among travelers.

#### African trypanosomiasis

Infection with *Trypanosoma brucei gambiensiae* or *Trypanosoma b. rhodesiensiae* causes a febrile syndrome due to circulating trypanosomes. The disease is transmitted by the bite of the tse-tse fly in Africa. Occasionally, a chancre can be seen at the site of inoculation during acute infection. Lymphadenopathy is common, particularly in the posterior cervical chain. Later, the trypanosomes invade the central nervous system. Lumbar puncture must be performed to determine which treatment regimen should be administered. If disease has progressed to the central nervous system, treatment with arsenicals or dimethyl-fluoro-ornithine is recommended. Otherwise, less toxic treatment with pentamidine or suramin is preferred (Chapter 40). African trypanosomiasis is uncommon among travelers.

#### Visceral leishmaniasis (kala-azar)

This disorder is characterized by hepatosplenomegaly, severe wasting, and fevers. Leishmania are transmitted by the bite of the sandfly. The kala-azar syndrome is usually caused by *Leishmania donovani*, which is endemic in areas of the Mediterranean, the Middle East, the Indian subcontinent, and Africa. Although visceral leishmaniasis is extremely uncommon among travelers, *L. tropica* was recently reported to cause a febrile syndrome in U.S. soldiers who were stationed in the Persian Gulf. This clinical syndrome, while not as severe as kala-azar, was associated with leishmanial forms in bone marrow biopsy specimens obtained from affected soldiers. Serology for leishmaniasis was most often negative in this group. Treatment with pentavalent antimonials has led to apparent cure.

*Leishmania basiliensis* is endemic in South America and usually causes cutaneous or mucocutaneous disease. Visceral disease with fever may occur, however, in the setting of immunosuppression and is a complication of HIV infection. Treatment of visceral leishmaniasis is with pentavalent antimonial drugs (e.g., stibogluconate sodium) or pentamidine isethionate (see Chapter 40). Therapy with human recombinant gamma interferon in combination with pentavelent antimony may be effective in patients refractory to conventional treatment.

#### Toxoplasmosis

Primary infection with *Toxoplasma gondii* can cause an acute febrile syndrome usually associated with generalized lymphadenopathy and hepatitis, which may be acquired by travelers via the consumption of undercooked meat. Transmission may be common in more developed countries, such as France, because of the popular ingestion of uncooked meat (e.g., steak tartar). The acute toxoplasmosis syndrome is a distinct disorder from relapsing disease producing ophthalmitis or encephalitis (see Chapter 74).

#### Strongyloidiasis

This disorder, usually acquired when larvae in contaminated soil penetrate the skin, rarely causes a febrile illness in travelers. However, immunocompromised hosts can develop a life-threatening hyperinfection syndrome, frequently complicated by significant disseminated strongyloidiasis outside of the gastrointestinal tract. Treatment is with thiabendazole or ivermectin (see Chapter 40).

#### Echinococcosis

Ingestion of the larvae of either *Echinococcus granulosus* or *E. multilocularis* (or, rarely, *E. vogeli* ) causes hydatid cyst disease involving the lungs or liver. Fever is usually absent unless the cyst(s) become secondarily infected. This disorder is most prevalent in southern South America, parts of southern Europe and the former Soviet Union, the Middle East, East Africa, and Alaska, especially in herding regions where domestic dogs are fed the entrails of slaughtered sheep. Traditionally, surgical excision of echinococcal cysts was the only therapeutic option, but recent studies have reported promising results with albendazole treatment.

## Bacteria

### Tuberculosis

Tuberculosis is an uncommon disease among short-term travelers (Table 92.1). It is more likely to occur among those going abroad to perform medical service or others abroad for prolonged lengths of time (see Chapter 57).

### Meningococcal disease

Meningococcal disease occurs sporadically in travelers to endemic areas (sub-Saharan Africa and Nepal) and in epidemics during times of crowding. Purpuric lesions and signs of meningismus are helpful, but individuals may present with only fever and respiratory symptoms. Diagnosis is established by culture, and treatment with penicillin or chloramphenicol is effective. Contacts of documented cases should receive prophylaxis with rifampin (see Chapter 73).

### Anthrax

Infection with *Bacillus anthracis* is common in Africa, the Middle East, and the Far East. Anthrax has been contracted following contact with imported contaminated animal hides and wool. It is usually associated with a local eschar and marked local edema. When bacteria proliferate and invade the bloodstream, systemic anthrax can develop with high mortality. Pulmonary anthrax, a fulminant hemorrhagic pneumonia, is a rare occurrence following inhalation or spores. Treatment is with penicillin, other $\beta$-lactams, or tetracycline.

### Leptospirosis

Infection with *Leptospira* species is acquired by contact with water contaminated by animal urine containing the responsible spirochetes. It is a common disorder in Oceania and the Far East, particularly in rice-growing regions where the spirochetes can be readily isolated from surface water. This disease may be contracted by abattoir workers, swimmers, and campers. Clinical illness ranges from relatively mild disease to fulminant hepatic failure (Weil's disease). Definitive diagnosis is based upon either serologic studies or the demonstration of leptospires in specimens of clinical fluids. Treatment involves supportive care for renal failure and coagulopathy and administration of penicillin or tetracycline.

### Brucellosis

Infection with *Brucella melitensis*, *B. suis*, *B. abortus*, or *B. canis* causes an illness which ranges from an indolent febrile syndrome to fulminant endocarditis. It is usually acquired by consumption of unpasteurized dairy products but may be encountered in abattoirs. Diagnosis is made by documenting a rise in specific agglutinins and/or isolation of the fastidious organism from normally sterile body fluids, including blood. Treatment is with streptomycin, other aminoglycosides, or tetracycline (see Chapter 38).

### Plague

This disease is reported to be epidemic in humans in certain regions of Vietnam. The etiologic agent, *Yersinia pestis*, is endemic in rodent populations in the southwestern United States and other areas of the world, where it is generally transmitted by infected rodent fleas. It causes a clinical syndrome of painful regional lymphadenitis (i.e., buboes) associated with necrotizing pneumonia and septicemia. *Y. pestis* can also be transmitted via the respiratory route, as demonstrated by the recent outbreak of pneumonic plague in India during 1995. Diagnosis is made by isolation of *Y. pestis* from blood, bubo, sputum, or other specimen. (Note: *Y. pestis* is a potential laboratory hazard.) Alternatively, fluorescent antibody staining of smears from clinical specimens can be used to confirm the diagnosis. Treatment is with streptomycin, gentamicin, tetracycline, or chloramphenicol.

### Melioidosis

Melioidosis is a systemic infection caused by *Pseudomonas pseudomallei*, which is characterized by a tuberculosis-like illness or septicemia. The disease is particularly prevalent in Southeast Asia, where it is especially common in rice paddy workers. Similar to tuberculosis, the bacteria may remain dormant for many years before reactivating and causing illness. Diagnosis is made by culture, and serologic testing may be helpful if cultures are negative. Whereas trimethoprim-sulfamethoxazole, chloramphenicol, tetracycline, and aminoglycosides have been employed in the past for treatment, ceftazidime is now the preferred treatment for melioidosis.

### Relapsing fever

This disease is caused by infection with a variety of *Borrelia* species. It is a worldwide tick-borne endemic disease, but louse-borne human–human transmission still occurs in epidemics in the highlands of Ethiopia, Sudan, Somalia, Chad, Bolivia, and Peru. Most short-term travelers rarely adopt the poor hygiene necessary to contact louse-borne disease. Diagnosis depends on the demonstration of extracellular spirochetes by blood smear and Giemsa staining. Treatment is with either tetracycline or erythromycin. Penicillin therapy is associated with slow spirochete clearance and possible relapses following treatment.

### Bartonellosis

Bartonellosis is caused by infection with *Bartonella bacilliformis*, which is transmitted by sand flies in river valleys with elevations between 2000 and 8000 feet in Peru, Ecuador, and Columbia. This infection can lead to acute hemolysis (Oroya fever) or chronic skin disease (verruga peruna). Penicillin, chloramphenicol, tetracycline, and aminoglycosides have all been used to treat acute infection. Because bacteremic salmonellosis frequently complicates acute bartonellosis, chloramphenicol is often chosen for treatment.

In developed countries, systemic *B. quintana* infection has been seen in outbreaks among homeless people. *B. henselae* is the etiologic agent of cat scratch disease in normal subjects (see Chapter 95) and bacillary angiomatosis in AIDS patients (see Chapter 100).

### Sexually transmitted diseases

Gonorrhea, syphilis, chlamydia, and *Haemophilus ducreyi* are all sexually transmitted diseases which may be contracted by travelers and give rise to fevers. These diseases are described in detail in Chapters 70 and 75.

## Viruses

Common respiratory and enteric viruses account for greater than 50% of cases of febrile illness in travelers. Hepatitis viruses are a relatively common cause of fever in travelers (100–200 per 100,000 travelers); prodromal symptoms such as fever, arthralgias, and a serum-sickness-like disease may precede the development of frank icterus. Hepatitis A occurs most frequently, followed by other enterically transmitted hepatitis viruses, such as hepatitis E. Hepatitis B and C may occur in health care workers, individuals with a history of sexual contact abroad, and patients who previously received blood transfusions (see Chapter 62). Acute HIV infection, resulting from sexual activity, blood transfusion, and intravenous drug use, has been reported among travelers.

Acute infection with Epstein-Barr virus (EBV) may be acquired abroad, especially by travelers in the 15–30-year-old age group. Hepatosplenomegaly, lymphadenopathy, and the presence of atypical lymphocytes on the blood smear are helpful clues. Heterophile antibody tests (e.g., Monospot) or specific EBV serologies are useful for diagnosis (see Chapter 53).

Rubeola (measles) remains an important cause of morbidity and mortality in developing countries and poses a substantial risk to travelers who have received inadequate immunization. Complications include progressive pneumonitis (especially in pregnant or immunocompromised patients), pulmonary bacterial superinfection, and encephalitis.

## Fungi (mycoses)

### Histoplasmosis

Although the incidence of infection is greatest in the Ohio and Mississippi river valleys of North America, histoplasmosis, due to *Histoplasma capsulatum* var. *capsulatum*, can be acquired on all inhabited continents. In contrast, the other pathogenic histoplasmosis species, *Histoplasma capsulatum* var. *duboisii*, is essentially restricted to tropical Africa. These organisms can remain dormant within the human host for years prior to reactivation. The majority of histoplasmosis cases are subclinical or self-limited, but clinically severe acute pulmonary or disseminated disease is possible. Metastatic skin involvement, characterized by subcutaneous abscesses or ulcerative lesions, is frequently seen in chronic, progressive histoplasmosis. Diagnosis is based on isolation of the fungus from body tissues or demonstration of the organism in tissue sections. Treatment with either fluconazole or itraconazole should be initiated in individuals with chronic active or progressive disease. Amphotericin B therapy is indicated for patients with life-threatening infection (see Chapters 41, 42).

### Coccidioidomycosis

Infection with *Coccidioides immitis* can be acquired throughout the lower Sonoran life zone, a desert region spanning the southwestern United States from the San Joaquin Valley of California to West Texas and including much of northern Mexico. Foci of endemic coccidioidomycosis exist in Central America and South America (especially Venezuela, Argentina, and Paraguay). Like *Histoplasma capsulatum*, *C. immitis* may remain dormant for prolonged periods inside the human host prior to reactivation. The majority of infections are asymptomatic. Symptomatic infection usually consists of a self-limited, flulike syndrome (e.g., "valley fever") which may be complicated by a maculopapular rash, arthralgias, or erythema nodosum. A small percentage of infections lead to severe pneumonitis or disseminated disease. Diagnosis is based on culture or histopathologic demonstration of the organism in body fluids or tissues. Treatment of disseminated or progressive disease consists of systemic fluconazole, itraconazole, or amphotericin B depending on the clinical circumstances (see Chapters 41, 42).

### Paracoccidioidomycosis (South American blastomycosis)

This is the most common respiratory mycosis in South America. The disease is acquired by inhalation of spores from the causative dimorphic fungus, *Paracoccioides brasiliensis*, which is widespread throughout Central and South America, from Mexico to Argentina. Although the majority of infections are either subclinical or self-limited, some infected individuals will develop disseminated disease, which is often characterized by the development of mucocutaneous lesions. Definitive diagnosis is based on cultivation of the fungus from clinical specimens. Presumptive diagnosis is often based on demonstration of suggestive morphologic features in tissue sections or body fluids. Amphotericin B, sulfonamides, and the systemic azoles appear to be effective agents for treatment (see Chapters 41, 42).

### Blastomycosis

Although most common in North America, blastomycosis has been acquired in Central and South America, Africa, Poland, India, and the Middle East. Clinical disease, which ranges from asymptomatic or mild to disseminated, fatal disease, is acquired by inhalation of spores of the causative dimorphic fungus, *Blastomyces dermatiditis.* Pneumonia is often complicated by pleurisy, and erythema nodosum is possible. Dissemination to the soft tissues and skin is relatively common, leading to the development of nodules and verrucous ulcerations. Diagnosis depends on isolation or histopathologic demonstration of the organism from tissues or body fluids. Itraconazole and amphotericin B are effective agents for the treatment of disseminated or chronic disease (see Chapters 41, 42).

## Approach to the Traveler with Fever

A directed but thorough evaluation, bearing in mind that most fevers are self-limited, is warranted for the traveler presenting with fever. A careful history including pretravel prophylaxis, itinerary, travel "style," exposures, apparent incubation period, fever pattern, symptoms, previous treatment, and diagnostic studies is essential. Laboratory tests to consider in the diagnostic evaluation include: blood smears (for detection of malaria, *Borrelia*, trypanosomes, *Babesia*, etc.), complete blood count and white cell differential, absolute eosinophil count, serum electrolytes, blood urea nitrogen and creatinine, glucose, bilirubin, hepatic transaminases, urinalysis, chest X ray, PPD skin test, hepatitis serologies, and bacterial cultures of blood, urine, and stool. In many instances, it is prudent to obtain and save an acute serum sample for future serologic studies.

Because the majority of travel-related febrile illnesses represent common self-limited viral syndromes, most fevers will spontaneously resolve. However, if fever persists for more than five days or if the patient's clinical condition deteriorates, repeat malarial smears and blood cultures may be warranted. Directed serologic studies to detect diseases compatible with the patient's history and physical examination should be considered. Imaging studies (e.g., abdominal CT or ultrasound) and biopsies (bone marrow, liver, lymph nodes, others) may be indicated. Hospitalization may be justified to expedite the work-up in certain circumstances. During the evaluation of perplexing cases of apparent travel-related illness, the clinician should bear in mind that noninfectious disorders, such as occult malignancies, systemic lupus erythematosus, and temporal arteritis, may present with fever (see Chapters 47, 49).

Presumptive empiric therapy directed against a likely pathogen may be justified, especially when either adequate diagnostic studies are not readily available or a patient is clinically deteriorating. Examples include oral quinine or intravenous quinidine for suspected infection with *Plasmodium falciparum*, chloramphenicol or quinolones for suspected typhoid fever, and doxycycline for suspected tick-borne, rickettsial, or spirochetal disease (Table 92.2). Early initiation of appropriate therapy may significantly reduce morbidity and potential mortality from these serious febrile illnesses of travelers.

## ANNOTATED BIBLIOGRAPHY


Centers for Disease Control and Prevention. Health Information for International Travel 1994. HHS publication # (CDC) 94-8280. GPO, Washington, DC, 1994.

*An important resource for physicians. Up-to-date, succinct discussions of recommendations for vaccination and prophylaxis of specific diseases. The source for information regarding current malaria risk and vaccinations required for entry into specific countries. Purchase from: Superintendent of Documents, US Govt Printing Office, Washington, DC 20402, (202) 783-3238.*

Jong EC, McMullen R, eds. The Travel and Tropical Medicine Manual, 2nd ed. WB Saunders, Philadelphia, 1995.

*A recently updated soft-bound manual (532 pages) with useful and practical information for physicians who provide care to international travelers. Manual is divided into six sections: the traveling patient; fever; diarrhea; skin lesions; sexually transmitted diseases; and worms.*

Strickland GT, ed. Hunter's Tropical Medicine, 7th ed. WB Saunders, Philadelphia, 1991.

*An outstanding, comprehensive textbook of tropical diseases. Authoritative discussions of the wide spectrum of infections that can be acquired by travelers to the underdeveloped world. The chapter on malaria is particularly noteworthy.*

Warren KS, Mahmoud AAF, eds. Tropical and Geographic Medicine, 2nd ed. McGraw-Hill, New York, 1990.

*A widely read and authoritative textbook.*

Wilson ME. A World Guide to Infections: Diseases, Distribution, Diagnosis. New York University Press, New York, 1991.

*A unique and practical textbook of tropical and travel medicine designed for the practicing clinician. Contains an enormous amount of information in a user-friendly format. This compendium is organized such that diseases endemic to a specific region or country can be quickly identified.*

Wolfe MS, ed. Health Hints for the Tropics, 11th ed. Northbrook, IL, American Committee on Clinical Tropical Medicine and Travelers' Health of the American Society of Tropical Medicine and Hygiene, 1993.

*Succinct, helpful discussions of travel-related issues such as immunizations, malaria prevention, and travelers' diarrhea. Designed as an informational pamphlet for lay travelers, but a handy, affordable resource for health care practitioners as well. Purchase from: The American Society of Tropical Medicine and Hygiene, 60 Revere Drive, Suite 500, Northbrook, IL 60062.*


### Telephone Numbers for Travel and Tropical Medicine Information Available from the United States Centers for Disease Control and Prevention (CDC)

| | | |
|---|---|---|
| CDC International Travelers Hotline | (404) 332-4559 | International health requirements and recommendations |
| CDC FAX Information | (404) 332-4565 | Regional information available by FAX |
| CDC Main Switchboard | (404) 639-3311 | Monday–Friday (8:00 AM–4:30 PM Eastern time) |
| CDC Emergency Consults | (404) 639-2888 | nights/weekends |
| CDC Parasitic Diseases Drug Service | (404) 639-3670 | Information and distribution of special drugs |

# 93

# Endemic and Traveler's Diarrhea in Tropical Countries

HERBERT L. DUPONT

In the developing tropical and semitropical world, microbial contamination of the environment and malnutrition among the local population commonly coexist, resulting in frequent enteric infection, diarrhea, and retarded growth of infants. The general microbial contamination also explains the common occurrence of diarrhea among persons traveling into these areas from industrialized countries such as the United States. In this chapter we will consider the enteric disease complications in the two population groups—local inhabitants and travelers to the region. Treatment of endemic and travelers' diarrhea will be considered in this chapter. Chapter 61 deals with gastroenteritis and diarrhea in developed countries.

## Endemic Diarrhea in the Local Population

In many areas of the developing world, diarrhea represents the most common cause of hospitalization and death among infants living in the region. Approximately one billion cases of diarrhea occur in these areas annually. The illness occurs most commonly in infants less than five years of age. Prolonged and recurrent diarrhea are commonplace among the affected children. Not only is diarrhea more common compared with developed regions, it is associated with high rates of mortality, particularly in infants and children. Nearly five million children die annually due to diarrhea and associated malnutrition. Diarrhea is less common in adults living in these regions, although its rate in adults exceeds that seen in industrialized countries.

The source of enteric infection among persons in developing countries is frequently foods and beverages given to infants early in life. Strict breast-feeding for the first few months of life serves an important protective role in the setting. Other factors relating to high rates of death associated with diarrhea include underlying malnutrition, failure to receive oral rehydration treatment, infection by certain pathogens (see below), and complications of enteric infection such as dehydration, pneumonia, and renal failure.

### Etiology and epidemiology

An etiologic agent can be detected in slightly more than half of pediatric diarrhea cases in these areas, if complete microbiologic evaluation is performed. In non-cholera-endemic areas, the most important definable pathogens are rotavirus, enterotoxigenic *Escherichia coli* (ETEC), *Shigella* spp., *Campylobacter jejuni*, and *Cryptosporidium parvum* (see Table 93.1). In certain areas *Vibrio cholerae* is an important cause of diarrhea. *Giardia lamblia* is a common pathogen, but symptomatic disease generally occurs only following the initial exposure to the organism. There is a subset of patients who develop chronic giardiasis. These persons characteristically suffer from IgA deficiency or another immunodeficiency. *Cryptosporidium parvum* is an important cause of acute and persistent diarrhea in developing regions, particularly among children. It shows a high frequency of secondary spread to household contacts. *Entamoeba histolytica* infection is found commonly among older children and adults living in areas where markedly reduced hygienic standards exist. Symptoms may be persistent or recurrent. The organism is an important cause of hepatic abscess in infected persons. This complication is much more likely in men than women (see Chapter 63).

Certain enteric pathogens produce a high rate of complications. Rotavirus, *V. cholerae*, and *Shigella dysenteriae* type 1 are associated with the highest mortality rates. Rotavirus, *V. cholerae*, and ETEC are important causes of dehydration. *S. dysenteriae* 1 is a cause of febrile dysentery with a high frequency of systemic complications (e.g., pneumonia and hemolytic uremic syndrome). In cases of persistent diarrhea the most frequently identified pathogens are enteroaggregative or enteroadherent *E. coli*, as well as *Shigella* spp., ETEC, *C. jejuni*, *Cr. parvum*, *Cyclospora*, and *E. histolytica*. Most patients fail to have a defined etiologic agent despite complete evaluation.

### Clinical features

There are five important enteric syndromes involving local persons living in developing regions: (*1*) infantile gastroenteritis; (*2*) acute watery diarrhea including cholera-like profuse diarrhea; (*3*) febrile and often dysenteric disease ("invasive" diarrhea); (*4*) persistent diarrhea; and (*5*) enteric fever. The specific syndrome often suggests one or more potential etiologic agents (Table 93.2). Enteric (typhoidal) fever will be considered elsewhere in this text (see Chapter 92) since diarrhea is not usually the prominent clinical finding in this disease which is characterized by the presence of systemic toxicity and fever. Oral electrolyte-fluid therapy (ORT) has been successful in reducing complications and mortality from infant gastroenteritis and acute watery diarrhea. Persistent diarrhea is associated with half of the fatal cases in these areas. The other major causes of death are the invasive bacterial agents causing dysenteric disease and enteric fever.

### Treatment

Diet and fluid-electrolyte replacement are fundamental therapies for all patients with enteric disease/diarrhea. Additional recommended treatment is otherwise determined by clinical illness (see Table 93.2). During a bout of diarrhea, it is important to feed the patient to provide calories (energy) and to facilitate enterocyte renewal. For infants, breast milk or lactose-free formula should be given. For older children and adults, boiled starches/cereals (potatoes, noodles/rice, wheat, oat) with some salt is indicated. Crackers, bananas, yogurt, soup, and boiled vegetables can also be administered. When stools are formed, diet may return to normal as tolerated. Milk products are excluded for older children or adults until clinically improved, because of possible transient lactase deficiency.

Oral rehydration treatment (ORT) is the mainstay of diarrhea management. It is effective regardless of etiology of diarrhea and is safe as long as the water used is not excessively contaminated. The concept of ORT is based on the principle that sodium is absorbed with glucose at the intestinal brush border, both serving as osmotic pulls to water. Other organic molecules such as peptides and amino acids also facilitate the absorption of sodium and water. The rate of administration of rehydration solution is based on the degree of dehydration found (Table 93.3).

Antimicrobial therapy is indicated for certain enteric infections. Invasive bacterial diarrheas associated with fever and/or dysentery or systemic toxicity suggesting bacteremia should be treated with antibacterial drugs. A valuable laboratory marker for invasive bacterial diarrhea is the fecal leukocyte test. Patients with fecal leukocytes usually will have their illness shortened by antibacterial therapy. Adults with diarrhea in this setting should be given one of the fluoroquinolones for 3–5 days if available. If typhoid fever is suspected, the antimicrobial should be given for 10–14 days. For children with febrile dysenteric disease or with toxicity amdinicillin, nalidixic acid, or trimethoprim-sulfamethoxazole plus erythromycin (if prevalent strains are likely to be trimethoprim-susceptible) may be used for 3–5 days depending upon severity. For milder cases of invasive illness in children, furazolidone may be used.

## Control and prevention

A number of interventions are known to be keys to minimizing the occurrence of diarrhea and the complications of illness that does occur. The two most fundamental in developing regions are promotion of strict breast-feeding of all children for at least the first six months of life with consequent delayed introduction of supplemental foods and the implementation of ORT programs in all regions for the management of illness when it does occur.

Other preventive measures have value and should be pursued as resources permit. They include introduction of water and san-

**Table 93.1** Etiology of diarrhea in endemic diarrhea and travelers' diarrhea occurring in developing regions

| Etiologic agent | Endemic diarrhea | Travelers' diarrhea |
|---|---|---|
| Enterotoxigenic *Escherichia coli* | Important in children <3 years of age | The most common cause, shows seasonal occurrence |
| *Shigella* spp. | Major cause of "invasive" diarrhea, important cause of persistent diarrhea and death with high rates of secondary spread | Second most common definable cause of illness |
| *Campylobacter jejuni* | Important cause of "invasive" diarrhea in infants <2 years of age | An occasional cause of diarrhea with seasonal occurrence |
| *Vibrio cholerae* | Important cause of epidemic disease in children and adults in well-defined areas | A rare cause of travelers' diarrhea |
| Rotavirus | Major cause of infantile gastroenteritis, may be implicated in up to one million deaths a year among local infants (<2 years of age) | Not uncommon in travelers to Mexico, uncommon in other areas |
| *Giardia lamblia* | A cause of symptomatic diarrhea when an infant is first exposed; a common cause of asymptomatic infection in endemic regions | A common cause of persistent diarrhea |
| *Cryptosporidium parvum* | Important cause of diarrhea in children, showing high rates of secondary spread | An occasional cause of diarrhea |
| *Entamoeba histolytica* | Important cause of acute, chronic or recurrent diarrhea in older children and adults in areas with markedly reduced levels of hygiene; an important cause of liver abscess | A rare cause of diarrhea |

**Table 93.2** Endemic diarrhea in developing regions: clinical syndromes, common causes, and guide to treatment

| Clinical syndrome | Common etiology | Recommended therapy |
|---|---|---|
| Infantile gastroenteritis (vomiting is predominant symptom) | Viral gastroenteritis (rotavirus, adenovirus, small round virus) or preformed toxin in food (food poisoning) | Oral rehydration treatment (ORT) and diet modification (see text) |
| Acute watery diarrhea | Enterotoxigenic *Escherichia coli*, *Vibrio cholerae*, any enteric pathogen | ORT and diet modification (see text) |
| Febrile/dysenteric disease | *Shigella* spp., *Campylobacter jejuni*; occasionally *Salmonella* spp., *Aeromonas* spp., *Yersinia enterocolitica* noncholera *Vibrio*, *Entamoeba histolytica* | Antimicrobial therapy |
| Persistent (≥14 days) diarrhea | Enteroaggregative, enteroadherent or enterotoxigenic *E. coli*, *Shigella* spp., *C. jejuni*, *C. parvum*, *E. histolytica*, lactase deficiency, small bowel bacterial overgrowth syndrome, spruelike syndrome, trace mineral or vitamin deficiency | Treatment is directed to any etiologic agent detected. If no etiology identified, calories, proteins, and micronutrients should be administered along with ORT. |
| Enteric or typhoidal fever | *Salmonella typhi*, *S. paratyphi*, occasionally other *Salmonella* spp. | Antimicrobial therapy |

itation systems into communities; education of households on principles of food and personal hygiene; improvements in the construction of the home; food and nutrient supplementation in areas where malnutrition is common; making available health care, particularly administration of ORT to cases of watery diarrhea and antimicrobial therapy for invasive diarrheal disease; family planning (larger families have more enteric disease); selected control of fly populations during peak diarrhea seasons, and measles vaccine programs.

Applied research is needed in specific areas to see which interventions are cost effective for the region. Also, enteric disease vaccine programs should be pursued in view of the importance

**Table 93.3** Administration of rehydration solutions based on degree of patient dehydration

| Degree of dehydration | Clinical findings | Fluid therapy |
|---|---|---|
| Mild (loss of 3%–5% of body weight) | Slightly dry mucous membranes, increased thirst, and concentrated urine | Oral rehydration treatment (ORT) 50 ml/kg for a period of four hours together with about 1 cup of ORT per diarrheal stool passed |
| Moderate (6%–9% reduction of body weight) | Dry mucous membranes, sunken eyes and fontanelle, loss of skin turgor | ORT 100 ml/kg for four hours with about 1 cup of ORT per diarrheal stool passed |
| Severe (10% or more reduction of body weight) | Rapid and weak pulse, lethargy, rapid shallow breathing, coma, cold extremities, and/or cyanosis | Intravenous fluids; if available, Ringer's lactate at a level of 20 ml/kg/hr until there is improvement in circulation and mentation |

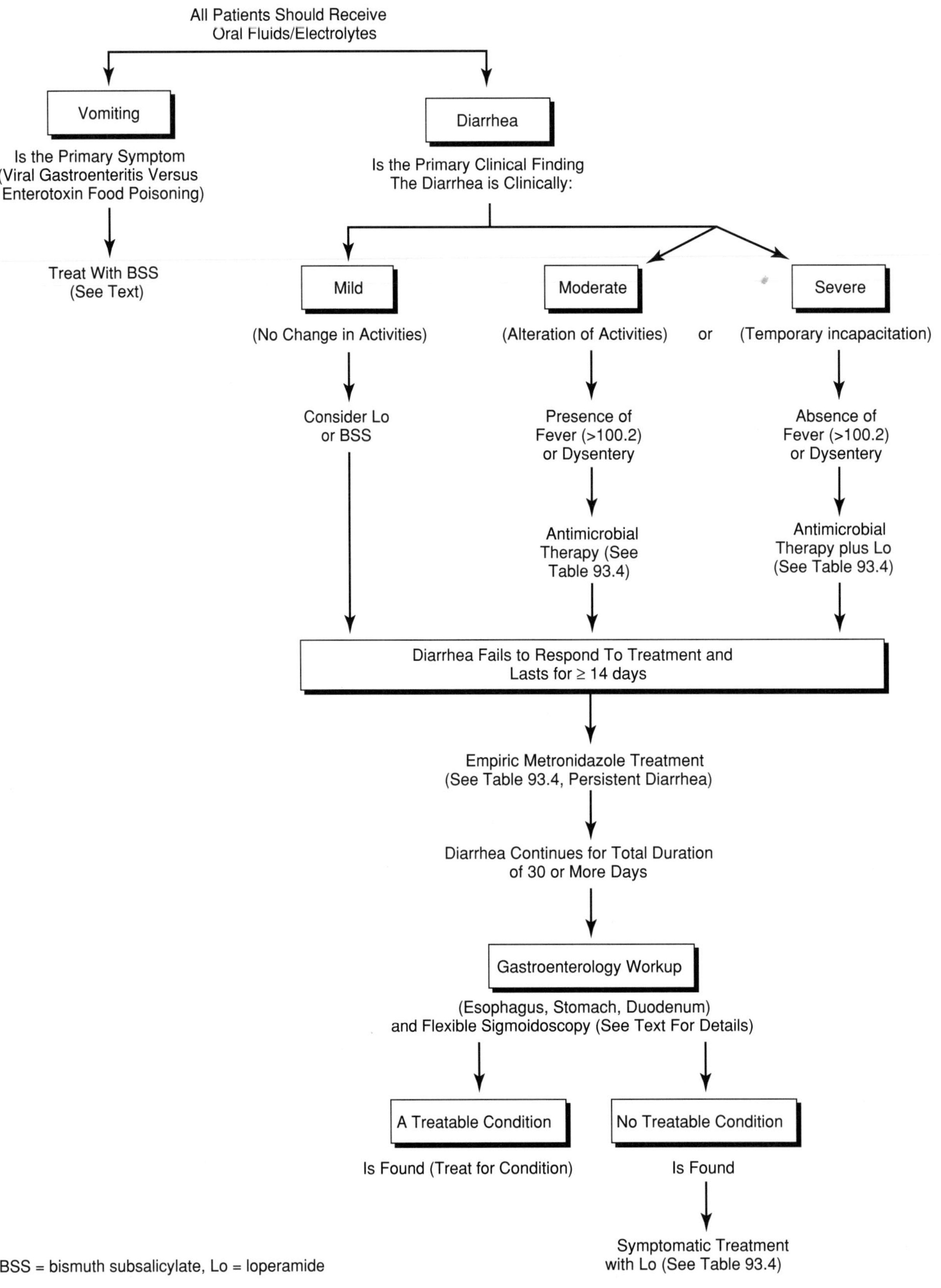

All Patients Should Receive
Oral Fluids/Electrolytes
Vomiting
Is the Primary Symptom
(Viral Gastroenteritis Versus
Enterotoxin Food Poisoning)
Treat With BSS
(See Text)
Diarrhea
Is the Primary Clinical Finding
The Diarrhea is Clinically:
Mild
(No Change in Activities)
Consider Lo
or BSS
Moderate
(Alteration of Activities)
or
Severe
(Temporary incapacitation)
Presence of
Fever (>100.2)
or Dysentery
Antimicrobial
Therapy (See
Table 93.4)
Absence of
Fever (>100.2)
or Dysentery
Antimicrobial
Therapy plus Lo
(See Table 93.4)
Diarrhea Fails to Respond To Treatment and
Lasts for ≥ 14 days
Empiric Metronidazole Treatment
(See Table 93.4, Persistent Diarrhea)
Diarrhea Continues for Total Duration
of 30 or More Days
Gastroenterology Workup
(Esophagus, Stomach, Duodenum)
and Flexible Sigmoidoscopy (See Text For Details)
A Treatable Condition
Is Found (Treat for Condition)
No Treatable Condition
Is Found
Symptomatic Treatment
with Lo (See Table 93.4)
BSS = bismuth subsalicylate, Lo = loperamide

**Fig. 93.1** Flow chart for the management of travelers' diarrhea.

of certain enteric infectious diseases that may one day be controlled by immunologic measures: rotavirus, cholera, ETEC diarrhea, and shigellosis.

## Travelers' Diarrhea

### Epidemiology

Persons from industrialized countries visiting developing tropical regions frequently experience diarrhea. The illness typically develops during the first week after arrival in the high-risk region. Immunity to subsequent enteric infection and diarrhea occurs after remaining in the region for several weeks, although the risk of subsequent illness is never completely eliminated. The customary source of the enteric disease is ingested food. Contaminated water is occasionally the source of the infection.

### Etiology

The most important causes of diarrhea among travelers from industrialized countries to developing tropical regions are the bacterial enteropathogens. The most important single cause is ETEC, found in just under half of the cases in most areas. In Mexico and Morocco, two semitropical regions, ETEC diarrhea is primarily a summertime pathogen. During the fall and winter in these areas when ETEC becomes unusual, *Campylobacter jejuni* is an important cause of illness. In Table 93.1, a summary of the important pathogens in travelers' diarrhea is provided.

### Clinical features

Travelers' diarrhea is highly variable in terms of clinical severity. The average illness consists of passage of 13 unformed stools over a five-day period of time. Approximately 15% of cases of travelers' diarrhea are associated with the passage of bloody stools (dysentery) with variable degrees of fever. Ten percent of the cases of enteric disease of travelers are best classified as gastroenteritis, in view of the prominence of the symptom of vomiting. In approximately 2% of the diarrhea cases, illness will last more than two weeks and in 1% the diarrhea lasts longer than one month. Some of these cases may have diarrhea for more than one year.

### Treatment

In Figure 93.1 a perspective on the management of travelers' diarrhea is provided. The key points in the algorithm are: administration of oral fluid and electrolytes to all persons; administration of bismuth subsalicylate to those with vomiting as the primary feature of the illness (see dose Chapter 61); administration of fluids and possibly symptomatic treatment for mild disease and antimicrobial drugs for moderate to severe disease; use of combined treatment with an antimicrobial drug and loperamide in moderate-to-severe disease without fever or dysentery; empiric metronidazole therapy for *Giardia* and bacterial overgrowth suspected in illness persisting for two weeks or longer; and a gastroenterology evaluation for diarrhea lasting for a month or longer after receiving empiric antibacterial and antiparasitic treatment. The endoscopy exam should include examination of the duodenum with biopsy of lesions found looking for inflammation, *Giardia*, *Microsporidia* and *Cryptosporidium* infection, and flexible sigmoidoscopy with biopsy of abnormal tissue to look for inflammation and enteric infection. Those with a negative work-up should be further managed with symptomatic treatment with loperamide. The patients should be reassured since the outcome is generally good, although the diarrhea may last for as long as a year. In Table 93.4, drug dosages are provided.

### Prevention

All travelers should attempt to minimize exposure to enteric pathogens by selecting the safest foods and beverages (Table 93.5). For those with certain underlying illnesses, prophylactic drugs (antibacterial drugs or bismuth subsalicylate) may be used to prevent diarrhea during brief periods of high risk. Antibacterial drugs are more effective in reducing the frequency of diarrhea (reduced by approximately 90%) than bismuth subsalicylate (frequency reduced by approximately 60%).

A subset of travelers have itineraries during periods of high risk where an illness lasting only six to eight hours may destroy the purpose of the trip. Potential examples of this sort of travel include a honeymoon couple, a long-weekend scuba diver, or a political leader involved in international negotiations during stays in high-risk areas. Only the traveler knows how important it is to remain disease free during travel. They must understand that

**Table 93.4** Chemotherapy of travelers' diarrhea occurring in adults

| Drug | Indications | Dose and duration |
|---|---|---|
| Fluoroquinolone: norfloxacin (NF), ciprofloxacin (CI), ofloxacin (OF), or fleroxacin (FL) | Travel in any area during any season | NF 400 mg BID, CI 500 mg BID, OF 300 mg BID or FL 400 QD for 1–3 days (depending upon severity) |
| Metronidazole | Empiric therapy of persistent diarrhea | 250 mg QID for 7–10 days |
| Loperamide | For improvement of symptoms in persons without fever or dysentery or for symptomatic treatment of patients with prolonged diarrhea without an identifiable and treatable cause | 4 mg initially followed by 2 mg after each unformed stool not to exceed 16 mg/day. For acute diarrhea, the agent is given for no more than 48 hours |

**Table 93.5** Prevention of travelers' diarrhea

| Category of traveler | Recommendations for prevention |
|---|---|
| All travelers | Education on consuming safe foods: i.e. those served steaming hot, dry foods (bread), citrus, syrups, and jellies. Chemoprophylaxis not routinely recommended unless as noted below. |
| Persons with significant underlying disease: diabetics on insulin; those with AIDS, advanced malignancy, cirrhosis, advanced cardiovascular disease; those taking regular omeprazole | Offer chemoprophylaxis as an option for trips of two weeks or less. Antimicrobials include one of the following: norfloxacin 400 mg, ciprofloxacin 500 mg, ofloxacin 300 mg, or fleroxacin 400 mg QD or bismuth subsalicylate 2 tablets QID (with meals and at bedtime). Begin the first day in the country of risk, continue for two days after leaving the region. |
| Persons on a critical mission or trip where an acute illness would produce serious problems | Offer chemoprophylaxis as an option for trips of two weeks or less. Bismuth subsalicylate is the safest prophylactic agent, where antibacterials are usually reserved for therapy of illness. |

as many as 1 in 10,000 may experience a potentially fatal reaction if they utilize an antibacterial drug, in this case to prevent a nonfatal disease. Also, treatment of the rare diarrhea that does occur when prophylactic antibacterial drugs are being employed may be difficult. The organism is likely to be resistant to conventional antibacterial treatment.

Prophylaxis is *not* advisable for persons planning to spend three weeks or longer in an area of risk (e.g., students) because of drug cost, the greater likelihood of an adverse reaction, and because of the interference with the development of protective immunity by using preventive drugs.

## ANNOTATED BIBLIOGRAPHY


Bhan M, Rai P, Levine M, et al. Enteroaggregative *Escherichia coli* associated with persistent diarrhea in a cohort of rural children in India. J Infect Dis 1989; 159:1061–1064.

*Fecal excretion of HEp-2-cell-adherent* E. coli *was shown to be associated with persistent diarrhea in infants and children in rural India.*

Black R, Brown K, Becker S, et al. Longitudinal studies of infectious diseases and physical growth of children in rural Bangladesh. II: Incidence of diarrhea and association with known pathogens. Am J Epidemiol 1982; 115:315–324.

*The relative importance of specific enteropathogens and their association with the occurrence of dehydration are reported in a study in rural Bangladesh. Rotavirus, enterotoxigenic* E. coli, *and* Shigella *spp. were found to be particularly important.*

Black R, Lopez de Romana G, Brown K, et al. Incidence and etiology of infantile diarrhea and major routes of transmission in Huascar, Peru. Am J Epidemiol 1989; 129:785–799.

*The relative importance of enteric pathogens found in childhood diarrhea in rural Peru was reported. Contaminated foods served in the homes were felt to be particularly important sources of diarrhea.*

Butler T, Islam M, Azad A, et al. Causes of death in diarrhoeal diseases after rehydration therapy: an autopsy study of 140 patients in Bangladesh. Bull WHO 1987; 65:317–321.

*The importance of invasive bacteria (especially* Shigella *spp.) as causes of fatal diarrhea in Bangladesh is reported.*

DuPont H. The importance of collaborative research to improve world health. J Infect Dis 1991; 163:946–950.

*International collaboration between investigators from industrialized regions working with colleagues in developing regions is presented as a means of solving world health problems.*

DuPont H. Diarrheal diseases in the developing world. Infect Dis Clin North Am 1995; 9:313–324.

*A review of the epidemiology and etiology of acute and persistent diarrhea in the developing world is provided.*

Huilan S, Zhen L, Mathan M, et al. Etiology of acute diarrhea among children in developing countries: a multicentre study in five countries. Bull WHO 1991; 69:549–555.

*Identical laboratory methods are employed to determine the cause of acute pediatric diarrhea in five regions of the developing world. The importance of enterotoxigenic* E. coli *and rotavirus is confirmed.*

Stanton B, Clemens J. An educational intervention for altering water-sanitation behaviors to reduce childhood diarrhea in urban Bangladesh. II: A randomized trial to assess the impact of intervention on hygienic behaviors and rates of diarrhea. Am J Epidemiol 1987; 125:292–301.

*Regular maternal handwashing was shown to reduce the frequency of infantile diarrhea.*

U.S. Department of Health and Human Services, Centers for Disease Control and Prevention (CDC). The management of acute diarrhea in children: oral rehydration, maintenance and nutritional therapy. October 16, 1992, Vol 41, No RR-16.

*The review includes current recommendations on the fluid and dietary management of acute diarrhea.*

Usha N, Sankaranarayanan A, Walla B, et al. Assessment of preclinical vitamin A deficiency in children with persistent diarrhea. J Pediatr Gastroenterol Nutr 1991; 13:168–175.

*Vitamin A deficiency has been shown to be an important cause of acute and persistent diarrhea in the developing world.*

# 94

# Eosinophilia in Travelers to Tropical Countries

ADEL A. F. MAHMOUD

An increase in peripheral blood eosinophil count is a significant finding in a traveler returning from a visit to developing countries. Eosinophilia is associated with multiple etiologies; most important among these are allergic, infectious, connective tissue, and malignant conditions. It is important to realize that eosinophilia is a specific finding which is usually related to a specific etiology. Infectious causes of eosinophilia have been associated with worm infections in which one stage or another migrates in host tissues or with systemic fungal infections such as aspergillosis. In spite of this clear association with migratory worm infections, there are several case reports describing other associations with most parasitic infections. None of these have been conclusively documented in an epidemiological or etiological significance.

## Approach to Evaluation of Eosinophilia

Eosinophilia is a common finding in returning travelers. Factors which should figure prominently in assessing such a finding include:

- *Level and duration of eosinophilia:* Eosinophilia of clinical significance in an individual returning from an overseas trip should be above 500 cells/mm$^3$. For purposes of initiating a work-up plan, high cell counts should be demonstrated on two separate occasions. It is also important to determine the duration of the overseas visit, when eosinophilia was first noted, and the relationship of its duration to the known incubation period or migratory phase of helminths.
- *Specific geographic areas visited:* Knowledge of the countries and specific locations visited overseas is essential, as the geographic distribution of worm infections in any particular country is sometimes limited only to known foci (see Chapter 5).
- *Dietary and other environmental exposures:* Most worm infections that are associated with peripheral blood eosinophilia are acquired either by ingestion, exposure to the ground or to bodies of fresh water, or the bites of mosquitos and other insect vectors. It is essential, therefore, to ask about these activities and any other indulgences in local dietary habits.
- *Associated symptoms, signs, and laboratory tests:* Migratory worms that are known to be associated with peripheral blood eosinophilia usually cause additional pulmonary, gastrointestinal, hepatic, or central nervous system symptoms and signs. These could be helpful in pointing toward the correct diagnostic procedure.

## Etiology

Eosinophilia in a traveler returning from an overseas trip that lasted several days to several weeks is usually related to the acute stage of helminthic infections. This is particularly the case in worm infections that undergo migratory phases in their early stages. The major worm infections that may be associated with early eosinophilia are outlined in Table 94.1.

In contrast, well-established helminthic infections may be associated with eosinophilia (usually of less degree). This occurs with worm infections in which adults or their progenies reside in host tissues (e.g., filariasis, schistosomiasis). The worm infections that are associated with eosinophilia during their established or chronic phase are summarized in Table 94.2.

Because there are multiple etiologies for eosinophilia seen in clinical practice, other causes should also be taken into consideration (Table 94.3).

## Biology of Eosinophils

The polymorphonuclear eosinophils were originally described in blood smears stained with differential acidic and basic stains. The cells are produced in the bone marrow, which contains a significant pool of stored mature eosinophils. Peripheral blood eosinophils circulate for a short period (one or two days), although in certain pathological combinations their presence in blood may extend to one or two weeks. Eosinophils are considered tissue cells; they migrate from peripheral blood to sites in the body including the submucosa of the gastrointestinal tract and the bronchial tree and to subcutaneous tissues. The cells survive in these locations for approximately two weeks, although our understanding of this aspect of eosinophil life cycle is fragmentary. Eosinophil production by bone marrow progenitor cells is influenced by several mediators. Eosinophilia in vivo has been shown to depend on an intact cellular immune response. In vitro, eosinophil production can be induced by IL-3, GM-CSF, and IL-5. During the past several years IL-5 has been demonstrated to be a specific meditor of eosinophil and basophil production. IL-5 is a disolphide-linked homodimeric glycoprotein. The human dimer has a molecular weight of 24,000. Recent studies have demonstrated that IL-5 has a characteristic four $\propto$-helices and a gross tertiary structure that is similar to IL-3 and GM-CSF. IL-5 exerts its effect on eosinophils through interaction with specific cell surface receptors. Human eosinophils exhibit a single population of high-affinity receptors each consisting of an alpha and a beta chain. Interestingly, the genes encoding IL-3, IL-4, IL-5, and GM-CSF form a cluster on chromosome 5 in humans and on chromosome 11 in mice.

The biological effects of IL-5 have been studied both in vitro and in vivo indicating its eosinophilopoietic activity. This cytokine is incapable, however, of stimulating the production of eosinophil precursors in vitro. Current evidence points to a network of cytokines, rather than a single molecule, which is responsible for the chain of events involved in eosinophilopoiesis. Enhanced activity of IL-5 in vivo, either by introducing a re-

**Table 94.1** Helminthiases associated with eosinophilia in the early phases of infection*

| Infection | Acquisition | Associated clinical features |
|---|---|---|
| Ascariasis | Ingestion of eggs | Loeffler's-like symptoms |
| Hookworms | Larva penetration of skin | Loeffler's-like symptoms |
| Strongyloidiasis | Larva penetration of skin | Loeffler's-like symptoms |
| Visceral larva migrans | Ingestion of eggs | Pulmonary and abdominal complaints |
| Trichinosis | Ingestion of muscle larvae | Gastrointestinal and muscle complaints; allergic reactions |
| Schistosomiasis | Cercarial penetration of skin | Serum-sickness-like symptoms |
| Fascioliasis | Ingestion of metacercaria on aquatic plants | Abdominal pain |

*Symptoms are due to migratory larvae.

combinant retro virus containing the cytokine gene or in transgenic mice, is associated with increased numbers of peripheral-blood as well as tissue eosinophils. In other studies, increased levels of IL-5 have been associated with high eosinophilia seen in helminth-infected experimental animals and humans. The effect of IL-5 on eosinophils extends beyond stimulating their production and maturation. The cytokine has been shown to prolong the survival of eosinophils in vitro from one or two days up to two weeks. This enhanced survival is associated with metabolic activation of the oxidative burst of eosinophils, leading to increased cytotoxicity to multiple targets.

## Functional Studies of Eosinophils

The known association between eosinophilia and two specific pathological conditions, worm infection and allergic diseases, has contributed significantly to our current understanding of eosinophil function. Studies in vitro have demonstrated the ability of human, mouse, rat, and guinea pig eosinophils to kill the larval stage of multiple helminths, including schistosomes and filariae. The reaction is enhanced in the presence of parasite-specific antibody or complement and may also be accentuated by the addition of IL-5. This antibody-dependent cell-mediated cy-

**Table 94.2** Worm infections associated with eosinophilia in their established phase

| Infection | Stages of helminth in host | Associated clinical features |
|---|---|---|
| Strongyloidiasis | Adult worms | Abdominal pain, malabsorption |
| Visceral larva migrans | Migrating larvae | Abdominal pain, hepatomegaly |
| Lymphatic filiarisis | Adult worm, microfilaria | Lymphadenopathy, elephantiasis |
| Tropical pulmonary eosinophilia | Occult microfilaria | Cough, tightness of chest |
| Onchocerciasis | Adult worm, microfilaria | Onchocercoma, recurrent skin irritation, eye symptoms |
| Loaisis | Adult worm, microfilaria | Calabar swelling, worms across eye |
| Dracunculiasis | Adult worms | Cutaneous vesicle with protruding worms |
| Trichinosis | Larvae in muscles | Muscle pain |
| Schistosomiasis haematobia | Adult worms, eggs in tissues | Hematuria, dysuria, hydroureter, hydronephrosis |
| Other schistosome species | Adult worms, eggs in tissues | Colicky, abdominal pain, hepatosplenomegaly |
| Paragonimiasis | Adult worms, eggs in sputum | Cough, hemoptysis |
| Cysticercosis | Cysticerci in tissues | Space-occupying lesions |
| Echinococcosis | Cysts in tissues | Cysts in liver, lungs |
| Angiostrongyliasis | Adult worms in brain | Headache, meningitis |

**Table 94.3** Conditions, other than worm infections, frequently associated with eosinophilia*

| |
|---|
| COMMON |
| Allergies: hay fever, urticaria, asthma, dermatitis herpetiformis |
| Drug reactions: iodides, erythromycin, sulfonamide, nitrofurantoin, others |
| Collagen vascular: allergic angitis, fasciitis, polyarteritis nodosa |
| Gastrointestinal: eosinophilic gastroenteritis |
| Hypereosinophilic syndromes |
| Miscellaneous: pulmonary infiltrate with eosinophilia |
| OCCASIONAL |
| Fungal infections: aspergillosis, coccidioidomycosis |
| Malignancies: lymphomas, solid tumors of lungs, stomach, postirradiation |
| Miscellaneous: chronic peritoneal dialysis, hereditary eosinophilia |

*Adapted from Warren KS, Mahmoud AAF, eds., Tropical and Geographical Medicine, 2nd ed. McGraw-Hill, New York, 1990, p. 66

totoxicity against multicellular targets is mediated by both the oxidative and nonoxidative machinery of eosinophils. The biological relevance of these observations was obtained in depletion studies in which the use of specific antieosinophil serum resulted in elimination of eosinophils and loss of acquired resistance to helminthic infection.

## Clinical Correlates

Eosinophilia due to specific helminthiasis usually presents either during the acute phase of infection or with established disease. Table 94.1 summarizes the main clinical features of acute helminthiases that are associated with eosinophilia. Of particular significance is the Loeffler's-like presentation seen during the larval migratory phase in the lungs of individuals with ascariasis, hookworms, or strongyloidiasis. This syndrome is typically transient and self-limited except in cases of disseminated strongyloidiasis. Patients usually present with dry cough and chest tightness. Multiple focal infiltrate may be seen on chest radiography. Laboratory investigations usually demonstrate eosinophils in sputum and high peripheral blood cell counts. Another mechanistically different clinical presentation is seen in acute schistosomiasis (Katayama fever). The syndrome is mainly seen in infection with either *Schistosoma haematobium* or *S. japonicum*. It occurs four to six weeks after exposure, and its severity may be related to intensity of infection (worm load and associated egg production). Individuals usually present with a travel history and exposure to bodies of fresh water in endemic areas. Clinically, the syndrome is manifest as fever, malaise, lymphadenopathy, and hepatosplenomegaly. A high peripheral blood eosinophil count is the hallmark of this clinical presentation. Acute schistosomiasis is considered a serum-sickness-like syndrome due to formation and deposition of antigen-antibody complexes.

Eosinophilia seen during the established phases of helminthic infection is usually associated with the specific clinical syndromes (Table 94.2). Examples include: *S. mansoni* intestinal or hepatic disease, *S. haematobium* bladder-associated pathology, and lymphadenitis and elephantiasis seen in individuals with chronic lymphatic filariasis.

## Diagnosis and Management

Eosinophilia detected in peripheral blood or tissue samples must be approached in a systematic manner. The observation must be confirmed by repeating blood examination on two separate occasions. Recording a detailed history, including travel experiences, and clinical examination are necessary steps if an infectious etiology is suspected. Knowledge of the possible pathogens and the correct diagnostic tests are the next challenges for practicing physicians. Consultation with experienced clinicians or the Parasitic Diseases Branch of the Centers for Disease Control and Prevention may be of significant help. Therapy is only indicated when a specific etiology is confirmed. For helminthic infections, details of the chemotherapeutic agents are given in Chapter 40. In most circumstances, no additional therapeutic interventions are needed. In rare cases, such as cerebral cysticerosis, steroids may be used as adjunct therapy to reduce chemotherapy-associated enhancement of tissue pathology.

### ANNOTATED BIBLIOGRAPHY


Mahmoud AAF. Eosinophilia. In: Tropical and Geographical Medicine, 2nd ed. McGraw-Hill, New York, pp 65–70, 1990.

*A summary of the biology, differential diagnosis, and function of eosinophils.*

Sanderson CJ. Interleukin-5, eosinophils and disease. Blood 1992; 79:3101–3109.

*A review of IL-5, its receptors, and functional correlates of eosinophils and tissue responses.*

Weller PF. Eosinophilia in travelers. Med Clin North Amer: Trav Med 1992; 76:1413–1432.

*A useful guide to appreciating the differential diagnosis and work-up plans.*

# 95

# Infections after Animal Bites and Scratches

STEPHEN J. GLUCKMAN

There are an estimated two million animal bites and scratches in the United States each year, although only about half are reported. Most are trivial, but because of their frequency, they account for 1% of all emergency room visits, and 1% of those visits result in hospitalization. Of the two million bites annually, 70%–90% are dog bites, 3%–15% cat bites, and 4% rodent bites, both pet and wild. Wild animals comprise less than 1% of reported bites. Greater than one-third of U.S. households own at least one dog, and most bites are thus from domestic offenders. Children less than ten years of age are the most often injured. Fatalities from animal bites are extremely rare and in this country are almost exclusively due to the trauma resulting from a large dog's attack rather than infection.

## Microbiology

Though some bacteria are particularly associated with animal bites, most infections are polymicrobial, averaging two to three species per wound culture in careful studies. The organisms cultured from an infected bite generally reflect the oral flora of the biting animal, which include many aerobes and anaerobes. Bite wound infections are most commonly due to streptococcal species, staphylococcal species, and anaerobes, including bacteroides and fusobacteria. In addition, *Pasteurella multocida* is found in up to 25% of infections from dog bites and over 50% from cat bites. *Capnocytophaga canimorsus* (DF-2) is an uncommon but important potential pathogen particularly associated with dog bites. There have also been case reports of group IIj, actinomycosis, blastomycosis, and tuberculosis acquired via bites. Virtually all of the pathogens associated with animal bites have also been reported to cause infection due to animal scratches. Infections occur less frequently after a scratch, most likely due to the more superficial injury and smaller number of organisms inoculated.

Certain bacteria are associated with particular settings or animals (Table 95.1). *Francisella tularensis* should be considered after exposure to multiple sylvatic animals, most commonly rabbits, hares, or muskrats in the United States. In addition to those of domestic cats, other feline bites also present a risk of *P. multocida* infections. Bites or scratches associated with salt water should raise the concern of *Vibrio vulnificus* infection. The bites of rats and other rodents may result in rat bite fever, either from *Streptobacillus moniliformis* or *Spirillum minus*. Monkey bites raise the concern of *Herpesvirus simiae* infection. Finally, the possibility of tetanus and rabies must always be considered when evaluating an animal bite.

## Clinical Presentation

It is unusual for infections from animal bites to become clinically apparent earlier than 8 hours after a bite, and two-thirds appear within 8–24 hours. Most commonly there is a cellulitis with a malodorous discharge. Lymphadenitis and lymphangitis are rare. Local complications include septic arthritis, tenosynovitis, and osteomyelitis. Sepsis and meningitis can also follow animal bite infections, but are rare in normal hosts.

## Management of an Animal Bite

The management of an animal bite is outlined in Table 95.2. As with most clinical problems the management begins with a careful history. This should include: (*1*) the time since the bite; (*2*) the type of animal; (*3*) the circumstances of the bite—provoked or unprovoked; (*4*) comorbid conditions such as diabetes, peripheral vascular disease, prior splenectomy, or an immunocompromised state—all of which may predispose a patient to a more severe infection; (*5*) tetanus immunization history; and (*6*) drug allergies. Physical examination should include diagramming the extent of the injuries and inflammation with particular attention to blood vessel, nerve, tendon, and joint involvement and function. The jaws of large dogs can exert pressures of 200–450 lb/in$^2$, so tissue damage and hematomata can complicate the situation. Simple puncture wounds should not be dismissed. Cats have needlelike teeth that can puncture tendons, bones, and joints. A gram strain and culture should be done on purulent drainage from the bite wound. However, a gram stain and culture of a clinically uninfected wound is generally not useful in predicting the presence of microorganisms or the risk of subsequent infection and therefore should not be done. An X ray should be done if a fracture or a foreign body is suspected.

### Local wound care

The wound should be irrigated copiously with sterile saline. Puncture wounds may require the insertion of small catheters to accomplish this properly. Necrotic tissue should be debrided and foreign material removed. Infected bites should not be sutured. The suturing of an uninfected wound from an animal bite is controversial and must be considered on an individual basis. In general, wounds that are seen in less than 8 hours, are clearly not infected, and are well debrided and irrigated can be closed. Wounds that are more than 24 hours old or are already infected should be left open.

### Antibiotics

The role of prophylactic antibiotics is also controversial. The few randomized trials that have been conducted are small and none have shown benefit from prophylactic antibiotics. However, a meta-analysis of the eight double-blind, randomized trials re-

**Table 95.1** Pathogens and the treatment of common animal bites and scratches

| | Pathogen | Treatment |
|---|---|---|
| Dog | *Streptococci, staphylococci,* anaerobes, *Pasteurella multocida* | Amoxicillin-clavulanate or cefuroxime |
| | *Caprocytophaga canimorsus* | Penicillin |
| Cat | *P. multocida* | Penicillin |
| Rat | *Streptobacillus moniliformis, Sprillum minus* | Penicillin |
| Monkey | *Herpesvirus simiae* | Acyclovir |
| | Mixed aerobes & anaerobes | Amoxicillin/clavulanate |
| Water | *Vibrio vulnificus, V. alginolyticus* | Tetracycline |
| | *Aeromonas hydrophila* | Floroquinolone |
| | *Erysipelothrix rhusiopathiae* | Penicillin |
| | *Mycobacterium marinum* | Rifampin-ethambutol or clarithromycin |
| Rabbits, hares, muskrats, ticks | *Francisella tularensis* | Streptomycin or gentamicin |
| | C. perfringens | Amoxicillin/clavulanate |

ported in the literature suggested that prophylaxis can decrease the relative risk of infections from dog bite by 40%. Though this sounds clinically important, the general use of prophylaxis for dog bites remains unclear since the infection incidence in the control groups was 16%. This means that approximately 14 bitten persons would need to receive prophylaxis to prevent one infection. Therefore, the prophylactic use of antibiotics for dog bites must be weighed against the cost and potential side effects of such treatment. Puncture wounds, especially from cats, wounds greater than eight hours old, wounds resulting in extensive crush injury, wounds that may involve a bone or joint, wounds of the hands and face, and patients with comorbid conditions that increase the risk of a severe infection should probably be given a three- to five-day course of antimicrobial prophylaxes. Antibiotics should, of course, be prescribed for all infected wounds.

**Table 95.2** Management of an animal bite

1. Obtain a history
   Time since the bite
   Type of animal
   Circumstances of the bite—provoked or unprovoked?
   Comorbid conditions
   Tetanus immunization history
   Drug allergies
2. Physical examination
   Life-threatening complications
   Extent of tissue damage with particular attention to nerves, blood vessels, tendons, joints
   Extent of inflammation
3. Gram stain and culture of purulent material
4. Copious irrigation
5. Debridement
6. Consider suturing (see text)
7. Give antibiotics, if infected; consider antibiotics, if not (see text)
8. Consider X ray
9. Consider hospitalization
   Toxemic?
   Joint or tendon involvement?
   Comorbid condition?
   Not responding to outpatient regimen
   Unreliable patient
10. Elevate and immobilize, if infected
11. Evaluate the need for tetanus and rabies prophylaxis
12. Report to health department
13. Arrange follow-up
14. Document well

Infections following animal bites, whether domestic or wild, generally reflect the flora of the oral cavity of the animal. This usually means a mixture of aerobes and anaerobes. Unusual pathogens associated with specific animal bites or scratches are listed in Table 95.3. For dogs and cats this should include coverage for streptococci, *Staphylococcus aureus*, *Pasteurella multocida*, and anaerobes. Amoxicillin-clavulanate and cefuroxime each offer good coverage in these situations. Tetracyclines are an acceptable alternative for patients with beta-lactam allergies, though they may not be active against some streptococci and staphylococci. Penicillin and ampicillin alone do not cover most *S. aureus* strains, while first-generation cephalosporins, vancomycin, clindamycin, dicloxacillin, and oral erythromycin do not predictably provide coverage for *P. multocida* and must be used with caution, if at all, in this setting. In vitro information suggest that floroquinolones are active against *P. multocida*, but, there is little clinical experience with these drugs and, other than trovafloxacin, they do not offer anaerobic coverage. Trimethoprim-sulfamethoxazole is similarly active against *P. multocida*, but not anaerobes. Complete coverage in beta-lactam-allergic children and pregnant women requires combination therapy. Intravenous treatment could be provided by a number of single agents including ampicillin-sulbactam, ticarcillin-clavulanate, cefuroxime, or imipenem. In a patient with a beta-lactam allergy, combination therapy is necessary.

In an asplenic patient serious consideration must be given to possible sepsis with *Capnocytophaga canimorsus*. Fortunately, this organism is susceptible to most antibiotics, including penicillins, cephalosporins, erythromycin, and tetracycline.

Antibiotic prophylaxis after wild animal bites is unstudied, but probably should follow the guidelines suggested for domestic-animal bites. As with dog and cat bites, patients with severe injury, long intervals before medical attention, or immunosuppression, and those with bites on the face and hand, should receive prophylaxis.

### Need for hospitalization

Patients with infected animal bites can generally be treated as outpatients. Hospitalization should be considered when (*1*) the patient is toxemic; (*2*) there is definite or suspected tendon, joint, or bone involvement; (*3*) the patient has diabetes mellitus, asplenia, severe peripheral vascular disease, or is immunosuppressed; (*4*) the infection has not responded to outpatient therapy; or (*5*) there is an issue of patient competence or adherence.

### Duration of antibiotic therapy

The proper duration of therapy, as for most infections, has not been "proven" with controlled studies. Patients with cellulitis generally are treated for one to two weeks. Bone, tendon, and joint infections require longer courses, often two to four weeks.

### Elevation and physical therapy

Elevation of the infected area is an important component of therapy. This must be stressed to the patient, and appropriate devices should be used to insure maintainence of elevation. If the hand is involved, it is often splinted in a position of function until the infection resolves; aggressive physical therapy should then be used to rehabilitate the hand. Consultation with a hand surgeon is usually appropriate to guide these decisions.

**Table 95.3** Unusual pathogens associated with specific animal bites and scratches*

| Animal | Pathogen |
|---|---|
| Alligator | *Aeromonas hydrophila, Citrobacter diversus, Enterobacter agglomerans, Pseudomonas, Serratia* |
| Coyote | *Francisella tularensis* |
| Cougar | *Pasteurella multocida* |
| Gerbil | *Streptobacillus moniliformis* |
| Hamster | *Acinetobacter anitratus* |
| Lion | *Pasteurella multocida, Staphylococcus aureus, Escherichia coli* |
| Opossum | *Pasteurella multocida* |
| Panther | *Pasteurella multocida* |
| Piranha | *Aeromonas hydrophila* |
| Pig | *Francisella tularensis, Pasteurella multocida, Streptococcus agaliaciae, Streptococcus milleri, Streptococcus equisimilis, Proteus* spp. *Escherichia coli, Bacteroides* spp. |
| Polar bear | Agent of seal finger |
| Rat | *Streptobacillus moniliformis, Sprillum minus, Leptospira interrogans, Pasteurella multocida* |
| Rooster | *Streptococcus bovis, Clostridium tertium, Aspergillus niger* |
| Shark | Marine vibrios |
| Squirrel | *Francisella tularensis* |
| Tiger | *Pasteurella multocida, Acinetobacter, Escherichia coli,* streptococci, staphylococci |
| Wolf | *Pasteurella multocida* |

*From Weber and Hansen.

### Tetanus and rabies prevention

Tetanus immunization should be updated if necessary, and the need for rabies prophylaxis should be considered. This will depend on the prevalence of rabies in the area, the animal involved, and the nature of the attack (see Chapter 48). Consultation with the local health department is often necessary.

If the bite wound is not infected, the patient should be taught the signs of infection and told to follow up immediately should any appear. Finally, if required, the bite should be reported to the health department.

## Specific Important Pathogens

### Pasteurella multocida

*Pasteurella multocida* is a coccobacillary gram-negative rod that is a prominent part of the oral flora of many animals. It can be found in 70%–90% of cats, 50%–60% of dogs, 50% of pigs, 15% of rats, and in many other animals. When it causes bite wound infections, the syndrome is typically one of rapid onset, generally within 24 hours of the injury. Intense pain and swelling are present in all, and a purulent drainage is present, in 40% of bites infected with this organism. Lymphangitis and adenitis are uncommon, occurring in 20% and 10%, respectively. Septic arthritis, tenosynovitis, and osteomyelitis are potential complications, resulting from direct inoculation at the time of the bite or by local extension. Cat bites are particularly at risk for these sequelae because of the potential for a deep puncture. The diagnosis can be suspected by the clinical setting and confirmed by culture of the wound drainage. It is important to remember that this organism is not effectively treated with oral erythromycin, first-generation cephalosporins, vancomycin, clindamycin, semisynthetic penicillins, or aminoglycosides, but is susceptible to penicillin, ampicillin, tetracycline, and second- or third-generation cephalosporins.

### *Capnocytophaga canimorsus* (DF-2)

*C. canimorsus*, an oxidase-positive, slow-growing, gram-negative rod, is an uncommon cause of infection after animal bites. However, it produces a characteristic and potentially devastating syndrome and must be recognized early. Most patients report an antecedent dog bite (50%) or dog exposure (20%). Less commonly cat and other animal bites have been implicated. Most of the reported infections have been in patients with a predisposing condition, particularly prior splenectomy. Other reported associations have been with Hodgkin's disease, alcoholism, and steroid therapy.

Infection with this organism typically results in sepsis and has a case fatality rate of 25%. When a patient presents with a sepsis syndrome after an animal bite, especially if the patient has had a splenectomy and there is evidence of disseminated intravascular coagulation, this diagnosis should be considered. A gram stain of the buffy coat may reveal the organism. Because *C. canimorsus* is fastidious, antibiotic susceptibilities have been difficult to determine with certainty. Penicillin is considered to be the drug of choice.

It has also been shown to be susceptible to cephalosporins, clindamycin, erythromycin, tetracycline, and floroquinolones.

### *Bartonella henselae*

Infection with *B. henselae* is associated with the scratch or bite of a cat. There are several different clinical syndromes that can result. The most common is cat scratch disease, a common cause of chronic, benign adenopathy in children and young adults (see Chapter 53). It is characterized by localized lymphadenopathy, which is usually preceded by an erythematous papule or pustule at the site of a cat, often a kitten, scratch. Fever and other systemic symptoms occur in one-third of patients. The adenopathy can vary from mildly tender to intensely inflamed with spontaneous purulent drainage. In immunocompetent patients 2% develop complications involving the central nervous system, liver, spleen, lung, bone, and skin. The diagnosis can be suspected by the characteristic histology of the lymph node, including stellate caseating granulomas, microabscesses, and follicular hyperplasia. It can be confirmed by identifying the organism with a Warthin-Starry stain of the lymph node. Recently developed serological tests and cultures are also available. The disease usually resolves spontaneously over weeks to several months. There is no established therapy for this syndrome, though ciprofloxacin has been reported to have some efficacy.

Infection with *B. henselae* in immunosuppressed hosts, primarily those with HIV infection, may result in several other syndromes, including cutaneous bacillary angiomatosis, fever with bacteremia, and bacillary peliosis hepatis (Chapter 100).

*B. henselae* can be isolated from blood cultures. Lysis-centrifugation is the most efficient method. It can also be grown by directly plating tissue. Bacillary peliosis hepatis should be suspected in an HIV-positive patient with an elevated alkaline phosphatase and hypodense ringlike lesions in the liver on CT scan. It can only be confirmed by biopsy.

Unlike cat scratch disease, treatment for bacillary angiomatosis, fever with bacteremia, and bacillary peliosis hepatis with either erythromycin or tetracycline is effective.

The demographics of dog and cat bites are somewhat different. Dogs typically bite the lower extremities and hands. Most dogs involved in bites are pets, and the bite occurs as the result of some interaction with the animal such as feeding or playing. These bites can result in tissue tears, avulsions, punctures, and superficial abrasions. Male German shepherds are far and away the most frequent offenders. Cats typically bite women in the 20–35 age range. The animals are most commonly stray females. The bites are usually punctures or abrasions, so there is often less tissue damage than with a dog bite, though the punctures are often difficult to clean adequately and more commonly enter joints or bone.

The risk of infection after a dog bite is reported to be between 2% and 29%, though most series put the risk in the 10%–15% range. The risk after a cat bite is higher; about 50% become infected. This risk is increased by puncture wounds, age greater than 50, and delay in treatment.

## Specific Infections after Other Animal Bites

### Rat bite fever

Infection following the bite of a rat can result in the syndrome of rat bite fever due to either *Streptobacillus moniliformis* in the United States or *Spirillum minor* in Asia. The former is a fastidious, microaerophilic, gram-negative rod that after an incubation period of less that one week produces a disease characterized by fever, rigors, myalgias, headache, and a diffuse morbilliform rash that often involves the palms and soles. In addition, polyarticular arthritis and/or arthralgias are very common. The bite site usually heals without signs of local inflammation. Infection with *S. minor* produces a disease called sodoku. The incubation period is typically longer at two to four weeks. Again chills and fever are present, however the bite site, after initially healing, develops a necrotic lesion that results in an eschar with lymphangitis. A blotchy macular rash often develops. Arthralgias and arthritis are infrequent. Both the bacillary and the spirillary forms of rat bite fever can resolve spontaneously and then relapse multiple times over the subsequent months. The organisms associated with both types of rat bite fever are sensitive to penicillin and tetracyclines.

### Water-associated infections

There are a number of organisms that may cause infection associated with water contact. When a person is bitten or scratched in the water, infections with these organisms should be considered. *Vibrio vulnificus* and *V. alginolyticus* cause a rapidly progressing cellulitis characterized by severe toxemia, hemorrhagic bullae, and extensive tissue necrosis. Treatment requires rapid extensive surgical debridement and, occasionally, amputation. Tetracyclines are generally considered the drugs of choice, though third-generation cephalosporins or chloramphenicol are also effective. *Aeromonas hydrophila* can cause a similar syndrome after water exposure. Floroquinolones, third-generation cephalosporins, or trimethoprim-sulfamethoxazole can be used for this organism. *Erysipelothrix rhusiopathiae* primarily produces an indolent, nonpyogenic, nodular cellulitis and, occasionally, disseminated disease and endocarditis. This organism is sensitive to penicillins and cephalosporins but resistant to vancomycin. *Mycobacterium marinum* can also produce infection after injury associated with the water, generally resulting in chronic nodular skin lesions. Rifampin and ethambutol are considered the standard therapy today, though the new macrolides will probably have an important role in treating infection with bacterium.

### Seal finger

Seal finger is a distinctive infection associated with a seal bite or other injury involving seals. Typically, after an incubation period of four to seven days a furuncle develops at the site of the injury. This is associated with extreme pain and swelling without lymphangitis or fever. Though the cause of this syndrome is unknown, it responds to tetracycline. Penicillin and erythromycin are ineffective.

### Infections from monkey bites

Infection with *Herpesvirus simiae* (*herpes B virus*) may result after the bite of an infected old world monkey. The disease is characterized by herpetiform vesicles or ulcerations at the site of the bite and an ascending myelitis leading to encephalitis that is fatal if untreated. Experimental infection, tissue culture data, and anecdotal case reports in humans all support the use of acyclovir for the treatment of this infection. The role of acyclovir for post-exposure prophylaxis is uncertain because its efficacy is unproven, and, though many cynomolgus monkeys carry the virus, transmission to humans after a bite is very uncommon.

Simian bites may also be the source of serious bacterial infections. Management should be similar to that of human bites. Wounds should be thoroughly cleaned and debrided. Antibiotics should be considered and should cover streptoccoci, staphylococci, enterococci, *Eikenella corrodens*, enterobacteriaceae, and anaerobes.

## Infections from snakebites

Although snake venom is sterile, the bacterial flora in the mouth of snakes reflects the fecal content of their prey. These organisms, which include *Clostridium perfringens*, *Bacteroides fragilis*, and enteric organisms including salmonella, can cause infection after a snakebite. Though it has been strongly discouraged, the practice of using the mouth to attempt to suck out venom after a bite adds the infection risk of human oral flora. Routine antibacterial prophylaxis is advised for all snake bites, generally with amoxicillin-clavulanate or cefuroxime.

### ANNOTATED BIBLIOGRAPHY

Adal KA, Cockerell CJ, Petri WA Jr, Cat scratch disease, bacillary angiomatosi, and other infections due to *Rochalimaea*. N Engl J Med 1994; 330:1509–1515.

*Review of the taxonomy, epidemiology, and clinical presentations of this organism.*

Cummings P. Antibiotics to prevent infection in patients with dog bite wounds: a meta-analysis of randomized trials. Ann Emerg Med 1994; 23:535–540.

*Eight trials were identified and analyzed by meta-analysis. The relative risk for infection in patients given antibiotics compared with controls was 0.56 (0.38–0.82). About 14 patients must be treated to prevent one infection. An editorial by Michael Callaham addressed this article in the same issue.*

Davenport DS, Johnson DR, Holmes GP, et al. Diagnosis and management of herpes B virus (*Herpesvirus simiae*) infections in Michigan. Clin Infect Dis 1994; 19:33–41.

*Clinical presentations, diagnostic options, and treatment.*

Goldstein EJC. Bite wounds and infection. Clin Infect Dis 1992; 14:633–640.

*Microbiology and management of dog, cat, and human bites. Short state-of-the-art paper covering primarily dog and cat bites and their management.*

Goldstein EJ, Pryor EP III, Citron DM. Simian bites and bacterial infection. Clin Infect Dis 1995; 20:1551–1552.

Janda DH, Verghese A, Alvarez S. Dysgonic fermenter-2 septicemia. Rev Infect Dis 1987; 9:884–890.

*Case report with review of the literature of the pathophysiology, clinical presentation, and management of this organism, now known as C. canimorsus*

Holley HP. Successful treatment of cat-scratch disease with ciprofloxacin. JAMA 1991; 265:1563–1565.

*Report of five patients with cat scratch disease who appeared to respond to treatment with oral ciprofloxacin 500 mg BID.*

Holmes GP, Chapman LE, Steward JA, Straus SE, Hilliard JK, Davenport DS, et al. Guidelines for the prevention and treatment of B-virus infections in exposed persons. Clin Infect Dis 1995; 20:421–439.

*Comprehensive summary of a CDC sponsored conference on the topic.*

Holroyd KJ, Reiner AP, Dick JD. *Streptobacillus moniliformis* polyarthritis mimicking rheumatoid arthritis: an urban case of rat bite fever. Am J Med 1988; 85:711–714.

*Comments in this article are a good clinical and microbiological review of streptobacillary rat bite fever.*

Klontz KC, Lieb S, Schreiber M, et al. Syndromes of *Vibrio vulnificus* infections. Ann Intern Med 1988; 109:318–323.

*Clinical and epidemiological review of 62 patients covering the three clinical syndromes associated with infection with this organism.*

Markham RB, Polk BF. Seal finger. Rev Infect Dis 1979; 1:567–569. Case report and discussion of the clinical features, pathology, and management of this entity.

McDonough JJ, Stern PJ, Alexander JW. Management of animal and human bites and resulting human infections. In: Current Clinical Topics in Infectious Diseases, vol 8. Remington JS, Swartz MN, eds. McGraw-Hill, New York, pp 11–36, 1987.

*General review of the topic with some attention to the surgical options.*

Ordog GJ. The bacteriology of dog bite wounds on initial presentations. Ann Emerg Med 1986; 15:1324–1329.

*A prospective study of the microbiology of over 400 dog bite wounds seen in a large urban emergency room.*

Weber DJ, Wolfson JS, Swartz MN. *Pasteurella multocida* infections. Medicine 1984; 63:133–154.

*Report of 34 cases from the Massachusetts General Hospital with a review of the literature.*

Weber DJ, Hansen AR. Infections resulting from animal bites. Infect Dis Clin North Am 1991; 5:663–680.

*Comprehensive review of epidemiology, evaluation, management, and prevention of animal bites.*

# 96

## Ectoparasite-Related Diseases

DAVID H. SPACH AND KAREN M. VAN DE VELDE

The term *ectoparasite* refers to an organism that infests the skin of another animal. These organisms derive sustenance from the host they infest, including those ectoparasites that take a brief blood meal and those that burrow into the skin and remain there for prolonged periods. Arthropods and helminths are the major organisms that act as ectoparasites. The major classes of arthropods associated with human ectoparasitic diseases include arachnids (ticks, mites, and spiders) and insects (lice, chiggers, and flies) (Table 96.1). The key distinguishing feature between these two classes of arthropods is that adult insects have six legs and adult arachnids have eight. Arthropods can cause human disease in one of three ways: by directly infesting the skin; by injecting antigenic secretions into the skin; and by transmitting infectious microorganisms to the host. This chapter will focus on selected important arthropod-related ectoparasitic diseases.

### Tick-Borne Diseases

Ticks are eight-legged blood-sucking arachnids that serve as the critical vector for an array of infectious organisms (Table 96.2). In addition, ticks can, on rare occasion, cause human disease by transmitting a neurotoxin to the host. Depending on the structure of their dorsal shield, ticks are classified as either hard ticks (family *Ixodidae*) or soft ticks (family *Argasidae*). Three major genera of hard ticks commonly transmit infectious pathogens to humans: *Ixodes* (deer and western black-legged ticks), *Dermacentor* (dog and wood ticks), and *Amblyomma* (lone star tick). Among the soft ticks, only the *Ornithodoros* ticks are known to cause human disease. These various hard and soft ticks inhabit predictable geographic regions that correspond with highly endemic regions for tick-borne diseases.

Individuals who venture into outdoor areas where tick-borne diseases occur—especially in highly endemic regions—should take precautions to minimize their risk of acquiring such a disease. In order to diminish the risk for tick attachment, one should cover as much of the body as comfortably possible with clothing, avoid walking through brushy vegetation (except on a path), and wear a tick repellant. If a tick is found attached to the body, it should be removed with tweezers by grasping the tick as close to the skin as possible and pulling in a perpendicular direction (straight out) with slow, steady pressure.

### Lyme disease

Lyme disease, also known as Lyme borreliosis, has emerged as the most common vector-borne disease in the United States, with an average of more than 8000 cases per year (in recent years). In Europe, Lyme borreliosis is the most common tick-borne disease. Although the true worldwide incidence remains unknown, scattered reports suggest a very broad geographic distribution that includes North America, Europe, Scandinavia, the former Soviet Union, China, Japan, Australia, and North Africa. The causative agent for this disease is *Borrelia burgdorferi*, a spirochete transmitted by *Ixodes* ticks. Recently, investigators have discovered several distinct subspecies of *B. burgdorferi* that occur in different regions of the world. These include *B. garinii* (Europe), *B. afzelli* (Europe), V5116 (Switzerland, United Kingdom), PotiB2 (Portugal), and *B. japonica* (Japan).

Although Lyme disease can occur in almost all regions of the United States, most cases are reported from the northeast, the upper Midwest, or northern California. In Europe, Lyme borreliosis has been reported from 19 countries. Patients from either North America or Europe typically develop the onset of disease during the summer months. Analogous to the stages described with syphilis, Lyme disease is often described as developing in three different stages: stage 1 (early-localized), onset days to weeks after infection; stage 2 (early-disseminated), onset days to months after infection; and stage 3 (late), onset months to years after infection. In clinical practice, however, individual presentations vary and patients usually do not sequentially pass through each of these three stages. With North American Lyme disease, approximately 70% of patients develop an erythematous, expanding skin rash known as erythema migrans (Plate 45), typically 7 to 10 days after the tick bite. Less than 50% of patients actually recall the tick bite. Patients from Europe generally have a decreased incidence of arthritis, but an increased incidence of neurologic symptoms (meningoencephalitis) and chronic cutaneous lesions (acrodermatitis chronica atrophicans). Multiple other clinical manifestations can develop, as highlighted in Table 96.3.

Because of problems with the laboratory diagnosis of Lyme disease, the diagnosis should predominantly be based on the combination of clinical findings and a history of a probable tick exposure, with the laboratory tests regarded as providing supplemental information. Although serologic testing suffers from lack of standardization, interlaboratory variability, and frequent false-positive results, it remains the most practical and widespread laboratory test used to assist in the diagnosis of Lyme disease. The enzyme-linked immunosorbent assay (ELISA) is usually ordered as the initial test, with subsequent Western immunoblotting used to clarify borderline-positive ELISA results. Unfortunately, most patients do not develop significant antibody titers until at least six weeks after their initial infection. With stage 3 Lyme disease, nearly all patients have positive serologies. Future advances in laboratory testing for Lyme disease will likely include improved standardization of serologic tests, antigen-based testing, and polymerase chain reaction (PCR) to detect *B. burgdorferi* genetic material. The treatment of Lyme disease depends on the stage of the disease and the severity of

**Table 96.1** Classification of selected ectoparasitic-related diseases

| Arthropod class | Family | Genus | Species |
|---|---|---|---|
| ARACHNIDS | | | |
| Ticks | Ixodidae (hard ticks) | Dermacentor | *D. variabilis* |
| | | | *D. andersoni* |
| | | Ixodes | *I. scapularis* |
| | | | *I. pacificus* |
| | | | *I. ricinus* |
| | | | *I. persulcatus* |
| | | Amblyomma | *A. americanum* |
| | Argasidae (soft ticks) | Ornithodorus | *Ornithodorus* spp. |
| Mites | Sarcoptidae | Sarcoptes | *Sarcoptes scabiei* |
| | Trombiculidae | Eutrombicula | *E. alfreddugesi* |
| INSECTS | | | |
| Lice | Pediculidae | Pediculus | *P. humanis* var. *capitus* |
| | | | *P. humanis* var. *corporis* |
| | | Ptheris | *Phthirus pubis* |
| Flies | Cuterebridae | Dermatobia | *D. hominis* |
| | | Cuterebra | *Cuterebra* spp. |
| | Calliphoridae | Cordylobia | *C. anthropophaga* |

the manifestations (Table 96.4). Early Lyme disease is generally treated with a two- to three-week course of oral antimicrobials (doxycycline or amoxicillin), whereas late Lyme disease usually requires a two- to three-week course of intravenous drugs (ceftriaxone or penicillin).

## Relapsing fever

Tick-borne relapsing fever is caused by infection with one of more than 15 species of *Borrelia*, including *B. hermsii*, *B. turicatae*, and *B. parkerii*. These spirochetes, which are distinct from the borrelia spirochete that causes Lyme disease, can change their surface antigens to evade host immune responses. Humans acquire relapsing fever via bites of infected *Ornithodoros* ticks, a type of soft tick that inhabits remote forested, mountainous regions at elevations generally above 3000 feet. Cases of relapsing fever have been reported worldwide. Many patients describe a visit to a rustic lodge, mountain cabin, shelter, or cave, typically about one week prior to the onset of their illness. Because the *Ornithodoros* ticks typically feed for less than 20 minutes, most patients do not recall a tick bite, although some may notice a small eschar at the inoculation site. Most individuals who develop relapsing fever have abrupt onset of symptoms, namely fever, chills, malaise, headache, myalgias, arthralgias, and abdominal pain. At the initial presentation, laboratory studies usually show leukocytosis and thrombocytopenia. Without treatment, patients typically have resolution of the primary febrile episode after three to six days, followed by an afebrile period for approximately one week. This cycle can repeat and three to five of these relapsing episodes will occur if the patient does not receive appropriate therapy.

To make a rapid and reliable diagnosis of relapsing fever, one should examine a Wright- or Giemsa-stained peripheral blood smear for the presence of spirochetes (Fig. 96.1). Serologic tests are primarily used to confirm smear-negative cases. Although treatment data remain limited, most authorities recommend a 7- to 10-day course of tetracycline or doxycycline, with erythromycin generally recommended for the treatment of young chil-

**Table 96.2** Major tick-borne diseases in the United States*

| Disease | Causative agent | Classification | Major vector(s)[a] | Endemic regions |
|---|---|---|---|---|
| Lyme disease | *Borrelia burgdorferi* | Bacteria (spirochete) | *Ixodes* spp. | Northeast, Wisconsin, Minnesota, California |
| Relapsing fever | *Borrelia* spp. | Bacteria (spirochete) | *Ornithodorus* spp. | West |
| Tularemia | *Francisella tularensis* | Bacteria | *Dermacentor* spp., *Amblyomma* spp. | Arkansas, Missouri, Oklahoma |
| RMSF | *Ricketsia rickettsii* | Rickettsia | *Dermacentor* spp. | Southeast, West South-central |
| Ehrlichiosis | *Ehrlichia chaffeensis* | Rickettsia | ?*Dermacentor* spp., ?*Amblyomma* spp. | South-central, South Atlantic |
| | *Ehrlichia* spp. | Rickettsia | ?*Ixodes* spp. | Upper midwest |
| Colorado tick fever | *Coltivirus* spp. | Virus | *Dermacentor* spp. | West |
| Babesiosis | *Babesia* spp. | Protozoa | *Ixodes* spp. | Northeast |
| Tick paralysis | Toxin | Neurotoxin | *Dermacentor* spp., *Amblyomma* spp. | Northwest, South |

*This table is reproduced and modified with permission from Spach DH et al. (p. 937).

a. The genera of the tick vectors are listed in this table; the individual species of ticks are described in the text.

dren or pregnant women (Table 96.4). Shortly after administering the first treatment dose, approximately 20%–30% of patients will develop a Jarisch-Herxheimer reaction characterized by chills, fever, tachycardia, and hypotension. Among all patients treated for relapsing fever, fatalities rarely occur.

## Rocky Mountain spotted fever

The causative organism for Rocky Mountain spotted fever (RMSF) is *Rickettsia rickettsii*, a small, pleomorphic, obligate intracellular pathogen. Humans acquire this disease via bites of *Dermacentor* ticks, most commonly in rural or suburban environments during late-spring and summer months. Manifestations of RMSF typically begin 5 to 7 days (range: 2 to 14 days) after the tick bite, most often with symptoms that include fever, malaise, severe frontal headache, and myalgias. In most patients, the classic RMSF rash appears 4 to 10 days into the illness and initially develops as macular lesions on the wrists and ankles that subsequently spread to involve the trunk, face, palms, and soles. Because *R. rickettsii* may infect vascular endothelial cells and induce a widespread vasculitis, patients can develop life-threatening cardiac, pulmonary, or central nervous system manifestations. The classic triad of RMSF, which consists of fever, rash, and history of tick exposure, is present in only 60%–70% of patients when they first seek medical care; approximately 10% of patients never develop a rash.

Common laboratory abnormalities include thrombocytopenia, hyponatremia, and elevated serum hepatic transaminases. In addition, patients may have a normal or decreased white blood cell count with a high proportion of bands. Because antibodies against *R. rickettsii* are not usually detectable until 7 to 10 days after the onset of illness, the initial diagnosis of RMSF is made on a clinical basis; medical providers must promptly initiate appropriate antimicrobial therapy in suspected cases. For adults, the recommended treatment is either tetracycline or doxycyline for 5 to 7 days (Table 96.4). For the treatment of children less than eight years of age, chloramphenicol is generally used and is considered an effective alternative agent. Antimicrobial therapy has reduced the mortality associated with RMSF from 25% to 5%.

## Ehrlichiosis

*Ehrlichia chaffeensis*, the causative agent of most cases of ehrlichiosis in the United States, is a small, *Rickettsia*-like coccobacillus. A distinct *ehrlichia* species, *E. sennetsu*, was previously isolated in 1953 from a patient in Japan who presented with a mononucleosis-like illness. Recently, investigators have identified a third ehrlichia species, which causes a clinical illness, termed human granulocytic ehrlichiosis; this illness appears to be similar to the illness caused by *E. chaffeensis*. The vector(s) for ehrlichiosis remains unconfirmed, but hard ticks have been implicated in almost every case. In the United States, cases caused by *E. chaffeensis* have predominantly occurred in the south-central and southern Atlantic states, particularly Oklahoma, Missouri, and Georgia. Several reports from Europe (Portugal and Spain) and Africa (Mali) have described patients with serologic evidence of *E. chaffeensis* infection and a compatible clinical illness. Cases of *E. sennetsu* have been described only in Asia. Patients with human granulocytic ehrlichiosis have been reported predominantly from the Northeast and upper Midwest of the United States.

More than 60% of patients with ehrlichiosis recall a tick bite. Ehrlichiosis typically occurs during the summer months; patients usually present 10 to 14 days after a tick bite with a nonspecific febrile illness that resembles RMSF or influenza. A maculopapular or petechial rash ultimately develops in about one-third of patients. This rash most commonly involves the trunk, legs, or arms, but, distinct from RMSF, it rarely involves the palms

**Table 96.3** Major manifestations of Lyme disease*

| System | Early | | Late |
|---|---|---|---|
| | Stage 1 localized | Stage 2 disseminated | Stage 3 chronic |
| Skin | Erythema migrans | Secondary annular lesions | Acrodermatitis chronica atrophicans |
| Musculoskeletal | Myalgias | Migratory pain in joints, bone, muscle; brief arthritis attacks | Prolonged arthritis attacks, chronic arthritis |
| Neurologic | Headache | Meningitis, Bell's palsy, cranial neuritis, radiculoneuritis | Encephalopathy, polyneuropathy, leukoencephalitis |
| Cardiac | | Atrioventricular block, myopericarditis, pancarditis | |
| Constitutional | Flulike symptoms | Malaise, fatigue | Fatigue |
| Lymphatic | Regional lymphadenopathy | Regional or generalized lymphadenopathy | |

*Adapted and reproduced with permission from Steere AC (p. 589).

and soles. Severe complications of the infection include disseminated intravascular coagulation, acute renal failure, cardiomegaly, encephalopathy, and a toxic-shock-like syndrome.

During the first several days of the patient's illness, laboratory studies generally remain normal, except for elevated serum hepatic transaminases. Subsequently, patients usually develop transient leukopenia, anemia, and thrombocytopenia. Several reports have demonstrated ehrlichial inclusion bodies (morulae) within leukocytes on standard Wright's stain of a peripheral blood smear; these inclusion bodies appear as 1–3 $\mu$m clusters of blue coccobacillary organisms. Patients with *E. chaffeensis* predominantly have involvement of monocytic cells, whereas patients with human granulocytic ehrlichiosis, as the name implies, have inclusions within granulocytes. If the diagnosis of ehrlichiosis is suspected, appropriate antimicrobial therapy should be initiated. For practical purposes, it is not necessary to immediately distinguish ehrlichiosis from RMSF since the treatment is the same. The diagnosis of *E. chaffeensis* infection is confirmed by using an indirect immunofluorescent antibody (IFA) assay that detects antibodies against this organism, with a positive test considered as a fourfold (or greater) rise (or fall) in antibody titer along with a minimum titer of 1:64. Recently developed tests using PCR appear promising. For diagnosing cases of human granulocytic ehrlichiosis, an IFA titer greater than or equal to 1:80 is considered a positive test. Retrospective data suggest that tetracycline (or doxycycline) is the drug of choice for either type of ehrlichial infection, with chloramphenicol viewed as a less effective alternative (Table 96.4). With appropriate antimicrobial therapy, less than 2% of patients die.

## Tularemia

*Francisella tularensis*, a small, gram-negative coccobacillus that causes tularemia, can be transmitted by multiple vectors, including rabbits, hares, and hard ticks. In the United States, approximately 50% of the reported tularemia cases result from tick transmission. Tularemia has been reported to occur in Canada, the Middle East, Europe, the former Soviet Union, and Japan. Tick-borne tularemia typically occurs during the summer and fall months, with most patients having the sudden onset of nonspecific symptoms following an incubation period of three to five days. Most commonly, patients subsequently develop either ulceroglandular disease (presence of an ulcer at the site of the tick bite associated with painful regional adenopathy), or glandular disease (presence of regional adenopathy without an ulcerative skin lesion). On rare occasions patients develop typhoidal disease—a systemic illness characterized by fever, headache, chills, and abdominal pain.

Routine laboratory studies are not helpful in making the diagnosis of tularemia, and serologic studies, although accurate,

**Table 96.4** Therapy for adults with tick-borne diseases*

| Disease | Therapy | Route | Dose | Duration |
|---|---|---|---|---|
| Lyme disease | | | | |
| Early (erythema migrans) | 1. Doxycycline[a] | PO | 100 mg BID | 14–21d |
| | 2. Amoxicillin | PO | 500 mg TID | 14–21d |
| | 3. Cefuroxime axetil | PO | 500 mg BID | 14–21d |
| | 4. Azithromycin | PO | 500 mg d1, 250 mg QD | 5d (total) |
| Arthritis | 1. Doxycycline[a] | PO | 100 mg BID | 30d |
| | 2. Amoxicillin | PO | 500 mg TID | 30d |
| | 3. Ceftriaxone | IV | 2g QD | 14–21d |
| Cardiac | | | | |
| Mild (AV block with PR ≤ 0.3s) | Doxycycline[a] | PO | 100 mg BID | 21d |
| Serious | Ceftriaxone | IV | 2g QD | 21d |
| Neurologic | | | | |
| Mild (facial palsy) | 1. Doxycycline[a] | PO | 100 mg BID | 30d |
| | 2. Amoxicillin | PO | 500 mg TID | 30d |
| Serious | Ceftriaxone | IV | 2g IV QD | 14–21d |
| Relapsing fever | 1. Doxycycline[a] | PO or IV | 100 mg BID | 7–10d |
| | 2. Erythromycin | PO or IV | 500 mg QID | 7–10d |
| Rocky Mountain spotted fever | 1. Doxycycline[a] | PO or IV | 100 mg BID | 7–10d |
| | 2. Chloramphenicol | PO or IV | 15 mg/kg Q6h | 7–10d |
| Ehrlichiosis | 1. Doxycycline[a] | PO or IV | 100 mg BID | 7–10d |
| | 2. Chloramphenicol | PO or IV | 15 mg/kg Q6h | 7–10d |
| Tularemia | 1. Streptomycin | IM | 1 gm Q12h | 10–14d |
| | 2. Gentamicin | IV | 1.5 mg/kg Q8h | 10–14d |
| Babesiosis | Clindamycin | PO or IV | 600 mg TID | 7–10d |
| | plus | | | |
| | quinine | PO | 650 mg TID | 7–10d |
| Colorado tick fever | Supportive | NA | NA | NA |
| Tick paralysis | Tick removal | NA | NA | NA |

*This table is reproduced with permission from: Spach DH, Liles WC. (p 34).

a. Tetracycline (500 mg QID) can be substituted for doxycycline. In most instances neither doxycycline nor tetracycline should be given to pregnant women, lactating women, or children 8 years old or younger. In life-threatening cases of tick-borne diseases, however, administering doxycycline (or tetracycline) would be reasonable.

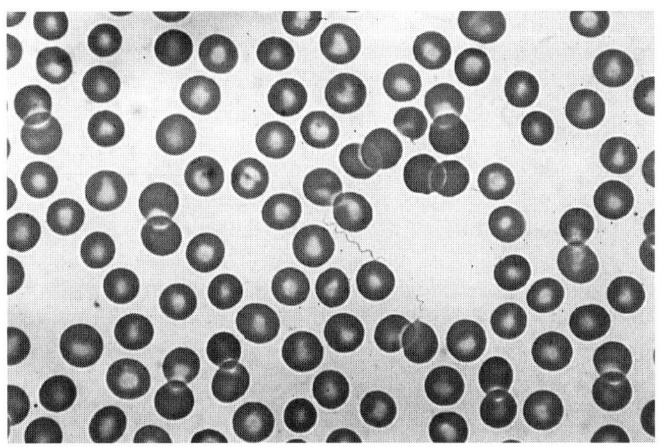

**Fig. 96.1** Wright stain of peripheral blood smear showing *Borrelia spirochete*. [Reproduced with permission from Spach et al.]

usually require obtaining acute and convalescent specimens four to six weeks apart. Thus, the immediate diagnosis should be based on clinical grounds, with treatment initiated empirically for patients with suspected tularemia. A fourfold rise in antitularemia antibody titer between acute and convalescent specimens is diagnostic, with an isolated titer ≥1:160 highly suggestive of active infection. The treatment of choice for all forms of tularemia remains streptomycin, given for 10 to 14 days (Table 96.4). Gentamicin and tetracycline are considered reasonable alternative agents, but have lower rates of cure. With appropriate antimicrobial therapy, the mortality associated with tularemia is approximately 1%–3%.

## Babesiosis

The most common species of *Babesia* to infect humans in the United States is *B. microti*, a protozoan parasite that is transmitted by the same *Ixodes* ticks that transmit *B. burgdorferi*. Similar to Lyme disease, patients usually acquire this infection during summer months, most frequently in the northeastern United States. Although most cases of babesiosis in Europe have involved splenectomized patients, reports in the United States have primarily described patients with intact spleens who were older or chronically ill. The true frequency with which babesiosis occurs remains unknown but is probably far underestimated; several seroprevalence studies have documented that infections with *B. microti* are often asymptomatic. Among those patients who develop a clinically apparent illness, symptoms typically begin approximately one week after a tick bite, with some patients having a mild to moderate self-limited illness, whereas others develop a more serious, potentially fatal course. Patients most often describe the initial symptoms as gradual and nonspecific. In the more serious cases, patients develop more pronounced symptoms, such as drenching sweats, myalgia, and headache. The serious sequelae of this disease result from the organism's ability to infect and hemolyze erythrocytes; specifically, patients may develop anemia, thrombocytopenia, hemoglobinuria, renal failure, and hypotension.

To rapidly diagnose babesiosis, one should examine a Giemsa-stained thick or thin peripheral blood smear. Because *Babesia* organisms appear as small ring forms present within erythrocytes, patients are often initially misdiagnosed as having malaria. Observation of a classic tetrad ("Maltese cross") configuration strongly supports the diagnosis of babesiosis. The diagnosis can be confirmed using an IFA serologic test, with a titer of ≥1:64 considered positive. Although treatment data remain limited, most authorities recommend quinine plus clindamycin for seven days (Table 96.4).

## Colorado tick fever

The causative agent of Colorado tick fever (CTF), an RNA virus of the genus *Coltivirus*, is transmitted to humans predominantly by *Dermacentor* ticks. Most cases in the United States occur in mountainous regions of the western states during the late spring or early summer. This infection causes a biphasic illness in approximately 50% of patients. The primary phase persists for approximately seven days and is characterized by the abrupt onset of fever, chills, headache, photophobia, and myalgias. Several days after the symptoms associated with the primary phase abate, patients may experience a secondary phase of illness that resembles the primary phase, except that it persists for only two to four days.

The most common laboratory abnormalities include leukopenia and thrombocytopenia. A presumptive clinical diagnosis of CTF is difficut, mainly because of the nonspecific nature of the illness. Most often, providers diagnose this disease retrospectively, using serologic studies. The mainstay of therapy consists of supportive care. Despite the lack of specific therapy for CTF, most patients have good outcomes. In some instances, however, patients have a prolonged convalesence.

## Tick paralysis

Tick paralysis results from transmission of a neurotoxin produced in the tick's salivary glands. Multiple species of ticks can produce this neurotoxin and transmit it to humans. In the United States, most reports of tick paralysis have come from the Pacific Northwest and the Rocky Mountain states, with cases predominantly occurring in spring and summer months. The typical presentation involves a patient who develops symmetrical lower extremity weakness two to seven days after tick attachment; if the tick is not removed, the patient rapidly develops an ascending flaccid paralysis. Despite the profound involvement of

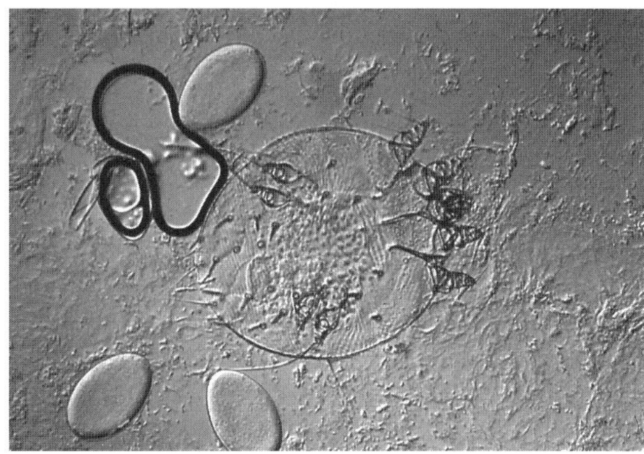

**Fig. 96.2** Adult scabies mite with 3 eggs visible in field (dark black circle represents air bubble). [Reproduced with permission from Spach DH, Fritsche TR, Norwegian scabies in a patient with AIDS. N Engl J Med 1994; 331:777.]

neurologic motor function, the sensory and mental status examinations are generally normal. An immediate diagnosis can be made by finding an embedded tick on the patient, most frequently on the scalp. Treatment consists of carefully removing the embedded tick. Following tick removal, most patients have resolution of their neurologic symptoms within hours to days.

## Diseases Caused by Mites

### Scabies

The causative agent of human scabies, *Sarcoptes scabiei*, is a 0.4 mm–long, round-bodied, eight-legged mite (Fig. 96.2). Most of the clinical symptoms associated with scabies result from infestation with the adult female. Following mating with the smaller adult male, the female burrows into the epidermis and lays two to three eggs daily until she dies approximately one month later; the male dies shortly after mating. The eggs hatch in three to four days, releasing larvae that emerge to the skin surface. The larvae then pass through a nymphal stage, mature into adult mites in two to three weeks, and mate. Human scabies infestation predominantly results from person-to-person contact, with fomite transmission playing a much less important role. Intimate interpersonal contact with a scabies-infested individual, especially sexual contact, poses a greater risk of transmission than does casual contact. Other risk factors associated with acquiring scabies include poor hygiene and overcrowding.

Scabies commonly manifests as a highly pruritic skin eruption that presumably results from the host immune response to the mite excreta. In general, pruritis is particularly troublesome at night and after the patient showers. Studies have demonstrated that symptomatic disease typically begins an average of four weeks after initial infestation, but almost immediately if reinfestation occurs. Among immunocompetent adults, infestation generally occurs below the neck and the average number of mites per patient is less than 15. Accordingly, mites are difficult to find. Nevertheless, they can often be found by a diligent search for burrows in high-yield areas, namely the fingerweb spaces, wrists, elbows, periumbilical region, feet, and genitalia. The burrows typically appear as slightly elevated, linear or wavy dark lines that measure 5–20 mm (Plate 47). Frequently, a vesicle or black dot at one end of the burrow can be seen; this corresponds with the location of the mite. Other helpful findings on physical examination include the presence of vesicles, small erythematous papules, and nodules. The scabetic nodules, which appear as 3–10 mm reddish-brown nodules, are most often located on male genitalia, the groin, or axillae. All types of scabies lesions can become secondarily infected, especially following overvigorous scratching.

Three unusual and difficult-to-diagnose types of scabies can occur: crusted (Norwegian) scabies, bullous scabies, and scabies incognita. Crusted scabies is a severe form of scabies characterized by hyperkeratotic lesions that predominantly occur among patients who are immunosuppressed or have a neurologic illness that interferes with itching and scratching. Patients with crusted scabies generally develop nonpruritic widespread erythroderma and deeply fissured, gray-white, hyperkeratotic plaques, often with involvement of the face and scalp (Plate 46). These altered clinical features result from the diminished host immune response and often lead to misdiagnosis. Because patients with crusted scabies are infested with thousands (or millions) of mites, they are highly contagious. Bullous scabies is characterized by the presence of tense bullae on an erythematous base, often mimicking bullous pemphigoid. Scabies incognito is a type of scabies that becomes unrecognizable as a result of treatment with systemic or potent topical steroids.

A definitive diagnosis of scabies requires finding a mite, egg, or scybala (barrel-shaped brown fecal pellets) on a skin scraping of a burrow. To more readily identify a burrow, one can spread ink from a black fountain pen over a suspect area, wipe the skin with an alcohol pad, then look for ink outlining the burrow. The burrow should be scraped with a scapel blade (or a similar device) followed by transfer of the material to a glass slide. Mineral oil or 10%–20% potassium hydroxide is then added. With Norwegian scabies, scraping any hyperkeratotic area will yield multiple mites.

First-line therapy for scabies usually consists of using 5% permethrin cream. The patient should thoroughly massage it into the skin from the neck down and then wash it off 8 to 12 hours later. Because the hands and fingernails are frequently infected, patients should trim their nails prior to the scabicide treatment and make certain that they have applied an adequate amount of medication to the hands, fingers, and area under the fingernails. The patient should be informed that itching will likely persist for several days after treatment. Second-line therapy consists of 1% lindane cream or lotion given in the same way as described for permethrin. Lindane-associated neurotoxicity can occur, especially after use in infants, repeated use, improper use, or in patients with significant skin damage. Therefore, lindane should not be used for children less than two years of age, pregnant or lactating women, persons with extensive dermatitis, or following a bath. The recommended treatment for pregnant women, nursing mothers, and infants is 5%–10% precipitated sulfur in petrolatum. This therapy, however, requires applying the precipitated sulfur three consecutive nights, leaving it on for 8 to 12 hours each night. Some authorites recommend that all patients with scabies receive a second treatment one week after the initial treatment, whereas others recommend limiting re-treatment to those instances when mites are observed on follow-up examinations.

**Table 96.5** Selected ectoparasitic disorders caused by mites

| Disease | Causative organism | Clinical features | Diagnostic studies | Treatment |
|---|---|---|---|---|
| Human scabies | *Sarcoptes scabiei* | Pruritis, rash, burrows | Scraping of burrow | Permethrin 5% cream |
| Animal scabies | *Sarcoptes* spp. | Erythematous papular eruption | Animal exposure, clinical | Antihistamines, topical steroids, treat animal |
| Chiggers | *Eutrombicular alfreddugesi* | Pruritis, erythematous papules | Clinical | Antihistamines, topical steroids |
| Demodicidosis | *Demodex* spp. | Acne rosacea, pustular folliculitis | Clinical | Permethrin 5% cream |

To avoid reinfection, bed linens and recently worn clothes should be washed using the hot cycle of the machine (or dry cleaned). If objects cannot be laundered or dry cleaned, they should be placed in a tightly closed plastic bag for at least seven days. In addition, close contacts should receive simultaneous treatment, even if they have no symptoms. Treatment of crusted scabies requires the removal of the thick hyperkeratotic crusts with keratolytics plus repeated (usually a minimum of three) head-to-toe applications of permethrin.

Transient infestation with animal scabies may occur in individuals who come into close contact with a scabies-infested animal. Most often, zoonotic scabies involves contact with a dog, cat, or horse. Patients generally develop an irritant or allergic response characterized by a pruritic, erythematous papular eruption. In almost all instances, the animal mite cannot propagate on the human host, thus infestation is self-limited. Treatment for the human generally requires only symptomatic relief with oral antihistamines and topical corticosteroids. Because animal infestation, manifested as mange, is not self-limited, it should be treated with scabicide therapy. In addition, the animal should receive treatment to prevent reinfecting humans.

### Chiggers

Infestation with the common chigger, the larval form of the trombiculid (harvest) mite, can occur worldwide but is particularly common in tropical and subtropical areas. Most cases of infestation occur in the summer or autumn. The larva, which live on low-lying vegetation, can attach to a warm-blooded host and pierce the skin with a tubelike structure, allowing them to digest tissue, lymph, and blood. After feeding, the mites usually drop off. Within 24 hours, the human host develops pruritus and erythematous papules; scratching generally kills the rare mite that remains attached. The skin lesions most commonly develop on the feet or ankles. Itching and burning may last for weeks, despite the abscence of any remaining viable chiggers on the skin. Because chiggers are very difficult to find on the skin, the diagnosis of chigger-induced dermatitis mainly relies on the patient's clinical history and the appearance of the cutaneous lesions. Treatment consists of providing symptomatic relief with oral antihistamines and topical corticosteroids. In addition to causing direct infestation, chiggers can serve as the vector for *Rickettsia tsutsugamushi*, the rickettsial organism that causes scrub typhus in regions of Asia.

### Demodex mites

Demodicidosis refers to infestation with 0.3–0.4 mm long, transparent, wormlike mites, namely *Demodex folliculorum* and *D. brevis*. Asymptomatic parasitism is common and becomes more prevalent with increasing age, with 90%–100% of elderly individuals infected in the United States. *D. folliculorum* typically resides in hair follicles, whereas *D. brevis* prefers the sebaceous glands. After the females are fertilized, they move headfirst into the follicle or sebaceous gland where they feed on sebum. These mites live on the face, neck, and chest. Although the demodex mites' pathogenicity remains controversial, they may play a role in several disorders, including acne rosacea, pustular folliculitis, pityriasis folliculorum, and blepharitis. Treatment options for demodicidosis include the use of 5% permethrin cream, 1% lindane, benzoyl benzoate, and 5% precipitate sulfur in 5% benzoyl peroxide.

## Lice Infestation (Pediculosis and Diseases Caused by Lice

Lice are blood-requiring, six-legged, wingless insects that cause human disease by either directly infesting the skin or by injecting antigenic secretions into the skin. In addition, they can serve as a vector for transmitting infectious microorganisms. Lice have a worldwide distribution and traditionally flourish in conditions associated with overcrowding, poor hygiene, and poverty. Transmission predominantly occurs by person-to-person contact, although, in some instances, fomites may play a role. In general, lice live about two months, but if away from the host for more than 10 days, they will die of starvation. Three different subspecies of lice commonly infect humans, with each type having a predilection for distinct body locations: *Pediculus humanus* var. *capitus*, or the head louse, which prefers the scalp; *Pediculus humanus* var. *corporis*, or the body louse, which prefers the trunk, axillae, and groin; and *Phthirus pubis*, also known as the pubic louse, which prefers short hairs found at the pubis, trunk, axillae, beard, eyebrows, eyelashes, and occiput.

### Head lice

Although *Pediculus humanus* var. *capitus*, the head louse, most often affects children, individuals of any age can become infested. The infestation can result from either direct person-to-person contact or by indirect means, such as by sharing contaminated grooming devices. Infested patients typically develop an intense pruritus of the scalp, although rare patients remain asymptomatic. As a result of the pruritus and subsequent scratching, patients can develop impetigo or furunculosis. When searching for head lice on a patient, one should carefully look at the base of hair shafts near the ears or neck. When found, the adult head lice appear elongated and small (1–3 mm). The adult female louse can lay up to three eggs (nits) per day, cementing each egg to the base of a hair shaft. In general nits are found more readily than the adult lice. As the hair grows, the nit remains firmly attached, allowing one to estimate the duration of infestation (the average hair grows 1 cm per month).

Control of head lice requires killing of both the adult and egg forms. Permethrin 1% liquid is the generally accepted treatment of choice, mainly because it is safe and it kills both the eggs and the lice. Before applying this medication, patients should wash, rinse, and towel dry their hair. Next they should apply the permethrin, leave it on for 10 minutes, then rinse it off. The other most commonly used and effective treatment consists of vigorously massaging lindane 1% shampoo into the scalp for four to five minutes, followed by thorough rinsing. Lindane does not kill eggs and must be reapplied one week later to kill hatching nymphs. In addition, reports have described lindane-resistant head lice. To remove the empty egg cases that will remain attached to the hair shaft, the patient should soak his or her hair for one hour in a solution of equal parts vinegar and water, then comb the nits out with a fine-toothed comb; shaving the hair is not necessary. The comb used to remove the nits should be discarded.

### Body lice

The body louse, or *Pediculus humanus* var. *corporis*, is the only type of louse known to serve as a vector for infectious microorganisms. This louse is capable of transmitting *Borrelia* species (louse-borne relapsing fever), *Ricksettsia prowazekii* (epidemic

**Table 96.6** Selected ectoparasitic diseases caused by insects

| Disease | Causative organism | Clinical features | Diagnostic studies | Treatment |
|---|---|---|---|---|
| LICE (PEDICULOSIS) | | | | |
| Head lice | *Pediculus humanus* var. *capitis* | Scalp pruritis | Finding lice or nits | Permethrin 1% liquid |
| Body lice | *Pediculus humanus* var. *corporis* | Pruritis, erythematous macules | Finding lice in clothing | Pyrethrins with piperonyl butoxide |
| Pubic lice | *Phthirus pubis* | Pruritis, blue macules | Finding lice or nits | Lindane 1% shampoo |
| FLIES (MYIASIS) | | | | |
| Furuncular | *Dermatobia hominis*<br>*Cordylobia anthropophaga*<br>*Cuterebra* spp. | Subcutaneous nodule(s) | Clinical | Noninvasive: bacon therapy, petrolatum<br>Invasive: surgical removal |
| Wound | *Callitroga americana*<br>*Chrysomyia bezziana* | Necrotic tissue | Find larvae in wound | Extract larvae |
| FLEAS | | | | |
| Plague | *Yersinia pestis* | Regional adenopathy, sepsis | Gram stain of aspirate, blood culture, serology | Streptomycin |
| Murine typhus | *Ricettsia typhi*<br>ELB | Fever, headache, rash | Serology | Tetracycline (or doxycycline) |

typhus), and *Bartonella quintana* (trench fever) (see Chapter 54). Unlike head lice or pubic lice, body lice do not live on their host, but rather live in the seams of clothing and bedding, travelling to the skin only to feed. Consequently, one rarely finds body lice on the skin. They are, however, easily identified in the seams of clothing, particularly at pressure sites such as belt lines. In addition to their ability to transmit infectious microorganisms, the body louse can directly irritate the skin; patients frequently develop generalized pruritis, often accompanied by erythematous macules or papules at feeding sites, and in some instances, urticarial wheals. As a result of the pruritis and consequent scratching, one may find linear scratch marks, thickening, and pigmentary changes. Secondary infection, manifested as impetigo or furunculosis, can also develop. Chronic infestation may result in marked hyperpigmentation and thickening of the skin, often referred to as vagabond's disease.

Effective treatment generally consists of applying pyrethrins with piperonyl butoxide, followed 10 minutes later by thorough bathing of the patient with soap and water. Because this therapy does not kill eggs, the patient should repeat the treatment one week later to kill hatching nymphs. Because body lice predominantly live in clothing and bedding, it is critical to launder the patient's clothes and bedding. Washing in water of at least 125 °F for 10 minutes or tumble drying will kill both eggs and lice.

### Pubic lice (crabs)

Transmission of *Phthirus pubis*, also known as pubic lice or crabs, predominantly occurs through sexual intercourse, although fomite transmission can occur. The diagnosis of pubic lice should lead one to investigate concomitant sexually transmitted diseases. Likewise, the presence of pubic lice in the eyelashes of a child should serve as a marker for possible sexual abuse. Pubic lice, which are broader than body or head lice, clasp onto hairs with their large hind-leg claws. Typically, they attach to the base of short body hairs located on the trunk, thighs, axillae, beard, eyebrows, eyelashes, or occiput. The nits cement themselves to the base of the hair shaft and grow out with the hair. Clinically, patients tend not to manifest symptoms during the incubation period (30 days), but subsequently will develop pruritus and 2–3 mm blue macules (maculae ceruleae).

The treatment of pubic lice requires applying lindane 1% shampoo to the affected area, leaving it on for 4 minutes, and then thoroughly washing it off. Alternatively, permethrin 1% cream rinse can be used in a similar manner, except that it is left on for 10 minutes. The presence of lice or nits on the eyelashes requires application of a thick coat of an occlusive eye ointment twice daily for 10 days.

## Diseases Caused by Flies

### Myiasis

Myiasis, the invasion of animal tissue by fly larvae (maggots), can occur worldwide, but most frequently develops in persons living in or traveling to the tropics. Myiasis may be produced by several different species of flies that commonly cause disease by either burrowing into tissue, known as furuncular myiasis, or by invasion of necrotic, decaying tissue, known as wound myiasis.

#### Furuncular myiasis

Although many species of fly larva can cause furuncular myiasis, human-associated disease most commonly occurs with one of three species: *Dermatobia hominis*, a botfly indigenous to Central and South America; *Cordylobia anthropophaga*, the Tumbu fly, present in Africa; or *Cuterebra* spp., a botfly that causes North American myiasis. Each of these species of flies has a distinct life cycle. The *D. hominis* life cycle begins with the adult female attaching her eggs onto the underside of an intermediate carrier, such as a blood-sucking fly, mosquito, or tick. When this intermediate carrier ingests a warm blood meal, the botfly larva becomes stimulated, emerges from its egg, and penetrates the skin. Within several days, a small erythematous nodule (warble) develops where the larva has penetrated (Fig. 96.3). At this point, and until it emerges, the larva anchors itself in the subcutaneous tissues and extends its breathing tube to the skin surface, creating a central pore in the lesion. When the larva has matured in 6 to 12 weeks, it works its way out of the skin, drops to the ground, and slowly develops into an adult fly. The entire cycle from egg to adult requires about three to four months.

Unlike *D. hominis*, *C. anthropophaga* does not incorporate an intermediate carrier in its life cycle. The female adult fly lays approximately 300 eggs in shaded areas of sandy ground or beaches. The female prefers to lay her eggs in an area contaminated by animal or human feces, but in some instances, they will lay their eggs on clothes. The larvae hatch and, upon coming into contact with human skin, quickly and painlessly penetrate it. The remaining life cycle is similar to that of *D. hominis*, except that the total time in the host skin ranges from 8 to 12 days (as opposed to 6 to 12 weeks). Similar to *C. anthropophaga*, *Cuterebra* sp. does not incorporate an intermediate carrier in its life cycle. The cuterebrid larvae normally infect rodents, rabbits, or hares. Adult *Cuterebra* spp. lay their eggs near trails or burrows made by these natural hosts; occasionally, these eggs will adhere to an unsuspecting human that has accidentally come into contact with vegetation or debris that harbor these eggs. Humans may also become infected by petting or kissing an egg-infested dog or cat. Stimulated by the warmth of the human host, the larvae hatch from the eggs, seek entry via a mucosal portal, and if none is found, they directly penetrate the host skin. The remaining aspects of the life cycle remain poorly characterized, but appear to resemble the *D. hominis* life cycle. Most cases occur in August

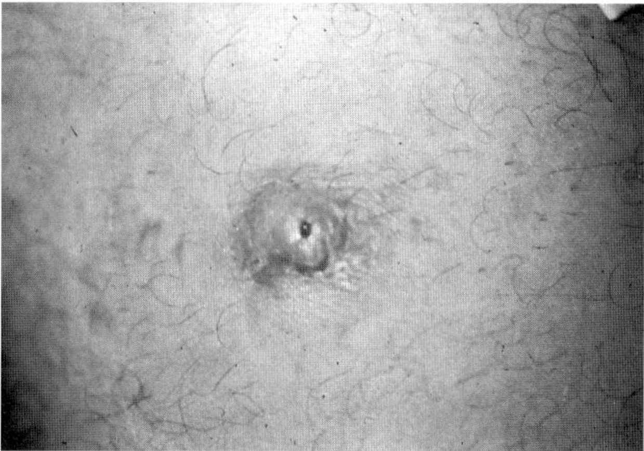

**Fig. 96.3** Furuncular myiasis: cutaneous nodular lesion with central pore present on a patient infected with *Dermatobia hominis*. [Slide courtesy of Dr. Marshall Welch.]

through October, predominantly in the northeastern United States.

Regardless of the type of infecting fly larva, patients usually present with one (or several) subcutaneous nodule(s) and symptoms that include a subcutaneous prickling sensation, pain, or awareness of movement within the skin. In some instances, patients may actually observe movement of the larva within the cutaneous lesion. Lesions can develop on any area of the body, including the chest, back, arms, legs, face, scalp, and genital region. Visualizing the larval posterior spiracles within the nodule confirms the diagnosis. Conjunctival infestation (ophthalmomyiasis) may result from infection with *D. hominis*; in rare instances, these larvae have migrated to the brain via an open anterior fontanelle. Patients infected with *Cuterebra* spp. may develop atypical manifestations that include cutaneous creeping eruption, infection of the vitreous humor, or involvement of the upper respiratory tract.

Although furuncular myiasis is a self-limited disorder, most patients decide, given the unsettling thought of having larvae under their skin, to have the larvae removed as soon as possible. Noninvasive treatment options consist of occluding the breathing orifice of the larva with petrolatum, beeswax, or occlusive dressings; if this measure is successful, the larva will die of suffocation or will crawl out of the skin nodule. One recent report described bacon therapy as a succesful noninvasive means of removing larvae. Specifically, this involved applying the fatty portion of raw bacon over a subcutaneous lesion, leaving it on for approximately three hours (to allow time for the larvae to migrate into the bacon), then quickly extracting the larvae with a pair of tweezers. In the event that noninvasive measures do not work, one can surgically extract the larvae (Fig. 96.4). For the rare cases of ophthalmomyiasis, treatment options include the use of topical corticosteroids, photocoagulation, and vitrectomy.

### Wound myiasis

Wound myiasis can be caused by numerous fly species, including *Callitroga americana*, the New World screwworm fly, and *Chrysomyia bezziana*, the Old World screwworm fly. In wound myiasis, flies lay eggs on necrotic tissue and these eggs rapidly hatch. The soft-bodied larvae that hatch have a voracious appetite and begin to ingest necrotic debris. Some species will, unfortunately, attack and destroy normal healthy tissue. Treatment involves applying chloroform (mixed with 10% vegetable oil to make it less irritating) under anesthesia followed by extraction of the larvae.

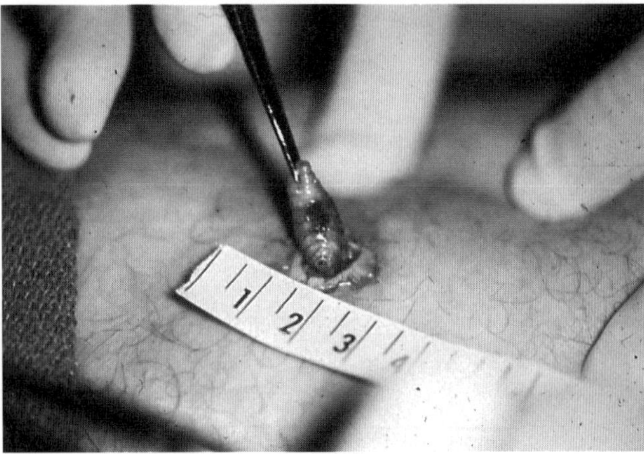


**Fig. 96.4** Removal of *D. hominis* botfly larvae following surgical incision of cutaneous furuncular lesion. [Slide courtesy of Dr. Marshall Welch.]

## Diseases Caused by Fleas

Fleas are directly implicated as the major vector in both plague and murine typhus. Worldwide, urban and domestic rats serve as the major reservoir for *Yersinia pestis*, the causative agent of plague. The oriental rat flea, *Xenopsylla cheopis*, acts as the most efficient vector for transmitting *Y. pestis*. Fleas become infected by ingesting a blood meal from a bacteremic animal. Once *Y. pestis* enters the flea, it secretes a coagulase that causes blood to clot in the foregut, thus blocking the flea's ability to swallow. When the flea attempts to partake in a blood meal from another host, it regurgitates thousands of organisms into the skin, thus infecting the host.

In most regions of the world the causative agent of murine typhus, *Rickettsia typhi*, is transmitted by *X. cheopis*. However, in southern Texas and southern California, the common cat flea, *Ctenocephalides felis*, plays a major role in the transmission of *R. typhi*. In recent years investigators have isolated a second rickettsial organism, ELB, that is transmitted by fleas and can also cause murine typhus. With both of these rickettsia, transmission occurs when infected flea feces are inoculated into the skin by the scratching of a pruritic flea bite wound. Infected fleas harbor *R. typhi* for the duration of their life.

Recently, the causative agent of cat scratch disease, *Bartonella henselae*, has been isolated from fleas. Although the exact mechanism of transmission of *B. henselae* from cats to humans remains unknown, fleas could possibly have a direct or indirect role in the transmission of *B. henselae*.

## ANNOTATED BIBLIOGRAPHY

Burns DA. The treatment of human ectoparasite infection. Br J Dermatol 1991; 125:89–93.

*Detailed recommendations are given for the treatment of lice and scabies. Practical tips are given in addition to a detailed discussion of the available medications.*

Dumler JS, Bakken JS. Ehrlichial diseases of humans: emerging tick-borne infections. Clin Infect Dis 1995; 20:1102–1110.

*The authors provide a thorough up-to-date review of ehrlichiosis.*

Dworkin MS, Anderson DE Jr, Schwan TG, et al. Tick-borne relapsing fever in the Northwestern United States and Southwestern Canada. Clin Infect Dis 1998; 3:122–131.

*This retrospective study examined 182 cases (133 confirmed and 49 probable) of tick-borne relapsing fever, the largest series of its kind. In this study, the authors found that many infections were not initially recognized and that the Jarisch-Herxheimer reaction occurred in about 50% of patients following initiation of therapy.*

Elgart ML. Pediculosis. Dermatol Clin 1990; 8:219–228.

*In this article, head, body, and pubic lice are discussed in detail, with emphasis on the clinical setting, symptomatology, and treatment.*

Elgart ML. Flies and myiasis. Dermatol Clin 1990; 8:237–244.

*This article discusses the biting flies (mosquitos and flies), followed by a detailed discussion of myiasis. The section on myiasis covers both wound myiasis and cutaneous (furuncular) myiasis. Several excellent photographs supplement the text of the article.*

Elgart ML. Scabies. Dermatol Clin 1990; 8:253–263.

*This is a comprehensive article on scabies that discusses epidemiology, clinical presentations (common and unusual), diagnosis, pathology, and treatment. The article concludes with a brief discussion of animal scabies.*

Spach DH, Liles WC, Campbell GL, et al. Tick-borne diseases in the United States. N Engl J Med 1993; 329:936–947.

*This review article begins by discussing the biology of ticks and includes photographs of the common North American ticks. Subsequently, the article covers the eight major tick-borne diseases in the United States with respect to their microbiology, epidemiology, diagnosis, and treatment.*

Steere AC. Lyme disease. N Engl J Med 1989; 321:586–596.

*This excellent review article covers the history, pathogenesis, clinical manifestations, diagnosis, and treatment of Lyme disease. Although several years old, it remains one of the best review articles on Lyme disease.*

Weber DJ, Walker DH. Rocky Mountain spotted fever. Infect Dis Clin North Am 1991; 5:19–35.

*This article provides an excellent overview of the major aspects of Rocky Mountain spotted fever, including details on the causative organism, epidemiology, pathogenesis, clinical features, laboratory features, diagnosis, and treatment.*

# VII

## HUMAN IMMUNODEFICIENCY VIRUS AND AIDS

# 97

# Epidemiology and Prevention

FRANÇOIS CRABBÉ, MARIE LAGA, AND PETER PIOT

The first cases of AIDS (acquired immunodeficiency syndrome) were recognized in 1981, prior to the identification of the etiologic agent. Thus the initial case definition of this new syndrome was based on available clinical and laboratory data.

For purposes of surveillance, the initial AIDS case definition by the Centers for Disease Control (CDC) required CD4 cell depletion accompanied by one or more specific opportunistic infections and/or tumors that became known as "AIDS-defining conditions." The CDC surveillance case definition was modified in 1985 and 1987 as more information became available about the spectrum of illnesses associated with HIV (human immunodeficiency virus) infection and as specific HIV antibody tests were developed.

Patients with HIV infection were categorized as having AIDS, AIDS-related complex (ARC), or asymptomatic disease. However, as more information has been gathered regarding the natural history of HIV infection, these terms have become outdated. It is now recognized that infection with HIV results in a progressive loss of immune system function, with individual cases progressing along a continuum from asymptomatic to increasingly severe clinical manifestations resulting from opportunistic infections and malignancies known as AIDS.

## Definition of AIDS

Several studies have shown the value of the absolute CD4 cell count as an important indicator of HIV disease. In January 1993 the CDC further expanded the definition of AIDS to include HIV-infected adolescents and adults with a CD4 count under 200/$\mu$L irrespective of clinical manifestations, as well as HIV-infected persons with pulmonary tuberculosis, recurrent pneumonia, and invasive cervical cancer (Table 97.1).

The epidemiologic definition of AIDS used in European countries is presented in Table 97.2. The major difference between authorities in the United States (CDC) and Europe is the omission of asymptomatic HIV-infected subjects with CD4 count below 200 cells in the European definition.

It should be remembered that this classification system has been designed primarily as an epidemiologic tool, rather than a clinical staging system. Other staging systems that have been designed for clinical purposes are described in subsequent chapters.

## Laboratory Diagnosis of HIV Infection

The most commonly used laboratory diagnostic assays for HIV infection are based on the detection of antibodies formed against HIV viral antigens. Antibody assays have been primarily designed for detection of antibodies in human serum, although some of the tests have been able to detect HIV antibodies on whole blood or saliva. Antibody testing is used not only to support the individual diagnosis of HIV infection but also for public health purposes, such as blood bank screening and surveillance of the epidemic, as well as research. More than 100 HIV antibody tests, some of them already outdated, have been developed since 1985 by more than 40 different companies. Techniques for detecting HIV have evolved rapidly, to reduce the costs, achieve earlier diagnosis, eliminate uninterpretable results, and simplify the lab procedure.

### Serologic diagnosis

Serologic tests are divided in two broad categories: *screening tests*, with the highest sensitivity, and *confirmatory tests*, with the highest specificity.

#### Screening tests

##### *Enzyme-linked immunosorbent assays*

These tests, commonly called ELISAs, are the most frequently used immunoassays for the detection of antibodies formed against HIV. They are called first-, second-, or third-generation tests, depending on the type of antigen—viral lysate, recombinant proteins, or synthetic peptides—and the type of conjugate used, with corresponding increases in specificity.

The advantages of ELISA include the high sensitivity and specificity, with differences in quality between various commercial brands, as well as the ease of performance for large numbers of samples. Among the disadvantages are the need for trained personnel, the cost and maintenance of equipment, and the duration of the procedure compared with rapid enzyme immunoassay (EIA) tests.

##### *Rapid EIA tests*

Based on the use of recombinant proteins or synthetic peptides fixed on a membranous support, rapid EIA tests have been designed for certain testing situations such as emergency wards, blood banks, or autopsy rooms, as well as field testing. Among the advantages are the quick performance—in general, under 30 minutes—and minimal equipment, as well as the ability for some of them to directly test blood rather than serum. Some of these tests are stable for up to 12 months, even at room temperature. Rapid tests are considered rather expensive, although costs vary widely (US <\$1–\$4), and they are not fit for processing large batches of samples. Sensitivity and specificity do not differ significantly from ELISA.

**Table 97.1** Revised classification system of HIV disease

| CD4 T-cell category (count/μL) | Clinical category A | B | C |
|---|---|---|---|
| ≥500 | A1 | B1 | C1 |
| 200–499 | A2 | B2 | C2 |
| <200 | A3 | B3 | C3 |

CATEGORY A

Asymptomatic HIV infection
Persistent generalized lymphadenopathy
Acute retroviral syndrome

CATEGORY B (FORMERLY ARC)

Bacillary angiomatosis
Candidiasis
  Oral
  Recurrent vaginal
Cervical dysplasia
Constitutional symptoms
(e.g., fever or diarrhea >1 month
Hairy leukoplakia, oral
*Herpes zoster*
Idiopathic thrombocytopenic purpura
Listeriosis
Pelvic inflammatory disease
Peripheral neuropathy

CATEGORY C (AIDS-DEFINING CONDITIONS)

CD4 count less than 200 cells/mm$^3$
Candidiasis
  Pulmonary
  Esophageal
Cervical cancer
Coccidioidomycosis
Cryptococcosis extrapulmonary
Cryptosporidiosis
Cytomegalovirus
Encephalopathy, HIV
Herpes simplex
  Chronic (>1 mo)
  Esophageal
Histoplasmosis
Isosporiasis
Kaposi's sarcoma
Lymphoma
*Mycobacterium avium*
*Mycobacterium kansasii*
*Mycobacteria tuberculosis*
*Pneumocystis carinii*
Pneumonia, recurrent
Progressive multifocal leukemia
*Salmonellosis*
Toxoplasmosis of brain
Wasting syndrome

Source: Centers for Disease Control. 1993 Revised Classification System for HIV Infection and Expanded Surveillance Case Definition for Aids among Adolescents and Adults.

The high sensitivity of screening tests does not overcome the problem of the "window" period, which is the time between exposure to HIV and the production of antibodies. However, with the newer tests this period has been reduced to a matter of days for most patients. Nevertheless, a period of up to 6 months is still considered necessary before an individual suspected of HIV infection is declared HIV-negative.

## Confirmatory tests

Confirmatory tests are used for their high specificity.

### *Western blot test*

The Western blot is currently the most commonly used method to confirm specific antibody responses to HIV viral proteins. It

**Table 97.2** Expanded European AIDS Surveillance Case Definition (1993)

Candidiasis
  Pulmonary
  Esophageal
Cervical cancer
Coccidioidomycosis
Cryptococcosis extrapulmonary
Cryptosporidiosis
Cytomegalovirus
Encephalopathy, HIV
Herpes simplex
  Chronic (>1 mo)
  Esophageal
Histoplasmosis
Isosporiasis
Kaposi's sarcoma
Lymphoma
*Mycobacterium avium*
*Mycobacterium kansasii*
*Mycobacteria tuberculosis*
*Pneumocystis carinii*
Pneumonia, recurrent
Progressive multifocal leukemia
*Salmonellosis*
Toxoplasmosis of brain
Wasting syndrome

is based on the detection of antibodies directed at nine specific viral proteins produced by the three major HIV structural genes, ENV, GAG, and POL. It has demonstrated greater than 99% sensitivity and specificity.

The Western blot is considered the "gold standard"—that is, the most widely accepted serologic confirmatory tests—because of the specific detection of antibodies against multiple HIV viral antigens. Aside from the basic positivity or negativity of samples, a qualitative evaluation of the recognized viral antigens can be performed. However, the limitations of the Western blot technique are numerous. The procedure is time-consuming, labor-intensive, and subjective. Its high sensitivity and specificity depend critically on the standardization of the technique, therefore requiring a high level of staff training and laboratory organization. Even commercial Western blots have shown a lack of consistency between batches, because of the varying antigen preparation, therefore making interpretation of results difficult. The World Health Organization (WHO) has made efforts to standardize the interpretation criteria for the Western blot. The cost of commercialized Western blots remains very high, approaching US$20 per test.

The Western blot's use is especially important in populations with a low prevalence of infection, since the risk of false-positive results with screening tests is high. In some high-risk populations, the predictive value of a positive enzyme immunoassay is greater than 99%, but the Western blot is still used as the confirmatory test.

#### *Line immunoassay*

The line immunoassay is a second-generation assay, having the potential to replace the Western blot. Recombinant proteins and/or synthetic peptides are applied in band patterns on nylon support strips and tested in a way similar to the Western blot. The line immunoassay has the advantage of being more easily standardized than the Western blot. It is also a less expensive alternative for confirmation and differentiation of viral strains because protein bands representing more than one virus can be applied to the strip. This may be an important consideration when both HIV-1 and HIV-2 are present or suspected.

#### *Other tests*

Other serologic techniques include the immunofluorescence (IF) and the radioimmunoprecipitation assay (RIPA). These techniques are confined to research settings.

### HIV testing strategies

Since no single test is 100% sensitive and specific, serologic tests need to be combined, depending on the purpose of HIV detection and the prevalence of infection in the population targeted. The conventional testing strategy—used for diagnosis of HIV infection in individual patients—recommends the use of an ELISA, possibly followed by a repeat ELISA on reactive samples in order to discard laboratory errors, and then a Western blot. The use of a differently formatted ELISA as the repeat test helps reduce the risk of producing false-positive results and limits the costs of Western blot controls.

Because of the limits of the Western blot, WHO has recommended alternative testing strategies for resource-poor settings in the developing world. However, these new approaches are still being widely debated.

### Virus detection techniques

Although the detection of HIV antibodies is the most conventional technique for HIV diagnosis, direct demonstration of virus, viral antigen, or viral DNA may be useful for clinical research situations.

Laboratory techniques have been developed for the detection of HIV p24 antigen in serum samples. It has been shown that viral antigenemia can be detected in HIV-1–infected individuals early in infection and in the late stages of the disease. Viral antigen detection is commercially available, and convenient, but it is not very sensitive. Its highest sensitivity is in acute HIV seroconversion.

Virus isolation is used for the direct demonstration of the virus-infected status. Detection of viral replication in peripheral blood mononuclear cell cultures relies on several techniques, such as measurement of released p24 viral antigen in the culture supernatant, measurement of reverse transcriptase activity, or HIV DNA detected by polymerase chain reaction (PCR) in cultured cells.

Polymerase chain reaction for HIV-1 DNA or RNA has a very high sensitivity and specificity, but it is still a complex and expensive procedure. Virus isolation and PCR are used for specific research questions. They are employed to detect HIV-1 in the interval between exposure and seroconversion, or for confirming indeterminate Western blot test results. They have proven useful in providing relevant information in perinatal transmission studies of HIV, where the presence of passive antibodies of the mother precludes the serodiagnosis of active infection of the exposed infant. Besides specific diagnostic situations, these techniques have also proved useful in monitoring the success of AIDS therapies.

## Status of HIV/AIDS Worldwide

### Global HIV/AIDS estimates

UNAIDS and WHO estimate that over 30 million people were living with HIV infection at the end of 1997 (see Fig. 97.1). That is one in every 100 adults in the sexually active ages of 15 to 49 worldwide. Included in the 30 million figure are 1.1 million children under the age of 15. The overwhelming majority of HIV-infected people—more than 90%—live in the developing world, and most of these do not know that they are infected.

These latest estimates also point up the continuing rapid spread of HIV. Altogether, 5.8 million people are believed to have acquired HIV infection in 1997, 590,000 of them children. Overall, that is equivalent to nearly 16,000 new infections every day of the year, including those in children infected at birth or through breastfeeding. Assuming that currently unbroken trends in many parts of the world will continue, it is estimated that more than 40 million people will be living with HIV in the year 2000.

An estimated 2.3 million people died of AIDS in 1997. These deaths represent a fifth of the total 11.7 million AIDS deaths since the beginning of the epidemic in the late 1970s. Of the people who died of AIDS this year, 46% were women and 460,000 were children.

### The regional epidemics

The regional distribution of global HIV/AIDS cases in adults and children is shown in Figure 97.2. North America, Europe, and Australasia are estimated to have a total of more than 1.5 mil-

| | | |
|---|---|---|
| **People newly infected with HIV in 1997** | **Total** | **5.8 million** |
| | Adults | 5.2 million |
| | *Women* | *2.1 million* |
| | Children <15 years | 590 000 |
| **No. of people living with HIV/AIDS** | **Total** | **30.6 million** |
| | Adults | 29.5 million |
| | *Women* | *12.1 million* |
| | Children <15 years | 1.1 million |
| **AIDS deaths in 1997** | **Total** | **2.3 million** |
| | Adults | 1.8 million |
| | *Women* | *820 000* |
| | Children <15 years | 460 000 |
| **Total no. of AIDS deaths since the beginning of the epidemic** | **Total** | **11.7 million** |
| | Adults | 9.0 million |
| | *Women* | *4.0 million* |
| | Children <15 years | 2.7 million |
| Total no. of AIDS orphans[a] since the beginning of the epidemic | | **8.2 million** |

[a] Defined as HIV-negative children who lost their mother or both parents to AIDS when they were under the age of 15

**Fig. 97.1** Global summary of the HIV/AIDS epidemic, December 1997.

lion infections. The spread of HIV infection among homosexual men appears to have decreased markedly, although increases in infection have been demonstrated in the United States because of older gay men returning to risk behavior or new gay generations engaging in unsafe sex. Transmission through injecting drug use and heterosexual intercourse increased during the latter half of the 1980s and the early 1990s.

The magnitude of the HIV/AIDS problem in eastern Europe and central Asia remains poorly defined. As of late 1997, an estimated 150,000 adults and children are infected with HIV in this region, and drug injection accounts for the majority of the new infections.

Two-thirds of all cumulative HIV infections have occurred in sub-Saharan Africa, with about half of these 20.8 million infected adults being women. About 1 million African children are estimated to have been infected as a result of mother-to-child transmission. Although central and eastern Africa remain the hardest hit by the epidemic, there is increasing spread in West Africa, southern Africa, and parts of North Africa. In some urban populations in central and eastern Africa, it is estimated that up to one in three adults is now infected. In eastern and central Africa HIV prevalences among female prostitutes may reach 80%, while it is common to find infection rates greater than 50% among sexually transmitted disease (STD) clinic patients. (See HIV/AIDS surveillance database from the U.S. Bureau of Census, Center for International Research, for a complete inventory of seroprevalence data on African populations.)

By contrast with sub-Saharan Africa, limited data are available on North Africa and the Middle East. As of late 1997, HIV was estimated at more than 210,000 for the region, mainly among homosexual and bisexual communities.

South and southeast Asia are currently experiencing a rapidly expanding HIV epidemic. Whereas in early 1991 WHO estimated that there were around 500,000 HIV infections in the region, as of late 1997 it was conservatively estimated that more than 6 million adults had been infected. At this pace, Asia will soon surpass Africa in the annual number of new infections.

Significant levels of HIV infection have recently been detected among injecting drug users (IDUs) in countries like Vietnam, Malaysia, Thailand, and China. Sexual transmission of HIV has been expanding at the same time, leading to significant levels of infection in female sex workers in various countries. In Thailand, HIV infection is now spreading to the general population, as demonstrated by surveys in young military recruits or antenatal clinic attenders.

As of late 1997, HIV prevalence in adults was estimated at 1.3 million in Latin America and the Caribbean. Brazil already has more AIDS cases than any developing country outside Africa. This region illustrates the diversity of epidemiologic patterns across the continent, with a combination of heterosexual, homosexual, bisexual, and drug-injection behaviors. Throughout this region, the proportion of AIDS cases among women is increasing, reflecting the importance of heterosexual transmission.

All these prevalence figures reveal little about the actual spread of HIV, except that it continues to increase at a staggering rate. In 1997 alone, it is estimated that 5.8 million people became infected. The majority of the new infections have occurred in sub-Saharan Africa, India, and Southeast Asia. Although there is still much uncertainty about the future spread of HIV and about the ultimate global dimensions of the epidemic, since it has not yet reached its equilibrium, a conservative estimate is that by the year 2000 there will be a minimal cumulative total of 40 million cases of HIV infection, with 10 million adult AIDS cases. Since approximately 90% of infections will have occurred in developing countries, it is becoming clear that the epidemic is turning into a mainly heterosexually transmitted disease of the developing world, and of marginalized populations within the industrialized world.

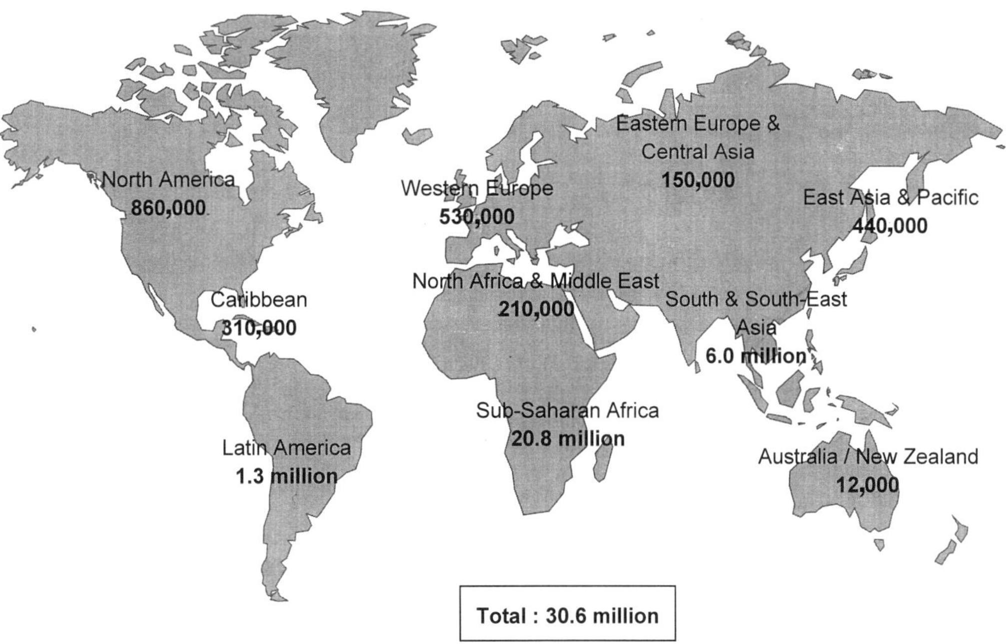


**Fig. 97.2** Adults and children estimated to be living with HIV/AIDS as of end 1997

## Modes of Transmission

The modes of transmission have not changed beyond those described or predicted early in the epidemic, and they are identical throughout the world. The vast majority of cases of HIV infection and AIDS throughout the world can be attributed to sexual contact, bloodborne transmission, or perinatal transmission.

Bloodborne transmission includes needle-sharing by drug users; receipt of infected blood, blood products, or organs and tissues; and percutaneous or mucosal occupational exposure.

### Sexual transmission

In a global sense HIV infection is primarily a sexually transmitted disease, since 75% of cases worldwide are estimated by WHO to be acquired by sexual contact. Receptive anal intercourse appears to be the most efficient mode of sexual transmission of HIV, explaining the prevalence of HIV infection among homosexual and bisexual male communities. Homosexual transmission still accounts for the majority of sexually transmitted AIDS cases in North America and most of Europe and Oceania, although heterosexual transmission is growing in importance.

Vaginal heterosexual intercourse is a fairly inefficient mode of transmission of HIV, particularly from woman to man. For Western countries, estimated per-contact probabilities of HIV infection range from 0.001 to 0.002. These figures contrast sharply with recent figures from Thailand reporting probabilities of 0.03 to 0.05. It is now known that the efficiency of heterosexual transmission can be greatly enhanced in the presence of well-defined risk factors, including a more advanced immunodeficiency of the infecting partner; anal intercourse; sex during menses; and the presence of ulcerative or nonulcerative STDs in either partner. The combination of such amplifying factors, in addition to high-risk sexual behavior patterns, may explain the widespread heterosexual epidemic in the Third World.

### Bloodborne transmission

Some 10%–15% of HIV infections are estimated to be acquired by bloodborne (or parenteral) transmission worldwide. This mode of transmission includes needle-sharing by drug users; receipt of infected blood, blood products, or organs and tissues; and percutaneous or mucosal occupational exposure.

Transmission of HIV through sharing of injection equipment among IDUs accounted for 5%–10% of HIV infections worldwide in 1993, but for 25% in developed countries. It is the main cause of bloodborne transmission in Asia, Latin America, and the Caribbean. In the United States, more than 20% of AIDS cases are attributed to injecting drug use. In Europe, Italy, Spain, France, and Switzerland report the highest percentages of drug-use–associated AIDS cases. The use of noninjecting drugs, such as crack cocaine, has also been associated with increased rates of HIV infection through the exchange of sex for money or drugs.

Transmission via contaminated blood or blood products is a very efficient form of transmission, approaching 100%. Fortunately, bloodborne routes of acquisition now account for only about 5% of HIV infections in the world. The proportion of AIDS cases attributable to blood transfusion has been steadily declining in the Western world thanks to rigorous screening techniques for blood donors. However, the risk of HIV infection by contaminated blood remains high in the developing world, as a result of the failing health care system. Although HIV infection has also been transmitted through donated organs and tissues, most cases occurred before 1985, when organ donors started to be routinely screened for HIV.

The risk of occupational HIV transmission in the health care setting is small. Occupational HIV transmission usually refers to health care worker exposure to patient or laboratory specimens through percutaneous injury.

The CDC have been collecting documented reports on occupational HIV transmission in a limited number of health care workers. Overall, the risk of infection from a needle stick appears to be around 0.3% of such exposures.

### Perinatal or "vertical" transmission

Transmission of HIV from mother to child during or after pregnancy accounts to 5%–10% of acquired HIV infections worldwide. It is by far the major source of infection in children. It has become a major public health problem in much of Africa, where around 1 million children had been infected as of late 1993. Transmission occurs before birth, during delivery, and through breastfeeding, with rates ranging from about 14% to 40%, the highest figures being observed in African studies. The differences in rates may be explained by the stage of infection of the mother, the risk of transmission being greater in early or advanced stages of infection, and by breastfeeding practices. In this case the risk is particularly great when the mother becomes infected during late pregnancy or while breastfeeding. Recently zidovudine (AZT) administered during pregnancy, at delivery, and in the first 6 weeks of life to the infant has reduced transmission by over two-thirds (from 25% to 8%).

There is no evidence so far that HIV is spread through casual contact. Studies of household contacts of HIV-infected persons have revealed only a single instance of transmission among persons who were not sex or needle-sharing partners of the index case. In that situation there appeared to be repeated blood contact from the index case with an active dermatitis in the recipient. There is no evidence that HIV can be transmitted by food, inanimate objects, skin contact such as handshaking, animals, or water. Although HIV has been isolated from saliva, suggesting the theoretical risk that HIV could be transmitted by deep kissing, biting, or other direct contact of infected saliva with nonintact skin or a mucous membrane, transmission by such route seems rare or nonexistent. Finally, HIV transmission by insects has been the subject of much speculation, yet it has not been corroborated by any evidence, even in developing countries where malaria and HIV are both endemic.

## Determinants of HIV Spread

The spread of HIV infection in a population can be characterized by four types of variables: behavioral, biologic, demographic, and socioeconomic/political.

### Behavioral variables

Sexual behavior is the most important determinant for the spread of HIV, its heterogeneity significantly influencing the dynamics of HIV infection among and between populations in the world. In particular, high rates of sexual partner change and contacts with highly infected core groups such as sex workers play a key role in the spread of HIV into the general population. The rate of sexual transmission of HIV is also affected by the rate of sexual practices such as anal intercourse, or by the rate of condom use.

### Biologic variables

It has been demonstrated that the risk of sexual transmission of HIV is greatly enhanced in the presence of ulcerative as well as nonulcerative STDs, since they increase both the infectiousness of the infected individual and the susceptibility of the noninfected sex partner. The efficiency of sexual transmission of HIV also increases with higher viral load, as in longer infected individuals, particularly those with overt AIDS.

### Demographic variables

Since HIV is primarily a sexually transmitted disease, young and sexually more active age groups are more affected by the epidemic.

Family separation and disintegration of social norms, which occur with large concentrations of migrant labor, as in mining areas or industrial plantations, create an imbalance between supply and demand of sexual contact between men and women. This in turn favors prostitution and its consequent contact with HIV-infected commercial sex workers.

### Socioeconomic/political factors

As in other epidemics, poverty is one of the major driving forces behind AIDS, generating family separation, prostitution, and drug addiction. In the developing world, crises in many health care systems have led to reduced access to health services, poor STD case management, and few resources for preventive activities. In addition, war and civil conflicts have generated large refugee flows and economic disarray, thus placing populations at higher risk of STDs or HIV infection.

Women's lack of personal power also correlates with the rapid spread of HIV infection, since women in this situation do not have the means to minimize the risks of heterosexual transmission of HIV.

## Epidemiology of HIV-2

Human immunodeficiency virus 2 is distinct from HIV-1 but also belongs to the family of retroviruses. Epidemiologic features characteristic of HIV-2 are briefly reviewed here. Further information can be found in Kanki and De Cock's review on epidemiology and natural history of HIV-2 (see References).

Although HIV-2 infection has been documented in Africa, Europe, the Americas, and Asia, its spread has remained very limited. It occurs predominantly in West Africa, and to some extent in Angola and Mozambique, and in Portugal. Guinea-Bissau is the major focus of HIV-2, with prevalence rates as high as 13.4% in the male general population. In most other countries of the region, HIV-2 seroprevalence rates of around 2.5% have been documented, with significant variations between countries and population groups.

The epidemiology, risk groups, and routes of transmission of HIV-2 are similar to those of HIV-1. There are, however, several distinctive features of HIV-2 epidemiology that differ from HIV-1. The age of acquisition of HIV-2 appears to be higher than for HIV-1, the prevalence of HIV-2 increases much more slowly than that of HIV-1, and infection in infants and young children is unusual. This supports the hypothesis that the risk of transmission and virulence of HIV-2 is much lower than of HIV-1. Many areas of West Africa are facing double epidemics of HIV, with both HIV-1 and HIV-2 cocirculating in the population. Patients coinfected with both viruses do occur. In countries with dual infections, it appears that the rate of HIV-1 spread is greater than that of HIV-2.

## Prevention of HIV Infection

No single intervention offers the "magic bullet" that will reduce the spread of HIV-1. However, multiple coordinated approaches can be effective. They include educational programs to encourage behavior change, condom promotion, and STD case management. In addition, risk reduction among injecting drug users (e.g., by needle exchange programs), as well as blood donor referral and HIV testing of blood donations, are essential components of a prevention package. Undeniably AIDS prevention interventions have produced long-term risk-behavior reduction in some populations. However, resources need to be sufficient to foster widespread behavior changes, and continued risk reduction depends on sustainable behavior-change programs.

It is essential that preventive interventions be integrated in national AIDS programs, which in turn provide technical support and coordination for all those who work in the field. Interventions are briefly reviewed next. Further information on prevention of HIV infection is noted in the References at the end of the chapter.

## Education

Education refers to interventions aimed at preventing people from engaging in risk behavior by improving their knowledge of the transmission of HIV infection. It must not be aimed only at individuals whose risk of infection is particularly high because they have multiple sex partners, but at all sexually active men and women, and at adolescents before they become sexually active. Educational issues include the reduction of the number of sex partners and/or high-risk practices, the use of barrier methods in high-risk sexual encounters, and women's responsibility to refuse sexual activity that places them at risk of infection. Among the educational channels or techniques are the use of mass media, peer educators, and face-to-face education through testing and counseling.

Mass media include newspapers, magazines, radio or TV programs, and telephone hot lines, aimed at various segments of the general population. Mass media campaigns in Switzerland, using mail and other supports to promote condom use, nonexchange of syringes, and monogamy, demonstrated that both sales and use of condoms increased significantly. In Thailand, "100% condom use" programs were implemented nationwide among sex workers and their clients. Within a short period, condom use among sex workers was shown to increase markedly, while at the same time reported STDs among the same group decreased dramatically (Fig. 97.3).

Peer educators are people of the same background and social standing as their target audiences, who speak the same language and share the same values. Peer education is essential for groups that are stigmatized by mainstream society, like gay men or sex workers, and are therefore suspicious of initiatives from outside. In several American cities peer educators were trained to deliver AIDS risk-reduction messages to fellow gay men. As a result, behavioral change could be demonstrated, at least for the short term.

Another example of peer education is provided by the community-based intervention program of Ciudad Juárez, Mexico. As a result of the program, involving sex workers as peer educators, significant changes in knowledge and practices related to STDs and HIV/AIDS were achieved. Peer educators are also used in community-based programs aimed at reaching at-risk groups like schoolchildren or out-of-school children. Limited experience among high school students in the United States shows that peer-led sex education can help teenagers to postpone the onset of sexual life.

The combination of testing for HIV and counseling both before and after the test aims at changing risk behavior. In their extensive review of counseling and testing, Higgins and coworkers (1991) concluded that this method was fairly effective in reducing high-risk behavior in the gay population, as well as in drug treatment centers, regarding sharing of injecting equipment and sexual behavior among drug users. More recently, counseling and testing were also demonstrated to be effective among discordant couples in the United States. However, limited studies in the United States have indicated only modest impact with STD patients. While short-term impact on condom use could be demonstrated in one study, marked increase in STD incidence was observed in other studies among STD patients counseled about a negative HIV test.

## Promotion of condom use and other barrier methods

However important it is to give people the full range of options for preventing sexual transmission, including abstinence, mutual

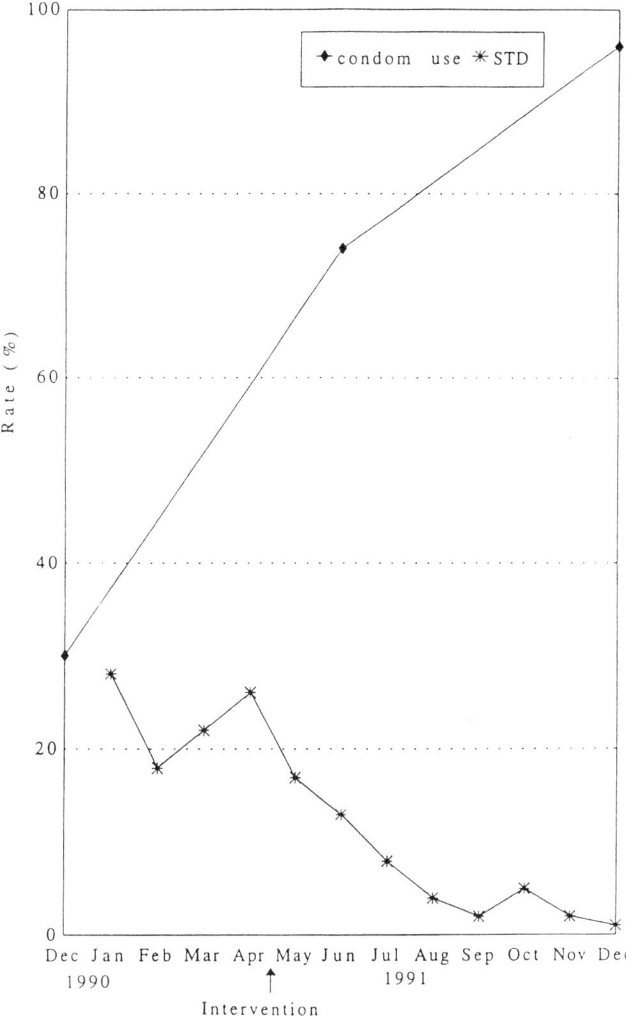


**Fig. 97.3** Increase in condom use and decrease in sexually transmitted diseases (STDs) among sex workers following introduction of 100% condom use, Pitsanuloke, Thailand.

fidelity, and nonpenetrative sex, it is essential to promote condom use and to make it available and inexpensive. In many developing countries, condoms have been distributed effectively through social marketing techniques. The experience of Zaire illustrates the successes of a vigorous condom social marketing program; between 1987 and 1991, condom sales soared from less than half a million to more than 18 million. Similar social marketing programs in several African countries also demonstrate marked increases in condom sales. Overall, condom use has increased in special-risk groups (gays, sex workers, IDUs) wherever preventive interventions have been conducted.

Efforts are still under way to develop barrier methods that can be used by women when they are unable to get their partner to use a condom, or when they otherwise wish to control the prevention process. One of the methods is the "female condom"—essentially a pouch that women can insert into the vagina before intercourse—which is now on the market in several countries, including Switzerland, Great Britain, and the United States. It offers effective protection, but it is expensive. There is an intensive research effort to develop chemical methods that can be applied by a woman without her partner's knowledge, and that can inactivate HIV locally and reduce the risk of acquisition of infection.

### Control of sexually transmitted diseases

Since conventional STDs are recognized risk factors of HIV transmission, STD diagnosis and treatment are key issues in the prevention of sexual transmission of HIV. The efficacy of STD control in preventing HIV was clearly shown in a community-based intervention trial in Mwanza, Tanzania. In those communities where STD control was strengthened HIV incidence was reduced by 42% compared to the control communities. Even outside the context of AIDS, the high burden of mortality and morbidity associated with classic STDs in the developing world and the relatively low cost of treatment justify STD control as a public health priority measure. Last but not least, since the target audiences are identical, STD clinical services offer unique opportunities of conveying credible educational messages regarding both STDs and HIV at the individual level.

### Reduction of vertical transmission

Results from a multicenter randomized double-blind clinical trial in the United States and France in 1995 showed that treatment of HIV-positive mothers and their infants with AZT may reduce by two-thirds the risk for perinatal HIV transmission. In this trial HIV-positive women took AZT during pregnancy, labor, and delivery; their newborns were given 6 weeks of treatment. The full treatment was demanding: 100 mg AZT 5 times/day during pregnancy; intravenous administration of 2 mg/kg followed by 1 mg/kg/hr during labor and delivery; 2 mg/kg every 6 hours in newborns for 6 weeks. No major side effects were observed, but long-term effects are still being assessed. This regimen is now recommended by the U.S. Public Health Service. Unfortunately, because of its cost and complexity, this approach may be of limited accessibility in the developing world, where most cases of mother-to-infant transmission occur.

When safe alternatives to breastfeeding are available, HIV-infected mothers should be advised not to breastfeed, in order to keep their infants uninfected. Yet in developing countries, where no safe alternative exists, WHO and the United Nations Children's Fund (UNICEF) recommend that the risk of HIV infection through breastfeeding be weighed against the benefits of breastfeeding in reducing the infant's risk of dying from infectious diseases or malnutrition.

### Prevention of HIV transmission through blood transfusions

Securing safety of blood supplies is of paramount importance, as the risk of infection through administration of a single contaminated blood transfusion exceeds 90%. In the United States and most Western countries blood safety was effectively accomplished by mid-1985. As part of the safety strategy, reduction of blood utilization in clinical therapeutics and the practice of autotransfusion have been encouraged. However, as reported above, in many developing countries systematic blood testing, as well as recruiting regular voluntary blood donors, has been of limited success.

### Reduction of transmission among injecting drug users

While the main prevention goal should be effective treatment of addiction, harm reduction programs including the distribution of clean needles and syringes have been demonstrated to reduce the HIV threat. These programs have been successful in several countries, including the United States, Australia, New Zealand, Sweden, the Netherlands, and the United Kingdom, in spite of strong political opposition at the beginning, on the grounds that these programs encouraged drug use and undermined the "war on drugs." In addition to providing safe equipment, these programs are effective entry points to other services for previously marginalized people. No evidence of increased drug use has emerged.

### Prevention of HIV transmission in the health care setting

Human immunodeficiency virus as well as other bloodborne pathogens can be transmitted within the health care setting from patient to patient, from patient to health care worker, and, rarely, from health care worker to patient. Transmission by these three routes can be minimized, although not eliminated, through the application of effective infection control practices based on the concept of "universal precautions." This concept assumes that all blood and body fluids are potentially infectious, regardless of whether they are from a patient or health care worker, and regardless of the laboratory test result. This concept is applied through numerous guidelines which include handwashing, careful handling of needles and other sharp objects, use of gloves and other protective barriers as indicated by the nature of the procedure, and sterilization or disposal of instruments as appropriate. Detailed recommendations can be found in Chapter 8.

Accidental occupational exposure to HIV cannot, however, be totally eliminated. Postexposure care includes immediate postexposure interventions, such as decontamination of the exposure site and consideration of chemoprophylaxis with AZT. Follow-up care for exposed persons includes education and counseling until infection is diagnosed or excluded with certainty and careful evaluation of the case. Detailed recommendations on the management of occupational exposure to HIV were published by the Public Health Service.

## ANNOTATED BIBLIOGRAPHY

Centers for Disease Control. 1993 revised classification system for HIV infection and expanded surveillance case definition for AIDS among Adolescents and Adults. MMWR 1992; 41(RR-17):1–19.
*Revised classification of HIV infection, emphasizing the clinical importance of CD4 cell count; primarily intended for public health practice.*

Centers for Disease Control. Zidovudine for the prevention of HIV transmission from mother to infant. MMWR 1994; 43:285–287.
*Results from a double-blind clinical trial suggest that treatment with zidovudine may significantly reduce the risk for perinatal transmission.*

Choi KH, Coates TJ. Prevention of HIV infection. Editorial review. AIDS 1994; 8:1371–1389.
*Review of literature on AIDS prevention programs, attempting to determine the efficacy of interventions on risk behavior.*

Constantine NT. Serologic tests for the retroviruses: approaching a decade of evolution. AIDS 1993; 7:1–13.
*Review of current serologic tests for the retroviruses, including features of newer assays.*

Higgins DL, Galavotti C, O'Reilly KR, et al. Evidence for the effects of HIV-antibody counseling and testing on risk behaviors. JAMA 1991; 266:2419–2429.
*Review of 1986–1990 literature for evidence of counseling and testing on risk behavior.*

Kanki PJ, De Cock KM. Epidemiology and natural history of HIV-2. AIDS 1994; 8(suppl 1):S85–S93.
*A comprehensive review of the virology, epidemiology, and diagnosis of HIV-2, highlighting its differences with HIV-1.*

Laga M, Diallo M, Buvé A. Inter-relationship of sexually transmitted diseases and HIV; where are we now? AIDS 1994; 8(suppl 1):S119–S124.
*Report of recent findings and issues concerning the interaction between HIV and STDs and its public health implications.*

Piot P, Laga M, et al. The global epidemiology of HIV infection: continuity, heterogeneity, and change. J AIDS 1990;3:403–412.
*Review of the changing trends in HIV epidemiology and the impact on health and society.*

World Health Organization. Proposed criteria for interpreting results from Western blot assays for HIV-1, HIV-2, and HTLV-I/HTLV-II. WHO Wkly Epidemiol Rec 1990; 37:281–283.
*Report of a meeting of experts to propose interpretation criteria for positive, negative, and indeterminate results of Western blot for retroviruses.*

World Health Organization/GPA. Consensus statement from the WHO/UNICEF consultation on HIV transmission and breastfeeding. WHO Wkly Epidemiol Rec 1992; 67:177–179.
*Joint WHO and UNICEF statement on weighed risks and benefits of breastfeeding by HIV-infected mothers.*

World Health Organization/GPA. Effective Approaches to AIDS Prevention. Report of a meeting. Geneva, 26–29 May 1992.
*Review of evidence of success of selected interventions, and identification of key elements to share with policymakers involved in AIDS programs in the world.*

UNAIDS/WHO. Report on the global HIV/AIDS epidemic; December 1997.
*UNAIDS Global HIV/AIDS and STD Surveillance.*

# 98

## AIDS Pathogenesis: Molecular Biology and Virology of HIV

J. MICHAEL KILBY AND GEORGE M. SHAW

In 1981, the first published reports of unusual opportunistic infections occurring in otherwise healthy homosexual men from urban centers of the United States led to widespread speculation among the scientific community about the etiology of this apparently rare syndrome. Three years later, the retrovirus that causes the acquired immunodeficiency syndrome (AIDS) was identified. Since that time, a great deal of knowledge about the human immunodeficiency virus (HIV) and its interactions with the immune system has accumulated, although the pathogenic mechanisms of the infection remain incompletely understood. Meanwhile, the scope of AIDS has grown from occasional case reports involving young men in U.S. cities to a worldwide epidemic affecting men, women, and children.

Several recent developments have rapidly altered the landscape of HIV research and are already having a significant impact on the clinical care of HIV-infected patients. Utilizing molecular methods for the quantification of plasma HIV RNA ("viral load") provides reliable estimates of prognosis and allows relatively rapid, dynamic assessments of therapeutic interventions. Highly active antiretroviral therapy ("HAART") regimens containing HIV-1 protease inhibitors have resulted in unprecedented antiviral potency and clinical benefits for many patients, while important insights into viral and cellular dynamics have been derived from scientific analyses of the effects of these potent therapies. The discovery of chemokine co-receptors for HIV entry into cells, which are variably expressed in the population, has contributed to our understanding of HIV cellular tropism as well as host immunogenetic factors which influence the rate of disease progression. This chapter will review how these evolving concepts have helped to shape our current knowledge regarding the pathogenesis of HIV infection.

### Overview of Retroviruses

Retroviruses had been studied for decades prior to the AIDS epidemic, and many were well known to induce solid tumors and leukemia in animals. In 1970, researchers (Temin and Mizutani; Baltimore) independently described the complex life cycle of retroviruses, including the enzyme reverse transcriptase (RT) which has the unique ability to transcribe viral RNA into complementary DNA.

In 1978, Gallo and colleagues discovered the first known human retrovirus, human T-cell leukemia virus (HTLV-1), using novel lymphocyte cell culture techniques. HTLV-I is now known to cause adult T-cell leukemia and a neurologic disease known as tropical spastic paraparesis, or HTLV-associated myelopathy. A second human retrovirus, HTLV-II, was isolated by Gallo et al. in 1982 from a patient with hairy cell leukemia, although this agent has not been definitively linked to any human diseases (see Table 98.1).

Because early epidemiologic investigations suggested that AIDS might be due to an infectious disease spread by blood transfusions and sexual contact, and because affected individuals had progressive declines in their T-lymphocytes, there was interest in searching for a retroviral agent as the cause of the syndrome. In 1983 and 1984, groups led by Gallo at the National Institutes of Health and Montagnier at the Pasteur Institute in Paris first isolated a retrovirus from patients with AIDS. First called lymphadenopathy-associated virus (LAV) and later HTLV-III, further characterization of the virus revealed that it was distinct from oncogenic retroviruses including HTLV-1 and HTLV-II. Instead, the virus resembled members of the lentivirus family in genomic organization, ultrastructure, and general biological properties and it was given the name human immunodeficiency virus type 1 or HIV-1. While HTLV-1 and HTLV-2 cause immortalization and malignant transformation of lymphocytes, HIV-1 is cytopathic for human T lymphocytes *in vitro* and induces (by poorly understood means) a slowly progressive loss of the subset of T cells expressing the CD4 marker *in vivo*.

Complete nucleotide sequencing of HIV-1 was published in 1985. Subsequently, lentiviruses similar to HIV-1 in morphology and genomic organization were found in immunodeficient rhesus macaques in U.S. primate centers. These viruses, designated the simian immunodeficiency viruses (SIV), are now known to infect a variety of African primates without causing obvious pathology, whereas they induce immunodeficiency when inoculated into unnatural primate hosts including Asian macaques and man. The following year a related retrovirus (in fact, phylogenetically more closely related to SIV than to HIV-1) was recovered from humans in West Africa. This was first called HTLV-IV, then LAV-2, and finally HIV-2. HIV-2 also causes lymphopenia leading eventually to AIDS in humans, although it appears to be less infectious and progresses clinically at a slower rate than HIV-1. Controversy remains about the precise phylogenetic relationship among HIV-1, HIV-2, and the many distinct groups of SIV now recognized in different primate species—but it is clear that HIV-1 and HIV-2 both evolved from primate ancestral viruses as a result of zoonotic (subhuman primate to human) spread. The least well-characterized retroviruses that have been occasionally isolated from humans are the "foamy viruses" which belong to the group of spumaviruses and have no proven disease association.

There is overwhelming evidence to indicate that HIV causes AIDS. While the risk factors for AIDS have been present for decades, patients with AIDS-like syndromes were very rare prior

*Acknowledgment:* The authors thank Jennifer Wilson for expert assistance with tables and figures.

**Table 98.1** Human retroviruses

ONCOVIRUSES

Human T-cell Leukemia Virus Type I (HTLV-I)
Associated with tropical spastic paraparesis (TSP), also called HTLV-I-associated myelopathy (HAM), and adult T-cell leukemia.
Human T-cell Leukemia Virus Type II (HTLV-II)
Unknown pathogenic potential—possible association with atypical T-cell hairy leukemia.

LENTIVIRUSES

Human Immunodeficiency Virus Type 1 (HIV-1)—previously called HTLV-III and LAV
Etiologic agent of the acquired immunodeficiency syndrome (AIDS).
Human Immunodeficiency Virus Type 2 (HIV-2)—previously called HTLV-IV or LAV-2
Etiologic agent of some AIDS cases, particularly in West Africa.

SPUMAVIRUSES

Human Foamy Virus
Unknown pathogenic potential—unverified reports of association with thyroiditis, amyotrophic lateral sclerosis, and certain neoplasms.

to the appearance of HIV. HIV can be detected in virtually all patients with AIDS, and with rare exceptions patients who meet clinical criteria for AIDS (including CD4+ lymphocyte depletion) have antibodies specific for HIV in their serum. Studies of transfusion-acquired and perinatally acquired HIV have consistently demonstrated HIV infection in both the "donor" and the "recipient," including cases in which the "recipient" had no other risk factors for HIV infection. Previously healthy laboratory workers, denying other risk factors for HIV infection, have been accidentally exposed to HIV, have become infected with strains of HIV virtually identical in genetic sequence to the laboratory strains to which they were exposed, and have then progressed to AIDS.

Recent technological advances have revealed high levels of viral replication in asymptomatic HIV-infected individuals at times when the virus could not be detected by previous methods. A series of studies clearly demonstrate that baseline viral load levels are highly predictive of the relative risk of disease progression. For example, the proportion of subjects who develop AIDS within a 5-year period increases with increasing baseline viral load (the risk of progression was 8%, 26%, 49%, and 62% among a group of largely untreated subjects who had <4530, 4,531–13,020, 13,021–36,270, and >36,270 HIV RNA copies/mL, respectively, around the time of initial infection). Viral load declines in response to therapy are also predictive of more favorable clinical outcomes. These findings have resulted in the general therapeutic principle that viral load should be suppressed as low as possible for as long as possible.

## General Characteristics of HIV-1

Lentiviruses, like other retroviruses, share a common structure—two copies of a single-stranded RNA genome linked together as a dimer are located inside of a conical core which in turn is surrounded by a bilayered lipid envelope. Each virion is 100–120 nm in diameter, which is comparable to the size of Herpesviruses and less than one-tenth that of a typical bacterium (see Figure 98.1).

The lipid envelope is derived from the host cell membrane as intact virions bud out from infected cells. Therefore, host cell proteins are exposed on the outer surface of the virion along with proteins encoded by the viral genome. Protruding from the surface of the envelope are the viral glycoproteins, gp120 and gp41. It is conventional to designate proteins (p) and glycoproteins (gp) by their mass expressed in kilodaltons. The gp120/gp41 complex plays a crucial role in viral interactions with cells and with all arms of the immune system. The gp120 subunit is known as the external glycoprotein and is responsible for the specific high-affinity interactions with the CD4 molecule as well as the newly characterized chemokine co-receptors expressed on lymphocytes and macrophages. The gp41 subunit is known as the transmembrane glycoprotein and is responsible for anchoring the envelope gp120/gp41 complex, which exists as an oligomer, to the surface of the virion. These subunits are initially translated as a single unit (gp160) which is cleaved by a cellular protease. Associated with the envelope is a layer of matrix protein (p17). The cone-shaped core of HIV is surrounded by the major capsid protein, p24. The core capsid contains two copies of single-stranded RNA and the associated enzymes necessary for replication—reverse transcriptase (RT) and integrase.

The life cycle of HIV (Figure 98.2) parallels that of other retroviruses: (1) invasion of the host cell, (2) reverse transcription of viral RNA into double-stranded DNA, (3) integration of viral DNA into the host DNA to form the provirus, (4) transcription of proviral DNA into messenger RNA (mRNA), (5) translation of mRNA into viral proteins using host cellular machinery, and (6) assembly of viral proteins and nucleic acid into infectious virions which then bud from the cell membrane. Understanding this unique life cycle and the corresponding natural history of HIV infection in greater detail requires a review of the genomic organization and gene regulation of the lentiviruses.

## Organization of the Genome

The genome of HIV-1 is comprised of a single strand of plus sense RNA (that is, corresponding in sequence to the subsequent mRNA strand which will be translated into viral proteins). The complete viral genome is approximately 9,750 base pairs (9.75 kilobases) long (Figure 98.3). This is similar in length but more complicated in organization compared to oncogenic retroviral genomes. HIV-1, HIV-2, and the SIVs contain additional regulatory genes and complex splicing patterns of overlapping reading frames not pre-

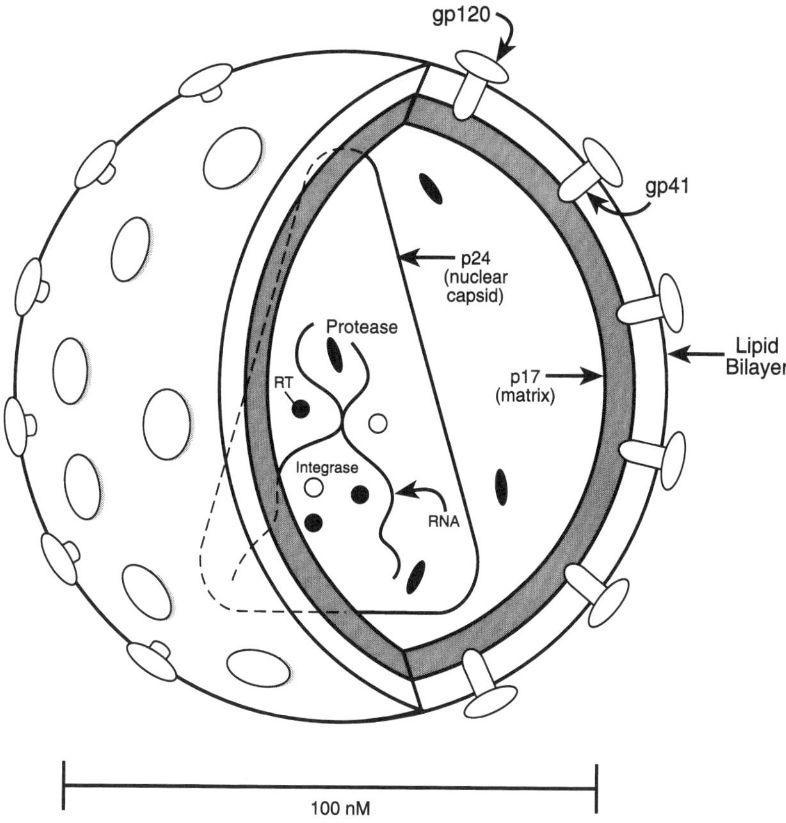


**Fig. 98.1** Schematic representation of the HIV virion.

sent in other retroviruses. Utilization of overlapping reading frames by alternative splicing means that the same genetic sequence can yield different protein products depending on the specific starting point and "reading frame" of translation. In addition, the various mRNAs that are produced can subsequently be spliced into smaller segments or the entire length of the viral genome can be translated into proteins without post-transcriptional splicing. There are more than 30 unique spliced forms of viral mRNA derived from the same proviral DNA genome in HIV. The "early" products of HIV-1 replication (regulatory proteins) are derived primarily from multiply spliced RNA transcripts and the "late" products from unspliced or single-spliced messages. The complex regulation of this differential expression of gene products is critical to the natural history of HIV infection, and ongoing research

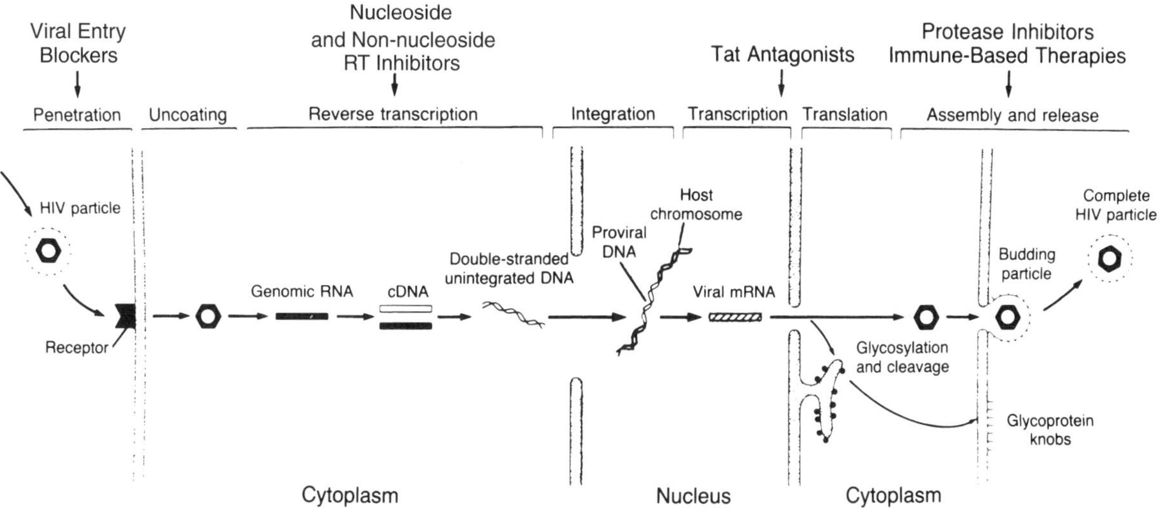


**Fig. 98.2** Diagram of the life cycle of HIV-1, showing the sites of action of some antiviral agents. (Adapted with permission from Hirsch therapy for human immunodeficiency virus infection. N Engl J Med 1993; 328:1687.)

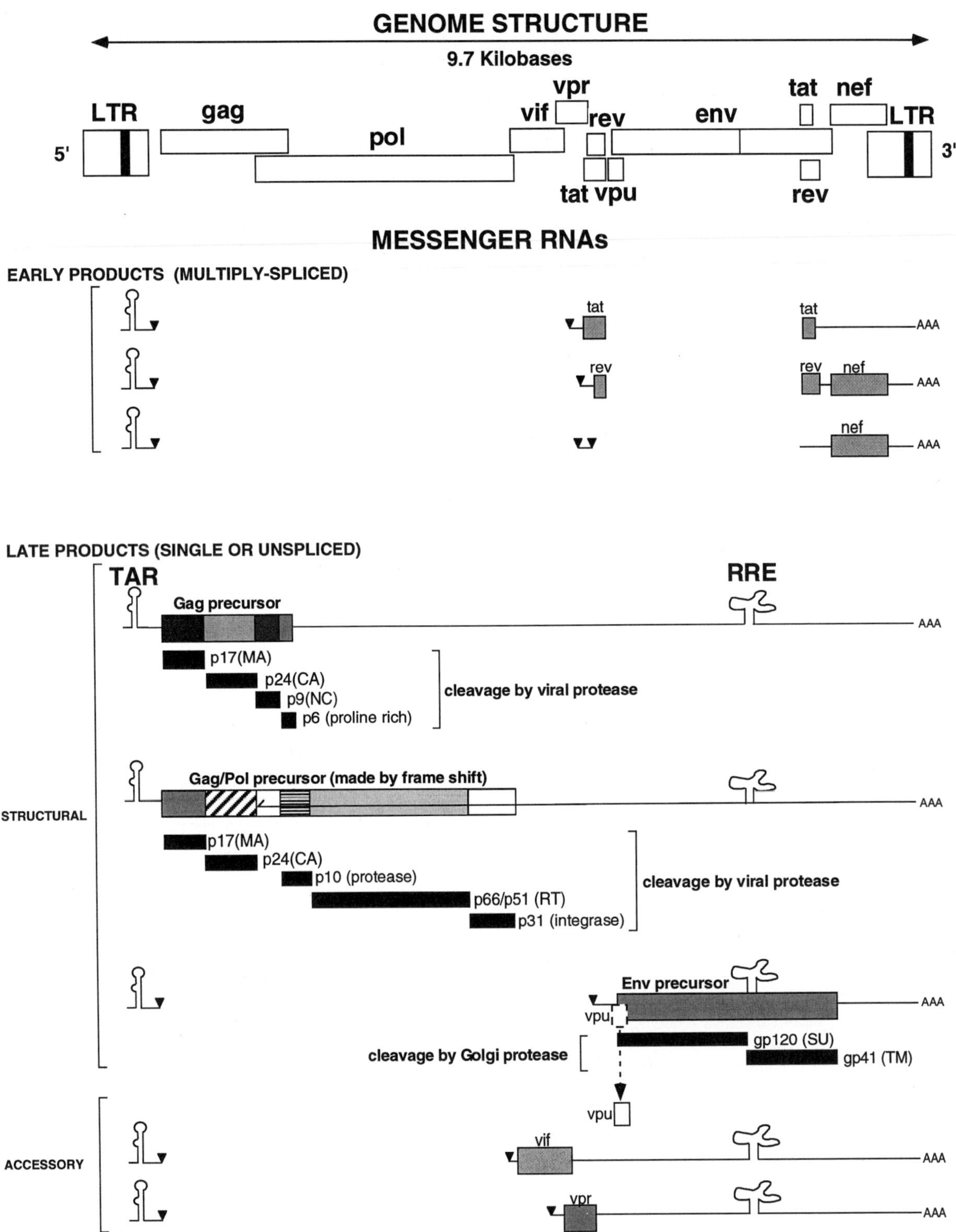


**Fig. 98.3** Genome structure and mRNAs produced by HIV-1. *Triangles* represent major splice sites. See text for abbreviations and further description. (Adapted with permission from Hahn, 1994. Copyright 1994 by Williams and Wilkins.)

in this area may provide important clues toward the development of logical therapeutic interventions.

There are three different types of gene products (Table 98.2) that are produced in varying ratios during the life cycle of HIV-1: (1) structural proteins (GAG,POL,ENV), which form the physical structure of the virion; (2) regulatory proteins (TAT,REV), which regulate transcription and translation but are not major structural components of the viral particle, and (3) accessory proteins (VPR, VIF, VPU, NEF, and in HIV-2, VPX), which may or may not be incorporated into the virion and generally play im-

**Table 98.2** Some HIV-1 genes and their products

| Gene | Size | Function |
|---|---|---|
| VIRAL STRUCTURAL PROTEINS | | |
| *gag | p17<br>p24 | Matrix protein<br>Nuclear capsid |
| *pol | p66/p51<br>p32<br>p10 | Reverse transcriptase<br>Integrase<br>Protease |
| *env | gp120<br>gp41 | External envelope glycoprotein<br>Transmembrane envelope glycoprotein |
| EARLY REGULATORY PROTEINS | | |
| *tat | p14 | Transcriptional and Post-transcription Regulator of gene expression |
| *rev | p19 | Pos-transcriptional regulator of gene expression |
| nef | p27 | Down-regulator CD4 expression |
| LATE REGULATORY PROTEINS | | |
| vif | p23 | Virus infectivity factor |
| vpu | p15 | Inhances assembly and export of new virions, degrades CD4 |
| ACCESSORY PROTEINS | | |
| vpr | p15 | Nuclear localization signals |

*Essential genes for productive *in vivo* infection.

portant but incompletely understood roles in viral replication *in vivo*.

The DNA provirus is flanked on either end (the 5′ or "left-hand side" and the 3′ or "right-hand side" of the genetic sequence) by long terminal repeat (LTR) segments which do not encode proteins but serve to initiate, regulate, and terminate steps of replication. As described below, part of the 5′ LTR region helps to coordinate the translocation of the forming mRNA strands and serves as the starting point for all mRNA transcripts. In the same region is a loop sequence (transactivation response element or TAR) which is the binding site for the regulatory gene product, TAT. In addition to the actions of viral regulatory proteins, there are also important interactions between host cell factors and the LTR region which regulate viral transcription. The 3′ LTR regulates the termination of transcription.

The first gene products formed by an invading virus are derived from multiply spliced messages that constitute the early regulatory elements TAT and REV. TAT, or the trans-activating transcription factor, is derived from a number of differently spliced mRNAs. When the "trans" element (TAT) binds to a "cis" element (TAR in the LTR region), it stimulates RNA transcription. TAT also has other effects including regulation of posttranscriptional events and complex interactions with host cell factors that influence virus replication.

The REV gene product is a second trans-activating element which is an early regulatory gene essential for viral replication; it binds to a "cis" element (the REV response element or RRE) located within the *env* region of the viral RNA. When REV accumulates in the nucleolus, an interaction with the RRE region of the viral mRNA facilitates the nuclear export of unspliced or single-spliced mRNAs. This results in a switch from the production of early regulatory proteins (REV,TAT) to the larger structural proteins (GAG,POL,ENV). Like TAT, REV may have additional posttranscriptional effects and interactions with cellular proteins. Mutant viruses that lack REV are unable to produce infectious progeny, and gene therapy strategies under investigation have been designed to interfere with REV signalling.

The *gag* gene, which is transcribed as a full-length unspliced viral RNA message, encodes the structural proteins of the viral capsid. A polyprotein precursor is cleaved by the viral protease enzyme into subunits corresponding to the matrix protein (p17), the major capsid protein (p24), and smaller proteins (p6 and p9). In addition to facilitating viral assembly, the p17 *gag* product is also involved, along with VPR, in the nuclear import of the viral preintegration complex immediately following infection of a cell by the virus.

The products of the *pol* gene are the enzymes essential to replication. Formation of these products involves translation of part of the *gag* message, and then a frameshift occurs followed by translation of all of the *pol* message, so that a GAG/POL polyprotein precursor results. This polyprotein is then processed by the viral protease into the enzyme products reverse transcriptase (RT), which is comprised of a p66/p51 heterodimer, integrase (p32), and protease itself (p10). Protease is a dimer of two identical subunits which has been structurally characterized by crystallography studies. Detailed analysis of this enzyme, integral for the processing of the viral capsid and transcriptional enzymes into functional proteins, has led to the synthesis of specific protease inhibitors which have dramatically improved antiretroviral treatment outcomes in recent years.

Reverse transcriptase (RT) is also a dimer encoded by the *pol* gene, but one subunit of the dimer (p51 of the p66/p51 heterodimer) has the portion containing RNAse activity trimmed away. RT has at least three important functions: (1) RNA-dependent DNA polymerization, (2) DNA polymerization from a single-stranded DNA intermediate, and (3) RNAse H activity, which degrades the RNA intermediates of reverse transcription. The nucleoside analog RT inhibitors (AZT,ddI,ddC,d4T, 3TC), which were the first approved antiretroviral therapies, compete with natural nucleosides (for example, zidovudine or AZT is an analog of thymidine) and cause premature termination of the elongating DNA chain during reverse transcription. Other inhibitors which block RT function noncompetitively by binding directly to the reverse transcription enzyme (nonnucleoside RT inhibitors such as nevirapine and delavirdine) have become available for clinical use more recently. "HAART" regimens made up of RT inhibitors and protease inhibitors in combination have the potential to lower virus load by as much as 1,000-fold and may significantly alter the natural history of HIV infection.

The remaining essential enzyme, integrase, facilitates the integration of viral DNA into host DNA, an essential step in the viral life cycle. It is capable of cleaving both viral and host DNA so that the provirus can be ligated into the host genome where the cellular DNA repair system completes the integration process. Inhibitors of this enzyme are under investigation.

The envelope proteins are initially translated from a single-spliced mRNA resulting in a gp160 precursor protein. This precursor contains a sequence which signals the protein is to be directed into a secretory pathway where it undergoes significant modification including the addition of many complex sugar moieties (over 50% of the weight of the resulting envelope glycoprotein is carbohydrate). gp160 is then cleaved into gp120 and gp41 by a cellular protease (not by the HIV-1 encoded protease). Nucleotide sequencing of the envelope glycoproteins has revealed highly conserved as well as hypervariable regions which are involved in the many processes carried out by this virus surface protein including cell targeting to CD4 receptors, entry, and syncytium formation.

An early accessory gene product, NEF, is required for viral replication in primary T-lymphocytes *in vitro* and during *in vivo* infection. Adult animals inoculated with SIV defective in NEF become infected, but do not develop immunodeficiency as do animals infected with wild-type virus. NEF was initially labeled as a negative regulator of transcription, but is now known to enhance viral replication in primary cells and to down-regulate CD4 receptor expression, possibly by inducing endocytosis and lysosomal destruction of the CD4 molecule. Deletions in the NEF region result in viral strains with attenuated virulence and an individual with long-term nonprogression (persistently low viral load over many years) has been characterized as having a NEF-deleted strain of HIV. A NEF-deleted mutant retrovirus has been proposed as a potential live attenuated HIV vaccine for humans, but the safety of this approach remains unknown.

A late accessory protein, VPU, is derived from a portion of the genome which overlaps with the *env* region, and its product is an integral membrane protein. This protein increases the rate of assembly and export of new virions out of the infected cell. Another effect of the VPU protein is to induce the degradation of the CD4 molecule inside the cell. Theoretically, the effects of both NEF and VPU on CD4 receptors could prevent superinfection of lymphocytes, limit the destruction of individual T cells, and thereby allow persistent infection to occur. VIF is also the product of a late accessory gene which confers infectivity to HIV-1 virions. Its mechanism of action is unknown, but it is thought to influence virus particle assembly and maturation.

The accessory proteins encoded by *vpr* and *vpx* are unique in that they are packaged into the completed virion in amounts equivalent to the structural proteins. VPR is present in all lentiviruses, while VPX is only found in HIV-2 and some SIV subtypes. The functions of these proteins are not clearly defined, although evidence suggests two effects shared by both—directing the entry of the viral preintegration complex into the nucleus and regulation of cellular differentiation. VPR mediates a cell cycle arrest which may result in increased viral expression in the face of rapid killing of target lymphocytes, thus resulting in viral persistence and a selective advantage over mutant viruses which lack the protein.

## HIV-1 Life Cycle

The entry of HIV-1 into the host cell marks a convenient albeit arbitrary starting point for describing the life cycle of HIV-1 (Figure 98.2). Attachment of HIV to the cell surface is mediated by specific sequences of the gp120 envelope protein that bind to the human CD4 receptor, which normally functions as a receptor for the major histocompatibility complex class II molecules (MHC-II). MHC-II molecules on antigen-presenting cells normally present foreign antigens to CD4+ cells in the process of generating immune responses. Multiple noncontiguous portions of the viral gp120 are brought together by a complex folding pattern to result in a three-dimensional CD4-binding structure. The importance of this gp120-CD4 interaction is supported by evidence that anti-CD4 antibodies can block infection and cell fusion *in vitro*, and that soluble CD4 competes with gp120 for cellular CD4 receptors so that HIV infection is inhibited.

The recent discoveries of several HIV-1 co-receptors help to explain why expression of CD4 is necessary but not sufficient for HIV entry *in vitro*. There is growing evidence that HIV binds to both the CD4 receptor and at least one co-receptor which is present in close proximity to CD4 on the cellular membrane. These co-receptors belong to a class of chemokine receptors which have in common seven membrane-spanning domains. One co-receptor, designated CKR5, tends to bind more selectively to the monocyte-tropic strains of virus which are often transmitted from person to person, while another, CXCR4, binds more readily to the syncytium-inducing, T lymphocyte-tropic virus strains associated with more rapidly progressive disease. As will be discussed further below, these co-receptors, which are variably expressed on different cell types as well as within individual hosts, are providing important insights into the host factors which determine disease progression. Preliminary *in vitro* investigations are already demonstrating the potential for blocking virus entry by inhibiting HIV-1/co-receptor interactions.

The binding of gp120 with cellular receptors appears to trigger conformational changes in the tertiary structure of the transmembrane protein gp41 which then facilitates fusion of the virus particles with the cell membrane. Studies suggest that interfering with these gp41 conformational changes, from a compact helical bundle to a "fusogenic" extended position and back again, provides potent antiretroviral effects *in vitro*. Results from a phase I/IIB clinical trial demonstrate that T-20, a peptide inhibitor of gp41-mediated fusion, substantially suppresses HIV replication in humans and raises the possibility of a new class of antiviral agents.

Cell-derived transfer RNA (tRNA), incorporated into viral particles during assembly, serves as a primer for reverse transcription. There are multiple copies of replication enzymes (RT and integrase) packaged into each virion. RT initiates reverse transcription by binding to a site near the 5′ end of the template and forming the minus strong stop DNA product in the 3′ to 5′ direction with respect to the plus-sense viral RNA strand. The redundant sequences at either end of the genome then mediate the elongating minus-sense DNA strand to the 3′ end of the template where transcription of the remainder of the genome (3′ to 5′ direction) is completed, resulting in a (+)RNA/(−) DNA hybrid. The RNAse H portion of the RT then degrades the original RNA strand as well as the attached tRNA. The DNA-dependent DNA polymerase activity of RT then completes the double stranded DNA provirus. VPR and the p17 GAG matrix proteins play an essential role in early replication events by facilitating the transport of the RNA/DNA/RT/integrase/GAG p17/VPR preintegration complex to the nucleus where reverse transcription is completed and integration of the viral DNA genome into the host cell chromosome is completed. Integrase specifically cleaves small portions from the terminal proviral sequences and from the chromosomal target DNA in order to facilitate integration of viral DNA into the host genome. At this point, transcription and translation of the viral genome are dependent on the cellular machinery as well as TAT and REV.

Once cellular RNA polymerases initiate the formation of viral mRNA transcripts, gene regulation is set in motion with amplification of early regulatory gene products preceding the structural components of the viral particle. The structural proteins are then expressed and processed, eventually leading to assembly of mature virions at the cell membrane. In this final step of virus replication, envelope glycoproteins are arrayed in characteristic fashion on the host membrane, where they are incorporated into the outer viral envelope as the virus buds from the cell surface.

## Viral Phenotype and Cellular Tropism

A pathognomonic laboratory feature of HIV-1 infection is a single-cell cytopathic effect or the formation of multinucleated giant syncytial cells which are short-lived. Syncytium induction has many similarities to the fusion between infecting viruses and cellular membranes, and both processes are orchestrated by interactions between CD4, possibly other cellular proteins, and the gp120/gp41 envelope glycoprotein complex. Both single-cell cytopathic effect and syncytium induction have been postulated to play a role in the destruction of infected cells. Additional mechanisms likely include the targeting of virus-expressing cells for destruction by virus-specific cytotoxic T lymphocytes (CTL) or natural killer (NK) cells.

As described above, the characterization of the chemokine coreceptors has resulted in a better understanding of the determinants of cellular tropism among HIV strains. For example, some naturally occurring strains of HIV-1 efficiently infect primary activated CD4+ lymphocytes and monocyte-macrophages but cannot infect immortalized human CD4+ lymphoblastoid cell lines. Conversely, other naturally occurring strains of HIV-1 efficiently infect primary human CD4+ lymphocytes as well as lymphoblastoid cell lines, where they cause massive syncytium induction but are less able to infect monocyte-macrophages. CKR5 tends to be the co-receptor for the non-syncytium-inducing (NSI) HIV isolates, while syncytium-inducing (SI) isolates primarily bind to the CXCR4 co-receptor. In patients with early, asymptomatic HIV infection, NSI viral variants usually predominate. Patients with advanced AIDS are more likely to be infected with SI viral strains. Precipitous declines in CD4 counts have been associated with the transition from NSI to SI phenotype in some patients. An analagous evolution of HIV-1 co-receptor usage appears to occur during disease progression as well. While the clinical utility of determining NSI/SI and co-receptor phenotypes remains uncertain, it is clear that ongoing study of these issues will contribute to our understanding of the host determinants for HIV progression.

## Viral and Cellular Dynamics

Because surrogate markers of HIV-1 infection such as the CD4+ cell count were imperfect in measuring the clinical response to antiretroviral therapies or in calculating the risk of disease progression, a more direct assay of viral burden within an individual was critically needed for the study of HIV pathogenesis-based clinical trials, determining prognosis, and monitoring responses to therapeutic interventions. Polymerase chain reaction (PCR) methods allow detection of HIV-1 RNA with 60,000-fold the sensitivity of quantitative microculture techniques, and they provide a much better marker of viral load than serum p24 antigen. PCR and branched DNA (bDNA) amplification methods can now be used to demonstrate large numbers of HIV particles in plasma of patients during all phases of HIV infection. Based on the evidence that viral load is tightly correlated with disease progression and changes in plasma viremia correlate with clinical responses to antiretroviral therapy, PCR-based viral load determinations have become a standard tool in the clinical care of HIV-infected patients. Although the widespread availability of viral load assays is relatively new, interim recommendations for their utilization in clinical practice have been published.

HIV-1 can be routinely detected and quantified as cell-free virus in plasma; within lymphocytes and monocyte-macrophages in the blood (primarily in lymphocytes); and in secondary lymphoid organs such as lymph nodes, the spleen, and gut-associated lymphoid tissue. Figure 98.4 shows the general relationship that exists between virus in these tissue compartments and the observed declines in CD4+ lymphocytes in HIV-1-infected individuals.

Investigations of changes in viral replication rates and the rapid selection for drug-resistant strains among patients receiving potent antiretroviral regimens provided important new perspectives on the viral and cellular dynamics characterizing HIV infection. These and subsequent studies revealed that plasma HIV has a very short half-life and that a large number of CD4+ lymphocytes undergo de novo infection on a daily basis. One interpretation of these studies is that the constant and tremendous viral replication which is occurring even in stable, asymptomatic individuals is counter-balanced by constant production of new uninfected lymphocytes, perhaps by peripheral expansion of existing cells.

Alternatively, it has also been proposed that the rise in CD4 cell counts observed following successful antiviral therapy is at least in part a matter of trafficking . A large decrease in viral antigen production could result in less antigen-trapping of activated lymphocytes in the lymphoid tissues so that a much larger proportion of lymphocytes are measurable in the circulation. This theory is based on evidence that in adults the number of CD4+ cells is relatively fixed, that these cells are long-lived unless they become activated (which typically triggers apoptosis), and that there is little capacity to rapidly replenish depleted or destroyed lymphocytes. This is supported by a study of lymphocytes obtained from HIV-infected individuals over the course of HIV progression which concluded that while CD8+ cells show telomere-shortening which is characteristic of ongoing high cellular turnover, CD4+ cells do not. While it is clear that patients benefit from the "T-cell reconstitution" that occurs when HAART

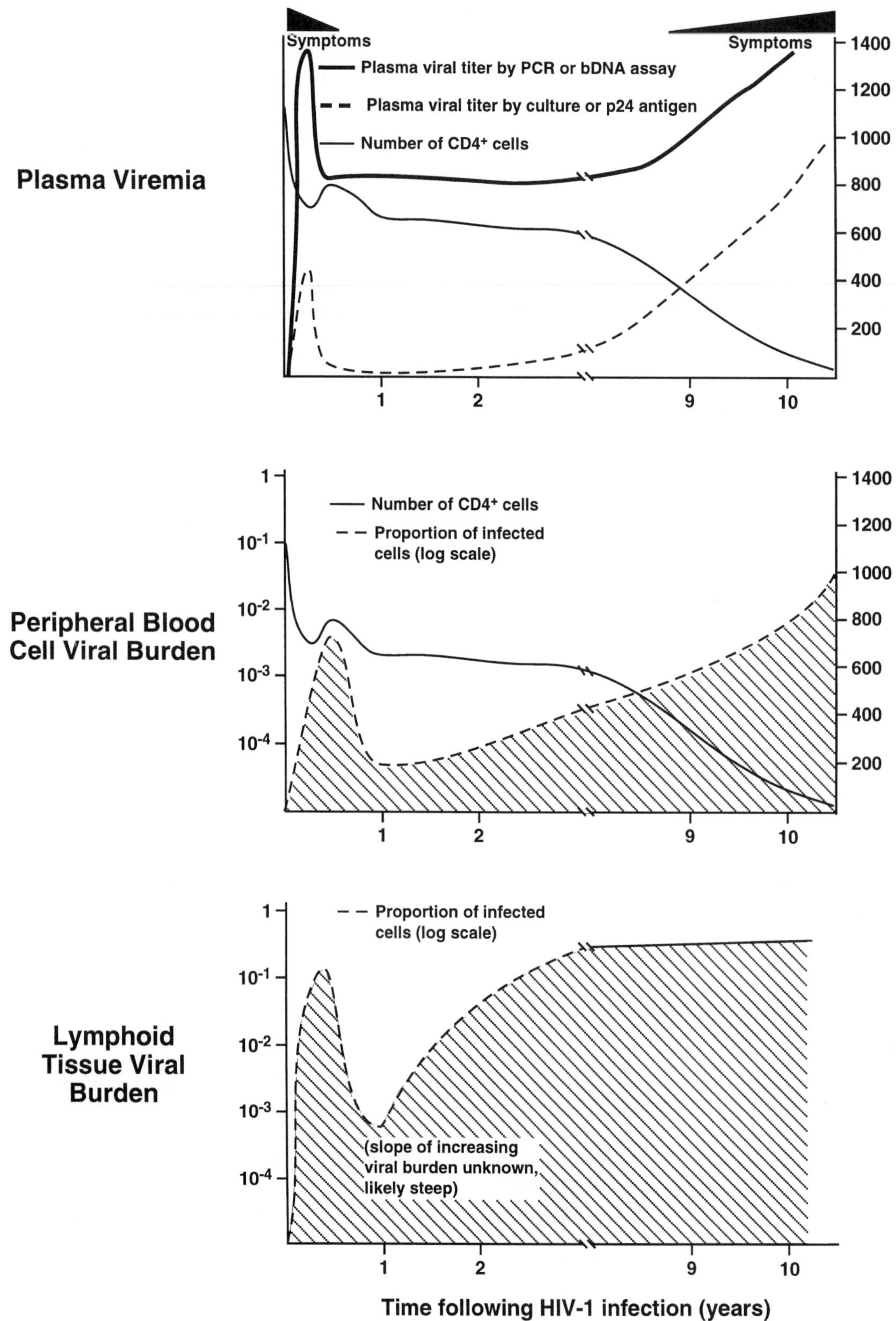


**Fig. 98.4** Representation of the natural history of HIV-1 infection. In the top graph, relative plasma viral load is depicted over time along with typical symptomatic periods and the progressive loss of CD4+ cells. The middle and bottom graphs depict the estimated proportion (expressed in log scale) of peripheral blood cells and lymphoid tissue cells, respectively, which are infected with HIV-1 over the same time period following initial exposure.

is initiated, the true nature of the cellular dynamics during HIV infection and treatment remain controversial and incompletely understood.

The prolonged suppression of viral load below detectable levels in some patients receiving antiretroviral regimens has led to speculation about the prospects of complete eradication of HIV infection from a patient. Two recent reports demonstrate, however, that patients who have had undetectable plasma viremia for as many as 30 months still have latently HIV-infected lymphocytes. By utilizing techniques to activate quiescent T cells, these two studies found that replication-competent virus could still be produced from resting lymphocytes. The frequency of latently infected cells appears to be quite low (roughly one per million cells) but, at least in a cross-sectional analysis, this reservoir does not decrease over time on therapy.

Now that HAART has apparently achieved complete suppression of viral replication in the bloodstream of some patients, the next frontier in HIV therapeutics may be to explore the role of immunomodulation in attempting to clear latently infected cells from the body. Clinical events or interventions that alter the activation state of the cellular immune system are known to influence viral load. Activation of the immune system, for example, may at least transiently increase plasma viremia during opportunistic infections, following the administration of vaccines, or when intravenous interleukin-2 is administered. At the opposite extreme, when immunosuppressive corticosteroid therapy is given to advanced AIDS patients with paradoxical immunoactivation and wasting syndrome, temporary declines in viral load are seen. Randomized clinical trials are currently being designed to explore the effects of immunoactivating interventions (IL-2 and vaccinations) on the frequency of latently infected cells in HIV-infected patients.

## HIV Variability and Antiretroviral Resistance

RNA viruses in general replicate with less fidelity than the more familiar DNA genomes present in other viruses, bacteria, and animals. Eigen and others theorized that self-replicating fragments of RNA were the predecessors to the first life on earth. These error-prone RNA's would rapidly form swarms of mutant progeny resulting in an ever-changing pool of variants with great genetic diversity termed "quasispecies." This concept of the quasispecies has been applied to HIV infection. The reverse transcriptase (RT) enzyme in retroviruses is particularly prone to errors during transcription, in part because it lacks a system to recognize and correct mistakes in base pair matching as they occur during DNA polymerization. The absence of viral DNA proofreading mechanisms combined with the innumerable replication cycles required to sustain HIV-1 infection *in vivo* over years results in the development of substantial viral genetic complexity in infected patients over time.

Studies of the variable regions of the HIV-1 envelope have shown that the rates of mutation during viral replication may be as much as one-million-fold more than that seen in cellular DNA systems. The coexistence of multiple genetic sequences (genotypes) as well as the rapid evolution of viral subtypes within a single infected individual have been convincingly demonstrated. Thus, it is a misconception to state that a patient is infected by a single viral isolate; instead, each individual harbors a dynamic, complex population of related but distinct viruses. A virtually imperceptible selective advantage can drive the evolution of this pool of viruses because they replicate so rapidly and mutate so frequently. Therefore, the influence of host immune responses or antiviral drugs, for example, on the make-up of the viral population in a single patient may be enormous. The same population of viruses may behave differently under one set of circumstances (in an *in vitro* assay) than it does in another (in the complex milieu of a recently infected, immunocompetent individual), because of genetic drift that occurs due to the selective advantage of one mutational variant over another. *In vitro* cultivation selects for a more homogenous viral population than that which is found in patients, thus underestimating the potential for *in vivo* evolution of a diversity of viral subtypes.

The diverse viral pool within an infected patient is not a random assortment, but instead represents branches derived from progenitor viruses responsible for the initial infection of that individual. Understanding patterns of retroviral evolution has moved researchers closer to mapping phylogenetic trees describing the origins of the lentiviruses. Similar strategies can be used to help resolve epidemiologic issues, such as providing evidence of the genetic relatedness of HIV strains obtained from an HIV-infected dentist and his patients in a highly publicized case of HIV-1 transmission.

The greatest variability in the HIV-1 genome occurs in the envelope sequence, while the *gag* and *pol* regions are relatively more conserved. *Env* mutations are of many types (deletions, insertions, duplications, and single-base substitutions) while *gag* and *pol* mutations more often are single-point mutations. This reflects the more strict structural limitation in GAG and POL proteins. Serial viral isolates may vary by approximately 1% each year in the *env* region, so that a single patient may have *env* sequences that vary from one another by 10% or more. HIV-1 isolates obtained from individuals in geographically distinct areas, in comparison, have been found to vary by as much as 25% in the envelope sequence. The envelope glycoproteins are made up of conserved regions interspersed with hypervariable loop regions which serve as antigenic epitopes.

There is great interest in finding effective neutralizing antibodies and cytotoxic T-cell responses directed at these crucial antigenic envelope sites, but genetic drift may occur in response to the selective forces of the immune system making effective vaccines difficult to develop. For example, serial isolates obtained from a patient with primary HIV infection show that the initial antiviral pressure exerted by cytotoxic T cells which are HIV-1-specific is lost over time as mutated "escape virus" is selected out which is no longer recognized by the host CTL. Thus, viral escape from immune responses may be comparable to the evolution of drug-resistant virus.

Vaccine efforts and some gene therapy strategies must also take into account predominant virus strains that circulate in particular geographic areas of interest. Virus strains which have highly similar genetic sequences have been categorized into "clades" or genetically related subtypes. An extreme example of HIV-1 heterogeneity is the HIV-1 group O, which was not sufficiently homologous to other HIV-1 (or HIV-2) subtypes to be consistently detected by previous HIV-1 or HIV-2 ELISA diagnostic tests. HIV-1 group O appears to have originated in Cameroon (West Africa), but numerous cases have been identified in Europe.

Attention continues to be focused on efficient methods to characterize the susceptibility of virus strains to antiretroviral drugs. The ideal system would allow the isolation of viral strains that are representative of the different tissue compartments and of virus expressing the range of cytopathicity (NSI and SI) present *in vivo*. A method was developed which utilized an immortalized epithelial cell line (HeLa) expressing the CD4 receptor (HeLa-T4 cells) as a cell target for quantifying drug-sensitive and drug-resistant viruses. HeLa cells predictably form plaques or syncytia within three days of *in vitro* infection by SI virus, and further cultivation of these infected cells in the presence of varying dosages of drug (i.e., AZT) permits a quantitative measurement of susceptibility based on the relative reduction of plaque formation. This method is reproducible and effective, but is limited only to SI phenotypes, which make up about one-third of clinical HIV isolates.

Another assay has therefore been developed which is not dependent on syncytium formation. This method, based on cocultivation of HIV-infected PBMCs from infected patients with PHA-stimulated PBMCs from normal donors, entails the measurement of p24 antigen levels in order to quantitate viral replication in the presence or absence of drug. Approximately 2 weeks are necessary to generate a standardized virus inoculum of the clinical isolate, which can then be assayed for drug susceptibility in the third week. This assay is thus more time-consuming and labor-intensive, but it is applicable to a wider range of viral isolates.

Understanding the molecular biology of the RT and the protease sequences within the *pol* gene has been crucial to studies of the development of antiretroviral resistance. For example, patients on prolonged AZT monotherapy develop characteristic point mutations in the RT region that confer *in vitro* resistance to AZT. The development of predominantly resistant HIV-1 virus strains *in vivo* correlates with clinical progression and lack of responsiveness to therapy. While complete sequencing of the protease and RT regions of viral isolates serves as an important research tool and has become available in some clinical settings, it is not clear whether treatment decisions should be based on these investigational results. Methods are also in development which utilize computer chip technology to rapidly probe viral isolates for the presence of resistance-conferring mutations.

Drug resistance occurs when there is inadequate viral suppression, and therefore single-agent therapy is no longer recommended for HIV management. Until recently, antiretroviral therapies which could completely suppress viral replication were not available, and eventual selection of drug-resistant viral strains seemed inevitable for all treated patients. The development of clinically significant viral resistance appears to be delayed when potent combination antiretroviral therapy is administered to treatment-naive patients. The virus isolates produced by the *in vitro* activation of latently infected cells derived from patients with long-term antiretroviral suppression do not contain mutations commonly associated with drug resistance. This suggests that while viral eradication is not achieved in these patients, viral suppression is possible to the extent that there is little or no evolution of drug-resistant virus over years in these individuals.

## Natural History of HIV Infection

The natural history of (untreated) HIV infection consists of (1) high plasma viremia following initial infection, (2) a clinically quiescent phase of variable length (average of 10 years) during which viral replication continues but at a lesser degree and the CD4 lymphocytes decline gradually, and finally (3) progressive, inexorable CD4 depletion which correlates with a return to very high levels of viral replication in the bloodstream and a greater risk for opportunistic infections and malignancies (see Figure 98.4).

### Primary HIV infection

Early studies of homosexual men at risk for HIV-1 infection demonstrated that several patients developed a mononucleosis-like syndrome that preceded HIV-1 seroconversion. These individuals noted onset of malaise, fever, arthralgias, headache, sore throat, diarrhea, lymphadenopathy, and a transient erythematous macular rash, all of which occurred 6 to 56 days following a likely exposure to the virus. Approximately half of HIV-infected patients can recall a similar viral syndrome antedating seroconversion. Subsequent studies have evaluated patients who developed symptomatic primary HIV-1 infection by in-depth virologic and molecular analyses. High titers of infectious virus could be cultured from both the plasma and PBMC of patients during the first 2 weeks after onset of symptoms. This impressive viral load, confirmed by PCR techniques, decreased precipitously within 2 to 4 weeks as symptoms resolved, consistent with the hypothesis that an initially effective host response was suppressing viral replication. The decrease in plasma viremia (and often the resolution of clinical symptoms) occurs coincidentally with an expansion of HIV-specific CD8+ cytotoxic T cells as well as the development of specific antibodies. The relative contributions of the humoral and cellular responses in at least temporarily curtailing viral replication is further discussed in the chapter on Immunology.

The development of antibodies to virtually all HIV structural proteins forms the basis of the current ELISA and confirmatory Western immunoblot. A variable "window" of time thus exists following initial exposure to virus during which patients are viremic and highly infectious but have false negative HIV-1 serologies. These patients often have very high viral loads (~1 million HIV RNA copies/mL) and detectable p24 antigen. The acute viral syndrome is variably characterized by a temporary decrease in CD4+ cells which is rarely associated with opportunistic infections such as *Pneumocystis* pneumonia or *Candida* esophagitis typically seen in much later stages of AIDS. CD4+ cells generally rebound to normal levels within months, although they seldom return to the values seen prior to infection.

There is intriguing evidence that some individuals who have been exposed repeatedly to HIV-1 express HIV-specific, cell-mediated immunity without developing any of the typical serological markers of active HIV infection and without having culturable virus in their blood. These findings suggest that it may be possible for the immune system to successfully eradicate virus following exposure under some circumstances. Individuals who remain uninfected with HIV despite high-risk exposures are more likely to express an uncommon homozygous deletion of the CKR5 receptor which renders their cells less susceptible to entry of HIV. Heterozygotes for this CKR5 defect, which can occur in up to 20% of caucasians in the United States, are overrepresented among patients with long-term nonprogressive HIV infection as compared with patients with more typical HIV disease progression. Similar associations are being explored for other putative chemokine HIV-1 co-receptors. At the other extreme, there are patients whose CD4+ counts remain markedly depressed after acute infection, leading to higher morbidity or earlier mortality. Prolonged symptoms during primary HIV-1 infection have been associated with more rapid progression to AIDS.

### HIV and the lymphoid organs

It has been theorized that primary HIV infection with a monocyte-tropic NSI virus could infect specialized monocyte/

macrophages such as Langerhans cells located in skin or mucosal tissues. These cells would then migrate to lymphoid tissues to serve as antigen-presenting cells. In this manner, lymphoid organs could be the critical site where the initial waves of CD4+ lymphocytes are first infected as they circulate through the tissues.

Most patients who become infected by HIV-1 experience a prolonged period of clinical quiesence following seroconversion (whether or not a symptomatic acute viral syndrome was noted) lasting for years in which they have no or very minimal symptoms of infection. Typically, PCR and bDNA methods demonstrate relatively lower levels of HIV-1 in plasma compared with late stage patients, although in most infected individuals plasma virus titers range from $10^2$ to $10^7$ virions per milliliter. *In situ* hybridization methods have generally demonstrated 10- to a 100-fold more virus DNA and RNA in lymphoid tissues than in peripheral blood cells during the asymptomatic period, suggesting that there is significant ongoing viral replication not detected by more routine clinical studies. It is thus believed that much of the pathophysiology of HIV-1 infection occurs within the secondary lymphoid organs where viral trapping, *de novo* cell infection, and virus production are all known to occur throughout infection. Image analysis of lymphoid tissue biopsies reveals a large proportion of follicular dendritic cell-associated extracellular viral material and a smaller population of productively infected mononuclear cells. In the presence of HAART, the amount of both FDC-trapped virus and productively infected cells appears to diminish markedly along with declines in plasma viremia. Our colleagues have developed a novel integrated approach to tissue analysis which suggests that the proportion of FDC-trapped extracellular virus in lymph node tissue is quite variable from patient to patient. Productively infected T cells generate a remarkably constant amount of viral replication (about 4,000 HIV RNA copies per infected cell) regardless of the stage of HIV disease and the presence or absence of treatment.

In the late stages of HIV infection, involution of the lymph node germinal center occurs and the node takes on a characteristic "burned out" appearance. This destruction of the lymph node architecture could lead to decreased effectiveness of cellular and humoral immunity, resulting in the unchecked viremia seen in late-stage AIDS.

## HIV and the brain

Some form of central nervous system pathology has been reported at all stages of HIV infection. During the primary HIV syndrome, occasional patients have neurologic complications such as aseptic meningitis, encephalitis, cranial neuropathies, a Guillian-Barre-like syndrome, or peripheral neuropathies. These are typically self-limited and may be comparable to other neurologic syndromes attributed to virus infection. However, even in asymptomatic patients who lack signs of neurologic dysfunction, HIV can be cultured or detected by PCR in cerebrospinal fluid. Many patients have mild CSF pleocytosis and elevated protein levels even though they are clinically asymptomatic.

CNS disease is more common later in HIV infection and is generally correlated (at postmortem examination) with the degree of multinucleated giant cell encephalitis and accompanying HIV-1 expression in these macrophage-derived cells. Neuronal loss appears to correlate with overall viral load as well. Patients with HIV dementia often have demonstrable improvement when AZT is administered and viral burden in the bloodstream decreases. Encephalopathy or subcortical dementia are frequent complications of AIDS, but the pathology seen on brain biopsies is somewhat heterogenous. The most common histopatholgic finding is multinucleated giant cell encephalitis. Some patients have a vacuolar myelopathy or diffuse white matter disease in which productive HIV infection may not be seen. Cells of true neuroectodermal origin have been infected *in vitro*, but infection of these cells *in vivo* does not appear to occur. The mechanism by which HIV-1 infection of macrophage-derived cells causes dementia is unknown, but it is presumably due to an indirect effect of macrophage products (including viral glycoproteins) on neurons and other cellular elements within the brain parenchyma.

Viruses isolated from the brain of patients with AIDS typically demonstrate macrophage tropism, which explains the infection of microglia and multinucleated giant cells, both of which are derived from monocyte-macrophage precursors.

## HIV clinical latency and "nonprogressors"

Even in the era before HAART, the average HIV-1-infected individual exhibited a period of 10 to 12 years following primary HIV infection during which there were no obvious signs of illness, although the duration of clinical latency in any one patient is quite variable. There is typically a very gradual decrease in CD4 levels (approximately 50 cells/mm$^3$ or less per year) prior to the first overt manifestations of immunosuppression. The factors that contribute to an acceleration of disease progression after such a prolonged latency are poorly understood. There is immense interest in the rare HIV-infected individuals, labeled "long-term nonprogressors," who have maintained stable CD4 cell counts after as many as 15 years. These patients represent more than statistical "outliers" since in some cases the viruses obtained from them have been shown to be genetically defective, such as the well-characterized individual with NEF-deleted HIV infection. In other cases, particular host factors may be determinants of survival, such as the chemokine co-receptor mutations previously described or genetically determined immune responses related to the major histocompatibility complex (MHC).

Rare individuals have been described who have delayed or absent HIV seroconversion and who experience a much more rapid decline in CD4+ lymphocyte counts, progressing to AIDS within a year of infection. Although virulence factors associated with the virus *per se* have also been postulated, none except for the SI phenotype have been conclusively identified. However, SI phenotype is not required for rapid disease progression to occur. Host factors or coinfections could play a role in triggering the more rapid pace of immunosuppression and disease that occurs late in HIV infection. Coinfections with other pathogens may accelerate HIV pathogenesis, for example, by increasing the susceptibility of cells to infection or by activating latently infected T cells so that replication of proviral material is accelerated.

## CD4 depletion

The fundamental question of how HIV infection leads to depletion of CD4 cells remains a major obstacle to more fully understanding the pathogenesis of AIDS. Recent evidence linking ongoing virus replication closely with CD4+ cell declines indicates that virus may play a direct role in cell killing. In addition, the much more rapid turnover of virus-expressing cells as compared with uninfected or latently infected CD4+ lymphocytes shown in the same studies suggests that virus expression *per se*, rather than an "innocent bystander" or "autoimmune" effect, is primarily involved in cell destruction. It is widely believed that cytopathic effects of the virus itself and virus-specific cell killing by cytotoxic T cells plays a dominant role in CD4+ cell destruction. Apoptosis, or programmed cell death, has also been suggested as a specific mechanism of cell killing.

## Conclusion

The various models of HIV pathogenesis outlined here are not mutually exclusive. A number of host and viral factors likely contribute to the ultimate development of immunodeficiency and corresponding high-level viremia that characterize the end stages of AIDS. Much progress has been made in understanding this complex infection, and continued efforts to explore basic virology and molecular biology, in conjunction with clinical trials, should bring our view of HIV pathogenesis into clearer focus.

### ANNOTATED BIBLIOGRAPHY

Barre-Sinoussi F, Chermann JC, Rey F, et al. Isolation of a T-lymphotropic retrovirus from a patient at risk for acquired immune deficiency syndrome (AIDS). Science 1983; 220:868–870.

Popovic M, Sarngadharan MG, Read E, Gallo RC. Detection, isolation, and continuous production of cytopathic retroviruses (HTLV-III) from patients with AIDS and pre-AIDS. Science 1984; 224:497–500.

*These two articles by investigative groups at the Pasteur Institute in Paris and the National Institutes of Health describe the initial isolation of the retrovirus that causes AIDS. The series of* Science *articles by Gallo and colleagues beginning with the one by Popovic et al. above further characterize the virus, the T-cell culture technique employed to isolate it, and the correlation with serologic tests.*

Clark SJ, Saag MS, Decker WD, et al. High titers of cytopathic virus in plasma of patients with symptomatic primary HIV-1 infection. N Eng J Med 1991; 324:954.

Daar ES, Moudgil T, Meyer RD, Ho DD. Transient high levels of viremia in patients with primary HIV-1 infection. N Eng J Med 1991; 324:961.

*These two groups independently followed groups of patients at risk for HIV and were able to characterize in detail the "acute retroviral syndrome" from the molecular, virologic, and immunologic standpoints.*

Dean M, Carrington M, Winkler C, et al. Genetic restriction of HIV-1 infection and progression to AIDS by a deletion of the CKR5 structural gene. Science 1996; 273:1856–1862.

*This article provided strong evidence that ongoing studies of chemokine coreceptors by a number of independent investigators could have clinically relevant applications.*

Ho DD, Moudgil T, Alam M. Quantitation of HIV-1 in the blood of infected persons. N Eng J Med 1989; 321:1621–1625.

*This article describes the technique of quantitative microculture, which helped to confirm the presence of the virus throughout all stages of HIV infection.*

Mellors JW, Kingsley LA, Rinaldo CR, et al. Prognosis in HIV-1 infection predicted by the quantity of virus in plasma. Science 1996; 272:1167–1170.

*First in a series of articles that demonstrated the tight link between virus load and progression of HIV disease.*

Pantaleo G, Graziosi C, Demarest JF, et al. HIV infection is active and progressive in lymphoid tissue during the clinically latent stage of disease. Nature 1993; 362:355–358.

*At a time when the concept that HIV was the cause of AIDS was being called into question by some outspoken critics, this article revealed the importance of ongoing tissue viral burden among asymptomatic patients without severe immunodeficiency. The analysis of lymphoid tissue has now become a major focus for many investigations into the pathogenesis of AIDS.*

Piatak M, Saag MS, Yang LC, et al. High levels of HIV in plasma during all stages of infection determined by QC-PCR. Science 1993; 259:1749.

*Advancements in the polymerase chain reaction provided the foundation for a practical tool to measure viral load in research and clinical practice settings.*

Wei X, Ghosh SK, Taylor ME, et al. Viral dynamics in HIV-1 infection. Nature 1995; 373:117–122.

Ho DD, Neumann AU, Perelson AS, Chen W, Leonard JM, Markowitz M. Rapid turnover of plasma virions and CD4 lymphocytes in HIV-1 infection. Nature 1995; 373:123–126.

*These two articles mathematically modeled the responses to potent antiretroviral therapies to characterize the high level of viral replication and turnover that occurs even in stable, asymptomatic HIV-infected patients.*

Wong JK, Hezareh M, Gunthard HF, Havlir DV, Ignacio CC, Spina CA, Richman DD. Recovery of replication-competent HIV despite prolonged suppression of plasma viremia. Science 1997; 278:1291–1295.

Finzi D, Hermankova M, Pierson T, et al. Identification of a reservoir for HIV-1 in patients on highly active antiretroviral therapy. Science 1997; 278:1295–1300.

*These investigations demonstrate the good news and the bad news about recent advancements in antiretroviral therapy. While there has been unprecedented success in suppressing the plasma viremia which appears to drive the clinical progression to AIDS, long-lived latently infected T cells can still be stimulated to produce replication-competent HIV under the right immunoactivating conditions.*

# 99

# AIDS Immunology

SHARON A. STRANFORD AND JAY A. LEVY

Infection by the human immunodeficiency virus (HIV) results in severe disruptions to the homeostasis of the host immune system. Some of these disruptions, such as enhanced antibody production and a decrease in the $CD4^+/CD8^+$ cell ratio, are universal features of this infection. Other immune alterations, such as lymph node architecture damage and the magnitude of $CD4^+$ cell depletion, are more variable (see Table 99.1 for a list of immunologic abnormalities associated with HIV infection). Differences in these less predictable clinical markers are most likely a result of diversity in host immune response and/or specific substrains of the virus encountered. In this chapter we discuss the effects that infection with HIV-1 has on the cells and tissues of the immune system, the range of potential antiviral immunologic responses generated by the host, and some autoimmune or oncogenic sequelae.

## Effects of HIV Infection on the Immune System

### Changes in lymphocyte subsets

Two clinical features which are consistently observed following HIV infection are a decrease in the number of cells expressing the CD4 molecule and an increase in overall immune activation. This latter finding is evidenced by an elevation in the $CD8^+$ cell subset of peripheral blood mononuclear cells (PBMCs), hypergammaglobulinemia (see below), and increased expression of cell surface activation markers. These cell surface indicators of immune activation, such as major histocompatibility complex (MHC) class II (DR), CD38, and interleukin 2 (IL-2) receptor (CD25), are normally elevated in HIV-infected individuals, especially within the $CD8^+$ lymphocyte subset. Determinations of these and other immunologic markers are routinely performed using flow cytometry and can be evident very early, even during the acute stage of HIV infection.

Although there are no clear correlations of cell surface markers with prognosis, certain changes are consistently noted over time. Progression to acquired immunodeficiency syndrome (AIDS) is frequently accompanied by rapidly decreasing $CD4^+$ cell numbers (especially those expressing the $CD29^+$ memory cell molecule), increasing numbers of $CD8^+$ $DR^+$ $CD38^+$ memory-type cells (CD45RO), and a loss of $CD8^+$ lymphocytes bearing the costimulatory molecule CD28. This loss of $CD4^+$ memory cells results in impaired antigenic stimulation responses and therefore increased susceptibility to common pathogens. With disease progression there is a stepwise decrease in proliferative responses to (*1*) recall antigens, (*2*) alloantigens, and finally (*3*) mitogens, which is most likely due to loss of this particular cell phenotype. Similarly, a reduction in the number of $CD8^+$ lymphocytes bearing the CD28 molecule translates into a loss of cells capable of receiving the costimulatory signals required for full antigenic activation. Thus the observed loss of important T-cell functions during disease development is mirrored by changes within specific lymphocyte subsets (i.e., cell surface molecule expression) as well as in the overall PBMC percentages of these key mediators of protective immune responses.

Recently, studies have been undertaken to evaluate the specific T-cell receptor (TCR) $V\beta$ repertoire expression of the initial $CD8^+$ cell population which expands immediately after HIV infection. Several HIV-exposed individuals were studied soon after the onset of acute viral symptoms (days 16–136). There were three general patterns of TCR repertoire expression observed within this group: prolific expansion of cells expressing a single $V_\beta$ gene segment, modest increases in cells expressing several different $V_\beta$ genes, and no significant expansion of clones bearing specific $V_\beta$ molecules. The most profound TCR repertoire alterations were observed at the earliest time points, with this phenomenon no longer evident by 4 months after the onset of symptoms. Preliminary studies suggest that individuals exhibiting expansions within a very limited $CD8^+$ $V_\beta$ repertoire are more likely to progress rapidly to AIDS, whereas those demonstrating a greater diversity within this initial repertoire have a more favorable prognosis. Finally, data showing the binding of these proliferating $CD8^+$ populations to HIV-specific antigens is lacking. However, their coincident appearance and disappearance with decreases and elevations in viral replication suggest that they may have a role in the early control of HIV infection (see below).

### B-Cell abnormalities

Dysregulation of B-cell function, presumably due to virally induced polyclonal activation, is another hallmark of HIV infection. B cells from infected subjects have been found to spontaneously secrete immunoglobulin (Ig) at titers substantially higher than those seen in uninfected individuals. A majority of these secreted antibodies are HIV-specific and are primarily directed against the gp120 and gp41 components of the viral envelope. One suggested mechanism for this phenomenon is the elevated production of IL-6 by macrophages. This cytokine has been found to enhance HIV-specific antibody production in vitro. Likewise, the viral envelope protein gp41 is also capable of polyclonal B-cell activation in an antigen-nonspecific manner, inducing the secretion of Ig without necessarily inducing B-cell proliferation. Therefore, both idiotype-specific and nonspecific mechanisms of B-cell activation can contribute to the observed state of hypergammaglobulinemia seen following HIV infection.

**Table 99.1** Immunologic abnormalities associated with HIV infection

B-LYMPHOCYTE COMPARTMENT

Polyclonal activation
Hyperagammaglobulinemia

T-LYMPHOCYTE COMPARTMENT

*$CD4^+$ CELLS*

Decrease in $CD4^+$ cell numbers (elevated CD8/CD4 ratio)
Decreased proliferation to antigen (recall, alloantigen, mitogen)
Reduced production of IL-2
Decreases in memory cell (CD45RO) numbers and functions
Alterations in cytokine profile production

*$CD8^+$ CELLS*

Increased cell numbers
Increased expression of activation markers (DR, CD25, CD38)
Decreased proliferation to antigen
Reduced antigen-specific cytotoxic activity
Decrease in anti-HIV responses

ANTIGEN PRESENTING CELLS

Reduced capacity for phagocytosis
Decreased chemotaxis
Decreased antimicrobial activity
Reduced production of IL-1
Reduced antigen-presenting potential

OTHER ACCESSORY CELLS

*NK CELLS*

Decreased cytotoxic activity

## Altered T-cell functions

One of the most prominent immunologic features of HIV infection is a reduction in the number of $CD4^+$ cells and their constituent percentage of total lymphocytes in the blood. However, even before substantial reductions in the numbers of these cells are noted, abnormalities in their functional abilities can be observed. The $CD4^+$ cells from infected individuals have a diminished ability to proliferate and produce cytokines (e.g., IL-2) in response to stimuli. As noted, studies of individuals at various times after infection show that responses to recall antigens (i.e., tetanus and influenza A) are lost first, followed by alloantigen (anti-HLA [human leukocyte antigen]) and finally mitogen-induced responses (PHA [phytohemagglutinin]). These results are coincident with reductions in the numbers of $CD4^+$ cells bearing the CD45RO molecule, a surface marker associated with the memory cell phenotype.

Impaired hematopoiesis of naive $CD4^+$ cells from bone marrow–derived precursors may also contribute to the observed lack of this particular cell subset in seropositive individuals. Some studies have found that the viral proteins gp120 and gp160 can block the in vitro growth of $CD34^+$ stem cells, the progenitor cell phenotype responsible for replenishing $CD4^+$ lymphocytes. However, actual evidence of stem cell infection in vivo, and/or their elimination due to virus infection, remains controversial. Apoptosis of $CD4^+$ cells remains the leading theory for the loss of this cell phenotype.

In addition to the processes just mentioned, HIV infection of $CD4^+$ cells may interfere with their ability to transduce intracellular signals. Protein products of HIV which have been implicated in perturbing signal transduction pathways include Env, Nef, and Tat. These components have been shown to cause dysfunctions such as decreased mobilization of intracellular free calcium and inhibition in the production of inositol phosphate, part of the activation-induced intracellular signal transduction system. The binding of TCR and costimulatory molecules with their ligands, along with the conjugation of cytokines with their respective receptors, normally leads to intracellular cascades of protein kinase activity and ligand-specific phosphorylation patterns. Inappropriate signaling of this second messenger system in the HIV-infected host likely contributes to the observed immunocompromised status.

## Antigen-presenting cells

A subset of hematopoietic cells, commonly referred to as antigen-presenting cells (APCs), have been so named for their proficiency at alerting other more antigen-specific cells in the immune system to the presence of a potential pathogen. Examples of APC types include dendritic cells (DCs), macrophage/monocytes, and B lymphocytes. Acquired immune responses depend on T-cell recognition of antigen–MHC complexes on APCs as well as the costimulatory signals provided by these cells (see Fig. 99.1). Any block in this process could result in a decreased ability to respond to many different antigens and therefore to many potential pathogens. In addition to functional changes, these cell types are also susceptible to virus-induced cytotoxicity. The mechanism for this could be either the destruction of infected cells by cytotoxic T lymphocytes (*discussed later*) or the direct cytopathic effects of the virus. One example of such a virus-induced event is the formation of cell syncytium. Typically, the development of syncytium-inducing (SI) virus strains occurs late in HIV infection and may be related to the substantial depletion of APCs observed in the lymph nodes of individuals progressing to AIDS.

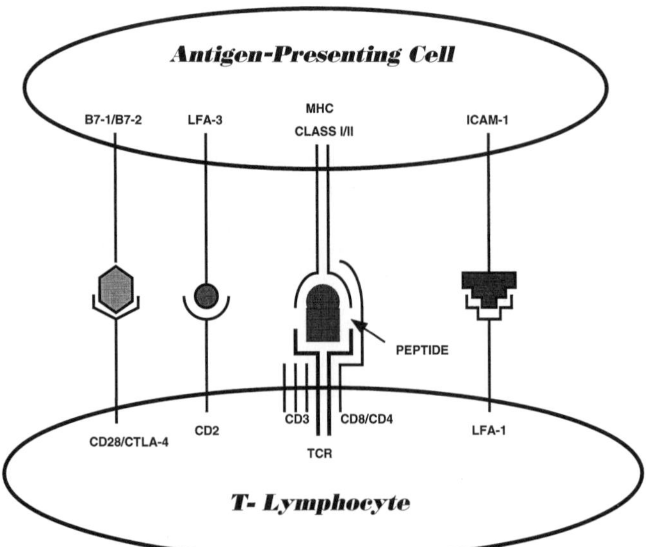


**Fig. 99.1** T-lymphocyte surface markers and their corresponding ligands on the antigen-presenting cell. Cell-to-cell contact between a $CD8^+$ (MHC class I–restricted) or a $CD4^+$ (MHC class II–restricted) T lymphocyte and an APC involve the binding of several surface molecules with their specific ligands on the APC surface. APC, antigen-presenting cell; ICAM, intracellular adhesion molecule; LFA, lymphocyte functional antigen; MHC, major histocompatibility complex; TCR, T-cell receptor.

## Dendritic cells

The dendritic cell, often referred to as a "professional" APC, is the premier mediator of antigen presentation. This is based on the DC's ability to elicit responses from naive lymphocytes, a cell type which is typically very stringent in its requirements for immune activation. For this reason, the DC is an early and key player in initiating a cellular immune response to antigen. Dendritic cells are primarily located in secondary lymphoid organs such as the lymph node, although they can also be found in small numbers in peripheral blood. These cells are known to express high levels of MHC class I and II, as well as the costimulatory molecule B7. This surface marker expression pattern provides them with an enhanced means of signaling antigen-specific T cells. It is this property which makes DCs uniquely suited for presenting antigen to naive lymphocytes, as well as being more efficient than B cells or macrophages at stimulating secondary immune responses.

The follicular dendritic cells (FDCs) of the lymph node use their long cell surface processes to trap passing antigen. Normally the antigen collected by these cells is internalized, processed, and presented to effector cells as an antigen–MHC complex. Recognition of this complex by antigen-specific lymphocytes along with the delivery of costimulatory signals lead to T-cell activation. However, FDCs either isolated from HIV-infected individuals or infected in vitro have been shown to trap and hold infectious virus at their cell surface. This particular cell type may act as a viral reservoir by supplying a localized source for the continued infection of passing target cells (e.g., $CD4^+$ cells and activated macrophages) which normally traffic through the lymph node compartment.

Following HIV infection, some of the antigen-presenting cell functions of DCs are impaired. As mentioned previously, DCs are normally characterized by their efficiency at stimulating naive T-cell proliferation. However, this ability is greatly weakened in cells that have been isolated from HIV-infected individuals. This is true even though only a small fraction of the cells may actually harbor virus. The mechanism for this dysfunction is not understood. However, the observed alterations in cytokine secretion patterns by $CD4^+$ cells in HIV-infected individuals may prove to be a contributing factor.

Studies aimed at evaluating the percentage of infected DCs in seropositive subjects have yielded conflicting results. However, one consistent finding is an increase in the numbers of infected DCs isolated from individuals in the later stages of disease. This finding, combined with the observed depletion of DCs in the lymph nodes of patients with AIDS, may account for the loss of immune functions typically associated with this cell type following disease progression.

## Macrophage/monocytes

Blood monocytes and their macrophage tissue counterparts are also capable of presenting antigen to T lymphocytes in the context of MHC class I and II molecules. Unlike DCs, there is little evident destruction of this cell type concomitant with HIV infection. Instead, the functional properties of these cells appear to be impaired. A reduced capacity for phagocytosis, chemotaxis and microbial killing has been observed in several different studies in which macrophages from seropositive individuals were used. Alterations in the production of such immune response–initiating cytokines as IL-1, IL-6, IL-12, and tumor necrosis factor alpha (TNF-$\alpha$) following macrophage/monocyte infection with HIV have been reported, although these observations remain controversial. Elevated levels of IL-10, a cytokine produced by T cells, have also been observed in some individuals during disease progression. This particular cytokine is capable of inhibiting the ability of macrophages and monocytes to present antigen by inducing decreased expression levels of several cell surface markers (e.g., B7 and MHC class II) and suppressing IL-12 secretion.

## Natural killer cells

As observed with many other cells within the immune system, the functional abilities of natural killer (NK) cells are impaired following HIV infection. Although there is no evidence for a decrease in NK cell numbers in HIV-infected individuals, the data show decreases in the production of lytic molecules, an inability to recognize and become activated by target cells, and reduced TNF-$\alpha$ and interferon gamma (IFN-$\gamma$) production by this cell type. Because of the ability of IFN-$\gamma$ to induce such type 1 immune responses as IL-12 production by macrophages, aberrations in NK cell secretion of cytokines can adversely affect many other immune responses. However, the issue of whether any of these observed impairments result from the direct infection of NK cells with virus still remains controversial.

## Apoptosis

The progressive loss of lymphocytes expressing the CD4 molecule is one of the most salient features of HIV infection. Although the direct infection of $CD4^+$ T lymphocytes and macrophages can lead to cell death, the observed magnitude of cell depletion in seropositive subjects cannot be accounted for when only 0.01% or less of the $CD4^+$ cells are infected with virus, as is often seen during the asymptomatic stages of disease. Instead, the induction of programmed cell death (PCD) via either cell-to-cell contact or interactions with viral proteins may be an important mechanism by which the elimination of large numbers of $CD4^+$ cells occurs in seropositive individuals.

Unlike neutralizing antibodies, which coat infected cells and induce APC-mediated lysis, PCD involves the mobilization of intracellular messengers which lead to DNA fragmentation and cell death from within. This process, commonly referred to as apoptosis, can disrupt immune cell homeostasis via the random destruction of uninfected T lymphocytes. The mechanism of apoptosis involves the delivery of signals, usually by virally infected cells, which then initiate PCD in a target cell. Examples of these signals include the secretion of cytotoxic substances (e.g., TNF), increased surface expression of Fas (target cell) or Fas ligand (effector cell), or the crosslinking of molecules on the target cell surface by viral proteins (see Table 99.2). Also noteworthy are decreases in the secretion of IL-1 and surface expression of B7 by virally infected macrophages. This altered pattern of cell features has been shown to lead to the apoptosis of responding cells. Therefore, the $CD4^+$ lymphocytes with receptors specific for HIV antigens presented by such cells would become antigen-specific targets for apoptotic destruction.

Apoptosis of $CD8^+$ cells has also been shown to occur in HIV seropositive individuals. Although the mechanism for this event is unknown, proposed routes include altered APC functions, the production of toxic cytokines following activation, and the withdrawal of cytokines essential to the survival of activated cells. In support of this latter mechanism, up to 50% of the $CD8^+$ cells

**Table 99.2** Possible factors leading to cell apoptosis in HIV-infected individuals

| |
|---|
| Immune hyperactivation |
| Crosslinking of the CD4 molecule by viral proteins followed by antigen stimulation |
| Increased expression of Fas (target) or Fas ligand (effector) on the cell surface |
| Reduced expression of B7 and decreased secretion of IL-1 by antigen-presenting cells |
| Production of toxic cytokines by neighboring cells (e.g., TNF) |
| Withdrawal of cytokines necessary for survival (e.g., IL-2) |

from HIV-infected subjects were found to be extremely sensitive to IL-2 withdrawal, dying in culture without the addition of this type 1 cytokine (see $CD4^+$ T Cells below).

In vitro activation of T cells isolated from seropositive donors can lead to apoptosis of both infected and uninfected $CD4^+$ cells. Elucidation of the possible reason for this comes from studies showing that the in vitro crosslinking of the CD4 molecule by gp120 before activation can result in apoptosis, mediating destruction of infected and uninfected cells alike. These findings could have clinical relevance, as serum levels of gp120 can reach concentrations equivalent to those used in the above experiments.

## Immune Responses to HIV Infection

### Humoral immunity

Diagnosis of HIV infection is routinely established by detection of antibodies to the virus. This humoral immune response normally persists throughout the course of the infection, waning only in the final stages of disease. Antibody responses specific to HIV are directed against several different viral proteins, including gp160, gp120, p66, p55, gp41, p32, p24, and p17. Many research studies have focused on identifying antibodies specific for various viral envelope proteins in hopes of defining a pattern of protective epitopes for use in vaccine design. However, rapid viral mutation rates in the sequences coding for these envelope proteins and the apparent lack of any identified correlates to protection have confounded these efforts. The various types of antibodies recognizing determinants on HIV and their potential role in disease resolution or propagation are discussed in this section.

### Neutralizing antibodies

Neutralizing antibodies are those immunoglobulins that are capable of binding to and inactivating a pathogen. In the case of HIV, these are antibodies that once attached to the virus will prevent it from infecting susceptible cells. The primary neutralizing epitopes of HIV are found in the external region of gp41 and in the viral envelope on the gp120 molecule. Neutralization of gp41 likely involves inactivation of domains involved in fusion of the viral and cellular membranes. The principal neutralizing domain on gp120 is found on the outermost crown of the variable region 3 (V3) loop structure (see Fig. 99.2). The consensus amino acid sequence GPGRAF, shared by many HIV isolates, is located within this region. This sequence is strain-specific, differing considerably among nonrelated strains. Similar regions have been proposed but not confirmed for HIV-2. Importantly, sera isolated from HIV-1–infected individuals can often neutralize HIV-2 strains, although the converse pattern of cross-reactivity is rare.

The CD4 binding region of HIV, located between V4 and V5 of the envelope protein, is another important neutralization epitope. Antibodies bound to this epitope are both protein sequence and conformation-dependent. The importance of the CD4 binding region is revealed by the ability of many different virus strains with widely varying V3 regions to be neutralized by antibodies directed against this one domain.

Although neutralizing antibodies to HIV can be found using in vitro assays and laboratory virus strains (especially early after infection), the sera from infected individuals rarely show high levels of antibodies capable of neutralizing autologous virus. Longitudinal studies have found that the ability to neutralize later stage autologous virus strains is diminished when compared with neutralization of virus isolates from earlier time points. This finding probably reflects the emergence over time of virus "escape" mutants which are resistant to antibody neutralization. Although the appearance of these viral subspecies is believed to adversely affect disease progression, the actual clinical benefit of neutralizing antibodies remains unclear.

### Enhancing antibodies

Unlike neutralizing antibodies, antibodies which enhance HIV infection are most often seen in individuals who are in the later stages of disease. These Ig molecules are capable of augmenting the ability of virions to which they have bound to infect cells. The postulated mechanism is through directed cellular targeting once bound to either the Fc or complement receptors present on such cell types as macrophages and NK cells.

This enhancing antibody phenotype is often observed at serum dilutions below which neutralizing antibody effects are normally seen. This finding could be due to the existence of high-titer, low-affinity enhancing antibodies. Thus the balance between these two antibody-mediated effects may be crucial to the final clinical outcome. Over time, as either nonneutralizable viral vari-

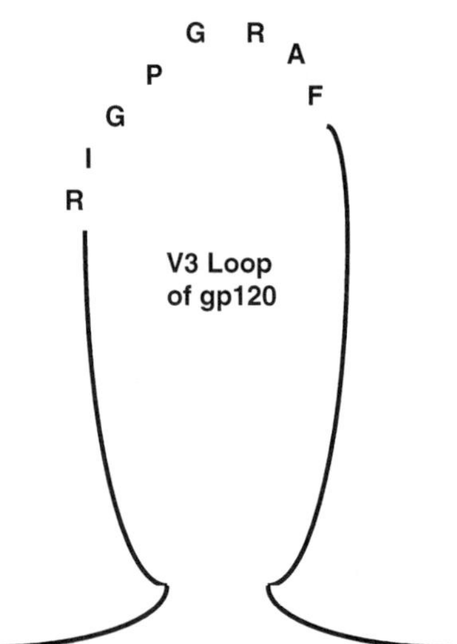


**Fig. 99.2** The V3 loop of gp120 showing the principal neutralizing domain. This region, in the crown of the V3 loop, can differ among viral isolates.

ants emerge or the levels of neutralizing Ig decrease, enhancing antibodies could predominate and favor enhanced virus spread.

## Antibody-dependent cellular cytotoxicity

As mentioned, the complement and Fc receptors (type I and III) present on effector cells can bind to the antibody-coated viral antigens present on the surface of infected cells. This process, referred to as antibody-dependent cell cytotoxicity (ADCC), occurs when effector cells bearing Fc and/or complement receptors, namely macrophages, monocytes, and NK cells, bind to the constant domain of antibody-coated target cells. Alternatively, effector cells may be "armed" with antibody bound to their Fc receptor prior to target cell encounter. Cell killing is then mediated by effector cells following the release of lytic particles such as perforin or by cytokine-induced (i.e., TNF-$\alpha$) apoptosis. Antibodies with specificity for epitopes contained within the gp120 and gp41 envelope proteins can induce lysis of infected cells. However, not all anti-envelope antibodies are equally capable of arming effector cells to mediate this function. In fact, only those Ig specific for particular envelope epitopes are known to induce this response.

The titer of HIV-specific antibodies in serum has been shown to correlate with the extent of ADCC activity observed within an individual. Seropositive subjects with fewer than 200 CD4$^+$ cells/$\mu$L were found to exhibit the lowest level of antibodies capable of mediating ADCC. In contrast, most asymptomatic subjects maintain relatively high levels of virus-specific, ADCC-mediating antibody titers.

It is important to note that with progression to disease both the numbers and functional abilities of ADCC-mediating effector cells (i.e., macrophages and NK cells) are reduced. In the case of NK cells, antibody-independent lysis of sensitive target cells is impaired in the later stages of disease. Loss of this activity may be due to the frequently observed decline in production of IFN-$\gamma$, IL-2, and IL-12, all of which are type 1 cytokines known to enhance NK cell activity.

Macrophages are also capable of mediating ADCC responses, primarily through the ligation of specific cellular receptors with the Fc portion of antibodies. These cells, like NK cells, are responsive to the augmenting effects of type 1 cytokines. Specifically, IFN-$\gamma$ treatment of macrophages enhances their efficiency at killing antibody-coated target cells. Any reductions in the secretion in this cytokine could therefore translate into the impaired ability of macrophages to mediate ADCC. For all of these reasons, reductions in ADCC responses to HIV are most likely due to the suppressed functions of the cellular mediators rather than merely to the loss of the antigen-specific antibodies.

## Complement

Components of the complement cascade (C1–C9) present in serum are capable of inactivating virus through both antibody-dependent and independent pathways. In antibody-dependent lysis, the C5–C9 compounds responsible for pore formation combined with subneutralizing concentrations of HIV-specific antibody can reduce the titers of free infectious virus. This process occurs upon binding of envelope-specific antibodies to their antigenic targets, initiating destruction of virus membrane integrity and the subsequent exposure of capsid molecules.

There are two antibody-independent mechanisms of complement activation and viral lysis. In the first, complement is activated by gp120 and lysis proceeds via the classical complement pathway. The level of gp120 on the surface of virally infected cells, which can be enhanced by treatment with TNF-$\alpha$, is directly proportional to the ability of these cells to be lysed by complement. The second mechanism involves complement fixation and utilizes the alternative pathway, where the cascade is activated after the binding of complement components to a virion or infected cell. Depressed levels of inhibitors to this reaction, such as decay-accelerating factor, can be found in seropositive individuals and may enhance this process during HIV infection. This second method of complement-mediated HIV destruction is believed to be the primary mechanism accounting for the relatively short half-life of free virus in the blood.

## Cellular immunity

As with any viral infection, cell-mediated immune responses are crucial for ultimate elimination of the pathogen. Although humoral immunity can play a role in helping to limit de novo infection by destruction of free virus, the recognition and/or removal of virally infected cells by T lymphocytes is essential. Cells infected with virus will often display peptide fragments derived from the infectious agent bound in the groove of self MHC molecules on their cell surface. These complexes are then ligands for specific T-cell receptor binding and serve as initiators of a range of cellular immune responses (see Fig. 99.1).

## Natural killer (NK) cells

As noted previously, NK cells are one constituent of the innate arm of the immune response. As suggested by their name, NK cells recognize and kill virally infected cells in a non-MHC, antigen-independent fashion. In this way, they are one of the earliest cell types mobilized toward virus resolution. Natural killer cells are most efficient at killing HIV-infected cells either in the presence of HIV-specific antibodies (by ADCC) or following treatment with such cytokines as IL-2 and IL-12, normally made by T lymphocytes and macrophages, respectively. When NK cells are isolated from seropositive individuals, they show a reduced ability to lyse HIV-infected targets. Moreover, after treatment in culture with the above two cytokines, they can be induced to secrete elevated concentrations of lytic molecules, although these levels are still reduced when compared with NK cells isolated from seronegative controls.

Natural killer cells also posses the unique ability to initiate type 1 immunity by secreting IFN-$\gamma$ very early in the immune response. In vitro treatment with IFN-$\gamma$ has been shown to enhance the levels of IL-12 generated by macrophages, thus enhancing NK cell activity and promoting type 1 responses. Further studies with IL-12 in vitro have demonstrated the reestablishment of normal T-cell responses to recall antigens in treated PBMC isolated from infected individuals. This cytokine was also found to block mitogen- and antigen-induced T-cell death in cells from infected subjects. These studies have prompted several phase I clinical trails using IL-12 therapy for HIV-infected patients. As with IL-2, this type 1 cytokine is typically used in moderate, intermittent doses due to the narrow concentration range of therapeutic benefit and the potential for drug-related side effects.

## T lymphocytes

T lymphocytes are important both as effectors in carrying out immune functions and for their ability to secrete and respond to cytokines. In this way, these cells control the direction of the ongoing immune response network. Fluctuations in T-cell numbers or functional abilities will therefore lead to profound effects on the entire immune system. As mentioned earlier, even cells from seropositive individuals which are not infected with virus will often display abnormal, most frequently diminished, activity patterns when exposed to stimuli. This observation may explain why a state of chronic virus infection exemplifies HIV. The following section deals with cellular immune responses which ensue during HIV infection.

### $CD4^+$ T cells

Based on their patterns of cytokine production, T-helper cells can be broadly divided into two types. Among other cytokines, T-helper type 1 (TH1) cells generally produce IL-2, TNF-$\beta$, and IFN-$\gamma$ following an encounter with stimuli. These cytokines are involved in propagating further cell-mediated immune activity. Conversely, T-helper type 2 (TH2) cells secrete IL-4, IL-5, IL-6, and IL-10, cytokines important for helping B cells to make antibody. The different immunologic outcomes represented by these two arms of cellular immunity are therefore often referred to as type 1 and type 2 responses, respectively (see Table 99.3).

Besides encouraging alternative pathways of subsequent activity, the cytokines secreted by these cells have the property of inversely regulating one another. For example, IFN-$\gamma$ made in a type 1 response can downregulate the generation of cytokines by cells specific for type 2 immunity, resulting in reduced levels of IL-4 and IL-10. In turn, these type 2 interleukins have the ability to dampen type 1 cytokine secretion.

Conflicting data exist concerning the relationship of type 1 *versus* type 2 cytokines to disease progression. Recent studies of individuals with AIDS have found reduced levels of IL-2 and increased production of IgE when compared to seropositive, asymptomatic subjects. This suggests a correlation of type 2 responses with disease development. Other groups have found that the in vitro production of type 1 as opposed to type 2 cytokines by lymphocytes from patients is predictive of a positive clinical prognosis. Moreover, the in vitro addition of the type 1 cytokine IL-2 to purified $CD8^+$ cells from HIV-infected individuals has been found to enhance the ability of these cells to suppress virus replication in infected $CD4^+$ cells. If, instead, these same cells are cultured in the presence of IL-10, a type 2 cytokine, elimination or reduction of this suppressing activity is observed. Thus, a shift in cellular responses from type 1 to type 2 has been postulated to explain disease progression in seropositive individuals. However, some more recent studies have failed to confirm any in vivo differences in the levels of type 1 versus type 2 cytokines between rapid progressors and long-term survivors, bringing into question the validity of this hypothesis

**Table 99.3** Cytokine secretion profiles of TH1, TH2, and CTLs

| Cytokine | TH1 | TH2 | CTL[a] |
|---|---|---|---|
| IL-2 | ++ | | +/− |
| IL-3 | ++ | ++ | + |
| IL-4 | − | ++ | − |
| IL-5 | − | ++ | − |
| IL-6 | − | ++ | − |
| IL-10 | − | ++ | ? |
| IFN-$\gamma$ | ++ | − | ++ |
| TNF-$\alpha$ | ++ | + | + |
| TNF-$\beta$ | ++ | − | + |
| GMCSF | ++ | + | ++ |

[a]This $CD8^+$ cell subset may also contain two or more subtypes based on cytokine secretion profiles.

Some $CD4^+$ lymphocytes exhibit cytotoxic properties which can be directed against either infected or uninfected target cells. This type of response is usually found within a subset of type 1 cytokine-secreting $CD4^+$ cells and is often directed against non-$CD4^+$ cells bearing MHC-II molecules associated with viral proteins. These $CD4^+$ cells are capable of mediating the lysis of infected cells but may contribute to HIV-associated pathogenesis by destroying uninfected "bystander" cells as well.

### $CD8^+$ cytotoxic T lymphocytes

Cytotoxic T lymphocytes (CTLs) kill virally infected cells via antigen and MHC-I–specific mechanisms. Most CTLs are present in the $CD8^+$ subset of T cells, although cytotoxic $CD4^+$ cells restricted by class II molecules have also been reported (see above). Cytotoxic T lymphocytes lyse cells in a contact-dependent fashion, either by the production of perforin or by inducing apoptosis in their targets. Traditionally, CTLs have represented a formidable arm of the immune response to virus infection. This status is based on the ability of CTLs to specifically recognize and kill infected cells which express viral antigens in the groove of their class I molecule, a surface marker present on most cell types in the body.

Cytotoxic T lymphocytes have been isolated from the blood, lung, and at times the cerebrospinal fluid of HIV-infected individuals. These lymphocytes express TCRs specific for a wide range of HIV-derived proteins, both structural and regulatory. In fact, the HIV-specific CTL responses of infected individuals are generally very strong, as would be expected with a chronic viral presence. Noteworthy is the finding that following isolation of these cells from infected individuals no in vitro priming is required to activate cytolytic potential. As this phenomenon has not been noted with CTLs specific for other pathogens, it represents a unique feature of infection with HIV.

The percentage of naive human CTLs with potential to develop into HIV-specific effectors is high. This population of cells, referred to as precursor CTL (pCTL), has been defined in seronegative individuals. The frequency of pCTLs in peripheral blood which are specific for HIV antigens can be as high as 66/10,000 (or 0.66%). This value is comparable to the normal pCTL frequency found against alloantigens, which are typically found at higher frequencies than cells specific for foreign antigens, suggesting the possible cross-reactivity of a viral antigen with some component encoded within the MHC loci.

Over the course of infection, HIV-specific CTL activity is normally found to wane. Generally, anti-HIV CTL activity peaks early during the acute phase, when it may represent a major mechanism by which HIV-infected, virus-producing cells are eliminated. Further, CTLs from seropositive individuals have been found to possess activity against several regions of the Gag protein, yet only three distinct epitopes have been identified within the Env protein. This limited anti-envelope response pattern may be relevant to the control of HIV infection. However, the observed decrease in CTL activity over time is not necessarily correlated with reduced capacities of noncytotoxic $CD8^+$ cells to mediate suppression. Likewise, depressed lytic activity can be observed against individual epitopes while others are spared and may therefore represent a selective loss of only certain antigen-specific CTL clones.

Also potentially relevant is the discovery of HIV-reactive CTLs in seronegative individuals who have been exposed to but not infected by HIV. Several different populations of these high-risk individuals have been studied, all with similar results. For example, in one study 26% of the uninfected children born to seropositive mothers were found to possess elevated levels of anti–HIV-specific CTL in their unstimulated PBMC. However, none of these children were diagnosed as HIV-infected after 50 months of follow-up studies. Likewise, studies involving the sexual partners of infected individuals, health care workers exposed to HIV-infected blood, and a cohort of Gambian prostitutes have all demonstrated that these populations possess higher levels of HIV-specific CTL activity than control populations. These populations represent examples of instances where CTL reactivity is found in the absence of antibody to the virus (seronegative), suggesting that perhaps protective immune responses could be elicited without humoral immunity.

### Suppression of HIV replication by CD8$^+$ cells

Some CD8$^+$ cells can mediate noncytolytic suppression of HIV replication in infected CD4$^+$ cells. This discovery was made early in the AIDS epidemic when virus could be isolated from CD8$^+$ cell-depleted but not the unseparated lymphocyte cultures prepared from infected individuals. Unlike most CD8$^+$ cell responses, this suppression is not MHC-restricted, although it is enhanced with MHC matching. Cell-to-cell contact is not required for this form of viral inhibition, although the magnitude of the response is often increased when cell contact is allowed. For this reason, the virus-suppressing activity is believed to be mediated, at least partially, by a soluble factor. The ratio of CD8$^+$ cells (effectors) to CD4$^+$ cells (targets) required to mediate this activity can be quite low, requiring as little as 1 effector per 20 target cells in healthy individuals. The mechanism of action appears to be a noncytotoxic inhibition of virus replication at a stage subsequent to virus entry and DNA integration. This is evidenced by a reduction in virus protein and RNA synthesis in infected CD4$^+$ lymphocytes cocultured in the presence of CD8$^+$ cells, with no concomitant decrease in infected cell numbers.

The soluble factor produced by CD8$^+$ cells and capable of inhibiting HIV replication appears to be an as yet uncharacterized cytokine. This compound, called CD8$^+$ cell antiviral factor (CAF), is a small protein (most likely less than 30 kD in size), heat stable, and resistant to low pH conditions. This CD8$^+$ cell antiviral factor (CAF) has been shown to inhibit virus replication in both naturally and acutely infected cells. The antiviral activity has been demonstrated in vitro against a range of HIV-1 isolates, including both syncytium- and non–syncytium-inducing strains, as well as several isolates of HIV-2 and simian immunodeficiency virus (SIV). Table 99.4 lists the characteristics of CAF which have been identified.

The extent of CD8$^+$ cell-mediated, nonlytic HIV suppression has been found to correlate with the clinical state of the patient. Healthy, seropositive individuals with peripheral blood CD4$^+$ cell counts above 500 cells/$\mu$L show the strongest pattern of this response. This conclusion is based on the relatively low number of CD8$^+$ cells required to suppress HIV replication in these individuals. Conversely, CD8$^+$ lymphocytes from subjects who have progressed to AIDS show either a poor response at the highest cell inputs or, frequently, a complete lack of this antiviral activity. The reason for this loss of suppressive activity is not known. However, studies showing a shift in the TH cell cytokine profile, from type 1 to type 2, with progression to disease suggest that the CD4$^+$ and/or CD8$^+$ cells in later stages are not capable of producing the cytokines necessary to sustain this antiviral activity. In vitro studies have shown a loss of HIV suppression by CD8$^+$ cells taken from asymptomatic individuals when these cells are cultured in the presence of IL-4 or IL-10, both type 2 cytokines. In contrast, the addition of IL-2 to CD8$^+$ cells cultured from these same individuals enhanced their ability to suppress virus in acutely infected cells. In some cases, activation of cultured CD8$^+$ cells from symptomatic patients in the presence of IL-2 has restored a previously undetectable antiviral response.

**Table 99.4** Properties of the CD8$^+$ cell antiviral factor

| |
|---|
| Secreted by activated CD8$^+$ CD28$^+$ lymphocytes, but not CD4$^+$ cells, NK, or macrophages |
| Blocks HIV replication without cell lysis |
| Active against a range of HIV-1 and HIV-2 isolates (NSI and SI) and SIV |
| Arrests HIV replication at RNA transcription stage |
| Non–HLA dependent |
| Heat stable |
| Resistant to low pH conditions |
| Positively charged |
| Lacks identity with all known cytokines and chemokines |

## Chemokines and their receptors

A recent focus in the immunology of HIV has been the study of chemokines, substances defined by their ability to induce chemotaxis in a range of target cells. Chemokines can be divided into two major subfamilies, $\alpha$ and $\beta$. The $\alpha$ chemokines contain *N*-terminal cysteines separated by one amino acid (CXC) while the $\beta$ chemokines express adjacent cysteines (CC). These substances, produced by a wide range of cell types (i.e., lymphocytes, macrophages, endothelial cells), have been shown to induce the migration of many different cell types, including neutrophils, eosinophils, basophils, monocytes, muscle cells, and fibroblasts. In general, the $\alpha$ chemokines tend to attract neutrophils while the $\beta$ chemokines exert their effects on monocytes and, in some cases, T lymphocytes.

Besides chemotaxis, chemokines can also modulate cellular functions in cells expressing the appropriate receptor. In vitro these substances can induce enzyme secretion, adhesion, and cytotoxicity. Chemokines will also initiate degranulation and tumor-specific lytic activity in NK cells and CTL. Finally, recent studies have suggested that these compounds may be able to provide the costimulatory signals required to induce proliferation and IL-2 secretion by T lymphocytes following activation. The role of chemokines in HIV infection is still unclear, although they are currently receiving the attention of many research groups. Initially, the combined use of recombinant forms of three $\beta$ chemokines, macrophage inflammatory protein MIP-1$\alpha$, MIP-1$\beta$, and RANTES (for regulation-upon-activation, normal T expressed, and secreted), was found to inhibit the entry of some primary HIV-1 isolates into susceptible target cells. Later, this observation was found to be due to the fact that some macrophage tropic strains of HIV-1 utilize a chemokine receptor (CCR-5) as a cofactor along with the CD4 molecule for virus-cell fusion. In this way, the $\beta$ chemokines could function by blocking the cofactor site and inhibiting HIV infection of the cells. Recent evidence demonstrates that the resistance of $CD4^+$ cells from some individuals to acute infection correlates with a lack of expression of CCR-5 on the cell surface.

Another chemokine receptor, initially called Fusin/LESTR and now referred to as CXCR-4, has been identified as a cofactor for T-cell line tropic strains of HIV-1. Its natural ligand was previously identified as a chemoattractant called stromal cell-derived factor (SDF-1). Both CXCR-4 and CCR-5 belong to the 7-transmembrane G protein–coupled receptor family. Following ligand binding, this group of receptors transduce intracellular signals leading to calcium mobilization and the initiation of functional activity by the cell (i.e., migration to sites of inflammation).

There is some redundancy in chemokine receptor specificity, allowing the CCR-5 molecule to serve as ligand for all three of the aforementioned $\beta$ chemokines, MIP-1$\alpha$, MIP-1$\beta$, and RANTES. Because of the role of this receptor as a cofactor for HIV entry into cells, it was of particular interest to study the CCR5 molecule in a group of high-risk individuals who appeared to be resistant to infection. In one such recent research study, two high-risk participants were found to carry a homozygous mutation which results in the lack of expression of the CCR-5 molecule on the cell surface. Concomitantly, $CD4^+$-enriched lymphocyte subsets isolated from these patients demonstrated a total absence of in vitro susceptibility to several different primary strains of HIV-1. However, the remainder of the more than 20 high-risk subjects in the study all carried one or more copies of the wild-type receptor, suggesting that other mechanisms of protection from HIV infection may exist.

In HIV-infected individuals, genetic polymorphisms in chemokine and/or chemokine receptor genes may have a role in mediating protection from disease progression. One study of infected subjects evaluated the role of three known polymorphisms, CCR5-$\Delta$32, CCR2-64I, and SDF1-3′A, in five different subject cohorts. They found that SDF1-3′A homozygous individuals, especially those also carrying the CCR5-$\Delta$32 and CCR2-64I alleles, were partially protected from disease progression.

## Autoimmune Disorders and Neoplasms Associated with HIV Infection

With the myriad of immune cell alterations that occur following HIV infection, it is no surprise that both autoimmune conditions and malignancies can be associated with seropositivity. For example, continual overstimulation of the immune system (i.e., hypergammaglobulinemia) could lead to autoimmune phenomena. Likewise, impaired immune functions, such as a lack of surveillance (i.e., NK cells), may predispose an individual to cancer. The following section includes a discussion of the most common autoimmune and malignant diseases associated with HIV infection.

### Autoimmunity

Autoimmunity arises when the host immune system fails to discriminate some normal cellular constituent as "self" and instead launches an immune attack against this component. Autoantibodies to a range of different cellular proteins including the CD4 molecule and HLA class I and II proteins have been described in seropositive individuals. The production of these self-reactive antibodies may result from the carryover and the incorporation of HIV proteins into the cell membrane during virus budding. Among the most common autoimmune disorders associated with HIV infection are Reiter's syndrome, systemic lupus erythematosus, Sjögren's syndrome, polymyositis, and vasculitis. This latter disease likely represents a manifestation of the immune complexes generated during an HIV infection, while the other syndromes result from pathogenesis induced by autoantibodies or autoreactive lymphocytes.

Several theories exist to explain the development of autoimmunity following HIV infection. These include B-cell proliferation, molecular mimicry, the carrier-hapten phenomenon, and anti-idiotypic antibody production. In the first case, unchecked proliferation of activated B cells is believed to result from the dysregulation of T lymphocytes normally responsible for the control of B-cell responses. The initial B-cell activation event may be caused by viral proteins, stimulatory cytokines (i.e., IL-6, IL-7, TNF-$\alpha$), or HIV-infected APCs. This hypothesis would be consistent with observations of enhanced type 2 cytokine production observed in some seropositive individuals.

Molecular mimicry describes the situation in which foreign proteins share similar amino acid sequences with normal cellular constituents. When this occurs any immune response to the foreign peptide can also lead to immunologic attacks against self-antigens. Data supporting this theory to explain HIV-associated autoimmunity come from studies of sequence similarities between host and viral proteins. Sequences with homology to IL-1, the IL-2 receptor, MHC class I and II molecules, and IFN coding regions have all been found within the HIV genome. Likewise, similarities between the sequences for gp120 and the human Fas gene have also been identified. These sequence similarities could result in the production of anti-Fas antibodies theoretically capable of nonspecifically inducing apoptosis.

A third potential mechanism of autoimmunity following HIV infection is the complexing of HIV proteins as a carrier with host molecules serving as the hapten. In this way, the autoantigen could suddenly become immunogenic. However, no such virus–cellular complexes have been identified and this event may therefore prove not to be salient to the induction of HIV-associated autoimmune disorders.

Finally, the development of anti-idiotypic antibodies directed against virus-specific antibodies may be involved in the development of autoimmunity. For instance, the antigen binding region of Ig specific for gp120 epitopes could structurally resemble the CD4 molecule, with anti-idiotypic antibodies directed against this domain possessing binding affinities for CD4. However, the anti-CD4 Ig from infected donors thus far described has not been directed against epitopes responsible for HIV binding and so is unlikely to be involved in this scenario of autoantibody production.

In conclusion, no one mechanism has been defined which predisposes HIV seropositive individuals to autoimmune susceptibility. The theories described here represent potential cofactors to HIV pathogenesis and the development of autoimmunity. It should also be noted that data from research studies involving the plasmaphoresis of seropositive individuals do not support a role for autoantibodies to the CD4 molecule in the loss of this cell type following infection.

## Kaposi's sarcoma

The form of cancer most frequently associated with HIV and specifically linked with progression to AIDS is Kaposi's sarcoma (KS). First described in 1872 by Moritz Kaposi, KS is an angioproliferative, often multifocal, neoplasia manifesting most commonly on the skin of the feet. This disorder is not uncommon in men over the age of 50, especially if they are of eastern European or Mediterranean descent. Endemically, KS is found in areas of sub-Saharan Africa, and more often in men than women. Most typical is the nonaggressive form of this cancer, which is rarely lethal.

Individuals infected with HIV are 20,000 times more likely to develop KS than uninfected subjects. In its association with HIV, KS is observed most frequently in young men, and with a much more aggressive, visceral manifestation than in the endemic form of the disease. Skin lesions can consist of a mixture of endothelial cells, macrophages, dendritic cells, mast cells, fibroblasts, and finally spindle-shaped cells in advanced tumors. However, much controversy still surrounds the identity of the cell origin, although vascular endothelium remains the leading candidate.

One common denominator for both endemic and HIV-associated forms of KS appears to be immune suppression. This cancer has been noted in conjunction with advancing age, reactivation of latent virus (specifically Epstein-Barr virus [EBV] and cytomegalovirus [CMV]), and immune-compromised conditions (i.e., transplant recipients on immunosuppressive therapy). These associations support the prevailing theory of KS induction arising from defects in cellular immune regulation, a prominent feature of HIV seropositivity.

A putative etiologic agent causing KS has recently been identified using the technique of representational difference analysis. DNA sequences detected within the KS lesions of $HIV^+$ as well as $HIV^-$ individuals have been characterized and found to contain regions of similarity with two other herpesviruses, *Herpesvirus saimiri* and EBV. This newly discovered virus species has been designated human herpesvirus 8 (HHV8) and represents a member of the $\gamma$ Herpesvirinae subfamily, the members of which are known both to infect lymphocytes and to have transforming properties. Moreover, HHV8 has been found associated with B-cell lymphomas present in the abdominal cavity. This finding is not unexpected as the virus has been detected in the $CD19^+$ (B-cell) fraction of PBMC from KS subjects. The genome size of HHV8 is estimated at 150 kb, with several regions of cellular homology identified. For example, HHV8 has been found to carry sequences resembling cyclin D, a cell cycle initiator, IL-6, MIP-1$\alpha$, and the bcl-2 gene, which encodes a protein involved in blocking apoptosis.

In strong support of a role for HHV8 in KS, virus-induced antibodies to both lytic and latent antigens have been identified in individuals with this malignancy. Antibody responses to latent, nonreplicative antigens were found to be strongly predictive of the development of either KS or B-cell lymphomas and therefore may represent antitumor antibodies. Approximately 1%–2% of a random control population possess antibodies to these latent HHV8 antigens. When investigating antigens expressed during the lytic, replicative stage of the virus cycle, up to 25% of the general population was found to be antibody positive. This observation contrasts with KS patients, 100% of whom are positive, and $HIV^+$ homosexual males with a 90% seropositivity against lytic antigens. Also, HHV8 sequences have been detected in the semen and saliva of KS patients. These data along with other studies, especially those demonstrating high levels of anti-HHV8 antibodies in patients visiting sexually transmitted disease (STD) clinics, suggest that this virus is transmitted through sexual contact, particularly receptive anal intercourse. However, the presence of HHV8 in young children and individuals without evidence of sexual exposure suggests the existence of additional routes of infection.

## B-Cell lymphomas

Another form of cancer associated with HIV infection is B-cell lymphoma (BCL). As noted earlier, increased levels of B-cell proliferation are common in seropositive populations. This increase is most likely due to polyclonal stimulation by HIV antigens and/or the overproduction of cytokines which encourage B-cell division, such as IL-6 and IL-10. This state of elevated proliferation may serve as a prelude to chromosomal aberrations which result in cellular transformation and ultimately malignancy.

Histologically, BCL are diffuse and aggressive, with extranodal involvement common (i.e., intestine, central nervous system, bone marrow, and liver). This cancer can be classified as either large-cell or Burkitt's lymphoma–like in nature. In seropositive individuals presenting with large-cell forms of BCL, there is a noted absence of *c-myc* rearrangements. Conversely, mutations in this gene are commonly found in Burkitt's lymphoma associated with HIV infection. Depending on cell type, genetic changes have been observed in the cellular oncogenes *myc* and *ras*, as well as in the p53 tumor suppressor gene.

Three types of HIV-associated BCL have been described: polyclonal, monoclonal, and monoclonal with EBV infection. Most of these tumors isolated from AIDS patients are of the monoclonal type, suggesting outgrowth from a single transforming event. Unlike Burkitt's lymphoma, however, HIV-associated BCL are frequently not EBV-positive. In cases where polyclonal BCL is observed, chronic B-cell activation secondary to aberrant cytokine production likely plays a significant role.

Only about 40% of non–brain B-cell lymphomas seen in AIDS patients are coinfected with EBV. This is in contrast to endemic Burkitt's and HIV-associated brain lymphomas, which are typically all EBV infected. One possible role for EBV in this form of cancer could be as a stimulus for cell proliferation, ultimately leading to karyotypic changes and transformation. In this way, the combination of EBV, HIV proteins, and B-cell stimulatory cytokines may encourage the outgrowth events required for development of this malignancy.

Impaired or dysregulated cell-mediated immunity may also play a role in the development of BCL. Evidence in support of this theory comes from the increased incidence of this malignancy noted in transplant patients under prolonged immunosuppressive therapy. Likewise, this type of cancer is 60 times more common in AIDS patients than in the general population. Again, this is most likely due to chronic B-cell stimulation by HIV and the enhanced production of particular cytokines. For instance, elevated levels of IL-10 have been observed in seropositive subjects. This cytokine is known to encourage B-cell growth and can lead to bcl-2 gene expression, reducing the rate of B-cell death due to apoptosis.

## Anal cell carcinoma

A rise in the rate of anal carcinoma has also been noted in association with HIV infection in both men and women. In seronegative populations, receptive anal intercourse and exposure to human papilloma virus (HPV) have been identified as risk factors for anal cell carcinoma. These events along with the immunosuppressed state of seropositive individuals are likely to be responsible for the initiation and propagation of this form of cancer in HIV-infected populations. In one study, up to 55% of HIV-infected homosexual men were found to be positive for HPV DNA and the associated anal cell dysplasia. Moreover, seropositive men with $CD4^+$ cell counts $<500/\mu L$ had a sixfold increased risk of anal cell dysplasia compared with infected men with counts $>500$ cells/$\mu$L. The presence of HPV sequences, cell dysplasia, and the development of this carcinoma appear to correlate with the extent of immune dysfunction in HIV-infected individuals.

## Conclusion

In this chapter we discussed the effects of HIV on the immune system, the immune responses generated against the virus, and HIV-associated immune sequelae. Shortly after infection, major disruptions are evident within the immune system, including decreases in $CD4^+$ cell numbers and elevations in the $CD8^+$ lymphocyte subset. The prevailing themes of these alterations are a state of immune activation and the destruction and/or impaired function of cells responsible for virus control. These immune disorders continue to escalate, ultimately leading to such impaired responsiveness to antigenic stimuli that life-threatening opportunistic infections ensue.

At early time points after infection, high levels of viremia are seen. With the appearance of $CD8^+$ cell-mediated antiviral responses and antibodies specific for viral proteins, viremia levels diminish to concentrations much lower than those observed during this initial burst. This new level of viremia, or "viral load set-point," is then generally maintained for the duration of the asymptomatic stage of infection. The efficiency of host anti-HIV immune responses in controlling de novo virus production most likely determines the magnitude of this set-point. This is evidenced by the direct correlation of a low viral load set-point with the length of the asymptomatic period. In this way, the viral load can be seen as a marker of the efficiency of the immune response against the virus.

A number of different immune system disruptions are most likely responsible for the eventual failure to control HIV. First, many of the cells capable of eliminating the virus (i.e., macrophages, dendritic cells, and $CD4^+$ lymphocytes) are also reservoirs of infection. Some of these cells are actually destroyed following infection while others fall prey to destruction via association either with viral proteins or with other cells of the immune system. The latter phenomenon is potentially mediated by apoptotic signals from infected cells. The loss of functional activity in these cells, most of which are not infected, leads to impaired initiation of further anti-HIV immunity and increased susceptibility to opportunistic pathogens. Finally, the emergence of HIV "escape mutants" into this environment of impaired immune capability can easily tip the host–pathogen balance in favor of the virus.

Two major goals remain in the struggle to understand host immune responses to HIV. First, truly protective immune parameters need to be defined. From the available data, strong anti-HIV $CD8^+$ cell responses, both CTL and noncytolytic suppression, appear to correlate with a prolonged asymptomatic clinical state. These $CD8^+$ cell-mediated responses are frequently seen without seropositivity, for example, in high-risk populations and during acute infection when HIV-specific antibodies are undetectable.

A clearer understanding of which antiviral mechanisms are protective is needed in order to make immunization against HIV a reality. Likewise, once beneficial immune mechanisms have been identified, therapeutic modalities which enhance these activities can be used in infected individuals. The elimination of free virus using current antiretroviral drugs, although it results in decreased viral loads, serves to control only de novo HIV infection. This effect becomes apparent with the emergence of drug-resistant viral strains. In order to make a dramatic impact on the presence of virus in the host, the cells which harbor the virus must be either eliminated or strictly controlled. To do this, a strong $CD8^+$ cell anti-HIV response is required. As long as cellular immunity to HIV is maintained, viral loads will stay low and cell destruction will be minimized, resulting in fewer naive cells becoming infected. In this way, the integrity of the immune system can be preserved in the face of long-term HIV infection.

## ANNOTATED BIBLIOGRAPHY


Alkhatib G, Combadiere C, Broder CC, et al. CC-CKR-5: a RANTES, MIP-1a, MIP-1b receptor as a fusion cofactor for macrophage-tropic HIV-1. Science 1996; 272:1955–1958.

*One of three concurrent articles describing the finding that primary macrophage tropic virus strains use the CCR5 beta chemokine receptor as a cofactor for target cell binding and fusion.*

Barker E, Barnett SW, Stamatatos L, et al. The human immunodeficiency viruses. Retroviridae 1994; 4:1–67.

*A comprehensive review of HIV including immune responses to the virus.*

Clerici M, Shearer GM. A TH1 to TH2 switch is a critical step in the etiology of HIV infection. Immunol Today 1993; 14:107–111.

Graziosi C, Pantaleo G, Gantt KR, et al. Lack of evidence for the dichotomy of Th1 and Th2 predominance in HIV-infected individuals. Science 1994; 265:248–252.

*The preceding two papers present conflicting views on the presence of type 1 versus type 2 cytokines in HIV-infected individuals, and their associations with disease.*

Knight SC. Bone-marrow–derived dendritic cells and the pathogenesis of AIDS. AIDS 1996; 10:807–817.

*An editorial review of the effect of HIV infection on various dendritic cell functions.*

Landay AL, Clerici M, Hashemi F, et al. *In vitro* restoration of T cell immune function in human immunodeficiency virus-positive persons: effects of interleukin (IL)-12 and anti–IL-10. J Infect Dis 1996; 173: 1085–1091.

*A study exploring the effects of IL-12 and anti–IL-10 in vitro on cells from HIV-infected individuals based on their $CD4^+$ cell counts. This study forms the basis for the scientific rationale behind IL-12 therapy in vivo.*

Levy JA. HIV and the Pathogenesis of AIDS. (1998). American Society for Microbiology, Washington, DC.

*Detailed text discussing all aspects of HIV and our current understanding of the development of disease.*

Oyaizu N, Pahwa S. Role of apoptosis in HIV disease pathogenesis. J Clin Immunol 1995; 15:217–231.

*A review of the mechanisms and importance of various inducers of apoptosis in the pathogenesis of AIDS.*

Pantaleo G, Demarest JF, Soudeyns H, et al. Major expansion of $CD8^+$ T cells with a predominant Vb usage during the primary immune response to HIV. Nature 1994; 370:463–467.

*A study of individuals undergoing acute viral syndrome, showing that for a limited time after infection mono/oligoclonal $CD8^+$ T-cell clones against HIV are detectable.*

Rowland-Jones SL, McMichael A. Immune responses in HIV-exposed seronegatives: have they repelled the virus? Curr Opin Immunol 1995; 7:448–455.

*A comprehensive review of our current knowledge about anti-HIV immune responses in various subpopulations exposed to but not infected with the virus.*

Winkler C, et al. Genetic restriction of AIDS pathogenesis by an SDF-1 chemokine gene variant. Science 1998; 279:389.

*A large, multi-cohort study evaluating the relative effect on disease progression of the three known chemokine/chemokine receptor polymorphisms.*

# 100

# Clinical Manifestations of HIV Infection and AIDS

ANN C. COLLIER, CHRISTINA M. MARRA, AND LILI A. SACKS

Persons with human immunodeficiency virus (HIV) type 1 infection have a broad spectrum of clinical conditions, which range from asymptomatic to life-threatening. Some clinical symptoms and signs are attributable to HIV infection, whereas others are due to infectious or malignant complications. Acquired immunodeficiency syndrome (AIDS) refers to a state of severe immunodeficiency caused by HIV infection, which is characterized by specific opportunistic diseases. More recently, the term *immunologic AIDS* has been used to refer to persons with HIV who have not had an opportunistic disease, but who have severe depletion of $CD4^+$ cells ($<200/\mu L$). Women with HIV infection have some gender-specific complications, although the majority of clinical conditions that occur in HIV-infected individuals occur in both men and women and with similar frequencies. Manifestations of HIV and AIDS in adults and children have many similarities, but there are also unique aspects of disease in each of these groups. Prevalence of certain HIV-associated opportunistic infections varies in different geographic regions of the world, and for selected conditions such as endemic mycoses, in different regions of the United States.

Since AIDS was first recognized in the early 1980s, knowledge about clinical manifestations has increased, and with improvements in preventive and therapeutic strategies, natural history of some HIV-related clinical conditions has changed. The clinical course and typical manifestations of HIV infection treated with aggressive, multidrug antiretroviral regimens is still being defined, and may differ from the presentations described prior to potent antiretrovirals. This chapter focuses on clinical manifestations of HIV infection and AIDS in adults in the developed world. Therapy for these conditions is discussed in Chapters 101 and 102.

## Stages of HIV Infection and Disease

Acquired immunodeficiency syndrome was first recognized from life-threatening opportunistic infections that can occur when persons with HIV develop severe immune suppression. Subsequently, it became clear that persons with HIV infection have a broad range of immunologic and clinical states. The most common clinical test used to categorize patients with HIV infection has been enumeration of $CD4^+$ cells in peripheral blood, also referred to as T4 counts. Persons with $CD4^+$ cells $<500/\mu L$ have evidence for immune impairment. The terms *early*, *midstage*, and *advanced* HIV infection have been used to describe asymptomatic adults with $CD4^+$ cells $>500/\mu L$, $200$–$499/\mu L$, and $<200/\mu L$, regardless of symptoms.

The Centers for Disease Control (CDC) developed the classification scheme most widely used in the United States to describe the spectrum of conditions associated with HIV infection. This was developed for public health and surveillance purposes, but it provides a useful overview of the spectrum of HIV-associated clinical conditions. The most recent CDC classification system for adults and adolescents ($\geq$13 years of age) is from 1993; it is a matrix of nine mutually exclusive categories based on clinical and immunologic criteria (Table 100.1). The classification system requires a confirmed diagnosis of HIV infection. It has three categories which describe a range of $CD4^+$ cell counts (1, 2, 3) and three clinical categories (A, B, C). The lowest $CD4^+$ cell count which an individual has had is used, even if it is not the most recent value. The system also allows for use of $CD4^+$ percentages.

The clinical categories of HIV infection are defined by occurrence of certain signs, symptoms, or specific diseases. Persons who have conditions that are part of multiple categories are assigned to the most advanced disease category. Category A includes persons who are asymptomatic, persons with persistent generalized lymphadenopathy, and persons with acute primary HIV. Category B includes symptomatic conditions of moderate severity that are not included in Category C, and that are indicative of a defect in cell-mediated immunity or have a clinical course or management that is complicated by HIV infection. Examples of category B conditions include oral candidiasis, persistent vaginal candidiasis, cervical dysplasia, oral hairy leukoplakia, recurrent or multidermatomal varicella zoster virus, and peripheral neuropathy. Category C includes all diseases and conditions included in CDC's AIDS surveillance definition (Table 100.2). This includes a wide variety of serious bacterial, fungal, parasitic, and viral infections, selected malignancies, and a few severe HIV-related conditions such as encephalopathy and wasting.

The important role which $CD4^+$ cell loss plays in the natural history of HIV disease is reflected in this and other classification systems. Table 100.3 shows $CD4^+$ cell counts at or below which common HIV-associated diseases usually occur. Information has become available about the prognostic value of quantitative measures of HIV, such as HIV RNA in plasma; higher HIV RNA values are associated with more rapid progression to AIDS and shorter survival. Levels of HIV RNA have not yet been specifically linked to various clinical manifestations or specific complications of HIV disease.

## Clinical Presentations

Symptoms and signs associated with HIV infection and diseases that complicate HIV may involve any body system and can be categorized as primarily involving systemic or disseminated diseases, the eye, nervous system, respiratory tract, gastrointestinal tract, and skin. Less frequent manifestations include endocrine,

**Table 100.1** Centers for Disease Control classification for HIV infection in adults and adolescents

| CD4+ T-cell category (cells/μL) | Clinical category (A) Asymptomatic, acute primary HIV or PGL[a] | (B) Symptomatic, not (A) or (C) conditions | (C) AIDS-indicator conditions[b] |
|---|---|---|---|
| (1) ≥500 | A1 | B1 | C1 |
| (2) 200–499 | A2 | B2 | C2 |
| (3) <200 | A3 | B3 | C3 |

[a]PGL refers to persistent generalized lymphadenopathy.

[b]See Table 100.2

cardiac, renal, genito-urinary and rheumatologic problems, which are not described in this chapter. Although HIV-associated diseases often involve more than one organ system, review of problems involving these major body systems provides a framework for discussion of clinical manifestations of HIV infection and AIDS. Primary HIV infection is discussed separately, since this diagnosis is relevant only in persons without HIV infection.

**Table 100.2** Conditions included in the 1993 Centers for Disease Control AIDS surveillance case definition

| |
|---|
| Candidiasis of bronchi, trachea, or lungs |
| Candidiasis, esophageal |
| Cervical cancer, invasive[a] |
| Coccidioidomycosis, disseminated or extrapulmonary |
| Cryptococcosis, extrapulmonary |
| Cryptosporidiosis, chronic intestinal (>1 month's duration) |
| Cytomegalovirus disease (other than liver, spleen, or nodes) |
| Cytomegalovirus retinitis (with loss of vision) |
| Encephalopathy, HIV-related |
| Herpes simplex: chronic ulcer(s) (>1 month's duration); or bronchitis, pneumonitis, or esophagitis |
| Histoplasmosis, disseminated or extrapulmonary |
| Isosporiasis, chronic intestinal (>1 month's duration) |
| Kaposi's sarcoma |
| Lymphoma, Burkitt's (or equivalent term) |
| Lymphoma, immunoblastic (or equivalent term) |
| Lymphoma, primary, of brain |
| *Mycobacterium avium* complex or *M. kansasii*, disseminated or extrapulmonary |
| *Mycobacterium tuberculosis*, any site (pulmonary[a] or extrapulmonary) |
| *Mycobacterium*, other species or unidentified species, disseminated or extrapulmonary |
| *Pneumocystis carinii* pneumonia |
| Pneumonia, recurrent[a] |
| Progressive multifocal leukoencephalopathy |
| *Salmonella* septicemia, recurrent |
| Toxoplasmosis of brain |
| Wasting syndrome due to HIV |

[a]Added in the 1993 expansion of the AIDS surveillance case definition.

## Primary HIV Infection

Acquisition of HIV may be asymptomatic or may be associated with clinical symptoms and signs, which range from mild to severe. Prevalence of symptoms in different cohorts of seroconvertors has varied from zero to 92%. Explanations for variability include differences in methods for identification of seroconvertors, for ascertainment of symptoms, and case definitions. Some investigators have suggested that symptomatic primary HIV infection is more frequently seen in persons acquiring HIV through sexual transmission than via injection drug use, although data are limited. Additionally, data suggest that the course of HIV in persons with symptomatic primary infection is more aggressive than in patients who have asymptomatic seroconversion. The incubation period is usually 2–6 weeks.

Among patients with symptomatic primary HIV infection, the illness often resembles a viral syndrome (Table 100.4) and may be mild or severe. Weight loss ranges from 1 kg to >10 kg.

Neurological manifestations were found in 17% of 125 symptomatic seroconverting patients from France, including meningitis in 6%, peripheral neuropathy in 9%, and acute encephalitis in 2%. Respiratory symptoms appear less frequently. Abnormal physical findings are common, including skin rash, lymphadenopathy, and splenomegaly. Skin rash is usually diffuse, erythematous, macular or maculopapular, and nonpruritic; it most often involves trunk, face, and/or arms. Lymphadenopathy may be generalized or involve cervical, axillary, inguinal, or epitrochlear regions. Oral lesions include erythema, oral ulcerations, and infrequently oral candidiasis. Genital ulcerations not attributable to other pathogens have also been described. Duration of symptoms ranges from <1 one week to >12 weeks.

Hematological abnormalities appear common; among 23 patients with symptomatic primary HIV infection, 74% had platelet counts <150,000/μL, 48% had white blood cells (WBC) < 4000/μL, 35% had neutrophils < 1500/μL, 30% had lymphocytes < 1000/μL, and 26% were anemic. Anti–HIV antibody tests are negative early after acquisition of HIV and can be used retrospectively for diagnosis of primary HIV infection if paired samples taken weeks or months apart demonstrate seroconversion from negative to a confirmed positive anti–HIV antibody profile. However, early (days to weeks) after acquisition of HIV, before the development of HIV antibodies, plasma HIV RNA and serum HIV p24 antigen assays are positive. Human immunodeficiency virus RNA assays are more sensitive than HIV p24 antigen assays. Diagnosis of primary HIV is certain if either of these tests is confirmed positive simultaneously with a negative anti–HIV antibody test.

**Table 100.3** Usual CD4$^+$ cell range of common HIV-associated diseases

| | CD4$^+$ cell count (cells/$\mu$L) | | | |
|---|---|---|---|---|
| Any | <500 | <200 | <100 | <50 |
| Lymphoma | Oral candidiasis | *P. carinii* pneumonia | Cryptococcal meningitis | *M. avium* complex |
| Syphilis | Oral hairy leukoplakia | HIV dementia | Cryptosporidium | Cytomegalovirus disease |
| Tuberculosis | Kaposi's sarcoma | Toxoplasmosis | Bacillary angiomatosis | Central nervous system lymphoma |
| Periodontitis | Xerotic eczema | Candida esophagitis | Histoplasmosis | |
| Herpes simplex virus | | Eosinophilic folliculitis | Progressive multifocal leukoencephalopathy | |
| Varicella zoster virus | | | Herpes simplex virus: esophagitis or severe anogenital disease | |
| Human papilloma virus | | | | |
| Seborrheic dermatitis | | | Aphthous ulcers | |
| Psoriasis | | | *Isospora belli* | |
| | | | Microsporidia | |

## Systemic Illnesses

Persons with HIV infection are at risk to develop a variety of opportunistic diseases that cause constitutional symptoms such as fever, night sweats, weight loss, and malaise. These illnesses include opportunistic infections and malignancies (Table 100.5). Although the clinical presentations of these illnesses have similarities, some have relatively unusual clinical features or epidemiologic aspects. Some diseases, such as disseminated *Mycobacterium avium* complex (MAC), rarely occur unless persons have severe immunosuppression (Table 100.3). Others illnesses, such as histoplasmosis and coccidiodomycosis, are uncommon unless patients have traveled to certain geographic areas. Some diseases, such as cytomegalovirus (CMV) and lymphoma, frequently involve specific organs as well as having systemic manifestations. In addition to entities that commonly cause systemic illness in persons with HIV and AIDS in developed countries, many other disseminated infections have been reported (Table 100.6).

## Nontuberculous Mycobacteria

The most frequent nontuberculous mycobacterial infection in patients with HIV infection is MAC. Manifestations include asymptomatic colonization, localized disease, bacteremia, and disseminated MAC. Presentations of disseminated MAC include bacteremia and an illness with prominent constitutional symptoms; this occurs in 15%–43% of patients with advanced AIDS. Postmortem studies of persons dying with AIDS suggest its true prevalence is even higher. Patients with symptomatic MAC usually have continuous high-level bacteremia. The major risk factor for development of disseminated MAC disease is severe immunosuppression. CD4$^+$ cell counts are usually between zero and 50 cells/$\mu$L and patients usually have other AIDS-defining illnesses. Other factors associated with disseminated disease are longer duration since an AIDS-defining illness, other past opportunistic infections, and severe anemia.

Common symptoms, signs, and laboratory findings that occur in patients with disseminated MAC are listed in Table 100.7. High temperatures, drenching night sweats, and significant weight loss are common. Lymphadenopathy can be generalized or localized, but it is often intra-abdominal or mediastinal and detectable only by imaging procedures. The most common method of diagnosing disseminated MAC is by blood culture; sensitivity of this test is 85%–90%. Alternative means for diagnosis of disseminated MAC or identification of patients at risk for disseminated disease include recovery of the organism from a normally sterile site. Average survival with untreated dissemi-

**Table 100.4** Common clinical manifestations of symptomatic primary HIV infection*

| Feature | Frequency (%) | Feature | Frequency (%) |
|---|---|---|---|
| Fever | 65–100 | Malaise | 26–67 |
| Lymphadenopathy | 50–92 | Skin rash | 20–67 |
| Fatigue | 51–90 | Headache | 38–61 |
| Sore throat | 37–77 | Nausea | 24–58 |
| Myalgias | 41–75 | Arthralgias | 29–49 |
| Weight loss | 13–70 | Diarrhea | 17–48 |

See Selected Bibliography.

*Less frequent manifestations include vomiting, oral ulcers, esophageal ulcers, cough, abdominal pain, oral candidiasis, esophageal candidiasis, chest pain, photophobia, rhabdomyolysis, and renal failure.

**Table 100.5** Major opportunistic diseases with systemic manifestations in HIV infection and AIDS

| |
|---|
| *Mycobacterium avium* complex infection (disseminated) |
| *Mycobacterium tuberculosis* infection (disseminated) |
| Nontuberculosis mycobacterial infection (disseminated) |
| Lymphoma |
| Cytomegalovirus disease |
| Bacillary angiomatosis |
| *Histoplasma capsulatum* infection (disseminated) |
| Syphilis |
| *Cryptococcus neoformans* infection (disseminated) |
| *Toxoplasma gondii* infection |
| *Coccidioides immitis* infection (disseminated) |
| *Pneumocystis carinii* infection (extrapulmonary) |

nated MAC infection was 3–4 months; with macrolide-containing treatment regimens it is 8–11 months.

Localized MAC disease is not as common as disseminated infection, but it can present with pulmonary infiltrates, soft-tissue abscesses, cervical lymphadenitis, skin lesions, pericarditis, hepatic disease, and brain or bone lesions. Infection with numerous other species of nontuberculous mycobacteria occurs in patients with AIDS, but much less frequently. Most of these organisms have clinical presentations similar to MAC.

## Lymphoma

Non-Hodgkin's lymphoma occurs in 5%–10% of patients with HIV infection, and incidence may increase as survival is prolonged by more effective treatments. Ninety-five percent of lymphomas that occur in persons with HIV are of B-cell origin; this diagnosis is considered an AIDS-defining illness, unlike T-cell lymphomas or Hodgkin's disease. Most AIDS-associated lymphomas are high grade or intermediate grade; histologically they are large cell immunoblastic, small noncleaved (Burkitt's-like), or diffuse large cell lymphomas. Biologically, however, these tend to all behave as aggressive lymphomas. Based on clinical characteristics, AIDS lymphomas can be categorized into two main groups, those with systemic disease and those with primary central nervous system disease. Persons who develop systemic lymphoma are heterogeneous with a wide range of $CD4^+$ cell counts; median in one series of 49 patients was 189 cells/$\mu$L (range 6–987). Only one-third have prior AIDS-defining illnesses. In contrast, patients with central nervous system lymphoma usually have marked immunosuppression; 75% have $CD4^+$ cell counts $< 50$ cells/$\mu$L, and most have other AIDS-defining illnesses. Prognosis of patients with systemic AIDS lymphoma is better if patients have the following characteristics: $CD4^+$ cell count $> 200$ cells/$\mu$L, no prior AIDS-defining diagnosis, no extranodal involvement, especially no bone marrow involvement, and Karnofsky performance score $> 70$. Median survival with untreated primary central nervous system lymphoma is very poor (1–2 months).

Clinical manifestions occurring with lymphoma depend on site and extent of disease. At least 90% of AIDS-associated lymphomas present with extranodal disease. Central nervous system, bone marrow, and liver are the most frequent extranodal sites, but almost every organ can be involved (Table 100.8). Constitutional symptoms (B symptoms) occur in >80% of patients with systemic and in >90% of patients with central nervous system lymphomas. Common presentations of central nervous system lymphoma include nonfocal symptoms such as decreased cognition or headaches, as well as new onset of seizures or cranial nerve palsies. Diagnosis of lymphoma should be considered in any patient with HIV who has constitutional symptoms, presents with a mass in any location, or has unexplained neurologic or gastrointestinal symptoms, including gastrointestinal bleeding. Diagnosis of lymphoma is made by histologic examination of tissue. Marked elevations in serum lactate dehydrogenase (LDH > 1000 U/L) are suggestive of lymphoma and warrant consideration of this diagnosis. Appearance of central nervous system lymphoma on head computed tomography (CT) or magnetic resonance (MR) scans is not pathognomic; lesions may be single or multiple, and they usually enhance with contrast. Lymphoma is a leading potential diagnosis for patients with ring-enhancing brain mass lesions who are seronegative for *Toxoplasma gondii* or who fail to respond to empiric therapy for toxoplasmosis. Management of patients with lymphoma includes staging to identify extent of disease and sites to evaluate response to therapy. Major complications of lymphoma therapy are related to opportunistic infections and cytopenias.

## Cytomegalovirus

An important cause of morbidity in immunosuppressed persons is CMV, a member of the herpesvirus group. Risk for CMV disease increases with advancing immunosuppression; CMV disease usually occurs with $CD4^+$ cell counts $< 50/\mu$L. Sight-

**Table 100.6** Less common disseminated opportunistic diseases with systemic manifestations in HIV infection and AIDS

| |
|---|
| FUNGAL |
| *Penicillium marneffei* |
| *Sporobolomyces salmonicolor* |
| *Fusarium* spp. |
| *Aureobasidium pullulans* |
| *Pseudallescheria boydii* |
| BACTERIAL |
| *GRAM POSITIVE* |
| *Corynebacterium jeikeium* |
| *Rhodococcus equi* |
| *Listeria monocytogenes* |
| *GRAM NEGATIVE* |
| *Salmonella arizonae* |
| *Protomonas extorquens* |
| *Shigella flexneri* |
| *Campylobacter cinaedi* |
| *MYCOBACTERIAL* |
| *M. malmoense* |
| Bacille Calmette-Guérin |
| VIRAL |
| Parvovirus B19 |
| Vaccinia virus |
| OTHER |
| *Leishmania donovani* |

Adapted from Gradon JD, Timpone JG, Schnittman SM. Emergence of unusual opportunistic pathogens in AIDS: a review. Clin Infect Dis 1992; 15:134–157.

**Table 100.7** Major clinical manifestations of disseminated *Mycobacterium avium* complex disease in AIDS

| Symptoms | Frequency (%) | Signs/laboratory findings | Frequency (%) |
|---|---|---|---|
| Fever | 75–88 | Weight loss/cachexia | 38–56 |
| Night sweats | 27–88 | Anemia | 60–90 |
| Weight loss | 30–77 | Lymphadenopathy | 38–45 |
| Fatigue/lethargy | 50–100 | Hepatosplenomegaly | 24–30 |
| Diarrhea | 40–63 | Elevated alkaline phosphatase (serum) | 28–60 |
| Nausea/vomiting | 25–42 | | |
| Abdominal pain | 22–37 | | |

See Selected Bibliography.

Adapted from Benson CA. Disease due to the *Mycobacterium avium* complex in patients with AIDS: epidemiology and clinical syndrome. Clin Infect Dis 1994; 18(suppl 3):S218–222.

threatening or life-threatening CMV disease develops in 20%–40% of those with AIDS and is even higher in autopsy studies. More than 90% of patients with CMV disease have other AIDS-defining illness(es); mean time from diagnosis of AIDS to CMV end-organ disease is 9–18 months.

Although CMV infection is systemic, the most frequent clinical manifestations in persons with HIV infection are from infection of target organs (discussed later). Cytomegalovirus disease affects several organ systems, most commonly eye and gastrointestinal tract (Table 100.9). However, systemic symptoms such as fever can occur before local involvement is evident. Typically, CMV biliary tract disease presents with prominent systemic symptoms, including fever and nausea, as well as abdominal pain, hepatomegaly, and elevated alkaline phosphatase.

## Bacillary angiomatosis

Bacillary angiomatosis (BA), a recently described infection that occurs primarily in persons with HIV, is caused by infection with *Bartonella* (formerly *Rochalimaea*) *henselae* and *B. quintana*. *Bartonella* species also cause cat scratch disease, relapsing fever, and endocarditis. Lesions of bacillary angiomatosis occur in a number of different organs (Table 100.10) and are characterized by localized vascular proliferation and the presence of organisms when appropriate stains are performed. Bacillary parenchymal peliosis (BPP; formerly called peliosis hepatitis) is associated with the same organisms but has a different histology from bacillary angiomatosis and may have a different pathogenesis. The prevalence and incidence of these conditions and organisms is unclear. Bacillary angiomatosis most often occurs in patients with $CD4^+$ cell counts $<100/\mu L$; median $CD4^+$ cell count in 42 affected patients was $21/\mu L$ (range 1–228).

Bacillary angiomatosis has many clinical presentations (Table 100.10). Constitutional symptoms are common; the majority of patients in one case series had fever (93%), decreased appetite (69%), lymphadenopathy (76%), and hepatomegaly (50%). Skin is the most commonly involved site, with lesions varying widely in appearance and number (one to hundreds). Cutaneous lesions can be red papules or dry, scaly, hyperkeratotic plaques. Subcutaneous nodules can be flesh-colored or have overlying erythema; they can be single or multiple (Fig. 100.1). Of note, 45% of patients in one series did not have cutaneous or subcutaneous involvement. Lymphadenopathy can occur in the regional lymph nodes draining involved skin or in the absence of skin lesions. Bacteremia with *B. henselae* and *B. quintana* can occur with or without localized tissue involvement. Bone lesions occur most often in long bones. Alternative diagnoses to cutaneous bacillary angiomatosis include Kaposi's sarcoma, an-

**Table 100.8** Extranodal sites of lymphoma in AIDS

| More common | Less common |
|---|---|
| Central nervous system/meninges | Lung/pleura |
| Bone marrow | Skin/soft tissue |
| Gastrointestinal tract (in total) | Small bowel |
| Liver | Bone |
| Spleen | Posterior pharynx |
| | Oral cavity |
| | Anorectum |
| | Stomach |
| | Large bowel/appendix |
| | Parotid gland |
| | Esophagus |
| | Bile duct |
| | Heart/pericardium |
| | Testes |
| | Conjunctiva |
| | Paranasal sinus |
| | Epidural space |

Adapted from Herndier BG, Kaplan LD, McGrath MS. Pathogenesis of AIDS lymphomas. AIDS 1994; 8:1025–1049.

**Table 100.9** Clinical manifestations of cytomegalovirus infection in HIV infection and AIDS

| | |
|---|---|
| OPHTHALMOLOGIC | CENTRAL NERVOUS SYSTEM |
| Retinitis | Encephalitis |
| | Myelitis |
| GASTROINTESTINAL | Peripheral neuropathy |
| Colitis | Polyradiculopathy |
| Esophagitis | |
| Gastritis | ADRENAL |
| Enteritis | Insufficiency |
| Hepatitis | |
| Biliary tract disease | RESPIRATORY |
| Cholecystitis | Pneumonia |
| Pancreatitis | |
| | SKIN |
| | Ulcers |
| | Rash |

**Table 100.10** Clinical manifestations of and involved organs with bacillary angiomatosis and bacillary parenchymal peliosis in HIV infection and AIDS

| More common | Less common |
|---|---|
| Skin (with fever) (BA) | Bone |
| Cutaneous (diverse lesions) | Painful osteolytic lesions (BA) |
| Subcutaneous nodules | |
| | Gastrointestinal tract |
| Hepatosplenomegaly (with fever) (BPP) | Nodular lesions (BA) |
| Abdominal pain/nausea/anorexia | |
| Elevated alkaline phosphatase | Respiratory tract |
| Increased transaminases (mild) | Nodular lesions (BA) |
| Lymphadenopathy (with fever) (BA) | Central nervous system |
| Single or multiple nodes | Mass lesions (BA) |
| Isolated fever (BA) | Bone marrow (BA) |
| | Bacteremia (BA) |
| | Endocarditis (BA) |

Abbreviations: BA, bacillary angiomatosis; BPP, bacillary parenchymal peliosis.

giosarcoma, pyogenic granuloma, subcutaneous tumors, and disseminated fungal and mycobacterial infections. Lymphoma and metastatic carcinoma are among the differential diagnoses for bacillary angiomatosis of lymph nodes. Diagnosis is usually made from characteristic histology and presence of organisms using a modified silver stain in tissue biopsies, or detection of one of these organisms in lysis-centrifugation blood cultures. Unlike some HIV-associated infections, response to appropriate antimicrobial therapy is excellent.

## Histoplasmosis

Histoplasmosis is an opportunistic fungal infection caused by *Histoplasma capsulatum*, which is endemic in soil in the Ohio and Mississippi river valleys, parts of Latin America, and the Caribbean. Histoplasmosis occurs in 2%–5% of persons with AIDS in endemic areas, and up to 25% in several midwestern cities during outbreaks. Histoplasmosis has been diagnosed in patients outside endemic areas, usually, but not exclusively, in persons who have traveled or lived in endemic areas. Risk factors for disseminated disease include immunosuppression; 90% of patients have $CD4^+$ cell counts $<100/\mu L$. Histoplasmosis is the initial AIDS-defining disease in nearly two-thirds of affected patients.

More than 95% of patients with HIV who develop histoplasmosis have disseminated disease, although local manifestations are also common (Table 100.11). Clinical presentation is most often subacute, with unexplained fever and progressive weight

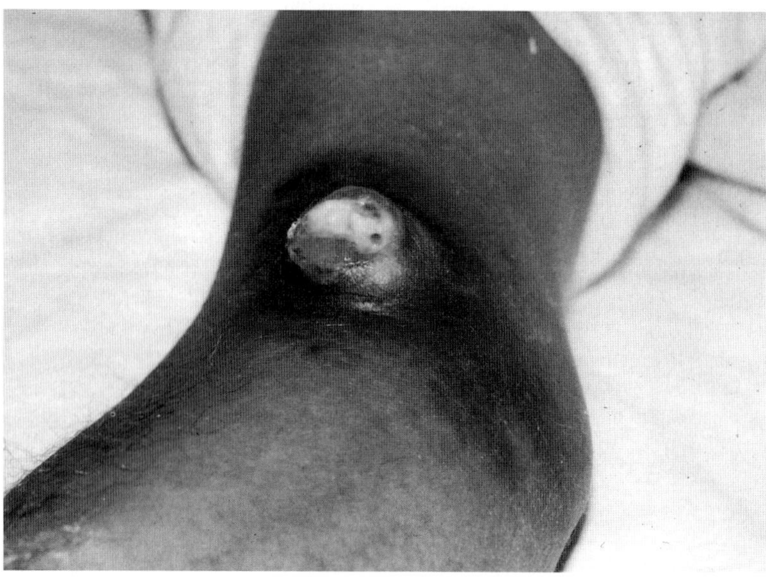

**Fig. 100.1** Large nodular bacillary angiomatosis lesion of the arm. [Credit: David Spach, MD.]

**Table 100.11** Major clinical manifestations of histoplasmosis in HIV infection and AIDS*

| Feature | Frequency (%) |
|---|---|
| Constitutional | |
| Fever | 90–96 |
| Weight loss | 60–96 |
| Lymphadenopathy | 16–37 |
| Respiratory | |
| Symptoms (cough, dyspnea) | 15–53 |
| Abnormal chest x-ray | 53–64 |
| Diffuse infiltrate | 44–46 |
| Local infiltrate | 7–11 |
| Gastrointestinal | |
| Splenomegaly | 13–35 |
| Hepatomegaly | 26–29 |
| Symptoms | 3–12 |
| Central nervous system | 5–20 |
| Septicemia syndrome[a] | 10–15 |
| Skin lesions | 1–18 |

See Selected Bibliography.

*Less common manifestations include oral lesions, colonic ulcers, mesentaric nodules, pericarditis, prostatitis, and thrombocytopenia.

[a]Hypotension, multiorgan failure, coagulopathy, pancytopenia, and/or rhabdomyolysis.

loss over several weeks; pulmonary symptoms are common. Neurologic manifestations include encephalopathy, meningitis, and focal brain lesions. Skin lesions can have a variety of appearances, including an erythematous maculopapular rash, pustules, papules, plaques, and crusted ulcers. Nonspecific laboratory abnormalities include pancytopenia and elevations in transaminases. Differential diagnosis includes other systemic opportunistic illnesses (Tables 100.5 and 100.6) and primary pulmonary pathogens such as *Pneumocystis carinii*. The most common methods to diagnose histoplasmosis are cultures (or less commonly stains) of blood or bone marrow; these cultures have sensitivities of >90%, although results may take up to 6 weeks. With localizing symptoms or signs, stains or cultures of bronchioalveolar lavage fluid, cerebrospinal fluid (CSF), and other sterile tissues and fluids may be useful (Fig. 100.2). Detection of histoplasma antigen allows for more rapid diagnosis than culture and can be used to monitor effects of therapy; antigen can be detected in urine, blood, bronchioalveolar lavage fluid, and CSF. Anti–*H. capsulatum* antibody assays are not as sensitive as culture or antigen detection, but they are positive in 50%–70%, depending on type of serological test.

## Syphilis

Syphilis, especially secondary syphilis, is well-known as an illness with protean systemic manifestations; this is also true in patients with HIV infection. Patients with syphilis and HIV infection have an increased likelihood of developing more florid or less common manifestations of syphilis. Although no unique manifestations of syphilis occur in patients with HIV, incidence of clinically symptomatic neurosyphilis, especially with hearing loss and ocular manifestations, appears greater. Neurologic manifestations of syphilis include acute or chronic meningitis, cranial nerve palsies, peripheral neuropathy, dementia, cerebrovascular disease, and myelopathy. Patients with HIV often have high nontreponemal serologic test titers, and patients who have received therapy for syphilis may have a delayed or inadequate serologic response to treatment. Patients with HIV infection and syphilis should be carefully evaluated for neurologic symptoms and signs and undergo further testing (e.g., ophthalmologic examination, lumbar puncture) if abnormalities are detected. A positive CSF VDRL is diagnostic of neurosyphilis, but

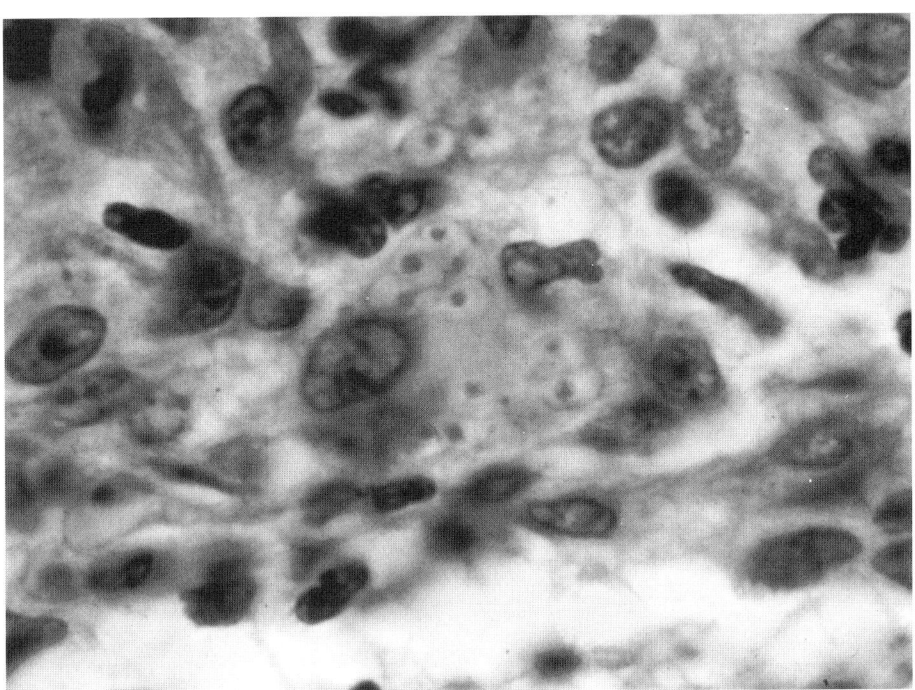

**Fig. 100.2** *Histoplasma capsulatum* in a liver biopsy stained with hematoxylin and eosin. [Credit: L. Joseph Wheat, MD.]

**Table 100.12** Major retinal and choroid manifestations in HIV infection and AIDS

| |
|---|
| DIFFERENTIAL DIAGNOSIS OF CMV RETINITIS |
| Cotton wool spots |
| Cytomegalovirus retinitis |
| Toxoplasmosis |
| Candidiasis |
| Syphilis |
| OTHER RETINAL MANIFESTATIONS |
| Acute retinal necrosis (ARN) |
| Progressive outer retinal necrosis (PORN) |
| Pneumocystis choroidopathy |
| Cryptococcus |
| Mycobacterial infection |
| Lymphoma |
| Histoplasmosis |

it is only 30%–70% sensitive. Treatment recommendations for syphilis in patients with HIV infection are similar to non–HIV-infected persons.

## Eye Disease

A variety of diseases can present with ophthalmologic manifestations, with CMV retinitis being the most frequent serious illness (Table 100.12). Cotton wool spots result from microvascular infarcts of the nerve fiber layer of the retina; they generally resolve over time. Unless recognized early and treated, CMV retinitis is a vision-threatening infection. It usually appears as perivascular yellow or white retinal infiltrate(s) with associated hemorrhage or with focal white, granular retinal infiltrates without hemorrhage. Lesions progress over days to weeks and result in atrophic, thinned areas with destruction of all layers of the retina and permanent visual loss. Lesions of CMV retinitis tend to expand in a "brushfire" pattern; there is minimal vitreous inflammation. In addition to irreversible necrosis that occurs in affected areas, surrounding areas may develop edema that is reversible if treatment is instituted. Symptoms of CMV retinitis and likelihood of visual impairment or loss depend on the location of the retinal lesion(s) (Table 100.13); persons with CMV retinitis can be asymptomatic. Eye pain, photophobia, and erythema are not characteristic. One or both eyes may be involved with CMV retinitis, with unilateral disease in about 60% at initial diagnosis. Up to 30% of patients may have subsequent retinal detachments; these patients often have acute ocular symptoms.

Diagnosis of CMV retinitis is a clinical one, based on characteristic appearance of the fundus in a patient with HIV and severe immunosuppression. Cytomegalovirus antibody assays, cultures, antigen, or viral DNA detection is not necessary for diagnosis, although the latter are being studied for use in prevention and management of CMV infection. A key principle in management of CMV retinitis is early diagnosis. Methods to add in recognition of CMV retinitis include educating patients about symptoms of CMV eye disease and regular use of the Amsler grid by patients to screen their vision. Once a diagnosis of CMV retinitis has been made, discussion of therapeutic options and prompt initiation of therapy is important. Even with successful initial therapy, recurrence of CMV retinitis is common.

## Neurologic Disease

A broad range of neurologic disorders can occur in association with HIV infection. Clinical manifestations of these entities can be broadly divided into disorders presenting primarily with dementia, focal central nervous system lesions, other central nervous system manifestations, myelopathy, peripheral neuropathy, and myopathy.

## Dementia

Dementia, confusion, or mental status changes can be a presenting feature of several HIV-associated diseases (Table 100.14). So-called HIV dementia—also called AIDS dementia complex, HIV encephalopathy, HIV-1–associated cognitive/motor complex, and subacute encephalitis—is the most common central nervous system complication of HIV, affecting an estimated 10%–20% of patients. Human immunodeficiency virus dementia is a subcortical disease whose specific pathogenesis is still under investigation, with theories suggesting direct or indirect effects of HIV, including toxic effects of viral gene products, neurotoxic cytokines, and activation of *N*-methyl-D-aspartate (NMDA) receptors. Most often HIV dementia occurs in patients with $CD4^+$ cell counts $< 200/\mu L$, who have had prior AIDS-defining diseases. Symptoms and signs of HIV dementia include cognitive, motor, and behavioral changes (Table 100.15); these usually have an insidious onset and are generally progressive if untreated.

Diagnosis of HIV dementia is a clinical diagnosis of exclusion. Evaluations to ensure other potential diagnoses are not present should include a neuroimaging study (preferably an MR scan), CSF examination, and blood studies for systemic infections (e.g., syphilis, cryptococcus). Neuroimaging studies often show cerebral atrophy, ventricular enlargement, and diffuse or patchy white matter increased signal. However, these findings are nonspecific, and scans may be normal. Abnormalities in CSF are common and similar to patients with HIV without dementia, including increased total protein, mild pleocytosis, oligoclonal bands, and intrathecal synthesis of anti-HIV immunoglobulin. Increased CSF $\beta_2$-microglobulin, neopterin, and quinolinic acid are more common in patients with HIV dementia than other patients with HIV, and levels may correlate with disease severity.

**Table 100.13** Major symptoms of cytomegalovirus retinitis in AIDS

| |
|---|
| POSTERIOR EYE LESIONS |
| Scotoma |
| Blindspots (visual defects) |
| Blurry vision or decreased visual acuity |
| Visual loss |
| Floaters[a] |
| ANTERIOR EYE LESIONS |
| No symptoms |
| Peripheral vision defects |
| Floaters[a] |
| RETINAL DETACHMENT |
| Flashing lights |
| Floaters[a] (multiple) |
| Scotoma |
| Visual (field) defects |
| Visual loss |

[a]From white blood cells or debris in vitreous.

**Table 100.14** Major disorders which commonly present with dementia, confusion, or mental status changes in HIV infection and AIDS

| Disorder | Clinical presentation | Fever |
|---|---|---|
| HIV dementia | Subacute | No |
| Toxoplasma encephalitis | Variable[a] | Often |
| Progressive multifocal leukoencephalopathy[b] | Subacute but progressive | No |
| Primary central nervous system lymphoma | Variable | Often |
| Cytomegalovirus encephalitis | Acute | Often |
| Neurosyphilis | Variable | Uncommon |
| Mood disorders | Variable | No |
| Delerium due to systemic illnesses | Acute | Often |
| Delerium due to medications | Acute | Uncommon |

[a]Subacute or acute

[b]Dementia, confusion, or mental status changes are rarely seen without concomitant focal findings.

One group has shown that a CSF $\beta_2$-microglobulin concentration of $\geq$3.8 mg/dL is very specific but insensitive for the diagnosis of HIV dementia. Patients with HIV dementia have abnormal results on neuropsychological testing; this may be useful in some patients to support the diagnosis and provide an objective measurement to follow during therapy.

## Cytomegalovirus encephalitis

Neurological involvement with CMV can manifest with several different clinical syndromes (Table 100.9). Histologic evidence of CMV infection is common in brains of persons with AIDS who have autopsies, but prevalence of clinically evident CMV encephalitis is unclear, because of the frequent presence of HIV or other opportunistic infections. Clinical presentation of CMV encephalitis has a more acute onset than HIV dementia and usually occurs in more immunocompromised patients (CD4$^+$ cell counts $< 50/\mu$L) who have CMV involvement of other organs. Diagnosis is suggested by detection of CMV DNA in CSF using a polymerase chain reaction (PCR) assay.

## Focal Central Nervous System Lesions

Focal intracerebral lesions are commonly found during evaluation of patients with neurological problems (Table 100.16). Patients may present with nonfocal or systemic symptoms such as headache, confusion, or fever; focal neurological complaints; or focal or generalized seizures. Physical examination findings that suggest presence of a focal lesion include hemiparesis, ataxia, aphasia, and mental status abnormalities.

## Toxoplasmosis

The most common cause of central nervous system mass lesions in patients with HIV is toxoplasma encephalitis, caused by the protozoa *T. gondii*. Toxoplasmosis occurs in 5%–40% of patients with AIDS and is almost always due to reactivation of chronic infection. Approximately 30% of United States adults and up to 90% in France and developing countries are infected with *T. gondii*. Toxoplasmosis generally occurs in patients with CD4$^+$ cell counts $<200/\mu$L and is the index AIDS-defining illness in 40%–50% of affected patients. Among persons seropositive for *T. gondii*, up to 25% will develop toxoplasma encephalitis within 2 years of severe immunosuppression, unless preventative therapy is used. Clinical manifestations of toxoplasma encephalitis are listed in Table 100.17; the most common presentation is an insidious onset of nonfocal symptoms followed by development of focal neurological problems over weeks to months. The illness can also present with acute symptoms and neurologic abnormalities, including confusion and coma. Overall, 75%–80% of patients have multiple symptoms. About half present with both

**Table 100.15** Major signs and symptoms of HIV dementia

| Cognitive | Motor | Behavioral | Other |
|---|---|---|---|
| | Early | | |
| Mental slowing<br>Decreased concentration<br>Forgetfulness | Motor slowing<br>Altered handwriting<br>Leg weakness<br>Unsteady gait | Apathy<br>Social withdrawal<br>Irritability | Decreased speech |
| | Later | | |
| Confusion<br>Disorientation<br>Memory loss | Decreased coordination<br>Leg weakness<br>Immobility<br>Spasticity<br>Psychomotor retardation | Mania<br>Psychosis<br>Psychomotor retardation<br>Alert but mute | Tremor<br>Frontal release signs<br>Seizures<br>Incontinence |

**Table 100.16** Neurological disorders associated with HIV and AIDS which present with focal central nervous system lesions

| More common | Less common |
|---|---|
| *Toxoplasma gondii* encephalitis | *Cryptococcus neoformans* meningitis |
| Central nervous system lymphoma | Bacterial brain abscess |
| Progressive multifocal leukoencephalopathy | Mycobacterial disease |
| | Neurosyphilis |
| | *Nocardia sp.* |
| | *Trypanosoma cruzi* |

nonfocal symptoms and focal neurologic findings, one-third with only focal complaints or findings, and the minority with only nonfocal symptoms.

Patients suspected of having toxoplasma encephalitis should undergo brain imaging and have a serological assay for anti–*Toxoplasma* immunoglobulin G (IgG). Brain CT scans show single or multiple ring or homogeneously contrast-enhancing lesions in >90% of patients. Since MR scans often show more lesions than CT scans, this is the preferred imaging procedure if available. If a CT scan shows only one lesion or is negative, MR scan should also be done. Single contrast-enhancing lesions on MR scan are more likely to be lymphoma than toxoplasmosis, although neither entity has a pathognomonic appearance. Rare patients may have diffuse encephalitis, without localized lesions. Anti–*Toxoplasma* IgG is detectable in serum in ≥95% of patients, using an enzyme-linked immunosorbent assay. Sensitivity of immunofluorescence assay is lower, approximately 85%. Detection of toxoplasma DNA in CSF by a polymerase chain reaction is being studied. Without this assay, the purpose of CSF evaluation is to exclude other diagnoses. Definitive diagnosis of toxoplasma encephalitis requires brain biopsy, but a presumptive diagnosis can be made by response to a treatment trial for toxoplasmosis. The best candidates for a treatment trial are patients with a characteristic clinical presentation, with more than one contrast-enhancing lesion on neuroimaging, detectable anti–*Toxoplasma* IgG, who are not using trimethoprim–sulfamethoxazole (for *Pneumocystis* prophylaxis), and who show no evidence of other more likely diagnoses. Brain biopsy should be considered in patients with negative toxoplasma serology, a single mass lesion on MR scan, patients taking trimethoprim–sulfamethoxazole, and in patients who fail to respond clinically or radiographically to anti-*Toxoplasma* therapy.

## Lymphoma

Primary central nervous system lymphoma is another common cause of mass lesions in persons with advanced HIV, as discussed previously.

## Progressive multifocal leukoencephalopathy

Progressive multifocal leukoencephalopathy (PML) is a demyelinating disease of the central nervous system caused by JC virus, a papovavirus which is often acquired in childhood and reactivates when severe immunosuppression occurs. It occurs in 4% of persons with HIV infection and is the initial AIDS-defining illness in about 30% of patients with PML. $CD4^+$ cell counts are usually $<100/\mu L$. The clinical presentation is not specific for PML. Symptoms include limb weakness or incoordination, confusion, speech problems, and less commonly headache. Common neurologic findings with PML include focal weakness or hemiparesis, altered mental status, visual field defects, dysarthria, and gait abnormalities. The usual course of illness is progressive neurologic impairment with a median survival of 2 to 4 months. However, approximately 10% of patients have a more benign course, with longer survival. Evaluation of patients with suspected PML should include a neuroimaging procedure, with MR scan being preferable to CT scanning. Magnetic resonance scans usually show multiple, often confluent, white matter lesions that do not enhance with contrast or show mass effect; lesions are

**Table 100.17** Major clinical manifestations of toxoplasma encephalitis in AIDS

| Symptoms | Frequency (%) | Signs | Frequency (%) |
|---|---|---|---|
| Headache | 49–73 | Altered mental status | 42–57 |
| Confusion | 15–56 | Hemiparesis | 28–51 |
| Fever | 6–56 | Cranial nerve findings | 7–37 |
| Lethargy | 11–52 | Aphasia | 6–22 |
| Seizures | 12–29 | Ataxia | 2–22 |
| Behavioral changes | 4–15 | Meningismus | 10–16 |
| | | Sensory changes | 10–12 |
| | | Visual field defect | 7–8 |
| | | Papilledema | 0–8 |

See Selected Bibliography.

low-intensity on T1-weighted images and high intensity on T2-weighted images (Fig. 100.3). Computed tomography scans of patients with PML may also show multiple, often confluent, hypodense, white matter lesions that do not enhance with contrast, and do not have mass effect, but CT scans may also be negative. Cerebrospinal fluid is usually normal in patients with PML but should be examined to ensure the patient does not have another concurrent central nervous system infection. Utility of polymerase chain reaction assays for JC virus in CSF is under study. Although brain biopsy is required to confirm a diagnosis of PML, a presumptive diagnosis can often be made in patients with typical clinical and neuroimaging characteristics, especially if CSF has detectable JC virus by PCR assay.

**Table 100.18** Initial presenting sites of *Cryptococcus neoformans* infection in HIV infection and AIDS

| Feature | Frequency (%) |
|---|---|
| Meningitis | 85–90 |
| Cryptococcemia (without meningitis) | 5–10 |
| Pneumonia (without meningitis) | 4–5 |
| Urinary tract | 1–2 |
| Cryptococcus antigenemia alone | <1 |
| Other[a] | <1 |

See Selected Bibliography.
[a]Includes bone marrow, peritoneal, hepatic infection.

## Other Central Nervous System Infections

### Cryptococcal disease

*Cryptococcus neoformans* is a ubiquitous fungus that causes life-threatening disease in immunocompromised patients. About 7% of persons with HIV develop extrapulmonary cryptococcal disease, which usually occurs in patients with $CD4^+$ cell counts $<100/\mu L$ and is the first AIDS-defining illness in approximately 50% of affected patients. Cryptococcal meningitis is the most frequent clinical presentation (Table 100.18). In patients with cryptococcal meningitis, extraneural disease occurs in up to 30%, with pulmonary and skin involvement being common. Clinical presentation of cryptococcal meningitis is nonspecific (Table 100.19). Findings consistent with meningeal inflammation, such as stiff neck and photophobia, occur in a minority and focal neurologic deficits occur in <20% of patients. Evaluation of patients with suspected cryptococcal meningitis should include neuroimaging, lumbar puncture with measurement of opening pressure, and CSF studies including cryptococcal antigen and fungal culture, as well as more routine studies, serum cryptococcal antigen, and fungal blood cultures. Diagnosis of cryptococcal meningitis is confirmed by isolation of the organism from CSF; >95% of patients will also have detectable CSF cryptococcal antigen. If cryptococcal antigen testing is unavailable, India ink staining can be performed, although it is less sensitive (80%). Head CT and MR scans are abnormal in approximately 30%, but findings are not specific. Some 50%–70% of patients with cryptococcal meningitis have cryptococcemia. In patients with cryptococcal meningitis, those who present with abnormal mental status, CSF WBC <20 cells/$\mu$L, CSF antigen >1:1024, or extraneural infection have a worse prognosis. Management strategies include prompt antifungal therapy. Measures to decrease intracranial pressure should be considered in patients with increased pressure. Patients who are found to have cryptococcal infection at an extraneural site should be evaluated for the presence of meningitis.

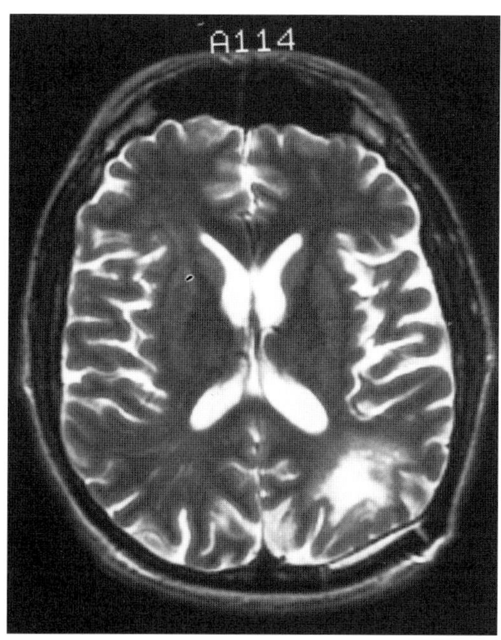


**Fig. 100.3** $T_2$-weighted magnetic resonance scan in an HIV-infected patient with biopsy-proven progressive multifocal leukoencephalopathy showing a focal area of increased signal in the left parietal white matter.

### Peripheral neuropathies

Peripheral neuropathy is characterized clinically by sensory loss, weakness, or diminished reflexes. Four main types of peripheral

**Table 100.19** Major clinical manifestations of cryptococcal meningitis in AIDS

| Feature | Frequency (%) |
|---|---|
| Headache | 67–100 |
| Fever | 61–88 |
| Malaise | 38–76 |
| Nausea/vomiting | 42–83 |
| Meningismus | 27–37 |
| Cough/dyspnea | 18–30 |
| Visual changes[a] | 30 |
| Mental status changes | 18–33 |
| Behavioral changes[a] | 23 |
| Photophobia | 18–19 |
| Skin lesions | 7–10 |
| Seizures | 4–11 |
| Syncope[a] | 7 |
| Psychosis/mania[a] | 4 |

See Selected Bibliography.
[a]Not specifically described in all series.

**Table 100.20** Characteristics of major types of peripheral neuropathies in HIV infection and AIDS

| Type | HIV stage | Onset | Symptoms | Signs |
|---|---|---|---|---|
| Distal sensory polyneuropathy | AIDS > earlier | Subacute for HIV-related<br>Acute for toxin-related | Progressive numbness, paresthesia, pain, burning in feet > hands | Symmetrical stocking/glove sensory abnormalities in feet > hands<br>Decreased or absent ankle reflexes |
| Inflammatory demyelinating polyneuropathy | Primary and early HIV | Variable[a] | Progressive weakness, mild sensory loss | Distal > proximal extremity weakness<br>Areflexia<br>Decreased vibration |
| Lumbosacral polyradiculopathy | AIDS<br>$CD4^+$ cells $< 200/\mu L$ | Variable[a] | Progressive leg weakness, urinary incontinence<br>Arm weakness later in course | Asymmetric leg weakness, paraparesis, or quadreparesis, sacral sensory loss<br>Asymmetric reflexes or areflexia<br>Urinary retention |
| Mononeuritis multiplex (2 forms) | Early | Acute | Self-limited numbness or weakness, pain | Multifocal or asymmetric sensory loss or weakness in nerve distribution or root, local decreased reflexes |
| | $CD4^+$ cells $< 50/\mu L$ | Acute | Progressive sensory loss, weakness, pain | Similar to above, but usually multiple nerves/roots and more severe[b] |

[a]Onset of illness may be acute or subacute.

[b]May be indistinguishable clinically from inflammatory demyelinating polyneuropathy.

**Table 100.21** Etiologies of distal sensory polyneuropathy in HIV infection and AIDS

| |
|---|
| HIV infection (direct or indirect effects such as cytokines) |
| B12 deficiency |
| Neurotoxins |
| Dapsone |
| Didanosine |
| Isoniazid |
| Ethambutol |
| Ethanol |
| Stavudine |
| Trimethoprim–sulfamethoxazole |
| Vincristine |
| Zalcitabine |
| Diabetes mellitis |
| Renal insufficiency |
| Hypothyroidism |

neuropathy occur in patients with HIV infection, and each has characteristic features (Table 100.20). Distal sensory polyneuropathy is the most common type of neuropathy, and pathologic evidence of this entity is present in the majority of patients dying of AIDS. Potential etiologies of distal sensory polyneuropathy are listed in Table 100.21. Usually HIV-related disease has a more subacute presentation than nucleoside-associated disease, but reversibility with discontinuation of neurotoxic therapy is the major means to differentiate etiology. Worsening of symptoms for several weeks after discontinuation of the offending therapy (called "coasting") may occur.

### Inflammatory demyelinating polyneuropathy

Inflammatory demyelinating polyneuropathy is similar to Guillain-Barre syndrome and is probably immune-mediated. Evaluation should include electromyography (EMG) and nerve conduction velocity (NCV) studies, which show electrophysiologic signs of demyelination and axonal loss. Lumbar puncture should be performed to evaluate the possibilities of CMV, syphilis, or malignancy. Cerebrospinal fluid typically shows elevated protein and mild pleocytosis.

### Lumbosacral polyradiculopathy

This has a fairly unusual clinical presentation. Rapid progression of deficits from distal to proximal is common. The most frequent etiology is CMV infection, although lymphoma, toxoplasmosis, neurosyphilis, and tuberculosis can cause similar findings. Lumbar puncture is the most important diagnostic procedure. Cerebrospinal fluid usually shows marked pleocytosis, with hundreds of neutrophils; fluid should be tested for CMV (culture, antigen, or PCR), cytology, VDRL, and *M. tuberculosis*. Cytomegalovirus culture is positive in about 50% of patients; a negative culture does not exclude the diagnosis. EMG/NCV studies show acute denervation. Presumptive therapy with antivirals effective against CMV is recommended in patients with typical clinical findings and CSF with neutrophils present and low glucose.

### Mononeuritis multiplex

Clinical course of mononeuritis multiplex varies in patients with early and advanced HIV infection. In early HIV infection, one or a few nerves are involved and the syndrome resolves spontaneously. In advanced HIV infection, the neuropathy is often rapidly progressive, may result in severe nerve involvement (e.g., quadraparesis or severe hoarseness with vocal cord paralysis), and appear similar to inflammatory demyelinating polyneuropathy. EMG/NCV studies can support the diagnosis; additionally, these studies can exclude entrapment neuropathies, which can have similar presentations. Anecdotal reports suggest that some patients with advanced HIV and mononeuritis multiplex may have CMV infection.

## Myopathy

Myopathy may occur at any stage of HIV infection and appears to be more frequent than in persons without HIV infection, although the prevalence is unknown. The most common clinical findings of myopathy are listed in Table 100.22. In the appropriate setting, elevated creatine phosphokinase (CPK) or aldolase can suggest the diagnosis, but EMG or muscle biopsy is required to confirm this diagnosis. Zidovudine has been implicated as a cause of myopathy.

## Pulmonary Disease

The lungs are the primary target organ for several serious complications of HIV infection (Table 100.23). At least 65% of AIDS-defining illnesses have pulmonary manifestations. Many systemic diseases involve the lungs (Tables 100.5 and 100.23). One important aspect of management of patients with HIV infection and unexplained pulmonary disease is to consider the need for respiratory isolation while diagnostic evaluations are undertaken, in order to minimize transmission of tuberculosis.

**Table 100.22** Major clinical manifestations of myopathy in HIV infection and AIDS

| Symptoms | Signs |
|---|---|
| Myalgias | Symmetric weakness: proximal > distal in UE and LE |
| Progressive weakness: proximal > distal in UE and LE | Elevated serum creatine kinase or aldolase |
| Weight loss | Abnormal (myopathic) electromyography |
| | Abnormal muscle biopsy: myofiber degeneration, myofiber necrosis, nemaline rod bodies, cytoplasmic bodies, mitochondrial abnormalities, inflammation |

**Table 100.23** Major pulmonary conditions in HIV infection and AIDS

| INFECTIONS | FUNGI |
|---|---|
| PROTOZOAN (FUNGI?)<br>*Pneumocystis Carinii* | *Histoplasma capsulatum*<br>*Cryptococcus neoformans*<br>*Coccidioides immitis* |
| MYCOBACTERIA<br>*M. tuberculosis*<br>*M. avium* complex<br>Other nontuberculosis mycobacteria | MALIGNANCIES<br>Kaposi's sarcoma<br>Lymphoma |
| BACTERIA<br>*Streptococcus pneumoniae*<br>*Haemophilus influenzae*<br>*Staphylococcus aureus*<br>*Branhamella catarrhalis*<br>*Legionella* species<br>*Mycoplasma pneumoniae*<br>*Rhodococcus equi* | IDIOPATHIC<br>Nonspecific interstitial pneumonitis |

Adapted from Meduri GU, Stein DS. Pulmonary manifestations of acquired immunodeficiency syndrome. Clin Infect Dis 1992; 14:98–113.

## *Pneumocystis carinii* pneumonia

*Pneumocystis carinii* pneumonia (PCP) was one of the first recognized manifestations of AIDS and is still among the most common. Infection with *P. carinii* commonly occurs in young children, but clinically evident disease is rare except with immune suppression. Generally PCP occurs in adults with $CD4^+$ cell counts $< 200/\mu L$. It usually presents with indolent onset of fever, malaise, nonproductive cough, and shortness of breath. Often symptoms are mild initially and progress over weeks, although fulminant respiratory failure may occur. Extrapulmonary *P. carinii* also occurs, with disease reported from diverse body locations, but it is not common. Physical examination of patients with PCP may show elevated respiratory rate, rhonchi or rales, but may be normal in up to 50%. Chest x-rays commonly reveal diffuse, bilateral interstitial infiltrates; nodules, apical disease, pneumothorax, and pleural effusions less commonly occur (Table 100.24 and Fig. 100.4). Chest x-rays may also be normal (6%–23%). Arterial blood gases are abnormal in 80% of patients. Exercise-induced oxygen desaturation may occur. Serum lactate dehydrogenase (LDH) levels are frequently elevated; however, this is nonspecific.

**Table 100.24** Common chest x-ray findings with pulmonary disease in HIV infection and AIDS

| DIFFUSE INTERSTITIAL INFILTRATES | PLEURAL EFFUSIONS |
|---|---|
| *P. carinii*<br>Tuberculosis<br>Histoplasmosis<br>Coccidioidomycosis<br>Kaposi's sarcoma<br>Nonspecific interstitial pneumonitis | Kaposi's sarcoma<br>Tuberculosis<br>Empyema (bacterial)<br>Cryptococcus<br>Lymphoma |
| FOCAL AIRSPACE DISEASE<br>Bacterial pneumonia<br>Cryptococcosis<br>*Mycoplasma* pneumonia<br>Legionellosis<br>Kaposi's sarcoma | NORMAL<br>PCP<br>*M. avium* complex (disseminated)<br>Histoplasmosis<br>*M. tuberculosis* |
| LYMPHADENOPATHY<br>Tuberculosis<br>*M. avium* complex (disseminated)<br>Kaposi's sarcoma<br>Lymphoma | |

Management of PCP includes prompt initiation of therapy when the diagnosis is suspected, studies to confirm the diagnosis, and general supportive measures for respiratory insufficiency. Definitive diagnosis of PCP requires demonstration of organisms with special stains in induced sputum, bronchioalveolar lavage (BAL), or transbronchial biopsy. Serologic studies and cultures are not clinically useful. If induced sputum is negative, or if the patient is severely ill and more expeditious diagnosis is needed, BAL should be performed. Lung biopsies may be helpful in selected patients since other pulmonary processes may require tissue for diagnosis. After initiation of therapy, patients may have clinical deterioration for 3–5 days before improving. Overall survival from PCP with appropriate therapy is about 80%, with lower mortality in patients with milder disease.

## Tuberculosis

*Mycobacterium tuberculosis* is a frequent copathogen in patients with HIV. Among HIV-infected patients with a positive tuberculin skin test (PPD, purified protein derivative), risk of developing active tuberculosis is 8%–10% per year. Active tuberculosis occurs in about 4% of patients in the United States and at much higher rates in developing countries. Tuberculosis often presents as an early manifestation of HIV infection, with median $CD4^+$ cell counts $> 300/\mu L$, although it may also occur later in the course of HIV disease.

Tuberculosis associated with HIV has two major presentations. The type that occurs relatively early in HIV infection, usually represents reactivation disease with well-formed granuloma and localized disease. The PPD skin test is usually positive, and dis-

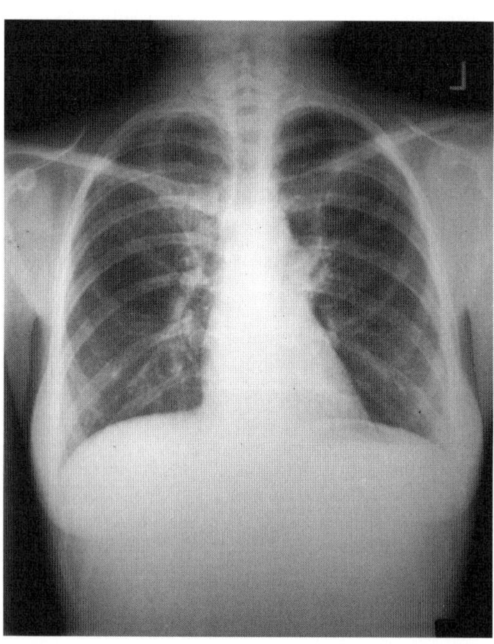

**Fig. 100.4** Chest x-ray in an HIV-infected patient with *Pneumocystis carinii* pneumonia, showing diffuse bilateral infiltrates.

ease is generally limited to the lung, presenting in a manner similar to that in non–HIV-infected individuals. Chest x-rays reveal localized apical infiltrates and cavitation similar to those seen in "typical" reactivation tuberculosis. The second form of tuberculosis occurs in patients with advanced HIV infection and often presents with nonapical pulmonary disease or at extrapulmonary sites. The PPD skin test is positive in only one-third of cases, and chest x-ray reveals features atypical for tuberculosis with lower lobe or diffuse infiltrates and hilar adenopathy. Extrapulmonary disease occurs in 25%–70% of patients with advanced HIV infection and tuberculosis, and it may involve lymph nodes, bone marrow, central nervous system, or other organs. Multi–drug-resistant tuberculosis often has a fulminant course in persons with advanced HIV infection.

Diagnosis of tuberculosis is made by identification of *M. tuberculosis* by culture, although use of PCR techniques appears promising. Specimens for mycobacterial stains and culture should be obtained from involved sites, for example, by sputum collection, BAL, or transbronchial biopsy; bone marrow aspirate and biopsy; or fine needle aspirate or biopsy of lymph nodes or other suspicious sites. Patients with positive acid-fast smears should receive presumptive antituberculosis chemotherapy until cultures are available to distinguish *M. tuberculosis* from other mycobacteria. Management of patients with active tuberculosis and HIV is similar to patients without HIV and involves prompt initiation of multidrug chemotherapy.

### Bacterial pneumonia

Bacterial pneumonias occur more commonly among HIV-infected individuals than among the general population and cause up to 10% of AIDS-associated pneumonias (Table 100.23). Clinical manifestations of bacterial pneumonia in patients with HIV infection are similar to patients without HIV and differ markedly from other more indolent pulmonary opportunistic infections. Patients with bacterial pneumonia generally present with acute onset of fever, productive cough, dyspnea, and pleuritic chest pain, and they have physical findings of lung consolidation. Duration of symptoms is usually a few days to a week. Chest x-rays usually have segmental or lobar consolidation; less commonly they have diffuse infiltrates (Table 100.24). White blood counts are usually elevated (in comparison to baseline) and have a left shift. Bacteremia is more common than in immune competent hosts.

### Other pulmonary pathogens

As discussed, many systemic opportunistic infections may have pulmonary manifestations. Pulmonary disease is often prominent with fungal infections, including histoplasmosis, cryptococcosis, and coccidioidomycosis. Symptoms are nonspecific, with fever, cough, dyspnea, and weight loss being common. *Mycobacterium avium* complex may have pulmonary manifestations in patients with AIDS, but disseminated disease is much more common. Viral infections, including CMV and other herpesviruses, are infrequent causes of pneumonia in patients with HIV infection, although recovery of CMV from BAL is common during PCP. When patients with pneumonia have histological evidence of CMV in the absence of other pathogens, CMV pneumonia should be considered.

## Gastrointestinal Disease

From oral cavity to anus, the gastrointestinal tract is a prime target for opportunistic diseases associated with HIV infection (Table 100.25). Serious gastrointestinal symptoms, particularly diarrhea, occur in 30%–50% of AIDS patients in the developed world, and virtually all persons with HIV infection will have gastrointestinal manifestations at some time.

### Oral disease

Oral lesions, which are extremely common, include increased frequency of common disorders and disease entities that are rare in normal hosts (Table 100.25; see also Chapter 60). Oral candidiasis and oral hairy leukoplakia are the most fre-

**Table 100.25** Major gastrointestinal pathogens and conditions in HIV infection and AIDS

| ORAL CAVITY | SMALL INTESTINE | LIVER/BILIARY TRACT |
|---|---|---|
| *Candida albicans* | *Cryptosporidium* | *M. avium* complex |
| Oral hairy leukoplakia | *Microsporidia* spp. | Cytomegalovirus |
| Herpes simplex virus | *Isospora belli* | *Cryptosporidium* |
| Aphthous ulceration | *M. avium* complex | Kaposi's sarcoma |
| Gingivitis | *Salmonella* spp. | *Cryptococcus neoformans* |
| Kaposi's sarcoma | *Campylobacter jejuni* | *Histoplasma capsulatum* |
| | Lymphoma | *M. tuberculosis* |
| ESOPHAGUS | Kaposi's sarcoma | Lymphoma |
| *Candida albicans* | Cytomegalovirus | Hepatitis A |
| Herpes simplex virus | | Hepatitis B |
| Cytomegalovirus | COLON | Hepatitis C |
| Aphthous ulceration | Cytomegalovirus | |
| Kaposi's sarcoma | *Cryptosporidium* | |
| Ulceration due to medication | *M. avium* complex | |
| Lymphoma | *Shigella flexneii* | |
| | *Campylobacter jejuni* | |
| STOMACH | *Clostridium difficile* | |
| Cytomegalovirus | *Histoplasma capsulatum* | |
| *M. avium* complex | Adenovirus | |
| Lymphoma | Herpes simplex virus | |
| Kaposi's sarcoma | (anorectum) | |

quent oral opportunistic infections (see also Chapters 86, 87 and 88).

### Oral candidiasis

Oral candidiasis (thrush) is frequently the first opportunistic infection that occurs in HIV-infected persons. Oral candidiasis occasionally occurs during acute HIV infection; however, generally it occurs when $CD4^+$ cell counts are $<500/\mu L$. Its frequency increases with increasing immunosuppression. Oral candidiasis is usually caused by *Candida albicans*, and less commonly by *Torulopsis glabrata*, *C. tropicalis* or other species. Lesions may be asymptomatic, although frequently patients complain of sore mouth, altered sense of taste, or a "grainy" sensation. Clinical features include white plaques on the oral mucosa (pseudomembranous candidiasis); diffuse erythema (erythematous candidiasis); hyperplastic, hyperkeratotic white patches (hyperplastic candidiasis); and painful ulceration/fissuring on the mouth corners (angular cheilitis). Diagnosis of oral candidiasis is based on typical clinical appearance and by finding hyphae and/or spores on potassium hydroxide prep. Cultures of lesions are unreliable for diagnosis, as many healthy persons are *C. albicans* carriers, but may be useful to determine antimicrobial resistance patterns in patients who do not respond to standard antifungal therapy.

### Oral hairy leukoplakia

Oral hairy leukoplakia is a white lesion found predominantly on sides of the tongue, generally in a fine corrugated pattern; the surface is irregular with prominent folds, giving it a "hairy" appearance. Epstein-Barr virus (EBV) has been shown to be present in these lesions. Oral hairy leukoplakia is seen in 25% of HIV-infected patients; most patients have $CD4^+$ cell counts $<500/\mu L$. Oral hairy leukoplakia is asymptomatic and does not require treatment; regression has been observed in patients on high-dose acyclovir for other reasons.

### Aphthous ulcers

Severe aphthous ulceration can occur in patients with HIV, usually in the setting of severe immunodeficiency. Prevalence and etiology of this condition are unclear, but single or multiple painful, enlarging, necrotic ulcers can occur in the mouth, hypopharynx, and esophagus. Lesions can interfere with eating and are often associated with malnutrition and weight loss. Diagnosis is made by biopsy of lesions for histopathology and viral and fungal culture (to exclude alternative diagnoses).

### Periodontal disease

Periodontitis occurs frequently at all stages of HIV infection. Gingivitis may occur where there is little plaque and no apparent explanation for gingivitis. Necrotizing periodontitis presents as rapid loss of soft tissue and bone with resultant loss of teeth.

## Esophageal disease

Dysphagia and odynophagia are common complaints among people with advanced HIV infection, generally signifying esophagitis (Table 100.25). Esophagitis generally occurs in patients with $CD4^+$ cell counts $<200/\mu L$.

### Esophageal candidiasis

Esophageal candidiasis is the most frequent cause of HIV-associated esophagitis and is usually caused by *C. albicans*, although other candidal strains occasionally cause disease. Patients typically complain of pain with swallowing (solids more than liquids); sometimes substernal chest pain occurs. Absence of oral thrush or use of topical antifungal therapy does not preclude the diagnosis. The entire esophagus is usually involved in a widespread, superficially erosive process. Most experts advocate empiric treatment with antifungal agents for all HIV-infected persons with symptoms of esophagitis. Upper endoscopy is reserved for patients who fail to respond to empiric treatment; it is preferred over barium swallow studies, because of higher sensitivity and need for tissue biopsies to diagnose other causes of esophagitis and drug-resistant fungi.

### Cytomegalovirus esophagitis

Generally CMV esophagitis occurs in patients with $CD4^+$ cell counts $<50/\mu L$. Patients often present with moderate to severe substernal pain with swallowing, but spontaneous substernal or midepigastric pain occurs frequently (50%). Nausea and weight loss are common. Diagnosis is made endoscopically, with one or more deep ulcers visualized in the distal esophagus. Biopsies reveal CMV intranuclear inclusion bodies in granulation tissue at the ulcer base.

### Herpes simplex virus esophagitis

Herpes simplex virus (HSV) is the least common specific infectious cause of esophagitis in patients with HIV infection; it generally occurs with $CD4^+$ cell counts $< 100/\mu L$. Symptoms tend to have an abrupt onset. Typically, HSV causes more widespread, shallow erosive ulceration than CMV.

### Aphthous ulceration of the esophagus

Idiopathic ulcerative esophagitis can occur in patients with advanced HIV infection and presents in a similar manner to CMV esophagitis. Aphthous ulcers are culture negative for CMV and HSV and lack inclusion bodies on histopathology.

### Other causes of esophagitis

Medications, including zalcitabine (and possibly other antiretrovirals), can cause ulcerative esophagitis. Kaposi's sarcoma and lymphoma may present with esophageal complaints, and other non–HIV-associated conditions such as reflux esophagitis can occur.

## Hepatobiliary disease

Liver disease is extremely common with HIV infection, ranging from asymptomatic transaminase elevation to severe right upper quadrant pain and biliary colic. Opportunistic infections and malignancies involving the liver usually reflect disseminated processes, but hepatic manifestations may be prominent.

Medications, although not specifically discussed, are a frequent cause of hepatic abnormalities in HIV-infected patients.

### *Mycobacterium avium* complex

*Mycobacterium avium* complex is a common hepatic opportunistic infection. Symptoms often include nausea and abdominal pain. Typically, patients develop elevated alkaline phosphatase, which is out of proportion to other liver function test abnormalities. Jaundice can occur if extrahepatic biliary obstruction occurs from enlarged peripancreatic lymph nodes. Biopsies classically reveal numerous acid fast bacilli with minimal granulomatous response.

### Cytomegalovirus

Evidence of hepatic involvement with CMV occurs in 30%–45% of AIDS autopsies. Cytomegalovirus produces two types of liver disease in patients with advanced HIV infection. Hepatitis is the more common form, with moderate elevations of serum transaminases and alkaline phosphatase. Jaundice is rare. Liver biopsies reveal CMV inclusion bodies in hepatocytes, vascular endothelial cells, and bile duct cells. Also, CMV may infect the biliary tree and produce a pattern similar to sclerosing cholangitis, with papillary stenosis or choledochal strictures. Patients typically have right upper quadrant pain, fever, and elevated serum alkaline phosphatase. Endoscopic retrograde cholangiopancreatography (ERCP) is usually necessary to diagnose these lesions, and sphincterotomy may provide symptomatic relief. Acalculous cholecystitis presenting with fever and right upper quadrant pain has also been attributed to CMV infection.

### Tuberculosis

Hepatic tuberculosis can occur in patients with HIV infection. Histopathology usually reveals well-formed granuloma with few acid fast bacilli.

### Cryptosporidium

Cryptosporidium, in addition to causing diarrhea (see below), can also cause sclerosing cholangitis and acalculous cholecystitis, clinically indistinguishable from CMV. The diagnosis can be made by biopsy or tissue resection.

### Other causes of liver disease in HIV infection

Several opportunistic infections, including *Cryptococcus neoformans*, *Histoplasma capsulatum*, and *Coccidioides immitis*, can also cause hepatitis in patients with HIV infection. Hepatitis A, B, and C are common; 10%–20% of patients with AIDS may have concurrent chronic hepatitis B infection. Kaposi's sarcoma and lymphoma may present as infiltrative hepatic lesions.

## Intestinal diseases

Certain diseases are more likely to affect small intestine or colon, while other conditions have generalized involvement (Table 100.25; see also Chapter 61). Diarrhea is an extremely common complaint in patients with advanced HIV infection, occurring in up to 50% of patients in developed countries and 90% of those in developing nations. In most cases (60%–85% of patients) a specific pathogen can be identified. Clinical presentation is rarely specific for a particular pathogen, although time course of illness, character of diarrhea, and associated symptoms or signs can narrow the diagnostic possibilities. Evaluation of any HIV-infected patient presenting with persistent or severe diarrhea should include assessment of hydration and nutritional status, as well as identification of specific pathogens through stool studies and sometimes intestinal biopsies.

### Cytomegalovirus

All parts of the gastrointestinal tract may be affected by CMV disease; colitis is the most frequent manifestation (Tables 100.9 and 100.25). Symptoms and signs that occur with CMV colitis include diarrhea, which may be severe and persistent or intermittent, fever, abdominal pain, weight loss, and less commonly hematochezia. Intestinal perforation can occur. Endoscopic findings can include erythema, ulceration (especially in the esophagus), hemorrhage, and edema, but the colonic mucosa can also appear normal to inspection. Diagnosis is made by histopathologic examination of gastrointestinal tissue showing large cytomegalic cells containing intranuclear inclusions and inflammatory infiltrates. Colonic involvement may be diffuse or localized and patchy, and it may involve only the right colon, suggesting that colonoscopy with multiple biopsies should be done when diagnosis of CMV colitis is under consideration.

### Cryptosporidium

Cryptosporidium is a protozoan that causes intractable watery diarrhea with severe abdominal cramping in advanced HIV infection. Less immunocompromised patients have less severe symptoms and a self-limited course. Cryptosporidium occurs in 10%–20% of AIDS patients with chronic diarrhea in the United States, and an even higher percentage in some developing nations. Malabsorption and weight loss are common. The diagnosis is usually made by microscopic identification of Cryptosporidium in stool specimens with a modified acid fast stain. It may also be identified in endoscopic biopsy samples, as it inhabits the brush border of intestinal epithelial cells. No specific effective therapy has been identified.

### *Isospora belli*

*Isospora belli* is a protozoan parasite that causes severe diarrhea in patients with advanced HIV infection, clinically similar to that caused by Cryptosporidium. *I. belli* is more common in tropical and subtropical climates than in the U.S., where it occurs in only 1%–3% of AIDS patients with diarrhea. Classically, it causes severe, watery, bloodless diarrhea, fever, and weight loss. Eosinophilia may be present. *Isospora belli* can be diagnosed on stool specimens using a modified acid fast stain or via small intestinal biopsy.

### Microsporidia

Microsporidia are obligate intracellular spore-producing protozoan parasites. There are several species of Microsporidia, although only two, *Enterocytozoon bieneusi* and *Septada intestinalis*, are known to directly infect the intestine. The role of Microsporidia in causing diarrhea in AIDS patients has been controversial. Up to 39% of small bowel biopsy specimens in HIV-infected patients with chronic unexplained diarrhea have revealed *E. bieneusi*. In contrast, one study reported *E. bieneusi* in small bowel biopsy samples of HIV-infected individuals without diarrhea, as well as with diarrhea; however, asymptomatic participants had higher $CD4^+$ cell counts than did those with diarrhea. It is possible that individuals become symptomatic only as $CD4^+$ cell counts fall. Most authorities believe that Microsporidia plays a role in chronic diarrhea in AIDS patients. Historically, these organisms have been detected only by electron microscopy. More recently, Microsporidia spores have been identified in stool specimens using light microscopy and modified trichrome or chromotropic stains.

### Other causes of intestinal disease

Another common cause of abdominal pain and diarrhea in advanced HIV infection is MAC infection, which typically occurs in the context of systemic illness, with fever, malabsorption, and weight loss. Diagnosis is based on visualization of acid fast organisms obtained from stool or biopsy samples, in the proper clinical setting. Generally, HSV proctitis presents with severe anorectal pain, tenesmus, and itching, as well as occasionally with hematochezia, sacral paresthesia, and fever; physical findings include severe tenderness, mild redness, edema, and shallow perianal ulcers. Infectious causes of diarrhea in immunocompetent hosts can also cause diarrhea in HIV-infected individuals. Bacterial infections such as *Salmonella*, *Shigella*, *Campylobacter*, and *Clostridium difficile* cause of diarrhea and fever in HIV-infected patients at all levels of $CD4^+$ cell counts. Patients with AIDS, however, are more likely to have bacteremia and recurrence of infection with these organisms. Parasitic infections such as *Giardia lamblia* and *Entamoeba histolytica* can also occur.

## Dermatologic Diseases

Cutaneous lesions are extremely common in HIV-infected individuals, affecting more than 90% of patients at some time (Tables 100.26 and 100.27). Most skin lesions are not specific for HIV infection, although they may occur more commonly or present with unusual or more severe manifestations than in persons without HIV. Other conditions, such Kaposi's sarcoma, are rarely seen in the absence of HIV infection. In general, the number and frequency of skin conditions is greater with increasing immunosuppression. The rash which occurs with primary HIV infection has been described.

**Table 100.26** Major cutaneous manifestations of infections in patients with HIV infection and AIDS

| VIRAL | BACTERIAL |
|---|---|
| Primary human immunodeficiency virus | Folliculitis |
| Herpes simplex virus | Abscesses |
| Varicella zoster virus | Impetigo |
| Molluscum contagiosum | Ecthyma |
| Human papillomavirus | Cellulitis |
| Common warts | Skin ulcers |
| Condylomata acuminata | Mycobacterial infections |
| Cytomegalovirus | Syphilis |
| | Bacillary angiomatosis |
| FUNGAL AND YEAST | Chancroid |
| Dermatophytosis | |
| Candidiasis | ARTHROPODS |
| Cryptococcus | *Sarcoptes scabiei* (scabies) |
| Histoplasmosis | Demodex folliculitis |
| Tinea versicolor | |

**Table 100.27** Major noninfectious conditions with cutaneous involvement in patients with HIV infection and AIDS

| |
|---|
| MALIGNANCIES |
| Kaposi's sarcoma |
| Lymphoma |
| Hodgkin's disease |
| Squamous cell carcinoma (anus) |
| PAPULOSQUAMOUS DISEASES |
| Xerotic eczema |
| Seborrheic dermatitis |
| Psoriasis |
| Reiter's syndrome |
| OTHER CONDITIONS |
| Drug-associated eruptions |
| Eosinophilic folliculitis |
| Pruritis |
| Pruritic papular eruption |
| Atopic dermatitis |
| Nail and hair disorders |

## Cutaneous infections

Infections comprise the largest category of skin disorders seen in HIV infection (Table 100.27). Microbial resistance to therapy is often relatively frequent with HIV-associated diseases.

### Herpes simplex virus

Early in the course of HIV infection, HSV infection presents in a manner similar to non–HIV-infected individuals. Lesions most typically present as grouped umbilicated vesicles on lip, genital, or perirectal areas; lesions may be primary or recurrent and usually crust and heal within 7–10 days.

With more advanced immunosuppression, symptomatic outbreaks and asymptomatic shedding become more frequent. Patients with profound immunosuppression may develop large, chronic, nonhealing ulcerative lesions. All ulcerative lesions in an HIV-infected patient should be examined for HSV infection; diagnosis is best made by examination of cells from the lesion base obtained by swab for herpesvirus culture and fluorescent antibody assay. Strains of HSV which are resistant to acyclovir, and less commonly to other antivirals, may occur. Lesions that do not respond to therapy should be recultured to detect virus for susceptibility testing.

### Varicella zoster virus

Zoster occurs in 3%–4% of HIV-infected patients and can occur at any stage of infection. Varicella zoster virus (VZV) infection in adults is most often from reactivation of latent virus. Typically, VZV presents with radicular pain followed by a vesicular eruption in a dermatomal distribution, although multidermatomal or disseminated infections can occur, especially with advanced

HIV infection. Acyclovir-resistant VZV can manifest as chronic localized or disseminated hyperkeratotic verrucous lesions. Diagnosis of VZV is confirmed by obtaining cells from the base of a lesion for fluorescent antibody assay and viral culture. The former test is more sensitive than culture.

#### Molluscum contagiosum

Molluscum contagiosum is caused by a poxvirus. Lesions are typically flesh colored, umbilicated papules, 2–5 mm in size, on the face, genitals, or trunk (Plate 48). Up to 20% of patients with AIDS develop molluscum, and lesions can enlarge and coalesce into larger ulcerative plaques. Molluscum lesions may be similar in appearance to lesions caused by disseminated histoplasmosis or cryptococcal infection. Unfortunately, recurrence is common.

#### Other cutaneous viral infections

Cutaneous cytomegalovirus is not common, but in severely immunosuppressed patients it can present with ulcers or small purpuric reddish papules and macules. Condylomata acuminata and common warts, associated with various subtypes of human papillomavirus (HPV), can occur with HIV infection and may be more refractory to therapy. HPV is commonly associated with cervical dysplasia in HIV-infected women.

#### Cutaneous bacterial and fungal infections

Bacterial infections of several types can occur with HIV infection; these include folliculitis, bullous impetigo, ecthyma, cellulitis, abscesses, and ulcers. Recurrent or chronic folliculitis, impetigo, and ecthyma are common. *Staphylococcus aureus* is the most common cause of cutaneous bacterial infections in HIV-infected patients, although *Streptococci* and other pathogens are sometimes involved. Folliculitis generally presents as erythematous, follicular pustules, or papules. Lesions typically occur in the hairy areas of the face, trunk, and groin; they are often intensely pruritic. Gram's stain and culture of a lesion should be obtained to confirm the diagnosis. Cutaneous mycobacterial infections are uncommon, but they may appear as folliculitis-like papules, indurated plaques, or abscesses. Appearance of skin lesions of syphilis vary with stage of syphilis, as is true in persons without HIV, and can mimic many other disorders.

A variety of fungal infections occur in HIV-infected individuals, including dermatophyte infections in up to 20% of patients and tinea versicolor (*Malassezia furfur*); both these conditions rarely respond to topical agents and often require systemic therapy. Lesions of cutaneous cryptococcus have a variety of appearances, including nodules, papules, pustules, plaques, and ulcers. However, these lesions commonly are multiple flesh-colored papules with central umbilication, similar to molluscum contagiosum. Skin biopsy for histologic examination and fungal culture is the means to diagnosis of cutaneous cryptococcus; patients should also have fungal blood cultures and serum cryptococcal antigen assay. Skin lesions found in bacillary angiomatosis and histoplasmosis have been described.

### Cutaneous malignancies

Kaposi's sarcoma is a neoplasm of endothelial cells whose pathogenesis has recently been linked to human herpesvirus 8, angiogenic growth factors, and cytokines (see Chapter 99). The most common malignancy in HIV-infected persons, Kaposi's sarcoma, has occurred in 15% of persons in the United States with AIDS. Although lymphoma sometimes presents with cutaneous involvement, and other cutaneous malignancies have been reported with HIV infection, Kaposi's sarcoma almost always presents with skin involvement. Incidence of Kaposi's sarcoma has decreased since the early 1980s, although prevalence remains high because of increases in numbers of persons with AIDS. Ninety-five percent of AIDS-associated Kaposi's sarcoma occurs in homosexual men. Most persons with Kaposi's sarcoma have $CD4^+$ cell counts $<500/\mu L$.

Skin lesions of Kaposi's sarcoma classically are violaceous, firm, palpable nodules, although morphology varies widely. Lesions may also present as asymptomatic small pink, red, brown, or black macules (Plate 49) or plaques or large tumor masses; pain and edema can occur with more advanced disease. Lesions can occur anywhere, number from one to several hundred, sometimes follow a skin fold distribution, and may have associated lymphedema. In addition to skin disease, the majority of patients with Kaposi's sarcoma also have internal involvement; frequent sites include hard palate, lymph nodes, and visceral organs, including gastrointestinal tract, lungs, liver, kidney, and spleen. Natural history of Kaposi's sarcoma varies widely; some individuals have stable, localized disease for prolonged periods while others have rapidly progressive, widespread disease. Patients with lower $CD4^+$ cell counts tend to have more aggressive disease.

Diagnosis is made by biopsy of involved skin or mucosa. It is important to establish the diagnosis, since Kaposi's sarcoma can resemble other skin disorders, including dermatofibroma, hemangioma, pyogenic granuloma, and bacillary angiomatosis. Biopsies of other tissues (e.g., lung) need to be performed with caution, because of potential for bleeding. Therapy is primarily aimed at controlling symptoms and for cosmetic reasons; lesions can be extremely disfiguring.

### Papulosquamous disorders

Generalized dry skin (xerotic eczema) occurs in 5%–20% of patients, most often with $CD4^+$ cell counts $<400/\mu L$. Seborrheic dermatitis is extremely common in all stages of HIV infection, with a prevalence of 20%–80%; it is characterized by pink or red scaly, flaky patches and plaques located in hairy areas of the face, eyebrows, nasolabial and retroauricular folds, scalp, and chest, and less commonly on the back, axilla, and groin. The spectrum of disease is broad, ranging from mild involvement to widespread erythroderma and plaques which can resemble psoriasis. Severity of disease often correlates with degree of immunosuppression. Diagnosis is usually made clinically, based on typical morphology.

Psoriasis is estimated to occur in 1%–5% of persons with HIV infection, compared to 1%–2% of the general population, and is often more severe. Psoriasis may occur as a new diagnosis in a patient with HIV, or it may present as worsening of a preexisting condition. Lesions may be discrete plaques or more diffuse dermatitis with thickening (keratoderma) of palms and soles.

Reiter's syndrome occurs among HIV-infected patients and may present with the classic triad of arthritis, urethritis, and conjunctivitis. Keratoderma blennorrhagicum, a condition characterized by areas of pustulation within hyperkeratotic plaques on hands and feet, is associated with Reiter's syndrome and also occurs with HIV infection.

**Table 100.28** Medications associated with cutaneous reactions in patients with HIV infection and AIDS

| |
|---|
| Amoxicillin–clavulanic acid |
| Atovaquone |
| Carbamazepine |
| Clindamycin |
| Delavirdine |
| Foscarnet (penile ulcers) |
| Ketoconazole |
| Nevirapine |
| Pentamidine |
| Phenytoin |
| Rifampin |
| Sulfadiazine–pyrimethamine |
| Thiacetazone |
| Trimethoprim–dapsone |
| Trimethoprim–sulfamethoxazole |

## Other skin disorders

Drug-associated eruptions are extremely common among HIV-infected patients and have been reported with a variety of medications commonly used for management of HIV infection and its associated complications (Table 100.28). Common offenders include trimethoprim–sulfamethoxazole, sulfadiazine, and pyrimethamine. Rashes are usually pruritic with fine erythematous macules or papules that can coalesce and become generalized; they usually resolve with discontinuation of the implicated therapy. Trimethoprim–sulfamethoxazole can often be continued in patients with mild reactions with concurrent use of systemic antihistamines. Other manifestations of drug reactions include fever, cytopenias, hepatitis, and less commonly interstitial pneumonitis. Stevens-Johnson syndrome and toxic epidermal necrolysis have also been associated with sulfonamide use in HIV-infected patients.

### Eosinophilic folliculitis

Eosinophilic folliculitis is the most frequent cause of non-staphylococcal folliculitis in HIV-infected patients. This skin eruption is characterized by a chronic, extremely pruritic folliculitis. Primary lesions consist of discrete, erythematous follicular papules measuring 3–5 mm in diameter. Excoriations are common and lesions are typically distributed along the trunk, forehead, neck, and proximal extremities. Eosinophilic folliculitis usually occurs in patients who have $CD4^+$ cell counts $< 300/\mu L$. Some patients have peripheral eosinophilia, as well as elevated serum IgE levels. Diagnosis is made by skin biopsy, which reveals inflammation with a predominance of eosinophils within and surrounding follicles.

## Conclusion

As this chapter demonstrates, the clinical manifestations of HIV and AIDS may involve systemic or focal processes, and a wide variety of conditions may occur simultaneously or sequentially. The likelihood of specific diagnoses varies with differing levels of immune suppression. Decreases in several opportunistic conditions traditionally associated with AIDS and some newer clinical presentations have been reported, temporally associated with the use of more potent antiretroviral therapies. The clinical presentations of HIV and AIDS in the setting of potent antiretroviral therapy remain to be characterized. HIV and AIDS will continue to challenge our clinical skills.

*Acknowledgments*—This work was supported in part by grants AI-27664 and 27757 from the National Institutes of Allergy and Infectious Diseases (NIAID); we are grateful to Linda Page for assistance in manuscript preparation.

## SELECTED BIBLIOGRAPHY

### Table 100.4

Dorrucci M, Rezza G, Vlahov D, et al. Clinical characteristics and prognostic value of acute retroviral syndrome among injecting drug users. AIDS 1995; 9:597–604.

Kinloch-de Loës S, de Saussure P, Saurat J-H, et al. Symptomatic primary infection due to human immunodeficiency virus type 1: review of 31 cases. Clin Infect Dis 1993; 17:59–65.

Kinloch-de Loës S, Hirschel BJ, Hoen B, et al. A controlled trial of zidovudine in primary human immunodeficiency virus infection. N Engl J Med 1995; 333:408–413.

Schacker T, Collier AC, Hughes J, et al. Clinical and epidemiologic features of primary HIV infection. Ann Intern Med 1996; 125:257–264.

Tindall B, Barker S, Donovan B, et al. Characterization of the acute clinical illness associated with human immunodeficiency virus infection. Arch Intern Med 1988; 148:945–949.

Vanhems P, Allard R, Cooper DA, et al. Acute human immunodeficiency virus type 1 disease as a mononucleosis-like illness: is the diagnosis too restrictive? Clin Infect Dis 1997; 24:965–970.

Vanhems P, Lambert J, Cooper DA, et al. Severity and prognosis of acute human immunodeficiency virus type 1 illness: a dose-response relationship. Clin Infect Dis 1998; 26:323–329.

### Table 100.7

Benson CA. Disease due to the *Mycobacterium avium* complex in patients with AIDS: epidemiology and clinical syndrome. Clin Infect Dis 1994;18(suppl 3):S218–222.

Chaisson RE, Benson CA, Dube MP, et al. Clarithromycin therapy for bacteremic *Mycobacterium avium* complex disease. Ann Intern Med 1994; 121:905–911.

Chiu J, Nussbaum J, Bozzette S, et al. Treatment of disseminated *Mycobacterium avium* complex infection in AIDS with amikacin, ethambutol, rifampin, and ciprofloxacin. Ann Intern Med 1990; 113:358–361.

Havlik JA, Horsburgh CR, Metchock B, et al. Disseminated *Mycobacterium avium* complex infection: clinical identification and epidemiologic trends. J Infect Dis 1992; 165:577–580.

Hoy J, Mijch A, Sandland M, et al. Quadruple-drug therapy for *Mycobacterium avium-intracellulare* bacteremia in AIDS patients. J Infect Dis 1990; 161:801–805.

Kemper CA, Havlir D, Haghighat D, et al. The individual microbiologic effect of three antimycobacterial agents, clofazimine, ethambutol, and rifampin, on *Mycobacterium avium* complex bacteremia in patients with AIDS. J Infect Dis 1994; 170:157–164.

Kemper CA, Meng T-C, Nussbaum J, et al. Treatment of *Mycobacterium avium* complex bacteremia in AIDS with a four-drug oral regimen. Ann Intern Med 1992; 116:466–472.

Modilevsky T, Sattler FR, Barnes PF. Mycobacterial disease in patients with human immunodeficiency virus infection. Arch Intern Med 1989; 149:2201–2205.

Young LS, Wiviott L, Wu M, et al. Azithromycin for treatment of *Mycobacterium avium-intracellulare* complex infection in patients with AIDS. Lancet 1991; 338:1107–1109.

### Table 100.11

American Thoracic Society. Fungal infection in HIV-infected persons. Am J Respir Crit Care Med 1995; 152:816–822.

Sharkey-Mathis PK, Velez J, Fetchick R, et al. Histoplasmosis in the acquired immunodeficiency syndrome (AIDS): treatment with itraconazole and fluconazole. J AIDS 1993; 6:809–819.

Wheat LJ, Connolly-Stringfield PA, Baker RL, et al. Disseminated histoplasmosis in the acquired immune deficiency syndrome: clinical findings, diagnosis and treatment, and review of the literature. Medicine 1990; 69:361–374.

### Table 100.17

Dannemann B, McCutchan JA, Israelski D, et al. Treatment of toxoplasmic encephalitis in patients with AIDS. Ann Intern Med 1992; 116:33–43.

Luft BJ, Hafner R, Korzun AH, et al. Toxoplasmic encephalitis in patients with the acquired immunodeficiency syndrome. N Engl J Med 1993; 329:995–1000.

Navia BA, Petito CK, Gold JWM, et al. Cerebral toxoplasmosis complicating the acquired immune deficiency syndrome: clinical and neuropathological findings in 27 patients. Ann Neurol 1986; 19:224–238.

Porter SB, Sande MA. Toxoplasmosis of the central nervous system in the acquired immunodeficiency syndrome. N Engl J Med 1992; 327:1643–1648.

Renold C, Sugar A, Chave J-P, et al. Toxoplasma encephalitis in patients with acquired immunodeficiency syndrome. Medicine 1992; 71:224–239.

### Table 100.18

Chuck SL, Sande MA. Infections with *Cryptococcus neoformans* in the acquired immunodeficiency syndrome. N Engl J Med 1989; 321:794–799.

Clark RA, Greer D, Atkinson W, et al. Spectrum of *Cryptococcus neoformans* infection in 68 patients infected with human immunodeficiency virus. Rev Infect Dis 1990; 12:768–777.

Zuger A, Louie E, Holzman RS, et al. Cryptococcal disease in patients with the acquired immunodeficiency syndrome. Ann Intern Med 1986; 104:234–240.

### Table 100.19

Chuck SL, Sande MA. Infections with *Cryptococcus neoformans* in the acquired immunodeficiency syndrome. N Engl J Med 1989; 321:794–799.

Clark RA, Greer D, Atkinson W, et al. Spectrum of *Cryptococcus neoformans* infection in 68 patients infected with human immunodeficiency virus. Rev Infect Dis 1990; 12:768–777.

Quagliarello VJ, Viscoli C, Horwitz RI. Primary prevention of cryptococcal meningitis by fluconazole in HIV-infected patients. Lancet 1995; 345:548–552.

Saag MS, Powderly WG, Cloud GA, et al. Comparison of amphotericin B with fluconazole in the treatment of acute AIDS-associated cryptococcal meningitis. N Engl J Med 1992; 326:83–89.

Zuger A, Louie E, Holzman RS, et al. Cryptococcal disease in patients with the acquired immunodeficiency syndrome. Ann Intern Med 1986; 104:234–240.

## ANNOTATED BIBLIOGRAPHY

American Thoracic Society. Fungal infection in HIV-infected persons. Am J Respir Crit Care Med 1995; 152:816–822.
*Overview of the major fungal infections which occur in persons with HIV, including epidemiology, clinical manifestations, diagnosis, and therapy.*

Bayard PJ, Berger TG, Jacobson MA. Drug hypersensitivity reactions and human immunodeficiency virus disease. J AIDS 1992; 5:1237–1257.
*Clinical review of major drug hypersensitivity reactions in persons with HIV infection.*

Berger TG, Koehler JE. Bacillary angiomatosis. AIDS Clin Rev 1993/1994; 43–60.
*Brief review of bacillary angiomatosis and the associated organisms; the clinical presentations, methods for diagnosis, and treatment.*

Centers for Disease Control. 1993 revised classification system for HIV infection and expanded surveillance case definition for AIDS among adolescents and adults. MMWR 1992; 41(RR-17):1–19.
*Description of the adult HIV infection classification scheme most frequently used in the United States, and the AIDS case definition used for public health reporting and disease surveillance.*

Dezube BJ. Clinical presentation and natural history of AIDS-related Kaposi's sarcoma. Hematol Oncol Clin North Am 1996; 10:1023–1029.
*Clinical review of the natural history and clinical manifestations of AIDS-associated Kaposi's sarcoma.*

Drew WL. Cytomegalovirus infection in patients with AIDS. Clin Infect Dis 1992; 14:608–615.
*Review of the major manifestations of CMV disease in patients with AIDS, diagnostic tests, and use of the first two available anti-CMV therapies.*

Gradon JD, Timpone JG, Schnittman SM. Emergence of unusual opportunistic pathogens in AIDS: a review. Clin Infect Dis 1992;15: 134–157.
*Comprehensive review of more unusual opportunistic pathogens that occur in patients with AIDS, organized by major organ system affected.*

Herndier BG, Kaplan LD, McGrath MS. Pathogenesis of AIDS lymphomas. AIDS 1994; 8:1025–1049.
*Review of epidemiology, clinical characteristics, and detailed discussion of diagnosis and pathogenesis of AIDS-associated lymphomas.*

Kemper CA, Deresinski SC. *Mycobacterium avium* complex infection in AIDS. AIDS Clin Rev 1995/1996; 155–204.
*Review of epidemiology, pathogenesis, clinical presentation, and patient management, including treatment, of MAC in patients with HIV.*

Kotler DP. Gastrointestinal manifestations of human immunodeficiency virus infection. Adv Intern Med 1995; 40:197–242.
*Clinical review of major gastrointestinal manifestations in patients with HIV infection, including an approach to diagnosis and brief discussion of therapies.*

Miller R. HIV-associated respiratory diseases. Lancet 1996; 348:307–312.
*Review of the major disorders causing respiratory tract disease in patients with HIV infection and AIDS. Includes brief discussion of idiopathic conditions and approach to diagnosis.*

Price RW. Neurologic complications of HIV infection. Lancet 1996; 348:445–452.
*Review of the clinical features, pathogenesis, and diagnosis of major neurologic diseases associated with HIV infection, with an emphasis on HIV dementia.*

Sha BE, Benson CA, Pottage JC Jr, et al. HIV infection in women: an observational study of clinical characteristics, disease progression, and survival for a cohort of women in Chicago. J AIDS 1995; 8:486–495.
*Descriptive study of the natural history and clinical manifestations of HIV-infected women.*

Whitcup SM. Ocular manifestations of AIDS. JAMA 1996; 275:142–144.
*Case discussion about three common ocular manifestations of AIDS, including a concise discussion of CMV retinitis and a list of other ocular disorders that occur in patients with AIDS.*

Zalla MJ, Su WPD, Fransway AF. Dermatologic manifestations of human immunodeficiency virus infection. Mayo Clin Proc 1992; 67:1089–1108.
*Clinical review of the major dermatologic manifestations of HIV infection and AIDS. Includes a comprehensive list of disorders and excellent pictures of several disorders.*

# 101

# Antiretroviral Therapy

LAWRENCE COREY

The last decade has brought continued advances in the use of agents that inhibit the human immunodeficiency viruses. It is now well established that antiretroviral therapy slows down the progression of acquired immunodeficiency syndrome (AIDS) and can prolong survival. However, the high replication rate of human immunodeficiency virus (HIV), the ability of the virus to develop resistance to antivirals, and the relatively low individual potency of many of the currently licensed agents has meant that combination chemotherapy must be utilized.

Figure 101.1 illustrates the life cycle of HIV. Two phases of the life cycle are of particular relevance to antiviral chemotherapy. The early events of replication, the viral functions which constitute the *establishment phase* of the HIV life cycle, include attachment, fusion, reverse transcription, and subsequent integration into the host cell chromosome. The later events of replication, called the *expression phase* of infection, start with the transcription and translation of viral proteins from proviral DNA and the subsequent packaging of these proteins into virions, which then are released by budding from the cell. To date, all licensed antiretrovirals inhibit either the viral reverse transcriptase (RT) or protease function. In vitro and in vivo combinations of RT inhibitors and protease inhibitors are at least additive in their antiviral effects.

## Inhibition of Reverse Transcription

The reverse transcriptase enzyme is a unique feature of animal retroviruses. Two major classes of RT inhibitors exist: competitive inhibitors, which currently are composed of dideoxynucleoside analogues (ddN), and noncompetitive reverse transcriptase inhibitors, which are nonnucleoside reverse transcriptase inhibitors (NNRTI). These latter compounds are allosteric inhibitors of the HIV RT binding site and are HIV-1 specific.

The dideoxynucleoside analogues differ from purine and pyramidine deoxynucleotides in that they lack the 3′-hydroxyl group. As such, they are essentially prodrugs, which must be metabolically activated to their respective 5′-triphosphates by kinases, nucleotides, or other cellular phosphorylating enzymes. The 5′-triphosphate competes with the corresponding endogenous 2′-deoxynucleoside-5′-triphosphate (NTP) for binding to the reverse transcriptase and/or acts as an alternative substrate to prevent formation of 3′5′-phosphodiester linkages that lead to premature termination of the elongating viral DNA chain. The viral reverse transcriptase has a greater affinity for the (DNTPs) than host DNA polymerases, a feature which contributes to their selective action. The antiviral activity of the nucleoside analogues is highly dependent on both activating and degrading cellular enzymes, the activity of which varies among cell types. The intracellular concentration of the ddN phosphate derivative compared to that of the corresponding endogenous deoxynucleoside triphosphate is an important factor in the relative activity of the compound in vitro. These interactions appear to account for the differences in the in vivo potency of these compounds on HIV replication. Differences in the intracellular metabolism and affinity for cellular polymerases of the different ddN also appear to be an important determinant in the clinical toxicities of the agents and their potential use in combination. All the current ddNs have significant side effects which complicate their long-term use. In addition, in vitro and in vivo resistance have been described for all the drugs.

## Zidovudine

Zidovudine (3′-azido-3′-deoxythymidine, AZT) was the first antiretroviral compound demonstrated to be effective against HIV in vitro and the first antiretroviral shown to be effective for the treatment of HIV infection. Besides its importance as a therapy for HIV infection, zidovudine therapy has been shown to reduce the frequency of transmission of HIV from mother to infant and may decrease infectivity after severe needle stick exposure. Because of the development of resistance, zidovudine is recommended only in combination with other antiretrovirals such as didanosine, lamivudine, and the protease inhibitors.

### Pharmacology

Zidovudine is well absorbed orally and extensive first-pass glucuronidation through the liver makes the bioavailability of zidovudine about 60%. The intracellular half-life of the active triphosphate is about 3 hours and thus most authorities recommend zidovudine to be taken on a 3 times daily regimen.

### Toxicities

The major toxicities of zidovudine are listed in Table 101.1. Most of these toxicities are dose-dependent and also related to severity of HIV infection, being found much more frequently in persons with more advanced HIV infection. Zidovudine-associated anemia and neutropenia are infrequent in persons with CD4 cell counts $> 300/mm^3$ (e.g., <5%/yr). In patients with later stage disease, anemia and neutropenia are seen in 8%–20% of patients.

Zidovudine-related anemia can be treated with either transfusion of packed red blood cells or with the administration of recombinant erythropoietin. The responses to erythropoietin in AZT-treated patients are dependent on the endogenous serum erythropoietin level. Patients with erythropoietin levels <500 mU/mL should receive erythropoietin at a dose of 100 U/kg 3 times weekly. In such patients, erythropoietin has reduced AZT-associated transfusion requirements by almost 40%.

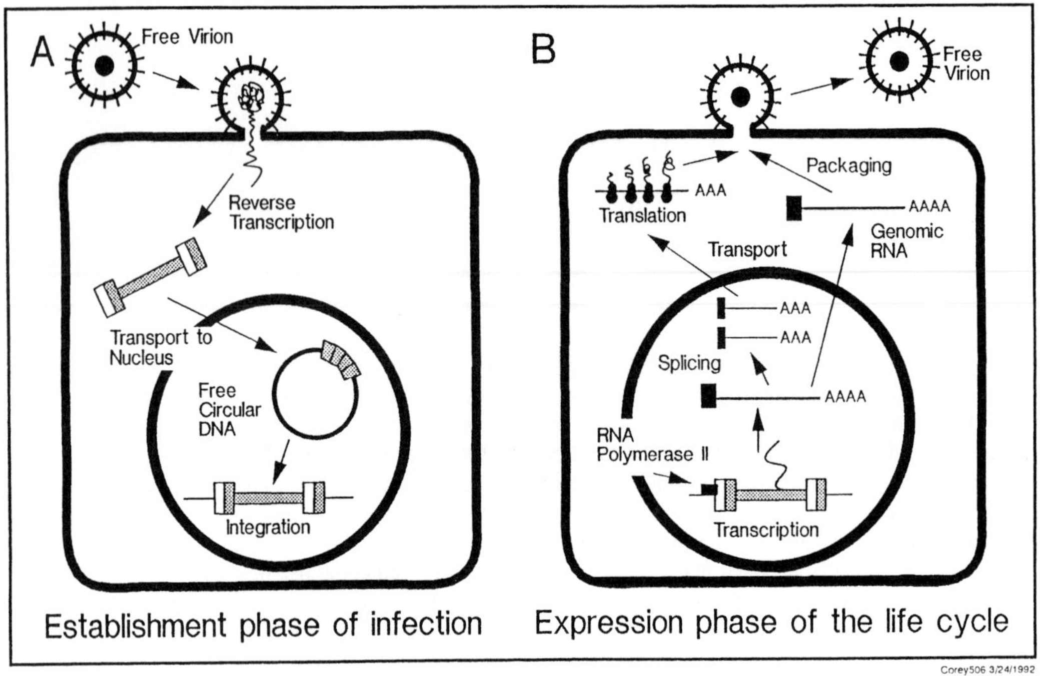


**Fig. 101.1** Life Cycle of the Retrovirus

Recombinant erythropoietin is not recommended for HIV-associated anemia due to iron or folate deficiencies, hemolysis, or gastrointestinal bleed. Zidovudine-associated neutropenia is usually reversible by reducing the dose or interrupting medication. In selected instances, granulocyte colony-stimulating factor (GCSF) and granulocyte-macrophage-stimulating factor (GMCSF) have been used. Myopathy has been associated with prolonged zidovudine therapy, an affect that may be related to depletion of muscle cell mitochondrial DNA. Nausea, vomiting, diarrhea, fatigue, malaise, myalgias, and headache are common. The initiation of therapy with lower doses such as 100 mg 3 times/day with gradual escalation to standard doses of 200 mg 3 times/day or 100 mg 5 times/day can mitigate against these side effects.

### Resistance

In 1987 Larder and Richman described the development of in vitro AZT resistance during the course of therapy. Resistance has been shown to be related to the development of several specific point mutations in the RT enzymes, which reduce the ability of AZT-TP to bind to the RT. Several of these mutations may be present at once. Two in particular, a change from methionine to leucine at amino acid 41 and threonine to tyrosine or phenylalanine at amino acid 215 confer a high grade (50 to 100-fold) change in in vitro susceptibility to HIV. Many of these changes appear stable as AZT-resistant strains have been transmitted between sexual partners and from mothers to infants. Zidovudine resistance is a factor in the continued progression of HIV replication that occurs while on zidovudine monotherapy. In vitro resistance to AZT occurs much sooner in those with AIDS than in those with earlier stages of infection. However, it is not the sole reason for the clinical failure of AZT.

**Table 101.1** Major toxicities of dideoxynucleosides

| Condition | AZT | ddI | ddC | D4T |
|---|---|---|---|---|
| Anemia | +++ | − | − | − |
| Leukopenia | +++ | − | − | − |
| Neutropenia | +++ | − | − | − |
| Thrombocytopenia | + | − | − | − |
| Peripheral neuropathy | − | + | ++ | ++ |
| Pancreatitis | − | +++ | + | ? |
| Hepatitis | +/− | +/− | +/− | ? |
| Myopathy | ++ | ? | ? | ? |
| Mucosal ulcerations | − | +/− | ++ | − |

## Lamivudine

Lamivudine (2′-deoxy-3′ thiacylidine, 3TC) is an antiretroviral that when given alone was associated with the rapid (2 to 4 weeks) development of in vivo resistance in the HIV RT gene. Molecular analyses indicated a point mutation codon 184 in the RT gene as the dominant mutation; nearly all circulating strains demonstrated this mutation. Once therapy was begun, Larder and colleagues noted that the presence of this lamivudine-associated mutation markedly increased the susceptibility of these isolates to zidovudine, especially in those isolates with codon changes that were associated with high-grade zidovudine resistance. Moreover, the viruses that emerged appear to have reduced replicative rates in vitro. Many of these observations have been borne out in vivo. Several phase II/III studies of AZT and 3TC dual therapy have indicated enhanced antiviral activity, as evidenced by greater and more sustained rise in CD4 cell counts and larger and more sustained suppression of HIV RNA than those who received either drug alone. Antiviral effects among previously untreated patients have averaged 1.5–2.0 log reduction in plasma RNA versus $\frac{1}{3}$–$\frac{1}{2}$ log reduction for AZT alone. Moreover, the time to development of AZT resistance is delayed. Zidovudine 400 mg to 500 mg twice a day and lamivudine 150 mg twice a day is now a commonly used regimen; a tablet containing the two preparations is now available.

## Didanosine

Didanosine (ddI) is an acid-labile compound, and in order to increase its bioavailability it is administered either in a buffered solution, concomitantly with antacids, or on an empty stomach. Drugs that may be affected by buffering of stomach acids should be administered at least 2 hours before ddI administration. The plasma elimination half-life of ddI is about 0.5 hours, however, the intracellular half-life of DDATP is 12–24 hours, and, as such, ddI is usually dosed in a twice daily regimen.

### Toxicities

The major toxicities of ddI are peripheral neuropathy and pancreatitis, the mechanism of which are poorly understood. Neuropathy can be reversed when recognized early by discontinuing treatment. Some cases of hemorrhagic pancreatitis occur spontaneously. In most cases, monitoring of serum amylase levels in patients can reduce the risk of severe pancreatitis. Concomitant use of medications which are associated with drug-induced pancreatitis as well as alcohol abuse appear to increase the frequency of ddI-associated pancreatitis. Whereas the background incidence of pancreatitis among patients with symptomatic HIV appears to be about 3%, didanosine-associated pancreatitis occurs in about 4%–5% of patients when used at the currently recommended dose of approximately 500 mg 4 times/day (400 mg 4 times/day for the pill form). The lack of overlapping toxicities between ddI and AZT has allowed the two medications to be used in combination. One of the major inconveniences of ddI therapy is the large tablet size and bitter taste of the current formulations. Use of sachet preparation or the pediatric formulation has benefited some patients.

### Resistance

Isolates with decreased sensitivity to ddI have been reported. The in vitro change in sensitivity to ddI appears to be a reduction of four- to fivefold. Isolates which demonstrate a reduced susceptibility to ddI in vitro also show reduced susceptibility to ddC (2′,3′-dideoxycytidine, zalcitabine). Fortunately, isolates which are resistant to zidovudine appear to be sensitive in vitro to ddI.

## Stavudine

3′-D4T stavudine (D4T) is a thymidine analogue whose 5′-triphosphate is also a potent in vitro inhibitor of the HIV RT. It is well absorbed, with an absolute bioavailability of 90% or greater, and its relatively long intracellular half-life allows twice daily dosing. Hematologic toxicity with D4T is uncommon, and its major clinical toxicity is peripheral neuropathy. Stavudine is a well-tolerated drug and does not cause the nausea, vomiting, and malaise seen with AZT. As such, it can be taken by AZT-intolerant patients. Recent trials suggest CD4 cell increases seen with D4T monotherapy may be more prolonged than those with AZT monotherapy. Recent studies show excellent tolerance and additive antiviral effects with D4T and 3TC dual therapy and this regimen is being used with increasing frequency. AZT and D4T appear to exert inhibitory effects and probably should not be utilized together.

## Zalcitabine

Zalcitabine (ddC) is well absorbed and has an oral bioavailability of approximately 80%. Renal excretion is the primary mode of elimination; dose reductions are recommended when the clearance is 40 mL/min or less. Dosing is generally given on a 3 times/day regimen (0.75 mg).

### Toxicities

The major dose-limiting side effect of ddC is a severe, painful peripheral neuropathy, which is reversible if detected early but which may be associated with long-term residual effects if ddC is continued. Pancreatitis, esophageal and penile ulcerations, and cardiomyopathy are also zalcitabine-associated toxicities.

### Uses

Because of its side effects and low potency, zalcitabine is an uncommonly used medication in current HIV treatment regimens.

## Nonnucleoside Reverse Transcriptase Inhibitors

The NNRTI drugs noncompetitively inhibit viral RT, presumably by binding to a site other than the nucleoside and template binding sites. This interaction between the NNRTI and the HIV-1 RT produces a conformational change that results in the inactivation of the viral RT. These drugs have great selectivity for the HIV-1 RT and have no antiretroviral activity against HIV-2 or other animal retroviruses. While they have potent in vivo antiviral activity, resistance with greater than 100-fold reduction in susceptibility may emerge within weeks after initiation of monotherapy. The NNRTI do appear to have an excellent safety profile; thus high concentrations of these compounds are being tested both alone and in combination with other antiretrovirals. Nevirapine, delavirdine, and efavirenz are the currently utilized NNRTIs.

## Nevirapine

Nevirapine inhibits HIV-1 RT in nanomole concentrations; it has >95% bioavailability and a half-life of 24–48 hours. While in vitro resistance does emerge, use of high concentrations of the compound (400 mg/d) reduces the frequency of these findings and concentrations above the ID90 of most clinical isolates still appear possible, especially when combined with other retrovirals. The most common adverse reaction to nevirapine has been rash, occurring most frequently at initiation of treatment. Nevirapine has recently been licensed for use in combination with other retrovirals such as AZT and 3TC. Its long half-life has led to its investigational use for the prevention of perinatal HIV-1 infection, especially in the developing world.

## Delavirdine

Delavirdine is a bisheteroarylpiperazine derivative that also inhibits replication in HIV in submicromolar concentrations, and both AZT- and ddI-resistant strains are susceptible to the compound. As with nevirapine, delavirdine and the dideoxynucleoside analogues are synergistic in vitro. Strains of HIV-1 that are resistant to delavirdine are not cross-resistant to other NNRTIs, and mutations at sites which confer delavirdine resistance produce isolates that are more sensitive to nevirapine. Phase III trials to evaluate the clinical utility of delavirdine have generally shown inconsistent efficacy and hence have limited its widespread use.

## Elfinavir

Elfinavir (DMP226) is a recently developed NNRTI with excellent potency. Rash appears to be its major toxicity. Its half-life allows twice a day dosing, clinical efficiency in combination regimens appears excellent, and this compound is being increasingly utilized in combination regimens.

## Foscarnet

Foscarnet, a licensed therapy for treatment of cytomegalovirus (CMV) retinitis, has in vitro and in vivo antiretroviral activity. In vitro foscarnet and zidovudine are synergistic, and foscarnet therapy is associated with a reduction in p24 antigen among persons on AZT. This antiretroviral effect likely accounts for the finding that foscarnet therapy prolonged survival over ganciclovir in a study comparing the two for CMV retinitis. As the anti-CMV activity of the two agents ganciclovir and foscarnet appeared similar, the difference in survival on foscarnet suggests its superiority was related to its anti-HIV activity. Unfortunately, the high cost, need for parenteral administration, time-consuming prehydration to decrease renal toxicity, and the substantial number of other toxicities associated with foscarnet administration severely limit its use as an antiretroviral.

## Interferon alpha

Parenterally administered interferon alpha has been widely used as a therapy for selected patients with AIDS-associated Kaposi's sarcoma, and favorable short-term effects on virologic markers such as HIV p24 antigen have been demonstrated among some patients. The toxicities of interferon alpha among HIV-infected persons are substantial and there is little compelling data about its clinical effectiveness.

## Proteinase Inhibitors

The HIV protease protein has been shown to be an essential part of the virion's life cycle; it is responsible for cleaving the Gag-Pol polyprotein into its component parts. Inhibition of the proteinase results in loss of the Gag (p24 protein), accumulation of unprocessed full-length Gag-Pol (p55), and emergence of "defective" particles of HIV. The HIV-1 protease belongs to the class of aspartyl proteases, and several inhibitors of this protease have been derived. The advantages of such agents is that they are able to inhibit HIV replication in cells that are chronically infected with HIV-1. In vitro these drugs appear to be more potent than most RT inhibitors and synergism exists between the RT inhibitors and the proteinase inhibitors. As such, clinical studies have employed combination therapy with these agents with excellent results. The major obstacle in the development of the protease inhibitors for HIV therapeutics has been their pharmacokinetic profiles. However, several compounds with reasonable bioavailability have been developed and recent data show their clinical effectiveness. At present, four protease inhibitors are available: saquinavir, ritonavir, indinavir and nelfinavir. These drugs reduce viral load and raise CD4 counts more than any of the current dideoxynucleoside derivatives. When used in combination with AZT or 3TC, 2 to $2\frac{1}{2}$ to 3 log reductions in virus load have been achieved. Greater than 80% of patients on combination therapy with protease inhibitors exhibit plasma RNA levels below 500 copies/mL by almost two-fold. Clinical trials have shown that ritonavir, indinavir, and saquinavir can prolong survival in persons with advanced HIV. Marked reductions in HIV-1-related mortality have been noted since the introduction of these drugs, and hospitalizations are reduced on persons who can comply with the triple-drug regimens.

Most authorities recommend one of these drug combinations (AZT/3TC and indinavir or D4T, 3TC and protease inhibitors) be utilized in persons with advanced HIV disease. Ritonavir has many drug interactions that preclude its concomitant use with rifabutin or clarithromycin. Indinavir and nelfinavir are, in this author's experience, better tolerated than ritonavir. Renal stones are an occasional complication of indinavir. Saquinavir is well tolerated but the least potent at present because of its limited bioavailability. New formulations with better bioavailability have recently been developed which may improve its potency and patient acceptability. Resistance to the proteinase inhibitors can occur and it appears there is cross-resistance between ritonavir and indinavir. Resistance appears promptly if compliance to medication is poor and viral load is already high. Monotherapy with protease inhibitors is discouraged. Dual protease therapy with ritonavir and saquinavir is under investigation due to the pharmacologic interactions between these two compounds.

## Guidelines for Therapy

It is now well established that combination antiretroviral therapy extends life and reduces the frequency of progression to AIDS. AIDS Clinical Trials Group (ACTG) 175 was a trial of more than 2000 persons with CD4 counts $<500\ \mu$L who were randomized to ddI vs. AZT vs. ddI and AZT or AZT and ddC. The most significant finding was that ddI monotherapy as well as combination therapy with either ddI and AZT or ddC and AZT were more effective than zidovudine monotherapy for reducing progression to AIDS and survival. The European Delta trial compared AZT with AZT and ddI and AZT and ddC and again showed combination therapy better than AZT monotherapy in reducing the time to AIDS progression and survival. These trials are important in that they confirm that the initiation of antiretroviral therapy in persons with CD4 counts $<500$ cells/mm$^3$, whether symptomatic or asymptomatic, prolongs survival. They help immensely in interpreting the previous trials of AZT monotherapy, which reduced progression to AIDS but not survival. It appears the added potency of combination therapy can result in greater clinical, true

**Table 101.2** Considerations for initiating antiretroviral therapy

| |
|---|
| Therapy is recommended for all patients with HIV RNA levels > 5000–10,000 copies/mL of plasma. |
| Therapy should be considered for all HIV-infected patients with detectable HIV RNA in plasma (>500 copies/mL). |
| For patients at low risk of progression (low plasma HIV RNA level and high CD4+ count), particularly those who are not committed to complex antiretroviral regimens, therapy might be safely deferred. These patients should be reevaluated every 3 to 6 months (see text). |

survival benefit. These trials also indicate that initial therapy for HIV-infected persons should begin with combination therapy. Recent studies indicate that starting therapy with potent antiretrovirals offers better long-term benefit than the sequential addition of the same antiretrovirals. Table 101.2 illustrates current guidelines for initiating HIV-1 therapy, and Table 101.3 lists currently recommended dosages of the most commonly used antiretrovirals. More and more, HIV-1 plasma RNA levels are being utilized as a means of defining initiation of therapy.

It is also clear that triple therapy (AZT, 3TC, and indinavir) prolonged survival more than twofold over AZT plus 3TC among persons with advanced HIV. Greater than 50% of persons with CD4 counts <200 cells/mm$^3$ can have their plasma virion RNAs driven below 500 copies/mL. Selected options for initial therapy of HIV-1 are presented in Table 101.4.

This success of three-drug therapy for initial HIV treatment has prompted the general utilization of viral load measurements as a means of guiding antiretroviral therapy. This goal is to utilize whatever drug combinations are needed to drive down viral titers to a predetermined level. Some authorities use <4000 copies/mL, some <500, and some <50 copies/mL as their "goal." Often two new agents are utilized among persons with advanced disease progression of infection and increasing viral loads. Lowering viral RNA titers to less than 50 copies/mL may also reduce the time to emergence of resistant viruses.

One of the major controversies at present is when to initiate antiretroviral therapy. While most studies have involved persons with <500 CD4 cells/mm$^3$, recent studies have suggested that plasma virus replication level is a predictor of disease progression independent of CD4 count. Persons with RNA levels of >34,000 copies/mL have a five times greater rate of progression to AIDS and death than those with levels <4000 copies/mL. Thus, many authorities feel that persons with CD4 counts >500 who have high viral loads (>5000 to 10,000 copies/mL) be treated. Table 101.4 illustrates the most commonly utilized combination therapy options.

Long-term studies to define whether this is the optimal strategy for therapy are as yet unavailable. But in this author's opinion, early therapy of all persons with HIV plasma RNA levels >5000 copies/mL should be initiated. Combination therapy should be utilized in all treated patients and posttreatment RNA levels should be at least 500 copies/ml and preferably <100 copies/mL. As HIV-1 is a chronic illness, compliance to medications is critical. How long combination therapy can hold back the tide of HIV-1 replication is unclear. However, early use of well-tolerated regimens among compliant patients markedly reduces the development of opportunistic infections. Rates of opportunistic infections such as CMV retinitis and disseminated MAC are markedly reduced among HIV-1 infected persons with low viral loads. Studies to define if immunoprophylaxis regimens can be redesigned based upon these new findings are underway.

**Table 101.3** Recommended dosages

| |
|---|
| NUCLEOSIDE ANALOGUES |
| Didanosine (ddI)/videx: Tablets: 200 mg PO every 12 h (for body weight < 60 kg, the recommended dose is 125 mg PO every 12 h); sachet: 250 mg PO every 12 h (for body weight < 60 kg, the recommended dose is 167 mg PO every 12 h) |
| Lamivudine (3TC)/epivir: 150 mg PO every 12 h (for body weight < 50 kg, the recommended dose is 2 mg/kg PO every 12 h) |
| Stavudine (d4T)/zerit: 40 mg PO every 12 h (for body weight < 60 kg, the recommended dose is 30 mg PO every 12 h) |
| Zalcitabine (ddC)/hivid: 0.75 mg PO every 8 h (for body weight < 60 kg, the recommended dose is 0.375 mg PO every 12 h) |
| Zidovudine (AZT)/retrovir: 200 mg PO every 8 h or 300 mg PO every 12 h |
| NONNUCLEOSIDE REVERSE TRANSCRIPTASE INHIBITORS |
| Nevirapine/virammune: 200 mg PO daily for 14 d, then increase to 200 mg PO every 12 h |
| Delavirdine/rescriptor: 400 mg PO 3 times/d |
| PROTEASE INHIBITORS |
| Indinavir/crixivan: 800 mg PO every 8 h |
| Ritonavir/norvir: start with 300 mg PO every 12 h for 1/d, then increase to 400 mg PO every 12 h for 2 d, then 500 mg PO every 12 h thereafter |
| Saquinavir/Invirase: 600 mg PO every 8 h |

**Table 101.4** Selected options for initial therapy

| Regimen | Advantages | Disadvantages |
|---|---|---|
| Two nucleoside RT inhibitors and PI | The regimen should be able to achieve plasma HIV RNA levels below limit of detection in large majority of drug-adherent patients | Strict adherence to this regimen is crucial; quality of life may be affected; durability of effect, long-term tolerance, and overall clinical benefit in antiretroviral-naive patients with early disease is not fully defined, however, early results are promising |
| Two nucleoside RT inhibitors and NNRTI | Many patients taking this regimen achieve plasma HIV RNA levels below limit of detection; it also permits deferral of a PI if this option is chosen | Strict adherence to this regimen is crucial; may not be as potent as a PI-containing regimen |

Abbreviations: NNRTI, nonnucleoside reverse transcriptase inhibitors; PI, protease inhibitor; RT, reverse transcriptase.

## ANNOTATED BIBLIOGRAPHY


Carpenter CCJ, Fischl MA, Hammer SM, et al. Antiretroviral therapy for HIV infection in 1997. JAMA 1997; 277:1962–1969.
*The latest International AIDS Society consensus panel recommendations for initiating, maintaining, or changing antiretroviral therapy.*

Connor EM, Sperling RS, Gelber R, et al. Reduction of maternal infant transmission of human immunodeficiency virus type 1 with zidovudine treatment. N Engl J Med 1994; 331:1173–1180.
*Sentinel article on the reduction of HIV transmission to the infant.*

Crumpacker CS. Molecular targets of antiviral therapy. N Engl J Med 1989; 321:163–172.
*Good review of antiviral drugs*

Eron JJ, Benott SL, Jemsek J, et al. Treatment with lamivudine, zidovudine, or both in HIV-positive patient with 200 to 500 CD4+ cells per cubic millimeter. N Engl J Med 1995; 333:1662–1669.
*Article describing the clinical utility of this commonly used combination of antiretrovirals.*

Ho DD, Neumann AU, Perelson AS, Chen W, et al. Rapid turnover of plasma virions and CD4 lymphocytes in HIV-1 infection. Nature 1995; 373:123–126.
*Sentinel article showing the high replication rate of HIV.*

Larder BA, Kemp SD. Multiple mutations in HIV-1 reverse transcriptase confer high-level resistance to zidovudine (AZT). Science 1989; 246:1155–1159.
*The original publication describing the importance of AZT resistance.*

Larder BA, Kemp SD, Harrigan PR. Potential mechanism for sustained antiretroviral efficacy of AZT-3TC combination therapy. Science 1995; 269:696–699.
*Important article showing 3TC/ZDV effectiveness.*

McLeod GX, Hammer SM. Zidovudine: five years later. Ann Intern Med 1992; 117:487–501.
*Good review of zidovudine.*

Mellors JW, Kingsley LA, Rinaldo CR Jr., et al. Quantitation of HIV-1 RNA in plasma predicts outcome after seroconversion. Ann Intern Med 1995; 122:573–579.
*Important article describing the association of HIV RNA and subsequent clinical course.*

O'Brien WA, Hartigan PM, Martin D, et al. Changes in plasma HIV-1 RNA and CD4+ lymphocyte count relative to treatment and progression to AIDS. N Engl J Med 1996; 334:426–431.
*Importance of lowering RNA and affecting clinical response.*

Richman DD. Zidovudine resistance of human immunodeficiency virus. Rev Infect Dis 1990; 12(suppl 5):S507–510.
*Excellent Review of ZDV resistance.*

Robins T, Plattner J. HIV protease inhibitors: their anti-HIV activity and potential role in treatment. J AIDS 1993; 6:162–170.
*Good review of the mechanism of action of these drugs.*

Saag MS, Holodniy M, Kuritzkes DR, et al. HIV viral load markers in clinical practice. Nat Med 1996; 2:625–630.
*Nice review of the use of these assays to manage patients with HIV infection.*

# 102

## Therapy of Opportunistic Infections

JASON I. N. TOKUMOTO AND HARRY HOLLANDER

Both opportunistic and nonopportunistic infections can complicate the course of human immunodeficiency virus (HIV) disease in the adult. In this chapter we review the ways in which the clinical presentation of infections is modified by underlying HIV. Infections are discussed in the context of common syndromes and of the progressive immunodeficiency due to HIV. Patients on highly active antiretroviral therapy have significantly decreased risk of these complications. Here, "early disease" refers to an immunologic status at which individuals are unlikely to develop life-threatening opportunistic infections. In HIV-infected adults, this usually means a CD4 lymphocyte count of greater than 200–300 cells/mm$^3$, but there is great variability between individuals. Nevertheless, knowledge of the CD4 count is extremely important in constructing a differential diagnosis for any of the syndromes discussed here. Specific treatment issues are reviewed in the text, and current antimicrobial regimens for the major opportunistic infections are outlined in Table 102.5.

### Pulmonary Infiltrates

Infectious, inflammatory, and neoplastic pulmonary complications are common at all stages of HIV disease and often account for mortality in late HIV infection. During early HIV infection, bacterial pneumonia is the predominant pulmonary complication, with a significantly increased incidence compared to age-matched controls. Bacterial pneumonia is a particular problem in the developing world and in injecting drug users. Pneumonia is often an indicator illness that leads to consideration of underlying HIV infection. Because of suboptimal responses to polysaccharide vaccines, HIV-infected adults may develop bacterial pneumonia despite appropriate immunization. The failure rate of this prophylactic measure has not yet been defined. In a subset of adults, episodes of bacterial pneumonia recur frequently; monthly intravenous immunoglobulin (400 mg/kg) may be of benefit in this setting.

The majority of bacterial pneumonias in early HIV disease are caused by encapsulated organisms; *Pneumococcus* is much more common than *Haemophilus influenzae. Staphylococcus aureus* is also overrepresented, consistent with the high nasopharyngeal carriage rate in this population. Legionnaires' disease is rarely encountered. The clinical presentation of pneumococcal pneumonia is no different in the presence of HIV infection (Chapter 56). Radiographically, focal infiltrates remain most common, but atypical findings such as diffuse interstitial disease can occur with underlying HIV infection. The rate of bacteremia with pneumococcal pneumonia exceeds 50%, but there is no evidence for a higher rate of bacterial endocarditis or other complications such as meningitis. Similarly, there appears to be no difference in treatment outcome whether or not HIV infection is present.

### Tuberculosis

Tuberculosis is another important pulmonary complication that may occur during early HIV disease. At normal or slightly depressed CD4 counts, the clinical presentation of pulmonary tuberculosis is no different from that in seronegative adults. However, the incidence of primary infection and disease is higher. In general, individuals with well-preserved CD4 counts have a typical radiographic appearance of pulmonary tuberculosis. With primary infection, the major manifestations are focal or lobar infiltrates with regional lymphadenopathy (Chapter 57). As the CD4 count falls, the chest x-ray tends to show fewer "classic" findings such as cavities, but more commonly shows a miliary or nonspecific pattern. Chest x-rays may also be completely normal when patients have a positive sputum smear and culture, but this occurs less than 5% of the time. In patients with advanced immunodeficiency, the clinical picture is often dominated by extrapulmonary disease, which occurs in approximately 60% of cases. The most common sites of involvement are the central nervous system (CNS), lymph nodes, and bone marrow. In individuals who are infected with sensitive *Mycobacterium tuberculosis* and who are compliant with therapy, the success rate of therapy is identical to that in HIV-seronegative individuals. For a complete discussion of tuberculosis and the issue of multiple drug resistance, see Chapter 57.

### Fungal pneumonias

Another diagnostic consideration for pulmonary infiltrates in early disease is fungal infection. In endemic areas, the incidence of histoplasmosis and coccidioidomycosis in HIV-infected individuals exceeds 25% over the course of illness. Blastomycosis has also been reported. The endemic mycoses present with a spectrum of findings, from asymptomatic seropositivity to fulminant, widely disseminated disease with high mortality. These infections are like tuberculosis in that the higher the CD4 count is, the more likely it is for the infection to be mild and self-limited. With CD4 counts below 200 cells/mm$^3$, diffuse pulmonary infiltrates are often present, but the clinical picture may be dominated by extrapulmonary disease. Histoplasmosis commonly affects bone marrow, gastrointestinal tract, liver, and spleen, while coccidioidomycosis more frequently involves skin, lymph nodes, and CNS. In individuals with coccidioidomycosis or histoplasmosis with well-preserved CD4 counts, pulmonary manifestations are the most important clinical problem; the findings mimic those seen in HIV-seronegative adults.

One confounding factor in establishing these diagnoses is the limited reliability of serologic testing. In the case of coccidioidomycosis, for example, HIV-infected individuals with isolated pulmonary or disseminated disease have a higher rate of false negative complement fixation serology. Thus definitive diagnosis often depends on histology or culture. It is easier to culture *H. capsulatum* than *Coccidioides immitis.* More than 50% of cases with disseminated histoplasmosis have positive blood cultures by lysis centrifugation. The diagnosis of disseminated histoplasmosis has also been aided by the development of a sensitive (>95%) antigen assay for urine. The therapeutic approach to isolated pulmonary histoplasmosis and coccidioidomycosis in this setting has not been well defined. Until further natural history data become available, it is prudent to treat all cases with at least a short course of antifungal therapy. This approach is strongly recommended when the CD4 count is <200 cells/mm$^3$ and the risk of disseminated disease is higher.

## Pneumonia in patients in late HIV disease

At CD4 counts <200 cells/mm$^3$, other opportunistic pulmonary infections increase in incidence. A common scenario is a subacute to acute onset of cough, dyspnea, fever, and diffuse interstitial infiltrates on the chest x-ray. Table 102.1 summarizes the infectious and noninfectious differential diagnosis. Besides the CD4 count, several pieces of clinical information may be helpful. Historical points include a detailed travel and exposure history and a medication history to elicit compliance with prophylactic antibiotics. Signs of extrapulmonary disease should be carefully sought. New neurologic findings, skin lesions, lymphadenopathy, or organomegaly may influence the differential diagnosis and provide other sources of diagnostic material. Routine laboratory tests may also provide evidence of multisystem disease. Often, however, other diagnostic clues are not present. One must then attempt to establish a specific diagnosis and decide whether to begin empiric therapy based on the individual's degree of illness.

### *Pneumocystis carinii* pneumonia

*Pneumocystis carinii* pneumonia (PCP) is still one of the most common etiologies of this pneumonia in the United States and Europe, although it remains uncommon in Africa. It is now more often seen in individuals who have not been under medical care, are noncompliant with a prophylactic regimen, or are taking less effective prophylactic agents such as dapsone or aerosolized pentamidine. The presentation of PCP is usually subacute, with symptoms present for several weeks. When cases occur despite prophylaxis, symptoms may be present longer before the diagnosis becomes clear. Dyspnea and cough are noted in a majority of cases, but in 15% of cases, pulmonary symptomatology may be absent or subtle. Nonspecific signs such as fever, tachycardia, and tachypnea are common, but the physical examination has poor specificity and sensitivity for PCP. In particular, the thoracic examination is usually normal; prominent pulmonary findings suggest alternative diagnoses.

The chest x-ray provides useful data for the diagnosis of PCP, but it has significant limitations. Typical findings include diffuse reticular interstitial or alveolar densities, most prominent in the perihilar regions. However, these findings are not specific. Furthermore, approximately 25% of cases present with a normal chest x-ray or with atypical findings such as predominant upper lobe disease, focal infiltrates, or nodules. Atypical x-rays are more common in individuals who have received aerosolized pentamidine. Radiographic findings that are are unusual for PCP are large pleural effusions and intratoracic adenopathy. Additional laboratory evaluation often shows other nonspecific findings. A sensitive marker is the serum lactate dehydrogenase (LDH), which is elevated in approximately 95% of documented cases. Thus a normal LDH has a high negative predictive value. Arterial blood gases commonly show a respiratory alkalosis and hypoxemia, but 10% of patients with PCP have a normal alveolar-arterial oxygen gradient at rest.

If an individual has had documented PCP and has a clinical and radiographic presentation identical to a prior episode, empiric therapy may cautiously be started without a definitive diagnosis. The presence of severe or rapidly progressive respiratory distress, an alveolar-arterial gradient of greater than 40 mm of mercury, development of disease despite trimethoprim–sulfamethoxazole prophylaxis, or intolerance of the available drugs argues for early definitive diagnosis. In individuals without prior PCP, specific microbiologic confirmation should be sought. Routine Wright-Giemsa staining of induced sputum has provided a valuable alternative to more invasive diagnostic techniques. The sensitivity exceeds 75% in experienced laboratories. Sensitivity may be increased through the use of immunofluorescent assay or monoclonal antibody tests. When examination of induced sputum fails to establish a diagnosis, bronchoscopy is indicated. Bronchoalveolar lavage without biopsy has an excellent yield for PCP (>95%). However, the yield may be decreased by prior prophylactic antimicrobial therapy. Thus if PCP is suspected despite prophylaxis and a negative sputum induction, or the clinical presentation and radiograph suggest other diagnoses, bronchoscopy with transbronchial biopsy should be considered. Bronchoscopy also allows inspection of the airways for lesions of Kaposi's sarcoma.

### Other pathogens

Several other pulmonary pathogens have become important in very late HIV disease with a CD4 count <50 cells/mm$^3$. Aspergillosis is increasing in frequency. Most cases have had no other classic risk factors for *Aspergillus* infection. The majority of HIV-infected individuals with this diagnosis have had CD4 counts

**Table 102.1** Causes of diffuse interstitial infiltrates in late HIV disease*

| Common | Uncommon |
|---|---|
| *Pneumocystis carinii* | *Toxoplasma gondii* |
| *Coccidioides immitis* | *Cryptosporidium parvum* |
| *Histoplasma capsulatum* | *Blastomyces dermatiditis* |
| *Mycobacterium tuberculosis* | *Aspergillus* spp |
| Bacterial pneumonia | *Mycobacterium avium* complex |
| Kaposi's sarcoma | *Mycobacterium kansasii* |
| | *Legionella* species |
| | Cytomegalovirus |
| | Adenovirus |
| | Lymphocytic or nonspecific pneumonitis |
| | Lymphoma |

*CD4 counts < 200 cells/mm$^3$.

<50 cells/mm$^3$. The course of pulmonary disease is variable. The spectrum of radiographic findings includes slowly progressive focal infiltrates, cavitary disease, and diffuse interstitial infiltrates. A unique form of pulmonary involvement is tracheobrchitis, which causes ulcerating airway lesions and presents with cough, chest pain, and airway obstruction rather than with pulmonary infiltrates. Disseminated disease may also occur. The mortality of all forms of aspergillosis in this setting is high.

*Pseudomonas aeruginosa* has also been increasingly reported with very advanced disease. Patients most often present with indolent pulmonary symptoms and focal radiographic abnormalities rather than with rapidly progressive pneumonia and sepsis. Unlike *Pseudomonas* pneumonia in other immunocompromised populations, this infection generally has a low rate of acute mortality, but the rate of relapse exceeds 50%. This syndrome is reminiscent of *Pseudomonas* pulmonary infection in patients with cystic fibrosis. In late HIV disease, *Pseudomonas* may also cause sinusitis, osteomyelitis, and catheter-related infection. As with aspergillosis, this infection identifies a population of HIV-infected individuals with a poor prognosis.

## Central Nervous System Complications

### Encephalopathy

Alterations in cognition and/or level of consciousness without focal neurologic deficits are common during HIV disease. Evaluation is frequently complicated by toxic/metabolic encephalopathy due to medications, sepsis, hypoxemia, or other acute medical problems. It is difficult to interpret fever accompanying encephalopathy in a patient with advanced HIV disease since there are often other explanations for fever. Individuals with early HIV disease have no obvious predisposition to nonopportunistic viral encephalitides. However, as the CD4 count falls, the presentation of *Herpes simplex* encephalitis may change, with less temporal localization and hemorrhage on imaging studies and fewer cerebrospinal fluid (CSF) abnormalities.

In patients with advanced HIV disease, the most common cause of subacute or chronic encephalopathy is the HIV-associated cognitive/motor complex (AIDS dementia complex). A fulminant course is unusual for this entity, as is a CD4 count higher than 200 cells/mm$^3$ at the time of diagnosis. Fever is not a presenting sign of the AIDS dementia complex. Thus if it is present, other CNS or peripheral infections should be considered. When individuals present with subacute or acute encephalopathy, cerebral imaging, preferably magnetic resonance imaging (MRI), should be performed to exclude the space-occupying lesions discussed below. Lumbar puncture is also commonly performed to exclude meningeal proccesses, particularly if headache or fever is also present.

Cytomegalovirus (CMV) encephalitis has been described more frequently in individuals with <100 CD4 cells/mm$^3$. The clinical presentation may be identical to other viral encephalitides, but the presence of CMV disease in another organ system or new cranial nerve abnormalities is suggestive of the diagnosis. Some documented cases have had intense periventricular enhancement on cerebral imaging studies. Hypoglycorhacchia and pleocytosis are common CSF findings, but these are variable. In the past, brain biopsy was required for diagnosis, but polymerase chain reaction or branched chain DNA assays of CSF are sensitive and specific. Some cases have responded to antiviral therapy.

### Focal neurologic deficits and space-occupying lesions

Since the differential diagnosis of focal intracerebral lesions is the same in early HIV disease as in nonimmunocompromised hosts (Chapter 26), the remainder of this discussion focuses on advanced disease. Table 102.2 outlines the etiologies of the intracerebral lesions encountered in this setting. Of these, toxoplasmosis is most common, accounting for more than half of the lesions. Because of this epidemiology, the approach to mass lesions is geared to the rapid diagnosis and treatment of this infection. Since most cases represent recrudescence of prior infection, the incidence of toxoplasmosis depends on the seroprevalence in a population. In countries such as Haiti and France, where seroprevalence exceeds 70%, cerebral toxoplasmosis is one of the most frequent presenting and subsequent opportunistic infection during the course of HIV disease. In HIV-infected individuals who have positive *Toxoplasma* IgG titers, the lifetime risk of cerebral toxoplasmosis ranges from 10% to 30%. The combination regimens of dapsone–pyrimethamine or trimethoprim–sulfamethoxazole decrease the prevalence when these agents are used for PCP prophylaxis.

The presentation of cerebral toxoplasmosis is usually acute or subacute. Headache, confusion, and fever are common complaints. Focal neurologic problems are noted by patients less

**Table 102.2** Causes of focal intracerebral lesions

| Common | Less common | Uncommon |
|---|---|---|
| *Toxoplasma gondii* | *Cryptococcus neoformans* | *Trypanosoma cruzii* |
| Bacterial brain abscess | *Aspergillus* spp. | Primary amebic meningoencephalitis due to *Acanthameba* |
| Lymphoma | *Mycobacterium tuberculosis* | |
| Progressive multifocal leukoencephalopathy | | *Histoplasma capsulatum*<br>*Coccidioides immitis*<br>Bacillary angiomatosis due to *Bartonella* spp<br>*Mycobacterium kansasii*<br>Cytomegalovirus<br>HIV<br>Solid tumor metastasis<br>Kaposi's sarcoma |

often. However, neurologic examination reveals focal findings in addition to encephalopathy in more than half the patients. The findings are variable and reflect the widespread distribution of lesions throughout the cerebral hemispheres and cerebellum. It is often difficult to clinically differentiate toxoplasmosis from other processes causing mass lesions. Rapid onset of disease, presence of focal findings, and depression of the level of consciousness favor the diagnosis of toxoplasmosis rather than the HIV-associated cognitive–motor complex. If headache is prominent, meningitis must also be considered.

Cerebral imaging is the cornerstone of presumptive or definitive diagnosis of toxoplasmosis. Comparative studies have established the superiority of MRI over computerized tomography. More than 85% of cases have contrast-enhancing, space-occupying lesions visualized; the majority have multiple lesions. Surrounding edema is often present. In contrast to toxoplasmic meningoencephalitis in other immunocompromised patients, negative imaging studies are rare. However, a minority of lesions of toxoplasmosis may have atypical radiographic patterns. If each lesion in a given individual is nonenhancing and causes no mass effect, the differential diagnosis shifts toward progressive multifocal leukoencephalopathy, other demyelinating processes, or vascular disease. When imaging studies show multiple enhancing lesions, this strongly favors toxoplasmosis, although 10% of patients may have several concomitant processes causing these findings.

Although early studies suggested that the false-negative rate of serologies is as high as 15%, more recent studies suggest that at least 95% of cases have positive *Toxoplasma* IgG serology by immunofluorescence, enzyme immunoassay (EIA), or dye test. In a patient with a compatible history, examination, and imaging findings, and a positive *Toxoplasma* IgG serology, toxoplasmosis should be diagnosed presumptively and therapy begun. Indications for early stereotactic brain biopsy rather than an empiric trial are listed in Table 102.3.

## Spinal cord disease and related conditions

Several important processes present late in the course of HIV disease with a constellation of paraparesis, lower extremity sensory deficits, and incontinence. When hyperreflexia and spastic paraparesis are present, the differential diagnosis comprises chronic myelopathies and infections or neoplasms causing spinal cord compression. Epidural abcess should be suspected in injecting drug users or others at risk for bacteremia. Lymphomatous cord compression is almost always seen in patients with previously diagnosed non-Hodgkin's lymphoma. Chronic myelopathy may have noninfectious etiologies such as vitamin $B_{12}$ deficiency, but it is more commonly attributable to chronic viral infection of the spinal cord. Vacuolar myelopathy often coexists with AIDS dementia and is a primary manifestation of HIV. The mechanism of disease is unknown. The other chronic viral myelopathy is associated with human T-cell leukemia virus (HTLV-1). Since neither vacuolar myelopathy nor HTLV-1–associated myelopathy is treatable, the diagnostic evaluation should aim to exclude spinal cord compression using MRI of the spine.

In individuals who present with hyporeflexic or flaccid paraparesis, cord compression is still a consideration, as are unusual intrinsic cord lesions caused by toxoplasmosis, tuberculosis, or lymphoma. If a mass lesion is excluded, the most likely diagnosis is myelitis or radiculomyelitis. Cases of acute transverse myelitis have been described with *H. simplex* and *H. zoster*. These may be amenable to antiviral therapy if treatment is initiated early. Cytomegalovirus radiculomyelitis or polyradiculopathy is an entity which mimics acute myelitis. This may be the initial manifestation of CMV disease or occur during therapy of other CMV disease. Typically, there is urinary retention, lower extremity pain, patchy sensory loss, and weakness that progress over days to weeks. Magnetic resonance imaging of the spine often shows meningeal enhancement and thickening of the nerve roots in the cauda equina. Analysis of CSF is helpful in differentiating this entity from other causes of infectious myelopathy. The CSF in HTLV-1–associated myelopathy and vacuolar myelopathy is usually acellular; in the case of herpesvirus myelitis, it shows a mild mononuclear pleocytosis. Patients with CMV polyradiculopathy have a striking CSF pleocytosis, with cell counts that may exceed 1000/mm$^3$. The differential cell count is also suggestive, since the leukocytes are predominantly polymorphonuclear. Hypoglycorhacchia and elevated CSF protein are also common. Routine culture of CSF yields CMV in approximately 50% of cases; polymerase chain reaction or branched chain DNA assays is more sensitive. When antiviral therapy is attempted, the outcome is best in individuals who can still ambulate and have less marked CSF abnormalities. Overall response rate is about 50% with either ganciclovir or foscarnet.

**Table 102.3** Relative indications to biopsy CNS mass lesions

| |
|---|
| 1. Rapid neurologic progression |
| 2. Mass effect necessitating the use of glucocorticoids |
| 3. Negative *Toxoplasma* IgG serology |
| 4. Single lesion by MRI |
| 5. Intolerance of antibiotics used to treat toxoplasmosis |
| 6. Development of lesions despite appropriate prophylaxis |

## Meningitis

During the early stages of HIV infection, CSF abnormalities due to CNS invasion by HIV are common, occurring in half of individuals with a CD4 count >400 cells/mm$^3$. These background CSF findings are most commonly low-grade lymphocytic pleocytosis (<50 cells/mm$^3$) and mild elevation of protein (<100 mg/dL). In addition to these findings in asymptomatic individuals, HIV has been associated with acute and chronic meningitis syndromes, with typical symptoms and signs of meningitis and more marked CSF abnormalities. The CSF abnormalities caused by HIV may lead to diagnostic confusion. For example, it may be impossible to differentiate the CSF formula due to HIV infection from that of neurosyphilis or other viral meningitides (Chapter 73).

Other etiological considerations for meningitis in early HIV disease include drug-induced meningitis, bacterial infection, tuberculosis, and coccidioidomycosis. As discussed earlier, there has not been convincing evidence for an increased incidence of bacterial meningitis due to *Pneumococcus* or *Haemophilus influenzae*. However, if they are not taking prophylactic trimethoprim-sulfamethoxazole, HIV-infected patients are predisposed to meningitis caused by *Listeria monocytogenes*. The clinical presentation, CSF findings, and outcome of bacterial meningitis are identical in HIV-seropositive and seronegative individuals. Tuberculous meningitis may also occur during early HIV infection, but the incidence rises with progressive immunodeficiency. Overall, about 10% of HIV-infected individuals with tuberculosis have CNS involvement. When tuberculosis is caused by multiple drug–resistant organisms, the incidence of meningitis exceeds 20%. As with bacterial meningitis, tuberculous meningitis does not differ in its clinical severity, tempo of disease, or response to therapy with underlying HIV infection. However, HIV-infected patients may have a higher incidence of intracranial tuberculomas. Cerebrospinal fluid abnormalities are comparable to those noted before the HIV epidemic, although there is probably a higher incidence of acellular CSF in HIV-infected individuals with tuberculous meningitis. Finally, coccidioidial meningitis may occur before there is profound immunodeficiency due to HIV. As with the other meningitides discussed previously, most studies suggest that one cannot differentiate the severity or outcome of this process from coccidioidal meningitis in HIV-uninfected people.

The most common pathogen causing meningitis in advanced HIV disease is *Cryptococcus neoformans.* Without antifungal prophylaxis, cryptococcal meningitis occurs in 5%–10% of AIDS patients in North America and Europe and probably a higher percentage of patients in sub-Saharan Africa. Prophylactic oral fluconazole decreases the incidence of invasive cryptococcal disease. The onset of cryptococcal meningitis is variable. The majority of patients with cryptococcal meningitis have a subacute presentation, but fulminant or more indolent courses are seen occasionally. Usually, headache is the presenting symptom, but this may be mild. Other constitutional symptoms, especially fever, are common, while localizing neurologic complaints are uncommon. The general physical examination is usually unrevealing. In rare cases, ulcerated skin lesions, abnormal pulmonary findings, or hepatosplenomegaly may be found. Meningeal signs are elicited in fewer than 20% of cases with HIV-related cryptococcal meningitis. The neurologic examination may be entirely normal or reveal a depressed level of consciousness. Cranial nerve findings are less common than in classic cryptococcal meningitis, and other focal findings due to cryptococcal disease are rare.

The diagnosis of cryptococcal meningitis is straightforward, utilizing fungal culture and the latex agglutination cryptococcal antigen test. Between 50% and 95% of individuals with HIV-related cryptococcal meningitis have a positive cryptococcal antigen titer in blood. Many individuals who are antigen positive also grow *Cryptococcus neoformans* from blood. In CSF, culture and antigen positivity are found in almost 100% of cases. False-negative antigen determinations have been reported with a high titer prozone phenomenon and with capsule-deficient strains unique to HIV-infected patients. Application of both antigen and culture techniques to CSF specimens is important, since routine CSF values may be normal in approximately 40% of patients. Cerebral imaging studies are not routinely required in the initial assessment of a patient with cryptococcal meningitis. If there is the suspicion of a complicating mass lesion or hydrocephalus, imaging should be performed. When imaging is done, nonspecific abnormalities such as punctate white matter lesions and meningeal enhancement are common. A rare but specific radiographic finding is a gelatinous pseudocyst, which is a low-density, nonenhancing lesion in the region of the basal ganglia. The pathologic correlate is large numbers of yeast in the Virchow-Robin spaces. When an enhancing, space-occupying lesion is found in a person with active cryptococcal meningitis, all other causes of focal lesions must still be considered since cryptococcomas are uncommon.

The prognosis of cryptococcal meningitis may be estimated from clinical and laboratory markers. The most powerful predictor of outcome is the level of consciousness. Individuals presenting with abnormal mental status have a mortality exceeding 40%. Laboratory markers of poor outcome include hyponatremia, absence of CSF pleocytosis, and CSF cryptococcal antigen titer greater than 1:512.

In addition to the choice of antimicrobial agents, management of increased intracranial pressure is also emerging as an important issue in therapy. Elevated intracranial pressure should be managed with a neurosurgical shunt if hydrocephalus has developed. If intracranial pressure is increased without hydrocephalus, the optimal management is unclear. The roles of repeated lumbar punctures, neurosurgical shunting, and medical therapy with acetazolamide are under investigation.

## Gastrointestinal Disease

### Diarrhea

Significant diarrhea occurs in as many as 90% of individuals over the course of HIV infection and is a particular problem in the developing world. The role of enteric viruses in causing diarrhea during early HIV disease is unknown, but bacterial enterocolitis may be caused by *Salmonella* species, *Shigella* (mainly *flexneri*), and *Campylobacter jejuni.* The incidence of these bacterial infections may be reduced with the widespread use of zidovudine and trimethoprim–sulfamethoxazole, two agents which have significant activity against gram-negative enteric pathogens. With each of these enteric pathogens, it is generally true that as immunosuppression progresses, there may be more prolonged illness, a higher rate of bacteremia, and more frequent relapse than in HIV-seronegative individuals. *Salmonella* enteritis is particularly problematic, with a 20- to 100-fold increased incidence in HIV-seropositive individuals, and a rate of accompanying bacteremia as high as 80% in one series. Bacteremia is often recurrent despite prolonged courses of appropriate antibiotics. This argues for routine therapy of any HIV-infected person found to harbor *Salmonella* species in the gastrointestinal tract. Therapy with ciprofloxacin may be more efficacious than other antibiotics to which the organisms appear sensitive. *Campylobacter fennelliae* and *Campylobacter cinaedi* are introduced through the gut and may cause a febrile illness with bacteremia, usually without significant diarrhea. Clostridium difficile is an important consideration since many patients have received broad spectrum antibiotics.

Enteric parasites may also cause diarrhea during early HIV infection in individuals who acquire these organisms via waterborne or sexual contact. The course of amebiasis and giardiasis is uneffected by underlying HIV infection, and therapy is not altered. There is some controversy about the role of *Blastocystis hominis* in causing diarrhea, but treatment with an amebicidal regimen should be considered if *Blastocystis* is the only pathogen discovered during evaluation of diarrhea. *Strongyloides stercoralis* may also be a cause of diarrhea in the developing world or other endemic areas. With progressive immunodeficiency, individuals with strongyloidiasis are at risk for the *Strongyloides* hyperinfection syndrome, although this risk has not been well quantified. Stool collection has a low sensitivity for *Strongyloides* (~30%); diagnostic yield can be increased by performing a duodenal aspirate or the Enterotest. When the hyperinfection syndrome infection is present, larvae can be identified in other involved organs. For gastrointestinal involvement, a routine course of thiabendazole should be given, but the optimal duration of antihelminthic therapy for the hyperinfection syndrome in HIV-infected patients is not known.

With progressive HIV disease, the infectious differential diagnosis for diarrhea includes the foregoing diseases plus other processes. *Cryptosporidium parvum* may cause diarrhea at any stage of HIV infection, but with a CD4 count <200 cells/mm$^3$, there is a higher likelihood of secretory diarrhea that does not resolve spontaneously. The diarrhea may be severe, causing volume depletion, and it may be associated with malabsorption and weight loss. Fever is uncommon. Extraintestinal involvement most commonly contributes to AIDS cholangiopathy, but pulmonary infiltrates have also been described. Cryptosporidiosis is diagnosed by examining stool specimens with a modified acid fast stain to identify oocysts. Rarely, small bowel biopsy is required to make the diagnosis. There is no definitive antimicrobial therapy. Treatment is palliative, aiming to decrease diarrhea with antimotility agents and to maintain nutritional and volume status.

Another group of organisms putatively associated with high-volume, secretory diarrhea is the microsporidia. The two genera most frequently described in the setting of HIV disease are *Enterocytozoon* and *Septata*. Clinically, microsporidiosis is virtually identical to cryptosporidiosis and it may also involve the biliary tree. A recent case control study also demonstrated frequent asymptomatic colonization of the gastrointestinal tract. Microsporidia can be identified in unconcentrated stool specimens using a modified chromotrope stain. There have been reports of successful therapy with paromomycin or albendazole, but the efficacy of antimicrobial agents remain in question.

At CD4 counts <50 cells/mm$^3$, enterocolitis due to *Mycobacterium avium* complex (MAC) and CMV become more important considerations in the person with diarrhea. At this level of immunosuppression, if routine stool studies do not establish an etiology, colonoscopy with biopsy should be performed. If colonoscopy is negative, some authors also advocate upper endoscopy with small bowel biopsy. Diarrhea due to MAC is associated with disseminated disease. Thus other symptoms of disseminated MAC infection are usually present. Often the diagnosis is established indirectly by blood culture. Cultures of stool are neither sensitive nor specific for enterocolitis. If endoscopy is performed, the most common findings are nonspecific mucosal erythema, edema, and whitish nodules. Biopsy may show numerous intracellular acid fast bacilli, but due to sampling error, this histologic finding is not as sensitive as blood culturing results. Unfortunately, when systemic MAC is treated, diarrhea often does not improve.

Cytomegalovirus enterocolitis is more common than upper gastrointestinal manifestations of this infection. Diarrhea, if present, is generally of low volume; hematochezia may occur. Abdominal cramping and pain are common, and CMV colitis may result in an acute surgical abdomen if perforation occurs. When this diagnosis is suspected or confirmed, a dilated funduscopic examination should be performed to exclude concurrent CMV retinitis. The diagnosis of CMV colitis must be made by colonoscopy. Diffuse mucosal ulceration is the most frequent finding, but CMV gastrointestinal disease may also present as an ulcerative mass that mimics a neoplasm. Biopsy of involved colon shows typical viral cytopathic effect, but the process is patchy. Thus multiple biopsies may be required to establish the diagnosis. Immunofluorescent staining may increase the diagnostic yield of biopsy specimens. Positive CMV cultures from biopsy specimens must be interpreted cautiously, since this may be a nonspecific finding in colonic inflammation of any etiology. Evaluation of efficacy of antiviral drugs for CMV colitis has been complicated by a significant rate of remission without specific therapy (~30%). Most authorities use the maximal "induction" dose of antiviral chemotherapy for initial therapy. Without maintenance antiviral therapy other CMV end organ disease usually occurs.

## Odynophagia and dysphagia

Esophageal disease usually presents during late HIV infection. In the individual with esophageal complaints, it is important to consider non–HIV-related processes, especially gastroesophageal reflux disease. However, most of the structural lesions diagnosed are opportunistic processes, mainly infectious esophagitis. *Candida* (usually *C. albicans*) accounts for 50%–80% of all cases of esophagitis. The absence of visible oral candidiasis does not exclude the possibility of *Candida* esophagitis. Thus when severity of esophageal symptoms does not mandate intravenous therapy for volume repletion, it is warranted to begin a 10–14 day empiric trial of an oral antifungal agent. Fluconazole is preferable to ketoconazole since individuals with low CD4 counts often have hypochlorhydria with impaired absorption ketoconazole. Upper endoscopy should be reserved for individuals who are severely ill, who develop symptoms despite systemic antifungal therapy, or who do not improve during an empiric azole trial. Azole-resistant *C. albicans* is becoming more frequent in the setting of HIV infection. If azole-resistant *Candida* esophagitis is diagnosed, parenteral amphotericin B (0.2 mg/kg/d) is indicated, usually for a duration of 10–14 days.

There are three viral etiologies of esophagitis. Human immunodeficiency syndrome can cause esophageal ulceration during primary infection. *Herpes simplex* also causes sporadic cases of esophagitis, but less commonly than in other immunocompromised patients. Cytomegalovirus is the major viral pathogen, occurring in individuals with very advanced disease. CMV esophagitis may coexist with gastritis or duodenitis. Thus in addition to substernal pain, nausea and vomiting may be prominent symptoms. The endoscopic appearance of CMV esophagitis is usually that of discrete, ulcerated lesions which must be differentiated histologically from idiopathic or dideoxycytidine-associated aphthous ulcerations. The limitations of endoscopic biopsy are identical to those discussed in the evaluation of CMV colitis. Antiviral therapy for CMV upper gastrointestinal disease may have a higher response rate than for CMV colitis. Although large comparative trials have not been reported, there is some evidence that foscarnet may have higher efficacy than ganciclovir for CMV upper gastrointestinal disease.

## Fever

In patients with advanced HIV disease, new or worsening fever is a common problem. With careful evaluation, an etiology can be identified in 80%–90% of episodes, suggesting that attribution of fever to HIV infection itself is most often mistaken. The initial evaluation should focus on localized processes such as sinusitis, bacterial pneumonia, PCP, and catheter-related infection. Often, the initial evaluation is unrevealing and the differential diagnosis shifts to that outlined in Table 102.4. In this situation, an appropriate microbiological evaluation includes several blood cultures for bacteria and mycobacteria, and a serum cryptococ-

**Table 102.4** Nonfocal diseases causing fever in late HIV infection*

| |
|---|
| *Pneumocystis carinii* |
| *Cryptococcus neoformans* |
| *Mycobacterium avium* complex |
| *Mycobacterium genavense* |
| *Bartonella* species |
| CMV |
| Drug fever |
| Lymphoma |

*CD4 count < 200 cells/mm$^3$.

cal antigen. The utility of CMV blood cultures is disputed since a positive result has poor predictive value for end-organ disease. There are no prospective studies that justify the use of computerized tomographic body scanning or other imaging modalities in the evaluation of fever in these patients. The role of lumbar puncture is unclear when there is no headache or neurologic findings.

Disseminated MAC infection is the most common etiology of nonfocal fever when the CD4 count is <50 cells/mm$^3$. The incidence of MAC in this group of patients exceeds 40% if prophylaxis is not offerred. This ubiquitous organism commonly colonizes the respiratory or gastrointestinal tracts, and dissemination occurs with progressive immunodeficiency. However, routine surveillance cultures identify fewer than 50% of those who will go on to develop disseminated disease. Conversely, in individuals with a positive stool or sputum culture, the risk of disseminated disease occurring within 1 year is approximately 60%.

The presentation of disseminated MAC is often dominated by constitutional complaints of intermittent or persistent fever, sweats, and weight loss. Diarrhea and abdominal pain are common. The physical examination may be normal except for evidence of recent weight loss, but new adenopathy or hepatosplenomegaly is seen in a minority of cases. Skin lesions are distinctly uncommon. Anemia is present in the majority of cases; other cytopenias are less common. Alkaline phosphatase elevation is observed in about 50% of cases as a result of infiltrative liver disease. Although sputum cultures are commonly positive, and MAC may on occasion cause pulmonary infiltrates, the lung parenchyma is most often spared. However, intrathoracic adenopathy may occur.

A diagnosis of disseminated MAC is established when the organism is cultured from normally sterile sites. Although the optimal number of blood cultures is not known, the overall sensitivity of lysis centrifugation blood cultures approaches 90%. Other sites from which MAC can be cultured less frequently include bone marrow, liver, and lymph nodes. Given the high prevalence of this infection, if other infectious processes have been excluded and the clinical picture is compatible with MAC, an empiric trial is often justified. With the broad-spectrum regimens that are utilized, an "antibiotic response" is not necessarily specific for MAC.

With the availability of macrolide-based regimens, the ability to treat disseminated MAC has dramatically improved (Chapters 37 and 57). Because there is rapid development of resistance during single-agent therapy, combination therapy is recommended. The most effective combination is not yet known. Even "successful" therapy of disseminated MAC is only partially successful unless patients are on effective antiretroviral therapy. Colony counts are decreased, but postmortem studies show persistence of the organism in tissue. Diminution of fever and malaise are the most common beneficial effects of therapy, and some patients are able to stabilize their weight. However, gastrointestinal symptoms and anemia tend not to improve with therapy. Between 50% and 70% of patients can expect some symptomatic improvement with currently available regimens. Response rates are lower in macrolide-resistant cases.

## Retinitis

Organisms that may occasionally cause retinal lesions in HIV-infected individuals include *Toxoplasma gondii*, *Pneumocystis carinii*, *Cryptococcus neoformans*, *Histoplasma capsulatum*, *Mycobacterium tuberculosis*, *Treponema pallidum*, *Herpes simplex*, and *Herpes zoster*. The combined incidence of these infections is overshadowed by CMV retinitis, which is diagnosed premortem in more than 30% of patients with late HIV disease. The incidence of disease is comparable to that of disseminated MAC in individuals with CD4 counts <50 cell/mm$^3$. Cytomegalovirus retinitis usually begins peripherally and may occasionally be diagnosed by dilated funduscopic examination at a presymptomatic stage. Invariably, there is progression of disease over days to weeks, with the development of visual floaters, scotomata, or decreased visual acuity. Nonspecific constitutional symptoms may accompany the onset of retinitis. The diagnosis is usually established by funduscopic examination performed by an experienced ophthalmologist. Typical ophthalmologic findings include vascular-based fluffy exudates with areas of hemorrhage. In a minority of cases, the optic disc may be swollen, reflecting retrobulbar involvement of the optic nerve. In most cases, only one eye is involved at the time of presentation, although without therapy, development of bilateral disease occurs in about 50% of cases. If the funduscopic examination is typical, other diagnostic tests are not needed. If retinitis occurs at a higher CD4 cell count or in an individual with negative CMV IgG serology, alternative diagnoses should be more strongly considered.

Foscarnet and ganciclovir have been shown to stabilize disease in 85% of individuals. One comparative study suggested a survival benefit conferred by foscarnet, but this was marred by the fact that individuals receiving ganciclovir were able to tolerate less antiretroviral therapy. A decision to treat with foscarnet commits individuals to more frequent subjective side effects, the inconvenience of daily infusions, and prolonged infusion times due to intravenous prehydration. With either drug regimen, breakthrough and progression of retinitis increase steadily over time. Both foscarnet- and ganciclovir-resistant strains of CMV have been described. Therefore, if progression of disease occurs after 3 to 6 months on therapy, a change alternative therapy is recommended. Combination therapy with ganciclovir and foscarnet, administration of systemic cidofavir, or intraocular implants of ganciclovir are options for patients with progressive disease.

## Antibiotic Hypersensitivity in HIV Infection

Table 102.5 lists preferred antimicrobials for prophylaxis or treatment of specific infections in HIV-infected patients. Table 102.6 lists some adverse effects that are increased in HIV-seropositive individuals. Early in the epidemic, an 85% rate of hypersensi-

**Table 102.5** Prophylaxis and therapy of major HIV-related infections*

| Organism | Primary prophylaxis | Acute infection | Maintenance |
|---|---|---|---|
| *Pneumocystis carinii* | FIRST LINE<br>Trimethoxazole-sulfamethoxazole 160–800 mg 3–7 times/wk PO<br>SECOND LINE<br>Dapsone 100 mg/PO<br>or<br>Pentamidine 300 mg inhaled 1–2 times/mo | Mild-Moderate Disease[a]<br>Trimethoprim–sulfamethoxazole 15 mg/kg/d PO of trimethoprim divided in 3–4 doses<br>or<br>Dapsone 100 mg PO plus trimethoprim 5 mg/kg PO every 8 h<br>or<br>Primaquine 15–30 mg base/d PO plus clindamycin 600 mg/8 h PO<br>or<br>Atovaquone 750 mg/8 h PO<br>Moderate-Severe Disease[b]<br>Trimethoprim–sulfamethoxazole<br>15 mg/kg/d of trimethoprim IV divided in 3–4 doses<br>or<br>Pentamidine 3 mg/kg/d IV plus prednisone 40 mg 2 times/d PO for 5 d, then 40 mg/d PO for 5 d, then 20 mg/day PO | See primary prophlyaxis |
| *Toxoplasma gondii*[c] | Avoidance of cat feces, contaminated soil, and undercooked meats if IgG serology if negative<br>Same as first-line PCP prophylaxis if IgG serology is positive; pyrimethamine 25 mg PO weekly is added if dapsone is used for PCP prophylaxis | Pyrimethamine 150–200 mg PO initially, then 50–75 mg/PO with leucovorin 5–10 mg/PO plus clindamycin 2.4–3.6 g/d PO or iv in 3–4 divided doses<br>or<br>Sulfadiazine 4.0–8.0 g/d PO in 4 divided doses<br>For failure or drug intolerance<br>Clarithromycin 1 g 2 times/d PO<br>or<br>Atovaquone 750 mg/PO alone, or in combination with pyrimethamine | Pyrimethamine 25 mg/d PO with leucovorin 5 mg 3–5 times/wk PO plus clindamycin 600 mg 1–2/d PO<br>or<br>Sulfadiazine 1 g/PO |
| *Cryptococcus neoformans*[d] | Fluconazole 200 mg/d PO | Amphotericin B 0.6–0.7 mg/kg/d IV alone or in combination with 5-flucytosine 100 mg/kg/d PO in 4 doses for 2 weeks, followed by fluconazole 200 mg 2 times/d PO | Fluconazole 200 mg/PO |
| *Histoplasma capsulatum* | None proven | Severe Disseminated Disease and/or CNS Involvement<br>Amphotericin B 0.6 mg/kg/d IV[e]<br>Mild–Moderate Disease<br>Itraconazole 200–400 mg/d PO in 1 or 2 doses | Itraconazole 200 mg/d PO |
| *Coccidioides immitis* | None proven | Severe Disseminated Disease and/or CNS Involvement<br>Amphotericin B 0.6 mg/kg/d IV[f]<br>Mild–Moderate Disease<br>Fluconazole 400–800 mg/d PO in 2 divided doses | Fluconazole 200 mg/d PO |
| *Candida albicans* | None | Fluconazole 100 mg for 10–14 d PO | Topical antifungals for frequent mucosal relapse<br>Avoid systemic therapy |

(*continued*)

**Table 102.5** Prophylaxis and therapy of major HIV-related infections* (*continued*)

| Organism | Primary prophylaxis | Acute infection | Maintenance |
|---|---|---|---|
| *Mycobacterium avium* complex[g] | Azithromycin 1200 mg weekly PO Clarithromycin 500 mg 2 times/d PO or Rifabutin 300 mg/d PO | Clarithromycin 750–1000 mg 2 times/d PO plus Ethambutol 15–20 mg/kg/d PO For severe disease can add one or more of the following: Ciprofloxacin 500–750 mg 2 times/d PO Rifampin 600 mg/d PO or rifabutin 300 mg PO qd Clofazamine 100 mg/d PO | Acute therapy is continued indefinitely; decrease dose of clarithromycin to 500 mg 2 times/d PO if adequate symptomatic control is achieved |
| *Bartonella henselae/quintana* | Minimize contact with young cats to decrease exposure to *B. henselae.* | Erythromycin 500 mg 4 times/d IV or POS or Doxycycline 100 mg 2 times/d PO | Erythromycin-optimal dose and duration unknown |
| Cytomegalovirus | Ganciclovir 1 g every 8 h PO | Ganciclovir 5 mg/kg every 12 h IV or Foscarnet 60 mg/kg every 8 h IV[h] (or 90 mg/kg every 12 h IV) or cidofovir 5 mg/kg every week IV with probenecid 500 mg PO before dosing | Ganciclovir 6 mg/kg/d 5 times a week IV or Foscarnet 90–120 mg/kg/d IV or cidofovir 5 mg/kg every 2 weeks IV with probenecid 500 mg PO before dosing or ganciclovir 1 gm every 8 h PO (for peripheral disease) |

*Infections not in the table either are treated with standard regimens used in other settings or have special considerations discussed in the text.

[a]Duration of therapy 14–21 days. Because of poor bioavailability and lower efficacy, atovaquone should be used only when there is intolerance to all other agents. G6PD should be checked in patients receiving dapsone or primaquine.

[b]If there is prompt improvement, the course can be completed with one of the oral regimens. Trimetrexate 45 mg/m$^2$/d IV plus leukovorin 80 mg/m$^2$/d PO have been used when the listed regimens have failed or cannot be used because of toxicity.

[c]For active disease, daily neurologic evaluation is essential, and cerebral imaging should be repeated by day 14 of therapy. Full-dose therapy is continued until there is maximal clinical and radiographic improvement, usually 4–8 weeks.

[d]For severe disease, amphotericin should be continued for approximately 6 weeks. For low-risk disease, amphotericin should be given for 10–14 days if tolerated before switching to fluconazole 200 mg twice daily PO to complete a 6 week course. Carefully selected individuals with normal neurological examination, low CSF antigen titer, and high compliance may be tried on fluconazole without amphotericin B lead-in. The adjunctive role of 5-flucytosine is being studied.

[e]In nonmeningeal disease, the course of amphotericin B can be shortened from the traditional 2.0–2.5 g, and therapy can be changed to itraconazole if there is a satisfactory clinical response.

[f]A subset of patients with mild meningitis may be controlled with high-dose fluconazole (600–800 mg/d). Patients with severe meningitis require adjunctive intraventricular amphotericin B.

[g]Amikacin 15 mg/kg/d IV in 2 doses can be used if a parenteral medication is needed, but it does not clearly add benefit to the available oral agents.

[h]Dosage decreased for renal insufficiency. Neutropenia due to ganciclovir may be reversed by filgrastim (GCSF) 300 $\mu$g SC or IV 3–5 times per week. HPMPC 5 mg/kg/wk IV with oral probenecid has been used experimentally for primary and salvage therapy.

**Table 102.6** Idiosyncratic side effects of antimicrobials in HIV-infected patients

| Drug | Toxicity |
|---|---|
| Trimethoprim–sulfamethoxazole | Rash, fever, hepatitis, leukopenia, thrombocytopenia |
| Dapsone | Rash, fever |
| Pyrimethamine | Leukopenia, rash |
| Clindamycin | Rash |
| Clarithromycin | Encephalopathy |
| Ciprofloxacin | Anaphylactoid reactions |
| Rifabutin | Rash, uveitis |
| Antituberculous drugs | Rash |

tivity to trimethoprim–sulfamethoxazole was recognized in AIDS patients. Subsequently, an increased rate of drug reactions has been shown for multiple classes of antibiotics and for other drugs such as anticonvulsants. The mechanism of these reactions is not completely understood, but in most cases it is not a classic IgE-mediated response. Thus true desensitization is not possible. Since individuals may develop multiple reactions, this can create significant difficulties in choosing an antimicrobial regimen that is effective and well tolerated.

## ANNOTATED BIBLIOGRAPHY

### Pulmonary Disease


Baron AD, Hollander H. *Pseudomonas aeruginosa* bronchopulmonary infection in late human immunodeficiency virus disease. Am Rev Respir Dis 1993; 148:992–996.

*Patients generally has a good outcome despite very low CD4 counts, but the rate of recurrence was greater than 80%.*

Dohn MN, Weinberg WG, Torres RA, et al. Oral atovaquone compared with intravenous pentamidine for Pneumocystis carinii pneumonia in patients with AIDS. Ann Intern Med 1994; 121:174–180.

*In this series, atovaquone was as effective and less toxic.*

Fichtenbaum CJ, Woeltje KF, Powderly WG. Serious *Pseudomonas aeruginosa* infections in patients with human immunodeficiency virus: a case-control study. Clin Infect Dis 1994; 19:17–22.

*In addition to pulmonary infection, sinusitis, bacteremia, and osteomyelitis occurred, again with a high recurrence rate.*

Fish DG, Ampel NM, Galgani JN, et al. Coccidioidomycosis during human immunodeficiency virus infection: a review of 77 patients. Medicine 1990; 69:384–391.

*Spectrum of illness depended on the CD4 count, with disseminated disease occurring at lower counts.*

Hughes W, Leoung G, Kramer F, et al. Comparison of atovaquone (566C80) with trimethoprim–sulfamethoxazole to treat *Pneumocystis carinii* pneumonia in patients with AIDS. N Engl J Med 1993; 328:1521–1527.

*Atovaquone was better tolerated but had a significantly higher failure rate than trimethoprim–sulfamethoxazole.*

Jones BE, Young SM, Antoniskis D, et al. Relationship of the manifestations of tuberculosis to CD4 cell counts in patients with human immunodeficiency virus infection. Am Rev Respir Dis 1993; 148:1292–1297.

*Typical radiographic patterns were seen with preserved CD4 count; otherwise, nonspecific patterns predominated, with a high prevalence of extrapulmonary disease.*

Lortholary O, Meyohas MC, Dupont B, et al. Invasive aspergillosis in patients with acquired immunodeficiency syndrome: report of 33 cases. French cooperative study group on aspergillosis in AIDS. Am J Med 1993; 95:177–187.

*Most individuals with positive respiratory cultures had invasive disease which varied in severity. A minority had disseminated infection.*

Markowitz N, Hansen NI, Wilcosky TC, et al. Tuberculin and anergy testing in HIV-seropositive and HIV-seronegative persons. Pulmonary complications of HIV infection study group. Ann Intern Med 1993; 119: 185–193.

*Skin test reactivity was most commonly seen in injecting drug users and declined with decreasing CD4 count.*

Toma E, Fournier S, Dumont M, et al. Clindamycin–primaquine versus trimethoprim–sulfamethoxazole as primary therapy for *Pneumocystis carinii* pneumonia in AIDS: a randomized, double-blind pilot trial. Clin Infect Dis 1993; 17:178–184.

*Both regimens had comparable degrees of success with a similar rate of adverse effects.*

Wallace JM, Rao AV, Glassroth J, et al. Respiratory illness in persons with human immunodeficiency virus infection. The pulmonary complications of HIV infection study group. Am Rev Respir Dis 1993; 148:1523–1529.

Wheat LJ, Hafner R, Wuffsohn M, et al. Prevention of relapse of histoplasmosis with itraconazole in patients with the acquired immunodeficiency sydrome. Ann Intern Med 1993; 118:610–611.

*Itraconazole was superior to weekly amphotericin in suppression of histoplasmosis.*


### CENTRAL NERVOUS SYSTEM INFECTIONS


Berenguer J, Moreno S, Laguna F, et al. Tuberculous meningitis in patients infected with the human immunodeficiency virus. N Engl J Med 1992; 326: 668–672.

*This complication occurred in about 10%of their HIV-infected patients with tuberculosis. CSF parameters and therapeutic outcome were the same as in seronegative patients.*

Dannemann B, McCutchan JA, Israelski D, et al. Treatment of toxoplasmic encephalitis in patients with AIDS. A randomized trial comparing pyrimethamine plus clindamycin to pyrimethamine plus sulfadiazine. The California collaborative treatment group. Ann Intern Med 1992; 116: 33–43.

*The success rate was similar for both regimens.*

Holland NR, Power C, Mathews VP, et al. Cytomegalovirus encephalitis in acquired immunodeficiency syndrome (AIDS). Neurology 1994; 44:507–514.

*Describes the major clinical laboratory and radiographic manifestations of this emerging complication.*

Kim YS, Hollander H. Polyradiculopathy due to cytomegalovirus: report of two cases in which improvement occurred after prolonged therapy and review of the literature. Clin Infect Dis 1993; 17:32–37.

*Patients with this diagnosis may deteriorate once antiviral therapy is initiated, but they may improve with long-term therapy.*

Luft BJ, Hafner R, Korzum AH, et al. Toxoplasmic encephalitis in patients with the acquired immunodeficiency syndrome. Members of the ACTG 077/ANRS 009 study team. N Engl J Med 1993; 329:995–1000.

*In patients who respond to therapy, the majority of clinical and radiographic improvement occus within the first 2 weeks.*

Powderly WG, Saag MS, Cloud GA. A controlled trial of fluconazole or amphotericin-B to prevent relapse of cryptococcal meningitis in patients with the acquired immunodeficiency syndrome. The NIAID AIDS clinical trials group and mycoses study group. N Engl J Med 1992; 326:793–798.

*Fluconazole was superior to amphotericin in preventing relapse of cryptococcal meningitis and had a favorable toxicity profile.*

Saag MS, Powderly WG, Cloud GA, et al. Comparison of amphotericin B with fluconazole in the treatment of acute AIDS-associated cryptococcal meningitis. The NIAID mycoses study group and the AIDS clinical trials group. N Engl J Med 1992; 326:83–89.

*Overall, the two regimens had equivalent efficacy. However, fluconazole sterilized the CSF more slowly.*

van der Horst CM, Saag MS, Cloud GA, et al. Treatment of cryptococcal meningitis associated with the acquired immunodeficiency syndrome. N Engl J Med 1997; 337:15–21.

*Patients receiving amphotericin-B plus flucytosine during the first two weeks of therapy had a trend toward lower mortality during that time frame and more rapid sterilization of cerebrospinal fluid.*

Von Einsiedel RW, Fife TD, Aksamit AJ, et al. Progressive multifocal leukoencephalopathy in AIDS: a clinicopathologic study and review of the literature. J Neurology 1993; 240:391–406.


### Gastrointestinal Complications


Dieterich DT, Lew EA, Kotler DP, et al. Treatment with albendazole for intestinal disease due to *Enterocytozoon bieneusi* in patients with AIDS. J Infect Dis 1994; 169:178–183.

*Reports significant improvement in diarrhea with albendazole therapy.*

Flanigan T, Whalen C, Turner J, et al. *Cryptosporidium* infection and CD4 counts. Ann Intern Med 1992; 116: 840–842.

*Individuals with CD4 counts >250 cells/mm$^3$ were much more likely to have benign, self-limited disease.*

Gruenewald R, Blum S, Chan J. Relationship between human immunodeficiency virus infection and salmonellosis in 20- to 59-year-old residents of New York City. Clin Infect Dis 1994; 18:358–363.

Kemper CA, Mickelsen P, Morton A, et al. *Helicobacter* (*Campylobacter*) *fennelliae*-like organisms as an important but occult cause of bacteraemia in a patient with AIDS. J Infect 1993; 26:97–101.

Kiehlbauch JA, Tauxe RV, Baker C, et al. *Helicobacter cinaedi*–associated bacteremia in the acquired immunodeficiency syndrome (AIDS). Ann Intern Med 1989; 110:1027–1029.

*The two preceding articles describe the major clinical manifestations and response to therapy of these* Campylobacter-*related organisms.*

Pol S, Romana CA, Richard S, et al. Microsporidia infection in patients with the human immunodeficiency virus and unexplained cholangitis. N Engl J Med 1993; 328:95–99.

Rabeneck L, Gyorkey F, Genta RM, et al. The role of microsporidia in the pathogenesis of HIV-related chronic diarrhea. Ann Intern Med 1993; 119:895–899.

*The first article finds microsporidia in association with AIDS cholangiopathy; however, the second study casts doubt on the role of these organisms in causing gastrointestinal symptomology.*

### Cytomegalovirus Disease

Dieterich DT, Kotler DP, Busch DF, et al. Ganciclovir treatment of cytomegalovirus colitis in AIDS: a randomized, double-blind, placebo-controlled multicenter study. J Infect Dis 1993; 167:278–282.

Dieterich DT, Poles MA, Dicker M, et al. Foscarnet treatment of cytomegalovirus gastrointestinal infections in acquired immunodeficiency syndrome patients who have failed ganciclovir induction. Am J Gastroenterol 1993; 88:542–548.

*The first paper suggests only modest improvement of CMV colitis with ganciclovir; the second reports on a small number of patients who appear to have a superior response to foscarnet therapy.*

Lalezari JP, Kupperman BD. Clinical experience with cidofovir in the treatment of cytomegalovirus retinitis. J Acq Immune Defic Synd Hum Retrovirol 1997; 14:S27–31.

Studies of Ocular Complications of AIDS Research Group, in collaboration with the AIDS Clinical Trials Group. Mortality in patients with the acquired immunodeficiency syndrome treated with either foscarnet or ganciclovir for cytomegalovirus retinitis. N Engl J Med 1992; 326: 213–220.

*Important study which showed equivalence of retinitis response rate for the two drugs but suggested a mortality adantage with foscarnet.*

### Mycobacterium avium Complex

Chin DP, Hopewell PC, Yajko DM, et al. *Mycobacterium avium* complex in the respiratory or gastrointestinal tract and the risk of *M. avium* complex bacteremia in patients with human immunodeficiency virus infection. J Infect Dis 1994; 169:289–295.

Chin DP, Reingold AL, Stone EN, et al. The impact of *Mycobacterium avium* complex bacteremia and its treatment on survival of AIDS patients—a prospective study. J Infect Dis 1994; 170;578–584.

*The preceding two papers prospectively evaluate the natural history of disseminated MAC and strongly point to the benefits of antimycobacterial therapy.*

Havlir DV, Dube MP, Sattler FR, et al. Prophylaxis against disseminated *Mycobacterium avium* complex with weekly azithromycin, daily rifabutin, or both. N Engl J Med 1996; 335:392–398.

*Demonstrates the superiority of azithromycin and the poor tolerance of the combination regimen.*

Nightingale SD, Cameron DW, Gordin FM, et al. Two controlled trials of rifabutin prophylaxis against *Mycobacterium avium* complex infection in AIDS. N Engl J Med 1993; 329:828–833.

*Rifabutin decreased MAC bacteremia by approximately 50% in individuals with <200 CD4 cells.*

Sepkowitz KA, Telzak EE, Carrow M, et al. Fever among outpatients with advanced human immunodeficiency virus infection. Arch Intern Med 1993; 153:1909–1912.

*Approximately 90% of patients have an etiology of fever elucidated, with MAC most comon if the presentation is nonfocal.*

### Bartonella

Koehler JE, Quinn FD, Berger TG, et al. Isolation of *Rochalimaea* species from cutaneous and osseous lesions of bacillary angiomatosis. N Engl J Med 1992; 327:1625–1631.

Koehler JE, Sanchez MA, Garrido CS, et al. Molecular epidemiology of *Bartonella* infections in patients with bacillary angiomatosis-peliosis. N Engl J Med 1997; 337:1876–1883.

Regnery RL, Anderson BE, Clarridge JE, et al. Characterization of a novel *Rochalimaea* species, *R. henselae* sp. nov., isolated from blood of a febrile, human immunodeficiency virus–positive patient. J Clin Microbiol 1992; 30:265–274.

*Both papers describe the biology of this new agent.*

Tappero JW, Mohle-Boetani J, Koehler JE, et al. The epidemiology of bacillary angiomatosis and bacillary peliosis. JAMA 1993; 269:770–775.

*An excellent early description of the epidemiology of this zoonotic infection.*

# 103

# Vaccines

DANI P. BOLOGNESI

Whereas basic public health and preventive measures have had a positive impact on the spread of human immunodeficiency virus (HIV) infection and new powerful antiviral therapies have prolonged and improved the quality of life of HIV infected individuals, the application of these interventions to impoverished nations has and continues to face imposing barriers. The ravaging effects of acquired immunodeficiency syndrome (AIDS) have caused enormous social and economic losses in the developing world to the point that the actual fabric of the affected populations is threatened.

While existing preventive measures can be improved and expanded upon and effective drugs to combat the virus made available to those in need, one common solution for stemming the tide of this pandemic is to develop a practical vaccine. There is ample historical precedent that vaccines represent the most effective, least costly, and safest approach to control infectious diseases (see Chapter 43), but the likelihood that a vaccine against HIV will be available soon is remote. This is because HIV presents a number of imposing, indeed unprecedented, obstacles for vaccine development. This chapter reviews the status of the HIV vaccine field and attempts to come to terms with the difficulties faced in meeting this vital goal.

## General Principles of Vaccine Development against Viruses

Antiviral vaccines are most successful against agents that exhibit a simple pathogenic profile and do not present complicating characteristics such as antigenic variation, latency, and immunopathogenicity. If the host recovers from such an infection, lifelong immunity to subsequent exposures to the pathogen generally results. This natural immunity provides the rationale for developing vaccines, since it signals that the pathogen harbors targets against which successful immune defenses can be mounted. It follows that most of the vaccines developed have been live attenuated or inactivated forms of the organism. Like the pathogen itself, the vaccine organisms would also be eliminated from the host after establishment of protective immunity, thus providing an important measure of safety. Such vaccines function not by preventing infection completely but by inducing antibodies that blunt the viremic phase and prevent the virus from reaching the target tissue in significant amounts. The limited infection that occurs is then cleared, most likely by the cellular arm of the immune system, and a long-term immunologic memory is established similar to that following host recovery from primary natural infection. In this group are viruses such as polio, measles, mumps, and rubella.

Infections in which natural immunity is ineffective in clearing virus, such as HIV, create several serious obstacles to developing an effective vaccination strategy: (*1*) correlates of protective immunity become difficult to establish; (*2*) the rationale for live attenuated or even whole inactivated vaccines is weakened because of concerns for safety; (*3*) the specter that all immune responses to the pathogen may not be beneficial must be resolved; and (*4*) the need to better understand virulence and how to overcome it becomes paramount. These issues are further complicated by several properties of HIV, such as variability, latency, and immunopathogenicity, which have thwarted vaccine development against other organisms. Thus empiricism, which historically has been so dominant in vaccine development against viruses, gives way to a concerted effort to understand the fine details of infection and pathogenesis and how this is correlated with the ensuing host responses.

## Correlates of Protection in Animal Models

Despite intensive studies in animal models where protection against HIV infection or attenuation of disease can be demonstrated, the correlates of protective immunity that apply to HIV-1 infection in humans remain ambiguous. Part of the problem stems from the diversity of the models, particularly the degree of virulence of the viruses used to challenge the vaccinated animals (Fig. 103.1). For example, in acute disease models, such as the simian immunodeficiency virus (SIV) mac251 isolate, the virus replicates rapidly and is highly pathogenic. Only live attenuated forms of the virus have produced solid protection against infection. With other strains of SIV, which replicate more slowly in their hosts and where the disease onset is protracted, one finds success with vaccine approaches that have failed in the more acute disease models. At the other extreme, there are infections that occur without disease progression, notably in chimpanzees infected with HIV-1. Here protection against infection can be achieved most frequently and with relatively simple vaccine candidates. These outcomes are not unexpected from studies with other retroviruses and suggest that the more effectively the host is able to control the virus, the more likely that the additional vaccine immunity will be beneficial. One issue raised by these studies is how to select animal models that are most representative of HIV infection in humans, where the pathogenic spectrum is also complex. Another is what the animal models are providing in terms of insights for correlates of protection. Here again the picture is complex. In nondisease models, particularly HIV-1 in chimpanzees, neutralizing antibodies appear to be the primary correlate of protection. In slow disease models, it appears that combinations of neutralizing antibodies and cellular immunity offer the best protection. In acute disease models, where protection is achieved by live attenuated vaccines, no clear correlates of immunity have been established, except that neu-

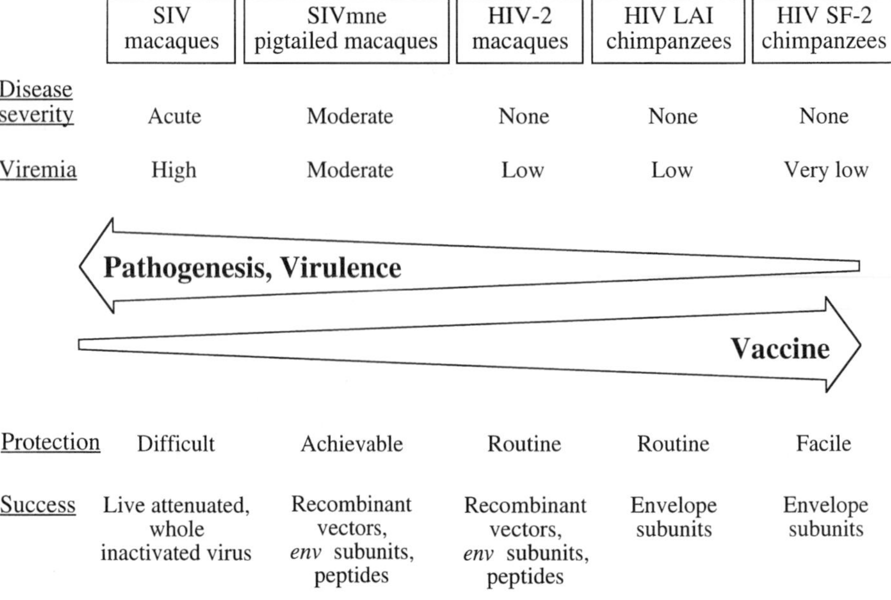


**Fig. 103.1** Relative vaccine efficacy in nonhuman primates infected with SIV, HIV-2, and HIV-1 suggests virulence correlates inversely with ease of vaccination.

tralizing antibodies appear to play an insignificant role. Cellular immunity and other factors that are associated with continuous replication of the live attenuated virus appear to be the protective mechanisms in this model.

A major question that remains unresolved in all animal model studies with vaccines to date is what the requirements for protection might be if acquisition of infection were through natural transmission. This considers not only the route of infection but also the nature of the infecting principle (i.e. free virus, virus infected cells, or both). Whereas no animal models of sexual transmission exist, approximations are possible by application of infectious material to mucosal surfaces that are associated with sexual transmission in humans.

In summary, whereas animal models of HIV infection have yet to provide clear insight about which vaccine candidates will likely have efficacy in humans, some of their limitations can be overcome by refinements in the models, and a clearer understanding of the questions that need to be addressed.

## Correlates of Immunity from Studies in Humans

While there are no natural immune mechanisms that can be linked directly to prevention of HIV infection or control of HIV replication, there are several indications that host responses to HIV may indeed play significant roles in both regards. Investigations in cohorts followed in natural history studies of HIV-1 infection, with particular attention to those which progress to disease vs. those that do not, have pointed out that immune mechanisms, particularly T-cell immunity are important for pathogenesis and control of HIV replication. Studies in acute HIV infection also favor the role of cellular immunity as the primary mechanism that suppresses the acute viremic phase of infection. There is no clear role for neutralizing antibodies. Perhaps the most enticing evidence of cellular immunity as a possible protective mechanism comes from studies of some HIV-1 exposed individuals who have resisted infection without seroconversion, but nonetheless harbor HIV specific cytotoxic lymphocytes. Similar findings come from mother-infant pairs that are discordant for HIV infection. On the other hand, both cellular and humoral immunity appear to be qualitatively superior in individuals where HIV-1 infection does not progress to disease.

Although the complex host response to HIV-1 infection precludes a clear dissection of which factors alone or in combination are responsible for a protective environment they do provide important insights that can be compared with experimental studies in animals and humans.

## Vaccine Studies in Humans

Based in large part on their ability to raise antibodies that effectively neutralize laboratory strains *in vitro* and the demonstration that defined thresholds of such antibodies prevented HIV infection in chimpanzees, envelope subunit vaccines emerged as the first candidates for development and proceeded quickly to studies in humans to determine safety and immunogenicity. These trials were highly successful and laid the foundation for a test of concept trial for neutralizing antibody as a correlate of immunity against HIV infection. However, for this to proceed it was important to demonstrate that the neutralizing antibody response would be active against viruses circulating in populations where the trial was to be conducted. When put to this test on laboratory assays which employ primary field viruses and target cells, no neutralizing activity was detectable in (Fig. 103.2). Because of this and the lack of experimental or conceptual evidence that these vaccines would generate a cytotoxic T-cell response and because breakthrough infections had been observed in Phase I and II vaccine trials, the expanded trials were suspended until more information could be obtained on these critical issues. [Expanded trials of subunit envelope vaccines have just begun under the sponsorship of Vax Gen.]

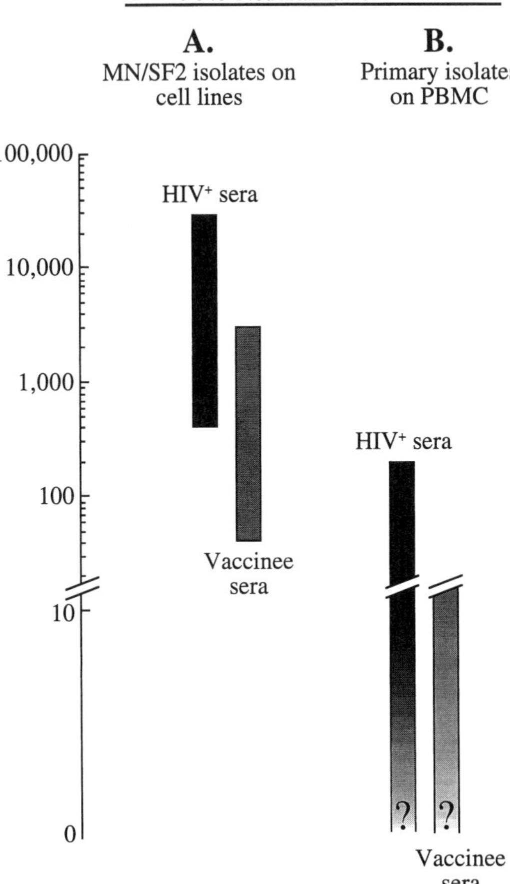


**Fig. 103.2** Neutralization of laboratory strains versus primary isolates. The bars indicate the range of neutralization titers of sera from HIV-1–infected individuals and uninfected volunteers that have been vaccinated with MN and SF2 envelope glycoproteins on (*A*) laboratory isolates grown on T-cell lines (MN, SF2) and (*B*) primary isolates (panel of 10) representative of clade B (origin of MN and SF2) passaged only on peripheral blood mononuclear cells (PBMCs). Note that sensitivity of neutralization of primary isolates drops dramatically with both sets of sera but while a fraction of sera HIV-1–infected individuals can still neutralize some of the isolates, none of the vaccinee sera tested register positive readings.

Why laboratory strains of HIV are sensitive to neutralization by antibodies, whereas primary viruses are resistant remains poorly understood. There seem to be substantive differences between the envelope structures of these two viral phenotypes, which also use different co-receptors for infectivity. But many researchers doubt that the simple substitution of one gp120 subunit for another will be enough to cause these constructs to act any differently from the early prototypes based on laboratory strains. Neither is there sufficient knowledge to design immunogens that can effectively induce neutralizing antibodies with sufficient potency and breadth against primary viruses. Insights to this end could emerge from increased understanding of the HIV envelope, its multimeric nature, the shielding of antibody targets by carbohydrate and its transitions during receptor-co-receptor binding, fusion and entry into the target cell.

The main vaccine concept currently under development is a combination of a multicomponent canarypox viral vector and one of the original gp120 envelope subunits. Such combined vaccines induce detectable cytotoxic T lymphocytes in about 60% of vaccinated people. These lymphocytes can recognize and lyse target cells infected by field strains, even from distantly related virus families (clades)—in contrast to the narrow specificity of the antibodies induced by the gp120 vaccines. However, there are some features of this vaccine candidate that could be improved. These include (*1*) the incomplete response rate for CTL induction, (*2*) the transient duration of CTL responses in some subjects and (*3*) the uneven responses to boosting. Several improvements in vector design have already been accomplished and are currently being evaluated in clinical trials.

The antibody responses induced by the canarypox vector alone are also limited, but they are substantially enhanced when combined with a gp120 subunit boost. Although these antibodies do not neutralize primary HIV isolates, they induce antibody-dependent cell cytotoxicity (which is detectable in 50%–70% of vaccinees). Moreover, T-cell proliferative responses are more potent and durable when the two vaccines are combined. The response of CD4-positive T-cells has been highlighted as a possible correlate for disease progression. Improvements in the subunits used for boosting such as inclusion of gp120 derived from primary HIV-1 isolates which are already in clinical trials (Table 103.1) may further enhance the outlook for this strategy and progress toward expanded trials.

Other vaccine concepts that have undergone preclinical evaluation and are entering clinical trials include DNA delivery of HIV-1 antigens, vaccines combined with cytokine adjuvants and strategies targeting mucosal immunity. None of these approaches will be ready for expanded trials within the next four to five years. Live attenuated vaccines face overwhelming safety concerns that may not be resolved for some time. There are also no vaccines based on whole inactivated HIV preparations currently slated for development.

## Conclusion

The HIV-vaccine field stands at a crossroads after more than ten years of concerted effort, awaiting the knowledge that will allow

**Table 103.1** Vaccine candidates based on primary virus envelopes

| Company | Subunit | Clade | Clinical trial | Status |
|---|---|---|---|---|
| Vax Gen | gp120 | B | Phase I/II-US | Started |
| Vax Gen | gp120 | E | Phase I/II—Thailand | Imminent |
| Chiron | gp120 | E | Phase I/II—Thailand | Imminent |

*Note*. In addition to the above, a number of primary isolate constructs are under study that include oligomeric gp140 and gp160 constructs, pseudovirions, virus-like particles, and DNA.

it to move forward in the right direction. Development of an effective vaccine entails a proper balance between the growing information about HIV and empirical principles that have guided the successful production of vaccines against other agents. Correlates of protection, although useful in guiding preclinical studies, can only be established retrospectively from the results of vaccine field trials. However, smaller trials with sufficient power to obtain indications of efficacy will enable dissection of the immunological and virological parameters that correlate with success or failure. Such experiments conducted with a promising vaccine candidate will be critical to the development of an effective vaccine against HIV.

*Acknowledgments*—This work is supported by NIH grant 2-P30-AI28662-05, Duke University Center for AIDS Research.

## ANNOTATED BIBLIOGRAPHY

Burton DR. A vaccine for HIV type 1; The antibody perspective. Proc Natl Acad Sci 1997; 94:10018–10023.

*A perspective on the nature of antibodies that may protect against HIV-1 infection as well as the existing barriers for design of immunogens to induce such antibodies.*

Cohen J. U.S. panel votes to delay real-world vaccine trials. Sci 1994; 264:1839.

*An editorial on the recommendation of an NIH panel to delay efficacy trials with two recombinant gp120 vaccine candidates.*

Connor RI et al. Immunological and virological analyses of persons infected by Human Immunodeficiency Virus Type 1 while participating in trials of recombinant gp120 subunit vaccines. J Virology 1998; 1552–1576.

Graham BS et al. Analysis of intercurrent HIV-1 infections in Phase I and II trials of candidate AIDS vaccines. J Infect Dis 1998; 176:384–397.

*Connor et al. and Graham et al. are companion reports dealing with HIV-1 infections in volunteers, participating in vaccine trials.*

Graham BS, Wright PF. Candidate AIDS vaccines. NEJM 1995; 333:1331–1339.

*A review of HIV vaccine concepts with emphasis on clinical studies of candidate vaccines.*

Liu MA, Vogel FR. Use of novel DNA vectors and immunologic adjuvants in HIV vaccine development. AIDS 1993; 7.

*In this review the progress with DNA vaccines as well as development of new adjuvants is updated.*

Matthews TJ. Dilemmas of neutralization resistance of HIV-1 field isolates and vaccine development. AIDS Res Hum Retro Viruses 1994; 10:631.

*An editorial comment on the difficulties facing vaccines with regard to neutralization of primary HIV isolates.*

Montelaro RC, Bolognesi DP. Vaccines against retroviruses. Retroviridae 1995; 4:605–645.

*A comprehensive review of vaccine studies from animal to human retroviruses.*

Schultz AM, Hu S-L. Primate models for HIV vaccines. AIDS 1993; 7(Suppl 1):S161.

*A comprehensive review of vaccine studies in nonhuman primate animal models.*

Walker MC, Fast PE. Clinical trials of candidate AIDS vaccines. AIDS 1993;(Suppl 1):S147.

*A detailed update of HIV vaccines in Phase I and Phase II clinical trials.*

Ferrari G et al. Clade B-based HIV-1 vaccines elicit cross-clade cytotoxic T lymphocyte reactivities in uninfected volunteers. Proc Natl Acad Sci 1997; 1396–1401.

*Documentation that vaccine induced CTL can lyse primary cells infected by viruses from different clades of HIV-1.*

# Index

Abdomen
in fever, 445
imaging of, 115–118
Abdominal drains, and infection, 785
Abdominal symptoms, with fever, 442
Abdominal viscera, infection of parasitic, 38–41, 40*t*
ABP. *See* Prostatitis, acute bacterial
Abscesses, 501–503
antimicrobial selection for, 235
brain, 723–727
definition of, 539, 606
epidural, 729–730
and fever of unknown origin, 462
intraabdominal, 613–619
pancreatic, definition of, 606
Absorption, 217
*Acanthamoeba*/infection
drug therapy for, 371*t*, 385
meningitis, 699
Acetaminophen (Paracetamol) for fever, 78*t*, 79
*N*-Acetylcysteine, 434
*Achromobacter xylosoxidans,*
antibiotic therapy for, 337
Acid-base disturbances, infection and, 133
Acid-fast stains, 149–150
*Acinetobacter*/infection
antibiotic therapy for, 337
of burns, 789
*Acinetobacter calcoaceticus*/infection of burns, 792
Acquired immunodeficiency syndrome (AIDS). *See also* Human immunodeficiency virus/infection
and chemotherapy research, 4
chest CT in, 115
clinical manifestations of, 937–957
definition of, 905, 906*t*
diseases included in, 938*t*
diarrhea in, 581–582
management of, 587–588, 588*t*
epidemiology of, 905–911
hemophagocytic syndrome associated with, 128
malignant lymphomas in, 129–130
ocular manifestations of, 739*t*, 739–740
opportunistic infections in
protozoal, drug therapy for, 382–384
therapy for, 965–975, 972*t*–973*t*
pathogenesis of, 915–926
pediatric, IGIV for, 412
prevalence of, 56
stages of, 937
Acridine orange (AO), 149
Acrodermatitis, infantile papular, 592
ACTH, and pyrogenic inhibition, 74
*Actinobacillus*/infection
antibiotic therapy for, 337
toxin, 24
*Actinobacillus actinomycetemcomitans*/infection, endocarditis, 623
antimicrobial therapy for, 630*t*, 631
*Actinomyces*/infection
antibiotic therapy for, 337
invasion of endocrine organs, 134
Actinomycosis
diagnosis of, 545
oral, 577
pathogenesis of, 545
pulmonary cavitation in, 545–546
treatment of, 545–546
Activating step loss, and antimicrobial resistance, 214
Active vaccines, 14
Acute inflammatory response, 83–90
PMN and, 89–90
Acute necrotizing ulcerative gingivitis (ANUG), 576
Acute-phase reactants, 135
Acute-phase reaction, associated with infectious diseases, 135–136
Acute-phase response, 74, 84–85
Acute respiratory distress syndrome (ARDS), 557–564
clinical manifestations of, 560–561
diagnosis of, 561*t*, 562
epidemiology of, 560
etiologies of, 558*t*, 558–560, 559*t*
extrapulmonary causes of, 559, 560*t*
host factors in, 560
infectious causes of, 558–560, 559*t*
laboratory studies in, 561–562
pathogenesis of, 557–558
pathology of, 557–558
with pulmonary fibroproliferation, and fever in hospitalized patient, 451
therapy for, 562–564
goals of, 562–563
Acute retroviral syndrome, rash in, 487
Acyclovir (Zovirax), 349–350, 351*t*
for herpes simplex virus prophylaxis, in bone marrow transplant recipients, 829–830, 831*f*
Acylureidopenicillins, 254
Adenovirus
hemophagocytic syndrome associated with, 128–129
and immune system, 33–34
vaccine for, 420*t*
Adherence, 7, 21–24
Adhesins, 7, 21

*Note.* The letter *t* following a number indicates *table*; the letter *f* indicates figure.

Adjunctive therapy
for brain abscess, 727
for meningitis, 695
for septic thrombophlebitis, 731
Adjuvants, 409–410, 434
Adnexa, infections of, 733–734
ADP-ribosyltransferases, 24
Adrenal insufficiency, and fever of unknown origin, 466
*Aeromonas hydrophilia,* antibiotic therapy for, 337
Aerosolization, 529
Agammaglobulinemia, vaccine use with, 424
Age
and antimicrobial selection, 234
and diarrhea, 583
and fever, 439
Agent, definition of, 53
AIDS. *See* Acquired immunodeficiency syndrome
AIHA. *See* Autoimmune hemolytic anemia
Air-borne transmission, 54
of nosocomial infection, 61
Albendazole, 366*t*, 385–386, 388
*Alcaligenes xylosoxidans,* antibiotic therapy for, 337
Alcohol abuse
and infection, 853–857
infectious complications of, 855–856, 856*t*
Alcoholic liver cirrhosis, 855
Alcoholism, immune effects of, 853–854
Alcohol-related diseases, and fever of unknown origin, 465
Allergic bronchopulmonary aspergillosis, 45
Allergic-hypersensitivity reactions, to antimicrobial agents, 225, 226*t*–227*t*
Allergic response, 104
Allergy, chronic fatigue syndrome and, 777
Allopurinol, 366*t*
for leishmaniasis, 384
Alphavirus/infection
arthritis, 760, 760*t*
encephalitis, 708
*Alternaria*/infection, 47–50
of burns, 793
Alternative pathway, 11, 83–84, 84*f*
and bacterial cell wall components, 473–474
Alveolar osteitis, 577
Amantadine (Symmetrel), 4, 353*t*, 360
mechanism of action, 32
Amdinocillin, 255
Amebiasis
drug therapy for, 381–382
in travelers to tropical countries, 870
Amikacin, 273, 330
dosage and administration, 283*t*, 329*t*
for children, 282*t*
drug interactions with, 333*t*
pharmacokinetics of, 331*t*
routes of elimination and adverse effects of, 332*t*
spectrum and mechanism of activity, 328*t*
Aminoglycoside-modifying enzymes, and antimicrobial resistance, 213
Aminoglycosides, 273–284, 274*t*
administration of, 274, 279–284
once-daily, 282*t*, 282–284, 283*t*
antimycobacterial uses of, 330
cochlear toxicity of, 279
distribution of, 274
excretion of, 274–275
indications for, 275–277
empiric therapy, 275*t*, 275–276
specific therapy, 276*t*, 276–277
intraperitoneal instillation of, for CAPD peritonitis, 281, 281*t*
mechanism of action, 273
multiple daily dosing, 280*t*, 280–282, 281*t*
nephrotoxicity of, 278
pathogenesis of, 277–278
risk factors for, 278*t*
pharmacokinetics of, 275
pharmacology of, 274–275
prophylactic, 277
resistance to, 277
spectrum of activity, 273–274
toxicity of, 277–279
Aminopenicillins, 253–254
Aminosalicylic acid
dosage and administration, 329*t*
drug interactions with, 333*t*
pharmacokinetics of, 331*t*
routes of elimination and adverse effects of, 332*t*
spectrum and mechanism of activity, 328*t*
Amoebae, free living, drug therapy for, 385
Amoebiasis, drug therapy for, 371*t*
Amoxicillin, 253–254
indications for, 252*t*
Amoxicillin-clavulanic acid, 255
Amphotericin B, 366*t*, 389–390
alternatives to, 397
for aspergillosis, 46
for candidemia, and deep-organ infection, 44
for cryptococcosis, 45
formulations of, 390
for free living amoebae infection, 385
indications for, 389–390, 391*t*
pharmacology of, 389, 390*t*
toxicity of, 389, 390*t*
Ampicillin, 253–254
indications for, 252*t*
Ampicillin-sulbactam, 255
Amplification methods, 141–142, 142*t*
Anal cell carcinoma, 935–936
Anal swabs, 181–186
*Ancylostoma duodenale*/infection
drug therapy for, 374*t*
and iron-deficiency anemia, 121
Anemia
hemolytic, 123–124
infectious diseases associated with, 124*t*
inflammatory, 121
iron-deficiency, 121
megaloblastic, 122
Aneurysms, mycotic, 641–642
Angiomatosis, bacillary, 201
antibiotic therapy for, 338
in HIV infection, 941–942, 942*t*, 942*f*
rash in, 494
*Angiostrongylus cantonensis*/infection
drug therapy for, 371*t*
meningitis, 699
*Angiostrongylus costaricensis*/infection, drug therapy for, 371*t*
Animal bites, infections from, 885–889
clinical presentation of, 885
management of, 885–887, 886*t*
microbiology of, 885, 886*t*
water-associated, 888
Animals, in viral culture, 161
Animal workers, vaccine use in, 425
Anisakiasis, drug therapy for, 371*t*
Antacids
drug interactions with, 300, 311
and gastric bacterial overgrowth, 66
Anthrax
antibiotic therapy for, 337
in travelers to tropical countries, 871
vaccine for, 416*t*
Antibiotic prophylaxis
for animal bites, 885–887
for bone marrow transplant recipients, 837
for burns, 794
for CMV in organ transplant recipient, 825, 825*t*
procedures recommended for, 634*t*
regimens for, 634*t*–635*t*
of surgical wounds
administration of, 785
agent selection for, 785
principles of, 785
timing of, 785
for traumatic injury, 796–797, 797*t*
Antibiotics. *See also* Antimicrobial agents
adverse effects of, 226*t*–227*t*
and candidiasis, 43
for eye infections, 740
hypersensitivity to, in HIV infection, 971–973, 973*t*
for meningitis
definitive, 694, 694*t*
dosage and administration, 694*t*
empiric, 692–694, 693*t*–694*t*
monitoring, 695

for osteomyelitis, 746–748, 748*t*
for pleural effusion, 571
for pneumonia, 535–536, 536*t*
for septic shock, 478–479, 479*t*
Antibodies
definition of, 11
enhancing, response to HIV, 930–931
and infection, 407
neutralizing, response to HIV, 930, 930*f*
and opsonization, 87
responses, in viral infection, 34–35
role in infection, 11–12
Antibody deficiency disorders, primary, 809, 810*t*
Antibody-dependent cellular cytotoxicity (ADCC), 11
response to HIV, 931
Antibody tests, 142–143, 143*t*
Anticoagulants
drug interactions with, 300–301, 303, 315
for infective endocarditis, 633
Antiendotoxin antibody preparations, 413
Antifungal agents, 389–395
for deep mycoses, 397–404
for rhinocerebral zygomycosis, 46
Antifungal prophylaxis, in bone marrow transplant recipients, 830, 833*t*, 837
Antifungal susceptibility testing, 178–179
guidelines for, 179*t*
recommendations for, 179*t*
Antigen, definition of, 91
Antigen detection
immunostains for, 164
specimen processing for, 161
Antigen presentation, 92–94
and B cell activation, 100–102, 101*f*
Antigen-presenting cells, 11
HIV's effects on, 928, 928*f*
Antigen-presenting molecules, 93–94, 94*f*
Antigen processing
pathways of, 33, 34*f*
viral inhibition of, 33–34
Antigen recognition, response to, 97–98
Antimalarial drugs, 365–381, 375*t*–376*t*
Antimicrobial action, mechanisms of, 209–210, 210*t*
Antimicrobial agents, 337–348
absorption of, 217
adjunctive approaches with, 236–237
administration of, route of, 235
for brain abscess, 725, 726*t*–727*t*
control of usage, 245–248
aims of, 245, 246*t*
economic issues in, 246
efficacy of, 245–246, 247*t*
personnel involved in, 245
setting for, 245
for diarrhea, 587, 587*t*
distribution of, 217–218
drug interactions of, 230*t*–231*t*, 230–232
for epidural abscess, 730
excretion of, 218–220
for infectious complications of pancreatitis, 607–609
for infective endocarditis, 628–631
metabolism of, 218
penetration into CNS, 221–222, 222*t*
for peritonitis, 615–616, 617*t*
changing, 616, 617*t*
pharmacodynamics of, 220–221
pharmacoeconomics of, 237–238, 238*t*
pharmacology of, 217–223
selection of, 233–239
for outpatient intravenous antibiotic therapy, 242–243, 243*t*
for septic thrombophlebitis, 731
serum concentrations of, monitoring, 222–223
for subdural empyema, 728
therapy with
duration of, 237
responses to, monitoring, 237
toxicities of, 225–232
Antimicrobial resistance
to acyclovir, 350
to amantadine, 360
to aminoglycosides, 277
to aztreonam, 269
to carbapenems, 265–266
to cephalosporins, 257–258
to cidofovir, 359
circumventing, 214
to clindamycin, 294
to didanosine, 961
to famiciclovir, 355–356
to fluoroquinolones, 305
to foscarnet, 358
to ganciclovir, 357
genes, detection of, 142
to glycopeptides, 285–287, 287*f*
in HIV, 923–924
to macrolides, 291
mechanisms of, 209–215, 211*t*
multiple, 214
and nosocomial infections, 67–68
in nosocomial infections, 62
to penems, 265–266
to penicillins, 250
public health response to, 57
to rimantadine, 361
to sulfonamides, 314
to tetracyclines, 299
to trimethoprim, 315
to trimethoprim/sulfamethoxazole, 316
to zidovudine, 960
Antimicrobial susceptibility testing, 233–234
Antimycobacterial drugs, 327–335
adverse effects of, 331–334, 332*t*
dosage and administration, 327–330, 329*t*
drug interactions with, 333*t*, 334
mechanism of action, 327, 328*t*
pharmacokinetics of, 330–331, 331*t*–332*t*
routes of elimination, 332*t*
spectrum of activity, 327
therapeutic drug monitoring with, 330
Antiparasitic agents, 365–388, 366*t*–379*t*
Antipyretic agents, 79
actions of, 72
Antiretroviral drugs, 959–964
guidelines for, 962–963, 963*t*–964*t*
$\alpha_1$-antitrypsin, 135–136
Antiviral agents, 4, 349–364, 351*t*–354*t*
for encephalitis, 713–714
Antiviral prophylaxis
for bone marrow transplant recipients, 837
for herpes simplex virus prophylaxis, 829–830, 831*f*–832*f*
ANUG. *See* Acute necrotizing ulcerative gingivitis
Aphthous ulcers
esophageal, in HIV infection, 952
oral, in HIV infection, 952
Apicomplexa, 37
Aplasia, pure red cell, 122–123
Apoptosis
HIV's effects on, 929*t*, 929–930
viral induction of, 34
Appendicitis, 617
imaging of, 117
Arbovirus/infection
encephalitis, 708
clinical presentation in, 708
diagnosis of, 712
epidemiology of, 708, 709*t*
host response in, 708
prevention of, 714
in travelers to tropical countries, 867–868, 869*t*
*Arcanobacterium haemolyticum*/infection
antibiotic therapy for, 337
rash in, 492
ARDS. *See* Acute respiratory distress syndrome
Arenaviruses/infection, encephalitis
clinical presentation in, 710
diagnosis of, 713
epidemiology of, 709
host response in, 710
pathogenesis of, 710
ARF. *See* Rheumatic fever, acute
Argentine hemorrhagic fever, 496, 869*t*
Arginine vasopressin (AVP), and pyrogenic inhibition, 74
Artemisinin (qinghaosu), 366*t*, 381
Arthritis
bacterial, 758–759, 759*t*
enteropathic, 765
fungal, 759
infectious, 757–766
clinical presentation in, 760–761
diagnosis of, 761–762
epidemiology of, 757

Arthritis (*continued*)
- etiology of, 758–760
- host factors in, 757
- laboratory findings in, 761
- pathogenesis of, 757–758
- prognosis and outcome in, 762
- treatment of, 762, 763*t*–764*t*
- postinfectious/reactive. *See* Reiter's syndrome
- rheumatoid (RA), 765
- viral, 759–760, 760*t*

Arthropathy, from fluoroquinolones, 311
Arthroplasty, infected, management of, 803–804, 805*f*
Ascariasis, drug therapy for, 371*t*
*Ascaris lumbricoides,* collection of, 187
Aspergilloma, 553*f*, 553–554
Aspergillosis, 45–46, 48*t*
- clinical manifestations of, 45
- diagnosis of, 45
- drug therapy for, 402, 403*t*
- in immunocompromised host, 43, 45
- invasive, 554
- pulmonary, 553–554
  - chronic necrotizing, 554
- treatment of, 46

*Aspergillus*/infection
- of burns, 793
- endocarditis, 623
- evasion of oxygen-dependent killing, 89
- examination of, 171, 175*f*
- in organ transplant recipient, 827

*Aspergillus fumigatus,* 45
*Aspergillus niger,* 45
Aspirates, specimen collection from, 188
Aspiration, and pneumonia, 529
Aspirin, for fever, 78*t*, 79
Asplenia, and vaccination, 415, 422*t*
Atovaquone, 366*t*
- for *Pneumocystic carinii* pneumonia, 383

Atrial myxoma, and fever of unknown origin, 464
Attenuation, 2
AUC/MIC ratio, 220–221
Australian X encephalitis, 708
Autoimmune disorders, associated with HIV infection, 934
Autoimmune hemolytic anemia (AIHA), 123
Autoinducers, 21
Avoparcin, 285
AVP. *See* Arginine vasopressin
Azathioprine, immunosuppression by, 821
Azithromycin, 291, 366*t*
- dosage and administration, 329*t*
- drug interactions with, 333*t*
- indications for, 293
- pharmacokinetics of, 331*t*
- routes of elimination and adverse effects of, 332*t*
- spectrum and mechanism of activity, 328*t*
- for toxoplasmosis, 383

Azlocillin, 254
Azoles, for aspergillosis, 46
Aztreonam, 268–270
- administration of, 269
- indications for, 269
- levels in tissue, 270, 270*t*
- mechanism of action, 269, 269*f*
- pharmacology of, 269–270
- resistance to, 269
- spectrum of action, 269
- toxicities of, 270

Babesiosis, 895, 895*f*
- antibiotic therapy for, 894*t*
- drug therapy for, 372*t*, 381
- and hemolytic anemia, 124
- hemophagocytic syndrome associated with, 128

Bacampicillin, 253–254
Bacille Calmette-Guérin, 418*t*
*Bacillus anthracis,* antibiotic therapy for, 337
*Bacillus cereus,* antibiotic therapy for, 337
*Bacillus subtilis,* evasion of oxygen-dependent killing, 88
Back pain, with fever, 442
Bacteremia, 471–481. *See also* Bloodstream infections
- definition of, 471, 472*t*
- epidemiology of, 471–472
- in intravenous drug user, 851
- and malnutrition, 843–844
- meningococcal, rash in, 493
- spontaneous, alcohol abuse and, 856

Bacteria
- anaerobic, imipenem for, 267
- by anatomic site, 22*t*–23*t*
- avoidance of host immune defenses, 25–26
- capsules of, 25
- cell wall components of, and humoral pathways, 473–475, 474*f*
- common, characteristics of, 151*t*–153*t*
- entry into host cells, 25
- gram-negative, imipenem for, 266
- gram-positive, imipenem for, 266
- immune response to, 96*t*
- macromolecular assembly by, 25
- nutrient acquisition in, 24
- other, characteristics of, 154*t*–155*t*
- pathogenicity of, 19
  - mechanisms of, 20–26
- secretion by, 25
- and sepsis, 472–473
- specimen categories, 145
- specimen transport, 145
- structure of, 19
- taxonomy, 19, 20*f*
- toxins of, 24–25
- virulence of, 19–26
  - regulation of, 20–21

Bacterial infections
- antibiotic therapy for, 337–348
- arthritis, 758–759, 759*t*
- in bone marrow transplant recipients, 829
  - treatment of, 836
- of burns, 792
- cutaneous, in HIV infection, 955
- cytokines and immunomodulators in, 427–429
- diagnostic methods for, 145–157
- and diarrhea, 582
- and fever of unknown origin, 460
- in intravenous drug user, 850–851
- meningitis, 689–695, 698–699
- myocarditis/pericarditis, 645
- oral, 573–577
- in organ transplant recipient, 827
- rash in, 489–492
- in travelers to tropical countries, 871

Bactericidal agents, 235, 236*t*
Bacteriology, clinical, 145–157
Bacteriostatic agents, 235, 236*t*
Bacteriuria, asymptomatic, treatment of, 655–656
*Bacteroides*/infection, antibiotic therapy for, 338
*Bacteroides bivius*/infection, vulvovaginitis, 681
*Bacteroides disidens*/infection, vulvovaginitis, 681
*Bacteroides fragilis*/infection
- antibiotic therapy for, 338
- of burns, 792

*Bacteroides melaninogenicus*/infection, of burns, 792
Balantidiasis, drug therapy for, 372*t*
Bannwarth's syndrome, 721
Barbiturates, drug interactions with, 300
Barium study, 117
*Bartonella henselae*/infection
- of animal bites, 888
- antibiotic therapy for, 338
- in bacillary angiomatosis, 201
- in cat scratch disease, 200
- endocarditis, 623

Bartonella, laboratory diagnosis of, 198*t*–199*t*, 200–201
*Bartonella quintana*/infection
- antibiotic therapy for, 338
- in bacillary angiomatosis, 201
- endocarditis, 623
- in trench fever, 200

Bartonellosis, 201
- and hemolytic anemia, 124
- in HIV infection, therapy for, 973*t*
- rash in, 496
- in travelers to tropical countries, 871

B cell growth factor (BCGF), 101
B-cell lymphomas, 935

B cells, 99, 101*f*
actions of, 92*f*
activation of, antigen presentation and, 100–102, 101*f*
HIV's effects on, 927
BCGF. *See* B cell growth factor
BDNA. *See* Branched DNA
Bell's palsy, 719–720
Benzimidazole, for trypanosomiasis, 385
Benzonidazole, 366*t*
Betacillin, 253
Beverage-borne transmission, and diarrhea, 582
Bilharziasis, drug therapy for, 377*t*
Biliary tract infections, pyogenic, 597–603
Biopsy material, collection and transportation, 188–189
*Bipolaris*/infection, 47–50
Bismuth subsalicylate, for diarrhea, 587
Bites
infections from, 885–889
soft-tissue infections associated with, 502–503
Bithionol, 366*t*, 387–388
BL. *See* Burkitt's lymphoma
Bladder biopsies, in diagnosis of parasitic infection, 188–189
*Blastocystis hominis*/infection, drug therapy for, 372*t*, 382
*Blastomyces dermatitides,* 50
examination of, 171, 176*f*
Blastomycosis, 49*t*, 50–51
drug therapy for, 400*t*, 401
pulmonary, 551–552
diagnosis of, 552
epidemiology of, 550*t*
treatment of, 552
South American, 49*t*, 51
in travelers to tropical countries, 872
*Blastoschizomyces capitatus,* 47
Bleeding, spontaneous, with fever in travelers to tropical countries, 863*t*
Blepharitis, 733–734
Bloodborne transmission
of HIV, 909–910
prevention of, 912
and nosocomial infections, 68
of pneumonia, 529–530
Blood-brain barrier, 221
Blood-CSF barrier, 221
Blood disease, parasitic, 38–41, 40*t*
Blood pressure, and fever, 443
Blood smears, in diagnosis of parasitic infection, 192
Blood specimens, 187
collection and transportation, 145–146, 161
Bloodstream infections (BSIs)
in bone marrow transplant recipients, 830–833
nosocomial, 65
pathogenesis of, 65
prevention of, 65
risk factors for, 64*t*, 65
Blood transfusions, fever associated with, 452–454
Body fluids, specimen collection from, 146, 161
Body lice, 898
Body sites
deep, closed, 145
deep communicating, 145
superficial, 145
Body Substance Isolation, 68
Body temperature
in fever, 72
normal ranges for, 71
Bolivian hemorrhagic fever, 496, 869*t*
Bone infections, fluoroquinolones for, 309
Bone marrow, aspirates from, specimen collection from, 188
Bone marrow-derived lymphocytes. *See* B cells
Bone marrow specimens, 187
Bone marrow transplant recipients
IGIV for, 412
infection in, 829–838
diagnosis of, 835–836
epidemiology of, 829–830, 830*f*
prevention of, 837–838
treatment of, 836–837
Bone scans, in osteomyelitis, 746
*Bordetella pertussis*/infection
adherence in, 24
antibiotic therapy for, 338
pathogenic strategies of, 20, 21*f*
toxin, 24
tracheal cytotoxin, 25
*Borrelia*/infection, antibiotic therapy for, 338
*Borrelia burgdorferi*/infection
antibiotic therapy for, 338
regulation of virulence in, 21
*Borrelia recurrentis*/infection, and hemolytic anemia, 124
Boutonneuse fever
laboratory diagnosis of, 196
rash in, 490
B/PI, in oxygen-independent killing, 89
Brain abscess, 723–727
clinical manifestations of, 724, 724*t*
diagnosis of, 724–725, 725*f*
epidemiology of, 723
etiology of, 723–724
pathogenesis of, 723
treatment of, 725–727, 726*t*–727*t*
Brain, HIV infection and, 925
Branched DNA (bDNA), 141–142, 142*t*
Brazilian purpuric fever, 496
Brill-Zinsser disease, rash in, 488
Bronchiectasis, 525–527
clinical manifestations of, 526
diagnosis of, 526
etiology of, 525, 525*t*
laboratory findings in, 526
pathophysiology of, 525–526
treatment of, 526–527
Bronchitis, 523–525
acute
clinical features of, 524
etiology of, 523, 524*t*
pathophysiology of, 523
treatment of, 524
chronic
clinical features of, 524
etiology of, 523
pathophysiology of, 523
treatment of, 524–525
definition of, 523
diagnosis of, 524
epidemiology of, 523
host factors in, 523
laboratory findings in, 524
Bronchoalveolar lavage, 159
Bronchoscopy, for pyogenic lung abscess with aspiration pneumonia, 542–543
*Brucella*/infection (Brucellosis)
antibiotic therapy for, 338
endocarditis, 623
meningitis, 699
rash in, 489
in travelers to tropical countries, 871
*Brugia malayi*/infection
collection of, 187
drug therapy for, 373*t*
BSIs. *See* Bloodstream infections
Bunyavirus infection, encephalitis, 708
*Burkholderia cepacia,* antibiotic therapy for, 338
Burkitt's lymphoma (BL), 129, 130*f*
Burn infections, 789–794
clinical features of, 790
diagnosis of, 790–791, 791*t*
epidemiology of, 789
etiology of, 789–790
nosocomial, 789, 791*f*
pathophysiology, 790
prophylaxis for, 793–794
treatment of, 791–792

California encephalitis, 708
*Calymmatobacterium granulomatis*
antibiotic therapy for, 338
in genital ulcer disease, 657
*Campylobacter*/infection
culturing, 150
and microangiopathic disorders, 127
and reactive arthritis, 764
*Campylobacter fetus*/infection, antibiotic therapy for, 339
*Campylobacter jejuni*/infection
antibiotic therapy for, 339
and diarrhea in residents of tropical countries, 875
incubating, 156

Canarypox, 409
Cancer, viral infection and, 27
Cancrum oris, 576, 576*f*
*Candida*/infection
  of burns, 789, 792–793
  characteristics of, 178
  endocarditis, 623
  examination of, 171, 175*f*
  in NICU nosocomial infections, 66
  opportunistic, emerging, 47
  in organ transplant recipient, 826
  vulvovaginitis, 681
*Candida albicans*/infection, 43
  arthritis, 759
  cervicitis, 382
  evasion of oxygen-dependent killing, 88
*Candida glabrata,* 43, 47
*Candida guillermondii,* 43, 47
*Candida krusei,* 43, 47
*Candida lipolytica,* 47
*Candida lusitaniae,* 47
*Candida parapsilosis,* 43, 47
  in nosocomial bloodstream infection, 65
*Candida pseudotropicalis,* 43, 47
*Candida rugose,* 47
*Candida stellatoidea,* 43, 47
*Candida tropicalis*/infection, 43, 47
  of surgical wounds, 784
*Candida zeylanoides,* 47
Candidemia, 44
  drug therapy for, 397
Candidiasis, 43–44, 48*t*
  central nervous system, drug therapy for, 398
  chronic mucocutaneous, infectious disease and, 134–135
  disseminated, rash in, 493–494
  drug therapy for, 397–399, 398*t*–399*t*
  esophageal, in HIV infection, 952
  in HIV infection, therapy for, 972*t*
  intra-abdominal, drug therapy for, 397–398
  mucocutaneous, 44
  mucocutaneous, chronic, drug therapy for, 397
  mucosal, drug therapy for, 397
  oral, 578
    in HIV infection, 952
    treatment of, 578
  osteoarticular, drug therapy for, 399
  pathogenesis of, 43–44
  prevention of, 44
  pulmonary, 554
CAPD. *See* Continuous ambulatory peritoneal dialysis
Capillariasis, drug therapy for, 372*t*
*Capnocytophaga canimorsus*/infection
  of animal bites, 887–888
  antibiotic therapy for, 339
*Capnocytophaga ochracea*/infection, antibiotic therapy for, 339
Capreomycin, 330
  dosage and administration, 329*t*
  drug interactions with, 333*t*
  pharmacokinetics of, 331*t*
  routes of elimination and adverse effects of, 332*t*
  spectrum and mechanism of activity, 328*t*
Carbamazepine, drug interactions with, 293
Carbapenems, 265–268
  indications for, 267
  mechanism of action, 265
  pharmacology of, 267–268
  resistance to, 265–266
  spectrum of action, 266–267
  structure of, 265, 266*f*
  toxicity, 268
Carbenicillin, 254
Carboxypenicillins, 254
Carbuncles, 501
*Cardiobacterium hominis*/infection
  antibiotic therapy for, 339
  endocarditis, 623
    antimicrobial therapy for, 630*t*, 631
Cardiomyopathy, definition of, 643
Cardiovascular management, for septic shock, 479
Caries, 573
Carrier state, 12
Carrion's disease, rash in, 496
Catch-up growth, 839
Catheterization, and nosocomial UTIs, 63–64
Catheters
  complications associated with, 637–642
  and fever in hospitalized patient, 451
  infections associated with
    diagnosis of, 638
    epidemiology of, 637
    management of, 639*t*, 639–640
    microbiology of, 638–639, 639*t*
    pathogenesis of, 637–638
    prevention of, 640–641
    of urinary tract, 656
  material of, and infection, 641
  specimen collection from, 148
  type of, and infection, 638
Cat-scratch disease, 200–201
  antibiotic therapy for, 338
  rash in, 494
Cavitary lesions, in immunocompromised host, 815, 817*f*
Cavitary pulmonary diseases, 539*t*, 539–555
  differential diagnosis of, radiographic, 539–541, 540*t*
  etiologies of, 539, 540*t*
  infectious causes of, 541–545
  noninfectious causes of, 541
CBP. *See* Prostatitis, chronic bacterial
CDC. *See* Centers for Disease Control and Prevention
CD4 cells
  depletion of, in HIV infection, 925–926
  ranges, in HIV-associated diseases, 939*t*
  response to HIV, 932, 932*t*
CD8 lymphocytes, 93
Cefaclor, 259
Cefamandole, 259
Cefazolin, 259
Cefixime, 260
Cefmetazole, 259
Cefodroxil, 259
Cefonicid, 259
Cefoperazone, 260
Ceforanide, 259
Cefotaxime, 260
Cefotetan, 259
Cefoxitin, 259
Cefpodoxime, 260
Cefprozil, 259
Ceftazidime, 260
Ceftizoxime, 260
Ceftriaxone, 260
Cefurixime axetil, 259
Cefuroxime, 259
Cell culture, in virology, 161–163
  modified methods in, 163
Cell membranes
  antimicrobial action and, 210
  and antimicrobial resistance, 212
Cellular immune cascade, 95–97, 96*f*–97*f*
Cellular immune response, 91–106
Cellular immunity, 12
  theories of, 3
Cellular pathways, and sepsis/septic shock, 475*f*, 475–476
Cellulitis, 501–503
  clostridial, 767–768
  definition of, 501
  nonclostridial anaerobic, 768
  orbital, 734, 734*f*, 738, 738*f*
  preseptal, 734
  treatment of, 502–503
Cell wall active agents, and antimicrobial action, 209
Cell wall biosynthesis, and antimicrobial resistance, 210–212
Cell wall-derived muramyl peptides, 25
Centers for Disease Control and Prevention (CDC), 56
  telephone numbers for travel and tropical medicine information, 873
Central nervous system
  antimicrobial penetration into, 221–222, 222*t*
  candidiasis of, drug therapy for, 398
  complications of, in HIV infection, therapy for, 967–969
  cryptococcosis of, 45
    drug therapy for, 399–400
  dysfunction, fever associated with, 454

imaging of, 111–112, 112*f*
infection of
in bone marrow transplant recipients, 835
focal, 723–731, 945–947, 946*t*
in HIV infection, 945–947, 946*t*, 947–949
parasitic, 41, 41*t*
post-traumatic, 798–799
reactions of, to fluoroquinolones, 311
Central venous catheters, and infection, 638
Cephalexin, applications, 259
Cephalosporins, 257–263
adverse reactions to, 260–262
chemistry of, 257, 258*f*
discovery of, 4
first generation, 257, 258*f*
clinical applications of, 259
indications for, 261*t*
spectrum of activity, 258–259
mechanism of action, 257
nomenclature of, 257
resistance to, 257–258
second generation, 257, 258*f*
clinical applications of, 259
indications for, 261*t*
spectrum of activity, 259
third generation, 257, 258*f*
clinical applications of, 259–260
indications for, 260, 261*t*
Cephalothin, applications, 259
Cephamycins, 259
Cephapirin, applications, 259
Cephradine, applications, 259
Cerebrospinal fluid (CSF)
aspirates from, specimen collection from, 188
evaluation of, in encephalitis, 711
infection of, detection of, 140*t*
prosthetic devices for, infections associated with, 801–802
specimen collection from, 161
specimens, 146
Cervicitis
clinical manifestations of, 683
control of, 686–687
diagnosis of, 683
epidemiology of, 682
etiology of, 682
host factors in, 682
laboratory studies in, 683, 684*t*
management of, 683
pathogenesis of, 682
pathology of, 682–683
Cestodeproglottids, in stool, key to, 192*t*
Cestodes
classification of, 39*t*
drug therapy for, 387–388
CF. *See* Cystic fibrosis
CFS. *See* Chronic fatigue syndrome
Chagas' disease
rash in, 496
in travelers to tropical countries, 870
Chain, 4
Chalazion, 733
Chancroid
antibiotic therapy for, 341
clinical manifestations of, 662, 662*f*
epidemiology of, 658–659
pathogenesis of, 660
treatment of, 666, 666*t*
ulceration in, 657
Chaperones, 25
Cheilitis, angular, 578
Chemokines, response to HIV, 933–934
Chemotherapy, history of, 3–4, 4*t*
Chest
in fever, 442–443
imaging, in immunocompromised host, 114–115
imaging of, 114, 114*f*
infectious-disease indications for, 114, 114*f*
Chest pain, with fever, 442
Chiggers, 897, 897*f*
Chikungunya fever, 497, 760, 760*t*, 868, 869*t*
Children
adverse reactions to antibiotics in, 228*t*, 229
AIDS in. *See* Acquired immunodeficiency syndrome, pediatric
aminoglycoside dosages for, 281, 282*t*
osteomyelitis in, 744
Chinese liver fluke, drug therapy for, 373*t*
*Chlamydia*/infection, 201–205
differential diagnosis of, 203*t*
evasion of phagocytosis, 88
microbiological characteristics of, 201–202
prevalence of, 56
rash in, 488–489
*Chlamydia pneumoniae,* 201
antibiotic therapy for, 339
culture of, 202
diagnosis of, 204–205
*Chlamydia psittaci,* 201
antibiotic therapy for, 339
culture of, 202
diagnosis of, 205
*Chlamydia trachomatis*/infection, 201
antibiotic therapy for, 339
cervicitis, 382
conjunctivitis, 735
culture of, 202–204
diagnosis of, 202–204
in men, 202*t*
in women, 203*t*
in genital ulcer disease, 657
and reactive arthritis, 757, 764
salpingitis, 684
urethritis, 669
Chloramphenicol, 299, 301–303
adverse effects of, 302–303
drug interactions with, 303
indications for, 302, 302*t*
mechanism of action, 301
pharmacology of, 301
resistance to, mechanisms of, 214
Chloroguanide. *See* Proguanil
Chloroquine, 366*t*
for amebiasis, 382
Chloroquine phosphate, 365
Chlorpropamide, drug interactions with, 303
Chlortetracycline, 299
Cholangitis, acute, 599–600
clinical manifestations of, 599–600
diagnosis of, 600
epidemiology of, 599
etiology of, 599
laboratory studies in, 600
pathogenesis of, 599
treatment of, 600
Cholecystitis, acute, 597–599
clinical features of, 598
diagnosis of, 598
epidemiology of, 597
etiology of, 597
imaging in, 117
laboratory studies in, 598
pathogenesis of, 597–598
treatment of, 598–599
Cholera
antibiotic therapy for, 346
vaccine for, 416*t*
Cholera toxin, 24
Choriomeningitis, lymphocytic, rash in, 487
Christmas tree methods, 165
*Chromobacterium violaceum,* antibiotic therapy for, 339
Chromomycosis. *See* Phaeohypomycosis
Chronic fatigue syndrome (CFS), 773–779
allergy and, 777
clinical course of, 778
clinical manifestations of, 775–777
comorbid conditions, 777–778
definition of, 773, 774*t*
diagnosis of, 777
epidemiology of, 774–775
etiology of, 773–774
host factors in, 775
immunological tests in, 776
laboratory studies in, 776
neuroendocrine abnormalities in, 777
pathophysiology, 773–774, 774*f*
physical examination in, 775–776
prognosis, 778
symptoms of, 775, 776*t*
treatment of, 778
virological assays in, 776–777
Chronic obstructive airway disease (COAD), 523
Chronic obstructive pulmonary disease (COPD), 523

Cidofovir (Vistide), 351*t*, 359
Cierny-Mader staging system, 741, 742*t*
Ciliophora, 37
Ciprofloxacin
  dosage and administration, 329*t*
  drug interactions with, 311, 333*t*
  indications for, 309
  pharmacokinetics of, 331*t*
  spectrum and mechanism of activity, 328*t*
  spectrum of action, 307, 307*t*, 308
*Citrobacter*/infection
  antibiotic therapy for, 339
  antimicrobial resistance in, 213
Clarithromycin, 291
  dosage and administration, 329*t*
  drug interactions with, 333*t*
  indications for, 293
  pharmacokinetics of, 331*t*
  routes of elimination and adverse effects of, 332*t*
  spectrum and mechanism of activity, 328*t*
Classical pathway, 11, 83–84, 84*f*
Classic pathway, and bacterial cell wall components, 473–474
Clavulanic acid, 255
CLCP, in oxygen-independent killing, 89
Clean-contaminated procedures, 64
Clean procedures, 64
Clindamycin, 291, 294–296, 366*t*
  administration of, 296
  drug interactions with, 295
  indications for, 296
  mechanism of action, 294
  for *Pneumocystic carinii* pneumonia, 383
  resistance to, 294
    mechanisms of, 214
  spectrum of activity, 294
  toxicity of, 294–296
Clioquinol, for amebiasis, 382
CLL. *See* Leukemia, chronic lymphocytic
Clofazimine
  dosage and administration, 329*t*
  drug interactions with, 333*t*
  pharmacokinetics of, 331*t*
  routes of elimination and adverse effects of, 332*t*
  spectrum and mechanism of activity, 328*t*
Clonal abortion, 94
*Clonorchis sinensis*/infection, drug therapy for, 373*t*
Clostridial toxins, 9, 25
*Clostridium difficile*/infection
  antibiotic therapy for, 340
  multiplication of, 8
*Clostridium perfringens*/infection
  antibiotic therapy for, 339
  cellulitis, 767–768
  dissemination of, 9
*Clostridium septicum*/infection
  antibiotic therapy for, 339
  in spontaneous gas gangrene, 770–771
*Clostridium tetani*/infection, antibiotic therapy for, 339
*Clostridium welchii*/infection, and hemolytic anemia, 124
Cloxacillin, 253
CMV. *See* Cytomegalovirus/infection
COAD. *See* Chronic obstructive airway disease
Coagulation cascade, and septic shock, 474
Coagulation disorders, and infection, 126–128, 127*t*-128*t*
Coagulopathy, with septic shock, management of, 479
Coasting, 949
*Coccidioides immitis,* 50
  examination of, 171
Coccidioidomycosis, 48*t*, 50
  arthritis, 759
  diagnosis of, 50
  drug therapy for, 400*t*, 401–402
  in HIV infection, therapy for, 972*t*
  meningitis, 699
  pathogenesis of, 50
  pulmonary, 552*f*, 552–553
    diagnosis of, 552–553
    epidemiology of, 550*t*
    treatment of, 553
  in travelers to tropical countries, 872
Cold agglutinins, 123
  diseases associated with, 123*t*
Cold agglutinin syndrome, 123
Cold-reactive antibodies, 123
Colebrook, 3
Colitis
  hemorrhagic, 56
  imaging, 116–117, 117*f*
Collagen vascular disorders, and fever of unknown origin, 464, 464*t*
Colonization, 7–8
Colony-stimulating factors (GCSF; GMCSF), 10
Colorado tick fever, 895
  rash in, 488
  therapy for, 894*t*
Combination therapy, 235–236
  for septic shock, 478–479
Common vehicle transmission, 54
  definition of, 54
  of nosocomial infection, 61
Complement system, 83–84, 84*f*
  activation of, 11
  deficiencies in, 809
    vaccine use with, 424
  malnutrition and, 841
  response to HIV, 931
Complete blood count, in diagnosis of diarrhea, 585
Computed tomography
  abdominal, 115–118, 116*f*–117*f*
  of chest, 114, 114*f*
    in immunocompromised host, 114–115
    infectious-disease indications for, 114, 114*f*
  of CNS, 111–112
  of enteritis and colitis, 116–117, 117*f*
  of head, 112
    in encephalitis, 711
  musculoskeletal, 113–114
  of neck, 112
  of sinuses, 112–113
  of spine, 113
Condoms, for prevention of HIV spread, 912
Condyloma latum, 489
Confirmatory tests, in diagnosis of HIV infection, 906–907
Congenital rubella syndrome, 493
Congo-Crimean hemorrhagic fever, 496
Conjunctivitis, 734–736, 735*t*
  differential diagnosis of, 735*t*
  nonpurulent, 734–736
  purulent, 734
  viral, 734–735
Connective tissue diseases, rash in, 490
Contact, 7
  definition of, 53
Contact lenses, and keratitis, 736
Contact transmission, 53–54
  of nosocomial infection, 61
Contaminated procedures, 64
Continuous ambulatory peritoneal dialysis (CAPD), infections in, 802–803
  treatment of, 802–803, 803*t*
COPD. *See* Chronic obstructive pulmonary disease
Corneal infections, 736–737
Corticosteroids
  for ARDS, 564
  and subsequent anti-infective drug penetration into CNS, 222
  therapeutic indications for, 431*t*
Corticosteroid therapy, and vaccination, 415
*Corynebacterium*/infection
  endocarditis, 623
  of surgical wounds, 783
*Corynebacterium diphtheriae*/infection
  antibiotic therapy for, 340
  and microangiopathic disorders, 127
  toxin of, 9
*Corynebacterium jeikeium,* antibiotic therapy for, 340
*Corynebacterium minutissimum,* antibiotic therapy for, 340
*Corynebacterium ulcerans,* antibiotic therapy for, 340
Coumadin, drug interactions with, 323
Country of origin, and infection, 441*t*
*Coxiella burnetii*/infection
  antibiotic therapy for, 340
  endocarditis, 623
  in Q fever, 198–199
  vaccine for, 418*t*

Coxiella, laboratory diagnosis of, 198–199, 199*t*–200*t*
Crabs, 898
Cranberry juice, 322
C-reactive protein (CRP), 135–136
Creatinine, drug interactions with, 315
Creutzfeld-Jakob disease, 27
Crick, James, 1
Crimean-Congo hemorrhagic fever, 869*t*
Crohn's disease
  and fever of unknown origin, 464–465
  and joint inflammation, 765
Croup (laryngotracheitis), 519–521
  clinical manifestations of, 519
  diagnosis of, 519, 520*f*
  epidemiology of, 519
  etiology of, 519
  pathophysiology of, 519
  therapy, 519–521
Cryptic abscesses, and fever of unknown origin, 462
Cryptococcosis, 44–45, 48*t*
  central nervous system, drug therapy for, 399–400
  clinical manifestations of, 44–45
  diagnosis of, 44
  disseminated, rash in, 494
  drug therapy for, 399–401, 400*t*
  extraneural, drug therapy for, 400–401
  hemophagocytic syndrome associated with, 128
  in HIV infection, 947, 947*t*
  in immunocompromised host, 43
  pathogenesis of, 44
  pulmonary, 553
    epidemiology of, 550*t*
  treatment of, 45
*Cryptococcus*/infection, 44
  examination of, 171, 175*f*
  meningitis, 699
*Cryptococcus neoformans*/infection, 44
  in HIV infection, therapy for, 972*t*
Cryptosporidiosis
  drug therapy for, 372*t*
  hepatitic, in HIV infection, 953
*Cryptosporidium parvum*/infection, and diarrhea in residents of tropical countries, 875
CT. *See* Computed tomography
CTL. *See* Cytotoxic T lymphocytes
Culture, 143
  of bacteria, 150–156
  in diagnosis of diarrhea, 586
  fungal, 171–177
  viral, 161–164
    modified, 163
    specimen processing for, 161
*Curvularia*/infection, 47–50
Cushing's syndrome, infectious disease and, 134
Cutaneous ulcers, aspirates from, specimen collection from, 188
Cyclacillin, 253–254
Cyclophosphamide
  drug interactions with, 303
  immunosuppression by, 821
Cycloserine
  dosage and administration, 329*t*
  drug interactions with, 333*t*
  pharmacokinetics of, 331*t*
  routes of elimination and adverse effects of, 332*t*
  spectrum and mechanism of activity, 328*t*
Cyclospora, drug therapy for, 372*t*
Cyclosporin
  drug interactions with, 293
  immunosuppression by, 821
*Cysticercus cellulosae*/infection, drug therapy for, 378*t*
Cystic fibrosis (CF), 527
  aminoglycoside dosages for, 281–282
Cystitis, acute uncomplicated
  clinical manifestations of, 652
  treatment of, 654, 655*t*
Cytokines, 12, 97, 427–435, 428*t*–429*t*
  actions of, 407, 408*t*
  in bacterial and fungal infections, 427–429
  definition of, 427
  in inflammation, 84
  in inflammatory anemia, 121, 122*f*
  in modulation of immune response, 105
  proinflammatory, in septic shock, 480
  therapeutic indications for, 430*t*–431*t*
  in viral infections, 429
Cytomegalovirus/infection (CMV)
  in bone marrow transplant recipients, ganciclovir prophylaxis and, 830, 832*f*
  of burns, 793
  cervicitis, 382
  encephalitis
    clinical presentation in, 707
    diagnosis of, 113
    epidemiology of, 706–707
    in HIV infection, 945
    host response in, 707
    pathogenesis of, 707
  esophagitis, in HIV infection, 952
  and hematologic malignancies, 129
  hemophagocytic syndrome associated with, 128–129
  hepatitis, in HIV infection, 953
  in HIV infection, 940–941, 941*t*
    therapy for, 973*t*
  and immune system, 34
  mononucleosis, rash in, 487
  oral, 579
  in organ transplant recipient, 824–825
    antibiotic prophylaxis for, 825, 825*t*
  and polyradiculitis, 721
  retinitis, in HIV infection, 944, 944*t*
Cytomegalovirus IGIV, 413
Cytotoxicity, antibody-dependent cellular, response to HIV, 931
Cytotoxic T lymphocytes (CTL), 92
  response to HIV, 932–933
  viral evasion of, 33
Cytovene. *See* Ganciclovir

Dacryoadenitis, 733
Dacryocystitis, 733
Dapsone, 366*t*
  dosage and administration, 329*t*
  drug interactions with, 333*t*
  pharmacokinetics of, 331*t*
  for *Pneumocystic carinii* pneumonia, 383
  routes of elimination and adverse effects of, 332*t*
  spectrum and mechanism of activity, 328*t*
Day care centers
  diarrhea in, 581
  infections acquired in, 54*t*
Deep venous thrombosis (DVT), and fever, in hospitalized patient, 451
Defense mechanisms, 10–12
  acute inflammatory, 10–11
  alcohol abuse and, 853, 854*t*
  avoidance of, by bacteria, 25–26
  local, 10
  redundancy in, 33
Defensins, in oxygen-independent killing, 89
Delavirdine, 962
  dosage and administration, 963*t*
Delayed-type hypersensitivity, 99
Demeclocycline, 299
Dementia, in HIV infection, 944, 945*t*
Demography, and HIV spread, 910
Dendritic cells, HIV's effects on, 929
Dengue fever, 867–868, 869*t*
  rash in, 487
Dengue hemorrhagic fever (DHF)
  adverse effects of immune response in, 35
  rash in, 487–488
Deoxyribonucleic acid (DNA), 1
Dermatitis-arthritis syndrome, 493
Dermodex mites, 897
Detection systems, in viral diagnosis, 165, 166*t*
Detoxifying enzymes, and antimicrobial resistance, 213–214
Developing countries, malnutrition in children in, 841
  diagnosis and management of, 845–846
DGI. *See* Gonococcal infection, disseminated
DHF. *See* Dengue hemorrhagic fever
Diabetes, juvenile-onset, viral infection and, 35
Diabetes mellitus, vaccine use with, 424, 424*t*
Diapedesis, 10

Diarrhea, 581–588
acute, and malnutrition, 842
in bone marrow transplant recipients, 834
clinical manifestations of, 584–585
diagnosis of, 585*t*, 585–586
epidemiology of, 581–582
etiology of, 582*t*, 582–583, 583*t*
febrile dysenteric, 584
in HIV infection, therapy for, 969–970
host factors in, 583–584
laboratory studies in, 585–586
management of, 586–588
in parasitic infections, 37
pathogenesis of, 583
persistent, 585
and malnutrition, 843
in residents of tropical countries, 875–879
clinical features of, 875, 877*t*
control and prevention of, 876–879
epidemiology of, 875
etiology of, 875, 876*t*
treatment of, 875–876
in travelers, 875, 879–880
Diarrheal disease, 584
Dibekacin, 273
DIC. *See* Disseminated intravascular coagulation
Dicloxacillin, 253
indications for, 252*t*
Didanosine, 961
dosage and administration, 963*t*
resistance to, 961
toxicities of, 961
*Dientamoeba fragilis*/infection, drug therapy for, 373*t*, 382
Diethylcarbamazine, 366*t*
for tissue nematodes, 386
Diethyldithiocarbamate (DTC), 434
Differential media, 150–156
Diffuse alveolar damage, 557
DiGeorge's syndrome, 94
Diloxanide, for amebiasis, 382
Diloxanide furoate, 366*t*
Dilution tests, 234
Diphtheria
alcohol abuse and, 856
pathogenesis of, 27
vaccine for, 416*t*
Diphtheria toxin, 24
*Diphyllobothrium latum*/infection
drug therapy for, 378*t*
and megaloblastic anemia, 122
*Dipylidium caninum*/infection, drug therapy for, 378*t*
Direct detection
of viral nucleic acids, 164
of viruses, 164
Direct fluorescent antibody tests, 139
Direct microscopic examination
of bacterial specimens, 148
of fungal specimens, 171
Dirty procedures, 64
Disc diffusion test, 233–234
Disseminated intravascular coagulation (DIC), 127, 128*t*
Dissemination, 8–9
Distribution, 217–218
Diverticulitis, 617–618, 618*f*
DNA. *See* Deoxyribonucleic acid
DNA probes, 139–141, 140*t*
for direct detection of organisms in clinical samples, 141, 141*t*
Döhle bodies, 124, 125*f*
Domagk, 3
Donath-Landsteiner antibodies, 123
Donovan bodies, 657
Donovanosis, 657
clinical manifestations of, 662
pathogenesis of, 660
Douglas, 3
Doxycycline, 299, 367*t*
*Dracunculus medinensis*/infection, drug therapy for, 373*t*, 387
Drug abuse. *See* Intravenous drug abuse
Drug fever, and fever of unknown origin, 465, 465*t*
Drug resistance, 4
DTC. *See* Diethyldithiocarbamate
Duncan syndrome, 129
Duodenal drainage, specimen collection from, 186
DVT. *See* Deep venous thrombosis
Dysentery, 585
Dysphagia, in HIV infection, therapy for, 970
Dysuria, causes of, 652*t*

Ear drainage, with fever, 442
Ear pain, with fever, 442
Ears, in fever, 444
Eastern equine encephalitis (EKE), 708
Ebola virus/infection, 868, 869*t*
rash in, 497
Echinococcosis, 495
in travelers to tropical countries, 870
*Echinococcus granulosus*/infection
collection of, 187
drug therapy for, 378*t*
*Echinococcus multilocularis*/infection, drug therapy for, 378*t*
Echocardiography, in myocarditis/pericarditis, 646–647, 647*f*
Echovirus, and antibody responses, 34
Eclipse interval, 31
Ectoparasites
definition of, 891
diseases associated with, 891–901, 892*t*
Education, for prevention of HIV spread, 911–912
effectiveness of, 911, 911*f*
*Edwardsiella tarda,* antibiotic therapy for, 340
Effector T cells, and infection, 407–408
Eflornithine, 367*t*
for trypanosomiasis, 384–385
*Ehrlichia*/infection
laboratory diagnosis of, 199, 199*t*–200*t*
rash in, 488, 490–491
*Ehrlichia chaffeensis*
antibiotic therapy for, 340
in ehrlichiosis, 199
Ehrlichiosis, 893–894
antibiotic therapy for, 894*t*
hemophagocytic syndrome associated with, 128
laboratory diagnosis of, 199
Ehrlich, Paul, 209
*Eikenella corrodens*/infection
antibiotic therapy for, 340
arthritis, 758
endocarditis, 623
antimicrobial therapy for, 630*t*, 631
EKE. *See* Eastern equine encephalitis
Elderly
adverse reactions to antibiotics in, 229, 229*t*
vaccine use in, 425*t*
Electrocardiography, in myocarditis/pericarditis, 646, 647*f*
Electroencephalography, in encephalitis, 112
Electrolyte disturbances, infection and, 134
Elevation, for infected animal bites, 887
Elfinavir, 962
ELISA. *See* Enzyme-linked immunosorbent assay
ELVIS. *See* Enzyme-linked virus inducible system
Emetine, 367*t*
for amebiasis, 382
Empyema, 565–572
definition of, 565
management of, 571–572
subdural. *See* Subdural empyema
Encephalitis, 703–714, 704*f*
definition of, 703
diagnosis of, 711–713, 712*t*
diagnostic studies in, 711
etiology of, 703, 705*t*
host response in, 703
Japanese B, vaccine for, 420*t*
pathogenesis of, 703
postinfectious, 703–704
postvaccination, 703–704
tick-borne, vaccine for, 420*t*
in travelers to tropical countries, diseases causing, 865*t*
treatment of, 713*t*, 713–714
Encephalopathy, in HIV infection, therapy for, 967
Endarteritis, 621
Endemic, definition of, 53
Endocarditis
candidal, drug therapy for, 398

enterococcal, antimicrobial therapy for, 628, 631*t*
and fever of unknown origin, 462–463
infective, 621–635
anticoagulant therapy for, 633
antimicrobial therapy for, 628–632
clinical manifestations of, 624*t*, 624–625
diagnosis of, 626, 627*t*
epidemiology of, 623–624
etiology of, 621–623, 622*t*
extracardiac complications of, 633
host factors in, 623–624
laboratory studies in, 625–626
prevention of, 633*t*, 633–635, 634*t*–635*t*
surgical intervention for, 632, 632*t*
treatment of, 626–628
in intravenous drug user, 850*t*, 850–851
nonbacterial thrombotic (NBTE), 621
staphylococcal native valve, antimicrobial therapy for, 628*t*, 628–631
staphylococcal prosthetic valve, antimicrobial therapy for, 630*t*, 631
streptococcal, antimicrobial therapy for, 628, 629*t*-630*t*
subacute bacterial, rash in, 493
Endocrine disorders, 133–136, 135*t*
and fever of unknown origin, 466
and hyperthermia, 76
infectious diseases complicating, 134–135
Endocrine organs, invasion of, 134
Endophthalmitis, 737–738
candidal, drug therapy for, 398–399
Endoscopy, in diagnosis of diarrhea, 586
Endosomes, 95
Endothelial cells, and sepsis, 475
Endotoxins, 10, 25
in septic shock, inhibition of, 480
Enoxacin, drug interactions with, 311
*Entamoeba histolytica*/infection, 186*f*
collection of, 187
and diarrhea in residents of tropical countries, 875
drug therapy for, 371*t*
toxins produced by, 41
*Entamoeba polecki*/infection, drug therapy for, 373*t*
Enteric pathogens, detection of, 139*t*
Enteritis, imaging, 116–117
*Enterobacter*/infection
antibiotic therapy for, 340
antimicrobial resistance in, 213
arthritis, 758
in nosocomial pneumonia, 66
prostatitis, 676–677
of surgical wounds, 783
*Enterobacter cloacae,* in nosocomial bloodstream infection, 65
*Enterobacteriaceae*/infection, endocarditis, 623
*Enterobius vermicularis*/infection, drug therapy for, 373*t*
*Enterococcus*/infection
antibiotic therapy for, 340–341
endocarditis, antimicrobial therapy for, 628, 631*t*
nosocomial, 62
in nosocomial UTIs, 63
osteomyelitis, 742*t*
prostatitis, 676–677
in surgical site infections, 64
of urinary tract, 650
vancomycin-resistant, in nosocomial infections, 62, 67
*Enterococcus casseliflavus,* antimicrobial resistance in, 212
*Enterococcus faecalis*/infection
antimicrobial resistance in, 212, 292
endocarditis, 623
*Enterococcus faecium*/infection
antimicrobial resistance in, 212
endocarditis, 623
*Enterococcus floweschers,* antimicrobial resistance in, 212
*Enterococcus gallinarum,* antimicrobial resistance in, 212
EnteroTest, 186
in diagnosis of diarrhea, 586
Enterotoxigenic *Escherichia coli* heat-labile toxin, 24
Enterovirus/infection
encephalitis
clinical presentation in, 711
diagnosis of, 713
epidemiology of, 711
pathogenesis of, 711
prevention of, 714
myocarditis/pericarditis, 645
rash in, 486–487
Environment, definition of, 53
Enzyme immunoassay, 139
Enzyme-linked immunosorbent assay (ELISA), 164
in diagnosis of HIV infection, 905
Enzyme-linked virus inducible system (ELVIS), 163
Eosinophilia
biology of, 881–882
in travelers to tropical countries, 881–883
clinical correlates in, 883
diagnosis of, 883
etiology of, 881, 882*t*–883*t*
evaluation of, 881
management of, 883
tropical pulmonary, drug therapy for, 374*t*
Eosinophilic folliculitis, in HIV infection, 956
Eosinophils, 11
functional studies of, 882–883
and infection, 125–126
Epicillin, 253–254
Epidemic, definition of, 53
Epidemiological factors, 7
Epidemiology
definition of, 53
of infectious diseases, 53–59
Epididymitis, 673–675
clinical manifestations of, 674–675
diagnosis of, 675
epidemiology of, 674
etiologies of, 674, 674*t*
host factors in, 674
laboratory studies in, 675
pathogenesis of, 674
treatment of, 675
Epidural abscess, 729–730
clinical manifestations of, 729
definition of, 729
diagnosis of, 729, 729*f*
epidemiology of, 729
pathogenesis of, 729
treatment of, 730
Epiglottitis, 519–521
clinical manifestations of, 519
diagnosis of, 519, 520*f*
epidemiology of, 519
etiology of, 519
pathophysiology of, 519
therapy, 519–521
Epitope, 105
Epstein-Barr virus/infection
and chronic fatigue syndrome, 773
encephalitis
clinical presentation in, 707
epidemiology of, 707
pathogenesis of, 707
and hematologic malignancies, 129
hemophagocytic syndrome associated with, 128–129
and immune system, 33
lymphocytes in, 125, 126*f*
oral, 579
in organ transplant recipient, 825
Ergot-derivatives, drug interactions with, 293
Erlich, Paul, 3
Erysipelas, 502, 502*f*
*Erysipelothrix rhusiopathiae,* antibiotic therapy for, 341
Erythema, annular, systemic infections with, 486*t*, 495
Erythema infectiosum, 122
rash in, 487
Erythema multiforme, rash in, 490–491
Erythema nodosum, rash in, 494–495
Erythrocytes, and infections, 121–124
Erythrocyte sedimentation rate (ESR), 136
Erythroderma, diffuse
noninfectious causes of, 492–493
systemic infections with, 485*t*, 492–493

Erythromycin
indications for, 293
resistance to, mechanisms of, 214
*Escherichia coli*/infection
antibiotic therapy for, 341
antimicrobial resistance in, 213–214
arthritis, 758
D1:H1, 57, and microangiopathic disorders, 127
enterohemorrhagic, virulence of, 19
enteropathogenic EaeA, adherence in, 24
enterotoxigenic, and diarrhea in residents of tropical countries, 875
evasion of oxygen-dependent killing, 88
gram stain and, 149, 150*f*
0157:H7, 56
α-hemolysin toxin, 24
intracellular digestion of, 89
K12, virulence of, 19
meningitis, 689
in NICU nosocomial infections, 66
nosocomial, 62
in nosocomial UTIs, 63
osteomyelitis, 742*t*
prostatitis, 676–677
of urinary tract, 650
Esophageal disease, in HIV infection, 952
Esophagitis, in HIV infection, 952
therapy for, 970
*Esxerohilum*/infection, 47–50
E test, 234
Ethambutol
dosage and administration, 329*t*
drug interactions with, 333*t*
pharmacokinetics of, 331*t*
routes of elimination and adverse effects of, 332*t*
spectrum and mechanism of activity, 328*t*
for tuberculosis, 327
Ethionamide
dosage and administration, 329*t*
drug interactions with, 333*t*
pharmacokinetics of, 331*t*
routes of elimination and adverse effects of, 332*t*
spectrum and mechanism of activity, 328*t*
Ethnicity, and chronic fatigue syndrome, 775
Exanthem subitum, rash in, 487
Excretion, 218–220
Exotoxins, 24
Explant systems, in viral culture, 161
Exposures, 13–14
Exudates, specimen collection from, 146
Eyelids, infections of, 733–734
Eyes, in fever, 444
Eye symptoms, with fever, 442
FA. *See* Fluorescent antibody tests
Famiciclovir (Famvir), 352*t*, 355–356
Familial Mediterranean fever (FMF), and fever of unknown origin, 465–466
Family history, and fever, 443
Famvir. *See* Famiciclovir
Fascial spaces, around jaw and face, 574, 575*f*
Fasciitis, 767–771
necrotizing, 768
clinical course of, 768, 769*f*
*Fasciola hepatica*/infection, drug therapy for, 374*t*
*Fasciolopsis buski*/infection, drug therapy for, 374*t*
Fc regions, 11
Fecal leukocytes, in diagnosis of diarrhea, 586
Fecal specimens, 147, 159, 181
Fermentation, 1
Ferrous sulfate administration of, drug interactions with, 311
Fever, 71–81
chronic, etiologies of, 440*t*
common infectious causes of, 440*t*
definition of, 71
with diarrhea, 584
differential diagnosis of, 439–447, 447*f*
laboratory studies in, 446
diseases causing, 72*t*
factitious, 466
in HIV infection, 970–971, 971*t*
therapy for, 970–971
hospital-acquired
differential diagnosis of, 456*t*
epidemiology of, 454–455
management of, 455–458, 457*t*
in hospitalized patients, 449–458
etiologies of, 449–454, 450*t*
of infectious causes, 449–450
of noninfectious causes, 450–454
procedure-related, 451–452
and host-microbe interactions, 74*t*, 74–75
versus hyperthermia, 459
induction of, sequence in, 72, 73*f*
in intravenous drug user, evaluation of, 849, 850*t*
management of, 446–447, 447*f*
medical history in, 439–443
with neutropenia
empiric therapy for, 814
imipenem for, 267
pathogenesis of, 72–74
physiologic events of, 72, 72*t*
remittent, 440
timing of, and etiology of, 454, 455*f*
in travelers to tropical countries, 859–873
approach to, 872–873
clinical characteristics of, 860–861, 863*t*
epidemiology of, 859
exposures and, 859, 862*t*
history in, 859
nosocomial transmission of, 861*t*
potentially fatal causes of, 861*t*
risk of, 860*t*
spontaneous bleeding in, 863*t*
telephone numbers for information on, 873
treatment of, 78*t*, 78–80
patient selection for, 78–79
physical, 79–80
of unknown origin, 459–469
clinical features of, 460
country and, 462*t*
definition of, 459, 460*t*
etiologies of, 459–460, 461*t*–462*t*
evaluation of, 466–468
history in, 466–467
HIV-associated, 469
laboratory and imaging studies in, 467
neutropenic, 469
nosocomial, 468–469
pathogenesis of, 459
physical examination in, 467
special tests in, 467–468
therapeutic trials for, 468
Fibrin, 801
Fibrinolysis, 474
Fibrinolytic therapy, intrapleural, 571
Fibromyalgia, and chronic fatigue syndrome, 777
Fibronectin, 801
Fifth disease. *See* Erythema infectiosum
Filariasis
drug therapy for, 373*t*
lymphatic, rash in, 496
specimen collection in, 187
in travelers to tropical countries, 868
Fimbria, 21
Finlay, Carlos, 5
Fish tape worm *(Diphyllobothrium latum)*, 37
FK-506 (tacrolimus), immunosuppression by, 821
Flagyl. *See* Metronidazole
Flamazine. *See* Silver sulfadiazine
Flavivirus infection, encephalitis, 708
*Flavobacterium meningosepticum*, antibiotic therapy for, 341
Fleas, diseases associated with, 899*t*, 900
Fleming, Alexander, 3–4, 249
Flies, diseases associated with, 898–900, 899*t*
Florey, Howard W., 4, 249
Flucloxacillin, 253
Fluconazole, 393–394
candidal minimal inhibitory concentrations and, 43
for cryptococcosis, 45
indications for, 393*t*, 394
pharmacokinetics of, 392*t*
toxicity of, 393*t*, 394

Flucytosine, 391–392
  dosage and administration, with renal insufficiency, 391
  indications for, 391*t*, 391–392
  pharmacology of, 390*t*, 391
  toxicity of, 390*t*, 391
Flukes, drug therapy for, 373*t*–374*t*
Flumadine. *See* Rimantadine
Fluorescent antibody tests (FA), 164
5-Fluorocytosine. *See* Flucytosine
Fluoroquinolones, 305–312, 306*t*
  adverse effects of, 311
  antimycobacterial uses of, 330
  blood and tissue levels of, 308
  clearance of, 308
  drug interactions with, 311
  indications for, 309–311, 310*t*
  mechanism of action, 305
  pharmacokinetics of, 308*t*, 308–309
  resistance to, 305
  spectrum of action, 307*t*, 307–308
  structure of, 305, 306*f*
  toxicities of, 311
FMF. *See* Familial Mediterranean fever
Folic acid
  metabolism of, and antimicrobial resistance, 212–213
  synthesis of, antimicrobial action and, 210
Folliculitis, 501
  eosinophilic, in HIV infection, 956
  eosinophilic pustular, rash in, 490
Fomites, 7, 54
Food-borne transmission, and diarrhea, 582
Formaldehyde, drug interactions with, 322
Fort Bragg fever, 489
Fosariosis, 48*t*
Foscarnet (Foscavir), 353*t*, 357–358, 962
Fosfomycin, resistance to, mechanisms of, 214
Fosfomycin trometamol, 322
Fournier's gangrene, 768
Fowlpox viruses, as vectors, 409
*Francisella tularensis*/infection
  antibiotic therapy for, 341
  rash in, 491
  vaccine for, 419*t*
Fungal infections, 43–51
  arthritis, 759
  in bone marrow transplant recipients, 830, 833–834
    treatment of, 836–837
  of burns, 792–793
  and cavitary lung disease, 550–554
  clinical recognition of, 169
  cutaneous, in HIV infection, 955
  cytokines and immunomodulators in, 427–429
  and diarrhea, 583
  drug therapy for, 389–395
  emerging, 47–50
  drug therapy for, 403, 403*t*
  endemic, 50–51
  and fever of unknown origin, 463
  filamentous, of burns, 793
  in HIV infection, therapy for, 965–966
  in intravenous drug user, 850–851
  keratitis, 736
  laboratory diagnosis of, 169–178
    approaches to, 170*t*
  meningitis, 699
  opportunistic, 43–50, 48*t*–49*t*
  oral, 578
  of orbit, 738–739
  in organ transplant recipient, 826–827
  osteomyelitis, therapy for, 754
  in travelers to tropical countries, 872
Fungal serology, 177–178
Fungi
  characteristics of, 173*t*–174*t*, 178
  demonstration of, 171, 172*t*, 175*f*–176*f*
  immune response to, 97*t*
Furazolidone, 367*t*
  for giardiasis, 382
*Fusarium*/infection, 50
  of burns, 793
  drug therapy for, 403*t*
  examination of, 171, 176*f*

GALT. *See* Gut-associated lymphoid tissue
Gamma interferon, 11
Ganciclovir (Cytovene), 352*t*, 356–357
  for cytomegalovirus prophylaxis, ganciclovir prophylaxis and, 830, 832*f*
Gangrene
  Fournier's, 768
  gas. *See* Gas gangrene
  Meleney's synergistic, 767
  pulmonary, 545
Gantanol. *See* Sulfamethoxazole
Gantrisin. *See* Sulfisoxazole
*Gardnerella vaginalis*/infection
  antibiotic therapy for, 341
  vulvovaginitis, 681
Gas gangrene
  post-traumatic
    clinical manifestations of, 769
    diagnosis of, 769–770
    pathogenesis of, 769
    prevention of, 770
    prognosis in, 770
    treatment of, 770
  spontaneous, non-traumatic
    clinical manifestations of, 770*f*, 770–771
    diagnosis of, 771
    pathogenesis of, 771
    prognosis, 771
    treatment of, 771
Gastroenteritis, definition of, 584
Gastrointestinal disease
  in bone marrow transplant recipients, 834
  fluoroquinolones for, 309
  in HIV infection, 951*t*, 951–954
    therapy for, 969–970
  and malnutrition, 842–843
  parasitic, 37–38, 40*t*
  trimethoprim/sulfamethoxazole for, 317
Gastrointestinal reactions
  to antimicrobial agents, 225–227
  to fluoroquinolones, 311
Gastrointestinal tract
  imaging of, in patient with HIV infection, 117
  specimen collection from, 159, 181–186
GCSF. *See* Granulocyte colony-stimulating factor
General medical patients, hospital-acquired fever in, 454
General surgical patients, hospital-acquired fever in, 454, 455*f*
Genetic factors, and diarrhea, 584
Genital herpes, 657–667
  clinical manifestations of, 660–661, 661*t*
  epidemiology of, 658, 658*f*
  etiology of, 657
  pathogenesis of, 660
  treatment of, 664–665, 665*t*
Genitalia, in fever, 445
Genital pathogens, detection of, 139*t*
  by DNA probe, 141*t*
Genital tract, specimen collection from, 147–148
Genital ulcer disease, 657–667
  clinical manifestations of, 660–663
  control of, 666
  diagnosis of, 663–664
  differential diagnosis of, 660–663
  epidemiology of, 657–659
  etiology of, 657, 658*t*
  history and examination in, 663
  host factors in, 659
  laboratory evaluation of, 663*t*, 663–664
  pathogenesis of, 660
  prevention of, 666
  treatment of, 664–666
Genitourinary specimens, 186–187
Gentamicin, 273
  dosage and administration, 282*t*
    for children, 282*t*
*Geotrichum capitatum,* 47
Germ theory of disease, 1
Gianotti-Crosti syndrome, 592
*Giardia lamblia*/infection
  cysts, 192*f*
  and diarrhea in residents of tropical countries, 875
  drug therapy for, 374*t*, 382
Gingivitis, acute necrotizing ulcerative (ANUG), 576

Glucocorticosteroids, for fever, 78*t*, 79
Glucose metabolism, infection and, 133
Glycopeptides, 285–289
  dosage and administration, 288
  indications for, 287–288
  mechanism of action, 285
  pharmacology of, 288
  resistance to, 285–287, 287*f*
  spectrum of action, 285
  structure of, 285, 286*f*
  toxicity of, 288
GMCSF. *See* Granulocyte-macrophage colony-stimulating factor
Gnathostomiasis, drug therapy for, 374*t*
Gonococcal infection, disseminated (DGI), rash in, 493
Gonorrhea
  oral, 577
  prevalence of, 56
  ulceration in, 657
Graft-versus-host disease (GVHD), 829
Gram-negative bacterial sepsis, 472
Gram stain, 148–149, 149*f*–150*f*
Granulocyte colony-stimulating factor (GCSF), 428*t*, 432
  therapeutic indications for, 430*t*
Granulocyte-macrophage colony-stimulating factor (GMCSF), 428*t*, 432
  therapeutic indications for, 430*t*
Granulocytes
  and infection, 124–125
  transfusions of, for infection in bone marrow transplant recipients, 836
Granuloma inguinale
  epidemiology of, 659
  ulceration in, 657, 663
Granulomatous diseases, and fever of unknown origin, 464–465
Granulomatous liver disease, 595–596, 596*t*
Gray syndrome, 303
Grepafloxacin
  indications for, 309
  spectrum of action, 307
Griffith, 1
Growth factors, 427–435
  for infection in bone marrow transplant recipients, 836
  myelopoietic, 429–432
Guillain-Barré syndrome, 719
Gut-associated lymphoid tissue (GALT), 95
Gynecologic patients, hospital-acquired fever in, 455

Habits
  and fever, 443
  and HIV spread, 910
*Haemophilus aphrophilus*/infection
  antibiotic therapy for, 341
  endocarditis, 623
    antimicrobial therapy for, 630*t*, 631
*Haemophilus ducreyi*
  antibiotic therapy for, 341
  in genital ulcer disease, 657
*Haemophilus influenzae*/infection
  antibiotic therapy for, 341
  antimicrobial resistance in, 210
  cervicitis, 382
  Gram stain and, 149, 149*f*
  osteomyelitis, 742*t*
  type b
    arthritis, 757–758
    meningitis, 689
    vaccine for, 416*t*
  vulvovaginitis, 681
*Haemophilus parainfluenzae*/infection
  antibiotic therapy for, 341
  endocarditis, 623
    antimicrobial therapy for, 630*t*, 631
Hairy cell leukemia, HTLV-II and, 130
Hairy leukoplakia (HL), 579
  oral, in HIV infection, 952
Halofantrine, 367*t*, 381
Hand-foot-and-mouth disease (HFM), 580
  rash in, 491
Hansen's disease, 721
Hantavirus/infection, 868, 869*t*
  rash in, 497
Hantavirus pulmonary syndrome, 559–560, 869*t*
H-2 blockers, and gastric bacterial overgrowth, 66
HBO. *See* Hyperbaric oxygen therapy
Headache, with fever, 441
Head, imaging of, 112
Head lice, 898
Health care setting, HIV transmission in, prevention of, 912–913
Health care workers
  and nosocomial infections, 68–69
  risk of blood-borne pathogens, 68
  risk of tuberculosis, 68
  vaccine use in, 425*t*
Hearing loss, with fever, 442
Heart
  abnormalities of, in pericarditis and myocarditis, 643
  in fever, 445
Heart disease, chronic, vaccine use with, 424
Heat dissipation, 71–72
Heat exhaustion, 75
Heat generation, 71–72
Heatstroke, 75
  classic, 75–76
  management of, 80
*Helicobacter pylori,* antibiotic therapy for, 342
Helminth infections
  diagnosis of, 41*t*, 41–42
  drug therapy for, 385–388
  and eosinophilia, 882*t*
  organ-specific, 37–41
  in travelers to tropical countries, 868–870
Helminths
  classification of, 37, 38*t*–39*t*
  global burden of illness due to, 38*t*
  ova, in stool, 191*t*
  parasitic, 37–42
  pathogenesis of, 41
Helper cells, 11
Hematologic alterations, 121–131
Hematologic laboratory tests, for coagulation disorders associated with infectious disease, 127*t*
Hematologic malignancies, secondary to infection, 129–130, 130*t*
Hematologic toxicity, of chloramphenicol, 302–303
Hematoma, and fever, in hospitalized patient, 451
Hematopoietic reactions, to antimicrobial agents, 227–228
Hematopoietic stem cell transplantation, 829–838
Hemolytic anemia, 123–124
  pathogenesis of, 123–124
Hemolytic uremic syndrome (HUS), 127, 128*f*
Hemorrhagic fever, 868, 869*t*
Henoch-Schönlein purpura, rash in, 493
Hepatic abscess, 600–602
  clinical manifestations of, 601
  diagnosis of, 602, 602*f*
  epidemiology of, 600
  etiology of, 600, 601*f*
  laboratory studies in, 601–602
  pathogenesis of, 600–601
  treatment of, 602
Hepatic failure
  antimicrobial dosages in, 218, 219*t*
  aztreonam dosages in, 270
  fluoroquinolone dosages in, 309
  penem/carbapenem dosages in, 268
Hepatic infections, pyogenic, 597–603
Hepatitis, 589–596
  granulomatous, and fever of unknown origin, 464–465
  viral
    versus alcohol- or drug-induced, 595
    cholestatic, 592
    chronic, 595
    clinical manifestations of, 590–591
    diagnosis of, 592–594, 593*t*
    epidemiology of, 589–591
    etiology of, 589, 590*t*
    fulminant, 592
    host factors in, 590
    immunoprophylaxis of, 594*t*, 594–595
    laboratory studies in, 592
    monitoring, 594
    in organ transplant recipient, 826
    prevention of, 594–595
    treatment of, 594

Hepatitis A virus/infection
 diagnosis of, 593
 epidemiology of, 589
 pathogenesis of, 590
 prevalence of, 56
 relapsing, 592
 vaccine for, 419*t*
Hepatitis B virus/infection
 arthritis, 759, 760*t*
 diagnosis of, 593
 encephalitis
  clinical presentation in, 707–708
  diagnosis of, 113
  epidemiology of, 707
  pathogenesis of, 707
 epidemiology of, 589
 and immune system, 33
 pathogenesis of, 590
 prevalence of, 56
 rash in, 487
 vaccine for, 419*t*
Hepatitis C virus, 5
 diagnosis of, 593
 epidemiology of, 589–590
 pathogenesis of, 590
Hepatitis D virus
 diagnosis of, 593–594
 epidemiology of, 590–591
 pathogenesis of, 590
Hepatitis E virus, 594
 epidemiology of, 590
 pathogenesis of, 590
Hepatobiliary disorders
 in bone marrow transplant recipients, 834
 esophageal, 952–953
Herald plaque, 490–491
Herpangina, 580
Herpes, genital. *See* Genital herpes
Herpes simplex virus/infection (HSV)
 in bone marrow transplant recipients, acyclovir prophylaxis and, 829–830, 831*f*
 of burns, 793
 cervicitis, 382
 disseminated, rash in, 491
 encephalitis, 703, 704*f*, 704–706
  clinical presentation of, 705–706, 706*t*
  diagnosis of, 112–113
  epidemiology of, 704
  host response in, 706
  prevention of, 714
  treatment of, 713*f*, 713–714
 encephalitis (HSE), pathogenesis of, 704
 esophagitis, in HIV infection, 952
 genital, treatment of, 665*t*
 and hematologic malignancies, 129
 hemophagocytic syndrome associated with, 128–129
 inhibition of antigen processing by, 33–34
 keratitis, 736–737
 oral, 579
 of skin, in HIV infection, 954
 type 2, sacral radiculitis, 721
Herpesviruses
 assembly of, 33
 drug therapy for, 349–356
 in organ transplant recipient, 824
Herpes zoster ophthalmicus (HZO), 737
Herpes zoster, rash in, 491
Herpetic keratitis, 35
Hetacillin, 254
Heterotropic ossification, and fever, in hospitalized patient, 451
HFM. *See* Hand-foot-and-mouth disease
HHC. *See* Home health care
HHV-8. *See* Human herpesvirus 8
Histamine ($H_2$) antagonists, drug interactions with, 311
*Histoplasma capsulatum,* 50
 evasion of phagocytosis, 87
 examination of, 171, 176*f*
 and mononuclear phagocytes, 126
*Histoplasma,* in immunocompromised host, 43
Histoplasmosis, 49*t*, 50
 drug therapy for, 400*t*, 401
 hemophagocytic syndrome associated with, 128
 in HIV infection, 942–943, 943*t*, 943*f*
  therapy for, 972*t*
 meningitis, 699
 oral, 578
 progressive disseminated (PDH), rash in, 494
 pulmonary
  clinical manifestations of, 551, 551*f*
  diagnosis of, 551
  epidemiology of, 550*t*
  treatment of, 551
 in travelers to tropical countries, 872
HIV dementia, 944, 945*t*
HL. *See* Hairy leukoplakia
Holmes, Oliver Wendell, 1
Home health care (HHC), nosocomial infections in, 67
Homosexual men, diarrhea in, 581
Hookworm
 drug therapy for, 374*t*
 and iron-deficiency anemia, 121
Hordeolum, 733
Horizontal transmission, 53
Hospitalization
 for infected animal bites, 887
 for malnutrition, 845, 845*t*
 for pneumonia, 536
Host, definition of, 53
Host factors, and antimicrobial selection, 234
HSE. *See* Herpes simplex virus/infection, encephalitis
HSV. *See* Herpes simplex virus/infection
HTLV. *See* Human T lymphotropic virus
Human herpesvirus 8 (HHV-8), 27
 and Kaposi's sarcoma, 129
Human immunodeficiency virus/infection (HIV). *See also* Acquired immunodeficiency syndrome
 arthritis, 760
 autoimmune disorders and neoplasms associated with, 934–936
 and brain, 925
 clinical manifestations of, 937–957
 clinical presentation of, 937, 939*t*
 and endocrine abnormalities, 135
 fever of unknown origin associated with, 469
 health care workers' exposure to, 68
 HIV-1
  cellular tropism in, 921
  characteristics of, 916, 917*f*
  dynamics of, 921–923, 922*t*
  gene products of, 918–919, 919*t*
  genome organization in, 916–920, 918*f*
  life cycle of, 916, 917*f*, 920–921, 959, 960*f*
  viral phenotype of, 921
 HIV-2, epidemiology of, 910–911
 imaging of gastrointestinal tract in, 117
 immune responses to, 930–934
 and immune system, 927–930
 immunology of, 927–936, 928*t*
 in intravenous drug user, 851
 laboratory diagnosis of, 905–907
  strategy for, 907
 latency in, 925
 and lymphoid organs, 924–925
 and lymphoma, 129–130
 and malnutrition, 844–845
 and microangiopathic disorders, 127
 and myelopathy, 718–719
 natural history of, 924–926
 oral, 579–580
 in organ transplant recipient, 826
 prevalence of, 907, 908*f*
 prevention of, 911–913
 primary, 924, 938, 939*t*
 regional epidemics of, 907–908, 909*f*
 replication of, suppression by CD8 cells, 933, 933*t*
 resistance to antiretroviral drugs by, 923–924
 spread of, factors affecting, 910
 stages of, 937, 938*t*
 systemic illnesses in, 939–943, 940*t*
 therapy guidelines for, 962–963, 963*t*–964*t*
 transmission of, 909–910
  bloodborne, 909–910, 912
  in health care setting, 912–913
  sexual, 909
  vertical, 812, 910
 and vaccination, 415, 422*t*
 vaccines for, 977–980, 979*t*

Human immunodeficiency virus/infection (*continued*)
correlates of immunity in humans, 978
correlates of protection in animal models, 977–978, 978*f*
mechanism of action, 979, 980*f*
studies in humans, 978–979, 979*f*
variability in, 923
Human leukocyte associated antigens (HLA antigens), 93–94, 94*f*
Human papillomavirus/infection, oral, 579
Human T lymphotropic virus
I
arthritis in, 760
malignancies associated with, 130
and myelopathy, 718
II
malignancies associated with, 130
and myelopathy, 718
Humoral immunity, 11, 99–104
and HIV infection, 930
malnutrition and, 841
and newborn period, 104
theories of, 3
HUS. *See* Hemolytic uremic syndrome
Hyalophyphomycosis, 50
Hydrocortisone, for fever, 78*t*
Hydroxychloroquine sulfate (Plaquenil), 365
Hygienic problems, and diarrhea, 583
*Hymenolepis nana*/infection, drug therapy for, 378*t*
Hyperbaric oxygen (HBO) therapy, adjunctive, for osteomyelitis, 754
Hyperkalemia, 134
Hypernatremia, 134
Hyperpyrexia, 72
management of, 80
Hypersensitivity
to antibiotics, in HIV infection, 971–973, 973*t*
delayed-type, 99
immediate, 102
Hypersensitivity vasculitis, rash in, 490
Hyperthermia, 75–77
caused by drug intoxication or withdrawal, 76
causes of, 75*t*
definition of, 71
exertional, 75
versus fever, 459
habitual, 466
malignant (MH), 76–77
treatment of, 78*t*, 78–80
Hyperthyroidism, and fever of unknown origin, 466
Hypochlorhydria, and diarrhea, 583–584
Hypoferremia, 75
Hypogammaglobulinemia, 811
vaccine use with, 424
Hyponatremia, 134
Hypothermia, 77–78
factors predisposing to, 77*t*
treatment of, 80
Hypothyroidism, infectious disease and, 135
HZO. *See* Herpes zoster ophthalmicus

ICDs. *See* Implantable cardioverter defibrillators
ICE. *See* IL-1$\beta$ converting enzyme
ICP47, 34
ICPs. *See* Infection-control practitioners
Idiotypes, 105
Idiotypic networks, 105, 106*f*
Idiotypic specificity, 100
Idoxuridine, 4
IF. *See* Immunofluorescence tests
IFA. *See* Indirect fluorescent antibody test
IGIV. *See* Immunoglobulin G, intravenous
IL-1$\beta$ converting enzyme (ICE), viral inhibition of, 33
IL-1 receptor antagonist protein (IL-1 RAP), 74
Imaging techniques, 111–120
Imidazoles, 392–394
Imipenem
administration of, 267
blood and tissue levels of, 267–268, 268*t*
excretion of, 268
mechanism of action, 265
spectrum of action, 266–267
Immediate hypersensitivity, 102
Immune cascade, cellular, 95–97, 96*f*–97*f*
Immune disorders, congenital, vaccine use with, 424
Immune hemolysis, 123
Immune response, 810*t*
to bacterial infection, 96*t*
to HIV infection, 930–934
and intracellular infection, 407–408, 408*t*
to nonbacterial infection, 97*t*
and nutritional status, 839–840, 840*t*
regulation of, 104–106
cytokines in, 105
immunoregulatory T cells in, 105–106, 106*f*
secondary, 99
trauma and, 785–786
to viral infection, adverse effects of, 35
Immune system
HIV infection and, 927–930
nutrition and, 839
and parasites, 41
and viruses, 33–35
Immunity, 14
cell-mediated
deficiency in, 811, 813
malnutrition and, 840–841
cellular
response to HIV, 931
theories of, 3
history of, 2
humoral. *See* Humoral immunity
theories of, 3
Immunization, history of, 2, 2*t*
Immunocompromised persons
aspergillosis in, 45
chest imaging in, 114–115
cryptococcal meningitis in, 44
fungal infection in, 43
histoplasmosis in, 50
hospital-acquired fever in, 455
immune response in, 91
*Mycobacterium avium* complex in, antibiotic therapy for, 347
parasitic infections in, 41, 41*t*
pneumonia in, 531, 531*t*
management of, 537
vaccines in, 415–424
Immunodeficiency, 809–819
acquired, 810–811, 811*t*
cell-mediated, primary, 809, 809*t*
and diarrhea, 584
evaluation of, 813, 813*t*
infections in, 811–813, 812*t*
prevention of, 818–819
treatment of, 813–814
pathogenesis of, 809–811
primary, 411–412, 809–810
Immunodetection tests, solid-phase, 164
Immunofluorescence tests (IF), 164
Immunofluorescent stains, 150
Immunogen, definition of, 91
Immunogenetics, 92–93
Immunoglobulin(s), 11, 99–100, 100*f*–101*f*
for bone marrow transplant recipients, 837
functions of, 102–103
G. *See* Immunoglobulin G
IgA, 103, 103*f*
IgD, 102
IgE, 102
IgM, 102
Immunoglobulin G, 102–103
deficiency of, 811
intravenous (IGIV)
hyperimmune, 413
preparations of, 411, 412*t*
Immunomodulators, 427–435
in bacterial and fungal infections, 427–429
in viral infections, 429
Immunopotentiation, 409–410
Immunoprophylaxis, 407–410
passive, 411–414
Immunostains, for antigen detection, 164
Immunosuppression
mechanisms of, 829
nature of, 829

in organ transplantation, pathogenesis of, 821, 822*t*
Immunotherapy, passive, 411–414
Impetigo, 502
Implantable cardioverter defibrillators (ICDs), infections associated with, 804–806
Incubation, of bacterial cultures
conditions of, 156
detection times and procedures for, 156
India ink preparation, in diagnosis of cryptococcosis, 44
Indinavir, 962
dosage and administration, 963*t*
Indirect contact, 7
Indirect contact transmission, 54
Indirect fluorescent antibody test (IFA), in diagnosis of rickettsia, 195
Indomethacin, drug interactions with, 315
Industrialized countries, malnutrition in, 841–842, 842*t*
diagnosis and management of, 846–847
Infantile papular acrodermatitis, 592
Infarction, and fever, in hospitalized patient, 450
Infection
clinical manifestations of, 12–13
host responses to, 71–81
immune responses and, 407–408, 408*t*
and nutritional status, 839–840, 840*t*
nutrition and, 839
outcomes of, 12
prevention of, 14
sepsis and, 13, 13*f*
Infection-control practitioners (ICPs), 58
and nosocomial infections, 61
Infection site, and antimicrobial selection, 234–235
Infectious disease(s), 7–15
chronic, 12
classification of, 13
clinical assessment of, control strategies in, 57–58, 58*t*
control and prevention of, 54–55
practitioner's role in, 57–58
definition of, 7
diagnosis of, 13–14
diagnostic approach to, 441*f*
emerging, 56–57
public health response to, 56–57
surveillance and reporting, 57
epidemiology of, 53–59
and fever of unknown origin, 460–463, 461*t*–462*t*
history of, 1–6
most commonly reported, in U.S., 56
notifiable, 55*t*, 55–56
surveillance and reporting, 55*t*, 55–56
tempo of, 13
transmission of, 7
modes and patterns of, 53–54
treatment of, 14
Infectious mononucleosis. *See also* Epstein-Barr virus/infection
fatal, 129
Inflammation, 83, 810*t*
and fever, in hospitalized patient, 450
PMN and, 89–90
Inflammatory anemia, 121
pathogenesis of, 121, 122*f*
Inflammatory bowel disease, and joint inflammation, 765
Influenza virus
A
drug therapy for, 360–361
vaccine for, 420*t*
B, vaccine for, 420*t*
and immune system, 33
Insect bites, infections from, 502
Insensible loss, 71
Integrins, 86
Intensive care unit (ICU)
admission to, for pneumonia, 536
hospital-acquired fever in, 455
IGIV prophylaxis in, 412–413
Interferon(s), 4, 432–433
alpha, 354*t*, 362–363, 429*t*, 433, 962
therapeutic indications for, 430*t*
beta, 429*t*, 433
class I, and viruses, 33
gamma, 433
and sepsis, 475–476
therapeutic indications for, 431*t*
Interleukin(s), 74, 433–434
IL-1, 97–98, 428*t*
$\alpha$, 74
$\beta$, 74
and sepsis, 475
therapeutic indications for, 430*t*
IL-2, 97, 428*t*
therapeutic indications for, 430*t*
IL-3, 106, 428*t*
therapeutic indications for, 430*t*
IL-4, 101, 428*t*
IL-5, 101, 428*t*
IL-6, 428*t*
IL-8, 428*t*
IL-9, 106
IL-11, 428*t*
IL-12, 428*t*
Intestinal fluke, drug therapy for, 374*t*
Intoxication, acute, immune effects of, 853
Intraabdominal abscesses, 613–619
clinical manifestations of, 614, 614*f*
diagnosis of, 614
microbiology of, 615, 615*t*
outcome in, 616
pathogenesis of, 613–614
specific causes of, 617–618
treatment of, 614–616
Intraabdominal infections, post-traumatic, 798
Intramuscular injections, and fever, in hospitalized patient, 451
Intraocular infections, 737–738
Intraoral infections, 573–580
Intrauterine contraceptive devices (IUDs), infections associated with, 806
Intravenous drug abuse
HIV transmission through, prevention of, 912
infectious complications of, 849–852
clinical manifestations of, 849–851
local, 849–850
prevention of, 851–852
treatment of, 849–850
long-term medical care for, 851–852
Intubation, and nosocomial pneumonia, 66
Invasion, 8
Invasive devices, and nosocomial infection, 61
Involucrum, 741
Iodoquinol, 367*t*
for amebiasis, 382
Iron, bacteria and, 24
Iron chelation, and zygomycosis, 47
Iron-deficiency anemia, 121
Isepamicin, 273
Isolation techniques, for bone marrow transplant recipients, 837
Isoniazid, 4
dosage and administration, 329*t*
drug interactions with, 333*t*
pharmacokinetics of, 331*t*
routes of elimination and adverse effects of, 332*t*
spectrum and mechanism of activity, 328*t*
for tuberculosis, 327
Isopinosine, 434
*Isospora belli*/infection
drug therapy for, 374*t*
hepatitic, in HIV infection, 953
Isotype, 11
Itraconazole, 394
for aspergillosis, 46
indications for, 393*t*, 394
pharmacokinetics of, 392*t*
toxicity of, 393*t*, 394
IUDs. *See* Intrauterine contraceptive devices
Ivermectin, 367*t*
for tissue nematodes, 386–387

Jaccoud's arthropathy, 765
Jamestown Canyon encephalitis, 708
Japanese B encephalitis, 708
vaccine for, 420*t*
Jaundice
in bone marrow transplant recipients, 834
and fever, 443–444
Jenner, Edward, 2
Jesty, Benjamin, 2

Joint infections, fluoroquinolones for, 309
Joint pain, with fever, 442

Kala-azar. *See Leishmania*/infection
Kallikrein, 474–475
Kanamycin, 273, 330
  contraindications to, 281
  dosage and administration, 283*t*, 329*t*
  drug interactions with, 333*t*
  pharmacokinetics of, 331*t*
  routes of elimination and adverse effects of, 332*t*
  spectrum and mechanism of activity, 328*t*
Kaposi's sarcoma, 935, 955
  HHV-8 and, 129
Kaposi's sarcoma-associated herpesvirus (KSHV), 27
  and immune system, 33
Katayama fever, drug therapy for, 377*t*
Kawasaki disease, 505
  rash in, 490, 492–493
Kenya tick fever, rash in, 490
Keratitis, 736–737
Keratoderma blennorrhagicum, in HIV infection, 955
Ketoconazole, 367*t*, 392–393
  for ARDS, 564
  for free living amoebae infection, 385
  indications for, 392–393, 393*t*
  pharmacokinetics of, 392, 392*t*
  toxicity of, 392, 393*t*
Kidneys, in metabolism of antimicrobial agents, 218
*Kingella*/infection
  antibiotic therapy for, 342
  endocarditis, 623
    antimicrobial therapy for, 630*t*, 631
Kinyoun stain, 149–150
Kitasato, 3, 5
*Klebsiella*/infection
  acute bacterial prostatitis, 676
  arthritis, 758
  of burns, 789
  of urinary tract, 650
*Klebsiella oxytoca,* antibiotic therapy for, 342
*Klebsiella ozaenae,* antibiotic therapy for, 342
*Klebsiella pneumoniae*/infection
  antibiotic therapy for, 342
  antimicrobial resistance in, 213–214
  meningitis, 689
*Klebsiella rhinoscleromatis,* antibiotic therapy for, 342
Koch, Robert, 1, 853
Koplik's spots, 580
Korean hemorrhagic fever, 497
KSHV. *See* Kaposi's sarcoma-associated herpesvirus

LaCrosse encephalitis, 708
β-Lactam antibiotics, 265–271
  drug interactions with, 303
β-Lactamase inhibitors, 255
  indications for, 252*t*, 253
β-Lactamases
  and antimicrobial resistance, 213–214
  structural classes of, 213*t*
Lactic acidosis, 133
*Lactobacillus*/infection, antibiotic therapy for, 342
Laminin, 801
Lamivudine, 960–961
  dosage and administration, 963*t*
Laparotomy, exploratory, in evaluation of fever of unknown origin, 468
Larva, cutaneous, drug therapy for, 372*t*
Larva migrans, visceral, drug therapy for, 379*t*
Laryngitis, 519–521
  clinical manifestations of, 519
  diagnosis of, 519
  epidemiology of, 519
  etiology of, 519
  pathophysiology of, 519
  therapy, 519–521
Laryngotracheitis. *See* Croup
Lassa fever, 868, 869*t*
  treatment of, 714
Latency, 27
Latent state, 12
Latex agglutination tests, 139
Lazear, 5
LBP. *See* Lipopolysaccharide-binding protein
LCR. *See* Ligase chain reaction
Leeuwenhoek, Anton van, 1
*Legionella*/infection, antibiotic therapy for, 342
*Legionella pneumophila,* evasion of oxygen-dependent killing, 88–89
*Leishmania*/infection, 186*f*
  drug therapy for, 375*t*, 384
  and mononuclear phagocytes, 126
  specimen collection in, 187
  visceral
    rash in, 496
    in travelers to tropical countries, 870
*Leishmania donovani,* collection of, 187
Leprosy, 721
Leptospirosis
  antibiotic therapy for, 342
  and hemolytic anemia, 124
  rash in, 489
  in travelers to tropical countries, 871
*Leptotrichia buccalis,* antibiotic therapy for, 342
*Leuconostoc*/infection, antibiotic therapy for, 342
Leukemia
  chronic lymphocytic (CLL), IGIV for, 412
  and fever of unknown origin, 463
  hairy cell, HTLV-II and, 130
  viral infection and, 130
Leukocyte function antigen 1 (LFA-1), 96–97, 97*f*
Leukocytes, and infection, 124–126, 127*t*
Leukoencephalopathy, progressive multifocal (PML), in HIV infection, 946–947
Levamisole, therapeutic indications for, 431*t*
Levofloxacin
  dosage and administration, 329*t*
  drug interactions with, 333*t*
  indications for, 309
  pharmacokinetics of, 331*t*
  routes of elimination and adverse effects of, 332*t*
  spectrum and mechanism of activity, 328*t*
  spectrum of action, 307
LGV. *See* Lymphogranuloma venereum
Lice infestation, 897*f*, 897–898, 899*t*
Ligase chain reaction (LCR), 141–142, 142*t*
Ligation-activated transcription, 164–165
Lincomycin, resistance to, mechanisms of, 214
Line immunoassay, in diagnosis of HIV infection, 907
Lipid A, 25
Lipid metabolism, infection and, 134
Lipopolysaccharide-binding protein (LBP), 87
*Listeria*/infection
  entry into host cells, 25
  listeriolysin O, 25
*Listeria innocua,* virulence of, 19
*Listeria monocytogenes*/infection
  antibiotic therapy for, 342
  evasion of oxygen-dependent killing, 88
  incubating, 156
  meningitis, 689
  in organ transplant recipient, 827
  virulence of, 19
Lister, Joseph, 1, 14
Lithium, drug interactions with, 323
Liver aspirates, specimen collection from, 188
Liver cirrhosis, alcoholic, 855
Liver disease. *See also* Hepatitis
  granulomatous, 595–596, 596*t*
  parasitic, 37–38, 40*t*
Liver enzymes, elevated, in bone marrow transplant recipients, 834, 834*t*
Liver fluke, drug therapy for, 374*t*
Liver, in metabolism of antimicrobial agents, 218
*Loa loa*/infection
  collection of, 187
  drug therapy for, 373*t*

Loiasis, 495
Long, Perrin, 3
Long-term care, nosocomial infections in, 67
Loperamide, for diarrhea, 586–587
Ludwig's angina, 574, 574*f*, 768
Lung disease, chronic, vaccine use with, 424
Lung fluke, drug therapy for, 374*t*
Lungs
  in fever, 442–443
  infection of, parasitic, 40*t*, 41
Lyme disease, 891–892, 893*t*
  antibiotic therapy for, 338, 894*t*
  meningitis, 698–699
  ocular manifestations of, 740
  prevalence of, 56
  rash in, 489–490
Lyme radiculitis, 721
Lymphadenitis, infectious diseases with, 505–512
Lymphadenopathy
  axillary, 510–511
  cervical, 509–510, 510*f*
  clinical manifestations of, 509
  diagnosis of, 511–512
  distribution of, 508*t*
  epidemiology of, 505–506
  epitrochlear, 510–511
  etiology of, 505, 507*t*–508*t*
  with fever, 444
  generalized, 511
  host factors in, 506–507
  infectious causes of, 507*t*–508*t*
  infectious diseases with, 505–512
  inguinal, 511
  intraabdominal, 511
  intrathoracic, 511
  laboratory studies in, 511–512
  noninfectious causes of, 506*t*
  in travelers to tropical countries, diseases causing, 864*t*
  treatment of, 512
Lymphangitis, nodular, rash in, 494
Lymphatics, infection of, parasitic, 38–41, 40*t*
Lymph nodes, 94–95
  aspirates from, specimen collection from, 188
  biopsies of, in diagnosis of parasitic infection, 188
  cervical, 510*f*
  structure and function of, 506*f*
Lymphocytes
  HIV's effects on, 927
  and infection, 125
Lymphogranuloma venereum (LGV)
  clinical manifestations of, 662
  epidemiology of, 659
  pathogenesis of, 660
  ulceration in, 657
Lymphoid organs
  HIV infection and, 924–925
  secondary, 94–95
Lymphoma(s)
  B-cell, 935
  EBV infection and, 129
  and fever of unknown origin, 463
  in HIV infection, 940, 941*t*
  HIV infection and, 129–130
Lysogeny, 5

MAbs. *See* Monoclonal antibodies
MacConkey's agar, 156
Machupo virus, 868, 869*t*
Macrolides, 291–294
  administration of, 295*t*
  drug interactions with, 293
  indications for, 293–294
  mechanism of action, 291
  pharmacokinetics of, 292–293
  resistance to, 291
  spectrum of activity, 291–292
  structure of, 291
  toxicities of, 293
Macrophage colony-stimulating factor (MCSF), 428*t*
  therapeutic indications for, 430*t*
Macrophages, 10–11
  activation of, 11–12
  HIV's effects on, 929
Maculopapular lesions
  diffuse, systemic infections with, 485–490
  with herald plaque or initial eschar, 490–491
  systemic infections with, 484*t*
Mafenide acetate (Sulfamylon), 314
Magnetic resonance imaging
  of CNS, 111–112
  of head and neck, 112
  musculoskeletal, 113–114, 114*f*
  of sinuses, 112–113
  of spine, 113, 113*f*
Major histocompatibility complex (MHC), 11
Major histocompatibility loci, 93–94
Malaria, 3
  clinical manifestations of, 864
  diagnosis of, 864–866, 867*f*
  drug therapy for, 365–381, 375*t*–376*t*
  and fever in travelers to tropical countries, 861–867
  and hemolytic anemia, 124
  and malnutrition, 844
  parasites causing, differential diagnosis of, 190*t*
  prevention of, 381
  specimen collection in, 188
  treatment of, 866–867
*Malassezia*/infection, 47
*Malassezia furfur*/infection, 47, 48*t*
  drug therapy for, 403*t*
*Malassezia pachydermatis,* 47
Malignancies, cutaneous, in HIV infection, 955
Malnutrition
  epidemiology of, 841–842
  hospitalization for, 845, 845*t*
  and immune function, 840–841
  infectious complications of, 839–848
    diagnosis and management of, 845–847
    etiology and epidemiology of, 842–845
  protein-energy (PEM), 839
    public health and, 847, 847*t*
*Mansonella,* collection of, 187
*Mansonella ozzardi*/infection, drug therapy for, 373*t*
*Mansonella perstans*/infection, drug therapy for, 373*t*
Marburg virus, 497, 868, 869*t*
Mather, Cotton, 2
May-Hegglin bodies, 124, 125*f*
MCSF. *See* Macrophage colony-stimulating factor
Measles
  encephalitis
    clinical presentation in, 710
    epidemiology of, 710
    host response in, 710
  and malnutrition, 844, 844*f*
  oral sign of, 580
  rash in, 486
  vaccine for, 420*t*
Mebendazole (Vermox), 367*t*
  for intestinal nematodes, 385–386
Mechanical ventilation, for ARDS, 563
Media, for bacterial culture, 150–156
  liquid and solid, 156
Medications, and fever, 452, 452*t*–453*t*
Mediterranean spotted fever, laboratory diagnosis of, 196
Mefloquine, 365–380, 368*t*
Megaloblastic anemia, 122
Meglumine antimonate, 368*t*
  for leishmaniasis, 384
Melanocyte-stimulating hormone (MSH), and pyrogenic inhibition, 74
Melarsoprol, 368*t*
  for trypanosomiasis, 384–385
Meleney's synergistic gangrene, 767
Melioidosis, 496
  pulmonary cavitation in, 546
  in travelers to tropical countries, 871
Meningitis, 689–702
  amebic, aseptic, 697
  aseptic, 695–698, 696*t*
    clinical manifestations of, 697–698
    diagnosis of, 698
    epidemiology of, 697
    laboratory studies in, 698
    treatment of, 698
  bacterial, 689–695
    aseptic, 697

Meningitis (*continued*)
chronic, 698–699
clinical manifestations of, 690–691, 692*t*
diagnosis of, 691–692, 692*t*
epidemiology of, 689
etiology of, 689, 690*t*
laboratory studies in, 691
pathogenesis of, 689–690, 690*t*
therapy, 692–695, 693*f*
chronic, 698–701
clinical manifestations of, 700, 700*t*
diagnosis of, 700, 701*t*
etiologies of, 698–701
laboratory studies in, 700
treatment of, 701
*Coccidioides,* 50
cryptococcal, 44–45
etiologies of, 695–697
fungal, chronic, 699
in HIV infection, therapy for, 968–969
noninfectious, 697
chronic, 700
parasitic, chronic, 699
in travelers to tropical countries, diseases causing, 865*t*
viral, aseptic, 695–697
Meningococcal bacteremia, rash in, 493
Meningococcal disease, in travelers to tropical countries, 871
Meningococcemia
acute, rash in, 493
rash in, 489
Meningococcemia/meningitis syndrome, rash in, 489
Meningoencephalitis, amoebic, drug therapy for, 371*t*
Mentally retarded persons, residential institutions for, diarrhea in, 581
Mepacrine, 3
Meperidine, for fever, 78*t*
Meropenem, 267
Metabolic alterations, 133–134
Metabolism, 218
*Metagonimus yokogawai*/infection, drug therapy for, 374*t*
Metazoan infections, and eosinophilia, 126
Metchnikoff, Elie, 3
Methacycline, 299
Methenamine, 321–322
clinical experience with, 322
drug interactions with, 322
mechanism of action, 321
pharmacokinetics of, 321
physicochemical properties of, 321, 321*f*
spectrum of activity, 321
toxicity of, 321–322
Methicillin, 253
Methisazone, 4
Methotrexate, drug interactions with, 315
Methoxyflurane, drug interactions with, 301
Methylprednisolone, drug interactions with, 293
Metrifonate, 387
Metronidazole (Flagyl), 322–324, 368*t*
adverse effects of, 323
for amebiasis, 381–382
drug interactions with, 323
indications for, 323–324
mechanism of action, 322
pharmacokinetics of, 322–323
physicochemical properties of, 322, 322*f*
spectrum of activity, 323
for tissue nematodes, 387
toxicity of, 323
Mezlocillin, indications for, 252*t*
MH. *See* Hyperthermia, malignant
MHC. *See* Major histocompatibility complex
Miasmatists, 1
Miconazole, 393
for free living amoebae infection, 385
indications for, 393*t*
Microangiopathic disorder, 127
Microbial factors, 8*f*
and antimicrobial selection, 234
Microbial toxins, 9–10
Microfilaria, differential diagnosis of, 190*t*
Micronutrient deficiency, and immunity, 841
*Microspora*/infection, of burns, 793
Microsporidiosis
drug therapy for, 377*t*
hepatic, in HIV infection, 953–954
Microsulfon. *See* Sulfadiazine
MICs. *See* Minimal inhibitory concentrations
MIC testing, of aminoglycosides, 273–274
Minimal inhibitory concentrations (MICs), 220–221
of candidal organisms, to fluconazole, 43
Minocycline, 299
adverse effects of, 300
Mintezol. *See* Thiabendazole
Mites, diseases associated with, 896*t*, 896–897
*MMWR. See Morbidity and Mortality Weekly Report*
*Mobiluncus*/infection, vulvovaginitis, 681
Molds, characteristics of, 178
Molecular biology
of AIDS, 915–926
and pathophysiology, 5–6
Molecular viral detection tests, 164–167
in diagnosis of HIV infection, 907
specimen collection for, 161
Molluscum contagiosum
in HIV infection, 955
oral manifestations of, 580
Monkey bites, infections from, 888–889
Monobactams, 265, 268–270
Monoclonal antibodies (MAbs), 411, 412*t*
Monocytes, HIV's effects on, 929
Monocytic cells, and sepsis, 475–476
Mononeuritis multiplex, in HIV infection, 948*t*, 949
Mononuclear phagocytes
defects of, 810
and infection, 126
Mononucleosis
CMV. *See also* Cytomegalovirus/infection
rash in, 487
infectious, rash in, 487
Montagu, Mary Wortley, 2
*Moraxella catarrhalis,* antibiotic therapy for, 342
*Morbidity and Mortality Weekly Report (MMWR),* 56
*Morganella*/infection, antibiotic therapy for, 342
Morphine sulfate, for fever, 78*t*
Motility-inhibiting drugs, for diarrhea, 586–587
Moxalactam, applications, 260
MRI. *See* Magnetic resonance imaging
Mucocutaneous lesions, specimen collection from, 159–161
Mucocutaneous lymph node syndrome. *See* Kawasaki disease
*Mucor*/infection
of burns, 793
examination of, 171
Mucormycosis. *See* Zygomycosis
Mucous patches, 489
Multiple organ failure, 75
Multiplication, 8
of bacteria, in host cells, 25
Mumps, 580
arthritis in, 760, 760*t*
encephalitis
clinical presentation of, 710
epidemiology of, 710
host response in, 710
pathogenesis of, 710
vaccine for, 420*t*
Murine typhus, 197–198, 899*t*
antibiotic therapy for, 344
diseases associated with, 900
rash in, 488
Murray Valley encephalitis, 708
Muscle biopsies, in diagnosis of parasitic infection, 188
Musculoskeletal system
in fever, 445
imaging of, 113–114, 114*f*
Myalgia, 767
Mycobacteria
antibiotic therapy for, 347
atypical, and pulmonary disease, 549–550
imipenem for, 267
Mycobacterial infections
disseminated, rash in, 494
and fever of unknown origin, 460

nontuberculous, in HIV infection, 939–940, 941*t*
pulmonary cavitation in, 546–550
*Mycobacterium*/infection, and mononuclear phagocytes, 126
*Mycobacterium avium* complex
antibiotic therapy for, 347
drug therapy for, 334*t*
hepatic, in HIV infection, 953
in HIV infection, 939–940, 941*t*
therapy for, 972*t*–973*t*
in immunocompromised host, antibiotic therapy for, 347
*Mycobacterium avium-intracellulare* complex, 550
*Mycobacterium chelonae,* antibiotic therapy for, 347
*Mycobacterium fortuitum,* antibiotic therapy for, 347
*Mycobacterium kansasii*/infection, 550
antibiotic therapy for, 347
*Mycobacterium leprae,* antibiotic therapy for, 347–348
*Mycobacterium marinum,* antibiotic therapy for, 347
*Mycobacterium tuberculosis*/infection. *See also* Tuberculosis
antibiotic therapy for, 348
antimicrobial resistance in, 212
drug therapy for, 334*t*
evasion of phagocytosis, 87
incubating, 156
invasion of endocrine organs, 134
in organ transplant recipient, 827
osteomyelitis, 741
therapy for, 754
resistant, 57
salpingitis, 684
Mycology, clinical, 169–180
*Mycoplasma*/infection, 5
rash in, 488–489
*Mycoplasma hominis*/infection
antibiotic therapy for, 342
vulvovaginitis, 681
*Mycoplasma pneumoniae,* antibiotic therapy for, 343
Mycoses
deep, drug therapy for, 397–404
deep endemic, epidemiology of, 550*t*
pulmonary, 550–553
Myelodysplastic syndromes, and fever of unknown origin, 463
Myelopathy, 715–719, 716*t*
definition of, 715
infectious, 716–719, 717*t*
transverse, 715–716, 716*f*
Myelopoietic growth factors, 429–432
Myiasis, 898–900, 899*t*
furuncular, 898–900
Myocardial infarction, and fever, in hospitalized patient, 450
Myocarditis, 643–648
cardiac abnormalities in, 643
clinical manifestations of, 645–646, 646*t*
definition of, 643
epidemiology of, 645
etiology of, 643, 644*t*
laboratory studies in, 646–648
management of, 648
pathogenesis of, 643–645
prognosis for, 648
Myonecrosis, 769
Myopathy, in HIV infection, 949, 949*t*
Myopericarditis, 643
viral, 643–644
Myositis, 767–771
Myxoedematous coma, 135
Myxomatosis, 5
Myxoma virus, and immune system, 33

*Naegleria*/infection, drug therapy for, 371*t*, 385
Nafcillin, 253
indications for, 252*t*
*Nanophyetus salmincola*/infection, drug therapy for, 374*t*
Nasal wash, 159
NASBA. *See* Nucleic acid sequence-based amplification
Nasopharyngeal swab, 159
National Nosocomial Infections Surveillance system (NNIS), 57, 62
National Notifiable Diseases Surveillance System (NNDSS), 55
Natural killer (NK) cells, 107, 107*f*
HIV's effects on, 929
response to HIV, 931
viral infection and, 34
NBP. *See* Prostatitis, nonbacterial
NBTE. *See* Endocarditis, nonbacterial thrombotic
*Necator americanus*/infection
drug therapy for, 374*t*
and iron-deficiency anemia, 121
Neck
in fever, 444
imaging of, 112
Negative selection, 94
*Neisseria gonorrhoeae*/infection
antibiotic therapy for, 343
antimicrobial resistance in, 210
arthritis, 757–758
cervicitis, 382
culturing, 150
endocarditis, 623
pathogenic strategies of, 20
pili of, 7
resistant, 57
salpingitis, 684
urethritis, 669
*Neisseria meningitidis*/infection
antibiotic therapy for, 343
antimicrobial resistance in, 210
meningitis, 689
vaccine for, 417*t*
Nematodes, 38, 39*t*
intestinal, drug therapy for, 385–386
tissue, drug therapy for, 386–387
Neomycin, 273
for free living amoebae infection, 385
Neonatal intensive care units (NICUs), nosocomial infection in, 66–67
Neoplasms
associated with HIV infection, 935–936
and fever of unknown origin, 463–464, 464*t*
Neoplastic disease, and meningitis, 700
Nephrotoxic agents, aminoglycosides, 277–278
Netilmicin, 273
dosage and administration, 283*t*
for children, 282*t*
Neurocysticercosis
drug therapy for, 378*t*
meningitis, 699
Neuroendocrine abnormalities, chronic fatigue syndrome and, 777
Neuroleptic malignant syndrome (NMS), 76
Neurological symptoms, in fever, 446
Neurologic disease, in HIV infection, 944–945
therapy for, 967*t*, 967–968
Neurologic imaging, in encephalitis, 711
Neurologic reactions, to antimicrobial agents, 228
Neuromuscular blockade, aminoglycosides and, 279
Neuropathy, 716*t*, 719–721
definition of, 715
infectious, 720–721, 721*t*
peripheral, in HIV infection, 947–949, 948*t*–949*t*
Neurovirulence, 703
Neutropenia, febrile, empiric therapy in, 814, 836
Neutrophilia, 124
Neutrophils, and sepsis, 475
Nevirapine, 961–962
dosage and administration, 963*t*
Newborn
humoral immunity and, 104
IGIV prophylaxis in, 413
osteomyelitis in, 743–744
Nezelof's syndrome, 123
Niclosamide, 368*t*
for cestodes, 387
NICUs. *See* Neonatal intensive care units
Nifurtimox, 368*t*
for trypanosomiasis, 385
Nitric oxide (NO)
for ARDS, 564
and sepsis, 475
Nitrofurantoin, 319–321
adverse effects of, 320

Nitrofurantoin (*continued*)
drug interactions with, 320
indications for, 320–321
mechanism of action, 319
pharmacokinetics of, 319
physicochemical properties of, 319, 320*f*
spectrum of activity, 319
toxicity of, 319–320, 320*t*
NMS. *See* Neuroleptic malignant syndrome
NNDSS. *See* National Notifiable Diseases Surveillance System
NNIS. *See* National Nosocomial Infections Surveillance System
NO. *See* Nitric oxide
*Nocardia*/infection
clinical manifestations of, 546
diagnosis of, 546
gram stain and, 149, 150*f*
pathogenesis of, 546
pulmonary cavitation in, 546
treatment of, 546
*Nocardia asteroides*
antibiotic therapy for, 343
in organ transplant recipient, 827
*Nocardia brasiliensis,* antibiotic therapy for, 343
Nodular lesions, systemic infections with, 486*t*, 493–495
Noguchi, 5
Noma, 576, 576*f*
Nonimmune-mediated hemolysis, 124
Nonnucleoside analogue reverse transcriptase inhibitors, 4
Nonprogressors, 925
Nonself, 91
Norfloxacin, indications for, 309
Normal flora, 7, 8*t*
North Asian tick-borne rickettsiosis, 197
Nose, in fever, 444
Nosocomial infections, 61–70
and antimicrobial resistance, 57
control of, 67–69
definition of, 61
distribution of, by site and pathogen, 62*t*, 62–63, 63*f*
epidemiology of, 61
recent developments in, 67–69
risk factors for, 61
surveillance of, 61–62
transmission of, 61
in special settings, 66–67
NSAIDs, for fever, 78*t*, 79
Nuclear imaging, 118–119
of nonosseous infection, 119
of osseous infection, 118*f*, 119
Nucleic acid-amplification methods, 141–142, 142*t*
Nucleic acid-based tests, 139–141, 177–178
Nucleic acid-detection techniques, 150, 164
Nucleic acid metabolism, and antimicrobial resistance, 212–213
Nucleic acid probe, in pneumonia, 535
Nucleic acid sequence-based amplification (NASBA), 141–142, 142*t*, 164
Nucleic acid synthesis, enzymes of, antimicrobial action and, 210
Nucleoside analogue inhibitors, 4
Nutritional assessment, 845

Obstetric patients, hospital-acquired fever in, 455
Occupational settings, infections acquired in, 54*t*
Occupation, and fever, 439
Ockelbo disease, 760, 760*t*
Ocular infections, 733–740
in HIV infection, 943–944, 944*t*
Odynophagia, in HIV infection, therapy for, 970
Ofloxacin
drug interactions with, 311
indications for, 309
spectrum of action, 308
*Onchocerca volvulus*/infection, drug therapy for, 373*t*
Onchocerciasis, 495
O'nyong-nyong fever, 497, 760, 760*t*
OPAT. *See* Outpatient intravenous antibiotic therapy
Ophthalmia neonatorum, 736
*Opisthorchis viverrini*/infection, drug therapy for, 374*t*
Opportunistic pathogens, 7
in AIDS. *See* Acquired immunodeficiency syndrome, opportunistic infections in
Opsonization, 3, 86–87
in absence of antibody and complement, 87
antibodies and, 87
microbial resistance to, 87
Oral contraceptives, drug interactions with, 301
Oral fluid-electrolyte therapy, for diarrhea, 586
Oral infections, 573–580
in HIV infection, 951–952
intracranial spread of, 577
Oral rehydration treatment (ORT), for diarrhea, 876
administration of, 877*t*
Orbital infections, 738*f*, 738–739
Orchitis, 673–675
clinical manifestations of, 674–675
diagnosis of, 675
epidemiology of, 674
etiologies of, 674, 674*t*
host factors in, 674
laboratory studies in, 675
pathogenesis of, 674
treatment of, 675
Organomegaly, in travelers to tropical countries, diseases causing, 864*t*
Organ-specific infections, parasitic, 37–41
Organ transplantation, immunosuppression in, pathogenesis of, 821, 822*t*
Organ transplant recipients, infection in, 821–828
epidemiology of, 822, 822*t*
therapy for, 827–828
timetable of, 822–824, 823*t*
Oriental spotted fever, rash in, 490
Ornidazole, 368*t*
Oropouche, 869*t*
Orthomyxovirus encephalitis, 711
Orthopedic devices, infections associated with, 803–804
treatment and prophylaxis of, 803–804, 804*t*
Osteomyelitis, 741–756
classification of, 741, 742*t*, 753
clinical manifestations of, 743–746
definition of, 741
diagnosis of, 746
epidemiology of, 742
etiology of, 741, 742*t*
and fever of unknown origin, 463
history and physical examination in, 745
host factors in, 742*t*, 743
host improvement in, 745, 745*t*
imipenem for, 267
laboratory studies in, 745–746
microbiologic documentation in, 746
oral, 577
pathophysiology of, 743, 743*f*–744*f*
prevention of, 754
signs and symptoms of, 743–745, 745*f*
source of infection in, 741, 742*t*
stage 1, 741, 747*f*
treatment of, 747–748, 749*f*, 753
stage 2, treatment of, 748, 750*f*, 753
stage 3, treatment of, 748, 751*f*, 753
stage 4, treatment of, 748, 752*f*, 753
treatment of, 745*t*, 746–754
antimicrobial, 746–748, 748*t*
secondary to contiguous focus infection with vascular diseases, 753–754
surgical, 748–753
vertebral, 754–755
diagnosis of, 754–755
therapy, 755
Osteoradionecrosis, 577
Otitis, 521–522
clinical manifestations of, 521
diagnosis of, 521
epidemiology of, 521
etiology of, 521
pathogenesis of, 521
therapy for, 521–522
Ototoxic agents, aminoglycosides, 279

Outbreaks
definition of, 53
recognition of, practitioner's role in, 57
Outpatient intravenous antibiotic therapy (OPAT), 241–244
antibiotic selection for, 242–243, 243*t*
models for, 241–242, 242*t*
monitoring, 243–244, 244*t*
patient selection for, 241, 242*t*
types of infection and, 242
Oxacillin, indications for, 252*t*
Oxamniquine, 368*t*, 387
Oxygen-dependent killing, 88
microbial evasion of, 88–89
Oxygen-independent killing, 89
Oxygen therapy, for ARDS, 563
Oxytetracycline, 299

Pacemakers, infections associated with, 804–806
PAE. *See* Postantibiotic effect
*Paecilomyces lilacinus*/infection, drug therapy for, 403*t*
PAF. *See* Platelet activating factor
Pancreatic abscess, definition of, 606
Pancreatic fat necrosis, 495
Pancreatitis
diagnosis of, 605, 606*t*
infected versus uninfected, 606, 607*f*, 607*t*
infectious complications of, 605–611
antimicrobial treatment of, 607–609
management of, 608*f*, 610
microbiology of, 607, 609*f*
operative treatment of, 609–610
and nosocomial infections, 606
Pancytopenia, secondary to infection, 128
Pandemic, definition of, 53
Panniculitis, factitial, 495
Papulosquamous disorders, in HIV infection, 955
Paracetamol. *See* Acetaminophen
Paracoccidioidomycosis, 49*t*, 51
drug therapy for, 400*t*, 402
pulmonary, epidemiology of, 550*t*
rash in, 496
in travelers to tropical countries, 872
Paragonimiasis, in travelers to tropical countries, 868–870
*Paragonimus*/infection, collection of, 187
*Paragonimus westermani*/infection, drug therapy for, 374*t*
Parainfectious, definition of, 715
Paramyxoviruses, encephalitis, 710
diagnosis of, 713
prevention of, 714
Parapneumonic effusion, 565
Parasites, 37–42
characteristics of, 190*t*–192*t*
Parasitic infections
arthritis, 760
and cavitary lung disease, 554
diagnosis of, 182*t*–185*t*
diagnostic methods for, 181–193
and diarrhea, 582
drug therapy for, 365–388, 366*t*–379*t*
and fever of unknown origin, 463
intestinal, and malnutrition, 843
meningitis, 699
myocarditis/pericarditis, 645
oral, 580
rash in, 490
serologies in, 192
tests done at CDC, 189*t*
Parasitism, definition of, 37
Parasitology, clinical, 181–193
Paratyphoid fever, in travelers to tropical countries, 867
Paromomycin, 368*t*, 383–384
Paroxysmal cold hemoglobinuria (PCH), 123
Parvovirus $B_{19}$ infection, 122, 759, 760*t*
Parvoviruses, 122
Passive vaccines, 14
*Pasteurella multocida*/infection
of animal bites, 887
antibiotic therapy for, 343
*Pasteurella* toxin, 24
Pasteur, Louis, 1–3
Past illness, and fever, 442–443
Pathogens
discovery of, 1
interactions with host, fever and, 74*t*, 74–75
intracellular digestion of, 89
intracellular, imipenem for, 266–267
killing, by PMN, 88–89
specific tests for, 137–139
specific therapy for, 3–4
PBPs. *See* Penicillin-binding proteins
PCH. *See* Paroxysmal cold hemoglobinuria
PCR. *See* Polymerase chain reaction
PDH. *See* Histoplasmosis, progressive disseminated
Peak/MIC ratio, 220–221
Pediatric intensive care units (PICUs), nosocomial infections in, 67
Pediatric units, nosocomial infection in, 66
Pediculosis, 897–898
PEEP. *See* Positive end-expiratory pressure
Pelvic examination, in fever, 445
Pelvic infections, imipenem for, 267
Pelvic inflammatory disease (salpingitis), 683–686
classification of, 686, 686*t*
clinical features of, 685
control of, 686–687
diagnostic criteria for, 685
epidemiology of, 684
etiology of, 683–684
host factors in, 684
management of, 685–686, 686*t*
pathogenesis of, 684–685
PEM. *See* Malnutrition, protein-energy
Penems, 265–268
indications for, 267
mechanism of action, 265
pharmacology of, 267–268
resistance to, 265–266
spectrum of action, 266–267
structure of, 265, 266*f*
toxicity, 268
Penicillin(s), 249–256
adverse reactions to, 255–256
allergic-hypersensitivity reactions to, 225
chemistry of, 249, 250*f*
discovery of, 3–4, 249
G, 252–253
indications for, 252, 252*t*
mechanism of action, 249, 250*f*–251*f*
natural, 252–253
penicillinase-resistant, 253
pharmacokinetics of, 251
resistance to, 250
spectrum of activity, 252
Penicillin-binding proteins (PBPs), 257, 265
*Penicillium*/infection, 3, 50
*Penicillium marneffei*/infection, 50
drug therapy for, 403*t*
Pentamidine, 368*t*
for free living amoebae infection, 385
for leishmaniasis, 384
for *Pneumocystic carinii* pneumonia, 383
for trypanosomiasis, 384
Pentavalent antimony, for leishmaniasis, 384
Peptic ulcer, perforated, 618
Peptidoglycan, 19
synthesis of, 209
*Peptococcus*/infection, of burns, 792
*Peptostreptococcus*/infection, antibiotic therapy for, 343
Percutaneous needle aspirates, collection and transportation, 145
Perforated peptic ulcer, 618
Periapical disease, 573–574
Pericardial constriction, 643
Pericardial tamponade, 643
Pericarditis, 643–648
cardiac abnormalities in, 643
clinical manifestations of, 645–646, 646*t*
definition of, 643
epidemiology of, 645
etiology of, 643, 644*t*
laboratory studies in, 646–648
pathogenesis of, 643–645
prognosis for, 648
pyogenic, 644–645
treatment of, 648
treatment of, 646*t*, 648
tuberculous, 645
viral, treatment of, 648
Pericoronitis, 576

Perinatal transmission, of HIV, 910
reduction of, 912
Periocular infections, 733–740
Periodontal abscess, 576
Periodontal disease, 574–576
in HIV infection, 952
immunology in, 575
microbiology of, 575
prevention of, 576
treatment of, 575–576
Periorbital abscess, 574, 575*f*
Peripheral venous catheters, and infection, 638
Peritoneal abscess, computed tomography of, 116, 117*f*
Peritonitis, 613–619
CAPD, aminoglycosides for, 281, 281*t*
definition of, 613
primary
clinical manifestations of, 613
definition of, 613
pathogenesis of, 613
treatment of, 613
secondary
clinical manifestations of, 614, 614*f*
definition of, 613
diagnosis of, 614
outcome in, 616
pathogenesis of, 613–614
treatment of, 614–616, 617*t*
spontaneous, alcohol abuse and, 856
tertiary, 616–617
definition of, 613
Pertussis toxin, 24
Pertussis, vaccine for, 417*t*
Petechial-purpuric rash, systemic infections with, 485*t*, 493
*P. falciparum,* 186*f*
Pfeiffer's cells, 125, 126*f*
Phaeohypomycosis, 47–50
Phaeosporotrichosis. *See* Phaeohypomycosis
Phagocytes
disorders of
acquired, 810
and infection, 811–812
primary, 810
in host defense, 85*f*, 85–86
Phagocytosis, 87, 95
bacterial-secreted inhibitors of, 26
microbial evasion of, 87–88
Phagolysosomes, 95
Pharmacodynamics, 220–221
Pharmacoeconomics, 237–238, 238*t*, 246
Pharmacokinetics, definition of, 217
Pharyngitis, 517–518
clinical manifestations of, 517–518, 518*t*
diagnosis of, 518
epidemiology of, 517
etiology of, 517
pathophysiology of, 517
therapy for, 518
Phenazopyridine, 313
Phenobarbital, drug interactions with, 303
Phenytoin, drug interactions with, 300, 303, 315, 320
Pheochromocytoma
and fever of unknown origin, 466
and hyperthermia, 76
Phycomycosis, 738–739
Physical therapy, for infected animal bites, 887
Picornaviruses, encephalitis, 710–711
Pilus, 21
Pinworms *(Enterobius vermicularis),* 37
Piperacillin, 254
indications for, 252*t*
Piperacillin-tazobactam, 255
Piperazine, 368*t*
for intestinal nematodes, 386
Pityriasis rosea, rash in, 490
Pivampicillin, 253–254
PKR. *See* Protein kinase
Place of origin
and fever, 439–440
and infection, 441*t*
Plague, 899*t*
antibiotic therapy for, 347
diseases associated with, 900
in travelers to tropical countries, 871
vaccine for, 417*t*
Plaquenil. *See* Hydroxychloroquine sulfate
Plasma protein binding, and distribution of antimicrobials, 218
*Plasmodium*/infection, drug therapy for, 375*t*–376*t*
*Plasmodium malariae*/infection, nephrotic syndrome associated with, 41
Platelet activating factor (PAF), and sepsis, 475
Plate media, 156
Platyhelminths, classification of, 39*t*
*Plesiomonas shigelloides,* antibiotic therapy for, 343
Pleura
definition of, 565
parietal, 565
visceral, 565
Pleural effusions
clinical manifestations of, 567–568
definition of, 565
differential diagnosis of, 566*t*
epidemiology of, 565, 566*t*
exudative, 566–567, 567*f*
pathophysiology of, 565–567
transudative, 565–566
Pleural lavage, 571
Pleural space drainage, 571
Pleurisy, 565–572
clinical manifestations of, 567–568
definition of, 565
diagnosis of, 568–570
management of, 571
microbiological findings in, 569*t*, 569–570, 570*t*
physical findings in, 568
presentation of, 567–568
Pleuritis. *See* Pleurisy
PML. *See* Leukoencephalopathy, progressive multifocal
PMN. *See* Polymorphonuclear leukocytes
*Pneumococcus*/infection, gram stain and, 149, 149*f*
*Pneumocystic carinii*/infection, 186*f*
drug therapy for, 377*t*
examination of, 171
and fever of unknown origin, 463
invasion of endocrine organs, 134
*Pneumocystic carinii* pneumonia
in AIDS, 950, 950*t*, 950*f*
drug therapy for, 382–383, 965, 972*t*
in organ transplant recipient, 826
Pneumonia
acute, 529–537
antigen detection in, 534–535
aspiration, pyogenic lung abscess in, 541*f*, 541–543
bacterial
cavitary lung disease in, 541
in HIV infection, 951
in bone marrow transplant recipients, 833–834
burns and, 789
chest radiography in, 532, 533*f*–534*f*
clinical manifestations of, 531–532
community-acquired, 530
approach to, 530*f*
etiology of, 530, 531*t*
management of, 535–536
epidemiology of, 530–531
in HIV infection, therapy for, 965–967
host defenses and, 529
in immunocompromised host, 531, 531*t*
management of, 537
with T-cell deficiency, 814–818
in intravenous drug user, 851
isolation of organism in, 532–534
laboratory studies in, 532–535
management of, 535–537
necrotizing gram-negative
clinical manifestations of, 544, 544*f*
diagnosis of, 544–545
pathogenesis of, 544
treatment of, 545
nosocomial, 65–66, 530–531
management of, 536–537
risk factors for, 64*t*, 66
nucleic acid probe in, 535
nursing home, 531
pathogenesis of, 529–530
physical examination in, 532
pneumococcal, 545
post-traumatic, 799
prevention of, 537
serology in, 535

staphylococcal
clinical manifestations of, 543
diagnosis of, 543
pathogenesis of, 543
treatment of, 543
symptoms of, 531–532
Poliomyelitis
and myelopathy, 716–718
vaccination for, 5
Polioviruses, vaccine for, 420*t*–421*t*
Political factors, and HIV spread, 910
Polymerase chain reaction (PCR), 141–142, 142*t*, 164–165
in diagnosis of murine typhus, 198
in diagnosis of Rocky Mountain spotted fever, 196
Polymorphic rash, systemic infections with, 485*t*
Polymorphonuclear leukocytes (PMN), 10, 85*f*, 85–86
chemotaxis of, 86
defects of, 810
diapedesis of, 85–86, 86*f*
intracellular digestion of microbes, 89
killing of microorganisms, 88–89
kinetics of, 85
malnutrition and, 841
in phagocytosis, 87–88
in regulation of inflammatory response, 89–90
Polymyxins, 324
Polyneuropathy
distal sensory, in HIV infection, 947–949, 948*t*–949*t*
inflammatory demyelinating, in HIV infection, 948*t*, 949
Polypeptides, antimycobacterial uses of, 330
Polyradiculopathy, lumbosacral, in HIV infection, 948*t*, 949
Pore-forming proteins, 24–25
Portal of entry, 7
Positive end-expiratory pressure (PEEP), for ARDS, 563
Positive selection, 94
Postantibiotic effect (PAE), 221, 221*t*
Poverty, and HIV spread, 910
Practitioners
in control and prevention of infectious diseases, 57–58
relationship to other partners/organizations, 58
Praziquantel, 369*t*
for trematodes/cestodes, 387
Prednisone, immunosuppression by, 821
Pregnancy
and antimicrobial selection, 234
safety of antibiotics in, 229*t*, 229–230
vaccine use in, 424
Prekallikrein, 474–475
Preterm infants, vaccine use in, 425
Primaquine, 369*t*, 380–381
for *Pneumocystic carinii* pneumonia, 383
Probe amplification, 165
Probe amplification methods, 141–142, 142*t*
Probenecid, drug interactions with, 315
Proglottides, collection and transportation of, 189
Proguanil (chloroguanide), 369*t*, 380
Prontosil, 313
Prontosil red, 3
Proofreading, 209
Propamidine, 369*t*
for free living amoebae infection, 385
*Propionibacterium acnes,* antibiotic therapy for, 343
Prostaglandin $E_1$, for ARDS, 564
Prostatitis, 675–678, 676*t*
acute bacterial (ABP), 675, 676*t*, 676–677
chronic bacterial (CBP), 675, 676*t*, 677–678
host factors in, 675–676
nonbacterial, 675, 676*t*
nonbacterial (NBP), 678
pathogenesis of, 675–676
Prostatodynia, 675, 676*t*, 678
Prosthetic device infections, 801–808
Protease inhibitors, 4, 962
Protein kinase (PKR), 33
Protein metabolism, infection and, 134
*Proteus*/infection
acute bacterial prostatitis, 676
antimicrobial resistance in, 213
toxin, 24
of urinary tract, 650
*Proteus mirabilis*
antibiotic therapy for, 343
antimicrobial resistance in, 212
*Proteus vulgaris,* antibiotic therapy for, 344
Proton density-weighted magnetic resonance imaging, 111
Protozoa
classification of, 37, 38*t*
cysts of, characteristics of, 190*t*
global burden of illness due to, 38*t*
immune response to, 97*t*
infections of
diagnosis of, 41*t*, 41–42
organ-specific, 37–41
parasitic, 37–42
pathogenesis of, 38–41
Protozoal infections
intestinal
in AIDS, drug therapy for, 383–384
drug therapy for, 381–382
systemic, drug therapy for, 365–381
in travelers to tropical countries, 870
*Providencia*/infection, antibiotic therapy for, 344
*Pseudallescheria boydii,* 50
pulmonary infection of, 554
Pseudallescheriasis, drug therapy for, 403, 403*t*
Pseudocavitation, 540
Pseudocyst
definition of, 606
infected, definition of, 606
*Pseudomonas*/infection
antimicrobial resistance in, 213
of burns, 789, 792
exotoxin A, 24
prostatitis, 676–677
of urinary tract, 650
*Pseudomonas aeruginosa*/infection
antibiotic therapy for, 344
antimicrobial agents for, 254
antimicrobial resistance in, 214, 305
arthritis, 758
culturing, 156
dissemination of, 9
endocarditis, 623
nosocomial, 62
in nosocomial bloodstream infection, 65
in nosocomial pneumonia, 66
in nosocomial UTIs, 63
osteomyelitis, 742*t*
pathogenic strategies of, 20
rash in, 489, 492
*Pseudomonas aeruginosa* IGIV, 413
*Pseudomonas mallei,* antibiotic therapy for, 344
*Pseudomonas pseudomallei,* antibiotic therapy for, 344
Psittacosis, rash in, 488–489
Psoriasis
in HIV infection, 955
pustular, 492
Psychiatric disorders, and chronic fatigue syndrome, 775
Pubic lice, 898
Public health
and emerging infectious diseases, 56–57
and protein-energy malnutrition, 847, 847*t*
syndromes and agents affecting, 58*t*
Puerperal sepsis, 1, 3
Pulmonary diseases
cavitary, 539–555
in HIV infection, 949–951, 950*t*
Pulmonary embolism
and fever, in hospitalized patient, 451
septic, 543–544, 544*f*
Pulmonary fibroproliferation, complicating ARDS, and fever in hospitalized patient, 451
Pulmonary infections, alcohol abuse and, 855
Pulmonary infiltrates
diffuse, 557–564
in immunocompromised host, 815–818, 818*f*
infectious causes of, 558–560, 559*t*
in HIV infection, therapy for, 965
in immunocompromised host, 815, 816*f*

Pulmonary symptoms, with fever, 442
Pulpitis, 573
Pulse, and fever, 443
Pure red cell aplasia, 122–123
pathogenesis of, 122–123
Pustular psoriasis, 492
Pyelonephritis, acute
clinical manifestations of, 652
treatment of, 654, 655*t*
Pylephlebitis, 641
Pyoderma gangrenosum, 492
Pyogenic lung abscess, with aspiration pneumonia, 541–543
clinical manifestations of, 542
complications of, 542
diagnosis of, 542
pathogenesis of, 541*f*, 541–542
treatment of, 542
Pyomyositis, 767
Pyrantel pamoate, 369*t*
for intestinal nematodes, 386
Pyrazinamide
dosage and administration, 329*t*
drug interactions with, 333*t*
pharmacokinetics of, 331*t*
routes of elimination and adverse effects of, 332*t*
spectrum and mechanism of activity, 328*t*
for tuberculosis, 327
Pyrimethamine, 369*t*, 380
for toxoplasmosis, 383
Pyrogens, 71–74, 73*t*
endogenous, 73–74
exogenous, 73

Q fever, 198–199
rash in, 488
vaccine for, 418*t*
Qinghaosu. *See* Artemisinin
Q$\beta$ replicase system, 141–142, 142*t*
Queensland tick fever, 197
rash in, 490
Quinacrine, for giardiasis, 382
Quinacrine HCL, 369*t*
Quinidine, 369*t*, 380
Quinine, 369*t*, 380
Quinolones, drug interactions with, 320

RA. *See* Rheumatoid arthritis
Rabies
encephalitis
clinical presentation in, 709
diagnosis of, 712–713
epidemiology of, 708
host responses to, 709
pathogenesis of, 709
prevention of, 714
prophylaxis, for infected animal bites, 887
vaccine for, 420*t*
Race, and chronic fatigue syndrome, 775
Radiculopathy, 716*t*, 719–721
definition of, 715
infectious, 720*t*, 720–721
Radiography
in osteomyelitis, 746
in pleurisy, 568, 568*f*–569*f*
in pneumonia, 532, 533*f*–534*f*, 535
Radionuclide scanning, in evaluation of fever of unknown origin, 467
Ramsay Hunt syndrome, 720
Ranitidine, drug interactions with, 311
Rapamycin, immunosuppression by, 821
Rapid detection, 137–144, 164
of CSF pathogens, 140*t*
of enteric pathogens, 139*t*
of genital pathogens, 139*t*
of respiratory pathogens, 138*t*
Rapid EIA tests, in diagnosis of HIV infection, 905–906
Rash
infections with, 483–499
clinical manifestations of, 485–492
diagnosis of, 497–499
etiologies of, 483, 484*t*–487*t*
history in, 497, 498*t*
laboratory studies in, 498–499
physical examination in, 497–498
in travelers, 486*t*–487*t*, 495–497
pathogenesis of, 485
Rat-bite fever, 888
antibiotic therapy for, 345
rash in, 489
spirillum minus, rash in, 491
Receptor theory, 3
Rectal biopsies, in diagnosis of parasitic infection, 188–189
Rectal examination, in fever, 445
Rectal swab (RS), 159
Reduced accumulation, and antimicrobial resistance, 214
Reed, Walter, 5
Regulatory T cells, 92, 105–106, 106*f*
and infection, 407
Regulons, 20
Reiter's syndrome, 584, 762–765
in HIV infection, 955
host factors in, 757
Relapsing fever, 440, 892–893, 895*f*
antibiotic therapy for, 894*t*
rash in, 489
in travelers to tropical countries, 871
Renal disease, vaccines with, 423, 423*t*
Renal insufficiency
antimicrobial dosages in, 218–219, 219*t*–220*t*
aztreonam dosages in, 270
flucytosine dosages in, 391
fluoroquinolone dosages in, 308–309
penem/carbapenem dosages in, 268, 268*t*
Renal reactions, to antimicrobial agents, 228–229
Renoquid. *See* Sulfacytine
Reovirus infection, encephalitis, 708
Reservoir, 7
Residence, and fever, 439–440
Residential institutions for mentally retarded persons, diarrhea in, 581
Resolution, 12
Respiration, and fever, 443
Respiratory infections, and malnutrition, 843
Respiratory pathogens, detection of, 138*t*
Respiratory syncytial virus IGIV, 413
Respiratory tract infections
fluoroquinolones for, 309–311
lower, imipenem for, 267
trimethoprim/sulfamethoxazole for, 316–317
upper, 513–522
pathogens in, 514*t*
Respiratory tract, specimen collection from, 146–147, 159, 187
Response regulator proteins, 20–21
Retinitis, 737
in HIV infection, 944, 944*t*
therapy for, 971
viral, 737
Retroviruses, 915–916, 916*t*
and immune system, 33
infection of cells, 32
Reverse transcriptase inhibitors, 959–961
nonnucleoside, 961–962
Rewarming techniques, 80
Reye's syndrome, 79
Rheumatic fever
acute, 495
acute (ARF), 765
Rheumatoid arthritis (RA), 765
Rhinitis, acute, 513–515
clinical manifestations of, 514
diagnosis of, 514–515
epidemiology of, 513
etiology of, 513, 514*t*
host factors in, 513–514
pathophysiology of, 514
treatment of, 515
*Rhizopus*/infection
of burns, 793
examination of, 171, 175*f*
*Rhodococcus bronchialis*/infection, of surgical wounds, 784
*Rhodococcus equi,* antibiotic therapy for, 344
*Rhodotorula*/infection, 47
Ribavirin (Virazole), 354*t*, 361–362
Ribosome, bacterial
agents acting on, 209
and antimicrobial resistance, 212
*Rickettsia conorii,* in Boutonneuse fever, 196
Rickettsia, laboratory diagnosis of, 195, 196*t*–197*t*
Rickettsial disease, rash in, 488, 490–491
Rickettsial diseases
laboratory diagnosis of, 195–201

in travelers to tropical countries, 868
Rickettsial-like diseases, epidemiologic features of, 199*t*
Rickettsialpox, 197
rash in, 490
*Rickettsia prowazekii,* antibiotic therapy for, 344
*Rickettsia rickettsii*
antibiotic therapy for, 344
in Rocky Mountain spotted fever, 195
*Rickettsia tsutsugamushi*
antibiotic therapy for, 344
in scrub typhus, 198
*Rickettsia typhi*
antibiotic therapy for, 344
in murine typhus, 197–198
*Rickettsii prowazekii,* in epidemic typhus, 198
Rifabutin
dosage and administration, 329*t*
drug interactions with, 333*t*
pharmacokinetics of, 331*t*
routes of elimination and adverse effects of, 332*t*
spectrum and mechanism of activity, 328*t*
Rifampin
dosage and administration, 329*t*
drug interactions with, 293, 303, 333*t*
pharmacokinetics of, 331*t*
routes of elimination and adverse effects of, 332*t*
spectrum and mechanism of activity, 328*t*
spectrum of activity, 327
for tuberculosis, 327
Rifamycins, antimycobacterial uses of, 330
Rift Valley fever, 497
Rimantadine (Flumadine), 353*t*, 360–361
mechanism of action, 32
Risk factors, 13–14
Ritonavir, 962
dosage and administration, 963*t*
RMSF. *See* Rocky Mountain spotted fever (RMSF)
RNA viruses, positive single-stranded, infection of cells by, 32
Roberts, William, 3
Rocky Mountain spotted fever (RMSF), 893
antibiotic therapy for, 344, 894*t*
laboratory diagnosis of, 195–196
rash in, 488
Roseola infantum, rash in, 487
Ross River fever, 497
Rotavirus, vaccine for, 421*t*
Roxithromycin, 291
Royal Society, 2
RS. *See* Rectal swab
Rubella virus/infection
arthritis, 760, 760*t*
congenital syndrome of, 493
rash in, 485
vaccine for, 421*t*
in pregnancy, 424
Rush, Benjamin, 853

*Saccharomyces*/infection, 47
St. Louis encephalitis (SLE), 708
Salicylates, drug interactions with, 315
*Salmonella*/infection
antibiotic therapy for, 344
arthritis, 758
endocarditis, 623
entry into host cells, 25
evasion of phagocytosis, 87
and reactive arthritis, 757, 764
virulence of, 19
*Salmonella typhi,* antibiotic therapy for, 344
*Salmonella typhimurium,* evasion of oxygen-dependent killing, 88
Salmonellosis, prevalence of, 56
Salpingitis. *See* Pelvic inflammatory disease
Salvarsan, 3
Sandfly fever, 496
Saquinavir, 962
dosage and administration, 963*t*
Sarcoidosis
and fever of unknown origin, 464–465
and meningitis, 700
Sarcomastigophora, 37
Scabies, 895*f*, 896–897
Scarlet fever
rash in, 489, 492
staphylococcal, rash in, 492
*Scedosporium prolificans*/infection, 50
drug therapy for, 403*t*
*Schistosoma haematobium,* collection of, 187
*Schistosoma mansoni,* 187
Schistosomiasis, 495
drug therapy for, 377*t*
and iron-deficiency anemia, 121
in travelers to tropical countries, 868
SCID. *See* Severe combined immunodeficiency disorders
*Scopulariopsis*/infection, 50
Scrub typhus, 198
antibiotic therapy for, 344
rash in, 491
SDA. *See* Strand-displacement amplification
Seal finger, 888
Seborrheic dermatitis, in HIV infection, 955
Selectins, 86
Selective media, 150
Self, 91
Self antigens, 93
Self-sustaining sequence-replication reaction (3SR), 141–142, 142*t*, 164
Semmelweiss, 1, 62
Sensor protein, 20–21
Sepsis, 13, 13*f*, 471–481
bacterial components and, 472–473, 474*f*
clinical manifestations of, 476, 477*t*
definition of, 472*t*
epidemiology of, 471–472
etiology of, 472, 473*t*
host factors in, 472
laboratory studies in, 476–478
pathogenesis of, 472–476
severe, definition of, 472*t*
treatment of, 478–480
underlying conditions and, 472, 473*t*
Sepsis score, 13
Septic cannibalism, 134
Septic pulmonary embolism, 543–544, 544*f*
Septic shock, 13, 471–481
clinical manifestations of, 476, 477*t*
definition of, 472*t*
epidemiology of, 471–472
etiology of, 472, 473*t*
host factors in, 472
laboratory studies in, 476–478
pathogenesis of, 472–476
treatment of, 478–480
underlying conditions and, 472, 473*t*
*Serratia*/infection
acute bacterial prostatitis, 676
antimicrobial resistance in, 213
of burns, 789
*Serratia marcescens*/infection
antibiotic therapy for, 345
antimicrobial resistance in, 214, 305
arthritis, 758
endocarditis, 623
osteomyelitis, 742*t*
*Serratia* toxin, 24
Serum amyloid A protein (SAA), 135–136
Severe combined immunodeficiency disorders (SCID), 809
Sex, and chronic fatigue syndrome, 775
Sexually-transmitted diseases (STDs)
control of, 912
fluoroquinolones for, 309
in intravenous drug user, 851
oral, 577
preexisting, and HIV spread, 910
prevalence of, 56
in travelers to tropical countries, 871
Sexual practices
and fever, 443
and HIV spread, 910
Sexual transmission, of HIV, 909
Shaving, preoperative, and infection, 785
Sheep liver fluke, drug therapy for, 374*t*
*Shigella*/infection
antibiotic therapy for, 345
and diarrhea in residents of tropical countries, 875
and microangiopathic disorders, 127

*Shigella flexneri*/infection, and reactive arthritis, 757, 764
Shigellosis, prevalence of, 56
Shingles, rash in, 491
Showering, preoperative, and infection, 785
Sigmoidoscopic aspirates, specimen collection from, 181
Signal-amplification methods, 141–142, 142*t*
Silver sulfadiazine (Flamazine), 314
Sinuses, imaging of, 112–113
Sinusitis, 515–517
  in bone marrow transplant recipients, 834
  clinical manifestations of, 516
  diagnosis of, 516
  epidemiology of, 515–516
  etiologies of, 515
  pathogenesis of, 515–516
  treatment of, 516–517, 517*t*
SIRS. *See* Systemic inflammatory response syndrome
Sjogren's syndrome, and chronic fatigue syndrome, 778
Skeletal pain, with fever, 442
Skin biopsies, in diagnosis of parasitic infection, 188
Skin disorders
  in bone marrow transplant recipients, 834–835
  in HIV infection, 954*t*, 954–956
    drug-induced, 956, 956*t*
Skin infections, fluoroquinolones for, 309
Skin reactions, to fluoroquinolones, 311
Skin symptoms
  with fever, 444
  in travelers to tropical countries, diseases causing, 866*t*
Slapped cheek disease. *See* Erythema infectiosum
SLE. *See* St. Louis encephalitis
Sleep disturbances, and chronic fatigue syndrome, 778
Sleeping sickness, 490
Smallpox, 2
Smith, Salmon and Theobald, 2
SMX. *See* Sulfamethoxazole
Snakebites, infections from, 889
Snowshoe Hare encephalitis, 708
Socioeconomic factors, and HIV spread, 910
Soft-tissue infections
  associated with bites, 502–503
  associated with specific risk factors, 502*t*
  fluoroquinolones for, 309
  necrotizing, 767
Solid organ abscess, computed tomography of, 115–116, 116*f*
Solid-phase immunodetection tests, 164
Solid tumors, and fever of unknown origin, 464
Soluble TNF receptors (sTNFR), 74
Sonography
  in acute cholecystitis, 117
  in appendicitis, 117
Sore throat, with fever, 442
Source, 7
South African tick fever, rash in, 490
Space-occupying lesions, in HIV infection, therapy for, 967*t*, 967–968, 968*t*
Sparfloxacin
  indications for, 309
  spectrum of action, 307
Specific adaptive immune response, 407
Specific immune response, 83, 91–108
  cellular elements of, 92–106
Specific immunity, 11
Specimen collection, 137, 138*t*
  bacterial, 145–148
  fungal, 169–171
  parasitic, 181–189, 182*t*–185*t*
  viral, 159–161, 160*t*
    for molecular tests, 161
Specimen management, 137–144
Specimens, bacterial, direct microscopic examination of, 148
Specimen selection, for recovery of opportunistic fungi, 170, 170*t*
Specimen transport
  bacterial, 145
  parasitic, 181–189
  viral, 161
    packaging for, 161
Spinal cord disease, in HIV infection, therapy for, 968
Spine, imaging of, 113, 113*f*
Spiramycin, 369*t*
  indications for, 293
*Spirillum minor,* antibiotic therapy for, 345
Spirillum minus rat-bite fever, rash in, 491
Spleen, 94–95
  aspirates from, specimen collection from, 188
Splenectomy
  and immunodeficiency, 811
  infection following, 799–800
Spontaneous generation, 1
*Sporothrix schenkii*/infection, 51
  arthritis, 759
Sporotrichosis, 49*t*, 51
  drug therapy for, 400*t*, 402
  pulmonary, epidemiology of, 550*t*
  rash in, 494
Sports, competitive, infections acquired through, 54*t*
3SR. *See* Self-sustaining sequence-replication reaction
SSIs. *See* Surgical site infections
SSPE. *See* Subacute sclerosing panencephalitis
Stains
  for fungal specimens, 171, 172*t*
  for parasite specimens, 189–192
  for stool smears, 190–192
Staphylococcal native valve endocarditis, antimicrobial therapy for, 628*t*, 628–631
Staphylococcal prosthetic valve endocarditis, antimicrobial therapy for, 630*t*, 631
Staphylococcal scalded skin syndrome (SSSS), rash in, 492
Staphylococcal scarlet fever, rash in, 492
*Staphylococcus*/infection
  antibiotic therapy for, 345
  in bone marrow transplant recipients, 829
  of burns, 789–790
  coagulase-negative
    in NICU nosocomial infections, 66
    nosocomial, 62
    in pediatric nosocomial infections, 66
    in surgical site infections, 64
  gram stain and, 149, 149*f*
  of prosthetic devices, 802
*Staphylococcus aureus*/infection
  antibiotic therapy for, 345
  antimicrobial resistance in, 212–213, 292, 305
  arthritis, 757–758
  dissemination of, 9
  endocarditis, 621, 623
    rash in, 493
  folliculitis, 501
  in hordeolum and chalazion, 733
  methicillin-resistant
    antibiotic therapy for, 345
    antimicrobial resistance in, 211
    of burns, 792
    in nosocomial infections, 62, 67
  in NICU nosocomial infections, 66
  nosocomial, 62
  in nosocomial pneumonia, 66
  osteomyelitis, 742*t*
  in pediatric nosocomial infections, 66
  of prosthetic devices, 801–802
  resistant, 57
  in surgical site infections, 64
  of surgical wounds, 783
  and toxic shock syndrome, 473
  toxin of, 10
  vulvovaginitis, 681
*Staphylococcus epidermis*/infection
  arthritis, 758
  osteomyelitis, 742*t*
  of prosthetic devices, 801
  of surgical wounds, 783–784
  of urinary tract, 650
*Staphylococcus lugdunensis*/infection, endocarditis, 623
*Staphylococcus saprophyticus*/infection
  chronic bacterial prostatitis, 677
  of urinary tract, 650
Starvation, and immune system, 839, 840*f*

Stavudine, 961
dosage and administration, 963*t*
STDs. *See* Sexually-transmitted diseases
*Stenotrophomonas maltophilia,* antibiotic therapy for, 345
Stevens-Johnson syndrome, 491
genital ulceration in, 663
Stibogluconate sodium, 369*t*
Still's disease, rash in, 490
Stokes, Adrian, 5
Stool smears, 190–192
Stool wet mounts, in diagnosis of parasitic infections, 189
Strand-displacement amplification (SDA), 141–142, 142*t*, 165
*Streptobacillus moniliformis*/infection
antibiotic therapy for, 345
rash in, 489
Streptococcal endocarditis, antimicrobial therapy for, 628, 629*t*–630*t*
Streptococcal toxic shock syndrome, 768
rash in, 492
*Streptococcus*/infection
of burns, 789, 792
group B, in pediatric nosocomial infections, 66
Viridans group, antibiotic therapy for, 346
vulvovaginitis, 681
*Streptococcus adjacens*/infection, endocarditis, 623
*Streptococcus agalactiae*/infection
antibiotic therapy for, 345
meningitis, 689
*Streptococcus bovis*/infection
antibiotic therapy for, 346
endocarditis, 623
*Streptococcus defectivus*/infection, endocarditis, 623
*Streptococcus oralis,* antimicrobial resistance in, 211
*Streptococcus pneumoniae*/infection
antibiotic therapy for, 346
antimicrobial resistance in, 210–211
fever and, 74
meningitis, 689
resistant, 57
vaccine for, 418*t*
*Streptococcus pyogenes*/infection
antibiotic therapy for, 346
antimicrobial resistance in, 292
dissemination of, 9
osteomyelitis, 742*t*
and toxic shock syndrome, 473
toxin of, 10
*Streptococcus sanguis,* antimicrobial resistance in, 211
*Streptococcus viridans,* dissemination of, 8–9
*Streptomyces erythreus,* 291
*Streptomyces nodosus,* 389
Streptomycin, 4, 330
contraindications to, 281
dosage and administration, 283*t*, 329*t*
drug interactions with, 333*t*
pharmacokinetics of, 331*t*
routes of elimination and adverse effects of, 332*t*
spectrum and mechanism of activity, 328*t*
for tuberculosis, 327
String test. *See* EnteroTest
Stroke, and fever, in hospitalized patient, 451
*Strongyloides stercoralis,* collection of, 187
Strongyloidiasis
drug therapy for, 377*t*
in travelers to tropical countries, 870
Subacute sclerosing panencephalitis (SSPE), 27
Subdural empyema, 727–729
clinical manifestations of, 728
definition of, 727
diagnosis of, 728, 728*f*
epidemiology of, 727
etiology of, 727–728
pathogenesis of, 727
treatment of, 728–729
Sucralfate, for stress bleeding prophylaxis, 66
Sulfacytine (Renoquid), 313
Sulfa derivatives, drug interactions with, 322
Sulfadiazine (Microsulfon), 313
for toxoplasmosis, 383
Sulfamethizole (Thiosulfil), 313
Sulfamethoxazole (SMX; Gantanol), 313
Sulfamylon. *See* Mafenide acetate
Sulfisoxazole (Gantrisin), 313
Sulfonamides, 313–315, 369*t*
adverse effects of, 314–315
allergic-hypersensitivity reactions to, 225
drug interactions with, 315
indications for, 314
mechanism of action, 313, 314*f*
pharmacology of, 313, 314*t*
preparations of, 313–314
resistance to, 314
spectrum of activity, 314
Sulphanilamide, 3
Superantigens, 10, 25, 73, 104
Supportive care, 14
for meningitis, 695
for septic shock, 479
Suppressor cells, 11
Suramin, 3, 370*t*
for trypanosomiasis, 384
Surfactant replacement, for ARDS, 564
Surgical procedures, and fever, 451–452
Surgical site infections (SSIs), 64–65
pathogenesis of, 65
prevention of, 65
risk factors for, 64*t*, 64–65
Surgical wound infections, 783–787, 798
deep, definition of, 783
incisional, definition of, 783
pathogens causing, 783–784, 784*t*
prevention of, 784–785
risk of, patient-related factors and, 785–786
treatment of, 786, 786*t*
Surveillance
definition of, 61
of nosocomial infections, 61–62
practitioner's role in, 57
Sweet's syndrome, 495
rash in, 490
Swimming pool granuloma, rash in, 494
Symmetrel. *See* Amantadine
Synergy, definition of, 628
Syphilis, 3
antibiotic therapy for, 346
clinical manifestations of, 661–662, 662*f*
epidemiology of, 658, 659*f*
in HIV infection, 943
meningitis, 698
ocular manifestations of, 739
oral, 577
pathogenesis of, 660
prevalence of, 56
secondary, rash in, 489
serologic tests for, 664
treatment of, 665*t*, 665–666
ulceration in, 657
Systemic inflammatory response syndrome (SIRS), 13, 13*f*, 75, 83, 471
definition of, 472*t*

Tacrolimus (FK-506), immunosuppression by, 821
*Taenia saginata*/infection, drug therapy for, 378*t*
*Taenia solium*/infection, drug therapy for, 378*t*
Tahyna encephalitis, 708
Talampicillin, 253–254
Tapeworm, drug therapy for, 378*t*
Target alterations, and antimicrobial resistance, 210–212
Target amplification, 164–165
Target sign, 116, 116*f*
TAS. *See* Transcription-based amplification system
T cell antigen receptor, 11
T cells, 92
actions of, 92*f*
deficiency of, and pneumonia, 814–818
HIV's effects on, 928
maturation of, 94
migration into tissues, 95
response to HIV, 931–933
selection in thymus, 94, 95*f*
T4 cells, 92

TDM. *See* Therapeutic drug monitoring
Teicoplanin, 285, 286*t*
dosage and administration, 288
indications for, 287–288
toxicity of, 288
TEN. *See* Toxic epidermal necrolysis
Terfonyl. *See* Trisulfapyrimidines
Tetanus prophylaxis
for burns, 793–794
for infected animal bites, 887
Tetanus toxin, 25
Tetanus, vaccine for, 416*t*
Tetracycline(s), 299–301, 370*t*
adverse effects of, 300
dosage and administration, 299
drug interactions with, 300–301
indications for, 299–300, 300*t*–301*t*
for malaria, 381
pharmacology of, 299
resistance to, 299
Tetrahydrofolic acid (THF), 313
Theophylline, drug interactions with, 293, 311
Therapeutic drug monitoring (TDM), with antimycobacterial drugs, 330
Thermoregulation, 71–72
*Thermus aquaticus (Taq)* polymerase, 165
THF. *See* Tetrahydrofolic acid
Thiabendazole (Mintezol), 370*t*
for intestinal nematodes, 385–386
Thiacetazone
dosage and administration, 329*t*
drug interactions with, 333*t*
pharmacokinetics of, 331*t*
routes of elimination and adverse effects of, 332*t*
spectrum and mechanism of activity, 328*t*
Thiosemicarbazones, 4
Thiosulfil. *See* Sulfamethizole
Thoracentesis, in pleurisy, 568–569
Throat
in fever, 444
sore, with fever, 442
Throat swab (TS), 159
Thrombocytopenia, infection and, 126–127, 127*t*
Thrombophlebitis
septic
clinical manifestations of, 730–731
diagnosis of, 731
epidemiology of, 730
etiology of, 730
pathogenesis of, 730
treatment of, 731
suppurative, 641
pelvic, 641
Thrombosis, septic, 641
Thrombotic thrombocytopenic purpura (TTP), 127
Thrush, 578
in HIV infection, 952
Thymus
development of, 94
T cell selection in, 94, 95*f*
Thymus atrophy, in malnutrition, 840
Thymus-derived lymphocytes. *See* T cells
Thyroid disorders, and body temperature, 71
Thyroiditis, subacute, and fever of unknown origin, 466
Thyroid storm, and hyperthermia, 76
Thyroxine ($T_4$), decreased, and infection, 135
Ticarcillin, 254
indications for, 252*t*
Ticarcillin-clavulanic acid, 255
Tick paralysis, 895–896
therapy for, 894*t*
Ticks, diseases associated with, 891–896, 892*t*
therapy for, 894*t*
Tinidazole, 324
Tissue biopsies, in evaluation of fever of unknown origin, 468
Tissue ischemia, and fever, in hospitalized patient, 450
Tissue perfusion by blood, and distribution of antimicrobials, 218
Tissue permeability, and distribution of antimicrobials, 218
Tissue tropism, 9
TMA. *See* Transcription-mediated amplification
TMP. *See* Trimethoprim
TMP/SMX. *See* Trimethoprim/sulfamethoxazole
TNF. *See* Tumor necrosis factor
Tobramycin, dosage and administration, 282*t*
for children, 282*t*
Tolbutamide, drug interactions with, 303
*Torulopsis glabrata. See Candida glabrata*
Toxic epidermal necrolysis (TEN), 492
Toxic granulation, 124, 125*f*
Toxic shock syndrome (TSS), 473
staphylococcal, rash in, 492
streptococcal, 768
rash in, 492
Toxocariasis, ocular, 737
*Toxoplasma gondii*
evasion of phagocytosis, 87
and mononuclear phagocytes, 126, 126*f*
Toxoplasmosis
of central nervous system, in HIV infection, 945–946, 946*t*
drug therapy for, 378*t*, 383
in HIV infection, therapy for, 972*t*
rash in, 490
retinitis, 737
in travelers to tropical countries, 870
Tracheal aspirates, 159
Trachoma, 735–736
Transcription-based amplification system (TAS), 164
Transcription-mediated amplification (TMA), 141–142, 142*t*
Transmission-Based Precautions, 68
Transmission, modes and patterns of, 53–54
Transplantation, vaccines with, 423, 424*t*
Trauma, and keratitis, 736
Traumatic injury
and altered host immunity, 785–786
infections complicating, 795–800
diagnosis of, 797–798
prevention of, 796–797, 797*t*
Travelers
diagnosis of parasitic infection in, 42
diarrhea in, 875, 879–880
antibiotic therapy for, 341
clinical features of, 879
epidemiology of, 879
etiology of, 876*t*, 879
management of, 587
prevention of, 879–880, 880*t*
therapy for, 309
treatment of, 878*f*, 879, 879*t*
eosinophilia in, 881–883
fever in, 859–873
infections acquired by, 55*t*
infections with rash in, 486*t*–487*t*, 495–497
Travel history, and fever, 439–440
Trematodes, drug therapy for, 387–388
Trench fever, 200
antibiotic therapy for, 338
rash in, 496
*Treponema pallidum,* 3
adherence in, 24
antibiotic therapy for, 346
fever and, 74
in genital ulcer disease, 657
Tretrexate, for *Pneumocystis carinii* pneumonia, 383
Triazoles, 392–394
*Trichinella spiralis*/infection, drug therapy for, 379*t*
Trichinosis
drug therapy for, 379*t*
and iron-deficiency anemia, 121
rash in, 490
in travelers to tropical countries, 870
*Trichomonas vaginalis*/infection
cervicitis, 382
collection of, 186–187
drug therapy for, 379*t*
vulvovaginitis, 681
Trichomoniasis, drug therapy for, 382
*Trichosporon*/infection, 47
*Trichosporon asahii,* 47
*Trichosporon asteroides,* 47
*Trichosporon beigelii*/infection, drug therapy for, 403*t*
*Trichosporon capitatum,* 47
*Trichosporon cutaneum,* 47

*Trichosporon inkin,* 47
*Trichosporon mucoides,* 47
Trichosporonosis, 48*t*
*Trichosporon ovoides,* 47
Trichostrongylus infection, drug therapy for, 379*t*
Trichuriasis, drug therapy for, 379*t*
Triiodothyronine ($T_3$), decreased, and infection, 135
Trimethoprim (TMP), 313, 370*t*
  adverse effects of, 315
  drug interactions with, 315
  indications for, 315
  mechanism of action, 313, 314*f*
  pharmacology, 315
  for *Pneumocystis carinii* pneumonia, 383
  resistance to, 315
  spectrum of action, 315
Trimethoprim/sulfamethoxazole (TMP/SMX), 315–317
  adverse effects of, 317
  indications for, 316–317
  pharmacology of, 315
  for *Pneumocystis carinii* pneumonia, 382–383
  resistance to, 316
  spectrum of activity, 315–316, 316*t*
Trimetrexate, 370*t*
Trisulfapyrimidines (Terfonyl), 313
Tropical countries
  and diarrheal illnesses, 875–879
  and eosinophilic illnesses, 881–883
  and febrile illnesses, 859–873
Tropical diseases, history of, 5
Tropical pulmonary eosinophilia, drug therapy for, 374*t*
Trovafloxacin
  indications for, 309
  spectrum of action, 307
*Trypanosomes brucei,* 187
Trypanosomiasis, 3
  African
    and hemolytic anemia, 124
    in travelers to tropical countries, 870
  American, in travelers to tropical countries, 870
  drug therapy for, 379*t*, 384–385
  rash in, 490, 496
  specimen collection in, 188
Tryparsamide, 370*t*
  for trypanosomiasis, 385
TS. *See* Throat swab
TSS. *See* Toxic shock syndrome
Tsutsugamushi disease. *See* Scrub typhus
TTP. *See* Thrombotic thrombocytopenic purpura
Tuberculosis, 4. *See also Mycobacterium tuberculosis*/infection
  alcohol abuse and, 855–856
  clinical manifestations of, 547, 547*f*
  diagnosis of, 547–548
  hemophagocytic syndrome associated with, 128
  in HIV infection, 950–951
    therapy for, 965
  and malnutrition, 843
  meningitis, 698
  miliary, rash in, 490
  nosocomial, 68
  oral, 577
  pathogenesis of, 546–547
  pericarditis, 645
  prevalence of, 56
  prevention of, 548–549, 549*t*
  pulmonary cavitation in, 546–549
  in travelers to tropical countries, 871
  treatment of, 548
  vaccine for, 418*t*
  vertebral, 755
Tularemia, 894–895
  antibiotic therapy for, 341, 894*t*
  rash in, 491
  vaccine for, 419*t*
Tumor necrosis factor (TNF), 74, 429*t*, 434
  alpha, and sepsis, 475
  therapeutic indications for, 430*t*
T1-weighted magnetic resonance imaging, 111
T2-weighted magnetic resonance imaging, 111
Tyndall, John, 3
Typhoid, 4
  in travelers to tropical countries, 867
Typhoid fever
  rash in, 489
  therapy for, 309
  vaccine for, 418*t*–419*t*
Typhus, 5
  epidemic, 198
    antibiotic therapy for, 344
  murine. *See* Murine typhus
  rash in, 488
  scrub, 198
    antibiotic therapy for, 344
    rash in, 491

Ulcerative colitis, and joint inflammation, 765
Universal Precautions, 68, 912
*Ureaplasma urealyticum*/infection
  antibiotic therapy for, 346
  and reactive arthritis, 764
  urethritis, 669
  vulvovaginitis, 681
Ureidopenicillins, 254
Urethritis, 669–673
  asymptomatic, diagnosis of, 672
  clinical manifestations of, 670–671
  definition of, 669
  epidemiology of, 670
  etiologies of, 669–670, 670*t*
  host factors in, 670
  laboratory studies in, 671–672
  pathogenesis of, 670
  symptomatic, diagnosis of, 672, 673*f*
  treatment of, 672–673, 673*f*
Urinary trace, specimen collection from, 147
Urinary tract infections, 649–656
  antibiotics for, 319–325
  bacterial factors in, 651
  candidal, drug therapy for, 398
  catheter-associated, 656
    prevention of, 656
    treatment of, 656
  clinical manifestations of, 651–652
  complicated
    clinical manifestations of, 652
    treatment of, 655*t*
  diagnosis of, 653
  epidemiology of, 649–651, 650*f*
  etiology of, 649, 650*t*
  and fever of unknown origin, 463
  fluoroquinolones for, 309
  host factors in, 651
  imipenem for, 267
  nosocomial, 63–64
    pathogenesis of, 64
    prevention of, 64
    risk factors for, 63–64, 64*t*
  pathogenesis of, 651
  prophylaxis of, 654–655
  treatment of, 653–654, 655*t*
  trimethoprim/sulfamethoxazole for, 316
Urine, specimen collection from, 159
Urticaria, annular, systemic infections with, 486*t*, 495
Ushers, 25
Uveitis, 737

Vaccination, 14
  encephalitis following, 703–704
  history of, 2, 2*t*, 5
  requirements for, 408
Vaccines, 415–426, 416*t*–421*t*
  active versus passive, 14
  for bone marrow transplant recipients, 837–838
  development of, 407–410, 977
    new approaches to, 409, 409*t*
  efficacy of, 407
  formulations of, 409
  for HIV, 977–980
  as immunotherapy, 408–409
  use
    with asplenia, 415, 422*t*
    in immunocompromised host, 415–424
    with malignancies, 422–423
    with renal disease, 423, 423*t*
    with transplants, 423, 424*t*
Valacyclovir (Valtrex), 350–355, 352*t*
Valley fever, 50
Valproate, drug interactions with, 293
Valtrex. *See* Valacyclovir

Vancomycin, 285–289, 286*t*
  dosage and administration, 288
  indications for, 287
  resistance to, mechanisms of, 211–212, 212*t*
  toxicity of, 288
Varicella, rash in, 491
Varicella-zoster virus/infection
  in bone marrow transplant recipients, 834
  encephalitis
    clinical presentation in, 706
    diagnosis of, 113
    epidemiology of, 706
    pathogenesis of, 706
  and myelopathy, 718
  oral, 579
  in organ transplant recipient, 825
  and radiculopathy/neuropathy, 720–721
  of skin, in HIV infection, 954–955
  vaccine for, 421*t*
Variolation, 2
Vascular catheters, specimen collection from, 148
Vascular diseases
  and fever of unknown origin, 465
  with osteomyelitis, 753–754
Vascular grafts, infections associated with, 806–807
Vasculitis, hypersensitivity, rash in, 490
Vector-borne transmission, 54
  of nosocomial infection, 61
VEE. *See* Venezuelan equine encephalitis
Vegetation, 621
Venezuelan equine encephalitis (VEE), 708
Venezuelan hemorrhagic fever, 496
Venous thromboembolism, and fever, in hospitalized patient, 451
Ventilatory support, for septic shock, 479
Ventriculoperitoneal shunts, 801
Vermox. *See* Mebendazole
Vertical transmission, 53
  of HIV, 812, 910
Vesicular-bullous eruptions
  noninfectious causes of, 492
  systemic infections with, 485*t*, 491–492
Veterinarians, vaccine use in, 425
*Vibrio cholerae*/infection
  antibiotic therapy for, 346
  and diarrhea in residents of tropical countries, 875
*Vibrio parahaemolyticus,* antibiotic therapy for, 347
*Vibrio vulnificus*
  antibiotic therapy for, 347
  rash in, 492
Viral diseases, 27–35
Viral genome
  exposure of, 32
  replication of, 32–33
Viral infections
  antiviral therapy for, 349–364
  arthritis, 759–760, 760*t*
  in bone marrow transplant recipients, 829–830, 831*f*, 833
    treatment of, 836
  of burns, 793
  chronic, and fever of unknown origin, 463
  conjunctivitis, 734–735
  cytokines and immunomodulators in, 429
  diagnostic methods for, 159–167
  and diarrhea, 582–583
  and diffuse maculopapular lesions, 485–488
  history of, 4–5
  immune response to, adverse effects of, 35
  in intravenous drug user, 851
  myocarditis/pericarditis, 645
  oral, 579–580
  in organ transplant recipient, 824*t*, 824–825
  rash in, 490–491
  retinitis, 737
  serology in, 165–167
    specimen processing for, 161
  temporal patterns of, 27, 28*f*
  in travelers to tropical countries, 867–868, 869*t*, 872
Viral isolates
  blind passage of, 163
  identification of, 163
Viral latency, 5
Virazole. *See* Ribavirin
Viremia, 29–30
Viroids, 27
Virology
  of AIDS, 915–926
  clinical, 159–167
  history of, 4–5, 27
Virulence, 7
  of bacteria, 19–26
  regulation of, 20–21
Virus-associated hemophagocytic syndrome, 128–129
Viruses
  assembly of, 33
  cells infected with, killing, 98*f*, 98–99, 99*f*
  characteristics of, in culture, 162*t*, 163
  differential diagnosis of
    in culture, 163
    strategies for, 160*f*
    tests for, 166*t*
  entry into host cells, 28, 30*f*
  enveloped, infection of cells, 32
  immune response to, 97*t*
  and immune system, 33–35
  infection of cells, 32–33
  internalization, receptors in, 31, 31*t*
  medically important families of
    characteristics of, 29*t*
    morphology of, 30*f*
  pathogenesis of
    cellular events in, 31–32
    at organism level, 28–31
  pathophysiology of, 27–35
  shedding, 28, 30*f*, 30–31
  spread in body, 28–29, 30*f*
  structure of, 28, 30*f*
  taxonomy of, 28
Virusoids, 27
Vision, rhinocerebral zygomycosis and, 46
Vistide. *See* Cidofovir
Visual symptoms, with fever, 442
Vitamin K, drug interactions with, 303
Vomiting, with diarrhea, 584–585
Vulvovaginitis
  clinical manifestations of, 681–682
  control of, 686–687
  diagnosis of, 682
  epidemiology of, 681
  etiology of, 681
  host factors in, 681
  laboratory studies in, 682
  management of, 682
  pathogenesis of, 681
  pathology of, 681

Warfarin, drug interactions with, 293, 303
Warm-reactive autoantibodies, 123
Water-borne transmission, and diarrhea, 582
Waterhouse, Benjamin, 2
Watson, Francis, 1
Weber-Christian disease, 495
WEE. *See* Western equine encephalitis
Wegener's granulomatosis, and fever of unknown origin, 464–465
Weil-Felix agglutination reaction
  in diagnosis of rickettsia, 195
  in diagnosis of rickettsial diseases, 198*t*
Western blot test, in diagnosis of HIV infection, 906–907
Western equine encephalitis (WEE), 708
West Nile fever, 496–497
Whipple's disease, and joint inflammation, 765
Whooping cough, antibiotic therapy for, 338
Wollman, Eugene and Elisabeth, 5
Worms
  immune response to, 97*t*
  infections of, and eosinophilia, 882*t*
  mature, collection and transportation of, 189
*Wuchereria bancrofti*/infection, 37
  collection of, 187
  drug therapy for, 373*t*

*Xanthomonas maltophilia,* antimicrobial resistance in, 214

X-linked lymphoproliferative syndrome, 129

Yeast organisms, non-albicans, 47
Yeasts, characteristics of, 178
Yellow fever, 5, 868, 869*t*
  rash in, 496
  vaccine for, 421*t*
*Yersinia*
  entry into host cells, 25
  secretion in, 25
*Yersinia enterocolitica*/infection
  antibiotic therapy for, 347
  and reactive arthritis, 757, 764
*Yersinia pestis,* antibiotic therapy for, 347
*Yersinia pseudotuberculosis,* antibiotic therapy for, 347
Yersin, J. E., 3, 5

Zalcitabine, 961
  dosage and administration, 963*t*
  toxicities of, 961
  uses of, 961
Zidovudine, 959–960
  adverse effects of, 68
  dosage and administration, 963*t*
  pharmacology of, 959
  postexposure, for HIV prophylaxis, 68
  resistance to, 960
  toxicities of, 959–960, 960*t*
Ziehl-Neelsen stain, 149–150
Zovirax. *See* Acyclovir
Zygomycetes, pulmonary infection of, 554
Zygomycosis, 43, 46–47, 48*t*
  clinical manifestations of, 46–47
  cutaneous, 47
  drug therapy for, 402, 403*t*
  pathogenesis of, 46
  pulmonary, 46–47
  rhinocerebral, 46
  treatment of, 46–47